PRAISE FOR THE BESTSELLING HOME EDITION OF
THE MERCK MANUAL OF MEDICAL INFORMATION

"Merck has accomplished what I had thought was impossible—to produce a clear, readable explanation of the normal and diseased functions of the human body. . . . This is a remarkable contribution. . . . Doctors should encourage their patients to own it."
  —Sherwin Nuland, M.D., clinical professor of surgery, Yale School of Medicine; author of *How We Die, Doctors,* and *The Wisdom of the Body*

"The manual is comprehensive, thorough, well written, and understandable."
  —Bernadine Healy, M.D., dean, Ohio State University College of Medicine; former director of the National Institutes of Health; author of *A New Prescription for Women's Health*

"Essential for all medical, consumer health, and public libraries."
  —*Library Journal* (starred review)

"Consumers can use the manual as a 'first step' in answering an array of health and medical questions."
  —Susan G. Braun, CEO, the Susan G. Komen Breast Cancer Foundation

"The biggest and best buy in bookstores this week."
  —*USA Today*

"Merck's *HOME EDITION* is the goods. . . . An invaluable reference work."
  —*The Boston Sunday Globe*

THE

MERCK MANUAL

OF

MEDICAL INFORMATION

HOME EDITION

Robert Berkow, M.D., EDITOR-IN-CHIEF

Mark H. Beers, M.D., ASSOCIATE EDITOR

Robert M. Bogin, M.D., SENIOR ASSISTANT EDITOR and EDITOR, ELECTRONIC VERSIONS

Andrew J. Fletcher, M.B., B.Chir., SENIOR ASSISTANT EDITOR

POCKET BOOKS
New York   London   Toronto   Sydney   Singapore

Editorial and Production Staff

Executive Editor	**Keryn A.G. Lane**
Senior Staff Editor	**William J. Kelly**
Senior Staff Editor	**Susan T. Schindler**
Staff Editor	**Julie Kostecky**
Staff Editor	**Sandra J. Masse**
Production Editor	**Debra G. Share**
Design Director	**Lynn Foulk**
Illustrator	**Michael Reingold**
Indexer	**Ann Cassar**
Textbook Production Coordinator	**Diane C. Zenker**
Medical Textbook Coordinator	**Dorothy A. Bailey**
Executive Assistant	**Diane C. Bobrin**
Publisher	**Gary Zelko**
Advertising and Promotional Supervisor	**Pamela J. Barnes**

POCKET BOOKS, a division of Simon & Schuster, Inc.
1230 Avenue of the Americas, New York, NY 10020

Copyright © 1997 by Merck & Co., Inc.

Published by arrangement with Merck & Company, Inc.

ISBN: 0-671-02726-3

First Pocket Books trade paperback printing September 2000

10 9 8 7 6 5 4 3 2 1

POCKET and colophon are registered trademarks of Simon & Schuster, Inc.

Printed in Canada

Preface

The *Merck Manual of Medical Information– Home Edition* has been published to meet a growing demand by the general public for highly detailed, sophisticated medical information. This book is based almost entirely on the text of *The Merck Manual of Diagnosis and Therapy*, commonly referred to as *The Merck Manual*.

First published in 1899, *The Merck Manual* is the oldest continuously published general medical textbook in the English language and the most widely used medical textbook in the world. It covers almost every disease that affects humans in specialties such as pediatrics, obstetrics and gynecology, psychiatry, ophthalmology, otolaryngology, dermatology, and dentistry, and special situations such as burns, heat disorders, radiation reactions and injuries, and sports injuries. No other medical textbook covers as wide a range of disorders.

Many fine books have been published during the last two decades to help meet the needs of the public for medical information. At the same time, more and more laypersons have been buying *The Merck Manual* for personal use, even though it is not advertised to the general public, and many find the book difficult to understand. We concluded that people who have a serious desire to understand medical issues want access to the same information that doctors have. This led us to translate *The Merck Manual* into language the general public can understand.

The Merck Manual–Home Edition contains nearly all the information in *The Merck Manual.* Some information, such as descriptions of heart murmurs and the appearance of diseased tissue under a microscope, hasn't been retained because lay readers aren't likely to listen to heart murmurs or examine such tissue specimens. Some details of drug treatments have also been deleted, because drug selection and dosing instructions vary far too much among specific situations to provide such information reliably. However, a great deal of treatment information is given in relation to each disease discussed, and a chapter on over-the-counter drugs has been added to the Drugs section.

Overviews of anatomy and physiology have been added to each section to help orient readers to the structure and function of specific organs. In-depth information about diseases, their causes, their recognition, and their treatment has been retained, and the harsh realities pertaining to incurable diseases and the risks of therapy have not been softened. The text acknowledges the actualities of what disease can do and what modern medicine can accomplish.

The strength of this book lies in the knowledge, experience, and judgment of its outstanding authors, consultants, and editorial board members. Their names are listed on the pages that follow the table of contents. They deserve a degree of thanks that cannot be adequately expressed here, but we know they will feel sufficiently rewarded if their efforts serve the reader's needs. Like *The Merck Manual,* this book is published by Merck Research Laboratories, a division of Merck & Co., Inc., on a not-for-profit basis.

The format and sequence of this book have some unique characteristics. Readers are urged to spend a few minutes reviewing the Guide for Readers (page xxiii), the Table of Contents, and the Index. An examination of the chapters in each section, headings in each chapter, and terms in boldface type will reveal a pattern of outlining intended to help readers locate information quickly and easily. Cross-references help direct readers to additional related information.

No book can replace the expertise and advice of health care practitioners who have direct contact with a patient. *The Merck Manual–Home Edition* is not intended to do so, nor is it meant to be a self-help book. Rather, we hope the medical information it provides will help readers communicate more effectively with their health care practitioners and, as a result, understand more completely their situations and choices. Suggestions for improvements will be warmly welcomed and carefully considered.

Robert Berkow, M.D.
Editor-in-Chief

Special Note to Readers

The authors, reviewers, editors, and publisher have made extensive efforts to ensure that the information is accurate and conforms to the standards accepted at the time of publication. However, constant changes in information resulting from continuing research and clinical experience, reasonable differences in opinions among authorities, unique aspects of individual situations, and the possibility of human error in preparing such an extensive text require that the reader exercise judgment when making decisions and consult and compare information from other sources. In particular, the reader is advised to discuss information obtained in this book with a doctor, pharmacist, nurse, or other health care practitioner.

Contents

Contents

Children's Health Issues (Continued)

Section 24
Accidents and Injuries 1335

Appendixes 1367

Index 1403

Editor-in-Chief

Robert Berkow, M.D.
Executive Director of Medical Literature
Merck & Co., Inc.
and
Clinical Professor of Medicine and Psychiatry
Allegheny University of the Health Sciences

Associate Editor

Mark H. Beers, M.D.
Senior Director of Geriatrics
Merck & Co., Inc.
and
Associate Clinical Professor of Medicine
Allegheny University of the Health Sciences

Senior Assistant Editors

Robert M. Bogin, M.D.
and
Andrew J. Fletcher, M.B., B.Chir.
Adjunct Professor of Pharmaceutical
Health Care
Temple University

Editorial Board

Consultants

Stephen Barrett, M.D. (Retired)
Allentown, PA
Nutrition

Ralph E. Cutler, M.D.
Professor of Medicine and Pharmacology, Loma Linda
University; Chief of Nephrology, Pettis Memorial VA
Medical Center
*Kidney and Urinary Tract Disorders; Men's Health
Issues*

Walter G. Larsen, M.D.
Clinical Professor of Dermatology, Oregon Health
Sciences University
Skin Disorders

Mortimer Lorber, D.M.D., M.D.
Associate Professor of Physiology and Biophysics,
Georgetown University
Mouth and Dental Disorders

Gregory J. Matz, M.D.
Professor and Chairman, Department of
Otolaryngology, Loyola University
Ear, Nose, and Throat Disorders

Hal B. Richerson, M.D.
Professor of Internal Medicine, University of Iowa
Immune Disorders

Melvin I. Roat, M.D.
Clinical Assistant Professor of Ophthalmology,
University of Maryland
Eye Disorders

H. Ralph Schumacher, Jr., M.D.
Professor of Medicine, University of Pennsylvania;
Director, Arthritis-Immunology Center, VA Medical
Center, Philadelphia
Bone, Joint, and Muscle Disorders

Ruth W. Schwartz, M.D.
Professor of Obstetrics and Gynecology, University of
Rochester
Women's Health Issues

Contributors

Hagop S. Akiskal, M.D.
Professor of Psychiatry, University
of California at San Diego
Depression and Mania

James K. Alexander, M.D.
Professor of Medicine, Baylor
University
Pulmonary Embolism

Chloe G. Alexson, M.D.
Professor of Pediatrics, University of
Rochester
Birth Defects (Heart Defects)

Roy D. Altman, M.D.
Professor of Medicine and Chief
(Acting), Arthritis, University of
Miami; Director of Clinical
Research, Geriatric Research,
Education, and Clinical Center,
Miami VA Medical Center
Paget's Disease of Bone

Karl E. Anderson, M.D.
Professor of Preventive Medicine
and Community Health, Internal
Medicine and Pharmacology and
Toxicology, The University of Texas
Medical Branch at Galveston
Porphyrias

Brian R. Apatoff, M.D., Ph.D.
Assistant Professor of Neurology,
Cornell University; Director, Multiple
Sclerosis Clinical Care and
Research Center, Department of
Neurology and Neuroscience, The
New York Hospital–Cornell Medical
Center
*Multiple Sclerosis and Related
Disorders*

Noel A. Armenakas, M.D.
Clinical Assistant Professor, Cornell
University; Attending Physician, The
New York Hospital–Cornell Medical
Center and Lenox Hill Hospital
Injury to the Urinary Tract

Hervy E. Averette, M.D.
American Cancer Society Professor
of Clinical Oncology and Sylvester
Professor and Director, Division of
Gynecologic Oncology, Sylvester
Comprehensive Cancer Center,
University of Miami
*Cancers of the Female
Reproductive System*

Zuhair K. Ballas, M.D.
Professor of Internal Medicine,
University of Iowa
Biology of the Immune System

John G. Bartlett, M.D.
Professor of Medicine and Chief,
Division of Infectious Diseases,
Johns Hopkins University
Pneumonia; Lung Abscess

Mark H. Beers, M.D.
Associate Editor, THE MERCK
MANUALS; Associate Clinical
Professor of Medicine, Allegheny
University of the Health Sciences
Anatomy; The Aging Body

Robert Berkow, M.D.
Editor-in-Chief, THE MERCK
MANUALS; Clinical Professor of
Medicine and Psychiatry, Allegheny
University of the Health Sciences
*Placebos; Psychosomatic
Disorders; Somatoform Disorders*

Richard W. Besdine, M.D.
Professor of Medicine and Director,
Travelers Center on Aging,
University of Connecticut; Director
of Health Standards and Quality
Bureau and Chief Medical Officer,
Health Care Financing
Administration
Drugs and Aging

John H. Bland, M.D.
Professor of Medicine–
Rheumatology (Emeritus),
University of Vermont
Osteoarthritis

M. Donald Blaufox, M.D., Ph.D.
Professor and Chairman of Nuclear
Medicine, Albert Einstein College of
Medicine
Radiation Injury

Philip K. Bondy, M.D.
Professor of Medicine (Retired),
Yale University
*Endocrine System and Hormones;
Adrenal Gland Disorders;
Polyglandular Deficiency Syndrome*

Roger C. Bone, M.D.
Professor of Medicine, Rush
University; President and CEO,
Medical College of Ohio
Bacteremia and Septic Shock

Sallyann M. Bowman, M.D.
Associate Professor of Clinical
Medicine, Allegheny University of
the Health Sciences
*Disorders of the Stomach and
Duodenum*

Thomas G. Boyce, M.D.
Medical Epidemiologist, Centers for
Disease Control and Prevention
Gastroenteritis

Lewis E. Braverman, M.D.
Professor of Medicine and
Physiology and Director, Division of
Endocrinology, University of
Massachusetts Medical Center
Thyroid Gland Disorders

Peter C. Brazy, M.D.
Professor of Medicine, University of
Wisconsin at Madison
*Metabolic and Congenital Kidney
Disorders*

George R. Brown, M.D.
Associate Chairman of Psychiatry,
East Tennessee State University;
Chief of Psychiatry, Mountain Home
VA Medical Center
*Sexuality and Psychosexual
Disorders*

John F. Burke, M.D.
Helen Andrus Benedict Professor of
Surgery, Harvard University; Chief
of Trauma Services (Emeritus),
Massachusetts General Hospital
Burns

Ronald W. F. Campbell, M.B.,
Ch.B., F.R.C.P., F.E.S.C.
British Heart Foundation Professor
of Cardiology, University of
Newcastle upon Tyne; Honorary
Consultant Cardiologist, Freeman
Hospital
Abnormal Heart Rhythms

John Caronna, M.D.
Professor of Clinical Neurology,
Cornell University; Attending
Neurologist, The New York
Hospital–Cornell Medical Center
Stroke and Related Disorders

C. Thomas Caskey, M.D.
Senior Vice President, Merck
Research Laboratories
Genetics

Alan S. Cohen, M.D.
Distinguished Professor of
Medicine, Boston University
Amyloidosis

Robert B. Cohen, D.M.D.
Senior Tutor, Harvard University;
Director, General Dentistry
Residency, Keesler Medical Center
(USAF)
Mouth and Dental Disorders

Sidney Cohen, M.D.
Richard Laylord Evans Professor of
Medicine and Assistant Vice
President, Health Sciences Center,
Temple University
Disorders of the Esophagus

Eugene L. Coodley, M.D.
Professor of Medicine, University of
California at Irvine; Chief, Internal
Medicine, VA Medical Center, Long
Beach
Common Medical Tests

Mary Ann Cooper, M.D.
Associate Professor of Emergency
Medicine, University of Illinois at
Chicago
Electrical Injuries

John K. Crane, M.D., Ph.D.
Assistant Professor of Medicine,
State University of New York at
Buffalo
Bacillary Infections (Gram-Negative)

Ralph E. Cutler, M.D.
Professor of Medicine and
Pharmacology, Loma Linda
University; Chief of Nephrology,
Pettis Memorial VA Medical Center
*Male Reproductive System; Biology
of the Kidneys and Urinary Tract;
Kidney Failure; Nephritis; Blood
Vessel Disorders of the Kidneys;
Urinary Tract Infections*

David C. Dale, M.D.
Professor of Medicine, University of
Washington
*Infections in People With Impaired
Defenses*

Patricia A. Daly, M.D.
Instructor in Medicine, Harvard
University
*Multiple Endocrine Neoplasia
Syndromes*

Anne L. Davis, M.D.
Associate Professor of Clinical
Medicine, New York University;
Attending Physician, Bellevue
Hospital
Bronchiectasis and Atelectasis

Norman L. Dean, M.D.
Geriatrician-Pulmonologist, Health
Services Division, North Carolina
Department of Corrections
Near Drowning

Ronald Dee, M.D.
Associate Clinical Professor of
Surgery, Albert Einstein College of
Medicine; Associate Attending
Surgeon, St. Joseph's Hospital,
Stamford
Venous and Lymphatic Disorders

Richard D. Diamond, M.D.
Professor of Medicine and
Research Professor of
Biochemistry, Boston University
Fungal Infections

Preston V. Dilts, Jr., M.D.
Professor of Obstetrics and
Gynecology (Emeritus), University
of Missouri at Kansas City
*Female Reproductive System;
Pregnancy; Complications of
Pregnancy; Labor and Delivery;
Complications of Labor and
Delivery; Postdelivery Period*

Eugene P. DiMagno, M.D.
Professor of Medicine, Mayo
Medical School; Director,
Gastroenterology Research Unit,
Mayo Clinic
Disorders of the Pancreas

George E. Downs, Pharm.D.
Professor of Clinical Pharmacy and
Dean of Pharmacy, Philadelphia
College of Pharmacy and Science
*Some Trade Names of Generic
Drugs*

Jeffrey M. Drazen, M.D.
Parker B. Francis Professor of
Medicine, Harvard University; Chief,
Pulmonary Critical Care Division,
Brigham & Women's Hospital
*Obstructive Airway Diseases
(Asthma)*

Douglas A. Drossman, M.D.
Professor of Medicine and
Psychiatry, University of North
Carolina at Chapel Hill
*Biology of the Digestive System;
Diagnostic Tests for Digestive
Disorders; Indigestion*

Carolyn P. Dukarm, M.D.
Instructor and Fellow in Pediatrics,
University of Rochester
*Puberty and Problems in
Adolescents*

Felton J. Earls, M.D.
Professor of Child Psychiatry,
Harvard University
Mental Health Disorders

David Eidelberg, M.D.
Director, Movement Disorders
Center, North Shore University
Movement Disorders

Sherman Elias, M.D.
Henry and Emma Meyer Chair in Obstetrics and Gynecology, Professor of Obstetrics and Gynecology, and Professor of Molecular and Human Genetics, Baylor University
Tests for Genetic Disorders

Stefan S. Fajans, M.D.
Professor Emeritus (Active) of Internal Medicine, University of Michigan
Diabetes Mellitus; Hypoglycemia

Wayne S. Fenton, M.D.
Medical Director, Chestnut Lodge Hospital; Director, Chestnut Lodge Research Institute
Schizophrenia and Delusional Disorder

Michael R. Foley, M.D.
Director, Obstetric Intensive Care and Associate Director, Maternal-Fetal Medicine, Good Samaritan Regional Medical Center; Associate Director, Phoenix Perinatal Associates
Drug Use During Pregnancy

Noble O. Fowler, M.D.
Professor of Medicine (Emeritus), University of Cincinnati
Pericardial Disease

Howard R. Foye, Jr., M.D.
Clinical Associate Professor of Pediatrics, University of Rochester
Developmental Problems in Young Children (Behavioral Problems, Eating Problems, Sleep Problems, Toilet Training Problems, Phobias, Hyperactivity)

Eugene P. Frenkel, M.D.
Professor of Internal Medicine and Radiology, Patsy R. and Raymond D. Nasher Distinguished Chair in Cancer Research, and A. Kenneth Pye Professorship in Cancer Research, Division of Hematology-Oncology, Department of Medicine, The University of Texas Southwestern Medical Center at Dallas
Biology of Blood; Anemias; Cancer and the Immune System; Diagnosis of Cancer; Complications of Cancer; Cancer Treatment

Mitchell H. Friedlaender, M.D.
Director, Cornea and Refractive Surgery, Scripps Clinic and Research Foundation
Eye Disorders

Steven M. Fruchtman, M.D.
Director, Stem Cell Transplant Program, Mount Sinai Hospital, New York
Myeloproliferative Disorders

Glen O. Gabbard, M.D.
Callaway Distinguished Professor, The Menninger Clinic
Overview of Mental Health Care

Marc Galanter, M.D.
Professor of Psychiatry and Director of the Division of Alcoholism and Drug Abuse, The New York University–Cornell Medical Center
Drug Dependence and Addiction

Robert H. Gelber, M.D.
Clinical Professor of Medicine and Dermatology, University of California at San Francisco
Leprosy

Ray W. Gifford, Jr., M.D.
Professor of Internal Medicine, Ohio State University; Consultant, Cleveland Clinic Foundation
High Blood Pressure

Robert Ginsburg, M.D.
Professor of Medicine, University of Colorado
Peripheral Arterial Disease

Barry Steven Gold, M.D.
Assistant Professor of Medicine, Johns Hopkins University
Venomous Bites and Stings

M. Jay Goodkind, M.D.
Clinical Associate Professor of Medicine, University of Pennsylvania; Chief (Retired), Department of Cardiology, Mercer Medical Center
Heart Tumors

Joe Graedon, M.S.
Lecturer, University of North Carolina at Chapel Hill; Graedon Enterprises, Inc., Durham, North Carolina
Over-the-Counter Drugs

Teresa Graedon, Ph.D.
Graedon Enterprises, Inc., Durham, North Carolina
Over-the-Counter Drugs

John H. Greist, M.D.
Clinical Professor of Psychiatry, University of Wisconsin; Distinguished Senior Scientist, Dean Foundation for Health, Research and Education
Anxiety Disorders

Richard L. Guerrant, M.D.
Thomas H. Hunter Professor of International Medicine, University of Virginia
Bacillary Infections (Gram-Negative)

John Gunderson, M.D.
Professor of Psychiatry, Harvard University; Director, Outpatient Personality Disorder Services, McLean Hospital
Personality Disorders

John W. Hallett, Jr., M.D.
Professor of Surgery, Mayo Clinic
Aortic Aneurysms and Dissection

Joan K. Harrold, M.D.
Instructor in Health Care Sciences and Medicine, The George Washington University; Research Scientist, The Center to Improve Care of the Dying
Death and Dying

I. Craig Henderson, M.D.
Adjunct Professor of Medicine, University of California at San Francisco; CEO, Sequus Pharmaceuticals, Inc.
Breast Disorders

Susan L. Hendrix, D.O.
Assistant Professor of Obstetrics and Gynecology, Wayne State University at Detroit
Menopause; Common Gynecologic Problems

Robert A. Hoekelman, M.D.
Professor of Pediatrics, University of Rochester
Pinworm Infection

Paul D. Hoeprich, M.D.
Professor of Medicine (Emeritus),
University of California at Davis

*Coccal Infections; Bacillary
Infections (Gram-Positive)*

Charles S. Houston, M.D.
Professor of Medicine (Emeritus),
University of Vermont

*Heat Disorders; Cold Injuries;
Mountain Sickness*

Daniel A. Hussar, Ph.D.
Remington Professor of Pharmacy,
Philadelphia College of Pharmacy
and Science

Factors Affecting Drug Response

Michael Jacewicz, M.D.
Associate Professor of Neurology,
University of Tennessee

*Vertigo; Muscle Weakness; Smell
and Taste Disorders; Infections of
the Brain and Spinal Cord*

George Gee Jackson, M.D.
Professor of Medicine (Emeritus),
University of Illinois at Chicago;
Clinical Professor of Medicine,
University of Utah

Viral Infections

Harry S. Jacob, M.D.
Clark Professor of Medicine and
Vice Chairman, Department of
Internal Medicine, and Head,
Division of Hematology, University
of Minnesota

Spleen Disorders

James W. Jefferson, M.D.
Clinical Professor of Psychiatry,
University of Wisconsin;
Distinguished Senior Scientist, Dean
Foundation for Health, Research
and Education

Anxiety Disorders

Nicholas Jospe, M.D.
Associate Professor of Pediatrics,
University of Rochester

*Metabolic Disorders; Hormonal
Disorders*

Fran E. Kaiser, M.D.
Professor of Medicine and
Associate Director, Division of
Geriatric Medicine, St. Louis
University

Impotence

Harold S. Kaplan, M.D.
Professor and Director, Transfusion
Medicine, The University of Texas
Southwestern Medical Center

Blood Transfusion

Stephen I. Katz, M.D., Ph.D.
Director, National Institute of
Arthritis and Musculoskeletal and
Skin Diseases, National Institutes of
Health

Skin Disorders

Donald Kaye, M.D.
Professor of Medicine, Allegheny
University of the Health Sciences;
President and CEO, Allegheny
University Hospitals

Anti-infective Drugs

**B. J. Kennedy, M.D., M.Sc.,
M.A.C.P.**
Regents' Professor of Medicine
(Emeritus) and Masonic Professor
of Oncology (Emeritus), University
of Minnesota

Causes and Risks of Cancer

Thomas Killip, M.D.
Professor of Medicine, Albert
Einstein College of Medicine;
Executive Vice President for
Medical Affairs, Beth Israel Medical
Center

Coronary Artery Disease

Richard P. Kluft, M.D.
Clinical Professor of Psychiatry,
Temple University

Dissociative Disorders

Calvin H. Knowlton, Ph.D.
Associate Professor of Pharmacy,
Philadelphia College of Pharmacy
and Science

Compliance With Drug Treatment

Arthur E. Kopelman, M.D.
Professor of Pediatrics and Head,
Neonatology, East Carolina
University

*Problems in Newborns and Infants;
Sick Children and Their Families*

David N. Korones, M.D.
Assistant Professor of Pediatrics,
University of Rochester

Childhood Cancers

John N. Krieger, M.D.
Professor of Urology, University of
Washington

*Disorders of the Penis, Prostate,
and Testes*

Douglas R. Labar, M.D., Ph.D.
Director, Comprehensive Epilepsy
Center, The New York Hospital–
Cornell Medical Center

Seizure Disorders

Jules Y.T. Lam, M.D., F.R.C.P.(C)
Associate Professor of Medicine,
University of Montreal; Montreal
Heart Institute

Atherosclerosis

Lewis Landsberg, M.D.
Irving S. Cutter Professor and
Chairman, Northwestern University

*Multiple Endocrine Neoplasia
Syndromes*

Edward H. Lanphier, M.D.
Senior Scientist (Emeritus),
Department of Preventive Medicine,
University of Wisconsin at Madison

Diving Injuries

Ruth A. Lawrence, M.D.
Professor of Pediatrics, Obstetrics
and Gynecology, University of
Rochester

*Normal Newborns and Infants;
Poisoning in Children*

Harvey Lemont, D.P.M.
Chairman, Department of Medicine,
Pennsylvania College of Podiatric
Medicine

Foot Problems

Joseph R. Lentino, M.D., Ph.D.
Professor of Medicine and Chief,
Section of Infectious Diseases,
Loyola University; Hines VA
Hospital

Anaerobic Bacterial Infections

Daniel Levinson, M.D.
Associate Professor of Family and
Community Medicine, University of
Arizona

Air Travel and Medical Problems

Robert I. Levy, M.D.
President, Wyeth-Ayerst Research

*Disorders of Cholesterol and Other
Fats*

James L. Lewis, III, M.D.
Assistant Professsor of Medicine
and Director, Nephrology Fellowship
Training Program, University of
Alabama at Birmingham
*Water Balance; Salt Balance; Acid-
Base Balance*

Lawrence M. Lichtenstein, M.D.,
Ph.D.
Professor of Medicine, Johns
Hopkins University; Director, Johns
Hopkins Asthma and Allergy Center
Allergic Reactions

Harold I. Lief, M.D.
Professor of Psychiatry (Emeritus),
University of Pennsylvania; Clinical
Professor of Psychiatry, Thomas
Jefferson University
Disorders of Sexual Function

James H. Liu, M.D.
Professor of Obstetrics and
Gynecology, University of Cincinnati
*Endometriosis; Infertility; Pituitary
Gland Disorders*

Elliot M. Livstone, M.D.
Attending Physician, Sarasota
Memorial Hospital
*Cancer and Other Growths of the
Digestive System*

Robert G. Loudon, M.B., Ch.B.
Professor of Medicine (Emeritus),
University of Cincinnati
Biology of the Lungs and Airways

Frank E. Lucente, M.D.
Professor and Chairman,
Department of Otolaryngology,
State University of New York Health
Science Center at Brooklyn
Ear, Nose, and Throat Disorders

Joanne Lynn, M.D., M.A.
Professor of Health Care Sciences
and Medicine, The George
Washington University; Director,
The Center to Improve Care of the
Dying
Death and Dying

Gerald L. Mandell, M.D.
Professor of Medicine, Owen R.
Cheatham Professor of the
Sciences, University of Virginia;
Chief, Division of Infectious
Diseases, University of Virginia
Health Sciences Center
*Biology of Infectious Disease;
Infections of the Skin and
Underlying Tissue; Abscesses;
Bone and Joint Infections; Charcot's
Joints*

Alfonse T. Masi, M.D., Dr.P.H.
Professor of Medicine and
Epidemiology, University of Illinois
*Disorders of Muscles, Bursas, and
Tendons*

Richard G. Masson, M.D.
Associate Professor of Medicine,
University of Massachusetts; Co-
Chief, Pulmonary Medicine and
Critical Care, Columbia Metrowest
Medical Center
*Diagnostic Tests for Lung and
Airway Disorders*

Alvin M. Mauer, M.D.
Professor of Medicine, University of
Tennessee
Leukemias

Elizabeth R. McAnarney, M.D.
Professor and Chair, Department of
Pediatrics, University of Rochester
Medical Center
*Puberty and Problems in
Adolescents*

Daniel J. McCarty, M.D.
Will and Cava Ross Professor of
Medicine and Director, Arthritis
Institute, Medical College of
Wisconsin
Gout and Pseudogout

J. Allen McCutchan, M.D.
Professor of Medicine, Division of
Infectious Disease, University of
California at San Diego
*Human Immunodeficiency Virus
Infection; Sexually Transmitted
Diseases*

Geralyn M. Meny, M.D.
Assistant Professor and Associate
Director, Transfusion Medicine, The
University of Texas Southwestern
Medical Center
Blood Transfusion

Gabe Mirkin, M.D.
Associate Clinical Professor of
Pediatrics, Georgetown University
*Sports Injuries; Exercise and
Fitness*

Daniel R. Mishell, Jr., M.D.
Lyle G. McNeile Professor and
Chairman, Department of Obstetrics
and Gynecology, University of
Southern California
Family Planning

W.K.C. Morgan, M.D.
Professor of Medicine, The
University of Western Ontario;
Chest Diseases Service, London
Health Sciences Centre, University
Campus, London, Ontario, Canada
Occupational Lung Diseases

Gary J. Myers, M.D.
Professor of Pediatrics and
Neurology, University of Rochester
Birth Defects

John C. Nemiah, M.D.
Professor of Psychiatry, Dartmouth
Medical School; Professor of
Psychiatry (Emeritus), Harvard
University
Anxiety Disorders

John D. Norante, M.D.
Clinical Associate Professor of
Otolaryngology, University of
Rochester
*Ear, Nose, and Throat Disorders in
Children*

Robert E. Olson, M.D., Ph.D.
Professor of Pediatrics, University of
South Florida
*Overview of Nutrition; Malnutrition;
Vitamins and Minerals; Nutritional
Disorders*

Joseph G. Ouslander, M.D.
Director, Division of Geriatric
Medicine and Gerontology and
Chief of Medicine, Wesley Woods
Geriatric Center at Emory
University; Director, Atlanta VA
Rehabilitation Research and
Development Center
Urinary Incontinence

Lawrence L. Pelletier, Jr., M.D.
Professor of Internal Medicine,
University of Kansas at Wichita
Endocarditis

Hart Peterson, M.D.
Professor of Neurology in Pediatrics
(Emeritus), Cornell University
Cerebral Palsy

Sidney F. Phillips, M.D.
Professor of Medicine, Mayo
Medical School; Consultant, Mayo
Clinic
Bowel Movement Disorders

Willy F. Piessens, M.D.
Professor of Tropical Public Health
and Associate Professor of
Medicine, Harvard University
Parasitic Infections

Fred Plum, M.D.
University Professor and Chairman
of Neurology (Emeritus), Cornell
University; Attending Neurologist,
The New York Hospital–Cornell
Medical Center
*Biology of the Nervous System;
Neurologic Examination and Tests;
Headaches; Sleep Disorders; Head
Injuries; Delirium and Dementia;
Stupor and Coma*

Russell K. Portenoy, M.D.
Associate Professor, Cornell
University; Co-Chief, Pain and
Palliative Care Service, Memorial
Sloan-Kettering Cancer Center
Pain

Glenn M. Preminger, M.D.
Professor of Urologic Surgery, Duke
University; Director, Duke
Comprehensive Kidney Stone
Center, Duke University Medical
Center
Urinary Tract Obstruction

Douglas J. Pritchard, M.D.
Professor of Orthopedics and
Oncology, Mayo Clinic
Bone Tumors

Lawrence G. Raisz, M.D.
Professor of Medicine and Head,
Division of Endocrinology and
Metabolism; Program Director,
General Clinical Research Center,
University of Connecticut
Osteoporosis

Robert W. Rebar, M.D.
Professor and Chair, Department of
Obstetrics and Gynecology,
University of Cincinnati
*Hormones and Reproduction;
Absent or Abnormal Uterine
Bleeding; Polycystic Ovary
Syndrome; Endometriosis; Infertility;
Pituitary Gland Disorders*

Hal B. Richerson, M.D.
Professor of Internal Medicine,
University of Iowa
Allergic Diseases of the Lungs

Jean E. Rinaldo, M.D.
Professor of Medicine, Vanderbilt
University
*Acute Respiratory Distress
Syndrome*

Melvin I. Roat, M.D.
Clinical Assistant Professor of
Ophthalmology, University of
Maryland
Eye Disorders in Children

William O. Robertson, M.D.
Professor of Pediatrics, University of
Washington; Medical Director,
Washington Poison Center
Poisoning

Beryl J. Rosenstein, M.D.
Professor of Pediatrics, Johns
Hopkins University
Cystic Fibrosis

G. Victor Rossi, Ph.D.
Leonard and Madlyn Abramson
Professor of Pharmacology,
Philadelphia College of Pharmacy
and Science
*Overview of Drugs;
Pharmacodynamics; Adverse Drug
Reactions*

Fred H. Rubin, M.D.
Clinical Associate Professor of
Medicine, University of Pittsburgh;
Chairman, Department of Medicine,
Shadyside Hospital
Immunizations to Prevent Infection

Michael Rubin, M.D.
Associate Professor of Clinical
Neurology, Cornell University;
Director of Neuromuscular Service,
The New York Hospital–Cornell
Medical Center
*Muscular Dystrophy and Related
Disorders; Spinal Cord Disorders;
Peripheral Nerve Disorders; Cranial
Nerve Disorders*

Paul S. Russell, M.D.
John Homans Professor of Surgery,
Harvard University; Visiting
Surgeon, Massachusetts General
Hospital
Transplantation

David B. Sachar, M.D.
Director, Division of
Gastroenterology, The Mount Sinai
Medical Center, New York
*Inflammatory Bowel Diseases;
Antibiotic-Associated Colitis*

Olle Jane Z. Sahler, M.D.
Adjunct Professor of Pediatrics,
University of Rochester
*Problems in Newborns and Infants
(Failure to Thrive); Gastrointestinal
Disorders in Children*

Jay P. Sanford, M.D. (*Deceased*)
Professor of Medicine, The
University of Texas Southwestern
Medical Center
Spirochetal Infections

James W. Sayre, M.D.
Clinical Professor of Pediatrics,
University of Rochester; Attending
Pediatrician, St. Mary's Hospital
Child Abuse and Neglect

Kurt Schapira, M.D., F.R.C.P.,
F.R.C.Psych.
Honorary Senior Research
Associate, Department of
Psychiatry, University of Newcastle
upon Tyne, England; Consultant
Psychiatrist (Emeritus), Royal
Victoria Infirmary
Suicidal Behavior

Albert P. Scheiner, M.D.
Professor of Pediatrics (Emeritus),
University of Massachusetts
Mental Retardation

H. Ralph Schumacher, Jr., M.D.
Professor of Medicine, University of Pennsylvania; Director, Arthritis-Immunology Center, VA Medical Center, Philadelphia
Bones, Joints, and Muscles; Disorders of Joints and Connective Tissue; Musculoskeletal Disorders in Children

Ronald W. Schworm, Ph.D.
Educational Consultant, The Reading and Learning Disorders Center, Rochester
Developmental Problems in Young Children (Attention Deficit Disorder, Learning Disabilities, Dyslexia)

Charles H. Scoggin, M.D.
Chairman and CEO, Rodeer Systems
Lung Cancer

Eldon A. Shaffer, M.D., F.R.C.P.(C), F.A.C.P.
Professor and Head, Department of Medicine, University of Calgary, Calgary, Alberta, Canada
Diagnostic Tests for Liver and Gallbladder Disorders; Fatty Liver, Cirrhosis, and Related Disorders; Blood Vessel Disorders of the Liver

William R. Shapiro, M.D.
Chairman, Division of Neurology, Barrow Neurological Institute/St. Joseph's Hospital, Phoenix
Tumors of the Nervous System

Harold Silverman, Pharm.D.
Director, Interscience, Washington, DC
Generic Drugs

Jerome B. Simon, M.D., F.R.C.P.(C)
Professor of Medicine, Queen's University, Kingston, Ontario, Canada
Biology of the Liver and Gallbladder; Clinical Manifestations of Liver Disease; Hepatitis; Liver Tumors

Arthur T. Skarin, M.D.
Associate Professor of Medicine, Harvard University; Attending Physician, Medical Oncology, Dana-Farber Cancer Institute
Lymphomas

Gordon L. Snider, M.D.
Professor of Medicine and Vice Chairman, Department of Medicine, Boston University; Chief, Medical Service, VA Medical Center, Boston
Bronchitis; Obstructive Airway Diseases (Chronic Obstructive Pulmonary Disease); Pleural Disorders

Norman Sohn, M.D.
Clinical Assistant Professor of Surgery, Cornell University
Disorders of the Anus and Rectum

David R. Staskin, M.D.
Assistant Professor of Urology, Harvard University; Director of Urodynamics and Incontinence, Beth Israel Hospital
Neurogenic Bladder

William W. Stead, M.D.
Professor of Medicine, University of Arkansas; Director, Tuberculosis Program, Arkansas Department of Health
Tuberculosis

E. Richard Stiehm, M.D.
Chief, Division of Pediatric Immunology/Allergy, University of California at Los Angeles
Immunodeficiency Disorders

Bradford G. Stone, M.D.
Clinical Associate Professor of Medicine, University of Minnesota
Gallbladder Disorders

Marvin J. Stone, M.D.
Chief of Oncology and Director, Baylor-Sammons Cancer Center, Baylor University
Plasma Cell Disorders

Albert J. Stunkard, M.D.
Professor of Psychiatry, University of Pennsylvania
Obesity; Eating Disorders

David A. Swanson, M.D.
Professor and Deputy Chairman, Department of Urology, The University of Texas, M.D. Anderson Cancer Center
Kidney and Urinary Tract Tumors and Cancers

Jan Peter Szidon, M.D.
Professor of Medicine, Section of Pulmonary Medicine, Rush University
Infiltrative Lung Diseases

Paul H. Tanser, M.D., F.R.C.P.(C)
Professor of Medicine, McMaster University; Senior Cardiologist, St. Joseph's Hospital, Hamilton, Ontario, Canada
Biology of the Heart and Blood Vessels; Diagnosis of Heart Disease; Heart Failure; Cardiomyopathy; Heart Valve Disorders

Mary Territo, M.D.
Professor of Medicine, Division of Hematology/Oncology, University of California at Los Angeles
White Blood Cell Disorders

Ronald G. Tompkins, M.D., Sc.D.
Professor of Surgery, Harvard University; Surgeon, Massachusetts General Hospital
Diverticular Disease; Gastrointestinal Emergencies

Courtney M. Townsend, Jr., M.D.
Professor and John Woods Harris Distinguished Chairman, Department of Surgery, The University of Texas Medical Branch at Galveston
Carcinoid

Thomas N. Tozer, Ph.D.
Professor of Biopharmaceutical Sciences and Pharmaceutical Chemistry (Emeritus), University of California at San Francisco
Drug Administration, Distribution, and Elimination

Stephen K. Urice, Ph.D., J.D.
Philadelphia, PA
Legal Issues

Elise W. van der Jagt, M.D.
Associate Professor of Pediatrics and Critical Care, University of Rochester
Injuries

Jack A. Vennes, M.D.
Professor of Medicine (Retired), University of Minnesota
Gallbladder Disorders

Elliot S. Vesell, M.D., Sc.D.
Evan Pugh Professor and Chair,
Department of Pharmacology,
Pennsylvania State University
*Factors Affecting Drug Response
(Genetics)*

Jacob Walfish, M.D.
Assistant Clinical Professor of
Medicine, The Mount Sinai School
of Medicine
*Inflammatory Bowel Diseases;
Antibiotic-Associated Colitis*

Wendy Watson, M.D.
Assistant Professor of Pediatrics,
University of Rochester
*Viral Infections in Children;
Infections in Newborns and Infants*

**William C. Watson, M.D., Ph.D.,
F.R.C.P.**
Professor (Emeritus), University of
Western Ontario, London,
Ontario, Canada
Malabsorption Syndromes

John M. Weiler, M.D.
Professor, University of Iowa
Biology of the Immune System

Geoffrey A. Weinberg, M.D.
Assistant Professor of Pediatrics,
University of Rochester; Attending
Physician, Pediatric Service and
Director, Maternal/Pediatric HIV
Program, Strong Memorial Hospital
*Bacterial Infections in Children;
Disorders Likely Caused by
Infection; Human Immunodeficiency
Virus Infection in Children*

Allan B. Weingold, M.D.
Professor of Obstetrics and
Gynecology and Vice President for
Medical Affairs, The George
Washington University
*High-Risk Pregnancy; Diseases
That Can Complicate Pregnancy*

Harvey J. Weiss, M.D.
Professor of Medicine, Columbia
University; Chief, Division of
Hematology-Oncology, St. Luke's–
Roosevelt Hospital
Bleeding Disorders

Claude E. Welch, M.D. *(Deceased)*
Clinical Professor of Surgery
(Emeritus), Harvard University;
Senior Surgeon, Massachusetts
General Hospital
*Diverticular Disease;
Gastrointestinal Emergencies*

Nanette K. Wenger, M.D.
Professor of Medicine (Cardiology),
Emory University; Director, Cardiac
Clinics, Grady Memorial Hospital;
Consultant, Emory Heart Center
Low Blood Pressure

**Theodore E. Woodward, M.D.,
M.A.C.P.**
Professor of Medicine (Emeritus),
University of Maryland
Rickettsial Infections

Acknowledgments

We wish to acknowledge the contributions of Shirley Claypool, who supervised and coordinated the initial editing and production of the book. We also wish to acknowledge the contributions of Project House, Inc., whose editorial skills were invaluable. Among those who merit special thanks are Stephanie Phillips, Marcye B. White, Bari Samson, Claudia Piano, Bea Dickstein, Anthony Greco, Marcia Ringel, and Lynn Atkinson.

Those who assisted with initial editing include Amy Crawford-Faucher, M.D., and Cathy Glew, M.D. We are grateful for the assistance of the following people who provided us with critical reviews of specific chapters: Sarah Atkinson, M.D., Ronald J. Brogan, Melvin Horwith, M.D., Irwin Reich, and Eric A. Voth, M.D.

A Guide for Readers

The Merck Manual of Medical Information—Home Edition is organized in a way that should facilitate its use. Topics of interest may be quickly located by consulting the Table of Contents or Index, but an understanding of the organization of sections and chapters will help the reader navigate through the book and find the most information.

Sections

The book is divided into sections. Some sections encompass organ systems, such as the eye, skin, or heart and blood vessels. Organization by sections means that related information is nearby. For example, in the Heart and Blood Vessel Disorders section, atherosclerosis is immediately followed by coronary artery disease, which is caused by atherosclerosis. Other sections correspond to medical specialties, such as hormonal disorders or infectious diseases. Three separate sections cover health issues of men, women, and children.

Most sections devoted to an organ system begin with a chapter describing the organ's normal structure and function. Reading about how the heart works or looking at illustrations of the heart, for example, may make a specific heart disorder more understandable. Many sections also include a chapter describing medical tests used to diagnose the diseases discussed in that section. Reading about coronary artery disease may prompt a referral to the chapter that describes tests, such as cardiac catheterization, used to diagnose heart disease.

Chapters

Some chapters describe a single disease, such as osteoporosis. Other chapters encompass related diseases or disorders, such as spinal cord disorders. In either case, a discussion generally starts with a definition of the disease or disorder, printed in italics. The information that follows is often organized under headings, such as causes, symptoms, diagnosis, prevention, treatment, and prognosis. Bold-faced type within the text indicates topics of major importance.

Some chapters cover a symptom or a problem caused by a disease. For example, a chapter in the Skin Disorders section discusses itching and its many causes. More information about the specific causes of itching can be found elsewhere in the book. A chapter in the Disorders of Nutrition and Metabolism section explains the complex ways the body maintains its acid-base balance and the many causes and consequences of abnormal balance.

Cross-references

Throughout the book are cross-references that identify other important or related discussions of a subject. Cross-references are marked with a symbol within the text (▲, ■, ★, ●, ◆, ♥); corresponding symbols, along with the page number where more information can be found, are located at the bottom of the page.

Medical Terms

Medical terms are often provided, usually in parentheses after the lay term. On page xxv is a list of prefixes, roots, and suffixes used in medical terminology; this list can help take the mystery out of medicine's multisyllabic vocabulary.

Sidebars

The book contains many sidebars, including tables and illustrations. They help explain material in the text or give additional, related information.

Drug Information

The Drugs section, beginning on page 23, provides comprehensive information on drugs. Individual drugs are almost always referred to by their generic names rather than by their brand or trade names. Appendix IV contains a list of most of the generic drugs mentioned in the book along with some of their corresponding trade names.

The book does not provide drug doses, because doses can vary dramatically, depending on individual circumstances. Factors such as age, sex, weight, height, the presence of more than one disease, and the use of other drugs modify what constitutes a safe, effective dose. Therefore, the dose of a drug, as well as the choice of drug, must always be tailored to the individual.

Diagnostic Tests

Diagnostic tests are mentioned throughout the book. Usually, an explanation is provided the first time a test is mentioned in a chapter. In addition, Appendix III lists many common diagnostic tests and procedures, explains what they are used for, and provides cross-references to where the major text discussions of a test can be found.

Resources for Help and Information

Appendix V lists the telephone numbers and addresses of many organizations that help people who have specific diseases. These organizations can provide additional information about a disease or help locate support services.

The authors, reviewers, and editors have worked hard to ensure that information in this book is accurate and that treatments conform to the standards accepted at the time of publication. However, because of constant changes in information resulting from continuing research and clinical experience, reasonable differences in opinions among authorities, unique aspects of individual people and situations, and the possibility of human error in preparing such an extensive text, information in this book may not apply to an individual situation. The reader is advised to discuss information learned here with a health professional.

Understanding Medical Terms

At first glance, medical terminology can seem like a foreign language. But often the key to understanding medical terms is focusing on their components (prefixes, roots, and suffixes). For example, *spondylolysis* is a combination of "spondylo," which means vertebra, and "lysis," which means dissolve, and so means dissolution of a vertebra.

The same components are used in many medical terms. "Spondylo" plus "itis," which means inflammation, forms *spondylitis,* an inflammation of the vertebrae. The same prefix plus "malacia," which means soft, forms *spondylomalacia,* a softening of the vertebrae.

Knowing the meaning of a small number of components can help with interpretation of a large number of medical terms. The following list defines many commonly used medical prefixes, roots, and suffixes.

a(n)	absence of
acou, acu	hear
aden(o)	gland
aer(o)	air
alg	pain
andr(o)	man
angi(o)	vessel
ankyl(o)	crooked, curved
ante	before
anter(i)	front, forward
anti	against
arteri(o)	artery
arthr(o)	joint
articul	joint
ather(o)	fatty
audi(o)	hearing
aur(i)	ear
aut(o)	self
bi, bis	double, twice, two
brachy	short
brady	slow
bucc(o)	cheek
carcin(o)	cancer
cardi(o)	heart
cephal(o)	head
cerebr(o)	brain
cervic	neck
chol(e)	bile, or referring to gallbladder
chondr(o)	cartilage
circum	around, about
contra	against, counter
corpor	body
cost(o)	rib
crani(o)	skull
cry(o)	cold
cut	skin
cyan(o)	blue
cyst(o)	bladder
cyt(o)	cell
dactyl(o)	finger or toe
dent	tooth
derm(ato)	skin
dipl(o)	double
dors	back
dys	bad, faulty, abnormal
ectomy	excision (removal by cutting)
emia	blood
encephal(o)	brain
end(o)	inside
enter(o)	intestine
epi	outer, superficial, upon
erythr(o)	red
eu	normal
extra	outside
gastr(o)	stomach
gen	become, originate
gloss(o)	tongue
glyc(o)	sweet, or referring to glucose
gram, graph	write, record
gyn	woman
hem(ato)	blood
hemi	half
hepat(o)	liver
hist(o)	tissue
hydr(o)	water
hyper	excessive, high

hypo	deficient, low		pharmaco	drug
hyster(o)	uterus		pharyng(o)	throat
iatr(o)	doctor		phleb(o)	vein
infra	beneath		phob(ia)	fear
inter	among, between		plasty	repair
intra	inside		pleg(ia)	paralysis
itis	inflammation		pnea	breathing
lact(o)	milk		pneum(ato)	breath, air
lapar(o)	flank, abdomen		pneumon(o)	lung
latero	side		pod(o)	foot
leuk(o)	white		poie	make, produce
lingu(o)	tongue		poly	much, many
lip(o)	fat		post	after
lys(is)	dissolve		poster(i)	back, behind
mal	bad, abnormal		presby	elder
malac	soft		proct(o)	anus
mamm(o)	breast		pseud(o)	false
mast(o)	breast		psych(o)	mind
megal(o)	large		pulmon(o)	lung
melan(o)	black		pyel(o)	pelvis of kidney
mening(o)	membranes		pyr(o)	fever, fire
my(o)	muscle		rachi(o)	spine
myc(o)	fungus		ren(o)	kidneys
myel(o)	marrow		rhag	break, burst
nas(o)	nose		rhe	flow
necr(o)	death		rhin(o)	nose
nephr(o)	kidney		scler(o)	hard
neur(o)	nerve		scope	instrument
nutri	nourish		scopy	examination
ocul(o)	eye		somat(o)	body
odyn(o)	pain		spondyl(o)	vertebra
oma	tumor		steat(o)	fat
onc(o)	tumor		sten(o)	narrow, compressed
oophor(o)	ovaries		steth(o)	chest
ophthalm(o)	eye		stom	mouth, opening
opia	vision		supra	above
opsy	examination		tachy	fast, quick
orchi(o)	testes		therap	treatment
osis	condition		therm(o)	heat
osse(o)	bone		thorac(o)	chest
oste(o)	bone		thromb(o)	clot, lump
ot(o)	ear		tomy	incision (operation by cutting)
path(o)	disease		tox(i)	poison
ped(o)	child		uria	urine
penia	deficient, deficiency		vas(o)	vessel
peps, pept	digest		ven(o)	vein
peri	around		vesic(o)	bladder
phag(o)	eat, destroy		xer(o)	dry

Fundamentals

CHAPTER 1

Anatomy

Biology includes the study of the anatomy and physiology of living organisms. Anatomy is the study of structure, and physiology is the study of function.

Because the structure of living organisms is complex, anatomy is organized by levels, from the smallest components of cells to the largest organs and their relationships to other organs. Gross anatomy is the study of the body's organs as seen with the naked eye during visual inspection and dissection. Cellular anatomy is the study of cells and their components, which require special instruments such as microscopes and special techniques for observation.

Cells

Often thought of as the smallest unit of living organisms, a cell is made up of many even smaller parts, each with its own function. Human cells vary in size, but all are quite small. The largest, a fertilized egg, is too small to be seen with the naked eye.

Human cells have a membrane that holds the contents together. However, this membrane is not just a sac. It has receptors that identify the cell to other cells. The receptors also react to sub-stances produced in the body and to drugs taken into the body, selectively allowing these sub-stances or drugs to enter and leave the cell. Reactions that take place at the receptors often alter and control a cell's functions.

Within the cell membrane are two major compartments, the cytoplasm and the nucleus. The cytoplasm contains structures that consume and transform energy and carry out the cell's functions; the nucleus contains the cell's genetic material and the structures that control cell division and reproduction.

The body is composed of many different types of cells, each with its own structure and function. Some, such as white blood cells, move freely, unattached to other cells. Others, such as muscle cells, are firmly attached one to another. Some cells, such as skin cells, divide and reproduce quickly; nerve cells, on the other hand, don't reproduce at all. Some cells, especially glandular cells, have as their primary function the production of complex substances, such as a hormone or an enzyme. For example, cells in the breast produce milk, those in the pancreas produce insulin, those in the lining of the lungs produce mucus, and those in the mouth produce saliva. Other cells have primary functions that are not related

Inside the Torso

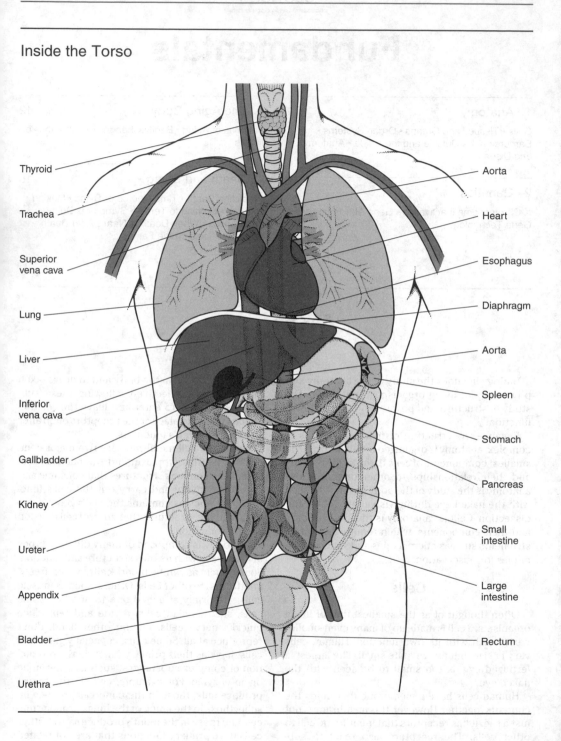

Thyroid

Trachea

Superior
vena cava

Lung

Liver

Inferior
vena cava

Gallbladder

Kidney

Ureter

Appendix

Bladder

Urethra

Aorta

Heart

Esophagus

Diaphragm

Aorta

Spleen

Stomach

Pancreas

Small
intestine

Large
intestine

Rectum

Inside a Cell

Although there are different types of cells, most cells have the same components. A cell consists of a nucleus and cytoplasm and is contained within the cell membrane, which regulates what passes in and out. The nucleus controls the production of proteins. It contains chromosomes, which are the cell's genetic material, and a nucleolus, which produces ribosomes. The cytoplasm consists of a fluid material and organelles, which could be considered the cell's organs. The endoplasmic reticulum transports materials within the cell. Ribosomes produce proteins, which are packaged by the Golgi apparatus so that they can leave the cell. Mitochondria generate energy for the cell's activities. Lysosomes contain enzymes that can break down particles entering the cell. For example, certain white blood cells engulf bacteria, which are then broken down by enzymes in lysosomes. Centrioles participate in cell division.

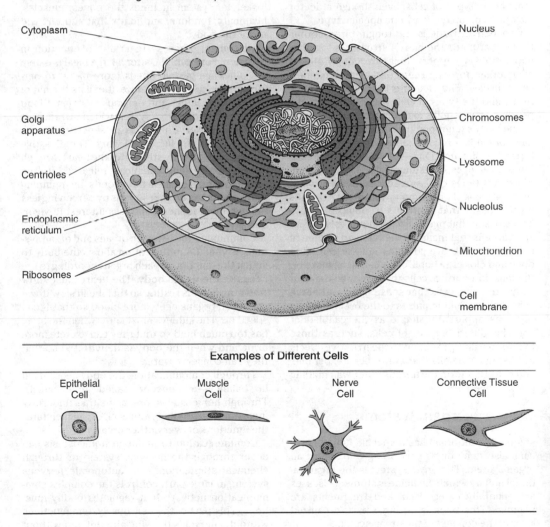

Cytoplasm
Golgi apparatus
Centrioles
Endoplasmic reticulum
Ribosomes
Nucleus
Chromosomes
Lysosome
Nucleolus
Mitochondrion
Cell membrane

Examples of Different Cells

| Epithelial Cell | Muscle Cell | Nerve Cell | Connective Tissue Cell |

to the production of substances—for example, cells in the muscles and heart contract. Nerve cells conduct electrical impulses, allowing communication between the central nervous system (brain and spinal cord) and the rest of the body.

Tissues and Organs

Related cells joined together are collectively referred to as a tissue. The cells in a tissue are not identical, but they work together to accomplish specific functions. A sample of tissue removed for examination under a microscope (biopsy) contains many types of cells, even though a doctor may be interested in only one specific type.

Connective tissue is the tough, often fibrous tissue that binds the body's structures together and provides support. It is present in almost every organ, forming a large part of skin, tendons, and muscles. The characteristics of connective tissue and the types of cells it contains vary, depending on where it's found in the body.

The body's functions are conducted by organs. Each organ is a recognizable structure that performs specific functions—for example, the heart, lungs, liver, eyes, and stomach. An organ is made of several types of tissue and therefore several types of cells. For example, the heart contains muscle tissue that contracts to pump blood, fibrous tissue that makes up the heart valves, and special cells that maintain the rate and rhythm of heartbeats. The eye contains muscle cells that open and close the pupil, clear cells that make up the lens and cornea, cells that produce the fluid within the eye, cells that sense light, and nerve cells that conduct impulses to the brain. Even an organ as apparently simple as the gallbladder contains different types of cells, such as those that form a lining resistant to the irritative effects of bile, muscle cells that contract to expel bile, and cells that form the fibrous outer wall holding the sac together.

Organ Systems

Although an organ has a specific function, organs also function as part of a group, called an organ system. The organ system is the organizational unit by which medicine is studied, diseases are generally categorized, and treatments are planned. This book is, in large part, organized around the concept of the organ system.

An example of an organ system is the cardiovascular system, which includes the heart (cardio) and blood vessels (vascular). The cardiovascular system is responsible for pumping and circulating the blood. The digestive system, extending from the mouth to the anus, is responsible for receiving and digesting food and excreting waste. This system includes not only the stomach, small intestine, and large intestine, which move food, but also associated organs such as the pancreas, liver, and gallbladder, which produce digestive enzymes, remove toxins, and store substances necessary for digestion. The musculoskeletal system includes the bones, muscles, ligaments, tendons, and joints that support and move the body.

Of course, organ systems do not function in isolation. For example, after a large meal is eaten, the digestive system needs more blood to perform its functions. Therefore, it enlists the aid of the cardiovascular and nervous systems. Blood vessels of the digestive system widen to transport more blood. Nerve impulses are sent to the brain, notifying it of the increased work. The digestive system even directly stimulates the heart through nerve impulses and chemicals released into the bloodstream. The heart responds by pumping more blood; the brain responds by perceiving less hunger, more fullness, and less interest in vigorous activity.

Communication between organs and organ systems is vital. Communication allows the body to adjust the function of each organ according to the needs of the whole body. The heart must know when the body is resting so that it can slow down and when organs need more blood so that it can speed up. The kidneys must know when the body has too much fluid so that they can excrete more urine and when the body is dehydrated so that they can conserve water.

Through communication, the body keeps itself in balance—a concept called homeostasis. Through homeostasis, organs neither underproduce nor overproduce, and each organ facilitates the functions of every other organ.

Communication to maintain homeostasis can occur through the nervous system or through chemical stimulation. The autonomic nervous system, in large part, controls the complex communication network that regulates bodily functions. This part of the nervous system functions without a person's thinking about it and without

Major Organ Systems

System	Organs in the System	System	Organs in the System
Cardiovascular	• Heart • Blood vessels (arteries, capillaries, veins)	Digestive	• Mouth • Esophagus • Stomach • Small intestine • Large intestine • Liver • Gallbladder • Pancreas (the part that produces enzymes)
Respiratory	• Nose • Mouth • Pharynx • Larynx • Trachea • Bronchi • Lungs	Endocrine	• Thyroid gland • Parathyroid gland • Adrenal glands • Pancreas (the part that produces insulin)
Nervous	• Brain • Spinal cord • Nerves	Urinary	• Kidneys • Ureters • Bladder • Urethra
Skin	• Skin		
Musculoskeletal	• Muscles • Tendons and ligaments • Bones • Joints	Male reproductive	• Penis • Prostate gland • Seminal vesicles • Vasa deferentia • Testes
Blood	• Blood cells and platelets • Plasma (liquid part of blood) • Bone marrow (where blood cells are produced) • Spleen • Thymus	Female reproductive	• Vagina • Cervix • Uterus • Fallopian tubes • Ovaries

much noticeable indication that it is working. Chemicals used to communicate are called transmitters. Transmitters that are produced by one organ and travel to other organs through the bloodstream are called hormones. Transmitters that conduct messages between parts of the nervous system are called neurotransmitters.

One of the best known transmitters is the hormone epinephrine (adrenaline). When a person is suddenly stressed or frightened, the brain instantly sends a message to the adrenal glands, which quickly release epinephrine. Within moments, this chemical has the entire body on alert, a response sometimes called preparation for fight or flight. The heart beats more rapidly and powerfully, the eyes dilate to allow more light in, breathing quickens, and the activity of the digestive system decreases to allow more blood to go to the muscles. The effect is rapid and intense.

Other chemical communications are less dramatic but equally effective. For example, when the body becomes dehydrated and needs more water, the volume of blood circulating through the cardiovascular system decreases. This decreased blood volume is perceived by receptors in the arteries in the neck. They respond by sending impulses through nerves to the pituitary gland, at the base of the brain, which then produces antidiuretic hormone. This hormone signals the kidneys to produce less urine and retain more water. Simultaneously, the brain senses thirst, stimulating a person to drink.

The body also has a group of organs—the endocrine system—whose primary function is to produce hormones that regulate the function of other organs. For example, the thyroid gland produces thyroid hormone, which controls the metabolic rate (the speed at which the body's chemical functions proceed); the pancreas produces insulin, which controls the use of sugar; and the adrenal glands produce epinephrine, which stimulates many organs to prepare the body for stress.

Barriers on the Outside and the Inside

As strange as it may seem, defining what's outside and what's inside the body isn't always easy because the body has many surfaces. The skin, which is actually an organ system, is one obvious surface, forming a barrier that prevents many harmful substances from entering the body. Although covered by a thin layer of skin, the ear canal is usually thought of as inside the body because it penetrates deep into the head. The digestive system is a long tube that begins at the mouth, winds through the body, and exits at the anus. Is food that's partially absorbed as it passes through this tube inside or outside of the body? Nutrients and fluid aren't really inside the body until they are absorbed into the bloodstream.

Air passes through the nose and throat into the windpipe (trachea), then into the extensive, branching airways of the lungs (bronchi). At what point does this passageway stop being outside and become inside the body? Oxygen in the lungs isn't useful to the body until it enters the bloodstream. To enter the bloodstream, oxygen must cross through a thin layer of cells lining the lungs. This layer acts as a barrier to viruses and bacteria, such as those that cause tuberculosis, which may be carried into the lungs with air. Unless these organisms penetrate the cells or enter the bloodstream, they don't cause disease. Because the lungs have many protective mechanisms, such as antibodies to fight infection and cilia to sweep debris out of the airways, most infectious organisms never cause disease.

Body surfaces not only separate the outside from the inside, but also keep structures and substances in their proper place so that they can function properly. For example, internal organs don't float in a pool of blood; blood is normally confined to blood vessels. If blood leaks out of the vessels into other parts of the body (hemorrhage), it not only fails to bring oxygen and nutrients to tissues but also can cause severe harm.

For example, a very small hemorrhage into the brain destroys brain tissue because there is no room for expansion within the confines of the skull. On the other hand, a similar amount of blood leaking into the abdomen doesn't destroy tissue.

Saliva, so important in the mouth, can cause severe damage if inhaled into the lungs. The hydrochloric acid produced by the stomach rarely causes harm there. However, the acid can burn and damage the esophagus if it flows backward and can damage other organs if it leaks through the stomach wall. Feces, the undigested part of food expelled through the anus, can cause life-threatening infections if it leaks through the intestinal wall into the abdominal cavity.

Anatomy and Disease

The human body is remarkably well designed. Most of its organs have a great deal of extra capacity or reserve: They can still function adequately even though damaged. For example, more than two thirds of the liver must be destroyed before serious consequences occur, and a person can survive after an entire lung is surgically removed as long as the other lung is functioning normally. Other organs can tolerate little damage before they malfunction. For example, if a stroke destroys a small amount of vital brain tissue, a person may be unable to speak, move a limb, or maintain balance. A heart attack, which destroys heart tissue, may slightly impair the heart's ability to pump blood, or it may result in death.

Disease affects anatomy, and changes in anatomy can cause disease. Abnormal growths, such as cancer, can directly destroy normal tissue or produce pressure that ultimately destroys it. If the blood supply to a tissue is blocked or cut off, the tissue dies (infarction), as in a heart attack (myocardial infarction) or stroke (cerebral infarction).

Because of the relationship between disease and anatomy, methods of seeing into the body have become a mainstay of the diagnosis and treatment of disease. The first breakthrough came with x-rays, which enabled doctors to see into the body and examine organs without surgery. Another major advance was computed tomography (CT), in which x-rays are linked with computers. A CT scan produces detailed, two-dimensional images of the body's interior.

Other methods of producing images of internal structures include ultrasound scanning, which uses sound waves; magnetic resonance imaging (MRI), which uses the movement of atoms in a magnetic field; and radionuclide imaging, which uses radioactive chemicals injected into the body. These are noninvasive ways to see into the body, in contrast to surgery, which is an invasive procedure.

Anatomy in This Book

Because anatomy is so important to medicine, almost every section of this book begins with a description of the anatomy of an organ system. Illustrations throughout the book focus on the part of the anatomy being discussed.

CHAPTER 2

Genetics

The body's genetic material is contained within the nucleus of each of its cells. The genetic material consists of coils of DNA (deoxyribonucleic acid) arranged in a complex way to form chromosomes. Human cells contain 46 chromosomes in pairs, including one pair of sex chromosomes.

Each DNA molecule is a long double helix that resembles a spiral staircase. The steps of the staircase, which determine a person's genetic code, consist of pairs of four types of molecules called bases. In the steps, adenine is paired with thymine, and guanine is paired with cytosine. The genetic code is written in triplets, so each group of three steps of the staircase codes the production of one of the amino acids, which are the building blocks of proteins.

When a part of the DNA molecule is actively controlling some function of the cell, the DNA helix splits open along its length. One strand of the open helix is inactive; the other strand acts as a template against which a complementary strand of RNA (ribonucleic acid) forms. The RNA bases are arranged in the same sequence as bases of the inactive strand of the DNA, except that RNA contains uracil and DNA contains thymine. The RNA copy, called messenger RNA (mRNA), separates from the DNA, leaves the nucleus, and travels into the cytoplasm of the cell. There, it attaches to ribosomes, the cell's factories for manufacturing proteins. The messenger RNA instructs the ribosome as to the sequence of amino acids for constructing a specific protein. Amino acids are brought to the ribosome by transfer RNA (tRNA), a much smaller type of RNA. Each molecule of transfer RNA brings one amino acid to be incorporated into the growing chain of protein.

A gene consists of the code required to construct one protein. Genes vary in size, depending on the size of the protein. Genes are arranged in a precise sequence on the chromosomes; the location of a particular gene is called its locus.

The two sex chromosomes determine whether a fetus becomes male or female. Males have one X and one Y sex chromosome; females have two X chromosomes, only one of which is active. The Y chromosome carries relatively few genes, one of which determines sex. In males, virtually all of the genes on the X chromosome, whether dominant or recessive, are expressed. Genes on the X chromosome are referred to as sex-linked, or X-linked, genes.

X-Chromosome Inactivation

Because a female has two X chromosomes, she has twice as many X-chromosome genes as does a male. This would seem to result in an overdose of some genes. However, one of the two X chromosomes in each cell of the female—except in the eggs in the ovaries—is thought to be inactivated early in the life of the fetus. The inactive X chromosome (the Barr body) is visible under a microscope as a dense lump in the nucleus of the cell.

The inactivation of the X chromosome explains certain observations. For example, extra X chromosomes cause far fewer developmental abnormalities than extra nonsex (autosomal)

Structure of DNA

DNA (deoxyribonucleic acid) is the cell's genetic material, found in jumbled, loosely coiled threads called chromatin in the nucleus of each cell. Just before a cell divides, the chromatin becomes tightly coiled, forming chromosomes.

The DNA molecule is a long, coiled double helix that resembles a spiral staircase. In it, two strands, composed of sugar (deoxyribose) and phosphate molecules, are connected by pairs of four molecules called bases, which form the steps of the staircase. In the steps, adenine is paired with thymine, and guanine with cytosine. Each pair of bases is held together by a hydrogen bond. A gene is a segment of DNA that has a particular function and consists of a specific sequence of bases.

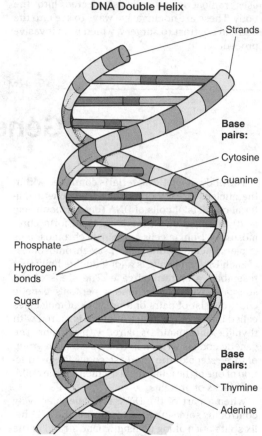

DNA Double Helix

Strands

Base pairs:

Cytosine

Guanine

Phosphate

Hydrogen bonds

Sugar

Base pairs:

Thymine

Adenine

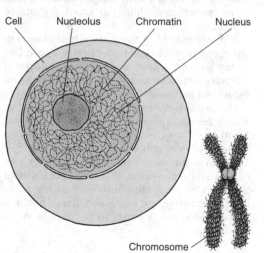

Cell   Nucleolus   Chromatin   Nucleus

Chromosome

chromosomes, because no matter how many X chromosomes a person has, all but one seem to be inactivated. Women with three X chromosomes (triple X syndrome) are often physically and mentally normal.▲ In contrast, an additional autosomal chromosome can be fatal during early fetal development. A baby born with an additional autosomal chromosome (a trisomy disorder) usually has many severe physical and mental abnormalities.■ Similarly, the absence of an autosomal chromosome is invariably fatal to the fetus, but the absence of one X chromosome usually results in relatively less severe abnormalities (Turner's syndrome).★

▲ see page 1239

■ see box, page 1239

★ see page 1239

Gene Abnormalities

Abnormalities of one or more genes, particularly recessive genes, are fairly common. Every

Examples of Genetic Disorders

Gene	Dominant	Recessive
Non–X-linked	Marfan's syndrome, Huntington's disease	Cystic fibrosis, sickle cell anemia
X-linked	Familial rickets, hereditary nephritis	Red-green color blindness, hemophilia

human being carries six to eight abnormal recessive genes. However, these genes don't cause cells to function abnormally unless two similar recessive genes are present. In the general population, the chance of a person's having two similar recessive genes is very small, but in children of close relatives, the chances are higher. Chances are also high among groups that intermarry, such as the Amish or Mennonites.

A person's genetic makeup is called a **genotype.** The body's response to having those genes—that is, the expression of the genotype—is called the **phenotype.**

All inherited characteristics (traits) are encoded by genes. Some characteristics, such as hair color, simply distinguish people from one another; they aren't considered abnormal. However, abnormal characteristics expressed by an abnormal gene may cause a hereditary disease.

Single-Gene Abnormalities

The effects of a single-gene abnormality depend on whether the gene is dominant or recessive and whether it's located on an X chromosome (X-linked). Because each gene directs the production of a particular protein, an abnormal gene produces an abnormal protein or an abnormal amount of protein, which may cause an abnormality in cell function and ultimately in physical appearance or bodily function.

Non–X-Linked Genes

The effect (trait) produced by an abnormal dominant gene on an autosomal chromosome may be a deformity, a disease, or a tendency to develop certain diseases.

The following principles generally apply to traits determined by a **dominant gene:**
• People with the trait have at least one parent with the trait, unless it's caused by a new mutation.

• Abnormal genetic traits are often caused by new genetic mutations rather than by inheritance from the parents.
• When one parent has an abnormal trait and the other does not, each child has a 50 percent chance of inheriting the abnormal trait and a 50 percent chance of not inheriting it. However, if the parent with the abnormal trait has two copies of the abnormal gene—a rare occurrence—all of their children will have the abnormal trait.
• A person who doesn't have the abnormal trait, even though his siblings have it, doesn't carry the gene and can't pass the trait on to his offspring.
• Males and females are equally likely to be affected.
• The abnormality can, and usually does, appear in every generation.

The following principles generally apply to traits determined by a **recessive gene:**
• Virtually everyone with the trait has parents who both have the gene, but neither parent may have the trait.
• Mutations are highly unlikely to result in expression of the trait.
• When one parent has the trait and the other has one recessive gene but doesn't have the trait, half of their children are likely to have the trait; the others will be carriers with one recessive gene. If the parent without the trait doesn't have the abnormal recessive gene, none of their children will have the trait, but all of their children will inherit an abnormal gene that they can pass on to their offspring.
• A person who doesn't have the abnormal trait but whose siblings do have it is likely to carry one abnormal gene.
• Males and females are equally likely to be affected.
• The abnormality can appear in every generation but usually doesn't unless both parents have the trait.

Inheriting Abnormal Recessive Genes

Some diseases result from an abnormal recessive gene. To have the disease, a person must receive two genes for it, one from each parent. If both parents carry one abnormal gene and one normal gene, they don't have the disease but they can pass the abnormal gene to their children. Each child has a 25 percent chance of inheriting two abnormal genes (and thus of developing the disease), a 25 percent chance of inheriting two normal genes, and a 50 percent chance of inheriting one normal and one abnormal gene (thus becoming carriers of the disease like the parents).

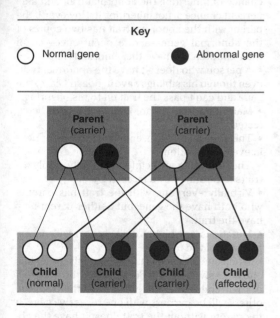

Key

◯ Normal gene   ● Abnormal gene

| Parent (carrier) | Parent (carrier) |

| Child (normal) | Child (carrier) | Child (carrier) | Child (affected) |

Dominant genes that cause severe diseases are rare. They tend to disappear because the people who have them are often too ill to have children. However, there are a few exceptions, such as Huntington's disease,▲ which causes severe deterioration in brain function that usually begins after

▲ see page 313

age 35. By the time symptoms occur, the person may already have had children.

Recessive genes are expressed only when a person has two such genes. A person with one recessive gene doesn't have the trait but is a carrier of the trait and can pass the gene on to his children.

X-Linked Genes

Because the Y chromosome in males has very few genes, the genes on the single X chromosome (X-linked, or sex-linked, genes) are virtually all unpaired and therefore expressed, whether they're dominant or recessive. But because females have two X chromosomes, the same principles apply to X-linked genes that apply to genes on autosomal chromosomes: Unless both genes in a pair are recessive, only dominant genes are expressed.

If an abnormal X-linked gene is dominant, affected males transmit the abnormality to all of their daughters but none of their sons. The sons of the affected male receive his Y chromosome, which doesn't carry the abnormal gene. Affected females with only one abnormal gene transmit the abnormality to half their children, male or female.

If an abnormal X-linked gene is recessive, nearly everyone with the trait is male. Men transmit the abnormal gene only to their daughters, all of whom become carriers. Carrier mothers do not have the trait but transmit the gene to half their sons, who usually have the trait. None of their daughters have the trait, but half are carriers.

Red-green color blindness, caused by a common X-linked recessive gene, affects about 10 percent of males but is unusual among females. In males, the gene for color blindness comes from a mother who is color-blind or who has normal vision but is a carrier of the color-blind gene. It never comes from the father, who instead supplies the Y chromosome. Daughters of color-blind fathers are rarely color-blind but are always carriers of the color-blind gene.

Codominant Inheritance

In codominant inheritance, both genes are expressed. An example is sickle cell anemia: If a person has one normal gene and one abnormal gene, both normal and abnormal red blood cell pigment (hemoglobin) is produced.

Abnormal Mitochondrial Genes

Inside every cell are mitochondria, tiny structures that provide the cell with energy. Each

Inheriting Abnormal Recessive X-Linked Genes

If a gene is X-linked, it appears on the X chromosome and not on the Y chromosome. Diseases that result from an abnormal recessive X-linked gene usually develop only in males. This is because males have only one X chromosome. Females have two X chromosomes, so they usually receive a normal gene on the second X chromosome. The normal gene is dominant, preventing females from developing the disease.

If the father has an abnormal recessive gene on his X chromosome and the mother has two normal genes, all of their daughters receive one abnormal gene and one normal gene, making them carriers. None of their sons receive the abnormal gene.

If the mother is a carrier and the father has the normal gene, any son has a 50 percent chance of receiving the abnormal gene from the mother. Any daughter has a 50 percent chance of receiving one abnormal gene and one normal gene (becoming carriers) or of receiving two normal genes.

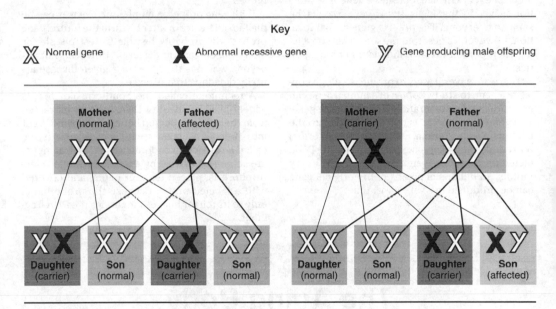

mitochondrion contains a circular chromosome. Several rare diseases are caused by abnormal genes carried by the chromosome inside a mitochondrion.

When an egg is fertilized, only mitochondria from the egg become part of the developing fetus; all mitochondria from the sperm are discarded. Therefore, diseases caused by abnormal mitochondrial genes are transmitted by the mother. A father with abnormal mitochondrial genes can't transmit any such diseases to his children.

Genes That Cause Cancer

Cancer cells may contain oncogenes, which are genes that cause cancer (also called tumor genes).▲ Sometimes oncogenes are abnormal versions of the genes responsible for growth and development before birth, which normally are permanently deactivated after birth. These on-

▲ see page 789

cogenes may be reactivated later in life and may cause cancer. How they are reactivated isn't known.

Gene Technology

Rapidly changing technology is improving the detection of genetic diseases, both before and after birth. Knowledge is expanding especially rapidly in the field of DNA technology.

One effort currently under way, called the Human Genome Project, is the identification and mapping of all the genes on human chromosomes. A genome is a person's entire set of genes. At each locus of every chromosome lies a gene. The function served by that locus, such as eye color, is the same in everyone. The precise gene at that location, however, varies from person to person, giving each person his own individual characteristics.

There are several ways to produce enough copies of a gene to study. Copies of a human gene can be produced in a laboratory by cloning the gene. The gene to be copied is usually spliced into the DNA inside a bacterium. Each time the bacterium reproduces, it makes an exact copy of all its DNA, including the spliced gene. Bacteria multiply very rapidly, so billions of copies of the original gene can be produced in a very short time.

Another technique for copying DNA uses the polymerase chain reaction (PCR). A specific segment of DNA, including a specific gene, can be copied (amplified) more than 200,000 times in a matter of hours in a laboratory. The DNA from a single cell is sufficient to start a polymerase chain reaction.

A gene probe can be used to locate a specific gene in a particular chromosome. A gene that has been cloned or copied becomes a labeled probe when a radioactive atom is added to it. The probe will seek out its mirror-image segment of DNA and bind to it. The radioactive probe can then be detected by sophisticated photographic techniques.

With gene probes, a number of diseases can be diagnosed before or after birth. In the future, gene probes will probably be able to test people for many major genetic diseases. However, not everyone who has the gene for a given disease actually develops that disease.

A technique called the Southern blot test is widely used to identify DNA. DNA is extracted from the cells of a person being studied and is cut into precise fragments with a type of enzyme called a restriction endonuclease. The fragments are separated in a gel by a technique called electrophoresis, placed on filter paper, and covered with a labeled probe. Because the probe binds only to its mirror image, it identifies the DNA fragment.

CHAPTER 3

The Aging Body

The average life expectancy has increased dramatically in the United States. A male child born in 1900 could expect to live only 46 years, whereas one born today can expect to live more than 72 years. A female child born in 1900 could expect to live 48 years, whereas one born today can expect to live about 79 years.

Despite the increase in average life expectancy, the maximum life span—the oldest age to which people can live—has changed little since records have been kept. Despite the best genetic makeup and medical care, no one seems to live much beyond 120 years.

Theories of Aging

Every species ages, undergoing noticeable changes from birth to death. Scientists have developed theories for why people age, although no theory has been proven. Ultimately, parts of each theory may explain why people grow old and die.

With the programmed senescence theory, the rate at which a species grows old is predetermined by its genes. Genes determine how long cells live. As cells die, organs begin to malfunction and eventually cannot maintain the biologic functions necessary to sustain life. Programmed senescence helps preserve a species; older members die at a rate that allows room for the young.

The free-radical theory says that cells age as a result of accumulated harm from ongoing chemical reactions within cells. During these ongoing chemical reactions, toxins called free radicals are produced. The free radicals ultimately damage the cells and cause a person to age. With age, more and more damage is done until many cells cannot function normally or have died. When that happens, the body dies. Different species age at different rates depending on how cells produce and respond to free radicals.

Bodily Changes

The human body changes in many noticeable ways with age. Perhaps the first sign of aging occurs when the eye cannot focus easily on close objects (presbyopia). Often by age 40 or so, many people find it difficult to read without using glasses. Hearing also changes with age. People tend to lose some ability to hear the highest pitched tones (presbycusis). Therefore, older people may find that violin music no longer sounds as exciting as it did when they were younger. Also, because most of the closed consonants of speech are high tones (sounds such as k, t, s, p, and ch), older people may think that others are mumbling.

In most people, the proportion of body fat increases by more than 30 percent with age. The distribution of fat also changes: There is less fat under the skin and more in the abdominal area. Thus, skin becomes thinner, wrinkled, and more fragile, and the shape of the torso changes.

Not surprisingly, most internal functions also decline with age. These functions generally peak shortly before age 30 and then begin a gradual but straightline decline. Even with this decline, however, most functions remain adequate throughout life, because most organs have considerably more functional capacity than the body needs (functional reserve). For example, even if half the liver is destroyed, more than enough liver tissue remains to maintain normal function. Disease, rather than normal aging, usually accounts for loss of function in old age. Even so, the decline in function means that older people are more likely to experience adverse effects from drugs, changes in the environment, toxins, and illness.

Although the decline in function of many organs has little effect on how people live, the de-

How the Body Changes With Age

- Blood flow to the kidneys, liver, and brain decreases

- The kidneys' ability to clear toxins and drugs decreases

- The liver's ability to clear toxins and metabolize most drugs decreases

- Maximum heart rate decreases, but resting heart rate doesn't change

- Maximum output of blood from the heart decreases

- Glucose tolerance decreases

- The lungs' air-moving capacity decreases

- Amount of air trapped in the lungs after exhaling increases

- Infection-fighting function of cells decreases

cline in some organs can greatly affect health and well-being. For example, although the amount of blood that the heart can pump at rest is not greatly reduced in old age, the heart cannot pump as much when pushed to its maximum. This means that older athletes will not be able to perform as well as younger athletes. Changes in kidney function can dramatically affect how well older people are able to eliminate certain drugs from their body.▲

Determining which changes are purely age related and which are the result of how a person has lived is often difficult. A sedentary lifestyle, poor diet, cigarette smoking, and alcohol and drug abuse can damage many body organs over time, often more so than aging alone. People who have been exposed to toxins may experience a more significant or more rapid decline in the function of some organs, especially the kidneys, lungs, and liver. People who worked in loud environments are likely to lose more of their hearing.

▲ see page 39

Disorders That Affect Mainly the Elderly

Disease or Condition	Explanation
Alzheimer's disease and other dementias	Brain disorders that lead to progressive loss of memory and other intellectual functions
Bedsores	Breakdown of skin from prolonged pressure
Benign prostatic hyperplasia	Enlargement of the prostate gland (in men), which blocks the flow of urine
Cataracts	Opacities in the lens of the eye that impair vision
Chronic lymphocytic leukemia	A type of leukemia
Diabetes, type 2 (adult onset)	A type of diabetes that may not require insulin treatment
Glaucoma	Elevation of the pressure in one of the chambers of the eye that can decrease vision and lead to blindness
Monoclonal gammopathies	A group of diverse conditions in which abnormal proliferation of a single type of cell produces high levels of an immunoglobulin

Disease or Condition	Explanation
Osteoarthritis	Degeneration of the cartilage that lines the joints, causing pain
Osteoporosis	Loss of calcium from the bones, which makes the bones fragile and can lead to fractures
Parkinson's disease	Slowly progressive degenerative brain disease that leads to tremor, muscle rigidity, difficulty moving, and postural instability
Prostate cancer	A cancer of the prostate gland (in men)
Shingles (herpes zoster)	A reawakening of the dormant chickenpox virus, which causes a skin rash and can cause prolonged pain
Stroke	A blockage or bleeding of a blood vessel in the brain that leads to weakness, loss of sensation, difficulty talking, or other neurologic problems
Urinary incontinence	Inability to control urination

Some changes can be prevented by changing to a healthier lifestyle. For example, stopping smoking at any age, even in one's 80s, helps improve lung function and decrease the chance of developing lung cancer. Weight-bearing exercise helps maintain muscle and bone strength regardless of age.

Implications of Illness

Geriatrics is the medical care of elderly people. Gerontology is the study of aging. There is no specific age at which a person becomes "elderly," although traditionally that age has been set at 65, because that is when working adults have tended to retire.

A number of disorders, sometimes called the geriatric syndromes or geriatric diseases, occur almost exclusively in older adults. Other disorders affect people of all ages but are more common or more severe or cause different symptoms or complications in the elderly.

Elderly people often experience illness differently than do younger adults. A disease may cause different symptoms in elderly people. For example, an underactive thyroid gland usually causes younger people to gain weight and feel sluggish. In the elderly, an underactive thyroid gland may also produce confusion that can be mistaken for dementia. An overactive thyroid usually causes younger people to become agitated and lose weight; in the elderly, it may cause them to become sleepy, withdrawn, depressed, and confused. Depression usually causes younger adults to become tearful, withdrawn, and noticeably unhappy. In the elderly, depression sometimes causes confusion, loss of memory, and apathy, all of which may be mistaken for dementia.

Acute illnesses such as heart attacks, hip fractures, and pneumonia were once likely to result in death for older adults. Now these illnesses are often treatable and controllable even when they are not curable. In turn, a chronic illness no longer necessarily means disability. Many people with diabetes, kidney problems, heart disease, and other chronic illnesses now find that they can remain functional, active, and independent.

Sociologic and economic factors often change the way the elderly seek and receive care. Many elderly people tend to conceal minor problems and don't seek medical care until the problems become major. Elderly people tend to have more than one disease at a time, and those diseases may have an impact on each other. For example, depression may make dementia worse, and diabetes may make an infection more severe.

Sociologic factors often complicate disease in the elderly. If illness leads to some temporary or permanent loss of independence, an older person may become depressed and need both social services and psychologic help. For these reasons, geriatricians often recommend multidisciplinary care. With this type of care, a team of medical personnel, which may consist of doctors, nurses, social workers, therapists, pharmacists, and psychologists, plan and implement care under the leadership of a primary doctor.

CHAPTER 4

Death and Dying

A century ago, most people who suffered traumatic injuries or contracted serious infections died soon afterward. Even those who developed heart disease or cancer had little expectation of a long life after the disease was diagnosed. Death was a familiar experience, and most people expected little more than comfort care from doctors.

Today, death is often seen as an event that can be deferred indefinitely rather than as an intrinsic part of life. The leading causes of death for people over age 65 years are heart disease, cancer, stroke, chronic obstructive pulmonary disease, pneumonia, and dementia. Medical procedures commonly extend the lives of people who have these diseases, often giving people many years in which quality of life and function are quite good. Other times, procedures extend life, but the quality of life and function decline. Death often seems unexpected even though the family knew that the person who died had a serious illness.

To say that a person is dying typically means that the person's death is expected to occur in hours or days. Also, people who are very old and frail or who have a fatal disease such as AIDS are often said to be dying. Most people with chronic diseases—such as heart disease, certain cancers, emphysema, liver or kidney failure, Alzheimer's disease, and other dementias—live for years, although they become limited in physical activity.

Predicting Death

Predicting when a person will die of a chronic disease is sometimes necessary. Health insurance often does not cover comfort care for chronic disease, except for hospice care, which usually requires a prognosis of less than 6 months—an arbitrary time that may be difficult to predict accurately.

Doctors can make a fairly accurate short-term prognosis for an average patient with certain conditions, based on statistical analyses of large groups of patients with similar conditions. For example, they may accurately estimate that 5 out of 100 patients with similar critical conditions will survive and leave the hospital. But predicting how long a particular person will survive is much more difficult. The best prediction a doctor can make is based on odds and the degree to which the doctor is confident in those odds. If the odds of survival are 10 percent, people should acknowledge the 90 percent likelihood of dying and should make plans accordingly.

When statistical information isn't available, a doctor may be unable to predict a prognosis or may make one on the basis of personal experience, which may be less accurate. Some doctors prefer to offer hope by describing remarkable recoveries without also mentioning the high likelihood that most people who have such a condition will die. However, gravely ill people and their families are entitled to the most complete information available and the most realistic prognosis possible.

Often the available choices are between dying sooner but remaining comfortable and living slightly longer by receiving aggressive therapy, which may prolong the dying process, increase discomfort and dependence, and decrease the quality of life. Nevertheless, patients and their families may feel that they must try such therapies if any chance of survival exists, even when hope of cure is unrealistic. Questions of philosophy, values, and religious beliefs come into play when such decisions are made by and for a dying patient.

Time Course of Dying

Dying may be marked by deterioration over a long period of time, punctuated with bouts of complications and side effects, as in some people who have cancer. Usually about 1 month before death, energy, function, and comfort decrease substantially. The person is visibly failing, and the fact that death is near becomes obvious to all.

Dying follows other time courses. Sometimes, a person being treated aggressively for a serious illness in a hospital abruptly worsens and is known to be dying only a few hours or days before death. Increasingly common, however, is dying with a slow decline in capabilities over a long period of time, perhaps with episodes of severe symptoms. Neurologic diseases such as Alzheimer's disease follow this pattern, as do emphysema, liver failure, kidney failure, and other chronic conditions. Severe heart disease disables people over time and causes severe symptoms intermittently, but it usually kills suddenly with a disturbance in the heart's rhythm (arrhythmia).

Knowing the likely time course of a disease enables a person who has the disease and the family to make plans. When death from an arrhythmia is likely, they should be prepared for death at any time. For people who have cancer, the decline that precedes death usually gives some warning that the final days have arrived.

Making Choices

Honest, open communication between patient and doctor about the patient's preferences for care at the end of life is essential for the best possible quality of life during a fatal illness. The doctor provides a candid assessment of the likelihood of recovery and disability during and after various treatment options, and the patient tells the doctor and his family what he wants and doesn't want to experience. The patient should state his preferences for treatment, the limits he wants placed on that treatment, and his wishes concerning where he wants to die and what he wants done when death is expected.

When choosing a doctor, a person should ask about care at the end of life: Does the doctor have substantial experience caring for dying patients? Does the doctor care for the patient until death in all settings—hospital, nursing home, or home? Does the doctor treat symptoms fully (palliative care) at the end of life? Is the doctor familiar with the home health, physical therapy, and occupational therapy services in the community—who qualifies for them, how they are paid for, and how to help patients and families get more intensive services when needed?

A system of care includes a financing system, such as insurance policies and managed care, and a care delivery system, such as a hospital, a nursing home, and home health care agencies. Asking questions of doctors, nurses, other patients and families, social workers, and case managers can help a person find a good system of care.

• What treatments are available in the system?
• What information is available about the merits of possible treatments? How can a patient talk to

other patients and families who have been treated there?

• What experimental treatments are available? How have other patients done with these treatments? How are these treatments paid for?

Having asked these questions, patients and families should ask themselves the following:

• Do they feel they are getting honest answers to their questions?

• Will they be medically, emotionally, and financially supported in this system?

• Will this system accommodate their specific preferences and plans?

Durable Power of Attorney for Health Care

A patient should name a trusted person as a proxy or surrogate in a legal document called a durable power of attorney for health care.▲ The proxy is given authority to make health care decisions for the patient in case the patient becomes unable to do so. If the patient doesn't name a proxy, the next of kin usually makes such decisions. But in some jurisdictions and for some decisions, the next of kin must go to court to obtain this authority. Having a durable power of attorney avoids court costs and delays and is especially important when the next of kin is not the best proxy or the relationship with the proxy is not legally recognized.

Advance Directives and Living Wills

A patient can give directions about the type of care he wants before he needs it. These advance medical directives are important if the patient becomes incapable of making decisions.■ The directives may be general statements of goals and philosophy, but they should become more specific as the illness progresses. Advance directives may be documented as living wills, but a letter written by the patient or documentation of the patient's directives in the medical chart may be all that's needed.

In making decisions about advance directives, patients must fully understand their circumstances and choices. Talking with a doctor is essential to making a specific, usable advance directive. In addition, the directives must be given to caregivers in all settings. Thoughtful decisions made at a nursing home are irrelevant if caregivers at a hospital know nothing about them. A person who wants to die at home and does not wish

Services to Know About

Home care is medically supervised care in a person's home by professional caregivers, who may help with administration of drugs, assess the person's condition, and provide baths and other personal services.

Hospice care is care at the end of life that emphasizes relief of symptoms and provides psychologic and social support for a dying person and the family. The setting may be the person's home, a hospice facility, or a hospital. To obtain hospice care, a person usually has to have a prognosis of less than 6 months.

Nursing home care is residential care in a licensed facility with nurses and support workers.

Respite care is temporary care at home, in a nursing home, or in a hospice facility that enables family members or other caregivers to travel, rest, or attend to other matters. It may last days or weeks, depending on the care delivery system and funding.

Voluntary organizations provide a variety of financial and support services to people who are ill and their families. Such organizations usually focus on people who have a certain disease.

to be resuscitated should ask the doctor to issue an order for emergency personnel not to transfer him to a hospital or attempt resuscitation. Family members should be instructed not to call 911 to request such interventions.

Planning Care

Patients and families may feel swept along by the illness and treatments, as if they have nothing to say about what's happening. Sometimes, this sense of having no control is preferable to taking responsibility for thinking about what else might be done. Patients and families vary in the amount

▲ see page 1369

■ see page 1368

of information and involvement in decision making that they want and should be able to have the amount they want. Then, all can be satisfied that everything was done to enable the patient to live as well and with as much dignity as possible while dying.

The patient, family, and professional caregivers should be realistic about the likelihood of death, discuss the likely complications, and plan to manage them. However, gaining perspective can be difficult when unexpected events happen and emotional responses confuse the decisions. Some decisions, such as whether to allow resuscitation—the only treatment provided automatically in the hospital—are less significant than they seem. An order against resuscitation attempts makes sense for most patients expected to die, and such a decision need not weigh heavily on the family. The patient is not likely to benefit from a resuscitation attempt. Resuscitation can be prohibited in advance directives. Food and water given through tubes (artificial nutrition and hydration) are not often useful to a dying patient and can also be prohibited in advance directives.

Other decisions may affect the patient and family more substantially and deserve more attention. For instance, the family may want to have the patient at home—a familiar, supportive setting—and not in a hospital. Family members should insist that doctors and other caregivers help make specific plans for these preferences and honor them. Hospitalization may be explicitly declined.

A patient nearing death is sometimes persuaded to try one last treatment, which often sacrifices the patient's last few days to side effects without gaining quality time. The patient and family should be skeptical of such treatments. As a patient nears death, the focus of care should shift entirely to providing comfort measures ensuring that he doesn't suffer.

Suicide

Many dying patients and their families consider suicide—even more so as the public debate grows. Those talking about suicide are largely motivated by loneliness, a sense of worthlessness, or uncontrolled symptoms. Discussing suicide with a doctor may help; the doctor can increase efforts to control pain, assure the patient and family that they are cherished, and help them find

meaning. Nevertheless, some patients and their families opt for suicide either as relief of an intolerable situation or as an exercise of autonomy in determining precisely when and how they wish to die.

Patients can ordinarily refuse treatments that might prolong life, including feeding tubes and respirators. Making such decisions isn't considered suicide.

Coming to Terms

People commonly experience denial when told that they will likely die of their illness. They may feel confused, distraught, angry, or sad, and they may withdraw. As these reactions abate, they begin to prepare for death—which often means finishing a life's work, setting things right with family and friends, and making peace with the inevitable.

Spiritual and religious issues are important to some patients and their families. Members of the clergy are part of the care team in some hospice and hospital facilities, and professional caregivers can help patients and their families find appropriate spiritual assistance if they don't have a relationship with a minister or other spiritual leader.

Preparing for death is hard work, with many emotional ups and downs. However, for most people, it's a time of new understanding and growth. By dealing with past hurts and mending relationships, a dying person and the family can achieve a profound sense of peace.

Symptoms During a Fatal Illness

Many fatal illnesses produce similar symptoms, including pain, shortness of breath, gastrointestinal problems, skin breakdown, and fatigue. Depression, anxiety, confusion, delirium, unconsciousness, and disability may also occur.

Pain

Most people fear pain as they confront dying. However, pain can usually be controlled while allowing the person to remain awake, involved in the world, and comfortable.

Radiation can control certain types of cancer pain. Physical therapy or analgesics, such as acetaminophen and aspirin, are used to control mild pain. For some people, hypnosis or biofeedback—approaches that have no notable adverse effects—effectively relieves pain. However, narcotics such as codeine and morphine are often needed.▲ Narcotics given by mouth can relieve pain effectively for many hours, and stronger narcotics can be given by injection. Drug addiction should not be a concern, and adequate medication should be given early, rather than held off until the pain is intolerable. There is no usual dose; some patients need small doses, whereas others need much larger doses.

Shortness of Breath

Struggling to breathe is one of the worst ways to live or die; it is also avoidable. Various methods can usually ease breathing—for example, relieving fluid buildup, changing the patient's position, providing supplemental oxygen, or shrinking a tumor that obstructs the airways with radiation or corticosteroids. Narcotics may help patients who have mild, persistent shortness of breath breathe more easily, even if they don't have pain. Taking narcotics at bedtime can promote comfortable sleep by preventing a patient from waking up frequently, fighting to breathe.

When these treatments aren't effective, most doctors who work in hospices agree that a patient suffering in this way should be given a narcotic in a dose that's high enough to relieve shortness of breath, even if the patient becomes unconscious. A patient who wants to avoid shortness of breath at the end of life should make sure that the doctor will treat this symptom fully, even if such treatment leads to unconsciousness or hastens death somewhat.

Gastrointestinal Problems

These problems, including a dry mouth, nausea, constipation, an intestinal obstruction, and loss of appetite, are common in people who are very sick. Some of these problems are caused by the disease. Others, such as constipation, are side effects of drugs.

A **dry mouth** can be relieved with wet mouth swabs or hard candy. Various commercially available products can soothe chapped lips. To prevent dental problems, a person should brush the teeth or use mouth sponges to clean the teeth, mouth, and tongue. A mouthwash that contains little or no alcohol should be used, because alcohol and petroleum-based products can be very drying.

Nausea and vomiting may be caused by drugs, an intestinal obstruction, or advanced disease. A doctor may have to change drugs or prescribe an antiemetic (antinausea) drug. Nausea caused by an intestinal obstruction may also be treated with antiemetics, and other comfort measures can be taken.

Constipation is very uncomfortable. A limited intake of food, a lack of physical activity, and certain drugs cause the intestine to be sluggish. Abdominal cramping may occur. A regimen of stool softeners, laxatives, and enemas may be needed to relieve constipation, especially when caused by narcotics. Relief of constipation is usually beneficial, even at late stages of a disease.

An **intestinal obstruction** may require surgery. However, depending on the patient's overall condition, his likely life span, and the reason for the obstruction, the use of drugs to paralyze the intestine, sometimes with nasogastric suction to keep the stomach clear, may be preferable. Narcotics are useful for pain relief.

Loss of appetite eventually occurs in most patients who are dying. A decrease in appetite is natural, doesn't cause additional physical problems, and probably plays a role in dying comfortably, although it may distress the patient and family. Patients won't keep their strength up by forcing themselves to eat, but they may enjoy eating small amounts of favorite home-cooked dishes.

If death is not expected to occur within hours or days, nutrition or hydration—given intravenously or via a tube inserted through the nose into the stomach—may be tried for a limited time to see if better nutrition improves the patient's comfort, mental clarity, or energy. The patient and family should have an explicit agreement with the doctor about what they are trying to accomplish with these measures and when the measures should be stopped if they aren't helping.

Reduced food or liquid intake does not cause suffering. In fact, as the heart and kidneys fail, a normal intake of liquids often causes shortness of breath as the fluid accumulates in the lungs. A reduced food and liquid intake may lessen the need for suctioning because of less fluid in the throat and may reduce pain because of less pres-

▲ see page 291

sure on tumors. It may even help the body release larger amounts of the body's natural pain-relieving chemicals (endorphins). Therefore, patients should not be forced to eat or drink, especially if doing so requires restraints, intravenous tubes, or hospitalization.

Skin Breakdown

Dying patients are susceptible to skin breakdown, which causes discomfort. Those who move very little, are confined to bed, or sit much of the time are at greatest risk. Ordinary pressure on the skin from sitting or moving across sheets may tear or damage the skin. Every effort should be made to protect the skin, and reddened or broken skin should be reported to the doctor promptly.▲

Fatigue

Most fatal illnesses produce fatigue. A person who is dying can try to save energy for activities that really matter. Often, making a trip to the doctor's office or continuing an exercise that's no longer helping is not essential, especially if doing so saps the energy needed for more satisfying activities.

Depression and Anxiety

Feeling sad when contemplating the end of life is a natural response, but this sadness is not depression. A person who is depressed may lack interest in what's going on, see only the bleak side of life, or feel no emotions.■ A dying person and his family should talk to the doctor about such feelings so that depression can be diagnosed and treated. Treatment, usually combining drugs and counseling, is often effective, even in the last weeks of life, improving the quality of the time remaining.

Anxiety is more than normal worry: Anxiety is feeling so worried and fearful that it interferes with daily activities.★ Feeling uninformed or overwhelmed can cause anxiety, which may be relieved by asking caregivers for more information or help. A person who typically feels anxiety during periods of stress may be more likely to feel anxiety when dying. Strategies that have helped

the person in the past—including reassurance, drugs, and channeling worry into productive endeavors—will probably help him when dying. A dying person troubled by anxiety should get help from counselors and may need antianxiety drugs.

Confusion, Delirium, and Unconsciousness

Patients who are very sick become confused easily. Confusion may be precipitated by a drug, a minor infection, or even a change in living arrangements. Reassurance and reorientation may relieve the confusion, but the doctor should be notified so that treatable causes can be sought. A patient who is very confused may need to be mildly sedated or constantly attended by a caregiver.

A dying person who is delirious or mentally disabled will not understand dying. Near death, a delirious person sometimes has surprising periods of clearheadedness. These episodes may be very meaningful to family members but can be misunderstood as improvement. The family should be prepared for such episodes but should not expect them.

Almost half of the people who are dying are unconscious most of the time during their last few days. If family members believe that a dying person who is unconscious is still able to hear, they can say their good-byes as if the person hears them. Drifting off while unconscious is a peaceful way to die, especially if the person and family are at peace and all plans have been made.

Disability

Progressive disability often accompanies fatal illnesses. People may gradually become unable to tend to a house or an apartment, prepare food, handle financial matters, walk, or care for themselves. Most people who are dying need help in their last weeks. Such disability should be anticipated, perhaps by choosing housing that's accessible to wheelchairs and close to family caregivers. Services such as occupational or physical therapy and home health nursing may help a person remain at home, even if the disability progresses. Some people choose to remain at home even though they know that it's unsafe, preferring an earlier death to institutionalization.

▲ see page 969

■ see page 403

★ see page 395

When Death Is Near

The prospect of dying raises questions about the nature and meaning of life and the reasons for suffering and dying. No easy answers to these fundamental questions exist. In their pursuit of answers, seriously ill patients and families can use their own resources, religion, counselors, friends, and research. They can talk, participate in religious or family rituals, or engage in meaningful activities. As death nears, the most important antidote to despair is often feeling cherished by another person. The torrents of medical diagnoses and treatments should not be allowed to obliterate the larger questions and the importance of human relationships.

Predicting the exact time of death is usually hard. Families are advised not to press for exact predictions or to rely on those that are offered. Very fragile patients sometimes live a few days, well past what seemed possible. Other patients die quickly. If a patient wants a particular person there at the time of death, arrangements should be made to accommodate that person for an indefinite time.

Often, there are characteristic signs that death is near. Consciousness may decrease. The limbs may become cool and perhaps bluish or mottled. Breathing may become irregular.

Secretions in the throat or the relaxing of the throat muscles can lead to noisy breathing, sometimes called the death rattle. Repositioning the patient or using drugs to dry secretions can minimize the noise. Such treatment is aimed at the comfort of the family or caregivers, because noisy breathing occurs at a time when the patient is unaware of it. This breathing can continue for hours.

At the time of death, a few muscle contractions may occur and the chest may heave as if to breathe. The heart may beat a few minutes after breathing stops, and a brief seizure may occur. Unless the dying person has a rare infectious disease, family members should be assured that touching, caressing, and holding the body of a dying person, even for a while after the death, are acceptable. Generally, seeing the body after death is helpful to those close to the person. Doing so seems to counter the irrational fear that the person really did not die.

After Death Occurs

Death must be pronounced by an authorized person, usually a licensed doctor, and the cause and circumstances of death must be certified. Ful-

filling these requirements varies substantially in different parts of the country. If a person plans to die at home, the family should know ahead of time what to expect and do. When a person has hospice care, the hospice nurse generally explains all of this. If police or other public officials must be called, they should be notified in advance that the person is dying at home and the death is expected. Hospices and home care programs often have routines for notifying officials that spare the family uncomfortable encounters. If no hospice or home care agency is involved, the family should contact the medical examiner or funeral home director to learn what to expect.

The need for a death certificate is often underestimated. It's necessary for making insurance claims, getting access to financial accounts, conveying real property titled to the deceased, and settling the estate. The family should obtain enough copies.

The family may be reluctant to ask for or approve an autopsy. Although it will not help the deceased, an autopsy may help the family and other people who have the same disease by revealing more about the disease process. After the autopsy, the body can be prepared by the funeral home or family for burial or cremation. Incisions made during the autopsy are usually hidden by clothing.

Effects on the Family

The family and close friends are fellow travelers with the dying person, and they too suffer. As the person is dying, the family should be told what's happening and what's likely to happen.

A family should also investigate the cost of a family member's death. Family members, often women at or past middle age, provide most of the care at the end of life for free. They should explore how professional caregivers can help them so that the burdens are tolerable. There are costs of giving up employment as well as of drugs, home care, and travel. One study showed that one third of families deplete most of their savings in caring for a dying relative. The family should talk openly about costs with the doctor, insisting on reasonable attention to costs and planning ahead to limit or prepare for them.

Even before the death, the family and loved ones begin to grieve. Building a life after bereavement depends on the nature of the relationship with the deceased, the age of the deceased, the kind of dying that was experienced, and the emotional and financial resources available. Also, the family needs to feel sure that they did what they should. Having a talk with the doctor a few weeks after the death can help answer lingering questions. The loneliness, disorientation, and unreality felt during the period near the death improve with time, but the sense of loss persists. People do not "get over" a death as much as they make sense of it and go on with life.

After the death, the family must settle the estate. Although discussing property and financial issues is hard to do when death is impending, it is a good idea. Doing so often reveals things that could be signed or arranged by the patient, easing the burden on the family.

Drugs

CHAPTER 5

Overview of Drugs

People in every civilization in recorded history have used drugs of plant and animal origin to prevent and treat disease. The quest for substances to combat sickness and to alter mood and consciousness is nearly as basic as the search for food and shelter. Many drugs obtained from plants and animals are still highly valued, but most drugs used in modern medicine are the products of advances in synthetic organic chemistry and biotechnology made since the end of World War II.

Under United States law, a drug is any substance (other than a food or device) intended for use in the diagnosis, cure, relief, treatment, or prevention of disease, or intended to affect the structure or function of the body. Oral contraceptives are examples of drugs that affect the structure or function of the body, as opposed to altering a disease process. Although this comprehensive definition is important for legal purposes, it isn't practical for everyday use. A simple but workable definition of a drug is *any chemical that affects the body and its processes.*

Traditional Cures, Modern Uses

Drug	Source	Condition Treated
Digitalis	Purple foxglove	Heart failure
Quinine	Cinchona bark	Malaria
Vinca alkaloids	Periwinkle plant	Cancer
Insulin	Pig, cow, and genetically engineered human insulin	Diabetes
Urokinase	Cultures of human kidney cells	Blood clots
Opium	Poppy plant	Pain

Prescription and Nonprescription Drugs

By law, drugs are divided into two categories: prescription drugs and nonprescription drugs. Prescription drugs—those considered safe for use only under medical supervision—may be dispensed only with a written prescription from a licensed professional (for example, a physician, dentist, or veterinarian). Nonprescription drugs—those considered safe for use without medical supervision—are sold over the counter without a prescription. In the United States, the Food and Drug Administration (FDA) is the government agency that decides which drugs require a prescription and which may be sold over the counter.

After many years of use under prescription regulation, drugs with excellent safety records may be approved by the FDA for over-the-counter sale.▲ The pain-relieving drug ibuprofen is one former prescription drug now available over the

▲ see box, page 54

■ see page 48

counter. Often, the amount of active ingredient in each tablet, capsule, or caplet of a drug approved for over-the-counter sale is substantially lower than the amount in a dose of the drug available by prescription.

In the United States, the inventor or discoverer of a new drug is given a patent that grants the person exclusive rights to the drug formula for 17 years, although usually many of those years have already passed by the time the drug is approved for sale. While the patent is in effect, the drug is a proprietary drug. A generic (nonproprietary) drug is not protected by patent. After the patent expires, the drug can be legally marketed under the generic name by any FDA-approved manufacturer or vendor, but the original holder of the copyright still controls the rights to the drug's trade name.■ Generic versions are usually sold at lower prices than the original drug.

Drug Names

Some understanding of how drugs are named can help in deciphering drug product labels. Every proprietary drug has at least three names— a chemical name, a generic (nonproprietary) name, and a trade (proprietary or brand) name.

The chemical name describes the atomic or molecular structure of the drug. Although the chemical name describes and identifies the product precisely, it's usually too complex and cumbersome for general use, except in the case of some simple, inorganic drugs such as sodium bicarbonate.

In the United States, the generic name is assigned by an official body—the United States Adopted Names (USAN) Council. The trade name is chosen by the pharmaceutical company that manufactures it. The company tries to choose a unique name that's short and easy to remember so doctors will prescribe it and consumers will look for it by name. For this reason, trade names sometimes link the drug to its intended use, for example, Diabinese for diabetes and Flexeril for muscle cramps.

The FDA requires that generic versions of drugs have the same active ingredients as the original and that they be absorbed into the body at the same rate. The manufacturer of a generic version may or may not decide to give the drug its own trade name, depending on whether it thinks its "branded" version will sell better.

What's in a Name?

Chemical Name	Generic Name	Trade Name
N-(4-hydroxyphenyl) acetamide	acetaminophen	Tylenol
7-chloro-1,3-dihydro-1-methyl-5-phenyl-2H-1,4-benzodiazepin-2-one	diazepam	Valium
4-[4-(p-chlorophenyl)-4-hydroxypiperidino]-4'-fluorobutyrophenone	haloperidol	Haldol
DL-threo-2-(methylamino)-phenylpropan-1-ol	pseudoephedrine hydrochloride	Sudafed
N''-cyano-N-methyl-N'-[2-[[(5-methyl-1H-imidazol-4-yl) methyl]thio]ethyl]guanidine	cimetidine	Tagamet

Drug Dynamics and Kinetics

Two primary medical considerations influence drug selection and use: pharmacodynamics (what the drug does to the body) and pharmacokinetics (what the body does to the drug). In addition to *what* the drug does (for example, relieve pain, lower blood pressure, reduce plasma cholesterol level), pharmacodynamics describes *where* (the site) and *how* (the mechanism) a drug acts on the body. Although what a drug does is readily apparent, the precise site and mechanism of action may not be understood until years after the drug has proved its worth many times over. For example, opium and morphine have been used for centuries to relieve pain and distress, but the brain structures and brain chemistry involved in the pain relief and euphoria they produce were discovered only recently.

For a drug to work, it has to get to the place in the body where the problem lies, and that's why the science of pharmacokinetics is important. Enough of the drug has to stay at the site of action until the drug does its job, but not so much that it produces severe side effects or toxic reactions. Every doctor knows that selecting the right dose is a tricky balancing act.

Many drugs get to their site of action through the bloodstream. How much time these drugs need to work and how long their effects last often depend on how fast they get into the bloodstream, how much of them gets into the blood-stream, how fast they leave the bloodstream, how efficiently they're broken down (metabolized) by the liver, and how quickly they're eliminated by the kidneys and intestines.▲

Drug Action

Much of the mystery surrounding drug action can be cleared up by recognizing that drugs affect only the *rate* at which biologic functions proceed; they do not change the basic nature of existing processes or create new functions. For example, drugs can speed up or slow down the biochemical reactions that cause muscles to contract, kidney cells to regulate the volume of water and salts retained or eliminated by the body, glands to secrete substances (such as mucus, gastric acid, or insulin), and nerves to transmit messages. How well the drug works generally depends on how well the targeted processes respond.

Drugs can alter the rate of existing biologic processes. For example, some antiepileptic drugs reduce seizures by sending the brain an order to slow down production of certain brain chemicals. However, drugs can't restore systems already damaged beyond repair. This fundamental limitation of drug action underlies much of the current frustration in trying to treat tissue-destroy-

▲ see page 28

ing or degenerative diseases such as heart failure, arthritis, muscular dystrophy, multiple sclerosis, and Alzheimer's disease.

Response to Drugs

Everyone responds to drugs differently. A large person generally needs more of a drug than a smaller person needs for the same effect. Newborn babies and elderly people metabolize drugs more slowly than children and young adults do. People with kidney or liver disease have a harder time getting rid of drugs once they've entered the body.

A standard or average dose is determined for every new drug on the basis of laboratory testing in animals and trials in humans. But the concept of an average dose is like "one size fits all" in clothing: It fits a range of individuals well enough, but it fits almost no one perfectly.

Adverse Reactions

In the early 1900s, the German scientist Paul Ehrlich described an ideal drug as a "magic bullet"; such a drug would be aimed precisely at a disease site and wouldn't harm healthy tissues. Although many new drugs are more selective than their predecessors, the perfect drug doesn't yet exist. Most drugs fall short of the precision envisioned by Ehrlich. Although they work against diseases, they also have some undesired effects.

Unwanted drug effects are called side effects or adverse reactions. If drugs had cruise control, they could automatically maintain a desired level of action. For example, they could maintain a normal blood pressure in someone with high blood pressure or a normal blood sugar level in someone with diabetes. However, most drugs can't maintain a specific level of action. Rather, a drug may produce too strong an effect, causing low blood pressure in a person being treated for high blood pressure or a low blood sugar level in a person with diabetes. Nevertheless, with good communication between a patient and doctor,

---

▲ see box, page 41

unwanted effects can often be reduced or avoided. The patient tells the doctor how the drug is affecting him, and the doctor adjusts the dosage.

A drug may affect several functions, even though it's targeted at only one. For example, antihistamines can help relieve allergy symptoms such as a stuffy nose, watery eyes, and sneezing. But because most antihistamines affect the nervous system, they can also cause sleepiness, confusion, blurred vision, dry mouth, constipation, and problems with urination. ▲

Whether a particular drug action is called a side effect or a desired effect depends on why the drug is being taken. For instance, antihistamines are the usual active ingredient in over-the-counter sleep aids. When they're taken for this purpose, their ability to produce sleepiness is a beneficial effect rather than an annoying side effect.

Effectiveness and Safety

The two goals of drug development are effectiveness (efficacy) and safety. Since all drugs can harm as well as help, safety is relative. The wider the margin of safety (therapeutic window)—the spread between the usual effective dose and a dose that produces severe or life-threatening side effects—the more useful the drug. If a drug's usual effective dose is also toxic, doctors aren't willing to use the drug except in serious situations in which there's no safer alternative.

The best drugs are both effective and, for the most part, safe. Penicillin is such a drug. Except in people who are allergic to it, penicillin is virtually nontoxic, even in large doses. On the other hand, barbiturates, which were commonly used as sleep aids, can interfere with breathing, disturb the heart rhythm, and even cause death if taken in excess. Newer sleep aids such as triazolam and temazepam have better safety margins.

Some drugs must be used despite their having a very narrow margin of safety. For example, warfarin, which is taken to prevent blood clotting, can cause bleeding. People who take warfarin need frequent checkups to see whether the drug is having too much or too little effect on blood clotting.

Clozapine is another example. This drug often helps people with schizophrenia when all other drugs have failed. But clozapine has a serious side effect: It can decrease the production of white blood cells needed to protect against infection. Because of this risk, people who take clozapine must have their blood tested frequently for as long as they take the drug.

When people know what to expect from a drug, both good and bad, they and their doctors can better judge how well the drug is working and whether potentially serious problems are developing. Anyone taking a drug shouldn't hesitate to ask a doctor, nurse, or pharmacist to explain the goals of treatment, the types of adverse drug reactions and other problems that may arise, and the extent to which they can participate in the treatment plan to help ensure the best outcome.▲ People should also keep their health care practitioners well informed about their medical history, current medications, and any other relevant information.

Drug Interactions

When two or more drugs are taken in the same general time period, they may interact in ways that are good or bad. Together they may be more effective in treating a problem, or they may increase the number or severity of adverse reactions. Drug interactions may occur between prescription and nonprescription (over-the-counter) drugs.■ If someone is receiving care from more than one doctor, each doctor needs to know all of the drugs being taken. Preferably, people should obtain all their prescription drugs from the same pharmacy, one that maintains a complete drug profile for each patient. The pharmacist can then check for the possibility of interactions. People should also consult their pharmacist when selecting over-the-counter drugs (for example, laxatives, antacids, and cough or cold remedies), particularly when they're also taking prescription drugs.

Although many people don't consider alcohol a drug, it affects body processes and is often responsible for drug interactions. Doctors or pharmacists can provide answers to questions about possible alcohol and drug interactions.

Drug interactions aren't always bad. For example, some drugs used for treating high blood pressure are prescribed in combination to reduce the

Let Them Know

To assist health care practitioners in developing a safe and effective treatment plan, people must be sure that their doctor, nurse, or pharmacist has the following information:
• What medical problems they have
• What drugs (both prescription and nonprescription) they have taken in the previous few weeks
• Whether they are allergic to or have had an unusual reaction to any drug, food, or other substance
• Whether they have special diets or food restrictions
• Whether they are pregnant or plan to become pregnant or are breastfeeding

side effects that could develop if a single drug were prescribed at a higher dose.

Drug Abuse

Through the ages, drugs have been enormously beneficial in relieving suffering and in preventing and treating diseases. However, to some people, the word *drug* means a substance that alters the brain's function in ways considered pleasurable. There has always been a dark side to the discovery and use of drugs, especially those that alleviate anxiety or alter mood and behavior in ways that satisfy people's emotional needs. Drug abuse—the excessive and persistent use of mind-altering substances without medical need—has accompanied the appropriate medical use of drugs throughout recorded history. Commonly abused drugs include alcohol, marijuana, cocaine, barbiturates, benzodiazepines, methaqualone, heroin and other narcotics, amphetamines, LSD (lysergic acid diethylamide), and PCP (phencyclidine).★

▲ see page 46

■ see pages 36 and 65

★ see page 440

CHAPTER 6

Drug Administration, Distribution, and Elimination

Drug treatment requires getting a drug into the body (administration) so it can move into the bloodstream (absorption) and travel to the specific site where it is needed (distribution). The drug leaves the body (elimination) either in the urine or by conversion to another substance.

Administration

Drugs can be taken by several routes. They can be taken by mouth (oral route) or by injection into a vein (intravenous), into a muscle (intramuscular), or beneath the skin (subcutaneous). They can be placed under the tongue (sublingual), inserted in the rectum (rectal), instilled in the eye (ocular), sprayed into the nose (nasal) or mouth (inhalation), or applied to the skin for a local (topical) or systemic (transdermal) effect. Each route has specific purposes, advantages, and disadvantages.

Oral Route

Oral administration is the most convenient, usually the safest, the least expensive, and therefore the most common route. However, it has limitations. Many factors, including other drugs and food, affect how drugs are absorbed after they're taken orally. Thus, some drugs should be taken on an empty stomach while others should be taken with food; still others can't be taken orally at all.

Drugs administered orally are absorbed from the gastrointestinal tract. Absorption begins in the mouth and stomach but takes place mostly in the small intestine. To reach the general circulation, the drug must pass through first the intestinal wall and then the liver. The intestinal wall and liver chemically alter (metabolize) many drugs, decreasing the amount absorbed. In contrast, drugs injected intravenously reach the general circulation without passing through the intestinal wall and liver, so they have a quicker and more consistent response.

Some orally administered drugs irritate the gastrointestinal tract; for example, aspirin and most other nonsteroidal anti-inflammatory drugs can harm the lining of the stomach and small intestine and can cause ulcers. Other drugs are absorbed poorly or erratically in the gastrointestinal tract or are destroyed by the acidic environment and digestive enzymes in the stomach. Despite these limitations, the oral route is used much more frequently than other routes of drug administration. Other routes are generally reserved for situations in which a person can't take anything by mouth, a drug must be administered rapidly or in a precise dose, or a drug is poorly and erratically absorbed.

Injection Routes

Administration by injection (parenteral administration) includes the subcutaneous, intramuscular, and intravenous routes. With the **subcutaneous route,** a needle is inserted beneath the skin. After being injected subcutaneously, the drug moves into small blood vessels and is carried away by the bloodstream. The subcutaneous route is used for many protein drugs, such as insulin, which would be digested in the gastrointestinal tract if taken by mouth. Drugs can be prepared in suspensions or in relatively insoluble complexes so that their absorption is prolonged for hours, days, or longer, and they don't need to be administered as often.

The **intramuscular route** is preferred to the subcutaneous route when larger volumes of a drug are needed. Because the muscles lie deeper than the skin, a longer needle is used.

With the **intravenous route,** a needle is inserted directly into a vein. An intravenous injection can be more difficult to administer than other parenteral injections, especially in people who are obese. Intravenous administration, whether in a single dose or a continuous infusion, is the best way to give drugs quickly and precisely.

Sublingual Route

Some drugs are placed under the tongue (given sublingually) so they can be absorbed directly into the small blood vessels that lie beneath the tongue. The sublingual route is especially good for nitroglycerin, which is used to relieve angina (chest pain), because absorption is rapid and the drug immediately enters the general circulation without first passing through the intestinal wall and liver. However, most drugs can't be given this way because absorption is often incomplete and erratic.

Rectal Route

Many drugs that are administered orally can also be administered rectally in suppository form. In this form, a drug is mixed with a waxy substance that dissolves after it's inserted into the rectum. With the rectum's thin lining and rich blood supply, the drug is readily absorbed. A suppository is prescribed when a person can't take a drug orally because of nausea, an inability to swallow, or a restriction on eating, as after surgery. Some drugs are irritating in suppository form; for such drugs, the parenteral route may have to be used.

Transdermal Route

Some drugs can be given by applying a patch to the skin. These drugs, sometimes mixed with a chemical that enhances penetration of the skin, pass through the skin to the bloodstream without injection. The transdermal route allows the drug to be delivered slowly and continuously over many hours or days, or even longer. However, some people develop irritation where the patch touches the skin. In addition, the transdermal route is limited by how quickly the drug can move through the skin. Only drugs to be given in relatively small daily doses can be delivered transdermally. Examples of such drugs include nitroglycerin (for angina), scopolamine (for motion sickness), nicotine (for smoking cessation), clonidine (for hypertension), and fentanyl (for pain relief).

Inhalation

Some drugs, such as gases used for anesthesia and aerosolized asthma drugs in metered-dose containers, are inhaled. These drugs travel through airways directly to the lungs, where they're absorbed into the bloodstream. Relatively few drugs are taken this way because inhalation must be carefully monitored to ensure that a person gets the right amount of drug within a specified time. Metered-dose systems are useful for drugs that act directly on the channels carrying air to the lungs. Because absorption into the bloodstream is highly variable with aerosol inhalation, this method is seldom used to administer drugs that act on tissues or organs other than the lungs.

Absorption

Bioavailability refers to the rate and extent to which a drug is absorbed into the bloodstream. Bioavailability depends on a number of factors, including the way a drug product is designed and manufactured, its physical and chemical properties, and the physiology of the person taking the drug.

A drug product is the actual dosage form of a drug, such as a tablet, capsule, suppository, transdermal patch, or solution. It usually consists of the drug combined with other ingredients. For example, tablets are a mixture of drug and additives that function as diluents, stabilizers, disintegrants, and lubricants. The mixtures are granulated and compressed into tablet form. The type and amount of additives and the degree of compression affect how quickly the tablet dissolves. Drug manufacturers adjust these variables to optimize the rate and extent of the drug's absorption.

If a tablet dissolves and releases the drug too quickly, it may produce a blood level of the active drug that provokes an excessive response. On the other hand, if the tablet doesn't dissolve and release the drug quickly enough, much of the drug may pass into the feces without being absorbed. Laxatives and diarrhea, which speed up passage through the gastrointestinal tract, may reduce drug absorption. Therefore, food, other drugs, and gastrointestinal diseases can influence drug bioavailability.

Consistency of bioavailability among drug products is desirable. Drug products that are chemically equivalent contain the same active drug but may have different inactive ingredients that can affect the rate and extent of absorption. The drug's effects, even at the same dose, may not be the same from one drug product to another. Drug products are bioequivalent when they not only contain the same active ingredient but also produce virtually the same blood levels over time. Bioequivalence thereby ensures therapeutic equivalence, and bioequivalent products are interchangeable.

Some drug products are specially formulated to release their active ingredients slowly—usually over 12 hours or more. These **controlled-release dosage forms** slow or delay the rate at which a drug is dissolved. For example, drug particles in a capsule may be coated with a polymer (a chemical substance) of varying thicknesses designed to dissolve at different times in the gastrointestinal tract.

Some tablets and capsules have protective (enteric) coatings that are intended to prevent irritants, such as aspirin, from harming the stomach lining or from decomposing in the acidic environment of the stomach. These dosage forms are coated with a material that doesn't begin to dissolve until it comes in contact with the less acidic environment or digestive enzymes of the small intestine. Such protective coatings don't always dissolve properly though, and many people, especially the elderly, pass such products intact in their feces.

Many other properties of solid dosage forms (tablets or capsules) affect absorption after oral administration. Capsules consist of drugs and other substances within a gelatin shell. The gelatin swells and releases its contents when it becomes wet. The shell usually erodes quickly. The size of the drug particles and other substances affects how fast the drug dissolves and is absorbed. Drugs from capsules filled with liquids tend to be absorbed more quickly than those from capsules filled with solids.

Distribution

After a drug is absorbed into the bloodstream, it rapidly circulates through the body, as blood has an average circulation time of 1 minute. However, the drug may move slowly from the bloodstream into the body's tissues.

Drugs penetrate different tissues at different speeds, depending on their ability to cross membranes. For example, the anesthetic thiopental rapidly enters the brain, but the antibiotic penicillin does not. In general, fat-soluble drugs can cross cell membranes more quickly than water-soluble drugs can.

Once absorbed, most drugs don't spread out evenly through the body. Some drugs tend to stay within the watery tissues of the blood and muscle while others concentrate in specific tissues such as the thyroid gland, liver, and kidneys. Some drugs bind tightly to blood proteins, leaving the bloodstream very slowly, while others escape from the bloodstream quickly into other tissues. Some tissues build up such high levels of a drug that they serve as reservoirs of extra drug, thereby prolonging the drug's distribution. In fact, some drugs, such as those that accumulate in fatty tissues, leave these tissues slowly and consequently circulate in the bloodstream for days after a person has stopped taking the drug.

Distribution of a given drug may also vary among different persons. For instance, people with large body frames, who have greater amounts of tissue and circulating blood, may require larger amounts of a drug. Obese people may store large amounts of drugs that concentrate in fat, while very thin people may store relatively little. This distribution is also seen in older people, because the proportion of body fat increases with age.

Elimination

All drugs are either metabolized or excreted intact. **Metabolism** is the process by which a drug is chemically altered by the body. The liver is the principal, but not the only, site of drug metabolism. The products of metabolism, metabolites, may be inactive, or they may have similar or different degrees of therapeutic activity or toxicity than the original drug. Some drugs, called prodrugs, are administered in an inactive form; their metabolites are active and achieve the desired effects. These active metabolites are either excreted (mainly in the urine or feces) or converted further to other metabolites, which are ultimately excreted.

The liver has enzymes that facilitate chemical reactions such as oxidation, reduction, and hydrolysis of drugs. It has other enzymes that attach substances to the drug, producing reactions called conjugations. The conjugates (drug molecules with the attached substances) are excreted in the urine.

Because metabolic enzyme systems are only partially developed at birth, newborns have difficulty metabolizing many drugs; therefore they require less drug in proportion to body weight than adults do. On the other hand, young children (2 to 12 years of age) require *more* drug in proportion to body weight than adults do. Like newborns, the elderly also have reduced enzymatic activity and aren't able to metabolize drugs as well as younger adults and children do. Consequently, newborns and the elderly often need smaller, and children larger, doses per pound of body weight.

Excretion refers to the processes by which the body eliminates a drug. The kidneys are the major organs of excretion. They are particularly effective in eliminating water-soluble drugs and their metabolites.

The kidneys filter drugs from the bloodstream and excrete them into the urine. Many factors can affect the kidneys' ability to excrete drugs. A drug or metabolite must be soluble in water and not bound too tightly to plasma proteins. The acidity of the urine affects the rate at which some acidic and alkaline drugs are excreted. The kidneys' ability to excrete drugs also depends on urine flow, blood flow through the kidneys, and the condition of the kidneys.

As people age, kidney function decreases. The kidney of an 85-year-old person is only about half as efficient in excreting drugs as that of a 35-year-old. Many diseases—especially high blood pressure, diabetes, and recurring kidney infections—and exposure to high levels of toxic chemicals can impair the kidneys' ability to excrete drugs.

If the kidneys aren't functioning normally, a doctor may adjust the dosage of a drug that's eliminated primarily through the kidneys. The normal decrease in kidney function with age can help the doctor determine an appropriate dosage based solely on a person's age. However, a more accurate way to determine an appropriate dosage is to assess kidney function with a blood test (measuring the amount of creatinine in serum), either alone or in combination with a urine test (measuring the amount of creatinine in urine collected for 12 to 24 hours).

The liver excretes some drugs through bile. These drugs enter the gastrointestinal tract and end up in the feces if they aren't reabsorbed into the bloodstream or decomposed. Also, small amounts of some drugs are excreted in saliva, sweat, breast milk, and even exhaled air. The administration of a drug eliminated primarily by metabolism in the liver may need to be adjusted for a person with liver disease. There are no simple measures of liver function (for drug metabolism) comparable to those for kidney function.

CHAPTER 7

Pharmacodynamics

Pharmacodynamics describes the many ways drugs affect the body. After being swallowed, injected, or absorbed through the skin, most drugs enter the bloodstream, circulate throughout the body, and interact with a number of target sites. However, depending on its properties or route of administration, a drug may act in only a specific area of the body (for example, the action of antacids is largely confined to the stomach). Interaction with the target site usually produces the desired therapeutic effect, whereas interaction with other cells, tissues, or organs may result in side effects (adverse drug reactions).▲

Selectivity of Drug Action

Some drugs are relatively nonselective; they act on many different tissues or organs. For example, atropine, a drug given to relax muscles in the gastrointestinal tract, may also relax muscles of the eye and the respiratory tract as well as decrease sweat and mucous gland secretion. Other drugs are highly selective and affect mainly a single or-

▲ see page 42

A Perfect Fit

A cell surface receptor has a configuration that allows a specific chemical, such as a drug, a hormone, or a neurotransmitter, to bind to it because the chemical has a configuration that perfectly fits the receptor.

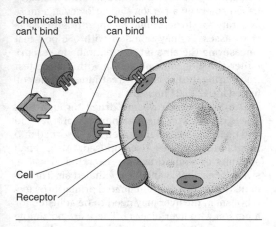

Chemicals that can't bind

Chemical that can bind

Cell

Receptor

gan or system. For example, digitalis, a drug given to people with heart failure, acts primarily on the heart to increase its pumping efficiency. Sleep aids target certain nerve cells of the brain. Non-steroidal anti-inflammatory drugs such as aspirin and ibuprofen are relatively selective because they act wherever inflammation is present.

How do drugs know where to exert their effects? The answer lies in how they interact with cells or substances such as enzymes.

Receptors

Many drugs attach (bind) to cells by means of receptors on the cell surface. Most cells have many surface receptors, which allow the activity of the cell to be influenced by chemicals such as drugs or hormones located outside the cell. A receptor has a specific configuration, which allows only a drug that fits precisely to attach to it—like a key fits in its lock. A drug's selectivity can often be explained by how selectively it attaches to receptors. Some drugs attach to only one type of receptor; others are like a master key and can attach to several types of receptors throughout the body.

Nature probably didn't create receptors so that drugs would someday be able to attach to them. Receptors have natural (physiologic) purposes, but drugs take advantage of them. For example, morphine and related pain-relieving drugs attach to the same receptors in the brain that endorphins (naturally produced chemical substances that alter sensory perception and reaction) attach to.

A class of drugs called **agonists** activates or stimulates their receptors, triggering a response that either increases or decreases the cell's function. For example, the agonist carbachol attaches to receptors in the respiratory tract called cholinergic receptors, causing smooth muscle cells to contract, producing bronchoconstriction (narrowing of the airways). Another agonist, albuterol, attaches to other receptors in the respiratory tract called adrenergic receptors, causing smooth muscle cells to relax, producing bronchodilation (widening of the airways).

Another class of drugs called **antagonists** blocks the access or binding of agonists to their receptors. Antagonists are used primarily to block or diminish cell responses to agonists (usually neurotransmitters) normally present in the body. For example, the cholinergic receptor antagonist ipratropium blocks the bronchoconstrictor effect of acetylcholine, the natural transmitter of cholinergic nerve impulses.

Agonists and antagonists are used as different but complementary approaches to the treatment of asthma. The adrenergic receptor agonist albuterol, which relaxes bronchiolar smooth muscle, may be used together with the cholinergic receptor antagonist ipratropium, which blocks the bronchoconstrictor effect of acetylcholine.

A widely used group of antagonists is the beta-blockers such as propranolol. These antagonists block or diminish the cardiovascular excitatory response to the stress hormones adrenaline and noradrenaline; they're used to treat high blood pressure, angina, and certain abnormal cardiac rhythms. Antagonists are most effective when the local concentration of an agonist is high. They work in much the same way that a roadblock affects a major highway. More vehicles are stopped by a roadblock during the 5:00 P.M. rush hour than at 3:00 A.M. Similarly, beta-blockers, in doses that have little effect on normal heart function, may protect the heart against sudden surges of stress hormones.

Enzymes

In addition to cell receptors, other important targets for drug action are enzymes, which help transport vital chemicals, regulate the rate of chemical reactions, or serve other transport, regulatory, or structural functions. While drugs targeted at receptors are classified as agonists or antagonists, drugs targeted at enzymes are classified as inhibitors or activators (inducers). For example, the drug lovastatin, used to treat some people who have high blood cholesterol levels, inhibits the enzyme HMG-CoA reductase, which is critical in the body's production of cholesterol.

Most interactions between drugs and receptors or drugs and enzymes are reversible—after awhile the drug disengages, and the receptor or enzyme resumes normal function. Sometimes an interaction is largely irreversible (as with omeprazole, a drug that inhibits an enzyme involved in the secretion of stomach acid), and the drug effect persists until the body manufactures more enzyme.

Affinity and Intrinsic Activity

Two drug properties important to a drug's action are affinity and intrinsic activity. Affinity is the mutual attraction or strength of the bond between a drug and its target, whether it's a receptor or an enzyme. Intrinsic activity is a measure of the drug's ability to produce a pharmacologic effect when bound to its receptor.

Drugs that activate receptors (agonists) have both properties; they must bind effectively (have an affinity) to their receptors, and the drug-receptor complex must be capable of producing a response in the target system (have an intrinsic activity). In contrast, drugs that block receptors (antagonists) bind effectively (have an affinity to them) but have little or no intrinsic activity—their function is to prevent agonist molecules from interacting with their receptors.

Potency and Efficacy

Potency refers to the amount of drug (usually expressed in milligrams) needed to produce an effect, such as relief of pain or reduction of blood pressure. For instance, if 5 milligrams of drug B relieves pain as effectively as 10 milligrams of drug A, then drug B is twice as potent as drug A. Greater potency does not necessarily mean that one drug

is better than another. Doctors consider many factors when judging the relative merits of drugs, such as their side effect profile, potential toxicity, duration of effectiveness (and, consequently, number of doses needed each day), and cost.

Efficacy refers to the potential maximum therapeutic response that a drug can produce. For example, the diuretic furosemide eliminates much more salt and water through the urine than does the diuretic chlorothiazide. Thus, furosemide has a greater efficacy, or therapeutic effectiveness, than chlorothiazide. As with potency, efficacy is only one factor that doctors consider when selecting the most appropriate drug for an individual patient.

Tolerance

Repeated or prolonged administration of some drugs results in tolerance—a diminished pharmacologic response. Tolerance occurs when the body adapts to the continued presence of the drug. Two mechanisms are usually responsible for tolerance: (1) Drug metabolism speeds up (most often because activity of the liver's drug-metabolizing enzymes increases), and (2) the number of receptors or their affinity for the drug decreases. The term resistance is used to describe the situation in which a person no longer responds well to an antibiotic, antiviral, or cancer chemotherapeutic drug. Depending on the degree of tolerance or resistance that develops, a doctor may increase the dose or select an alternative drug.

Drug Design and Development

Many of the drugs in current use were discovered by experimental trial and observation in animal and human subjects. Newer approaches to drug development are based on a determination of the abnormal biochemical and cellular changes caused by disease and the design of compounds that may specifically prevent or correct these abnormalities. When a new compound shows promise, it's usually modified many times to optimize its selectivity, potency, receptor affinity, and therapeutic efficacy. Other factors, such as whether the compound is absorbed through the intestinal wall and whether it's stable in body tissues and fluids, are also considered in drug development.

Ideally, a drug should be effective when taken orally (for the convenience of self-administration), well absorbed from the gastrointestinal tract, and reasonably stable in body tissues and fluids so that one dose a day is adequate. The drug should be highly selective for its target site, so that it has little or no effect on other body systems (minimal or no side effects). Further, the drug should have a high potency and a high degree of therapeutic efficacy, so that it's effective at low doses even for conditions that are difficult to treat.

No drugs are perfectly effective and completely safe. Therefore, doctors assess potential drug benefits and risks with every therapeutic situation that requires prescription drug treatment. However, sometimes conditions are treated without a doctor's supervision; for example, people treat themselves with over-the-counter drugs for minor pain, insomnia, and coughs and colds. In such cases, they should read the information provided in the drug package insert and follow the directions for drug use explicitly.▲

CHAPTER 8

Factors Affecting Drug Response

The speed with which drugs move in and out of the body varies widely among different people. Many factors can affect a drug's absorption, distribution, metabolism, excretion, and ultimate effect. Among other reasons, people respond to drugs differently because of genetic differences, because they may be taking two or more drugs that interact with each other, or because they have diseases that influence the drug's effects.

Genetics

Genetic (inherited) differences among individual people affect drug kinetics, the rate at which drugs move through the body. The study of genetic differences in the response to drugs is called pharmacogenetics.

Because of their genetic makeup, some people metabolize drugs slowly; a drug may accumulate in the body and cause toxicity. Other people have a genetic makeup that causes them to metabolize drugs quickly; a drug may be metabolized so quickly that drug levels in the blood never become high enough for the drug to be effective. Sometimes genetic differences affect drug metabolism in other ways. For example, at usual dose

levels, a drug may be metabolized at normal speed; but in some people, if a drug is given at a high dose or with another drug that uses the same system to metabolize it, the system may be overwhelmed and the drug may reach toxic levels.

To make sure a person gets enough drug for a therapeutic effect with little toxicity, doctors must individualize therapy: They must select the right drug; consider the age, sex, size, diet, race, and ethnic origin of the person; and adjust the dose carefully. The presence of disease, use of other drugs, and limited knowledge about interactions of these factors complicate this process.

Genetic differences in the way drugs affect the body (pharmacodynamics) are much less common than differences in the way the body affects drugs (pharmacokinetics). Even so, genetic differences are particularly important in certain ethnic groups and races.

About half the people in the United States have low activity of *N*-acetyltransferase, a liver enzyme that helps metabolize some drugs and many toxins. People with low activity of this enzyme metabolize many drugs slowly, and these drugs tend to reach higher blood levels and remain in the body longer than in people with high activity of *N*-acetyltransferase.

About 1 in 1,500 people have low levels of pseudocholinesterase, a blood enzyme that inactivates drugs such as succinylcholine, which is

▲ see box, page 64

Many Factors Influence Drug Response

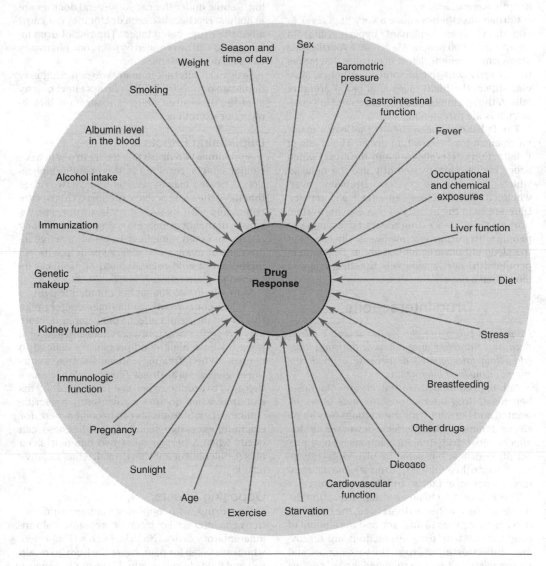

given with anesthesia to temporarily relax muscles. Although this enzyme deficiency isn't common, its consequences are important. If succinylcholine isn't inactivated, it leads to paralysis of muscles, including those involved in breathing. This may require prolonged use of a ventilator.

Glucose-6-phosphate dehydrogenase, or G6PD, is an enzyme normally present in red blood cells that protects these cells from certain toxic chemicals. About 10 percent of black men and fewer black women have G6PD deficiency. Some drugs (for example, chloroquine, pamaquine, and primaquine, used to treat malaria, and aspirin, probenecid, and vitamin K) destroy the red blood cells in people with G6PD deficiency, causing hemolytic anemia.▲

Certain anesthetics cause a very high fever (a condition called malignant hyperthermia) in about 1 in 20,000 people. Malignant hyperthermia stems from a genetic defect in muscles that makes them overly sensitive to some anesthetics. Muscles stiffen, the heart races, and blood pressure falls. Although malignant hyperthermia isn't common, it is life threatening.

The P-450 enzyme system is the liver's major mechanism for inactivating drugs. The levels of P-450 activity determine not only the rate at which drugs become inactivated but also the point at which the enzyme system becomes overwhelmed. Many factors can alter P-450 activity. Differences in the activity of this enzyme system profoundly influence drug effects. For example, in people with normal enzyme levels, the effects of the sleep aid flurazepam last about 18 hours; in people with low enzyme levels, the effects can last more than 3 days.

Drug Interactions

Drug interactions are changes in a drug's effects because of another drug taken at the same time (drug-drug interactions) or because of food consumed (drug-food interactions).

Although combined drug effects are sometimes beneficial, drug interactions are most often unwanted and harmful. Drug interactions may intensify or diminish a drug's effects or worsen its side effects. Most drug-drug interactions involve prescription drugs, but some involve nonprescription (over-the-counter) drugs■—most commonly, aspirin, antacids, and decongestants.

The risk of developing a drug interaction depends on the number of drugs used, the tendency of particular drugs to interact, and the amount of drug taken. Many drug interactions are discovered during testing of drugs. Doctors, nurses, and pharmacists can reduce the incidence of serious problems by keeping informed about potential drug interactions. Reference books and computer software programs can help. The risk of a drug interaction increases when drug prescribing isn't coordinated with drug dispensing and counseling. People under the care of several doctors are at highest risk because each doctor may not know all of the drugs being taken. The risk of drug interactions can be reduced by using one pharmacy to fill all prescriptions.

Drugs can interact in many ways. A drug may duplicate or oppose another drug's effect or may alter the other drug's rate of absorption, metabolism, or excretion.

Duplicating Effects

Sometimes two drugs taken concurrently have similar effects, resulting in therapeutic duplication. A person may inadvertently take two drugs that have the same active ingredient. This occurs commonly with over-the-counter drugs. For example, diphenhydramine is an ingredient of many allergy and cold remedies; it's also the active ingredient of many sleep aids. Aspirin may be an ingredient of cold remedies and of products intended for pain relief.

More often, two similar but not identical drugs are taken concurrently. Sometimes doctors plan this to obtain greater effect. For example, doctors may prescribe two antihypertensive drugs for a person whose high blood pressure is difficult to control. When treating cancer, doctors sometimes give several drugs (combination chemotherapy) to produce a better effect. But problems can arise when doctors inadvertently prescribe similar drugs. Side effects can become severe; for example, excessive sedation and dizziness can occur when a person takes two different sleep aids (or alcohol or another drug that has sedative effects).

Opposing Effects

Two drugs with opposing (antagonistic) actions can interact. For example, nonsteroidal antiinflammatory drugs (NSAIDs) such as ibuprofen, which are taken for pain, cause the body to retain salt and fluid; diuretics help rid the body of excess salt and fluid. If these drugs are taken together, the NSAID decreases (opposes or antagonizes) the diuretic's effectiveness. Some drugs taken to control high blood pressure and heart disease (for example, beta-blockers such as propranolol and atenolol) counteract certain drugs taken for asthma (for example, beta-adrenergic stimulant drugs such as albuterol).

▲ see page 746

■ see page 65

Changes In Absorption

Drugs taken by mouth must be absorbed through the lining of either the stomach or the small intestine. Sometimes food or a drug can reduce another drug's absorption. For example, the antibiotic tetracycline isn't absorbed properly if taken within an hour of ingesting calcium or foods containing calcium, such as milk and other dairy products. Following specific directions—such as avoiding food for 1 hour before or several hours after taking a drug, or taking drugs at least 2 hours apart—is important.

Changes in Metabolism

Many drugs are inactivated by metabolic systems in the liver, such as the P-450 enzyme system. The drugs circulate through the body and pass through the liver, where enzymes work to inactivate the drugs or to change their structure so that the kidneys can filter them. Some drugs can alter this enzyme system, causing the inactivation of another drug to proceed more quickly or more slowly than usual. For example, because barbiturates such as phenobarbital increase the liver's enzyme activity, drugs such as warfarin become less effective when taken during the same period. Therefore, doctors may need to increase the doses of certain drugs to compensate for this effect. However, if phenobarbital is later stopped, the levels of other drugs may increase dramatically, leading to potentially serious side effects.

Chemicals in cigarette smoke can increase the activity of some liver enzymes. This is why smoking decreases the effectiveness of some analgesics (such as propoxyphene) and some drugs used for lung problems (such as theophylline).

The antiulcer drug cimetidine and the antibiotics ciprofloxacin and erythromycin are examples of drugs that may slow liver enzyme activity, prolonging the action of the drug theophylline. Erythromycin affects the metabolism of the antiallergy drugs terfenadine and astemizole, leading to a potentially serious buildup of these drugs.

Changes in Excretion

A drug may affect the rate at which the kidneys excrete another drug. For example, some drugs alter the urine's acidity, which in turn affects the excretion of other drugs. In large doses, vitamin C can do this.

How to Reduce the Risk of Drug Interactions

- Consult your primary care doctor before taking any new drugs

- Keep a list of all drugs being taken and periodically discuss this list with the doctor

- Keep a list of all medical illnesses and periodically discuss this list with the doctor

- Select a pharmacist who provides comprehensive services and have all prescriptions filled with this pharmacist

- Learn about the purpose and actions of all prescribed drugs

- Learn about the drugs' possible side effects

- Learn how to take the drugs, what time of day they should be taken, and whether they can be taken at the same time as other drugs

- Review the use of nonprescription (over-the-counter) drugs with the pharmacist and discuss any medical conditions and prescription drugs being taken

- Follow the recommended instructions for taking drugs

- Report to the doctor or pharmacist any symptoms that might be related to the use of a drug

Drug-Disease Interactions

Most drugs circulate throughout the body; although they exert most of their effects on a specific organ or system, they also affect other organs and systems. A drug taken for a lung condition may affect the heart, and a drug taken to treat a cold may affect the eyes. Because drugs can affect medical conditions other than the disease being targeted, doctors should be made aware of all conditions before they prescribe a new drug. Diabetes, high or low blood pressure, glaucoma, an enlarged prostate, poor bladder control, and insomnia are particularly important.

Placebo: I Shall Please

In Latin, *placebo* means "I shall please." In 1785, the word placebo first appeared in a medical dictionary as "a commonplace method or medicine." Two editions later, the placebo had become "a make-believe medicine," allegedly inert and harmless. We now know that placebos can have profound effects, both good and bad.

Placebos

Placebos are substances that are prescribed like drugs but contain no active chemicals.

A true placebo is made to look exactly like a real drug but is made up of an inactive chemical such as a starch or sugar. Placebos are used in research studies for comparison with active drugs. In addition, a placebo may be prescribed under very limited circumstances to relieve symptoms if the doctor doesn't think that a drug with an active chemical is appropriate.

A placebo effect—a modification in symptoms after receiving a treatment with no proven effect—may occur with any type of therapy, including drugs, surgery, and psychotherapy.

Placebos can cause or be associated with a remarkable number of changes, both desirable and undesirable. Two factors tend to influence a placebo effect. One is the *anticipation* of results (usually optimistic) from taking a drug, sometimes called suggestibility, faith, hope, or optimism. The second factor, *spontaneous change,* is at times even more important. Sometimes people experience spontaneous improvement; they get better without any treatment. If spontaneous improvement occurs after a placebo is taken, the placebo may incorrectly be given credit for the result. Conversely, if a headache or rash develops spontaneously after taking a placebo, the placebo may incorrectly be blamed.

Studies to determine whether people with certain personality characteristics are more likely to respond to placebos have led to vastly different conclusions. Placebo reactivity is a matter of degree, since virtually everyone is influenced by

suggestion under some circumstances. However, some people seem more susceptible than others. Some people who respond strongly to placebos show many of the characteristics of drug addiction: a tendency to need dose increases, a compulsive desire to take the drug, and the development of withdrawal symptoms when deprived of it.

Use in Research

Any drug can have a placebo effect—good or bad effects unrelated to the active chemical ingredients. To sort out a true drug effect from a placebo effect, investigators compare drugs with placebos in experimental trials. In such studies, half the participants are given the test drug and half are given an identical-looking placebo. Ideally, neither the participants nor the investigators know who received the drug and who received the placebo (the study is thus called a double-blind trial).

When the study is completed, all changes observed for the test drug are compared with those for the placebo. To estimate the test drug's true chemical effects, the placebo's effects are subtracted from the results found for the test drug. A test drug must perform significantly better than the placebo to justify its use. For example, in studies of new drugs to relieve angina (chest pain from inadequate blood supply to the heart muscle), relief with a placebo commonly exceeds 50 percent. For this reason, demonstrating the effectiveness of new drugs is a significant challenge.

Use in Therapy

Every treatment has a placebo effect, making effects attributed to drugs vary from person to person and doctor to doctor. A person with a positive opinion of drugs, doctors, nurses, and hospitals is more likely to respond favorably to placebos or to have a placebo response to active drugs than is a person with a negative orientation—who may deny benefit or experience adverse effects.

A positive effect is more likely when both patient and doctor believe that the placebo will be beneficial. An active drug with no known therapeutic effect for the disorder being treated (for example, vitamin B_{12} for arthritis) may provide relief, or a mildly active drug (for example, a mild pain reliever) may have an enhanced effect.

Doctors generally avoid deliberate, secret placebo use (as opposed to use in research trials) because deception may hurt the doctor-patient relationship. Also, the doctor may misinterpret the patient's response, mistakenly believing that the patient's symptoms aren't based on bodily illness or are exaggerated. When other doctors or nurses are involved (as in a group practice or hospital setting), their attitudes and behaviors toward the patient may be adversely affected, and the potential for discovery of the deception is increased.

However, doctors have a simple, direct way to prescribe placebos. For instance, if a patient with chronic pain is becoming too dependent on a potentially addictive analgesic, the doctor may suggest a trial of placebos. In essence, the patient and doctor agree on an experiment to see if the risky drug is really needed.

Although doctors rarely prescribe placebos, most doctors see patients who are *totally convinced* that use of some substance either prevents or relieves their illnesses, even with no scientific evidence to support this belief. For example, people who perceive benefit from taking vitamin B_{12} or other vitamins as a tonic often feel ill and can become upset if denied their medication. Some people who are told that their weak pain relievers are strong often get excellent pain relief and are convinced that the drugs are stronger than anything they used before. Because of cultural beliefs or psychologic attitudes, some people seem to require and benefit from either a scientifically unproven medication or a particular dosage form (for example, an injection when a tablet should suffice). Doctors generally are troubled in these situations because they view these effects as unscientific and, considering the potential disadvantages to the doctor-patient relationship, are uncomfortable recommending or prescribing these drugs. However, most doctors realize that some patients are so dependent on placebos that depriving them may do more harm than good (assuming that the placebo used has a high margin of safety).

CHAPTER 9

Drugs and Aging

Because elderly people are more likely to have chronic diseases, they take more medications than younger adults. On the average, an elderly person takes four or five prescription drugs and two over-the-counter drugs. Elderly people are more than twice as susceptible to adverse drug reactions as younger adults.▲ Reactions are also likely to be more severe.

As people age, the amount of water in the body decreases. Since many drugs dissolve in water, and since less water is available to dilute them, these drugs reach higher levels of concentration in the elderly. Also, the kidneys are less able to excrete drugs into the urine, and the liver is less able to metabolize many drugs. For these reasons, many drugs tend to stay in an elderly person's body much longer than they would in a younger person's body. As a result, doctors often should prescribe smaller doses of many drugs for elderly people or perhaps fewer daily doses.

The elderly body is also more sensitive to the effects of many drugs. For example, elderly people tend to become sleepier and are more likely to become confused when using antianxiety drugs or sleep aids. Drugs that lower blood pressure by relaxing arteries and reducing stress on the heart tend to lower the pressure much more dramatically in the elderly than in the young. The brain, eyes, heart, blood vessels, bladder, and intestines become considerably more sensitive to

▲ see page 42

Drugs That Pose Increased Risk to the Elderly

Analgesics

Propoxyphene offers no more pain relief than acetaminophen and has narcotic side effects. It may cause constipation, drowsiness, confusion, and (rarely) slowed breathing. Like other narcotics (opioids), it may be addictive.

Of all the nonsteroidal anti-inflammatory drugs, **indomethacin** most affects the brain. It sometimes causes confusion or dizziness. When injected, **meperidine** is a strong analgesic, but when taken orally, it's not very effective for pain and often causes confusion.

Pentazocine is a narcotic analgesic that is more likely to cause confusion and hallucinations than are other narcotics.

Anticlotting drugs

Dipyridamole can cause light-headedness upon standing (orthostatic hypotension) in the elderly. For most people, it offers little advantage over aspirin in preventing blood clots.

Ticlopidine is no more effective than aspirin for most people in preventing blood clots and is considerably more toxic. It may be useful as an alternative for people who can't take aspirin.

Antiulcer drugs

Typical doses of some histamine blockers (especially **cimetidine,** but also to some extent **ranitidine, nizatidine,** and **famotidine**) may cause adverse effects, especially confusion.

Antidepressants

Because of its strong anticholinergic and sedating properties, **amitriptyline** usually isn't the best antidepressant for the elderly. **Doxepin** is also strongly anticholinergic.

Antinausea drugs (antiemetics)

Trimethobenzamide is one of the least effective drugs for nausea and can cause adverse effects, including abnormal movements of the arms, legs, and body.

Antihistamines

All nonprescription and many prescription antihistamines have potent anticholinergic effects. The drugs include **chlorpheniramine, diphenhydramine, hydroxyzine, cyproheptadine, promethazine, tripelennamine, dexchlorpheniramine,** and combination cold remedies. Although sometimes helpful for allergic reactions and seasonal allergies, antihistamines are generally not appropriate for a runny nose and other symptoms of a viral infection. When antihistamines are needed, those without anticholinergic effects (terfenadine, loratadine, and astemizole) are preferable. Cough and cold remedies that don't include antihistamines are generally safer for the elderly.

Antihypertensives

Methyldopa, alone or in combination with other drugs, may slow the heartbeat and worsen depression. **Reserpine** is risky, as it can induce depression, impotence, sedation, and dizziness upon standing.

Antipsychotics

Although antipsychotics such as **chlorpromazine, haloperidol, thioridazine,** and **thiothixene** are effective in treating psychotic disorders, their effectiveness in treating behavioral disturbances associated with dementia (such as agitation, wandering, repeated questioning, throwing, and hitting) hasn't been established. These drugs are often toxic, producing sedation, movement disorders, and anticholinergic side effects.

Elderly people should use antipsychotics in small doses, if at all. The need for treatment should be reassessed often, and the drugs should be discontinued as soon as possible.

Gastrointestinal antispasmodics

Gastrointestinal antispasmodics, such as **dicyclomine, hyoscyamine, propantheline, belladonna alkaloids,** and **clidinium-chlordiazepoxide,** are given to treat stomach cramps and pain. They are highly anticholinergic, and their usefulness—especially at the low doses tolerated by the elderly—is questionable.

Antidiabetic drugs (hypoglycemics)

Chlorpropamide has long-lasting effects, which are exaggerated in the elderly, and can cause prolonged low blood sugar levels (hypoglycemia). Because chlorpropamide causes the body to retain water, it can also lower the level of sodium in the blood.

Iron supplements

Doses of **ferrous sulfate** exceeding 325 milligrams daily don't greatly improve absorption and are likely to cause constipation.

Muscle relaxants and antispasmodics

Most muscle relaxants and antispasmodics, such as **methocarbamol, carisoprodol, oxybutynin, chlorzoxazone, metaxalone,** and **cyclobenzaprine,** lead to anticholinergic side effects, sedation, and weakness. The usefulness of all muscle relaxants and antispasmodics at the low doses tolerated by the elderly is questionable.

Sedatives, antianxiety drugs, and sleep aids

Meprobamate offers no advantages over benzodiazepines and has many disadvantages.

Chlordiazepoxide, diazepam, and **flurazepam**—benzodiazepines used to treat anxiety and insomnia—have extremely long-lasting effects in the elderly (often more than 96 hours). These drugs, alone or in combination with others, can cause prolonged drowsiness and increase the risk of falls and fractures.

Diphenhydramine, an antihistamine, is the active ingredient in many over-the-counter sedatives. However, diphenhydramine has potent anticholinergic effects.

Barbiturates, such as **secobarbital** and **phenobarbital,** cause more adverse effects than other drugs used to treat anxiety and insomnia. They also interact with many other drugs. Generally, the elderly should avoid barbiturates except for the treatment of seizure disorders.

Anticholinergic: What Does It Mean?

Acetylcholine is one of the body's many neurotransmitters. A neurotransmitter is a chemical substance that nerve cells use to communicate with each other, with muscles, and with many glands. Drugs that block the action of the neurotransmitter acetylcholine are said to have anticholinergic effects. Most of these drugs aren't designed to block acetylcholine; their anticholinergic effects are side effects. Elderly people are particularly sensitive to drugs with anticholinergic effects because the amount of acetylcholine in the body decreases with age and because their bodies are less able to use what's there. Drugs that have anticholinergic effects can cause confusion, blurred vision, constipation, dry mouth, light-headedness, and difficulty with urination or loss of bladder control.

the anticholinergic side effects of some commonly used drugs. Drugs with anticholinergic effects block the normal action of part of the nervous system called the cholinergic nervous system.

Certain drugs tend to cause adverse reactions more often and more intensely in the elderly and should be avoided by them. In almost all cases, safer substitutes are available.

Failure to follow a doctor's directions in taking a drug can be risky; however, noncompliance with medical directions is no more common among the elderly than among younger people.▲ Not taking a drug or taking too little or too much of a drug can cause problems. For example, an illness may result, or a doctor may change the therapy, thinking that the drug hasn't worked. An elderly person who doesn't wish to follow a doctor's directions should discuss the matter with the doctor rather than act alone.

▲ see page 47

CHAPTER 10

Adverse Drug Reactions

A common misperception is that a drug's effects can be clearly divided into two categories: desired or therapeutic effects and undesired or side effects. Actually, most drugs produce several effects, but a doctor usually wants a patient to experience only one (or a few) of them; the other effects may be regarded as undesired. Although most people, including health care practitioners, use the term *side effect,* the term *adverse drug reaction* is more appropriate for effects that are undesired, unpleasant, noxious, or potentially harmful.

Not surprisingly, adverse drug reactions are common. About 10 percent of hospital admissions in the United States are estimated to be for treatment of adverse drug reactions. Some 15 to 30 percent of hospitalized patients have at least one adverse drug reaction. Although many of these reactions are relatively mild and disappear when the drug is stopped or the dose is changed, others are more serious and last longer.

Types of Adverse Reactions

Adverse drug reactions may be divided into two major types. The first type is reactions that represent an excess of the drug's known and desired pharmacologic or therapeutic effects. For example, a person taking a drug to reduce high blood pressure may feel dizzy or light-headed if the drug reduces the blood pressure too much. A person with diabetes may develop weakness, sweating, nausea, and palpitations if insulin or a hypoglycemic drug reduces the blood sugar excessively. This type of adverse drug reaction is usually predictable but sometimes unavoidable. An adverse reaction may occur if a drug dose is too high, if the person is unusually sensitive to the drug, or if another drug slows the metabolism of the first drug and thus increases its blood levels.

The second major type is reactions resulting from mechanisms that aren't currently understood; this type of adverse drug reaction is largely unpredictable until doctors become aware of other people who have had similar reactions. Examples of such adverse reactions include skin rashes, jaundice (liver damage), anemia, a fall in the white blood cell count, kidney damage, and nerve injury with possible visual or hearing impairment. These reactions typically develop in a very small number of people. Such people may have a drug allergy or hypersensitivity to the drug because of genetic differences in drug metabolism or in their body's response to drugs.

Some adverse drug reactions don't fit easily into one category or the other. These reactions are usually predictable, and the mechanisms involved are largely understood. For example, stomach irritation and bleeding often occur when people chronically use aspirin or other nonsteroidal anti-inflammatory drugs such as ibuprofen, ketoprofen, and naproxen.

Severity of Adverse Reactions

No universal scale exists for describing or measuring the severity of an adverse drug reaction; the assessment is largely subjective. Since most drugs are taken orally, gastrointestinal disturbances—loss of appetite, nausea, a bloating sensation, and constipation or diarrhea—account for a high percentage of all reported reactions.

Doctors usually consider gastrointestinal disturbances as well as headaches, fatigue, vague muscle aches, malaise (a general feeling of illness or discomfort), and changes in sleep patterns to be **mild reactions** and of minor significance. But such reactions can be a real concern to the person who experiences them. In addition, a person who perceives a reduction in the quality of life may not cooperate with the prescribed drug plan, which may be a major problem if the goals of treatment are to be achieved.

Moderate reactions include those listed as mild if a person considers them to be distinctly annoying, distressing, or intolerable. Added to this list are such reactions as skin rashes (especially if they're extensive and persistent), visual disturbances (especially in people who wear corrective lenses), muscle tremor, difficulty with urination (common with many drugs in elderly men), any perceptible change in mood or mental function, and certain changes in blood components (such as fats or lipids).

Testing the Safety of New Drugs

Before a new drug can be approved by the Food and Drug Administration (FDA) for marketing in the United States, it is subjected to rigorous study in animals and humans. Much of the testing is directed toward evaluating the drug's effectiveness (efficacy) and relative safety. Studies are conducted first in animals to gather information on drug kinetics (absorption, distribution, metabolism, elimination), drug dynamics (actions and mechanisms),and safety, including possible effects on reproductive capacity and health of the offspring. Many drugs are rejected at this stage because they fail to demonstrate beneficial activity or are found to be too toxic.

If animal testing is successful, the FDA approves the researchers' Investigational New Drug application, and the drug is then studied in humans. These studies progress through several phases. In the premarketing phases (phases I, II, and III), the new drug is studied first in a small number of healthy volunteers, and then in increasingly larger numbers of people who have or are at risk for the disease that the drug is intended to treat or prevent. In addition to determining therapeutic effectiveness, studies in humans focus on the type and frequency of adverse reactions and on factors that make people susceptible to these reactions (such as age, sex, complicating disorders, and interactions with other drugs).

Data from the animal and human tests, together with intended drug manufacturing procedures, package insert information, and product labeling, are submitted in a New Drug Application to the FDA. In most cases, the review and approval process takes 2 to 3 years after a New Drug Application is submitted, although the FDA may shorten the time for a drug that represents a major therapeutic advance.

Even after a new drug is approved, the manufacturer must conduct a postmarketing surveillance (phase IV) and promptly report any additional or previously undetected adverse drug reactions. Doctors and pharmacists are encouraged to participate in the ongoing monitoring of the drug. Such monitoring is important, because even the comprehensive premarketing studies can detect adverse reactions that occur only about once in every 1,000 doses. Important adverse reactions that occur once in every 10,000 doses or even once in every 50,000 doses can be detected only when a large number of people use the drug after it's on the market. The FDA may withdraw approval if new evidence indicates that a drug poses a significant hazard.

Mild or moderate adverse drug reactions do not necessarily mean that a drug must be discontinued, especially if no suitable alternative is available. However, a doctor will likely reevaluate the dosage, frequency of administration (number of doses a day), timing of doses (before or after meals; in the morning or at bedtime), and possible use of other agents that may relieve distress (for example, the doctor may recommend using a stool softener if a drug causes constipation).

Sometimes drugs cause **severe reactions** that are potentially life-threatening, although they are relatively rare. People who develop a severe reaction usually must stop using the drug and have the reaction treated. However, sometimes doctors must continue administering high-risk drugs (for example, chemotherapeutic drugs to cancer patients or immunosuppressant drugs to patients undergoing organ transplantation). They'll use every possible means to cope with the serious adverse reaction. For example, doctors may give antibiotics to patients with an impaired immune system to combat infection; they may give high-potency liquid antacids or H_2-receptor blockers such as famotidine or ranitidine to prevent or heal stomach ulcers; they may infuse platelets to treat serious bleeding problems; or they may inject erythropoietin in patients with drug-induced anemia to stimulate red blood cell production.

Benefits Versus Risks

Every drug has the potential to cause harm as well as to do good. Whenever doctors consider prescribing a drug, they must weigh the possible risks against the expected benefits. Use of a drug

Some Serious Adverse Drug Reactions

Adverse Reaction	Drugs
Peptic ulcers or bleeding from the stomach	• Corticosteroids (such as prednisone or hydrocortisone) taken orally or by injection (not applied to the skin in creams or lotions) • Aspirin and other nonsteroidal anti-inflammatory drugs (such as ibuprofen, ketoprofen, and naproxen) • Anticoagulants (such as heparin, warfarin)
Anemia (decreased production or increased destruction of red blood cells)	• Certain antibiotics (such as chloramphenicol) • Some nonsteroidal anti-inflammatory drugs (such as indomethacin, phenylbutazone) • Antimalarial and antituberculotic drugs in patients with G6PD enzyme deficiency
Decreased production of white blood cells, with increased risk of infection	• Certain antipsychotic drugs (such as clozapine) • Anticancer drugs • Some antithyroid drugs (such as propylthiouracil)
Liver damage	• Acetaminophen (repeated use of excessive doses) • Some antituberculotic drugs (such as isoniazid) • Excessive amounts of iron compounds • Many other drugs, especially in people with preexisting liver disease or those who consume large amounts of alcoholic beverages
Kidney damage (risk of drug-induced kidney damage is increased in the elderly)	• Nonsteroidal anti-inflammatory drugs (repeated use of excessive doses) • Aminoglycoside antibiotics (such as kanamycin and neomycin) • Some anticancer drugs (such as cisplatin)

isn't justified unless the expected benefits outweigh the possible risks. Doctors must also consider the likely outcome of withholding the drug. Potential benefits and risks can seldom be determined with mathematical precision.

When assessing the benefits and risks of prescribing a drug, doctors consider the severity of the disorder being treated and the impact it's having on the patient's quality of life. For example, the relatively minor discomforts of coughs and colds, muscle strains, or infrequent headaches can be relieved with over-the-counter drugs, and only a very low risk of adverse effects is acceptable. Over-the-counter drugs for treating minor disorders have a wide safety margin when used according to directions. However, the risk of an adverse drug reaction rises sharply when a person is taking other over-the-counter or prescrip-

tion drugs. In contrast, when a drug is being used to treat a serious or life-threatening disease or condition (for example, a heart attack, stroke, cancer, organ transplant rejection), it's necessary to accept a higher risk of a severe drug reaction.

Risk Factors

Many factors can increase the likelihood of an adverse drug reaction. They include the simultaneous use of several drugs, very young or old age, pregnancy, certain diseases, and hereditary factors.

Multiple Drug Therapy
Taking several prescription and over-the-counter drugs contributes to the risk of having an adverse drug reaction. The number and severity of adverse reactions increase disproportionately

with the number of drugs taken. The use of alcohol, which is also a drug, increases the risk. Having a doctor or pharmacist periodically review all the drugs a person is taking can reduce the risk of an adverse drug reaction.

Age

Infants and very young children are at special risk of adverse drug reactions because their capacity to metabolize drugs is not fully developed. For example, newborns can't metabolize and eliminate the antibiotic chloramphenicol; those who are given the drug could develop gray baby syndrome, a serious and often fatal reaction. Tetracycline, another antibiotic, given to infants and young children during the period when their teeth are being formed (up to about age 7) may permanently discolor tooth enamel. Children under age 15 are at risk of Reye's syndrome if they are given aspirin while they have influenza or chickenpox.

Elderly people are also at high risk of having an adverse drug reaction, primarily because they're likely to have many health problems and thus to be taking several prescription and over-the-counter drugs. Some elderly people may be prone to confusion regarding instructions for the proper use of drugs. Kidney function and the ability to eliminate drugs from the body decline with age; these problems are often further complicated by malnourishment and dehydration. Elderly people who take drugs that may cause light-headedness, confusion, and impaired coordination are at risk of falling and fracturing a bone. Among the drugs that can cause such problems are many of the antihistamines, sleep aids, and antianxiety and antidepressant drugs.▲

Pregnancy

Many drugs pose a risk to the normal development of a fetus. To the extent possible, pregnant women shouldn't take drugs, especially during the first trimester. A doctor should supervise the use of any prescription and over-the-counter drugs during pregnancy. Social and illicit drugs (alcohol, nicotine, cocaine, and narcotics such as heroin) also pose risks to the pregnancy and fetus.

Other Factors

Diseases can alter drug absorption, metabolism, and elimination and the body's response to drugs.■ Heredity may make some people more

susceptible to the toxic effects of certain drugs. The realm of mind-body interactions, including such aspects as mental attitude, outlook, and belief in self and confidence in health care practitioners, remains largely unexplored.

Drug Allergies

In general, the number and severity of adverse drug reactions increase as the dose increases. However, this dose-response relationship doesn't apply to people who are allergic or hypersensitive to a drug. For these people, even small amounts of the drug can trigger an allergic reaction, ranging from minor and simply annoying to severe and life-threatening.★ Allergic reactions may include skin eruptions and itching; fever; constriction of the airways and wheezing; swelling of tissues, such as the larynx and glottis, which would impair breathing; and a fall in blood pressure, sometimes to dangerously low levels.

Drug allergies are unpredictable because reactions occur after a person has been previously exposed to the drug (whether it was applied to the skin, taken orally, or injected) one or more times without any allergic reaction. A mild reaction may require treatment with only an antihistamine; a severe or life-threatening reaction may require an injection of adrenaline (also called epinephrine) or corticosteroids (such as hydrocortisone).

Doctors usually ask if a person has any known drug allergies before prescribing a new drug. People who have had severe allergic reactions, who have serious medical problems, or who are taking high-risk drugs should wear a Medic Alert necklace or bracelet. Information inscribed in the bracelet (for example, penicillin allergy, insulin-dependent diabetic, taking warfarin) will alert medical and paramedical personnel in case of an emergency.

Overdose Toxicity

Overdose toxicity refers to serious, often injurious, and possibly fatal toxic reactions to acci-

---

▲ see box, page 40

■ see page 37

★ see page 823

dental overdosage of a drug (because of a doctor's, pharmacist's, or patient's error) or intentional overdosage (homicide or suicide).

A lower risk of overdose toxicity is often the reason doctors prefer one drug to another when both drugs are equally effective. For example, if a sedative, antianxiety drug, or sleep aid is needed, doctors usually prescribe benzodiazepines such as diazepam and triazolam rather than barbiturates such as pentobarbital. Benzodiazepines are not more effective than barbiturates, but they have a wider margin of safety and are much less likely to cause severe toxicity in case of an accidental or intentional overdosage. Safety is also the reason why newer antidepressants such as fluoxetine and paroxetine have largely replaced older but equally effective antidepressants such as imipramine and amitriptyline.

Young children are at high risk of overdose toxicity. Most of the brightly colored tablets and capsules that attract the attention of toddlers and young children are adult-dose formulations. Federal regulations require that all oral prescription drugs in the United States be dispensed in childproof containers unless a person signs a waiver to the effect that such a container presents a handicap.

Most metropolitan areas in the United States provide information services on chemical and drug poisoning, and most telephone directories list the number of the local Poison Control Center. This number should be copied and placed near a telephone or programmed into an automatic dialing telephone.

CHAPTER 11

Compliance With Drug Treatment

The medical profession defines compliance as the degree to which a patient follows a treatment plan.

Studies of patient behavior show that only about half the people who leave a doctor's office with a prescription take the drug as directed. Among the many reasons people give for not complying with a treatment plan, forgetfulness is the most common. However, the key question is, why do people forget? Often, the psychologic mechanism of denial is at work. Something about the treatment may greatly concern the person, resulting in a repression of the desire to follow the plan. Being ill is a cause for concern, and having to take a drug is a constant reminder of the illness. Other reasons for not complying with a medical treatment plan include the cost of treatment, inconvenience, and possible adverse effects.

Results of Noncompliance

Even the best treatment plan will fail if it isn't followed. The most obvious consequence of noncompliance is that a person's illness may not be relieved or cured.

According to an estimate from the Office of the United States Inspector General, every year noncompliance with drug treatment results in 125,000 deaths from cardiovascular disease such as heart attack and stroke. In addition, up to 23 percent of nursing home admissions, 10 percent of hospital admissions, many doctor visits, many diagnostic tests, and many unnecessary treatments could be avoided if people took their drugs as directed.

Not only does noncompliance add to the cost of medical care, it can worsen the quality of life. For example, missed doses of a glaucoma drug can lead to optic nerve damage and blindness; missed doses of a heart drug may lead to an erratic heart rhythm and cardiac arrest; missed doses of a high blood pressure drug can lead to stroke; and failure to take prescribed doses of an antibiotic can cause an infection to flare up again and can lead to the emergence of drug-resistant bacteria.

Compliance Among Children

Children are even less likely than adults to follow a treatment plan. A study of children with streptococcal infections who were prescribed a 10-day course of penicillin showed that 56 percent stopped taking the drug by the third day, 71 percent by the sixth day, and 82 percent by the ninth day. Compliance with a treatment plan is even worse with chronic diseases such as juvenile diabetes and asthma that require complex therapy over a long period of time.

Sometimes parents don't clearly understand instructions. Studies show that parents forget about half the information 15 minutes after meeting with a doctor. Parents remember the first third of the discussion best and remember more about diagnosis than about the details of the treatment plan. That's why pediatricians try to keep the treatment plan simple and often provide written instructions.

Compliance Among the Elderly

Older people may be taking several drugs, making it harder for them to remember when to take each of them and more likely that they will have an adverse drug interaction.▲ Some of their drugs may have been prescribed by different doctors, and they may also be taking nonprescription drugs. Therefore, all doctors involved need to know about all the drugs a person is taking. Good communication can help the doctor develop a simpler treatment plan as well as avoid the dangers of unforeseen drug interactions. Older people are generally more sensitive to drugs, and they may need different doses.■ Good communication helps ensure that they don't decrease the drug dose on their own in order to decrease side effects.

Purchasing all drugs from one pharmacist can also help, as most pharmacists keep computerized records of the drugs a person is taking and can monitor them for possible drug duplication or interactions.

Ways to Improve Compliance

People usually have an easier time complying with their treatment plan if they have a good relationship with their doctor. Two-way communication works best; most people want to be a part of the decision-making process. When people participate in their health care planning, they also assume responsibility for it and are more likely to

Reasons for Not Complying With a Treatment Plan

- Not understanding or misinterpreting the instructions

- Forgetting to take the drug

- Experiencing adverse effects (the treatment may be perceived as worse than the disease)

- Denying illness (repressing the diagnosis or its significance)

- Not believing that the drug will help

- Mistakenly believing that the illness has been sufficiently treated (for example, with an infection, the fever may disappear before all the infectious bacteria are eradicated)

- Fearing adverse consequences or becoming dependent on the drug

- Worrying about the expense

- Not caring about getting better (apathy)

- Confronting obstacles (for example, having difficulty swallowing tablets or capsules, having problems opening bottles, finding the treatment plan inconvenient, being unable to obtain the drug)

stay with the plan. Receiving clear explanations and understanding the rationale for the treatment also help ensure compliance.

People are also more likely to comply if they believe that their doctor, nurse, physician assistant, or pharmacist cares whether or not they stick with the plan. Studies show that people who receive explanations from a concerned doctor are more satisfied with the help they receive and like the doctor more; the more they like the doctor, the better they follow a treatment plan. Written instructions help people avoid mistakes caused by poor recall of what the doctor said.

▲ see page 42

■ see page 39

Why a Treatment Plan Can Go Astray

Drug errors
- Failing to fill a prescription
- Filling the prescription but taking it incorrectly
- Taking a drug that isn't prescribed

Inadequate contact with the doctor
- Delay in seeking care
- Refusing or being unable to enter a treatment program
- Having no treatment facility accessible, convenient, or affordable
- Not keeping appointments
- Quitting a treatment plan early
- Not bringing a problem to the doctor's attention

Behavioral resistance to treatment
- Not taking recommended preventive steps
- Not following instructions completely
- Not participating in recommended health programs

Creating a two-way relationship between patient and doctor can start with an information exchange. By asking questions, a person can come to terms with the severity of an illness and intelligently weigh the advantages and disadvantages of a treatment plan. Misunderstandings can often be clarified simply by talking to an informed professional. Good communication also ensures that all caregivers understand the plan prescribed by other health care practitioners.

People who take responsibility for helping to monitor the good and bad effects of the treatment and discussing concerns with health care practitioners will likely have better results with a treatment plan. They should inform the doctor, pharmacist, or nurse about unwanted or unexpected effects before adjusting or stopping the treatment on their own. A person often has good reasons for not following a plan, and a doctor can make an appropriate adjustment after a frank discussion of the problem.

Support groups are often available for people with similar conditions. These groups can often reinforce treatment plans and provide suggestions for coping with problems. Names and telephone numbers of support groups can be obtained through local hospitals and community councils.

CHAPTER 12

Generic Drugs

The term *generic* is used to describe the less expensive copycat versions of well-known and widely used brand-name products. For some foods and household products, the term generic implies paying less but settling for a lower standard of quality and effectiveness. With pharmaceuticals, this is generally not the case.

Drugs are often known by a variety of names.▲ When first discovered, a drug is given a **chemical name,** a shorthand version of the chemical name, or a code name developed for easy reference

among researchers. If the Food and Drug Administration (FDA), the government agency responsible for ensuring that drugs in the United States are safe and effective, approves the drug for general prescribing, it's given two additional names: a **generic name** (official name) and a **trade name** (also called **proprietary** or **brand name**), which identifies it as the exclusive property of a particular company. The government, doctors, researchers, and others who write about the new compound use the drug's generic name because it refers to the drug itself, not a particular company's brand of that drug or a specific product. However, written prescriptions usually use a trade name.

▲ see box, page 25

Generic names are usually more complicated and harder to remember than trade names. Many generic names are a kind of shorthand for the drug's chemical name, structure, or formula. The most important characteristic of a generic name is its uniqueness. Trade names also must be unique and are usually catchy and relatively easy to remember. They often indicate a particular characteristic of the drug. For example, Lopressor lowers blood pressure, Vivactil is an antidepressant that might make a person more vivacious, Glucotrol controls high blood sugar (glucose), and Skelaxin is a skeletal muscle relaxant. The trade name Minocin, on the other hand, is simply a shortened version of minocycline, the drug's generic name.

Authorities must be certain that trade and generic names are unique and can't be mistaken for other drugs. Names too similar to those of other drugs can lead to mistakes in drug prescribing or dispensing.

Patent Protection

In the United States, a company that develops a new drug can be granted a patent for the drug itself, the way it's made, or how it's to be used. A manufacturer often owns more than one patent for a drug and may even own a patent on the system that delivers and releases the drug into the bloodstream. Patents grant the company exclusive rights to a drug for 17 years. However, usually about 10 years elapse between the time a drug is discovered and the time it's approved for human or veterinary use, leaving the manufacturer only about 7 years to exclusively market a new drug. (AIDS drugs and other new drugs for life-threatening illnesses often receive faster approval.)

After a patent has expired, other companies may sell a generic version of the drug, typically at a much lower price than the original brand. Not all off-patent drugs have generic versions; sometimes a drug is too hard to duplicate or adequate tests aren't available to prove that the generic drug acts the same as the trade-name drug. However, generic drugs generally can be assumed to work as well. A generic drug may be sold under a brand name (a branded generic drug) or only under its generic name. In any case, the FDA must approve all generic versions of a drug.

Evaluation and Approval Procedures

The FDA's approval of a generic drug is based on scientific evidence that the generic drug produces an effect in humans that's essentially identical to that of the original product. The FDA tests new generic drugs to ensure that they contain appropriate amounts of active (drug) ingredients, that they're being manufactured according to federal standards (Good Manufacturing Practices), and that they're released into the body at the same rate and to the same extent as the original trade-name drugs.

Researchers at companies that make generic drugs conduct studies, usually among relatively small numbers (15 to 50) of healthy volunteers, solely to determine if the generic version of a drug releases its active ingredients into the bloodstream in the same manner as the original brand. These research studies are called bioequivalence studies. In comparison, new drugs require larger, more complex, and much more expensive studies to prove that the drugs are safe and effective.▲

Manufacturers of trade-name drugs use bioequivalence study techniques when they develop new dosage forms or strengths of their drugs. Often the tablet or capsule used during clinical trials and product development must be modified for commercial reasons. Tablets may be made sturdier, flavoring or coloring may be added or changed, or inactive ingredients may be changed to increase consumer acceptance. Whenever a new form of a drug is developed, it must be proved bioequivalent to the form that was originally used to establish the drug's safety and effectiveness.

The rules are different for timed-release (long-acting, sustained-release) drugs. Since these drugs are subject to much more variation than regular tablets and capsules, federal regulators require the extensive testing involved in preparing a *full* New Drug Application before a company can market a timed-release version of any drug. This requirement applies even if another timed-release version of the drug is already on the market. Although this requirement has slowed the

---

▲ see box, page 43

availability of generic versions of some timed-release drugs, the required research is in the consumer's best interest.

Comparing Generic and Trade-Name Drugs

Developing and manufacturing prescription drugs isn't like following a cookbook. Many different routes may be taken to produce a drug that's safe and effective.

When a company decides to develop a generic version of a drug, the company's experts in drug formulation figure out how to design their product. While they use active ingredients that are identical to those of the original drug, they are likely to use different inactive ingredients. Inactive ingredients are added for specific reasons, for example, to provide bulk so that a tablet is large enough to handle, to keep a tablet from crumbling between the time it's manufactured and the time it's used, to help a tablet dissolve in the stomach or intestine, or to provide a pleasant taste and color.

Inactive ingredients are generally harmless substances that don't affect the body. However, in a few people inactive ingredients can cause unusual and sometimes severe allergic reactions, making one brand or generic version of a drug more acceptable than another. For example, the bisulfites (such as sodium metabisulfite), which are used as preservatives in many products, cause asthmatic allergic reactions in a large number of people. Consequently, drug products containing bisulfites are now prominently labeled. Ironically, people with asthma are likely to have been exposed to bisulfites because these preservatives are found in many sprays and solutions used to treat asthma.

For legal reasons, a generic drug differs from its trade-name counterpart in size, color, and shape. Therefore, consumers usually find that a generic version looks very different from the trade-name drug they are familiar with.

Generally, bioequivalence of different versions of a drug can vary by as much as 20 percent without any noticeable difference in effectiveness. These variations can occur between trade and generic versions of a drug or between different batches (lots) of a manufacturer's trade-name or generic drug. For example, a batch of a drug manufactured in company X's plant in New Jersey may not be identical to a batch of the drug manufactured in company X's plant in Puerto Rico. Nor will either be the same as a generic version of the drug manufactured in company Y's plant in Boston. All these versions must be tested to ensure that they produce a similar effect in the human body.

Actual differences between FDA-approved generic and trade-name drugs taken by mouth are much smaller than the allowable 20 percent. The observed variations are only about 3.5 percent overall and rarely exceed 10 percent in any single study.

Sometimes generic versions are available but can't be freely substituted for the original drug because no standards for comparison have been established. These products may be sold but shouldn't be considered equivalent. An example is the thyroid hormones. All versions are acceptable for treating underactive thyroid glands. However, they shouldn't be substituted for one another because no standards have been set for comparing them. Pharmacists and doctors can explain which generic drugs are acceptable substitutes and which are not.

Choosing a Generic Drug

Each year, the FDA publishes *Approved Drug Products With Therapeutic Equivalence Evaluations*, also known as "the orange book" because it has a bright orange cover. The book is available to anyone but is intended for use by doctors and pharmacists. It provides guidance about which generic drugs can be considered identical to their trade-name counterparts and which cannot. Generic drugs that are identical to the trade-name drug may be freely substituted in any prescription, unless a doctor indicates otherwise. To verify that the generic drug dispensed is equivalent to a previous prescription, consumers can check the label of the drug for the generic name of its active ingredient. The pharmacist is responsible for accurately dispensing and labeling prescriptions.

Consumers can choose between a trade-name drug and a generic version unless their doctor has written on the prescription that no substitution can be made. However, consumers may have

When Generic Substitution May Not Be Appropriate

Drug Category	Examples	Comments
Drugs for which the toxic dose is only slightly higher than the therapeutic dose	Warfarin, digoxin (for heart failure); phenytoin, carbamazepine, valproic acid, and other antiseizure drugs	The margin of safety is relatively small (narrow therapeutic range); too little drug may not work and too much drug may cause side effects
Drugs on the market before the 1938 amendments to the Food, Drug, and Cosmetic Act	Digoxin and other digitalis derivatives (for heart failure); thyroid hormone and thyroid hormone derivatives such as levothyroxine, liothyronine, liotrix, and thyroglobulin (for hypothyroidism and Graves' disease)	These drugs are exempt from generic drug requirements, although few pre-1938 drugs are still prescribed. Switching among different versions is unwise because no standards are available by which to compare these drugs
Corticosteroid creams, lotions, and ointments	Alclometasone, amcinonide, betamethasone, clocortolone, desonide, desoximetasone, dexamethasone, diflorasone, fluocinolone, fluocinonide, flurandrenolide, fluticasone, halcinonide, halobetasol, hydrocortisone, mometasone, triamcinolone	These products are standardized by tests of skin response. Many have been rated as equivalent by the FDA. But response can vary, and different drug vehicles (creams, ointments, gels) also can cause variable effects. Response is so unpredictable that a product that's effective shouldn't be switched for another
Corticosteroid tablets	Dexamethasone, some brands of prednisone	Many generic versions are not equivalent to trade-name drugs and shouldn't be freely substituted for them
High blood pressure drugs	Reserpine, reserpine plus hydrochlorothiazide, reserpine plus hydroflumethiazide, hydralazine	Generic versions are not equivalent to trade-name drugs
Aerosol drugs, especially those for asthma	Metaproterenol and terbutaline (widely used bronchodilators); some aerosol corticosteroid preparations	Any of the versions may be effective, but standards for comparing them are still under development
Oral asthma drugs	Theophylline, dyphilline, some brands of aminophylline	Products are generally not equivalent. Someone doing well with a particular brand should avoid switching unless absolutely necessary
Antidepressant drugs	A few brands of amitriptyline, one brand of amitriptyline-perphenazine combination	Not all brands are substitutable. A pharmacist can advise whether a particular generic drug is considered equivalent by the FDA
Diabetes drugs	Glyburide (for adult-onset diabetes)	One brand of glyburide (Glynase) may not be interchanged with the others
Antipsychotic drugs	Chlorpromazine tablets	Generic versions are not equivalent to the trade-name version
Gout drugs	Probenecid, colchicine	Generic versions are not equivalent to the trade-name version

(continued)

When Generic Substitution May Not Be Appropriate (Continued)

Drug Category	Examples	Comments
Hormones	Esterified estrogen (for estrogen replacement therapy in postmenopausal women); some brands of medroxyprogesterone; most generic versions of methyltestosterone	The two brands of esterified estrogen are not equivalent. Since hormones are generally taken in extremely small doses, differences could produce major swings in patient response
Potassium	Most long-acting potassium replacement products in *tablet* form	The long-acting potassium replacement *capsules* are considered equivalent and may be freely substituted
Other drugs	Disulfiram Fluoxymesterone Mazindol Nicotine patches Phenytoin, prompt Promethazine tablets and suppositories Rauwolfia serpentina Trichlormethiazide	Generic versions of these drug products are not equivalent. Although any brand can be effective, brands should not be interchanged

to take whichever generic version the pharmacist has decided to stock. Many insurance plans and health maintenance organizations (HMOs) require that generic drugs be prescribed and dispensed whenever possible to save money.

State laws that control certain aspects of the practice of medicine and pharmacy vary regarding how much the consumer can participate in these prescribing decisions. In some states, the consumer has no say; if the doctor prescribes a generic drug, the pharmacist must dispense a generic drug. In other states, consumers may insist on a trade-name drug even if the doctor and pharmacist have recommended a generic drug. If the doctor prescribes a trade-name drug but the consumer wants a generic version, the consumer can discuss this matter with the doctor, who can write a prescription authorizing a generic version.

Critics of widespread generic drug use have raised other concerns, such as the possible increase to the person's health care bill resulting from extra visits to the doctor, new laboratory tests, and other aspects of being restabilized on a new brand of prescription drug. Critics wonder

how much money is really saved by switching to a generic version after these additional costs are paid. Another concern is whether differences in a generic drug's color, size, or shape may reduce a person's motivation to follow the doctor's instructions for taking it.

Generic Nonprescription Drugs

Generic versions of the most popular nonprescription (over-the-counter) drugs are often sold as house brands by drug chains or cooperatives. These drugs are evaluated in the same way that generic prescription drugs are evaluated and must meet the same requirements.

Selecting a house brand or generic version of an over-the-counter drug can probably save money. Pharmacists can advise which generic over-the-counter drug products should be as effective as the original. However, individual product preference is often related to appearance, taste, consistency, and other product characteristics. Although the active ingredients are the same, other characteristics may differ.

Over-the-Counter Drugs

Over-the-counter (OTC) drugs are those available without a prescription. They allow people to relieve many annoying symptoms and cure some diseases simply and without the cost of seeing a doctor. However, the self-care revolution of the past few decades, encouraged by the availability of safe and effective OTC drugs, calls for common sense and responsibility.

Historical Background

Once most drugs were available without a prescription. Before the federal Food and Drug Administration (FDA) existed, just about anything could be put in a bottle and sold as a sure-fire cure. Alcohol, cocaine, marijuana, and opium were included in some OTC products without notification to users. The enactment of the Food, Drug, and Cosmetic (FD&C) Act in 1938 gave the FDA some authority to issue regulations, but no clear guidelines were provided as to which drugs should be sold by prescription only and which could be sold over the counter.

The FD&C Act was amended in 1951 in an effort to resolve safety problems and clarify the difference between OTC and prescription drugs. Prescription drugs were compounds that could be habit forming, toxic, or unsafe for use except under medical supervision. Anything else could be sold over the counter.

As noted by the FD&C Act of 1962, OTC drugs were required to be both safe *and* effective. However, what works for one person may not work for another. What's more, any drug may cause adverse effects. (Some people refer to adverse effects as side effects, but this term doesn't make it clear that the additional effects are usually unwanted.) With no organized system for reporting the adverse effects of OTC drugs, the FDA and drug manufacturers have virtually no way of knowing how common or serious they are.

Finally, an important change in recent years has been the reclassification of many prescription drugs to OTC status.

Safety Considerations

Safety is a primary concern when the FDA considers whether a drug previously available only by prescription should be switched to OTC status. All drugs have benefits and risks; some degree of risk has to be tolerated if people are to receive a drug's benefits. However, defining an acceptable degree of risk is a judgment call.

Safety depends on using an OTC drug properly. Proper use often relies on consumer self-diagnosis, which leaves room for error. For example, most headaches are not dangerous, but in rare cases a headache may be an early warning sign of a brain tumor or hemorrhage. Similarly, what seems like severe heartburn might be a warning of an impending heart attack. Ultimately, a person must use common sense in determining when a symptom or ailment is minor and when it requires medical attention.

In establishing appropriate doses of OTC drugs, manufacturers and the FDA try to balance safety and efficacy. People who purchase OTC drugs should read and follow the instructions carefully. Since the same brand name may be applied to an immediate-release or controlled-release (slow release) formulation, the label should be checked each time a product is purchased. It isn't safe to assume that the dose is the same.

Brand inflation has occurred in recent years, so it's also important to check the ingredients and not just rely on familiar brand names. For example, more than a dozen different Tylenol formulations with a vast array of ingredients are available. Not all Maalox products contain the same ingredients—some contain aluminum and magnesium oxides, others contain calcium carbonate. When selecting a product, a person must know which ingredient is most appropriate for the particular problem.

Some people experience adverse effects from OTC drugs even when using them properly. For example, a severe, rare allergic reaction (anaphylaxis)▲ to analgesics such as aspirin, ketoprofen,

▲ see page 828

Some Drugs Reclassified to Over-the-Counter Status

Generic Name	Selected Brand Names	Generic Name	Selected Brand Names
Acetaminophen	Tylenol	Ketoconazole	Nizoral Shampoo
Acetaminophen, pseudoephedrine, dextromethorphan, doxylamine	Vicks NyQuil	Ketoprofen	Actron, Orudis KT
		Loperamide	Imodium A-D, Maalox Anti-Diarrheal, Pepto Diarrhea Control
Brompheniramine, phenylpropanolamine	Dimetapp	Miconazole	Micatin, Monistat 7
Chlorpheniramine	Chlor-Trimeton	Minoxidil	Rogaine
Cimetidine	Tagamet HB	Naproxen	Aleve
Clemastine	Tavist	Nizatidine	Axid
Clotrimazole	Gyne-Lotrimin, Lotrimin AF, Mycelex OTC Cream, Mycelex-7 Vaginal Cream	Oxymetazoline	Afrin, Dristan 12 Hour Nasal, Duration, Neo-Synephrine 12 Hour, Sinex Long-Acting
Diphenhydramine	Benadryl, Nytol, Sominex, Unisom Maximum Strength SleepGels	Permethrin	Nix
		Phenylephrine	Neo-Synephrine, Sinex
Doxylamine	Unisom Nighttime Sleep-Aid	Pseudoephedrine	Afrin Tablets, Efidac/24, Sudafed
Ephedrine	Bronkaid, Primatene	Pyrantel	Antiminth, Pin-Rid, Pin-X
Famotidine	Pepcid AC	Ranitidine	Zantac 75
Fluoride	ACT, Fluorigard, Listermint with Fluoride	Tolnaftate	Tinactin
Hydrocortisone	Cortaid, Cortizone	Triprolidine, pseudoephedrine	Actifed
Ibuprofen	Advil, Bayer Select Pain Relief, Midol 200, Motrin IB, Nuprin	Xylometazoline	Otrivin

naproxen, or ibuprofen may lead to hives, itching, breathing problems, and cardiovascular collapse. Such drugs can also irritate the digestive tract and may cause ulcers.

Often the labels of OTC drugs don't list the full range of possible adverse reactions. As a result, many people assume that these drugs have few, if any, adverse effects. For example, the package insert for one analgesic only cautions people not to take the drug for more than 10 days for pain. Information on the box, bottle, and package insert that accompany the drug doesn't describe its possible serious adverse effects with long-term use. Consequently, people with chronic pain or inflammation may take the drug for a long time without realizing that such use could lead to problems.

Analgesics and Anti-inflammatory Drugs

Over-the-counter analgesics (pain relievers) such as aspirin, ibuprofen, ketoprofen, naproxen, and acetaminophen are reasonably safe to take for short periods of time. All except acetaminophen also reduce inflammation and are classified as nonsteroidal anti-inflammatory drugs (NSAIDs). Their labels caution against use for more than 7 to 10 days for pain. A doctor should be consulted if symptoms get worse or don't go away.

Aspirin

The oldest and least expensive OTC analgesic is aspirin (acetylsalicylic acid). Aspirin and other nonsteroidal anti-inflammatory drugs block the enzyme cyclooxygenase, which is crucial to the creation of prostaglandins. Prostaglandins are hormonelike substances that alter the diameter of blood vessels, raise body temperature in response to infection, and play a crucial role in blood clotting, among other effects. The body's release of prostaglandins in response to an injury—burn, break, sprain, or strain—leads to inflammation, redness, and swelling.

Because prostaglandins play a role in protecting the digestive tract from stomach acid, taking aspirin or a similar drug can cause gastrointestinal upset, ulcers, and even bleeding. All nonsteroidal anti-inflammatory drugs, including aspirin, can cause heartburn, indigestion, and peptic ulcers.

Buffered compounds may diminish the direct irritating effects of aspirin. Such products contain an antacid, which creates an alkaline environment that enhances the dissolving of aspirin and may reduce the time aspirin is in contact with the stomach lining. However, because buffering can't counteract the diminished prostaglandin formation, buffered aspirin can irritate the stomach too.

Enteric-coated aspirin is designed to pass through the stomach intact and dissolve in the small intestine, minimizing direct irritation. However, coated aspirin may be absorbed erratically. Eating food is likely to delay stomach emptying and therefore slow enteric-coated aspirin absorption and pain relief.

Because aspirin can interfere with blood clotting, people who take aspirin have an increased risk of bleeding. People who bruise easily may be

especially vulnerable. Anyone who has ever had a bleeding disorder or uncontrolled high blood pressure should avoid taking aspirin except under medical supervision. Using both aspirin and anticoagulants (such as warfarin) could lead to life-threatening bleeding. Generally, aspirin shouldn't be used in the week before scheduled surgery.

Aspirin can also aggravate asthma. People with nasal polyps are likely to develop wheezing if they take aspirin. Allergy to aspirin can lead to a rash or severe breathing difficulties. Large doses of aspirin can cause ringing in the ears (tinnitus).

Children and teenagers who have, or may have, influenza or chickenpox must not take aspirin because they could develop Reye's syndrome. Al-

---

Considerations in Reclassifying a Drug

Margin of safety
- What harmful effects may the drug produce?
- Is the product used in a way that requires the assistance of a health care professional?
- Could the product have harmful effects (including from misuse)?
- Is the product habit forming?
- What is the potential for abuse?
- Do the benefits of OTC status outweigh the risks?

Ease of diagnosis and treatment
- Can the average person self-diagnose the condition that calls for the drug?
- Can the average person treat that condition without a doctor?

Labeling
- Can adequate directions for use be written?
- Can warnings against unsafe use be written?
- Can the labeling be understood by the average person?

Reprinted with permission from "FDA's Review of OTC Drugs," the *Handbook of Nonprescription Drugs*, tenth edition, page 29, © 1993 by the American Pharmaceutical Association.

though rare, Reye's syndrome can have serious consequences, including death.▲

Ibuprofen, Ketoprofen, and Naproxen

Ibuprofen was reclassified from prescription to OTC status in 1984. Prescription-strength ibuprofen comes in 300-, 400-, 600-, and 800-milligram tablets; OTC ibuprofen is available only in 200-milligram tablets.

Ketoprofen was approved for OTC sale in 1995. Prescription-strength ketoprofen comes in 25-, 50-, and 75-milligram capsules, and in 100-milligram sustained-release capsules. OTC ketoprofen is available only in a 25-milligram formulation.

Naproxen was approved for OTC sale in 1994. Prescription-strength naproxen comes in 250-, 375-, and 500-milligram formulations; OTC naproxen is available only in a 200-milligram formulation. Dosing instructions for OTC naproxen caution people not to exceed 3 caplets in 24 hours unless directed by a doctor. Adults over age 65 are cautioned not to take more than 1 caplet every 12 hours unless directed by a doctor.

Ibuprofen, ketoprofen, and naproxen are generally believed to be gentler on the stomach than aspirin, although few studies have actually compared the drugs. Like aspirin, ibuprofen, ketoprofen, and naproxen can cause indigestion, nausea, diarrhea, heartburn, stomach pain, and ulcers.

Other adverse effects include drowsiness, dizziness, ringing in the ears, visual disturbances, fluid retention, and shortness of breath. Although ibuprofen, ketoprofen, and naproxen generally don't impair blood clotting as much as aspirin does, people shouldn't combine these drugs with anticoagulants such as warfarin (Coumadin) except under close medical supervision. Likewise, medical supervision is needed before ibuprofen, ketoprofen, or naproxen is used by people with kidney or liver problems, heart failure, or high blood pressure. Some prescription heart and blood pressure drugs may not work as well when combined with these analgesics. People who regularly drink alcoholic beverages may be at greater risk of stomach upset, ulcers, and impaired liver function.

People who are allergic to aspirin may also be allergic to ibuprofen, ketoprofen, and naproxen.

▲ see page 1280

A rash, itching, or breathing difficulties require immediate medical attention.

Acetaminophen

Originally introduced in 1955 for children's fever and pain, acetaminophen became available over the counter in 1960. Acetaminophen is roughly comparable to aspirin in its pain-relieving potential and fever-lowering action, but it has less anti-inflammatory activity than aspirin, ibuprofen, ketoprofen, or naproxen. An understanding of how acetaminophen works remains elusive.

New research suggests that acetaminophen is often beneficial against the pain of osteoarthritis. In one study, acetaminophen was as effective as ibuprofen in relieving arthritis symptoms in the knee.

Acetaminophen has almost no adverse effects on the stomach. People who can't tolerate aspirin, ibuprofen, ketoprofen, or naproxen often do well with acetaminophen. Perhaps the lack of stomach problems has led some people to assume that acetaminophen has no adverse effects. However, taking large doses of acetaminophen for long periods may carry some risks, including damage to the kidneys. Regular use of other nonsteroidal anti-inflammatory drugs, although not aspirin, may also increase the risk of developing kidney disease.

An overdose of more than 15 grams of acetaminophen can lead to irreversible liver disease. Whether smaller doses over long periods of time harm the liver is less certain. People who consume large amounts of alcohol are probably at highest risk of developing liver problems from overuse of acetaminophen. Fasting may also contribute to liver toxicity. Additional research is needed, but the implications are that people who take acetaminophen and stop eating because of a bad cold or influenza could be more vulnerable to liver damage.

Many OTC products, such as remedies for the symptoms of allergy, cold, cough, flu, pain, and sinus problems, contain acetaminophen. People should be careful not to take many drugs containing acetaminophen simultaneously.

Cold Remedies

More than 100 viruses are responsible for the misery attributed to the common cold, and a cure remains elusive. People spend billions of dollars every year trying to relieve cold symptoms. How-

Some Over-the-Counter Pain Relievers

Brand Names	Concentration of Ingredient (mg = milligrams)	Uses	Potential Problems
Products containing aspirin			
Halfprin	162 mg aspirin	Lowering risk of heart attack (enteric coated)	Gastrointestinal irritation and bleeding from prolonged use, ringing in the ears (tinnitus), allergic reaction in sensitive people, complications of labor in pregnant women, Reye's syndrome in children and teenagers with chickenpox or flu
8-Hour Bayer Timed-Release Caplets	650 mg aspirin	Pain and inflammation (timed release)	
Alka-Seltzer with Aspirin Ascriptin A/D Aspirin Bufferin Ecotrin Tablets Empirin Genuine Bayer Aspirin Tablets Regular Strength Ascriptin	325 mg aspirin	Fever, pain, inflammation	
Arthritis Pain Formula Bufferin Extra Strength Ecotrin Maximum Strength Tablets Maximum Bayer Aspirin Tablets	500 mg aspirin	Fever, pain, inflammation	
Aspergum	227.5 mg aspirin	Fever, mild to moderate pain (gum tablets)	
Bayer Children's Aspirin	81 mg aspirin	Fever, pain (chewable)	
Bayer Low Adult Strength Halfprin 81 St. Joseph Adult Chewable Aspirin	81 mg aspirin	Lowering risk of heart attack	
Products containing Ibuprofen, ketoprofen, or naproxen			
Advil Bayer Select Pain Relief Formula Excedrin IB Haltran Ibuprin Ibuprofen Medipren Midol IB Motrin IB Nuprin Pamprin-IB Trendar	200 mg ibuprofen	Fever, inflammation, menstrual cramps, mild to moderate pain	Digestive tract irritation, ulcers from prolonged use, kidney damage in elderly and other susceptible people, allergic reaction in sensitive people
Aleve	220 mg naproxen sodium	Fever, mild to moderate pain, inflammation, menstrual cramps	

(continued)

Some Over-the-Counter Pain Relievers (Continued)

Brand Names	Concentration of Ingredient (mg = milligrams)	Uses	Potential Problems
Products containing ibuprofen, ketoprofen, or naproxen (continued)			
Actron Orudis KT	25 mg ketoprofen	Fever, mild to moderate pain, inflammation, menstrual cramps	See previous page
Products containing acetaminophen			
Acetaminophen (APAP) Anacin-3 Tylenol Caplets	325 mg acetaminophen	Fever, mild to moderate pain	Liver damage from repeated high doses on an empty stomach or with alcohol, risk of kidney problems from prolonged use, allergic reaction in sensitive people
Anacin-3, Children's St. Joseph Aspirin-Free Fever Reducer for Children Tempra Tylenol, Children's	80 mg acetaminophen	Fever, headache or other mild pain	
Arthritis Pain Formula Aspirin Free Aspirin Free Anacin Maximum Strength Datril Extra Strength Panadol Tylenol Extra Strength	500 mg acetaminophen	Fever, mild to moderate pain	
Feverall Sprinkle Caps Junior Strength Panadol Liquiprin Elixir St. Joseph Aspirin-Free Fever Reducer for Children Tempra Tylenol Junior Strength	160 mg acetaminophen	Fever, mild to moderate pain	
Products containing salicylate			
Arthropan	870 mg choline salicylate per 5 milliliters	Arthritis pain, inflammation	Ringing in the ears (tinnitus)
Backache Maximum Strength Relief	467 mg magnesium salicylate	Mild to moderate pain	
Bayer Select Maximum Strength Backache	580 mg magnesium salicylate	Mild to moderate pain	
Original Doan's	325 mg magnesium salicylate	Mild to moderate pain	

ever, some authorities say that a person can take nothing at all and the cold will disappear in about a week, or a person can take a drug and feel better in about 7 days. Children are especially likely to get colds and be given cold remedies, even though the effectiveness of such drugs for pre-school children hasn't been proved.

Ideally, each cold symptom should be treated with a single drug. In reality, single-ingredient cold remedies are hard to find. Most remedies contain a variety of drugs—antihistamines, decongestants, analgesics, expectorants, and cough suppressants—designed to treat a wide range of symptoms.

Taking a cough suppressant, an expectorant, or an analgesic won't relieve a congested nose. If a cough is the problem, why take an antihistamine or a decongestant? If a sore throat is the only symptom, an analgesic (acetaminophen, aspirin, ibuprofen, or naproxen) is likely to work. Throat lozenges, especially those with a local anesthetic such as dyclonine or benzocaine, or a saltwater gargle (half a teaspoon of salt in 8 ounces of warm water) may also be helpful. Finding the appropriate treatment for individual symptoms can be a challenge. Reading the labels or consulting a pharmacist should help.

Occasionally, a cold or cough may be a sign of a more serious condition. A doctor should be consulted if symptoms linger for more than a week, especially if chest pain occurs or a cough produces dark sputum. Fever and pain are unlikely to accompany a common cold and may indicate influenza or a bacterial infection.

Antihistamines

Many experts believe that antihistamines shouldn't be included in OTC cold remedies. The concern is that antihistamines can cause drowsiness and make people feel sluggish. Driving, operating heavy equipment, and engaging in other activities that require alertness could become dangerous. The elderly are particularly susceptible to the adverse effects of antihistamines and may develop blurred vision, light-headedness, dry mouth, difficulty in urinating, constipation, and confusion.▲ Children are occasionally stimulated by antihistamines and may experience insomnia or hyperactivity. Despite widespread concern about these risks, most cold remedies contain antihistamines. Again, reading labels or seeking advice from a pharmacist is helpful.

Some Over-the-Counter Antihistamines

Brompheniramine

Chlorpheniramine

Dexbrompheniramine

Diphenhydramine

Doxylamine

Phenindamine

Pheniramine

Pyrilamine

Triprolidine

Decongestants

When viruses invade mucous membranes, especially in the nose, blood vessels dilate and cause swelling. Decongestants constrict vessels to provide some relief. Active ingredients in oral decongestants include pseudoephedrine, phenylpropanolamine, and phenylephrine. Phenylpropanolamine is also the primary ingredient of many OTC diet products.

Adverse effects of decongestants may include nervousness, agitation, palpitations, and insomnia. Because these drugs circulate throughout the body, they constrict other blood vessels—not just those in the nose—possibly raising the blood pressure. For this reason, people with high blood pressure or heart disease should take decongestants only under a doctor's supervision or not at all. Other conditions that require medical supervision when using decongestants include diabetes, heart trouble, and hyperthyroidism.

In an attempt to avoid such complications, people often turn to nasal sprays, which relieve swollen nasal tissues without affecting other organ systems. However, nasal sprays work so fast and so well that many people are tempted to use them longer than the 3-day limit listed on the label. This could lead to the vicious circle of rebound nasal

▲ see box, page 41

Cough Suppressants Containing Only Dextromethorphan

Benylin DM

Children's Hold

Delsym Extended Release

Hold DM

Robitussin Cough Calmers

Robitussin Pediatric Cough

St. Joseph Cough Suppressant

Scot-Tussin DM Cough Chasers

Sucrets Cough Control

congestion. As the effect wears off, small blood vessels in the nose can expand, causing congestion and stuffiness. This feeling may be so uncomfortable that use of the nasal spray is continued. Such use may lead to a drug dependency that lasts months or years. Sometimes withdrawal may have to be supervised by a doctor specializing in ear, nose, and throat disorders.

Long-acting nasal sprays include the drugs oxymetazoline and xylometazoline, which may provide relief for as long as 12 hours. Some long-acting nasal sprays are Afrin, Allerest 12 Hour Nasal, Duration 12 Hour Nasal Spray, 4-Way Long Lasting Nasal Spray, Neo-Synephrine Maximum Strength 12 Hour, Otrivin, and Vicks Sinex 12-Hour Nasal Decongestant Spray. They should also be used for no more than 3 days at a time.

Cough Remedies

Coughing is a natural reflex to lung irritation; it rids the lungs of excess secretions or mucus.▲ If a person is congested and can cough up phlegm, suppression of such a productive cough is unwise.

Single-ingredient cough suppressants are hard to find. Expectorants are often added to cough

▲ see page 152

suppressants in cold and cough remedies. Combining a drug that makes phlegm easier to cough up with a drug that suppresses coughing seems senseless to some experts. Guaifenesin, the only approved expectorant on the market, is supposed to help loosen lung secretions and make them easier to cough up. Products with guaifenesin include Anti-Tuss, Naldecon Senior EX, Organidin NR, Robitussin, Triaminic Expectorant, and others. The drug's actual benefit, however, has been hard to establish.

An unproductive or dry cough can be very irritating, especially at night; a cough suppressant can provide relief and contribute to restful sleep. Codeine, a highly effective cough suppressant, can be helpful at bedtime because of its slight sedative effect. Because codeine is a narcotic, some people fear it may be addicting. In reality, addiction is uncommon, but many states require that codeine be sold only by prescription. Other states permit pharmacists to sell cough medicine containing codeine only if the customer signs for it. Examples of codeine-containing products include Cheracol Cough Syrup, Guiatuss AC, Mytussin AC Cough Syrup, Robitussin A-C Cough Syrup, and Tussi-Organidin NR Liquid.

Codeine causes nausea, vomiting, and constipation in some people. Because light-headedness, drowsiness, or dizziness may also occur, cough medicine containing codeine shouldn't be taken by anyone who is about to drive a vehicle or perform a task that requires concentration. Allergy to codeine is uncommon. Adverse effects may increase when central nervous system depressants such as alcohol, sedatives, sleep aids, antidepressants, or antihistamines are taken at the same time as codeine. Consequently, the combination should be taken only under medical supervision.

Dextromethorphan is the most common ingredient in OTC cough remedies. Its cough-suppressing potential is roughly comparable to that of codeine. Adverse effects are rare, although an upset stomach or drowsiness can occur.

Diet Aids

Nonprescription diet aids are supposed to suppress hunger and make a low-calorie diet easier to follow. Two ingredients are approved for this purpose: phenylpropanolamine, which also acts as a decongestant in many cold and allergy remedies, and benzocaine, a local anesthetic that's supposed to numb the taste buds. Benzocaine's most logical form is gum, candy, or lozenges that are held in the mouth before a meal.

In one study, phenylpropanolamine helped dieters lose more weight than did an identical-appearing placebo. However, the difference in weight lost was unimpressive—about 5 pounds. Phenylpropanolamine's effectiveness has been proved for only about 3 to 4 months. Phenylpropanolamine is likely to be most helpful when it's part of a program that includes exercise and modified eating habits.

The dose of phenylpropanolamine in diet aids is higher than the dose generally found in cold or allergy remedies. Adverse effects such as nervousness, insomnia, dizziness, restlessness, headache, and nausea may occur if more than the recommended dose is taken. In rare cases, people experience adverse effects with the usual dose. Some people may also become restless or agitated and experience hallucinations within a few hours of taking phenylpropanolamine.

The most worrisome potential adverse effect is a significant increase in blood pressure. Strokes and other cardiovascular problems may occur if susceptible people take high doses of phenylpropanolamine alone or in combination with other drugs, or if they use the drug for a long time.

Because drug interactions are possible, checking with a doctor or pharmacist is important before taking any drug containing phenylpropanolamine. Labels warn people with diabetes, thyroid disease, high blood pressure, or heart disease not to take diet aids without medical supervision. Monoamine oxidase inhibitors, drugs that may be prescribed for depression, could interact with phenylpropanolamine to cause a dangerous rise in blood pressure.

Antacids and Indigestion Aids

Heartburn, indigestion, and sour stomach are a few of the many terms used to describe gastrointestinal distress. Self-diagnosing indigestion is risky because causes vary from a minor dietary indiscretion to peptic ulcer disease or even stomach cancer. Sometimes symptoms of heart disease resemble acute indigestion. Although many people treat their own heartburn, they'd be better off seeking medical attention for symptoms that last longer than 2 weeks.

Some Over-the-Counter Diet Aids

Brand Name	Active Ingredient
Acutrim 16 Hour Steady Control	75 mg phenylpropanolamine
Acutrim Maximum Strength	75 mg phenylpropanolamine
Appedrine Caplets	25 mg phenylpropanolamine
Control Capsules	75 mg phenylpropanolamine
Dexatrim Maximum Strength Caffeine-Free Caplets	75 mg phenylpropanolamine
Dexatrim Plus Vitamins Caplets	75 mg phenylpropanolamine

The goal of treatment is to prevent the production of stomach acid or to neutralize it. Histamine$_2$ blockers, including cimetidine, famotidine, nizatidine, and ranitidine, reduce the amount of acid produced in the stomach and help prevent heartburn. Antacids are neutralizing agents and work more quickly. While they can't completely neutralize the extremely acidic pH of the stomach, antacids can raise the pH level from 2 (very acidic) to between 3 and 4. This neutralizes almost 99 percent of stomach acid and significantly relieves symptoms for most people.

Most antacid products contain one or more of four primary ingredients: aluminum salts, magnesium salts, calcium carbonate, and sodium bicarbonate. All ingredients work in a minute or less, but the products work for different lengths of time. Some products provide relief for only about 10 minutes, while others are effective for more than an hour and a half. Histamine blockers take longer to work but produce a more sustained effect.

Antacids can interact with many different prescription drugs, so a pharmacist should be consulted about drug interactions before they're taken. Anyone who has heart trouble, hypertension, or kidney problems should consult a doctor before selecting an antacid. Cimetidine may also interact with some prescription drugs, and there-

Antacids That Have a High Calcium Content

Brand Name	Active Ingredient
Alka-Mints	850 mg calcium carbonate in a tablet
Calcium Rich Rolaids	550 mg calcium carbonate in a tablet
Chooz	500 mg calcium carbonate in a gum tablet
Maalox Antacid Caplets	1,000 mg calcium carbonate in a caplet
Mylanta Lozenges	600 mg calcium carbonate in a lozenge
Titralac Plus Liquid	1,000 mg calcium carbonate in 2 teaspoons
Tums E-X Extra Strength	750 mg calcium carbonate in a tablet
Tums Ultra	1,000 mg calcium carbonate in a tablet

fore its use needs to be monitored carefully by a doctor or pharmacist.

Aluminum and Magnesium

Antacids that contain both aluminum and magnesium salts once seemed ideal because each ingredient complemented the other. Aluminum hydroxide dissolves slowly in the stomach and starts to work gradually but provides long-lasting relief. It also causes constipation. Magnesium salts work fast and neutralize acids effectively but can also act as a laxative. Antacids with both aluminum and magnesium seem to offer the best of both worlds: quick, long-lasting relief with less risk of diarrhea or constipation.

However, the long-term safety of antacids containing aluminum has been questioned. Prolonged use may weaken bones by depleting the body of phosphorus and calcium.

▲ see page 678

Calcium Carbonate

Chalk (calcium carbonate) has been a mainstay of antacids for a long time. Calcium carbonate acts fast and neutralizes acids for a relatively long time. Another benefit is that it provides an inexpensive source of calcium. However, a person can overdose on calcium. The maximum daily amount shouldn't exceed 2,000 milligrams unless a doctor has directed otherwise.

Sodium Bicarbonate

One of the least expensive and most readily available antacids is no farther away than the kitchen cabinet. Baking soda (sodium bicarbonate) has provided fast acid-neutralizing action for decades. The baking soda burp is caused by the liberation of carbon dioxide gas.

Sodium bicarbonate is an excellent short-term solution to indigestion, but too much bicarbonate can wreak havoc with the body's acid-base balance and lead to metabolic alkalosis.▲ Its high sodium content may also cause problems for people with heart failure or high blood pressure.

Motion Sickness Drugs

The drugs used to prevent motion sickness are antihistamines. They are occasionally prescribed but are also available over the counter. Motion sickness drugs are most likely to be effective if taken 30 to 60 minutes before a trip.

Motion sickness drugs often make a person drowsy and less alert. In fact, one motion sickness drug, diphenhydramine, is the active ingredient in most OTC sleep aids. Anyone who drives a car, boat, or other vehicle, or who performs an activity that requires close attention shouldn't take these drugs. Motion sickness drugs shouldn't be taken with alcohol, sleep aids, or tranquilizers, since the effects may add up unexpectedly. Adverse effects are more common in the elderly.

Other adverse effects, such as blurred vision, confusion, headache, stomachache, constipation, palpitations, or difficulty with urination, are less common. Babies and very young children may become agitated and shouldn't be given these drugs except under a doctor's supervision. Too high a dose in a young child could lead to hallucinations or even convulsions, which might prove fatal.

People with narrow-angle glaucoma, an enlarged prostate gland, or constipation should take motion sickness drugs only if a doctor recommends or approves their use.

Sleep Aids

Over-the-counter sleep aids are intended to ease an occasional sleepless night, not chronic insomnia, which could signal a serious underlying problem.▲ Taking an OTC sleep aid for more than a week to 10 days isn't recommended.

Two ingredients, the antihistamines diphenhydramine and doxylamine, are used as OTC sleep aids. These drugs tend to make people drowsy or groggy and can interfere with concentration or coordination. Not everyone reacts that way, though. Asians seem to be less sensitive to the sedative effects of diphenhydramine than are people from Western countries.

Some people react in the opposite way (a paradoxical reaction) and find that diphenhydramine or doxylamine makes them feel nervous, restless, and agitated. Older people, those with brain damage, and young children are apparently more susceptible to this response than others. Some people also occasionally experience adverse effects such as dry mouth, constipation, blurred vision, and ringing in the ears.

Elderly people, pregnant women, and breast-feeding women should probably avoid these drugs unless directed to use them by a doctor. People with narrow-angle glaucoma, angina, arrhythmias, or an enlarged prostate gland should consult a doctor before using an antihistamine for sleeping or any other purpose.

Special Precautions

Common sense is a critical element of self-care. Certain people are more vulnerable than others to potential harm from drugs. The very young, the very old, and the very sick should be given drugs only with extreme care, which may include professional supervision. To avoid dangerous interactions, people should consult a pharmacist or doctor before combining prescription drugs and OTC drugs. OTC drugs aren't designed to treat serious illnesses and can actually make some conditions worse. An unanticipated reaction, such as a rash or insomnia, should serve as a signal to stop taking the drug immediately and obtain medical advice.

Motion Sickness Drugs: Precautions for Children

Brand Name	Active Ingredient	Children Who Should Not Take the Drug
Marezine	Cyclizine	Under 6 years old
Calm-X	Dimenhydrinate	Under 2 years old
Dramamine	Dimenhydrinate	Under 2 years old
Marmine	Dimenhydrinate	Under 2 years old
Benadryl	Diphenhydramine	Weigh less than 22 pounds
Nordryl	Diphenhydramine	Weigh less than 22 pounds
Meclizine	Meclizine	Under 12 years old
Dramamine II	Meclizine	Under 12 years old
Bonine	Meclizine	Under 12 years old

Children

Children's bodies metabolize and react to drugs differently from the way adults' bodies do. A drug may be in wide use for many years before its hazards to children are discovered. For example, 5 years passed before researchers confirmed that the risk of Reye's syndrome was linked to the use of aspirin in children with chickenpox or influenza. Doctors and parents alike are often surprised to learn that most OTC drugs, even

▲ see page 300

Guidelines for Choosing and Using Over-the-Counter Drugs

• Make sure that a self-diagnosis is as accurate as possible. Don't assume the problem is "something that's going around."

• Select products on the basis of rational planning and ingredients, not because they're labeled with a familiar brand name.

• Choose a product with the fewest appropriate ingredients. Remedies that attempt to relieve every possible symptom are likely to expose people to unnecessary drugs, pose additional risks, and cost more.

• When in doubt, check with a pharmacist or doctor for the most appropriate ingredient or product.

• Have a pharmacist check for potential interactions with other drugs being used.

• Read the label carefully to determine the proper dose and precautions. Find out what conditions would make the drug a poor choice.

• Ask the pharmacist to write down possible adverse effects.

• Do not exceed the recommended dose.

• Never take an OTC drug longer than the maximum time suggested on the label. Stop taking the drug if symptoms get worse.

• Keep all drugs, including OTC drugs, out of the reach of children.

those with recommended pediatric dosages, haven't been thoroughly tested in children. The effectiveness of cough and cold remedies in particular is unproved, especially for children, so that using these drugs may be a waste of money and may unnecessarily expose children to toxicity.

Giving a child a correct drug dose can be tricky. Although children's doses are often expressed in terms of age ranges (for example, children age 2

▲ see page 39

to 6 or 6 to 12), age isn't the best criterion. Children can vary enormously in size within any age range, and experts don't agree on whether the best measurement for determining drug dose is weight, height, or total body surface. A recommended dose expressed in terms of the child's weight may be the easiest to interpret and administer.

If the label doesn't give instructions on how much drug to give the child, a parent shouldn't guess. When in doubt, consult a pharmacist or doctor. Taking precautions may prevent a child from receiving a dangerous drug or a dangerously high dose of a potentially helpful one.

Many drugs for treating children come in liquid form. While the label should give clear guidelines about the dose, sometimes the adults in charge may give the wrong dose because they use an ordinary teaspoon. Kitchen spoons other than measuring spoons aren't accurate enough to measure liquid drugs. A cylindrical measuring spoon is far better for a child's dose, and an oral syringe is preferred for squirting a precise amount of drug into a baby's mouth. The cap should always be removed from the tip of an oral syringe before use. A child can choke if a cap is accidentally propelled into the windpipe.

Several children's drugs come in more than one form. Adults must read labels carefully every time a new children's drug is brought into the house.

Elderly People

Aging changes the speed and ways in which the body handles drugs.▲ The changes in liver and kidney function that occur naturally with aging can affect how drugs are metabolized or eliminated. Elderly people may be more vulnerable than younger ones to adverse effects or drug interactions. More and more prescription drug labels specify whether different doses are needed for the elderly, but such warnings are rarely printed on OTC drug labels.

Many OTC drugs are potentially hazardous for the elderly. The risk increases when drugs are taken regularly at the maximum dose. For example, an elderly person who suffers from arthritis may be inclined to use an analgesic or anti-inflammatory drug frequently, with potentially serious consequences. A bleeding ulcer is a life-threatening complication for an elderly person and can occur without warning symptoms.

Antihistamines, such as diphenhydramine, also pose special risks for elderly people. Nighttime pain relief formulas, sleep aids, and many cough and cold remedies often contain antihistamines. Besides possibly worsening asthma, narrow-angle glaucoma, or an enlarged prostate gland, antihistamines can make a person dizzy or unsteady, leading to falls and broken bones. Antihistamines can sometimes cause confusion or delirium in elderly people, particularly at a high dose or in combination with other drugs.

Elderly people may be more susceptible to the possible adverse effects of digestive tract drugs. Antacids containing aluminum are more likely to cause constipation, while magnesium-based antacids are more likely to lead to diarrhea and dehydration. Even taking vitamin C can cause stomach upset or diarrhea in elderly people.

During visits to the doctor, elderly people should mention any OTC product they're taking, including vitamins and minerals. This information helps the doctor evaluate the entire drug regimen and determine whether or not the OTC drug may be responsible for certain symptoms.

Drug Interactions

Many people neglect to mention their use of OTC drugs to their doctor or pharmacist. Drugs taken intermittently, as for colds, constipation, or an occasional headache, are mentioned even less often. Health care practitioners may not think of asking about OTC drugs when prescribing or filling a prescription. Yet many OTC products have the potential to interact adversely with a wide range of drugs.

Some of these interactions can be serious. For example, as little as one aspirin tablet can reduce the effectiveness of enalapril (Vasotec) in the treatment of severe heart failure. This may also occur with other angiotensin converting enzyme (ACE) inhibitors. Taking aspirin with the anticoagulant warfarin (Coumadin) can increase the risk of abnormal bleeding. People with heart disease may not realize that taking an antacid containing aluminum or magnesium can reduce the absorption of digoxin (Lanoxin). Even taking a multiple vitamin and mineral supplement can interfere with the action of some prescription drugs. The antibiotic tetracycline may be ineffective if swallowed with calcium, magnesium, or iron.

No systematic research has been devoted to OTC drug interactions. Many serious problems have been discovered accidentally, after adverse reactions or deaths were reported. Although some OTC drugs have interaction warnings on the label, the language may be meaningless to most consumers. For example, some diet aids and cold remedies that contain phenylpropanolamine caution against using the product either with a prescription monoamine oxidase inhibitor (given for depression) or for 2 weeks after discontinuing the prescription. For the many people who don't realize the antidepressant they're taking is a monoamine oxidase inhibitor, this important warning isn't helpful.

The best way to reduce the risk of drug interactions is to ask the pharmacist to check for incompatibility. Additionally, the doctor should be told about all other drugs being taken, both prescription and OTC.▲

Drug Overlap

Another potential problem is drug overlap. Unless people read the labels on everything they take, they can accidentally overdose themselves. For example, a person who takes a diet aid as well as a cold remedy, both containing phenylpropanolamine, may take double the dosage considered safe. Acetaminophen is commonly found in sinus medications. A person simultaneously taking a sinus medication and acetaminophen for a headache might exceed the recommended dose.

Chronic Conditions

A number of chronic conditions can become worse if an OTC drug is taken inappropriately. Antihistamines, which are found in OTC sleep aids, allergy medications, and cough and cold or influenza remedies, shouldn't be taken by anyone with asthma, emphysema, or chronic lung problems unless directed by a doctor. Taking an antihistamine can also complicate glaucoma and an enlarged prostate gland.

People with high blood pressure, heart disease, diabetes, hyperthyroidism, or an enlarged prostate gland should consult a doctor or pharmacist

---

▲ see box, page 37

before taking OTC decongestants or antihistamines, as their adverse effects can be dangerous in such conditions.

A person of any age with a serious medical condition should consult a health care practitioner before purchasing OTC products. People with diabetes, for example, may need help locating a cough syrup that doesn't contain sugar. Recovering alcoholics need to be vigilant about avoiding cold medicines containing alcohol; some products contain as much as 25 percent alcohol.

People with heart disease may need advice on treating a cold or even an upset stomach with a product that won't interact with their prescription drugs.

Because OTC drugs are intended primarily for occasional use by people who are essentially healthy, a medical consultation is wise for anyone who is chronically ill or who plans to take the drug every day. Such use is beyond the normal boundaries of self-care and calls for the advice of an expert.

Heart and Blood Vessel Disorders

CHAPTER 14

Biology of the Heart and Blood Vessels

The heart, a hollow muscular organ, lies in the center of the chest. The right and the left sides of the heart each have an upper chamber (atrium), which collects blood, and a lower chamber (ventricle), which ejects blood. To ensure that blood flows in only one direction, the ventricles have an inlet and an outlet valve.

The heart's primary functions are to supply oxygen to the body and to rid the body of waste products (carbon dioxide). In short, the heart performs these functions by collecting oxygen-depleted blood from the body and pumping it to the lungs, where it picks up oxygen and drops off carbon dioxide; the heart then collects the oxygen-enriched blood from the lungs and pumps it to the tissues of the entire body.

Function of the Heart

During each heartbeat, each heart chamber relaxes as it fills, a period called diastole, and then contracts as it pumps blood, a period called systole. The two atria relax together and contract together, and the two ventricles relax together and contract together.

Here's how blood moves through the heart. First, oxygen-depleted, carbon dioxide–laden blood from the body flows through the two largest veins (the venae cavae) into the right atrium. When this chamber fills, it propels the blood into the right ventricle. When the right ventricle fills, it pumps the blood through the pulmonary valve into the pulmonary arteries, which supply the lungs. The blood then flows through tiny capillaries, which surround the air sacs in the lungs, absorbing oxygen and giving up carbon dioxide, which is then exhaled. The now oxygen-rich blood flows through the pulmonary veins into the left atrium. This circuit between the right side of the heart, the lungs, and the left atrium is called the pulmonary circulation. When the left atrium fills, it propels the oxygen-rich blood into the left

ventricle. When this chamber fills, it pumps the blood through the aortic valve into the aorta, the largest artery in the body. This oxygen-rich blood supplies all of the body except the lungs.

Blood Vessels

The rest of the circulatory (cardiovascular) system is composed of arteries, arterioles, capillaries, venules, and veins. The arteries, which are strong and flexible, carry blood away from the heart and bear the highest blood pressures. Their resilience helps maintain blood pressure while the heart is between beats. The smaller arteries and arterioles have muscular walls that adjust their diameter to increase or decrease blood flow to a particular area. Capillaries are tiny, extremely thin-walled vessels that act as bridges between arteries, which carry blood away from the heart, and veins, which carry blood back to the heart. The capillaries allow oxygen and nutrients to pass from the blood into the tissues and allow waste products to pass from the tissues into the blood. They drain into the venules, which in turn drain into the veins that lead back to the heart. Because veins are thin-walled but generally larger in diameter than arteries, they carry the same volume of blood at a lower speed and under much less pressure.

Heart's Blood Supply

The heart muscle (myocardium) itself receives a fraction of the large volume of blood flowing through the atria and ventricles. A system of arteries and veins (coronary circulation) supplies the myocardium with oxygen-rich blood and then returns oxygen-depleted blood to the right atrium. The right coronary artery and the left coronary artery branch off the aorta to deliver blood; the cardiac veins empty into the coronary sinus, which returns blood to the right atrium. Because

A Look Into the Heart

This cross-sectional view of the heart shows the direction of normal blood flow.

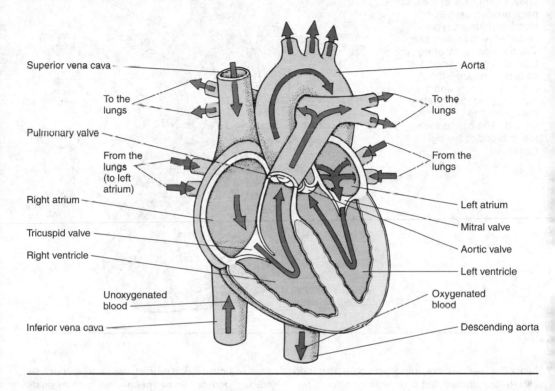

Superior vena cava

To the lungs

Pulmonary valve

From the lungs (to left atrium)

Right atrium

Tricuspid valve

Right ventricle

Unoxygenated blood

Inferior vena cava

Aorta

To the lungs

From the lungs

Left atrium

Mitral valve

Aortic valve

Left ventricle

Oxygenated blood

Descending aorta

of the great pressure exerted in the heart as it contracts, most blood flow through the coronary circulation takes place while the heart is relaxing between beats (during ventricular diastole).

Symptoms of Heart Disease

No single symptom unmistakably identifies heart (cardiac) disease, but certain symptoms suggest the possibility, and several symptoms together may make the diagnosis almost certain. A doctor begins the diagnostic process with an interview (a history) and a physical examination. Often, tests are ordered to confirm the diagnosis, to assess the severity of the problem, or to help in planning treatment.▲ However, sometimes even serious heart disease may have no symptoms until it reaches a late stage. Routine health checkups or a visit to the doctor for another reason may uncover such asymptomatic heart disease.

The symptoms of heart disease include certain types of pain, shortness of breath, fatigue, palpitations (an awareness of a slow, fast, or irregular heartbeat), light-headedness, and fainting. However, these symptoms don't necessarily indicate

▲ see page 72

Heart's Blood Supply

Like any other tissue in the body, the muscle of the heart must receive oxygen-rich blood and have oxygen-depleted blood taken away. The right coronary artery and the left coronary artery with its two branches—the circumflex artery and the left anterior descending artery—deliver blood to the heart muscle. The cardiac veins return blood to the right atrium.

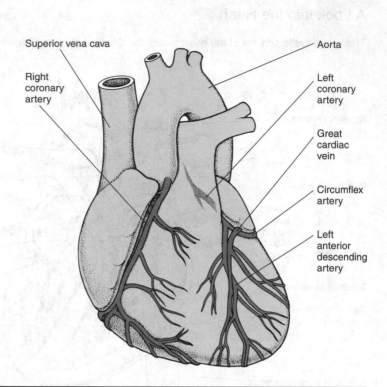

Superior vena cava

Right coronary artery

Aorta

Left coronary artery

Great cardiac vein

Circumflex artery

Left anterior descending artery

heart disease. For example, chest pain may indicate heart disease, but it may also indicate respiratory disease or gastrointestinal disease.

Pain

When muscles don't get enough blood (a condition called ischemia), inadequate oxygen and excessive waste products cause cramping. Angina, a tightness or squeezing sensation in the chest, results when the heart muscle doesn't receive enough blood. However, the type and de-

▲ see page 121

■ see page 133

★ see page 104

gree of pain or discomfort varies tremendously among people. Some people with inadequate blood supply have no pain at all (a condition called silent ischemia).▲

If too little blood flows to other muscles, particularly the calf muscles, a person usually feels a tightening and fatiguing pain in the muscle during exercise (claudication).■

Pericarditis, an inflammation or injury to the sac that surrounds the heart, causes pain that gets worse when lying down and gets better when sitting up and leaning forward.★ Exertion doesn't make the pain worse. Inhaling or exhaling may make it better or worse because pleuritis, an inflammation of the membrane surrounding the lungs, may also occur.

When an artery tears or ruptures, a person may feel a sharp pain that comes and goes fairly quickly and may be unrelated to physical activity. Sometimes the major arteries, especially the aorta, become damaged. A stretched-out, bulging portion of the aorta (aneurysm) may suddenly leak, or the lining may tear slightly, permitting blood to seep between the layers of the aorta (dissection of the aorta). These events produce sudden, severe pain that may come and go with further damage such as tearing or with movement of blood outside its normal channel. Pain from the aorta is often felt in the back of the neck, between the shoulder blades, down the back, or in the abdomen.▲

The valve between the left atrium and left ventricle may bulge back into the left atrium when the left ventricle contracts (mitral valve prolapse). People with this condition sometimes have brief episodes of stabbing or needle-like pain. Usually, the pain is centered below the left breast regardless of the person's position or physical activity.■

Shortness of Breath

Shortness of breath is a common symptom of heart failure. The shortness of breath results from fluid seeping into the air spaces of the lung, a condition called pulmonary congestion or pulmonary edema. Ultimately, this process is similar to drowning. In the early stages of heart failure, a person may be short of breath only during physical exertion. As heart failure worsens, shortness of breath occurs with less and less activity, until it occurs at rest. People are short of breath mostly when they lie down because fluid seeps throughout the lung tissue. When they sit up, gravity causes fluid to collect at the base of the lungs, which is less of a problem. Nocturnal dyspnea is shortness of breath that occurs when a person is lying down at night; it's relieved by sitting up.

Shortness of breath isn't limited to heart disease; people with lung disease, disease of the respiratory muscles, or diseases of the nervous system that interfere with breathing can also be short of breath. Any disorder that upsets the normal, delicate balance between oxygen supply and oxygen requirement, such as inadequate oxygen-carrying capacity of the blood from anemia or increased overall metabolism in the body from an overactive thyroid, can make a person short of breath.

Fatigue

When the heart pumps inefficiently, blood flow to the muscles may be inadequate during exercise, causing the person to feel weak and tired. Symptoms are often subtle. People compensate by gradually diminishing activity, or they may blame the symptoms on increasing age.

Palpitations

Ordinarily, people don't notice the beating of their heart. But under certain circumstances— when even healthy people exercise strenuously or have a dramatic emotional experience, for example—they may become aware of their heartbeat. They may feel the heart beating very forcefully or rapidly or sense an irregular heartbeat. A doctor can confirm these symptoms by checking the pulse and listening to the heartbeat through a stethoscope placed on the chest. Whether the palpitations are abnormal depends on answers to a number of questions, such as whether anything seems to bring them on, whether they started suddenly or gradually, how fast the heart beats, and whether and to what extent the beat seems to be irregular. Palpitations that occur together with other symptoms such as shortness of breath, pain, weakness and fatigue, or fainting are more likely to result from an abnormal heart rhythm or a serious underlying disease.

Light-headedness and Fainting

Inadequate blood flow resulting from an abnormal heart rate or rhythm or poor pumping ability may cause light-headedness, faintness, and fainting.★ These symptoms can also result from brain or spinal cord disease, or they may have no serious cause. For instance, soldiers may feel faint when standing still for long periods because the leg muscles have to be active to help return blood to the heart. Strong emotion or pain, which activates part of the nervous system, also can cause fainting. Doctors must distinguish fainting caused by heart disease from epilepsy, in which a loss of consciousness results from a brain disorder.

▲ see page 139

■ see page 95

★ see page 108

Diagnosis of Heart Disease

A doctor usually can tell whether someone has heart disease on the basis of the medical history and the physical examination. Diagnostic tests are used to confirm the diagnosis, determine the extent and consequence of the disease, and help in planning treatment.

Medical History and Physical Examination

A doctor first asks about symptoms such as chest pain, shortness of breath, swelling of the feet and ankles, and palpitations, which suggest the possibility of heart disease. A doctor then asks if the person has other symptoms such as fever, weakness, fatigue, lack of appetite, and a general malaise, which may point to heart disease. Next, the person is questioned about past infections; previous exposure to chemicals; use of medications, alcohol, and tobacco; home and work environments; and recreational activity. The doctor also questions the person about whether family members have had heart disease and other diseases and whether the person has any diseases that may affect the cardiovascular system.

During the physical examination, a doctor notes the person's weight and overall physique and looks for paleness, sweating, or drowsiness, which may be subtle indicators of heart disease. The person's general mood and feeling of well-being, which also may be affected by heart disease, are noted.

Assessing skin color is important because pallor or cyanosis (a bluish coloration) may indicate anemia or poor blood flow. These findings can indicate that the skin is receiving inadequate oxygen from the blood because of lung disease, heart failure, or various circulatory problems.

A doctor feels the pulse in arteries in the neck, beneath the arms, at the elbows and wrists, in the abdomen, in the groin, at the knees, and in the ankles and feet to assess whether blood flow is adequate and equal on both sides of the body. The blood pressure and body temperature are also checked. Any abnormalities may suggest heart disease.

A doctor inspects the veins in the neck because they're directly connected to the right atrium of the heart and give an indication of the volume and pressure of blood entering the right side of the heart. For this part of the examination, the person lies down with the upper part of the body elevated at a 45-degree angle. Sometimes the person sits, stands, or lies flat.

The doctor presses the skin over the ankles and legs and sometimes over the lower back to check for fluid accumulation (edema) in the tissues beneath the skin.

An ophthalmoscope (an instrument that allows a doctor to examine the inside of the eye) is used to view the blood vessels and nerve tissues of the retina (the light-sensitive membrane on the inner surface of the back of the eye). Visible abnormalities in the retina are common in people with high blood pressure, diabetes, arteriosclerosis, and bacterial infections of the heart valves.

A doctor observes the chest to determine if the breathing rate and movements are normal and then taps (percusses) the chest with the fingers to determine if the lungs are filled with air, which is normal, or if they contain fluid, which is abnormal. Percussion also helps determine whether the sac surrounding the heart (pericardium) or the membrane layers covering the lungs (pleura) contain fluid. Using a stethoscope, a doctor also listens to the breathing sounds to determine whether airflow is normal or obstructed and whether the lungs contain fluid as a result of heart failure.

A doctor places a hand on the chest to determine the heart size and the type and force of contractions during each heartbeat. Sometimes abnormal, turbulent blood flow within vessels or between heart chambers causes a vibration that can be felt with the fingertips or palm.

A doctor listens to the heart with a stethoscope (a procedure called auscultation), noting the distinctive sounds caused by the opening and closing of the heart valves. Abnormalities of the valves and heart structures create turbulent blood flow that causes characteristic sounds called murmurs. Turbulent blood flow typically occurs as blood moves through narrowed or leaking valves. Not all heart diseases cause murmurs, and not all murmurs indicate heart disease. Pregnant women usually have heart murmurs because of the normal increase in blood flow. Harmless heart murmurs also are common in infants and children because of the rapid flow of blood through small structures in the heart. As vessel walls, valves, and other tissues gradually stiffen in the elderly, blood may flow turbulently, even without serious underlying heart disease.

Placing the stethoscope over arteries and veins elsewhere in the body, a doctor may listen for sounds of turbulent blood flow, called bruits, caused by narrowing of the vessels or abnormal connections between vessels.

A doctor feels the abdomen to determine if the liver is enlarged from a backup of blood in the major veins leading to the heart. Abnormal abdominal swelling from fluid retention may indicate heart failure. The pulse and size of the abdominal aorta also are checked.

Diagnostic Tests

Doctors have access to a wide array of tests and procedures for making rapid, precise diagnoses. The technology includes electrical measurements, x-rays, echocardiography, magnetic resonance imaging (MRI), positron emission tomography (PET) scans, and cardiac catheterization.

Most cardiac diagnostic procedures carry only a tiny risk, but the risk increases with the complexity of the procedure and the severity of the underlying heart disease. With cardiac catheterization and angiography, the chance of a major complication—such as stroke, heart attack, or death—is 1 in 1,000. Exercise testing has a 1 in 5,000 risk of heart attack or death. Virtually the only risk of radionuclide studies comes from the tiny dose of radiation the person receives, which is less radiation than a person receives from most x-rays.

Electrocardiography

Electrocardiography is a quick, simple, painless procedure in which electrical impulses in the heart are amplified and recorded on a moving strip of paper. The electrocardiogram (ECG) allows a doctor to analyze the pacemaker of the heart that triggers each heartbeat, the nerve conduction pathways of the heart, and the rate and rhythm of the heart.

To obtain an ECG, an examiner places small metal contacts (electrodes) on the skin of the person's arms, legs, and chest. These electrodes measure the flow and direction of electric currents in the heart during each heartbeat. The electrodes are connected by wires to a machine, which produces a tracing for each electrode. Each tracing represents a particular "view" of the heart's electrical patterns; these views are called leads.

Most people suspected of having heart disease have an ECG taken. This test can help doctors identify a number of heart problems, including abnormal heart rhythms, inadequate blood and oxygen supply to the heart, and an excessive thickening (hypertrophy) of heart muscle, which can result from high blood pressure. An ECG also can reveal when the heart muscle is thin or absent because it's been replaced by nonmuscular tissue; this condition can result from a heart attack (myocardial infarction).

Exercise Tolerance Testing

A person's exercise endurance can tell a doctor a lot about the existence and severity of coronary artery disease and other heart disorders. An exercise tolerance test (stress test), which monitors a person's ECG and blood pressure during exercise, can reveal problems that wouldn't appear at rest. If the coronary arteries are partially blocked, the heart may have a sufficient blood supply when the person is resting but not when the person exercises. Simultaneous pulmonary function testing can distinguish between exercise limitation from heart or lung disease and limitation from heart and lung disease together.

During the test, the person pedals an exercise bicycle or walks on a treadmill at a given pace; gradually, the pace is increased. The ECG is monitored continuously, and blood pressure is measured at intervals. Generally, people taking the exercise tolerance test are asked to keep going until their heart rate reaches between 80 and 90 percent of the maximum for their age and sex. If

ECG: Reading the Waves

An electrocardiogram (ECG) represents the electrical current moving through the heart during a heartbeat, and each part of the ECG is given an alphabetical designation. Each heartbeat begins with an impulse from the heart's main pacemaker (sinoatrial node). This impulse first activates the upper chambers of the heart (atria). The P wave represents this activation of the atria.

Next, the electrical current flows down to the lower chambers of the heart (ventricles). The QRS complex represents the activation of the ventricles.

The T wave represents the recovery wave, as the electrical current spreads back over the ventricles in the opposite direction.

Many kinds of abnormalities show up on an ECG. The easiest to understand are abnormalities of the heartbeat rhythm: too fast, too slow, or irregular. By reading the ECG, a doctor can usually determine where in the heart the abnormal rhythm starts and can begin to determine its cause.

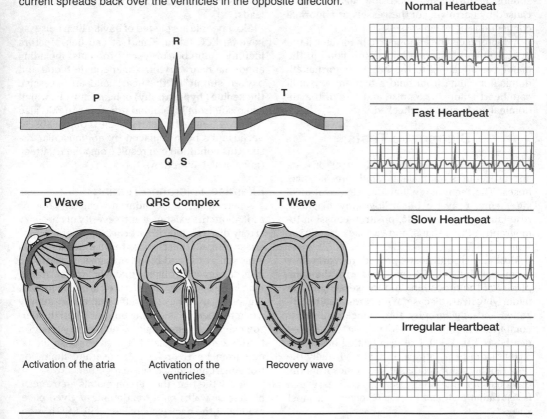

Normal Heartbeat

Fast Heartbeat

Slow Heartbeat

Irregular Heartbeat

P Wave
Activation of the atria

QRS Complex
Activation of the ventricles

T Wave
Recovery wave

symptoms, such as shortness of breath or chest pain, become too uncomfortable, or if significant abnormalities appear in the ECG or blood pressure recordings, the person stops sooner.

People who can't exercise for any reason may undergo stress electrocardiograms, which provide similar information to exercise tolerance tests but don't involve exercise. Instead, a drug that increases the blood supply to normal heart tissue but further decreases the supply to abnormal tissue, such as dipyridamole or adenosine, is injected to simulate the effects of exercise.

An exercise tolerance test suggests coronary artery disease when certain ECG abnormalities appear, the person develops angina, or the blood pressure decreases.

No test is perfect. Sometimes these tests show abnormalities in people who don't have coronary artery disease (a false-positive result), and sometimes no abnormalities are found in people who actually have angina (a false-negative result). In people without symptoms, especially younger people, the likelihood of coronary artery disease is low, despite an abnormal test result. Nevertheless, exercise testing is often used for screening purposes in apparently healthy people—for example, before an exercise program is begun or during an evaluation for life insurance. The many false-positives that result may cause considerable worry and medical expense. Because of this, most experts discourage routine exercise testing in people without symptoms.

Continuous Ambulatory Electrocardiography

Abnormal heart rhythms and insufficient blood flow to the heart muscle may occur only briefly or unpredictably. To detect such problems, a doctor may use a continuous ambulatory ECG recording. With this test, the person carries a small battery-powered device (Holter monitor) that records the ECG for 24 hours. While wearing the monitor, the person notes in a diary the time and type of any symptoms. Subsequently, the recording is run through a computer, which analyzes the rate and rhythm of the heart, looks for changes in electrical activity that could indicate inadequate blood flow to the heart muscle, and reproduces a record of every heartbeat during the 24 hours. Symptoms recorded in the diary then can be correlated with changes in the ECG.

If necessary, the ECG can be transmitted by telephone to a computer at the hospital or doctor's office for an immediate reading as soon as symptoms occur. Sophisticated ambulatory units can simultaneously record ECGs and electroencephalograms (measures of the brain's electrical activity) in people who have episodes of losing consciousness. Such recordings may help to differentiate between epileptic seizures and cardiac rhythm abnormalities.

Electrophysiologic Testing

Electrophysiologic testing is used to evaluate serious rhythm or electrical conduction abnor-

Holter Monitor: Continuous ECG Readings

A person wears the small monitor over one shoulder. With the electrodes attached to the chest, the monitor continuously records the electrical activity of the heart.

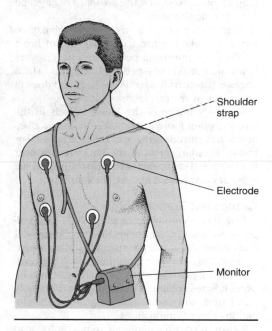

Shoulder strap

Electrode

Monitor

malities. In the hospital, a doctor inserts tiny electrodes through veins and sometimes arteries directly into the heart chambers to record the ECG from within the heart and identify the precise location of the electrical conduction pathways.

Sometimes a doctor intentionally provokes an abnormal heart rhythm during testing to find out whether a particular drug can stop the disturbance or whether an operation will help. If necessary, a doctor can quickly bring back a normal rhythm with a brief electrical shock to the heart (cardioversion). Though electrophysiologic testing is an invasive procedure and the patient requires anesthesia, the test is very safe: The risk of death is 1 in 5,000.

Radiologic Tests

Anyone thought to have heart disease has chest x-rays taken from the front and the side. The x-rays show the shape and size of the heart and outline the blood vessels in the lungs and chest. Abnormal heart shape or size and abnormalities such as calcium deposits within heart tissue are readily seen. Chest x-rays also can reveal the condition of the lungs, particularly the lung blood vessels, and the presence of any fluid in or around the lungs.

Heart failure or an abnormal heart valve often tends to make the heart grow larger. But heart size may be normal in people who have severe heart disease. In constrictive pericarditis, which encases the heart in scar tissue, the heart doesn't enlarge even as heart failure occurs.

The appearance of the blood vessels in the lungs is often more important in making a diagnosis than the appearance of the heart itself. For instance, enlargement of the lung arteries near the heart and narrowing of them in the lung tissue suggest enlargement of the right ventricle.

Computed Tomography

Ordinary computed tomography (CT) isn't often used in diagnosing heart disease; however, it can detect structural abnormalities of the heart, pericardium, major vessels, lungs, and supporting structures in the chest. With this test, a computer creates cross-sectional images of the whole chest from x-ray scans, showing the precise location of any abnormalities.

Newer ultrafast–computed tomography, also called cine–computed tomography, provides a three-dimensional moving display of the heart. This test may be used to assess structural and motion abnormalities.

Fluoroscopy

Fluoroscopy is a continuous x-ray procedure that shows the heart beating and the lungs inflating and deflating on a screen. However, fluoroscopy, which involves a relatively high dose of radiation, has been largely replaced by echocardiography and other tests.

Fluoroscopy is still used as a component of cardiac catheterization and electrophysiologic testing. It can be helpful in some difficult diagnoses

involving heart valve disease and birth defects of the heart.

Echocardiography

Echocardiography is one of the most widely used techniques in diagnosing heart disease because it is noninvasive, uses no x-rays, and provides excellent imaging. The test is harmless, painless, relatively inexpensive, and widely available.

Echocardiography uses high-frequency ultrasound waves emitted by a recording probe (transducer) and bounced off structures in the heart and blood vessels to produce a moving image. The image appears on a video screen and is recorded on a videocassette or paper. By varying the placement and angle of the probe, a doctor can view the heart and major blood vessels from various angles to get an accurate picture of heart structure and function. To obtain greater clarity or to analyze structures at the back of the heart, a doctor can pass a probe down the patient's throat into the esophagus and record signals from right behind the heart; this is known as transesophageal echocardiography.

Echocardiography can detect abnormalities in heart wall motion, the volume of blood being pumped from the heart with each beat, thickening and diseases of the sac around the heart (the pericardium), and an accumulation of fluid between the pericardium and the heart muscle.

The main types of ultrasound tests are M-mode, two-dimensional, Doppler, and color Doppler. In M-mode ultrasound, the simplest technique, a single beam of ultrasound is aimed at the part of the heart being studied. Two-dimensional ultrasound, the most widely used technique, produces realistic two-dimensional images in computer-generated "slices." Doppler ultrasound detects the movement and turbulence of blood and can be displayed in color (color Doppler). Color Doppler and Doppler echocardiography can determine and display the direction and velocity of blood flow in the heart chambers and vessels. The images allow a doctor to see if the heart valves open and close properly, if and how much they leak when closed, and if blood flows normally. Abnormal connections between blood vessels or heart chambers can be detected, and the structure and function of the vessels and chambers can be determined.

Magnetic Resonance Imaging

Magnetic resonance imaging (MRI) is a technique that uses a powerful magnetic field to create detailed images of the heart and chest. This extremely expensive and sophisticated imaging technique is still in a developmental stage for use in diagnosing heart disease.

The person is placed inside a large electromagnet that causes atomic nuclei in the body to vibrate and give out characteristic signals, which are converted into two- and three-dimensional images of cardiac structures. Usually, contrast agents (radiopaque dyes) aren't needed. Occasionally, however, paramagnetic contrast agents are given intravenously to help identify areas of poor blood flow in the heart muscle.

One disadvantage of MRI is that each image takes longer to produce than with computed tomography (CT). Because of the movement of the heart, the images obtained with MRI are fuzzier than those obtained with CT. In addition, some people become claustrophobic during MRI because they must lie still in a narrow space in a giant machine.

Radionuclide Imaging

In radionuclide imaging, minute amounts of radioactively labeled substances (tracers) are injected into a vein, yet this testing exposes a person to less radiation than most x-rays. The tracers are quickly distributed through the body, including the heart. Then they are detected by a gamma camera. An image is displayed on a screen and stored on computer disk for further analysis.

Different types of radiation recording cameras may record a single image or may produce a series of computer-enhanced cross-sectional images, a technique known as single photon emission computed tomography. The computer can also generate a three-dimensional image.

Radionuclide imaging is particularly useful in diagnosing people with chest pain of unknown cause. In those who have coronary artery narrowing, it's used to learn how the narrowing is affecting the heart's blood supply and function. Radionuclide imaging also is used to assess the improvement in blood supply to the heart muscle after bypass surgery or similar procedures and to determine a person's prognosis after a heart attack (myocardial infarction).

Blood flow through heart muscle is usually examined by injecting thallium-201 into a vein and obtaining images while the person performs an exercise test. The amount of thallium-201 absorbed by the heart muscle cells depends on the blood flow. At peak exercise, an area of heart muscle that has a poor blood supply (ischemia) shows less radioactivity—and produces a fainter image—than neighboring muscle with a normal supply. In people unable to exercise, an intravenous injection of the drug dipyridamole or adenosine may be used to simulate the effects of exercise on the blood flow. These drugs divert the blood supply from abnormal to normal vessels.

After the person rests for a few hours, a second scan is done. A doctor can then see which areas of the heart have a reversible lack of flow, which usually results from coronary artery narrowing, and which areas have irreversible scarring of the heart muscle, which usually results from a previous heart attack.

If an acute heart attack is suspected, tracers containing technetium 99m are used as an alternative to thallium-201. Unlike thallium, which accumulates primarily in normal tissue, technetium accumulates primarily in abnormal tissue. However, because technetium also accumulates in bone, the ribs obscure the heart image to some extent.

Technetium scanning is used to diagnose a heart attack (myocardial infarction). The damaged area of the heart absorbs the technetium, and the test can detect a heart attack for about 1 week beginning 12 to 24 hours after it occurs.

Positron Emission Tomography

In positron emission tomography (PET), a nutrient necessary for heart cell function is labeled with a substance that gives off radioactive particles called positrons and then is injected into a vein. In a few minutes, when the labeled nutrient reaches the area of the heart being examined, a detector scans the area and records sites of high activity. A computer constructs a three-dimensional image of the area, revealing how actively the different regions of heart muscle are using the labeled nutrient. Positron emission tomography scans produce clearer images than other nuclear medicine studies. However, these scans are very expensive and not widely available. They are used as research tools and in cases in which simpler, less expensive tests are inconclusive.

Cardiac Catheterization

In cardiac catheterization, a thin catheter (tube) is inserted through an artery or vein, usually in an arm or leg, and advanced into the major vessels and heart chambers. To reach the right side of the heart, a doctor inserts the catheter into a vein; to reach the left side, a doctor inserts it into an artery. Catheters can be placed in the heart either for diagnosis or treatment. The person receives local anesthesia before the procedure, which is performed in the hospital.

A catheter often contains a measuring instrument or another device at its tip. Depending on the type, catheters can be used to measure pressure, view the inside of blood vessels, widen a narrowed heart valve, or clear a blocked artery. Catheters are used extensively in evaluating the heart because they can be inserted without major surgery.

A specially designed catheter with a balloon at its tip can be inserted into a vein in the arm or neck and threaded through the right atrium and right ventricle of the heart to the opening of the pulmonary artery; this procedure is called pulmonary artery catheterization. The catheter is used to measure blood pressure in the major vessels and heart chambers. The heart's output of blood to the lungs can also be measured. Samples of blood can be drawn through the catheter for analysis of oxygen and carbon dioxide content. Because inserting a catheter into the pulmonary artery may cause abnormal heart rhythms, the heart is monitored with an electrocardiogram. Usually, a doctor can correct abnormal rhythms by moving the catheter to another position. If that doesn't help, the catheter is removed.

A doctor can use the catheter to obtain blood specimens for metabolic studies. Using a catheter, a doctor also can instill dyes that show up on movie x-rays of blood vessels and heart chambers. Anatomic abnormalities and abnormal blood flow can be seen and filmed while x-rays are taken. Using instruments passed through the catheter, a doctor can obtain heart muscle tissue

samples for microscopic examination (biopsy) from inside the heart chambers. Blood pressures in the heart chambers and major blood vessels can be measured separately at each site, and the oxygen and carbon dioxide content of the blood can be sampled in different parts of the heart.

A doctor also can evaluate the pumping ability of the heart by analyzing the motion of the left ventricle wall and calculating the efficiency with which blood is pumped out (ejection fraction). This analysis provides one measure of how much injury the heart has sustained from ischemic coronary artery disease or other disease.

Coronary Angiography

Coronary angiography is a study of the coronary arteries using a catheter. A doctor threads a slender catheter into an artery in the arm or groin toward the heart and into the coronary arteries. During insertion, a doctor may use fluoroscopy (a continuous x-ray procedure) to monitor the progress of the catheter. The catheter tip is positioned appropriately, a dye that can be seen on x-rays is injected through the catheter into the coronary arteries, and the outline of the arteries appears on a video screen. Movie x-rays (cineangiography) provide clear pictures of the heart chambers and coronary arteries. Coronary artery disease shows up because the inner walls of the coronary arteries look irregular or narrowed. If a person has coronary artery disease, a catheter can be used to treat it by relieving the blockage; this procedure is called percutaneous transluminal coronary angioplasty.▲

Minor side effects of coronary angiography occur immediately after the injection. Usually, the patient has a temporary feeling of warmth, especially in the head and face, as the dye spreads through the bloodstream. The heart rate increases, and blood pressure falls slightly. Rarely, mild reactions such as nausea, vomiting, and coughing occur. Serious reactions, which are very rare, may include shock, convulsions, kidney problems, and a cessation of the heartbeat (cardiac arrest). Allergic reactions range from skin rashes to a rare life-threatening condition called anaphylaxis. Abnormal heart rhythms may occur if the catheter touches the heart wall. The team performing the procedure is equipped and trained to treat any of the side effects immediately.

▲ see page 125

Abnormal Heart Rhythms

The heart is a muscular organ with four chambers designed to work efficiently, reliably, and continuously over a lifetime. The muscular walls of each chamber contract in a precise sequence, pushing along the most blood while expending the least possible energy during every heartbeat.

The contraction of the muscle fibers in the heart is controlled by an electrical discharge that flows through the heart in a precise manner along distinct pathways and at a controlled speed. The rhythmic discharge that begins each heartbeat originates in the heart's pacemaker (sinoatrial node), which lies in the wall of the right atrium. The rate of discharge is influenced by nerve impulses and by levels of hormones circulating through the bloodstream.

The part of the nervous system that regulates the heart rate automatically is the autonomic nervous system, which consists of the sympathetic and parasympathetic nervous systems. The sympathetic system speeds up the heart rate; the parasympathetic system slows it down. The sympathetic system supplies the heart with a network of nerves, the sympathetic plexus. The parasympathetic system supplies the heart through a single nerve, the vagus nerve.

Heart rate is also influenced by the sympathetic system's circulating hormones—epinephrine (adrenaline) and norepinephrine (noradrenaline)—which speed up the heart rate. Thyroid hormone influences heart rate as well. With too much thyroid hormone, the heart beats too fast; with too little, it beats too slowly.

The normal heart rate at rest is usually between 60 and 100 beats per minute. However, much lower rates may be normal in young adults, particularly those who are physically fit. Variations in heart rate are normal. The heart rate responds not only to exercise and inactivity but also to stimuli such as pain and anger. Only when the heart rate is inappropriately fast (tachycardia) or slow (bradycardia) or when the electrical impulses travel in abnormal pathways is the heartbeat considered to have an abnormal rhythm (arrhythmia). Abnormal rhythms may be regular or irregular.

Electrical Pathway

The electrical discharge from the pacemaker flows first through the left and right atria, causing muscle tissue to contract in sequence and blood to be ejected from the atria to the ventricles. The electrical discharge then reaches the atrioventricular node between the atria and the ventricles. This node delays transmission of the electrical discharge to allow the atria to contract completely and the ventricles to fill with as much blood as possible during ventricular diastole, the period of ventricular relaxation.

After passing through the atrioventricular node, the electrical discharge travels down the bundle of His, a group of fibers that divide into a left bundle for the left ventricle and a right bundle for the right ventricle. The discharge then spreads in an orderly manner over the surface of the ventricles, initiating ventricular contraction (systole), during which blood is ejected from the heart.

Various problems can occur with this flow of electrical current, resulting in arrhythmias ranging from harmless to life threatening. Each type of arrhythmia has its own cause, but some causes can trigger a variety of arrhythmias. Minor arrhythmias may be triggered by excessive alcohol consumption, smoking, stress, or exercise. Overactive and underactive thyroid function and some drugs, especially those used to treat lung disease and some used to treat high blood pressure, may affect the rate and rhythm of the heart. The most common cause of arrhythmias is heart disease, particularly coronary artery disease, abnormal heart valve function, and heart failure. Sometimes arrhythmias occur without any detectable underlying heart disease or other cause.

Symptoms

The awareness of one's heartbeat (called palpitations) varies widely among people. Some people can feel even normal heartbeats. At times when lying on the left side, most people can feel the heart beating. Also, people may be aware of abnormal heartbeats. Often, the awareness of one's heartbeat is disturbing, but usually it

Tracing the Heart's Electrical Pathway

The sinoatrial node (1) initiates an electrical impulse that flows over the right and left atria (2), making them contract. When the electrical impulse reaches the atrioventricular node (3), it's delayed slightly. The impulse then travels down the bundle of His (4), which divides into the right bundle branch for the right ventricle (5) and the left bundle branch for the left ventricle (5). The impulse then spreads over the ventricles, making them contract.

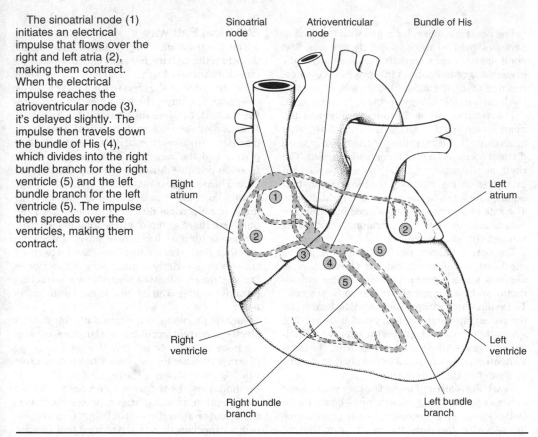

Sinoatrial node
Atrioventricular node
Bundle of His
Right atrium
Left atrium
Right ventricle
Left ventricle
Right bundle branch
Left bundle branch

---

doesn't result from an underlying disease. Rather, it results from unusually strong contractions that occur periodically for a variety of reasons.

A person who has a certain type of arrhythmia tends to have that same arrhythmia repeatedly. Some types of arrhythmias cause few or no symptoms but eventually cause problems. Other arrhythmias never cause serious problems but do cause symptoms. Often, the nature and severity of the underlying heart disease are more important than the arrhythmia itself.

▲ see page 108

When arrhythmias affect the heart's ability to pump blood, they can produce light-headedness, dizziness, and fainting (syncope).▲ Arrhythmias that produce these symptoms require prompt attention.

Diagnosis

A person's description of symptoms often can help a doctor make a preliminary diagnosis and determine the severity of the arrhythmia. The most important considerations are whether a person with palpitations describes the heartbeats as fast or slow, regular or irregular, brief or prolonged; whether the person feels dizzy, light-headed, or faint or even loses consciousness; and whether chest pain, shortness of breath, or other unusual sensations occur along with the palpitations. A doctor also needs to know whether the palpitations occur at rest or only during strenuous or unusual activity and whether they start and stop suddenly or gradually.

Usually, some additional testing is needed to determine the exact nature of the condition. Electrocardiography▲ is the main diagnostic procedure for detecting arrhythmias. This test provides a graphic representation of the arrhythmia.

However, an electrocardiogram (ECG) shows the heart rhythm over only a very brief time, and often arrhythmias are intermittent. Thus, a portable monitor (Holter monitor),■ which is worn for 24 hours, can provide more information. This monitor can record sporadic arrhythmias as the person goes about a normal daily routine. The person also keeps a diary of symptoms during the 24-hour period. People with suspected life-threatening arrhythmias are generally hospitalized for monitoring.

When a sustained, life-threatening arrhythmia is suspected, electrophysiologic studies may be helpful. A catheter containing wires is threaded through a vein and into the heart. Electrical stimulation and sophisticated monitoring are combined to determine the type of arrhythmia and the most likely response to treatment. Most serious arrhythmias can be detected by this technique.

Prognosis and Treatment

The prognosis depends in part on whether an arrhythmia begins in the heart's normal pacemaker, the atria, or the ventricles. In general, those starting in the ventricles are more serious, although many of them aren't harmful.

Most arrhythmias neither cause symptoms nor interfere with the pumping action of the heart, so they pose little or no risk. Nevertheless, arrhythmias can cause considerable anxiety if a person becomes aware of them. Understanding their harmlessness may be reassurance enough. Sometimes, when a doctor changes a person's medications or adjusts the dosages, or when a person avoids alcohol or strenuous exercise, arrhythmias occur less often or even stop.

Antiarrhythmic drugs are useful for suppressing arrhythmias that cause intolerable symptoms or pose a risk. No single drug cures all arrhythmias in all people. Sometimes several drugs must

be tried until a satisfactory one is found. Antiarrhythmic drugs can produce side effects and can worsen or even cause arrhythmias.

Artificial pacemakers, electronic devices that act in place of the heart's own pacemaker, are programmed to imitate the normal conduction sequence of the heart. Usually, they're implanted surgically under the skin of the chest and have wires running to the heart. Because of low-energy circuitry and new battery designs, these units now last about 8 to 10 years. New circuitry has almost completely eliminated the risk of interference from automobile distributors, radar, microwaves, and airport security detectors. Some equipment—such as machines used in magnetic resonance imaging (MRI) and diathermy (physical therapy used to bring heat to muscles)—may, however, interfere with pacemakers.

The most common use of pacemakers is to treat abnormally slow heart rates. When the heart slows below a set threshold, the pacemaker begins to fire off electrical impulses. Very rarely, a pacemaker is used to deliver a series of impulses to stop an abnormally fast rhythm and slow the heart rate. Such pacemakers are used only for fast rhythms that start in the atria.

Sometimes an electric shock to the heart can stop an abnormal rhythm and restore a normal one; using an electric shock for this purpose is called cardioversion, electroversion, or defibrillation. Cardioversion may be used for arrhythmias starting in the atria or the ventricles. Usually, a large machine that delivers the shock (a defibrillator) is used by a team of doctors and nurses to stop a life-threatening arrhythmia. However, a defibrillator about the size of a pack of cards can be implanted surgically. These small devices, which automatically sense life-threatening arrhythmias and deliver a shock, are used in people who would otherwise die when their heart suddenly stops. Because these defibrillators don't prevent arrhythmias, the person usually takes drugs as well.

Certain types of arrhythmias can be corrected by surgical and other invasive procedures. For example, arrhythmias caused by coronary artery disease may be controlled by angioplasty or cor-

---

▲ see box, page 74

■ see box, page 75

onary artery bypass surgery.▲ When an arrhythmia is caused by an irritable spot in the electrical system of the heart, the spot can be destroyed or removed. Most often, the spot is destroyed by catheter ablation (delivery of radiofrequency energy through a catheter inserted in the heart). After a heart attack (myocardial infarction), some people have life-threatening episodes of an arrhythmia called ventricular tachycardia. This arrhythmia may be triggered by an injured area of heart muscle that can be identified and removed during open heart surgery.

Atrial Ectopic Beats

An atrial ectopic beat is an extra heartbeat caused by electrical activation of the atria before the normal heartbeat.

Atrial ectopic beats occur as additional heartbeats in healthy people and rarely cause symptoms. Sometimes they're caused by or worsened by alcohol, cold remedies containing drugs that stimulate the sympathetic nervous system (such as ephedrine or pseudoephedrine), or drugs used to treat asthma.

Diagnosis and Treatment

Atrial ectopic beats may be detected by physical examination and are confirmed by an electrocardiogram (ECG). If treatment is necessary because ectopic beats occur frequently and cause intolerable palpitations, a doctor may prescribe a beta-blocker to slow the heart rate.

Paroxysmal Atrial Tachycardia

Paroxysmal atrial tachycardia is a regular, fast (160 to 200 beats per minute) heart rate that occurs suddenly and is triggered in the atria.

Several mechanisms can produce paroxysmal atrial tachycardias. The fast rate may be triggered by a premature atrial beat that sends an impulse on an abnormal path to the ventricles.

The fast heart rate tends to start and stop suddenly and may last anywhere from a few minutes to many hours. It's almost always experienced as an uncomfortable palpitation and is often associated with other symptoms, such as weakness.

▲ see page 125

Usually, the heart is otherwise normal, and the episodes are more unpleasant than dangerous.

Treatment

Episodes of the arrhythmia often can be stopped by one of several maneuvers that stimulate the vagus nerve and thus slow the heart rate. These maneuvers, which are usually conducted by a doctor, include having the person strain as if having a difficult bowel movement, rubbing the person's neck just below the angle of the jaw (which stimulates a sensitive area on the carotid artery called the carotid sinus), and plunging the person's face into a bowl of ice-cold water. These maneuvers work best when they're used shortly after the arrhythmia starts.

If these maneuvers don't work, the episode will usually stop if the person simply goes to sleep. However, most people seek medical intervention to end the episode. A doctor can usually stop an episode promptly by giving an intravenous dose of the drug verapamil or adenosine. Rarely, the drugs don't work, and cardioversion (delivery of a shock to the heart) may be used.

Prevention is more difficult than treatment, but several drugs may be effective when used alone or in combination. In rare cases, an abnormal pathway in the heart may need to be destroyed by catheter ablation (delivery of radiofrequency energy through a catheter inserted in the heart).

Atrial Fibrillation and Flutter

Atrial fibrillation and atrial flutter are very fast electrical discharge patterns that make the atria contract extremely rapidly, thus causing the ventricles to contract faster and less efficiently than normal.

These abnormal rhythms may occur sporadically or may persist. During fibrillation or flutter, the contractions of the atria are so fast that the atrial walls simply quiver, so blood isn't pumped effectively to the ventricles. In fibrillation, the atrial rhythm is irregular, so the ventricular rhythm is also irregular; in flutter, the atrial and ventricular rhythms usually are regular. In both cases, the ventricles beat more slowly than the atria because the atrioventricular node and the bundle of His can't conduct electrical impulses at such a fast rate, and only every second to fourth impulse gets through. Still the ventricles beat too fast to fill completely. Therefore, inadequate amounts of blood are pumped out of the heart, blood pressure falls, and heart failure may occur.

The heart may go into atrial fibrillation or flutter with no other sign of heart disease, but more often the cause is an underlying problem, such as rheumatic heart disease, coronary artery disease, high blood pressure, alcohol abuse, or too much thyroid hormone (hyperthyroidism).

Symptoms and Diagnosis

Symptoms of atrial fibrillation or flutter depend largely on how fast the ventricles beat. A modest ventricular rate—less than about 120 beats per minute—may produce no symptoms. Higher rates cause unpleasant palpitations or chest discomfort. With atrial fibrillation, the person may be aware of the rhythm irregularities.

The diminished pumping ability of the heart may make the person feel weak, faint, and short of breath. Some people, especially the elderly, develop heart failure, chest pain, and shock.

In atrial fibrillation, the atria don't empty completely into the ventricles with each beat. Over time, some blood inside the atria may stagnate and clot. Pieces of the clot may break off, pass into the left ventricle, and continue into the general circulation, where they may block a smaller artery. (Pieces of a clot that block an artery are called emboli.) Most often, the pieces of a clot break off shortly after atrial fibrillation converts to a normal rhythm, either spontaneously or with treatment. Blockage of an artery in the brain may cause a stroke. Rarely, a stroke is the first sign of atrial fibrillation.

The diagnosis of atrial fibrillation or flutter is suspected from the symptoms and confirmed by an electrocardiogram (ECG). With atrial fibrillation, the pulse is irregular. With atrial flutter, the pulse is more likely to be regular but rapid.

Treatment

Treatments for atrial fibrillation and flutter are designed to control the rate at which the ventricles contract, treat the disorder responsible for the abnormal rhythm, and restore the normal rhythm of the heart. With atrial fibrillation, treatment is also usually given to prevent clots and emboli.

The first step in treating atrial fibrillation or flutter is usually to slow the ventricular rate to improve the heart's efficiency in pumping blood. Contractions of the ventricles usually can be slowed and strengthened with digoxin, a drug that slows the conduction of impulses to the ventricles. When digoxin alone doesn't help, giving a second drug—a beta-blocker such as propranolol or atenolol or a calcium channel blocker such as diltiazem or verapamil—usually does.

Treatment of the underlying disease rarely alleviates atrial arrhythmias unless the disease is hyperthyroidism.

Though occasionally atrial fibrillation or flutter spontaneously reverts to a normal rhythm, more often it must be converted to normal. Sometimes such a conversion can be achieved with certain antiarrhythmic drugs. However, electric shock (cardioversion) is often the most effective approach. Success by any means is less likely the longer the atria have been in their abnormal rhythm (especially after 6 months or more), the more the atria are enlarged, and the more severe the underlying heart disease has become. When conversion is successful, the risk that the arrhythmia will return is high, even if the person takes preventive drugs such as quinidine, procainamide, propafenone, or flecainide.

If all other treatments fail, the atrioventricular node can be destroyed by catheter ablation (delivery of radiofrequency energy through a catheter inserted in the heart). This procedure interrupts conduction from the fibrillating atria to the ventricles, but a permanent artificial pacemaker is required for the ventricles afterward.

The risk of developing blood clots is highest in people with atrial fibrillation who have an enlarged left atrium or who have mitral valve disease.▲ The risk that a clot will be dislodged and cause a stroke is particularly high in people who have intermittent but persistent episodes of atrial fibrillation or whose fibrillation is converted to the normal rhythm. Because anyone with atrial fibrillation is at risk of a stroke, anticoagulant therapy generally is recommended to prevent clots unless there's a specific reason not to give it, such as high blood pressure. However, anticoagulant therapy itself carries a risk of excessive bleeding that can lead to hemorrhagic stroke and other bleeding complications. Therefore, a doctor balances the potential benefits and risks for each person.

▲ see page 93

Wolff-Parkinson-White Syndrome

Wolff-Parkinson-White syndrome is an abnormal heart rhythm in which electrical impulses are conducted along an extra pathway from the atria to the ventricles, causing episodes of a rapid heart rate.

Wolff-Parkinson-White syndrome is the most common of several disorders that involve such extra (accessory) pathways. This extra pathway is present at birth but seems to conduct impulses through the heart only occasionally. It may become apparent as early as the first year of life or as late as age 60.

Symptoms and Diagnosis

Wolff-Parkinson-White syndrome can cause sudden episodes of a very rapid heart rate with palpitations.

In the first year of life, babies may develop heart failure if the episode is prolonged. They sometimes seem out of breath or lethargic, stop eating well, or have rapid, visible pulsations of the chest.

The first episodes may occur in the teens or early twenties. Typical episodes begin suddenly, often during exercise. They may last for only a few seconds or may persist for several hours, rarely more than 12 hours. In a young and otherwise physically fit person, the episodes usually cause few symptoms, but very rapid heart rates are uncomfortable and distressing and can cause fainting or heart failure. The rapid heart rate sometimes changes to atrial fibrillation. Atrial fibrillation is particularly dangerous in about 1 percent of people with Wolff-Parkinson-White syndrome because the extra pathway can conduct the rapid impulses to the ventricles much more successfully than the normal pathway can. The result is an extremely rapid ventricular rate that may be life threatening. Not only is the heart very inefficient when it beats so rapidly, but this extremely rapid heart rate may progress to ventricular fibrillation, which is immediately fatal.

The diagnosis of Wolff-Parkinson-White syndrome with or without atrial fibrillation is made using an electrocardiogram (ECG).

Treatment

Episodes of the arrhythmia often can be stopped by one of several maneuvers that stimulate the vagus nerve and thus slow the heart rate. These maneuvers, which are usually conducted by a doctor, include having the person strain as if having a difficult bowel movement, rubbing the person's neck just below the angle of the jaw (which stimulates a sensitive area on the carotid artery called the carotid sinus), and plunging the person's face into a bowl of ice-cold water. The maneuvers work best when they're used shortly after the arrhythmia starts. When these maneuvers don't work, drugs such as verapamil or adenosine usually are given intravenously to stop the arrhythmia. Other antiarrhythmic drugs are then used for long-term prevention of episodes of rapid heart rate.

In infants and children under age 10, digoxin may be given to suppress episodes of rapid heart rate. Adults must not take digoxin because it can speed up conduction in the extra pathway and increase the risk of developing fatal ventricular fibrillation. For this reason, the drug is usually stopped before a person reaches puberty.

Destruction of the extra conduction pathway by catheter ablation (delivery of radiofrequency energy through a catheter inserted in the heart) is successful more than 95 percent of the time. The risk of death during the procedure is less than 1 in 1,000. Catheter ablation is particularly useful for young people who might otherwise face a lifetime of taking antiarrhythmic drugs.

Ventricular Ectopic Beats

A ventricular ectopic beat (premature ventricular contraction) is an extra heartbeat caused by electrical activation of the ventricles before the normal heartbeat.

Ventricular ectopic beats occur commonly and don't indicate danger in people who don't have heart disease. However, when they occur frequently in a person who has heart failure or aortic stenosis or who has had a heart attack, they may be followed by more dangerous arrhythmias such as ventricular fibrillation, which can cause sudden death.

Symptoms and Diagnosis

Isolated ventricular ectopic beats have little effect on the pumping action of the heart and usually don't cause symptoms, unless they're extremely frequent. The main symptom is the perception of a strong or skipped beat.

Ventricular ectopic beats are diagnosed using an electrocardiogram (ECG).

Treatment

In an otherwise healthy person, no treatment is needed other than decreasing stress and avoiding alcohol and over-the-counter cold remedies containing drugs that stimulate the heart. Drug therapy is usually prescribed only if symptoms are intolerable or the pattern of ectopic beats suggests danger. Beta-blockers are usually tried first because they're relatively safe drugs. However, many people don't want to take them because of the sluggishness they can cause.

After a heart attack, a person who is experiencing frequent ventricular ectopic beats may reduce the risk of sudden death by taking beta-blockers and undergoing angioplasty or coronary artery bypass surgery▲ to relieve the underlying coronary artery blockage. Antiarrhythmic drugs can suppress ventricular ectopic beats, but they also may increase the risk of a fatal arrhythmia. Therefore, they're used very carefully in selected patients after sophisticated cardiac studies and risk evaluation.

Ventricular Tachycardia

Ventricular tachycardia is a ventricular rate of at least 120 beats per minute triggered in the ventricles.

Sustained ventricular tachycardia (ventricular tachycardia lasting at least 30 seconds) occurs in various heart diseases that damage the ventricles. Most commonly, it occurs weeks or months after a heart attack.

Symptoms and Diagnosis

A person with ventricular tachycardia almost always has palpitations. Sustained ventricular tachycardia can be dangerous and often requires emergency treatment because the ventricles can't fill adequately and pump blood normally. Blood pressure tends to fall, and heart failure follows. Sustained ventricular tachycardia is also dangerous because it can worsen until it becomes ventricular fibrillation—a form of cardiac arrest. Sometimes, ventricular tachycardia causes few symptoms, even at rates of up to 200 beats per minute, but it may still be extremely dangerous.

The diagnosis of ventricular tachycardia is made with an electrocardiogram (ECG).

Treatment

Treatment is given for any episode of ventricular tachycardia that causes symptoms and for episodes that last more than 30 seconds even without symptoms. If episodes cause blood pressure to fall below normal, cardioversion is needed immediately. Lidocaine or similar drugs are given intravenously to suppress ventricular tachycardia. If episodes of ventricular tachycardia persist, a doctor may conduct an electrophysiologic study and try other drugs. The one that works best during electrophysiologic testing can be continued to help prevent recurrences. Sustained ventricular tachycardia is usually triggered by a small abnormal area in the ventricles, and this trigger area can sometimes be removed surgically. In some people with ventricular tachycardia that doesn't respond to drug therapy, a device called an automatic cardioverter-defibrillator may be implanted.

Ventricular Fibrillation

Ventricular fibrillation is a potentially fatal, uncoordinated series of very rapid ineffective contractions throughout the ventricles caused by multiple chaotic electrical impulses.

Ventricular fibrillation is electrically similar to atrial fibrillation, but it has a much graver prognosis. In ventricular fibrillation, the ventricles merely quiver and don't carry out coordinated contractions. Because no blood is pumped from the heart, ventricular fibrillation is a form of cardiac arrest and is fatal unless treated immediately.

The causes of ventricular fibrillation are the same as those of cardiac arrest. The most common cause is inadequate blood flow to the heart muscle because of coronary artery disease or a heart attack. Other causes are shock and very low levels of potassium in the blood (hypokalemia).

Symptoms and Diagnosis

Ventricular fibrillation leads to unconsciousness in seconds. If untreated, the person usually has convulsions and develops irreversible brain damage after about 5 minutes because oxygen is no longer reaching the brain. Death soon follows.

A doctor considers a diagnosis of ventricular fibrillation when a person suddenly collapses. On examination, no pulse or heartbeat is detected,

▲ see page 125

and blood pressure can't be measured. The diagnosis is confirmed by an electrocardiogram (ECG).

Treatment

Ventricular fibrillation must be treated as an emergency. Cardiopulmonary resuscitation (CPR) must be started within a few minutes and then followed as soon as possible by cardioversion (an electric shock delivered to the chest). Drugs are then given to help maintain the normal heart rhythm.

When ventricular fibrillation occurs within a few hours of a heart attack and the person isn't in shock or doesn't have heart failure, prompt cardioversion has a 95 percent success rate, and the prognosis is good. Shock and heart failure are signs of major damage to the ventricles; if they're present, even prompt cardioversion has only a 30 percent success rate, and 70 percent of resuscitated survivors die.

Heart Block

Heart block is a delay in electrical conduction through the atrioventricular node, which lies between the atria and the ventricles.

Heart block is graded as first-degree, second-degree, or third-degree, depending on whether conduction to the ventricles is slightly delayed, intermittently delayed, or completely blocked.

In **first-degree heart block,** every impulse from the atria reaches the ventricles, but it's slowed for a fraction of a second as it moves through the atrioventricular node. This conduction problem produces no symptoms. First-degree heart block is common among well-trained athletes, teenagers, young adults, and people with a highly active vagus nerve. However, the condition also occurs in rheumatic fever and sarcoid heart disease and may be caused by drugs. The diagnosis is made by observing the conduction delay on an electrocardiogram (ECG).

In **second-degree heart block,** not every impulse from the atria reaches the ventricles. This block results in the heart beating slowly or irregularly. Some forms of second-degree block progress to third-degree heart block.

In **third-degree heart block,** impulses from the atria to the ventricles are completely blocked, and the heart rate and rhythm are paced from either the atrioventricular node or the ventricles

themselves. Without stimulation from the heart's normal pacemaker (sinoatrial node), the ventricles beat very slowly, less than 50 beats per minute. Third-degree heart block is a serious arrhythmia that can affect the heart's pumping ability. Fainting (syncope), dizziness, and sudden heart failure are common. When the ventricles beat faster than 40 beats per minute, symptoms are less severe but include tiredness, low blood pressure when the person stands up, and shortness of breath. The atrioventricular node and the ventricles are not only slow as substitute pacemakers but they're frequently irregular and unreliable.

Treatment

First-degree block requires no treatment even when it's caused by heart disease. Some cases of second-degree block may require an artificial pacemaker. Third-degree block almost always requires an artificial pacemaker. A temporary pacemaker may be used in an emergency until a permanent one can be implanted. Most people need an artificial pacemaker for the rest of their lives, although normal rhythms sometimes return after recovery from an underlying cause, such as a heart attack.

Sick Sinus Syndrome

Sick sinus syndrome includes a wide variety of abnormalities of natural pacemaker function.

This syndrome may result in a persistently slow heartbeat (sinus bradycardia) or a complete blockage between the pacemaker and the atria (sinus arrest) in which the impulse from the pacemaker fails to make the atria contract. When this happens, an escape pacemaker lower in the atrium or even in the ventricle usually takes over.

An important subtype of the sick sinus syndrome is the bradycardia-tachycardia syndrome, in which rapid atrial rhythms, including atrial fibrillation or flutter, alternate with prolonged periods of slow heart rhythms. All types of sick sinus syndrome are particularly common in the elderly.

Symptoms and Diagnosis

Many types of sick sinus syndrome cause no symptoms, but persistent slow heart rates commonly cause weakness and tiredness. Fainting may occur if the rate becomes very slow. Rapid heart rates are often perceived by the person as palpitations.

A slow pulse, especially an irregular one, or a pulse that varies greatly without any change in the person's activity leads a doctor to consider a diagnosis of sick sinus syndrome. Characteristic electrocardiogram (ECG) abnormalities—particularly abnormalities recorded over a 24-hour period and considered along with accompanying symptoms—usually help a doctor make a diagnosis.

Treatment

People with symptoms usually are given a permanent artificial pacemaker. These pacemakers are used to accelerate the heart rate, rather than slow it down. In people who sometimes have a fast rate, drugs also may be needed. Therefore, the best therapy is often an implanted pacemaker together with a heart-slowing drug such as a beta-blocker or verapamil.

CHAPTER 17

Heart Failure

Heart failure (congestive heart failure) is a serious condition in which the quantity of blood pumped by the heart each minute (cardiac output) is insufficient to meet the body's normal requirements for oxygen and nutrients.

Although some people mistakenly believe that the term heart failure means the heart has stopped, the term actually refers to the diminished ability of the heart to keep up with its workload. Heart failure has many causes, including a number of diseases; heart failure is much more common in older people because they are more likely to have the diseases that cause it. Although the condition usually worsens slowly over time, people with heart failure can live for years. In the United States, about 400,000 new cases of heart failure are diagnosed yearly, and 70 percent of people with heart failure die of the disease within 10 years.

Causes

Any disease that affects the heart and interferes with the circulation can lead to heart failure. Diseases may selectively affect the heart muscle, impairing its ability to contract and pump blood. By far, the most common of these is coronary artery disease, which limits blood flow to the heart muscle and can cause a heart attack. Myocarditis (an infection of heart muscle caused by bacteria, viruses, or other microscopic organisms) may damage the heart muscle as may diabetes, an overactive thyroid gland, or extreme obesity. Heart valve disease may obstruct blood flow between the heart's chambers or between the heart and the major arteries. Alternatively, a valve that leaks may allow blood to flow backward. These conditions increase the heart muscle's workload, which eventually weakens the force of the heart's contractions. Other diseases primarily affect the heart's electrical conduction system, resulting in slow, fast, or irregular heartbeats that can't pump blood effectively.

If the heart has to work unusually hard over months or years, it gets larger, just as biceps do after months of exercise. At first, this enlargement provides a stronger contraction, but eventually an enlarged heart may result in decreased pumping ability and heart failure. High blood pressure (hypertension) can make the heart work harder. The heart also works harder when it has to force the blood through a narrowed exit from the heart, usually a narrowed aortic valve. The resulting condition is similar to the extra burden on a water pump when it's forced to push water through narrow pipes.

In some people, the pericardium—the thin, transparent covering of the heart—stiffens. This stiffening prevents the heart from fully expanding between beats and thus keeps it from filling adequately with blood. Much less often, diseases affecting other parts of the body greatly increase the demand for oxygen and nutrients, so that an otherwise normal heart is unable to meet this increased demand. The result is heart failure.

The causes of heart failure vary around the world because of the different varieties of disease that develop in different countries. For instance, in tropical countries certain parasites can lodge in the heart muscle; this typically causes heart failure at a much younger age than in developed countries.

Compensatory Mechanisms

The body has a number of response mechanisms to compensate for heart failure. The initial, short-term (within minutes to hours) emergency response mechanism is the fight-or-flight reaction caused by the release of adrenaline (epinephrine) and noradrenaline (norepinephrine) from the adrenal gland into the bloodstream; noradrenaline is also released from nerves. Adrenaline and noradrenaline are the body's first-line defenses against any sudden stress. In compensated heart failure, adrenaline and noradrenaline cause the heart to work harder, helping it to increase its output of blood and compensate to some degree for the pumping problem. Cardiac output may return to normal, although usually with an increased heart rate and a more forceful heartbeat.

In a person without heart disease who has a short-term need for increased heart function, these responses are beneficial. In a person who has chronic heart failure, these responses may produce long-term increased demands on an already damaged cardiovascular system. Over time, this increased demand leads to a deterioration of heart function.

As another corrective mechanism, the kidneys retain salt (sodium). To keep the blood's sodium concentration constant, the body simultaneously retains water. This additional water increases the volume of blood in the circulation and, at first, improves the heart's performance. One of the major consequences of fluid retention is that the larger volume of blood stretches the heart muscle. This stretched muscle contracts more forcefully, much as an athlete's muscle stretched before exercise does. This is one of the heart's main mechanisms for increasing its performance in heart failure. As heart failure progresses, however, the excess fluid escapes from the circulation and accumulates in various body sites, causing swelling (edema). Where the fluid accumulates depends on the amount of excess fluid held in the body and the effects of gravity. If the person is standing, the fluid sinks into the legs and feet. If the person is lying down, the fluid usually accumulates on the back or in the abdomen. Weight gain caused by the body's retention of sodium and water is common.

The other major mechanism by which the heart compensates is enlargement of the heart muscle (hypertrophy). The enlarged heart muscle can contract with greater force, but eventually it malfunctions, making the heart failure worse.

Symptoms

People with uncompensated heart failure feel tired and weak when performing physical activities because their muscles aren't getting an adequate amount of blood. The swelling also causes many symptoms. Besides being influenced by gravity, the location and effects of swelling are influenced by which side of the heart is predominantly impaired.

Although disease on one side of the heart always causes failure of the whole heart, the symptoms of disease on one side or the other often predominate. Right-sided disease tends to result in a buildup of blood flowing into the right side of the heart. This buildup leads to swelling in the feet, ankles, legs, liver, and abdomen. In contrast, left-sided disease leads to a buildup of fluid in the lungs (pulmonary edema), which causes extreme shortness of breath. At first, it happens during exertion, but as the disease progresses, it also occurs at rest. Sometimes, the shortness of breath happens at night while the person is lying down because fluid moves into the lungs. The person often wakes up, gasping for breath or wheezing. Sitting up causes the fluid to drain from the lungs, which makes breathing easier. People with heart failure may have to sleep in a sitting position to avoid this effect. A severe buildup of fluid (acute pulmonary edema) is a life-threatening emergency.

Diagnosis

These symptoms alone are usually enough for a doctor to make a diagnosis of heart failure. The following findings can confirm a doctor's initial diagnosis: a weak and often rapid pulse rate, reduced blood pressure, certain abnormalities in heart sounds, an enlarged heart, swollen neck veins, fluid in the lungs, an enlarged liver, rapid weight gain, and a swollen abdomen or legs. A chest x-ray can show an enlarged heart and fluid accumulated in the lungs.

The heart's performance is often evaluated with further tests, such as echocardiography, which uses sound waves to create an image of the heart, and electrocardiography, which examines the electrical activity of the heart.▲ Other tests may be carried out to determine the underlying cause of the heart failure.

Treatment

Much can be done to make physical activity more comfortable, improve the quality of life, and prolong life, but for most people with heart failure, no cure exists. Doctors approach therapy from three angles: treating the underlying cause, removing contributing factors that can worsen heart failure, and treating the heart failure itself.

Treating the Underlying Cause

Surgery can correct a narrowed or leaking heart valve, an abnormal connection between heart chambers, or a blockage of the coronary arteries, all of which may lead to heart failure. Sometimes the cause can be eliminated completely without surgery. For example, antibiotics can cure an infection. Drugs, surgery, or radiation therapy can correct an overactive thyroid gland. Similarly, drugs can reduce and control high blood pressure.

Removing Contributing Factors

Smoking, eating salt, being overweight, and drinking alcohol all aggravate heart failure as do extremes of room temperature. Doctors may recommend a program to help a person stop smoking, make appropriate dietary changes, stop drinking alcohol, or perform regular, moderate exercise to improve overall fitness. For those with more severe heart failure, bed rest may be prescribed as an important part of treatment for a few days.

Excess dietary salt (sodium) can cause fluid retention that counteracts the medical treatment. The amount of sodium in the body usually goes down if table salt, salt in cooking, and salted foods are limited. People with severe cases of heart failure are usually given detailed information on how to limit salt intake. People with heart failure can check the salt content of packaged foods by reading the labels carefully.

A simple, reliable way to check on the body's retention of fluid is to check body weight daily. Fluctuations of more than 2 pounds per day are almost certainly because of fluid retention. A consistent, rapid weight gain (2 pounds per day) is a clue that the heart failure is getting worse. For this reason, doctors often ask people with heart failure to weigh themselves as accurately as possible every day, typically upon arising in the morning, after urinating, and before eating breakfast. Trends are easier to spot when people use the same scale, wear a similar amount of clothing, and keep a written record of their daily weight.

Treating Heart Failure

The best treatment for heart failure is prevention or early reversal of the underlying cause. But even when prevention or early reversal isn't possible, major advances in treatment can prolong life and improve the quality of life for people with heart failure.

Chronic Heart Failure: When salt restriction alone doesn't reduce fluid retention, a doctor may prescribe diuretic drugs to increase urine formation and remove sodium and water from the body through the kidneys. Fluid reduction decreases the volume of blood entering the heart and so reduces the amount of work the heart has to do. Diuretics are most commonly taken by mouth on a long-term basis, but in an emergency they are very effective given intravenously. Because certain diuretics can cause an undesired loss of the body's potassium, a potassium supplement or a potassium-sparing diuretic may be given as well.

Digoxin increases the power of each heartbeat and slows a heart rate that's too rapid. Heart rhythm irregularities (arrhythmias)—in which the heartbeat is too fast, too slow, or erratic—can be treated with drugs or with an artificial pacemaker. Drugs that relax (dilate) the blood vessels (vasodilators) often are used. A vasodilator may dilate arteries, veins, or both. Arterial dilators expand arteries and lower blood pressure, which in turn reduces the work required of the heart. Venous dilators expand the veins, providing more room for the blood that has accumulated and is unable to enter the right side of the heart. This extra room relieves congestion and reduces the load on the heart. The most widely used vasodilators are the ACE (angiotensin converting enzyme) inhibitors. These drugs not only improve symptoms but also prolong life. The ACE inhibitors dilate both arteries and veins; many of the older drugs dilate one much more than the other.

▲ see page 73

For example, nitroglycerin dilates veins, and hydralazine dilates arteries.

Dilated and poorly contracting heart chambers may allow blood clots to form in them. The danger here is that these clots can break off, travel through the circulation, and cause damage in other vital organs such as the brain, causing a stroke. Anticoagulant drugs are important because they help prevent clots from forming in the heart chambers.

A number of new drugs are under investigation. Like the ACE inhibitors, milrinone and amrinone dilate both arteries and veins; like digoxin, they also increase the power of the heart. These new drugs are used only for short periods in patients who are closely monitored in the hospital because the drugs can cause dangerous heart rhythm irregularities.

Heart transplantation may be recommended for some otherwise healthy people whose worsening heart failure doesn't respond sufficiently to medications. Temporary, partial, or complete mechanical hearts are still largely experimental. Problems of effectiveness, infection, and blood clots are still being worked out.

Cardiomyoplasty is one experimental operation in which a large muscle taken from the person's back is wrapped around the heart and then stimulated by an artificial pacemaker to contract rhythmically. A newer experimental operation is showing promise for selected patients with severe heart failure—flabby, nonfunctioning heart muscle is simply cut out.

Acute Heart Failure: If fluid accumulates suddenly in the lungs (acute pulmonary edema), the person with heart failure has to gasp for breath. High concentrations of oxygen are given through a face mask. Intravenous diuretics and drugs such as digoxin can produce rapid, dramatic improvement. Nitroglycerin given intravenously or placed under the tongue (sublingually) dilates the veins, thereby reducing the amount of blood flowing through the lungs. If these measures fail, a tube is inserted into the person's airway so breathing can be assisted by a mechanical ventilator. In rare situations, tourniquets can be applied to three of the four limbs to trap blood in them temporarily, reducing the blood volume returning to the heart. These tourniquets are rotated between limbs every 10 to 20 minutes to avoid damaging the limbs. Morphine relieves the anxiety that generally accompanies acute pulmonary edema, decreases the rate of breathing, slows the heart rate, and thereby reduces the heart's workload.

Drugs similar to adrenaline and noradrenaline, such as dopamine and dobutamine, are used to stimulate heart contractions in hospitalized patients who need short-term relief. However, if stimulation by the body's internal emergency response system is too great, drugs that have the opposite action (beta-blockers) sometimes are used instead.

CHAPTER 18

Cardiomyopathy

Cardiomyopathy is a progressive disorder that alters the structure or impairs the function of the muscular wall of the lower chambers of the heart (ventricles).▲

Cardiomyopathy can be caused by many known diseases, or it may have no identifiable cause.

Dilated Congestive Cardiomyopathy

Dilated congestive cardiomyopathy is a group of heart disorders in which the ventricles enlarge but aren't able to pump enough blood for the body's needs, resulting in heart failure.

In the United States, the most common identifiable cause of dilated congestive cardiomyopathy is widespread coronary artery disease.■ Such coronary artery disease results in inadequate blood supply to the heart muscle, which can lead

▲ see box, page 69

■ see page 121

to permanent injury. The remaining uninjured heart muscle then stretches to compensate for the lost pumping action. When this stretching doesn't adequately compensate, dilated congestive cardiomyopathy develops.

An acute inflammation of the heart muscle (myocarditis) from a viral infection may weaken the heart muscle and produce dilated congestive cardiomyopathy (sometimes called viral cardiomyopathy). In the United States, infection with coxsackievirus B is the most common cause of viral cardiomyopathy. Certain chronic hormonal disorders such as diabetes and thyroid disease can eventually result in dilated congestive cardiomyopathy. Dilated congestive cardiomyopathy also can be caused by drugs such as alcohol, cocaine, and antidepressants. Alcoholic cardiomyopathy may develop after about 10 years of heavy alcohol abuse. Rarely, pregnancy or connective tissue diseases such as rheumatoid arthritis may cause dilated congestive cardiomyopathy.

Symptoms and Diagnosis

The usual first symptoms of dilated congestive cardiomyopathy—becoming short of breath on exertion and tiring easily—result from a weakening of the heart's pumping action (heart failure).▲ When cardiomyopathy results from an infection, the first symptoms may be a sudden fever and flulike symptoms. Whatever the cause, the heart rate speeds up, blood pressure is normal or low, fluid is retained in the legs and abdomen, and the lungs fill with fluid. The enlargement of the heart causes the heart valves to open and close improperly, and those leading to the ventricles (the mitral and tricuspid valves) often leak. Improper valve closure causes murmurs, which a doctor can hear with a stethoscope. Damage to and stretching of the heart muscle may make the heart rhythm abnormally fast or slow. These abnormalities interfere further with the heart's pumping action.

The diagnosis is based on the symptoms and a physical examination. Electrocardiography (a test that examines the electrical activity of the heart) may show characteristic changes. Echocardiography (a test that uses ultrasound waves to create an image of the heart structures)■ and magnetic resonance imaging (MRI) may be used to confirm the diagnosis. If the diagnosis remains in doubt, a catheter that measures pressures is inserted into the heart for more precise evalua-

tion. During catheterization, a tissue sample can be removed for microscopic examination (biopsy) to confirm the diagnosis and often to detect the cause.

Prognosis and Treatment

About 70 percent of people with dilated congestive cardiomyopathy die within 5 years of when their symptoms begin, and the prognosis worsens as the heart walls become thinner and heart function decreases. Abnormal heart rhythms also indicate a worse prognosis. Overall, men survive only half as long as women, and blacks half as long as whites. About 50 percent of the deaths are sudden, probably resulting from an abnormal heart rhythm.

Treating specific underlying causes such as alcohol abuse or an infection can prolong life. If alcohol abuse is the cause, the person must abstain from alcohol. If a bacterial infection causes sudden inflammation of the heart muscle, it's treated with an antibiotic.

In a person with coronary artery disease, the poor blood supply may cause angina (chest pain caused by heart disease),★ requiring treatment with a nitrate, beta-blocker, or calcium channel blocker. Beta-blockers and calcium channel blockers may reduce the force of heart contractions. Getting enough rest and sleep and avoiding stress help reduce strain on the heart.

Pooling of blood in the swollen heart may cause clots to form on the chamber walls. Anticoagulant drugs are usually given to prevent clotting. Most drugs used to prevent abnormal heart rhythms are prescribed in small doses, and the doses are adjusted in small increments because the drugs may reduce the force of heart contractions. Heart failure also is treated with drugs—an angiotensin converting enzyme inhibitor, often with a diuretic. However, unless a specific cause of the dilated congestive cardiomyopathy can be treated, the heart failure is likely to eventually be fatal. Because of this poor prognosis, dilated congestive cardiomyopathy is the most common reason for heart transplants.

▲ see page 87

■ see page 76

★ see page 121

Hypertrophic Cardiomyopathy

Hypertrophic cardiomyopathy is a group of heart disorders in which the walls of the ventricles thicken.

Hypertrophic cardiomyopathy may occur as a birth defect. It also may occur in adults with acromegaly, a condition resulting from excessive growth hormone in the blood, or in people who have pheochromocytoma, a tumor that produces adrenaline. People with neurofibromatosis, a hereditary condition, may also develop hypertrophic cardiomyopathy.

Usually, any thickening of the muscular walls of the heart represents the muscle's reaction to an increased workload. Typical causes include high blood pressure, narrowing of the aortic valve (aortic valve stenosis), and other conditions that increase resistance to blood flow from the heart. But people who have hypertrophic cardiomyopathy don't have these conditions. Instead, the thickening in hypertrophic cardiomyopathy usually results from an inherited genetic defect.

The heart becomes thicker and stiffer than normal and more resistant to filling with blood from the lungs. One result is back pressure in the lung veins, which can cause fluid to accumulate in the lungs, so the person is chronically short of breath. Also, as the ventricle walls thicken, they may block the flow of blood, preventing the heart from filling properly.

Symptoms and Diagnosis

Symptoms include faintness, chest pain, palpitations produced by irregular heartbeats, and heart failure with shortness of breath. Sudden death may result from irregular heartbeats.

A doctor can usually identify hypertrophic cardiomyopathy by physical examination. For instance, the heart sounds heard through a stethoscope are usually characteristic. The diagnosis usually is confirmed by an echocardiogram, electrocardiogram (ECG), or chest x-ray. Cardiac catheterization to measure pressures within the heart may be necessary if surgery is being considered.

Prognosis and Treatment

About 4 percent of people with hypertrophic cardiomyopathy die each year. Death is usually sudden. Death from chronic heart failure is less common. People who learn that they've inherited this disorder may wish to obtain genetic counseling when planning a family.

Treatment is aimed primarily at reducing the heart's resistance to filling with blood between heartbeats. Taken alone or together, beta-blockers and calcium channel blockers are the main treatment. Surgery to remove some heart muscle improves the outflow of blood from the heart, but it's performed only on people whose symptoms are incapacitating despite drug therapy. Surgery can relieve symptoms, but it doesn't lower the risk of death.

Before dental work or a surgical procedure, antibiotics may be given to reduce the risk of infection of the inside lining of the heart (infective endocarditis).

Restrictive Cardiomyopathy

Restrictive cardiomyopathy is a group of disorders of the heart muscle in which the walls of the ventricles become stiff, but not necessarily thickened, and resist normal filling with blood between heartbeats.

The least common form of cardiomyopathy, restrictive cardiomyopathy shares many features with hypertrophic cardiomyopathy. Its cause is usually unknown. In one of its two basic types, the heart muscle is gradually replaced by scar tissue. In the other, the heart muscle is infiltrated by abnormal material, such as white blood cells. Other causes of infiltration include amyloidosis and sarcoidosis. If the body contains too much iron, it may accumulate in the heart muscle, as in iron overload (hemochromatosis). The cause may also be a tumor invading the heart tissue.

Because the heart resists filling with blood, the amount of blood pumped out is adequate when the person is resting but not when the person is exercising.

Symptoms and Diagnosis

Restrictive cardiomyopathy causes heart failure with shortness of breath and tissue swelling (edema). Chest pain and fainting are less likely than in hypertrophic cardiomyopathy, but abnormal heart rhythms and palpitations are common.

Restrictive cardiomyopathy is one of the possible causes investigated when a person has heart failure. The diagnosis is based largely on a physical examination, an electrocardiogram (ECG), and an echocardiogram. Magnetic resonance imaging (MRI) can provide additional information about the structure of the heart. A precise diagnosis usually requires catheterization of the heart to measure pressures and a biopsy of the heart muscle (removal and microscopic examination of a specimen), which may enable the doctor to identify the infiltrating substance.

Prognosis and Treatment

About 70 percent of people with restrictive cardiomyopathy die within 5 years of when symptoms begin. For most, no therapy is satisfactory. For instance, diuretics, which normally are used to treat heart failure, may reduce the amount of blood entering the heart, worsening the condition instead of improving it. Drugs normally used in heart failure to reduce the heart's workload usually aren't helpful because they may reduce blood pressure too much.

Sometimes the cause of restrictive cardiomyopathy can be treated to prevent heart damage from getting worse or even to partially reverse it. For example, removing blood at regular intervals reduces the stored iron in people with iron overload. Those who have sarcoidosis may take corticosteroids.

CHAPTER 19

Heart Valve Disorders

The heart has four chambers—two small upper chambers (atria) and two large lower chambers (ventricles).▲ Each ventricle has a one-way inlet valve and a one-way outlet valve. The tricuspid valve opens from the right atrium into the right ventricle, and the pulmonary valve opens from the right ventricle into the pulmonary arteries. The mitral valve opens from the left atrium into the left ventricle, and the aortic valve opens from the left ventricle into the aorta.

The heart valves can malfunction either by leaking (valve regurgitation) or by failing to open adequately (valve stenosis). Either problem can seriously interfere with the heart's ability to pump blood. Sometimes a valve has both problems.

Mitral Valve Regurgitation

Mitral valve regurgitation (mitral incompetence, mitral insufficiency) is leakage back through the mitral valve each time the left ventricle contracts.

As the left ventricle pumps blood out of the heart and into the aorta, some blood leaks back into the left atrium, increasing the volume and pressure there. This, in turn, increases blood pressure in the vessels leading from the lungs to the heart, resulting in fluid buildup (congestion) in the lungs.

Rheumatic fever used to be the most common cause of mitral valve regurgitation. But today, rheumatic fever is rare in countries that have good preventive medicine. In North America and Western Europe, for instance, the use of antibiotics for strep throat (streptococcal infection of the throat) now largely prevents rheumatic fever. In these regions, rheumatic fever is a common cause of mitral valve regurgitation only among elderly people who didn't have the benefit of antibiotics in their youth. In countries that have poor preventive medicine, however, rheumatic fever is still common, and it's a common cause of mitral valve regurgitation.

In North America and Western Europe, a more common cause of mitral valve regurgitation is a heart attack, which can damage the supporting structures of the mitral valve. Another common cause is myxomatous degeneration, a condition in which the valve gradually becomes floppy.

Symptoms

Mild mitral valve regurgitation may not produce any symptoms. The problem may be recognized only if a doctor, listening through a stethoscope, hears a distinctive heart murmur caused by blood leaking back into the left atrium when the left ventricle contracts.

Because the left ventricle has to pump more blood to make up for the blood leaking back to the left atrium, it gradually enlarges to increase the force of each heartbeat. The enlarged ventricle may cause palpitations (an awareness of force-

---

▲ see box, page 69

Understanding Stenosis and Regurgitation

The heart valves can malfunction either by failing to open properly (stenosis) or by leaking (regurgitation). These illustrations depict the two problems at the mitral valve, though they can occur at the other heart valves as well.

Normal Valve Mechanisms

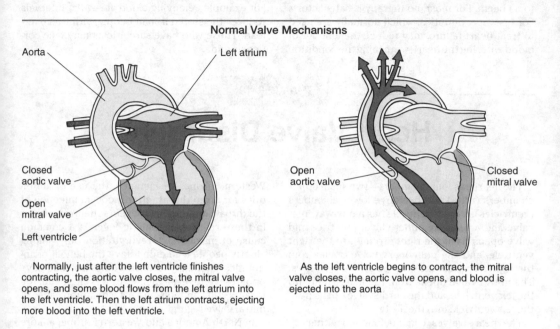

Normally, just after the left ventricle finishes contracting, the aortic valve closes, the mitral valve opens, and some blood flows from the left atrium into the left ventricle. Then the left atrium contracts, ejecting more blood into the left ventricle.

As the left ventricle begins to contract, the mitral valve closes, the aortic valve opens, and blood is ejected into the aorta

Mitral Valve Stenosis

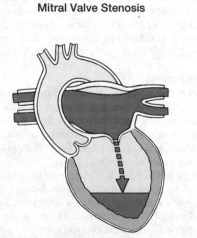

In mitral valve stenosis, the mitral valve doesn't open as wide as it should, and blood flow from the left atrium to the left ventricle is partially restricted.

Mitral Valve Regurgitation

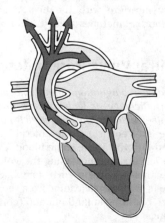

In mitral valve regurgitation, the mitral valve leaks when the left ventricle contracts, and some blood flows backward into the left atrium.

ful heartbeats), particularly when a person lies on the left side.

The left atrium also tends to enlarge to accommodate the extra blood leaking back from the ventricle. A very enlarged atrium often beats rapidly in an irregular disorganized pattern (atrial fibrillation),▲ which reduces the heart's pumping efficiency. A fibrillating atrium is really just quivering, not pumping, and the lack of proper blood flow through it allows blood clots to form. If a clot becomes detached, it's pumped out of the heart and may block a smaller artery, possibly causing a stroke or other damage.

Severe regurgitation reduces the forward flow of blood enough to cause heart failure, which may produce coughing, shortness of breath on exertion, and swollen legs.

Diagnosis

Doctors can usually recognize mitral valve regurgitation by its characteristic murmur—a sound heard through a stethoscope when the left ventricle contracts. An electrocardiogram (ECG) and chest x-rays indicate that the left ventricle is enlarged. The most informative test is echocardiography, an imaging technique that uses ultrasound waves. This test can produce an image of the faulty valve and indicate the severity of the problem.■

Treatment

If regurgitation is severe, the valve needs to be repaired or replaced before the left ventricle becomes so abnormal that the problem can't be corrected. Surgery may be performed to repair the valve (valvuloplasty) or to replace it with a mechanical one or one made partly from a pig's valve. Repairing the valve eliminates the regurgitation or reduces it enough to make the symptoms tolerable and prevent damage to the heart. Each type of replacement valve has advantages and disadvantages. Although mechanical valves are usually effective, they increase the risk of blood clots, so anticoagulants usually are taken indefinitely to reduce this risk. Pig valves work well and don't pose a risk of blood clots, but they don't last as long as mechanical valves. If a replacement valve fails, it must be replaced immediately.

Atrial fibrillation also may require treatment. Drugs such as beta-blockers, digoxin, and verapamil can slow the heart rate and help control the fibrillation.

The surfaces of damaged heart valves are susceptible to serious infection (infective endocarditis).★ Anyone with a damaged or artificial valve should take antibiotics before a dental or surgical procedure to prevent infection.

Mitral Valve Prolapse

In mitral valve prolapse, the valve leaflets bulge into the left atrium during ventricular contraction, sometimes allowing leakage (regurgitation) of small amounts of blood into the atrium.

About 2 to 5 percent of the population has mitral valve prolapse. It rarely causes serious heart problems.

Symptoms and Diagnosis

Most people with mitral valve prolapse have no symptoms. Others have symptoms that are difficult to explain on the basis of the mechanical problem alone; these include chest pain, palpitations, migraine headaches, fatigue, and dizziness. In some people, blood pressure may fall below normal when they stand up; in others, slightly irregular heartbeats may cause palpitations (an awareness of the heartbeat).

A doctor diagnoses the condition after hearing the characteristic clicking sound through a stethoscope. Regurgitation is diagnosed if a murmur is heard during ventricular contraction. Echocardiography, an imaging technique that uses ultrasound waves, allows a doctor to view the prolapse and determine the severity of any regurgitation.●

Treatment

Most people with mitral valve prolapse need no treatment. If the heart is beating too fast, a beta-blocker may be taken to slow the heart rate and to reduce palpitations and other symptoms.

If there's regurgitation, the person should take antibiotics before dental or surgical procedures because of the small risk that bacteria released during such procedures might infect the heart valve.

▲ see page 82

■ see page 76

★ see page 101

● see page 76

Mitral Valve Stenosis

Mitral valve stenosis is a narrowing of the mitral valve opening that increases resistance to blood flow from the left atrium to the left ventricle.

Mitral valve stenosis almost always results from rheumatic fever, which is rare today in North America and Western Europe. Thus, in these parts of the world, mitral valve stenosis occurs mostly in older people who had rheumatic fever during childhood. In the rest of the world, rheumatic fever is common, and it leads to mitral valve stenosis in adults, teenagers, and sometimes even children. Typically, when rheumatic fever is the cause of mitral valve stenosis, the mitral valve leaflets are partially fused together.

Mitral valve stenosis also can be congenital. Infants born with the disorder rarely live beyond age 2, unless they have surgery. Myxoma (a noncancerous tumor in the left atrium) or a blood clot can obstruct the flow of blood through the mitral valve, producing the same effect as mitral valve stenosis.

Symptoms and Diagnosis

If stenosis is severe, blood pressure increases in the left atrium and in the veins in the lungs, resulting in heart failure, in which fluid accumulates in the lungs (pulmonary edema). If a woman with severe mitral valve stenosis becomes pregnant, heart failure may develop rapidly.▲ A person with heart failure easily becomes fatigued and short of breath. At first, shortness of breath may develop only during physical activity. Later, the symptoms may occur even during rest. Some people can breathe comfortably only when they're propped up with pillows or sitting upright. A plum-colored flush in the cheeks suggests that a person has mitral valve stenosis. High pressure in the veins in the lung may cause a vein or capillaries to burst and bleed slightly or massively into the lungs. Enlargement of the left atrium can result in atrial fibrillation—a rapid, irregular heartbeat.

Using a stethoscope, a doctor can hear a characteristic heart murmur as the blood rushes through the narrowed valve from the left atrium.

▲ see page 1160

■ see page 76

Unlike a normal valve, which opens silently, the valve often makes a snapping sound as it opens to allow blood into the left ventricle. The diagnosis is usually confirmed by electrocardiography, a chest x-ray showing an enlarged atrium, or echocardiography (an imaging technique that uses ultrasound waves).■ Sometimes cardiac catheterization is necessary to determine the extent and characteristics of the blockage.

Prevention and Treatment

Mitral valve stenosis can be prevented only by preventing rheumatic fever, a childhood illness that sometimes occurs after untreated strep throat (streptococcal throat infection).

Drugs such as beta-blockers, digoxin, and verapamil can slow the heart rate and help control atrial fibrillation. Digoxin also strengthens the heartbeat if heart failure occurs. Diuretics can reduce the blood pressure in the lungs by reducing the volume of circulating blood.

If drug therapy doesn't reduce the symptoms satisfactorily, valve repair or replacement may be needed. A doctor may be able to simply stretch the valve opening using a procedure called balloon valvuloplasty. In this procedure, a balloon-tipped catheter is threaded through a vein and eventually into the heart. Once inside the valve, the balloon is inflated, separating the valve leaflets where they have fused together. Alternatively, heart surgery may be carried out to separate the fused leaflets. If the valve is too badly damaged, it may be surgically replaced with a mechanical valve or one made partly from a pig's valve.

People with mitral valve stenosis are given preventive antibiotics before any dental or surgical procedure to reduce the risk of a heart valve infection.

Aortic Valve Regurgitation

Aortic valve regurgitation (aortic incompetence, aortic insufficiency) is leakage of the aortic valve each time the left ventricle relaxes.

In North America and Western Europe, the most common causes used to be rheumatic fever and syphilis—both now rare because of the widespread use of antibiotics. In other regions, damage to the valve from rheumatic fever is still common. Aside from these infections, the most common cause of aortic valve regurgitation is a weakening of the valve's usually tough, fibrous material because of myxomatous degeneration, a birth defect, or other unknown factors. Myxomatous degeneration is an inherited connective tissue disorder that weakens the heart valve tissue, allowing it to stretch abnormally and rarely to tear. Other causes are bacterial infection and injury. About 2 percent of boys and 1 percent of girls are born with a valve containing two leaflets instead of the usual three, which can cause mild regurgitation.

Symptoms and Diagnosis

Mild aortic valve regurgitation produces no symptoms other than a characteristic heart murmur that can be heard with a stethoscope each time the left ventricle relaxes. With severe regurgitation, the left ventricle carries an increasingly large load of blood, which leads to enlargement of the ventricle and eventually to heart failure. The heart failure causes shortness of breath on exertion or when lying flat, especially at night. Sitting up allows backed-up fluid to drain out of the upper part of the lungs, restoring normal breathing. The person also may have palpitations (an awareness of strong heartbeats) caused by forceful contractions of the enlarged ventricle. Chest pains may occur, especially at night.

A doctor can usually make the diagnosis after hearing the characteristic heart murmur, observing other indications of aortic valve regurgitation during a physical examination (such as certain pulse abnormalities), and noting heart enlargement on an x-ray. An electrocardiogram may show changes in the heart's rhythm and signs of an enlarged left ventricle. Echocardiography can produce an image of the faulty valve and indicate the severity of the problem.▲

Treatment

Antibiotics are given before dental or surgical procedures to prevent infection of the damaged heart valve. This precaution is taken even with mild aortic valve regurgitation.

A person who develops symptoms of heart failure should have surgery before the left ventricle becomes irreversibly damaged. In the weeks before surgery, the heart failure is treated with digoxin and angiotensin converting enzyme inhibitors or other drugs that dilate blood vessels and reduce the work of the heart. Usually, the valve is replaced with a mechanical one or one made partly from a pig's valve.

Aortic Valve Stenosis

Aortic valve stenosis is a narrowing of the aortic valve opening that increases resistance to blood flow from the left ventricle to the aorta.

In North America and Western Europe, aortic valve stenosis is mainly a disease of the elderly— the result of scarring and calcium accumulation in the valve leaflets. Aortic valve stenosis from this cause begins after age 60 but doesn't usually produce symptoms until age 70 or 80. Aortic valve stenosis also may result from rheumatic fever contracted in childhood. When rheumatic fever is the cause, aortic valve stenosis is usually accompanied by mitral valve disease producing stenosis, regurgitation, or both.

In younger people, the most common cause is a birth defect.■ The narrowed aortic valve may not be a problem in infancy but becomes one as a person grows. The valve remains the same size as the heart enlarges and tries to pump increasing amounts of blood through the small valve. The valve may have only two leaflets instead of the usual three, or it may have an abnormal funnel shape. Over the years, the opening of such a valve often becomes stiff and narrow from accumulated calcium deposits.

Symptoms and Diagnosis

The left ventricle wall thickens as the ventricle attempts to pump enough blood through the narrow aortic valve, and the enlarged heart muscle requires an increasing blood supply from the coronary arteries. Eventually, the blood supply becomes insufficient, causing chest pain (angina)★ on exertion. This insufficient blood supply can damage the heart muscle, so that the output of blood from the heart becomes inadequate for the body's needs. The resulting heart failure causes fatigue and shortness of breath on exertion. A person with severe aortic stenosis may faint on exertion because the narrow valve prevents the ventricle from pumping enough blood to the arteries of the muscles, which have dilated to accept more oxygen-rich blood.

▲ see page 76

■ see page 1224

★ see page 121

A doctor usually bases the diagnosis on a characteristic heart murmur heard through a stethoscope, pulse abnormalities, abnormalities on an electrocardiogram, and heart wall thickening revealed on a chest x-ray. For people who experience angina, shortness of breath, or faintness, echocardiography (an imaging technique that uses ultrasound waves) and possibly cardiac catheterization may be used to identify the cause and determine the severity of the stenosis.▲

Treatment

In any adult with fainting, angina, and shortness of breath on exertion caused by aortic valve stenosis, the aortic valve is surgically replaced, preferably before the left ventricle is irreparably damaged. The replacement valve may be a mechanical one or one made partly from a pig's valve. Anyone with a replacement valve must take antibiotics before undergoing dental or surgical procedures to prevent a heart valve infection.

In children, surgery may be performed even before symptoms develop if the stenosis is severe. Early treatment is important because sudden death may occur before any symptoms appear. For children, safe, effective alternatives to valve replacement are surgical valve repair and balloon valvuloplasty (in which a balloon-tipped catheter is inserted into the valve and the balloon is inflated to expand the valve opening). Balloon valvuloplasty is also used in frail elderly patients who aren't able to have surgery, even though the stenosis tends to recur. Valve replacement is usually the best treatment for adults of all ages, however, and it provides an excellent prognosis.

Tricuspid Valve Regurgitation

Tricuspid valve regurgitation (tricuspid incompetence, tricuspid insufficiency) is leakage of the tricuspid valve each time the right ventricle contracts.

With tricuspid valve regurgitation, when the right ventricle contracts, it not only pumps blood forward to the lungs, it also pushes some blood back into the right atrium. The valve leakage increases the pressure in the right atrium, causing it to enlarge. This high pressure is transmitted to

the veins that enter the atrium, creating resistance to the flow of blood from the body to the heart.

The usual cause of tricuspid valve regurgitation is resistance to the outflow of blood from the right ventricle caused by severe lung disease or a narrowing of the pulmonary valve (pulmonary valve stenosis). To compensate, the right ventricle enlarges to pump harder, and the valve opening stretches.

Symptoms and Diagnosis

Besides vague symptoms, such as weakness and fatigue caused by a low output of blood from the heart, the only symptoms are usually discomfort in the right upper part of the abdomen from an enlarged liver and pulsations in the neck. These symptoms result from the backflow of blood into the veins. Enlargement of the right atrium can result in atrial fibrillation—a rapid, irregular heartbeat. Eventually, heart failure occurs, and the body retains fluids, mainly in the legs.

The diagnosis is based on the person's medical history, physical examination, electrocardiogram, and chest x-ray. The valve leakage creates a murmur that a doctor can hear with a stethoscope. Echocardiography can produce an image of the leakage and measure the severity.■

Treatment

Usually, tricuspid valve regurgitation itself requires little or no treatment. However, the underlying lung disease or pulmonary valve disease may require treatment. Problems such as irregular heart rhythms and heart failure are usually treated without performing surgery on the tricuspid valve.

Tricuspid Valve Stenosis

Tricuspid valve stenosis is a narrowing of the tricuspid valve opening that increases resistance to blood flow from the right atrium to the right ventricle.

Over many years, tricuspid valve stenosis causes the right atrium to enlarge and the right ventricle to shrink. The amount of blood returning to the heart is reduced and pressure on the veins bringing blood back to the heart is increased.

Nearly all cases are caused by rheumatic fever, which has become rare in North America and

▲ see page 78

■ see page 76

Western Europe. Rarely, the cause is a tumor in the right atrium, a connective tissue disease, or, even more rarely, a birth defect.

Symptoms, Diagnosis, and Treatment

Symptoms are generally mild. The person may have palpitations (an awareness of heartbeats) or a fluttering discomfort in the neck and may feel generally tired. Abdominal discomfort may result if the increased pressure on the veins leads to liver enlargement.

A doctor may hear the murmur of tricuspid valve stenosis through a stethoscope. A chest x-ray reveals that the right atrium is enlarged, and an echocardiogram can produce an image of the stenosis and measure its severity. An electrocardiogram shows changes indicating that the right atrium is strained.▲

Tricuspid valve stenosis is rarely severe enough to require surgical repair.

Pulmonary Valve Stenosis

Pulmonary valve stenosis is a narrowing of the pulmonary valve opening that increases resistance to blood flow from the right ventricle to the pulmonary arteries.

Pulmonary valve stenosis, which is rare in adults, is usually a birth defect.■

CHAPTER 20

Heart Tumors

A tumor is any type of abnormal growth, whether cancerous (malignant) or noncancerous (benign). Tumors that originate in the heart are called primary tumors and may develop in any of the heart tissues. They may be cancerous or noncancerous and are rare. Secondary tumors originate in some other part of the body—usually the lung, breast, blood, or skin—and then spread (metastasize) to the heart; they are always cancerous. Secondary tumors are 30 to 40 times more common than primary tumors but are still uncommon.

Heart tumors may cause no symptoms or may cause life-threatening heart malfunction that imitates other heart diseases. Examples of such heart malfunctions include sudden heart failure, sudden onset of irregular heartbeats, and a sudden drop in blood pressure caused by bleeding into the pericardium (the sac surrounding the heart). Heart tumors are difficult to diagnose because they're relatively uncommon and because their symptoms resemble those of many other conditions. To make the diagnosis, a doctor usually has to have reason to suspect that a heart tumor is present. For example, if a person has cancer elsewhere in the body but comes to a doctor with symptoms of heart malfunction, the doctor may suspect a heart tumor.

Myxomas

A myxoma is a noncancerous tumor, usually irregular in shape and jellylike in consistency.

Half of all primary heart tumors are myxomas. Three quarters of myxomas are found in the left atrium, the chamber of the heart that receives oxygen-rich blood from the lungs.

Myxomas in the left atrium often grow from a stalk and can swing freely with the flow of blood like a tetherball. As they swing, they may move in and out of the nearby mitral valve—the pathway from the left atrium to the left ventricle. This swinging may plug and unplug the valve over and over again, so that the blood flow stops and starts intermittently. Fainting or episodes of lung congestion and shortness of breath can develop when the person is standing because gravity pulls the tumor down to the valve opening; lying down relieves the symptoms.

The tumor may damage the mitral valve, so that blood leaks through it, creating a heart murmur that a doctor may hear with a stethoscope. Based

---

▲ see page 73

■ see page 1227

How a Myxoma Can Block Blood Flow in the Heart

A myxoma in the left atrium may grow from a stalk and swing freely with the flow of blood. As it swings, the myxoma may move in and out of the nearby mitral valve—the pathway from the left atrium to the left ventricle.

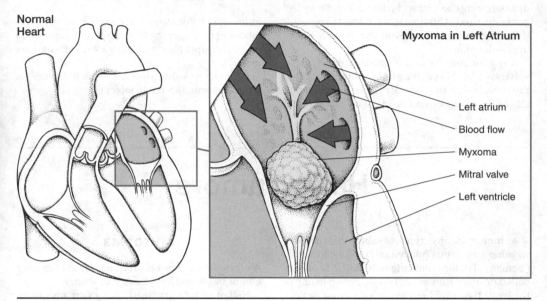

Normal Heart

Myxoma in Left Atrium

Left atrium

Blood flow

Myxoma

Mitral valve

Left ventricle

on the way a murmur sounds, a doctor must consider whether it results from a leak caused by damage from a tumor, a very rare cause, or from a more common cause, such as rheumatic heart disease.

Pieces of a myxoma or blood clots that form on the surface of the myxoma may break off, circulate to other organs, and block blood vessels there. Symptoms depend on which vessel is blocked. For example, a blocked vessel in the brain may produce a stroke; a blocked vessel in the lung may cause pain and coughing up of blood. Other symptoms of myxomas include fever, weight loss, cold and painful fingers and toes on exposure to cold (Raynaud's phenomenon), anemia, low blood platelet count (because platelets are involved in blood clotting), and symptoms suggesting severe infection.

Other Primary Tumors

Less common noncancerous heart tumors, fibromas and rhabdomyomas, may grow directly from the heart's fibrous tissue cells and muscle cells. Rhabdomyomas, the second most common type of primary tumors, develop in infancy or childhood, usually in a rare childhood disease called tuberous sclerosis. Other primary heart tumors, including primary cancerous tumors, are extremely rare, and no good treatment exists. The children who get them usually live less than 1 year.

Several tests are used to diagnose heart tumors. Often, echocardiography (a test that uses sound waves to outline structures) is used to outline the tumors. The sound waves may be passed through the chest wall or from inside the esophagus (a procedure called transesophageal echocardiography). A catheter inserted through a vein to the heart can be used to inject substances that can outline a heart tumor on x-rays; however, this procedure is needed less often.▲ Computed tomography (CT) and magnetic resonance imaging (MRI) scans also are used. If a tumor is found, a small sample can be removed with a special catheter; the sample is used to identify the type of tumor and help in selecting the proper treatment.

A single noncancerous primary heart tumor usually can be removed by surgery, which usually cures the person. Typically, doctors don't treat primary tumors when several are present or treat tumors that are so large that they can't be removed. Primary and secondary cancerous tumors are incurable; only their symptoms can be treated.

CHAPTER 21

Endocarditis

Endocarditis is inflammation of the smooth interior lining of the heart (the endocardium), most often resulting from a bacterial infection.

Infective Endocarditis

Infective endocarditis is an infection of the endocardium and the heart valves.

Bacteria (less often, fungi) that either enter the bloodstream or, in rare instances, contaminate the heart during open heart surgery can lodge on heart valves and infect the endocardium. Abnormal or damaged valves are most susceptible to infection, but normal valves can be infected by some aggressive bacteria, especially those present in large numbers. Accumulations of bacteria and blood clots on the valves (called vegetations) can break loose and travel to vital organs, where they can block arterial blood flow. Such obstructions are very serious: They can cause stroke, heart attack, and infection and damage in the area where they lodge.

Infective endocarditis can come on suddenly and become life threatening within days (called acute infective endocarditis), or it can develop gradually and subtly over a period of weeks to several months (called subacute infective endocarditis).

Causes

Although bacteria aren't normally found in the blood, an injury to the skin, lining of the mouth, or gums (even an injury from a normal activity such as chewing or brushing the teeth) can allow a small number of bacteria to invade the blood-

stream. Gingivitis (infection and inflammation of the gums), minor skin infections, and infections elsewhere in the body may allow bacteria to enter the bloodstream, increasing the risk of endocarditis. Certain surgical, dental, and medical procedures also may introduce bacteria into the bloodstream—for example, the use of intravenous lines to provide fluids, nutrition, or medications; cystoscopy (insertion of a viewing tube to examine the bladder); and colonoscopy (insertion of a viewing tube to examine the large intestine). In people with normal heart valves, no harm is done, and the body's white blood cells destroy these bacteria. Damaged heart valves, however, may trap the bacteria, which then lodge on the endocardium and start to multiply. Rarely, when a heart valve is replaced with an artificial (prosthetic) valve, bacteria may be introduced; these bacteria are more likely to be resistant to antibiotics. People with a birth defect or abnormality that allows blood to leak from one part of the heart to another (for instance, from one ventricle to the other) also have an increased risk of endocarditis.

A few bacteria in the blood (bacteremia) may not cause immediate symptoms, but bacteremia may develop into septicemia, a severe blood infection typically causing high fever, chills, shaking, and low blood pressure. A person with septicemia is particularly at risk of developing endocarditis.

▲ see page 78

An Inside View of Infective Endocarditis

This cross-sectional view shows vegetations (accumulations of bacteria and blood clots) on the four valves of the heart.

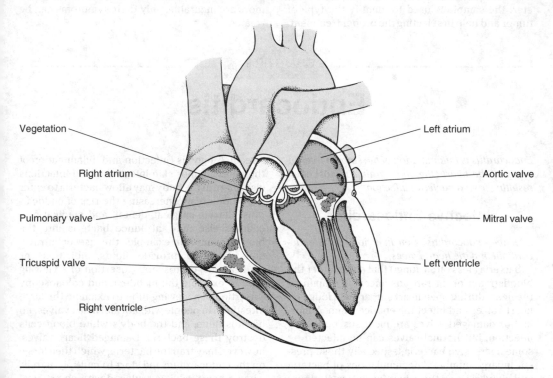

The bacteria that cause acute bacterial endocarditis are sometimes aggressive enough to infect normal heart valves; the bacteria that cause subacute bacterial endocarditis nearly always infect abnormal or damaged valves. In the United States, most cases of endocarditis occur in people with birth defects of the heart chambers and valves, people with artificial heart valves, and elderly people with valve damage from childhood rheumatic fever or with heart valve changes associated with aging. Injecting drug users are at high risk of developing endocarditis because they often inject bacteria directly into their bloodstream through dirty needles, syringes, or drug solutions.

In injecting drug users and people who develop endocarditis from prolonged catheter use, the inlet valve to the right ventricle (the tricuspid valve) is most often infected. In most other cases of endocarditis, the inlet valve to the left ventricle (the mitral valve) or the outlet valve from the left ventricle (the aortic valve) is infected. For a person with an artificial valve, the risk of infective endocarditis is greatest during the first year after surgery; after that the risk diminishes but remains slightly higher than normal. For unknown reasons, the risk always is greater with an artificial aortic valve than with an artificial mitral valve and with a mechanical valve rather than with one transplanted from a pig.

Symptoms

Acute bacterial endocarditis usually begins suddenly with a high fever (102° F. to 104° F.), fast heart rate, tiredness, and rapid and extensive heart valve damage. Dislodged endocardial vegetations (emboli) can travel to other areas and create additional infection sites. Collections of pus (abscesses) may develop at the base of infected heart valves or wherever infected emboli settle. Heart valves may be perforated, and major leaks may develop within a few days. Some people go into shock, and their kidneys and other organs stop functioning (a condition called sepsis syndrome). Arterial infections can weaken blood vessel walls, causing them to rupture. The rupture can be fatal, particularly if it's in the brain or near the heart.

Subacute bacterial endocarditis may produce symptoms for months before heart valve damage or emboli make the diagnosis clear to the doctor. Symptoms may include tiredness, mild fever (99° F. to 101° F.), weight loss, sweating, and a low red blood cell count (anemia). A doctor may suspect endocarditis in a person with a fever and no obvious source of infection if the person has a new heart murmur or if the sound of an existing murmur has changed. A doctor may note an enlarged spleen. Very small spots resembling tiny freckles may appear on the skin, and similar spots may appear in the whites of the eyes or under the fingernails. These spots are areas of minuscule bleeding caused by tiny emboli that have broken off the heart valves. Larger emboli may cause stomach pain, sudden blockage of an artery to an arm or leg, a heart attack, or stroke.

Other symptoms of acute and subacute bacterial endocarditis may include chills, joint pain, pale skin, rapid heartbeat, painful nodules under the skin, confusion, and blood in the urine.

Endocarditis of an artificial heart valve may be an acute or subacute infection. Compared with infection of a natural valve, infection of an artificial valve is more likely to spread to the heart muscle at the base of the valve and loosen the valve. Emergency surgery is then needed to replace the valve because heart failure from severe valvular leaks can be fatal. Alternatively, the heart's electrical conduction system may be interrupted, resulting in slowing of the heartbeat, which may lead to a sudden loss of consciousness or even death.

Diagnosis

People suspected of having acute bacterial endocarditis usually are hospitalized promptly for diagnosis and treatment. Because the symptoms of subacute bacterial endocarditis are initially vague, the infection may damage heart valves or spread to other sites before it's diagnosed. Untreated subacute endocarditis is just as life threatening as acute endocarditis.

A doctor may suspect endocarditis based on the symptoms alone, particularly when they occur in someone with a predisposing condition. Echocardiography, which uses reflected sound waves to create an image of the heart,▲ can identify heart valve vegetations and damage. To identify the disease-causing bacteria, a doctor may have blood samples drawn and cultured. Because bacteria are only intermittently released into the bloodstream in large enough numbers to be identified, three or more samples are taken at different times to increase the likelihood that at least one will contain enough bacteria to be grown in the laboratory. Various antibiotics are tested against the bacteria to determine the best one to use.

Sometimes bacteria can't be cultured from blood samples. The reason may be that special techniques are needed to grow the particular bacteria, or the patient may have taken antibiotics that didn't cure the infection but did reduce the number of bacteria enough to hide their presence. Another possibility: The patient doesn't have endocarditis but has one of several conditions very similar to endocarditis, such as a heart tumor.

Prevention and Treatment

As a preventive measure, people with heart valve abnormalities, artificial valves, or congenital defects are given antibiotics before dental and surgical procedures; this is why dentists and surgeons need to know if a person has had a heart valve disorder. Although the risk of endocarditis

---

▲ see page 76

isn't very high for surgical procedures and preventive antibiotics aren't always effective, the consequences of endocarditis are so severe that most doctors believe that giving antibiotics before these procedures is a reasonable precaution.

Because treatment usually consists of at least 2 weeks of high-dose intravenous antibiotics, people with bacterial endocarditis are almost always treated in the hospital. Antibiotics alone don't always cure an infection on artificial valves. Heart surgery may be needed to repair or replace damaged valves and remove vegetations.

Noninfective Endocarditis

Noninfective endocarditis is a condition in which blood clots develop on damaged heart valves.

People most at risk include those with systemic lupus erythematosus (an immune system disease); lung, stomach, or pancreatic cancer; tuberculosis; pneumonia; bone infection; or diseases causing a marked weight loss. As with infective endocarditis, the heart valves may leak or fail to open properly. The risk of emboli causing a stroke or heart attack is high. Drugs that prevent clotting may be used, but studies have not yet confirmed their benefits.

CHAPTER 22

Pericardial Disease

The pericardium is a flexible, stretchable, two-layered sac that envelops the heart. It contains just enough lubricating fluid between the two layers for them to slide easily over one another. The pericardium keeps the heart in position, prevents the heart from overfilling with blood, and protects the heart from chest infections. However, the pericardium isn't essential to life; if the pericardium is removed, there's no measurable effect on the heart's performance.

In rare cases, the pericardium is missing at birth, or it has weak spots or holes in it. These defects can be dangerous because the heart or a major blood vessel might bulge (herniate) through a hole in the pericardium and become trapped, which could cause death in minutes. Therefore, these defects are usually surgically repaired; if such repair isn't feasible, the whole pericardium may be removed. Aside from birth defects, diseases of the pericardium can come from infections, injuries, and widespread tumors.

Acute Pericarditis

Acute pericarditis is inflammation of the pericardium that begins suddenly and is often painful; the inflammation causes fluid and blood products such as fibrin, red blood cells, and white blood cells to pour into the pericardial space.

Acute pericarditis has many causes, ranging from viral infections (which may be painful but are short-lived and usually have no lasting effects) to life-threatening cancer. Other causes include AIDS, heart attack (myocardial infarction), heart surgery, systemic lupus erythematosus, rheumatoid disease, kidney failure, injury, radiation treatment, and leakage of blood from an aortic aneurysm (a balloonlike weakening of the aorta). Acute pericarditis also may result as a side effect of certain drugs, such as anticoagulants, penicillin, procainamide, phenytoin, and phenylbutazone.

Symptoms and Diagnosis

Usually, acute pericarditis causes fever and chest pain, which typically extends to the left shoulder and sometimes down the left arm. The pain may be similar to that of a heart attack, except that it tends to be made worse by lying down, coughing, or even deep breathing. Pericarditis may cause cardiac tamponade, a potentially fatal condition.

Cardiac Tamponade: The Most Serious Complication of Pericarditis

Tamponade most commonly follows fluid accumulation or bleeding into the pericardium that results from a tumor, injury, or surgery. Viral and bacterial infections and kidney failure are other common causes. The blood pressure may fall rapidly, reaching abnormally low levels when the person breathes in. To confirm the diagnosis, a doctor may use echocardiography (a test that uses ultrasound waves to create an image of the heart).

Cardiac tamponade is often a medical emergency. Doctors treat it immediately by performing surgical drainage or by puncturing the pericardium with a long needle and removing fluid to relieve the pressure. A doctor uses a local anesthetic to prevent the patient from feeling pain when the needle goes through the chest wall. When time permits, fluid removal is closely monitored using echocardiography. With pericarditis of unknown origin, a doctor may surgically drain the pericardium and remove a specimen to help with the diagnosis.

After the pressure is relieved, the patient is usually kept in the hospital in case the tamponade recurs.

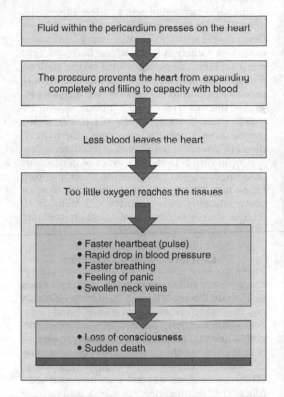

Fluid within the pericardium presses on the heart

⬇

The pressure prevents the heart from expanding completely and filling to capacity with blood

⬇

Less blood leaves the heart

⬇

Too little oxygen reaches the tissues

⬇

- Faster heartbeat (pulse)
- Rapid drop in blood pressure
- Faster breathing
- Feeling of panic
- Swollen neck veins

⬇

- Loss of consciousness
- Sudden death

A doctor can diagnose acute pericarditis by the patient's description of the pain and by listening through a stethoscope placed on the patient's chest. Pericarditis can produce a crunching sound similar to the creaking of a leather shoe. A chest x-ray and echocardiography (a test that uses ultrasound waves to create an image of the heart)▲ may show too much fluid in the pericardium. Echocardiography also may reveal the underlying cause—for example, a tumor—and show the pressure of the pericardial fluid on the right chambers of the heart; high pressure is a possible warning sign of cardiac tamponade. Blood tests can detect some of the conditions that cause pericarditis—for example, leukemia, AIDS, infections, rheumatic fever, and increased blood levels of urea resulting from kidney failure.

Prognosis and Treatment

The prognosis depends on the cause. When pericarditis is caused by a virus or when the cause isn't apparent, recovery usually takes 1 to 3 weeks. Complications or recurrences can slow recovery. People with cancer that has invaded the pericardium rarely survive beyond 12 to 18 months.

Doctors usually hospitalize people with pericarditis, give them drugs that reduce inflammation and pain (such as aspirin or ibuprofen), and watch them for complications (particularly car-

▲ see page 76

diac tamponade). Intense pain may require an opiate, such as morphine, or a corticosteroid. The most commonly used drug for intense pain is prednisone.

Further treatment of acute pericarditis varies, depending on the underlying cause. Cancer patients may respond to chemotherapy (anticancer drugs) or radiation therapy, but these patients often undergo surgical removal of the pericardium. People on dialysis because of kidney failure usually respond to changes in their dialysis programs. Doctors treat bacterial infections with antibiotics and surgically drain the pus from the pericardium. Drugs that may cause the pericarditis are discontinued whenever possible.

People with repeated episodes of pericarditis resulting from a virus, an injury, or an unknown cause may get relief from aspirin, ibuprofen, or corticosteroids. In some cases, colchicine is effective. If drug treatment fails, usually the pericardium is removed surgically.

Chronic Pericarditis

Chronic pericarditis is inflammation that results in fluid accumulation or thickening of the pericardium and that begins gradually and is long-lasting.

In **chronic effusive pericarditis,** fluid slowly accumulates in the pericardium. Usually the cause is unknown, but the condition may be caused by cancer, tuberculosis, or low thyroid function. When possible, known causes are treated; if heart function is normal, doctors take a wait-and-see approach.

Chronic constrictive pericarditis is a rare disease that usually results when fibrous (scarlike) tissue forms around the heart. The fibrous tissue tends to contract over the years, compressing the heart and making it smaller. Compression increases the pressure in the veins that return blood to the heart because higher pressure is needed to fill the heart. Fluid backs up and then leaks out and accumulates under the skin, in the abdomen, and sometimes in spaces around the lungs.

Causes

Any condition that causes acute pericarditis can cause chronic constrictive pericarditis, but usually the cause is unknown. The most common known causes of chronic constrictive pericarditis are viral infections and radiation treatment for breast cancer or lymphoma. Chronic constrictive pericarditis also may result from rheumatoid arthritis, systemic lupus erythematosus, a previous injury, heart surgery, or a bacterial infection. Previously, tuberculosis was the most common cause in the United States, but today tuberculosis accounts for only 2 percent of cases. In Africa and India, tuberculosis is still the most common cause of all forms of pericarditis.

Symptoms and Diagnosis

Symptoms of chronic pericarditis include shortness of breath, coughing (because high pressure in the veins of the lungs pushes fluid into the air sacs), and fatigue (because the heart becomes inefficient). Otherwise, the condition is painless. Fluid in the abdomen and the legs is also common.

Symptoms provide important clues that a person has chronic pericarditis, particularly if there's no other reason for reduced heart performance—such as high blood pressure, coronary artery disease, or heart valve disease. In chronic constrictive pericarditis, the heart usually doesn't look abnormally large on chest x-rays, whereas in most other heart diseases, the heart is enlarged. Nearly half of those with chronic constrictive pericarditis have calcium deposits in the pericardium that show up on x-rays.

Two types of procedures may confirm the diagnosis. Cardiac catheterization can be used to measure blood pressure in the heart chambers and major blood vessels. Alternatively, a magnetic resonance imaging (MRI) scan or a computed tomography (CT) scan can be used to measure the thickness of the pericardium.▲ Normally the pericardium is less than an eighth of an inch thick, but in chronic constrictive pericarditis it's usually a quarter of an inch thick or more.

Treatment

Although diuretics (drugs that remove excess fluid) may improve symptoms, the only possible cure is surgical removal of the pericardium. Surgery cures about 85 percent of people who undergo it. However, because the risk of death from this operation is 5 to 15 percent, most people don't have the operation unless the disease substantially interferes with daily activities.

▲ see pages 76 and 77

Low Blood Pressure

Low blood pressure (hypotension) is blood pressure low enough to cause symptoms, such as dizziness and fainting.

Maintaining the pressure of blood as it leaves the heart and circulates throughout the body, like maintaining water pressure in the pipelines throughout a home, is essential. The pressure must be high enough to deliver oxygen and nutrients to all cells in the body and remove waste products from them. But if the blood pressure is too high, it can rupture a blood vessel and cause bleeding in the brain (hemorrhagic stroke) or other complications. If the blood pressure is too low, the blood can't supply enough oxygen and nutrients to the cells and properly remove wastes from them. However, healthy people with low normal blood pressure at rest tend to live longer.

Compensatory Mechanisms

Three factors help determine blood pressure: the amount of blood pumped from the heart, the volume of blood in the blood vessels, and the capacity of the blood vessels.

The more blood pumped from the heart (cardiac or heart output) per minute, the higher the blood pressure. The amount of blood pumped may be reduced if the heart beats slower or its contractions are weakened, as may happen after a heart attack (myocardial infarction). An extremely rapid heartbeat, which can reduce the efficiency of the heart's pumping action, may also reduce the cardiac output, as may other types of abnormal heart rhythms.

The more blood in the circulation, the higher the blood pressure. A loss of blood from dehydration or bleeding can reduce the blood volume and decrease the blood pressure.

The smaller the capacity of the blood vessels, the higher the blood pressure. So widening (dilating) the blood vessels makes the blood pressure fall, and constricting them makes the blood pressure rise.

Sensors, particularly those in the neck and chest, constantly monitor the blood pressure. When they detect a change caused by one of these three factors, the sensors trigger a change in one of the other factors to compensate and so maintain a steady blood pressure. Nerves carry signals from these sensors and from brain centers to several key organs:

• The heart, to modify the rate and strength of heartbeats (thus changing the amount of blood pumped)

• The kidneys, to regulate the excretion of water (thus changing the volume of blood in circulation)

• The blood vessels, to cause constriction or dilation (thus changing the capacity of the blood vessels)

Therefore, if the blood vessels dilate, which tends to reduce blood pressure, sensors immediately send signals through the brain and to the heart to increase the heart rate, which increases the heart's output of blood. As a result, blood pressure changes little, if at all.

These compensatory mechanisms have limitations, however. For example, when a person bleeds, the heart rate increases, increasing the heart's output, and the blood vessels contract, reducing the capacity of the blood vessels. Nevertheless, if the person loses a lot of blood quickly, the compensatory mechanisms are insufficient, and blood pressure falls. If the bleeding is stopped, fluids from the rest of the body move into the circulation to begin restoring the volume and thus the blood pressure. Eventually, new blood cells are manufactured, and the blood volume is fully restored. Receiving a blood transfusion ▲ restores blood volume quickly.

Low blood pressure also may result from a malfunction in the mechanisms that maintain blood pressure. For instance, if the ability of the nerves to conduct signals is impaired by any disease, the compensatory control mechanisms may not function properly.

▲ see page 738

Selected Causes of Low Blood Pressure

Change in Compensatory Mechanism	Causes
Decreased cardiac output	Abnormal heart rhythms
	Heart muscle damage, loss, or malfunction
	Heart valve disorders
	Pulmonary embolus
Decreased volume of blood	Excessive bleeding
	Diarrhea
	Excessive sweating
	Excessive urination
Increased capacity of blood vessels	Septic shock
	Exposure to heat
	Vasodilator drugs (nitrates, calcium blockers, angiotensin converting enzyme inhibitors)

Fainting

Fainting (syncope) is a sudden brief loss of consciousness.

Fainting is a symptom of an inadequate supply of oxygen and other nutrients to the brain, usually caused by a temporary decrease in blood flow. Such a decrease in blood flow can occur whenever the body can't quickly compensate for a drop in blood pressure. For instance, if a person has an abnormal heart rhythm, the heart may be unable to increase its output of blood enough to compensate for the decrease in blood pressure. People with such conditions may feel fine when resting, but they feel faint when exercising because the body's demand for oxygen increases suddenly; this fainting is called exertional or effort syncope. Often, the person faints *after* exercising. The reason: The heart is barely able to maintain adequate blood pressure during exercise; when the exercise stops, the heart rate begins to fall, but the blood vessels from the muscles remain dilated to remove metabolic waste products. Be-

cause of the combination of reduced heart output and increased capacity of the vessels, blood pressure falls and the person faints.

Obviously, blood volume decreases when a person bleeds. But it also may decrease when a person becomes dehydrated from conditions such as diarrhea, excessive sweating, and excessive urination, which often occurs with untreated diabetes or Addison's disease.

Fainting also can result when the compensatory mechanisms are affected by signals sent via the nerves from other parts of the body. For example, an intestinal cramp may send a signal to the heart via the vagus nerve that slows the heart rate enough to cause a person to faint. Such fainting is called vasomotor or vasovagal syncope. Many other signals—including other pains, fear, and the sight of blood—can lead to this type of fainting.

Fainting from coughing (cough syncope) or urinating (micturition syncope) usually results when the amount of blood flowing back to the heart decreases during straining. Fainting caused by urinating is particularly common in the elderly. Swallowing syncope can accompany diseases of the esophagus.

Fainting may also result from a decrease in the number of red blood cells (anemia), a decrease in the level of blood sugar (hypoglycemia), or a decrease in the level of carbon dioxide in the blood (hypocapnia) caused by overbreathing (hyperventilation). Sometimes, anxiety leads to hyperventilation. When the carbon dioxide level decreases, the blood vessels in the brain contract, and the person may feel faint but not actually lose consciousness. Weight lifter's syncope may result from hyperventilating before lifting.

In rare cases, typically in the elderly, fainting may be part of a mild stroke in which the blood flow to a part of the brain suddenly decreases.

Symptoms

Dizziness or light-headedness may precede fainting, especially when a person is standing. After a person falls, the blood pressure increases, partly because the person is lying down and often because the cause of the fainting has passed. Getting up too quickly may cause the person to faint again.

When the cause is an abnormal heart rhythm, fainting begins and ends suddenly. Sometimes the person experiences palpitations (an awareness of the heart beating) just before fainting.

Orthostatic fainting occurs when a person sits up or stands too quickly.▲ A related form of fainting, called parade ground syncope, occurs when a person stands still for a long time on a hot day. Because the leg muscles aren't being used, they don't push blood up toward the heart; therefore, blood pools in the leg veins, and blood pressure falls.

Vasovagal syncope may occur when a person is sitting or standing and is often preceded by nausea, weakness, yawning, blurring of vision, and sweating. The person becomes ghostly pale, the pulse becomes very slow, and the person faints.

Fainting that begins gradually with warning symptoms and also disappears gradually suggests changes in blood chemistry, such as decreased levels of blood sugar (hypoglycemia) or decreased levels of carbon dioxide in the blood (hypocapnia) caused by hyperventilating. Hypocapnia is often preceded by a pins-and-needles sensation and chest discomfort.

Hysterical fainting is not a true faint. The person only appears to be unconscious but doesn't have a heart rate or blood pressure abnormality and doesn't sweat or turn pale.

Diagnosis

A doctor tries to determine the underlying cause of fainting because some causes are more serious than others. Heart disease, such as an abnormal heart rhythm or aortic valve stenosis, can be fatal; other causes are much less worrisome.

Factors that help a doctor make a diagnosis include the person's age when the fainting episodes began, the circumstances under which fainting occurs, any warning signs before a fainting episode, and the steps that help the person recover—such as lying down, holding the breath, or drinking orange juice. Descriptions from witnesses of the fainting episode may be helpful. A doctor also needs to know whether the person has any medical conditions and whether the person is taking any prescription or nonprescription drugs.

A doctor may be able to re-create a fainting spell under safe conditions by asking the patient to breathe quickly and deeply. Or while monitoring the heartbeat with an electrocardiogram (ECG),■ a doctor may press gently over the carotid sinus (a portion of the internal carotid artery containing sensors that monitor blood pressure).

An electrocardiogram may indicate an underlying heart or lung disease. To find the cause of fainting, a doctor may have a person wear a Holter monitor, a small device that records the heart's rhythms for 24 hours as the person engages in ordinary activities.★ If an irregular heart rhythm coincides with an episode of fainting, it's probably—but not necessarily—the cause.

Other tests, such as echocardiography (an imaging technique that uses ultrasound waves),● can determine whether the heart has a structural or functional abnormality. Blood tests may show that the person has low blood sugar levels (hypoglycemia) or low numbers of red blood cells (anemia). To diagnose epilepsy (which may occasionally be confused with fainting), a doctor may use electroencephalography, a test that shows patterns of electrical brain waves.◆

Treatment

Usually, lying flat is all that's needed for a person to regain consciousness. Raising the legs can speed up recovery by increasing blood flow to the heart and brain. If the person sits up too rapidly or is propped up or carried in an upright position, another fainting episode may occur.

In young people who don't have heart disease, fainting usually isn't serious, and extensive diagnostic investigations and treatment rarely are necessary. However, in older people, fainting may result from several interrelated problems that prevent the heart and blood vessels from adjusting appropriately to a decrease in blood pressure. Treatment depends on the cause.

A heartbeat that's too slow can be corrected by surgically implanting a pacemaker, an electronic device that stimulates heartbeats. Drug therapy can be used to slow a heart rate that's too rapid. A defibrillator can be implanted to jolt the heart back into the normal rhythm if the heart beats irregularly from time to time. Other causes of fainting—such as hypoglycemia, anemia, or low

▲ see page 110

■ see page 73

★ see page 75

● see page 76

◆ see box, page 348

blood volume—can be treated. Surgery is considered for problems with heart valves, regardless of the person's age.

Orthostatic Hypotension

Orthostatic hypotension is an excessive decrease in blood pressure when a person stands up, resulting in reduced blood flow to the brain and fainting.

Orthostatic hypotension isn't a specific disease but an inability to regulate blood pressure quickly. It has many causes.

When a person stands up suddenly, gravity causes some blood to pool in the veins of the legs and lower body. The pooling slightly reduces the amount of blood that returns to the heart and the amount of blood pumped by the heart. As a result, blood pressure falls. The body quickly responds: The heart beats faster, and the contractions are stronger. The blood vessels constrict, so their capacity is smaller. If these compensatory responses fail or are sluggish, orthostatic hypotension occurs.

Most episodes of orthostatic hypotension result as a side effect of drugs, particularly certain drugs given for cardiovascular problems and particularly in elderly people. For example, diuretics, especially powerful ones in high doses, can reduce blood volume by removing fluid from the body and so reduce the blood pressure. Drugs that dilate the blood vessels—such as nitrates, calcium blockers, and angiotensin converting enzyme inhibitors—increase the capacity of the vessels, also lowering blood pressure.

Blood volume can be reduced by bleeding or an excessive loss of fluid from severe vomiting, diarrhea, excessive sweating, untreated diabetes, or Addison's disease.

The sensors within the arteries that trigger compensatory responses can be impaired by certain drugs, including barbiturates, alcohol, and drugs used to treat high blood pressure and depression. Diseases that damage the nerves that regulate blood vessel diameter can also cause orthostatic hypotension. Such damage is a common complication of diabetes, amyloidosis, and spinal cord injuries.

Symptoms and Diagnosis

Most people with orthostatic hypotension experience some faintness, light-headedness, dizziness, confusion, or blurred vision when they get out of bed abruptly or stand up after sitting for a long time. Fatigue, exercise, alcohol, or a heavy meal can make the symptoms worse. A severe decrease in blood flow to the brain can cause the person to faint and even to have convulsions.

When these symptoms occur, a doctor can diagnose orthostatic hypotension. The diagnosis can be confirmed if the blood pressure falls significantly when the person stands, and it returns to normal when the person lies down. A doctor then looks for the cause of the person's orthostatic hypotension.

Prognosis and Treatment

A diabetic person with high blood pressure is likely to have a worse prognosis if he also has orthostatic hypotension. When the cause of orthostatic hypotension is low blood volume or a particular drug or drug dosage, the condition can be corrected rapidly.

When the cause of orthostatic hypotension can't be treated, often the symptoms can be reduced or eliminated. Susceptible people should not sit up or stand up rapidly or remain standing still for long periods. If low blood pressure results from pooling of blood in the legs, fitted elastic hose may help. When orthostatic hypotension results from prolonged bed rest, a person may improve the condition by sitting up for a longer period of time each day.

Ephedrine or phenylephrine may be taken to help keep blood pressure from falling. Blood volume can also be expanded by increasing salt intake and, if necessary, by taking hormones that cause salt retention, such as fludrocortisone. People who don't have heart failure or high blood pressure are often told to salt their food liberally or to take salt tablets. Elderly people with orthostatic hypotension should drink plenty of fluids and little or no alcohol. Because of the salt and fluid retention, a person may quickly gain 3 to 5 pounds, and the high-salt diet can lead to heart failure, particularly in the elderly. If these measures are ineffective, other drugs—including propranolol, dihydroergotamine, indomethacin, and metoclopramide—may help relieve orthostatic hypotension, but there's a significant risk of adverse effects.

Shock

Shock is a life-threatening condition in which blood pressure is too low to sustain life.

Shock results when a low blood volume, an inadequate pumping action of the heart, or excessive relaxation (dilation) of the blood vessel walls (vasodilation) causes severe low blood pressure. This low blood pressure, which is much more severe and prolonged than in fainting (syncope), ▲ causes an inadequate blood supply to body cells. The cells can be quickly and irreversibly damaged and die.

Low blood volume may result from severe bleeding, an excessive loss of body fluids, or inadequate fluid intake. Blood may be rapidly lost because of an accident or internal bleeding, such as that caused by an ulcer in the stomach or intestine, a ruptured blood vessel, or a ruptured ectopic pregnancy (pregnancy outside the uterus). An excessive loss of other body fluids can occur with major burns, inflammation of the pancreas (pancreatitis), perforation of the intestinal wall, severe diarrhea, kidney disease, or excessive use of strong drugs that increase the output of urine (diuretics). Despite feeling thirsty, people may not drink enough fluid to compensate for fluid losses if a physical disability (such as severe joint disease) prevents them from obtaining water without assistance.

An inadequate pumping action of the heart also can result in less than normal amounts of blood being pumped out with every heartbeat. The inadequate pumping action may result from a heart attack, pulmonary embolism, failure of a heart valve (particularly an artificial valve), or an irregular heartbeat.

Excessive dilation of the blood vessel walls may result from a head injury, liver failure, poisoning, overdoses of certain drugs, or severe bacterial infection. (Shock caused by such an infection is called septic shock.)■

Symptoms and Diagnosis

Symptoms of shock are similar, whether the cause is low blood volume or inadequate pumping action of the heart. The condition may begin with tiredness, sleepiness, and confusion. The skin becomes cold and sweaty and often bluish and pale. If the skin is pressed, color returns much more slowly than normal. A bluish network of lines may appear under the skin. The pulse is weak and rapid, unless a slow heartbeat is causing the shock. The person usually breathes rapidly, but breathing and the pulse may both slow down if death is imminent. The blood pressure drops so low that it often can't be measured with a blood pressure cuff. Eventually, the person can't sit up without passing out and may die.

When shock results from excessive dilation of blood vessels, the symptoms are somewhat different. For instance, the skin may be warm and flushed, particularly at first.★

In the earliest stages of shock, especially septic shock, many symptoms may be absent or undetected unless they're specifically looked for. The blood pressure is very low. Urine flow is also very low, and waste products build up in the blood.

Prognosis and Treatment

If untreated, shock is usually fatal. If shock is treated, the outlook depends on the cause, other illnesses the person has, the amount of time before treatment begins, and the type of treatment given. Regardless of treatment, the likelihood of death from shock after a massive heart attack or from septic shock in an elderly patient is high.

The first person to arrive on the scene should keep the victim warm and raise the legs slightly to facilitate the return of blood to the heart. Any bleeding should be stopped, and breathing should be checked. The victim's head should be turned to the side to prevent inhalation of vomit. Nothing should be given by mouth.

▲ see page 108

■ see page 860

★ see page 860

Emergency medical personnel may provide mechanically assisted breathing. Any drugs are given intravenously. Narcotics, sedatives, and tranquilizers generally aren't given because they tend to decrease blood pressure. Attempts may be made to increase blood pressure with military (or medical) antishock trousers (MAST). These pants apply pressure to the lower body, thus driving blood from the legs to the heart and brain. Fluid is given intravenously. Usually, blood is cross-matched before a blood transfusion, but in an urgent situation when there's no time for cross-matching, type O negative blood can be given to anyone.

The intravenous fluid and blood transfusion may be too little to counteract the shock if bleeding or fluid loss continues or if the shock is caused by a heart attack or another problem unrelated to blood volume. Drugs that constrict the blood vessels may be given to boost blood flow to the brain or heart, but they should be used as briefly as possible because they can reduce blood flow to the tissues.

When shock is caused by an inadequate pumping action of the heart, efforts are made to improve the heart's performance. The rate and rhythm abnormalities of the heartbeat are corrected, and blood volume is increased if necessary. Atropine may be used to increase a slow heartbeat, and other drugs may be given to improve the ability of the heart muscle to contract.

In those with a heart attack, a balloon pump can be inserted into the aorta to reverse shock temporarily. After this procedure, emergency coronary artery bypass surgery or surgery to correct heart defects may be needed.

In some cases of shock after a heart attack, emergency percutaneous transluminal coronary angioplasty to open the blocked artery▲ can improve the damaged heart's inadequate pumping action and the resulting shock. Before this procedure, patients usually receive intravenous drugs to break up clots (thrombolytic drugs). If emergency percutaneous transluminal coronary angioplasty or cardiac surgery is *not* performed, a thrombolytic drug is given as soon as possible, unless it could worsen other medical problems the patient has.

Shock caused by excessive dilation of the blood vessels is treated primarily with drugs that constrict the vessels while the underlying cause of the excessive dilation is being corrected.

CHAPTER 25

High Blood Pressure

High blood pressure (hypertension) is generally a symptomless condition in which abnormally high pressure in the arteries increases the risk of problems such as stroke, aneurysm, heart failure, heart attack, and kidney damage.

To many people, the word hypertension suggests excessive tension, nervousness, or stress. In medical terms, however, hypertension refers to a condition of elevated blood pressure, regardless of the cause. It has been called "the silent killer" because it usually doesn't cause symptoms for many years—until a vital organ is damaged.

▲ see page 125 and box, page 126

The number of Americans who have high blood pressure is estimated to be more than 50 million. It occurs more often in blacks—38 percent of black adults have high blood pressure, compared with 29 percent of whites. At any given blood pressure level, the consequences of high blood pressure are worse in blacks.

In the United States, only an estimated two out of three people with high blood pressure have been diagnosed. Of these people, about 75 percent receive drug treatment, and of these, about 45 percent receive adequate treatment.

When blood pressure is checked, two values are recorded. The higher one occurs when the heart contracts (systole); the lower occurs when the heart relaxes between beats (diastole). Blood pressure is written as the systolic pressure followed by a slash followed by the diastolic pressure—for example, 120/80 mm Hg (millimeters of mercury). This reading would be referred to as "one-twenty over eighty."

High blood pressure is defined as a systolic pressure at rest that averages 140 mm Hg or more, a diastolic pressure at rest that averages 90 mm Hg or more, or both. In high blood pressure, usually both the systolic and the diastolic pressures are elevated.

In **isolated systolic hypertension,** the systolic pressure is 140 mm Hg or more, but the diastolic pressure is less than 90 mm Hg—that is, the diastolic pressure is in the normal range. Isolated systolic hypertension is increasingly common with advancing age. In almost everyone, blood pressure increases with age, with systolic pressure increasing until at least age 80 and diastolic pressure increasing until age 55 to 60, then leveling off or even falling.

Malignant hypertension is a particularly severe form of high blood pressure that, if left untreated, usually leads to death in 3 to 6 months. It's fairly rare, occurring in only about 1 in every 200 people who have high blood pressure, but it's several times more common in blacks than in whites, in men than in women, and in people of lower socioeconomic status than in those of higher socioeconomic status. Malignant hypertension is a medical emergency.

Control of Blood Pressure

The pressure in the arteries can be increased in various ways. For one, the heart can pump with more force, putting out more fluid each second. Another possibility is that the large arteries can lose their normal flexibility and become stiff, so that they can't expand when the heart pumps blood through them. Thus, the blood from each heartbeat is forced through less space than normal, and the pressure increases. That's what happens in elderly people whose arterial walls become thickened and stiff because of arteriosclerosis. Blood pressure is similarly increased in vasoconstriction—when the tiny arteries (arterioles) are temporarily constricted as a result of stimulation by nerves or by hormones in the blood. A third way in which the pressure in the

<table>
<tr><td>

Ups and Downs of Blood Pressure

Blood pressure varies naturally over a person's life. Infants and children normally have much lower blood pressure than adults. Activity also affects blood pressure, which is higher when a person is active and lower when a person rests. Blood pressure varies with the time of day, too: It's highest in the morning and lowest at night during sleep.

</td></tr>
</table>

arteries can be increased is for more fluid to be added to the system. This happens when the kidneys malfunction and aren't able to remove enough salt and water from the body. The volume of blood in the body increases, so the blood pressure increases.

Conversely, if the heart's pumping activity diminishes, if the arteries are dilated, or if fluid is removed from the system, the pressure falls. Adjustments of these factors are governed by changes in kidney function and in the autonomic nervous system—the part of the nervous system that regulates many body functions automatically.

The sympathetic nervous system, which is part of the autonomic nervous system, temporarily increases blood pressure during the fight-or-flight response (the body's physical reaction to a threat). The sympathetic nervous system increases both the speed and force of the heartbeats. It also narrows most arterioles, but it expands those in certain areas, such as in skeletal muscle, where an increased blood supply is needed. In addition, the sympathetic nervous system decreases the kidney's excretion of salt and water, thereby increasing the body's blood volume. The sympathetic nervous system also releases the hormones epinephrine (adrenaline) and norepinephrine (noradrenaline), which stimulate the heart and blood vessels.

The kidneys control blood pressure in several ways. If blood pressure rises, they increase their

Regulating Blood Pressure: The Renin-Angiotensin-Aldosterone System

A fall in blood pressure (1) causes the release of renin—a kidney enzyme.

Renin (2) in turn activates angiotensin (3), a hormone that causes the muscular walls of the small arteries (arterioles) to constrict, increasing blood pressure.

Angiotensin also triggers the release of the hormone aldosterone from the adrenal gland (4), which causes the kidney to retain salt (sodium) and excrete potassium. The sodium retains water, thus expanding the blood volume and increasing blood pressure.

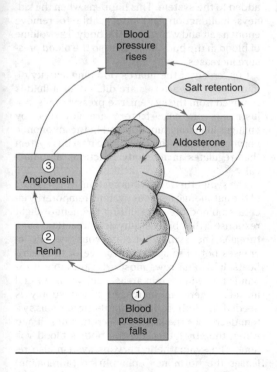

excretion of salt and water, which lowers blood volume and brings the blood pressure back down to normal. Conversely, if blood pressure falls, the kidneys decrease their excretion of salt and water, so that blood volume increases and blood pressure returns to normal. The kidneys also can in-

crease blood pressure by secreting an enzyme called renin, which triggers the production of a hormone called angiotensin, which in turn triggers the release of a hormone called aldosterone.

Because the kidneys are important in controlling blood pressure, many kidney diseases and abnormalities can cause high blood pressure. For example, a narrowing of the artery supplying one of the kidneys (renal artery stenosis) can cause hypertension. Kidney inflammation of various types and injury to one or both kidneys can also cause blood pressure to rise.

Whenever a change causes an increase in blood pressure, a compensatory mechanism is triggered to counteract it and keep the pressure at normal levels. So an increase in the volume of blood pumped out by the heart, which tends to increase blood pressure, causes the blood vessels to dilate and the kidneys to increase their excretion of salt and water, which tends to reduce blood pressure. However, the presence of arteriosclerosis makes arteries stiff and prevents the dilation that would otherwise lower blood pressure back to normal. Arteriosclerotic changes in the kidney can impair the kidneys' ability to excrete salt and water, which tends to increase blood pressure.

Causes

In about 90 percent of people with high blood pressure, the cause isn't known and the condition is referred to as essential or primary hypertension. Essential hypertension probably has more than one cause. Several changes in the heart and blood vessels probably combine to elevate the blood pressure.

When the cause is known, the condition is called secondary hypertension. In 5 to 10 percent of the people with high blood pressure, the cause is kidney disease. In 1 to 2 percent, the cause is a condition such as a hormonal disorder or the use of certain drugs such as oral contraceptives (birth control pills). A rare cause of high blood pressure, pheochromocytoma is a tumor of the adrenal gland that produces the hormones epinephrine (adrenaline) and norepinephrine (noradrenaline).

Obesity, a sedentary lifestyle, stress, and excessive amounts of alcohol or salt in food all can play a role in the development of high blood pressure in people who have an inherited sensitivity.

Stress tends to cause the blood pressure to increase temporarily, but blood pressure usually returns to normal once the stress is over. This explains "white coat hypertension," in which the stress of visiting a doctor's office causes the blood pressure to rise high enough to be diagnosed as high blood pressure in someone who, at other times, has normal blood pressure. In susceptible people, these brief increases in blood pressure are thought to cause damage that eventually results in permanently high blood pressure, even though the stress may no longer be present. This theory that temporary high blood pressure can give rise to permanent high blood pressure hasn't been proved.

Symptoms

In most people, high blood pressure causes no symptoms, despite the coincidental occurrence of certain symptoms that are widely—but erroneously—believed to be associated with high blood pressure: headaches, nosebleeds, dizziness, flushed face, and tiredness. Although people with high blood pressure may have these symptoms, they occur just as frequently in those with normal blood pressure.

If a person has high blood pressure that's severe or long-standing and untreated, symptoms such as headache, fatigue, nausea, vomiting, shortness of breath, restlessness, and blurred vision occur because of damage to the brain, eyes, heart, and kidneys. Occasionally, people with severe high blood pressure develop drowsiness and even coma caused by brain swelling. This condition, called hypertensive encephalopathy, requires emergency treatment.

Diagnosis

Blood pressure is measured after the person sits or lies for 5 minutes. A reading of 140/90 mm Hg or more is considered high, but a diagnosis can't be based on a single high reading. Sometimes, even several high readings aren't enough to make the diagnosis. If a person has an initial high reading, the blood pressure is measured again and then measured twice on at least two other days to make sure that the high blood pressure persists. The readings not only determine the presence of high blood pressure but also are used to classify its severity.

After high blood pressure has been diagnosed, its effects on key organs, especially the blood vessels, heart, brain, and kidneys, are usually evaluated. The retina (the light-sensitive membrane on the inner surface of the back of the eye) is the only place where a doctor can directly view the effects of high blood pressure on arterioles. The assumption is that the changes in the retina are similar to changes in blood vessels elsewhere in the body, such as the kidneys. To examine the retina, a doctor uses an ophthalmoscope (an instrument that provides a view of the inside of the eye). By determining the degree of damage to the retina (retinopathy), a doctor can classify the seriousness of the high blood pressure.

Changes in the heart—particularly enlargement because of the increased work required to

Classifying Blood Pressure in Adults

When a person's systolic and diastolic pressures fall into different categories, the higher category is used to classify blood pressure.

For instance, 160/92 is classified as stage 2 hypertension, and 180/120 is classified as stage 4 hypertension.

The optimal blood pressure for minimizing the risk of cardiovascular problems is below 120/80 mm Hg. However, unusually low readings must be evaluated.

Category	Systolic Blood Pressure	Diastolic Blood Pressure
Normal blood pressure	Below 130 mm Hg	Below 85 mm Hg
High normal blood pressure	130–139	85–89
Stage 1 (mild) hypertension	140–159	90–99
Stage 2 (moderate) hypertension	160–179	100–109
Stage 3 (severe) hypertension	180–209	110–119
Stage 4 (very severe) hypertension	210 or higher	120 or higher

pump blood at the increased pressure—can be detected by electrocardiography▲ and chest x-rays. In the early stages, such changes are best detected by echocardiography (a test that uses ultrasound waves to create an image of the heart).■ An abnormal heart sound, called the fourth heart sound, which can be heard with a stethoscope, is one of the earliest heart changes caused by high blood pressure.

Early indications of kidney damage are detected primarily by examining the person's urine. The presence of blood cells and albumin (a type of protein) in the urine, for example, can indicate such damage.

A doctor also looks for the cause of the high blood pressure, especially in a younger person, even though a cause is identified in less than 10 percent of people. The higher the blood pressure

and the younger the patient, the more extensive the search for a cause is likely to be. The evaluation may include x-ray and radioisotope studies of the kidney, a chest x-ray, and examinations of blood and urine for certain hormones.

To detect a kidney problem, a doctor first takes a medical history, asking about previous kidney problems. Then during the physical examination, the area of the abdomen over the kidneys is checked for tenderness. A stethoscope is placed over the abdomen to listen for a bruit (the sound caused by blood rushing through a narrowing in the artery supplying the kidney). A urine specimen may be sent to the laboratory for analysis, and x-rays or ultrasound scans of the kidney's blood supply and other tests of the kidneys are performed, if necessary.

When pheochromocytoma is the cause, breakdown products of the hormones epinephrine (adrenaline) and norepinephrine (noradrenaline) show up in the urine. Usually, these hormones also produce various combinations of severe headache, anxiety, an awareness of a rapid or

▲ see page 73

■ see page 76

irregular heart rate (palpitations), excessive perspiration, tremor, and paleness.

Other rare causes of high blood pressure may be detected by certain routine tests. For example, measuring the potassium level in the blood can help detect hyperaldosteronism,▲ and measuring the blood pressure in both arms and legs can help detect coarctation of the aorta.

Prognosis

Untreated high blood pressure increases a person's risk of developing heart disease (such as heart failure or heart attack), kidney failure, and stroke at an early age. High blood pressure is the most important risk factor for stroke. It's also one of the three major risk factors for heart attack (myocardial infarction) that a person can do something about; the other two are smoking and high blood cholesterol levels. Treatment that lowers high blood pressure greatly decreases the risk of stroke and heart failure. Such treatment may also decrease the risk of heart attack, although not as dramatically. Without treatment, fewer than 5 percent of people with malignant hypertension survive for a year.

Treatment

Essential hypertension can't be cured, but it can be treated to prevent complications. Because high blood pressure itself has no symptoms, doctors try to avoid treatments that make people feel bad or interfere with their lifestyle. Before any drugs are prescribed, alternative measures are usually tried.

Overweight people with high blood pressure are advised to reduce their weight to ideal levels. Changes in diet for those with diabetes, obesity, or high blood cholesterol levels also are important for overall cardiovascular health. Cutting down to less than 2.3 grams of sodium or 6 grams of sodium chloride a day (while maintaining an adequate intake of calcium, magnesium, and potassium) and reducing daily alcohol intake to less than 24 ounces of beer, 8 ounces of wine, or 2 ounces of 100-proof whiskey may make drug therapy for high blood pressure unnecessary. Moderate aerobic exercise is helpful. People with essential hypertension don't have to restrict their activities as long as their blood pressure is controlled. Smokers should stop smoking.

Often, doctors recommend that people with high blood pressure should monitor their blood pressure at home. Those who monitor their own blood pressure are probably more likely to follow a doctor's recommendations regarding treatment.

Drug Therapy

Virtually any person with high blood pressure can get it under control with the wide variety of drugs available, but treatment has to be tailored to the individual. Treatment is most effective when patients and doctors communicate well and collaborate on the treatment program.

Experts don't agree on how much blood pressure should be lowered during treatment or on when and how stage 1 (mild) high blood pressure should be treated. But there is agreement that the higher the blood pressure, the greater the risks—even within the normal blood pressure range. So some experts point out that any elevation, however small, should be treated and that the more the blood pressure is lowered, the better. Other experts say that treatment of blood pressures below a certain level may actually increase the risks of heart attack and sudden death rather than reduce them, particularly in people with coronary artery disease.

Different types of drugs reduce blood pressure by different mechanisms. Some doctors use a stepped approach to drug therapy: They start with one type of drug and add others as necessary. Other doctors prefer a sequential approach: They prescribe one drug; if it's ineffective, they discontinue it and prescribe another type of drug. In choosing a drug, a doctor considers such factors as the person's age, sex, and race; the severity of the high blood pressure; the presence of other conditions, such as diabetes or high blood cholesterol levels; the potential side effects, which vary from drug to drug; and the costs of the drugs and of tests needed to monitor their safety.

Most people tolerate their prescribed antihypertensive drugs without problems. But any antihypertensive drug can cause side effects. So if side effects do develop, a person should tell the doctor, who can adjust the dose or switch to another drug.

▲ see page 715

A **thiazide diuretic** is commonly the first drug given to treat high blood pressure. Diuretics help the kidneys eliminate salt and water, which decreases fluid volume throughout the body, thus lowering blood pressure. Diuretics also cause blood vessels to dilate. Because diuretics cause a loss of potassium in the urine, potassium supplements or potassium-retaining drugs sometimes must be taken along with the diuretics. Diuretics are particularly useful in blacks, the elderly, obese people, and people with heart failure or chronic kidney failure.

Adrenergic blockers—a group of drugs that includes the alpha-blockers, beta-blockers, and the alpha-beta blocker labetalol—block the effects of the sympathetic nervous system, the system that may rapidly respond to stress by raising blood pressure. The most commonly used adrenergic blockers, the beta-blockers are particularly useful in whites, young people, and people who have had a heart attack or who have rapid heart rates, angina pectoris (chest pain), or migraine headaches.

Angiotensin converting enzyme inhibitors lower blood pressure by dilating arteries. They are particularly useful in whites, young people, people with heart failure, people with protein in their urine because of chronic kidney disease or diabetic kidney disease, and men who are impotent as a side effect of taking another drug.

Angiotensin II blockers lower blood pressure by a mechanism similar to—but more direct than—the one used by angiotensin converting enzyme inhibitors. Because of the way they work, angiotensin II blockers appear to cause fewer side effects.

Calcium antagonists cause blood vessels to dilate by a completely different mechanism. They are particularly useful in blacks, the elderly, and people with angina pectoris (chest pain), certain types of rapid heart rates, or migraine headaches. Recent reports suggest that people using short-acting calcium antagonists may have an increased risk of death from heart attacks, but there are no reports suggesting such effects for long-acting calcium antagonists.

Direct vasodilators dilate blood vessels by yet another mechanism. A drug of this class is almost never used alone; rather, it's added as a second drug when another drug alone doesn't lower blood pressure sufficiently.

Hypertensive emergencies—for example, malignant hypertension—require rapid lowering of the blood pressure. Several drugs can lower blood pressure quickly; most of them are given intravenously. These drugs include diazoxide, nitroprusside, nitroglycerin, and labetalol. Nifedipine, a calcium antagonist, is very fast acting and can be given orally; however, it can cause hypotension, so the patient must be monitored closely.

Secondary Hypertension Treatment

Treatment of secondary hypertension depends on the underlying cause of the high blood pressure. Treating kidney disease can sometimes normalize the blood pressure or at least lower it, so that drug therapy is more effective. A narrowed artery to the kidney may be dilated by inserting a balloon-tipped catheter and inflating the balloon. Or the narrowed part of the artery supplying the kidney can be bypassed; often such surgery cures the high blood pressure. Tumors that cause high blood pressure, such as pheochromocytoma, usually can be removed surgically.

CHAPTER 26

Atherosclerosis

Arteriosclerosis is a general term for several diseases in which the wall of an artery becomes thicker and less elastic. The most important and most common of these diseases is atherosclerosis, in which fatty material accumulates under the inner lining of the arterial wall.

Atherosclerosis can affect the arteries of the brain, heart, kidneys, other vital organs, and the arms and legs. When atherosclerosis develops in the arteries that supply the brain (carotid arteries), a stroke may occur; when it develops in the arteries that supply the heart (coronary arteries), a heart attack may occur.

In the United States and most other Western countries, atherosclerosis is the leading cause of illness and death. In the United States alone, it caused almost 1 million deaths in 1992—twice as many as from cancer and 10 times as many as from accidents. Despite significant medical advances, coronary artery disease (which results from atherosclerosis and causes heart attacks) and atherosclerotic stroke are responsible for more deaths than all other causes combined.

Causes

Atherosclerosis begins when white blood cells called monocytes migrate from the bloodstream into the wall of the artery and are transformed into cells that accumulate fatty materials. In time, these fat-laden monocytes accumulate, leading to a patchy thickening in the inner lining of the artery. Each area of thickening (called an atherosclerotic plaque or atheroma) is filled with a soft cheeselike substance consisting of various fatty materials, principally cholesterol, smooth muscle cells, and connective tissue cells. Atheromas may be scattered throughout the medium and large arteries, but usually they form where the arteries branch off—presumably because the constant turbulence at these areas injures the arterial wall, making it more susceptible to atheroma formation.

Arteries affected with atherosclerosis lose their elasticity, and as the atheromas grow, the arteries narrow. With time, the atheromas collect calcium deposits, may become brittle, and may rupture. Blood may then enter a ruptured atheroma, making it larger, so that it narrows the artery even more. A ruptured atheroma also may spill its fatty contents and trigger the formation of a blood clot (thrombus). The clot may further narrow or even occlude the artery, or it may detach and float downstream where it causes an occlusion (embolism).

Symptoms

Usually, atherosclerosis doesn't produce symptoms until it severely narrows the artery, or until

How Atherosclerosis Develops

Atherosclerosis begins when white blood cells called monocytes migrate from the bloodstream into the wall of the artery and are transformed into cells that accumulate fatty materials. In time, a patchy thickening (plaque) develops in the inner lining of the artery.

Cross Section of an Artery

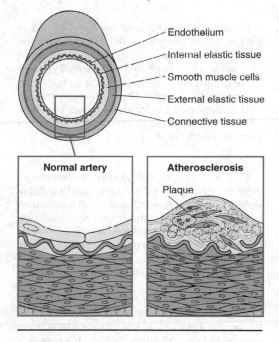

- Endothelium
- Internal elastic tissue
- Smooth muscle cells
- External elastic tissue
- Connective tissue

Normal artery

Atherosclerosis

Plaque

it causes a sudden obstruction. Symptoms depend on where the atherosclerosis develops; thus, they may reflect problems in the heart, the brain, the legs, or almost anywhere in the body.

As atherosclerosis severely narrows an artery, the areas of the body it serves may not receive enough blood, which carries oxygen to the tissues. The first symptom of a narrowing artery may be pain or cramps at times when the blood flow can't keep up with the body's demand for oxygen. For instance, during exercise, a person

What Is Arteriolosclerosis?

Arteriolosclerosis is a less common type of arteriosclerosis that primarily affects the inner and middle layers of the walls of small muscular arteries (arterioles). This disease occurs mainly in people who have high blood pressure.

may feel chest pain (angina) because of a lack of oxygen to the heart, or while walking, a person may feel leg cramps (intermittent claudication) because of a lack of oxygen to the legs. Typically, these symptoms develop gradually as the atheroma slowly narrows the artery. However, when an obstruction occurs suddenly—for example, when a blood clot lodges in an artery—the symptoms come on suddenly.

Risk Factors

The risk of developing atherosclerosis increases with high blood pressure, high blood cholesterol levels, cigarette smoking, diabetes, obesity, a lack of exercise, and advancing age. Having a close relative who developed atherosclerosis at an early age also puts a person at risk. Men have a higher risk than women, though after menopause, the risk increases in women and eventually equals that in men.

People with the inherited disease homocystinuria develop extensive atheroma formation, particularly at a young age. The disease affects many arteries but doesn't primarily affect the coronary arteries, which supply the heart. In contrast, in the inherited disease familial hypercholesterolemia, extremely high levels of blood cholesterol cause atheromas to form in the coronary arteries much more than in other arteries.

▲ see page 681

■ see page 117

★ see page 272

Prevention and Treatment

To help prevent atherosclerosis, a person needs to eliminate the controllable risk factors—high blood cholesterol levels, high blood pressure, cigarette smoking, obesity, and lack of exercise. So depending on a particular person's risk factors, prevention may consist of lowering cholesterol levels, ▲ lowering blood pressure, ■ quitting smoking, losing weight, and beginning an exercise program.★ Fortunately, taking steps to achieve some of these goals helps achieve others. For instance, starting an exercise program helps a person lose weight, which in turn helps lower cholesterol levels and blood pressure. Quitting smoking helps lower cholesterol levels and blood pressure.

In people who already have a high risk of heart disease, smoking is particularly dangerous. Cigarette smoking decreases the level of good cholesterol (high-density lipoprotein cholesterol or HDL cholesterol) and increases the level of bad cholesterol (low-density lipoprotein cholesterol or LDL cholesterol). Smoking also raises the level of carbon monoxide in the blood, which may increase the risk of injury to the lining of the arterial wall, and smoking constricts arteries already narrowed by atherosclerosis, further decreasing the amount of blood reaching the tissues. Plus, smoking increases the blood's tendency to clot, so it increases the risk of peripheral arterial disease, coronary artery disease, stroke, and obstruction of an arterial graft after surgery.

A smoker's risk of coronary artery disease is directly related to the number of cigarettes smoked daily. People who quit smoking have only half the risk of those who continue to smoke—regardless of how long they smoked before quitting. Quitting also decreases the risk of death after coronary artery bypass surgery or a heart attack. Additionally, quitting decreases illness and the risk of death in those who have atherosclerosis in arteries other than those that supply the heart and brain.

In short, the best treatment for atherosclerosis is prevention. When atherosclerosis becomes severe enough to cause complications, a doctor must treat the complications themselves—angina, heart attack, abnormal heart rhythms, heart failure, kidney failure, stroke, or obstructed peripheral arteries.

Coronary Artery Disease

Coronary artery disease is a condition in which fatty deposits accumulate in the cells lining the wall of a coronary artery and obstruct the blood flow.

Fatty deposits (called atheromas or plaques) build up gradually and are scattered in the large branches of the two main coronary arteries, which encircle the heart and supply it with blood; this gradual process is known as atherosclerosis.▲ Atheromas bulge into the arteries, narrowing them. As the atheromas enlarge, portions may rupture and enter the bloodstream, or small blood clots may form on their surfaces.

For the heart to contract and pump blood normally, the heart muscle (myocardium) requires a continuous supply of oxygen-enriched blood from the coronary arteries. But as an obstruction of a coronary artery worsens, ischemia (inadequate blood supply) to the heart muscle can develop, causing heart damage. The most common cause of myocardial ischemia is coronary artery disease. The major complications of coronary artery disease are angina and heart attack (myocardial infarction).

Coronary artery disease affects people of all races, but the incidence is extremely high among whites. However, race itself doesn't seem to be as important a factor as a person's lifestyle: Specifically, a high-fat diet, smoking, and a sedentary lifestyle increase the risk of coronary artery disease.

In the United States, cardiovascular disease is the leading cause of death among both sexes, and coronary artery disease is the major cause of cardiovascular disease. The death rate is higher for men than for women, especially between the ages of 35 and 55. After age 55, the death rate for men declines, and the rate for women continues to climb. Compared with the death rates for whites, those for black men are higher until age 60 and those for black women are higher until age 75.

Angina

Angina, also called angina pectoris, is temporary chest pain or a sensation of pressure that occurs while heart muscle isn't receiving enough oxygen.

The heart's oxygen needs are determined by how hard the heart is working—how fast the heart

is beating and how strong the beats are. Physical exertion and emotions make the heart work harder and thus increase the heart's oxygen needs. When the arteries are narrowed or blocked so that blood flow to the muscle can't increase to meet the need for more oxygen, ischemia may occur, resulting in pain.

Causes

Usually, angina results from coronary artery disease. But it can result from other causes, including abnormalities of the aortic valve, especially aortic valve stenosis (narrowing of the aortic valve), aortic valve regurgitation (leakage of the aortic valve), and hypertrophic subaortic stenosis.■ Because the aortic valve is near the entrance to the coronary arteries, these abnormalities reduce blood flow through the coronary arteries. Arterial spasm (sudden temporary constriction of an artery) may also cause angina, and severe anemia may reduce the supply of oxygen to the heart muscle, triggering angina.

Symptoms

Not everyone with ischemia experiences angina. Ischemia without angina is called silent ischemia. Doctors don't understand why ischemia is sometimes silent.

Most commonly, a person feels angina as a pressure or ache beneath the sternum (breastbone). Pain also may occur in the left shoulder or down the inside of the left arm; through the back; in the throat, jaw, or teeth; and occasionally down the right arm. Many people describe the feeling as discomfort rather than pain.

Typically, angina is triggered by physical activity, lasts no more than a few minutes, and subsides with rest. Some people experience angina predictably with a certain degree of exertion. In other people, episodes occur unpredictably. Often, angina is worse when exertion follows a meal. And it's usually worse in cold weather. Walking into the wind or moving from a warm room into

---

▲ see page 118

■ see pages 96–97

Fatty Deposits in a Coronary Artery

As fatty deposits accumulate in a coronary artery, blood flow is reduced and the heart muscle is deprived of oxygen.

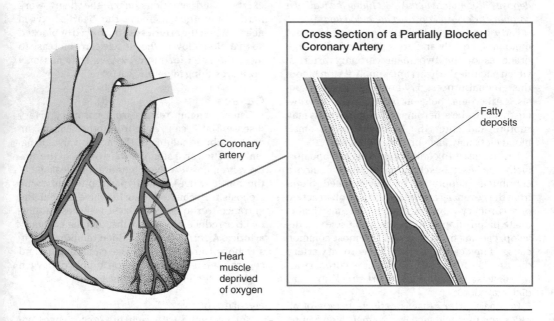

Cross Section of a Partially Blocked Coronary Artery

Coronary artery

Fatty deposits

Heart muscle deprived of oxygen

the cold air may start an angina attack. Emotional stress may also cause or worsen angina. Sometimes, experiencing a strong emotion while resting or experiencing a bad dream during sleep can cause angina.

Variant angina results from a spasm of the large coronary arteries on the surface of the heart. It's called variant because it's characterized by pain while *at rest*, not on exertion, and by certain changes in the electrocardiogram (ECG) during an episode of angina.

Unstable angina refers to angina in which the pattern of symptoms changes. Because the characteristics of angina in a given person usually remain constant, any change—such as more severe pain, more frequent attacks, or attacks occurring with less exertion or during rest—is serious. Such changes in symptoms usually reflect a rapid progression of coronary artery disease, with an increasing obstruction of a coronary artery be-

cause an atheroma has ruptured or a clot has formed. The risk of a heart attack is high. Unstable angina is a medical emergency.

Diagnosis

A doctor diagnoses angina largely by a person's description of the symptoms. Between and even during attacks of angina, a physical examination or an ECG may reveal little, if anything, abnormal. During an attack, the heart rate may increase slightly, blood pressure may go up, and a doctor may hear a characteristic change in the heartbeat while listening with a stethoscope. During an attack of typical angina, a doctor may detect changes in the ECG, but the ECG may be normal between episodes, even in a person with extensive coronary artery disease.

When symptoms are typical, the diagnosis is usually easy for a doctor. The kind of pain, its location, and its association with exertion, meals, weather, and other factors may help a doctor make the diagnosis. Certain tests may help determine the severity of the ischemia and the presence and extent of coronary artery disease.▲

Exercise tolerance testing (a test in which the person walks on a treadmill while being monitored by an ECG) can help in evaluating the severity of coronary artery disease and the ability of the heart to respond to ischemia. The results also may help determine the need for coronary arteriography or surgery.

Radionuclide imaging combined with exercise tolerance testing may provide a doctor with valuable information about a person's angina. Radionuclide imaging not only confirms the presence of ischemia but also identifies the region and amount of heart muscle affected and shows the amount of blood flow reaching the heart muscle.

Exercise echocardiography is a test in which images (echocardiograms) are obtained by bouncing ultrasound waves off the heart. The test is harmless and shows heart size, movement of the heart muscle, blood flow through the heart valves, and valve function. Echocardiograms are obtained at rest and at peak exercise. When ischemia is present, the pumping motion of the wall of the left ventricle is abnormal.

Coronary arteriography may be performed when a diagnosis of coronary artery disease or ischemia isn't certain. However, most commonly, this test is used to determine the severity of coronary artery disease and to help evaluate whether the person needs a procedure to improve blood flow—either coronary artery bypass surgery or angioplasty.

In a few people with typical symptoms of angina and an abnormal exercise tolerance test, coronary arteriography doesn't confirm the presence of coronary artery disease. In some of these people, the small arteries in the heart muscle are abnormally constricted. Many questions remain about this condition, which some experts call syndrome X. Usually, symptoms improve when people with this syndrome take nitrates or beta-blocker drugs. The prognosis for someone with syndrome X is good.

Continuous ECG monitoring with a Holter monitor (a portable, battery-powered ECG recorder) reveals abnormalities indicating silent ischemia in some patients. Doctors debate the significance of silent ischemia, but generally the severity of coronary artery disease determines the extent of

Cholesterol and Coronary Artery Disease

The risk of coronary artery disease increases with elevated levels of total cholesterol and low-density lipoprotein cholesterol (LDL cholesterol or bad cholesterol) in the blood. The risk of coronary artery disease decreases with elevated levels of high-density lipoprotein cholesterol (HDL cholesterol or good cholesterol).

Diet influences the total cholesterol level—and thus the risk of coronary artery disease. The typical American diet increases total cholesterol levels. Changing the diet (and taking prescribed drugs if needed) can lower cholesterol levels. Lowering levels of total cholesterol and bad cholesterol slows or reverses the progress of coronary artery disease.

The benefits of lowering levels of bad cholesterol are greatest in patients with other risk factors of coronary artery disease. These risk factors include cigarette smoking, high blood pressure, obesity, inactivity, high triglyceride levels, a genetic predisposition, and male steroids (androgens). Quitting smoking, lowering blood pressure, losing weight, and increasing exercise decrease the risk of coronary artery disease.

silent ischemia and therefore the prognosis. An ECG also helps diagnose variant angina by detecting certain changes that occur when angina develops during rest.

Angiography (movie-type x-rays of arteries taken after a dye is injected) sometimes can detect spasm in coronary arteries that don't have an atheroma. Sometimes, certain drugs are given to produce the spasm during angiography.

Prognosis

Key factors in predicting what may happen to people who have angina include age, the extent

▲ see page 73

of coronary artery disease, the severity of symptoms, and, most of all, the degree of normal heart muscle function. The more coronary arteries affected or the worse the blockage of the arteries, the poorer the prognosis. The prognosis is surprisingly good in a person with stable angina and normal pumping ability (ventricular muscle function). Reduced pumping ability dramatically worsens the outlook.

Treatment

Treatment begins with attempts to prevent coronary artery disease, to slow its progression, or to reverse it by dealing with its known causes (risk factors). Primary risk factors, such as elevated blood pressure and elevated cholesterol levels, are treated promptly. Cigarette smoking is the most important preventable risk factor in coronary artery disease.

Treatment of angina depends partially on the severity and stability of the symptoms. When symptoms are stable and mild to moderate, reducing risk factors and using drugs may be most effective. When symptoms get worse rapidly, immediate hospitalization and drug treatment are usual. If the symptoms don't markedly subside with drug treatment, diet, and lifestyle changes, angiography may be used to determine if coronary artery bypass surgery or angioplasty is feasible.

Stable Angina Treatment

Treatment is designed to prevent or reduce ischemia and minimize symptoms. Four types of drugs are available: beta-blockers, nitrates, calcium antagonists, and antiplatelet drugs.

Beta-blockers interfere with the effects of the hormones epinephrine (adrenaline) and norepinephrine (noradrenaline) on the heart and other organs. The drugs reduce the resting heart rate. During exercise, they limit the increase in heart rate and so reduce the demand for oxygen. Beta-blockers and nitrates have been shown to reduce heart attacks and sudden death, improving the long-term outcome in people with coronary artery disease.

Nitrates, such as nitroglycerin, dilate the walls of the blood vessels. Either short-acting or long-acting nitrates can be taken. A tablet of nitroglycerin placed under the tongue (sublingual administration) usually relieves an episode of angina in 1 to 3 minutes; the effects of this short-acting nitrate last 30 minutes. People with chronic stable angina should keep nitroglycerin tablets or spray with them at all times. Taking a tablet just before reaching a level of exertion known to induce angina also may be useful. Nitroglycerin may also be taken by placing a tablet next to the gum or by inhaling an oral spray, but sublingual administration is most common. Long-acting nitrates are taken 1 to 4 times a day. Nitrate skin patches and paste, in which the drug is absorbed through the skin over many hours, are also effective. Long-acting nitrates taken regularly can soon lose their ability to provide relief. Most experts recommend 8- to 12-hour periods without taking the drug to maintain long-term effectiveness.

Calcium antagonists prevent the blood vessels from constricting and can counter coronary artery spasm. These drugs also are effective in treating variant angina. Some calcium antagonists, such as verapamil and diltiazem, may slow the heart rate. This effect can be useful in some people, and these drugs may be combined with a beta-blocker to prevent episodes of tachycardia (an excessive heart rate).

Antiplatelet drugs, such as aspirin, also may be given. Platelets are cell fragments circulating in the blood that are important in clot formation and the blood vessel's response to injury. But when platelets collect on arterial wall atheromas, the resulting clot formation (thrombosis) can narrow or block the artery and result in a heart attack. Aspirin binds irreversibly to platelets and keeps them from clumping on blood vessel walls; thus, aspirin reduces the risk of death from coronary artery disease. For most people with coronary artery disease, one baby aspirin, one half of an adult aspirin, or one full adult aspirin daily is recommended. People with an allergy to aspirin may take ticlopidine as an alternative.

Unstable Angina Treatment

Frequently, people with unstable angina are hospitalized, so that drug therapy can be closely monitored and other therapies can be used if necessary. These patients receive drugs to reduce the clotting tendency of blood. Heparin (an anticoagulant that decreases blood clotting), a glycoprotein IIb/IIIa inhibitor (such as abciximab or tirofiban), and aspirin may be prescribed. Also, beta-blockers and intravenous nitroglycerin are given to reduce the workload of the heart. If drugs aren't effective, coronary arteriography and angioplasty or bypass surgery may be necessary.

Coronary Artery Bypass Surgery: This surgery, commonly called bypass surgery, is highly effective in people who have angina and coronary artery disease that's not widespread. It can improve exercise tolerance, reduce symptoms, and decrease the number or dose of drugs needed. Bypass surgery is most likely to benefit a person who has severe angina that hasn't improved with drug therapy, a normally functioning heart, no previous heart attacks, and no other conditions that would make surgery hazardous (for example, chronic obstructive pulmonary disease). In such a person, nonemergency surgery carries a risk of death of 1 percent or less and a chance of heart damage (for example, heart attack) during surgery of less than 5 percent. About 85 percent of patients have complete or dramatic relief of symptoms with surgery. The risk from surgery is somewhat higher in people with decreased pumping ability of the heart (poor left ventricular function), damaged heart muscle from a previous heart attack, or other cardiovascular problems.

Bypass surgery consists of grafting veins or arteries from the aorta (a major artery that takes blood from the heart to the rest of the body) to the coronary artery, thus skipping over (bypassing) the obstructed area. The veins are usually taken from the leg. Most surgeons also use at least one artery as a graft. The artery is usually taken from beneath the sternum (breastbone). These arteries rarely develop coronary artery disease, and more than 90 percent of them still work properly 10 years after the bypass surgery. Vein grafts may gradually become obstructed, and after 5 years one third or more may be completely obstructed. Besides improving angina symptoms, bypass surgery improves the prognosis in certain people, especially those with severe disease.

Coronary Angioplasty: The reasons people with angina have angioplasty are similar to the reasons they have bypass surgery. Not all coronary artery obstructions are suited to angioplasty because of their location, length, degree of calcification, or other conditions. Thus, doctors carefully determine if a person is a good candidate for the procedure.

The procedure begins with a puncture of a large peripheral artery, usually the femoral artery in the leg, with a large needle. Then a long guide wire is threaded through the needle and into the arterial system, through the aorta, and into the obstructed coronary artery. A catheter with a balloon attached to the tip is threaded over the guide wire and into the diseased coronary artery. The catheter is positioned so that the balloon is at the level of the obstruction. The balloon is then inflated for several seconds. Inflation and deflation may be repeated several times. The person is closely monitored during the procedure because balloon inflation momentarily obstructs the coronary artery blood flow. This obstruction can produce ECG changes and ischemic symptoms in some people. The inflated balloon compresses the obstructing atheroma, distends the artery, and partially tears the inner layers of the arterial wall. When angioplasty is successful, the obstruction is greatly reduced. Between 80 and 90 percent of obstructed arteries that are reached are opened.

About 1 to 2 percent of people die during angioplasty, and 3 to 5 percent have nonfatal heart attacks. Coronary artery bypass surgery becomes necessary immediately after angioplasty in 2 to 4 percent of people. In about 20 to 30 percent, the coronary artery becomes obstructed again within 6 months—often within the first few weeks after the procedure. Angioplasty often is repeated and may successfully control coronary artery disease over the long term. To keep the artery open after angioplasty, a doctor may use a newer procedure in which a device made of wire mesh (a stent) is inserted into the artery. This procedure appears to cut the risk of a subsequent arterial obstruction in half.

Few studies have compared the results of angioplasty with drug therapy. Success rates of angioplasty are thought to be similar to those of bypass surgery. In a study comparing bypass surgery with angioplasty, recovery time was shorter after angioplasty, and the risk of death and heart attack remained about the same over the $2\frac{1}{2}$ years of the study.

Newer techniques to remove atheromas, many of which are still being evaluated, include the use of devices to ream out thick, fibrous, and calcified obstructions. However, these techniques, coronary artery bypass surgery, and angioplasty are all only mechanical measures for correcting the immediate problem; they don't cure the underlying disease. To improve the overall prognosis, a person needs to modify risk factors.

Understanding Angioplasty

After puncturing a large artery (usually the femoral artery), a doctor threads a balloon-tipped catheter through the arterial system and into the obstructed coronary artery. Then the doctor inflates the balloon to force the plaque against the arterial wall and thus open the artery.

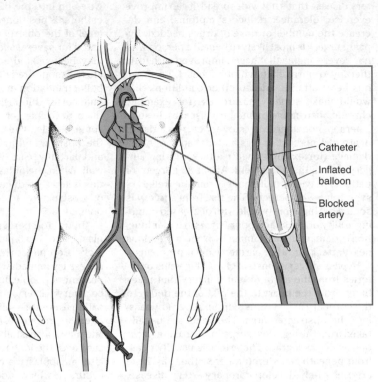

Catheter

Inflated balloon

Blocked artery

Heart Attack

Heart attack (myocardial infarction) is a medical emergency in which some of the heart's blood supply is suddenly severely restricted or cut off, causing heart muscle (myocardium) to die from lack of oxygen.

Some people use the term *heart attack* loosely, applying it to other heart conditions. But in this chapter, the term refers specifically to a myocardial infarction.

Causes

A heart attack usually occurs when a blockage in a coronary artery severely restricts or cuts off the blood supply to a region of the heart. If the supply is cut off or greatly reduced for more than a few minutes, heart tissue dies.

The heart's ability to keep pumping after a heart attack is directly related to the extent and location of the damaged tissue (infarction). Because each coronary artery supplies a specific section of the heart, the location of the damage is determined by which artery is blocked. If more than half of the heart tissue is damaged, the heart generally can't function, and severe disability or death is likely. Even when damage is less extensive, the heart may be unable to pump adequately, resulting in heart failure or shock—an even more serious condition. The damaged heart may enlarge, partly to compensate for the decrease in pumping ability (a larger heart beats more forcefully). The enlargement also may reflect the heart muscle damage itself. Enlargement after a heart attack suggests a worse prognosis than a normal heart size.

A blood clot is the most common cause of a blocked coronary artery. Usually, the artery is already partially narrowed by atheromas. As discussed, an atheroma may rupture or tear and create more blockage, which promotes clot formation. The ruptured atheroma not only restricts the flow of blood through an artery, but also makes platelets stickier, further encouraging clots to form.

An uncommon cause of a heart attack is a clot from part of the heart itself. Sometimes a clot (embolus) forms in the heart, breaks away, and lodges in a coronary artery. Another uncommon cause is a spasm of a coronary artery that stops blood flow. Spasm may be caused by drugs such as cocaine or by smoking, but sometimes the cause is unknown.

Symptoms

About two out of three people who have heart attacks experience intermittent chest pain, shortness of breath, or fatigue a few days beforehand. The episodes of pain may become more frequent even after less and less physical exertion. Such unstable angina may culminate in a heart attack. Usually, the most recognizable symptom is pain in the middle of the chest that may spread to the back, jaw, or left arm; less often, it spreads to the right arm. The pain may occur in one or more of these places and not in the chest at all. The pain of a heart attack is similar to the pain of angina but is generally more severe, lasts longer, and isn't relieved by rest or nitroglycerin. Less often, pain is felt in the abdomen, where it may be mistaken for indigestion, especially because belching may bring partial or temporary relief.

Other symptoms include a feeling of faintness and a heavy pounding of the heart. Irregular heartbeats (arrhythmias) may seriously interfere with the heart's pumping ability or may cause the heart to stop pumping effectively (cardiac arrest), leading to a loss of consciousness or death.

During a heart attack, a person may become restless, sweaty, and anxious and may experience a sense of impending doom. The lips, hands, or feet may turn slightly blue. An elderly person may become disoriented.

Despite all the possible symptoms, as many as one out of five people suffering a heart attack have only mild symptoms or none at all. Such a silent heart attack may be recognized only on a routine electrocardiogram (ECG) some time afterward.

Diagnosis

Whenever a man over age 35 or a woman over age 50 complains of chest pain, a doctor usually considers the possibility of a heart attack. But several other conditions can produce similar pain: pneumonia, a blood clot in the lung (pulmonary embolism), inflammation of the membrane that surrounds the heart (pericarditis), rib fracture, spasm of the esophagus, indigestion, or chest muscle tenderness after injury or exertion. An ECG▲ and certain blood tests can usually confirm the diagnosis of a heart attack in a few hours.

The ECG is the most important initial diagnostic test when a doctor suspects a heart attack. In many instances, it immediately shows that a person is having a heart attack. Several abnormalities may show up on the ECG, depending mainly on the size and location of the heart muscle damage. If a person has had previous heart problems that altered the ECG, the current muscle damage may be harder for doctors to detect. If a few ECGs over several hours are normal, a doctor considers a heart attack unlikely, but certain blood and other tests help in this determination.

The levels of certain enzymes in the blood can be measured to help diagnose a heart attack. An enzyme called CK-MB is normally found in heart muscle and is released into the blood when heart muscle is damaged. Elevated levels show up in the blood within 6 hours of a heart attack and persist for 36 to 48 hours. Levels of CK-MB are usually checked when the person is admitted to the hospital and at 6- to 8-hour intervals for the next 24 hours.

When ECG and CK-MB test results don't provide enough information, an echocardiogram or radionuclide imaging may be done. Echocardiograms may show reduced motion in part of the wall of the left ventricle (the heart chamber that pumps blood to the body), suggesting damage from a heart attack. Radionuclide imaging may show a persistent reduction in blood flow to a region of the heart muscle, suggesting a scar (dead tissue) caused by a heart attack.

Treatment

A heart attack is a medical emergency. Half of the deaths from heart attacks occur in the first 3

▲ see page 73 and box, page 74

or 4 hours after symptoms begin. The sooner treatment begins, the better the chances of survival. Anyone having symptoms that might indicate a heart attack should get prompt medical attention.

A person suspected of having a heart attack is usually admitted to a hospital that has a cardiac care unit. In the unit, the person's heart rhythm and blood pressure and the amount of oxygen in the blood are closely monitored to assess heart damage. Nurses in these units are specially trained to care for people with heart problems and to handle cardiac emergencies.

Initial Treatment

Usually, a person is immediately given an aspirin tablet to chew. This therapy improves the chances of survival by reducing the clot in the coronary artery. Because decreasing the heart's workload also helps limit tissue damage, a beta-blocker may be given to slow the heart rate and make the heart work less hard to pump blood through the body.

Often, oxygen is given through a face mask or a tube with prongs inserted into the nostrils. This therapy increases the oxygen pressure in the blood, which provides more oxygen to the heart and keeps heart tissue damage to a minimum.

If a blocked coronary artery can be cleared quickly, heart tissue may be saved. Blood clots in an artery often can be dissolved by thrombolytic therapy, using drugs such as streptokinase, urokinase, and tissue plasminogen activator. To be effective, the drugs are given intravenously within 6 hours of the start of heart attack symptoms. After 6 hours, some damage is permanent, and removing the blockage probably doesn't help. Early treatment increases blood flow in 60 to 80 percent of people and keeps heart tissue damage to a minimum. Aspirin, which prevents platelets from forming blood clots, or heparin, which also stops clotting, may enhance the effectiveness of thrombolytic therapy.

Because thrombolytic therapy can cause bleeding, it generally isn't given to people who have gastrointestinal bleeding, have severe high blood pressure (hypertension), have had a recent stroke, or have had surgery during the month before the heart attack. Elderly people who don't have any of these conditions can safely receive thrombolytic therapy.

Some cardiovascular treatment centers use angioplasty or coronary artery bypass surgery right after the heart attack instead of thrombolytic therapy.

If the drugs used to increase coronary artery blood flow don't also relieve the patient's pain and distress, morphine is usually injected. This drug also has a calming effect and reduces the work of the heart. Nitroglycerin can relieve pain by reducing the work of the heart. Usually, it's first given intravenously.

Subsequent Treatment

Because excitement, physical exertion, and emotional distress place stress on the heart and make it work harder, a person who has just had a heart attack should stay in bed in a quiet room for a few days. Visitors are usually limited to family members and close friends. Watching television may be permitted if the programs don't cause stress. Smoking is a major risk factor for coronary artery disease and heart attack. Smoking is prohibited in most hospitals and is certainly prohibited in cardiac care units. Moreover, a heart attack is a compelling reason to stop smoking.

Stool softeners and gentle laxatives may be used to prevent constipation. If the person can't pass urine or if the doctors and nurses must keep track of the precise amount of urine produced, a bladder catheter is used.

Nervousness and depression are common after a heart attack. Because severe nervousness can stress the heart, a mild tranquilizer may be prescribed. To deal with mild depression and denial of illness, which are common after a heart attack, patients and their families and friends are encouraged to talk about their feelings with doctors, nurses, and social workers.

Drugs called angiotensin converting enzyme (ACE) inhibitors can reduce heart enlargement in many patients who suffer a heart attack. Therefore, these drugs are routinely given to patients a few days after a heart attack.

Prognosis and Prevention

Most people who survive for a few days after a heart attack can expect a full recovery, but about 10 percent die within a year. Most deaths occur in the first 3 or 4 months, typically in people who continue to have angina, ventricular arrhythmias, and heart failure.

To estimate whether a person will have more heart problems or needs additional treatment, a doctor may order certain tests. For instance, a

Complications of a Heart Attack

A person who has a heart attack may experience any of these complications: myocardial rupture, blood clots, irregular heartbeats (arrhythmias),▲ heart failure■ or shock,★ or pericarditis.●

Myocardial Rupture

Because damaged heart muscle is weak, it sometimes ruptures under the pressure of the heart's pumping action. Two parts of the heart are particularly susceptible to rupture during or after a heart attack: the heart muscle wall and the muscles that control the opening and closing of one of the heart's valves—the mitral valve. If these muscles rupture, the valve can't function—the result is sudden and severe heart failure.

The heart muscle may rupture in the wall separating the two ventricles (septum) or on the external heart wall. Although ruptures of the septum can sometimes be repaired surgically, ruptures of the external heart wall almost always lead to rapid death.

More often, heart muscle damaged by a heart attack doesn't contract properly even if it isn't torn or ruptured. The damaged muscle is replaced by tough, fibrous scar tissue that contracts very little or not at all. Sometimes part of the heart wall expands or bulges when it should contract. Angiotensin converting enzyme (ACE) inhibitors can reduce the extent of these abnormal areas.

The damaged muscle may form a thin bulge (aneurysm) on the heart wall. A doctor may suspect an aneurysm from an abnormal electrocardiogram (ECG) pattern but needs to use an echocardiogram to be sure. These aneurysms don't rupture, but they may cause episodes of irregular heartbeats and may diminish the heart's pumping ability. Because blood flows more slowly through aneurysms, blood clots can form in the heart's chambers.

Blood Clots

Clots form in the heart in 20 to 60 percent of people who've had a heart attack. In about 5 percent of these people, parts of the clots can break off, travel through the arteries, and lodge in smaller blood vessels throughout the body, blocking the blood supply to part of the brain (causing a stroke) or to other organs. An echocardiogram may be taken to detect clots forming in the heart or to see if a person has predisposing factors, such as an area of the heart's left ventricle that isn't beating as well as it should. Doctors often prescribe anticoagulants such as heparin and warfarin to help prevent clot formation. These medications are usually taken for 3 to 6 months after a heart attack.

person may have to wear a Holter monitor, which records the ECG for 24 hours, so a doctor can see if arrhythmias or episodes of silent ischemia are occurring. An exercise tolerance test (a test in which the person runs on a treadmill while being monitored by an ECG)◆ before or shortly after discharge can help determine how well the person is doing after the heart attack and whether ischemia is continuing. If these tests reveal arrhythmias or ischemia, drug therapy may be recommended. If ischemia persists, a doctor may recommend coronary arteriography to evaluate the possibility of angioplasty or bypass surgery to restore blood flow to the heart.

Many doctors recommend one baby aspirin, one half of an adult aspirin, or one full adult aspirin daily after a heart attack. Because aspirin prevents platelets from forming clots, it reduces the risk of death and the risk of a second heart attack by 15 to 30 percent. People with an allergy to aspirin may take ticlopidine as an alternative. Doctors also prescribe beta-blockers because they reduce the risk of death by about 25 percent. The more serious the heart attack, the more ben-

▲ see page 79

■ see page 87

★ see page 111

● see page 104

◆ see page 73

efit these drugs provide. However, some people can't tolerate the side effects, and not everyone benefits.

Rehabilitation

Cardiac rehabilitation is an important part of recovery. Remaining in bed for longer than 2 or 3 days leads to physical deconditioning and sometimes to depression and a sense of helplessness. Barring complications, heart attack patients usually progress to chair rest, passive exercise, walking to the bathroom, and nonstressful work or reading by the third or fourth day after the heart attack. Most people go home after a week or less in the hospital.

Over the next 3 to 6 weeks, a person should slowly increase activity. Most people can safely resume sexual activity 1 or 2 weeks after leaving the hospital. If shortness of breath and chest pain don't occur, a full range of normal activity can be resumed after about 6 weeks.

After a heart attack, a doctor and patient should discuss risk factors that contribute to coronary artery disease, especially ones the patient can change. Quitting smoking, losing weight, controlling blood pressure, reducing blood cholesterol levels through diet or medication, and performing daily aerobic exercises all help reduce the risk of coronary artery disease.

CHAPTER 28

Peripheral Arterial Disease

Occlusive arterial disease includes both coronary artery disease, which can lead to a heart attack,▲ and peripheral arterial disease, which may affect the abdominal aorta and its major branches as well as the arteries of the legs. Other peripheral arterial diseases are Buerger's disease, Raynaud's disease, and acrocyanosis.

Most people with peripheral arterial disease have atherosclerosis, a disease process in which fatty material accumulates under the lining of the arterial wall, gradually narrowing the artery.■ However, a partial or complete occlusion of an artery can result from other causes, such as a blood clot. When an artery narrows, the parts of the body it serves may not receive enough blood. The resulting decrease in oxygen supply (ischemia) can come on suddenly (acute ischemia) or gradually (chronic ischemia).

To help prevent peripheral arterial disease, a person should reduce the number of risk factors

for atherosclerosis, such as smoking, obesity, high blood pressure, and high cholesterol levels.★ Diabetes also is a major cause of peripheral arterial disease, and appropriate treatment of diabetes may delay the arterial disease. Once peripheral arterial disease appears, treatment is directed at its complications—severe leg cramps while walking, angina, abnormal heart rhythms, heart failure, heart attack, stroke, and kidney failure.

Abdominal Aorta and Branches

Obstruction of the abdominal aorta and its major branches may be sudden or gradual. A sudden, complete obstruction usually results when a clot carried by the bloodstream lodges in an artery (embolism), a clot forms (thrombosis) in a narrowed artery, or the artery wall tears (aortic dissection). An obstruction that develops gradually usually results from atherosclerosis; less often, it results from an abnormal growth of muscle in the artery wall or pressure from an expanding mass, such as a tumor, outside the artery.

Symptoms

A sudden, complete obstruction of the superior mesenteric artery, a major branch of the abdom-

▲ see page 126

■ see page 118

★ see page 120

When Blood Supply to the Intestine Is Blocked

The superior mesenteric artery supplies a large part of the intestine with blood. When this artery is blocked, intestinal tissue begins to die.

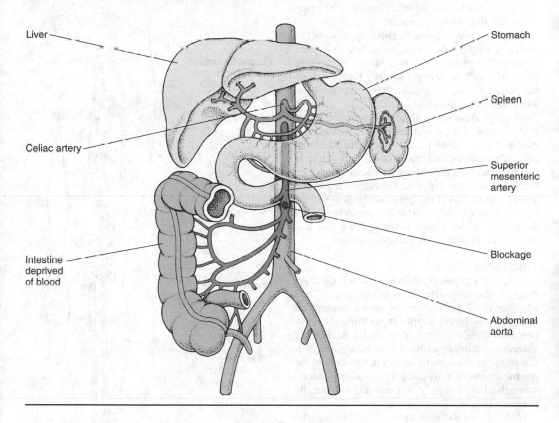

Liver

Celiac artery

Intestine deprived of blood

Stomach

Spleen

Superior mesenteric artery

Blockage

Abdominal aorta

inal aorta that supplies a large part of the intestine, is an emergency. A person with such an obstruction becomes seriously ill and has severe abdominal pain. Initially, vomiting and urgent bowel movements usually occur. Although the abdomen may feel tender when a doctor presses on it, the severe abdominal pain is usually worse than the tenderness, which is widespread and vague. The abdomen may be slightly distended. Through a stethoscope, a doctor initially hears fewer bowel sounds than normal in the abdomen. Later, no bowel sounds can be heard. Blood appears in the stool, though at first it can be detected only by laboratory tests. Soon the stool looks bloody. Blood pressure falls, and the person goes into shock as the intestine becomes gangrenous.

A gradual narrowing of the superior mesenteric artery typically causes pain 30 to 60 minutes after eating because digestion requires an increased blood flow to the intestine. The pain is steady, severe, and usually centered on the navel. This pain makes people afraid to eat, and they may lose considerable weight. Because of the reduced blood supply, nutrients may be poorly absorbed into the bloodstream, contributing to the weight loss.

When a clot lodges in one of the renal arteries, the branches that supply the kidneys, a sudden pain occurs in the side, and the urine becomes bloody. Gradual obstruction of the arteries to one or both kidneys usually results from atherosclerosis and may lead to high blood pressure (renovascular hypertension), which accounts for 5 percent of all high blood pressure.

When the lower aorta is abruptly obstructed where it divides into two branches that pass through the pelvis to deliver blood to the legs (iliac arteries), both legs suddenly become painful, pale, and cold. No pulse can be felt in the legs, which may become numb.

When gradual narrowing occurs in the lower aorta or one of the iliac arteries, the person feels muscle tiredness or pain in the buttocks, hips, and calves while walking. In men, impotence is common with narrowing of the lower aorta or both iliac arteries. If the narrowing occurs in the artery that begins at the groin and goes down the leg to the knee (femoral artery), a person typically feels pain in the calves while walking and has weak or no pulses below the obstruction.

Treatment

Whether a person survives a sudden obstruction of the superior mesenteric artery and whether the intestine can be saved depend on how fast the blood supply is restored. To save precious time, a doctor may send a patient for emergency surgery without even taking x-rays. If the superior mesenteric artery is blocked as the doctor suspects, only immediate surgery can restore the blood supply fast enough to save the person's life.

With a gradual obstruction of blood flow to the intestine, nitroglycerin may relieve the abdominal pain, but only surgery can relieve the obstruction. Doctors use Doppler ultrasound and angiography▲ to determine how extensive the obstruction is and whether to operate.

Blood clots in the hepatic and splenic arteries, the branches supplying the liver and spleen, generally aren't as dangerous as obstructed blood flow to the intestine. Even though an obstruction can cause injury to parts of the liver or spleen, surgery is rarely needed to correct the problem.

▲ see pages 76 and 78

Arteries of the Leg

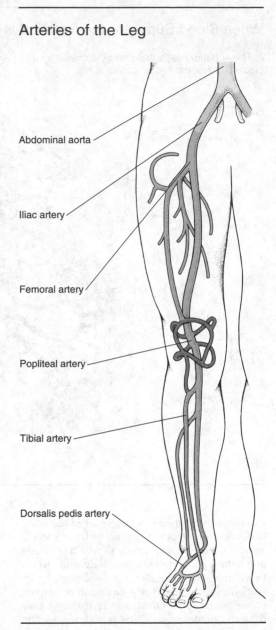

Abdominal aorta

Iliac artery

Femoral artery

Popliteal artery

Tibial artery

Dorsalis pedis artery

Early surgical removal of a clot from a renal artery may restore kidney function. With a gradual obstruction of a renal artery, doctors can sometimes use angioplasty (a procedure in which a balloon is inserted into the artery and inflated to clear the obstruction), but usually they must remove or bypass the blockage surgically.

Emergency surgery can clear a sudden obstruction of the lower aorta where it divides into two branches to deliver blood to the legs. Sometimes doctors can dissolve the clot by injecting a thrombolytic drug, such as urokinase, but surgery is more likely to be successful.

Arteries of the Legs and Arms

With a gradually narrowing leg artery, the first symptom is a painful, aching, cramping, or tired feeling in leg muscles during physical activity; this feeling is called intermittent claudication. Muscles hurt when the person walks, and the pain comes on faster and is more severe when the person walks quickly or uphill. Most commonly, the pain is in the calf, but it can also be in the foot, thigh, hip, or buttocks, depending on the location of the narrowing. The pain can be relieved by resting. Usually, after 1 to 5 minutes of sitting or standing, the person can walk the same distance already covered before feeling pain again. The same kind of pain on exertion is also caused by narrowing of the arteries in the arms.

As the disease gets worse, the distance the person can walk without pain gets shorter. Eventually, the muscles may ache even at rest. The pain usually begins in the lower leg or foot, is severe and unrelenting, and gets worse when the leg is elevated. The pain often prevents sleep. For relief, a person may hang the feet over the side of the bed or rest sitting up with the legs hanging down.

A foot with a severely reduced blood supply is usually cold and numb. The skin may be dry and scaly, and the nails and hair may not grow well. As the obstruction worsens, a person may develop sores, typically on the toes or heel and occasionally on the lower leg, especially after an injury. The leg may shrink. A severe obstruction may cause tissue death (gangrene).

With a sudden, complete obstruction of a leg or arm artery, a person feels severe pain, coldness, and numbness. The person's leg or arm is either pale or bluish (cyanotic). No pulse can be felt below the obstruction.

Diagnosis

A doctor suspects an obstruction based on the symptoms the patient describes and a pulse that's diminished or absent below a certain point in the leg. Doctors estimate blood flow to a person's legs in several ways, including comparing blood pressure at the ankle with blood pressure in the arm. Normally, the ankle pressure is at least 90 percent of the arm pressure, but with severe narrowing it may be less than 50 percent.

The diagnosis may be confirmed by certain tests. With Doppler ultrasound, a probe is placed on the person's skin over the obstruction, and the sound of the blood flow indicates the degree of obstruction.▲ A more sophisticated ultrasound technique, color Doppler produces a picture of the artery that shows different flow rates in different colors. Because it doesn't require an injection, it's used instead of angiography whenever possible.

In angiography, a solution that's opaque to x-rays is injected into the artery. Then x-rays are taken to show the rate of blood flow, the diameter of the artery, and any obstruction.■ Angiography may be followed by angioplasty to open up the artery.

Treatment

People with intermittent claudication should walk at least 30 minutes a day, if possible. When they feel pain, they should stop until it subsides and then walk again. By doing this, they can usually increase the distance they can walk comfortably, probably because the exercise improves muscle function and makes other blood vessels supplying the muscles grow larger. People with obstructions shouldn't use tobacco in any form. Elevating the head of the bed with 4- to 6-inch blocks may help by increasing blood flow to the legs.

Doctors may prescribe a drug such as pentoxifylline in an effort to improve oxygen delivery to the muscles. Other drugs, such as calcium antagonists or aspirin, also may be helpful. Beta-blockers, which help people with coronary artery obstructions by slowing the heart and reducing its need for oxygen, sometimes worsen symptoms in people with leg artery obstructions.

Foot Care

The goal of foot care is to protect circulation to the foot and prevent complications of poor cir-

▲ see page 76

■ see page 78

Performing Foot Care

A person with poor circulation to the feet should use these self-care measures and precautions:

- Inspect feet daily for cracks, sores, corns, and calluses.

- Wash feet daily in lukewarm water with mild soap and dry them gently and thoroughly.

- Use a lubricant, such as lanolin, for dry skin.

- Use unmedicated powder to keep the feet dry.

- Cut toenails straight across and not too short. (A podiatrist may have to cut the nails.)

- Have a podiatrist treat corns or calluses.

- Don't use adhesive or harsh chemicals.

- Change socks or stockings daily and shoes often.

- Don't wear tight garters or stockings with tight elastic tops.

- Wear loose wool socks to keep the feet warm.

- Don't use hot water bottles or heating pads.

- Wear shoes that fit well and have wide toe spaces.

- Ask the podiatrist about a prescription for special shoes if the foot is deformed.

- Don't wear open shoes or walk barefoot.

---

culation. A person with foot ulcers requires meticulous care to prevent further deterioration that would make amputation of the foot necessary. The ulcer must be kept clean: It should be washed daily with mild soap or salt solution and covered with clean, dry dressings. A person with a foot ulcer may need complete bed rest with the head of the bed raised. A person who has diabetes also

▲ see box, page 126

must control blood sugar levels as well as possible. As a rule, anyone with poor circulation to the feet or with diabetes should have a doctor check any foot ulcer that isn't healing after about 7 days. Many times, a doctor prescribes an antibiotic ointment. If the ulcer becomes infected, the doctor generally prescribes antibiotics to be taken by mouth. Healing may take weeks or even months.

Angioplasty

Doctors often perform angioplasty immediately after they perform angiography. Angioplasty consists of inserting a catheter with a balloon on its tip into the narrowed part of the artery and then inflating the balloon to clear the obstruction.▲ Angioplasty may require only 1 or 2 days in the hospital and may help the person avoid a major operation. The procedure isn't painful but may be somewhat uncomfortable because the person has to lie still on a hard x-ray table. A mild sedative, but not general anesthesia, is given. Afterward, the patient may be given heparin to prevent blood clots from forming in the treated area. Many doctors prefer giving patients a platelet inhibitor such as aspirin to prevent clotting. A doctor can use ultrasound to check on the outcome of the procedure and make sure that the narrowing doesn't recur.

Angioplasty can't be performed if the narrowing is widespread, if it extends for a long distance, or if the artery is severely and extensively hardened. Surgery may be needed if a blood clot forms over the narrowed area, a piece of the clot breaks off and blocks a more distant artery, blood seeps into the lining of the artery causing it to bulge and close off blood flow, or the person has bleeding (usually from heparin given to prevent clotting).

Besides balloons, devices—including lasers, mechanical cutters, ultrasonic catheters, stents, and rotational sanders—are used to relieve obstructions. No one device has proved superior.

Surgery

Surgery very often relieves symptoms, heals ulcers, and prevents amputation. A vascular surgeon can sometimes remove a clot if only a small area is blocked. Alternatively, a surgeon may put in a bypass graft, in which a tube made of a synthetic material or a vein from another part of the body is joined to the obstructed artery above and below the obstruction. Another approach is to remove the blocked or narrowed section and insert a graft in its place. Cutting the nerves near the obstruction (an operation called a sympathectomy) prevents the arteries from having spasms and can be very helpful in some cases.

When amputation is needed to cut out infected tissue, relieve unrelenting pain, or stop worsening gangrene, surgeons remove as little of the leg as possible, particularly if the person plans to wear an artificial limb.

Buerger's Disease

Buerger's disease (thromboangiitis obliterans) is the obstruction of small and medium-sized arteries and veins by inflammation triggered by smoking.

Men ages 20 to 40 who smoke cigarettes get Buerger's disease more than anyone else. Only about 5 percent of people with the disease are women. Although no one knows what causes Buerger's disease, only smokers get it, and continuing to smoke makes it worse. Because only a small number of smokers get Buerger's disease, some people must be more susceptible than others. Why and how cigarette smoke causes the problem aren't known.

Symptoms

Symptoms of reduced blood supply to the arms or legs develop gradually, starting at the fingertips or toes and progressing up the arms or legs, eventually causing gangrene. About 40 percent of people with this disease also have episodes of inflammation in the veins, particularly the superficial veins, and the arteries of the feet or legs. People may feel coldness, numbness, tingling, or burning before their doctor sees any signs. They often have Raynaud's phenomenon▲ and get muscle cramps, usually in the arches of their feet or in their legs but rarely in their hands, arms, or thighs. With more severe obstruction, the pain is worse and lasts longer. Early in the disease, ulcers, gangrene, or both may appear. The hand or foot feels cold, sweats a lot, and turns bluish, probably because the nerves are reacting to severe, persistent pain.

Diagnosis

In more than 50 percent of people with Buerger's disease, the pulse is weak or absent in one or more arteries of the feet or wrists. Often, the affected hands, feet, fingers, or toes become pale when raised above the heart and red when low-

ered. People may develop skin ulcers and gangrene, usually of one or more fingers or toes.

Ultrasound tests reveal a severe decrease in blood pressure and blood flow in the affected feet, toes, hands, and fingers. Angiograms (x-rays of the arteries) show obstructed arteries and other circulation abnormalities, especially in the hands and feet.

Treatment

A person with this disease must stop smoking, or it will relentlessly worsen, and ultimately an amputation may be necessary. Also, the person should avoid exposure to the cold; injuries from heat, cold, or substances such as iodine or acids used to treat corns and calluses; injuries from poorly fitting shoes or minor surgery (such as trimming calluses); fungal infections; and drugs that can narrow blood vessels.

Walking 15 to 30 minutes twice a day is recommended, except for people with gangrene, sores, or pain at rest; they may need bed rest. People should protect their feet with bandages that have heel pads or with foam-rubber booties. The head of the bed can be raised on 6- to 8-inch blocks so gravity helps blood flow through the arteries. Doctors may prescribe pentoxifylline, calcium antagonists, or platelet inhibitors such as aspirin, especially when the obstruction results from spasm.

For people who quit smoking but still have arterial occlusion, surgeons may improve blood flow by cutting certain nearby nerves to prevent spasm. They seldom perform bypass grafts, because the arteries affected by this disease are too small.

Functional Peripheral Arterial Disorders

Most of these disorders result from a spasm of arteries in the arms or legs. They may be caused by a fault in the blood vessels or by disturbances in the nerves that control the widening and narrowing of arteries (sympathetic nervous system).

▲ see page 136

Such nerve defects may themselves be a consequence of blockage from atherosclerosis.

Raynaud's Disease and Raynaud's Phenomenon

Raynaud's disease and Raynaud's phenomenon are conditions in which small arteries (arterioles), usually in the fingers and toes, go into spasm, causing the skin to become pale or a patchy red to blue.

Doctors use the term Raynaud's disease when no underlying cause is apparent and the term Raynaud's phenomenon when a cause is known. Sometimes, the underlying cause can't be diagnosed at first, but usually it becomes apparent within 2 years.

Between 60 and 90 percent of the cases of Raynaud's disease occur in young women.

Causes

Possible causes include scleroderma, rheumatoid arthritis, atherosclerosis, nerve disorders, decreased thyroid activity, injury, and reactions to certain drugs, such as ergot and methysergide. Some people with Raynaud's phenomenon also have migraine headaches, variant angina, and high blood pressure in their lungs (pulmonary hypertension). These associations suggest that the cause of the arterial spasms may be the same in all these disorders. Anything that stimulates the sympathetic nervous system, such as emotion or exposure to cold, can cause arterial spasms.

Symptoms and Diagnosis

Spasm of small arteries in the fingers and toes comes on quickly, most often triggered by exposure to cold. It may last minutes or hours. The fingers and toes turn white, usually in a spotty fashion. Only one finger or toe or parts of one or more may be affected, turning a patchy red and white. As the episode ends, the affected areas may be pinker than usual or bluish. The fingers or toes usually don't hurt, but numbness, tingling, a pins-and-needles sensation, and a burning sensation are common. Rewarming the hands or feet restores normal color and sensation. However, when people have long-standing Raynaud's phenomenon (especially those with scleroderma), the skin of the fingers or toes may change permanently—appearing smooth, shiny, and tight.

Small painful sores may appear on the tips of the fingers or toes.

To distinguish between arterial blockage and arterial spasm, doctors perform laboratory tests before and after someone is exposed to cold.

Treatment

People can control mild Raynaud's disease by protecting their trunk, arms, and legs from cold and by taking mild sedatives. They must stop smoking because nicotine constricts blood vessels. For a few people, relaxation techniques, such as biofeedback, may reduce the spasms. Raynaud's disease is commonly treated with prazosin or nifedipine. Phenoxybenzamine, methyldopa, or pentoxifylline occasionally helps. When people have progressive disability and other treatment doesn't work, sympathetic nerves may be cut to relieve the symptoms, but the relief may last only 1 to 2 years. This operation, called a sympathectomy, generally is more effective for people with Raynaud's disease than for those with Raynaud's phenomenon.

Doctors treat Raynaud's phenomenon by treating the underlying disorder. Phenoxybenzamine may help. Drugs that may constrict blood vessels (such as beta-blockers, clonidine, and ergot preparations) may make Raynaud's phenomenon worse.

Acrocyanosis

Acrocyanosis is a persistent, painless blueness of both hands and, less commonly, the feet, caused by unexplained spasm of the small blood vessels of the skin.

The disorder usually occurs in women, not necessarily those with occlusive arterial disease. The fingers or toes and hands or feet are constantly cold and bluish and sweat profusely; they may swell. Cold temperatures usually intensify the blue coloring, and warming reduces it. The condition isn't painful and doesn't damage the skin.

Doctors diagnose the disorder based on persistent symptoms limited to the person's hands and feet along with normal pulses. Treatment is usually unnecessary. Doctors may prescribe drugs that dilate the arteries, but they usually don't help. Very rarely, sympathetic nerves are cut to relieve symptoms.

Aortic Aneurysms and Dissection

The aorta, the largest artery, receives all the blood ejected from the left ventricle for distribution to the entire body except the lungs. Like a large river, the aorta branches into smaller tributaries along its route from the left ventricle to the lower abdomen at the top of the hipbone (pelvis).

Problems with the aorta include weak spots in its walls that allow bulges (aneurysms) to develop, external ruptures and hemorrhage, and separation of the layers of the wall (dissection). Any of these conditions can be immediately fatal, but most take years to develop.

Viewing the Aorta and Its Major Branches

The blood that leaves the heart by way of the aorta reaches every part of the body except the lungs.

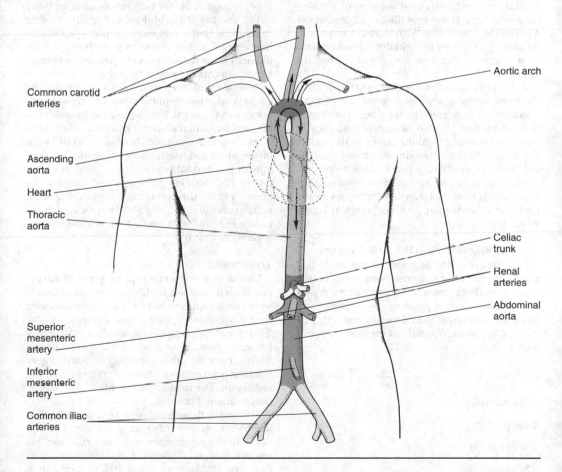

Common carotid arteries

Ascending aorta

Heart

Thoracic aorta

Superior mesenteric artery

Inferior mesenteric artery

Common iliac arteries

Aortic arch

Celiac trunk

Renal arteries

Abdominal aorta

Aneurysms

An aneurysm is a bulge (dilation) in the wall of an artery, usually the aorta.

The bulge generally occurs in a weak area in the wall. Although aneurysms can develop anywhere along the aorta, three quarters of them develop in the segment that runs through the abdomen. Aneurysms are either round (saccular) or tubelike (fusiform) swellings. Most are fusiform.

Aortic aneurysms result primarily from arteriosclerosis,▲ which weakens the wall of the aorta enough that the pressure inside forces it to balloon outward. A blood clot (thrombus) often develops in the aneurysm and may spread along its entire wall. High blood pressure and cigarette smoking increase the risk of an aneurysm. Trauma, inflammatory diseases of the aorta, hereditary connective-tissue disorders such as Marfan's syndrome,■ and syphilis can all predispose a person to aneurysms. With Marfan's syndrome, an aneurysm is most likely in the ascending aorta (the segment that emerges directly from the heart).

Aneurysms also can develop in arteries other than the aorta. Many result from a congenital weakness or arteriosclerosis; others result from injuries caused by stab or gunshot wounds or from bacterial or fungal infections in the wall of the artery. Infection usually starts elsewhere in the body, typically in a heart valve.★ Infected aneurysms of the arteries to the brain are particularly dangerous, making early treatment important. Treatment often involves surgical repair, which is very risky.

ABDOMINAL AORTIC ANEURYSMS

Aneurysms in the segment of the aorta that passes through the abdomen tend to run in families. Many times, these aneurysms occur in people with high blood pressure. Such aneurysms often become larger than 3 inches and may rupture. (The normal diameter of the aorta is $^3/_4$ to 1 inch.)

▲ see box, page 120

■ see page 1306

★ see page 101

● see page 111

Symptoms

A person with an abdominal aortic aneurysm often becomes aware of a pulsing sensation in the abdomen. The aneurysm may cause pain, typically a deep, penetrating pain mainly in the back. The pain can be severe and is usually steady, although changing position may relieve it.

The first sign of a rupture is usually excruciating pain in the lower abdomen and back and tenderness over the aneurysm. With severe internal bleeding, a person may rapidly go into shock.● A ruptured abdominal aneurysm is often fatal.

Diagnosis

Pain is a useful but late clue. However, many people with aneurysms have no symptoms and are diagnosed by chance during routine physical examinations or when x-rays are taken for some other reason. A doctor may feel a pulsating mass in the midline of the abdomen. Rapidly growing aneurysms that are about to rupture frequently hurt or feel tender when pressed during an abdominal examination. In obese people, even large aneurysms may not be detected.

Several laboratory procedures help diagnose aneurysms. An abdominal x-ray may show an aneurysm that has calcium deposits in its wall. Usually, an ultrasound scan clearly reveals the size of an aneurysm. A computed tomography (CT) scan of the abdomen, particularly if performed after injecting a dye intravenously, is even more accurate in determining the size and shape of an aneurysm, but this test is more expensive. A magnetic resonance imaging (MRI) scan is also accurate but more expensive than ultrasound and is rarely necessary.

Treatment

Unless an aneurysm is rupturing, treatment depends on its size. An aneurysm less than 2 inches wide rarely ruptures, but if the aneurysm is wider than $2^1/_2$ inches, rupture is much more common. Therefore, doctors usually recommend surgery for aneurysms more than 2 inches wide, unless it's too risky for other medical reasons. Surgery consists of inserting a synthetic graft to repair the aneurysm. The death rate from this type of surgery is about 2 percent.

Rupture or threatened rupture of an abdominal aneurysm requires emergency surgery. The risk of death during an operation for a ruptured aneurysm is about 50 percent. When an aneurysm ruptures, the kidneys are at risk of injury from disrupted blood supply or from shock related to blood loss. If kidney failure develops after the operation, the chances of survival are very poor. An untreated ruptured aneurysm is always fatal.

THORACIC AORTIC ANEURYSMS

Aneurysms in the segment of the aorta that runs through the chest (thorax) account for one quarter of all aortic aneurysms. In one particularly common form of thoracic aortic aneurysm, the aorta widens where it leaves the heart. This enlargement may cause a malfunction of the valve between the heart and the aorta (aortic valve), allowing blood to leak back into the heart when the valve is closed. About 50 percent of people with this problem have Marfan's syndrome or a variation of it. In the other 50 percent, the condition has no apparent cause, although many of these people have high blood pressure.

Symptoms

Thoracic aortic aneurysms may become huge without causing symptoms. Symptoms result from the pressure of the enlarging aorta against nearby structures. Typical symptoms are pain (usually high in the back), cough, and wheezing. The person may cough up blood because of pressure on or erosion of the windpipe (trachea) or nearby airways. Pressure on the esophagus, the channel that carries food to the stomach, may make swallowing difficult. Hoarseness may come from pressure on the nerve to the voice box (larynx). A person may develop a group of symptoms (Horner's syndrome) that consists of a constricted pupil, drooping eyelid, and sweating on only one side of the face. Chest x-rays may show a displaced windpipe. Abnormal chest wall pulsations also may be a sign of a thoracic aortic aneurysm.

When a thoracic aortic aneurysm ruptures, excruciating pain usually begins high in the back. It may radiate down the back and into the abdomen as the rupture progresses. The pain also may be felt in the chest and arms, simulating a heart attack (myocardial infarction). The person can quickly go into shock▲ and die from a loss of blood.

Diagnosis

A doctor may diagnose a thoracic aortic aneurysm from its symptoms or may discover the aneurysm by chance during an examination. A chest x-ray done for another reason may reveal an aneurysm. Computed tomography (CT), magnetic resonance imaging (MRI), or transesophageal ultrasound is used to determine the precise size of the aneurysm. Aortography (an x-ray procedure performed after injecting a dye that outlines the aneurysm) usually is used to help a doctor determine what type of surgery, if any, is needed.

Treatment

If a thoracic aortic aneurysm is 3 inches wide or more, surgical repair using a synthetic graft is generally performed. Because a rupture is more likely in people with Marfan's syndrome, doctors may recommend that they have a surgical repair even for smaller aneurysms. The risk of death during repair of thoracic aortic aneurysms is high—about 10 to 15 percent. Therefore, drug therapy with a beta-blocker may be given to reduce the heart rate and blood pressure enough to lessen the risk of a rupture.

Aortic Dissection

An aortic dissection (dissecting aneurysm, dissecting hematoma) is an often fatal event in which the inner lining of the aortic wall tears while the outer lining remains intact; blood surges through the tear, dissecting the middle layer, creating a new channel in the aorta's walls.

Deterioration of the arterial wall is responsible for most aortic dissections. The most common cause of such deterioration is high blood pressure, found in more than two thirds of people who develop aortic dissections. Other causes include hereditary disorders of connective tissue, especially Marfan's and Ehlers-Danlos syndromes; birth defects of the heart and blood vessels such as coarctation of the aorta, patent ductus arteriosus, and defects of the aortic valve;■ arteriosclerosis; and injury. In rare instances, a dissection occurs accidentally when a doctor is inserting a catheter into an artery (as in aortography or angiography) or is performing surgery on the heart and blood vessels.

▲ see page 111

■ see page 1224

Understanding Aortic Dissection

In an aortic dissection, the inner lining of the aortic wall tears, and blood surges through the tear, dissecting (splitting) the middle layer and creating a new channel in the wall.

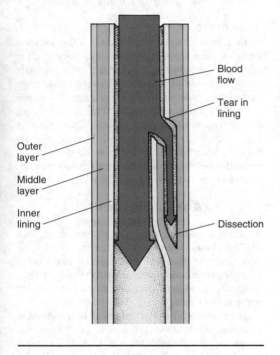

Blood flow

Tear in lining

Outer layer

Middle layer

Inner lining

Dissection

Symptoms

Virtually everyone who has an aortic dissection experiences pain—typically sudden, excruciating pain. Most commonly, people feel the pain, often described as tearing or ripping, over the chest. It's also often in the back between the shoulder blades. The pain frequently follows the path of the dissection as it extends along the aorta.

As the dissection advances, it can close off a point where one or more arteries are connected to the aorta. Depending on which arteries are blocked, the consequences include stroke, heart attack, sudden abdominal pain, nerve damage that causes tingling, and an inability to move a limb.

Diagnosis

The distinctive symptoms of an aortic dissection generally make the diagnosis obvious to a doctor. When examined, about two thirds of people with aortic dissection have diminished or absent pulses in their arms and legs. A dissection that's moving backward toward the heart may cause a murmur that can be heard through a stethoscope. Blood may accumulate in the chest. Blood leaking from a dissection around the heart may prevent the heart from beating properly and cause cardiac tamponade▲—a life-threatening condition.

Chest x-rays show widened aortas in 90 percent of people with symptoms. Ultrasound scans can usually confirm the diagnosis even when the aorta isn't enlarged. Computed tomography (CT) performed after injecting a dye is reliable and can be done quickly, which is important in an emergency.

Treatment

People with aortic dissections are admitted to intensive care units, where their vital signs (pulse, blood pressure, and rate of breathing) are closely monitored. Death can occur a few hours after an aortic dissection begins. Therefore, as soon as possible, doctors give drugs to reduce the heart rate and blood pressure to the lowest level that will maintain a sufficient blood supply to the brain, heart, and kidneys. Soon after drug therapy begins, a doctor must decide whether to recommend surgery or to just continue the drug therapy.

Doctors almost always recommend surgery for dissections that involve the first few inches of the aorta closest to the heart, unless complications of the dissection make the risk of surgery too great. For dissections farther from the heart, doctors usually continue drug therapy—except for dissections that cause the artery to leak blood and dissections in people with Marfan's syndrome. In these cases, surgery is necessary.

During surgery, the surgeon removes the greatest possible area of dissected aorta, prevents blood from entering the false channel, and rebuilds the aorta with a synthetic graft. If the aortic valve is leaking, the surgeon repairs or replaces it.

▲ see box, page 105

Prognosis

About 75 percent of people with aortic dissections who aren't treated die within the first 2 weeks. In contrast, 60 percent of people who are treated and survive the first 2 weeks are still alive 5 years after treatment; 40 percent live at least 10 years. Of people who die after the first 2 weeks, about a third die of complications of the dissection; the other two thirds die of other diseases.

The death rate from surgery in specialized major medical centers is now about 15 percent for aortic dissections closer to the heart and some-what higher for those farther away. Doctors give all people with aortic dissections, including those treated surgically, long-term drug therapy to keep their blood pressure down and thus place less stress on the aorta.

Doctors watch closely for late complications, the three most important of which are another dissection, development of aneurysms in the weakened aorta, and progressive leakage back through the aortic valve. Any of these complications may require surgical repair.

CHAPTER 30

Venous and Lymphatic Disorders

The veins return blood to the heart from all the organs of the body. The main problems of the veins include inflammation, clotting, and defects that lead to distention and varicose veins. The lymphatic system consists of thin-walled vessels that drain fluid, proteins, minerals, nutrients, and other substances from all organs of the body into the veins. The system passes the fluid through lymph nodes, where protection against the spread of infection or cancer is provided, and finally empties the contents into the venous system in the neck. The main problems of the lymphatic system occur when the vessels are unable to handle the amount of fluid that drains into them and when the vessels become blocked by a tumor or inflamed.

The legs contain two major groups of veins: the superficial veins, located in the fatty layer under the skin, and the deep veins, located in the muscles. Short veins connect the superficial and deep veins. Blood pressure in all veins is normally low, and in the leg veins, this low pressure can pose a problem. Blood has to flow from the leg veins upward to reach the heart when a person is standing. The deep veins play a major role in propelling blood upward. Located within the powerful calf muscles, these veins are forcefully compressed with every step. Just as squeezing a toothpaste tube ejects the toothpaste, compressing the deep veins pushes the blood upward. These veins carry 90 percent or more of the blood from the legs toward the heart.

To keep the blood flowing up, not down, the deep veins contain one-way valves. Each valve consists of two halves (cusps) with edges that meet. The blood pushes the cusps open like a pair of swinging doors, but blood forced in the opposite direction by gravity pushes the cusps closed.

Superficial veins have the same type of valves, but these veins don't get squeezed because they aren't surrounded by muscles. So blood in the superficial veins flows more slowly than blood in the deep veins. Much of the blood that flows up the superficial veins is diverted into the deep veins through the many short veins that connect the two systems.

Deep Vein Thrombosis

Deep vein thrombosis is blood clotting in the deep veins.

A clot that forms in a blood vessel is called a thrombus. Although thrombi can occur in either the superficial or deep leg veins, only those in the deep veins are potentially dangerous. Deep vein thrombosis is dangerous because all or part of the thrombus can break loose, float along in the bloodstream, and lodge in a narrow artery in the lung, obstructing blood flow. A moving thrombus is called an embolus. The less inflammation around a thrombus, the less tightly it adheres to the vein wall and the more likely it will become an embolus. The squeezing action of the calf mus-

One-way Valves in the Veins

These two illustrations show how the valves in the veins work. The illustration on the left shows the valves opened by normal blood flow; the illustration on the right shows the valves closed by a backflow of blood.

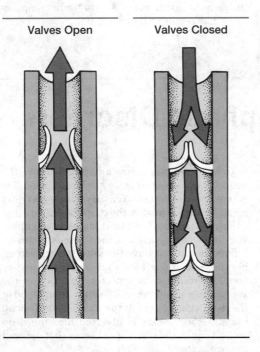

| Valves Open | Valves Closed |

cles can dislodge the thrombus, especially as a convalescing person becomes more active.

Because blood in the leg veins travels to the heart and then to the lungs, emboli originating in the leg veins will obstruct one or more arteries in the lungs, a condition called pulmonary embolism.▲ The seriousness of pulmonary embolism depends on the size and number of emboli. A large pulmonary embolus can block all or nearly all of the blood traveling from the right side of the heart to the lungs, quickly causing death. Fortunately, such massive emboli aren't common, but no one can predict which case of deep vein thrombosis,

▲ see page 165

if untreated, will lead to a massive embolus. Thus, doctors are greatly concerned about every patient with deep vein thrombosis.

Deep vein thrombosis shouldn't be confused with phlebitis in varicose veins, which is painful but comparatively harmless.

Causes

Three factors can contribute to deep vein thrombosis: injury to the lining of the vein; an increased tendency for blood to clot, as can happen with some cancers and rarely with oral contraceptive use; and slowing of the blood flow in the veins, as happens during prolonged bed rest because the calf muscles aren't contracting and squeezing the blood toward the heart. For example, deep vein thrombosis can occur in heart attack patients who lie in hospital beds for several days with little leg movement or in paraplegics who sit for long periods and whose muscles don't function. Injury or major surgery also can increase the tendency for blood to clot. Thrombosis can even occur in healthy people who sit for long periods, for instance, during lengthy drives or plane flights.

Symptoms

About half the people with deep vein thrombosis have no symptoms at all. In these people, chest pain caused by pulmonary embolism may be the first indication that something is wrong. When deep vein thrombosis causes substantial inflammation and blood flow obstruction, the calf swells and may be painful, tender to the touch, and warm. The ankle, foot, or thigh may also swell, depending on which veins are involved.

Some thrombi heal by being converted to scar tissue, which may damage the valves in the veins. The resulting accumulation of fluid (edema) can make the leg swell. The edema can extend up the leg and even affect the thigh, if the obstruction is high enough in the vein. Edema is worse toward the end of the day because of the effect of gravity when standing or sitting. Overnight the edema subsides because the veins empty well when the legs are horizontal.

A late symptom of deep vein thrombosis is brown skin discoloration, usually above the ankle. The discoloration is from red blood cells that escape from distended veins into the skin. The discolored skin is vulnerable, and even a minor injury such as a scratch or bump can break it open, resulting in an ulcer.

Diagnosis

Deep vein thrombosis may be difficult for a doctor to detect because there's a lack of pain and often either no swelling or only very slight swelling. When this disorder is suspected, ultrasound examination of the leg veins (duplex scanning) can confirm the diagnosis. If the person has symptoms of pulmonary embolism, a doctor orders radioactive scans of the chest to confirm the diagnosis and duplex scanning to check the legs.

Prevention and Treatment

Although the risk of deep vein thrombosis can't be entirely eliminated, it can be reduced in several ways. People at risk for deep vein thrombosis—people who have just had major surgery or those taking long trips, for example—should flex and extend the ankles about 10 times every 30 minutes.

Wearing **elastic stockings** (support hose) continuously makes the veins narrow slightly and the blood flow more rapidly, making clotting less likely. However, elastic stockings provide minimal protection and may give a false sense of security, discouraging more effective methods of prevention. If not worn correctly, they may bunch up and aggravate the problem by obstructing blood flow in the legs.

Anticoagulant therapy before, during, and sometimes after surgery reduces blood clotting much more effectively.▲

Pneumatic stockings are another effective way to prevent clots. Usually made of plastic, these stockings are automatically pumped up and emptied by an electric pump, thereby repeatedly squeezing the calves and emptying the veins. The stockings are put on before surgery and kept on during the operation and the postoperative period until the person can walk again.

Swelling of the Legs

Swelling can be eliminated either by resting in bed and elevating the legs or by wearing compression bandages. These bandages must be applied by an experienced doctor or nurse, and they must be kept on for several days. During this time, walking is important. If the swelling doesn't completely subside, the bandages must be reapplied.

The veins never recover after deep vein thrombosis develops, and surgery to correct the problem is experimental. After the compression bandages are removed, elastic stockings are worn every day to prevent swelling from recurring. The stockings don't have to be worn above the knee; swelling above the knee is of little concern and causes no complications. Leotard-type elastic stockings or strong elastic pantyhose generally is not needed.

Skin Ulcers

If painful skin ulcers develop, properly applied compression bandages can help. Applied once or twice a week, these bandages almost always heal the ulcer by improving the blood flow in the veins. Skin creams, balms, or skin medications of any kind have little effect. The ulcers are almost always infected, and pus and a foul-smelling discharge appear on the bandage each time it's changed. The pus and discharge can be washed off the skin with soap and water; they don't substantially delay healing.

Once blood flow in the veins has improved, the ulcer will heal by itself. After it has healed, wearing an elastic stocking daily can prevent a recurrence. The stocking must be replaced as soon as it becomes too loose. If finances permit, the person should purchase seven stockings (or seven pairs of stockings, if both legs are involved). These should be labeled for each day of the week, worn only on that day, then washed and put away for the following week. This way, the stockings last considerably longer.

Rarely, ulcers that don't heal require skin grafting.

Superficial Phlebitis

Superficial phlebitis (thrombophlebitis, phlebitis) is inflammation and clotting in a superficial vein.

Phlebitis can occur in any vein in the body, but it most often affects the leg veins. Usually, phlebitis occurs in people with varicose veins; however, most people with varicose veins do not develop phlebitis.

▲ see page 167

Even a slight injury can cause a vein to become inflamed. Unlike deep vein thrombosis, which causes very little inflammation and is often painless, superficial phlebitis involves a sudden (acute) inflammatory reaction that causes the thrombus to adhere firmly to the vein wall and lessens the likelihood that it will break loose. Unlike the deep veins, superficial veins have no surrounding muscles to squeeze and dislodge a thrombus. For these reasons, superficial phlebitis rarely causes an embolism.

Symptoms and Diagnosis

Localized pain, swelling, and skin redness over the vein develop rapidly, and the area feels warm. Because blood in the vein is clotted, the vein feels like a hard cord under the skin, not soft like a normal or varicose vein. This hard cord feeling may extend for the length of the vein. The diagnosis is usually obvious to a doctor just from examining the painful area.

Treatment

Most often, superficial phlebitis subsides by itself. Taking an analgesic, such as aspirin or ibuprofen, may help relieve pain. Although the phlebitis generally improves in a matter of days, several weeks may pass before the lumps and tenderness subside completely. To provide early relief, a doctor may inject a local anesthetic, remove the thrombus, and then apply a compression bandage, which the person wears for several days.

When superficial phlebitis occurs in the groin, where the main superficial vein joins the main deep vein, a thrombus may extend into the deep vein and break away. To prevent this, some surgeons recommend emergency surgery to tie off the superficial vein. Usually, this surgery can be done using a local anesthetic and without admitting the person to the hospital; normal activities may be resumed afterward.

Varicose Veins

Varicose veins are enlarged superficial veins in the legs.

The precise cause of varicose veins isn't known but is probably a weakness in the walls of the superficial veins. This weakness may be inherited. Over time, the weakness causes the veins to lose their elasticity. They stretch and become longer and wider. To fit in the same space that they occupied when they were normal, the elongated veins become tortuous, with a snakelike appearance if they cause a bulge in the skin over them. More important than the elongation is the widening, which causes the valve cusps to separate. As a result, the veins rapidly fill with blood when the person stands, and the thin-walled, tortuous veins enlarge even more. The enlargement also affects some of the connecting veins, which normally allow blood to flow only from the superficial veins into the deep veins. If the valves of these connecting veins fail, blood squirts backward into the superficial veins when the muscles squeeze the deep veins, causing the superficial veins to stretch further.

Symptoms and Complications

Besides being unsightly, varicose veins commonly ache and make the legs feel tired. Many people, however, even some with very large veins, may have no pain. The lower part of the leg and ankle may itch, especially if the leg is warm after the person removes socks or stockings. Itching can lead to scratching and cause redness or a rash, which is often incorrectly attributed to dry skin. The symptoms are sometimes worse when varicose veins are developing than when they're fully stretched.

Only a small percentage of people with varicose veins have complications, such as dermatitis, phlebitis, or bleeding. The dermatitis produces a red, scaling, itchy rash or brown area, usually on the inside of the leg above the ankle. Scratching or a minor injury can cause a painful ulcer that doesn't heal.

Phlebitis may occur spontaneously or result from an injury. Though usually painful, phlebitis that occurs with varicose veins is rarely harmful.

If the skin over a varicose vein or spider veins is thin, a minor injury, particularly from shaving or scratching, can cause bleeding. Ulcers may also cause bleeding.

Diagnosis

Varicose veins usually can be seen bulging under the skin, but a person may have symptoms before the veins become visible. When varicose veins aren't visible, a doctor experienced in checking for them can palpate the leg to determine the full extent of the problem.

Some doctors order x-rays or ultrasound tests to assess the functioning of the deep veins. Usually, such testing is necessary only if changes in the skin suggest a malfunction of the deep veins or if the person's ankle is swollen because of edema (fluid accumulation in the tissue under the skin). Varicose veins alone don't cause edema.

Treatment

Because varicose veins can't be cured, treatment mainly relieves symptoms, improves appearance, and prevents complications. Elevating the legs—by lying down or using a footstool when sitting—relieves the symptoms of varicose veins but doesn't prevent varicose veins. Varicose veins that appear during pregnancy usually get much better during the 2 or 3 weeks after delivery; during this time, they shouldn't be treated.

Elastic stockings (support hose) compress the veins and prevent them from stretching and hurting. People who don't want surgery or injection therapy or who have a medical condition that prevents them from having these treatments may choose to wear elastic stockings.

Surgery

Surgery aims to remove as many of the varicose veins as possible. The largest superficial vein is the long saphenous vein, which extends from the ankle to the groin, where it joins the main deep vein. The saphenous vein can be removed by a procedure called stripping. The surgeon makes two incisions, one at the groin and one at the ankle, and opens the vein at each end. A flexible wire is then threaded through the entire vein and pulled on to remove the vein. To remove as many other varicose veins as possible, the surgeon makes more incisions in other areas. Because the superficial veins play a less significant role than the deep veins in returning blood to the heart, their removal doesn't impair circulation if the deep veins are functioning normally. This procedure is lengthy, so the person is usually given a general anesthetic. Although surgery relieves the symptoms and prevents complications, the procedure leaves scars. The more extensive the surgery, the longer the time before new varicose veins develop. However, surgery doesn't cure the tendency to develop new varicose veins.

Injection Therapy

In injection therapy, an alternative to surgery, the veins are sealed, so that no blood can flow

Valves in Varicose Veins

In the normal vein, the cusps of the valves close to prevent a backflow of blood. In a varicose vein, the cusps can't close because the vein is abnormally widened, and blood can flow in the wrong direction.

Normal Vein	Varicose Vein

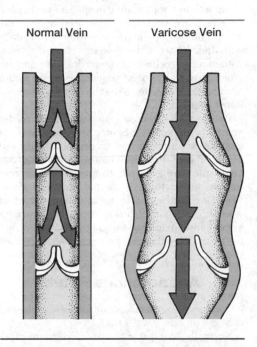

through them. A solution is injected to irritate the vein and cause a thrombus. In essence, this procedure produces a harmless kind of superficial phlebitis. Healing of the thrombus leads to scar tissue, which blocks the vein. However, the thrombus may dissolve instead of becoming scar tissue, and the varicose vein then reopens.

Injection therapy was common in the United States between the 1930s and 1950s but fell into disrepute because of poor results and complications. Many of the medications used weren't adequately tested and caused unpleasant or even dangerous side effects. Because the procedure seemed simple, many doctors attempted it without adequate experience. Current techniques have an improved likelihood of success and are safe for varicose veins of all sizes.

If the diameter of the injected vein is reduced by compression with a special bandaging technique, the size of the thrombus is reduced, and it's more likely to form scar tissue, as desired. A further advantage of the newer technique is that adequate compression virtually eliminates the pain usually associated with superficial vein phlebitis.

Although injection therapy is more time-consuming than surgery, anesthesia isn't necessary, new varicose veins can be treated as they develop, and people can go about their normal daily activities between treatments. However, even with modern techniques, some doctors consider injection therapy only when varicose veins return after surgery or when a person desires cosmetic improvement.

People with varicose veins often have spider veins as well, sometimes incorrectly called burst capillaries. Although spider veins may be caused by back pressure from blood in the varicose veins, they are generally thought to result from poorly understood hormonal factors, which would explain why they most commonly affect women, particularly during pregnancy. If spider veins cause pain or a burning sensation or are unsightly, they also may be treated with injection therapy.

Arteriovenous Fistula

An arteriovenous fistula is an abnormal channel between an artery and a vein.

Normally, blood flows from arteries into capillaries and then into veins. With an arteriovenous fistula, blood flows directly from an artery into a vein, bypassing the capillaries. A person may be born with an arteriovenous fistula (a congenital fistula), or it may develop after birth (an acquired fistula).

Congenital arteriovenous fistulas are uncommon. Acquired arteriovenous fistulas can be caused by any injury that damages an artery and a vein lying side by side. Typically, the injury is a piercing wound, as from a knife or bullet. The fistula may appear immediately or may develop after a few hours. The area can swell quickly if blood escapes into the surrounding tissues.

Some medical treatments—kidney dialysis, for example—require that a vein be pierced each time. With such repeated piercing, the vein becomes inflamed and clotting can develop; eventually the vein can become obliterated with scar tissue. To avoid this problem, a doctor may deliberately create an arteriovenous fistula, usually between an adjoining vein and artery in the arm. This procedure widens the vein, making needle insertion easier, and the faster flowing blood is less likely to clot. Unlike some large arteriovenous fistulas, these small fistulas don't cause heart problems, and they can be closed when no longer needed.

Symptoms and Diagnosis

When congenital arteriovenous fistulas are near the surface of the skin, they may appear swollen and reddish blue. In conspicuous places, such as the face, they appear purplish and may be unsightly.

If a large acquired arteriovenous fistula isn't treated, a large volume of blood flows under high pressure from the artery into the vein network. Vein walls aren't strong enough to resist such high pressure, so the walls stretch and the veins enlarge and bulge (sometimes resembling varicose veins). The abnormally rapid return of blood to the heart via the arteriovenous shortcut may strain the heart, causing heart failure.▲ The larger the fistula, the faster heart failure can develop.

With a stethoscope placed over a large acquired arteriovenous fistula, a doctor can hear a distinctive to-and-fro sound, like that of moving machinery (machinery murmur). To confirm the diagnosis and to determine the extent of the problem, a doctor injects the blood vessels with a dye that shows up on x-rays. The dye showing the pattern of blood flow is revealed on the x-ray images (angiograms).

Treatment

Small congenital arteriovenous fistulas can be cut out or destroyed by laser coagulation therapy. This procedure must be done by a skilled vascular surgeon because the fistulas are sometimes more extensive than they appear to be on the surface. Arteriovenous fistulas near the eye, brain, or other major structures can be especially difficult to treat.

Acquired arteriovenous fistulas are corrected by a surgeon as soon as possible after diagnosis.

▲ see page 87

Lymph, Lymph Nodes, and the Lymphatic System

How do oxygen, nutrients, and other life-sustaining substances reach the tissues? They're dissolved in fluid that diffuses through the very thin walls of capillaries. Some of the fluid is reabsorbed into the capillaries; the remainder of the fluid (lymph) flows into small vessels (lymphatic vessels). The lymphatic vessels are larger than capillaries but smaller than the smallest veins. Most of the lymphatic vessels have valves like those in the veins to keep the lymph, which can clot, flowing in the right direction—toward two large lymph ducts located in the neck. These lymph ducts then empty the lymph back into the blood by way of the veins.

As the lymph flows through the lymphatic vessels, it passes through strategically placed lymph nodes (sometimes called lymph glands), which play a major part in the body's immune defenses. Lymph nodes filter out foreign particles that get into the lymph—for example, cancer cells that have separated from a nearby cancerous growth. Doctors evaluate lymph nodes when a cancer is diagnosed to determine if it has spread. Lymph nodes also produce essential components of the immune system, including white blood cells that make antibodies to destroy foreign organisms.

Bacteria trapped by lymph nodes may cause them to swell and become tender, producing a condition called lymphadenitis. Occasionally, the bacteria cause the lymphatic vessels to become inflamed, producing a condition called lymphangitis. The person has tender, red streaks along the skin and usually a fever and chills. Staphylococci and streptococci are the bacteria that most frequently cause lymphangitis.

If the surgeon can't reach the fistula easily—for example, if it's in the brain—it may be treated by blocking the artery using complex injection techniques that cause thrombi that stop the flow of blood into the fistula.

Lymphedema

Lymphedema is swelling caused by interference with the normal drainage of lymph back into the blood.

Rarely, lymphedema is obvious at birth. More often, it appears later in life from either congenital or acquired causes.

Congenital lymphedema results from having so few lymphatic vessels that they can't handle all the lymph. The problem almost always affects the legs; rarely, it affects the arms. Women are much more likely than men to have congenital lymphedema.

The swelling may already be obvious at birth, but usually the lymphatic vessels can handle the small amount of lymph produced in an infant. More often, the swelling appears later as the volume of lymph increases and overwhelms the small number of lymph vessels. The swelling starts gradually in one or both legs. The first sign of lymphedema may be puffiness of the foot, making the shoe feel tight at the end of the day; the shoe may leave marks in the skin. In the early stages of the condition, the swelling goes away when the leg is elevated. (Many people who don't have lymphedema experience swelling after they stand for prolonged periods.) Congenital lymphedema gets worse with time; the swelling becomes more obvious and doesn't disappear completely, even after a night's rest.

Acquired lymphedema is more common than congenital lymphedema. It typically appears after major surgical treatment, especially after cancer treatment in which lymph nodes and lymphatic vessels are removed or irradiated with x-rays. For example, the arm may become prone to swelling after removal of a cancerous breast and the associated lymph nodes. Scarring of repeatedly infected lymphatic vessels also may cause lymphedema, but this is very uncommon except in infection by the tropical parasite *Filaria*.

In acquired lymphedema, the skin looks healthy but is puffy or swollen. Pressing the area with a finger doesn't leave an indentation, as it does when swelling caused by an accumulation of fluid (edema) results from inadequate blood flow in the veins. In rare instances, the swollen limb is extremely large and the skin is so thick and ridged that it looks almost like elephant skin (elephantiasis).

Treatment

Lymphedema has no cure. For people with mild lymphedema, compression bandages can reduce the swelling. People who are more severely affected may wear pneumatic stockings every day for an hour or two to reduce the swelling. Once the swelling has been reduced, the person must wear elastic stockings up to the knee every day from the moment of rising until bedtime. This controls the swelling to some degree. For lymphedema in the arm, pneumatic sleeves—like pneumatic stockings—can be used every day to reduce the swelling; elastic sleeves are also available. For elephantiasis, an extensive operation may be performed to remove most of the swollen tissues under the skin.

Lipedema

Lipedema is an abnormal collection of fat under the skin, most often in the lower part of the leg between the calf and ankle.

Lipedema is much more common in females and is present at birth. Though it looks similar to lymphedema, it's a distinct disorder.

Both legs are affected. The lower legs and ankles lose their normal contour, but the enlargement stops just below the ankle bones and doesn't include the feet. The legs look swollen and may ache. Pressing on the leg with a finger doesn't leave an indentation. The skin of the legs looks normal but may be tender, possibly because of the underlying collection of fat.

Liposuction may greatly improve the shape of the legs.

Lung and Airway Disorders

Biology of the Lungs and Airways

The respiratory system begins with the nose and mouth and continues through airways to the lungs, where oxygen from the atmosphere is exchanged for carbon dioxide from the body's tissues. The lungs, the largest parts of the respiratory system, look like large pink sponges that almost fill the chest. The left lung is a little smaller than the right lung because it shares space with the heart in the left side of the chest. Each lung is divided into sections (lobes): three in the right lung and two in the left.

Air enters the respiratory system through the nose and mouth and passes down the throat (pharynx) and through the voice box (larynx). The entrance to the larynx is covered by a small flap of muscular tissue (epiglottis) that closes when swallowing, thus preventing food from entering the airways.

The largest airway is the windpipe (trachea), which branches into two smaller airways (bronchi) to supply the two lungs. The bronchi themselves divide many times before evolving into smaller airways (bronchioles). These are the narrowest airways—one fiftieth of an inch across. The airways look like an upside-down tree, which is why this part of the respiratory system is often called the bronchial tree.

At the end of each bronchiole are dozens of bubble-shaped, air-filled cavities (alveoli) that resemble bunches of grapes. Each lung contains millions of alveoli, and each alveolus is surrounded by a dense network of capillaries. The extremely thin walls of the alveoli allow oxygen to move from the alveoli into the blood in the capillaries and allow the waste product called carbon dioxide to move from the blood in the capillaries into the alveoli.

The pleura is a slippery membrane that helps the lungs move smoothly during each breath. It covers the lungs and comes back around to line the inside of the chest wall. Normally, the two lubricated layers of the pleura have almost no space between them and glide smoothly over each other as the lungs expand and contract.

The lungs and other organs in the chest are protected by a bony cage, which is formed by the breastbone (sternum), ribs, and spine. The 12 pairs of ribs curve around the chest. At the back of the body, each pair is joined to the bones (vertebrae) of the spine. In the front of the body, the upper seven pairs of ribs are joined directly to the sternum by the costal cartilages. The eighth, ninth, and tenth pairs of ribs join the cartilage of the pair above; the last two pairs (floating ribs) are shorter and don't join in the front.

The intercostal muscles, which lie between the ribs, help move the rib cage and thus assist in breathing. The most important muscle used for breathing is the diaphragm, a bell-shaped sheet of muscle that separates the lungs from the abdomen. The diaphragm is attached to the base of the sternum, the lower parts of the rib cage, and

Inside the Lungs and Airways

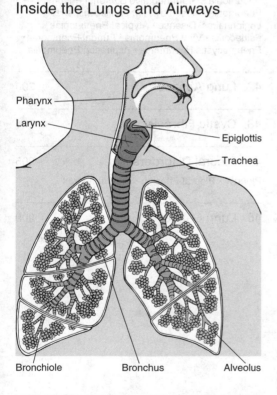

Pharynx

Larynx

Epiglottis

Trachea

Bronchiole   Bronchus   Alveolus

Gas Exchange Between Alveoli and Capillaries

The function of the respiratory system is to exchange two gases: oxygen and carbon dioxide. The exchange takes place between the millions of alveoli in the lungs and the capillaries that surround them. As shown below, inhaled oxygen moves from the alveoli to the blood in the capillaries, and carbon dioxide moves from the blood in the capillaries to the alveoli.

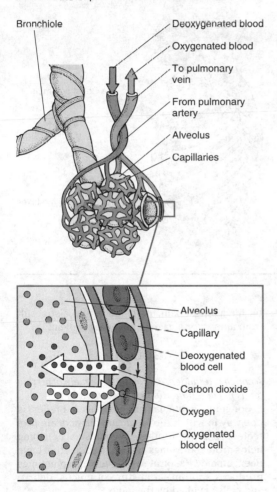

Bronchiole

Deoxygenated blood

Oxygenated blood

To pulmonary vein

From pulmonary artery

Alveolus

Capillaries

Alveolus

Capillary

Deoxygenated blood cell

Carbon dioxide

Oxygen

Oxygenated blood cell

the spine. When the diaphragm contracts, it increases the size of the chest cavity and thus expands the lungs.

Respiratory System Function

The primary functions of the respiratory system are to bring oxygen into the lungs, transfer the oxygen to the blood, and expel the waste product called carbon dioxide. Inhaled oxygen enters the lungs and reaches the alveoli. The walls of the alveoli and of the surrounding capillaries are only one cell thick and are in very close contact with each other. Oxygen passes easily through the thin walls of the alveoli and into the blood in the capillaries, and carbon dioxide passes from the blood into the alveoli and is exhaled through the nose and mouth. Oxygenated blood travels from the lungs through the pulmonary veins and into the left side of the heart, which pumps the blood to the rest of the body. Oxygen-depleted, carbon dioxide–rich blood returns to the right side of the heart through two large veins, the superior and inferior vena cavae, and is pumped through the pulmonary artery to the lungs, where it picks up oxygen and releases carbon dioxide.▲

Control of Breathing

Breathing is usually automatic, controlled subconsciously by the respiratory center at the base of the brain. The brain and small sensory organs in the aorta and carotid arteries sense when oxygen levels are too low or carbon dioxide levels are too high, and the brain increases the speed and depth of breathing. Conversely, when carbon dioxide levels get too low, breathing is slowed. In quiet breathing, the average adult inhales and exhales about 15 times a minute. Because the lungs have no muscles of their own, the work of breathing is done primarily by the diaphragm and, to a lesser extent, by the muscles between the ribs (intercostal muscles). During forced or labored breathing, other muscles in the neck, chest wall, and abdomen also participate.

As the diaphragm contracts, it moves down, enlarging the chest cavity. This reduces pressure in the chest. Air rushes into the lungs to equalize

▲ see box, page 69

Diaphragm's Role in Breathing

When the diaphram contracts, the chest cavity enlarges, reducing the pressure inside. To equalize the pressure, air rushes into the lungs. When the diaphragm relaxes, the chest cavity contracts, raising the pressure, thus pushing air out of the lungs.

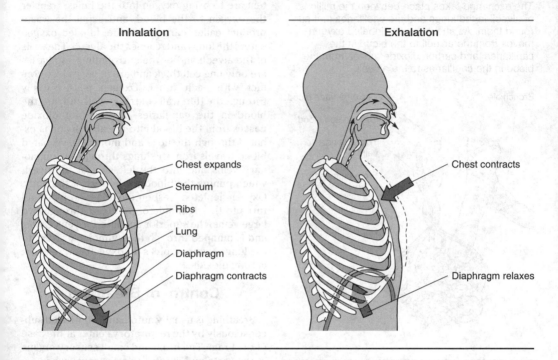

Inhalation	Exhalation
Chest expands	Chest contracts
Sternum	
Ribs	
Lung	
Diaphragm	
Diaphragm contracts	Diaphragm relaxes

the pressure. The diaphragm then relaxes and moves up; the chest cavity contracts and raises the air pressure. Air is pushed out of the lungs because of their elasticity. The intercostal muscles participate in this process, especially if breathing is deep or rapid.

Respiratory Symptoms

Among the most common symptoms of respiratory disorders are a cough, shortness of breath, chest pain, wheezing, stridor (a crowing sound when breathing), hemoptysis (coughing up of blood), cyanosis (bluish discoloration), finger clubbing, and respiratory failure. Some of these symptoms don't always indicate a respiratory problem. Chest pain, for instance, may also result from a heart or a gastrointestinal problem.

Cough

A cough is a sudden, explosive movement of air that tends to clear material from the airways.

Coughing, a familiar but complicated reflex, is one way in which the lungs and airways are protected. Along with other mechanisms, coughing helps protect the lungs against particles that have been inhaled (aspirated). Coughing sometimes produces sputum—a mixture of mucus, debris, and cells expelled by the lungs.

Coughs vary considerably. A cough may be distressing, especially if coughing episodes are accompanied by chest pain, shortness of breath, or unusually large amounts of sputum, also called phlegm. However, if coughing develops over decades, as it may in a smoker with chronic bronchitis, the person may hardly be aware of it.

Information about a cough helps a doctor determine its cause. Therefore, a doctor may ask
- How long it's been present
- What time of day it occurs
- Which factors—such as cold air, posture, talking, eating, or drinking—influence it
- Whether it's accompanied by chest pain, breathlessness, hoarseness, dizziness, or other symptoms
- Whether it brings up sputum

A person may produce sputum without coughing, or a person may have a dry cough without sputum. The appearance of the sputum helps a doctor make a diagnosis. A yellowish, green, or brown appearance may point to a bacterial infection. Clear, white, or watery sputum doesn't indicate a bacterial infection, but a virus, allergy, or irritant may be present. A doctor may examine the sputum microscopically; bacteria and white blood cells seen under the microscope are additional indications of infection.

Treatment

Because coughing plays an important role in bringing up sputum and clearing the airways, a cough that produces a lot of sputum generally shouldn't be suppressed. Treating the underlying cause—such as an infection, fluid in the lungs, or an allergy—is more important. For example, antibiotics can be given for an infection, or antihistamines can be taken for an allergy.

Cough medicines can be used to suppress a dry cough (one that doesn't produce sputum) if it's disturbing. Also, in certain circumstances, such as when a person is exhausted but unable to sleep, cough medicines may be used to reduce a cough, even if it's bringing up sputum. A cough can be treated by two groups of drugs: antitussives and expectorants.

Antitussive Therapy

Antitussive drugs suppress a cough. **Codeine,** a narcotic, is a painkiller (analgesic) that suppresses coughs by suppressing the cough center in the brain, but it can make people drowsy. It may also cause nausea, vomiting, or constipation. If codeine is taken for a prolonged period, the dose needed to suppress a cough may increase.

Many other narcotics that can be used to suppress coughing have similar side effects.

Dextromethorphan isn't an analgesic, but it effectively suppresses the cough center in the brain. An ingredient in many over-the-counter cough medications, it isn't addictive, and it doesn't produce drowsiness.

Demulcents form a protective coating over the irritated lining. They're useful for coughs caused by an irritation above the larynx. Demulcents come in lozenges and syrups.

Local anesthetics, such as benzocaine, inhibit the cough reflex. These medications are sprayed into the back of the throat before the doctor begins a procedure that would be disrupted by coughing, such as bronchoscopy (an examination using a viewing tube passed into the bronchi).

Steam inhalation, for example from a vaporizer, can help stop a cough by reducing irritation in the pharynx and airways. The moisture from the steam also loosens secretions, making them easier to cough up. A cool-mist humidifier can achieve the same result.

Expectorants

Expectorants help loosen mucus by making bronchial secretions thinner and easier to cough up. Iodides are commonly used expectorants, and guaifenesin and terpin hydrate are ingredients in many over-the-counter preparations. A small dose of syrup of ipecac may help in children, especially those with croup. Drugs that reduce the thickness of mucus (called mucolytics) are sometimes used when thick, sticky bronchial secretions are a major problem, as in cystic fibrosis.

Antihistamines, Decongestants, and Bronchodilators

Antihistamines, which dry the respiratory tract, have little or no value in treating a cough, except when it's caused by an allergy or when a common cold is in its early stages. With coughs from other causes, however, the drying action of the antihistamines can be harmful, thickening the respiratory secretions and making them difficult to cough up.

Decongestants such as phenylephrine that relieve a stuffy nose aren't useful in relieving a cough, unless it's caused by postnasal drip.

Bronchodilators such as inhaled sympathomimetic agents or oral theophylline may be prescribed if a cough occurs with airway narrowing, as happens in bronchial asthma and emphysema.

Shortness of Breath

Shortness of breath (dyspnea) is the unpleasant sensation of difficulty in breathing.

A healthy person breathes faster during exercise and at high altitudes. Although the faster breathing is rarely uncomfortable, it may limit the amount of exercise that can be performed. With dyspnea, the faster breathing is accompanied by the sensation that the person is running out of air and that the person can't breathe fast enough or deeply enough. Dyspnea limits the amount of exercise that can be performed.

Other sensations related to dyspnea include an awareness of increased muscular effort to expand the chest when breathing in or to expel air when breathing out, the uncomfortable sensation that an inspiration is urgently needed before expiration is completed, and various sensations most often described as tightness in the chest.

Types of Dyspnea

The most common type of dyspnea accompanies physical exertion. During exercise, the body makes more carbon dioxide and uses more oxygen. The respiratory center in the brain accelerates breathing when blood levels of oxygen are low or blood levels of carbon dioxide are high. If the lungs and heart aren't functioning properly, even a little exertion can lead to dramatic increases in breathing rates and dyspnea. In the most severe forms, dyspnea may even occur at rest.

Lung-related (pulmonary) dyspnea may result from restrictive or obstructive defects. In restrictive dyspnea, the work of breathing increases either because the lungs are damaged and stiff or because a deformed chest wall or a thickened pleura limits expansion during breathing. The volume of air in the lungs, as measured by pulmonary function tests,▲ is low. People with restrictive dyspnea are usually comfortable at rest but become very short of breath when they're active because their lungs can't expand enough to take in the needed volume of air.

▲ see page 159

■ see page 87

Obstructive dyspnea involves increased resistance to airflow because the airways are narrowed. Usually, air can be pulled in, but that air can't be forced from the lungs as fast as normal because the airways become smaller on exhalation. Breathing is labored, especially on expiration. Pulmonary function testing can measure the degree of obstruction. A respiratory problem may include both restrictive and obstructive defects.

Because the heart pumps the blood through the lungs, the heart must function properly for the lungs to function properly.■ If the heart is pumping inadequately, fluid may accumulate in the lungs, a condition called pulmonary edema. This condition causes shortness of breath that's often accompanied by a feeling of smothering or heaviness in the chest. The fluid accumulation in the lungs may also lead to airway narrowing and wheezing—a condition called cardiac asthma.

Some people whose heart pumps inadequately experience orthopnea—shortness of breath when lying down that's relieved by sitting up. Paroxysmal nocturnal dyspnea is a sudden, often terrifying, attack of shortness of breath during sleep. The person awakens gasping and must sit or stand to take a breath. This condition is a form of orthopnea and a sign of heart failure.

In periodic or Cheyne-Stokes respiration, periods of fast breathing (hyperpnea) alternate with periods of slow breathing (hypopnea) or no breathing (apnea). Possible causes include heart failure and reduced efficiency of the breathing control center in the brain.

Circulatory dyspnea, a serious condition that comes on suddenly, occurs when the blood can't carry enough oxygen to the tissues, for example, because of severe bleeding or anemia. The person breathes rapidly and deeply, trying to obtain adequate oxygen.

Increased blood acidity, such as occurs in diabetic acidosis, may produce a pattern of slow, deep respirations (Kussmaul's respiration), but the person doesn't feel short of breath. In contrast, someone with severe kidney failure feels out of breath and may begin to pant quickly because of a combination of acidosis, heart failure, and anemia.

Sudden brain injury from a cerebral hemorrhage, trauma, or other condition may cause intense, rapid breathing (hyperventilation).

Many people have episodes of feeling that they can't get enough air, and they breathe heavily and rapidly. These episodes, called hyperventilation syndrome, are commonly caused by anxiety rather than a physical problem. Many people who experience this syndrome are frightened and may believe they're having a heart attack. The symptoms result from changes in the blood gas levels (mostly from a lowering of the carbon dioxide level) caused by the overbreathing. The person may experience a change in consciousness usually described as a feeling that events occurring around them are far away. The person also has a tingling feeling in the hands and feet and around the mouth.

Chest Pain

Pain in the chest may arise from the pleura, lungs, chest wall, or internal structures that aren't part of the respiratory system, especially the heart.

Pleuritic pain, a sharp pain arising from an irritation in the lining of the lungs, is made worse by deep breathing and coughing. The pain can be reduced by keeping the chest wall still—for instance, by holding the side that hurts and avoiding deep breathing or coughing. Usually, the site of the pain can be pinpointed, although it may move over time. Pleural effusion,▲ a fluid buildup in the space between the two layers of pleura, may produce pleuritic pain at first, but the pain often subsides as the two layers are separated by accumulating fluid.

Pain arising from other respiratory structures is usually more difficult to describe than pleuritic pain. A lung abscess or tumor, for example, may cause a vague, deep-seated ache in the chest.

Pain can also originate in the chest wall itself. This pain may worsen with deep breathing or coughing and often is confined to one area in the chest wall, which also feels sore when pressed. The most common causes are chest wall injuries, such as broken ribs and torn or injured muscles between the ribs. A tumor growing into the chest wall may cause pain in just that spot or, if it grows into an intercostal nerve, may cause referred pain (pain along the whole area supplied by that nerve). Shingles, caused by the varicella-zoster

virus, sometimes causes chest wall pain during each breath before the telltale rash appears.

Wheezing

Wheezing is a whistling, musical sound during breathing that results from partially obstructed airways.

Wheezing results from an obstruction somewhere in the airways. It may be caused by a general narrowing of the airways (as in asthma or chronic obstructive pulmonary disease), by a local narrowing (as with a tumor), or by a foreign particle lodged in an airway. The most common cause of recurring wheezing is asthma, although many people who have never had asthma wheeze at some time in their lives.

A doctor usually is able to detect wheezing by listening with a stethoscope as the person breathes. Pulmonary function testing■ may be needed to help measure the extent of airway narrowing and to assess the benefits of treatment.

Stridor

Stridor is a crowing sound heard during breathing, mainly during inhalation, that results from a partial blockage of the throat (pharynx), voice box (larynx), or windpipe (trachea).

Stridor is usually loud enough to be heard at some distance, but it may be audible only during a deep breath. The sound is caused by turbulent airflow through a narrowed upper airway. In children, the cause may be an infection of the epiglottis★ or an inhaled foreign object. In adults, it may be a tumor, an abscess, swelling (edema) in the upper airway, or a malfunction of the vocal cords.

Stridor can be a symptom of a life-threatening emergency. In such cases, a tube may be inserted through the person's mouth or nose (tracheal intubation) or directly into the trachea (tracheostomy) to allow air to get past the blockage and to save the person's life.

▲ see page 206

■ see page 159

★ see page 1264

Selected Causes of Hemoptysis

Respiratory tract infections
- Bronchitis
- Pneumonia
- Tuberculosis
- Fungal infection (for example, *Aspergillus* infection)
- Lung abscess
- Bronchiectasis

Circulation problems
- Heart failure
- Mitral valve stenosis
- Arteriovenous malformations

Foreign object in airways

Bleeding disorders

Trauma

Injury during a medical procedure

Pulmonary embolism

Tumor

Hemoptysis

Hemoptysis is the coughing up of blood from the respiratory tract.

Blood-streaked sputum is rather common and usually not serious. Infections such as acute or chronic bronchitis cause about half the cases. However, a large amount of blood in the sputum requires quick evaluation by a doctor.

Tumors, especially lung cancer, account for 20 percent of cases of hemoptysis. Doctors check for lung cancer in smokers over age 40 who develop hemoptysis, even if the sputum is only blood streaked. A pulmonary infarction (death of lung tissue from blockage of the artery supplying the tissue) may also cause hemoptysis. Blockage of a pulmonary artery, called pulmonary embolism, can result when a blood clot travels through the bloodstream and lodges in the artery.

Bleeding may be severe if a pulmonary vessel is accidentally damaged by a catheter. Such a catheter may be inserted into the pulmonary artery or vein to measure pressures in the heart and the blood vessels to and from the lungs. High blood pressure in the pulmonary veins, as may occur in heart failure, may also cause hemoptysis.

Diagnosis

If hemoptysis causes significant blood loss or recurs often, it may be life threatening, so the source must be found and the bleeding stopped. Bronchoscopy (an examination using a viewing tube passed into the bronchi) may identify the bleeding point. A scan using a radioactive marker (perfusion scan) may reveal pulmonary embolism. Despite testing, the cause of hemoptysis isn't found in 30 to 40 percent of cases; however, the cause of severe hemoptysis usually is found.

Treatment

Mild hemoptysis may require no treatment or only antibiotics to clear an infection. Bleeding may produce clots that block the airways and lead to further breathing problems; therefore, coughing is important to keep the airways clear and shouldn't be suppressed with antitussive medications. Breathing steam or cold mist from a vaporizer or humidifier may help the person expel a clot. Respiratory therapy may be needed. If a large clot blocks a major bronchus, the clot can be removed using a bronchoscope.

Bleeding from smaller vessels usually stops by itself. However, bleeding from a major vessel usually requires treatment. A doctor may try to close off the bleeding vessel using a procedure called bronchial artery embolization. Using x-rays for guidance, the doctor passes a catheter into the vessel and then injects a chemical that causes the blood vessel to close. Bleeding caused by an infection or heart failure usually subsides if the underlying disorder is treated successfully. Sometimes bronchoscopy or surgery may be needed to stop bleeding, or surgery may be needed to remove a diseased portion of the lung. These high-risk procedures are used only as last resorts. If clotting abnormalities are contributing to the bleeding, a transfusion of plasma, clotting factors, or platelets may be needed.

Cyanosis

Cyanosis is a bluish discoloration of the skin resulting from an inadequate amount of oxygen in the blood.

Cyanosis occurs when oxygen-depleted blood, which is bluish rather than red, circulates through the skin. Cyanosis restricted to the fingers and toes usually occurs because blood flows through the limbs very slowly. It may result when the pumping action of the heart is weak or when a person is exposed to cold. Cyanosis that occurs throughout the body can be caused by many types of severe lung disease and by certain blood vessel and heart malformations that shunt blood from the venous to the arterial side of the circulation.

The amount of oxygen in the blood can be determined by arterial blood gas analysis.▲ X-rays, blood flow studies, and lung and heart function tests may be needed to determine the cause of decreased oxygen in the blood and the resulting cyanosis. Supplemental oxygen is often the first treatment given.

Finger Clubbing

Finger clubbing is an enlargement of the tips of the fingers or toes and a loss of the angle where the nails emerge.

Clubbing of the fingers, which poses no medical danger, is often caused by lung disease, although many other diseases can cause it. Finger clubbing unrelated to any disease is inherited in some families.

Respiratory Failure

Respiratory failure is a condition in which the level of oxygen in the blood becomes dangerously low or the level of carbon dioxide becomes dangerously high.

Respiratory failure results from an inadequate exchange of oxygen and carbon dioxide between the lungs and the blood or from an inadequate movement of air (ventilation) in and out of the lungs.

Almost any condition that affects breathing or the lungs can lead to respiratory failure. An overdose of narcotics or alcohol can cause such profound sleepiness that a person stops breathing and suffers respiratory failure. Obstruction of the airways, injury to the lung tissues, damage to the bones and tissues around the lungs, and weakness of the muscles that normally inflate the lungs are also common causes. Respiratory failure can occur if blood flow through the lungs becomes abnormal, as occurs in pulmonary embolism. This disorder doesn't stop air from moving in and out of the lung, but without blood flow to a portion

Recognizing Finger Clubbing

Finger clubbing is characterized by enlarged fingertips and a loss of the normal angle at the nail bed.

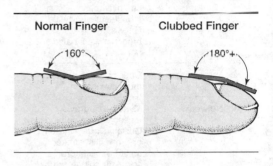

Normal Finger   **Clubbed Finger**

of the lung, the oxygen isn't properly extracted from the air, and carbon dioxide isn't transferred to it. Other causes of abnormal blood flow, such as congenital disorders that send blood directly to the rest of the body without its first going through the lungs, can also lead to respiratory failure.

Symptoms and Diagnosis

Some symptoms of respiratory failure vary with the cause. However, low oxygen levels cause cyanosis (a blue tinge to the skin), and high carbon dioxide levels cause confusion and sleepiness. A person with an obstructed airway may gasp and struggle for breath; someone who is intoxicated or weak will quietly slip into a coma. No matter what the cause of respiratory failure, eventually low levels of oxygen make the brain and heart malfunction, resulting in deteriorating consciousness and abnormal heart rhythms (arrhythmias) that can lead to death. The buildup of carbon dioxide causes the blood to become acidic, further affecting all the organs, especially the heart and brain. The body tries to rid itself of carbon dioxide by deep, rapid breathing, but if the lungs can't function normally, this breathing pattern may not help.

▲ see page 160

What Causes Respiratory Failure?

Underlying Reason	Cause
Airway obstruction	Chronic bronchitis, emphysema, bronchiectasis, cystic fibrosis, asthma, bronchiolitis, inhaled particles
Poor breathing	Obesity, sleep apnea, drug intoxication
Muscle weakness	Myasthenia gravis, muscular dystrophy, polio, Guillain-Barré syndrome, polymyositis, stroke, amyotrophic lateral sclerosis, spinal cord injury
Abnormality of lung tissue	Acute respiratory distress syndrome, drug reaction, pulmonary fibrosis, fibrosing alveolitis, widespread tumors, radiation, sarcoidosis, burns
Abnormality of chest wall	Kyphoscoliosis, chest wound

If respiratory failure develops slowly, pressure in the blood vessels through the lungs increases, a condition called pulmonary hypertension. If left untreated, this condition damages the blood vessels, further impairs the transfer of oxygen to the blood, and stresses the heart, causing heart failure.

Treatment

Almost always, oxygen is given initially. Usually, the amount given is more than is needed, unless the person has chronic respiratory insufficiency. Such people tend to slow their breathing when they're overtreated with oxygen.

The underlying cause also must be treated. Antibiotics are used to fight infection, and bronchodilators are used to open the airways. Other medications may be given to decrease inflammation or prevent blood clots.

Some very ill patients need mechanical ventilation to aid breathing. A plastic tube is inserted through the nose or mouth and into the trachea; this tube is attached to a machine that forces air into the lungs. Exhalation occurs passively because of the elastic recoil of the lungs. Many types of ventilators and modes of operation may be used, depending on the underlying disorder. If the lungs aren't functioning well, additional oxygen may be delivered through the ventilator. Mechanical ventilation can be lifesaving whenever patients aren't able to move enough air in and out of their lungs.

The amount of fluid in the body must be carefully monitored and adjusted to maximize lung and heart function. The acidity of the blood must be kept in balance both by adjusting the rate of breathing and using medications that buffer acidity. Medications are given to keep the person calm, thereby reducing the body's oxygen demands and making lung inflation easier.

When the lung tissue is severely damaged, as in acute respiratory distress syndrome, doctors often consider giving corticosteroids, medications that decrease inflammation. However, the routine use of these medications isn't justified. Corticosteroids can cause many complications, including loss of muscle strength. In general, they're most beneficial to those suffering from conditions known to cause inflammation of the lungs or airways, such as vasculitis, asthma, and allergic reactions.

Respiratory Therapy

Respiratory therapists use several different techniques to help treat lung disease, including postural drainage, suctioning, breathing exercises, and pursed-lip breathing. The choice of therapy is based on the underlying disease and the patient's overall condition.

Postural Drainage

In postural drainage, the person is tilted or propped at an angle to help drain secretions from the lungs. Also, the chest or back may be clapped with a cupped hand to help loosen secretions—a technique called chest percussion. Alternatively, the therapist may use a mechanical vibrator.

These techniques are used at intervals on patients with conditions that produce a great deal of sputum, such as cystic fibrosis, bronchiectasis, and lung abscess. The techniques may also be used when a person can't cough up sputum effectively, as may happen with elderly people, people who have muscular weakness, and people recovering from surgery, an injury, or a severe illness.

Suctioning

Respiratory therapists and nurses may use suctioning to help remove secretions from the airways. To perform suctioning, they usually pass a small plastic tube through the nose and a few inches into the airway. A gentle vacuum sucks out the secretions that can't be coughed up. Suctioning is also used to clear secretions in someone who has a tracheostomy or a breathing tube inserted through the nose or mouth and into the trachea.

Breathing Exercises

Breathing exercises may promote a sense of well-being, improve the quality of life, and help strengthen the muscles that inflate and deflate the lungs, but they don't directly improve lung function. Still, breathing exercises decrease the likelihood of lung complications after surgery in heavy smokers and others with lung disease. Such exercises are particularly helpful for sedentary people who have chronic obstructive pulmonary disease or who have been put on a ventilator.

Often, these exercises involve using an instrument called an incentive spirometer. A person sucks as hard as possible on a tube attached to a plastic device. The device houses a ball, and each sucking breath lifts the ball. These devices are used routinely in hospitals before and after surgery. However, deep breathing exercises encouraged by nurses and respiratory therapists may be more effective than breathing exercises using an incentive spirometer.

Pursed-Lip Breathing

This technique may be helpful to people with chronic obstructive pulmonary disease who overinflate their lungs during attacks of airway narrowing, panic, or exercise. Pursed-lip breathing also provides an additional breathing exercise for people undergoing respiratory training.

The person is taught to exhale against partially closed (pursed) lips, as if preparing to whistle. This increases pressure in the airways and helps prevent them from collapsing. The exercise causes no ill effects, and some people adopt the habit without instruction.

CHAPTER 32

Diagnostic Tests for Lung and Airway Disorders

Tests for respiratory disease are designed to give an accurate assessment of how well the lungs are working. Each test assesses a different aspect of lung function.

One group of tests called pulmonary function tests measure the lungs' capacity to hold air as well as their ability to move air in and out and to exchange oxygen and carbon dioxide. These tests are better at detecting the type and severity of lung disorders than at defining the specific cause of problems. The tests are used to diagnose some diseases, however, including asthma. Pulmonary function tests include lung volume and flow rate measurements, flow volume testing, muscle strength assessment, and diffusing capacity measurement.

Lung Volume and Flow Rate Measurements

The assessment of respiratory disease often involves testing how much air the lungs can hold as well as how much and how quickly air can be exhaled. These measurements are made with a spirometer, which consists of a mouthpiece and tubing connected to a recording device. A person inhales deeply, then exhales vigorously and as quickly as possible through the tubing while measurements are taken. The volume of air inhaled or exhaled and the length of time each breath takes are recorded and analyzed. Often, the tests are repeated after a person takes a drug that opens the airways of the lungs (a bronchodilator).

Using a Spirometer

A spirometer consists of a mouthpiece, tubing, and a recording device. To use a spirometer, a person inhales deeply, then exhales vigorously and as quickly as possible through the tubing. The recording device measures the volume of air inhaled or exhaled and the length of time each breath takes.

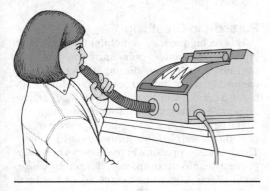

A simpler device for measuring how quickly air can be exhaled is the peak flow meter. After inhaling deeply, a person blows into this small, handheld device as hard as possible. This inexpensive device helps asthmatic patients monitor the severity of their disease at home.

Lung volume measurements reflect the stiffness or elasticity of the lungs and the rib cage. The measurements are abnormally low in disorders such as pulmonary fibrosis and curvature of the spine (kyphoscoliosis). Disorders that cause stiff lungs or that reduce the movement of the rib cage are called restrictive disorders.

Flow rate measurements reflect the degree of narrowing or obstruction of the airways. The measurements are abnormal in disorders such as bronchitis, emphysema, and asthma. This type of disorder is called an obstructive disorder.

Flow Volume Testing

Most newer spirometers can continuously display lung volumes and flow rates during a forced breathing maneuver. These flow rates can be particularly helpful in detecting abnormalities that partially block the voice box (larynx) and windpipe (trachea).

Muscle Strength Assessment

The strength of the respiratory muscles can be measured by having a person forcibly inhale and exhale against a pressure gauge. A disease that weakens the muscles, such as muscular dystrophy, makes breathing more difficult and causes low inspiratory and expiratory pressures. This test also helps predict whether a person on a ventilator will be able to breathe independently after being taken off it.

Diffusing Capacity Measurement

A diffusing capacity test for carbon monoxide can estimate how efficiently oxygen is transferred from the air sacs of the lungs (alveoli) to the bloodstream. Because the diffusing capacity of oxygen is difficult to measure directly, a person inhales a small amount of carbon monoxide, holds the breath for 10 seconds, and then exhales into a carbon monoxide detector.

If the lungs are normal, carbon monoxide is very well absorbed from inspired air. If the test shows that carbon monoxide isn't well absorbed, oxygen won't be exchanged normally between the lungs and the bloodstream either. The diffusing capacity is characteristically abnormal in people with pulmonary fibrosis, emphysema, and disorders affecting the blood vessels of the lungs.

Sleep Studies

Breathing is usually automatic and controlled by centers in the brain that respond to the levels of oxygen and carbon dioxide in the blood. If this control is abnormal, breathing may stop for prolonged periods, especially during sleep—a condition called sleep apnea.▲ The test for sleep apnea consists of placing an electrode on the finger or earlobe to measure the oxygen concentration in the blood, placing an electrode in one nostril to measure airflow, and placing an electrode or gauge on the chest to measure the motion of breathing.

Arterial Blood Gas Analysis

Arterial blood gas tests measure the concentrations of oxygen and carbon dioxide in the arterial blood. These concentrations are important indicators of lung function because they reflect how

▲ see page 304

well the lungs are getting oxygen into the blood and getting carbon dioxide out of it.

Oxygen concentrations can be monitored using an electrode placed on a finger or an earlobe—a procedure called oximetry. When a person is seriously ill or a doctor also needs a carbon dioxide measurement, however, a blood sample is necessary. Usually, it's taken from the radial artery at the wrist. With an arterial blood sample, the laboratory can determine the oxygen and carbon dioxide concentrations as well as the acidity of blood, something that can't be measured on blood taken from a vein.

Chest Imaging

Routinely, **chest x-rays** are taken from the back to front, but sometimes this view is supplemented with a side view. Chest x-rays provide a good outline of the heart and major blood vessels and usually can reveal a serious disease in the lungs, the adjacent spaces, and the chest wall including the ribs. For example, chest x-rays can clearly show pneumonias, lung tumors, a collapsed lung (pneumothorax), fluid in the pleural space (pleural effusion), and emphysema. Although chest x-rays seldom give enough information to determine the exact cause of the abnormality, they can help a doctor determine which other tests are needed to make a diagnosis.

Computed tomography (CT) scanning of the chest provides more detail than a plain x-ray. With CT scanning, a series of x-rays is analyzed by a computer, which then provides several cross-sectional views. During CT scanning, a dye may be injected into the bloodstream or given by mouth. The dye helps clarify certain abnormalities in the chest.

Magnetic resonance imaging (MRI) also produces highly detailed pictures that are especially useful when a doctor suspects blood vessel abnormalities in the chest, such as an aortic aneurysm. Unlike CT scanning, MRI doesn't use radiation. Instead, it records the magnetic characteristics of atoms within the body.

Ultrasound scanning creates a picture on a monitor from the reflection of sound waves in the body. Ultrasound is often used to detect fluid in the pleural space (the space between the two layers of pleura covering the lung). Ultrasound also can be used for guidance when using a needle to aspirate the fluid.

Nuclear lung scanning uses minute amounts of short-lived radioactive materials to show the flow of air and blood through the lungs. Usually, the test is done in two stages. In the first stage, a person inhales a radioactive gas, and a scanner creates a picture of how the gas is distributed throughout the airways and the air sacs (alveoli). In the second stage, a radioactive substance is injected into a vein, and a scanner creates a picture of how it's distributed throughout the blood vessels of the lung. This type of imaging is particularly useful in detecting blood clots in the lungs (pulmonary emboli); it also may be used during the preoperative assessment of lung cancer patients.

Angiography accurately shows the blood supply to the lungs. Dye that can be seen on x-rays is injected into a blood vessel, and pictures are taken of the arteries and veins in the lungs. Angiography is used most often when pulmonary embolism is suspected, usually on the basis of abnormal lung scan results. Pulmonary artery angiography is considered the definitive test (gold standard) for diagnosing and for ruling out pulmonary embolism.

Thoracentesis

In thoracentesis, pleural effusion (fluid that has collected abnormally in the pleural space)▲ is removed with a needle and syringe, so it can be analyzed. The two principal reasons to perform thoracentesis are to relieve shortness of breath caused by lung tissue compression and to obtain a fluid sample for diagnostic testing.

During the procedure, the patient sits comfortably and leans forward, resting the arms on supports. A small area of skin on the back is cleaned and numbed with a local anesthetic. Then a doctor inserts a needle between two ribs and withdraws some fluid into a syringe. Sometimes a doctor uses ultrasound for guidance while inserting the needle. The collected fluid is analyzed to assess its chemical makeup and to determine whether bacteria or cancerous cells are present.

If a large volume of fluid has accumulated, causing shortness of breath, more fluid can be removed to allow the lung to expand and the person

▲ see page 206

Understanding Bronchoscopy

To view the airways directly, a doctor passes a flexible, fiber-optic bronchoscope through a patient's nostril and down into the airways. The circular inset here shows the doctor's view.

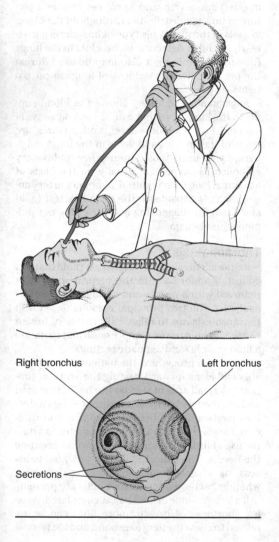

Right bronchus   Left bronchus

Secretions

to breathe more easily. During thoracentesis, a doctor can also insert substances into the pleural space to prevent a reaccumulation of fluid.

After the procedure, a chest x-ray is taken to document the amount of fluid removed, to get a clearer look at the lung that was previously obscured by fluid, and to ensure that the procedure hasn't caused any complications.

The risk of complications during and after thoracentesis is low. Occasionally, a patient may feel some pain as the lung fills with air and expands against the chest wall. Also, a patient may briefly feel light-headed and short of breath. Other possible complications include a lung collapse (pneumothorax), bleeding into the pleural space or chest wall, fainting, infection, puncture of the spleen or liver, and very rarely, accidental entry of air bubbles into the bloodstream (air emboli).

Needle Biopsy of the Pleura

If thoracentesis doesn't uncover the cause of a pleural effusion or if a tissue specimen from a tumor is needed, a doctor may perform a needle biopsy. First, the skin is anesthetized as for thoracentesis. Then using a larger bore needle, a doctor takes a small sample of tissue from the pleura and sends it to a laboratory to be examined for signs of cancer or tuberculosis. About 85 to 90 percent of the time, a pleural biopsy is accurate in diagnosing these diseases. Complications are similar to those for thoracentesis.

Bronchoscopy

Bronchoscopy is a direct visual examination of the voice box (larynx) and airways through a fiber-optic viewing tube (a bronchoscope). A bronchoscope has a light at the end that allows a doctor to look down through the larger airways (bronchi) into the lung.

Bronchoscopy can help a doctor make a diagnosis and treat certain conditions. A flexible bronchoscope can be used to remove secretions, blood, pus, and foreign bodies; to place medications in specific areas of the lung; and to investigate the source of bleeding. If a doctor suspects lung cancer, the airways can be examined and specimens can be taken from any suspicious areas. Bronchoscopy is used for collecting the organisms that are causing pneumonia and that are difficult to collect and identify in other ways. Bronchoscopy is especially helpful for obtaining specimens in people who have AIDS and other immune deficiencies. When people have been burned or have inhaled smoke, bronchoscopy helps doctors assess the condition of the larynx and airways.

For at least 4 hours before bronchoscopy, the person shouldn't eat or drink. A sedative is often given to ease anxiety, and atropine is given to reduce the risks of a spasm of the voice box and a slowing of the heart rate, which sometimes occur during the procedure. The throat and nasal passage are anesthetized with an anesthetic spray, and then the flexible bronchoscope is passed through the nostril and into the airways of the lungs.

Bronchoalveolar lavage is a procedure doctors can use to collect specimens from the smaller airways that can't be seen through the bronchoscope. After wedging the bronchoscope into a small airway, a doctor instills salt water (saline) through the instrument. The fluid is then suctioned back into the bronchoscope, bringing cells and any bacteria with it. Examination of the material under the microscope helps in diagnosing infections and cancers; culturing the fluid is a better way to diagnose infections. Bronchoalveolar lavage also can be used to treat pulmonary alveolar proteinosis▲ and other conditions.

Transbronchial lung biopsy involves obtaining a specimen of lung tissue through the bronchial wall. A doctor removes pieces of tissue from a suspicious area by passing a biopsy instrument through a channel in the bronchoscope and then through the wall of a small airway and into the suspicious area of lung. A doctor may use a fluoroscope for guidance in identifying the suspicious area. Such guidance can also decrease the risk of accidentally perforating the lung and causing a lung collapse (pneumothorax). Although transbronchial lung biopsy increases the risk of complications, it often provides additional diagnostic information and may make major surgery unnecessary.

After bronchoscopy, the person is observed for several hours. If a tissue specimen was removed, chest x-rays are taken to check for complications.

Thoracoscopy

Thoracoscopy is the visual examination of the lung surfaces and pleural space through a viewing tube (a thoracoscope). A thoracoscope also may be used in treating accumulations of fluid in the pleural space (pleural effusions).

The patient usually is given general anesthesia for this procedure. Then a surgeon makes up to three small incisions in the chest wall and passes a thoracoscope into the pleural space; this allows

air to enter, collapsing the lung. Besides being able to view the lung surface and pleura, a doctor may take samples of tissue for microscopic examination and may give drugs through the thoracoscope to prevent a reaccumulation of fluid in the pleural space. After the thoracoscope is removed, a chest tube is inserted to remove air that entered the pleural space during the procedure, enabling the collapsed lung to reinflate.

Complications are similar to those for thoracentesis and needle biopsy of the pleura. However, this procedure is more invasive, leaves a small wound, and requires hospitalization and general anesthesia.

Mediastinoscopy

Mediastinoscopy is the direct visual examination of the area of the chest between the two lungs (the mediastinum) through a viewing tube (mediastinoscope). The mediastinum contains the heart, trachea, esophagus, thymus, and lymph nodes. Nearly all mediastinoscopies are used to diagnose the cause of enlarged lymph nodes or to evaluate how far lung cancer has spread before chest surgery (thoracotomy).

Mediastinoscopy is performed in an operating room with the patient under general anesthesia. A small incision is made in the notch just above the breastbone (sternum). The instrument then is passed down into the chest, allowing the doctor to observe all the contents of the mediastinum and to obtain specimens for diagnostic tests if necessary.

Thoracotomy

Thoracotomy is an operation in which the chest wall is opened to view the internal organs, to obtain samples of tissue for laboratory examination, and to treat diseases of the lungs, heart, or major arteries.

Although thoracotomy is the most accurate means of assessing lung diseases, it's a major operation and therefore is used less often than other diagnostic techniques. Thoracotomy is used when procedures such as thoracentesis, bronchoscopy, or mediastinoscopy fail to provide

▲ see page 192

adequate information. The lung problem is identified in more than 90 percent of people who undergo this operation because the sample site can be seen and selected and because large tissue samples can be taken.

Thoracotomy requires general anesthesia in an operating room. An incision is made in the chest wall, and tissue samples of the lung are removed for microscopic examination. If specimens are to be taken from areas in both lungs, the breastbone is often split. If necessary, a lung segment, a lung lobe, or an entire lung can be removed.

A chest tube is inserted and left in place for 24 to 48 hours afterward. The patient usually stays in the hospital for several days.

Suctioning

Suctioning is used to obtain secretions and cells from the trachea and large bronchi. It's used to obtain specimens for microscopic examination or a sputum culture and to help patients clear secretions from their airways when their cough is ineffective.

One end of a long, flexible, clear plastic tube is attached to a suction pump; the other end is passed through a nostril or the mouth and into the trachea. When the tube is in position, suction is applied in intermittent bursts lasting 2 to 5 seconds. With people who have an artificial opening directly into the trachea (tracheostomy), the tube can be inserted directly into the trachea.

CHAPTER 33

Acute Respiratory Distress Syndrome

Acute respiratory distress syndrome (also called adult respiratory distress syndrome) is a type of lung failure resulting from many different disorders that cause fluid accumulation in the lungs (pulmonary edema).

Acute respiratory distress syndrome is a medical emergency that can occur in people who previously had normal lungs. Despite the fact that it's sometimes called adult respiratory distress syndrome, this condition can occur in children.

Causes

The cause can be any disease that directly or indirectly injures the lungs. About a third of the people with the syndrome develop it as a consequence of a severe, widespread infection (sepsis).

When the small air sacs (alveoli) and capillaries of the lung are injured, blood and fluid leak into the spaces between the alveoli and eventually into the alveoli themselves. The inflammation

that follows can lead to scar tissue formation. As a result, the lungs can't function normally.

Symptoms and Diagnosis

Acute respiratory distress syndrome usually develops within 24 to 48 hours of the original injury or illness. The person first experiences shortness of breath, usually with rapid, shallow breathing. Through a stethoscope, a doctor may hear crackling or wheezing sounds in the lungs. Because of low oxygen levels in the blood, the skin may become mottled or blue, and other organs such as the heart and brain may malfunction.

Arterial blood gas analysis indicates low levels of oxygen in the blood,▲ and chest x-rays show fluid filling spaces that should be filled with air. Further tests may be needed to ensure that heart failure isn't the cause of the problem.

Complications and Prognosis

The oxygen deprivation caused by this syndrome can produce complications in other organs soon after the condition starts or, if the situation doesn't improve, days or weeks later.

▲ see page 160

Prolonged oxygen deprivation can cause such serious complications as kidney failure. Without prompt treatment, the severe oxygen deprivation from this syndrome causes death in 90 percent of patients. However, with appropriate treatment, about half of all people with severe acute respiratory distress syndrome survive.

Because people with acute respiratory distress syndrome are less able to fight lung infections, they commonly develop bacterial pneumonia sometime during the course of the illness.

Treatment

People with acute respiratory distress syndrome are treated in an intensive care unit. Oxygen therapy is vital to correct low oxygen levels. If oxygen delivered by a face mask doesn't correct the problem, a ventilator must be used. The ventilator delivers oxygen under pressure through a tube inserted into the nose, mouth, or trachea; this pressure helps force oxygen into the blood. The pressure can be adjusted to help keep the small airways and alveoli open and to ensure that the lungs don't receive an excessive concentration of oxygen—an important consideration because an excessive concentration can damage the lungs and worsen acute respiratory distress syndrome.

Other supportive treatment, such as intravenous fluid or food, is also important because dehydration or malnutrition can increase the likelihood that several organs will stop functioning, a condition called multiple organ failure. Additional treatments crucial to success depend on the un-

Causes of Acute Respiratory Distress Syndrome

- Severe, widespread infection (sepsis)
- Pneumonia
- Severe low blood pressure (shock)
- Aspiration (inhalation) of food into the lung
- Several blood transfusions
- Injury to the lungs from breathing high concentrations of oxygen
- Pulmonary embolism
- Chest injury
- Burns
- Near drowning
- Cardiopulmonary bypass surgery
- Inflammation of the pancreas (pancreatitis)
- Overdose of a drug, such as heroin, methadone, propoxyphene, or aspirin

derlying cause of acute respiratory distress syndrome. For example, antibiotics are given to fight infection.

Those who respond promptly to treatment usually recover completely with few or no long-term lung abnormalities. Those whose treatment involves long periods on a ventilator are more likely to develop lung scarring. Such scarring may improve over a few months after the patient is taken off the ventilator.

CHAPTER 34

Pulmonary Embolism

An embolus is usually a blood clot (thrombus), but may also be fat, amniotic fluid, bone marrow, a tumor fragment, or an air bubble that travels through the bloodstream until it blocks a blood vessel. Pulmonary embolism is the sudden blocking of an artery of the lung (pulmonary artery) by an embolus.

Usually, unobstructed arteries can send enough blood to the affected part of the lung to prevent tissue death. However, when very large vessels are blocked or the person has a preexist-

ing lung disease, the amount of blood supplied may be insufficient to prevent tissue death. About 10 percent of people with pulmonary embolism suffer some lung tissue death, called pulmonary infarction.

If the body breaks up small clots quickly, damage is kept to a minimum. Large clots take much longer to disintegrate, so more damage is done. Large clots may cause sudden death.

What Predisposes Someone to Clotting?

The cause of clotting in the veins may not be discernible, but many times predisposing conditions are obvious. These conditions include
• Surgery
• Prolonged bed rest or inactivity (such as sitting during a long car or plane trip)
• Stroke
• Heart attack
• Obesity
• Hip or leg fracture
• Increased tendency of blood to clot (for example, in certain cancers, with oral contraceptive use, and with a hereditary deficiency of a blood clotting inhibitor)

Causes

The most common type of pulmonary embolus is a blood clot, usually one that begins in a leg or pelvic vein.▲ Blood clots tend to form when the blood is flowing slowly or not at all, as may occur in the leg veins when a person stays in one position for a long time. When the person starts moving again, the clot can break loose. Far less often, clots begin in the veins of the arms or in the right side of the heart. Once a clot in a vein breaks free into the bloodstream, it usually travels to the lungs.

Another type of embolus may form from fat that escapes into the blood from the bone marrow when a bone is fractured. An embolus also may form from amniotic fluid during childbirth. However, both fat and amniotic fluid emboli are rare. They generally lodge in small vessels like arterioles and capillaries of the lung; if many of these vessels become obstructed, acute respiratory distress syndrome may develop.■

Symptoms

Small emboli may not cause any symptoms, but most cause shortness of breath. This may be the

only symptom, especially if infarction doesn't develop. Often, the breathing is very rapid, and the person may feel anxious or restless and appear to have an anxiety attack. Sharp pain may be felt in the chest, especially when the person breathes deeply; the pain is called pleuritic chest pain.

In some people, the first symptoms may be light-headedness, fainting, or convulsions. These symptoms usually result from a sudden decrease in the heart's ability to deliver enough well-oxygenated blood to the brain and other organs. Irregular heartbeats may also occur. People with an occlusion of one or more large vessels of the lungs may have a blue skin color (cyanosis) and can die suddenly.

Pulmonary infarction produces coughing, blood-stained sputum, sharp chest pain on breathing, and fever. The symptoms of pulmonary embolism usually develop abruptly, whereas the symptoms of pulmonary infarction develop over a period of hours. Symptoms of infarction often last several days but usually become milder every day.

In people who have recurring episodes with small pulmonary emboli, symptoms such as chronic shortness of breath, swelling of ankles or legs, and weakness tend to develop progressively over weeks, months, or years.

Diagnosis

A doctor suspects pulmonary embolism based on a person's symptoms and predisposing factors. However, certain procedures are often needed to confirm the diagnosis.

A **chest x-ray** may reveal subtle changes in the blood vessel patterns after embolism and signs of pulmonary infarction. However, chest x-rays often are normal, and even when they are abnormal, they rarely confirm pulmonary embolism.

An **electrocardiogram** may show abnormalities, but often they're transient and can only support the possibility of pulmonary embolism.

A lung **perfusion scan** is often performed. A small amount of radioactive substance injected into a vein travels to the lungs, where it outlines the blood supply (perfusion) of the lung. Areas without normal blood supply appear dark on the scan because no radioactive particles can reach them. Normal scan results indicate that the person doesn't have a significant blood vessel obstruction, but abnormal scan results may reflect causes other than pulmonary embolism.

▲ see page 141

■ see page 164

Usually, the perfusion scan is coupled with a lung **ventilation scan**. The person inhales a harmless gas containing a trace of radioactive material, which is distributed throughout the small air sacs (alveoli) in the lungs. The areas where oxygen is being exchanged can then be seen on a scanner. By comparing this scan to the pattern of blood supply shown on the perfusion scan, a doctor can usually determine whether the person has pulmonary embolism: An area of embolism shows normal ventilation but decreased perfusion.

Pulmonary arteriography is the most accurate means of diagnosing pulmonary embolism, but it poses some risk and is more uncomfortable than other tests. A dye that can be seen on x-rays is injected into an artery and flows into the arteries of the lung. On an x-ray, pulmonary embolism shows up as a blockage in an artery.

Additional tests may be performed to find out where the embolus originally developed.

Prognosis

The likelihood of dying from pulmonary embolism depends on the size of the embolus, the size and number of pulmonary arteries blocked, and the person's overall health. Anyone with a serious heart or lung problem is in greater peril from embolism. A person with normal heart and lung function will usually survive unless the embolus blocks half or more of the pulmonary vessels. Fatal pulmonary embolism usually causes death within 1 to 2 hours.

About half of all people with untreated pulmonary embolism will have another embolism in the future. As many as half of these recurrences may be fatal. Therapy with drugs that inhibit blood clotting (anticoagulants) can reduce the rate of recurrence to about 1 in 20.

Prevention

Attempts are made to prevent clots from forming in the veins of people at risk of pulmonary embolism. For postoperative patients—especially the elderly—wearing elastic stockings, doing leg exercises, getting out of bed, and becoming active as soon as possible reduce the risk of clot formation. Leg compression stockings designed to keep blood moving lower the rate of clot formation in the calf, thereby lowering the rate of pulmonary embolism.

The most widely used therapy for reducing the likelihood of clots in calf veins after surgery is heparin, an anticoagulant. Small doses are injected just under the skin immediately before the operation and for 7 days afterward. Heparin can cause bleeding and retard healing, so it's given only to people at high risk of developing clots, including those who are in heart failure or shock, have chronic lung disease, are obese, or have had clots. Heparin isn't used for operations involving the spine or brain because the danger of hemorrhage in these areas is too great. Hospitalized people at high risk of developing pulmonary embolism may be given small doses of heparin even if they're not undergoing surgery.

Dextran, which must be injected intravenously, also helps prevent clots. Like heparin, it may cause bleeding. With certain kinds of surgery that are particularly likely to cause clots, such as hip fracture repair or joint replacement, the drug warfarin may be given orally. Warfarin therapy may be continued for several weeks or months.

Treatment

Treatment of pulmonary embolism begins with the administration of oxygen and, if necessary, analgesics. Anticoagulants such as heparin are given to prevent existing blood clots from enlarging and additional clots from forming. The heparin is given intravenously to achieve a rapid effect, and the dose must be carefully regulated. Warfarin, which also inhibits clotting but takes longer to start working, is given next. Because warfarin can be taken orally, it's suitable for long-term use. Heparin and warfarin are given together for 5 to 7 days, until blood tests show that the warfarin is effectively preventing clotting.

The duration of anticoagulation treatment depends on the patient's situation. If pulmonary embolism is caused by a temporary predisposing factor, such as surgery, treatment continues for 2 to 3 months. If the cause is some longer-term problem, treatment usually continues for 3 to 6 months, but sometimes it must continue indefinitely. While taking warfarin, the person periodically has a blood test to determine if the dose needs to be adjusted.

People who appear to be in danger of dying of a pulmonary embolus may benefit from two other treatment approaches—thrombolytic therapy and surgery. Thrombolytics (drugs that break up the clot) such as streptokinase, urokinase, or tissue plasminogen activator may be helpful.

However, these drugs can't be given to people who have had surgery in the preceding 10 days, are pregnant, have had a recent stroke, or have a propensity to bleed excessively. Surgery may be needed to save someone with severe embolism. Pulmonary embolectomy (removal of the embolus from the pulmonary artery) may be lifesaving.

If emboli recur despite all preventive treatment or if anticoagulants cause significant bleeding, a filter can be surgically placed in the main vein from the legs and pelvis to the right side of the heart. Clots generally originate in the legs or pelvis, and this filter prevents them from being carried into the pulmonary artery.

CHAPTER 35

Bronchitis

Bronchitis is an inflammation of the bronchi usually caused by an infection.

The condition is usually mild and eventually heals completely. But bronchitis may be serious in chronically ill people with heart or lung disease and in the elderly.

Causes

Infectious bronchitis occurs most often in winter. It may be caused by viruses, bacteria, and especially the bacteria-like organisms *Mycoplasma pneumoniae* and *Chlamydia.* Smokers and people who have chronic lung or airway diseases that interfere with clearing inhaled particles from the bronchi may have repeated attacks.▲ Recurring infections may result from chronic sinusitis, bronchiectasis, allergies, and, in children, enlarged tonsils and adenoids.

Irritative bronchitis may be caused by various kinds of dust; fumes from strong acids, ammonia, some organic solvents, chlorine, hydrogen sulfide, sulfur dioxide, and bromine; the air pollution irritants ozone and nitrogen dioxide; and tobacco and other smoke.

Symptoms and Diagnosis

Infectious bronchitis often starts with symptoms of a common cold: runny nose, tiredness, chills, back and muscle aches, slight fever, and sore throat. The start of a cough usually signals the beginning of bronchitis. The cough is dry at first and may remain so, but a person often coughs up small amounts of white or yellow sputum after a day or two. Later, a person may cough up much more sputum, which may be yellow or green. Someone with severe bronchitis may have a high fever for 3 to 5 days, after which most symptoms improve. The cough, however, may last several weeks. If the airways are obstructed, the person may be short of breath. Wheezing, especially after coughing, is common. Pneumonia may develop.

A diagnosis of bronchitis is usually made on the basis of the symptoms, especially the appearance of the coughed-up sputum. If symptoms persist, a chest x-ray may be needed to be sure the person hasn't developed pneumonia.

Treatment

Adults may take aspirin or acetaminophen to reduce fever and general feelings of illness, but children should take only acetaminophen. Resting and drinking plenty of fluids help.

Antibiotics are used for people with symptoms that suggest their bronchitis results from a bacterial infection (such as those who cough up yellow or green sputum and those whose fever remains high) and for people with preexisting lung disease. Adults may receive trimethoprim-sulfamethoxazole, tetracycline, or ampicillin. Often when a *Mycoplasma pneumoniae* infection is suspected, erythromycin is given. For children, amoxicillin is the usual choice. Antibiotics don't help if the infection is caused by a virus.

When symptoms persist or recur or when bronchitis is unusually severe, a laboratory culture of coughed-up sputum may show whether a different antibiotic is needed.

▲ see page 177

Bronchiectasis and Atelectasis

Both bronchiectasis and atelectasis result from damage to a portion of the respiratory tract. In bronchiectasis, the bronchi (the airways that branch off the trachea) are damaged. In atelectasis, part of a lung contracts because of a loss of air.

Bronchiectasis

Bronchiectasis is an irreversible widening (dilation) of portions of the bronchi resulting from damage to the bronchial wall.

Bronchiectasis isn't a single disease; it's produced in several ways and results from several conditions that injure the bronchial wall either directly or indirectly by interfering with its defenses. The condition may be diffuse, or it may appear in only one or two areas. Typically, bronchiectasis causes dilation in medium-sized bronchi, but often the smaller bronchi below them become scarred and obliterated. Occasionally, a form of bronchiectasis affecting larger bronchi occurs in allergic bronchopulmonary aspergillosis, a condition caused by an immune response to the *Aspergillus* fungus.▲

Normally, the bronchial wall is made up of several layers that vary in thickness and composition in different parts of the airways. The inner lining (mucosa) and the region below it (submucosa) contain cells that help protect the airways and lungs from potentially harmful substances. These cells include mucus-secreting cells, ciliated cells with hairlike projections that help sweep particles and mucus up and out of the airways, and many other cells that play a role in immunity and the defense of the body against invading organisms and other harmful substances. Elastic and muscle fibers and a cartilage layer give the airways structure, yet allow the diameter to vary as needed. Blood vessels and lymphoid tissue aid in nourishing and defending the bronchial wall.

In bronchiectasis, areas of the bronchial walls are destroyed and chronically inflamed, the ciliated cells are damaged or destroyed, and mucus production increases. Also, the normal tone of the wall is lost: The affected area becomes wider and flabby and may develop outpouchings or sacs that resemble tiny balloons. The increased mucus promotes the growth of bacteria, often obstructs the bronchus, and leads to pooling of infected secretions and further damage to the bronchial wall. The inflammation can extend to the small air sacs of the lungs (alveoli) and produce bronchopneumonia, scarring, and a loss of functioning lung tissue. In severe cases, scarring and a loss of blood vessels in the lung ultimately can strain the heart. Also, inflammation and an increase in blood vessels in the bronchial wall can cause a person to cough up blood. Blockage of the damaged airways can lead to abnormally low levels of oxygen in the blood.

Many conditions can cause bronchiectasis. The most common cause is infection—either chronic or recurring. Abnormal immune responses, birth abnormalities affecting the structure of the airways or the ability of cilia to clear mucus, and mechanical factors such as bronchial obstruction may predispose a person to infections that lead to bronchiectasis. A small number of cases probably result from inhaling toxic substances that injure the bronchi.

Symptoms and Diagnosis

Although bronchiectasis can develop at any age, most often the process begins in early childhood. However, symptoms may not appear until much later, or they may never appear. Symptoms begin gradually, usually after a respiratory tract infection, and tend to worsen over the years. Most people develop a long-standing cough that produces sputum; the amount and type of sputum depend on how extensive the disease is and whether there's a complicating infection. Often the person has coughing spells only early in the morning and late in the day. Coughing up blood is common and may be the first or only symptom.

Frequent bouts of pneumonia may also be a clue that a person has bronchiectasis. People with widespread bronchiectasis may develop wheezing or shortness of breath; they also may have chronic bronchitis, emphysema, or asthma. Very severe disease, which occurs more com-

▲ see page 188

Understanding Bronchiectasis

In bronchiectasis, some areas of the bronchial wall are destroyed and chronically inflamed, the cilia are destroyed or damaged, and mucus production increases.

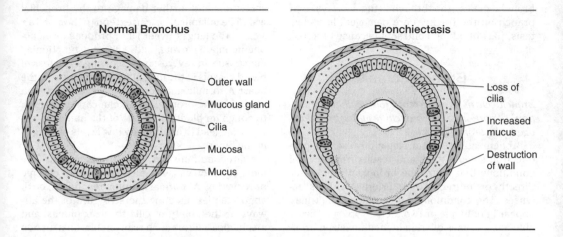

Normal Bronchus

- Outer wall
- Mucous gland
- Cilia
- Mucosa
- Mucus

Bronchiectasis

- Loss of cilia
- Increased mucus
- Destruction of wall

monly in less developed countries, may strain the heart and lead to heart failure—a condition that may cause swelling (edema) of the feet or legs, fluid accumulation in the abdomen, and more difficult breathing, especially when the person is lying down.

Bronchiectasis may be suspected because of a person's symptoms or the presence of another condition associated with it. However, x-ray studies are needed to confirm the diagnosis and assess the extent and location of the disease. Standard chest x-rays may be normal, but sometimes they detect the lung changes caused by bronchiectasis. High resolution computed tomography (CT) can usually confirm the diagnosis and is especially helpful in determining the extent of the disease when surgical treatment is being considered.

After bronchiectasis is diagnosed, tests often are performed to check for diseases that may be causing it. Such tests may include measuring the immunoglobulin levels in blood, measuring the salt levels in sweat (which are abnormal in cystic fibrosis), and examining nasal, bronchial, or sperm specimens to determine if the cilia are structurally or functionally defective. When bronchiectasis is limited to one area—for example, a lung lobe or segment—doctors often perform fiber-optic bronchoscopy (an examination using a viewing tube passed into the bronchi) to determine whether an inhaled foreign object or lung tumor is the cause. Other tests may be performed to identify underlying diseases, such as allergic bronchopulmonary aspergillosis.

Prevention

Childhood immunizations against measles and whooping cough have helped reduce the number of people who develop bronchiectasis. Annual influenza vaccines help prevent the destructive damage of flu viruses. The pneumococcal vaccine can help prevent specific types of pneumococcal pneumonia with their severe complications. Taking antibiotics early in the course of infections such as pneumonia and tuberculosis may also prevent bronchiectasis or reduce its severity. Re-

Selected Causes of Bronchiectasis

Respiratory infections
Measles
Whooping cough
Adenoviral infection
Bacterial infection—for instance, by *Klebsiella*,
Staphylococcus, or *Pseudomonas*
Influenza
Tuberculosis
Fungal infection
Mycoplasma infection

Bronchial obstruction
Inhaled object
Enlarged lymph glands
Lung tumor
Mucus plug

Inhalation injuries
Injury from noxious fumes, gases, or particles
Aspiration of stomach acid and food particles

Genetic conditions
Cystic fibrosis
Ciliary dyskinesia, including Kartagener's
syndrome
Alpha$_1$-antitrypsin deficiency

Immunologic abnormalities
Immunoglobulin deficiency syndromes
White blood cell dysfunctions
Complement deficiencies
Certain autoimmune or hyperimmune
disorders, such as rheumatoid arthritis,
ulcerative colitis

Other conditions
Drug abuse, such as heroin abuse
Human immunodeficiency virus (HIV) infection
Young's syndrome (obstructive azoospermia)
Marfan's syndrome

ceiving immunoglobulin for an immunoglobulin deficiency syndrome may prevent complicating, recurring infections. Appropriate use of anti-inflammatory drugs such as corticosteroids, especially in those with allergic bronchopulmonary aspergillosis, may prevent the bronchial damage that results in bronchiectasis.

Avoiding the inhalation of noxious fumes, gases, smoke (including tobacco smoke), and injurious dusts (such as silica or talc) also helps prevent bronchiectasis or reduce its severity. Inhalation (aspiration) of foreign objects into the airways may be prevented by carefully checking to see what children put in their mouth, avoiding oversedation from drugs or alcohol, and seeking medical care for neurologic symptoms, such as impaired consciousness, or gastrointestinal symptoms, such as difficulty in swallowing or regurgitation or coughing after eating. Also, oily drops or mineral oil shouldn't be placed in the mouth or nose at bedtime because they can be inhaled into the lungs. Bronchoscopy can be used to detect and treat a bronchial obstruction before severe damage occurs.

Treatment
Drugs that suppress coughing may worsen the condition and generally shouldn't be used. For people with large amounts of secretions, postural drainage and chest percussion▲ several times a day help drain the mucus and are essential in managing bronchiectasis.

Infections are treated with antibiotics. Sometimes antibiotics are prescribed for a long period to prevent infections from recurring frequently. Anti-inflammatory drugs such as corticosteroids and mucolytics (drugs that thin the pus and mucus) may also be given. If the blood oxygen level is low, oxygen therapy may help prevent complications such as cor pulmonale (heart disease related to lung disease). If the person has heart failure, diuretics can alleviate some of the swelling. If the person has wheezing or shortness of breath, bronchodilator drugs often help.

▲ see page 158

Rarely, part of a lung is surgically removed. Such surgery is an option only if the disease is confined to one lung, or preferably to one lung lobe or segment. Surgery may be considered for people who have repeated infections despite treatment or who cough up large amounts of blood. Alternatively, a doctor may deliberately obstruct a bleeding vessel to control bleeding.

Atelectasis

Atelectasis is a condition in which part of the lung becomes airless and contracts.

The main cause of atelectasis is an obstruction of a bronchus, one of the two main branches of the trachea leading directly to the lungs. Smaller airways can also become blocked. The obstruction may be caused by a plug of mucus, a tumor, or an inhaled object inside the bronchus. Or the bronchus may be blocked by something pressing from the outside, such as a tumor or enlarged lymph nodes. When an airway becomes blocked, the air in the alveoli is absorbed into the bloodstream, causing the alveoli to shrink and retract. The collapsed lung tissue commonly fills with blood cells, serum, and mucus and becomes infected.

After surgery—especially chest or abdominal surgery—breathing is often shallow, and the lower parts of the lung don't expand properly. Surgery as well as other causes of shallow breathing can lead to atelectasis.

In **middle lobe syndrome,** a type of long-standing atelectasis, the middle lobe of the right lung contracts, usually because of pressure on the bronchus from a tumor or enlarged lymph glands but sometimes without bronchial compression. The blocked, contracted lung may develop pneumonia that fails to clear up completely and leads to chronic inflammation, scarring, and bronchiectasis.

In **acceleration atelectasis,** which occurs in jet fighter pilots, the high forces generated by high-speed flying close small airways, leading to the collapse of alveoli.

In **patchy** or **diffuse microatelectasis,** the surfactant system of the lung is impaired. Surfactant is the substance that coats the lining of the alveoli and reduces surface tension of the alveoli, preventing them from collapsing. When premature babies have a surfactant deficiency, they develop neonatal respiratory distress syndrome. Adults can also develop microatelectasis from excessive oxygen therapy, a severe generalized infection (sepsis), or many other factors that injure the lining of the alveoli.

Symptoms and Diagnosis

Atelectasis can develop slowly and cause only slight shortness of breath. People with middle lobe syndrome may have no symptoms at all, although many have a hacking cough.

If a large area of a lung develops atelectasis quickly, a person may become blue or ashen and have sharp pain on the affected side and extreme shortness of breath. If there's an accompanying infection, the person also may have a fever and a rapid heart rate; occasionally, the person may have seriously low blood pressure (shock).

Doctors suspect atelectasis based on a person's symptoms and the physical examination findings. A chest x-ray that shows the airless area confirms the diagnosis. A computed tomography (CT) scan or fiber-optic bronchoscopy may be performed to find the cause of the blockage.

Prevention and Treatment

People can take steps to avoid atelectasis after surgery. Although people who smoke have a greater risk of developing atelectasis, they can decrease the risk if they stop smoking 6 to 8 weeks before the operation. After an operation, people should be encouraged to breathe deeply, cough regularly, and move about as soon as possible. Breathing devices and exercises may help.

People with chest deformities or neurologic conditions that cause shallow breathing for long periods may benefit from mechanical devices that assist their breathing. The machines apply continuous pressure to the lungs so that even at the end of a breath, the airways can't collapse.

The main treatment for sudden, massive atelectasis is the removal of the underlying cause. If a blockage can't be removed by coughing or by suctioning the airways, it often can be removed by bronchoscopy. Antibiotics are given for any infection. Long-standing atelectasis often is treated with antibiotics because infection is almost inevitable. In certain cases, the affected part of the lung may be removed when recurrent or persistent infection becomes disabling or bleeding is significant. If a tumor is blocking the airway, alleviating the obstruction by surgery or other means may prevent atelectasis from progressing and recurrent obstructive pneumonia from developing.

Obstructive Airway Diseases

After entering the body through the mouth and nose, air passes through the throat (pharynx) into a series of tubelike channels beginning with the voice box (larynx) and the windpipe (trachea). The air then passes into the two main bronchi, each of which supplies one lung. The right and left main bronchi divide repeatedly into smaller and smaller branches (bronchioles) as they progress more deeply into the lungs. The bronchioles ultimately carry air to and from the clusters of air sacs (alveoli), where the exchange of oxygen and carbon dioxide takes place.▲

The bronchi and bronchioles are basically tubes with muscular walls. Their inner lining is a mucous membrane containing a few cells that produce mucus. Other cells lining the bronchi have three main types of specialized surface receptors that sense the presence of substances and stimulate the underlying muscles to contract and relax. When stimulated, beta-adrenergic receptors make the muscles relax, thereby widening the airways and making it easier for air to enter and exit. Cholinergic receptors when stimulated by acetylcholine and peptidergic receptors when stimulated by neurokinins make the muscles contract, thereby narrowing the airways and making it harder for air to enter and exit.

Airway obstruction may be reversible or irreversible. In asthma, airway obstruction is completely reversible. In chronic obstructive pulmonary disease caused by chronic bronchitis, it's partially reversible, and in chronic obstructive pulmonary disease caused by emphysema, it's irreversible.

Asthma

Asthma is a condition in which the airways are narrowed because hyperreactivity to certain stimuli produces inflammation; the airway narrowing is reversible.

Asthma affects about 10 million Americans and is becoming more common. Between 1982 and 1992, the number of people with asthma increased by 42 percent. The condition also seems to be becoming more serious, requiring more peo-

ple to be hospitalized. Between 1982 and 1992, the death rate from asthma in the United States increased by 35 percent.

Causes

In a person with asthma, the airways narrow in response to stimuli that don't affect the airways in normal lungs. The narrowing can be triggered by many stimuli, such as pollens, dust mites, animal dander, smoke, cold air, and exercise. In an asthma attack, the smooth muscles of the bronchi go into spasm, and the tissues lining the airways swell from inflammation and secrete mucus into the airways. These actions narrow the diameter of the airways (a condition called bronchoconstriction); the narrowing requires the person to exert more effort to move air in and out.

Certain cells in the airway, particularly the mast cells, are thought to be responsible for initiating the airway narrowing. Mast cells throughout the bronchi release substances such as histamine and leukotrienes that cause smooth muscle to contract, mucus secretion to increase, and certain white blood cells to migrate to the area. Mast cells can be triggered to release these substances in response to something they recognize as foreign (an allergen), such as pollen, house dust mites, or animal dander. However, asthma is also common and severe in many people without defined allergies. When someone with asthma exercises or breathes cold air, a similar reaction occurs. Stress and anxiety also can trigger mast cells to release histamine and leukotrienes. Eosinophils, another type of cell found in the airways of people with asthma, release additional substances including leukotrienes and other materials, contributing to airway narrowing.

Symptoms and Complications

Asthma attacks vary in frequency and severity. Some people with asthma are symptom-free most of the time, with an occasional, brief, mild episode

▲ see box, page 151

How Airways Narrow

During an asthma attack, the smooth muscle layer goes into spasm, narrowing the airway. The mucosa swells from inflammation and more mucus is produced, further narrowing the airway.

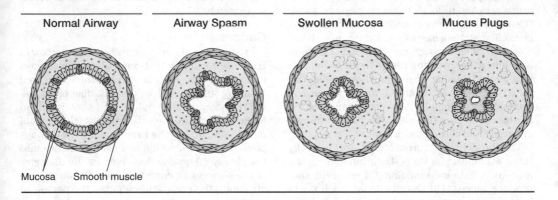

Normal Airway   Airway Spasm   Swollen Mucosa   Mucus Plugs

Mucosa   Smooth muscle

of shortness of breath. Others cough and wheeze most of the time and have severe attacks after viral infections, exercise, or exposure to allergens or irritants. Crying or hearty laughing may also bring on symptoms.

An asthma attack may begin suddenly with wheezing, coughing, and shortness of breath. Wheezing is particularly noticeable when the person breathes out. At other times, an asthma attack may come on slowly with gradually worsening symptoms. In either case, people with asthma usually first notice shortness of breath, coughing, or chest tightness. The attack may be over in minutes, or it may last for hours or days. Itching on the chest or neck may be an early symptom, especially in children. A dry cough at night or while exercising may be the only symptom.

During an asthma attack, shortness of breath may become severe, creating a feeling of anxiety. The person instinctively sits upright and leans forward, using the neck and chest muscles to help in breathing, but still struggles for air. Sweating is a common reaction to the effort and anxiety.

In a very severe attack, a person will be able to say only a few words without stopping for breath. However, wheezing may diminish because hardly

▲ see box, page 160

any air is moving in and out of the lungs. Confusion, lethargy, and blue skin color (cyanosis) are signs that the person's oxygen supply is severely limited, and emergency treatment is needed. Usually, a person recovers completely, even from a severe asthma attack.

Rarely, some of the lung's air sacs (alveoli) may rupture, allowing air to accumulate in the pleural space (the space between the membrane layers covering the lungs) or allowing air to gather around the organs in the chest. These complications worsen the shortness of breath.

Diagnosis

A doctor suspects asthma based largely on a patient's report of characteristic symptoms. A diagnosis of asthma can be confirmed when repeated spirometry tests ▲ performed over hours or days reveal that airway narrowing has improved and was therefore reversible. If the airways aren't narrowed at the time of the first test, a diagnosis can be confirmed by a test in which the person inhales aerosol bronchoconstrictors in doses too low to affect a normal person. If the person's airways narrow after inhalation, a diagnosis of asthma is made.

Spirometry also is used to assess the severity of the airway obstruction and to monitor treatment. Peak expiratory flow (the fastest rate at which air can be exhaled) can be measured using a small handheld peak flow meter. Often, this test is used to monitor the severity of asthma at home. Usually, peak flow rates are lowest between 4:00 and 6:00 A.M. and highest at 4:00 P.M. However, more than a 15 to 20 percent difference in rates at these times is considered evidence of moderate to severe asthma.

Determining what triggers a person's asthma is often difficult. Allergy skin testing can help identify allergens that may trigger asthma symptoms. However, an allergic response to a skin test doesn't necessarily mean that the allergen being tested is causing the asthma. The person still has to note whether attacks occur after exposure to this allergen. If a doctor suspects a particular allergen, a blood test that measures the level of antibody produced in response to the allergen can be performed to determine the degree of sensitivity.

If the diagnosis of asthma is in doubt or if identifying the substance that triggers the attacks is essential, an inhalational bronchial challenge test can be done. Because the test tries to provoke an episode of airway narrowing, there's a slight risk of a severe asthma attack. First, the examiner uses spirometry to measure the volume of air the person can force out of the lungs in 1 second by actively exhaling—a measurement known as the forced expiratory volume in 1 second (FEV_1). Next, the person inhales a very dilute solution of an allergen. About 15 to 20 minutes later, the spirometry measurements are repeated. If the forced expiratory volume in 1 second decreases by more than 20 percent after the allergen has been inhaled, the person's asthma can be triggered by the allergen.

To test for exercise-induced asthma, an examiner uses spirometry to measure forced expiratory volume in 1 second before and after exercise on a treadmill or stationary bicycle. If the forced expiratory volume in 1 second decreases more than 15 percent, the person's asthma can be induced by exercise.

Prevention and Treatment

Asthma attacks may be prevented if the factors that trigger them are identified and avoided. Often, attacks triggered by exercise can be avoided by taking medication beforehand.

Drug treatments allow most people with asthma to lead relatively normal lives. Immediate treatments to get asthma attacks under control

Avoiding Common Causes of Asthma Attacks

The most common indoor allergens are house dust mites, feathers, cockroaches, and animal dander. Anything that can be done to reduce exposure to these allergens may reduce the number or severity of attacks. Exposure to house dust mites can be reduced by removing wall-to-wall carpets and keeping the relative humidity low (preferably below 50 percent) in the summer by using air conditioning. Also, special pillow and mattress covers can help reduce exposure to these mites. Cats and dogs must be removed to significantly decrease animal dander.

Irritating fumes such as cigarette smoke should also be avoided. In some people with asthma, aspirin and other nonsteroidal anti-inflammatory drugs trigger attacks. Tartrazine, a yellow coloring used in some drug tablets and food, may also bring on an attack. Sulfites—commonly added to foods as a preservative—may trigger attacks after a susceptible person eats from a salad bar or drinks beer or red wine.

differ from continuous treatments designed to prevent attacks.

Beta-adrenergic receptor agonists are the best drugs for relieving sudden attacks of asthma and preventing attacks that might be triggered by exercise. These bronchodilators stimulate beta-adrenergic receptors to widen the airways. Bronchodilators that act on all beta-adrenergic receptors, such as adrenaline, cause side effects such as rapid heartbeat, restlessness, headache, and muscle tremors. Bronchodilators that act mainly on $beta_2$-adrenergic receptors, which are found primarily on cells in the lungs, have little effect on other organs. These bronchodilators, such as albuterol, cause fewer side effects than bronchodilators that act on all beta-adrenergic receptors.

Most bronchodilators act within minutes, but the effects last only 4 to 6 hours. New, longer-acting bronchodilators are available, but because they don't begin to act as quickly, they are used for prevention rather than for acute attacks of asthma. The bronchodilators can be taken orally, injected, or inhaled and are highly effective. Inhalation deposits the drug directly in the airways, so that it acts quickly, but the drug may not reach the airways that are severely obstructed. The oral and injected bronchodilators can reach these airways but are more likely to cause side effects and tend to work more slowly.

When a person with asthma feels the need to use more of a beta-adrenergic receptor agonist than is recommended, the person should get immediate medical attention. Overusing these drugs can be very dangerous. The need for continuous use indicates severe bronchospasm, which can lead to respiratory failure and death.

Theophylline is another drug that produces bronchodilation. Usually taken orally, theophylline comes in many forms, from short-acting tablets and syrups to longer-acting sustained release capsules and tablets. In a severe asthma attack, it can be given intravenously.

The amount of theophylline in the blood can be measured in a laboratory and must be closely monitored by a doctor, because too little drug in the blood may give little benefit, and too much drug may cause life-threatening abnormal heart rhythms or seizures. When first taking theophylline, a person with asthma may feel slightly nauseated or jittery. Both side effects usually disappear as the body adjusts to the drug. When people take larger doses, a rapid heartbeat or palpitations frequently occur. A person may also experience insomnia, agitation, vomiting, and seizures.

Corticosteroids block the body's inflammatory response and are exceptionally effective at reducing asthma symptoms. If taken for long periods, corticosteroids gradually reduce the likelihood of asthma attacks by making the airways less sensitive to a number of provocative stimuli.

However, long-term use of oral or injected corticosteroids may result in poor wound healing, stunted growth in children, loss of calcium from the bones, stomach bleeding, premature cataracts, elevated blood sugar levels, hunger, weight gain, and mental problems. Oral or injected corticosteroids may be used for 1 to 2 weeks to relieve a severe asthma attack. Usually for long-term use, inhalant corticosteroids are prescribed because inhaling delivers 50 times more drug to the lungs than to the rest of the body. Oral corticosteroids are prescribed on a long-term basis only when no other treatments can control the symptoms.

Cromolyn and **nedocromil** are thought to inhibit the release of inflammatory chemicals from mast cells and make the airways less likely to constrict. They're useful for preventing attacks but not for treating an attack. The drugs are especially helpful for children with asthma and for people who develop asthma from exercise. Cromolyn and nedocromil are very safe, but they're relatively expensive and must be taken regularly even when a person is free of symptoms.

Anticholinergic drugs, such as atropine and ipratropium bromide, block acetylcholine from causing smooth muscle contraction and from producing excess mucus in the bronchi. These drugs further widen the airways in people who have already been given beta$_2$-adrenergic receptor agonists. However, they're only marginally effective as asthma treatments.

Leukotriene modifiers, such as montelukast, zafirlukast, and zileuton, are the newest drugs available to help control asthma. They prevent the action or synthesis of leukotrienes, which are chemicals made by the body that cause asthma symptoms.

Treatment for Asthma Attacks

An asthma attack should be treated as quickly as possible to open the airways. Most of the same drugs used to prevent an attack are used but in higher doses or different forms. Beta-adrenergic receptor agonists are taken with a handheld inhaler or, when breathlessness is severe, with a nebulizer. The nebulizer directs air or oxygen under pressure through a solution of the drug, producing a mist for inhalation. Nebulizers produce a continuous mist, so the person doesn't have to coordinate breathing with the action of the nebulizer. Less effective ways of treating asthma attacks include injections under the skin of epinephrine or terbutaline and intravenous infusions of aminophylline, a type of theophylline. People having severe attacks and those who don't show improvement with other treatment may receive corticosteroid injections, usually intravenously.

Because people with severe asthma commonly have low blood oxygen levels, they may receive oxygen during attacks while they receive other treatment. Intravenous fluids may be needed if the person is dehydrated. Antibiotics also may be needed if a doctor suspects an infection.

During the treatment of severe asthma, a doctor may check the levels of oxygen and carbon dioxide in the person's blood.▲ A doctor may also check pulmonary function, usually with a spirometer or a peak flow meter. Usually, a chest x-ray is needed only in severe attacks. Generally, people with asthma are admitted to the hospital if their lung function doesn't improve after receiving a beta-adrenergic receptor agonist and aminophylline or if they have a seriously low blood oxygen level or a high blood carbon dioxide level. Patients with very severe asthma attacks may need to be placed on a respirator.

Long-term Asthma Therapy

One of the most common, effective asthma treatments is an inhaler that's filled with a beta-adrenergic receptor agonist. Most are metered-dose inhalers, handheld cartridges containing gas under pressure. The pressure turns the drug into a fine spray containing a measured amount of drug. For those who experience difficulty using a metered-dose inhaler, spacers or holding chambers can be used. With any type of inhaler, proper technique is vital; if the device isn't used properly, the drug won't reach the airways. Excessive use of inhalers suggests that the person has life-threatening asthma; the person may also have side effects from excessive use, such as irregular heart rhythms.

If a single metered-dose inhaler doesn't contain enough medication to relieve symptoms for 4 to 6 weeks, cromolyn or inhaled corticosteroids may be added to the daily regimen. Oral theophylline may be added as well if symptoms persist, especially at night.

Chronic Obstructive Pulmonary Disease

Chronic obstructive pulmonary disease (COPD) is persistent obstruction of the airways caused by emphysema or chronic bronchitis.

Emphysema is an enlargement of the tiny air sacs of the lungs (alveoli) and the destruction of their walls. Chronic bronchitis is a persistent chronic cough that produces sputum and is not due to a medically discernible cause such as lung cancer. In chronic bronchitis, bronchial glands are enlarged, causing excess secretion of mucus.

There are two causes for the airflow obstruction in chronic obstructive pulmonary disease. The first is emphysema. Normally, the clusters of alveoli connected to the small airways (bronchioles) provide a fairly rigid structure and hold the

---

How to Use a Metered-Dose Inhaler

1. Shake the inhaler.

2. Breathe out for 1 or 2 seconds.

3. Put the inhaler either in your mouth or 1 to 2 inches from it and start to breathe in slowly, like sipping hot soup.

4. While starting to breathe in, press the top of the inhaler.

5. Breathe in slowly until your lungs are full. (This should take about 5 or 6 seconds.)

6. Hold your breath for 4 to 6 seconds.

7. Breathe out and repeat the procedure 5 to 7 minutes later.

---

airways open. In emphysema, however, the alveolar walls are destroyed, so the bronchioles lose their structural support. Thus, the bronchioles collapse when air is exhaled. In emphysema, therefore, the airflow narrowing is structural and permanent. The second cause of airflow obstruction is inflammation of the small airways in chronic bronchitis. There is scarring of their walls, swelling of their lining, partial obstruction of their passages by mucus, and spasm of smooth muscle. The swelling, mucus obstruction, and smooth muscle spasm can vary in severity from time to time and may improve in response to bronchodilator drugs. This component of the airflow obstruction is partially reversible.

In the United States, about 14 million people suffer from chronic obstructive pulmonary disease. It's second only to heart disease as a cause of disability that makes people stop working, and it's the fourth most common cause of death. More than 95 percent of all deaths from chronic obstructive pulmonary disease occur in people over age 55. It affects men more frequently than women and is more often fatal in men. It's also fatal more often in whites than in nonwhites and in blue-collar workers than in white-collar workers.

▲ see page 160

Chronic obstructive pulmonary disease appears more frequently in some families, so there may be an inherited tendency. Working in an environment polluted by chemical fumes or nonhazardous dust may increase the risk of chronic obstructive pulmonary disease. However, smoking increases the risk much more than a person's occupation.

About 10 to 15 percent of smokers develop chronic obstructive pulmonary disease. Pipe and cigar smokers develop it more often than nonsmokers but not as often as cigarette smokers. Cigarette smokers have higher death rates from chronic bronchitis and emphysema than nonsmokers. With age, cigarette smokers lose lung function much more rapidly than nonsmokers. The more cigarettes a person smokes, the greater the loss of function.

Causes

Irritants cause inflammation of the alveoli. If such inflammation is long-standing, permanent damage may result. White blood cells collect in inflamed alveoli and release enzymes (especially neutrophil elastase) that damage connective tissue in the walls of the alveoli. Smoking further impairs the lung's defenses by damaging the tiny hairlike cells (cilia) lining the airways that normally carry mucus toward the mouth and help expel toxic substances.

The body produces a protein, called alpha$_1$-antitrypsin, whose main role is to prevent neutrophil elastase from damaging the alveoli. In a rare hereditary condition, there's little or no alpha$_1$-antitrypsin in the body, so emphysema develops by early middle age, especially in smokers.

All forms of chronic obstructive pulmonary disease cause air to become trapped in the lungs. The number of capillaries in the walls of the alveoli decreases. These abnormalities impair the exchange of oxygen and carbon dioxide between the alveoli and the blood. In the earlier phases of the disease, blood oxygen levels are decreased, but carbon dioxide levels remain normal. In the later stages, carbon dioxide levels are elevated, and blood oxygen levels fall even further.

▲ see box, page 160

Symptoms

The earliest symptom of chronic obstructive pulmonary disease, which may appear after as little as 5 to 10 years of smoking, is a cough and the raising of mucus, most commonly on arising. The cough is generally mild and is often dismissed as a "normal" smoker's cough, although of course, it is not normal. There is often a tendency for head colds to go down into the chest. During chest colds, sputum often becomes yellow or green because of pus in the sputum. As the years go by, these chest illnesses may become more frequent. They may be accompanied by wheezing, which is often more evident to family members than to the patient.

Around age 60, shortness of breath on effort often appears and is slowly progressive. Ultimately, the patient has shortness of breath on activities of daily living, such as toileting, washing, dressing, and preparing food. About one third of patients experience severe weight loss, which is due in part at least to worsening shortness of breath after eating. Swelling of the legs often develops, which may be due to heart failure. In the late stages of the disease, a chest illness that might have been easily tolerated early in the course of the disease may cause severe shortness of breath at rest, an indication of acute respiratory failure.

Diagnosis

In mild chronic obstructive pulmonary disease, a doctor may find nothing abnormal during a physical examination except for a few wheezes heard through the stethoscope. Usually, the chest x-ray is also normal. Using spirometry to measure forced expiratory volume in 1 second▲ is required to demonstrate airflow obstruction and to make the diagnosis. In a person who has chronic obstructive pulmonary disease, the test shows reduced airflow during a forceful exhalation.

As the disease progresses, chest movement diminishes during breathing, and the neck and shoulder muscles participate in the person's labored breathing. Breath sounds become harder to hear through the stethoscope.

If a person develops chronic obstructive pulmonary disease at a young age, alpha$_1$-antitrypsin deficiency is suspected, and the blood level of the protein is measured. It's also measured in family members of a person known to have the deficiency.

Treatment

Because cigarette smoking is the most important cause of chronic obstructive pulmonary disease, the main treatment is to stop smoking. Stopping smoking when the airflow obstruction is mild or moderate slows the development of disabling shortness of breath. However, stopping smoking at any point in the disease process provides some benefit. The person should also try to avoid exposure to other airborne irritants.

If the person contracts influenza or pneumonia, chronic obstructive pulmonary disease may worsen markedly. Therefore, a person with the disease should receive an influenza vaccination every year and a pneumococcal vaccination once every 6 or so years.

The reversible elements of airway obstruction include muscle spasm, inflammation, and increasing secretions. Improvement in any of these elements will generally lessen symptoms. Muscle spasm may be reduced by using bronchodilators, including beta-adrenergic receptor agonists (such as albuterol in a metered-dose inhaler) and a slowly absorbed form of oral theophylline. Inflammation may be reduced by using corticosteroids, but symptoms respond to corticosteroids in only about 20 percent of patients. There's no reliable therapy for thinning secretions so they can be coughed up more easily. However, avoiding dehydration may prevent thick secretions. A rule of thumb is to drink enough fluids to keep the urine pale except for that passed first in the morning. In severe chronic obstructive pulmonary disease, respiratory therapy▲ may help loosen secretions in the chest.

Flare-ups of chronic obstructive pulmonary disease sometimes result from bacterial infection, which can be treated with antibiotics. A 7- to 10-day course of treatment is often prescribed. Many doctors provide their patients with a supply of an antibiotic and advise them to start taking the drug early in a flare-up.

Long-term oxygen therapy prolongs the life of people who have severe chronic obstructive pulmonary disease and severely low oxygen levels in the blood. Although round-the-clock therapy is best, 12 hours of oxygen a day also has some benefit. This therapy reduces the excess of red blood cells caused by low blood oxygen levels, improves the person's mental functioning, and improves the heart failure caused by chronic obstructive pulmonary disease. Oxygen therapy may also improve shortness of breath during exercise.

People must never use oxygen therapy near open flames or while smoking. For oxygen use in the home, large tanks of compressed oxygen are expensive and inconvenient to deliver. Oxygen concentrators, which extract oxygen from room air and supply it to the person through a 50-foot length of tubing, are cheaper. Small, portable tanks of compressed oxygen also may be needed for brief periods outside the home. Refillable liquid oxygen tanks, while providing most portability both in and outside the home, are the most expensive system.

Exercise programs can be carried out in the hospital and at home. These programs can improve the person's independence and quality of life, decrease the frequency and length of hospital stays, and improve the ability to exercise even though lung function doesn't improve. Stationary bicycling, stair climbing, and walking are used to exercise the legs. Weight lifting is used for the arms. Often, oxygen is recommended during exercise. Special techniques are taught for improving function during activities such as cooking, engaging in hobbies, and sexual activity. As with any exercise program, gains in conditioning are quickly lost if the person stops exercising.

For people with a severe alpha$_1$-antitrypsin deficiency, the missing protein can be replaced. The treatment, which requires weekly intravenous infusions of the protein, is expensive. Lung transplantation may be used in selected patients under age 50.

An operation in the early stages of development known as lung volume reduction surgery can be carried out in people with severe emphysema. The procedure is complex, and it requires the person to stop smoking for at least 6 months before surgery and to undergo an intense training program. The operation improves lung function and the ability to exercise in some people, although the duration of the improvement isn't known.

▲ see page 158

Prognosis

The prognosis for patients with mild airway obstruction is favorable, little worse than the prognosis for smokers without chronic obstructive pulmonary disease. With moderate and severe airway obstruction, the prognosis becomes progressively worse. About 30 percent of people with the most severe airway obstruction die in 1 year; 95 percent die in 10 years. Death may result from respiratory failure, pneumonia, leakage of air into the pleural space around the lungs (pneumothorax), heart rhythm abnormalities (arrhythmias), or blockage of the arteries leading to the lungs (pulmonary embolism). People with chronic obstructive pulmonary disease also have an increased risk of lung cancer. Some people with severe chronic obstructive pulmonary disease may survive for 15 years or more.

CHAPTER 38

Occupational Lung Diseases

Occupational lung diseases are caused by harmful particles, mists, vapors, or gases inhaled while a person works. Where in the airways or lungs an inhaled substance ends up and what type of lung disease develops depend on the size and kind of particles inhaled. Larger particles may get trapped in the nose or large airways, but the smallest ones reach the lungs. There, some particles dissolve and may be absorbed into the bloodstream; most solid particles that don't dissolve are removed by the body's defenses.

The body has several means of getting rid of inhaled particles. In the airways, mucus coats particles so they can be coughed up more easily. In the lungs, special scavenger cells engulf most particles and render them harmless.

Different types of particles produce different reactions in the body. Some particles—plant pollens, for example—can cause allergic reactions such as hay fever or a type of asthma. Particles such as coal dust, carbon, and tin oxide don't produce much of a reaction in the lungs. Other particles, such as quartz dust and asbestos, may cause permanent scarring of lung tissue (pulmonary fibrosis). In large enough quantities, certain particles, such as asbestos, can cause cancer in smokers.

Silicosis

Silicosis is permanent scarring of the lungs caused by inhaling silica (quartz) dust.

Silicosis, the oldest known occupational lung disease, develops in people who have inhaled silica dust for many years. Silica is the main constituent of sand, so exposure is common among metal miners, sandstone and granite cutters, foundry workers, and potters. Usually, symptoms appear only after 20 to 30 years of exposure to the dust. However, in occupations such as sandblasting, tunneling, and manufacturing abrasive soaps, in which high levels of silica dust are produced, symptoms may appear in less than 10 years.

When inhaled, silica dust passes into the lungs, and scavenger cells such as macrophages engulf it.▲ Enzymes released by the scavenger cells cause the lung tissue to scar. At first, the scarred areas are tiny round lumps (simple nodular silicosis), but eventually they may aggregate into large masses (conglomerate silicosis). These scarred areas can't transfer oxygen into the blood normally. The lungs become less flexible, and breathing takes more effort.

Symptoms and Diagnosis

People with simple nodular silicosis have no trouble breathing, but they may cough and produce sputum because their large airways are ir-

▲ see page 810

ritated, a condition called bronchitis. Conglomerate silicosis may cause coughing, sputum production, and severe shortness of breath. At first, the shortness of breath may occur only during exercise, but eventually it occurs even during rest. Breathing may worsen for 2 to 5 years after the person stops working with silica. The lung damage strains the heart and can lead to heart failure, which can be fatal. Also, when exposed to the organism that causes tuberculosis (*Mycobacterium tuberculosis*), people with silicosis are three times more likely to develop tuberculosis than people without silicosis.

Silicosis is diagnosed when someone who has worked with silica has a chest x-ray that shows the distinctive patterns of scarring and nodules.

Prevention

Controlling the dust in the workplace can help prevent silicosis. When dust can't be controlled, as may be true in the sandblasting industry, workers should wear hoods that supply clean external air or masks that completely filter out the tiny particles. Such protection may not be available to all people working in a dusty area (for example, painters and welders), so whenever possible, abrasives other than sand should be used.

Workers exposed to silica dust should have regular chest x-rays—every 6 months for sandblasters and every 2 to 5 years for other workers—so that problems can be detected early. If the x-rays show silicosis, a doctor will probably advise the worker to avoid continued exposure to silica.

Treatment

Silicosis can't be cured. However, if a person with an early stage of the illness stops being exposed to silica, the progression of silicosis may stop. A person who has difficulty breathing may benefit from the treatments used for chronic obstructive pulmonary disease, such as drug therapy to keep the airways open and free of secretions.▲ Because people with silicosis have a high risk of developing tuberculosis, they should have regular checkups that include a tuberculosis skin test.

Black Lung

Black lung (coal workers' pneumoconiosis) is a lung disease caused by deposits of coal dust in the lungs.

Black lung results from inhaling coal dust over a long time. In simple black lung, coal dust collects around the small airways (bronchioles) of the lungs. Although coal dust is relatively inert and doesn't provoke much reaction, it spreads throughout the lungs and shows up as tiny spots on an x-ray. The coal dust doesn't block the airways. Nevertheless, every year 1 to 2 percent of the people with simple black lung develop a more serious form of the disease called progressive massive fibrosis, in which large areas of the lung (at least $1/2$ inch in diameter) become scarred. Progressive massive fibrosis may worsen even after a person is no longer exposed to coal dust. Lung tissue and the blood vessels in the lungs can be destroyed by the scarring.

In **Caplan's syndrome,** a rare disorder that can affect coal miners who have rheumatoid arthritis, large round nodules of scarring develop quickly in the lung. Such nodules may form in people who have had significant exposure to coal dust, even if they don't have black lung.

Symptoms and Diagnosis

Simple black lung usually doesn't cause symptoms. However, many people with this disease cough and easily become short of breath because they also have emphysema (from cigarette smoking) or bronchitis (from cigarette smoking or toxic exposure to other industrial pollutants). The severe stages of progressive massive fibrosis, on the other hand, cause coughing and often disabling shortness of breath.

A doctor makes the diagnosis after noting characteristic spots on the chest x-ray of a person who has been exposed to coal dust for a long time—usually someone who has worked underground at least 10 years.

Prevention and Treatment

Black lung can be prevented by adequately suppressing coal dust at a work site. Coal workers should have chest x-rays every 4 to 5 years, so that the disease can be detected at an early stage. If the disease is detected, the worker should be transferred to an area where coal dust levels are low to prevent progressive massive fibrosis.

▲ see page 179

Who Is at Risk for Occupational Lung Diseases?

Silicosis	• Lead, copper, silver, and gold miners • Certain coal miners (for example, roof bolters) • Foundry workers • Potters • Sandstone or granite cutters • Tunnel workers • Workers who make abrasive soaps • Sandblasters
Black lung	• Coal workers
Asbestosis	• Workers who mine, mill, or manufacture asbestos • Construction workers who install or remove materials that contain asbestos
Berylliosis	• Aerospace workers
Benign pneumoconiosis	• Welders • Iron miners • Barium workers • Tin workers
Occupational asthma	• People who work with grains, western red cedar wood, castor beans, dyes, antibiotics, epoxy resins, tea, and enzymes used in manufacturing detergent, malt, and leather goods
Byssinosis	• Cotton, hemp, jute, and flax workers
Silo filler's disease	• Farmers

Prevention is crucial because there's no cure for black lung. A person who can't breathe freely may benefit from the treatments used for chronic obstructive pulmonary disease, such as drug therapy to keep the airways open and free of secretions.▲

▲ see page 179

Asbestosis

Asbestosis is widespread scarring of lung tissue caused by breathing asbestos dust.

Asbestos is composed of fibrous mineral silicates of different chemical compositions. When inhaled, asbestos fibers settle deep in the lungs, causing scars. Asbestos inhalation also can cause the two layers of membrane covering the lungs (the pleura) to thicken.

People who work with asbestos are at risk of developing lung disease. Workers who demolish buildings that have insulation containing asbestos are also at risk, although the risk is small. The more a person is exposed to asbestos fibers, the greater the risk of developing an asbestos-related disease.

Symptoms

Symptoms of asbestosis appear gradually only after many scars have formed and the lungs lose their elasticity. The first symptoms are a mild shortness of breath and decreased ability to exercise. Heavy smokers who have chronic bronchitis along with asbestosis may cough and wheeze. Gradually, breathing becomes more and more difficult. In about 15 percent of people with asbestosis, severe shortness of breath and respiratory failure develop.

Inhaling asbestos fibers can occasionally cause fluid to accumulate in the space between the two pleural layers, called the pleural space. Rarely, asbestos causes tumors in the pleura, called mesotheliomas, or in the membranes of the abdomen, called peritoneal mesotheliomas. The mesotheliomas caused by asbestos are cancerous and can't be cured. Mesotheliomas most commonly appear after exposure to crocidolite, one of four types of asbestos. Amosite, another type, also causes mesotheliomas. Chrysotile probably doesn't cause mesotheliomas, but sometimes it's contaminated with tremolite, which does cause them. Mesotheliomas usually develop 30 to 40 years after exposure.

Lung cancer is related in part to the level of exposure to asbestos fibers; however, among people with asbestosis, lung cancer develops almost exclusively in those who also smoke cigarettes, particularly those who smoke more than a pack a day.

Diagnosis

In a person who has a history of exposure to asbestos, a doctor sometimes can diagnose asbestosis with a chest x-ray that shows characteristic changes. Usually, the person also has abnormal lung function, and a doctor listening with a stethoscope placed over the lungs can hear abnormal sounds called crackles. To determine if a pleural tumor is cancerous, a doctor must perform a biopsy (remove a small piece of pleura and examine it under a microscope). Fluid around the lungs may be removed with a needle and analyzed (a procedure called thoracentesis); however, this procedure isn't usually as accurate as performing a biopsy.

Prevention and Treatment

Diseases caused by asbestos inhalation can be prevented by minimizing asbestos dust and fibers in the workplace. Because industries that use asbestos have improved dust control, fewer people develop asbestosis today, but mesotheliomas are still occurring in people who were exposed as much as 40 years ago. Asbestos in the home should be removed by workers trained in safe removal techniques. Smokers who have been in contact with asbestos can reduce their risk of lung cancer by giving up cigarettes.

Most treatments for asbestosis ease symptoms—for example, oxygen therapy relieves shortness of breath. Draining fluid from around the lungs also may make breathing easier. Occasionally, lung transplantation has been successful in treating asbestosis. Mesotheliomas are invariably fatal; chemotherapy doesn't work well, and surgical removal of the tumor doesn't cure the cancer.

Berylliosis

Berylliosis is a lung inflammation caused by inhaling dust or fumes that contain beryllium.

In the past, beryllium was commonly mined and extracted for use in the electronics and chemical industries and in the manufacture of fluorescent light bulbs. Today, it's used mainly in the aerospace industry. Besides workers in these industries, a few people living near beryllium refineries also have developed berylliosis.

Berylliosis differs from other occupational lung diseases in that lung problems seem to occur only in people who are sensitive to beryllium—about 2 percent of those who come in contact with it. The disease can occur even in those who have had a relatively brief exposure to beryllium, and symptoms may not appear for 10 to 20 years.

Symptoms and Diagnosis

In some people, berylliosis develops suddenly (acute berylliosis), mainly as an inflammation of the lungs (pneumonitis). People with acute berylliosis have an abrupt onset of coughing, difficulty in breathing, and weight loss. Acute berylliosis also can affect the skin and eyes.

Other people have chronic berylliosis, in which abnormal tissue forms in the lungs and the lymph nodes enlarge. In these people, coughing, difficult breathing, and weight loss develop gradually.

The diagnosis is based on the person's history of exposure to beryllium, the symptoms, and characteristic changes on a chest x-ray. However, x-rays of berylliosis resemble those of another lung disease, sarcoidosis, and additional immunologic tests may be needed.

Prognosis and Treatment

Acute berylliosis may be severe—even fatal. However, most people recover, even though initially, they're very ill: Their lungs are stiff and function poorly. With appropriate treatment, such as ventilator support and corticosteroid drugs, people usually recover in 7 to 10 days and have no aftereffects.

If the lungs are severely damaged by chronic berylliosis, the heart may become strained, causing heart failure and death. Sometimes corticosteroid drugs such as oral prednisone are prescribed for chronic berylliosis, although they generally aren't very helpful.

Occupational Asthma

Occupational asthma is a reversible spasm of the airways caused by inhaling work-related particles or vapors that act as irritants or cause an allergic reaction.

Many substances in the workplace can cause spasms of the airways, which make breathing difficult. Some people are particularly sensitive to airborne irritants.

Symptoms

Occupational asthma may cause shortness of breath, a tightness in the chest, wheezing, coughing, sneezing, runny nose, and watery eyes. For some people, wheezing at night is the only symptom.

Symptoms may develop during work hours but often don't start until a few hours after work. In some people, symptoms begin as much as 24 hours after exposure. Also, symptoms may come and go for a week or more after exposure. Thus, the link between the workplace and the symptoms is often obscured. Symptoms often become milder or disappear on weekends or over holidays. They worsen with repeated exposure.

Diagnosis

To make a diagnosis, a doctor asks the person about the symptoms and exposure to a substance known to cause asthma. Occasionally, the allergic reaction can be detected with a skin test (patch test), in which a small amount of a suspected substance is placed on the skin. When making a diagnosis is more difficult, a doctor uses an inhalation challenge test, in which the person inhales small amounts of a suspected substance and is observed for wheezing and shortness of breath and tested for decreasing lung function.

Because the airways may begin to narrow before symptoms appear, a person with delayed symptoms may use a device to monitor the airways while at work. This device, a portable peak flow meter, measures the speed at which a person can blow air out of the lungs. When the airways narrow, the rate slows markedly, suggesting occupational asthma.

Prevention and Treatment

Industries using substances that can cause asthma follow dust and vapor control measures, but eliminating the dusts and vapors may be impossible. Workers with severe asthma should change jobs, if possible. Continued exposure often leads to more severe and persistent asthma.

Treatments are the same as for other types of asthma.▲ Drugs that open the airways (bronchodilators) may be given in an inhaler (for example, albuterol) or as a tablet (for example, theophylline). For severe attacks, corticosteroids

---

▲ see page 175

(such as prednisone) may be taken by mouth for a short time. For long-term management, inhaled corticosteroids are preferred.

Byssinosis

Byssinosis is a narrowing of the airways caused by inhaling cotton, flax, or hemp particles.

In the United States and Great Britain, byssinosis occurs almost exclusively in people who work with unprocessed cotton. Those who work with flax and hemp may also develop the condition. People who open bales of raw cotton or who work in the first stages of cotton processing seem to be most affected. Apparently, something in the raw cotton causes the airways of susceptible people to narrow.

Symptoms and Diagnosis

Byssinosis may cause wheezing and tightness in the chest, usually on the first day of work after a break. Unlike with asthma, the symptoms tend to diminish after repeated exposure, and the chest tightness may disappear by the end of the workweek. However, after a person has worked with cotton for many years, the chest tightness may last for 2 or 3 workdays or even the whole week. Prolonged exposure to cotton dust increases the frequency of wheezing but doesn't lead to permanent disabling lung disease.

The diagnosis is made by using a test that shows decreasing lung capacity over the course of a workday; usually, this decrease is greatest on the first day of the workweek.

Prevention and Treatment

Controlling dust is the best way to prevent byssinosis. Wheezing and chest tightness can be treated with the drugs used for asthma. Drugs that open the airways (bronchodilators) may be given in an inhaler (for example, albuterol) or as a tablet (for example, theophylline).

Gas and Chemical Exposure

Many types of gases—such as chlorine, phosgene, sulfur dioxide, hydrogen sulfide, nitrogen dioxide, and ammonia—may suddenly be released during industrial accidents and may severely irritate the lungs. Gases such as chlorine and ammonia easily dissolve and immediately irritate the mouth, nose, and throat. The lower parts of the lungs are affected only when the gas is inhaled deeply. Radioactive gases, which may be released in a nuclear reactor accident, may cause lung and other cancers that take many years to develop.

Some gases—for instance, nitrogen dioxide—don't easily dissolve. Therefore, they don't produce early warning signs of exposure, such as irritation of the nose and eyes, and they're more likely to be inhaled deeply into the lungs. Such gases can cause inflammation of the small airways (bronchiolitis) or lead to fluid accumulation in the lungs (pulmonary edema). In silo filler's disease, which results from inhaling fumes that contain nitrogen dioxide given off by moist silage, fluid may not develop in the lungs for up to 12 hours after exposure; the condition may temporarily improve and then recur 10 to 14 days later, even without further contact with the gas. A recurrence tends to affect the small airways (bronchioles).

In some people, exposure to small amounts of gas or other chemicals over a long period may result in chronic bronchitis. Also, exposure to some chemicals, such as arsenic compounds and hydrocarbons, is thought to cause cancer in some people. Cancer may develop in the lungs or elsewhere in the body, depending on the substance inhaled.

Symptoms and Diagnosis

Soluble gases such as chlorine cause severe burning in the eyes, nose, throat, windpipe, and large airways. They often produce a cough and blood in the sputum (hemoptysis). Retching and shortness of breath also are common. Less soluble gases such as nitrogen dioxide produce shortness of breath, sometimes severe shortness of breath, after a delay of 3 to 4 hours.

A chest x-ray can show whether pulmonary edema or bronchiolitis has developed.

Prognosis, Prevention, and Treatment

Most people recover completely from accidental exposure to gases. The most serious complication is lung infection.

The best way to prevent exposure is to use extreme care when handling gases and chemicals. Gas masks with their own air supply should be available in case of accidental spillage. Farmers need to know that accidental exposure to toxic gases in silos is dangerous.

Oxygen is the mainstay of treatment. If lung damage is severe, a person may need mechanical ventilation. Drugs that open the airways, intravenous fluids, and antibiotics may be helpful. Corticosteroids such as prednisone are often prescribed to reduce inflammation in the lungs.

Benign Pneumoconioses

Other substances occasionally cause the lungs to appear abnormal on x-rays. Siderosis results from inhalation of iron oxide, baritosis from inhalation of barium, and stannosis from inhalation of tin particles. Although these dusts are evident on a chest x-ray, they don't cause much of a reaction in the lung, so people exposed to them don't have any symptoms or functional impairment.

CHAPTER 39

Allergic Diseases of the Lungs

The lungs are particularly prone to allergic reactions because they're exposed to large quantities of airborne antigens, including dusts, pollens, and chemicals. Exposure to irritating dusts or airborne substances, often when a person is at work, increases the likelihood of allergic respiratory reactions. However, allergic reactions in the lungs don't result only from inhaling antigens. Such a reaction may also occur from eating a certain food or taking a drug.

Types of Allergic Reactions

The body reacts to an antigen by forming antibodies.▲ The antibodies bind to the antigen, usually rendering it harmless. Sometimes, however, when the antibody and antigen interact, inflammation and tissue damage occur. Allergic reac-

▲ see page 811

What Causes Hypersensitivity Pneumonitis?

Disease	Source of Dust Particles
Farmer's lung	Moldy hay
Bird fancier's lung, pigeon breeder's lung, hen worker's lung	Droppings from parakeets, pigeons, chickens
Air conditioner lung	Humidifiers, air conditioners
Bagassosis	Sugarcane waste
Mushroom worker's lung	Mushroom compost
Cork worker's lung (suberosis)	Moldy cork
Maple bark disease	Infected maple bark
Malt worker's lung	Moldy barley or malt
Sequoiosis	Moldy sawdust from redwoods
Cheese washer's lung	Cheese mold
Wheat weevil disease	Infested wheat flour
Coffee worker's lung	Coffee beans
Thatched roof worker's lung	Straw or reed used in roofing
Chemical worker's lung	Chemicals used in manufacturing polyurethane foam, molding, insulation, synthetic rubber, and packaging materials

tions are classified by the type of tissue damage that develops. Many allergic reactions are a mixture of more than one type of tissue damage. Some allergic reactions involve antigen-specific lymphocytes (a type of white blood cell) rather than antibodies.

Type I (atopic or anaphylactic) reactions occur when an antigen entering the body meets mast cells or basophils—types of white blood cells that have antibodies attached to their surfaces and that are part of the immune system. When the antigen binds to these cell-surface antibodies, the mast cells release substances, such as histamine, that cause the blood vessels to dilate and the airways to narrow. These substances also attract other white blood cells to the area. An example of a type I reaction is allergic bronchial asthma.

Type II (cytotoxic) reactions destroy cells because the antigen-antibody combination activates toxic substances. An example of a disease caused by a type II reaction is Goodpasture's syndrome.

Type III (immune complex) reactions occur when large numbers of antigen-antibody complexes accumulate. They may cause widespread inflammation that damages tissues, particularly blood vessel walls, a condition called vasculitis. Systemic lupus erythematosus is an example of a disease that results from a type III reaction.

Type IV (delayed or cell-mediated) reactions occur when an antigen interacts with antigen-specific lymphocytes that release inflammatory and toxic substances, attract other white blood cells, and injure normal tissue. The skin test for tuberculosis (tuberculin test) is an example of this type of reaction.

Hypersensitivity Pneumonitis

Hypersensitivity pneumonitis (extrinsic allergic alveolitis, allergic interstitial pneumonitis, organic dust pneumoconiosis) is an inflammation in and around the tiny air sacs of the lung (alveoli) caused by an allergic reaction to inhaled organic dusts or, less commonly, chemicals.

Causes

Many types of dust can cause allergic reactions in the lungs. Organic dusts that contain microorganisms or proteins as well as chemicals, such as isocyanates, may cause hypersensitivity pneumonitis. Farmer's lung, which results from repeated inhalation of heat-loving (thermophilic) bacteria in moldy hay, is a well-known example of hypersensitivity pneumonitis.

Only a small number of people who inhale these common dusts develop allergic reactions, and only a small proportion of those who develop allergic reactions suffer irreversible damage to the lungs. Generally, a person must be exposed to these antigens continuously or frequently over time before sensitivity and disease develop.

Lung damage appears to result from a combination of type III and type IV allergic reactions. Exposure to the dusts causes lymphocyte sensitization and antibody formation that lead to inflammation of the lungs and a buildup of white blood cells in the walls of the alveoli. Functioning lung tissue may be replaced or destroyed, leading to symptomatic disease.

Symptoms and Diagnosis

If a person has developed a hypersensitivity to an organic dust, a fever, cough, chills, and shortness of breath typically appear 4 to 8 hours after reexposure to it. Other symptoms may include a loss of appetite, nausea, and vomiting. Wheezing is unusual. If the person has no further contact with the antigen, symptoms usually improve within hours, but complete recovery may take weeks.

In a slower form of allergic reaction (subacute form), a cough and shortness of breath may develop over days or weeks and sometimes may be so severe that the person needs to be hospitalized.

With chronic hypersensitivity pneumonitis, a person repeatedly comes in contact with the allergen over months to years, and diffuse scars may form in the lungs, a condition called pulmonary fibrosis. Shortness of breath during exercise, coughing up of sputum, tiredness, and weight loss get worse over months or years. Eventually, the disease may lead to respiratory failure.▲

The diagnosis of hypersensitivity pneumonitis depends on identifying the dust or other substance causing the problem, which may be difficult. People exposed at work may not be sick until hours later, when they're at home. A good clue that the work environment may be the source is that a person is sick on workdays but not on weekends or holidays.

The diagnosis is often suspected because of an abnormal chest x-ray. Then pulmonary function tests■—which measure the lungs' capacity to hold air and their ability to move air in and out and to exchange oxygen and carbon dioxide—may help in making the diagnosis of hypersensitivity pneumonitis. Blood tests for antibodies may confirm exposure to the suspected antigen. When the antigen can't be identified and the diagnosis is in doubt, a lung biopsy (removal of a small piece of lung tissue for examination under a microscope) may be performed. The tissue may be removed during bronchoscopy (an examination of the airways using a viewing tube), thoracoscopy (an examination of the lung surface and pleural space using a viewing tube), or thoracotomy (an operation in which the chest wall is opened).★

Prevention and Treatment

The best prevention is to avoid exposure to the antigen, but this may be impractical if a person can't change jobs. Eliminating or reducing dust or wearing protective masks may help prevent a recurrence. Chemically treating hay or sugarcane waste and using good ventilation systems help prevent workers from being exposed and becoming sensitized to these materials.

People who have an acute episode of hypersensitivity pneumonitis usually recover if further contact with the substance is avoided. If the episode is severe, corticosteroids, such as prednisone, reduce symptoms and may help reduce severe inflammation. Prolonged or recurring episodes may lead to irreversible disease; pulmonary function can become so compromised that the person requires supplemental oxygen therapy.●

Eosinophilic Pneumonia

Eosinophilic pneumonia, also called pulmonary infiltrates with eosinophilia (PIE) syndrome, constitutes a group of lung diseases in which eosinophils, a specialized type of white blood cell, appear in increased numbers in the lungs and usually in the bloodstream.

Eosinophils participate in the immune defense of the lung. The number of eosinophils increases during many inflammatory and allergic reactions, including asthma, which frequently accompanies certain types of eosinophilic pneumonia. In eosinophilic pneumonias, the tiny air sacs of the lungs (alveoli) and often the airways fill with eosinophils. Blood vessel walls may also be invaded by

▲ see page 157

■ see page 159

★ see page 163

● see page 179

eosinophils, and the narrowed airways may become plugged with mucus if asthma develops.

The exact reason that eosinophils build up in the lungs isn't well understood, and often it isn't possible to identify the substance that's causing the allergic reaction. But some known causes of eosinophilic pneumonia include certain drugs, chemical fumes, and fungal and parasitic infections and infestations.

Symptoms and Diagnosis

Symptoms may be mild or life threatening. Simple eosinophilic pneumonia (Löffler's syndrome) and similar pneumonias may produce mild fever and mild respiratory symptoms, if any. A person may cough, wheeze, and feel short of breath but usually recovers quickly. Occasionally, an eosinophilic pneumonia can progress to severe respiratory failure in a few hours.

Chronic eosinophilic pneumonia is severe, and if untreated, often it gets worse. Life-threatening shortness of breath can develop.

With the eosinophilic pneumonias, tests show large numbers of eosinophils in the blood, sometimes as many as 10 to 15 times the normal number. A chest x-ray usually shows shadows in the lungs that are characteristic of pneumonia. However, unlike pneumonia caused by bacteria or viruses, eosinophilic pneumonias typically show rapidly appearing and disappearing shadows on serial x-rays. Microscopic examination of coughed-up sputum typically shows clumps of eosinophils rather than the sheets of granulocytes that are found in bacterial pneumonia. Other laboratory tests may be performed to search for a cause, especially an infection with fungi or parasites; these tests may include microscopic examination of stool specimens. A doctor also considers whether any medication the patient is taking may be the cause.

Treatment

Eosinophilic pneumonia may be mild and may get better without treatment. For severe cases, a corticosteroid such as prednisone is usually needed. If a person also has asthma, routine asthma treatment is given as well.▲ If worms or

other parasites are the cause, they're treated with appropriate drugs. Ordinarily, drugs that may be causing the illness are discontinued.

Allergic Bronchopulmonary Aspergillosis

Allergic bronchopulmonary aspergillosis is an allergic lung disorder that often mimics pneumonia and is characterized by asthma, airway and lung inflammation, and increased numbers of eosinophils in the blood; it's caused by an allergic reaction to a fungus, most commonly Aspergillus fumigatus.

Aspergillus is a fungus that flourishes in the soil, decaying vegetation, foods, dusts, and water. A person who inhales the fungus may become sensitized and develop allergic asthma. In some people, a more complex allergic reaction in the airways and lungs can eventually develop. Although the fungus doesn't actually invade the lungs or directly destroy tissue, it colonizes the asthmatic mucus in the airways and causes recurrent allergic inflammation in the lung. The tiny air sacs of the lungs (alveoli) become packed primarily with eosinophils. Increased numbers of mucus-producing cells may also appear. In advanced cases, inflammation may cause the central airways to widen permanently, a condition called bronchiectasis. Eventually, the lungs become scarred.

Other forms of aspergillosis can occur. *Aspergillus* can invade the lungs and cause serious pneumonia in people with suppressed immune systems. This is an infection, not an allergic reaction.■ The fungus can also form a fungus ball, called an aspergilloma, in cavities and cysts of lungs already damaged by another disease, such as tuberculosis.

Symptoms and Diagnosis

The first indications of allergic bronchopulmonary aspergillosis are usually progressive symptoms of asthma, such as wheezing and shortness of breath, and a mild fever. The person usually doesn't feel well. Brownish flecks or plugs may appear in coughed-up sputum.

Repeated chest x-rays show areas that look like pneumonia, but they move around, most commonly in the upper parts of the lungs. With long-standing disease, computed tomography (CT) may show widened airways. The fungus itself, along with excess eosinophils, may be seen when the sputum is examined under the microscope.

▲ see page 175

■ see page 199

The blood contains high levels of eosinophils and certain antibodies to *Aspergillus*. Skin testing can show whether the person is allergic to *Aspergillus*, but it doesn't distinguish between allergic bronchopulmonary aspergillosis and a simple allergy to *Aspergillus*, which may occur in allergic asthma without aspergillosis.

Treatment

Because *Aspergillus* appears in many places in the environment, it's difficult to avoid. Antiasthma drugs, especially corticosteroids, are used to treat allergic bronchopulmonary aspergillosis. Prednisone taken initially in high doses and over a long period of time in lower doses may prevent progressive lung damage. Because the ill effects aren't caused by infection, antifungal drugs aren't helpful. Receiving allergy shots (desensitization) isn't recommended.

Because the lung damage may worsen without causing any noticeable symptoms, a doctor regularly monitors the disease, using chest x-rays, pulmonary function tests,▲ and antibody measurements. As the disease is controlled, the antibody levels fall.

Pulmonary Wegener's Granulomatosis

Wegener's granulomatosis, a potentially fatal disease, is characterized by severe inflammation of blood vessel walls (granulomatous vasculitis), sinuses, lungs, kidneys, and skin with lumps called granulomas.■ In some cases, only the nasal passages, airways, and lungs are affected.

In this condition, blood vessels in the lungs become inflamed, and some lung tissue may be destroyed. The cause of Wegener's granulomatosis is unknown, but allergic reactions may be involved.

Symptoms and Diagnosis

Pulmonary Wegener's granulomatosis may not cause any symptoms. Or it may produce fever, weight loss, tiredness, cough, shortness of breath, and chest pain.

A chest x-ray may show cavities or dense areas in the lungs that look like cancer. A definite diagnosis can be made only by microscopic examination of a small piece of tissue, which may be taken from an affected area such as the skin, nasal passages, airways, or lungs. A distinctive antibody, called antineutrophil cytoplasmic antibody, often can be detected in the blood of people with Wegener's granulomatosis.

Treatment

Without treatment, the disease can worsen rapidly and cause death, so treatment should start immediately after the diagnosis is made. Pulmonary Wegener's granulomatosis may respond to corticosteroids alone, but many people also need another immunosuppressive drug, such as cyclophosphamide.

Goodpasture's Syndrome

Goodpasture's syndrome is an uncommon allergic disorder in which bleeding into the lungs and progressive kidney failure occur.

This disease usually affects young men. For unknown reasons, people with Goodpasture's syndrome produce antibodies against certain structures in the filtering apparatus of the kidneys and the tiny air sacs (alveoli) and capillaries of the lungs. These antibodies trigger inflammation that interferes with kidney and lung function. Presumably, they're the direct cause of the disease.

Symptoms and Diagnosis

A person with this disease typically develops shortness of breath and coughs up blood. Symptoms can quickly become severe: Breathing can fail, and large amounts of blood can be lost. At the same time, the kidneys can rapidly fail.★

Laboratory tests show the characteristic antibodies in the blood. Urine testing shows blood and protein in the urine. Anemia often is present. A chest x-ray shows abnormal areas in both lungs. A kidney tissue needle biopsy shows microscopic deposits of antibodies in a specific pattern.

▲ see page 159

■ see page 240

★ see page 593

Treatment

The disease may lead to death very rapidly. High doses of corticosteroids and cyclophosphamide may be given intravenously to suppress the activity of the immune system. The person may also undergo plasmapheresis—a procedure in which blood is removed from the circulation, the unwanted antibodies are removed from the blood, and the blood cells are returned to the circulation. The early use of this combination of treatments may help save kidney and lung function. Once damage occurs, it's permanent.

Many people may need supportive care until the disease runs its course. Treatment may require supplemental oxygen or a respirator. Blood transfusions may be needed. If the kidneys fail, kidney dialysis or a kidney transplant is needed.

CHAPTER 40

Infiltrative Lung Diseases

Several diseases with similar symptoms result from abnormal accumulations of inflammatory cells in lung tissue. Early in the course of these diseases, white blood cells and protein-rich fluid accumulate in the lungs' air sacs (alveoli), causing inflammation (alveolitis). If the inflammation persists, the fluid may solidify, and scarring (fibrosis) may replace lung tissue. Extensive scarring of the tissue around the alveoli can progressively destroy the functioning alveoli and leave cysts in their place.

Idiopathic Pulmonary Fibrosis

Pulmonary fibrosis can be caused by many diseases, especially those that involve immune system abnormalities. Yet, despite the many possible causes, in half the people who have pulmonary fibrosis, the cause is never identified. These people are said to have idiopathic pulmonary fibrosis (fibrosing alveolitis, usual interstitial pneumonia). The word *idiopathic* means of unknown cause.

Symptoms and Diagnosis

Symptoms depend on the extent of the lung damage, the rate at which the disease is progress-

ing, and the development of complications such as infections and heart failure. The main symptoms start insidiously as shortness of breath on exertion and diminished stamina. Common symptoms include coughing, loss of appetite, weight loss, tiredness, weakness, and vague chest pains. Late in the disease as the level of oxygen in the blood decreases, the skin may take on a bluish tinge, and the ends of the fingers may become thick or club-shaped.▲ Strain on the heart may cause heart failure. Heart failure caused by underlying lung disease is called cor pulmonale.

A chest x-ray may indicate lung scarring and cyst formation. However, a chest x-ray occasionally can be normal, even when symptoms are severe. Pulmonary function tests■ show that the amount of air the lungs can hold is below normal. Analysis of blood gases shows a low level of oxygen in the blood.

To confirm the diagnosis, a doctor may perform a biopsy (removal of a small piece of lung tissue for microscopic examination) using a bronchoscope.★ Many times, a larger specimen is needed and must be removed surgically.

Desquamative interstitial pneumonia, a variant of idiopathic pulmonary fibrosis, has the same symptoms, but the microscopic appearance of the lung tissue is distinctive.

Lymphoid interstitial pneumonia, another variant, involves mainly the lower lobes of the lung. About a third of the cases occur in people with Sjögren's syndrome. Lymphoid interstitial pneumonia also may develop in children and adults with HIV infection. The pneumonia progresses slowly but

▲ see box, page 157

■ see page 159

★ see page 162

may lead to the formation of cysts in the lungs and to lymphoma.

Treatment and Prognosis

If chest x-rays or a lung biopsy shows that scarring isn't extensive, the usual treatment is a corticosteroid, such as prednisone. A doctor evaluates the patient's response using chest x-rays and pulmonary function tests. A few people who aren't helped by prednisone may improve with azathioprine or cyclophosphamide.

Other treatments are aimed at relieving symptoms: oxygen therapy for low blood oxygen levels, antibiotics for infection, and drugs for heart failure. Several medical centers are using lung transplantation in people with severe idiopathic pulmonary fibrosis.

The prognosis varies greatly. Most people continue to get worse. Some survive for many years; a few die within several months.

Desquamative interstitial pneumonia responds better to corticosteroid treatment, and the survival time is greater and the death rate is lower for people with this variant. Lymphoid interstitial pneumonia is sometimes relieved by corticosteroids.

Histiocytosis X

Histiocytosis X is a group of disorders (Letterer-Siwe disease, Hand-Schüller-Christian disease, eosinophilic granuloma) in which abnormal scavenger cells called histiocytes and another immune system cell type called eosinophils proliferate, especially in the bone and lung, often causing scars to form.

Letterer-Siwe disease starts before age 3 and is usually fatal without treatment. The histiocytes damage not only the lungs but also the skin, lymph glands, bone, liver, and spleen. Collapse of a lung (pneumothorax) may occur.

Hand-Schüller-Christian disease usually begins in early childhood but can start in late middle age. The lungs and bones are most frequently affected. Rarely, damage to the pituitary gland causes bulging eyes (exophthalmos) and diabetes insipidus,▲ a condition in which large quantities of urine are produced, leading to dehydration.

Eosinophilic granuloma tends to start between ages 20 and 40. It usually affects the bones but also affects the lungs in 20 percent of people; sometimes only the lungs are involved. When the lungs are affected, the symptoms can include

> ### Common Causes of Pulmonary Fibrosis
>
> Immune system abnormalities (rheumatoid arthritis, scleroderma, polymyositis, and rarely, systemic lupus erythematosus)
>
> Infection (viruses, rickettsias, mycoplasmas, disseminated tuberculosis)
>
> Mineral dust (silica, carbon, metal dusts, asbestos)
>
> Organic dust (molds, bird droppings)
>
> Gases, fumes, and vapors (chlorine, sulfur dioxide)
>
> Therapeutic or industrial radiation
>
> Drugs and poisons (methotrexate, busulfan, cyclophosphamide, gold, penicillamine, nitrofurantoin, sulfonamides, amiodarone, paraquat)

coughing, shortness of breath, fever, and weight loss, but some people have no symptoms. Collapse of a lung (pneumothorax) is a common complication.

People with Hand-Schüller-Christian disease or eosinophilic granuloma may recover spontaneously. All three disorders may be treated with corticosteroids and cytotoxic drugs such as cyclophosphamide, although no therapy is clearly beneficial. The therapy for bone involvement is similar to that for bone tumors.■ Death usually results from respiratory failure or heart failure.

Idiopathic Pulmonary Hemosiderosis

Idiopathic pulmonary hemosiderosis (iron in the lungs) is a rare, often fatal, disease in which blood leaks from the capillaries into the lungs for unknown reasons.

This disease affects mainly children but can also affect adults. Some of the blood that leaks

▲ see page 703

■ see page 222

out of the capillaries is taken up by scavenger cells in the lung. The breakdown products of the blood irritate the lung and lead to scarring.

The main symptom is the coughing up of blood (hemoptysis). The frequency and severity depend on how often the capillaries bleed into the lungs. After the lungs become scarred, shortness of breath develops. Excessive blood loss leads to anemia; massive bleeding can cause death.

Treatment is aimed mostly at relieving symptoms. Corticosteroids and cytotoxic drugs such as azathioprine may help during flare-ups. Blood transfusions may be needed for blood loss, and oxygen therapy may be needed for a low level of oxygen in the blood.

Pulmonary Alveolar Proteinosis

Pulmonary alveolar proteinosis is a rare disease in which the air sacs of the lungs (alveoli) become plugged with a protein-rich fluid.

The disease generally affects people between ages 20 and 60 who aren't known to have lung disease. The cause of pulmonary alveolar proteinosis is unknown.

In rare instances, lung tissue becomes scarred. The disease may progress, remain stable, or disappear spontaneously.

Symptoms and Diagnosis

When the alveoli are filled, the lungs can't transfer oxygen to the blood. Consequently, most people with this disease experience shortness of breath when they exert themselves. Some have severe breathing difficulty, even at rest. Most also have a cough that doesn't usually produce sputum unless they're smokers.

A chest x-ray shows patchy shadowing in both lungs. Pulmonary function tests▲ reveal that the volume of air that the lungs can hold is abnormally small. Tests show low levels of oxygen in the blood, at first only during exercise but later at rest, too.

To make the diagnosis, a doctor obtains a sample of the fluid in the alveoli for examination. To

obtain a sample, a doctor uses a bronchoscope to wash segments of the lung with a salt solution and then collects the washings.■ Sometimes a doctor performs a biopsy (obtains a lung tissue sample for microscopic examination) during bronchoscopy. Occasionally, a larger specimen is needed and must be removed surgically.

Treatment

People who have few or no symptoms don't require treatment. For those with symptoms, the protein-rich fluid in the alveoli can be washed out with a salt solution during bronchoscopy. Sometimes only a small section of the lung must be washed, but if symptoms are severe and the levels of oxygen in the blood are low, the person is given general anesthesia, so that an entire lung can be washed. From 3 to 5 days later, the other lung is washed, again with the patient under general anesthesia. One washing is enough for some people, while others need washings every 6 to 12 months for many years.

People with pulmonary alveolar proteinosis often are short of breath indefinitely, but the disease rarely kills them as long as they have regular lung washings. The usefulness of other treatments, such as potassium iodide and enzymes that break up proteins, is unclear. Corticosteroids aren't effective and may actually increase the chances of infection.

Sarcoidosis

Sarcoidosis is a disease in which abnormal collections of inflammatory cells (granulomas) form in many organs of the body.

The cause of sarcoidosis is unknown. It may result from an infection or from an abnormal response of the immune system. Inherited factors may be important. Sarcoidosis develops predominantly between ages 20 and 40 and is most common among northern Europeans and American blacks.

Microscopic examination of a tissue specimen from a person with sarcoidosis reveals granulomas. These granulomas may eventually disappear completely or become scar tissue. Granulomas commonly appear in the lymph nodes, lungs, liver, eyes, and skin, and less often in the spleen, bones, joints, skeletal muscles, heart, and nervous system.

▲ see page 159

■ see page 163

Symptoms

Many people with sarcoidosis have no symptoms, and the disease is discovered during a chest x-ray that's being taken for other reasons. Most people develop minor symptoms that don't progress. Serious symptoms are rare.

The symptoms of sarcoidosis vary greatly according to the site and extent of the disease. Fever, weight loss, and aching joints may be the first indications of a problem. Enlarged lymph nodes are common but don't often cause symptoms. A fever may recur throughout the illness.

The organ most affected by sarcoidosis is the lung. Enlarged lymph nodes at the place where the lungs meet the heart or to the right of the trachea may be seen on a chest x-ray. Sarcoidosis produces inflammation in the lungs that may eventually lead to scarring and cyst formation, which can cause coughing and shortness of breath. Severe lung disease can eventually weaken the heart.

The skin is frequently affected by sarcoidosis. In Europe, sarcoidosis often starts as raised, tender, red lumps, usually on the shins (erythema nodosum), accompanied by a fever and joint pain, but this is less common in the United States. Prolonged sarcoidosis may lead to the formation of flat patches (plaques), raised patches, or lumps just under the skin.

About 70 percent of people with sarcoidosis have granulomas in their liver. They often have no symptoms, and the liver seems to function normally. Fewer than 10 percent of people with sarcoidosis have an enlarged liver. Jaundice caused by liver malfunction is rare.

The eyes are affected in 15 percent of people with sarcoidosis. Uveitis (inflammation of certain internal eye structures) makes the eyes red and painful and interferes with vision. Inflammation that persists for a long time may block fluid drainage from the eye, causing glaucoma, which can lead to blindness. Granulomas may form in the conjunctiva (the membrane over the eyeball and inside the eyelids). Such granulomas often don't cause symptoms, but the conjunctiva is an accessible site from which a doctor can take tissue samples for examination. Some people with sarcoidosis complain of dry, sore, and reddened eyes, probably caused by sluggish tear glands that have been affected by the disease and no longer produce enough tears to keep the eyes lubricated.

Granulomas that form in the heart may cause angina or heart failure. Those that form near the electrical conducting system of the heart can trigger potentially fatal irregularities in the heartbeat.

Inflammation can cause widespread pain in the joints. The joints in the hands and feet are most commonly affected. Cysts form in the bones and can make nearby joints swollen and tender.

Sarcoidosis can affect the cranial nerves (nerves of the head), causing double vision and making one side of the face droop. If the pituitary gland or the bones surrounding it are affected, diabetes insipidus▲ may result. The pituitary gland stops producing vasopressin, a hormone needed by the kidney to concentrate urine, causing frequent urination and excessive amounts of urine.

Sarcoidosis can cause high levels of calcium to accumulate in the blood and urine. These high levels occur because sarcoid granulomas produce activated vitamin D, which enhances calcium absorption from the intestine. High blood calcium levels lead to a loss of appetite, nausea, vomiting, thirst, and excessive urine production. If present for a long time, high blood calcium levels may lead to the formation of kidney stones or calcium deposits in the kidney and, eventually, to kidney failure.

Diagnosis

Doctors most often diagnose sarcoidosis by observing its distinctive shadowing on a chest x-ray. Sometimes, further testing isn't necessary. When it is, microscopic examination of a tissue specimen for inflammation and granulomas confirms the diagnosis. The most convenient sources of tissue specimens are skin abnormalities, enlarged lymph nodes close to the skin, and granulomas on the conjunctiva. Examination of a specimen from one of these tissues is accurate in 87 percent of cases. Occasionally, a specimen from the lungs, liver, or muscle is needed.

Tuberculosis can cause many changes similar to those caused by sarcoidosis. Therefore, a doctor also does a tuberculin skin test to make sure the problem isn't tuberculosis.

Other methods that can help a doctor diagnose sarcoidosis or assess its severity include measuring the level of angiotensin converting enzyme

▲ see page 703

in the blood, washing the lungs,▲ and using a whole-body gallium scan. In many people with sarcoidosis, the level of angiotensin converting enzyme in the blood is high. The washings from a lung with active sarcoidosis contain a large number of lymphocytes, but this isn't unique to sarcoidosis. Because gallium scanning shows abnormal patterns in the lungs or lymph nodes of a person with sarcoidosis in those places, this test is sometimes used when the diagnosis is uncertain.

In people with pulmonary scarring, pulmonary function tests show that the amount of air the lung can hold is below normal. Blood tests may reveal a low number of white blood cells. Immunoglobulin levels are often high, especially in blacks. The levels of liver enzymes, particularly alkaline phosphatase, may be high if the liver has been affected.

Prognosis

Commonly, sarcoidosis improves or clears up spontaneously. More than two thirds of people with lung sarcoidosis have no symptoms after 9 years. Even enlarged lymph nodes in the chest and extensive lung inflammation may disappear in a few months or years. More than three quarters of those with only enlarged lymph nodes and more than half of those with lung involvement recover after 5 years.

People who have sarcoidosis that hasn't spread beyond the chest do better than those who also have sarcoidosis elsewhere in the body. People with enlarged lymph nodes in the chest but no sign of lung disease have a very good prognosis. Those whose disease began with erythema nodosum have the best prognosis. About 50 percent of people who once had sarcoidosis have relapses.

About 10 percent of people with sarcoidosis develop a serious disability from damage to the eyes, respiratory system, or elsewhere. Lung scarring leading to respiratory failure is the most common cause of death, followed by bleeding from lung infection caused by the fungus *Aspergillus.*

Treatment

Most people with sarcoidosis don't need treatment. Corticosteroids are given to suppress severe symptoms such as shortness of breath, joint pain, and fever. These drugs also are given if tests show high levels of calcium in the blood; if the heart, liver, or nervous system is affected; if the sarcoidosis causes disfiguring skin lesions or eye disease that corticosteroid eyedrops fail to cure; or if lung disease continues to worsen. People who have no symptoms shouldn't take corticosteroids even if some of their laboratory test results are abnormal. Although corticosteroids control symptoms well, they don't prevent lung scarring over the years. About 10 percent of those who need treatment fail to respond to corticosteroids and are switched to chlorambucil or methotrexate, which may be very effective. Hydroxychloroquine is sometimes helpful in eliminating disfiguring skin lesions.

The success of treatment can be monitored with chest x-rays, pulmonary function tests, and measurements of calcium or angiotensin converting enzyme levels in blood. These tests are repeated regularly to detect relapses after treatment stops.

CHAPTER 41

Pneumonia

Pneumonia is an infection of the lungs that involves the small air sacs (alveoli) and the tissues around them.

▲ see page 163

In the United States, about 2 million people develop pneumonia each year, and 40,000 to 70,000 of them die. Often, pneumonia is the final illness in people who have other serious, chronic diseases. It's the sixth most common cause of death overall, and the most common fatal infection acquired in hospitals. In developing countries, pneumonia is either the leading cause of death or second only to dehydration from severe diarrhea.

Causes

Pneumonia isn't a single illness but many different ones, each caused by a different microscopic organism. Usually pneumonia starts after organisms are inhaled into the lungs, but sometimes the infection is carried to the lungs by the bloodstream or it migrates to the lungs directly from a nearby infection.

In adults, the most common causes are bacteria, such as *Streptococcus pneumoniae, Staphylococcus aureus, Legionella,* and *Hemophilus influenzae.* Viruses, such as influenza and chickenpox, can also cause pneumonia. *Mycoplasma pneumoniae,* a bacterialike organism, is a particularly common cause of pneumonia in older children and younger adults. Some fungi also cause pneumonia.

Some people are more susceptible to pneumonia than others. Alcoholism, cigarette smoking, diabetes, heart failure, and chronic obstructive pulmonary disease all predispose people to pneumonia. The very young and very old are also at higher than average risk. So are people whose immune system is suppressed by certain drugs (such as those used to treat cancer and those used to prevent the rejection of an organ transplant). People who are debilitated, bedridden, paralyzed, or unconscious or who have a disease that impairs the immune system, such as AIDS, are also at risk.

Pneumonia may follow surgery, particularly abdominal surgery, or an injury (trauma), particularly a chest injury, because of the resulting shallow breathing, impaired ability to cough, and retention of mucus. *Staphylococcus aureus,* pneumococci, *Hemophilus influenzae,* or a combination of these organisms is often the cause.

Symptoms and Diagnosis

Common symptoms of pneumonia are a cough that produces sputum, chest pain, chills, fever, and shortness of breath. These symptoms may vary, however, depending on how extensive the disease is and which organism is causing it. When a person appears to have pneumonia, a doctor listens to the chest with a stethoscope to evaluate the condition. Pneumonia usually produces distinctive changes in the way sounds are transmitted, which can be heard with the stethoscope.

Meeting Increasing Resistance

An increasing number of the bacteria that cause pneumonia are developing resistance to antibiotics. For example, many staphylococci produce enzymes (penicillinases) that prevent penicillin from killing them. Pneumococci are also becoming more resistant to penicillin by a different mechanism. Resistance to antibiotics is a serious problem, particularly with infections that are acquired in the hospital.

Resistant staphylococci infections can be treated with antibiotics that are effective in the presence of penicillinase, but some staphylococci are becoming resistant to these drugs, too. For these staphylococci, a drug called vancomycin is often used. Staphylococcal pneumonia tends to respond slowly to antibiotics, and the patient requires a long convalescence.

In most cases, the diagnosis of pneumonia is confirmed with a chest x-ray, which often helps determine which organism is causing the disease. Sputum and blood specimens also are examined in an attempt to identify the organism causing pneumonia. However, the precise organism can't be identified in up to half of people who have pneumonia.

Treatment

Deep-breathing exercises and therapy to clear secretions help prevent pneumonia in people at high risk, such as those who have had chest surgery and those who are debilitated. People with pneumonia also need to clear secretions.

Often, people who aren't very sick can take oral antibiotics and remain at home. The elderly and those who are short of breath or have preexisting heart or lung disease are generally hospitalized and given intravenous antibiotics. They may also need supplemental oxygen, intravenous fluids, and mechanical respiratory support.

Pneumococcal Pneumonia

Streptococcus pneumoniae (pneumococcus) is the most common bacterial cause of pneumonia. A person who has been infected with one of the

80 known types of pneumococcus develops partial immunity to reinfection with that type but no immunity to the others.

Pneumococcal pneumonia usually starts after an upper respiratory tract viral infection (a cold, sore throat, or influenza) damages the lungs enough to allow pneumococci to infect the area. Shaking and chills are followed by a fever, a cough-producing sputum, shortness of breath, and chest pain on the side of the affected lung when breathing. Nausea, vomiting, fatigue, and muscle aches are also common. The sputum is often rust-colored from blood.

A vaccine is available that protects up to 70 percent of people from serious pneumococcal infections. Vaccination is recommended for people at high risk of pneumococcal pneumonia—such as those with lung or heart disease, weakened immune systems, or diabetes, and those over age 65. The protection from vaccination usually lasts a lifetime, although people at highest risk are sometimes revaccinated after 5 to 10 years. About half the time, vaccinations cause redness and pain at the injection site. Only 1 percent of people develop a fever and muscle pain after vaccination. Even fewer have a severe allergic reaction.

Pneumococcal pneumonia may be treated with any of several antibiotics, including penicillin. People who are allergic to penicillin receive erythromycin or another antibiotic instead. The pneumococci that are resistant to penicillin may be treated with other drugs; however, these pneumococci are becoming more resistant to the other drugs as well.

Staphylococcal Pneumonia

Staphylococcus aureus causes only 2 percent of pneumonia cases acquired outside the hospital, but it causes 10 to 15 percent of those acquired in hospitals while people are being treated for another disorder. This type of pneumonia tends to develop in the very young, the very old, and people who are already debilitated by other illnesses. It also tends to occur in alcoholics. The death rate is about 15 to 40 percent—in part because those who develop staphylococcal pneumonia are usually already seriously ill.

Staphylococcus causes typical pneumonia symptoms, but the chills and fever are more persistent in staphylococcal pneumonia than in pneumococcal pneumonia. *Staphylococcus* may cause abscesses (collections of pus) in the lungs and may produce lung cysts that contain air (pneumatoceles), especially in children. Bacteria may be carried from the lung by the bloodstream and produce abscesses elsewhere. Collections of pus in the pleural space (empyema) are relatively common.▲ These collections are drained using a needle or a chest tube.

Gram-negative Bacterial Pneumonia

Bacteria are classified as either gram-positive or gram-negative based on how they look when stained on a microscope slide. Most cases of pneumonia are caused by pneumococci and staphylococci, which are gram-positive bacteria. Gram-negative bacteria, such as *Klebsiella* and *Pseudomonas*, cause pneumonia that tends to be extremely serious.

Gram-negative bacteria rarely infect the lungs of healthy adults. More commonly, they infect infants, the elderly, alcoholics, and people with chronic diseases, especially immune system abnormalities. Gram-negative infections are often acquired in a hospital or nursing home.

Gram-negative bacteria may rapidly destroy lung tissue, so gram-negative pneumonia tends to become serious quickly. Fever, coughing, and shortness of breath are common. The coughed-up sputum may be thick and red—the color and consistency of currant jelly.

Because of the seriousness of the infection, the person is treated intensively in the hospital with antibiotics, supplemental oxygen, and intravenous fluids. Sometimes the person must be put on a ventilator. Despite receiving excellent treatment, about 25 to 50 percent of people with gram-negative pneumonia die.

Pneumonia Caused by *Hemophilus influenzae*

Hemophilus influenzae is a bacterium; despite its name, it isn't the influenza virus that causes the flu. *Hemophilus influenzae* type b strains are the most virulent strains and cause serious diseases, including meningitis, epiglottitis, and pneumonia, usually in children under age 6. How-

▲ see page 206

ever, because of the widespread use of the *Hemophilus influenzae* type b vaccine, serious disease from this organism is becoming less common. The pneumonia is more common among Native Americans, Eskimos, blacks, people with sickle cell disease, and people with immune deficiency disorders. Most such cases are caused by strains other than those used in the *Hemophilus influenzae* type b vaccine.

Signs of the infection include sneezing and a runny nose followed by typical pneumonia symptoms, such as a fever, a cough that produces sputum, and shortness of breath. Fluid in the pleural space (the space between the membrane layers covering the lungs) is common; this condition is called pleural effusion.▲

Vaccination for type b strains of *Hemophilus influenzae* is recommended for all children. The vaccine is given in three doses—at ages 2, 4, and 6 months. Antibiotics are used to treat *Hemophilus influenzae* type b pneumonia.

Legionnaires' Disease

Legionnaires' disease, caused by the bacterium *Legionella pneumophila* and other species of *Legionella,* accounts for 1 to 8 percent of all pneumonias and about 4 percent of fatal pneumonias acquired in hospitals. It tends to strike in late summer and early fall. *Legionella* bacteria live in water, and outbreaks have occurred when the organism has spread through the air conditioning systems of hotels and hospitals. An outbreak of respiratory illness among American Legion members attending a convention in a hotel in 1976 led to the discovery—and naming—of the bacterium. No cases are known in which one person directly infected another.

Although Legionnaires' disease may occur at any age, people who are middle-aged and older have been affected most often. People who smoke tobacco, abuse alcohol, or take corticosteroids seem to be at greater risk. Legionnaires' disease can produce relatively minor symptoms or can be life threatening.

The first symptoms, appearing 2 to 10 days after the infection is transmitted, include fatigue, fever, headache, and muscle aches. A dry cough that later brings up sputum follows. People with serious infections can become extremely short of breath and commonly have diarrhea. Confusion and other mental disturbances are less common. Laboratory tests are performed on sputum,

blood, and urine specimens to confirm the diagnosis. Because people infected with *Legionella pneumophila* produce antibodies to fight the disease, blood tests show an increasing concentration of these antibodies. However, the results of antibody tests usually aren't available until after the pneumonia has run its course.

The antibiotic erythromycin is the first choice for treating this pneumonia. In less severe cases, erythromycin can be taken orally; otherwise, it's given intravenously. About 20 percent of the people who develop the disease die. The death rate is much higher among those who contract the disease in the hospital or have lowered immunity. Most people treated with erythromycin get better, but recovery can take a long time.

Atypical Pneumonias

Atypical pneumonias are pneumonias caused by organisms other than the so-called typical bacteria, viruses, or fungi. The most common causes are Mycoplasma *and* Chlamydia—*two bacterialike organisms.*

Mycoplasma pneumoniae is the most common cause of pneumonia in people ages 5 to 35, but it's an uncommon cause in others. Epidemics occur especially in confined groups such as students, military personnel, and families. The epidemics tend to spread slowly because the incubation period lasts 10 to 14 days. Most commonly, this type of pneumonia strikes in the spring.

Mycoplasmal pneumonia often starts with fatigue, a sore throat, and a dry cough. The symptoms slowly worsen. Attacks of severe coughing may produce sputum. About 10 to 20 percent of people develop a rash. Occasionally, anemia, joint pains, or neurologic problems develop. Symptoms often persist for 1 to 2 weeks, followed by slow improvement. Some people still feel weak and tired after several weeks. Although mycoplasmal pneumonia can be severe, it's usually mild, and most people recover without treatment.

Chlamydia pneumoniae is another common cause of pneumonia in people ages 5 to 35. It also affects some elderly people. The disease is transmitted from person to person in tiny airborne droplets spread by coughing. The symptoms are similar to those of mycoplasmal pneumonia. Most

▲ see page 206

people don't become seriously ill, although 5 to 10 percent of the elderly people who contract the disease die.

Diagnosis of both diseases is made by using blood tests to check for antibodies against the suspected organism and by using chest x-rays.

The antibiotics erythromycin and tetracycline are effective, but the response to treatment is slower in chlamydial pneumonia than in mycoplasmal pneumonia. If treatment is stopped too early, symptoms tend to return.

Psittacosis

Psittacosis (parrot fever) is a rare pneumonia caused by *Chlamydia psittaci*, a bacterium found mainly in birds such as parrots, parakeets, and lovebirds. It's also found in other birds, such as pigeons, finches, chickens, and turkeys. Usually, people are infected by inhaling dust from the feathers or the waste of infected birds. The organism also may be transmitted by a bite from an infected bird and, rarely, from person to person in cough droplets. Psittacosis is mainly an occupational disease of people who work in pet shops or on poultry farms.

About 1 to 3 weeks after being infected, a person develops a fever, chills, fatigue, and loss of appetite. A cough develops, which is initially dry but later brings up greenish sputum. The fever persists for 2 to 3 weeks and then slowly subsides. The disease may be mild or severe, depending on the person's age and the extent of lung tissue involved.

Blood antibody tests are the most reliable method for confirming the diagnosis.

Bird breeders and owners can protect themselves by avoiding the dust from the feathers and the cages of sick birds. Importers are required to treat susceptible birds with a 45-day course of tetracycline, which generally gets rid of the organism.

Psittacosis is treated with tetracycline for at least 10 days. Recovery may take a long time, especially in severe cases. The death rate may reach 30 percent in severe untreated cases.

▲ see page 914

Viral Pneumonia

Many viruses can infect the lungs, causing viral pneumonia. In infants and children, respiratory syncytial virus, adenovirus, parainfluenza virus, and influenza virus are the most common causes. The measles virus also may cause pneumonia, especially in malnourished children.

In healthy adults, two types of influenza virus, called types A and B, cause pneumonia.▲ The chickenpox virus can also cause pneumonia in adults. In elderly people, viral pneumonia is likely to be caused by influenza, parainfluenza, or respiratory syncytial virus. People of any age with impaired immunity may develop severe pneumonia from cytomegalovirus or the herpes simplex virus.

Most viral pneumonias aren't treated with drugs to kill the virus. However, certain severe viral pneumonias can be treated with antiviral drugs. For example, pneumonia caused by the chickenpox virus or herpes simplex virus may be treated with acyclovir. Annual influenza vaccinations are recommended for health care workers, the elderly, and people with chronic conditions such as emphysema, diabetes, heart disease, and kidney disease.

Fungal Pneumonia

Three types of fungi commonly cause pneumonia: *Histoplasma capsulatum*, which causes histoplasmosis, *Coccidioides immitis*, which causes coccidioidomycosis, and *Blastomyces dermatitidis*, which causes blastomycosis. Most people who become infected have only minor symptoms and don't know that they're infected. Some become gravely ill.

Histoplasmosis occurs worldwide but is prevalent in river valleys in temperate and tropical climates. In the United States, it occurs most commonly in the Mississippi and Ohio river valleys and in the river valleys of the East. More than 80 percent of those living in the Mississippi and Ohio river valleys have been exposed to the fungus. After being inhaled, the fungus causes no symptoms in many people. In fact, many people learn that they've been exposed only after having a skin test. Other people may have a cough, fever, muscle aches, and chest pain. The infection may cause acute pneumonia, or it may develop into chronic pneumonia with symptoms that persist for months. Rarely, the infection spreads to other areas of the body, especially the bone marrow, liver, spleen, and gastrointestinal tract. This disseminated form of the disease tends to occur in people with AIDS and other immune system disorders. Usually, the diagnosis is made by identifying the fungus in a sputum sample or by performing a blood test that identifies certain antibodies; the blood test, however, simply demonstrates exposure to the fungus and isn't proof that the fungus is causing disease. Treatment typically consists of giving an antifungal drug, such as itraconazole or amphotericin B.

Coccidioidomycosis occurs primarily in semi-arid climates, especially the southwestern United States and certain parts of South America and Central America. After being inhaled, the fungus may cause no symptoms, or it may cause either acute or chronic pneumonia. In some cases, the infection spreads beyond the respiratory system—typically to the skin, bones, joints, and lining of the brain (meninges). This complication is more common in men, especially Filipinos and blacks, and in people with AIDS and other immune system disorders. The diagnosis is made by identifying the fungus in a sputum sample or a sample taken from another infected area or by performing a blood test that identifies certain antibodies. Treatment typically consists of giving an antifungal drug, such as fluconazole or amphotericin B.

Blastomycosis occurs primarily in the southeastern, south central, and midwestern United States and in areas around the Great Lakes. After being inhaled, the fungus causes infection primarily in the lung; however, the infection usually produces no symptoms. Some people have a flu-like illness. Occasionally, symptoms of a chronic lung infection last for months. The disease may spread to other parts of the body, especially the skin, bones, joints, and prostate gland. Usually, the diagnosis is made by identifying the fungus in sputum. Treatment typically consists of giving an antifungal drug, such as itraconazole or amphotericin B.

Other fungal infections occur primarily in people with severely suppressed immune systems. These infections include **cryptococcosis,** caused by *Cryptococcus neoformans*; **aspergillosis,** caused by *Aspergillus*; **candidiasis,** caused by *Candida*; and **mucormycosis**. All four occur throughout the world. Cryptococcosis, the most common one, may occur in an otherwise healthy person but usually is severe only in people with underlying immune system disorders, such as AIDS. Crypto-

coccosis may spread, especially to the meninges, where the resulting disease is cryptococcal meningitis. *Aspergillus* causes pulmonary infections in people who have AIDS or have undergone organ transplantation. A rare infection, pulmonary candidiasis, occurs most often in patients with low white blood cell counts, such as people with leukemia who are undergoing chemotherapy. Mucormycosis, a relatively rare fungal infection, occurs most frequently in those with severe diabetes or leukemia. The four infections are treated with antifungal drugs, such as itraconazole, fluconazole, and amphotericin B. However, people with AIDS and other immune system disorders may not recover.

Pneumocystis Pneumonia

Pneumocystis carinii is a common organism that may reside harmlessly in normal lungs, usually causing disease only when the body's defenses are weakened because of cancer, cancer treatment, or AIDS. More than 80 percent of AIDS patients who don't receive standard prophylaxis develop pneumocystis pneumonia at some time. Often, it's the first indication that a person with human immunodeficiency virus (HIV) infection has developed AIDS.

Most people develop a fever, shortness of breath, and a dry cough. These symptoms usually arise over several weeks. The lungs may not be able to deliver sufficient oxygen to the blood, leading to severe shortness of breath.

The diagnosis is made by microscopic examination of a sputum specimen obtained by one of two techniques, sputum induction (in which water or water vapor is used to stimulate coughing) or bronchoscopy (in which an instrument is inserted into the airways to collect a specimen).▲

The usual antibiotic taken for pneumocystis pneumonia is trimethoprim-sulfamethoxazole. Side effects, which are particularly common in people with AIDS, include rashes, a reduced concentration of disease-fighting white blood cells, and fever. Alternative drug treatments are dapsone and trimethoprim, clindamycin and primaquine, trimetrexate and leucovorin, atovaquone, and pentamidine. People with a very low blood oxygen level may also be given corticosteroids.

▲ see page 162

Even when the pneumonia is treated, the overall death rate is 10 to 30 percent. AIDS patients who have been treated successfully for pneumocystis pneumonia generally take medications such as trimethoprim-sulfamethoxazole or aerosolized pentamidine to prevent the disease from returning.

Aspiration Pneumonia

Tiny particles from the mouth frequently dribble into the airways, but usually they're cleared out by normal defense mechanisms before they can get into the lungs or cause inflammation or infection. When such particles aren't cleared, they can cause pneumonia. People who are debilitated, intoxicated by alcohol or drugs, or unconscious from anesthesia or a medical condition are especially at risk for this type of pneumonia. Even a healthy person who inhales a large amount of material, as may happen during vomiting, can develop pneumonia.

Chemical pneumonitis occurs when the inhaled (aspirated) material is toxic to the lungs; the problem is more the result of irritation than infection. A commonly inhaled toxic material is stomach acid. The immediate result is sudden shortness of breath and a rapid heart rate. Other symptoms include a fever, pink frothy sputum, and a bluish tinge to the skin caused by poorly oxygenated blood (cyanosis).

Chest x-rays and measurements of oxygen and carbon dioxide concentrations in arterial blood may help a doctor make the diagnosis, but usually it's obvious from the sequence of events. Treatment consists of oxygen therapy and mechanical ventilation▲ if necessary. The trachea may be suctioned to clear secretions and aspirated particles out of the airways.

Sometimes, antibiotics are given to prevent infection. Generally, people with chemical pneumonitis either recover rapidly, progress to acute respiratory distress syndrome, or develop a bacterial infection. About 30 to 50 percent of people with chemical pneumonitis die.

Bacterial aspiration is the most common form of aspiration pneumonia. It's usually caused by bacteria swallowed and inhaled into the lungs.

Mechanical obstruction of the airways may be caused by aspiration of particles or objects. Young children are most at risk because they often put objects into their mouth and may aspirate small toys or parts of toys. Obstruction can also occur in adults, typically when meat is aspirated while eating. If an object becomes stuck high in the trachea, the person may be unable to breathe or speak. If the object isn't removed immediately, the person will quickly die. The Heimlich maneuver, performed to dislodge the object, can save the person's life. If an object gets stuck lower in the airways, an irritating chronic cough and recurring infections may result. The object is usually removed during bronchoscopy (a procedure using an instrument that allows a doctor to view the airway and remove samples and foreign material).■

CHAPTER 42

Lung Abscess

A lung abscess is a pus-filled cavity in the lung surrounded by inflamed tissue and caused by an infection.

Causes

The usual reason an abscess forms is that bacteria from the mouth or throat are inhaled into the lungs, causing an infection. The body has many defenses against such infections, so they occur only when these defenses are down—for instance, when a person is unconscious or very drowsy because of sedation, anesthesia, alcohol abuse, or a disease of the nervous system. Often, gum disease is the source of the bacteria, but if inhaled, even normal saliva contains enough bacteria to cause an infection. In some people, particularly those over age 40, a lung tumor may cause a lung abscess by blocking an airway.

▲ see page 158

■ see page 162

Pneumonia caused by certain bacteria, such as *Staphylococcus aureus* or *Legionella pneumophila*, or fungi may lead to a lung abscess. In people with a poorly functioning immune system, less common organisms may be the cause. Rare causes include infected pulmonary emboli and infections that are spread by the bloodstream.

Usually, a person develops only one lung abscess, but when more develop, they're typically in the same lung. If an infection reaches the lung through the bloodstream, many scattered abscesses may develop. This problem is most common among addicts who inject drugs using unclean needles.

Eventually, most abscesses rupture into an airway, producing a lot of sputum that needs to be coughed up. A ruptured abscess also leaves a cavity in the lung that's filled with fluid and air. Sometimes an abscess ruptures into the pleural space (the space between the membrane layers covering the lungs), filling it with pus, a condition called empyema. Rarely, a large abscess ruptures into a bronchus (a large airway that supplies the lung), and the pus spreads through the lung, causing pneumonia and acute respiratory distress syndrome. If an abscess destroys a blood vessel wall, serious bleeding may occur.

Symptoms and Diagnosis

The symptoms may start slowly or suddenly. Early symptoms resemble those of pneumonia: fatigue, loss of appetite, sweating, fever, and coughing that brings up sputum. The sputum may be streaked with blood. Often, the sputum smells foul because bacteria from the mouth or throat tend to produce foul odors. The person also may feel chest pain with breathing, especially if the pleura is inflamed.

Doctors can't diagnose a lung abscess based on the pneumonialike symptoms and examination findings alone. However, they do suspect a lung abscess when pneumonialike symptoms develop in people who have certain problems, such as a nervous system disorder, an alcohol or drug abuse problem, or a recent episode of unconsciousness for any reason.

Chest x-rays often reveal a lung abscess. However, when an x-ray only suggests an abscess, computed tomography (CT) scanning of the chest is usually needed. Cultures of sputum from the lungs may help identify the organism causing the abscess.

Treatment

Prompt, complete healing of a lung abscess requires antibiotics given intravenously or orally. This treatment continues until the symptoms disappear and a chest x-ray shows that the abscess has resolved. Such improvement usually takes several weeks or months of antibiotic therapy.

To help drain a lung abscess, a person must cough and receive respiratory therapy.▲ When the cause is thought to be a blocked airway, bronchoscopy is performed to remove the obstruction.

In about 5 percent of cases, the infection doesn't clear up. Occasionally, an abscess can be drained through a tube inserted through the chest wall and into the abscess. More often, infected lung tissue may have to be removed. Sometimes a whole lung lobe or even an entire lung has to be removed.

The death rate for people with a lung abscess is about 5 percent. The rate is higher when the person is debilitated or has a malfunctioning immune system, lung cancer, or a very large abscess.

CHAPTER 43

Cystic Fibrosis

Cystic fibrosis is a hereditary disease that causes certain glands to produce abnormal secretions, resulting in several symptoms, the most important of which affect the digestive tract and the lungs.

Cystic fibrosis is the most common inherited disease leading to death among white people in

the United States. It occurs in 1 of every 2,500 white babies and in 1 of every 17,000 black babies.

▲ see page 158

It's rare in Asians. Cystic fibrosis is equally common in boys and girls. Many people with cystic fibrosis die young, but 35 percent of Americans with cystic fibrosis reach adulthood.

About 5 percent of white people carry one defective gene responsible for cystic fibrosis, but the trait is recessive, and the disease develops only if a person has two defective genes.▲ People with only one defective gene have no noticeable symptoms. The gene controls the production of a protein that regulates the transfer of chloride and sodium (salt) across cell membranes. When both genes are abnormal, chloride and sodium transfer is disrupted, leading to dehydration and increased stickiness of secretions.

Cystic fibrosis affects nearly all the exocrine glands (glands that secrete fluids into a duct). The secretions are abnormal in different ways, and they affect gland function. In some glands, such as the pancreas and those in the intestines, the secretions are thick or solid and may block the gland completely. The mucus-producing glands in the airways of the lungs produce abnormal secretions that clog the airways and allow bacteria to multiply. The sweat glands, parotid glands, and small salivary glands secrete fluids containing more salt than normal.

Symptoms

The lungs are normal at birth, but breathing problems can develop at any time afterward. Thick bronchial secretions eventually block the small airways, which then become inflamed. As the disease progresses, the bronchial walls thicken, the airways fill with infected secretions, areas of the lung contract (a condition called atelectasis), and the lymph nodes enlarge. All these changes reduce the lung's ability to transfer oxygen to the blood.

Meconium ileus, a form of intestinal obstruction in newborns, occurs in 17 percent of those with cystic fibrosis. Meconium, the dark green substance that emerges as the newborn's first stool, is thick and passes more slowly than normal. If the meconium is too thick, it blocks the

intestine. Blockage may lead to perforation of the intestinal wall or a twisted intestine. Meconium may also form plugs in the large intestine or anus, causing a temporary blockage. Babies who have meconium ileus almost always develop other symptoms of cystic fibrosis later.

The first symptom of cystic fibrosis in an infant who doesn't have meconium ileus is often poor weight gain at 4 to 6 weeks. Inadequate amounts of the pancreatic secretions essential for proper digestion of fats and proteins lead to poor digestion in 85 to 90 percent of babies with cystic fibrosis. The baby has frequent, bulky, foul-smelling, oily stools and may have a protruding abdomen. Growth is slow despite a normal or large appetite. The baby is thin and has flabby muscles. Inadequate absorption of the fat-soluble vitamins—A, D, E, and K—may lead to night blindness, rickets, anemia, and bleeding disorders. In 20 percent of untreated infants and toddlers, the lining of the large intestine protrudes through the anus, a condition called rectal prolapse. Babies who have been fed soy protein formula or breast milk may develop anemia and swelling because they aren't absorbing enough protein.

About half the children with cystic fibrosis are first taken to the doctor because they keep coughing, wheezing, and having respiratory tract infections. Coughing, the most noticeable symptom, is often accompanied by gagging, vomiting, and disturbed sleep. As the disease progresses, the chest becomes barrel-shaped, and insufficient oxygen may make the fingers clubbed and the skin bluish. Polyps may form in the nose. The sinuses may fill with thick secretions.

Teenagers often have slowed growth, delayed puberty, and declining physical endurance. Complications in adults and adolescents include a collapsed lung (pneumothorax), coughing up of blood, and heart failure. Infection is also a major problem. Recurrent bronchitis and pneumonia gradually destroy the lungs. Death usually results from a combination of respiratory failure and a failing heart caused by the underlying lung disease.

About 2 to 3 percent of people with cystic fibrosis develop insulin-dependent diabetes because the scarred pancreas can no longer produce enough insulin. The blockage of bile ducts by

▲ see box, page 10

thick secretions can lead to inflammation of the liver and eventually to cirrhosis. Cirrhosis may cause increased pressure in the veins entering the liver (portal hypertension), leading to enlarged, fragile veins at the lower end of the esophagus (esophageal varices). These abnormal veins can bleed copiously.

People with cystic fibrosis often have impaired reproductive function. Among adult men, 98 percent produce no sperm or have a low sperm count because the vas deferens has developed abnormally. In women, cervical secretions are too thick, causing decreased fertility. Women with cystic fibrosis have a higher likelihood of complications during pregnancy than unaffected women, but many women with cystic fibrosis have had babies.

When the person sweats excessively in hot weather or has a fever, dehydration may result because of the increased loss of salt and water. A parent may notice the formation of salt crystals or even a salty taste on the child's skin.

Diagnosis

In newborns with cystic fibrosis, the level of the digestive enzyme trypsin in the blood is high. This level can be measured in a small drop of blood collected on a piece of filter paper. Although this technique is used in screening programs to test newborns, it's not a conclusive test for cystic fibrosis.

The quantitative pilocarpine iontophoresis sweat test measures the amount of salt in sweat. The drug pilocarpine is given to stimulate sweating in a small area of skin, and a piece of filter paper is placed against the skin to absorb the sweat. The concentration of salt in the sweat is then measured. A salt concentration above normal confirms the diagnosis in people who have symptoms of cystic fibrosis or who have family members with cystic fibrosis. Although the results of this test are valid any time after a baby is 24 hours old, collecting a large enough sweat sample from a baby younger than 3 or 4 weeks old may be difficult. The sweat test can also confirm the diagnosis in older children and adults.

Because cystic fibrosis can affect several organs, several other tests may help a doctor diagnose it. If pancreatic enzyme levels are reduced, an analysis of the person's stool may reveal de-creased or absent levels of the digestive enzymes trypsin and chymotrypsin or high levels of fat. If insulin secretion is reduced, blood sugar levels are high. Pulmonary function tests▲ may show that breathing is compromised. Also, a chest x-ray may suggest the diagnosis.

Relatives other than the parents of a child with cystic fibrosis may want to know if they're likely to have children with the disease. Genetic testing on a small blood sample can help determine who has a defective cystic fibrosis gene. Unless both parents have at least one such gene, their children will not have cystic fibrosis. If both parents carry a defective cystic fibrosis gene, each pregnancy has a 25 percent chance of producing a child with cystic fibrosis. During pregnancy, an accurate diagnosis of cystic fibrosis in the fetus is usually possible.

Prognosis

The severity of cystic fibrosis varies greatly from person to person regardless of age; the severity is determined largely by how much the lungs are affected. However, deterioration is inevitable, leading to debility and eventually death. Nonetheless, the outlook has improved steadily over the past 25 years, mainly because treatments can now postpone some of the changes that occur in the lungs. Half of the people with cystic fibrosis live longer than 28 years. Long-term survival is somewhat better in males, people who don't have pancreatic problems, and people whose initial symptoms are restricted to the digestive system. Despite their many problems, people with cystic fibrosis usually attend school or work until shortly before death. Gene therapy holds great promise for treating cystic fibrosis.

Treatment

Therapy includes prevention and treatment of lung problems, good nutrition, physical activity, and psychologic and social support. Much of the burden of treating a child with cystic fibrosis falls on the parents. They should receive adequate information so they can understand the condition

---

▲ see page 159

and the reasons for the treatments. The patient should have a comprehensive program of therapy directed by an experienced doctor and assisted by nurses, a dietitian, a social worker, and physical and respiratory therapists.

A certain type of enema can relieve an uncomplicated meconium ileus; if the enema isn't effective, surgery may be needed. Regularly taking drugs that draw fluid into the intestine, such as lactulose, may prevent stools from obstructing the intestinal tract.

With each meal, people who have pancreatic insufficiency must take enzyme replacements; a powder (for infants) and capsules are available. The diet should provide enough calories and protein for normal growth. The proportion of fat should be normal to high. Because people with cystic fibrosis don't absorb fats well, they need to consume higher than normal amounts of fat to ensure adequate growth. People with cystic fibrosis should double the usual daily dose of multivitamins and take water-soluble vitamin E. When they exercise, have a fever, or are exposed to hot weather, they should take supplemental salt. Special milk formulas containing protein and fats that are easy to digest may help infants with severe pancreatic problems. Children who can't maintain adequate nutrition may need supplementary feedings through a tube inserted into the stomach or small intestine.

The treatment of lung problems focuses on preventing airway blockage and controlling infection. The person should receive all routine immunizations and the influenza vaccine, because viral infections can increase lung damage. Respiratory therapy—consisting of postural drainage, percussion and vibration, and assisted coughing—is started at the first sign of lung problems.▲ Parents of a young child can learn these techniques and do them at home every day. Older children and adults can carry out respiratory therapy independently, using special breathing devices or compression vests.

Often, people are given drugs that help prevent airway narrowing (bronchodilators). People with severe lung problems and a low level of oxygen in the blood may need supplemental oxygen ther-

apy. In general, people with lung failure don't benefit from using a ventilator; however, occasional, short periods of mechanical ventilation may help people during severe infections if their lungs were functioning adequately before the infection.

Aerosol drugs that help thin the mucus (mucolytics), such as recombinant human DNase, are widely used because they make it easier to cough up sputum and they improve lung function. They also decrease the frequency of serious lung infections. Mist tents have no proven benefit. Corticosteroids can relieve symptoms in infants with severe bronchial inflammation and in people who have narrowed airways that can't be opened with bronchodilators. Sometimes, other nonsteroidal anti-inflammatory drugs, such as ibuprofen, are used to slow the deterioration in lung function.

Lung infections must be treated early with antibiotics. At the first sign of a lung infection, samples of coughed-up sputum are collected, so that the laboratory can identify the infecting organism and the doctor can choose the drugs most likely to destroy it. An antibiotic usually can be given by mouth, or the antibiotic tobramycin can be given in an aerosol mist. However, if the infection is severe, intravenous antibiotics may be needed. This treatment often requires hospitalization but may be given at home. Taking oral or aerosol antibiotics continuously helps some people prevent recurrences of infection.

Massive or recurrent bleeding in a lung can be treated by blocking off the bleeding artery.

Surgery may be needed for the collapse of a lung segment (pneumothorax), a chronic sinus infection, severe chronic infection in one area of the lung, bleeding from blood vessels in the esophagus, gallbladder disease, or obstruction of the intestine. Liver transplantation has been successful for severe liver damage. Transplantation of a heart and two lungs is being performed for severe heart and lung disease. These types of transplantation are becoming more routine and more successful with experience and improved techniques. One year after transplantation, about 75 percent of patients are alive, and their condition is much improved.

People with cystic fibrosis usually die of respiratory failure after many years of deteriorating lung function. A small number, however, die of liver disease, bleeding into the airway, or complications of surgery.

▲ see page 158

Pleural Disorders

The pleura is a thin, transparent membrane that covers the lungs and also lines the inside of the chest wall. The surface that covers the lungs lies in close contact with the surface that lines the chest wall. Between the two thin flexible surfaces is a small amount of fluid that lubricates them as they slide smoothly over one another with each breath. Air, blood, fluid, or other material can get between the pleural surfaces, creating a space. If too much material accumulates, one or both lungs may not be able to expand normally with breathing, resulting in the collapse of a lung.

Pleurisy

Pleurisy is an inflammation of the pleura.

Pleurisy develops when an agent (usually a virus or bacterium) irritates the pleura, resulting in inflammation. Fluid may accumulate in the pleural space (a condition called pleural effusion), or fluid may not accumulate (a condition called dry pleurisy). After the inflammation subsides, the pleura may return to normal, or adhesions may form that make the pleural layers stick together.

Symptoms and Diagnosis

The most common symptom of pleurisy is chest pain, which usually begins suddenly. The pain varies from vague discomfort to an intense stabbing pain. It may be felt only when the person breathes deeply or coughs, or it may be felt continuously but may be worsened by deep breathing and coughing. The pain results from inflammation of the outer pleural layer and is usually felt in the chest wall right over the site of the inflammation.

Two Views of the Pleura

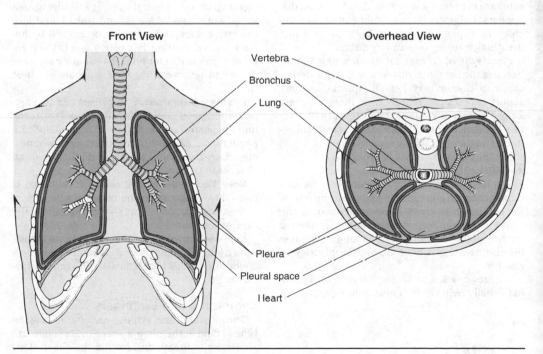

Front View   Overhead View

Vertebra
Bronchus
Lung
Pleura
Pleural space
Heart

Major Causes of Pleurisy

- Pneumonia
- Lung infarction caused by pulmonary embolism
- Cancer
- Tuberculosis
- Rheumatoid arthritis
- Systemic lupus erythematosus
- Infection with parasites, such as amebas
- Pancreatitis
- Injury, such as a rib fracture
- Irritants that reach the pleura from the airways or elsewhere, such as asbestos
- Allergic reactions caused by drugs, such as hydralazine, procainamide, isoniazid, phenytoin, chlorpromazine

However, the pain may be felt also or only in the abdomen or neck and shoulder as referred pain.▲

Breathing may be rapid and shallow because deep breathing induces pain; the muscles on the painful side move less than those on the normal side. If a large amount of fluid accumulates, it may separate the pleural layers, so the chest pain disappears. Large amounts of fluid can cause difficulty in expanding one or both lungs when breathing, causing respiratory distress.

Pleurisy is often easy for doctors to diagnose because the pain is so distinctive. Using a stethoscope, a doctor may hear a squeaky rubbing sound, called a pleural rub. Even though a chest x-ray won't show pleurisy, it may reveal a rib fracture, evidence of lung disease, or a small collection of fluid in the pleural space.

Treatment

The treatment of pleurisy depends on the particular cause. If the cause is a bacterial infection, for example, antibiotics are prescribed. If the cause is a viral infection, no treatment is needed for the infection. If the cause is an autoimmune disease, treating it often allows the pleurisy to resolve.

Analgesics such as acetaminophen or ibuprofen usually help relieve chest pain regardless of

▲ see page 288

the cause of the pleurisy. Codeine and other narcotics are stronger pain relievers, but they tend to suppress coughing, which isn't a good idea because deep breathing and coughing help prevent pneumonia. Thus, a person with pleurisy is encouraged to breathe deeply and cough when breathing becomes less painful. Coughing may be less painful if the person or a helper holds a pillow firmly against the part of the chest that hurts. Wrapping the entire chest in wide, nonadhesive elastic bandages helps relieve severe chest pain. However, binding the chest to reduce expansion during breathing increases the risk of pneumonia.

Pleural Effusion

Pleural effusion is the abnormal collection of fluid in the pleural space.

Normally, only a thin layer of fluid separates the two layers of the pleura. An excessive amount of fluid may accumulate for many reasons, including heart failure, liver cirrhosis, and pneumonia.

Other types of fluid that may collect in the pleural space include blood, pus, milky fluid, and high-cholesterol fluid.

Blood in the pleural space (hemothorax) usually results from a chest injury. Rarely, a blood vessel ruptures into the pleural space, or a bulging area in the aorta (aortic aneurysm) leaks blood into the space. Bleeding may also be caused by impaired blood clotting. Because blood in the pleural space doesn't clot fully, it's usually easy for a doctor to remove it through a needle or chest tube.

Pus in the pleural space (empyema) can accumulate when pneumonia or a lung abscess spreads into the pleural space. Empyema may complicate pneumonia, an infection from chest wounds, chest surgery, a rupture of the esophagus, or an abscess in the abdomen.

Milky fluid in the pleural space (chylothorax) is caused by an injury to the main lymphatic duct in the chest (thoracic duct) or by blockage of the duct by a tumor.

High-cholesterol fluid in the pleural space results from a long-standing pleural effusion caused by a condition such as tuberculosis or rheumatoid arthritis.

Symptoms and Diagnosis

The most common symptoms, regardless of the type of fluid in the pleural space or its cause, are shortness of breath and pain in the chest. However, many people with pleural effusion have no symptoms at all.

A chest x-ray, which shows the fluid, is usually the first step in making the diagnosis. Computed tomography (CT) more clearly shows the lung and the fluid and may show evidence of pneumonia, a lung abscess, or a tumor. An ultrasound scan may help a doctor determine the position of a small collection of fluid, so it can be drained.

A specimen of the fluid is almost always removed for examination using a needle, a procedure called thoracentesis.▲ The appearance of the fluid may help a doctor determine its cause. Certain laboratory tests evaluate the chemical composition and determine the presence of bacteria or fungi. The specimen is also examined for the number and types of cells and for the presence of cancerous cells.

If these tests can't identify the cause of the effusion, a biopsy of the pleura may be needed.■ Using a biopsy needle, a doctor removes a sample of the outer layer of pleura for analysis. If the specimen is too small for an accurate diagnosis, a tissue sample must be taken through a small incision in the chest wall, a procedure called an open pleural biopsy. Sometimes, a sample is obtained using a thoracoscope (a viewing tube that allows a doctor to examine the pleural space and obtain samples).★

Occasionally, bronchoscopy (a direct visual examination of the airways through a viewing tube)● helps the doctor find the source of the fluid. In about 20 percent of people with pleural effusions, the cause is never found, even after extensive testing.

Treatment

Small pleural effusions may require treatment of only the underlying cause. Larger effusions, especially those causing shortness of breath, may require fluid drainage. Usually, drainage dramatically relieves shortness of breath. Often, fluid can be drained using thoracentesis, a procedure in which a small needle (or catheter) is inserted into the pleural space. Although thoracentesis is usually performed for diagnostic purposes, a doctor can remove as much as 1.5 liters of fluid at a time using this procedure.

When larger amounts of fluid must be removed, a tube may be inserted through the chest wall. After numbing the area by injecting a local anes-

---

Common Causes of Pleural Effusion

- Heart failure
- Low blood protein levels
- Cirrhosis
- Pneumonia
- Blastomycosis
- Coccidioidomycosis
- Tuberculosis
- Histoplasmosis
- Cryptococcosis
- Abscess under the diaphragm
- Rheumatoid arthritis
- Pancreatitis
- Pulmonary embolus
- Tumors
- Systemic lupus erythematosus
- Heart surgery
- Injury to the chest
- Drugs such as hydralazine, procainamide, isoniazid, phenytoin, chlorpromazine, and rarely, nitrofurantoin, bromocriptine, dantrolene, procarbazine
- Improper placement of feeding tubes or intravenous catheters

---

thetic, a doctor inserts a plastic tube into the chest between two ribs. Then the doctor connects the tube to a water-sealed drainage system that prevents air from leaking into the pleural space. A chest x-ray is then taken to check the tube's position. Drainage can be blocked if the chest tube is incorrectly positioned or becomes kinked. If the fluid is very thick or full of clots, it may not flow out.

An accumulation of pus from an infection (empyema) requires intravenous antibiotics and fluid drainage. Tuberculosis or coccidioidomycosis re-

---

▲ see page 161

■ see page 162

★ see page 163

● see page 162

quires prolonged treatment with antibiotics. If the pus is very thick or if it has formed within fibrous compartments, drainage is more difficult, and part of a rib may have to be removed so a large drainage tube can be placed. Rarely, surgery to strip off the outer layer of pleura (decortication) may be needed.

Fluid accumulation caused by tumors of the pleura may be difficult to treat because fluid tends to reaccumulate rapidly. Draining the fluid and giving antitumor drugs sometimes prevents further fluid accumulation. But if fluid continues to accumulate, sealing the pleural space may be helpful. All fluid is drained through a tube, which is then used to administer a pleural irritant, such as a doxycycline solution or talc, into the space. The irritant seals the two layers of pleura together, so that no room remains for additional fluid to accumulate.

If blood has entered the pleural space, usually drainage through a tube is all that's needed—as long as the bleeding has stopped. Drugs that help break up blood clots, such as streptokinase and streptodornase, may be administered through the drainage tube. If the bleeding continues or if the collection can't be removed adequately with a tube, surgery may be needed.

Treatment of chylothorax focuses on repairing the damage to the lymphatic duct. Such treatment may consist of surgery or medication for a cancer that is blocking lymph flow.

Pneumothorax

A pneumothorax is a pocket of air between the two layers of pleura.

A pneumothorax may occur for no identifiable reason; doctors call this a spontaneous pneumothorax. A pneumothorax may also follow an injury or a medical procedure that introduces air into the pleural space, such as thoracentesis. Ventilators can cause pressure damage to the lungs that leads to a pneumothorax—most often in people with severe acute respiratory distress syndrome▲ who need high-pressure mechanical ventilation to survive.

▲ see page 164

Normally, the pressure in the pleural space is lower than that inside the lungs. When air enters the pleural space, the pressure in the pleura becomes greater than that in the lungs, and the lung collapses partially or completely. Sometimes most or all of the lung collapses, leading to immediate and severe shortness of breath.

Simple spontaneous pneumothorax is usually caused when a small weakened area of lung (bulla) ruptures. The condition is most common in tall men under age 40. Most incidents of simple spontaneous pneumothorax aren't caused by exertion. Some occur during diving or high-altitude flying, apparently because of pressure changes in the lungs. Most people recover fully.

Complicated spontaneous pneumothorax occurs in people with extensive lung disease. This type of pneumothorax most often results from the rupture of a bulla in older people who have emphysema. Complicated spontaneous pneumothorax may also occur in people with other lung conditions, such as cystic fibrosis, eosinophilic granuloma, lung abscess, tuberculosis, and *Pneumocystis carinii* pneumonia. Because of the underlying lung disease, the symptoms and outcome are generally worse in complicated spontaneous pneumothorax.

Tension pneumothorax is a serious and potentially life-threatening form of pneumothorax. In this condition, the tissues surrounding the area where air is entering the pleural space act as a one-way valve, allowing air to enter but not to escape. This situation causes such high pressure in the pleural cavity that the lung completely collapses, and the heart and other mediastinal structures are pushed over to the opposite side of the chest. If not relieved quickly, tension pneumothorax can cause death in minutes.

Symptoms and Diagnosis

Symptoms vary greatly depending on how much air enters the pleural space and how much of the lung collapses. They range from a little shortness of breath or chest pain to severe shortness of breath, shock, and life-threatening cardiac arrest. Most often, sharp chest pain and shortness of breath and occasionally a dry hacking cough begin suddenly. Pain may be felt in the shoulder, neck, or abdomen. Symptoms tend to be less severe in a slowly developing pneumothorax than in a rapidly developing one. Except with a very large pneumothorax or a tension pneumothorax, symptoms usually subside as the body adapts to the lung collapse, and the lung slowly begins to reinflate.

A physical examination can usually confirm the diagnosis. Using a stethoscope, a doctor may note that one part of the chest doesn't transmit the normal sounds of breathing. The trachea, the large airway that passes through the front of the neck, may be pushed to one side because of a collapsed lung. A chest x-ray shows the air pocket and the collapsed lung.

Treatment

A small pneumothorax usually requires no treatment. It usually doesn't cause serious breathing problems, and the air is absorbed in a few days. The full absorption of a larger pneumothorax may take 2 to 4 weeks; however, the air can be removed more quickly by inserting a chest tube into the pneumothorax. A chest tube is needed if the pneumothorax is large enough to impair breathing. The tube is connected to a water-sealed drainage system or a one-way valve that allows the air to exit without allowing any air

to get back in. A suction pump may have to be attached to the tube if air keeps leaking in from an abnormal connection (fistula) between an airway and the pleural space. Occasionally, surgery is necessary. Often the surgery is performed using a thoracoscope inserted through the chest wall and into the pleural space.

A recurring pneumothorax can cause considerable disability. For people at high risk—for example, divers and airplane pilots—surgery is considered after the first episode of pneumothorax. For people who have a pneumothorax that won't heal or a pneumothorax that occurs twice on the same side, surgery is performed to eliminate the cause of the problem. In a complicated spontaneous pneumothorax with a persistent air leak into the pleural space or with a recurring pneumothorax, the underlying lung disease may make surgery hazardous. Often, the pleural space can be sealed by giving doxycycline through a chest tube that's draining air from the space.

In tension pneumothorax, emergency removal of the air may prevent death. Air is immediately suctioned out, using a large syringe attached to a needle inserted into the chest. Then, a tube is inserted separately to drain the air continuously.

CHAPTER 45

Lung Cancer

Most lung cancer originates in the cells of the lungs; however, cancer may also spread (metastasize) to the lung from other parts of the body.

Lung cancer is the most common cancer in both men and women. More importantly, it's the most common cause of death from cancer in both men and women.

Causes

Cigarette smoking is the main cause of about 90 percent of lung cancer cases in men and about 70 percent of them in women. Lung cancer has become more common in women because more women are smoking cigarettes. The more ciga-

rettes a person smokes, the greater the risk of lung cancer.

A small proportion of lung cancers (about 10 to 15 percent in men and 5 percent in women) are caused by substances encountered or breathed in at work. Working with asbestos, radiation, arsenic, chromates, nickel, chloromethyl ethers, mustard gas, and coke-oven emissions has been linked with lung cancer, although usually only in people who also smoke cigarettes. The role of air pollution in causing lung cancer is still uncertain. Exposure to radon gas in homes may be important in a small number of cases. Occasionally, lung cancers, especially adenocarcinoma and alveolar cell carcinoma, develop in people whose lungs have been scarred by other lung diseases, such as tuberculosis and fibrosis.

Types of Lung Cancer

More than 90 percent of lung cancers start in the bronchi (the large airways that supply the lungs); such cancer is called bronchogenic carcinoma. The types are squamous cell carcinoma, small cell (oat cell) carcinoma, large cell carcinoma, and adenocarcinoma.

Alveolar cell carcinoma originates in the air sacs (alveoli) of the lung. Although this cancer can be a single growth, it often develops in more than one area of the lung at once.

Less common lung tumors are bronchial adenoma (which may be cancerous or noncancerous), chondromatous hamartoma (noncancerous), and sarcoma (cancerous). Lymphoma is a cancer of the lymphatic system. It may start in the lungs or spread to them.

Many cancers that start elsewhere in the body spread to the lungs. Cancers spread to the lungs most commonly from the breast, colon, prostate, kidney, thyroid, stomach, cervix, rectum, testis, bone, and skin.

Symptoms

The symptoms of lung cancer depend on its type, its location, and the way it spreads. Usually, the main symptom is a persistent cough. People with chronic bronchitis who develop lung cancer often notice that their coughing becomes worse. If sputum can be coughed up, it may be streaked with blood. If the cancer grows into underlying blood vessels, it may cause severe bleeding.

The cancer may cause wheezing by narrowing the airway in which or around which it's growing. Blockage of a bronchus may lead to the collapse of the part of the lung that the bronchus supplies, a condition called atelectasis. Another consequence may be pneumonia with coughing, fever, chest pain, and shortness of breath. If the tumor grows into the chest wall, it may produce persistent chest pain.

Symptoms that arise later include loss of appetite, weight loss, and weakness. Lung cancers often cause fluid accumulations around the lung (pleural effusions▲) that lead to shortness of breath. If cancer spreads within the lungs, severe shortness of breath, low levels of oxygen in the blood, and heart failure may develop.

The cancer may grow into certain nerves in the neck, causing a droopy eyelid, small pupil, sunken eye, and reduced perspiration on one side of the face—together these symptoms are known as Horner's syndrome. Cancers at the top of the lung may grow into the nerves that supply the arm, making the arm painful, numb, and weak. Nerves to the voice box may also be damaged, making the voice hoarse.

A cancer may grow directly into the esophagus, or it may grow near it and put pressure on it, leading to difficulty in swallowing. Occasionally, an abnormal channel (fistula) between the esophagus and bronchi develops, causing severe coughing during swallowing because food and fluid enter the lungs.

A lung cancer may grow into the heart, causing abnormal heart rhythms, an enlargement of the heart, or fluid in the pericardial sac surrounding the heart.■ The cancer may grow into or around the superior vena cava (one of the large veins in the chest). Obstruction of this vein causes blood to back up in other veins of the upper body. The veins on the chest wall enlarge. The face, neck, and upper chest wall—including the breasts—swell and become tinged with purple. The condition also produces shortness of breath, headache, distorted vision, dizziness, and drowsiness. These symptoms usually worsen when the person bends forward or lies down.

Lung cancer may also spread through the bloodstream to the liver, brain, adrenal glands, and bone. This may occur early in the disease, especially with small cell carcinoma. Symptoms—such as liver failure, confusion, seizures, and bone pain—may develop before any lung problems become evident, making an early diagnosis difficult.

Some lung cancers produce effects far from the lungs, such as metabolic, nerve, and muscle disorders (paraneoplastic syndromes). These syndromes aren't related to the size or location of the

▲ see page 206

■ see page 104

lung cancer and don't necessarily indicate that the cancer has spread outside the chest; rather, they are caused by substances secreted by the cancer. These symptoms may be the first sign of cancer or the first indication that cancer has returned after treatment. One example of a paraneoplastic syndrome is the Eaton-Lambert syndrome, characterized by extreme muscle weakness. Another example is the muscle weakness and soreness caused by inflammation (polymyositis), which may be accompanied by skin inflammation (dermatomyositis).

Some lung cancers secrete hormones or hormonelike substances, resulting in abnormally high hormone levels. For example, small cell carcinoma tumors may secrete corticotropin, causing Cushing's syndrome, or antidiuretic hormone, causing water retention and low levels of sodium in the blood. Excessive hormone production can also cause the carcinoid syndrome—flushing, wheezing, diarrhea, and heart valve problems. Squamous cell carcinoma may secrete a hormonelike substance that leads to very high blood levels of calcium. Other hormonal syndromes linked to lung cancers include breast enlargement in men (gynecomastia) and an excess of thyroid hormone (hyperthyroidism). Skin changes, including darkening of the skin in the armpit, may also occur. Lung cancer can even change the shape of the fingers and toes▲ and cause changes at the ends of long bones that can be seen on x-rays.

Diagnosis

A doctor explores the possibility of lung cancer when a patient, especially a smoker, has a persistent or worsening cough or other lung symptoms. Sometimes a shadow on a chest x-ray of someone with no symptoms provides the first clue.

A chest x-ray can detect most lung tumors, although it may miss small ones. However, an x-ray shows only a shadow in the lung, which isn't proof of cancer. Usually, a microscopic examination of a tissue specimen is needed. Sometimes a sample of coughed-up sputum can provide enough material for such an examination (called sputum cytology). Or bronchoscopy■ may be performed to obtain tissue. If the cancer is too deep in the lung

to be reached with a bronchoscope, a doctor can usually obtain a specimen by inserting a needle through the skin while using computed tomography (CT) for guidance; this procedure is called a needle biopsy. Sometimes, a specimen can be obtained only by a surgical procedure called a thoracotomy.★

CT scanning may show small shadows that don't appear on chest x-rays. The CT scans also can reveal whether the lymph nodes are enlarged; however, a biopsy (removal of a specimen for microscopic examination) often is needed to determine if the enlargement results from inflammation or cancer. CT scans of the abdomen or head may show that the cancer has spread to the liver, adrenal glands, or brain. A bone scan may show that it has spread to the bones. Because small cell carcinoma tends to spread to the bone marrow, a doctor sometimes performs a bone marrow biopsy (removal of a specimen for microscopic examination).

Doctors categorize cancers based on how large the tumor is, whether it has spread to nearby lymph nodes, and whether it has spread to distant organs. The different categories are called stages.● The stage of a cancer suggests the most appropriate treatment and enables a doctor to estimate the patient's prognosis.

Treatment

Noncancerous bronchial tumors are usually removed surgically because they may block the bronchi and may become cancerous over time. Often a doctor can't be sure if a tumor at the edge of the lungs is cancerous until it has been removed and examined microscopically.

For cancer other than small cell carcinoma that hasn't spread beyond the lung, surgery is sometimes possible. Although 10 to 35 percent of cancers can be removed surgically, removal doesn't always result in a cure. Among people who have

---

▲ see box, page 157

■ see page 162

★ see page 163

● see page 795 and box, page 796

an isolated, slow-growing tumor removed, 25 to 40 percent survive at least 5 years after the diagnosis. Survivors must have regular checkups because lung cancer recurs in 6 to 12 percent of people who have undergone surgery. The percentage is much higher for those who continue to smoke after surgery.

Before surgery, a doctor performs pulmonary function tests▲ to determine if the remaining lung can provide enough function. If the test results are poor, surgery may not be possible. The amount of lung to be removed is decided during surgery, with the amount varying from a small part of a lung segment to an entire lung.

Occasionally, cancer that begins elsewhere and spreads to the lungs is removed from the lungs after being removed at the source. This procedure is recommended rarely, and only about 10 percent of people who have it survive 5 years or more.

If the cancer has spread beyond the lungs, if the cancer is too close to the trachea, or if the person has other serious conditions (such as severe heart or lung disease), surgery isn't useful. Radiation therapy may be given to people who can't undergo surgery because they have another serious disease. In such cases, the radiation therapy isn't intended to cure but to slow the growth

▲ see page 159

of the cancer. Radiation therapy also is useful for controlling bone pain, superior vena cava syndrome, and spinal cord compression. However, the therapy can cause inflammation in the lungs (radiation pneumonitis), which produces coughing, shortness of breath, and fever. These symptoms may be relieved with corticosteroids, such as prednisone. For lung cancer other than small cell carcinoma, no chemotherapy regimens are particularly effective.

Because small cell carcinoma of the lung has almost always spread to distant parts of the body by the time of diagnosis, surgery isn't an option. Instead, this cancer is treated with chemotherapy, sometimes coupled with radiation treatment. In about 25 percent of patients, chemotherapy substantially prolongs survival. People with small cell carcinoma of the lung who have been responding well to chemotherapy may benefit from radiation treatment to the head to treat cancer that has spread to the brain.

Many people with lung cancer experience a substantial decrease in lung function, whether or not they undergo treatment. Oxygen therapy and drugs that widen the airways may ease breathing difficulties. Many people with advanced lung cancer develop such pain and difficulty in breathing that they require large doses of narcotics in the weeks or months before their death. Fortunately, narcotics can help substantially if used in adequate doses.

Bone, Joint, and Muscle Disorders

Bones, Joints, and Muscles

Bone is a constantly changing bodily tissue that has several functions. All the bones together make up the skeleton. The skeleton, muscles, tendons, ligaments, and other components of joints form the musculoskeletal system. The skeleton provides strength, stability, and a frame for muscles to work against in producing movement. Bones also serve as shields to protect delicate internal organs.

Bones have two main shapes: flat (such as the plates of the skull and the vertebrae) and long (such as the thighbones and arm bones). But their internal structure is essentially the same. The hard outer part consists largely of proteins, such as collagen, and a substance called hydroxyapatite. Composed mainly of calcium and other minerals, hydroxyapatite stores much of the body's calcium and is largely responsible for the strength of bones. The marrow in the center of each bone is softer and less dense than the rest of the bone and contains specialized cells that produce blood cells. Blood vessels run through a bone, and nerves surround it.

Bones come together to form joints. The configuration of a joint determines the degree and direction of possible motion. Some joints, such as those between the plates of the skull, called sutures, don't move in adults. Others allow a range of motion. For example, the shoulder joint, which has a ball-and-socket design, allows inward and outward rotation as well as forward, backward, and sideways motion of the arm. Hinge joints in the elbows, fingers, and toes allow only bending (flexion) and straightening (extension).

Other components of joints provide stability and reduce the risk of damage from constant use. In a joint, the ends of bones are covered with cartilage—a smooth, tough, protective tissue that acts as a shock absorber and reduces friction. Joints also have a lining (synovial tissue) that encloses them to form the joint capsule. Cells in the synovial tissue produce a clear fluid (synovial fluid) that fills the capsule, further reducing friction and facilitating movement.

Muscles are bundles of fibers that can contract. Skeletal muscles, which are responsible for posture and movement, are attached to bones and arranged in opposing groups around joints. For example, muscles that bend the elbow (biceps) are countered by muscles that straighten it (triceps).

Tendons, tough bands of connective tissue, attach each end of a muscle to a bone. Ligaments, which are similar tissues, surround joints and connect one bone to another. They help strengthen and stabilize joints, permitting movement only in certain directions. Bursas are fluid-filled sacs that provide extra cushioning, usually between adjacent structures that otherwise might rub against each other, causing wear and tear—for instance, between a bone and a ligament.

The components of a joint work together to facilitate movement that is balanced and causes no damage. For example, when the knee is bent to take a step, the hamstring muscles on the back of the thigh contract and shorten, pulling the lower leg in and bending the knee. At the same time, the quadriceps muscles on the front of the thigh relax, allowing the knee to bend. Within the knee joint, the cartilage and synovial fluid minimize friction. Five ligaments around the joint help keep the bones properly aligned. Bursas provide cushioning between structures such as the shinbone (tibia) and the tendon attached to the kneecap (patellar tendon).

Musculoskeletal Disorders

Disorders of the musculoskeletal system are major causes of chronic pain and physical disability. Although the components of this system thrive on use, they can become worn, injured, or inflamed.

Injuries to bones, muscles, and joints are very common, ranging in severity from mild pulled muscles to strained ligaments, dislocated joints, and broken bones (fractures). Although these injuries generally are painful and may lead to

Inside the Knee

The knee is designed for its own protection. It's completely surrounded by a joint capsule that's flexible enough to allow movement but strong enough to hold the joint together. The capsule is lined with synovial tissue, which secretes synovial fluid to lubricate the joint. Wear-resistant cartilage covering the ends of the thighbone (femur) and shinbone (tibia) helps reduce friction during movement. Pads of cartilage (menisci) act as cushions between the two bones and help distribute body weight in the joint. Fluid-filled sacs (bursas) provide cushioning as skin or tendons move across bone. Ligaments along the sides and the back of the knee reinforce the joint capsule, adding stability. The kneecap (patella) protects the front of the joint.

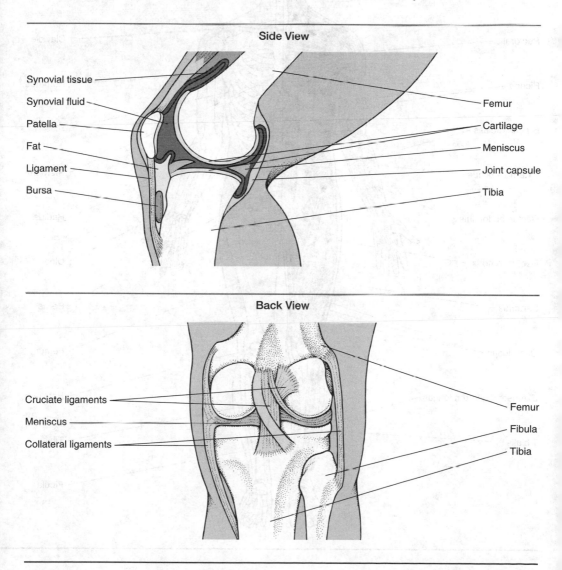

Side View

Synovial tissue
Synovial fluid
Patella
Fat
Ligament
Bursa

Femur
Cartilage
Meniscus
Joint capsule
Tibia

Back View

Cruciate ligaments
Meniscus
Collateral ligaments

Femur
Fibula
Tibia

Musculoskeletal System

Muscles

Bones

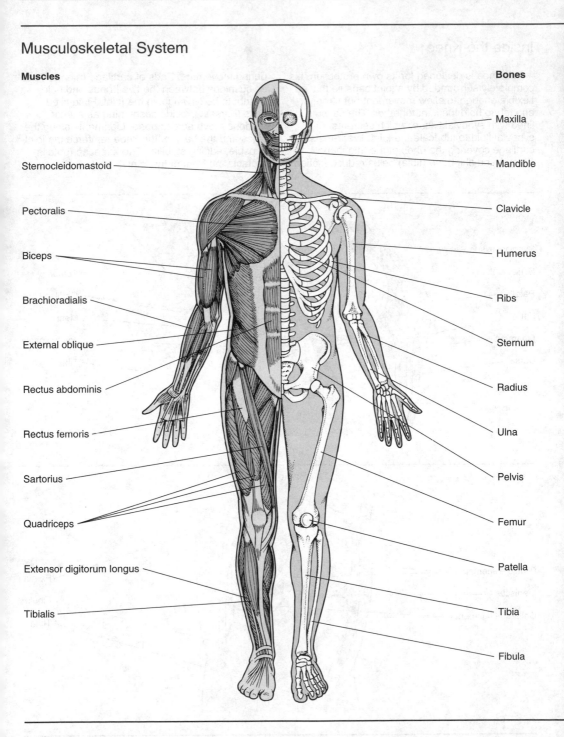

Sternocleidomastoid

Pectoralis

Biceps

Brachioradialis

External oblique

Rectus abdominis

Rectus femoris

Sartorius

Quadriceps

Extensor digitorum longus

Tibialis

Maxilla

Mandible

Clavicle

Humerus

Ribs

Sternum

Radius

Ulna

Pelvis

Femur

Patella

Tibia

Fibula

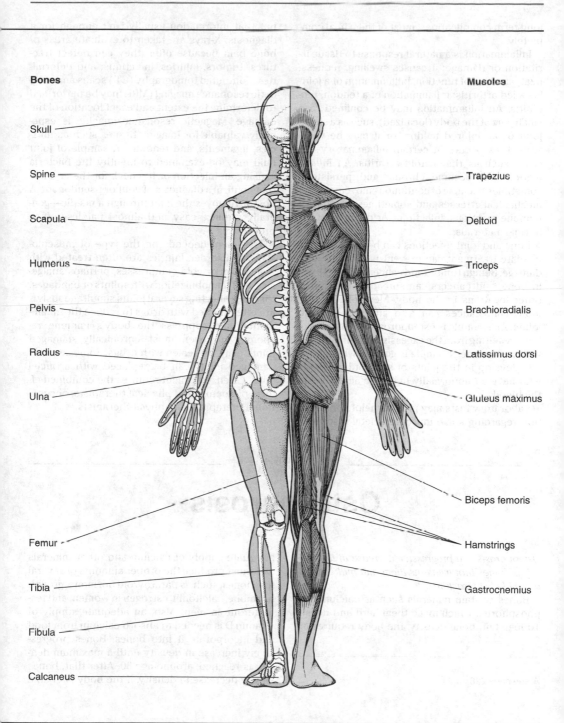

Bones

Skull

Spine

Scapula

Humerus

Pelvis

Radius

Ulna

Femur

Tibia

Fibula

Calcaneus

Muscles

Trapezius

Deltoid

Triceps

Brachioradialis

Latissimus dorsi

Gluteus maximus

Biceps femoris

Hamstrings

Gastrocnemius

long-term complications, most of them heal completely.

Inflammation is a natural response to tissue irritation or damage; it causes swelling, redness, heat, and loss of function. Inflammation of a joint is called arthritis; inflammation of a tendon, tendinitis. An inflammation may be confined to a small part of the body (localized), such as a single joint or an injured tendon, or it may be widespread, as occurs in certain inflammatory diseases such as rheumatoid arthritis. An inflammation can become chronic and persistent, sometimes because of continuous movement and mechanical stresses and sometimes because of immune reactions, infections, or deposits of abnormal materials.

Bone and joint infections can be crippling. Immediate treatment can prevent permanent joint damage. Benign tumors and cancers can originate in bone, and cancers can spread to bone from other locations in the body. Metabolic or hormonal imbalances can also affect bones and joints. An example is osteoporosis—a thinning of bone resulting from the excessive loss of minerals in bone. Another example is gout, in which crystals develop in the joints of susceptible people who have an abnormally high uric acid level in the blood.

Laboratory tests may provide helpful information regarding some musculoskeletal disorders, but that information usually isn't enough for a diagnosis. X-rays are taken to evaluate areas of bone pain because often they can detect fractures, tumors, injuries, infections, and deformities. Computed tomography (CT) scans and magnetic resonance imaging (MRI) may be performed to determine the extent and exact location of the damage. Magnetic resonance imaging is especially valuable for imaging tissues such as muscles, ligaments, and tendons. A sample of joint fluid may be examined to identify the bacteria causing an infection or to check for the crystals that confirm a diagnosis of gout or pseudogout. A doctor removes the fluid through a needle—generally a quick, easy, and almost painless office procedure.

Treatment depends on the type of musculoskeletal disorder. Injuries are often treated with rest, warm or cold compresses, perhaps analgesics, and immobilization with splints or bandages. Diseases affecting several joints simultaneously▲ are often treated with drugs to reduce the inflammation and suppress the body's immune response; however, most chronically damaged joints can't be healed with drugs. Some severely damaged joints can be replaced with artificial ones. Often, treatment requires the combined efforts of doctors and physical therapists, occupational therapists, and physiotherapists.

CHAPTER 47

Osteoporosis

Osteoporosis is a progressive decrease in the density of bones that weakens them and makes them more likely to fracture.

Bones contain minerals such as calcium and phosphorus, which make them hard and dense. To maintain bone density, the body requires an adequate supply of calcium and other minerals and must produce the proper amounts of several hormones, such as parathyroid hormone, growth hormone, calcitonin, estrogen in women, and testosterone in men. Also, an adequate supply of vitamin D is needed to absorb calcium from food and incorporate it into bones. Bones progressively increase in density until a maximum density is reached, around age 30. After that, bones slowly decrease in density. If the body isn't able

▲ see page 226

to regulate the mineral content of bones, they become less dense and more fragile, resulting in osteoporosis.

Types

There are several different types of osteoporosis.

Postmenopausal osteoporosis is caused by a lack of estrogen, the main female hormone, which helps regulate the incorporation of calcium into bone in women. Usually, symptoms develop in women between ages 51 and 75, but they can begin earlier or later. Not all women are at equal risk of developing postmenopausal osteoporosis. For example, white and Oriental women are more prone to the condition than black women.

Senile osteoporosis probably results from age-related calcium deficiency and an imbalance between the rate of bone breakdown and new bone formation. Senile means only that the condition occurs in the elderly. It usually affects people over age 70 and is twice as common in women as in men. Women often have both senile and postmenopausal osteoporosis.

Fewer than 5 percent of the people who have osteoporosis have **secondary osteoporosis,** which is caused by another medical condition or by drugs. It can be caused by conditions such as chronic renal failure and hormonal disorders (especially thyroid, parathyroid, or adrenal disorders) and by drugs such as corticosteroids, barbiturates, anticonvulsants, and excessive amounts of thyroid hormone. Excessive alcohol consumption and cigarette smoking may worsen the condition.

Idiopathic juvenile osteoporosis is a rare type whose cause hasn't been identified. It occurs in children and young adults who have normal hormone levels and function, normal vitamin levels, and no obvious reason to have weak bones.

Symptoms

Bone density decreases slowly, especially in people who have senile osteoporosis, so at first, osteoporosis produces no symptoms. Some people never have symptoms.

When bone density decreases so much that bones collapse or break, aching bone pain and deformities develop. Chronic back pain may oc-

---

Risk Factors for Osteoporosis in Women

Family members with osteoporosis

Insufficient calcium in the diet

Sedentary lifestyle

White or Oriental race

Thin build

No pregnancies

Use of certain drugs, such as corticosteroids and excessive amounts of thyroid hormone

Early menopause

Cigarette smoking

Excessive alcohol consumption

---

cur if vertebrae collapse (vertebral crush fractures). The weakened vertebrae may collapse spontaneously or after a slight injury. Usually, the pain starts suddenly, stays in a particular area of the back, and worsens when a person stands or walks. The area may be sore when touched, but usually the soreness goes away gradually after a few weeks or months. If several vertebrae break, an abnormal curvature of the spine (a dowager's hump) may develop, causing muscle strain and soreness.

Other bones may fracture, often because of minor stress or a fall. One of the most serious fractures is a hip fracture, a major cause of disability and loss of independence in the elderly. Fracture of the arm bone (radius) where it joins the wrist, called a Colles' fracture, is also common. In addition, fractures tend to heal slowly in people who have osteoporosis.

Diagnosis

In people who have a fracture, the diagnosis of osteoporosis is based on a combination of symptoms, physical examination, and bone x-rays. Further testing may be needed to rule out treatable conditions that might lead to osteoporosis.

Osteoporosis can be diagnosed before a fracture occurs with tests that assess bone density. The most accurate test is dual-energy x-ray absorptiometry (DXA). This test is painless and safe and can be performed in 5 to 15 minutes. It is useful for women at high risk of developing osteoporosis, those in whom the diagnosis is uncertain, or those in whom treatment results must be assessed accurately.

Prevention and Treatment

Prevention is more successful than treatment; it involves maintaining or increasing bone density by consuming adequate calcium, engaging in weight-bearing exercise, and for some people, taking drugs.

Consuming an adequate amount of calcium is effective, especially before maximum bone density is reached (around age 30) but also after. Drinking two glasses of milk and taking a vitamin D supplement daily help increase bone density in middle-aged women who previously weren't getting enough of these nutrients. However, most women need to take calcium in tablet form. Many preparations are available; some include supplemental vitamin D. About 1.5 grams of calcium daily is recommended.

Weight-bearing exercise, such as walking and stair-climbing, increases bone density. Exercises that don't involve weight bearing, such as swimming, don't increase bone density.

Estrogen helps maintain bone density in women; it is often taken with progesterone. Estrogen replacement therapy is most effective when started within 4 to 6 years after menopause, but starting it later can still slow bone loss and reduce the risk of fractures. Decisions about using estrogen replacement therapy after menopause are complex, because the treatment may have side effects and risks.▲ Raloxifene is a new estrogen-like drug that may be less effective than estrogen in preventing bone loss, but it does not have typical estrogen effects on the breast or uterus. Bisphosphonates, such as alendronate (see below), may be used alone or with hormone replacement therapy to prevent osteoporosis.

Treatment is aimed at increasing bone density. All women, especially those with osteoporosis, should take adequate calcium and vitamin D.

Postmenopausal women who have osteoporosis may also be given estrogen (usually with progesterone) or alendronate, which can slow or halt the progression of the disease.

Bisphosphonates are also useful in treating osteoporosis. Alendronate reduces the rate of bone resorption in postmenopausal women, increasing bone mass in the spine and hips and reducing the incidence of fractures. However, to make sure that alendronate is absorbed, it must be swallowed with a full glass of water the first thing on arising for the day, and no other food or drink should be taken for the next 30 minutes. Because alendronate can irritate the lining of the upper gastrointestinal tract, the person must not lie down after taking a dose for at least the next 30 minutes, until they have had something to eat. Certain people with difficulty swallowing or with certain disorders of the esophagus or stomach should not use it.

Many authorities recommend calcitonin, particularly for people who have painful fractures of the vertebrae. This drug can be taken by injection or nasal spray.

Fluoride supplements can increase bone density. However, because the resulting bone may be abnormal and fragile, they are not generally recommended. New forms of fluoride, which may not have adverse effects on bone quality, are being tested.

Men who have osteoporosis usually take calcium and vitamin D supplements, especially if tests show that their body isn't absorbing adequate amounts of calcium. Men don't benefit from estrogen, but may benefit from testosterone if their testosterone level is low.

Fractures resulting from osteoporosis must be treated. For hip fractures, usually part or all of the hip is replaced surgically. A wrist fracture is placed in a cast or reset surgically. When vertebrae collapse and cause severe back pain, supportive back braces, analgesics, and physical therapy are used, but the pain tends to last a long time. Heavy lifting and falls can make symptoms worse.

▲ see page 1078

Paget's Disease of Bone

Paget's disease is a chronic disorder of the skeleton in which areas of bone grow abnormally, enlarging and becoming soft.

The disorder can affect any bone, but those most commonly affected are the pelvis, thighbone (femur), skull, shin, spine (vertebrae), collarbone (clavicle), and upper arm bone (humerus).

In the United States, about 1 percent of the people over age 40 have the disorder, which rarely occurs in those under 40. Men are 50 percent more likely than women to develop it. Paget's disease is more common in Europe (excluding Scandinavia), Australia, and New Zealand than in the Americas, Africa, and Asia. It's particularly common in England.

Normally, cells that break down old bone (osteoclasts) and cells that form new bone (osteoblasts) work in balance to maintain bone structure and integrity. In Paget's disease, both osteoclasts and osteoblasts become overactive in some areas of bone, and the turnover rate in these areas increases tremendously. The overactive areas enlarge but are structurally abnormal and therefore weaker than normal areas.

The cause of Paget's disease isn't known. Although the disorder tends to run in families, no specific genetic pattern has been discovered. Some evidence suggests that a viral infection is involved.

Symptoms

Paget's disease usually produces no symptoms. When symptoms such as stiff joints and fatigue occur, they usually develop slowly and subtly. Bone pain, enlargement, or deformity may occur. Bone pain may be deep, aching, and occasionally severe and may worsen at night. The enlarging bones may compress nerves, adding to the pain. Sometimes Paget's disease leads to the development of painful osteoarthritis in adjacent joints.

Symptoms vary, depending on which bones are affected. The skull may enlarge, and the brow and forehead may look more prominent. A person may notice this enlargement when a larger-size hat is needed. Enlarged skull bones can cause hearing loss by damaging the inner ear (cochlea); headaches, by compressing nerves; and bulging veins on the scalp, by increasing blood flow to the skull. The vertebrae may enlarge, weaken, and buckle, resulting in loss of height. Damaged vertebrae may pinch the nerves of the spinal cord, causing numbness, tingling, weakness, or even paralysis in the legs. People whose hip or leg bones are affected may have bowed legs and take short, unsteady steps. The abnormal bone is more likely to break.

Rarely, heart failure develops because the increased blood flow through the abnormal bone puts extra stress on the heart. In fewer than 1 percent of the people who have Paget's disease, the abnormal bone becomes cancerous.

Diagnosis and Treatment

Paget's disease is often discovered accidentally when x-rays or laboratory tests are performed for other reasons. Otherwise, the diagnosis may be suspected on the basis of symptoms and the physical examination. The diagnosis can be confirmed by x-rays showing abnormalities characteristic of the disorder and by a laboratory test measuring blood levels of alkaline phosphatase, an enzyme involved in bone cell formation. A bone scan shows which bones are affected.

A person who has Paget's disease needs treatment only if the symptoms cause discomfort or if the risk of complications, such as hearing loss, arthritis, or deformity, is great. Aspirin, other nonsteroidal anti-inflammatory drugs, and common analgesics such as acetaminophen usually reduce bone pain. If one leg becomes bowed, heel lifts can help make walking easier. Sometimes surgery is needed to relieve pinched nerves or to replace an arthritic joint.

A bisphosphonate—etidronate, pamidronate, or alendronate—or calcitonin can be used to slow the progression of Paget's disease. These drugs are given before surgery to prevent or reduce bleeding during surgery; they're also given to treat severe pain caused by Paget's disease, to prevent or slow the progression of weakness or paralysis in people who can't have surgery, and to attempt to prevent arthritis, further hearing loss, or further deformity. Etidronate and alendronate usually are given orally, and pamidronate usually is given intravenously. Calcitonin is given as an injection under the skin or in muscle or as a nasal spray.

CHAPTER 49

Bone Tumors

Bone tumors are growths of abnormal cells in the bones.

Bone tumors may be noncancerous (benign) or cancerous (malignant). Noncancerous bone tumors are relatively common, but cancerous ones are rare. Also, bone tumors may be primary—noncancerous or cancerous tumors that originate in the bone itself—or metastatic—cancers that originate elsewhere in the body (for example, in the breast or prostate gland) and then spread to bone. In children, most cancerous bone tumors are primary; in adults, most are metastatic.

Bone pain is the most common symptom of bone tumors. In addition, a lump or mass may be noticeable. Sometimes a tumor, especially if cancerous, weakens a bone, causing it to fracture with little or no stress (pathologic fracture).

A persistently painful joint or limb should be x-rayed. However, x-rays show only an abnormality, usually without indicating whether a tumor is noncancerous or cancerous. Computed tomography (CT) and magnetic resonance imaging (MRI) often help determine the exact location and size of the tumor but usually don't provide a specific diagnosis.

Usually, removing a sample of the tumor for examination under a microscope (biopsy) is necessary for diagnosis. For many tumors, a sample may be taken by inserting a needle (aspiration biopsy) into the tumor and withdrawing some cells; however, a surgical procedure (open incisional biopsy) may be necessary to obtain an adequate sample for diagnosis. Prompt treatment, which may include some combination of drugs, surgery, and radiation therapy, is extremely important for cancerous tumors.

Noncancerous Bone Tumors

Osteochondromas (osteocartilaginous exostoses), the most common type of noncancerous bone tumors, usually occur in people aged 10 to 20 years. These tumors are growths on the surface of a bone that protrude as hard lumps. A person may have one or several tumors. The tendency to develop several tumors may run in families. At some point in their lives, about 10 percent of the people who have more than one osteochondroma develop a cancerous bone tumor called a chondrosarcoma; however, people who have only one osteochondroma are unlikely to develop a chondrosarcoma.

Benign chondromas, which usually occur in people aged 10 to 30 years, develop in the central part of a bone. These tumors often are discovered when x-rays are taken for other reasons and often can be diagnosed by their appearance on the x-ray. Some chondromas cause pain. If a chondroma doesn't cause pain, it doesn't have to be removed or treated. However, follow-up x-rays may be taken to monitor its size. If the tumor can't be diagnosed with certainty on x-rays or if it causes pain, a biopsy may be needed to determine whether it's noncancerous or cancerous.

Chondroblastomas are rare tumors that grow in the ends of bones. They usually occur in people aged 10 to 20 years. These tumors may cause pain, leading to their discovery. Treatment consists of surgical removal; occasionally, the tumors recur after surgery.

Chondromyxoid fibromas are very rare tumors, which occur in people under age 30. Pain is the usual symptom. These tumors have a distinctive appearance on x-rays. Treatment consists of surgical removal.

Osteoid osteomas are very small tumors that commonly develop in the arms or legs but can occur in any bone. They usually cause pain that worsens at night and is relieved by low doses of aspirin. Sometimes the muscles surrounding the tumor waste away (atrophy); this condition may improve after the tumor is removed. Bone scans using radioactive tracers help determine the exact location of the tumor. Sometimes the tumor is difficult to locate, and additional tests such as CT scans and special x-ray techniques may be needed. Surgically removing the tumor is the only way to eliminate the pain permanently. Rather than undergo surgery, some people prefer to take aspirin indefinitely.

Giant cell tumors usually occur in people in their 20s and 30s. These tumors most commonly originate in the ends of bones and may extend into adjacent tissue. They usually cause pain. Treatment depends on the tumor's size. A tumor can be surgically removed, and the hole can be filled with a bone graft or a synthetic bone cement to preserve the bone's structure. Occasionally, very extensive tumors may require removal of the affected segment of bone. About 10 percent of the tumors recur after surgery. Rarely, these tumors become cancerous.

Primary Cancerous Bone Tumors

Multiple myeloma, the most common type of primary cancerous bone tumor, originates in the bone marrow cells that produce blood cells.▲ It most commonly occurs in older people. This tumor may affect one or more bones, so pain may occur in one location or in several. Treatment is complex and may include chemotherapy drugs, radiation therapy, and surgery.

Osteosarcoma (osteogenic sarcoma) is the second most common type of primary cancerous bone tumor. Although most common in people aged 10 to 20 years, osteosarcomas can occur at any age. Older people who have Paget's disease sometimes develop this type of tumor. About half these tumors occur in or around the knee, but they can originate in any bone. They tend to spread to the lungs. Usually, these tumors cause pain and swelling. A biopsy is needed for diagnosis.

Osteosarcomas are usually treated with a combination of chemotherapy and surgery. Usually, chemotherapy is given first; pain often subsides during this phase of treatment. Then the tumor is surgically removed. About 75 percent of the people who have this type of tumor survive for at least 5 years after diagnosis. Because surgical procedures have improved, the affected arm or leg is usually saved today, whereas in the past, it often had to be amputated.

Fibrosarcomas and **malignant fibrous histiocytomas** are similar to osteosarcomas in appearance, location, and symptoms. Treatment also is the same.

Chondrosarcomas are tumors composed of cancerous cartilage cells. Many chondrosarcomas are slow-growing or low-grade tumors, which often can be cured with surgery. However, some are high-grade tumors, which tend to spread. A biopsy is needed for diagnosis. A chondrosarcoma must be completely removed surgically, because it doesn't respond to chemotherapy or radiation therapy. Amputation of the arm or leg is rarely necessary. More than 75 percent of the people who have a chondrosarcoma survive if the entire tumor is removed.

Ewing's tumor (Ewing's sarcoma) affects males more often than females and appears most commonly in people aged 10 to 20 years. Most of these tumors develop in the arms or legs, but they may develop in any bone. Pain and swelling are the most common symptoms. Tumors may become quite large, sometimes affecting the entire length of a bone. Although CT and MRI scans can help determine the exact size of the tumor, a biopsy is needed for diagnosis. Treatment consists of a combination of surgery, chemotherapy, and radiation therapy, which can cure more than 60 percent of the people who have Ewing's sarcoma.

Malignant lymphoma■ of bone (reticulum cell sarcoma) usually affects people in their 40s and 50s. It can originate in any bone or elsewhere in the body and spread to bone. Usually, this tumor causes pain and swelling, and the damaged bone is prone to fractures. Treatment usually consists of a combination of chemotherapy and radiation

---

▲ see page 779

■ see page 770

therapy, which appears to be as effective as surgical removal of the tumor. Amputation is rarely necessary.

Metastatic Bone Tumors

Metastatic bone tumors are cancers that have spread to bone from their original site elsewhere in the body.

Cancers most likely to spread to bone include breast, lung, prostate, kidney, and thyroid cancers. Cancer may spread to any bone but usually doesn't spread beyond the elbow and knee. A person who has or has had cancer and develops bone pain or swelling usually is examined for metastatic bone tumors. X-rays and bone scans using radioactive tracers can help locate these tumors. Occasionally, a metastatic bone tumor causes symptoms before the original cancer has been detected. Symptoms may consist of pain or a fracture where the tumor has weakened the bone. In these situations, a biopsy usually gives clues as to the location of the original cancer.

Treatment depends on the type of cancer.▲ Some types respond to chemotherapy, some to radiation therapy, some to both, and some to neither. Surgery to stabilize the bone can sometimes prevent fractures.

CHAPTER 50

Osteoarthritis

Osteoarthritis (degenerative arthritis, degenerative joint disease) is a chronic joint disorder characterized by degeneration of joint cartilage and adjacent bone that can cause joint pain and stiffness.

Osteoarthritis, the most common joint disorder, affects many people to some degree by age 70. Men and women are equally affected, but the disorder tends to develop at an earlier age in men. Osteoarthritis also occurs in almost all animals with a backbone—including fish, amphibians, and birds. Animals supported by water, such as dolphins and whales, can develop osteoarthritis, but the two animals that hang upside down, bats and sloths, don't develop it. Because the disorder is so widespread in the animal kingdom, some authorities think that osteoarthritis may have evolved from an ancient method of cartilage repair.

Many myths about osteoarthritis persist, for example, that it's an inevitable part of aging, like gray hair and skin changes; that it results in little disability; and that treatment isn't effective. Although osteoarthritis is more common in older people, it's not caused by the simple wear and tear that occurs with aging. Most people who have the disorder, especially younger ones, have few if any symptoms; however, some older people develop significant disabilities.

Causes

Normally, joints have such a low friction level that they don't wear out unless they are used excessively or are injured. Osteoarthritis probably begins most often with an abnormality of the cells that synthesize the components of cartilage, such as collagen (a tough, fibrous protein in connective tissue) and proteoglycans (substances that provide the cartilage's resilience). Next, the cartilage may grow too much, but it eventually thins and develops cracks on the surface. Tiny cavities form in the marrow of the bone beneath the cartilage, weakening the bone. Bone can overgrow at the edges of the joint, producing bumps (osteophytes), which can be seen and felt. These bumps may interfere with normal joint function, causing pain.

Ultimately, the smooth, slippery surface of the cartilage becomes rough and pitted, so that the joint can no longer move smoothly. All the components of the joint—bone, joint capsule (tissues that enclose some joints), synovial tissue (tissue lining the joint), tendons, and cartilage—fail in various ways, altering the joint.

Osteoarthritis is classified as **primary** (idiopathic) when the cause isn't known and **secondary** when the cause is another disease, such as

---

▲ see page 799

Paget's disease, or an infection, deformity, injury, or overuse of a joint. Some people who repetitively stress their joints, such as foundry workers, coal miners, and bus drivers, are particularly at risk. However, trained long-distance runners aren't at higher risk of developing the disorder. Obesity may be a major factor in the development of osteoarthritis, but the evidence is inconclusive.

Symptoms

By age 40, many people have some evidence of osteoarthritis on x-rays, especially in weight-bearing joints such as the hip, but relatively few have symptoms. Usually, symptoms develop gradually and affect only one or a few joints at first. Joints of the fingers, base of the thumbs, neck, lower back, big toes, hips, and knees are commonly affected. Pain, usually made worse by exercise, is the first symptom. In some people, the joint may be stiff after sleep or some other inactivity, but the stiffness usually subsides within 30 minutes after they start moving the joint.

As the damage from osteoarthritis worsens, the joint may become less movable and eventually may freeze in a bent position. The new growth of cartilage, bone, and other tissue can enlarge joints, and the roughened cartilage causes joints to grate or crackle when they are moved. Bony growths (Heberden's nodes) commonly develop in the joints at the ends of the fingers.

In some joints, such as the knee, the ligaments, which surround and support the joint, stretch so that the joint becomes unstable. Touching or moving the joint can be very painful. In contrast, the hip becomes stiffer, losing its range of motion; moving it is also painful.

Osteoarthritis frequently affects the spine. Back pain is the most common symptom. Usually, damaged joints in the spine cause only mild pain and stiffness. However, osteoarthritis in the neck or lower back can cause numbness, odd sensations, pain, and weakness in an arm or leg if the overgrowth of bone presses on nerves. Rarely, the blood vessels supplying the back of the brain are compressed, causing vision problems, a whirling sensation (vertigo), nausea, and vomiting. Sometimes bony growths compress the esophagus, making swallowing difficult.

Osteoarthritis most often continues to progress slowly after symptoms develop, and many people develop some degree of disability. Occasionally, however, joint degeneration stops or even reverses.

Treatment

Appropriate exercises—including stretching, strengthening, and postural exercises—help maintain healthy cartilage, increase a joint's range of motion, and strengthen surrounding muscles so that they absorb shock better. Exercise must be balanced with rest of painful joints, but immobilizing a joint is more likely to worsen osteoarthritis than to improve it. Using excessively soft chairs, recliners, mattresses, and car seats may worsen symptoms; using straight-backed chairs, firm mattresses, and bed boards is often recommended. For osteoarthritis of the spine, specific exercises sometimes help, and back supports or braces may be needed when problems are severe. Maintaining ordinary daily activities, a functional, independent role in the family, and job performance is important.

Physical therapy, often with heat treatment, can be helpful. For example, using hot paraffin wax mixed with mineral oil at temperatures of 118° to 126° F., dipping the hand in a paraffin bath, and taking hot or warm baths may be recommended for finger pain. Splints or supports can protect specific joints during painful activities. Massage by trained therapists, traction, and deep heat treatment with diathermy or ultrasound may be useful when certain types of osteoarthritis affect the neck.

Drugs are the least important aspect of the total treatment program. An analgesic such as acetaminophen may be all that's needed. A nonsteroidal anti-inflammatory drug such as aspirin or ibuprofen may be taken to lessen pain and swelling.▲ Cox-2 inhibitors, which control inflammation and relieve pain with fewer side effects, are in final studies. If a joint suddenly becomes inflamed, swollen, and painful, corticosteroids may be injected directly into the joint. This treatment usually provides only short-term relief.

Surgery may help when all other treatments have failed to bring relief. Some joints, most commonly the hip and knee, can be replaced with an artificial joint; replacement is usually very successful, almost always improving motion and function and dramatically decreasing pain. Thus, when function becomes limited, joint replacement should be considered.

▲ see page 55

Disorders of Joints and Connective Tissue

Disorders that affect joints and their components—muscles, bones, cartilage, and tendons—are considered **connective tissue diseases** because these structures contain large amounts of connective tissue. However, many are also a type of **autoimmune disease,** involving immune reactions in which something triggers the immune system to react against the body's own tissues and to produce abnormal antibodies that attack these tissues (autoantibodies).▲

Immune reactions are characterized by inflammation, which is normally a repair process and subsides when the repair is completed. However, in autoimmune diseases, the inflammation may be chronic, resulting in damage to normal tissues. For example, in rheumatoid arthritis, chronic inflammation damages the joint's cartilage. In rheumatoid arthritis and many autoimmune diseases, the inflammation affects several joints, probably because it's caused by antibodies that circulate throughout the body in the bloodstream.

Connective tissue in and around joints and elsewhere in the body can become inflamed. Commonly, muscles also become inflamed. The sac that surrounds the heart (pericardium), the membrane that covers the lungs (pleura), and even the brain can be affected. The type and severity of symptoms depend on which organs are affected.

Diagnosis

Each autoimmune disease is diagnosed on the basis of its particular symptom pattern, the findings during a physical examination, and the results of laboratory tests. Sometimes the symptoms of one disease overlap with another so much that a distinction can't be made, so undifferentiated connective tissue disease or overlap disease is diagnosed.

▲ see page 816

■ see page 742

★ see page 291

Anemia (an insufficient number of red blood cells)■ often accompanies connective tissue diseases. The erythrocyte sedimentation rate, which measures the rate at which red blood cells settle to the bottom of a test tube containing blood, is often above normal in these diseases. A rate that's above normal suggests that active inflammation is present, but this test alone can't identify the cause of the inflammation. Doctors may monitor the sedimentation rate when symptoms are mild to determine whether the disease is still active.

In some connective tissue diseases, unusual antibodies can be detected and measured in the blood. If the antibodies are virtually specific to a disease, their presence confirms the diagnosis. For example, antibodies to double-stranded DNA occur almost exclusively in systemic lupus erythematosus. However, in most diseases, antibodies are not specific to the disease. For example, 70 percent of the people with rheumatoid arthritis have antibodies called rheumatoid factor, but the rest do not, and rheumatoid factor can occur in several other diseases. In such cases, laboratory test results can help a doctor make a diagnosis but they can't confirm it.

When a disease affects a specific tissue or organ, a doctor may perform a biopsy, in which a sample of that tissue is removed and examined under a microscope for changes. The results may be helpful in confirming a suspected diagnosis or in following the progression of a disease.

Treatment

Treatment varies according to the type of disease and its severity. Drug treatment is aimed at reducing inflammation. When the inflammation can cause severe symptoms or can even be fatal, aggressive treatment must be started immediately.

Drugs that reduce inflammation include **nonsteroidal anti-inflammatory drugs** (NSAIDs), such as aspirin and ibuprofen,★ which are used for mild inflammation and minor flare-ups. These drugs also control pain. Certain nonsteroidal anti-inflammatory drugs can be purchased without a prescription, but high doses, which are generally needed to treat autoimmune diseases, require a prescription. Side effects, most commonly stomach upset, are generally minor when the drugs are taken in modest doses for short periods of time. However, side effects can be numerous and severe, especially when the drugs are taken in high doses for a long time.

Corticosteroids that are synthetic forms of natural hormones are very potent anti-inflammatory drugs that can be given by injection or by mouth. Prednisone is the most widely used corticosteroid given by mouth. Low doses of a corticosteroid may have to be taken for months or years after the inflammation has been controlled with higher doses. Compared with nonsteroidal anti-inflammatory drugs, corticosteroids produce many more severe side effects, such as high blood sugar levels, an increased risk of infection, osteoporosis, water retention, and fragility of the skin. To avoid these side effects, a doctor prescribes the lowest effective dose, especially for long-term treatment.

Immunosuppressive drugs, such as methotrexate, azathioprine, and cyclophosphamide, are used to suppress the immune response, thereby reducing inflammation. These drugs, some of which are also used to treat cancer, have potentially dangerous side effects. Long-term use of azathioprine and cyclophosphamide may increase the risk of developing some forms of cancer. Some immunosuppressive drugs may contribute to reproductive system dysfunction. Because the immune system is suppressed, common infections can become life threatening. Consequently, the most potent immunosuppressive drugs are generally used only in severe cases.

Rheumatoid Arthritis

Rheumatoid arthritis is an autoimmune disease in which joints, usually including those of the hands and feet, are symmetrically inflamed, resulting in swelling, pain, and often the eventual destruction of the joint's interior.

Rheumatoid arthritis can also produce a variety of symptoms throughout the body. Its exact cause isn't known, but many different factors, including genetic predisposition, may influence the autoimmune reaction. This disease develops in about 1 percent of the population, affecting women two to three times more often than men. Usually, rheumatoid arthritis first appears between 25 and 50 years of age, but it may occur at

any age. In some people, the disease resolves spontaneously, and treatment relieves symptoms in three out of four people; however, at least 1 out of 10 people eventually becomes disabled.

In this disease, the immune system attacks the tissue that lines and cushions joints. Eventually, the cartilage, bone, and ligaments of the joint erode, causing scars to form within the joint. The joints deteriorate at a highly variable rate.

Symptoms

Rheumatoid arthritis may start suddenly, with many joints becoming inflamed at the same time. More frequently, it starts subtly, gradually affecting different joints. Usually, the inflammation is symmetric: When a joint on one side of the body is affected, the corresponding joint on the other side is also affected. Typically, the small joints in the fingers, toes, hands, feet, wrists, elbows, and ankles become inflamed first. The inflamed joints are usually painful and often stiff, especially just after awakening or after prolonged inactivity. Some people feel tired and weak, especially in the early afternoon.

Affected joints enlarge and can quickly become deformed. Joints may freeze in one position (contractures) so that they can't extend or open fully. The fingers tend to bend toward the little finger on each hand, causing tendons in the fingers to slip out of place. Swollen wrists can result in carpal tunnel syndrome. Cysts, which may develop behind affected knees, can rupture, causing pain and swelling in the lower legs. About 30 to 40 percent of people with rheumatoid arthritis have hard bumps (nodules) just under the skin, usually near diseased areas.

Rheumatoid arthritis may produce a low-grade fever and occasionally an inflammation of blood vessels (vasculitis) that causes nerve damage or leg sores (ulcers). Inflammation of the membranes around the lungs (pleurisy) or the sac surrounding the heart (pericarditis) or inflammation and scarring of the lungs can lead to chest pain, difficulty in breathing, and abnormal heart function. Some people develop swollen lymph nodes, Sjögren's syndrome, or an eye inflammation.

Still's disease is a variation of rheumatoid arthritis in which high fever and other generalized symptoms develop first.

Diagnosis

Distinguishing rheumatoid arthritis from the many other conditions that can cause arthritis

---

Identifying Rheumatoid Arthritis

A person who has four of the following characteristics is likely to have rheumatoid arthritis:

- Stiffness in the morning that lasts for more than 1 hour (for at least 6 weeks)
- Inflammation (arthritis) in three or more joints (for at least 6 weeks)
- Arthritis in the hand, wrist, or finger joints (for at least 6 weeks)
- Rheumatoid factor in the blood
- Characteristic changes on x-rays

---

may be difficult. Conditions that resemble rheumatoid arthritis in some aspects include acute rheumatic fever, gonococcal arthritis, Lyme disease, Reiter's syndrome, psoriatic arthritis, ankylosing spondylitis, gout, pseudogout, and osteoarthritis.

Rheumatoid arthritis may produce a characteristic pattern of symptoms, but laboratory tests, an examination of a joint fluid sample obtained with a needle, and even a biopsy (removal of a tissue sample for examination under a microscope) of nodules may be needed to pin down the diagnosis. Characteristic changes in the joints may be seen on x-rays.

Some laboratory test results are typical of rheumatoid arthritis. For example, in 9 out of 10 people who have rheumatoid arthritis, the erythrocyte sedimentation rate is increased. Most people have mild anemia. Rarely, the white blood cell count becomes abnormally low. When a person has a low white blood cell count, an enlarged spleen, and rheumatoid arthritis, the condition is called Felty's syndrome.

Many people with rheumatoid arthritis have distinctive antibodies in their blood. Seven out of 10 people have an antibody called rheumatoid factor. (This factor also occurs in several other disorders, such as chronic liver disease and some infections; some people have this factor without

---

▲ see pages 55 and 291

any evidence of disease.) Usually, the higher the level of rheumatoid factor in the blood, the more severe the rheumatoid arthritis and the poorer the prognosis. The rheumatoid factor level may decrease when joints are less inflamed and increase when flare-ups occur.

Treatment

Treatments range from simple, conservative measures such as rest and adequate nutrition to drugs and surgery. Treatment starts with the least aggressive measures, moving to more aggressive ones if needed.

A basic principle of treatment is to rest the affected joints, because using them aggravates the inflammation. Regular rest periods often help relieve pain, and sometimes a short period of total bed rest helps relieve a severe flare-up in its most active, painful stage. Splints can be used to immobilize and rest one or several joints, but some systematic movement of the joints is needed to prevent stiffening.

A regular, healthy diet is generally appropriate. Some people have flare-ups after eating certain foods. A diet rich in fish and plant oils but low in red meat can have minor beneficial effects on the inflammation.

The main categories of drugs used to treat rheumatoid arthritis are nonsteroidal anti-inflammatory drugs (NSAIDs), slow-acting drugs, corticosteroids, and immunosuppressive drugs. Generally, the stronger the drug, the more severe its potential side effects, so that closer monitoring is needed.

Nonsteroidal Anti-inflammatory Drugs

The nonsteroidal anti-inflammatory drugs,▲ which include aspirin and ibuprofen, are the most widely used drugs. They reduce the swelling in affected joints and alleviate the pain. Aspirin is the traditional cornerstone of treatment for rheumatoid arthritis; the newer nonsteroidal anti-inflammatory drugs may have fewer side effects and are usually simpler to take, but they are more expensive.

People usually begin aspirin treatment with 2 tablets (325 mg) four times a day but may have to increase the dose for sufficient relief. Ringing in the ears is a side effect that indicates the dose is too high. Upset stomach, a common side effect of high doses, and ulcers can often be prevented by eating food or taking antacids or other drugs at the same time. Misoprostol may help prevent erosion of the stomach's lining and the formation of stomach (gastric) ulcers in people at high risk of developing such conditions, but it also may cause diarrhea and doesn't prevent the nausea or abdominal pain that can result from taking aspirin or other nonsteroidal anti-inflammatory drugs.

If aspirin can't be tolerated, other nonsteroidal anti-inflammatory drugs are tried. However, all such drugs can upset the stomach and can't be taken by anyone who has active gastrointestinal tract (peptic) ulcers. Other, less common side effects include headaches, confusion, increased blood pressure, swelling (edema), and sometimes kidney disease.

Slow-acting Drugs

Slow-acting drugs sometimes alter the course of the disease, although improvement may take several months and side effects can be dangerous. Their use must be closely supervised and monitored by a doctor. These drugs are usually added if nonsteroidal anti-inflammatory drugs have proved ineffective after 2 or 3 months or sooner if the disease is progressing rapidly. The slow-acting drugs currently in use are gold compounds, penicillamine, hydroxychloroquine, and sulfasalazine.

Gold compounds, which can slow the formation of bone deformities, may cause a temporary remission of the disease. Usually, the gold compound is given as a weekly injection, although a preparation given by mouth is available. The weekly injections are continued until a total of 1 gram has been given or until side effects or significant improvement occurs. If the drug is effective, the frequency of the injections can be gradually decreased. Sometimes improvement is sustained for years on maintenance doses.

Gold compounds can adversely affect several organs, and people who have severe liver or kidney disease or certain blood disorders can't take these drugs. Consequently, blood and urine samples are tested before treatment begins and frequently—up to once a week—during treatment. Side effects of these drugs include potentially dangerous rashes, itchy skin, and decreased numbers of blood cells. Less commonly, gold compounds can affect the liver, lungs, and nerves, and rarely, they cause diarrhea. Gold is usually discontinued if any of these severe side effects occurs.

Penicillamine has beneficial effects similar to those of gold and may be used when gold isn't effective or when it causes intolerable side effects. The dose is gradually increased until a person shows some improvement. Side effects include suppression of blood cell production in the bone marrow, kidney problems, muscle disease, rash, and a bad taste in the mouth. If any of these side effects occur, the drug must be discontinued. Penicillamine can also cause disorders such as myasthenia gravis, Goodpasture's syndrome, and a lupus-like syndrome. Blood and urine samples are tested as frequently as every 2 to 4 weeks during treatment.

Hydroxychloroquine is used rather than gold compounds or penicillamine to treat less severe rheumatoid arthritis. Side effects, which are usually mild, include rashes, muscle aches, and eye problems. However, some eye problems can be permanent, so people taking hydroxychloroquine must have their eyes checked by an ophthalmologist before treatment begins and every 6 months during treatment. If the drug hasn't helped after 6 months, it's discontinued. Otherwise, it can be continued as long as necessary.

Sulfasalazine is increasingly prescribed for rheumatoid arthritis. The dose is increased gradually, and improvement usually occurs within 3 months. Like the other slow-acting drugs, it can cause stomach upset, liver problems, blood cell disorders, and rashes.

Corticosteroids

Corticosteroids, such as prednisone, are the most dramatically effective drugs for reducing inflammation anywhere in the body. Although corticosteroids are effective for short-term use, they tend to become less effective over time, and rheumatoid arthritis is usually active for years. They generally don't slow the progression of the disease. Furthermore, the long-term use of corticosteroids invariably leads to many side effects, involving almost every organ in the body.

Common side effects are thinning of the skin, bruising, osteoporosis, high blood pressure, elevated blood sugar levels, and cataracts. Consequently, these drugs are usually reserved for the immediate treatment of flare-ups when several joints are affected or when all other drugs have been ineffective. They're also useful in treating inflammation outside of joints, for example, in the membrane covering the lungs (pleurisy) or the sac surrounding the heart (pericarditis). Because of the risk of side effects, the lowest effective dose is almost always used. Corticosteroids can be injected directly into the affected joints for fast, short-term relief but can actually contribute to long-term damage, especially when a person who receives frequent injections overuses the temporarily pain-free joint, hastening its destruction.

Immunosuppressive Drugs

Immunosuppressive drugs (methotrexate, azathioprine, and cyclophosphamide) are effective in treating severe rheumatoid arthritis. They suppress the inflammation so that corticosteroids can be avoided or lower doses of a corticosteroid can be given. But these drugs have potentially fatal side effects, including liver disease, lung inflammation, an increased susceptibility to infection, the suppression of blood cell production in the bone marrow, and, with cyclophosphamide, bleeding from the bladder. In addition, azathioprine and cyclophosphamide may increase the risk of developing cancer.

Methotrexate, given by mouth once a week, is being used increasingly to treat rheumatoid arthritis in its early stages because this drug can take effect quickly—sometimes after several weeks; it may be given before slow-acting drugs when the arthritis is severe. People tolerate this drug well but must be closely monitored. They must refrain from drinking alcohol to minimize the risk of liver damage. Cyclosporine, which suppresses lymphocytes (a type of white blood cell), may be used to treat severe arthritis when other drugs have been ineffective.

Other Therapies

Along with drugs to reduce joint inflammation, a treatment plan for rheumatoid arthritis can include exercise, physical therapy, the application of heat to inflamed joints, and sometimes surgery. Inflamed joints should be exercised gently so they don't freeze. As the inflammation subsides, regular, active exercises can help, although a person shouldn't exercise to the point of fatigue. For many people, exercise in water may be easier.

Treatment of frozen joints consists of intensive exercises and occasionally the use of splints to gradually extend the joint. If drugs haven't helped, surgery may be needed. Surgically replacing knee or hip joints is the most effective way to restore mobility and function when the joint dis-

ease is advanced. Joints can also be removed or fused, especially in the foot, to make walking less painful. The thumb can be fused to enable a person to grasp, and unstable vertebrae at the top of the neck can be fused together to prevent them from compressing the spinal cord.

People who are disabled by rheumatoid arthritis can use several aids to accomplish daily tasks. For example, specially modified orthopedic or athletic shoes can make walking less painful, and devices such as grippers reduce the need to squeeze the hand forcefully.

Psoriatic Arthritis

Psoriatic arthritis is a form of arthritis that occurs in people who have psoriasis▲ of the skin or nails.

The disease resembles rheumatoid arthritis but doesn't produce the antibodies characteristic of rheumatoid arthritis.

Symptoms and Diagnosis

Psoriasis (a skin condition causing flare-ups of red, scaly rashes and thickened, pitted nails) may precede or follow the joint inflammation. The arthritis usually affects joints of the fingers and toes, although other joints, including the hips and spine, are often affected as well. The joints may become swollen and deformed when inflammation is chronic. The skin and joint symptoms may appear and disappear together.

The diagnosis is made by identifying the characteristic arthritis in a person who has psoriasis or a family history of psoriasis.

Prognosis and Treatment

The prognosis for psoriatic arthritis is usually better than that for rheumatoid arthritis because fewer joints are affected. Nonetheless, the joints can be severely damaged.

Treatment is aimed at controlling the skin rash and alleviating the joint inflammation. Several drugs that are effective in treating rheumatoid arthritis are also used to treat psoriatic arthritis. They include gold compounds, methotrexate, cyclosporine, and sulfasalazine. Another drug, etretinate, is usually effective in severe cases, but its side effects may be serious; because it can cause birth defects, it should not be taken by pregnant women. Etretinate remains in the body for a long time, so women should not become pregnant while taking the drug or for at least 1 year after discontinuing it. The combination of taking me-

----

▲ see page 957

thoxsalen by mouth and undergoing ultraviolet light (PUVA) treatments alleviates the skin symptoms and most joint inflammation but not inflammation of the spine.

Discoid Lupus Erythematosus

Discoid lupus erythematosus is a chronic, recurring disorder characterized by clearly defined round, red patches on the skin.

Its cause is unknown. The disorder is more common in females, most often women in their 30s. The age range is much wider than the usual range for systemic lupus erythematosus.

Symptoms

The characteristic rash may persist or may come and go for years. The appearance of the patches changes over time. At first, they're red and round, about the diameter of a pencil eraser. Usually, they develop on the cheeks, bridge of the nose, scalp, and ears, but they can also develop on the upper trunk, back of the arms, and shins. Mouth sores are very common. If the disorder isn't treated, each patch gradually spreads outward. The central area degenerates, leaving a scar. In particularly scaly areas, the plugged hair follicles dilate, leaving pits shaped like carpet tacks. Scarring can cause widespread hair loss. The rash may be accompanied by achy joints and a decreased number of white blood cells but is only infrequently accompanied by the more severe symptoms of systemic lupus erythematosus.

Diagnosis and Treatment

The diagnosis isn't easy to confirm because the rash in discoid lupus erythematosus may be identical to the one in systemic lupus erythematosus and similar to rashes caused by diseases such as rosacea, seborrheic dermatitis, lymphoma, and sarcoidosis. A doctor takes a thorough medical history and performs a complete examination to make sure that no other organs are affected. Blood tests to measure the number of red and white blood cells and evaluate kidney function can help the doctor eliminate other possible diagnoses. Another laboratory test can be performed to look for antibodies to double-stranded DNA, which are found in many people who have systemic lupus erythematosus but in almost none who have discoid lupus erythematosus.

Treatment, if begun early, can prevent or reduce the severity of permanent scarring. Sunlight and ultraviolet light, as used in tanning salons, can make the rash worse and should be avoided. Sunscreen can be used as a preventive measure. Small patches of rash can usually be treated successfully with a corticosteroid cream. Larger, more resistant rashes often require a few months of treatment with corticosteroids given by mouth or with immunosuppressive drugs such as those used to treat systemic lupus erythematosus.

Systemic Lupus Erythematosus

Systemic lupus erythematosus (lupus) is an autoimmune disease that results in episodes of inflammation in joints, tendons, and other connective tissues and organs.

Different tissues and organs become inflamed in different people, and the severity of the disease ranges from mild to debilitating, depending on the number and variety of antibodies that appear and the organs affected. About 90 percent of the people who have lupus are young women in their late teens to 30s, but children, mostly girls, and older men and women can also be affected.

Occasionally, certain heart drugs (hydralazine, procainamide, and beta-blockers) can cause a lupus-like syndrome that disappears after the drug is discontinued.

Symptoms

The number and variety of antibodies that can appear in lupus are greater than those in any other disease, and they—along with other unknown factors—determine which symptoms develop. Therefore, symptoms, and their severity and gravity, vary greatly from person to person. Lupus can be quite mild, or it can be devastating, disabling, or fatal. For example, in people who have antibodies that affect only the skin, the skin symptoms may be mild—protecting the skin from sunlight may even prevent them—or they may be severe and disfiguring.

Because symptoms vary greatly, lupus may resemble many other diseases. For example, the connective tissue of joints is commonly affected in lupus, and the arthritis that results may resemble rheumatoid arthritis. Lupus may resemble epilepsy or some psychologic disorders when the brain is affected.

Although lupus can be chronic and ongoing, it usually flares up intermittently. What triggers a flare-up of lupus in people who are predisposed

Characteristics of Lupus

- Facial rash
- Skin rash
- Sensitivity to sunlight
- Mouth sores
- Fluid around the lungs, heart, or other organs
- Arthritis
- Kidney dysfunction
- Low white blood cell count or low platelet count
- Nerve or brain dysfunction
- Positive results of a blood test for antinuclear antibodies, followed in some cases by positive results of a more specific test for antibodies to double-stranded DNA
- Anemia

to it often isn't known, although sunlight seems to be one factor.

Lupus may begin with a fever. A high fever can occur abruptly, or episodes of fever and a generally sick feeling (malaise) can come and go, sometimes for years. About 90 percent of people with lupus have joint inflammation, which ranges from intermittent mild aches to severe arthritis in several joints. Years of joint symptoms may precede other symptoms. In fact, many people who have lupus recall having growing pains as children. Long-standing joint inflammation can lead to deformity and permanent damage to the joint and surrounding tissue, but the bone doesn't erode as it does in rheumatoid arthritis.

Skin rashes are common, often occurring on the face, neck, upper chest, and elbows. The most characteristic is a red, butterfly-shaped rash that appears across the bridge of the nose and on the cheeks. Circular, raised bumps may develop. These rashes rarely blister or become raw. Mouth sores are also common. Mottled, reddish-purple areas may appear on the sides of the palms and on the fingers; swelling and redness may develop around the nails. Hair loss is common when the disease is active. In almost half the people who

have lupus, the skin is highly sensitive to light; it may burn easily or a rash may develop after exposure to sunlight.

Occasionally, an inflammation develops and extra fluid accumulates in the membranes surrounding the lungs. This inflammation (pleurisy) can make deep breathing painful. Fluid may accumulate in the sac around the heart, resulting in pericarditis, which can cause severe, constant chest pain. Children, young adults, and blacks with lupus commonly develop swollen lymph nodes throughout the body, and about 10 percent of the people with lupus develop an enlarged spleen.

Sometimes the nervous system is affected, causing headaches, personality changes, seizures, and symptoms that resemble dementia, such as difficulty in thinking clearly. Strokes occur less often. Protein or red blood cells in the urine, detected by a laboratory test, indicate kidney damage caused by glomerulonephritis, an inflammation of the kidneys, which is a common consequence of lupus. If severe, progressive kidney disease develops, blood pressure can become dangerously high, and kidney failure, which may be fatal, can follow. Early detection and treatment of kidney damage in people who have lupus reduces the incidence of severe kidney disease.

Diagnosis

Lupus is diagnosed mainly on the basis of its symptoms, particularly if they occur in a young woman. Because of the wide range of symptoms, distinguishing lupus from similar diseases can be difficult at first.

Laboratory tests can help confirm the diagnosis. A blood test can detect antinuclear antibodies, which are present in almost all people who have lupus. However, these antibodies also occur in other diseases. Therefore, if antinuclear antibodies are detected, a test for antibodies to double-stranded DNA is also performed. A high level of these antibodies is almost specific for lupus, but not all people who have lupus have these antibodies. Blood tests to measure complement levels (a group of proteins that are part of the immune system) and to detect other antibodies may be performed to predict the activity and course of the disease.

Kidney damage from lupus may be detected by blood and urine tests. Sometimes a biopsy of kidney tissue must be performed to help the doctor plan treatment.

Prognosis and Treatment

Because the course of lupus is unpredictable, the prognosis varies widely. The disease tends to be chronic and relapsing, often with symptom-free periods that can last for years. Flare-ups rarely occur after menopause. The prognosis has improved markedly over the last two decades. Usually, if the initial inflammation is controlled, the long-term prognosis is good.

If the symptoms of lupus are caused by taking a drug, discontinuing the drug cures the lupus, although the recovery may take months.

Treatment depends on which organs are affected and whether the disease is mild or severe. Mild lupus is characterized by fever, arthritis, rash, mild heart and lung involvement, and headaches. Severe lupus may cause life-threatening blood disorders, massive heart and lung involvement, significant kidney damage, vasculitis of the arms and legs or gastrointestinal tract, or severe nervous system dysfunction.

Mild disease may require little or no treatment. Nonsteroidal anti-inflammatory drugs (NSAIDs) often can relieve joint pain. Aspirin is used in low doses if the person's blood has a tendency to clot, as happens in some people with lupus; doses that are too high can harm the liver. Hydroxychloroquine, chloroquine, or quinacrine, sometimes taken in combination, helps relieve joint and skin symptoms.

Severe disease is treated immediately with a corticosteroid such as prednisone. The dose and duration of treatment depend on which organs are affected. Sometimes an immunosuppressive drug such as azathioprine or cyclophosphamide is given to suppress the body's autoimmune attack. The combination of a corticosteroid and an immunosuppressive drug is most often used for severe kidney or nervous system disease and vasculitis.

Once the initial inflammation is controlled, a doctor determines the dose that most effectively suppresses the inflammation over the long term. Usually, the dose of prednisone is gradually decreased when symptoms are controlled and laboratory test results improve. Relapses or flare-ups can occur during this process. For most people who have lupus, the dose of prednisone can eventually be decreased or discontinued.

Surgical procedures and pregnancy are more complicated for people who have lupus, and they require close medical supervision. Miscarriages and flare-ups after childbirth are common.

Scleroderma

Scleroderma (systemic sclerosis) is a chronic disease characterized by degenerative changes and scarring in the skin, joints, and internal organs and by blood vessel abnormalities.

Its cause isn't known. The disorder is four times more common in women than in men and is rare in children. Scleroderma may occur as part of mixed connective tissue disease.

Symptoms

The usual initial symptoms are thickening and swelling of the ends of the fingers. Raynaud's phenomenon,▲ in which the fingers suddenly become very pale and tingle or become numb in response to cold or emotional upset, is also common. Fingers typically become blue as they warm up. Aches and pains in several joints often accompany early symptoms. Heartburn, difficulty in swallowing, and shortness of breath are occasionally the first symptoms of scleroderma, but usually they appear later, if the esophagus, heart, and lungs become damaged.

Scleroderma can damage large areas of skin or only the fingers (sclerodactyly). As the disease progresses, the skin becomes taut, shiny, and darker than usual. The skin on the face tightens, sometimes resulting in a masklike inability to change facial expressions. Spider veins (telangiectasia) appear on the fingers, chest, face, lips, and tongue. Bumps composed of calcium can develop on the fingers, on other bony areas, or at the joints.

Often, a grating sound can be heard as the inflamed tissues move over each other, particularly at and below the knees. The fingers, wrists, and elbows can become fixed in flexed (contracted) positions because of scarring in the skin. Sores can develop on the fingertips and knuckles.

Scarring commonly damages the lower end of the esophagus (the tube connecting the mouth and stomach). The damaged esophagus can no longer propel food to the stomach efficiently. Swallowing difficulties and heartburn eventually

---

▲ see page 136

develop in most people who have scleroderma. Abnormal cell growth in the esophagus (Barrett's syndrome) occurs in about a third of the people, increasing their risk of esophageal blockage or cancer. Damage to the intestines can interfere with food absorption (malabsorption) and cause weight loss. The drainage system from the liver may become blocked by scar tissue (biliary cirrhosis), resulting in liver damage and jaundice.

Scleroderma can cause scar tissue to accumulate in the lungs, resulting in abnormal shortness of breath during exercise. It can also cause several life-threatening heart abnormalities, including heart failure and abnormal rhythms.

Severe kidney disease can result from scleroderma. The first symptom of kidney damage is usually an abrupt, progressive rise in blood pressure. High blood pressure is an ominous sign, although treatment usually controls it.

The **CREST syndrome,** also called limited cutaneous sclerosis (scleroderma), is usually a less severe form of the disease that's less likely to cause serious internal organ damage. It's named for its symptoms: calcium deposits in the skin and throughout the body, Raynaud's phenomenon, esophageal dysfunction, sclerodactyly (skin damage on the fingers), and telangiectasia (spider veins). Skin damage is limited to the fingers. People who have the CREST syndrome can develop pulmonary hypertension, which can cause heart and respiratory failure.

Diagnosis

A doctor diagnoses scleroderma by the characteristic changes in the skin and internal organs. The symptoms may overlap with those of several other connective tissue diseases, but the whole pattern is usually distinctive. Laboratory tests alone can't identify the disease because test results, like the symptoms, vary greatly among people who have scleroderma. However, tests for an antibody to centromeres (part of a chromosome) may help distinguish limited cutaneous scleroderma from the more generalized form.

Prognosis and Treatment

The course of scleroderma is variable and unpredictable. Sometimes scleroderma worsens rapidly and becomes fatal. At other times, it af-

fects only the skin for decades before affecting internal organs, although some damage to internal organs such as the esophagus is almost inevitable, even in the CREST syndrome. The prognosis is worst for those who have early symptoms of heart, lung, or kidney damage.

No drug can stop the progression of scleroderma. However, drugs can relieve some symptoms and reduce organ damage. Nonsteroidal anti-inflammatory drugs (NSAIDs) or occasionally corticosteroids help relieve severe muscle and joint pain and weakness. Penicillamine slows the rate of skin thickening and may delay the involvement of additional internal organs, but some people can't tolerate this drug's side effects. Immunosuppressive drugs such as methotrexate may help some people.

Heartburn can be relieved by eating small meals and taking antacids and histamine-blocking drugs, which inhibit stomach acid production. Sleeping with the head of the bed elevated often helps. Surgery can sometimes correct severe stomach acid reflux problems.▲ Constricted areas of the esophagus can be dilated. Tetracycline or other antibiotics can help prevent intestinal malabsorption caused by the overgrowth of bacteria in the damaged intestine. Nifedipine may relieve the symptoms of Raynaud's phenomenon but may also increase acid reflux. Antihypertensive drugs, particularly angiotensin converting enzyme (ACE) inhibitors, are useful in treating kidney disease and high blood pressure.

Physical therapy and exercise can help maintain muscle strength but can't totally prevent joints from freezing in flexed positions.

Sjögren's Syndrome

Sjögren's syndrome is a chronic inflammatory disorder characterized by excessive dryness of the eyes, mouth, and other mucous membranes.

This syndrome is often associated with other symptoms more characteristic of rheumatoid arthritis or systemic lupus erythematosus (lupus). Sjögren's syndrome is thought to be an autoimmune disease, but its cause isn't known. It's less common than rheumatoid arthritis and more prevalent in women than in men.

White blood cells infiltrate the glands that secrete fluids, such as the salivary glands in the mouth and the tear glands in the eyes. The white blood cells injure the glands, resulting in a dry mouth and dry eyes—the hallmark symptoms of

▲ see page 491

this syndrome. Sjögren's syndrome can also dry out the mucous membranes lining the gastrointestinal tract, windpipe (trachea), vulva, and vagina.

Symptoms

In some people, only the mouth or eyes are dry (sicca complex, sicca syndrome). Dryness of the eyes may severely damage the cornea, and a lack of tears can cause permanent eye damage. Insufficient saliva in the mouth can dull taste and smell, make eating and swallowing painful, and can cause cavities.

In other people, many organs are affected. Dryness of the trachea and lungs can make them more susceptible to infection, leading to pneumonia. The protective sac surrounding the heart may be inflamed—a condition called pericarditis. Nerves may be damaged, especially in the face. The liver, pancreas, spleen, kidneys, and lymph nodes all may be affected. Arthritis occurs in about a third of the people, affecting the same joints that rheumatoid arthritis affects, but the arthritis of Sjögren's syndrome tends to be milder and usually isn't destructive.

Lymphoma, a cancer of the lymphatic system, is 44 times more common in people who have Sjögren's syndrome than in the general population.

Diagnosis

A person who has a dry mouth, dry eyes, and joint inflammation probably has Sjögren's syndrome. Various tests can help a doctor diagnose this disorder. The amount of tears produced can be estimated by placing a filter paper strip under each lower eyelid and observing how much of the strip is moistened (Schirmer test). A person who has Sjögren's syndrome may produce less than a third of the normal amount. An ophthalmologist can test for damage to the eye's surface.

More sophisticated tests to evaluate salivary gland secretion may be performed, and a doctor may order scans or a biopsy of the salivary glands. Blood tests can detect abnormal antibodies, including SS-B, an antibody that's highly specific for Sjögren's syndrome. Often, people with Sjögren's syndrome also have antibodies that are more characteristic of rheumatoid arthritis (rheumatoid factor) or lupus (antinuclear antibody). The erythrocyte sedimentation rate is elevated in about 7 out of 10 people, and 1 out of 3 has a

decreased number of red blood cells (anemia) or of certain types of white blood cells.

Prognosis and Treatment

The prognosis depends on the potential of the antibodies to damage vital organs. Rarely, pneumonia, kidney failure, or lymphoma is fatal.

No cure for Sjögren's syndrome is available, but symptoms can be relieved. Dry eyes can be treated with artificial tear drops.▲ A dry mouth is moistened by continuously sipping liquids, chewing sugarless gum, or using a mouth rinse. Drugs that reduce the amount of saliva, such as decongestants and antihistamines, should be avoided because they can worsen the dryness. The drug pilocarpine may help stimulate the production of saliva if the salivary glands are not too severely damaged. Fastidious dental hygiene and frequent dental visits can minimize tooth decay and loss. Painful, swollen salivary glands can be treated with analgesics. Because joint symptoms are usually mild, aspirin and rest are often sufficient treatment. When symptoms resulting from damage to internal organs are severe, corticosteroids such as prednisone given by mouth can be very useful.

Mixed Connective Tissue Disease

Mixed connective tissue disease is a collection of symptoms similar to those of several connective tissue diseases: systemic lupus erythematosus, scleroderma, polymyositis, and dermatomyositis.

About 80 percent of the people who have this disease are women. It affects people from ages 5 to 80. Its cause is unknown, but an autoimmune reaction is likely.

Symptoms

The typical symptoms are Raynaud's phenomenon (hands and feet that become white in spots and painful when chilled), joint aches or arthritis, swollen hands, muscle weakness, difficulty in swallowing, heartburn, and shortness of breath. Raynaud's phenomenon may precede other symptoms by many years. (However, Raynaud's phenomenon is more commonly an isolated

▲ see page 1039

symptom that's not part of a connective tissue disease.) Regardless of how this disease starts, it tends to worsen, and symptoms spread to several parts of the body.

The hands are frequently so swollen that the fingers look like sausages. A purplish butterfly-shaped rash on the cheeks and bridge of the nose, red patches on the knuckles, a violet discoloration of the eyelids, and red spider veins on the face and hands all may appear. The hair may thin. Skin changes similar to those in scleroderma also may occur.

Almost everyone with mixed connective tissue disease has aching joints, and three fourths of its victims develop the inflammation and pain typical of arthritis. Mixed connective tissue disease damages the muscle fibers, so the muscles may feel weak and sore, especially in the shoulders and hips.

Although the esophagus is usually affected, it seldom causes difficulty in swallowing and isn't painful. Fluid may collect in or around the lungs. In some people, lung dysfunction is the most serious problem, causing shortness of breath during exertion and heart strain.

Occasionally, the heart is weakened, leading to heart failure. Heart failure may result in fluid retention, shortness of breath, and fatigue. The kidneys and nerves are affected in only 10 percent of the people, and the damage is usually mild. Other symptoms may include a fever, swollen lymph nodes, abdominal pain, and persistent hoarseness. Sjögren's syndrome may develop. Over time, most people develop symptoms that are more typical of lupus or scleroderma.

Diagnosis

Doctors suspect mixed connective tissue disease when some symptoms from systemic lupus erythematosus, scleroderma, polymyositis, or rheumatoid arthritis overlap.

Blood tests are performed to detect an unusual antibody to ribonucleoprotein, which is present in almost all people who have mixed connective tissue disease. A high level of this antibody without the other antibodies seen in lupus is reasonably specific for this disease.

Treatment

The treatment is similar to that of lupus. Corticosteroids are usually effective, especially when the disease is diagnosed early. Mild cases can be treated with aspirin, other nonsteroidal anti-inflammatory drugs, quinacrine or similar drugs, or very low doses of corticosteroids. The more severe the disease, the higher the dose of corticosteroid needed. In severe cases, immunosuppressive drugs may also be needed.

In general, the more advanced the disease and the greater the organ damage, the less effective the treatment. Scleroderma-like damage to the skin and esophagus is least likely to respond to treatment. Symptom-free periods can last for many years with little or no continuing treatment with a corticosteroid. Despite treatment, the disease progresses in about 13 percent of the people, producing potentially fatal complications in 6 to 12 years.

Polymyositis and Dermatomyositis

Polymyositis is a chronic connective tissue disease characterized by painful inflammation and degeneration of the muscles; dermatomyositis is polymyositis accompanied by skin inflammation.

These diseases result in disabling muscle weakness and deterioration. The weakness typically occurs in the shoulders and hips but can affect muscles symmetrically throughout the body.

Polymyositis and dermatomyositis usually occur in adults from ages 40 to 60 or in children from ages 5 to 15 years. Women are twice as likely as men to develop either disease. In adults, these diseases may occur alone or as part of other connective tissue diseases, such as mixed connective tissue disease.

The cause is unknown. Viruses or autoimmune reactions may play a role. Cancer may also trigger the diseases—an autoimmune reaction against cancer may be directed against a substance in the muscles as well. About 15 percent of men over 50 who have polymyositis also have cancer; women who have polymyositis are a little less likely to have cancer.

Symptoms

The symptoms of polymyositis are similar for people of all ages, but the disease usually develops more abruptly in children than in adults. Symptoms, which may begin during or just after an infection, include muscle weakness (particularly in the upper arms, hips, and thighs), muscle and joint pain, Raynaud's phenomenon, a rash, difficulty in swallowing, a fever, fatigue, and weight loss.

Muscle weakness may start slowly or suddenly and may worsen for weeks or months. Because muscles close to the center of the body are affected most, tasks such as lifting the arms above the shoulders, climbing stairs, and getting out of a chair can become very difficult. If the neck muscles are affected, even raising the head from a pillow may be impossible. Weakness in the shoulders or hips can confine a person to a wheelchair or bed. Muscle damage in the upper part of the esophagus can cause swallowing difficulties and food regurgitation. The muscles of the hands, feet, and face, however, aren't affected.

Joint aches and inflammation occur in about a third of the people. The pain and swelling tend to be mild. Raynaud's phenomenon occurs most frequently in people who have polymyositis along with other connective tissue diseases.

Polymyositis usually doesn't affect internal organs other than the throat and esophagus. However, the lungs may be affected, causing shortness of breath and a cough. Bleeding ulcers in the stomach or intestine may cause bloody or black bowel movements, more commonly in children than in adults.

In dermatomyositis, rashes tend to appear at the same time as periods of muscle weakness and other symptoms. A shadowy red rash (heliotrope rash) can appear on the face. A reddish-purple swelling around the eyes is characteristic. Another rash, which may be scaly, smooth, or raised, may appear almost anywhere on the body but is especially common on the knuckles. The fingernail beds may redden. When the rashes fade, brownish pigmentation, scarring, shriveling, or pale depigmented patches may develop on the skin.

Diagnosis

Certain criteria are used to make the diagnosis: muscle weakness at the shoulders or hips, a characteristic rash, increased blood levels of certain muscle enzymes, characteristic changes in muscle tissue observed under a microscope, and abnormalities in the electrical activity of muscles measured by a device called an electromyograph. Special tests performed on muscle tissue samples may be needed to rule out other muscle disorders.

Laboratory tests are helpful but can't specifically identify polymyositis or dermatomyositis. Blood levels of certain muscle enzymes, including creatine kinase, are often higher than normal,

indicating muscle damage. These enzymes are measured repeatedly in blood samples to monitor the disease; the levels usually fall to normal or near normal with effective treatment. A physical examination and additional tests may be needed to determine whether cancer is also present.

Treatment and Prognosis

Restricting activities when the inflammation is most intense often helps. Generally, a corticosteroid, usually prednisone, given by mouth in high doses slowly improves strength and relieves pain and swelling, controlling the disease. After about 4 to 6 weeks, when the muscle enzyme levels have returned to normal and muscle strength has returned, the dose is gradually decreased. Most adults must continue taking a low dose of prednisone for many years or even indefinitely to prevent a relapse. After about a year, children may be able to stop taking the drug and stay symptom-free. Occasionally, prednisone actually worsens the disease or isn't fully effective. In these cases, immunosuppressive drugs are used instead of or in addition to prednisone. When other drugs are ineffective, gamma globulin (a substance that contains large quantities of many antibodies) may be given intravenously.

When polymyositis is associated with cancer, it usually doesn't respond well to prednisone. However, the condition usually improves if the cancer can be successfully treated.

Adults with severe, progressive disease who develop difficulty in swallowing, malnutrition, pneumonia, or respiratory failure may die.

Relapsing Polychondritis

Relapsing polychondritis is an uncommon disorder characterized by episodes of painful, destructive inflammation of the cartilage and other connective tissues in the ears, joints, nose, voice box (larynx), windpipe (trachea), bronchi, eyes, heart valves, kidneys, and blood vessels.

This disorder affects men and women equally, usually in middle age. Typically, both ears become red, swollen, and very painful. At the same time or later, a person can develop arthritis, which may be mild or severe. Any joint may be affected. The cartilage that connects the ribs to the breastbone may become inflamed. Cartilage in the nose is also a common site of inflammation. Other sites include the eyes, larynx, trachea, inside of the ears, heart, blood vessels, kidneys, and

Disorders Characterized by Vasculitis

Disorder	Description
Henoch-Schönlein purpura	Inflammation of small veins, causing hard, purple blotches on the skin
Erythema nodosum	Inflammation of blood vessels in the deep layers of the skin, causing deep, tender red bumps on the arms and legs
Polyarteritis nodosa	Inflammation of medium-sized arteries, impairing blood flow through vessels and to the surrounding tissues
Temporal (giant cell) arteritis	Inflammation of arteries in the brain and head, sometimes causing headaches and blindness
Takayasu's arteritis	Inflammation of large arteries, such as the aorta and its branches, causing blockages and loss of pulse

skin. Flare-ups of inflammation and pain last a few weeks, subside, then recur over a period of several years. Eventually, the supporting cartilage can be damaged, resulting in floppy ears, a sloping saddle nose, and vision, hearing, and balance problems.

People who have this disorder may die if their airways collapse or if their heart and blood vessels are severely damaged.

Diagnosis and Treatment

Relapsing polychondritis is diagnosed when a doctor observes at least three of the following symptoms developing over time: inflammation of both ears, painful swelling in several joints, inflammation of the cartilage in the nose, inflammation of the eye, cartilage damage in the respiratory tract, and hearing or balance problems.

A biopsy of the affected cartilage may show characteristic abnormalities, and blood tests can detect evidence of chronic inflammation.

Mild relapsing polychondritis can be treated with aspirin or other nonsteroidal anti-inflammatory drugs such as ibuprofen. In more severe cases, daily doses of prednisone are given, then tapered off rapidly as the symptoms begin to improve. Sometimes critical cases are treated with immunosuppressive drugs such as cyclophosphamide. These drugs treat the symptoms but haven't been shown to alter the ultimate course of the disorder.

Vasculitis

Vasculitis is an inflammation of blood vessels.

Vasculitis is not a disease but rather a disease process that occurs in a number of autoimmune connective tissue diseases, such as rheumatoid arthritis and systemic lupus erythematosus. Vasculitis can also occur without connective tissue involvement.

No one knows what triggers vasculitis in most people, but in some, hepatitis viruses are involved. Presumably, the inflammation occurs when the immune system mistakenly identifies blood vessels or parts of a blood vessel as foreign and attacks them. Cells of the immune system, which cause inflammation, surround and infiltrate the affected blood vessels, destroying them and possibly damaging the tissues they supply. The blood vessels can become leaky or clogged; either condition disrupts blood flow to nerves, organs, and other parts of the body. The areas deprived of blood (ischemic areas) can be damaged permanently. Symptoms may result from direct damage to the blood vessels or damage to tissues whose blood supply is impaired.

Any blood vessel may be affected. Vasculitis may be limited to veins, large arteries, small arteries, or capillaries, or it may be limited to vessels in one part of the body, such as the head, leg, or kidney. Disorders such as the Henoch-Schönlein syndrome, erythema nodosum, polyarteritis nodosa, temporal (giant cell) arteritis, and Takayasu's arteritis are characterized by vasculitis limited to blood vessels of a particular size or depth.

Polyarteritis Nodosa

Polyarteritis nodosa is a disease in which segments of medium-sized arteries become inflamed and damaged, reducing the blood supply to the organs they supply.

This disease is often fatal if not treated adequately. It usually develops at 40 to 50 years of age but can occur at any age. Men are three times more likely than women to develop it.

Its cause is unknown, but reactions to some drugs and vaccines may cause it. Viral and bacterial infections sometimes appear to trigger the inflammation, but most often no triggering event or substance can be found.

Symptoms

The disease can be mild at first but fatal within several months, or it can develop subtly as a chronic debilitating disease. Any organ or combination of organs in the body can be affected; the symptoms depend on which organs are affected. Polyarteritis nodosa often resembles other diseases in which inflammation of arteries (vasculitis) occurs. One such disease is Churg-Strauss syndrome, which unlike polyarteritis nodosa produces asthma.

A fever is the most common early symptom. Abdominal pain, numbness and tingling in the hands and feet, weakness, and weight loss can also develop early. Three fourths of the people who have polyarteritis nodosa develop kidney damage, which can cause high blood pressure, swelling from water retention, and the production of little or no urine. When blood vessels in the gastrointestinal tract are affected, areas of the intestines can become perforated, causing an abdominal infection (peritonitis), severe pain, bloody diarrhea, and a high fever. Chest pain and heart attacks can result if the blood vessels to the heart are affected. Damaged blood vessels in the brain can cause headaches, convulsions, and hallucinations. The liver can be extensively damaged. Muscle and joint pain is common, and joints may be inflamed. Blood vessels near the skin may feel bumpy and irregular to the touch, and occasionally ulcers form on the skin over the blood vessels.

Diagnosis and Treatment

No blood test can confirm the diagnosis of polyarteritis nodosa. Doctors suspect the disease when the combination of symptoms and laboratory test results can't be explained in any other way. They also suspect it when fever and neurologic symptoms such as patchy numbness, tingling, or paralysis develop in a previously healthy middle-aged man. The diagnosis can be confirmed by a biopsy of an affected blood vessel. A biopsy of the liver or kidney may also be needed. X-rays taken after a dye is injected into the arteries (arteriograms) may show abnormalities in the blood vessels.

Without treatment, only 33 percent of the people survive for 1 year; 88 percent die within 5 years. Aggressive treatment can prevent death. Any drugs that may have precipitated the disease are discontinued. High doses of a corticosteroid, such as prednisone, can prevent the disease from worsening and induce a symptom-free period in about a third of the people. Because long-term treatment with a corticosteroid is usually needed, the dose is reduced once symptoms have subsided. If corticosteroids don't reduce the inflammation adequately, they may be replaced or accompanied by drugs that suppress the immune system (immunosuppressive drugs), such as cyclophosphamide. Other treatments, such as those used to control high blood pressure, are often needed to prevent damage to internal organs.

Even with treatment, several vital organs may fail or a weakened blood vessel may rupture. Kidney failure is a common cause of death. Potentially fatal infections may occur because the long-term use of corticosteroids and immunosuppressive drugs reduces the body's ability to fight infections.

Polymyalgia Rheumatica

Polymyalgia rheumatica is a condition causing severe pain and stiffness in the muscles of the neck, shoulders, and hips.

Polymyalgia rheumatica occurs in people over age 50 and is twice as common in women as in men. Its cause isn't known. Although painful, polymyalgia rheumatica does not cause weakness or muscle damage. Sometimes, polymyalgia rheumatica occurs with temporal (giant cell) arteritis.

Symptoms and Diagnosis

Polymyalgia rheumatica causes severe pain and stiffness in the neck, shoulders, and hips. The stiffness is worse in the morning and after periods of inactivity. A fever, vague discomfort, weight loss, and depression may accompany the muscle symptoms. All these symptoms may develop suddenly or gradually.

A doctor makes the diagnosis on the basis of the physical examination and test results. Biopsies of muscle tissue are usually not needed but, if performed, show no evidence of muscle damage, and electromyograms▲ show no abnormalities. Blood tests may detect anemia. Blood tests, such as the erythrocyte sedimentation rate and C-reactive protein, are usually very high, indicating that the disease is active. Creatine kinase levels, which are elevated in polymyositis, are normal in polymyalgia rheumatica.

Treatment

Polymyalgia rheumatica usually improves dramatically with low doses of prednisone, a corticosteroid. When temporal arteritis also occurs, higher doses of a corticosteroid are needed. As the symptoms subside, the dose is gradually reduced to the lowest effective dose. Most people can stop taking prednisone in 2 to 4 years, although some need low doses for an even longer time. Aspirin or other nonsteroidal anti-inflammatory drugs may provide less complete relief.

Temporal Arteritis

Temporal (giant cell) arteritis is a chronic inflammatory disease of large arteries.

This disease affects about 1 out of 1,000 people over age 50 and slightly more women than men. Its cause is unknown. The symptoms overlap with those of polymyalgia rheumatica, and some authorities believe they are variations of the same disease.

Symptoms

The symptoms vary, depending on which arteries are affected. Typically, the large arteries to the head are affected, and a severe headache usually develops suddenly at the temples or back of the head. The blood vessels in the temple may feel swollen and bumpy to the touch. The scalp may

feel painful when the hair is brushed. Double vision, blurred vision, large blind spots, blindness of one eye, or other eye problems may develop. The greatest danger is permanent blindness, which can occur suddenly if the blood supply to the optic nerve is blocked. Characteristically, the jaw, chewing muscles, and tongue may hurt when eating or speaking. Other symptoms may include those of polymyalgia rheumatica.

Diagnosis and Treatment

Doctors base their diagnosis on the symptoms and a physical examination and confirm it by performing a biopsy of the temporal artery, located in the temple. Blood tests are also helpful, usually detecting a very high erythrocyte sedimentation rate and anemia.

Because temporal arteritis causes blindness in 20 percent of untreated people, treatment must begin as soon as the disease is suspected. Prednisone is effective. Initially, the dose is high—to stop the inflammation in the blood vessels; after several weeks, the dose is slowly tapered if the person is improving. Some people can stop taking prednisone within a few years, but many need very low doses for many years to control symptoms and prevent blindness.

Wegener's Granulomatosis

Wegener's granulomatosis is an uncommon disease that often begins with an inflammation of the lining of the nose, sinuses, throat, or lungs■ and may progress to an inflammation of blood vessels throughout the body (generalized vasculitis) or fatal kidney disease.

This disease can occur at any age and is twice as common in men as in women. Its cause is unknown. It resembles an infection, but no infecting organism can be found. Wegener's granulomatosis is thought to be caused by an allergic response to a trigger that hasn't yet been identified. The result is a potent, inappropriate immune response that damages many tissues in the body.

The disease produces vasculitis and an unusual type of inflammation called a granuloma, which ultimately destroys normal tissue.

Symptoms

The disease may begin suddenly or gradually. The first symptoms usually affect the upper res-

---

▲ see page 287

■ see page 189

piratory tract—the nose, sinuses, ears, and windpipe (trachea)—and may include severe nosebleeds, sinusitis, middle ear infections (otitis media), coughing, and coughing up of blood. The lining of the nose may become red and rough, bleeding easily. A fever, a generally sick feeling (malaise), loss of appetite, joint aches and swelling, and an eye or ear inflammation may develop. The disease may affect arteries to the heart, causing chest pain or a heart attack (myocardial infarction), or it may affect the brain or spinal cord, producing symptoms that resemble those of several neurologic diseases.

The disease may progress to a generalized (disseminated) phase, with inflammation of blood vessels throughout the body. As a result, sores appear on the skin and spread extensively; they can severely scar the skin. Kidney damage, common at this stage of Wegener's granulomatosis, ranges from mild impairment to life-threatening kidney failure. Severe kidney disease causes high blood pressure and symptoms resulting from the buildup of wastes in the blood (uremia).▲ Occasionally, the lungs are the only major organ affected. Granulomas may form in the lungs, impairing breathing. Anemia is common and can be severe.

Improvement can occur spontaneously, but without treatment, Wegener's granulomatosis more often progresses and can be fatal.

Diagnosis and Treatment

Wegener's granulomatosis must be diagnosed and treated early to prevent complications, including kidney disease, heart attacks, and brain damage. A doctor usually recognizes the distinctive pattern of symptoms but performs a biopsy of an affected area to confirm the diagnosis. Although blood test results can't specifically identify Wegener's granulomatosis, they can strongly support the diagnosis. One such test can detect antineutrophil cytoplasmic antibodies, which strongly suggest this disease. If the nose, throat, or skin is not affected, diagnosis can be difficult because the symptoms and x-rays can resemble those of several lung diseases.

The generalized form of the disease used to be universally fatal. The prognosis improved significantly with the use of immunosuppressive drugs such as cyclophosphamide and azathioprine, which control the disease by reducing the body's inappropriate immune reaction. Treatment is usually continued for at least a year after the symptoms disappear. Corticosteroids, given at the same time to suppress inflammation, can usually be tapered off and discontinued. Because these drugs reduce the body's ability to fight infections, antibiotics may be needed to treat pneumonia, which may develop when the lungs are damaged. Occasionally, anemia may become so severe that a blood transfusion is needed.

Reiter's Syndrome

Reiter's syndrome is an inflammation of the joints and tendon attachments at the joints, often accompanied by an inflammation of the eye's conjunctiva■ and the mucous membranes, such as those of the mouth, urinary tract, vagina, and penis, and by a distinctive rash.

Reiter's syndrome is called a reactive arthritis because the joint inflammation appears to be a reaction to an infection originating in an area of the body other than the joints. This syndrome is most common in men aged 20 to 40.

There are two forms of Reiter's syndrome. One occurs with sexually transmitted infections such as a chlamydial infection and occurs most often in young men; the other usually follows an intestinal infection such as salmonellosis. People who develop Reiter's syndrome after exposure to these infections appear to have a genetic predisposition to this type of reaction, related to the same gene found in people who have ankylosing spondylitis. However, most people who have these infections don't develop the syndrome.

Symptoms

Typically, symptoms begin 7 to 14 days after the infection. The first symptom is often an inflammation of the urethra (the channel that carries urine from the bladder to the outside of the body). In men, this inflammation causes moderate pain and a discharge from the penis. The prostate gland may be inflamed and painful. The genital and urinary symptoms in women, if any occur, are usually mild, consisting of a slight vaginal discharge or uncomfortable urination.

▲ see page 593

■ see page 1037

The conjunctiva (the membrane that lines the eyelid and covers the eyeball) can become red and inflamed, causing itching or burning and excessive tearing. Joint pain and inflammation may be mild or severe. Several joints are usually affected at once—especially the knees, toe joints, and areas where tendons are attached to bones, such as the heels. In more severe cases, the spine may also become inflamed and painful.

Small, painless sores develop in the mouth, on the tongue, and on the end of the penis. Occasionally, a distinctive rash of hard, thickened spots may develop on the skin, especially of the palms and soles. Yellow deposits may develop under the fingernails and toenails.

In most people, the initial symptoms disappear in 3 or 4 months. In half, however, the arthritis or other symptoms recur over several years. Joint and spinal deformities may develop if the symptoms persist or recur frequently. Very few people who have Reiter's syndrome become permanently disabled.

Diagnosis and Treatment

The combination of joint, genital, urinary, skin, and eye symptoms lead a doctor to suspect Reiter's syndrome. Because these symptoms may not appear simultaneously, the disease may not be diagnosed for several months. No simple laboratory tests are available to confirm the diagnosis. A sample taken from the urethra with a swab or a sample of joint fluid may be tested, or a biopsy (removal of tissue for examination under a microscope) of the joint may be performed to try to identify the infectious organism that triggered the syndrome.

First, antibiotics are given to treat the infection, but treatment is not always successful and its optimal duration isn't known. The arthritis is usually treated with nonsteroidal anti-inflammatory drugs. Sulfasalazine or methotrexate, an immunosuppressive drug, may be used, as in rheumatoid arthritis. Corticosteroids are generally not given by mouth but by direct injection into an inflamed joint, which sometimes helps. Conjunctivitis and skin sores don't need treatment, although a severe eye inflammation may require a corticosteroid ointment or eyedrops.

Behçet's Syndrome

Behçet's syndrome is a chronic, relapsing inflammatory disease that can produce recurring, painful *mouth sores, skin blisters, genital sores, and swollen joints.*

The eyes, blood vessels, nervous system, and gastrointestinal tract may also become inflamed.

This syndrome affects men twice as often as women. It usually appears in people during their 20s, but sometimes it develops in childhood. Behçet's syndrome is uncommon in the United States. People from Mediterranean countries, Japan, Korea, and the area along the silk route through China are at highest risk. The cause of Behçet's syndrome is unknown, but viruses and autoimmune diseases may play a role.

Symptoms

Almost everyone with this syndrome has recurrent, painful mouth sores, similar to canker sores, which are usually the first symptom. Sores on the penis, scrotum, and vulva tend to be painful; those in the vagina may be painless.

Other symptoms appear days to years later. A recurring inflammation of part of the eye (relapsing iridocyclitis) produces eye pain, sensitivity to light, and hazy vision. Several other eye problems can occur; one of them, uveitis, can cause blindness if untreated.

Skin blisters and pus-filled pimples develop in about 80 percent of the people. A minor injury, even a puncture from a hypodermic needle, can cause the area to become swollen and inflamed. About half the people develop a relatively mild, nonprogressive arthritis in the knees and other large joints. Inflammation of blood vessels (vasculitis) throughout the body can cause blood clot formation, aneurysms (bulges in weakened blood vessel walls), strokes, and kidney damage. When the gastrointestinal tract is affected, symptoms may range from mild discomfort to severe cramping and diarrhea.

The recurring symptoms of Behçet's syndrome can be very disruptive. The symptoms or the symptom-free periods (remissions) may last weeks, years, or decades. Paralysis is a potential complication. Occasionally, damage to the nervous system, gastrointestinal tract, or blood vessels is fatal.

Diagnosis and Treatment

The diagnosis is based on the physical examination because no laboratory tests can detect Behçet's syndrome. Confirming the diagnosis can take months. Symptoms resemble those of many other diseases, including Reiter's syndrome, Stevens-Johnson syndrome, systemic lupus erythematosus, Crohn's disease, and ulcerative colitis.

Although there is no cure, specific symptoms can usually be relieved by treatment. For example, a corticosteroid applied externally can help heal inflamed eyes and skin sores. Needle punctures should be avoided because they may become inflamed. People who develop a severe inflammation of the eyes or the nervous system may need to be treated with prednisone or another corticosteroid. Cyclosporine, an immunosuppressive drug, may be given when the eye problems are severe or when prednisone does not adequately control symptoms.

Ankylosing Spondylitis

Ankylosing spondylitis is a connective tissue disease characterized by an inflammation of the spine and large joints, resulting in stiffness and pain.

The disease is three times more common in men than in women, developing most commonly between the ages of 20 and 40. Its cause isn't known, but the disease tends to run in families, indicating that genetics plays a role. The disease is 10 to 20 times more common in people whose parents or siblings have it.

Symptoms and Diagnosis

Mild to moderate flare-ups of inflammation generally alternate with periods of almost no symptoms. The most common symptom is back pain, which varies in intensity from one episode to another and from one person to another. Pain is often worse at night. Early morning stiffness that's relieved by activity is also very common. Pain in the lower back and the associated muscle spasm are often relieved by bending forward. Therefore, people often assume a stooped posture, which can lead to a permanent bent-over position if not treated. In others, the spine becomes noticeably straight and stiff. Loss of appetite, weight loss, fatigue, and anemia can accompany the back pain. If the joints connecting the ribs to the spine are inflamed, the pain may limit the ability to expand the chest to take a deep breath. Occasionally, pain starts in large joints, such as the hips, knees, and shoulders.

A third of the people have recurring attacks of mild eye inflammation (acute iritis), which usually doesn't impair vision. In a few people, inflammation injures a heart valve. If the damaged vertebrae press against nerves or the spinal cord, numbness, weakness, or pain can develop in the area supplied by the affected nerves. The cauda equina (horse's tail) syndrome, a rare complication, consists of symptoms that develop when the inflamed spinal column compresses the group of nerves that extend below the end of the spinal cord. The symptoms include impotence, urinary incontinence at night, diminished sensation in the bladder and rectum, and the loss of reflexes in the ankle.

The diagnosis is based on the pattern of symptoms and on x-rays of the spine and affected joints, which show erosion at the joint between the spine and the hip bone (sacroiliac joint) and the formation of bony bridges between the vertebrae, making the spine stiff. The erythrocyte sedimentation rate tends to be high. In addition, a specific gene, HLA-B27, is found in about 90 percent of the people who have this disease.

Prognosis and Treatment

Most people don't develop disabilities and can lead normal, productive lives. In some, the disease is more progressive, causing severe deformities.

Treatment focuses on relieving back and joint pain and preventing or correcting spinal deformities. Aspirin and other nonsteroidal anti-inflammatory drugs can reduce the pain and inflammation. Indomethacin may be the most effective of these drugs; side effects, risks, and costs vary. Corticosteroids help only in the short-term treatment of iritis and in severe joint inflammation, usually treated by injection into the joint. Muscle relaxants and narcotic analgesics are usually used for only brief periods to relieve severe pain and muscle spasms. Surgery to replace a joint can relieve pain and restore function to the hips and knees when they become eroded or fixed in a bent position.

The long-range goals of treatment are to maintain proper posture and develop strong back muscles. Daily exercises strengthen the muscles that oppose the tendency to bend and stoop.

Gout and Pseudogout

Gout and pseudogout are both caused by crystal deposits in the joints, and both cause joint inflammation (arthritis) and pain. However, different types of crystals are deposited in the two disorders.

Gout

Gout is a disorder characterized by sudden, recurring attacks of very painful arthritis caused by deposits of monosodium urate crystals, which accumulate in the joints because of an abnormally high uric acid level in the blood (hyperuricemia).

Joint inflammation can become chronic and deforming after repeated attacks. Almost 20 percent of the people who have gout develop kidney stones.

Normally, some uric acid, a by-product of cell breakdown, is present in the blood because the body is continually breaking down cells and forming new ones and because familiar foods contain precursors of uric acid. The uric acid level becomes abnormally high when the kidneys can't eliminate enough in the urine. The body may also produce very large amounts of uric acid because of a hereditary enzyme abnormality or a disease such as blood cancer, in which cells multiply and are rapidly destroyed. Some types of kidney disease and certain drugs impair the kidneys' ability to eliminate uric acid.

Symptoms

Attacks of gout (acute gouty arthritis) occur without warning. They may be triggered by a minor injury, surgery, consumption of large quantities of alcohol or protein-rich food, fatigue, emotional stress, or illness. Typically, severe pain occurs suddenly in one or more joints, often at night; the pain becomes progressively worse and often is excruciating. The joint swells, and the skin over the joint appears red or purplish, tight, and shiny, and it feels warm. Touching the skin over the joint can be extremely painful.

The disorder most often affects the joint at the base of the big toe, causing a condition called podagra, but it also commonly affects the instep, ankle, knee, wrist, and elbow. Crystals may form in these peripherally located joints because they are cooler than the central part of the body and urate tends to crystallize at cooler temperatures. Crystals also form in the ears and other relatively cool tissues. In contrast, gout rarely affects the spine, hips, or shoulders.

Other symptoms of acute gouty arthritis can include fever, chills, a general sick feeling, and a rapid heartbeat. Gout tends to be more severe in people who develop symptoms before age 30. Usually, gout develops during middle age in men and after menopause in women.

The first few attacks usually affect only one joint and last for a few days. The symptoms gradually disappear, the joint's function returns, and no symptoms appear until the next attack. However, if the disorder progresses, untreated attacks last longer, occur more frequently, and affect several joints. Affected joints may be permanently damaged.

Severe, chronic gout that causes a deformity may develop. Urate crystals continually deposited in the joints and tendons cause damage that increasingly restricts joint motion. Hard lumps of urate crystals (tophi) are deposited under the skin around joints. Tophi also can develop in the kidney and other organs, under the skin on the ears, or around the elbow. If untreated, tophi on the hands and feet can erupt and discharge chalky masses of crystals.

Diagnosis

Gout is often diagnosed on the basis of its distinctive symptoms and an examination of the joint. A high uric acid level in the blood supports the diagnosis; however, this level is often normal during an acute attack. The diagnosis is confirmed when needle-shaped urate crystals are identified in a sample of joint fluid removed by suction (aspirated) with a needle and viewed under a special type of microscope that uses polarized light.

Treatment

The first step is to relieve pain by controlling the inflammation. Colchicine is a traditional treatment. Usually, joint pains begin to subside after

12 to 24 hours of treatment with colchicine and are gone within 48 to 72 hours. Colchicine usually is given orally but can be given intravenously if it upsets the digestive tract. This drug often causes diarrhea and can cause more serious side effects, including damage to the bone marrow.

Currently, nonsteroidal anti-inflammatory drugs (NSAIDs) such as ibuprofen and indomethacin are used more often than colchicine and effectively relieve pain and swelling in the joint.▲ Sometimes, corticosteroids such as prednisone are prescribed for the same purpose. If only one or two joints are affected, a corticosteroid crystal suspension can be injected through the same needle used to remove fluid from the joint. This treatment effectively terminates the inflammation caused by urate crystals. Rarely, additional analgesics such as codeine and meperidine are used to control pain. The inflamed joint may be immobilized to reduce pain.

The second step is to prevent recurrences. Drinking plenty of fluids, avoiding alcoholic beverages, and eating smaller amounts of protein-rich foods may be all that's needed. Many people who have gout are overweight. When they lose weight, uric acid levels in the blood often return to normal or near normal.

For some people—especially those who have repeated, severe attacks—long-term drug treatment is started when symptoms of the attack have disappeared and is continued between attacks. Low doses of colchicine may be taken daily and can prevent attacks or at least reduce their frequency. Routinely taking nonsteroidal anti-inflammatory drugs also can prevent some attacks. Sometimes, both colchicine and a nonsteroidal anti-inflammatory drug are needed. However, this combination doesn't prevent or heal progressive joint damage caused by crystal deposits, and it does pose some risks for people who have kidney or liver disease.

Drugs such as probenecid or sulfinpyrazone lower the uric acid level in the blood by increasing the excretion of uric acid in the urine. Aspirin blocks the effects of probenecid and sulfinpyrazone and should not be used at the same time. If pain medication is needed, acetaminophen or a nonsteroidal anti-inflammatory drug such as ibuprofen can be safely used instead. Drinking plenty of fluids—at least 3 quarts a day—may help reduce the risk of damage to the joints and kidneys when the excretion of uric acid is increased.

Allopurinol, a drug that blocks production of uric acid in the body, is especially helpful to people who have a high uric acid level and kidney stones or kidney damage. However, allopurinol can upset the stomach, cause a skin rash, decrease the number of white blood cells, and cause liver damage.

Most tophi on the ears, hands, or feet shrink slowly when the uric acid level in the blood is decreased, but extremely large tophi may have to be removed surgically.

People who have a high uric acid level in the blood but no symptoms of gout are sometimes treated with drugs to lower this level. However, because of the risk of adverse effects from these drugs, their use is probably not justified unless the amount of uric acid in the urine is very large. For such people, treatment with allopurinol may prevent kidney stones.

Pseudogout

Pseudogout (calcium pyrophosphate dihydrate crystal deposition disease) is a disorder characterized by intermittent attacks of painful arthritis caused by deposits of calcium pyrophosphate crystals.

The disorder usually occurs in older people and affects men and women equally. Ultimately, it causes degeneration of the affected joints.

Causes and Symptoms

The cause of pseudogout is unknown. It may occur in people who have other diseases, such as an abnormally high calcium level in the blood caused by a high level of parathyroid hormone (hyperparathyroidism), an abnormally high iron level in the tissues (hemochromatosis), or an abnormally low magnesium level in the blood (hypomagnesemia).

Symptoms vary widely. Some people have attacks of painful arthritis, usually in the knees, wrists, or other relatively large joints. Other people have lingering, chronic pain and stiffness in joints of the arms and legs, which doctors may confuse with rheumatoid arthritis. Acute attacks are usually less severe than those in gout. Some people have no pain between attacks, and some

▲ see pages 55 and 291

have no pain at any time despite large deposits of crystals.

Diagnosis and Treatment

Pseudogout is often confused with other joint disorders, especially gout. The diagnosis is made by taking fluid from an inflamed joint through a needle. Crystals composed of calcium pyrophosphate, rather than urate, are found in the joint fluid. X-rays also may support the diagnosis because calcium pyrophosphate crystals, unlike urate crystals, block x-rays and appear as white deposits on x-ray film.

Usually, treatment can stop acute attacks and prevent new attacks but can't prevent damage to the affected joints. Most often, nonsteroidal anti-inflammatory drugs (NSAIDs) such as ibuprofen are used to reduce the pain and inflammation. Occasionally, colchicine may be given intravenously to relieve the inflammation and pain during attacks and can be given orally in low doses daily to prevent attacks. Sometimes, excess joint fluid is drained and a corticosteroid crystal suspension is injected into the joint to reduce the inflammation. No effective long-term treatment is available to remove crystals.

CHAPTER 53

Bone and Joint Infections

Bones and the fluid and tissues of joints can become infected. Such infections include osteomyelitis and infectious arthritis.

Osteomyelitis

Osteomyelitis is a bone infection usually caused by bacteria but sometimes by a fungus.

When a bone is infected, the soft, inner part (bone marrow) often swells. As the swollen tissue presses against the rigid outer wall of the bone, the blood vessels in the marrow may be compressed, reducing or cutting off the blood supply to the bone. Without an adequate blood supply, parts of the bone may die. The infection also can spread outward from the bone to form collections of pus (abscesses) in adjacent soft tissues, such as the muscle.

Causes

Bones, which usually are well protected from infection, can become infected through three routes: the bloodstream, direct invasion, and adjacent soft tissue infections.

The bloodstream may carry an infection from another part of the body to the bones. An infection usually occurs in the ends of leg and arm bones in children and in the spine (vertebrae) in adults. People who undergo kidney dialysis and those who inject illegal drugs are particularly susceptible to an infection of the vertebrae (verte-

bral osteomyelitis). Infections also may occur where a piece of metal has been attached to a bone, as is done to repair hip or other fractures. The bacteria that cause tuberculosis also can infect the vertebrae (Pott's disease).

Organisms may invade the bone directly through open fractures, during bone surgery, or from contaminated objects that pierce the bone. An infection in an artificial joint, usually acquired during surgery, can spread to adjacent bone.

An infection in the soft tissues around a bone may spread to the bone after several days or weeks. A soft tissue infection may start in an area damaged by an injury, radiation therapy, or cancer or in a skin ulcer caused by poor circulation or diabetes. A sinus, gum, or tooth infection may spread to the skull.

Symptoms

In children, bone infections acquired through the bloodstream cause fever and, sometimes days later, pain in the infected bone. The area over the bone may be sore and swollen, and movement may be painful.

Infections of the vertebrae usually develop gradually, producing persistent back pain and tenderness when touched. Pain worsens with movement and isn't relieved by resting, applying heat, or taking analgesics. Fever, the usual sign of an infection, is often absent.

Bone infections resulting from infections in adjacent soft tissues or direct invasion cause pain and swelling in the area over the bone; abscesses may form in the surrounding tissue. These infections may not cause fever, and blood test results may be normal. A person who has an infected artificial joint or limb usually has persistent pain in that area.

If a bone infection isn't treated successfully, chronic osteomyelitis may develop. Sometimes, this type of infection is undetectable for a long time, producing no symptoms for months or years. More commonly, chronic osteomyelitis causes bone pain, recurring infections in the soft tissue over the bone, and constant or intermittent drainage of pus through the skin. Drainage occurs when pus from the infected bone breaks through the skin's surface and a passage (sinus tract) forms from the bone to the skin.

Diagnosis

Symptoms and findings during a physical examination may suggest osteomyelitis. The infected area almost always appears abnormal on bone scans (radionuclide scans using technetium), except in infants, but it may not appear on an x-ray until more than 3 weeks after the first symptoms occur. Computed tomography (CT) and magnetic resonance imaging (MRI) also can identify the infected area. However, these tests can't always distinguish infections from other bone disorders. To diagnose a bone infection and identify the bacteria causing it, doctors may take samples of blood, pus, joint fluid, or the bone itself. Usually, for an infection of the vertebrae, samples of bone tissue are removed with a needle or during surgery.

Treatment

For children or adults who have recently developed bone infections through the bloodstream, antibiotics are the most effective treatment. If the bacteria causing the infection can't be identified, then antibiotics effective against *Staphylococcus aureus,* the bacteria most commonly responsible, and in some cases against other bacteria are used. Depending on the severity of the infection, antibiotics may be given intravenously at first, but they may be given orally later during a 4- to 6-week course of treatment. Some people need months of treatment. If the infection is detected at an early stage, surgery usually isn't necessary. Occasionally, however, abscesses are drained surgically.

For adults who have infections of the vertebrae, the usual treatment is appropriate antibiotics for 6 to 8 weeks, sometimes with bed rest. Surgery may be needed to drain abscesses or to stabilize affected vertebrae.

When a bone infection results from an adjacent soft tissue infection, treatment is more complex. Usually, all the dead tissue and bone are removed surgically, and the empty space is packed with healthy bone, muscle, or skin. Then the infection is treated with antibiotics.

Usually, an infected artificial joint is removed and replaced. Antibiotics may be given several weeks before surgery, so that the infected artificial joint can be removed and a new one implanted at the same time. Rarely, treatment is not successful and the infection continues, requiring surgery to fuse the joint or amputate the limb.

Infections that spread to the bone from foot ulcers caused by poor circulation or diabetes often involve a variety of bacteria and are difficult to cure with antibiotics alone. Cure may require removing the infected bone.

Infectious Arthritis

Infectious arthritis is an infection in the fluid (synovial fluid) and tissues of a joint.

Infecting organisms, mainly bacteria, usually reach the joint through the bloodstream, but a joint can be infected directly if it's contaminated by surgery, an injection, or an injury. Different bacteria can infect a joint, but the bacteria most likely to cause infection depend on a person's age. Staphylococci, *Hemophilus influenzae,* and bacteria known as gram-negative bacilli most often infect babies and young children, whereas gonococci (bacteria that cause gonorrhea), staphylococci, and streptococci most often infect older children and adults. Viruses—such as the human immunodeficiency virus (HIV), parvoviruses, and those that cause rubella, mumps, and hepatitis B—can infect joints in people of any age. Chronic joint infections are most often caused by tuberculosis or fungal infections.

Symptoms

Infants usually have fever and pain and tend to be fussy. Generally, infants don't move the infected joint because moving or touching it is painful. In older children and adults who have bacterial or viral joint infections, symptoms usually begin very suddenly. The joint usually becomes red and warm, and moving or touching it is very painful. Fluid collects in the infected joint, causing it to swell and stiffen. Symptoms also include fever and chills.

The joints most commonly infected are the knee, shoulder, wrist, hip, finger, and elbow. Fungi or mycobacteria (bacteria that cause tuberculosis and similar infections) usually cause less dramatic symptoms. Most bacterial, fungal, and mycobacterial infections affect only one joint or, occasionally, several joints. For example, the bacteria that cause Lyme disease most often infect knee joints. Gonococcal bacteria and viruses can infect many joints at the same time.

Diagnosis

An infected joint can be destroyed within days unless antibiotic treatment is started promptly. For this reason, several diagnostic tests are performed immediately if an infection is suspected. Usually, a sample of joint fluid is removed. It's examined for white blood cells and tested for bacteria and other organisms. The laboratory can almost always grow and identify the infecting bacteria from the joint fluid, unless the person has recently taken antibiotics. However, the bacteria that cause gonorrhea, Lyme disease, and syphilis are difficult to recover from joint fluid.

A doctor generally orders blood tests because bacteria from joint infections often appear in the bloodstream. Phlegm, spinal fluid, and urine may also be tested for bacteria to help determine the source of infection.

Treatment

Antibiotic treatment is started as soon as an infection is suspected, even before the laboratory has identified the infecting organism. Antibiotics that kill the most likely bacteria are given first, then other antibiotics are given later, if necessary. Antibiotics are often given intravenously at first, to ensure that enough of the drug reaches the infected joint. Rarely, antibiotics are injected directly into the joint. If the antibiotics are appropriate, improvement usually occurs within 48 hours.

To prevent accumulation of pus, which may damage a joint, a doctor removes it with a needle. Sometimes a tube is inserted to drain the pus, especially if the joint is difficult to reach with a needle—a hip joint, for example. If drainage with a needle or tube is unsuccessful, arthroscopy (a procedure using a small scope to view the interior of the joint directly) or surgery may be needed to drain the joint. Splinting the joint can help ease pain at first, but physical therapy also may be needed to prevent stiffness and permanent loss of function.

Infections caused by fungi are treated with antifungal drugs, and a tuberculosis infection is treated with a combination of antibiotics. However, viral infections usually get better on their own. They require treatment only for pain and fever.

When an artificial joint becomes infected, antibiotics alone are usually inadequate. After several days of antibiotic treatment, surgery may be needed to replace the joint.

CHAPTER 54

Charcot's Joints

Charcot's joints (neuropathic joint disease) results from nerve damage that impairs a person's ability to perceive pain coming from a joint; consequently, repeated minor injuries and fractures go unnoticed until the accumulated damage permanently destroys the joint.

A variety of injuries, diseases, and conditions, such as diabetes mellitus, spinal diseases, and syphilis, can damage the nerves supplying sensation to the joints. As a result, a person can't feel pain in the affected joint.

Symptoms and Diagnosis

Many years may pass before enough damage occurs to cause joint dysfunction and symptoms. After symptoms develop, however, the disease can progress so rapidly that the joint is destroyed within a few months.

In its early stages, Charcot's joints is often confused with osteoarthritis. Stiffness and fluid in the joint are common. Usually, the joint isn't painful or is less painful than would be expected considering the amount of joint damage. However, if the disease progresses rapidly, the joint can become extremely painful. In these cases, the joint is usually swollen from excess fluid and new bony growths. It's often deformed because repeated fractures, with stretching of ligaments, allow it to slip out of place. Bone fragments may float around in the joint, causing a coarse, grating sound when the joint is moved.

Although the knee is most often affected, this disease can develop in almost any joint. The foot is most commonly affected in people who have diabetes. The joints affected—frequently only one and usually not more than two or three—depend on the location of the nerve damage.

The diagnosis is suspected when a person who has a neurologic disease develops relatively painless joint damage. Joint symptoms usually develop several years after the nerve damage. X-rays show the joint damage, which often includes calcium deposits and abnormal bone growth.

Prevention and Treatment

Sometimes, Charcot's joints can be prevented. Treatment of the underlying neurologic disease can slow or even reverse joint destruction. Diagnosing and immobilizing painless fractures and splinting unstable joints can help stop or minimize joint damage. Hips and knees may be surgically replaced if the neurologic disease isn't progressing, but artificial joints often loosen prematurely.

CHAPTER 55

Disorders of Muscles, Bursas, and Tendons

The muscles, bursas, tendons, and bones must be healthy and functioning properly for the body to move normally.▲ Muscles, which contract to produce movement, are connected to the bones by tendons. Bursas are fluid-filled cushions that reduce friction in areas where skin, muscles, tendons, and ligaments rub over bones. Injury, overexertion, infections, and occasionally other diseases can temporarily or permanently damage muscles, bursas, tendons, and bones. This damage can cause pain, limit control over movement, and reduce the normal range of motion.

Spasmodic Torticollis

Spasmodic torticollis is painful intermittent or continuous spasm of the neck muscles, forcing the head to rotate and tilt forward, backward, or sideways.

Torticollis occurs in 1 out of 10,000 people and is about $1^{1}/_{2}$ times more common in women than in men. The disorder can occur at any age but develops most frequently between ages 30 and 60. Usually, its cause is unknown. Occasionally, conditions such as hyperthyroidism, nervous system infections, tardive dyskinesia (abnormal facial movements resulting from taking antipsychotic drugs), and neck tumors cause torticollis.

Rarely, newborns have torticollis (congenital torticollis) as a result of neck muscle damage during a difficult delivery.■ Imbalanced eye muscles and bone or muscle deformities of the upper spine can cause torticollis in children.

Symptoms

Sharp, painful neck muscle spasms may start suddenly and may occur intermittently or continuously. Usually, only one side of the neck is affected. The direction in which the head tilts and rotates depends on which neck muscle is af-

---

▲ see page 214

■ see page 1233

fected. One third of the people who have this disorder also have spasms in other areas, usually in the eyelids, face, jaw, or hand. The spasms occur without warning and rarely during sleep.

Torticollis varies from mild to severe and unrelenting. About 10 to 20 percent of the people who have it—usually young people with mild cases—recover without treatment within 5 years. In most, however, the disorder gradually worsens for 1 to 5 years, then stabilizes. Torticollis may persist for life, producing continued pain, restricted movement of the neck, and postural deformities.

Diagnosis and Treatment

During a physical examination of an infant, a doctor can detect neck muscle damage that may cause torticollis. To diagnose the disorder in children and adults, the doctor asks detailed questions about past injuries and other neck problems. Various imaging tests, including x-rays, computed tomography (CT) scans, and magnetic resonance imaging (MRI), are sometimes used to look for specific causes of neck muscle spasms, although such causes are rarely found.

When a cause, such as abnormal bone growth, is identified, the torticollis can usually be treated successfully. However, treatment is less likely to control the spasms when the cause is a nervous system disorder or is unknown.

Sometimes the spasm can be temporarily relieved by physical therapy and massage. In one type of massage, slight pressure is applied to the jaw on the same side as the head rotation.

Drugs help reduce muscle spasms and involuntary movements in nearly a third of the people and usually help control the pain caused by the spasms. Anticholinergic drugs, which block specific nerve impulses, and benzodiazepines, which are mild sedatives, are commonly used. Less frequently, muscle relaxants and antidepressants are prescribed. Several injections of a small dose of the substance that causes botulism reduce pain and spasms, allowing the head to be held in a more natural (less tilted) position; this improvement may last for a few months. Surgically removing the nerves to the dysfunctional neck muscles is sometimes successful and may be tried if other treatments do not provide relief. If emotional problems contribute to the spasms, psychiatric treatment may help.

For congenital torticollis, intensive physical therapy to stretch the damaged muscle is begun within the first few months of life. If the physical therapy is unsuccessful or started too late, the muscle may have to be repaired surgically.

Fibromyalgia Syndromes

The fibromyalgia syndromes (myofascial pain syndromes, fibromyositis) are a group of disorders characterized by achy pain and stiffness in soft tissues, including muscles, tendons (which attach muscles to bones), and ligaments (which attach bones to each other).

The pain and stiffness (fibromyalgia) may occur throughout the body or may be restricted to certain locations, as in the myofascial pain syndromes. Fibromyalgia throughout the body is more common in women than in men. Men are more likely to develop myofascial pain or fibromyalgia in a particular area, such as a shoulder, from an occupational or recreational muscle strain. Fibromyalgia isn't dangerous or life threatening, but persistent symptoms can be very disruptive.

Causes

Although its cause is unknown, fibromyalgia may be triggered by physical or mental stress, inadequate sleep, an injury, exposure to dampness or cold, certain infections, and occasionally rheumatoid arthritis or a related disorder.

A common variation, the **primary fibromyalgia syndrome,** usually occurs in previously healthy young women who may be depressed, anxious, or stressed, often with interrupted and nonrestorative sleep. (Nonrestorative sleep does not refresh, leaving a person as tired as or more tired than before sleeping.) This syndrome may occur at any age, including adolescence; it usually affects girls. In older adults, it often occurs in conjunction with but unrelated to osteoarthritis of the spine.

Symptoms

Stiffness and pain usually develop gradually. In the primary fibromyalgia syndrome, the symptoms are usually aches; in fibromyalgia confined to a specific area, the pain may be more sudden and sharp. In both, the pain usually worsens with fatigue, straining, or overuse. Specific areas may be tender when pressure is applied. Muscle tightness and spasms may occur. Although any fibrous tissue or muscle may be affected, those of the neck, shoulders, chest and rib cage, lower back, and thighs are especially likely to be painful. In the primary fibromyalgia syndrome, pain may occur throughout the body and is accompanied by more general symptoms, such as nonrestorative sleep, anxiety, depression, fatigue, and irritable bowel syndrome.

Diagnosis and Treatment

The diagnosis of fibromyalgia syndromes is based on the pattern and location of the pain. Doctors determine whether pressure produces pain in one spot (tender points) or whether the pain seems to travel (refer) to other areas (trigger points).

Nondrug treatments are usually the most helpful. Reducing stress can alleviate some mild cases. Stretching and conditioning exercises, improvements in sleep, the application of heat, and gentle massage as well as keeping warm are usually beneficial.

Aspirin or other nonsteroidal anti-inflammatory drugs generally aren't very helpful. Occasionally, local anesthetics, alone or with corticosteroids, are injected directly into a particularly tender area. Doctors may prescribe low doses of antidepressants at bedtime to help promote deeper sleep and relieve symptoms.

Bursitis

Bursitis is the painful inflammation of a bursa (a flat sac containing synovial fluid that facilitates the normal movement of some joints and muscles and reduces friction).

Bursas are located at sites of friction, especially where tendons or muscles pass over bone. A bursa normally contains very little fluid. If injured, however, it becomes inflamed and may fill with fluid.

Bursitis can be caused by chronic overuse, injury, gout, pseudogout, rheumatoid arthritis, or infections; often, the cause is unknown. Although the shoulder is most susceptible to bursitis, bursas in the elbows, hips, pelvis, knees, toes, and heels commonly become inflamed.

Symptoms

Bursitis causes pain and tends to limit movement, but the specific symptoms depend on the location of the inflamed bursa. For example, when a bursa in the shoulder becomes inflamed, raising the arm out from the side of the body, as when putting on a jacket, is painful and difficult.

Trigger Finger

Trigger finger is a condition in which a finger becomes locked in a bent position. It occurs when one of the tendons that flex the finger becomes inflamed and swollen. Normally, the tendon moves smoothly in and out of its surrounding sheath as the finger straightens and bends. As the finger bends, the inflamed tendon moves out of the sheath, but when the tendon is too swollen or nodular, it can't easily move back in as the finger straightens. To straighten the finger, a person must force the swollen area into the sheath—which produces a popping sensation similar to that felt when pulling a trigger.

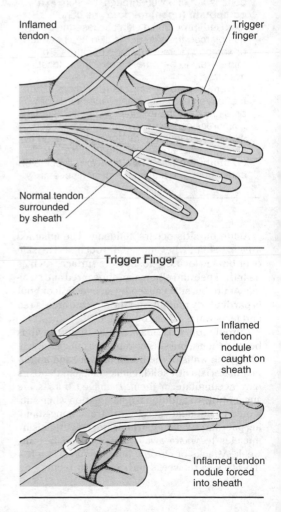

Inflamed tendon

Trigger finger

Normal tendon surrounded by sheath

Trigger Finger

Inflamed tendon nodule caught on sheath

Inflamed tendon nodule forced into sheath

Fractures

A fracture is a break in a bone, usually accompanied by injury to the surrounding tissues. Most fractures result from an injury, such as that caused by an automobile accident, sports, or a fall. A fracture occurs when the force against a bone is greater than the strength of the bone. The direction, speed, and power of the force affect the type and severity of the fracture, as do the age, resilience, and type of bone. Bones weakened by osteoporosis or tumors can be fractured with very light force.

In a **simple (closed) fracture,** the broken bone is not exposed through the skin. In a **compound (open) fracture,** the bone is exposed through the skin because the bone has pierced the skin or the skin has been torn or scraped (abraded). Open fractures are more likely to become infected than closed fractures.

Compression fractures result from forces that drive one bone against another or that press against the length of the bone. Compression fractures often occur in elderly women whose vertebral bones, weakened by osteoporosis, compress and then fracture. In **comminuted fractures,** a severe, direct force causes several breaks, producing several bone fragments. These fractures may heal very slowly if the blood supply to part of the bone is interrupted. **Avulsion fractures** are caused by strong muscle contractions pulling off sections of bone to which the muscle tendon is attached. These fractures most commonly occur in the shoulders and knees but can also occur in the legs and heels. **Pathologic fractures** occur where a tumor, usually a cancer, has grown into a bone and weakened it. The weakened bones may fracture even with a slight injury or no injury.

Symptoms and Diagnosis

Pain is usually the most obvious symptom. It may be severe and usually worsens with time and movement. Touching the area around the broken bone is also painful. Fractures usually cause swelling and bruising at the site. Depending on the type of fracture, a broken limb may appear deformed. The limb may not function properly, so that moving an arm, standing on a leg, or gripping with a hand is impossible. Blood may leak from a fractured bone, sometimes in large amounts, into the surrounding tissue or out of the wound made by the injury.

Acute bursitis occurs suddenly. The inflamed area is painful when moved or touched. The skin over bursas located close to the surface, such as near the knee and elbow, can appear red and swollen. Acute bursitis caused by an infection or gout is particularly painful, and the affected area is red and feels warm when touched.

Chronic bursitis may result from previous bouts of acute bursitis or repeated injuries. Eventually, the walls of the bursa thicken, and abnormal material with solid, chalky calcium deposits may accumulate in them. Damaged bursas are susceptible to additional inflammation when subjected to unusual exercise or strain. Long-standing pain and swelling can limit movement, causing muscles to waste away (atrophy) and become weak. Attacks of chronic bursitis may last a few days to several weeks and frequently recur.

Diagnosis and Treatment

A doctor suspects bursitis if the area around a bursa is sore when touched and specific joint movements are painful. If the bursa is noticeably swollen, the doctor may remove a sample of fluid from the bursa with a needle and syringe to test for causes of the inflammation, such as an infection or gout. X-rays are usually not helpful, unless they detect the typical calcium deposits.

Infected bursas must be drained, and appropriate antibiotics are given. Noninfectious acute bursitis is usually treated with rest, temporary immobilization of the affected joint, and a nonsteroidal anti-inflammatory drug such as indomethacin, ibuprofen, or naproxen. Occasionally, stronger analgesics are needed. Alternatively, a mixture of a local anesthetic and a corticosteroid can be injected directly into the bursa. The injection may have to be repeated.

X-rays can usually detect a fracture. However, other tests, such as a computed tomography (CT) scan or magnetic resonance imaging (MRI), are occasionally needed to view the damaged area more clearly. Once the bone has begun to heal, x-rays can be used to monitor healing.

Treatment

Fractures heal as new bone is formed to bridge the gap between the broken sections. So the goal of treatment is to position the broken ends near each other and to keep them aligned properly. Broken bones require at least 4 weeks to heal solidly, although in the elderly, healing often takes longer. Once completely healed, the bone is usually strong and fully functional.

For some fractures, splints that only restrict motion are used. Fractures of the collarbone (especially in children), shoulder blades, ribs, toes, and fingers generally heal well with such treatment.

Other fractures must be completely immobilized to heal. Fractures may be immobilized with a splint, brace, cast, traction, or internal (surgical) fixation.

- A splint or brace is a firm object that's affixed to the area surrounding the bone. For example, a firm plastic brace may be affixed to a broken finger.
- A cast is a firm material, either plastic or plaster, wrapped around the area that surrounds the broken bone. A layer of softer material is placed against the skin to protect it from injury.
- Traction, which uses a pulley and weights, holds a limb in alignment. Not commonly used anymore, it was once the main treatment for broken hips.
- Internal fixation requires surgery to attach a metal plate or rod to the pieces of broken bone. Internal fixation is often the best treatment for hip fractures and complicated fractures.

Immobilizing an arm or leg causes the muscles to become weak and tight. Therefore, most people who have broken a bone in an arm or leg need physical therapy. The therapy begins while the bone is immobilized and continues after the splint, cast, or traction has been removed. For certain types of fractures, especially hip fractures, full recovery may require 6 to 8 weeks of therapy or occasionally even longer.

People who have severe bursitis may be given a corticosteroid such as prednisone by mouth for a few days. As the pain subsides, performing specific exercises to increase the joint's range of motion can help.

Chronic bursitis is treated in a similar way, although rest and immobilization are less likely to help. Rarely, large calcium deposits in the shoulder may be irrigated through a wide-gauge needle or may be removed by surgery. Disabling bursitis in the shoulder may be relieved by several injections of corticosteroids along with intensive physical therapy to restore the joint's function. Exercises can help strengthen weakened muscles and reestablish the joint's full range of motion. Bursitis frequently recurs if the underlying cause, such as gout, rheumatoid arthritis, or chronic overuse, isn't corrected.

Tendinitis and Tenosynovitis

Tendinitis is the inflammation of a tendon; tenosynovitis is tendinitis accompanied by an inflammation of the protective sheath around the tendon.

Tendons are fibrous cords of tough tissue that connect muscles to bones. Tendon sheaths surround some tendons.

Most tendinitis occurs in middle or old age, as the tendons become more susceptible to injury. However, it also occurs in younger people who exercise vigorously and in people who perform repetitive tasks.

Certain tendons, especially those of the hand, are particularly susceptible to inflammation. An inflammation of the tendon that extends the thumb away from the hand is called de Quervain's disease. Inflammation can cause the tendons that close the other fingers to get caught, producing a popping feeling (trigger finger). Tendinitis above the biceps muscle in the upper arm causes pain when the elbow is bent or the forearm is rotated. The Achilles tendon in the heel▲ and a tendon that runs over the top of the foot also commonly become inflamed.

Tendon sheaths can also be affected by joint diseases, such as rheumatoid arthritis, systemic scleroderma, gout, and Reiter's syndrome. In young adults who contract gonorrhea, especially women, gonococcal bacteria can cause tenosynovitis, usually affecting the tendons of the shoulders, wrists, fingers, hips, ankles, and feet.

Symptoms

The inflamed tendons are usually painful when moved or touched. Moving the joints near the tendon, even a little, may cause severe pain. The tendon sheaths may be visibly swollen from the accumulation of fluid and inflammation, or they may remain dry and rub against the tendons, causing a grating sensation that may be felt or a sound that may be heard with a stethoscope when the joint is moved.

Treatment

Several forms of treatment may alleviate the symptoms of tendinitis. Rest, immobilization with a splint or cast, and application of heat or cold—whichever works—are often helpful. Nonsteroidal anti-inflammatory drugs such as aspirin or ibuprofen can reduce the pain and inflammation when used for 7 to 10 days.

Sometimes corticosteroids and local anesthetics are injected into the tendon sheath. This treatment is particularly helpful for treating a trigger finger. Rarely, the injection causes a flare-up that lasts for less than 24 hours; the flare-up can be treated with cold compresses and analgesics.

Treatments may have to be repeated every 2 or 3 weeks for a month or two before the inflammation subsides completely. Chronic, persistent tendinitis, as may occur in rheumatoid arthritis, may have to be treated surgically to remove inflamed areas, and physical therapy may be needed after surgery. Surgery is commonly needed to treat a chronic trigger finger or to remove calcium deposits from areas of long-standing tendinitis, such as the area around the shoulder joint.■

CHAPTER 56

Foot Problems

Some foot problems start in the foot itself, for instance, from a foot injury; others result from diseases that affect the whole body. Any bone, joint, muscle, tendon, or ligament of the foot can be affected.

Ankle Sprain

An ankle sprain is an injury to the ligaments (the tough elastic tissue that connects bones to one another) in the ankle.

Any of the ligaments in the ankle can be injured. Sprains usually occur when the ankle rolls out-

ward, causing the sole of the foot to face the other foot (invert). Loose ligaments in the ankle, weak or nerve-damaged leg muscles, certain types of shoes such as spiked heels, and certain walking patterns tend to allow the foot to roll outward, increasing the risk of a sprain.

Symptoms

The severity of the sprain depends on the degree of stretching or tearing of the ligaments. In a mild (grade 1) sprain, the ligaments may stretch, but they don't actually tear. The ankle usually doesn't hurt or swell very much, but a mild sprain increases the risk of a repeat injury. In a moderate (grade 2) sprain, a ligament tears partially. Obvious swelling and bruising are common, and walking is usually painful and difficult. In a severe (grade 3) sprain, a ligament tears completely, causing swelling and sometimes bleeding under

▲ see page 258

■ see page 271

the skin. As a result, the ankle is unstable and unable to bear weight.

Diagnosis and Treatment

Physical examination of the ankle can give clues to the extent of ligament damage. X-rays are often taken to determine whether a bone is broken, but they can't determine whether the ankle is sprained. Other tests are rarely needed.

Treatment depends on how severe the sprain is. Usually, mild sprains are treated by wrapping the ankle and foot with an elastic bandage or tape, applying ice packs to the area, elevating the ankle, and as the sprain heals, gradually increasing the amount of walking and exercise. For moderate sprains, a walking cast is usually applied and left in place for 3 weeks. It immobilizes the lower leg but allows a person to walk on the injured ankle. For severe sprains, surgery may be needed. However, whether to perform surgery is controversial; some surgeons believe that surgically reconstructing badly damaged and torn ligaments is no better than treatment without surgery. Physical therapy to restore movement, strengthen muscles, and improve balance and response time is very important before a person returns to strenuous activity.

For people who sprain their ankles easily, subsequent injuries may be prevented by wearing ankle braces and placing devices in the shoe to stabilize the foot and ankle.

Complications

Sometimes a moderate or severe sprain causes problems even after the ligament has healed. A small nodule can develop in one of the ankle's ligaments and cause constant friction in the joint, leading to chronic inflammation and eventually permanent damage. Injecting the ankle with a mixture of corticosteroids to reduce inflammation and a local anesthetic to numb the pain often produces improvement. Surgery is rarely needed.

A nerve that travels over one of the ankle's ligaments may also be damaged in a sprain. The resulting pain and tingling (neuralgia) are often relieved, sometimes permanently, by an injection of a local anesthetic.

People who have a sprained ankle may walk in a way that overuses the tendons (the strong, flexible cords of tissue connecting muscles to bone or muscle to muscle) on the outside of the ankle, resulting in inflammation. This condition, called peroneal tenosynovitis, can cause chronic swell-

Severe Ankle Sprain

An ankle sprain may occur when the ankle rolls outward (inverts), tearing the ligament along the outside of the ankle.

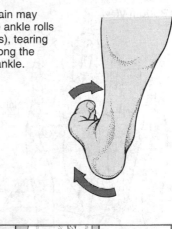

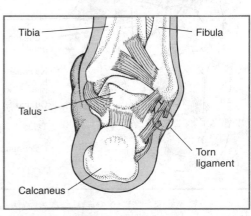

ing and tenderness of the outer ankle. Treatment consists of wearing ankle supports that limit movement of the ankle joint. Cortisone injections into the sheath of the tendon may also be effective but must not be overused.

Occasionally, the shock of a severe sprain causes blood vessels in the ankle to go into spasm, thereby reducing blood flow. As a result, areas of bone and other tissues may be damaged because they're deprived of blood and may begin to waste away. This condition, called reflex sympathetic dystrophy or Sudeck's atrophy, can cause the foot to swell painfully. Pain, often severe, can move from one location to another in the ankle and foot. Despite the pain, a person

Bones of the Foot

Bottom View

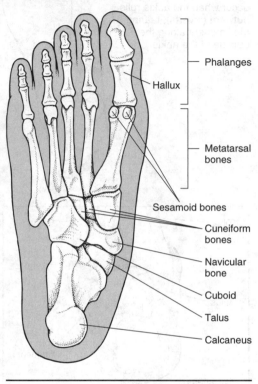

Phalanges

Hallux

Metatarsal bones

Sesamoid bones

Cuneiform bones

Navicular bone

Cuboid

Talus

Calcaneus

must continue to walk. Physical therapy and analgesics taken by mouth may help. A local anesthetic injected into or around the nerve (a nerve block) supplying the ankle, corticosteroids, and psychologic counseling can help people cope with the chronic, intense pain.

Sinus tarsi syndrome is persistent pain in the area between the heel bone (calcaneus) and the ankle bone (talus) after a sprain. It may be related to partial tearing of ligaments deep in the foot.

▲ see page 263

Injections of corticosteroids and local anesthetics often help.

Foot Fractures

Almost any bone in the foot can be broken (fractured). Many of these fractures don't require surgery; others must be surgically repaired to prevent permanent disability. The area over the site of a fractured bone is usually swollen and painful. Swelling and pain may extend beyond the fracture site if the soft tissues in the area are bruised.

Fractures in and around the ankle joint occur most commonly when the ankle rolls in so that the sole of the foot turns out (inversion ankle sprain) or when the ankle rolls out (eversion ankle sprain). Pain, swelling, and bleeding tend to occur. These fractures can be serious if not treated promptly. As a rule, all ankle fractures should be placed in a cast. Surgery may be needed for severe ankle fractures in which the bones are widely separated or misaligned.

Fractures of the metatarsal bones (bones of the midfoot) are common.▲ These fractures most commonly result from excessive walking or indirect stress from overuse, although they can result from a sudden, severe impact. In most instances, immobilization in a stiff-soled shoe rather than a cast is all that's needed to allow the bone to heal. Rarely, a below-the-knee cast is needed. If the bones are widely separated, surgery to align the fractured segments may be needed. A fracture of the metatarsal bone of the big or little toe tends to be more complicated, requiring a cast or surgery.

The sesamoid bones (two small round bones located under the end of the metatarsal bone of the big toe) may be fractured. Running, long walks, and sports involving coming down too hard on the ball of the foot, such as basketball and tennis, may cause these bones to fracture. Using padding or specially constructed orthoses (insoles) for the shoe helps relieve the pain. If pain continues, the sesamoid bone may have to be removed surgically.

Injuries to the toes, particularly the little toe, are common, especially when walking barefoot. Simple fractures of the four smaller toes heal without a cast. Splinting the toes with tape or Velcro to the adjacent toes for 4 to 6 weeks may help. Wearing stiff-soled or slightly wider shoes may help relieve the pain. If walking in normal shoes is too painful, specially fabricated boots can be fitted or prescribed by a doctor.

Generally, a fracture of the big toe (hallux) tends to be more severe, causing more intense pain, swelling, and bleeding under the skin. A big toe may be broken by stubbing it or dropping a heavy object on it. Fractures that affect the joint of the big toe may require surgery.

Heel Spurs

Heel spurs are growths of extra bone at the heel that may be caused by excessive pulling on the heel bone by tendons or fascia (the connective tissue attached to the bone).

Pain on the bottom of the heel can be caused by a heel spur. Flatfoot (an abnormal flatness of the sole and arch of the foot) and disorders in which the heel cord is always contracted may put excess tension on the fascia, increasing the risk of heel spurs.

Heel spurs are usually painful as they develop, especially when a person is walking. Occasionally, a fluid pocket (bursa) develops beneath the spur and becomes inflamed. This condition, called inferior calcaneal bursitis, usually adds a throbbing quality to the pain caused by the spur and can develop when no spur is present. Sometimes the foot adapts to the spur so that the pain actually diminishes as the spur enlarges. On the other hand, a painless spur may become painful after a slight injury to the area, as may occur during sports.

Usually, heel spurs can be diagnosed during a physical examination. Pressing the center of the heel causes pain if spurs are present. X-rays may be taken to confirm the diagnosis, but they may not detect newly formed spurs.

Treatment is aimed at relieving pain. A mixture of corticosteroids and a local anesthetic can be injected into the painful area of the heel. Wrapping the arch with padding and using orthotics (inserts for shoes) that help stabilize the heel can minimize stretching of the fascia and reduce pain. Most painful heel spurs resolve without surgery. Surgery to remove the spur should be performed only when constant pain interferes with walking. However, the results are not predictable. Occasionally, pain persists after surgery.

Heel Spur

A heel spur is a growth of extra bone on the heel bone (calcaneus). It may form when the plantar fascia, the connective tissue extending from the heel bone to the base of the toes, pulls excessively on the heel. Usually, the spur is painful as it develops, but it may become less painful as the foot adjusts to it. Most spurs can be treated without surgery.

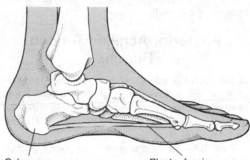

Calcaneus   Plantar fascia

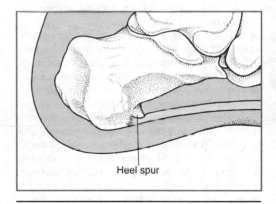

Heel spur

Sever's Disease

Sever's disease is heel pain in children caused by damage to the cartilage.

The heel bone (calcaneus) develops in two sections. Until the bone hardens completely between the ages of 8 and 16 years, the two parts are connected by cartilage, which is softer than bone. Occasionally, vigorous activity or excessive strain can break the cartilage, causing pain, usually along the edges of the heel.

Sever's disease is diagnosed when a child who has participated in athletics has pain along the sides of the heel. Sometimes the heel is mildly swollen and slightly warm to the touch. Because x-rays can't detect cartilage injury, they aren't helpful in the diagnosis, except to exclude a bone fracture as the cause of pain.

The broken cartilage eventually heals, usually after several months. Heel pads placed in the shoes can help by reducing the pressure on the heel bone. Immobilizing the foot in a cast sometimes helps as well.

Posterior Achilles Tendon Bursitis

Posterior Achilles tendon bursitis (Haglund's deformity) is an inflammation of the fluid-filled sac (bursa) located between the skin of the heel and the Achilles tendon (the tendon that attaches the calf muscles to the heel bone).

This disorder occurs mainly in young women but can develop in men. Walking in a way that repeatedly presses the soft tissue behind the heel against the hard back support of a shoe can worsen it.

At first, a mildly red, hardened, tender spot develops high on the back of the heel. When the inflamed bursa enlarges,▲ it appears as a red lump under the skin of the heel and causes pain at and above the heel. If the condition becomes chronic, the swelling may harden.

Treatment is aimed at reducing the inflammation and adjusting the foot's position in the shoe to relieve pressure on the heel. Foam rubber or felt heel pads can be placed in the shoe to eliminate pressure by elevating the heel. Stretching the back part of the shoe or placing padding around the inflamed bursa may help. Sometimes a special shoe is designed to help control abnormal heel motion. If these measures don't help, nonsteroidal anti-inflammatory drugs such as ibuprofen can temporarily relieve the pain and inflammation, as can injections of a mixture of corticosteroids and local anesthetics into the inflamed area. When these treatments aren't effective, part of the heel bone may be surgically removed.

▲ see page 251

Anterior Achilles Tendon Bursitis

Anterior Achilles tendon bursitis (Albert's disease) is an inflammation of the fluid-filled sac (bursa) in front of the attachment of the Achilles tendon to the heel bone (calcaneus).

Any condition that puts extra strain on the Achilles tendon, which attaches the calf muscles to the heel, can cause this disorder. Injuries to the heel, diseases such as rheumatoid arthritis, and even the rigid back support of shoes can cause it.

When the bursa becomes inflamed after an injury, symptoms usually develop suddenly; when the inflammation is caused by a disease, symptoms may develop gradually. Symptoms usually include swelling and warmth at the back of the heel.

Applying warm or cool compresses to the area may help reduce pain and inflammation. Injections of a corticosteroid mixed with a local anesthetic into the inflamed bursa also relieve the symptoms.

Posterior Tibial Neuralgia

Posterior tibial neuralgia is pain in the ankle, foot, and toes caused by compression of or damage to the nerve supplying the heel and sole (posterior tibial nerve).

This nerve runs along the back of the calf, through a bony canal near the heel, and into the sole of the foot. When tissues around this nerve become inflamed, they can compress it, causing pain.

Pain, the most common symptom of this condition, usually has a burning or tingling quality. It may occur when a person stands, walks, or wears particular types of shoes. Usually located around the ankle and extending to the toes, the pain worsens during walking and is relieved by rest. Occasionally, pain also occurs during rest.

To diagnose this condition, a doctor manipulates the foot during the physical examination. For example, tapping the injured or compressed area often causes tingling, which may extend to the heel, arch, or toes. Extensive tests may be needed to determine the cause of the injury, especially if foot surgery is being considered.

Injections of a mixture of corticosteroids and local anesthetics into the area may relieve pain. Other treatments include wrapping the foot and placing specially constructed devices in the shoe to reduce pressure on the nerve. When other treatments don't relieve the pain, surgery to relieve pressure on the nerve may be necessary.

Pain in the Ball of the Foot

Pain in the ball of the foot is usually caused by damage to the nerves between the toes or to the joints between the toes and foot.

NERVE DAMAGE

The nerves that supply the bottom of the foot and toes travel between the bones of the toes. Pain in the ball of the foot may be caused by noncancerous growths of nerve tissue (neuromas), usually between the base of the third and fourth toes (Morton's neuroma), although they may occur between any two toes. Neuromas usually develop in only one foot and are more common in women than in men.

In the early stages, the neuroma may cause only a mild ache around the fourth toe, occasionally accompanied by a burning or tingling sensation. These symptoms are generally more pronounced when a person wears certain types of shoes. As the condition progresses, a constant burning sensation may radiate to the tips of the toes, regardless of which shoes are worn. A person may also feel as if a marble or pebble were inside the ball of the foot. Doctors diagnose the condition by considering the history of the problem and examining the foot. X-rays, magnetic resonance imaging (MRI), and ultrasound scanning can't accurately identify this disorder.

Injecting the foot with corticosteroids mixed with a local anesthetic and wearing shoe inserts can usually relieve the symptoms. Repeating the injections two or three times at intervals of 1 or 2 weeks may be necessary. If these treatments don't help, surgical removal of the neuroma often relieves the discomfort completely but may cause permanent numbness in the area.

TOE JOINT PAIN

Pain involving the joints of the four smaller toes is a very common problem, usually caused by misalignment of the joints. This misalignment may result from high or low arched feet that cause the toes to stay in a bent position (hammer toes). Constant friction against the bent toes causes the skin over the joint to thicken, resulting in a corn. Treatment is directed at relieving the pressure caused by misalignment: Making the shoes

Bursitis in the Heel

Normally, only one bursa is found in the heel, between the Achilles tendon and the heel bone (calcaneus). This bursa may become inflamed, swollen, and painful, resulting in anterior Achilles tendon bursitis.

As a result of abnormal pressure and foot dysfunction, a protective (adventitious) bursa may form between the Achilles tendon and the skin. This bursa may also become inflamed, swollen, and painful, resulting in posterior Achilles tendon bursitis.

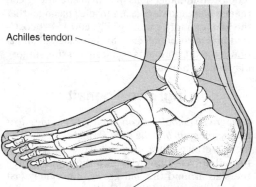

Achilles tendon

Calcaneus   Normal bursa

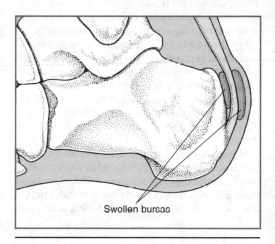

Swollen bursas

deeper, placing pads in the shoes, surgically straightening the toes, and paring down the corn may help.

Chronic arthritis (osteoarthritis) of the big toe, which is extremely common, can result from various standing and walking positions, including the tendency to roll the foot inward during walking (pronation). Occasionally, an injury to the big toe may also cause painful arthritis. Joint pain in the big toe is usually aggravated by wearing shoes. Later, a person may become unable to bend the big toe during walking. The area is not warm to the touch.

Fitting the shoe with devices to correct improper foot motion and relieve pressure on the affected joints is the mainstay of treatment. Pain in the big toe that started recently may be relieved by toe traction and exercises that move and extend the joint. Injections of a local anesthetic can relieve pain and decrease muscle spasm so that the joint can move more easily, and a corticosteroid may also be injected to decrease inflammation. If these treatments aren't successful, surgery may relieve the pain.

Ingrown Toenail

An ingrown toenail is a condition in which the edges of the nail grow into the surrounding skin.

An ingrown nail can result when a deformed toenail grows improperly into the skin or when the skin around the nail grows abnormally fast and engulfs part of the nail. Wearing narrow, ill-fitting shoes and trimming the nail into a curve with short edges rather than trimming it straight across can cause or worsen ingrown toenails.

Ingrown nails may produce no symptoms at first but eventually may become painful, especially when pressure is applied to the ingrown area. The area is usually red and may be warm; if not treated, it's prone to infection. If infected, the area becomes painful, red, and swollen, and pus-filled blisters (paronychia) may develop and drain.

Mildly ingrown toenails can be trimmed away, the free edge gently lifted, and sterile cotton placed under the nail until the swelling goes away. If an ingrown nail requires medical attention, a doctor usually numbs the area with a local anes-

thetic, then cuts away and removes the ingrown section of nail. The inflammation can then subside, and the ingrown nail usually doesn't recur.

Onychomycosis

Onychomycosis is a fungal infection of the nails.

The fungus can be acquired by walking barefoot in public places or, most commonly, as part of an athlete's foot infection.▲ Mild infections may produce few or no symptoms; in more severe infections, the nails turn whitish, thicken, and detach from the nail bed. Usually, debris from the infected nail collects under its free edge. A doctor usually confirms the diagnosis by examining a sample of the nail debris under a microscope and culturing it to determine which fungus is causing the infection.

Fungal infections are difficult to cure, so treatment depends on how severe or bothersome the symptoms are. The nails should be kept trimmed very short to minimize discomfort. Antifungal drugs, taken by mouth, may improve the condition and occasionally completely cure it. The infection often recurs when the drugs are discontinued. Applying antifungal drugs directly to the infected nail as the only treatment is generally not effective, except when the fungal infection is only superficial.

Nail Discoloration

Many conditions can cause changes in the color and texture of the nails. For example, an injury, such as that caused by a heavy object dropped on the toe, can cause blood to collect under the nail, making it look black. If the entire nail is affected, it may detach from the nail bed and fall off. Black discoloration under a nail should always be evaluated by a doctor to determine whether it's a melanoma, a skin cancer. Injuries can cause whitish spots or streaks on the nail. Overexposure to strong soaps, chemicals, or some drugs can cause nails to turn shades of black, gray, yellow, or brown. Fungal infections can also discolor the nails.

Treatment involves correcting the condition causing the discoloration and waiting for healthy nails to grow in. After removal, nails take about 12 to 18 months to grow back.

▲ see page 979

Sports Injuries

More than 10 million sports injuries are treated each year in the United States. The principles of sports medicine can be applied to the treatment of many musculoskeletal injuries, which resemble sports injuries but have different causes. For example, tennis elbow can be caused by carrying a suitcase, turning a screw, or opening a stuck door, and runner's knee can be caused by excessive inward rolling of the foot (pronation) while walking.

Causes

Sports injuries are caused by faulty training methods, structural abnormalities that stress certain parts of the body more than others, and weakness of muscles, tendons, and ligaments. Many of these injuries are caused by chronic wear and tear, which results from repetitive motion stressing susceptible tissue.

Faulty Training Methods

The most common cause of muscle and joint injuries is faulty training methods: The exerciser doesn't allow for adequate recovery after a workout or doesn't stop exercising when pain develops.

Every time muscles are stressed by an intensive workout, some muscle fibers are injured and others use up their available energy, which has been stored as the carbohydrate glycogen. More than 2 days are required for fibers to heal and glycogen to be replaced. Because only uninjured and adequately nourished fibers function properly, closely spaced, intensive workouts eventually require comparable work from fewer healthy fibers, increasing the likelihood of injury. Consequently, allowing at least 2 days between intensive workouts or alternating workouts that stress different parts of the body can help prevent chronic injury.

Most training programs alternate a hard workout one day with rest or an easy workout the next.▲ For example, many weight lifters alternate a hard workout on one day with no workout the next. A runner may run 5-minute miles one day and 6- to 8-minute miles the next. If an athlete trains twice a day, each hard workout should be followed by at least three easy ones. Only swimmers can perform both a hard and an easy workout every day without injury. The buoyancy of the water probably helps protect their muscles and joints.

Pain, which precedes most wear-and-tear injuries, first occurs when a limited number of muscle or tendon fibers start to tear. Stopping exercise at the first sign of pain limits the injury to these fibers, resulting in a quicker recovery. Continuing to exercise with pain tears more fibers, extending the damage and delaying recovery.

Structural Abnormalities

Structural abnormalities can make a person susceptible to a sports injury by stressing parts of the body unevenly. For example, when the legs are unequal in length, greater force is placed on the hip and knee of the longer leg. Habitually running along the sides of banked roads has the same effect; repeatedly hitting the slightly higher surface increases the risk of pain or injury on that side. A person who has an exaggerated curve in the spine may have back pain when swinging a baseball bat. In general, the pain disappears when the activity is stopped but recurs each time the same exercise intensity is reached.

The biomechanical factor that causes most foot, leg, and hip injuries is excessive pronation—an inward rolling of the feet after they strike the ground. Some degree of pronation is normal and prevents injuries by helping distribute the foot's striking force throughout the foot. However, excessive pronation can cause foot, knee, and leg pain. In people with excessive pronation, the ankles are so flexible that the arches of the feet touch the ground during walking or running, giving the appearance of flatfeet. A runner with excessive pronation may have knee pain when running long distances.

The opposite problem—too little pronation—can occur in people who have rigid ankles. In these people, the foot appears to have a very high arch and doesn't absorb shock well, increasing the risk of developing small cracks in the bones (stress fractures) of the feet and legs.

▲ see page 272

Muscle, Tendon, and Ligament Weakness

Muscles, tendons, and ligaments tear when subjected to forces greater than their inherent strength. For example, they may be injured if they're too weak or tight for the exercise being attempted. Joints are more prone to injury when the muscles and ligaments that support them are weak, as they are after a sprain. Bones weakened by osteoporosis may fracture easily.

Strengthening exercises help prevent injuries. Regular exercise neither enlarges nor strengthens muscles significantly. The only way to strengthen muscles is to exercise against progressively greater resistance, as in performing a sport more intensely, lifting progressively heavier weights, or using special strength training machines. Rehabilitation exercises to strengthen healed muscles and tendons are usually done by lifting or pressing against resistance, in sets of 8 to 12 repetitions, no more frequently than every other day.

Diagnosis

To diagnose a sports or other musculoskeletal injury, a doctor asks when and how the injury happened and what recreational and occupational activities the person has recently or routinely been engaged in. The doctor also examines the injured area. The person may be referred to a specialist for further testing. Diagnostic tests may include x-rays, computed tomography (CT) scans, magnetic resonance imaging (MRI), arthroscopy (viewing the injured joint through a small scope inserted into the joint), electromyography,▲ and computer-aided testing of muscle and joint function.

Prevention

Warming up before beginning strenuous exercise helps prevent injuries. Exercising at a relaxed pace for 3 to 10 minutes warms the muscles enough to make them more pliable and resistant to injury. This active method of warming up prepares muscles for strenuous exercise more effectively than passive methods such as warm water, heating pads, ultrasound, or an infrared lamp. Passive methods don't increase blood circulation significantly.

Cooling down—gradually slowing down before stopping exercise—prevents dizziness by keeping blood flowing. When strenuous exercise is stopped abruptly, blood may collect (pool) in the leg veins, temporarily reducing the flow of blood to the head. The result may be dizziness and even fainting. Cooling down also helps remove waste products such as lactic acid from the muscles, but it doesn't seem to prevent next-day muscle soreness, which is caused by damaged muscle fibers.

Stretching exercises don't seem to prevent injuries, but they do lengthen muscles so they can contract more effectively and perform better. To avoid damaging muscles when stretching, a person should stretch after warming up or exercising, and each stretch should be comfortable enough to hold for a count of 10.

Shoe inserts (orthotics) can often correct foot problems such as pronation. The inserts, which may be flexible, semirigid, or rigid and may vary in length, should be fitted into appropriate running shoes. Good running shoes have a rigid heel counter (the back part of the shoe that surrounds the heel) to control movement of the back of the foot, a support across the instep (saddle) to prevent excessive pronation, and a padded opening (collar) to support the ankle. The shoe must have adequate space for the insert. Orthotics usually reduce the shoe's width by one letter size: For example, a D width shoe with an orthotic becomes a C width.

Treatment

Immediate treatment for almost all sports injuries consists of rest, ice, compression, and elevation (RICE). The injured part is rested immediately to minimize internal bleeding and swelling and to prevent the injury from becoming worse. Ice causes blood vessels to constrict, helping limit inflammation and reduce pain. Wrapping the injured part with tape or an elastic bandage (compression) and raising the injured part above the heart (elevation) help limit swelling. A commercial ice pack or a bag of crushed or chipped ice—which conforms to body contours better than ice cubes—can be placed on a towel over the injured part for 10 minutes. An elastic bandage can be wrapped loosely around the ice bag and the injured part. The injured part is kept elevated, but the ice is removed for 10 minutes, then reapplied for 10 minutes over a period of 1 to $1^1/_2$ hours. This process can be repeated several times during the first 24 hours.

▲ see page 287

Ice reduces pain and swelling in several ways. The injured part swells because fluid leaks from blood vessels. By causing the blood vessels to constrict, cold reduces their tendency to leak, thus restricting the amount of fluid and swelling in the injured part. Lowering the temperature of the skin over the injury can reduce pain and muscle spasms. It also limits tissue destruction by slowing cellular processes.

Applying ice for too long, however, can damage tissue. The skin reacts reflexively when it reaches a low temperature (around 59° F.) by widening blood vessels in the area. The skin turns red, feels hot and itchy, and may hurt. These effects usually occur 9 to 16 minutes after the ice is applied and subside about 4 to 8 minutes after the ice has been removed. Therefore, the ice should be removed when these effects occur or after 10 minutes, whichever comes first, but it can be reapplied 10 minutes after removal.

Injections of corticosteroids into an injured joint or the surrounding tissue relieve pain, reduce swelling, and can sometimes be a useful addition to rest. However, these injections can delay healing, increase the risk of tendon and cartilage damage, and enable a person to use an injured joint before it's fully healed, perhaps worsening the injury.

Physical therapists may incorporate heat, cold, electricity, sound waves, traction, or exercising in water into a treatment plan in addition to therapeutic exercises. Special shoe inserts or other orthotics may be recommended. How long physical therapy is needed depends on the severity and complexity of the injury.

The activity or sport that caused the injury should be avoided until the injury has healed. Substituting activities that don't stress the injured part is preferable to abstaining from all physical activity because complete inactivity causes muscles to lose mass, strength, and endurance. For example, a week of rest requires at least 2 weeks of exercise to return to the level of fitness before the injury. Substitute activities include bicycling, swimming, skiing, and rowing when the lower leg or foot is injured; jogging in place or on a trampoline, swimming, and rowing when the upper leg is injured; bicycling and swimming when the lower back is injured; and jogging, skating, and skiing when the shoulder or arm is injured.

Common Sports Injuries

Common sports injuries include stress fractures, shin splints, tendinitis, runner's knee, hamstring injuries, weight lifter's back, tennis elbow, head injuries,▲ and foot injuries.■ They can be caused by many different activities.

Stress Fractures of the Foot

Stress fractures are small cracks in bones that often develop from chronic, excessive impact.

In runners, the bones of the midfoot (metatarsals) are especially prone to these fractures. The bones most likely to fracture are the metatarsal bones of the middle three toes. The metatarsal bone of the big toe is relatively immune to injury because of its strength and larger size, and the metatarsal bone of the little toe is usually protected because the greatest force from pushing off (toeing off) is exerted on the big toe and the one next to it.

Risk factors for stress fractures in the foot include high arches, running shoes with inadequate shock absorption, and a sudden increase in the intensity or amount of exercise. Postmenopausal women may be particularly susceptible to stress fractures because of osteoporosis.

The primary symptom is pain in the front part of the foot, usually during a long or intense workout. At first, the pain disappears within seconds of stopping exercise. If workouts are continued, however, the pain returns earlier in the workout and lasts longer after stopping exercise. Ultimately, severe pain may make running impossible, and pain may persist even during rest. The area around the fracture may swell.

A doctor can often make the diagnosis from a history of the symptoms and an examination of the foot. The fracture site hurts when touched. Stress fractures are so fine that x-rays often can't detect them immediately, but they can detect the tissue (callus) that forms around the broken bone 2 or 3 weeks after the injury, as the bone heals. A bone scan can confirm the diagnosis earlier but is rarely needed.

▲ see page 357

■ see page 254

Stress Fracture in the Foot

Stress fractures, small cracks caused by repetitive impact, commonly occur in the bones of the midfoot—the metatarsals.

Top View

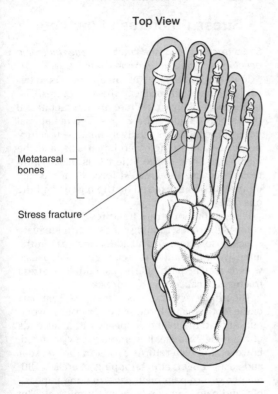

Metatarsal bones

Stress fracture

A person should not run until the stress fracture has healed, but other exercises can be substituted. After the fracture has healed, wearing athletic shoes with adequate shock-absorbing support and running on grass or other soft surfaces can help prevent a recurrence. A cast is rarely needed. When used, it's removed after a week or two to prevent the muscles from becoming weak. Healing generally takes 3 to 12 weeks but may take longer in the elderly or infirm.

Shin Splints

A shin splint is pain resulting from damage to the muscles along the shin.

The usual cause is long-standing, repeated stress to the lower leg. Two groups of muscles in the shin are susceptible to shin splints. The location of the pain depends on which group is affected.

Anterolateral shin splints affect the muscles in the front (anterior) and outside (lateral) parts of the shin. This type of injury results from a natural imbalance in the size of opposing muscles. The shin muscles pull the foot up, and the larger and stronger calf muscles pull the foot down each time the heel touches the ground during walking or running. The calf muscles exert so much force that they can injure the shin muscles.

The main symptom of anterolateral shin splints is pain along the front and outside of the shin. At first, the pain is felt only immediately after the heel strikes the ground during running. If running is continued, the pain occurs throughout each step, eventually becoming constant. Usually by the time the person sees a doctor, the shin hurts when touched.

To allow this type of shin splint to heal, the runner must stop running temporarily and do other kinds of exercise. Exercises to stretch the calf muscles are helpful. Once the shin muscles start to heal, exercises to strengthen them, such as the bucket-handle exercise, can be done in 3 sets of 10 every other day.

Posteromedial shin splints affect the muscles in the back (posterior) and inner (medial) parts of the shin, which are responsible for lifting the heel just before the toes push off. This type of shin splint often results from running on banked tracks or crowned roads and can be worsened by rolling the feet inward excessively or by wearing running shoes that don't adequately prevent such rolling.

The pain produced by this type of shin splint usually starts along the inside of the lower leg, about 1 to 8 inches above the ankle, and worsens when a runner rises up on the toes or rolls the ankle in. If the person continues to run, the pain moves forward, affecting the inner ankle, and may extend up the shin to within 2 to 4 inches of the knee. The severity of the pain increases as the shin splints progress. At first, only the muscle tendons are inflamed and painful, but if the person persists in running, the muscles themselves can be affected. Eventually, tension on the inflamed tendon can actually pull it from its attachment to bone, causing bleeding and further inflammation. Sometimes the part of the shinbone attached to the tendon is torn away.

The primary treatment is to stop running and do other types of exercise until running is no longer painful. Running shoes with a rigid heel counter (the back part of the shoe) and special arch supports can keep the foot from rolling in excessively. Avoiding running on banked surfaces can help prevent shin splints from recurring. Exercises to strengthen the injured muscles are useful. For severe cases in which a part of the shinbone has been torn away, treatment may include surgery to reattach it. Afterward, the person must not run for a long time. An experimental treatment consisting of calcitonin (a hormone that builds bone) injected daily or alendronate (a drug that slows bone loss) given by mouth has healed some shin splints that were unresponsive to other measures. Sometimes none of the available treatments are effective, and the runner must abandon running permanently.

Popliteus Tendinitis

Popliteus tendinitis is a tear in the popliteus tendon, which extends from the outer surface of the bottom of the thighbone (femur) diagonally across the back of the knee to the inner side of the top of the shinbone (tibia).

The popliteus tendon prevents the lower leg from twisting outward during running. Excessive inward rolling of the feet (pronation), as well as running downhill, tends to put excessive stress on this tendon, which can tear it.

Pain and soreness, particularly when running downhill, develop along the outside of the knee. A person shouldn't run until the area is free of pain and shouldn't run downhill for at least 3 weeks after resuming running. Bicycling is a good alternative exercise during healing. Shoe inserts, especially a triangular wedge (varus wedge) placed in front of the heel, can help keep the foot from rolling inward.

Achilles Tendinitis

Achilles tendinitis is an inflammation of the Achilles tendon, the tough band extending from the calf muscles to the heel.

The calf muscles and the Achilles tendon lower the forefoot after the heel touches the ground and raise the heel as the toes push off just before stepping to the other foot.

Achilles tendinitis occurs when stresses placed on the tendon are greater than the tendon's

Shin Splints

Shin splints may develop in the muscles in the front and outer parts of the shin (anterolateral shin splints) or in the muscles in the back and inner parts (posteromedial shin splints). Pain is felt in different areas, depending on which muscles are affected.

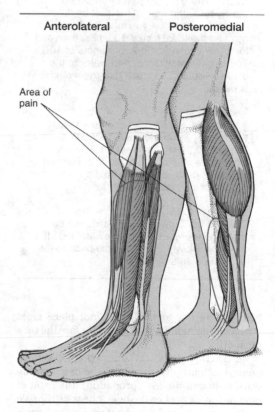

Anterolateral   Posteromedial

Area of pain

strength. Running downhill places extra stress on the Achilles tendon because the forefoot has farther to go before touching the ground. Running uphill also stresses this tendon because the calf muscles must exert greater force to raise the heel as the toes push off. A soft heel counter (the back part of the shoe that surrounds the heel) allows excessive movement of the heel, stressing the Achilles tendon unevenly and increasing the likelihood that it will tear. Stiff-soled shoes that don't

Strengthening the Shin Muscles

Bucket-handle exercise

Wrap a towel around the handle of an empty water bucket. Sit on a table or other surface high enough to prevent the feet from touching the floor. Place the bucket handle over the front part of one shoe. Slowly raise the front of the foot by flexing the ankle, then slowly extend the foot by pointing the toe. Repeat 10 times, then rest for a few seconds. Do 2 more sets of 10. To increase resistance, add water to the bucket—but not so much that the exercise is painful.

Toe raises

Stand up. Slowly rise up on the toes, then slowly lower the heels to the floor. Repeat 10 times, then rest for 1 minute. Do 2 more sets of 10. When this exercise becomes easy, do it while holding progressively heavier weights.

Outward rolls

Stand up. Slowly roll the ankle out so that the inner part of the sole is raised off the floor. Slowly lower the sole back to the floor. Do 3 sets of 10.

bend where the toes join the foot place great stress on the Achilles tendon just before the toes push off.

Various biomechanical factors predispose this tendon to injury. They include the excessive inward rolling of the feet (pronation), the habit of landing too far back on the heel (checking the sole of the running shoe can show where the heel is most worn), bowed legs, tight hamstring and calf muscles, high arches, tight Achilles tendons, and heel deformities.

Pain, the major symptom, is usually most severe when a person starts to move after sitting or lying down or starts to run or jog. It's often relieved by continuing to walk or run despite the pain and stiffness. The Achilles tendon is enclosed in a protective sheath; between the tendon and its sheath is a thin layer of fat, which enables the tendon to move freely. When the tendon is injured, scars form between it and its sheath,

causing the tendon to pull on the sheath with each movement. That's why movement is painful. Continuing to walk or run relieves the pain because it increases the temperature of the sheath, making it more pliable, so that the tendon can move more freely. Usually, pressing on the tendon also causes pain.

If the person ignores the pain and continues to run, rigid scar tissue replaces the elastic tendon, and the tendon will always hurt during exercise, with no chance of a cure.

Refraining from running and pedaling a bicycle as long as the pain persists is an important part of treatment. Other measures depend on the probable cause or predisposing conditions and include wearing shoes with flexible soles and placing inserts in running shoes to reduce tension on the tendon and stabilize the heel. Exercises to stretch the hamstring muscles can be started as soon as they can be done without pain. Exercises to strengthen the Achilles tendon, such as toe raises, are helpful. After running is resumed, the person shouldn't run uphill or downhill at a fast pace until the tendon is fully healed—which can be weeks to years later.

Runner's Knee

Runner's knee (patellofemoral stress syndrome) is a condition in which the kneecap (patella) rubs against the end of the thighbone (femur) when the knee moves.

The kneecap is a circular bone that's attached to ligaments and tendons around the knee. The kneecap normally moves up or down slightly without touching the thighbone during running.

Runner's knee may be caused by a structural defect, such as a kneecap located too high in the knee joint (patella alta), or tight hamstrings, tight Achilles tendons, and weak thigh muscles—which normally help stabilize the knee. The most common treatable cause is excessive inward rolling of the feet (pronation) when walking or running while the front thigh muscles (quadriceps) pull the kneecap outward. Together, these forces cause the kneecap to rub against the end of the thighbone.

Pain and sometimes swelling usually start during running and are concentrated on the undersurface of the kneecap. At first, only running downhill is painful, but later any running and eventually even other leg movements, particularly walking down steps, are painful.

Runner's Knee

Normally, the kneecap (patella) moves up or down slightly without touching the thighbone (femur) during running. If the feet roll in excessively (pronation), the lower leg twists inward, pulling the kneecap inward, while the quadriceps muscles pull the kneecap outward. These opposing forces cause the back of the kneecap to rub against the end of the thighbone, resulting in pain.

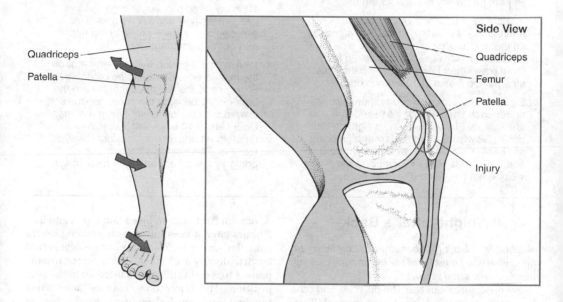

Quadriceps
Patella

Side View
Quadriceps
Femur
Patella
Injury

Refraining from running until it can be done without pain is important. Other exercises, such as riding a bicycle (if not painful), rowing, and swimming, can be continued to maintain physical fitness. Exercises to stretch the muscles in the back (hamstrings) and front (quadriceps) of the thigh and to strengthen the vastus medialis, an inner thigh muscle that pulls the kneecap inward, are helpful. Commercially available arch supports placed in both exercise and street shoes may help. Sometimes, shoe inserts have to be custom-made.

Hamstring Injury

A hamstring injury (posterior femoral muscle strain, hamstring tear) is any injury to the hamstring muscles, the muscles in the back of the thigh.

The hamstrings, which straighten the hip and bend the knee, are weaker than the opposing quadriceps (muscles in the front of the thigh). If the hamstrings are not at least 60 percent as strong as the quadriceps, the quadriceps overpower and injure them. A hamstring injury usually causes sudden pain in the back of the thigh when the hamstrings are contracted suddenly and violently.

Immediate treatment includes rest, ice, compression, and elevation. A person shouldn't run or jump but may jog in place, row, or swim—unless these activities cause pain—while the muscle heals. After healing begins, exercises to strengthen the hamstrings can help prevent a recurrence.

Strengthening the Vastus Medialis Muscle

1. Stand with both knees straight. Contract the quadriceps muscles (in the front of the thighs), raising the kneecaps. Hold this position for a count of 10, then relax. Repeat frequently throughout the day.

2. Sit on the floor with both knees straight and the legs far apart. Rotate legs outward so that the toes point as far to the side as possible. Slowly raise the injured leg from the hip and then lower it, keeping the knee straight. Do 3 sets of 10 every other day.

3. Sit on the floor with two or more pillows under each knee so that it's flexed at a 135° angle. Place a 5-pound weight on the ankle. Slowly raise the foot by straightening the knee, then slowly lower the foot. Do 3 sets of 10. Progress by increasing the weight, not the number of repetitions.

Strengthening the Hamstrings

1. Attach a 5-pound weight to the foot on the injured side and lie face down on a bed with the lower part of the body (from the waist down) off the bed and the toes touching the floor. Keeping the knee straight, slowly raise and lower the leg. Do 3 sets of 10 every other day. As strength returns, use increasingly heavier weights. This exercise strengthens primarily the upper part of the hamstrings.

2. Attach a 5-pound weight to the foot on the injured side. Stand on the other leg. Slowly raise the weighted foot toward the buttocks by bending the knee, and lower it toward the floor by straightening the knee. Do 3 sets of 10 every other day. As strength returns, use increasingly heavier weights. This exercise strengthens primarily the lower part of the hamstrings.

Weight Lifter's Back

Weight lifter's back (lumbar strain) is an injury to the tendons and muscles of the lower back causing muscle spasms and soreness.

Any great force can tear the muscles and tendons of the lower back (the lumbar region). This type of injury is common in sports that require pushing or pulling against great resistance, such as snatching a heavy weight from the ground in weight lifting or pushing against an opposing lineman in football. It also occurs in sports that require sudden twisting of the back: turning to dribble after a rebound in basketball, swinging a bat in baseball, and swinging a club in golf.

Risk factors for a lower back injury include an exaggerated curve of the lower spine, a pelvis (hipbone) that tilts forward, inflexible or weak back muscles, weak abdominal muscles, and tight, inflexible hamstrings. The back is also prone to injury when the spine is weakened by arthritis, misaligned vertebrae, slipped or ruptured disks, or a spinal bone tumor.

A lower back injury usually causes sudden pain in the lower back during twisting, pushing, or pulling. At first, the pain isn't severe enough to prevent further exercise. However, the torn muscle or tendon continues to bleed and swell, and 2 or 3 hours later, it goes into spasm, causing severe pain. Because muscle spasms can be aggravated by virtually any back movement, a person usually prefers to remain still, often curled up in the fetal position. The lower back may be sore when touched and may feel worse when the person bends forward.

As soon as possible after the injury, the person should rest and apply ice and compression to the sore back. Exercises to strengthen the abdominal muscles, which help stabilize the back, and to stretch and strengthen the back muscles are beneficial after healing begins. A rowing machine is excellent for strengthening the back if using it isn't painful.

An exaggerated curve of the lower spine, which tends to put additional stress on the muscles supporting the lower back, is determined largely by the tilt of the pelvis. So an exaggerated curve can be decreased with a variety of exercises that tilt the top of the pelvis backward to a more normal position. Such exercises include strengthening the abdominal muscles (to shorten them) and stretching the thigh muscles (to lengthen them). Wearing a weight-lifting belt may help prevent injury to the back.

Preventing Back Injuries

Pelvic tilt (to decrease an exaggerated curve of the lower spine)

Lie on the back with the knees bent, heels on the floor, and the weight on the heels. Lower the small of the back so that it touches the floor, raise the buttocks about half an inch from the floor, and contract the stomach muscles. Hold this position for a count of 10. Repeat 20 times. Do this exercise daily.

Abdominal curls (to strengthen abdominal muscles)

Lie on the back with the knees bent and feet on the floor. Place hands across abdomen. While keeping shoulders on the floor, slowly raise the head. Slowly raise shoulders 10 inches from the floor. Then slowly lower them. Do 3 sets of 10. When this exercise becomes too easy, wrap a weight in a towel and hold it behind the neck while doing the exercise. Increase the weight as strength improves.

Hip and quadriceps stretch

Stand with one foot on the floor and the knee of the other leg bent at a 90° angle. Hold the front of the ankle of the bent leg with the hand on the same side. Keeping the knees together, pull the ankle backward, bringing the heel toward the buttocks. Hold for a count of 10. Repeat with the other leg. Do this exercise 10 times.

Lower back stretches

Sitting toe touch

Sit on the floor with the knees straight and legs as far apart as possible. Place both hands on the same knee. Slowly slide both hands down that leg toward the ankle. Stop if pain is felt and go no farther than a position that can be held comfortably for 10 seconds. Slowly release the leg. Repeat with the other leg. Do this exercise 10 times with each leg.

Single leg lifts with arched spine

Lie on the back with the knees bent at a 90° angle and both heels on the floor. While keeping the knee bent, hold one knee in both hands and bring it to the chest. Hold for a count of 10. Slowly lower that leg and repeat with the other leg. Do this exercise 10 times.

Swan (to increase the back's flexibility)

Lie on the stomach with the elbows bent and hands touching the ears. Raise the shoulders and legs from the floor at the same time. Don't bend the knees. Hold this position for a count of 10 and repeat 20 times. Do this exercise daily.

Caution: Forcibly extending the spine can worsen many back conditions. Do this exercise with care and stop immediately if pain is felt.

Backhand Tennis Elbow

Backhand tennis elbow (lateral epicondylitis) is damage to the tendons that bend the wrist backward away from the palm, causing pain on the outer, back side of the forearm.

The forearm muscles that are attached to the outer part of the elbow become sore when excessive stress is placed on the point of attachment. Backhand tennis elbow is most often evident during a backhand return. The force of the racket hitting the ball can damage the tendons as they roll over the end of the elbow. Factors that increase the chances of developing backhand tennis elbow include using improper backhand strokes, having weak shoulder and wrist muscles, playing with a racket that's too tightly strung or too short, hitting the ball off center on the racket, and hitting heavy, wet balls.

The first symptom is pain during a backhand stroke or other similar repetitive movements. Pain is felt along the outer, back side of the elbow and forearm on the same side as the thumb when the hand is by the side with the thumb away from the body. Continuing to play can extend the area of pain from the elbow down to the wrist and result in pain even at rest. The elbow hurts when a person places the arm and hand palm down on a table and tries to raise the hand against resistance by bending the wrist.

Tennis Elbow

The two types of tennis elbow—backhand and forehand tennis elbow—cause pain in different areas of the elbow and forearm.

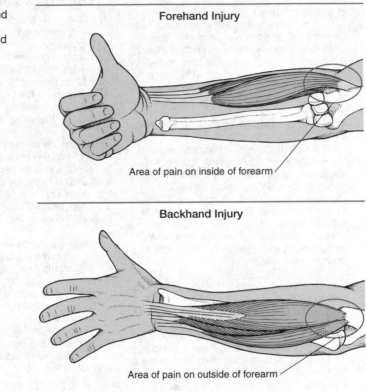

Forehand Injury

Area of pain on inside of forearm

Backhand Injury

Area of pain on outside of forearm

Treatment consists of avoiding any exercise that produces pain. Exercises that don't use the wrist primarily, such as jogging, cycling, or basketball, or even racquetball or squash—in which the ball hits the racket with less force than in tennis—can be substituted to maintain physical fitness. As the injury heals, strengthening exercises can be started. Generally, all the muscles that bend and straighten the wrist should be strengthened.

Forehand Tennis Elbow

Forehand tennis elbow (baseball elbow, suitcase elbow, medial epicondylitis) is damage to the ten-

dons that bend the wrist toward the palm, causing pain on the palm side of the forearm from the elbow toward the wrist.

This injury is caused by bending the wrist toward the palm with excessive force. Factors that produce such force include having weak shoulder or hand muscles; serving with great force in tennis; using a spin serve; hitting heavy, wet balls; using a racket that is too heavy, has a grip that's too small, or has strings that are too tight; pitching a baseball; throwing a javelin; and carrying a heavy suitcase. Continuing to exercise with pain can pull the tendons from the bone, causing bleeding.

Strengthening Wrist Muscles

For backhand tennis elbow

1. Sit on a chair next to a table. Place the injured forearm on the table, palm down, with the elbow straight and the wrist and hand hanging over the edge. Hold a 1-pound weight in the hand. Slowly raise and lower the hand by bending and straightening the wrist. Repeat 10 times. Rest 1 minute, then do 2 more sets of 10. If the exercise causes pain, stop immediately and try again the next day. Do this exercise every other day. Increase the weight as the exercise becomes easier.

2. With the palm down, hold a piece of wood the diameter of a broomstick with a 1-pound weight attached to it by a rope. Wind the weight up. Repeat 10 times. Stop if any pain is felt. Do this exercise every other day. Gradually increase the weight but not the number of repetitions.

For forehand tennis elbow

1. Sit on a chair next to a table. Place the injured forearm on the table, palm up, with the wrist and hand hanging over the edge. Hold a 1-pound weight in the hand. Slowly raise and lower the hand by bending and straightening the wrist. Repeat 10 times. Rest 1 minute, then do 2 more sets of 10. If the exercise causes pain, stop and try again the next day. As the exercise becomes easier, increase the weight.

2. With the palm up, hold a piece of wood the diameter of a broomstick with a 1-pound weight attached to it by a rope. Wind the weight up. Repeat 20 times. Stop if the exercise becomes painful. Gradually increase the weight but not the number of repetitions.

3. Several times a day, gently squeeze a soft sponge ball, then relax.

Pain is felt along the palm side of the elbow and forearm on the same side as the thumb when bending the wrist toward the palm against resistance or when squeezing a hard rubber ball. To confirm the diagnosis, a doctor asks the person to sit in a chair with the injured arm resting on a table, palm up. The doctor holds the wrist down and asks the person to raise the hand by bending the wrist. A person who has forehand tennis elbow feels pain at the elbow.

Any activity that causes pain when the wrist is bent toward the palm or turned so that the little finger is next to the body should be avoided. Surgery generally relieves persisting pain. After the injury has healed, a tennis player should strengthen the wrist and shoulder muscles, as well as the injured muscles.

Rotator Cuff Tendinitis

Rotator cuff tendinitis (swimmer's shoulder, tennis shoulder, pitcher's shoulder, shoulder impingement syndrome) is a tearing and swelling of the rotator cuff (the muscles and tendons that hold the upper arm in the shoulder joint).

These tendons are often injured in sports that require the arm to be moved over the head repeatedly, such as pitching in baseball, lifting heavy weights over the shoulder, serving the ball in racket sports, and swimming freestyle, butterfly, or backstroke. Repeatedly moving the arm over the head causes the top of the arm bone to rub against part of the shoulder joint and its tendons, tearing individual fibers. If the movement is continued despite the pain, the tendon can tear or actually pull off part of the bone.

Shoulder pain is the main symptom. Initially, the pain occurs only during activities that require lifting the arm over the head and forcibly bringing it forward. Later, pain can occur even when the arm is moved forward to shake hands. Usually, pushing objects away is painful, but pulling them in toward the body isn't.

The diagnosis is made when specific movements, especially raising the arm above the shoulder, cause pain and soreness. Sometimes arthrograms (x-rays taken after a substance visible on x-rays is injected into the joint) can detect

---

Strengthening the Shoulders

Bench press
Lie on the back. Use a special bench or ask a spotter to help lift the weight off when the exercise is finished. Hold the barbell in the hands with the thumbs facing each other. Slowly raise the weight from the chest and then slowly lower it. Do 3 sets of 10 repetitions, stopping immediately if pain is felt. As strength improves, increase the weight. *Caution:* This exercise should be started with a very light weight because it stresses the injured muscles.

complete tears of the rotator cuff tendon, but they usually aren't sensitive enough to detect partial tears.

Treatment consists of resting the injured tendons and strengthening the shoulder. Exercises that involve pushing something away or raising the elbows over the shoulder should be avoided. However, upright rowing with free weights (by bending, not raising, the elbows) and downward lat pulls on a weight machine, which exercise the latissimus muscle in the back and shoulders, can be continued if they aren't painful. Surgery is sometimes needed when the injury is particularly severe, the tendon is completely torn, or the injury doesn't heal within a year.

CHAPTER 58

Exercise and Fitness

Exercise is planned physical activity performed repetitively to develop or maintain fitness; fitness is the capacity to perform physical activities.

To become and stay fit, people need to exercise regularly. Exercise makes the heart stronger, enabling it to pump more blood with each heartbeat. The blood can then deliver more oxygen to the body, increasing the maximum amount of oxygen that the body can take in and use. This amount, called maximum oxygen uptake, can be measured to determine a person's fitness.

Exercise benefits the body in many other ways. Stretching can increase flexibility. Weight-bearing exercise strengthens bones and helps prevent osteoporosis. Exercise also helps prevent constipation, prevent and control some forms of diabetes, lower blood pressure, and reduce stress, body fat, and levels of total and low-density lipoprotein (LDL) cholesterol.

Exercise can benefit people of any age, including older people. Recent studies show that exercise can strengthen the muscles of frail elderly people living in nursing homes. Older men who continue to train and compete in long-distance running races can maintain their maximum oxygen uptake. Inactivity, rather than aging itself, is the main cause of the decline in older people's physical capabilities.

The benefits of exercise are lost soon after a person stops exercising. Heart strength and muscle strength decrease, as does the level of high-density lipoprotein (HDL) cholesterol—the good cholesterol—and blood pressure and body fat increase. Even former athletes who stop exercising don't retain measurable long-term benefits. They have no greater capacity to perform physical activities, no fewer risk factors for heart attacks, and no faster response to exercise than do those who have never exercised.

Starting an Exercise Program

The safest way to start an exercise program is to perform the chosen exercise or sport at a low intensity until the legs or arms ache or feel heavy. If muscles ache after just a few minutes, the first workout should last only that long. As fitness increases, a person should be able to exercise longer without feeling muscle pain or discomfort. When a person can exercise comfortably for 10 consecutive minutes, the workouts should be done every other day, gradually working up to 30 minutes of continuous exercise. Guidelines concerning how long and how often to exercise, how hard to exercise, and how to prevent injuries are the same for all types of exercise and sports.

How Long and How Often?

To achieve and maintain fitness, a person needs to exercise only 30 minutes three times a week. Exercising more than 30 minutes at a time isn't necessary for most people, because fitness, as measured by maximum oxygen uptake, increases very little with workouts that last longer than 30 minutes.

Improvement comes from stressing the muscles and allowing them to recover, not from doing the same workout every day. Although the heart can be exercised several times a day every day, skeletal muscles start to break down when exercised intensely more often than every other day. The day after intense exercise, bleeding and microscopic tearing can be seen in muscle fibers. That's why muscles feel sore the day after an adequate workout. Exercisers should allow about 48 hours for muscles to recover after exercise. When the muscles heal, they are stronger. Exercising two or three times a week, alternating exercise days with rest days, can help prevent injuries.

How Hard?

Fitness is determined more by the intensity of exercise than the duration. Workouts should be hard enough that the muscles are somewhat sore the next day but fully recovered the day after that.

To strengthen the heart, exercise must be performed at an intensity that increases heart rate (measured in beats per minute) at least 20 beats above the resting heart rate. The harder a person exercises, the faster the heart beats and the stronger the heart muscle becomes.

Heart rate is determined by how hard the skeletal muscles contract. When a person starts to exercise, the skeletal muscles contract and squeeze the veins near them, forcing blood toward the heart. When the skeletal muscles relax, these veins fill with blood. The alternating contraction and relaxation of skeletal muscles serve as a second heart, pumping extra blood to the heart. The increased blood flow causes the heart to beat faster and more forcefully. So the harder the skeletal muscles contract, the faster the heart beats.

The recommended heart rate for exercise (the training heart rate) is 60 percent of a person's estimated maximum heart rate, which is 220 minus the person's age. However, this calculation doesn't apply to older people who are physically fit. Maximum heart rate measures skeletal muscle strength, not heart strength, so a strong, fit older person will have a much higher maximum heart rate than a weak, out-of-shape younger person.

Measuring the heart rate isn't necessary as long as a person begins exercising slowly and increases the intensity gradually. The intensity should be increased until the training heart rate is reached: when the shoulders rise with each breath and breathing is faster and deeper, indicating that the person needs more oxygen. To become fit, a person doesn't have to exercise any more intensely than this. Only athletes training for competition need to exercise to the point of becoming short of breath.

As exercise intensity increases, skeletal muscles are more likely to be injured. They are far more likely to be injured during sustained intense exercise than during intermittent exercise. In intermittent exercise, a person warms up by starting slowly, then gradually increases the pace. When the muscles start to feel heavy, painful, or uncomfortable, the person slows down. When the muscles feel fresh again, the pace is increased. The person alternates between faster and slower movements until the muscle heaviness does not go away, then ends the workout. Improvement is made by increasing the time spent exercising intensely and decreasing the time spent slowing down.

People should feel good after exercise. If they don't, they've probably exercised too much. Overexercising makes joints, muscles, tendons, and bones ache, increases the risk of injury, and makes a person irritable.

Preventing Injuries

More than 6 out of 10 people who start an exercise program drop out in the first 6 weeks because of an injury. Injuries can be prevented by scheduling workouts 48 hours apart. On this type of schedule, a person can exercise every other day, or a person who wants to exercise every day can exercise different muscle groups on alternate days or exercise intensely one day and less intensely the next (the hard-easy principle). Exercising in the same way every day doesn't improve fitness but does increase the chances of an injury. In addition, people should stop exercising immediately if they feel pain.

Exercising Every Other Day

Waking up with stiff, sore muscles the day after playing a competitive sport or exercising vigorously is normal. The fastest way to recover is to rest—not to exercise at all that day. Prolonged, vigorous exercise can use up most of the stored sugar (glycogen) in muscles, which is the major source of energy during exercise. If glycogen levels are low, muscles feel heavy, weak, and tired. Eating carbohydrate-rich foods such as bread, pasta, fruit, cereals, whole grains, and most desserts fills the muscles with glycogen. Resting allows almost all the glycogen that enters the muscles to be stored and allows injured muscle fibers to heal.

Alternating Exercises

Different exercises stress different muscle groups. For example, running stresses primarily the lower leg muscles; landing on the heels and rising on the toes exert the greatest force on the ankle. Riding a bicycle stresses primarily the upper leg muscles; pedaling works the knees and hips. Rowing and swimming stress the upper body and back. An ideal schedule alternates exercise for the upper body on one day with exercise for the lower body on the next.

For people who exercise every day, alternating exercises allows the muscles to recover, prevents injuries, and promotes a higher level of fitness. Running 30 minutes one day and riding a bicycle for 30 minutes the next day is far less likely to cause injury than doing both every day for 15 minutes each.

Marathon runners are injured more frequently than triathletes, who compete in three sports, even though triathletes exercise more. Triathletes exercise different muscle groups on successive days: They may run one day and swim and cycle on the next.

Following the Hard-Easy Principle

To attain higher levels of fitness or compete in athletic events, a person must exercise intensely two or three times a week and less intensely on the other days (the hard-easy principle).

Competitive athletes train every day, and training is specific to the sport—a person doesn't become a better runner by riding a bicycle. So to protect themselves from injuries, athletes plan a hard workout one day, followed by an easy one the next day. In this way, the hard workouts cause less muscle damage.

Hard and easy refer to intensity, not quantity. For example, on an easy day, a marathon runner might run 20 miles but at a much slower pace than on a hard day. Weight lifters lift very heavy weights only once a week and lighter weights the rest of the week. Basketball players play long, exhausting practice games one day, then practice plays and shooting the next day.

To build strength, speed, and endurance, athletes exercise hard or long enough on one day to make the muscles feel heavy or burn slightly—a sign that the muscles are adequately worked. Usually, the muscles ache for about 48 hours. Then, athletes exercise less intensely the next few days, until their muscles stop aching. Exercising intensely when muscles ache causes injuries and decreases performance, whereas waiting for the muscles to stop aching before exercising intensely again strengthens muscles.

Two types of muscle discomfort may be felt after exercise. The desirable type, delayed-onset muscle soreness, doesn't start until several hours after exercising intensely, usually affects both sides of the body equally, goes away 48 hours later, and usually feels better after the warm-up for the next workout. On the other hand, the pain of injury is usually felt soon after it occurs, is worse on one side of the body, does not disappear 48 hours later, and becomes much more severe if a person tries to exercise.

Warming Up

Raising the temperature of muscles (warming up) before exercising or participating in a sport can help prevent injuries. Warm muscles are more pliable and less likely to tear than cold muscles, which contract sluggishly. The most effective warm-up—much better than passively heating the muscles with warm water or heating pads—is slowly going through the actual motions of the exercise or sport. Going through the motions increases blood flow to the muscles that will be used, warming them up and readying them for more vigorous exercise. Blood flow must increase substantially to protect the muscles from injury during exercise. Calisthenics (a series of movements that exercise an isolated muscle group, such as push-ups) aren't specific enough to warm up muscles for a particular sport.

Stretching

A person should stretch only after warming up or exercising, when the muscles are warm and less likely to tear. Stretching lengthens muscles and tendons, and longer muscles can generate more force around joints, helping a person jump higher, lift heavier weights, run faster, and throw farther. However, stretching, unlike exercising against resistance (as in weight training), doesn't strengthen muscles; strengthening muscles makes them less likely to tear. There's scant evidence that stretching prevents injuries or delayed-onset muscle soreness, which is caused by muscle fiber damage.

Cooling Down

Slowing down gradually (cooling down) at the end of exercise helps prevent dizziness. When the leg muscles relax, blood collects (pools) in the veins near them. To return the blood toward the heart, the leg muscles must contract. When exercise is suddenly stopped, blood pools in the legs and not enough blood goes to the brain, causing dizziness.

Cooling down also helps remove lactic acid, a waste product that builds up in the muscles after exercise. Lactic acid doesn't cause delayed-onset muscle soreness, so cooling down doesn't prevent this soreness.

Choosing the Right Exercise

Any exercise that increases the circulation of blood through the heart improves fitness. The safest exercises are walking, swimming, and pedaling a stationary bicycle. During walking, at least one foot is on the ground at all times, so the force with which the foot strikes the ground is never much more than the person's weight. During swimming, the muscles are supported by the water, so they rarely are subjected to the forces that cause muscles to tear. Bicycles are pedaled in a smooth circular motion that doesn't jolt the muscles.

Walking slowly won't make a person very fit. To walk faster, a person can take longer steps in addition to moving the legs faster. Steps can be lengthened by swiveling the hips from side to side so that the feet can reach further forward. Swiveling the hips tends to make the toes point outward when the feet touch the ground, so the toes don't reach as far forward as they would if they were pointed straight ahead. Therefore, a walker should always try to point the toes straight ahead. Moving the arms faster helps the feet move faster. To move the arms faster, a person bends the elbows to shorten the swing and reduce the time the arms take to swing back and forth from the shoulder.

Swimming exercises the whole body—the legs, arms, and back—without stressing the joints and muscles. Often, swimming is recommended for people who have muscle and joint problems. Swimmers, moving at their own pace and using any stroke, can gradually work up to 30 minutes of continuous swimming. If weight loss is one of the main goals of exercise, swimming isn't the best choice. Exercise out of water is more effective because air insulates the body, increasing body temperature and metabolism for up to 18 hours. This process burns extra calories after exercise as well as during exercise. In contrast, water conducts heat away from the body, so that body temperature doesn't rise and metabolism doesn't remain increased after swimming.

Riding a stationary bicycle is good exercise. The tension on the bicycle wheel should be set so that the rider can pedal at a cadence of 60 rotations a minute. As they progress, riders can gradually increase the tension and the cadence up to 90 rotations per minute.

A recumbent stationary bicycle is a particularly good choice for older people. Many older people have weak upper leg muscles because walking is their only exercise and walking on level ground barely uses these muscles. As a result, many older people have difficulty getting up from a chair without using their hands, rising from a squatting position, or walking up stairs without holding on to the railing. Pedaling a bicycle strengthens the upper leg muscles. However, some people can't maintain their balance even on a stationary bicycle, and others won't use one because the pressure of the narrow seat against the pelvis feels uncomfortable. In contrast, a recumbent stationary bicycle is both secure and comfortable. It has a contoured chair that even a person who has had a stroke can sit in. Also, if one leg is paralyzed, toe clips can hold both feet in place, so that the person can pedal with one leg.

Aerobic dancing, a popular type of exercise offered in many communities, exercises the whole body. People can exercise at their own pace with guidance from experienced instructors. Lively music and familiar routines make the workout fun, and committing to a schedule and exercising with friends can improve motivation. Aerobic dancing also can be done at home with videotapes. Low-impact aerobic dancing eliminates the jumping and pounding of regular aerobic dancing, thus decreasing stress on the joints. Step aerobics stresses primarily the muscles in the front and back of the upper legs (the quadriceps and hamstrings) as a person steps up and down a raised platform (a step) in a routine set to music at a designated pace. As soon as these muscles start to feel sore, exercisers should stop, do something else, and return to step aerobics a couple of days later. Water aerobics is an excellent choice for older people and those with weak muscles.

Cross-country skiing machines exercise the upper body and the legs. Many people enjoy using this equipment, but others find the motions difficult to master. Because using these machines requires more coordination than most types of exercise, a person should try out a machine before buying one.

Rowing machines strengthen the large muscles of the legs, shoulders, and back and help protect a healthy back from injury. However, a person who has back problems should not use one. The extra force of rowing, done primarily with the back, may aggravate already damaged back muscles and joints. All good rowing machines have sliding seats, and the best ones have a spinning wheel that allows exercisers to adjust the tension while rowing.

Exercisers who can do a 30-minute workout easily may want to add variety to their exercise programs. Race walking (walking as fast as possible while swinging the arms vigorously), jogging, running, cycling, ice-skating, roller-blading, cross-country skiing, racquetball, handball, and squash are excellent for fitness but require at least a moderate level of coordination and skill. They also have a higher risk of injury.

Brain and Nerve Disorders

CHAPTER 59

Biology of the Nervous System

The brain, the spinal cord, and the nerves throughout the body make up the nervous system. The nervous system has two distinct parts: the central nervous system and the peripheral nervous system. The **central nervous system** comprises the brain and spinal cord. The **peripheral nervous system** is a network of nerves that connects the brain and spinal cord to the rest of the body.

Brain

The brain's functions are both mysterious and remarkable. From the brain come all thoughts, beliefs, memories, behaviors, and moods. The brain is the site of thinking and the control center for the rest of the body. The brain coordinates the ability to move, touch, smell, hear, and see. It allows people to form words, understand and manipulate numbers, compose and appreciate music, see and understand geometric shapes, and communicate with others. The brain even has the capacity to plan ahead and fantasize.

The brain reviews all stimuli, whether from internal organs, the surface of the body, or the eyes, ears, and nose. It then reacts to these stimuli by correcting the position of the body, the move-

ment of limbs, and the rate at which the internal organs function. The brain can also adjust alertness and mood.

No computer has yet come close to matching the capabilities of the human brain. However, this sophistication doesn't come without a price. The brain needs constant nourishment; it demands an extremely high and continuous flow of blood and oxygen—about 20 percent of the blood flow from the heart. A loss of blood flow for more than about 10 seconds can cause loss of consciousness (syncope). Lack of oxygen, abnormally low blood sugar levels, or toxic substances can cause the brain to malfunction within seconds, but the brain is defended by mechanisms that are usually able to prevent these problems.

The brain has three major anatomic components: the cerebrum, the brain stem, and the cerebellum.

The **cerebrum** consists of dense, convoluted masses of tissue divided into two halves—the left and right cerebral hemispheres—that are connected in the middle by nerve fibers called the corpus callosum. The cerebrum is further divided into the frontal, parietal, occipital, and temporal lobes.

• The frontal lobes control skilled motor behavior, including speech, mood, thought, and plan-

Viewing the Brain

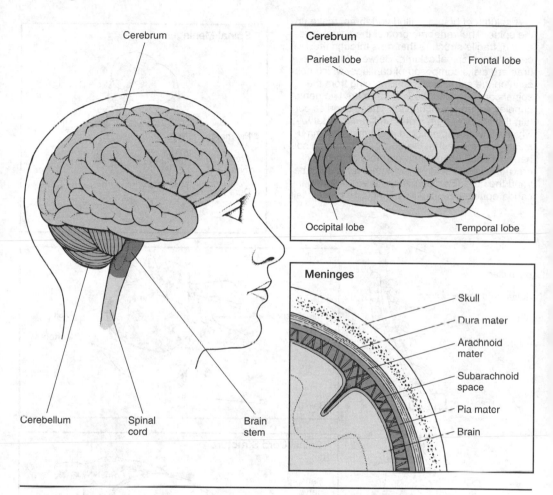

Cerebrum

Cerebellum   Spinal cord   Brain stem

Cerebrum

Parietal lobe   Frontal lobe

Occipital lobe   Temporal lobe

Meninges

Skull
Dura mater
Arachnoid mater
Subarachnoid space
Pia mater
Brain

ning for the future. In most people, control of language is situated predominantly in the left frontal lobe.

• The parietal lobes interpret sensory input from the rest of the body and control body movement.
• The occipital lobes interpret vision.
• The temporal lobes generate memory and emotions. They allow people to recognize other people and objects, process and retrieve long-term memories, and initiate communication or action.

Collections of nerve cells lie at the base of the cerebrum in structures called the basal ganglia, thalamus, and hypothalamus. The basal ganglia help to smooth out movements; the thalamus generally organizes sensory messages to and from the highest levels of the brain (cerebral cortex); and the hypothalamus coordinates some of the more automatic functions of the body, such as controlling sleep and wakefulness, maintaining body temperature, and regulating the balance of water within the body.

How the Spine is Organized

A column of bones, called vertebrae, make up the spine. The vertebrae protect the spinal cord, a long, fragile structure that runs through the center of the spinal column. Between the vertebrae are disks composed of cartilage, which help cushion the spinal column. Emerging from the spinal cord between the vertebrae are two nerve bundles called spinal nerves. These bundles contain the fibers of both motor and sensory nerves, which allow the spinal cord and brain to communicate with the rest of the body. Although the spinal cord ends about three quarters of the way down the spinal column, some nerves extend beyond the cord. This bundle of nerves is called the cauda equina because it resembles a horse's tail.

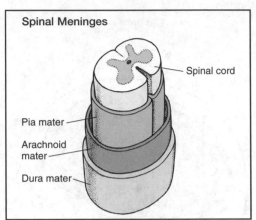

Spinal Meninges

Spinal cord

Pia mater

Arachnoid mater

Dura mater

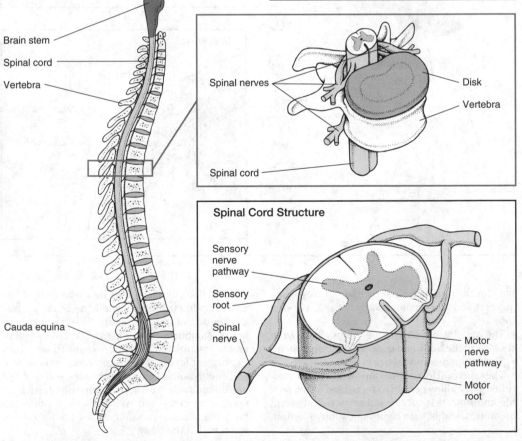

Brain stem

Spinal cord

Vertebra

Spinal nerves

Spinal cord

Disk

Vertebra

Cauda equina

Spinal Cord Structure

Sensory nerve pathway

Sensory root

Spinal nerve

Motor nerve pathway

Motor root

Other critical body functions are automatically regulated by the **brain stem.** The brain stem helps to adjust posture; regulates breathing, swallowing, and heartbeat; controls the rate at which the body burns foods; and increases alertness when needed. If the brain stem becomes severely damaged, these automatic functions cease and death soon follows.

The **cerebellum,** which lies beneath the cerebrum just above the brain stem, coordinates the body's movements. With information it receives from the cerebrum and with information about the position of the arms and legs and their degree of muscle tone, it helps the body make smooth, accurate movements.

Both the brain and spinal cord are wrapped in three layers of tissue (the **meninges**), as follows:
• The pia mater is the innermost layer that adheres to the brain and spinal cord.
• The delicate, spiderweb-like arachnoid mater is the middle layer that serves as a channel for cerebrospinal fluid.
• The leathery dura mater is the outermost and toughest layer.

The brain and its meninges are contained in a tough, bony protective structure, the skull. Additional protection is provided by the **cerebrospinal fluid,** which flows over the surface of the brain between the meninges, fills internal spaces within the brain (ventricles), and cushions the brain against sudden jarring and minor injury.

Spinal Cord

The spinal cord—a long, fragile structure that begins at the end of the brain stem and continues down almost to the bottom of the spine—carries both incoming and outgoing messages between the brain and the rest of the body. Just as the brain is protected by the skull bones, the spinal cord is protected by the back bones (vertebrae) that make up the spinal column.

The brain communicates with much of the body through nerves that run up and down the spinal cord. Each vertebra forms an opening between it and the vertebrae above and below it. Through this opening, a pair of spinal nerves branch out and carry messages from the spinal cord to the more distant parts of the body. Nerves at the front of the spinal cord, called **motor nerves,** carry information from the brain to the muscles; those at the back of the spinal cord, called **sensory nerves,** carry sensory information from distant

Typical Structure of a Nerve Cell

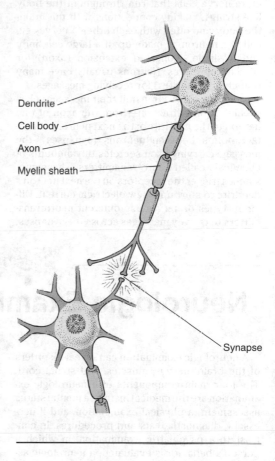

Dendrite
Cell body
Axon
Myelin sheath
Synapse

parts of the body to the brain. This network of nerves makes up the peripheral nervous system. Peripheral nerves are actually bundles of single nerve fibers. Some are very small (less than $\frac{1}{64}$ of an inch in diameter), and others are quite large (more than $\frac{1}{4}$ of an inch in diameter).

The peripheral nervous system also includes nerves that communicate between the brain stem and the body's internal organs. These nerves, called the **autonomic nervous system,** regulate internal body processes that require no conscious awareness, for example, the rate of heart contractions, the rate of breathing, the amount of stomach acid secreted, and the speed at which food passes through the digestive tract.

Nerves

The nervous system contains 100 billion or more nerve cells that run throughout the body like strings, making connections with the brain, the body, and often with each other. A nerve cell, called a neuron, is made up of a large cell body and a single, elongated extension (axon) for sending messages. Neurons usually have many branches (dendrites) for receiving messages.

Normally, nerves transmit their messages electrically in one direction—from the axon of one neuron to the dendrite of the next neuron. At contact points between neurons (synapses), the message-carrying axon secretes tiny amounts of chemicals called neurotransmitters. These substances trigger the receptors on the next neuron's dendrite to start up a new electrical current. Different types of nerves use different neurotransmitters to convey messages across the synapses.

Each large axon is surrounded by a kind of insulator, the myelin sheath, which functions much like the insulation around an electrical wire. When that insulation is interrupted or defective, nerve transmission slows or stops, resulting in such diseases as multiple sclerosis and Guillain-Barré syndrome.

The brain and nerves make up an extraordinarily complex communication system that can normally send and receive voluminous amounts of information simultaneously. But the system is vulnerable to diseases and injuries. For example, nerves can degenerate, causing Alzheimer's disease or Parkinson's disease. Bacterial or viral infections of the brain or spinal cord can cause meningitis or encephalitis. A blockage in the blood supply to the brain can cause a stroke. Injuries or tumors can cause structural damage to the brain or spinal cord.

CHAPTER 60

Neurologic Examination and Tests

A neurologic examination can reveal disorders of the brain, nerves, muscles, and spinal cord. The four main components of a neurologic examination are the medical history, a mental status assessment, a physical examination, and if necessary, diagnostic tests and procedures. In contrast to a psychiatric examination, in which a person's behavior is evaluated, a neurologic assessment requires a *physical* examination. Nevertheless, abnormal behavior often provides clues about the brain's physical condition.

Medical History

Before performing a physical examination and diagnostic tests, a doctor interviews a person to obtain his medical history. The doctor asks the person to describe current symptoms, telling precisely where and how often they occur, how severe they are, how long they last, and whether the person can still perform daily routines. Neurologic symptoms may include headaches, pain, weakness, poor coordination, diminished or abnormal sensations, fainting, and confusion.

The person should also tell the doctor about past or present illnesses or operations, serious illnesses in close blood relatives, allergies, and medications he is currently taking. In addition, the doctor may ask if the person has had work-related or home-related difficulties or has suffered any losses, since these circumstances may affect health and the ability to cope with illness.

Mental Status Assessment

The medical history gives the doctor a good idea of a person's mental status. However, more specific mental status testing is usually needed to diagnose a problem that's affecting the thought processes.

Mental Status Testing

What a Person May Be Asked to Do	What This Test Indicates	What a Person May Be Asked to Do	What This Test Indicates
Tell the current date and place and name specific people	Orientation to time, place, and person	Follow a simple command involving three different body parts that requires distinguishing right from left (such as "put your right thumb over your left ear and stick out your tongue")	Ability to follow simple commands
Repeat a short list of objects	Attention		
Recall three unrelated items after 3 or 5 minutes	Immediate recall	Name simple objects and body parts and read, write, and repeat certain phrases	Language function
Describe an event that happened in the last day or two	Recent memory	Identify small objects held in the hand and numbers written on the palm, and discriminate between being touched in one or two places (for example, on the palm and on the fingers)	How the brain processes information from sense organs
Describe events from the distant past	Remote memory		
Interpret a proverb (such as "a rolling stone gathers no moss") or explain a particular analogy (such as "why the brain is like a computer")	Abstract thinking		
		Copy simple and complex structures (for example, using building blocks) or finger positions and draw a clock, cube, or house	Spatial relationships
Describe feelings and opinions about the illness	Insight into illness		
Name the last five presidents and the state capital	Fund of knowledge	Brush the teeth or take a match out of a box and strike it	Ability to perform an action
Tell how he feels on this day and usually on other days	Mood	Perform simple arithmetic	Ability to perform math

Physical Examination

When performing a physical examination as part of a neurologic examination, a doctor usually examines all of the body systems but focuses on the nervous system. The cranial nerves, motor nerves, sensory nerves, and reflexes are examined, as well as the person's coordination, stance, and gait, his autonomic nervous system function, and blood flow to the brain.

Cranial Nerves

The doctor tests the function of the 12 cranial nerves that are connected directly to the brain. A cranial nerve may be damaged anywhere along its length as a result of an injury, a tumor, or an infection, and the exact site of the damage must be discovered.

Motor Nerves

Motor nerves activate the voluntary muscles (muscles that produce movement, such as the leg muscles used when walking). Damage to a motor nerve may cause weakness or paralysis of the muscle it serves. Lack of peripheral nerve stimulation also causes the muscle to shrivel or waste away (atrophy). A doctor looks for muscle wasting and then tests the strength of various muscles by asking the person to push or pull against resistance.

Cranial Nerve Testing

Cranial Nerve Number	Name	Function	Test
I	Olfactory	Smell	Items with very specific odors (such as soap, coffee, and cloves) are placed under the nose for identification
II	Optic	Vision	The ability to see near and far objects and to detect objects or movement from the corners of the eyes (peripheral vision) is tested
III	Oculomotor	Eye movement upward, downward, inward	The ability to look upward, downward, and inward is tested; the upper eyelid is checked for drooping (ptosis)
IV	Trochlear	Eye movement downward and inward	The ability to move each eye downward and inward from an upward and outward position is tested
V	Trigeminal	Facial sensation and movement	Sensation on affected areas of the face and weakness or paralysis of muscles that control the jaw's ability to clench the teeth are tested
VI	Abducens	Lateral eye movement	The ability to move the eye outward beyond the midline either spontaneously or while looking at a target is tested
VII	Facial	Facial movement	The ability to open the mouth and show the teeth and to close the eyes tightly is tested
VIII	Acoustic	Hearing and balance	Hearing is tested with a tuning fork. Balance is tested when the person walks a straight line, foot by foot
IX	Glossopharyngeal	Throat function	The voice is checked for hoarseness; the ability to swallow is tested; and the position of the uvula (at the back of throat in the center) is checked with the person saying "ah-h-h"
X	Vagus	Swallowing, heart rate	The voice is checked for hoarseness and nasality; the ability to swallow is tested
XI	Accessory	Neck and upper back movement	The shoulders are shrugged and observed for weakness or absence of movement
XII	Hypoglossal	Tongue movement	The tongue is extended and observed for deviation to one side or the other

Sensory Nerves

Sensory nerves carry information to the brain about such things as pressure, pain, heat, cold, vibration, the position of body parts, and the shape of things.

The surface of the body is tested for loss of feeling. Usually the doctor concentrates on an area where the person feels numbness, tingling, or pain, using a pin at first, then something blunt to see if the person can tell the difference between sharp and dull sensations. Sensory nerve function may also be tested by applying gentle pressure, heat, or vibration. To test position sense, the doctor tells the person to close his eyes and then moves the person's finger or toe up or down, asking the person to describe its position.

Reflexes

A reflex is an automatic response to a stimulus. For example, the lower leg jerks when the tendon below the kneecap is gently tapped with a small rubber hammer. This **knee jerk reflex** (one of the deep tendon reflexes) demonstrates that the sensory nerve to the spinal cord, the nerve connections in the cord, and the motor nerves back to the leg muscles are all functioning. The reflex arc follows a complete circuit, from the knee to the spinal cord and back to the leg; the brain isn't involved.

The reflexes most commonly tested are the knee jerk, a similar reflex at the elbow and ankle, and Babinski's reflex. **Babinski's reflex** is tested by firmly stroking the outer border of the sole of the foot with a blunt object. Normally the toes curl downward, except in infants 6 months or younger. Having the big toe go upward and the other toes spread out laterally may be a sign of an abnormality in the brain or in the motor nerves from the brain to the spinal cord. Many other reflexes can be tested to evaluate specific nerve functions.

Coordination, Stance, and Gait

To test coordination, a doctor asks a person first to touch his nose with a forefinger, next to touch the doctor's finger, and then to repeat these actions rapidly. The person may be asked to touch his nose, first with his eyes open, then with his eyes closed. The person may be asked to stand still with arms outstretched and eyes closed, then to open the eyes and begin to walk.

Reflex Arc: A No-Brainer

A reflex arc is the pathway that a nerve reflex follows. The knee jerk reflex is an example.

1. A tap on the knee stimulates sensory receptors, generating a nerve signal.
2. The signal travels along a nerve pathway to the spinal cord.
3. At the spinal cord, the signal is transmitted from the sensory nerve to a motor nerve.
4. The motor nerve sends the signal back to a muscle in the thigh.
5. The muscle contracts, causing the lower leg to jerk upward. The entire reflex occurs without involving the brain.

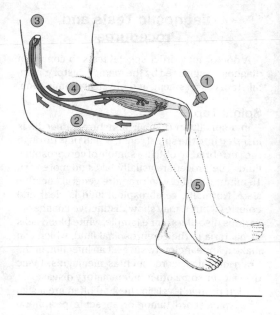

These actions test the motor and sensory nerves as well as brain function. Various other simple tests may also be performed.

Autonomic Nervous System

An abnormality of the autonomic (involuntary) nervous system may cause such problems as a fall in blood pressure upon standing, a lack of sweating, or sexual problems such as difficulty in initiating or maintaining an erection. Again, the doctor may perform a variety of tests, such as measuring blood pressure while the person is sitting and immediately after the person stands.

Blood Flow to the Brain

A severe narrowing of the arteries that carry blood to the brain puts a person at risk for a stroke. The risk is higher in people who are elderly or who have high blood pressure, diabetes, or diseases of the arteries or heart. To assess the arteries, the doctor places a stethoscope over the neck arteries and listens for sounds of blood being forced past a narrow area (called bruits). More sophisticated tests such as Doppler ultrasound scanning or cerebral angiography are needed for an accurate evaluation.

Diagnostic Tests and Procedures

A doctor may order special tests to confirm a diagnosis suggested by the medical history, mental status assessment, and physical examination.

Spinal Tap

In a spinal tap (lumbar puncture), a needle is inserted into the spinal canal, which runs through the vertebrae, to obtain a sample of cerebrospinal fluid. The procedure usually takes no more than 15 minutes and doesn't require general anesthesia.▲ Normally, cerebrospinal fluid is clear and colorless, but it may show distinctive changes in various disorders. For example, white blood cells or bacteria in the cerebrospinal fluid, which can make it appear cloudy, suggest an infection in the brain or spinal cord, such as meningitis, Lyme disease, or some other inflammatory disease.

High protein levels in the fluid often are a sign of a spinal cord tumor or an acute peripheral nerve disorder, such as a polyneuropathy or Guillain-Barré syndrome. Abnormal antibodies may suggest multiple sclerosis. Low glucose levels indicate an infection of the meninges or, in some cases, a cancer. Blood in the fluid may indicate a brain hemorrhage. A variety of diseases, including brain tumors and meningitis, can increase the fluid's pressure.

Computed Tomography

Computed tomography (CT) is a computer-enhanced scanning technique for analyzing x-ray pictures. A computer generates two-dimensional, high-resolution images that resemble anatomic slices of the brain or whatever organ is being imaged. A person must lie still during the procedure but experiences no discomfort. With CT, doctors can detect a wide range of brain and spinal abnormalities with such precision that the technique has revolutionized the practice of neurology and has greatly improved the quality of neurologic care. CT is used not only to diagnose neurologic disease but also to monitor the progress of treatment.

Magnetic Resonance Imaging

Magnetic resonance imaging (MRI) of the brain or spinal cord is performed by placing a person's head or entire body in a confined space and generating a very powerful magnetic field that produces exquisitely detailed anatomic images. No x-rays are involved, and MRI is extremely safe.

MRI is better than CT for detecting certain serious problems, such as previous strokes, most brain tumors, abnormalities of the brain stem and cerebellum, as well as multiple sclerosis. Sometimes a contrast agent (a substance that shows up clearly on an MRI image) is injected into a person's veins to further enhance the images. Newer MRI models can measure how the brain functions by special computer processing of the MRI images.

The major disadvantages of MRI are its expense and the time it takes (usually 10 to 45 minutes) to perform a procedure. MRI can't be used with people who are dependent on respirators, who are prone to severe claustrophobia, or who have a cardiac pacemaker or metallic clips or prostheses.

Echoencephalography

Echoencephalography creates an ultrasound image of the brain in children under 2 years of age. The procedure is simple, painless, and relatively inexpensive. It can be performed at the bedside to detect bleeding or enlargement of the chambers inside the brain (hydrocephalus). For older children and adults, CT or MRI scanning has replaced echoencephalography.

▲ see box, page 374

Positron Emission Tomography

Positron emission tomography (PET) uses positron emitters, special types of radioisotopes, to obtain images of the brain's inner structures and information about their function. A substance injected into the bloodstream works its way into brain structures to measure activity in the brain. For example, the technique may reveal which part of the brain is most active when a person is performing mathematical calculations. PET scanning can also provide information about epilepsy, brain tumors, and strokes. It is used mainly in research.

Single Photon Emission Computed Tomography

Single photon emission computed tomography (SPECT) uses radioisotopes to obtain general information about blood flow and metabolic function in the brain. The radioisotopes are inhaled or injected and then delivered to the brain by the blood. Once there, the intensity of the radioisotopes in different brain regions reflects the rate of blood flow or the density of functioning neurotransmitter receptors, which attract the radioisotopes. The technique isn't as accurate or specific as positron emission tomography.

Cerebral Angiography

Cerebral angiography (arteriography) is a technique used to detect blood vessel abnormalities in the brain, such as a bulge in an artery (aneurysm), an inflammation (arteritis), an abnormal configuration (arteriovenous malformation), or a blocked blood vessel (stroke). A radiopaque dye, a substance visible on x-rays, is injected into an artery that supplies the brain. The dye shows the brain's blood flow patterns on x-rays. MRI images also can be modified to show the blood flow patterns of arteries in the neck and at the base of the brain, but the images are less detailed than those of cerebral angiography.

Doppler Ultrasound Scanning

Doppler ultrasound scanning is used mainly to measure blood flow through the carotid arteries or through the arteries at the base of the brain to assess a person's risk of having a stroke. The technique displays different rates of blood flow in different colors on a monitor. Doppler ultrasound scanning is a painless technique that can be performed at the bedside and is relatively inexpensive.

Myelography

Myelography is a technique in which a CT or x-ray image of the spinal cord is taken after injection of a radiopaque dye, a substance that shows up on the image. Myelography can show abnormalities within the spinal column, such as a herniated disk or a cancerous growth. Extremely clear images are obtained when a CT scan is used. Most myelography has been replaced by MRI, which shows greater detail, is simpler, and is safer.

Electroencephalography

Electroencephalography (EEG) is a simple, painless procedure in which 20 wires (leads) are pasted on the scalp to trace and record the brain's electrical activity.▲ Recordings in the form of wave patterns help identify epilepsy and sometimes certain rare metabolic brain diseases. In some cases, such as epilepsy that is difficult to detect, a recording is made over a 24-hour period. Otherwise the test provides little specific information.

Evoked Responses

Evoked responses are indications of the brain's response to certain stimuli. Sight, sound, and touch each stimulate specific areas of the brain. For example, a flashing light stimulates the back part of the brain where vision is perceived. Normally, the brain's response to a stimulus is too slight to be picked up on an EEG, but responses to a series of stimuli can be averaged by a computer to show that the stimuli were received by the brain. Evoked responses are particularly useful if the person being tested can't talk. For example, a doctor can test an infant's hearing by checking for a brain response after a noise.

Evoked responses may reveal slight damage to the optic nerve (the nerve to the eyes) in a person with multiple sclerosis. In a person with epilepsy, they may also reveal abnormal electrical discharges triggered by deep and rapid breathing or by watching a flashing light.

Electromyography

Electromyography is a technique in which small needles are inserted into a muscle to record

---

▲ see box, page 348

the muscle's electrical activity. The activity is displayed on an oscilloscope and heard through a loudspeaker. Normal resting muscle produces no electrical activity. However, even a slight muscular contraction produces some electrical activity, which increases as the contraction grows stronger. In muscular, peripheral nerve, and spinal motor neuron diseases, the electrical activity is abnormal.

The speed at which motor nerves conduct impulses can be measured with nerve conduction studies. A motor nerve is stimulated with a small charge of electricity to trigger an impulse. The impulse moves along the nerve, eventually reaching the muscle and causing it to contract. By measuring the time the impulse takes to reach the muscle, a doctor can calculate the impulse speed.

Similar measurements can be made for sensory nerves. If muscle weakness is caused by a muscular disease, the nerve conduction speed remains normal. If muscle weakness is caused by a neurologic disease, the nerve conduction speed is usually slowed.

The weakness experienced by people who have myasthenia gravis ▲ is caused by a defect at the point where the nerve impulse crosses a synapse to the muscle. Repeated impulses sent along the nerve to the muscle lead to increasing resistance to the neurotransmitters at the synapse, resulting in a progressively weaker response over time.

CHAPTER 61

Pain

Pain is an unpleasant sensation signaling that the body is damaged or threatened with an injury.

Pain begins at special pain receptors scattered throughout the body. These pain receptors transmit messages as electrical impulses along nerves to the spinal cord and then upward to the brain. Sometimes the signal evokes a reflex response when it reaches the spinal cord; when this happens, a signal is immediately sent back along motor nerves to the original site of the pain, triggering the muscles to contract. An example of a reflex response is the immediate pull-away reaction upon inadvertently touching something very hot. The pain signal is also relayed to the brain. Only when the brain processes the signal and interprets it as pain does a person become consciously aware of it.

Pain receptors and their nerve pathways differ in different parts of the body. Because of this, pain sensation varies with the type and location of injury. For example, pain receptors in the skin are plentiful and capable of transmitting precise information, such as where an injury is located and whether the cause was sharp such as a knife wound or dull such as pressure, heat, or cold. In contrast, pain signals from the intestine are limited and imprecise. The intestine can be pinched, cut, or burned without generating a pain signal. However, stretching and pressure can cause severe intestinal pain, even from something as relatively harmless as a trapped gas bubble. The brain can't identify the precise source of intestinal pain; rather, the pain is difficult to locate and is likely to be felt over a large area.

Pain felt in some areas of the body may not accurately represent where the trouble is, because pain can be *referred* to another area. Referred pain happens because signals from several areas of the body often lead into the same nerve pathways going to the spinal cord and brain. For example, pain from a heart attack may be felt in the neck, jaws, arms, or abdomen, and pain from a gallbladder attack may be felt in the shoulder.

People differ remarkably in their ability to tolerate pain. One person may find the pain of a small cut or bruise intolerable, while another person can tolerate a major accident or knife wound with little complaint. Ability to withstand pain varies

▲ see page 333

according to mood, personality, and circumstance. In a moment of excitement during an athletic match, an athlete may not notice a severe bruise but will likely be very aware of the pain after the match, particularly if the team lost.

Pain may even change with age. As people age, they complain less of pain, perhaps because changes in the body decrease the sensation of pain. On the other hand, the elderly may simply be more stoic than younger people.

Evaluation of Pain

Pain may be sharp or dull, intermittent or constant, throbbing or consistent, at a single site or all over. Some pains are very difficult to describe in words. The intensity can vary from minor to intolerable. No laboratory test can prove the presence or severity of pain.

A doctor asks about the history of the pain to fully understand its characteristics. Sometimes a scale of 0 (none) to 10 (severe) is used to help people describe their pain. For children, drawings of faces in a series—from smiling to frowning and crying—serve the same purpose. Doctors always try to determine both the physical and psychologic causes of pain. Many chronic diseases (such as cancer, arthritis, or sickle cell anemia) and acute disorders (such as wounds, burns, torn muscles, broken bones, sprained ligaments, appendicitis, kidney stones, or a heart attack) cause pain. Yet, psychologic illness (such as depression and anxiety) can also cause pain, called psychogenic pain. Psychologic factors may also make the pain of a physical injury appear more or less intense. A doctor must consider these issues.

Doctors also consider whether pain is acute or chronic. **Acute pain** is pain that begins suddenly and usually doesn't last long. When severe, it may cause a rapid heartbeat, increased breathing rate, elevated blood pressure, sweating, and dilated pupils. **Chronic pain** is pain that lasts for weeks or months; the term usually describes pain that persists for more than 1 month beyond the usual course of an illness or injury, pain that recurs off and on over months or years, or pain that's associated with a long-term disease such as cancer. Chronic pain usually doesn't affect the heartbeat, breathing rate, blood pressure, or pupils, but it may disturb sleep, decrease appetite, and cause constipation, weight loss, loss of interest in sexual activity, and depression.

Phantom Limb Pain

A good example of neuropathic pain is phantom limb pain, in which someone who has lost an arm or leg senses pain in the missing limb. Clearly, the pain can't be caused by something in the limb; rather, it must be caused by the nerves above the site where the limb was amputated. The brain misinterprets the nerve signals as coming from the amputated limb.

Types of Pain

People suffer many different types of pain. Some of the major types include neuropathic pain, pain after surgery, cancer pain, and pain related to psychologic disorders. Chronic pain is also a major aspect of many diseases, such as arthritis, sickle cell anemia, inflammatory bowel disease, and AIDS.

Neuropathic Pain

Neuropathic pain is caused by an abnormality anywhere in a nerve pathway. An abnormality disrupts nerve signals, which are then abnormally interpreted in the brain. Neuropathic pain may cause a deep ache or burning sensation and other sensations such as hypersensitivity to touch.

Infections, such as herpes zoster▲ (shingles), can inflame nerves and produce **postherpetic neuralgia,** a chronic, burning type of neuropathic pain that continues in the area infected with the virus.

Reflex sympathetic dystrophy is a type of neuropathic pain in which pain is accompanied by swelling and sweating or changes in local blood flow or by changes in the tissues, such as atrophy or osteoporosis. Stiffening (contractures) of the joints makes them unable to bend or straighten completely. Similar to reflex sympathetic dystrophy is a syndrome called **causalgia,** which may follow an injury or disease of a major nerve. As with reflex sympathetic dystrophy, causalgia produces severe, burning pain along with swelling,

▲ see page 918

sweating, changes in blood flow, and other effects. The diagnosis of reflex sympathetic dystrophy or causalgia is important because some people will be helped dramatically by treatment with a special nerve block, called a sympathetic nerve block. This treatment isn't usually considered for other disorders.

Pain After Surgery

Almost everyone experiences pain after surgery. The pain is often both constant and intermittent, getting worse when the person moves, coughs, laughs, or breathes deeply or when the dressings over the surgical wound are changed.

Usually, opioid (narcotic) analgesics are prescribed after surgery. They are most effective when taken every few hours before pain becomes severe. The dose may be increased or supplemented with an additional drug if the pain temporarily worsens, if the person needs to exercise, or if the wound dressing is about to be changed. Too often, exaggerated concern about the addiction potential of opioids leads to pain being undertreated, but adequate doses should be taken as needed.

Nursing staff and family members must be vigilant for side effects of opioids, such as nausea, sedation, and confusion. When the pain eases, doctors reduce the dose and prescribe nonopioid analgesics such as acetaminophen.

Cancer Pain

Cancer can cause pain in several ways. The tumor can grow into bones, nerves, and other organs, causing mild discomfort or severe, unrelenting pain. Some cancer treatments, such as surgery and radiation therapy, can also cause pain. People with cancer often fear pain, yet patients and doctors too often avoid adequate doses of analgesics because of unfounded fears about addiction. Cancer pain can and should be controlled.

Whenever possible, pain is best relieved by treating the cancer. Pain may decrease when a tumor is removed by surgery or shrunk by radiation. However, other pain relief is generally needed.

Nonopioid drugs, such as acetaminophen or nonsteroidal anti-inflammatory drugs, often work well. If they don't, the doctor may prescribe an opioid analgesic. The longer-acting opioids are prescribed more often because they provide more hours of relief between doses and generally allow a better night's sleep.▲

Whenever possible, opioids are taken orally. Some people, such as those who can't tolerate oral drugs, are given opioids by another route, such as through the skin or a vein. Injections can be given every few hours, but repeated injections can become annoying. Multiple needle sticks can be avoided by using a continuous-infusion pump, which is connected to a catheter that has been placed in a vein or under the skin. The constant infusion can be supplemented with extra doses when needed. Sometimes the person can control release of the drug by pressing a button. In unusual circumstances, opioids can be administered directly into the spinal fluid through a pump, which provides high concentrations of drug to the brain.

Over time, some people need increasing doses of opioids to control pain because the cancer grows bigger or because they develop drug tolerance. Yet, people with cancer shouldn't fear that the drug will stop working. They also shouldn't fear becoming addicted. If the cancer is cured, most people will be able to withdraw from the opioid without serious difficulty. If the cancer can't be cured, being free of pain is essential.

Pain Related to Psychologic Disorders

Pain is usually caused by disease, so doctors search first for a treatable cause. Some people have persistent pain without evidence of a disease that would cause the pain. Many others have a degree of pain and disability out of proportion to what most people with a similar injury or disease experience. Psychologic processes often account for at least part of these complaints. The perceived pain may be predominantly psychogenic in origin, or it may be caused by a physical disorder and exaggerated in degree or duration because of psychologic stresses. Most often, psychologically produced pain appears as a headache, low back pain, facial pain, abdominal pain, or pelvic pain.

The fact that the pain stems (in part or entirely) from psychologic causes doesn't mean that it's

---

▲ see box, page 292

not real. Psychogenic pain requires treatment, sometimes by a psychiatrist. As with other kinds of treatment for chronic pain, the treatment for this type of pain varies from person to person, and a doctor will try to match the treatment with the person's needs. Some people are given treatment that emphasizes rehabilitation and psychologic therapies. Other people are given various types of drugs or other treatments.

Other Types of Pain

Some diseases, such as AIDS, can cause pain as severe and unrelenting as cancer. The treatment of pain related to these diseases is virtually identical to that of cancer.

Other disorders may or may not be progressive and have pain as the major problem. Arthritis, which may be caused by wear and tear on joints (osteoarthritis) or by a specific disease (such as rheumatoid arthritis), is one of the most common types of pain. A doctor may try to relieve arthritis pain with drugs, exercise, and other approaches while considering treatments for the underlying disease.

A pain is called idiopathic, meaning the cause is unknown, if doctors find no evidence of either a disease or a psychologic cause.

Treatment of Pain

Several types of analgesics (pain relievers) can help alleviate pain. These drugs fall into three categories: opioid (narcotic) analgesics, nonopioid analgesics, and adjuvant analgesics. Opioid analgesics are the most powerful pain relievers and are the mainstay for treating severe pain because they are so effective.

Opioid Analgesics

Opioid analgesics are all chemically related to **morphine,** a natural substance extracted from poppies, although some are extracted from other plants and others are produced in a laboratory. Opioid analgesics are very effective in controlling pain but have many side effects. With time, a person using them may need higher doses. In addition, before the long-term use of opioid analgesics can be stopped, the dose must be gradually tapered to minimize the development of withdrawal signs. Despite these drawbacks, people with se-

vere pain shouldn't avoid opioids. Using these drugs appropriately helps to avoid side effects.

Different opioid analgesics have different advantages and disadvantages. Morphine, the prototype of these drugs, is available in an injectable form, an oral form, and a sustained-release oral form. The sustained-release form provides relief for 8 to 12 hours and is widely used to treat chronic pain.

Opioid analgesics often cause constipation, especially in older people. Laxatives, usually stimulant laxatives such as senna or phenolphthalein, help prevent or treat constipation.

People who must take high doses of opioids often become sleepy. For some this sleepiness is welcome, but for others it's unwanted. Stimulant drugs, such as methylphenidate, can help keep a person awake and alert.

Sometimes people with pain feel nauseated, and opioid analgesics can increase the nausea. Antiemetic drugs taken by mouth, by suppository, or by injection help prevent or relieve nausea. Some commonly used antiemetics are metoclopramide, hydroxyzine, and prochlorperazine.

Too much of an opioid can cause serious reactions, including a dangerous slowing of breathing and even coma. These effects can be reversed with naloxone, an antidote given intravenously.

Nonopioid Analgesics

All of the nonopioid analgesics except acetaminophen are **nonsteroidal anti-inflammatory drugs (NSAIDs).** These drugs work in two ways: First, they interfere with the prostaglandin system, a system of interacting substances partially responsible for the sensation of pain. Second, most of these drugs reduce inflammation, swelling, and irritation that often surround a wound and worsen pain.

Aspirin, the prototype NSAID, has been used for about 100 years. It was first extracted from the bark of the willow tree. Only recently have scientists understood how aspirin works.▲ Aspirin is taken orally and provides 4 to 6 hours of moderate pain relief. It does have side effects, however. Aspirin can irritate the stomach, leading to peptic

▲ see page 55

Opioid Analgesics

Drug	Length of Effectiveness	Other Information
Morphine	Intravenous or intramuscular—2 to 3 hours By mouth—3 to 4 hours Sustained release—8 to 12 hours	Starts to work quickly. Oral form can be very effective for cancer pain
Codeine	By mouth—3 to 4 hours	Less potent than morphine. Sometimes taken with aspirin or acetaminophen
Meperidine	Intravenous or intramuscular—about 3 hours By mouth—not very effective	Can cause seizures, tremors, and muscle spasms
Methadone	By mouth—4 to 6 hours, sometimes longer	Also used for treating heroin withdrawal
Propoxyphene	By mouth—3 to 4 hours	Generally taken with aspirin or acetaminophen to treat mild pain
Levorphanol	Intravenous or intramuscular—4 hours By mouth—about 4 hours	Oral form is strong. Can be used instead of morphine
Hydromorphone	Intravenous or intramuscular—2 to 4 hours By mouth—2 to 4 hours Rectal suppository—4 hours	Begins to work quickly. Can be used instead of morphine. Helpful for cancer pain
Oxymorphone	Intravenous or intramuscular—3 to 4 hours Rectal suppository—4 hours	Starts to work quickly
Oxycodone	By mouth—3 to 4 hours	Usually combined with aspirin or acetaminophen
Pentazocine	By mouth—up to 4 hours	Can block painkilling action of other opioids. About as strong as codeine. Can cause confusion and anxiety, especially in the elderly

ulcers. By affecting the blood's ability to clot, aspirin also makes bleeding throughout the body more likely. In very high doses, aspirin can cause serious side effects such as abnormal breathing. One of the first signs of overdose is ringing in the ears (tinnitus).

The many NSAIDs available vary in how quickly they work and how long they relieve pain. Although they are about equally effective, people respond to NSAIDs differently, and one person may find a particular drug to be more effective or have fewer side effects than another.

▲ see page 1324

All NSAIDs can irritate the stomach and cause peptic ulcers, but most are less likely to do so than aspirin. Taking NSAIDs with food and using antacids may help prevent stomach irritation. The drug misoprostol can help prevent stomach irritation and peptic ulcers, but it can cause other problems, including diarrhea.

Acetaminophen is somewhat different from aspirin and the NSAIDs. It also works on the prostaglandin system but at a different point. Acetaminophen doesn't affect the blood's ability to clot and doesn't lead to peptic ulcers or bleeding. Acetaminophen is taken by mouth or suppository, and its effects generally last 4 to 6 hours. Very high doses can cause dangerous side effects, such as liver damage.▲

Adjuvant Analgesics

Adjuvant analgesics are drugs that are usually given for reasons other than pain but may relieve pain in certain circumstances. For example, some antidepressants are also nonspecific pain relievers and are used to treat many kinds of chronic pain, including low back pain, headaches, and neuropathic pain. Antiseizure drugs such as carbamazepine and oral local anesthetics such as mexiletine are used to treat neuropathic pain. Many other drugs are adjuvant analgesics, and a doctor may suggest repeated trials of different drugs for people who have poorly controlled chronic pain.

Local and Topical Anesthetics

Local anesthetics can be placed directly on or near a sore area to help reduce pain. For example, a doctor may inject a local anesthetic into the skin before performing minor surgery. The same technique can be used to control pain from an injury. When chronic pain is caused by an injury to a single nerve, a doctor may be able to inject a chemical directly into the nerve to permanently stop the pain.

Topical anesthetics, such as a lotion or ointment containing lidocaine, can be used to control the pain of some conditions. For example, certain topical anesthetics mixed in a mouthwash can relieve a sore throat.

A cream containing capsaicin, a substance found in hot peppers, is sometimes helpful in reducing the pain caused by herpes zoster, osteoarthritis, and other conditions.

Nondrug Pain Treatments

In addition to drugs, many other treatments can help relieve pain. Often, treating the underlying disease eliminates or minimizes the pain. For example, simply setting a broken bone in a cast or giving antibiotics for an infected joint helps reduce pain.

Treatments applied directly to the pain, such as **cold and warm compresses,** often help. Some new techniques may relieve chronic pain. **Ultrasound** provides deep heating and may relieve the pain of torn or damaged muscles and inflamed ligaments. With **transcutaneous electrical nerve stimulation (TENS),** a gentle electric current is applied to the skin's surface; some people find that this relieves pain.

Nonsteroidal Anti-inflammatory Drugs

Aspirin	Meclofenamate
Choline magnesium trisalicylate	Nabumetone
	Naproxen
Diclofenac	Oxaprozin
Diflunisal	Phenylbuta-
Fenoprofen	zone
Flurbiprofen	Piroxicam
Ibuprofen	Salsalate
Indomethacin	Sulindac
Ketoprofen	Tolmetin

Inflammation is the body's protective response to an injury. The blood supply to the injured area increases, which brings in fluids and white blood cells to wall off the damaged tissue and clean up the area. This process causes the swelling, redness, heat, tenderness, and pain of inflammation. Nonsteroidal anti-inflammatory drugs (NSAIDs) interrupt inflammation, decreasing these symptoms. Both NSAIDs and acetaminophen directly reduce pain and fever.

With **acupuncture,** tiny needles are inserted into specific areas of the body. The mechanisms by which acupuncture works are poorly understood, and some experts still doubt the technique's effectiveness. Yet, many people find substantial relief with acupuncture, at least for a time.

Biofeedback and other cognitive techniques (such as hypnosis or distraction) can help people relieve pain by changing the way they focus their attention. These techniques train people to control pain or reduce its impact.

The importance of **psychologic support** for people in pain shouldn't be underestimated. Because people in pain suffer, they should be watched carefully for signs of depression and anxiety that might require help from a mental health professional.

CHAPTER 62

Headaches

Headaches are among the most common medical problems. Some people have headaches often, while others hardly ever have them. Both chronic and recurring headaches may be painful and distressing but rarely reflect a serious medical condition. However, a change in the pattern or nature of headaches—for instance, from rare to frequent, or from mild to severe—could signal a serious problem and calls for prompt medical attention.

Most headaches are muscle tension headaches, migraines, or head pain with no obvious cause. Many headaches are related to problems with the eyes, nose, throat, teeth, and ears. Most chronic headaches attributed to eyestrain are actually tension headaches; a new, severe pain in or around the eyes may signal high fluid pressure (glaucoma) in the eye and is a medical emergency.▲ Consulting an ophthalmologist may lead to identifying the cause of and obtaining treatment for this type of pain. High blood pressure may produce a throbbing sensation in the head, but high blood pressure rarely causes chronic headaches.

Usually a doctor can determine the cause of a headache from the patient's medical history and a physical examination. However, occasionally blood tests may be needed to detect an underlying illness. A lumbar puncture (spinal tap), in which a small amount of fluid is taken from the spinal column and examined under a microscope,■ is performed when a doctor suspects that the headaches are caused by an infection (for example, meningitis). A bacterial or fungal infection that inflames the meninges (the membrane that surrounds the brain and spinal cord) is a rare cause of a distinctive, usually acute and unrelenting headache. Such an infection is also marked by fever and other signs of serious illness. A lumbar

▲ see page 1049

■ see box, page 374

★ see page 380

puncture may also be performed if the doctor suspects bleeding into the meninges.

Only rarely are chronic headaches caused by brain tumors, brain injuries, or lack of oxygen to the brain. If the doctor suspects a tumor, stroke, or other problem with the brain, computed tomography (CT) scanning or magnetic resonance imaging (MRI) may be ordered to provide images of the brain.

Tension Headaches

Tension headaches are caused by muscle tension in the neck, shoulders, and head; muscle tension may result from an uncomfortable body position, social or psychologic stress, or fatigue.

Symptoms and Diagnosis

Tension headaches generally begin in the morning or early afternoon and worsen during the day. A steady, moderately severe pain often occurs above the eyes or in the back of the head; a feeling of tight pressure, like a band around the head, may accompany the pain. Pain may spread over the entire head and sometimes down into the back of the neck and shoulders.

To distinguish tension headaches from more serious disorders, a doctor considers how long the pain lasts as well as the patient's description of where the pain occurs, what brings it on, what relieves it, and whether other symptoms such as dizziness, weakness, loss of feeling, or fever accompany it. Headaches that began more recently, wake a person from sleep, are unusually severe, continue relentlessly, follow a head injury, or coincide with other symptoms such as tingling, weakness, loss of coordination, changes in vision, or fainting are probably not tension headaches. They may have a serious cause that should be promptly evaluated by a doctor. For example, headaches from a brain tumor or another problem are more likely to be of recent onset, have a steady progression, be worse in the morning than late in the day, be unrelated to fatigue or work, be accompanied by decreased appetite and nausea, and get better or worse when the person shifts position (lies down or gets up).★

How Headaches Differ

Type or Cause	Characteristics*	Diagnostic Tests
Muscle tension	Headaches occur frequently; pain is intermittent, moderate, and felt on front and back of head, or person has a general feeling of tightness or stiffness	Tests to rule out physical disease; evaluation of psychologic factors and personality
Migraine	Pain begins in and around eye or temple, spreads to one or both sides, usually affects whole head but may be one-sided, throbs, and is accompanied by loss of appetite, nausea, and vomiting Person has similar periodic attacks over extended period; attacks are often preceded by mood changes, loss of appetite, flickering-edged holes in vision; rarely, a person has weakness on one side of body; often runs in families	If diagnosis is in doubt and headache is recent, MRI or CT scan; otherwise, a migraine drug to see if it works
Cluster headache	Attacks are brief (1 hour); pain is severe and felt on one side of head; attacks occur episodically in clusters (with periods of no headaches) and mainly in males Person has the following symptoms on same side as pain: swelling below eye, runny nose, watery eyes	Migraine drugs to see if they work—for example, sumatriptan, methysergide—or vasoconstrictor drugs, corticosteroids, indomethacin, or oxygen inhalation
High blood pressure (hypertension)	Rare cause of headache, except in people with severe on and off hypertension from a tumor in the adrenal gland; pain is throbbing, occurs in spasms, and is felt in back or top of head	Blood chemistry analysis, kidney tests
Eye problems (iritis, glaucoma)	Pain is at front of head or in or over eyes, is moderate or severe, and is often worse after using eyes	Eye examination
Sinus problems	Pain is acute or subacute (not chronic), is felt at front of head, is dull or severe, and is usually worse in morning, improved in afternoon, and worse in cold, damp weather Person has a history of upper respiratory infection, pain in one part of face, stuffy or runny nose	X-ray of sinuses
Brain tumor	Pain is of recent onset, intermittent, and mild to severe; can be in one spot or over whole head Person may have slowly increasing weakness on one side of body, convulsions, visual changes, loss of speech, vomiting, mental changes	MRI or CT scan
Brain infection (abscess)	Pain is of recent onset, intermittent, and mild to severe; can be in one spot or over whole head Person may have previous ear, sinus, or lung infection or rheumatic or congenital heart disease	MRI or CT scan

(continued)

How Headaches Differ (Continued)

Type or Cause	Characteristics*	Diagnostic Tests
Infection in tissues around brain (meningitis)	Pain is of recent onset, constant, severe, and over whole head; travels down neck Person feels ill, with fever, vomiting, and preceding sore throat or respiratory infection; has difficulty bending neck to rest chin on chest	Blood tests, spinal tap
Accumulation of blood around brain		
Subdural hematoma	Pain is of recent onset, intermittent or constant, and mild to severe; can be in one spot or over whole head; travels down neck Person has had previous injury; may drift in and out of consciousness	MRI or CT scan
Subarachnoid hemorrhage	Pain is of sudden onset, widespread, severe, and constant; occasionally may be felt in and around one eye; eyelid droops	MRI or CT scan; if result is negative, spinal tap (lumbar puncture)
Syphilis Tuberculosis Cryptococcosis Sarcoidosis Cancer	Pain is dull to severe and felt over whole head or over top of head Person has moderate fever and history of syphilis, tuberculosis, cryptococcosis, sarcoidosis, or cancer	Spinal tap

*A person may have one, some, or all of the characteristics listed.

Treatment

Tension headaches can often be prevented or controlled by avoiding or understanding and adjusting to the stresses that bring them on. Once a headache begins, gently massaging the muscles of the neck, shoulders, and head; lying down and relaxing for several minutes; or using biofeedback may help relieve it.▲

For most headaches, almost any nonprescription analgesic such as aspirin, acetaminophen, or ibuprofen can provide fast, temporary relief. Severe headaches may respond to stronger, prescription analgesics, some of which contain narcotics (for example, codeine or oxycodone).■ Some people find that caffeine, an ingredient of some headache preparations, enhances the effect of analgesics. However, too much caffeine may induce headaches.

For headaches caused by chronic stress or depression, analgesics alone won't provide a cure because they don't treat the underlying psychologic problems. People who have headaches caused by unresolved social or psychologic conflicts may benefit from professional counseling.

Migraine Headaches

A migraine headache is a recurring, throbbing, intense pain that usually affects one side of the head but sometimes affects both sides; the pain begins suddenly and may be preceded or accompanied by visual, neurologic, or gastrointestinal symptoms.

Although migraine headaches can start at any age, they usually begin in people between ages 10 and 30. Sometimes they disappear after age 50. Migraines are more common in women than in men. The fact that more than half the people who

▲ see page 293

■ see box, page 292

have migraines have close relatives who also have them suggests that the tendency may be genetically transmitted. Migraine headaches are generally more severe than tension headaches.

Migraine headaches occur when arteries to the brain become narrow (constrict) and then widen (dilate), which activates nearby pain receptors. What causes the blood vessels to constrict and dilate isn't known, but abnormally low blood levels of serotonin, a chemical substance involved in nerve cell communication (neurotransmitter), may trigger the contractions. Rarely a blood vessel malformation may be the underlying cause of migraine headaches; in such instances, the headaches almost always occur on the same side. However, in most people, the headaches occur randomly on either side.

Symptoms and Diagnosis

No laboratory test is available to help diagnose migraines, but usually the headaches' distinct pattern makes them easy to identify.

Some 10 to 30 minutes before the headache begins (a period called the **aura** or **prodrome**), symptoms of depression, irritability, restlessness, nausea, or loss of appetite occur in about 20 percent of the people. A similar percentage of people lose vision in a specific area (called a blind spot or scotoma) or see jagged, shimmering, or flashing lights. Less commonly, images are distorted; for instance, objects appear smaller or larger than they are. Some people experience tingling sensations or, rarely, weakness in an arm or leg. Usually these symptoms disappear shortly before the headache begins, but sometimes they merge with it.

The pain of a migraine may be felt on either side of the head or over the entire head. Occasionally, the hands and feet may get cold and turn blue. In most of those who have a prodrome, the pattern and headache location remain the same with each migraine. Migraine headaches may occur frequently for long periods but then disappear for many weeks, months, or even years.

Prevention and Treatment

Migraine attacks may last for several hours or days if not treated. For some people, the headaches are mild and easily relieved with nonprescription analgesics. Quite often, migraine headaches are severe and temporarily disabling,

especially when they're accompanied by nausea, vomiting, and discomfort from bright light (photophobia). In this case, common analgesics usually don't relieve the headaches, which may relent only after a period of rest and sleep. Some people feel irritable during migraine attacks and seek seclusion, often in a dark room.

Because the headache and major symptoms of the migraine don't occur until after the constricted artery dilates, the prodrome provides a warning period during which drugs may prevent the headache. The most commonly used drug is ergotamine (a vasoconstrictor), which narrows blood vessels and thus helps prevent them from dilating and causing pain. Caffeine in high doses also helps prevent blood vessels from dilating and is often given in combination with analgesics or ergotamine. New drugs, such as eletriptan, naratriptan, rizatriptan, sumatriptan, and zolmitriptan, enhance the effects of serotonin, low blood levels of which are thought to bring on migraine attacks. These drugs are more effective than aspirin or acetaminophen in relieving migraine symptoms, but they are much more expensive. *Ergotamine and the new drugs can be dangerous and must not be used more often than prescribed.*

Some drugs taken every day may prevent migraine attacks from recurring. The beta-blocker propranolol provides long-term relief for about half the people who have frequent migraine headaches. The calcium channel blocker verapamil is effective for a few people. Recently, the antiseizure drug divalproex has been found to reduce the frequency of migraine headaches when taken daily. Methysergide is one of the most effective preventive drugs, but it must be taken intermittently because it can unpredictably cause a serious complication called retroperitoneal fibrosis—the formation of scar tissue deep within the abdomen, which can block blood supply to vital organs. Therefore, the use of this drug must be closely supervised by a doctor.

Cluster Headaches

Cluster headaches are an extremely painful but uncommon type of migraine headache.

Cluster headaches affect mostly men over 30 years old. Alcohol may bring on attacks, as can insufficient oxygen (for example, in high altitudes). An attack almost always starts suddenly and ends within an hour. It often starts with itching or watery discharge from one nostril that proceeds to intense pain on that side of the head and spreads around the eye. After the attack, the eyelid on the same side may droop, and the pupil often constricts. Attacks come in groups, ranging from two attacks a week to several a day. Most episodes of cluster headaches last for 6 to 8 weeks, and occasionally longer, followed by headache-free intervals of several months before the episodes recur.

Prevention and Treatment

Ergotamine, corticosteroids, or methysergide may prevent attacks. Sumatriptan injections bring prompt relief but do not prevent future episodes. During an attack, inhaling oxygen sometimes relieves the pain.

CHAPTER 63

Vertigo

Vertigo is a false sensation of moving or spinning or of objects moving or spinning, usually accompanied by nausea and loss of balance.

Some people use the word **dizziness** to describe light-headedness, a vague spaced-out feeling, faintness, or weakness, but only true dizziness—what doctors call vertigo—causes a sense of moving or spinning. Vertigo may last for only a few moments or may continue for hours or even days. A person with vertigo sometimes feels better when lying still; however, vertigo may continue even when a person isn't moving at all.

Causes

The body senses position and controls balance through organs of equilibrium located in the inner ear.▲ These organs have nerve connections to specific areas of the brain. Vertigo can be caused by abnormalities in the ear, in the nerves connecting the ear to the brain, or in the brain itself. Vertigo may also be related to vision problems or to sudden changes in blood pressure.

Many conditions can affect the inner ear and cause vertigo. These conditions include infection with bacteria or viruses, tumors, abnormal pressure, nerve inflammation, or toxic substances.

The most common cause of vertigo is motion sickness, which may develop in anyone whose inner ear is sensitive to particular motions, such as swaying or sudden stops and starts. Such people may feel especially dizzy in a moving car or a rocking boat.

Meniere's disease produces sudden, episodic attacks of vertigo, along with ringing in the ears (tinnitus) and progressive deafness.■ Episodes usually last from several minutes to several hours and are often accompanied by severe nausea and vomiting. The cause is unknown.

Viral infections affecting the inner ear (labyrinthitis) can cause vertigo that usually comes on suddenly and worsens over several hours. Within several days, the condition disappears without treatment.

The inner ear communicates with the brain by way of nerves. An area in the back part of the brain controls balance and equilibrium. When the blood supply to this area of the brain is inadequate (a condition called vertebrobasilar insufficiency), the person may have several neurologic symptoms, including vertigo.

Headaches, slurred speech, double vision, weakness of an arm or leg, and uncoordinated movements are usually signs that vertigo is caused by a neurologic brain disorder rather than a problem limited to the ear. Such brain disorders include multiple sclerosis, skull fractures, seizures, infections, and tumors (especially those

▲ see page 996

■ see page 1009

growing in or near the base of the brain). Because the body's ability to maintain balance is linked to visual cues, poor vision, especially double vision, can produce a loss of balance and equilibrium.

Older people or those taking drugs for heart disease or high blood pressure may get dizzy or black out when they stand up suddenly. This type of dizziness results from a brief fall in blood pressure (orthostatic hypotension),▲ usually lasts for only a few seconds, and can sometimes be prevented by standing slowly or wearing support stockings.

Diagnosis

Before dizziness can be treated, a doctor must determine its nature and then its cause. Is the problem uncoordinated gait, faintness, vertigo, or something else? Did it originate in the inner ear or somewhere else? Details about when the dizziness began, how long it lasted, what triggered or relieved it, and what other symptoms—headaches, deafness, noises in the ear, or weakness—were present help to pinpoint the nature of the problem. Most cases of dizziness are not vertigo, nor are they a serious symptom.

A person's eye movements may provide the doctor with important clues. Abnormal eye movements indicate a possible dysfunction of the inner ear or its nerve connections to the brain. Nystagmus is a rapid flitting of the eyes, as though the person were watching a ping-pong ball bounce quickly from right to left or up and down. Since the direction of these movements can help with the diagnosis, the doctor may try to stimulate nystagmus by suddenly moving the person's head or by putting a few drops of cold water into the ear canal. Balance may be tested by asking the person to stand still and then to walk a straight line, first with the eyes open and then with the eyes closed.

Some laboratory tests can help determine the cause of dizziness and vertigo. Hearing tests often reveal ear disorders that affect both balance and hearing. Additional tests may include x-rays and computed tomography (CT) or magnetic resonance imaging (MRI) scans of the head. These tests can show bone abnormalities or tumors pressing on nerves. If an infection is suspected, a doctor may take a sample of fluid from the ear or sinus or from the spine by lumbar puncture (spinal tap). If the doctor suspects that not enough blood is reaching the brain, an angiogram (in which a dye is injected into the bloodstream and x-rays are taken to locate blockages in the blood vessels) may be ordered.■

Common Causes of Vertigo

Environmental condition
• Motion sickness

Drugs
• Alcohol
• Gentamicin

Circulatory problem
• Transient ischemic attack (temporary disturbances in brain function caused by insufficient blood supply to parts of the brain for brief periods) affecting the vertebral and basilar arteries

Abnormalities in the ear
• Calcium deposits in one of the semicircular canals in the inner ear (causing benign paroxysmal positional vertigo)
• Bacterial infection of the inner ear
• Herpes zoster
• Labyrinthitis (viral infection of the labyrinth in the ear)
• Inflamed vestibular nerve
• Meniere's disease

Neurologic disorders
• Multiple sclerosis
• Skull fracture with injury to the labyrinth, its nerve, or both
• Brain tumors
• Tumor compressing the vestibular nerve

Treatment

Treatment depends on the underlying cause of the vertigo. Drugs that relieve mild vertigo include meclizine, dimenhydrinate, perphenazine, and scopolamine. Scopolamine, which is partic-

▲ see page 110

■ see page 287

ularly helpful in preventing motion sickness, can be applied as a skin patch that works for several days. All of these drugs may cause drowsiness, especially in elderly people. Scopolamine in the patch form tends to produce the least drowsiness.

Benign Paroxysmal Positional Vertigo

Benign paroxysmal positional vertigo is a common disorder in which vertigo begins suddenly and lasts less than a minute. A change in head position—usually occurring when a person lies down, gets up, turns over in bed, or tips the head backward to look up—triggers most episodes. The disorder appears to be caused by deposits of calcium debris in one of the semicircular canals in the inner ear that sense position.

This type of vertigo can be frightening, but it's harmless, usually subsiding on its own in weeks or months. A doctor can teach the person maneuvers that will gradually dissolve the debris in the posterior semicircular canal, providing relief without using drugs. The person experiences no hearing loss or ringing in the ear.

CHAPTER 64

Sleep Disorders

Sleep disorders are disturbances in falling asleep, staying asleep, or duration of sleep or abnormal sleep behaviors such as night terrors or sleepwalking.

Sleep is necessary for survival and good health, but why sleep is needed or exactly how it benefits people is not fully understood. Individual requirements for sleep vary widely; healthy adults may need as few as 4 hours or as many as 9 hours of sleep every day. Most people sleep at night, but many must sleep during the day to accommodate work schedules. This situation often leads to sleep disorders. Most sleep disorders are common.

How long a person sleeps and how rested a person feels on waking can be influenced by many factors, including excitement or emotional distress. Medications also can play a part; some medications make a person sleepy while others make sleeping difficult. Even some food elements or additives such as caffeine, strong spices, and monosodium glutamate (MSG) may affect sleep.

Average Daily Sleep Requirements

Age	Total Number of Hours	REM Sleep (percentage of total)	Stage 4 Sleep (percentage of total)
Newborn	13 to 17	50%	25%
2 years	9 to 13	30 to 35%	25%
10 years	10 to 11	25%	25 to 30%
16 to 65 years	6 to 9	25%	25%
Over 65 years	6 to 8	20 to 25%	0 to 10%

Stages of the Sleep Cycle

Sleep normally cycles through distinct stages five or six times during the night. Relatively little time is spent in deep sleep (stages 3 and 4). More time is spent in rapid eye movement (REM) sleep as the night progresses, but this stage is interrupted by brief returns to light sleep (stage 1). Brief awakenings occur throughout the night.

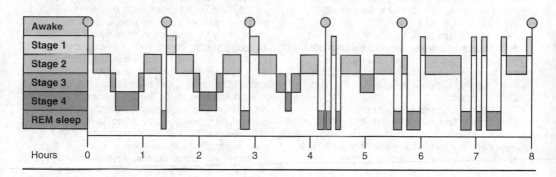

Sleep is not a uniform state; it has several distinct stages through which it normally cycles five or six times every night. Sleep progresses from stage 1 (the lightest level, during which the sleeper can be awakened easily) to stage 4 (the deepest level, during which waking the sleeper is difficult). In stage 4, the muscles are relaxed, the blood pressure is at its lowest, and the heart and breathing rates are at their slowest. Besides these four stages, there is a form of sleep accompanied by rapid eye movements (REM) and behavioral activity. During REM sleep, electrical activity in the brain is unusually high, somewhat resembling that of wakefulness. The eye movement and brain wave changes that accompany REM sleep can be recorded electrically on an electroencephalogram (EEG).

In REM sleep, the rate and depth of breathing increase, but the muscles are greatly relaxed—more so than during the deepest levels of non-REM sleep. Most dreaming occurs during REM and stage 3 sleep, while most talking during sleep, night terrors, and sleepwalking occur during stages 3 and 4. During a normal night's sleep, REM sleep immediately follows each of the five or six cycles of four-stage non-REM sleep, but it can occur at any of the stages.

Insomnia

Insomnia is difficulty in falling asleep or staying asleep or a disturbance in sleep that makes people feel as if they've had insufficient sleep when they awaken.

Insomnia isn't a disease—it's a symptom that has many different causes, including emotional and physical disorders and medication use. Difficulty in falling asleep is common among both the young and the old; it often occurs with emotional disturbances such as anxiety, nervousness, depression, or fear. Sometimes, people find it hard to fall asleep simply because their body and brain aren't tired.

As people get older, they tend to sleep less. Sleep stages also change: Stage 4 sleep becomes shorter and eventually disappears, and more awakenings occur during all stages. These changes, though normal, often make older people think they're not getting enough sleep. However, there's no proof that healthy older people need as much sleep as younger people or that they need sleep medications to remedy these normal, age-related changes.

An **early morning awakening** pattern is more common in the elderly. Some people fall asleep nor-

Sleep Medications: Not to Be Taken Lightly

Hypnotics (sedatives, minor tranquilizers, antianxiety drugs) are among the most commonly used drugs. Most are quite safe, but all can lose their effectiveness once a person becomes accustomed to them. Hypnotics may also produce withdrawal symptoms when use is discontinued. After more than a few days' use, discontinuing a hypnotic can make the original sleep problem worse (rebound insomnia) and increase anxiety. Doctors recommend reducing the dose slowly; complete withdrawal can take several weeks.

Most hypnotics require a doctor's prescription because they may be habit-forming or addictive, and overdose is possible. Hypnotics are particularly risky for the elderly and for people with breathing problems because they tend to suppress brain areas that control breathing. They also reduce daytime alertness, making driving or operating machinery hazardous. Hypnotics are especially dangerous when taken with alcohol, other hypnotics, narcotics, antihistamines, and antidepressants. All of these drugs cause drowsiness and can suppress breathing, making the combined effects more dangerous.

The most common and safest hypnotics are **benzodiazepines.** Because they don't decrease the total amount of REM sleep, they don't reduce dreaming. Some benzodiazepines remain in the body longer than others. The elderly, who can't metabolize and excrete drugs as well as younger people, may be more likely to experience daytime drowsiness, slurred speech, and falls. For this reason, doctors try to avoid prescribing long-acting benzodiazepines such as flurazepam, chlordiazepoxide, and diazepam.

Barbiturates, once the most commonly used hypnotics, and **meprobamate** aren't as safe as benzodiazepines. **Chloral hydrate** is relatively safe but is used much less often than benzodiazepines.

Some **antidepressants,** amitriptyline for instance, can relieve depression-associated insomnia or early morning awakening caused by panic attacks, but adverse effects can be a problem, especially in the elderly.

Diphenhydramine and **dimenhydrinate** are two inexpensive nonprescription (over-the-counter) drugs that can relieve mild or occasional sleeping problems, but they're not used primarily as sedatives and they have potential adverse effects, especially in the elderly.

mally but wake up several hours later and are unable to fall asleep again easily. Sometimes they drift in and out of a restless, unsatisfactory sleep. Early morning awakening at any age may be a sign of depression.

People whose sleep patterns have been disrupted may experience **sleep rhythm reversal:** They fall asleep at inappropriate times and then can't sleep when they should. These reversals often happen as a result of jet lag (especially when traveling from east to west), working irregular night shifts, frequent changes in work hours, or excessive alcohol use. Sometimes they're a side effect of medication. Damage to the brain's built-in clock (caused by encephalitis, stroke, or Alzheimer's disease, for example) can also disrupt sleep patterns.

Diagnosis

To diagnose insomnia, a doctor evaluates a person's sleep pattern; use of medications, alcohol, and illicit drugs; degree of psychologic stress; medical history; and level of physical activity. Some people need less sleep than others, so the diagnosis of insomnia is based on a person's individual needs. Doctors may classify insomnia as primary insomnia, a long-standing condition with little or no apparent relationship to any stress or life event, or secondary insomnia, a condition caused by pain, anxiety, medication, depression, or extreme stress.

Treatment

The treatment of insomnia depends on its cause and severity. Older people experiencing age-related sleep changes usually don't need treatment because the changes are normal. Since total sleeping time is likely to decrease with age, older people may find going to bed later or getting up earlier helpful. People with insomnia may benefit by staying calm and relaxed in the hour before bedtime and making the bedroom atmosphere conducive to sleep. Soft lighting, minimal noise, and a comfortable room temperature are necessary.

If emotional stress is causing the insomnia, treatment to relieve the stress is more useful than taking sleep medication. When insomnia occurs with depression, the depression should be thoroughly evaluated and treated by a doctor. Some antidepressant drugs can improve sleep because they have sedating properties.

When sleep disorders interfere with a person's normal activities and sense of well-being, the intermittent use of sleep medications (sedatives, hypnotics) may be helpful.

Hypersomnia

Hypersomnia is an increase in sleep by about one fourth of a person's regular sleep pattern.

Less common than insomnia, hypersomnia is a symptom that often indicates the possibility of a serious illness. Temporary hypersomnia may occur in healthy people for a few nights or days after a period of sustained sleep deprivation or unusual physical exertion. Hypersomnia that lasts for more than a few days may be a symptom of a psychologic disorder, such as severe anxiety or depression; overuse of hypnotic drugs; lack of oxygen and a buildup of carbon dioxide in the body as a result of sleep apnea; or a brain disorder. Chronic hypersomnia that begins at an early age may be a symptom of narcolepsy.

When excessive sleepiness is recent and sudden, the doctor asks about the person's mood, knowledge of current events, and any drugs the person may be taking. Since a disease may be the cause, the doctor examines the heart, lungs, and liver; laboratory tests can confirm the disease. Recent hypersomnia that can't be easily explained by a disease or excessive drug use may be caused by a psychiatric disorder (such as depression) or a neurologic problem (such as encephalitis, meningitis, or a tumor growing within the skull). A neurologic examination may point to depression, impaired memory, or abnormal neurologic signs. A computed tomography (CT) or magnetic resonance imaging (MRI) scan is ordered for a person who has signs of a neurologic problem, and the person is referred to a neurologist.

Narcolepsy

An uncommon sleep disorder, narcolepsy is marked by recurring, irrepressible attacks of sleep during normal waking hours, as well as by cataplexy, sleep paralysis, and hallucinations.

The cause of narcolepsy isn't known, but the disorder tends to run in families, suggesting a genetic predisposition. While narcolepsy has no serious medical consequences, it can be frightening and may increase the risk of accidents.

Symptoms

Symptoms usually begin in healthy adolescents or young adults and persist throughout life. A person with narcolepsy is overcome by sudden attacks of irrepressible sleepiness that can occur at any time. Falling asleep can be resisted only temporarily, but once asleep, the person usually can be easily aroused. A person may have many attacks in a single day or only a few, each usually lasting an hour or less. The attacks are most likely to occur in monotonous situations such as boring meetings or long periods of highway driving. The person may feel refreshed on awakening but may fall asleep again several minutes later.

A person with narcolepsy may become paralyzed momentarily without losing consciousness (a condition called **cataplexy**) in response to a sudden emotional reaction such as anger, fear, joy, laughter, or surprise. The person may become limp, may drop something being held, or may fall to the ground. The person may also have occasional episodes of **sleep paralysis;** when just falling asleep, or immediately on awakening, the person experiences a sense of wanting to move but is unable to do so. This experience can be terrifying. Vivid **hallucinations,** during which the person sees or hears things that aren't there, may occur at the beginning of sleep or, less often, on awakening. The hallucinations are similar to those of normal dreaming but more intense. Only about 10 percent of the people with narcolepsy have all of these symptoms; most have only a few.

Diagnosis

While the diagnosis is usually based on the symptoms, similar symptoms don't necessarily mean that a person has narcolepsy. Cataplexy, sleep paralysis, and hallucinations are all common in young children and occur occasionally in otherwise healthy adults. If a doctor is uncertain of the diagnosis, the person may be sent to a sleep study laboratory. An electroencephalogram (EEG), a recording of the brain's electrical activity, may show that REM-type sleep patterns occur as the person falls asleep, which is typical of narcolepsy. No structural changes in the brain have been noted, and no abnormalities have appeared in blood tests.

Treatment

Stimulant drugs, such as ephedrine, amphetamine, dextroamphetamine, and methylphenidate, may help relieve narcolepsy. The dose may need to be adjusted to prevent side effects such as jitteriness, overactivity, or weight loss, so doctors monitor patients closely when they begin drug treatment. Imipramine, an antidepressant drug, usually helps relieve cataplexy.

Sleep Apnea Syndromes

Sleep apnea is a group of serious sleep disorders in which a sleeping person repeatedly stops breathing (apnea) long enough to decrease the amount of oxygen in the blood and brain and to increase the amount of carbon dioxide.

Sleep apnea can be either obstructive or central. **Obstructive sleep apnea** is caused by a blockage in the throat or upper airway. **Central sleep apnea** is caused by a dysfunction in the part of the brain that controls breathing. Sometimes in obstructive sleep apnea, a combination of prolonged low levels of oxygen and high levels of carbon dioxide in the blood reduce the brain's sensitivity to these abnormalities, adding an element of central apnea to the problem.

Obstructive sleep apnea usually occurs in obese men, most of whom try to sleep on their back. The disorder is much less common in women. The obesity, perhaps in combination with aging body tissues and other factors, leads to narrowing of the upper airways. Tobacco smoking, excessive alcohol use, and lung diseases such as emphysema increase the risk of developing obstructive sleep apnea. A predisposition to sleep apnea—narrow throat and upper airways—may be inherited, affecting several members of a family.

Symptoms

Because symptoms occur during sleep, they must be described by someone who observes the person sleeping. The most common symptom is snoring associated with episodes of gasping, choking, pauses in breathing, and episodes of sudden awakening. In severe cases, people have repeated bouts of sleep-related obstructive choking, both at night and during the day. Eventually, these bouts interfere with daytime work and increase the risk of complications. Prolonged, severe sleep apnea can result in headaches, excessive daytime sleepiness, slowed mental activity, and eventually heart failure and pulmonary insufficiency, in which the lungs are unable to adequately provide oxygen and remove carbon dioxide.

Diagnosis

In its early stages, sleep apnea is often diagnosed on the basis of information provided by the person's sleep partner, who may describe loud snoring or gasping noises and frightened awakenings from sleep associated with choking, or worsening daytime fatigue. A confirmation of the diagnosis and an evaluation of its severity are best performed in a sleep study laboratory. Such analyses can help doctors distinguish between obstructive and central sleep apnea.

Treatment

For people with obstructive sleep apnea, quitting smoking, avoiding excessive use of alcohol, and losing weight are first steps. Heavy snorers and people who often choke in their sleep shouldn't take tranquilizers, sleep aids, and other sedating drugs. People with central sleep apnea are usually helped by an artificial breathing device used while sleeping. Changing the sleep position is important; people who snore are advised to sleep on their side or face down.

If such simple procedures don't eliminate sleep apnea, continuous positive airway pressure can be applied with a device worn like an oxygen mask that delivers a mixture of air and oxygen through the nose. Such a device keeps the airway open to assist regular breathing. Except for alcoholics, most people adapt quickly to these devices. Oral devices, made by dentists, can reduce apneas and snoring for many people.

Rarely, a person who has severe sleep apnea needs a tracheostomy, a surgical procedure that creates a permanent opening into the windpipe through the neck. Sometimes other surgical procedures are performed to widen the upper airway and alleviate the problem. However, such extreme measures are seldom needed and are usually performed by a specialist.

Parasomnias

Parasomnias are vivid dreams and physical activities that occur during sleep.

A variety of unconscious and largely unremembered movements can occur during sleep, more often in children than in adults. Just before falling asleep, almost all people occasionally experience brief, single, involuntary jerks of the entire body. Some people also experience sleep paralysis or brief hallucinations. During sleep, people normally have occasional leg jerks; adults may have furious teeth clenching, periodic movements, and nightmares. Sleepwalking, head-banging, night terrors, and nightmares are more common and very distressing in children. Epileptic seizures may occur in people of any age.

Restless legs (akathisia) is a relatively common disorder that often occurs just before falling asleep, particularly among people over age 50. Especially when they're under stress, people with akathisia have vaguely uncomfortable sensations in the legs, along with spontaneous, uncontrollable leg movements. The cause is unknown, but a family history of the disorder is found in a third or more of the people who have it. Benzodiazepine drugs taken at bedtime sometimes bring relief.

Night terrors are frightening episodes during which a person screams, flails about, and often sleepwalks. These episodes usually arise during non-REM phases of the sleep cycle. Treatment with benzodiazepines, such as diazepam, may be helpful.

Nightmares are vivid, frightening dreams that affect children and adults. The dreams are followed by sudden awakening. Nightmares occur during REM sleep and are more common during periods of stress, fever, or excessive fatigue or after alcohol consumption. No specific treatment is available.

Sleepwalking (somnambulism), most common in late childhood and adolescence, is walking in a semiconscious manner without being aware of it. People don't dream while sleepwalking—in fact, brain activity during sleepwalking, although abnormal, indicates more of a wakeful state than a sleeping one. Sleepwalkers may mumble repetitiously and can hurt themselves by walking into obstacles. Most sleepwalkers have no memory of sleepwalking.

No specific treatment is available for this sleep disorder, but the sleepwalker can be gently led back to bed. Leaving a light on in the bedroom or adjacent hall sometimes reduces the tendency to sleepwalk. Forcibly awakening the sleepwalker may provoke an angry reaction and is not advised. Obstacles or breakable objects in the sleepwalker's potential path should be removed, and low windows should be kept closed and locked.

CHAPTER 65

Muscle Weakness

Muscle weakness is a common problem, but it often means different things to different people. To some people, it means simply feeling tired or run down. With true muscle weakness, however, full effort doesn't generate normal strength. Weakness may involve the entire body, or it may be limited to an arm, a leg, or even a hand or finger. Although weakness can be caused by problems in the muscles, tendons, bones, or joints, most often muscle weakness is caused by problems in the nervous system. Some weakness always follows a period of disease and often occurs with aging (sarcopenia).

Causes of Muscle Weakness

Underlying Problem	Example	Major Consequences
Brain damage	Stroke or brain tumor	Weakness or paralysis on the side of the body opposite the brain damage. Speech, swallowing, personality, and thinking processes may be affected
Spinal cord damage	Trauma to the neck or back, spinal cord tumors, spinal canal narrowing, multiple sclerosis, transverse myelitis, vitamin B_{12} deficiency	Weakness or paralysis of the arms and legs below the level of injury, progressive loss of sensation below the level of injury, back pain. Bowel, bladder, and sexual function may be affected
Degeneration of nerves in the spinal cord	Amyotrophic lateral sclerosis	Progressive loss of muscle bulk and strength, but no loss of sensation
Spinal nerve root damage	Ruptured disk in the neck or lower spine	Pain in the neck and weakness or numbness in an arm, low back pain shooting down the leg (sciatica) and leg weakness or numbness
Damage to a single nerve (mononeuropathy)	Diabetic neuropathy, local pressure	Weakness or paralysis of muscles and loss of sensation in the area served by the injured nerve
Damage to many nerves (polyneuropathy)	Diabetes, Guillain-Barré syndrome, folate deficiency, other metabolic diseases	Weakness or paralysis of muscles and loss of sensation in the areas served by the affected nerves
Disease of the neuro-muscular junction	Myasthenia gravis, curare toxicity, Eaton-Lambert syndrome, insecticide poisoning	Paralysis or weakness of many muscles
Muscle disease	Duchenne's disease (muscular dystrophy)	Progressive muscle weakness throughout the body
	Infections or inflammatory disorders (acute viral myositis, polymyositis)	Muscles tender or painful and weak
Psychologic problems	Depression, imagined symptoms, hysteria (conversion reaction), fibromyalgia	Complaint of whole body weakness, paralysis with no evidence of nerve damage

Diagnosis

When doctors evaluate a person with muscle weakness, they look for clues to identify the cause of the problem, and they try to establish exactly which muscles are weak and how weak they are. The muscles are tested systematically, usually beginning with the face and neck, then the arms, and finally the legs. Normally, a person should be able to hold the arms extended for several minutes without their sagging or shaking. Inability to hold the arms steady may be a sign of weakness. Strength against resistance is tested by pushing or pulling while the doctor pushes and pulls in the opposite direction.

Functional testing—having a person perform various maneuvers while the doctor notes any deficiencies in the muscle groups involved—may also give clues to muscle weakness. For example, a doctor may check a person's ability to rise from a chair without using the arms, to squat and get up from a squatting position, to stand on the toes and heels, and to grip an object.

Doctors look for wasting away of muscle (atrophy), which can result from damage to either the muscle itself or its nerves. Muscle atrophy can also be caused by lack of use (disuse atrophy), as sometimes occurs from prolonged bed rest. Muscle enlargement (hypertrophy) normally occurs with exercise such as weight lifting. When a person is ill, hypertrophy results from one muscle working harder to compensate for the weakness of another. Muscles can also enlarge when normal muscle tissue is replaced by abnormal tissue, which occurs in amyloidosis and in certain inherited muscle disorders such as congenital myotonia.

During an examination, the doctor checks muscles for tenderness and texture. Normally, a muscle is firm but not hard, and smooth but not lumpy. Muscles are also checked for abnormal movements. Brief, fine, irregular muscle twitches visible just under the skin (fasciculations) usually indicate a nerve disease, although they sometimes develop in healthy people (especially when a person is nervous or cold) and commonly occur in the calf muscles of older people. A muscle's inability to relax (myotonia) usually indicates a problem with the muscle rather than with the nerves.

Getting to the Root of Muscle Weakness

Problem in the Nerves	Problem in the Muscles
Muscles may waste away but be stronger than they look	Muscles may be weaker than they look
Muscle twitches occur under the skin	Muscle twitches do not occur under the skin
Reflexes may be unexpectedly poor or missing altogether	Reflexes may be present even though muscles are very weak
Feeling may be lost in the general area of the muscle weakness	Sensations (such as touch and warmth) are normal, but muscles may be tender

A thorough neurologic examination helps to identify any abnormalities of sensation, coordination, fine motor movement, and reflexes.▲ Nerve studies, including measurements of nerve conduction, help determine if the nerves supplying the muscles are functioning normally. An electromyogram, a test in which electrical impulses from muscles are recorded, helps determine whether the muscles are normal. If the muscles are abnormal, an electromyogram can help distinguish between a primary nerve abnormality and a primary muscle abnormality.

If the problem lies in the muscle itself, the doctor may perform a muscle biopsy during which a small piece of muscle is removed and examined under a microscope. Blood tests may be used to measure the sedimentation rate of red blood cells, which may be elevated if inflammation is present, as well as the level of creatine kinase, a normal muscle enzyme that leaks out and is released into the bloodstream when muscle is damaged.

▲ see page 282

CHAPTER 66

Muscular Dystrophy and Related Disorders

Muscular dystrophies are a group of inherited muscle disorders that lead to muscle weakness of varying severity. Other inherited muscle disorders include myotonic myopathies, glycogen storage diseases, and periodic paralysis.

Duchenne's and Becker's Muscular Dystrophies

Duchenne's and Becker's muscular dystrophies— the most common muscular dystrophies—are diseases that cause weakness in the muscles closest to the torso.

The gene defect that causes Duchenne's muscular dystrophy is different from the one that causes Becker's muscular dystrophy, but both defects involve the same gene. The gene is recessive and is carried on the X chromosome.▲ While a female can carry the defective gene, she doesn't have the disease because the normal X chromosome compensates for the gene defect on the other X chromosome. However, any male who receives the defective X chromosome will have the disease.

Boys with Duchenne's muscular dystrophy lack almost totally the essential muscle protein, **dystrophin,** believed to be important for maintaining the structure of muscle cells. Of every 100,000 boys born, 20 to 30 have Duchenne's muscular dystrophy. Boys with Becker's muscular dystrophy produce dystrophin, but the protein is oversized and doesn't function properly. Becker's muscular dystrophy affects 3 of every 100,000 boys.

Symptoms

Duchenne's muscular dystrophy usually first occurs in boys between the ages of 3 and 7 as weakness in or around the pelvis. Weakness in the shoulder muscles usually follows and gets steadily worse. As the muscles weaken they also enlarge, but the abnormal muscle tissue isn't strong. In 90 percent of the boys with Duchenne's muscular dystrophy, the heart muscle also enlarges and weakens, causing problems with the heartbeat, which show up on an electrocardiogram.

Boys with Duchenne's muscular dystrophy generally waddle, fall often, have trouble climbing stairs, and have difficulty rising from a sitting position. The muscles of their arms and legs usually contract around the joints, so that the elbows and knees can't fully extend. Eventually, an abnormally curved spine (scoliosis) develops. By age 10 or 12, most children with the disease are confined to a wheelchair. The increasing weakness also makes them susceptible to pneumonia and other illnesses, and most die by the age of 20.

Though their symptoms are similar, boys with **Becker's muscular dystrophy** have a less severe illness. Symptoms first appear at about age 10. At age 16, very few are confined to a wheelchair, and more than 90 percent are still alive at age 20.

Diagnosis

Doctors suspect muscular dystrophy when a young boy becomes weak and grows weaker. An enzyme (creatinine kinase) leaks out of muscle cells, causing enzyme levels in the blood to be abnormally high. However, high blood levels of creatinine kinase don't necessarily mean that a person has muscular dystrophy; other muscle diseases may also cause elevated levels of this enzyme.

A doctor usually takes a muscle biopsy—in which a small piece of the muscle is removed for examination under a microscope—to be sure of the diagnosis. Under the microscope, the muscle generally shows dead tissue and abnormally large muscle fibers. In the late stages of muscular dystrophy, fat and other tissues replace the dead

---

▲ see box, page 11

muscle tissue. Duchenne's muscular dystrophy is diagnosed when special tests show extremely low levels of the protein dystrophin in the muscle. Tests to support the diagnosis include electrical studies of muscle function (electromyography) and nerve conduction studies.▲

Treatment

Neither Duchenne's nor Becker's muscular dystrophy can be cured. Physical therapy and exercise help prevent the muscles from contracting permanently around joints. Sometimes surgery is needed to release tight, painful muscles.

Prednisone, a corticosteroid drug, is being investigated as a means of temporarily relieving the muscle weakness. Also under investigation is gene therapy that would enable muscles to produce dystrophin.

Families with members who have either Duchenne's or Becker's muscular dystrophy are advised to consult a genetic counselor for help in evaluating the risk of passing the muscular dystrophy trait on to their children.

Other Muscular Dystrophies

Several much less common forms of muscular dystrophy, all inherited, also cause progressive muscle weakness.

Landouzy-Dejerine muscular dystrophy is transmitted by an autosomal dominant gene;■ therefore, only one abnormal gene can cause the disease, and the disease can appear in either males or females. Landouzy-Dejerine muscular dystrophy usually begins between the ages of 7 and 20. The facial and shoulder muscles are always affected, so that a person has difficulty raising the arms, whistling, or closing the eyes tightly. Some people with the disease also develop weakness in their lower legs, making it hard to bend the feet up at the ankle, which results in a footdrop (the foot flops down). The weakness of Landouzy-Dejerine muscular dystrophy is rarely severe, and people who have this disease have a normal life expectancy.

Limb-girdle muscular dystrophies cause weakness in the muscles of either the pelvis **(Leyden-Möbius muscular dystrophy)** or the shoulder **(Erb's muscular dystrophy)**. These inherited diseases usually don't appear until adulthood and rarely produce serious weakness.

Mitochondrial myopathies are muscle disorders inherited when faulty genes in mitochondria (the energy factories of cells) are passed down through the cytoplasm of the mother's egg. Mitochondria carry their own genes. Because sperm don't contribute mitochondria during fertilization, all mitochondrial genes come from the mother. Therefore, these diseases can never be inherited from the father. These rare disorders sometimes cause increasing weakness in only one muscle group, such as the eye muscles (ophthalmoplegia).

Diagnosis

Diagnosis requires taking a sample of the weak muscle tissue for biopsy and either examining it under a microscope or performing chemical tests on it. However, because specific treatments aren't available, a precise diagnosis of these less common forms of muscular dystrophy is rarely useful.

Myotonic Myopathies

Myotonic myopathies are a group of inherited disorders in which the muscles aren't able to relax normally after contraction, possibly leading to weakness, muscle spasms, and shortening of the muscles (contractures).

Myotonic dystrophy (Steinert's disease) is an autosomal dominant disorder affecting males and females. The disorder produces both weakness and tight, contracted muscles, especially in the hands. Drooping eyelids are also common. Symptoms can appear at any age and can range from mild to severe. People with the most severe form of the disease have extreme muscle weakness and many other symptoms including cataracts, small testes, premature balding, irregular heartbeats, diabetes, and mental retardation. They usually die by age 50.

Myotonia congenita (Thomsen's disease) is a rare autosomal dominant disorder that affects males and females. Symptoms usually start in infancy. The hands, legs, and eyelids become very stiff because of an inability to relax the muscles. Muscle weakness, however, is usually minimal. The

---

▲ see page 287

■ see page 9

diagnosis is made from the child's characteristic appearance, inability to relax the handgrip rapidly after opening and closing the hand, and prolonged contraction after the doctor taps a muscle. An electromyogram is needed to confirm the diagnosis. Thomsen's disease is treated with phenytoin, quinine, procainamide, or nifedipine to relieve muscle stiffness and cramping; however, all of these drugs have undesirable side effects. Regular exercise may be beneficial. People with Thomsen's disease have a normal life expectancy.

Glycogen Storage Diseases

Glycogen storage diseases are a related group of rare autosomal recessive inherited disorders in which muscles can't metabolize sugars normally, so they build up large stores of glycogen (a starch).

The most severe form of glycogen storage disease, **Pompe's disease,** usually begins in the first year of life. Glycogen accumulates in the liver, muscles, nerves, and heart, preventing them from functioning properly. The tongue, heart, and liver enlarge. Children with the disease are floppy as infants and become progressively weaker. They have difficulty swallowing and breathing. Pompe's disease can't be cured. Most infants with the disease die by age 2. Less severe forms of Pompe's disease can affect older children and adults, causing weakness of the arms and legs and diminished ability to breathe deeply.

People with other forms of glycogen storage disease suffer painful cramps and weakness, usually after exercise; these symptoms can range from very mild to severe. Avoiding exercise allows the symptoms to subside.

Damage to the muscles causes the protein myoglobin to be released into the blood. Because myoglobin is excreted in the urine, it can be measured with a urine test, which leads to the diagnosis of a glycogen storage disease. Myoglobin may harm the kidneys. The level of myoglobin is decreased by limiting exercise. Drinking plenty of water, especially after exertion, can dilute the level of myoglobin. When myoglobin levels are high, doctors may prescribe diuretics to prevent kidney damage. A liver transplant may help people with glycogen storage diseases other than Pompe's disease.

Periodic Paralysis

Periodic paralysis describes a group of rare related autosomal dominant inherited disorders that cause sudden attacks of weakness and paralysis.

During an attack of periodic paralysis, muscles don't respond to normal nerve impulses or even to artificial stimulation with an electronic instrument. Attacks are different from seizures because the person remains completely awake and alert. The precise form that the disease takes varies in different families. In some families, the paralysis is related to high levels of potassium in the blood (hyperkalemia); in others, the paralysis is related to low levels of potassium (hypokalemia).

Symptoms

On awakening the day after engaging in vigorous exercise, a person may feel some weakness in certain muscle groups or in the arms and legs. The weakness generally lasts 1 or 2 days. In the hyperkalemic form, the attacks often begin by age 10 and last 30 minutes to 4 hours. In the hypokalemic form, the attacks generally first appear during the 20s and always by age 30. They last longer and are more severe. Some people with the hypokalemic form are prone to attacks of paralysis the day after eating meals high in carbohydrates, but fasting also can precipitate attacks.

Diagnosis

A doctor's best clue to the diagnosis is a person's description of a typical attack. If possible, the doctor draws blood while an attack is in progress to check the level of potassium. Doctors usually check thyroid gland function and perform additional tests to be sure abnormal potassium levels in the blood aren't from other causes.

Prevention and Treatment

Acetazolamide, a drug that alters the blood's acidity, may prevent attacks that stem from either too much or too little potassium. People whose blood potassium levels drop during attacks can take potassium chloride in an unsweetened solution while the attack is in progress. Usually symptoms improve considerably within an hour.

Carbohydrate-rich meals and strenuous exercise should be avoided by those with the hypokalemic form of periodic paralysis. People with the hyperkalemic form can prevent attacks by eating frequent meals rich in carbohydrates and low in potassium.

CHAPTER 67

Movement Disorders

A movement as simple as raising a leg calls upon a complex communication system involving the brain, nerves, and muscles. When an area of the nervous system that regulates movement is damaged or abnormal, a person may experience any of a wide range of movement disorders.

Tremor

A tremor is an involuntary, rhythmic, shaking movement produced when muscles repeatedly contract and relax.

Everyone has some degree of tremor, called physiologic tremor, although in most people it is too slight to be noticed. Tremors are classified according to how fast and rhythmic the shaking is, where and how frequently it happens, and how severe it is. **Action tremors** occur when the muscles are active; **resting tremors** occur when the muscles are resting. Resting tremors can make an arm or leg shake even when a person is completely relaxed. These tremors may be a sign of Parkinson's disease.▲ **Intention tremors** occur when a person makes a purposeful movement. **Essential tremors** are tremors that usually begin in early adulthood, slowly become more obvious, and have no known cause. **Senile tremors** are essential tremors that begin in older people. Essential tremors that occur in families are sometimes called **familial tremors.**

Intention tremors may occur in people who have a disease of the cerebellum or its connections.■ Multiple sclerosis commonly causes this type of tremor. Other neurologic diseases, a stroke, or chronic alcoholism also can damage the cerebellum, resulting in intention tremors. These tremors may be present at rest and may increase with an activity, such as trying to maintain a posture or bringing the hand to a fixed target. Intention tremors are slower than essential tremors and involve broad, coarse movements.

Although essential tremors usually remain mild and don't indicate serious disease, they can become a nuisance. They can affect handwriting, can make it difficult to use utensils, and can be embarrassing. Emotional stress, anxiety, fatigue, caffeine, or stimulants prescribed by a doctor can intensify them. Many drugs, especially those for asthma and emphysema, can worsen an essential tremor. Although drinking alcohol in moderation may reduce the tremor in some people, heavy drinking and alcohol withdrawal can make the tremor worse.

Essential tremors generally stop when the arms or legs are at rest but become obvious when they are outstretched and may worsen when they are held in uncomfortable positions. The tremors are relatively fast, with little movement. Essential tremors may affect one side of the body more than the other but usually involve both sides. Sometimes the head trembles and bobs. If the vocal cords are affected, the voice shakes.

Diagnosis and Treatment

A doctor can usually distinguish an essential tremor from others. Sometimes laboratory tests show that a treatable condition such as an overactive thyroid gland is the cause.

Treatment usually isn't needed. Avoiding uncomfortable positions can help, as can using a firm, comfortable grip on objects and holding them close to the body.

Drugs may help people who have difficulty using utensils or who do work that requires steady hands. A beta-blocker such as propranolol is the drug most commonly prescribed; if it doesn't help, primidone is often tried. Brain surgery is reserved for severe, disabling tremors that do not respond to drugs.

Cramps

A cramp is a sudden, brief, usually painful contraction of a shortened muscle or group of muscles.

Cramps are common in healthy people, especially after vigorous exercise. Some people have leg cramps at night while sleeping. Cramps may be caused by inadequate blood flow to the muscles; for example, after eating, the blood flows primarily to the gastrointestinal tract rather than to the muscles. Cramps are usually harmless and

---

▲ see page 315

■ see page 281

don't need to be treated. They can usually be prevented by avoiding exercise after eating and stretching the muscles before exercising and sleeping.

Myoclonus

Myoclonus describes fleeting bursts of muscular excitation or relaxation, resulting in a synchronous quick jerk of the muscles involved.

Myoclonic jerks may affect most muscles at once, as commonly occurs when a person first falls asleep. They also may be confined to a single hand, a group of muscles in the upper arm or leg, or even a group of facial muscles. Multifocal myoclonus is caused by a sudden lack of oxygen to the brain, certain types of epilepsy, or degenerative late-life diseases.

If the myoclonic jerks are so severe that they require treatment, antiseizure drugs such as clonazepam or valproic acid are sometimes helpful.

Hiccups

Hiccups, a form of myoclonus, are repeated spasms of the diaphragm (the muscle that separates the chest from the abdomen), followed by quick, noisy closings of the glottis (the opening between the vocal cords that checks the flow of air to the lungs).

Hiccups can develop when a stimulus triggers the nerves that contract the diaphragm. The nerves involved may be those that lead to and from the diaphragm, or—because contraction of the diaphragm is responsible for each breath— they may be the nerves leading to and from the area in the brain that controls breathing.

Most bouts of hiccups are harmless. They begin suddenly, usually without an obvious cause, and they usually stop spontaneously after several seconds or minutes. Sometimes a bout of hiccups is triggered by swallowing hot or irritating food or liquids. Less common but more serious causes of hiccups include irritation of the diaphragm from pneumonia, chest or stomach surgery, or harmful substances in the blood (such as those that build up when a person has kidney failure). Rarely, hiccups develop when a brain tumor or stroke interferes with the breathing center in the brain. These more serious disorders may lead to long bouts of hiccups that are very hard to stop.

Treatment

Many home remedies have been used to cure hiccups. Almost all are based on the fact that when carbon dioxide accumulates in the blood, hiccups generally stop. Since holding the breath increases carbon dioxide in the blood, most cures for hiccups require holding the breath. Breathing into a paper bag also raises carbon dioxide levels. Because stimulating the vagus nerve that runs from the brain to the stomach may help, drinking water quickly or swallowing dry bread or crushed ice may stop the hiccups. Gently pulling on the tongue and *gently* rubbing the eyeballs are other ways to stimulate the vagus nerve. For most people with hiccups, any of these remedies will work.

Persistent hiccups require more intensive treatment. Several drugs have been used with varying success; they include scopolamine, prochlorperazine, chlorpromazine, baclofen, metoclopramide, and valproate. The very length of the list reflects the lack of consistent success.

Tourette's Syndrome

Tourette's syndrome is a disorder in which motor and vocal tics occur frequently throughout the day for at least one year.

Tourette's syndrome often begins with simple tics (repetitive, unwanted, purposeless, jerking muscle movements) in early childhood and progresses to bursts of complex movements, including vocal tics and sudden, spastic breathing. Vocal tics may start as grunting or barking noises and progress to compulsive, involuntary bouts of cursing.

Causes

Tourette's syndrome is a hereditary disorder that is three times more common in men than in women. The precise cause isn't known but is thought to be an abnormality in dopamine or other brain neurotransmitters (substances that nerve cells use to communicate).

Symptoms and Diagnosis

Many people have simple tics, such as repetitive eye blinks, that are nervous habits and may disappear with time. The tics in Tourette's syndrome are more complex than just a blink. A child with Tourette's syndrome may repeatedly move the head from side to side, blink the eyes, open the mouth, and stretch the neck. More complex tics include hitting and kicking, grunting, snorting, and humming. People with Tourette's syndrome may call out obscenities for no apparent reason, often in the midst of conversation. They may also repeat words immediately after hearing them (echolalia). Some people are able to suppress some of the tics, usually with difficulty; other people have trouble controlling the tics, especially during times of emotional stress.

People with Tourette's syndrome often have a difficult time in social situations. In the past, they were shunned, isolated, or even thought to be possessed by the devil. Many people with the disorder develop impulsive, aggressive, and self-destructive behaviors, and children often have difficulty in learning. Whether the disorder itself or the extraordinary stresses of living with the disorder cause these behaviors isn't known.

Treatment

Early diagnosis can help parents understand that the behaviors aren't voluntary or spiteful and that punishment can't stop them.

Antipsychotic drugs may help suppress the tics even though psychosis is not the problem. Haloperidol, the most commonly used antipsychotic drug, is effective but can cause side effects such as stiffness, weight gain, blurred vision, sleepiness, and dulled, slowed thinking. Side effects of pimozide, another antipsychotic drug, are usually less severe. Clonidine, which is not an antipsychotic, can help control anxiety and obsessive-compulsive behavior; its side effects are less severe than those of haloperidol and pimozide. Clonazepam is an antianxiety drug that has had limited success in the treatment of Tourette's syndrome.

Chorea and Athetosis

Chorea consists of repetitive, brief, jerky, large-scale, dancing-like, uncontrolled movements that start in one part of the body and move abruptly, unpredictably, and often continuously to another. Athetosis is a continuous stream of slow, sinuous, writhing movements, generally of the hands and feet. Chorea and athetosis can occur together (choreoathetosis).

Causes

Chorea and athetosis aren't diseases; rather they are symptoms that can result from several very different diseases. People with chorea and athetosis have abnormalities in the basal ganglia of the brain.▲ The basal ganglia's job is to smooth out the coarse movements that are initiated by commands from the brain. In most forms of chorea, an excess of the neurotransmitter dopamine in the basal ganglia disrupts its fine-tuning function. Drugs and illnesses that alter dopamine levels or the brain's ability to recognize dopamine can make chorea worse.

The disease that most often produces chorea and athetosis is **Huntington's disease,** but it is fairly rare, affecting fewer than 1 in 10,000 people. **Sydenham's disease** (also called St. Vitus' dance or Sydenham's chorea) is a complication of a childhood infection caused by certain streptococci; it can last for several months. Chorea sometimes develops in the elderly for no apparent reason and affects particularly the muscles in and around the mouth. It also can affect women in the first 3 months of pregnancy, but it disappears without treatment shortly after they give birth.

Treatment

Chorea that develops as a drug's side effect may improve if the drug is stopped, but the chorea doesn't always disappear. Drugs that block dopamine's action, such as antipsychotic drugs, may help control the abnormal movements.

Huntington's Disease

Huntington's disease (Huntington's chorea) is an inherited disease in which people in midlife begin having occasional jerks or spasms and gradual loss of brain cells, progressing to chorea, athetosis, and mental deterioration.

The gene for Huntington's disease is dominant; therefore, children of people who have this disease have a 50 percent chance of developing it. Because Huntington's disease begins subtly, the exact age of onset is difficult to determine. Symptoms usually begin between ages 35 and 40.

▲ see page 279

Genetic Testing for Huntington's Disease

The gene mutation that causes Huntington's disease has been identified. Of the 23 pairs of human chromosomes, chromosome 4 carries the defective gene; a person who has Huntington's disease carries the defective gene on one of the two copies of chromosome 4. But the crucial question is whether the normal or the abnormal chromosome 4 was passed on to a child— the odds are fifty-fifty.

People who have a parent with Huntington's disease can find out whether they have inherited the disease. Usually the DNA next to the Huntington's disease gene on the parent's abnormal chromosome 4 is different from the corresponding segment of DNA on the parent's normal chromosome 4. Blood tests can determine whether a person has inherited the neighboring DNA fragment from the abnormal or the normal chromosome 4. The odds are high that a person who has inherited the DNA next to the Huntington's disease gene has also inherited the defective gene. New tests make it possible to determine whether the Huntington's disease gene itself has been inherited.

Children with a parent who has Huntington's disease may or may not want to know whether they have inherited it. This issue should be discussed with an expert in genetic counseling.

Symptoms and Diagnosis

During the early stages of Huntington's disease, people can blend the spontaneous abnormal movements into intentional ones so that they're barely noticeable. However, with time, the movements become more obvious. Eventually, the abnormal movements involve the entire body so that eating, dressing, and even sitting still become nearly impossible. Distinct changes in the brain can be seen on a computed tomography (CT) scan.

▲ see page 279

Mental changes in Huntington's disease are subtle at first. People with the disease may gradually become irritable and excitable; they may lose interest in their usual activities. Later in the course of the disease, they may behave irresponsibly and often wander aimlessly. They may lose control over their impulses and become promiscuous. Over years or decades, they may lose their memory and the ability to think rationally. They may become severely depressed and attempt suicide. In advanced disease, almost all functions become impaired, and full-time assistance or nursing home care is needed. Death, often precipitated by pneumonia or a fatal falling injury, usually occurs 13 to 15 years after symptoms first appeared.

Treatment

Although drugs can help relieve symptoms and control behavior, no cure exists for Huntington's disease. For people with a family history of the disease, genetic counseling and testing can estimate their risk of passing the disease on to their children.

Dystonia

In dystonia, involuntary, slow, repetitive, sustained muscle contractions may cause "freezing" in the middle of an action, as well as twisting, turning, or torsion movements of the trunk, the entire body, or segments of the body.

Causes

Overactivity in several areas of the brain—the basal ganglia, thalamus, and cerebral cortex—seems to cause dystonia.▲ Most chronic dystonia has a genetic origin. Dystonia that isn't genetic in origin can be caused by a severe lack of oxygen to the brain either at birth or later in life. Dystonia can also be caused by Wilson's disease (a hereditary condition), certain metal poisons, and stroke. Sometimes dystonia can be an unusual reaction to antipsychotic drugs. In these cases, prompt administration of diphenhydramine by injection or by capsule usually stops the episode quickly.

Symptoms

Writer's cramp may be a form of dystonia. The symptom may involve a true involuntary cramping of the hand while writing, but it may be a more subtle deterioration of handwriting or an inability to hold a pen, rather than a cramp. Sometimes writer's cramp is the only symptom of dystonia, but half the people who have it develop a tremor of one or both arms and some develop generalized dystonia, which affects the whole body. Some dystonias are progressive—the movements may become more bizarre over time. Severe muscle contractions can force the neck and arms into odd, uncomfortable positions.

Golfers who have muscle spasms (yips) may actually be experiencing dystonia. Likewise, musicians who have bizarre spasms of the hands and arms that prevent them from performing may have dystonia.

Types of Dystonia

In **Idiopathic** (of unknown cause) **torsion dystonia,** episodes begin between ages 6 and 12. Early symptoms can be as mild as writer's cramp. The dystonia commonly starts in one foot or leg. It may remain limited to the trunk or a leg, but sometimes it affects the whole body, ultimately confining the child to a wheelchair. Adult-onset idiopathic torsion dystonia usually begins in face or arm muscles and generally doesn't progress to other parts of the body.

Blepharospasm is a type of dystonia in which the eyelids are repeatedly and involuntarily forced shut. Occasionally, only one eye is affected at first, but the other eye ultimately is affected too. It usually begins as excessive blinking, eye irritation, or extreme sensitivity to bright light. Many people with blepharospasm discover ways to keep their eyes open, such as yawning, singing, or opening the mouth wide. These techniques become less effective as the disorder progresses. The gravest consequence of blepharospasm is impairment of vision.

Torticollis is dystonia involving the muscles of the neck. The recurring spasms can twist the neck sideways, forward, or backward. **Spasmodic dysphonia** affects the muscles that control speech; people with this disorder usually have a tremor somewhere else as well. Spasms of the vocal cord muscles may block speech altogether or make speech sound strained, quivery, hoarse, jerky, creaky, staccato, or garbled and difficult to understand.

Treatment

The treatment for dystonia is limited. Drugs with anticholinergic properties, such as trihexyphenidyl, are sometimes helpful but also cause

Yips—Golfers' Dystonia

In the golf world, a bad case of dystonia is known as the yips. The muscles of the hands and wrists spontaneously contract, making it nearly impossible to putt. What was supposed to be a 3-foot putt can end up as a 15-foot putt when a golfer loses control because of the yips. The famous golfer Ben Hogan was afflicted with the yips; these muscle spasms are partly to blame for ending his career.

side effects, such as drowsiness, dry mouth, blurred vision, dizziness, constipation, difficulty with urination, or tremor, especially in older people. Injections of botulin (a bacterial toxin that paralyzes muscles) into the overactive muscles have been the most successful treatment.

Parkinson's Disease

A slowly progressing, degenerative disorder of the nervous system, Parkinson's disease has several distinguishing characteristics: tremor (shaking) when at rest, sluggish initiation of movements, and muscle rigidity.

Parkinson's disease affects about 1 in every 250 people over 40 years old and about 1 in every 100 people over 65 years old.

Causes

Deep within the brain is an area known as the basal ganglia.▲ When the brain initiates an action such as lifting an arm, nerve cells in the basal ganglia help smooth the movements and coordinate changes in posture. The basal ganglia process signals and transmit messages to the deep-lying thalamus, which relays the processed information back to the cerebral cortex. All these signals are transmitted by chemical neurotransmitters as electrical impulses along nerve pathways and between nerves. The main neurotransmitter of the basal ganglia is **dopamine.**

▲ see page 279

In Parkinson's disease, nerve cells in the basal ganglia degenerate, resulting in lower production of dopamine and fewer connections with other nerve cells and muscles. The cause of the nerve cell degeneration and dopamine loss usually isn't known. Genetics doesn't appear to play a major role, although the disease tends to occur in some families.

Sometimes the cause is known. In some cases, Parkinson's disease is a very late complication of viral encephalitis, a relatively rare but severe, flu-like infection that causes brain inflammation. In other cases, Parkinson's disease results when other degenerative diseases, drugs, or toxins interfere with or inhibit dopamine's action in the brain. For example, antipsychotic drugs used to treat severe paranoia and schizophrenia block the action of dopamine on nerve cells. Also, an illegal, street-synthesized form of opiate known as N-MPTP can cause severe Parkinson's disease.

Symptoms and Diagnosis

Parkinson's disease begins subtly and progresses gradually. In many people, it begins with a tremor in the hand while the hand is at rest; the tremor decreases when the hand is moving purposefully and disappears completely during sleep. Emotional stress or fatigue may increase the tremor, which has a smooth, rhythmic quality. Although the tremor starts in one hand, it may eventually progress to the other hand, the arms, and the legs. The jaw, tongue, forehead, and eyelids may also be affected by a tremor. In about one third of the people with Parkinson's disease, a tremor isn't the first symptom; in others, it becomes less obvious as the disease progresses; and in still others, a tremor never develops.

Initiating a movement is particularly difficult, and muscle stiffness (rigidity) develops as well, further impairing movement. When the forearm is bent back or straightened out by another person, the movement may feel stiff and ratchetlike. The rigidity and immobility can contribute to muscle ache and fatigue. The combination of stiffness and difficulty in initiating movements causes many difficulties. Because the small muscles of the hands are often impaired, daily tasks such as buttoning a shirt and tying shoelaces become increasingly harder.

Taking a step becomes an effort, and people often walk with a shuffling, short-stepped gait in which their arms don't swing with their stride. When some people start walking, they have difficulty in stopping or turning. Their steps may inadvertently quicken, forcing them to break into a short run to keep from falling. Posture becomes stooped, and balance is difficult to maintain, leading to a tendency to fall forward or backward.

A person's face becomes less expressive because the facial muscles that create expression don't move. Sometimes this lack of expression is mistaken for depression, although many people with Parkinson's disease do become depressed. Eventually the face can take on a blank stare with open mouth and infrequent blinking. Often a person drools or chokes because muscle stiffness in the face and throat makes swallowing difficult. People with Parkinson's disease often speak softly in a monotone and may stutter because they have difficulty articulating their thoughts. Most people maintain normal intellect, but many develop dementia.▲

Treatment

Parkinson's disease may be treated with a wide variety of drugs, including levodopa, bromocriptine, pergolide, selegiline, anticholinergics (benztropine or trihexyphenidyl), antihistamines, antidepressants, propranolol, and amantadine. None of these drugs cures the disease or stops its progression, but they make movement easier and they can prolong functional life for many years.

Levodopa is converted to dopamine in the brain. The drug reduces the tremor and muscle rigidity and improves movement. With levodopa, people who have mild Parkinson's disease can regain a nearly normal level of activity, and some people who are bedridden can regain their independence.

Levodopa-carbidopa is the foundation of treatment for Parkinson's disease, but finding the best dose for a particular person is a difficult balancing act. Carbidopa is added to increase levodopa's effectiveness in the brain and decrease levodopa's unwanted effects outside the brain. Certain possible side effects—involuntary movements of the mouth, face, and limbs—may limit the amount of levodopa that a person can tolerate. For many people, taking levodopa for several years means having to put up with some involuntary tongue and lip movements, grimacing, head bobbing, and twitching of the arms and legs. Some authorities

▲ see page 365

Drugs Used to Treat Parkinson's Disease

Drug	How or When Used	Comments
Levodopa (in combination with carbidopa)	The main treatment for Parkinson's disease. Given with carbidopa to increase effectiveness and reduce side effects. Started with low doses, which are increased until greatest effect is reached	After several years, effectiveness may lessen
Bromocriptine or pergolide	Often given in addition to levodopa early in treatment to enhance levodopa's action, or may be given later when levodopa's side effects become more of a problem	Rarely given alone
Selegiline	Often given in addition to levodopa	Action is modest at best. May increase levodopa's activity in the brain
Anticholinergic drugs: benztropine and trihexyphenidyl, certain antidepressants, antihistamines such as diphenhydramine	May be given without levodopa in early stages of disease, with levodopa in later stages. Started at low doses	Can produce a range of side effects
Amantadine	Used in early stages for mild disease. In later stages to enhance levodopa's effects	May become ineffective after several months if used alone

believe that adding or substituting bromocriptine for levodopa during the early years of treatment can delay the appearance of involuntary movements.

After several years, the period of relief following each dose of levodopa-carbidopa becomes shorter, and periods when initiating a movement is difficult alternate with periods of uncontrollable hyperactivity. Within seconds, a person's condition may change from being fairly mobile to being severely impaired (the on-off effect). Such abrupt changes affect more than half the people who take levodopa for 5 or more years and are usually controlled by taking lower, more frequent doses.

Dopamine-producing nerve cells taken from human fetal tissue and implanted in the brain of a person with Parkinson's disease may reverse the chemical abnormality, but not enough data are available to recommend this procedure. An earlier experimental procedure involved transplanting a piece of a person's adrenal gland into the brain; because the procedure proved to be risky

and only modestly beneficial, it has been abandoned.

Continuing to perform as many daily activities as possible and following a program of regular exercise can help people with Parkinson's disease maintain mobility. Physical therapy and mechanical aids such as wheeled walkers can also help them maintain independence. A nutritious diet rich in high-fiber foods can help counteract the constipation that may result from inactivity, dehydration, and some drugs. Dietary supplements and stool softeners can help keep bowel movements regular. Attention needs to be paid to the diet; because muscle rigidity may make swallowing extremely difficult, a person may become malnourished.

Progressive Supranuclear Palsy

Progressive supranuclear palsy, much rarer than Parkinson's disease, causes muscle rigidity, inability to move the eyes, and weakness of the throat muscles.

Progressive supranuclear palsy usually begins in late middle age with an inability to roll the eyes upward. As with Parkinson's disease, this disease progresses to severe stiffness and disability. The disease, which destroys the brain's basal ganglia and brain stem, has no known cause. No completely effective treatment exists, but the drugs used for Parkinson's disease sometimes provide some relief.

Shy-Drager Syndrome

Shy-Drager syndrome is a disorder of unknown cause in which many parts of the nervous system degenerate.

Shy-Drager syndrome (also called **idiopathic orthostatic hypotension**) is similar to Parkinson's disease in many ways. However, it also causes malfunction and destruction of the autonomic nervous system, which regulates blood pressure, heart rate, gland secretion, and eye focusing. Blood pressure drops dramatically when a person stands up; the amount of sweat, tears, and saliva diminishes; eyesight is poor; urination is difficult; constipation is common; and movement disorders are similar to those in Parkinson's disease. Degeneration of the cerebellum sometimes causes incoordination.

The treatment of Shy-Drager syndrome is the same as for Parkinson's disease but includes the drug fludrocortisone to help raise the blood pressure. People who don't take this drug need to add salt to their diet and drink a lot of water.

Coordination Disorders

The cerebellum is the part of the brain most responsible for coordinating sequences of movements; it also controls balance and posture.▲ Prolonged alcohol abuse is the most common cause of damage to the cerebellum. Other causes are strokes, tumors, certain diseases (such as multiple sclerosis), certain chemicals, and malnutrition. Several rare hereditary disorders, such as **Friedreich's ataxia** and **ataxia-telangiectasia**, also may damage the cerebellum.

Various types of incoordination may result from damage to the cerebellum. People with **dysmetria** are unable to control the accuracy of body movements. For example, in attempting to reach for an object, a person with dysmetria may reach beyond the object. People with **ataxia** can't control the position of their arms and legs or their posture, so they stagger and make broad, zigzag movements with their arms. Poor coordination of speech muscles causes **dysarthria**, marked by slurred speech and uncontrolled fluctuations in volume.■ A person with dysarthria may also exaggerate movement of the muscles around the mouth. Tremor also results from damage to the cerebellum.

CHAPTER 68

Multiple Sclerosis and Related Disorders

Nerve fibers inside and outside the brain are wrapped with many layers of insulation called the myelin sheath. Much like the insulation around an electrical wire, the myelin sheath permits electrical impulses to be conducted along the nerve fiber with speed and accuracy. When myelin is damaged, nerves don't conduct impulses properly.

When babies are born, many of their nerves lack mature myelin sheaths, so their movements are gross, jerky, and uncoordinated. The normal development of myelin sheaths is impaired in children born with certain inherited diseases, such as Tay-Sachs disease, Niemann-Pick disease, Gaucher's disease, and Hurler's syndrome. Such abnormal development can result in permanent, often extensive, neurologic defects.

▲ see page 281

■ see page 361

Stroke, inflammation, immune diseases, and metabolic disorders are among the forces that can destroy the myelin sheath in an adult, a process called **demyelination**. Poisons or drugs, such as alcohol used excessively, can also damage or destroy the myelin sheath. If the sheath is able to repair and regenerate itself, normal nerve function may return; if demyelination is extensive, the underlying nerve usually dies, causing irreversible damage.

Demyelination in the central nervous system (brain and spinal cord) occurs in several disorders of uncertain cause (**primary demyelinating diseases**). Multiple sclerosis is the best known.

Multiple Sclerosis

Multiple sclerosis is a disorder in which the nerves of the eye, brain, and spinal cord lose patches of myelin.

The term *multiple sclerosis* comes from the multiple areas of scarring (sclerosis) that represent many patches of demyelination in the nervous system. The possible neurologic signs and symptoms of multiple sclerosis are so diverse that doctors may miss the diagnosis when the first symptoms appear. While the disease often worsens slowly over time, affected people usually have periods of relatively good health (remissions) alternating with debilitating flare-ups (exacerbations). About 400,000 Americans, mostly young adults, have the disease.

Causes

The cause of multiple sclerosis is unknown, but a likely explanation is that a virus or some unknown antigen somehow triggers an autoimmune process, usually early in life.▲ Then the body, for some reason, produces antibodies against its own myelin; the antibodies provoke inflammation and damage the myelin sheath.

Heredity seems to have a role in multiple sclerosis. About 5 percent of the people with the disease have a brother or sister who is also affected, and about 15 percent have a close relative who is affected.

Environment also plays a role; multiple sclerosis occurs in 1 out of every 2,000 people who spend their first decade of life in a temperate climate but in only 1 out of every 10,000 people born in a tropical climate. Multiple sclerosis almost never occurs in people who grow up near the equator. The climate in which a person spent the

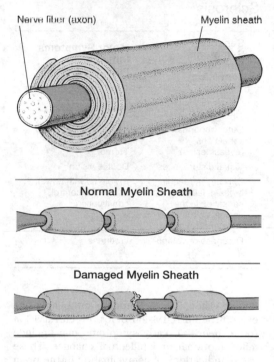

Nerve Fiber and Its Myelin Sheath

Nerve fiber (axon)   Myelin sheath

Normal Myelin Sheath

Damaged Myelin Sheath

first decade of life appears to be more important than that in which later years are spent.

Symptoms

Symptoms generally appear in people aged 20 to 40; women are more likely than men to have the disease. Demyelination can occur in any part of the brain or spinal cord, and the symptoms depend on the area affected. Demyelination in the nerve pathways that bring signals to muscles causes problems with movement (motor symptoms), while demyelination in the nerve pathways that carry sensations to the brain causes disturbances in sensation (sensory symptoms).

Common early symptoms are tingling, numbness, or other peculiar feelings in the arms, legs, trunk, or face. A person may lose strength or dexterity in a leg or a hand. Some people develop symptoms only in the eyes and may experience

▲ see page 816

Common Symptoms of Multiple Sclerosis

Sensory Symptoms (changes in sensation)	Motor Symptoms (changes in muscle function)
Numbness	Weakness, clumsiness
Tingling	Difficulty in walking or maintaining balance
Other abnormal sensations (dysesthesias)	Tremor
Visual disturbances	Double vision
Difficulty in reaching orgasm, lack of sensation in the vagina, sexual impotence in men	Problems with bowel or bladder control, constipation
Dizziness or vertigo	Stiffness, unsteadiness, unusual tiredness

double vision, partial blindness and pain in one eye, dim or blurred vision, or loss of central vision (optic neuritis). Early symptoms may include mild emotional or intellectual changes. These vague indications of demyelination in the brain sometimes begin long before the disease is recognized.

Multiple sclerosis follows a varied and unpredictable course. In many people, the disease starts with an isolated symptom, followed by months or years without further symptoms. In others, symptoms become worse and more generalized within weeks or months. Very warm weather, a hot bath or shower, or even a fever may intensify symptoms. A relapse (flare-up) of the disease can occur spontaneously or can be triggered by an infection such as influenza. As relapses become more frequent, disability worsens and may become permanent. Despite the disability, most people with multiple sclerosis have a normal life span.

▲ see box, page 374

Diagnosis

Doctors consider the possibility of multiple sclerosis in younger people who suddenly develop blurred vision, double vision, or motor and sensory abnormalities in different parts of the body. A pattern of relapses and recoveries strengthens the diagnosis.

When doctors suspect multiple sclerosis, they thoroughly evaluate the nervous system as part of the physical examination. Signs that the nervous system isn't functioning properly, such as uncoordinated eye movements, muscle weakness, or numbness in scattered parts of the body; other findings such as inflammation of the optic nerve; and symptoms that wax and wane make the diagnosis fairly certain.

No single test is diagnostic, but laboratory tests can distinguish between multiple sclerosis and other conditions with similar symptoms. Doctors may take a sample of cerebrospinal fluid by spinal tap (lumbar puncture).▲ People with multiple sclerosis may have a few more white blood cells and slightly more protein than normal in the fluid. The concentration of antibodies in the cerebrospinal fluid may be high, and specific types of antibody and other substances are present in up to 90 percent of the people with multiple sclerosis.

Magnetic resonance imaging (MRI) is the most sensitive diagnostic imaging technique, possibly revealing areas of the brain that have lost myelin. An MRI scan may even distinguish areas of active, recent demyelination from areas in which demyelination took place some time ago.

Evoked potentials is a test that records electrical responses in the brain when nerves are stimulated. For example, normally the brain responds to a flash of light or a noise with characteristic patterns of electrical activity; in people with multiple sclerosis, the response may be slower because signal conduction along demyelinated nerve fibers is impaired.

Treatment

Injectable beta-interferon, a relatively new treatment, reduces the frequency of relapses. Other promising treatments still under investigation include other interferons, oral myelin, and glatiramer to help keep the body from attacking its own myelin. The benefits of plasmapheresis and intravenous gamma globulins haven't been established, and these treatments aren't practical for long-term therapy.

Corticosteroids such as prednisone taken by mouth or methylprednisolone given intravenously for short periods to relieve acute symptoms have been the main form of therapy for decades. Although corticosteroids may shorten the duration of attacks, they don't stop progressive disability over the long term. The benefits of corticosteroids may be offset by the many potential side effects they cause with long-term use—increased susceptibility to infection, diabetes, weight gain, fatigue, osteoporosis (fragile bones), and ulcers. Other immunosuppressive therapies, such as azathioprine, cyclophosphamide, cyclosporine, and total lymphoid irradiation, haven't proved helpful and can cause significant complications.

People with multiple sclerosis can often maintain an active lifestyle, though they may tire easily and may not be able to keep up with a demanding schedule. Regular exercise such as riding a stationary bicycle, walking, swimming, or stretching reduces spasticity and helps maintain cardiovascular, muscular, and psychologic health. Physical therapy can help with maintaining balance, walking ability, and range of motion and can lessen spasticity and weakness.

The nerves that control urination or bowel movements can also be affected, leading to urinary or fecal incontinence or retention. Many people learn to catheterize themselves to empty the bladder and begin a regular program of stool softeners or laxatives to help move their bowels. People who become weak and unable to move easily may develop bedsores, so they and their caregivers must take extra care to prevent such skin damage.

Other Primary Demyelinating Diseases

Acute disseminated encephalomyelitis (postinfectious encephalomyelitis) is a rare type of inflammation leading to demyelination that generally follows a viral infection or vaccination.▲ It's thought to be a misguided immune reaction triggered by the virus. Guillain-Barré syndrome seems to be a similar disorder of the peripheral nerves.■

Diseases Causing Symptoms Similar to Those of Multiple Sclerosis

- Viral or bacterial infections of the brain (Lyme disease, AIDS, syphilis)
- Structural abnormalities of the base of the skull and spine (severe arthritis of the neck, ruptured spinal disk)
- Tumors or cysts of the brain and spinal cord (syringomyelia)
- Spinocerebellar degeneration and the hereditary ataxias (disorders in which muscle action is irregular or muscles fail to coordinate)
- Small strokes (especially in people with diabetes or hypertension who are prone to such strokes)
- Amyotrophic lateral sclerosis (Lou Gehrig's disease)
- Inflammation of the blood vessels in the brain or spinal cord (lupus, arteritis)

Adrenoleukodystrophy and **adrenomyeloneuropathy** are rare inherited metabolic disorders. Adrenoleukodystrophy affects young boys, usually by the age of 7, although a more slowly developing form of the disease can begin in young adults in their 20s. Adrenomyeloneuropathy affects adolescent boys. In these diseases, widespread demyelination is accompanied by abnormal adrenal gland function. Eventually the mental state deteriorates, and the child becomes spastic and blind. No cure is known. Dietary supplements with glycerol trioleate and glycerol trierucate (known as Lorenzo's oil) improve the blood's fatty acid composition but haven't been shown to improve the disease's course. Bone marrow transplantation is an experimental treatment.

Leber's hereditary optic atrophy causes demyelination leading to partial blindness. The disease is more common in men, and usually symptoms first

▲ see page 376

■ see page 338

appear in the late teens or early 20s. This disease is inherited from the mother and seems to be transmitted in mitochondria, the energy factories of cells.

Infection by the human T-cell lymphotropic virus (HTLV) can cause demyelination in the spinal cord **(HTLV-associated myelopathy).** This disease is most common in certain tropical countries and regions of Japan. The disease worsens over several years, leading to gradual spasticity and weakness of the legs as well as impaired bladder and bowel function.

CHAPTER 69

Spinal Cord Disorders

The **spinal cord,** the main pathway of communication between the brain and the rest of the body, is a soft tubelike structure of nerves that extends downward from the base of the brain. The cord is protected by the bones of the **spinal column** (vertebrae). Nerves enter and exit from the spinal cord throughout its length, passing through small openings between each vertebra.

The spinal cord is highly organized; rather than being grouped haphazardly, nerves are bundled so that related types run together. The side of the spinal cord that faces the front of the body contains **motor nerves** that transmit information to muscles and stimulate movement. The side of the spinal cord that faces the back and sides contains **sensory nerves** that transmit information to the brain about sensations such as touch, position, pain, heat, and cold.

The spinal cord can be damaged in many ways, producing various symptom patterns; these patterns enable a doctor to determine the location (level) of spinal cord damage. The spinal cord can be cut in an accident, compressed, destroyed by infection, damaged when its blood supply is cut off, or affected by diseases (such as spinal cord cysts, cervical spondylosis, or multiple sclerosis) that alter its nerve function.

Accident-Related Injuries

When the spinal cord is injured in an accident, function can be totally or partially destroyed in any part of the body below the level of the injury. For example, severe damage to the spinal cord in the middle of the back leaves the arms functioning normally but may leave the legs paralyzed. In addition, the site of the injury or the area above it may be painful, especially when the vertebrae have been injured.

Certain reflex movements that aren't controlled by the brain may remain intact or may even be increased below the site of the injury. For example, the knee-jerk reflex, in which a tap with a small hammer just below the knee causes the lower leg to extend upward, is preserved and may even be exaggerated. The increased reflex response leads to leg spasms. These preserved reflexes cause the affected muscles to tighten, resulting in a spastic type of paralysis. The spastic muscles feel tight and hard; they twitch from time to time, causing the legs to jerk.

Recovery is likely if movement or sensation returns the first week after the injury. Any dysfunction remaining after 6 months is likely to be permanent. Once spinal cord nerves have been destroyed, the damage is permanent.

Treatment

The first goal is to prevent further damage. Emergency personnel take great care when moving an accident victim with a possible spinal cord injury. Usually, the person is strapped to a firm board and carefully padded to prevent movement. Even slight shifting when the spinal cord has been damaged increases the possibility of permanent paralysis.

Doctors usually give corticosteroid drugs such as prednisone right away to help prevent swelling around the injury. Muscle-relaxing drugs and pain relievers may be given to reduce spasms. If the spinal column has been fractured or otherwise injured, a surgeon may implant steel rods to stabilize it, so that further movement doesn't do more harm to the cord. A neurosurgeon removes any blood that has accumulated around the spinal cord.

Expert nursing care is extremely important to prevent complications from weakness and paralysis while the spinal cord is healing. People with spinal cord injuries are especially vulnerable to bedsores.▲ Special beds can help minimize pressure on the skin. When necessary, a bed that can be turned to switch pressure from front to back and from side to side (a Stryker frame) is used.

People who have had a spinal cord injury need strong emotional support to combat the depression and depersonalization that can follow extensive loss of body functions. They want to know exactly what has happened and what to expect in the near and distant future. Physical and occupational therapy help preserve muscle function and teach special techniques to overcome lost functions. Most people are helped by compassionate, skilled nursing care and psychologic counseling. Family members and close friends may need counseling as well.

Spinal Cord Compression

Normally the spinal cord is protected by the bony spinal column, but certain disorders may put pressure on the spinal cord, disrupting its normal function. Pressure can come from a broken vertebra or other bone in the spinal column, a rupture of one or more of the cartilage disks that lie between the vertebrae, an infection (spinal cord abscess), or a tumor in the spinal cord or column. Sudden compression of the spinal cord is usually caused by an injury or bleeding but can be caused by an infection or tumor. An abnormal blood vessel (arteriovenous malformation) can also compress the cord.

If the compression is very great, nerve signals going up and down the spinal cord may be completely blocked. Less severe compression may disrupt only some signals. When the compression is discovered and treated before nerves are destroyed, the spinal cord's function usually returns completely.

Symptoms

The area of the spinal cord that's damaged determines which muscles and sensations are affected.■ Weakness or paralysis and either decreased or complete loss of sensation are likely to develop below the area (level) of the injury.

A tumor or infection in or around the spinal cord can slowly compress the cord, causing pain and tenderness at the site of the compression as well as weakness and changes in sensation. As the compression worsens, the pain and weakness progress to paralysis and loss of sensation, often over days or weeks. However, if the blood supply to the spinal cord is cut off, paralysis and loss of sensation can occur in minutes. The slowest spinal cord compression usually results from abnormalities in the bones caused by degenerative arthritis or very slow-growing tumors; the person has little or no pain, and changes in sensation (for example, tingling) and weakness progress over many months.

Diagnosis

Because the spinal cord nerves are organized in a specific way, doctors can tell which part of the spinal cord is affected by evaluating a person's symptoms and performing a physical examination. For example, damage to the midchest (thoracic) area of the spine may cause leg (but not arm) weakness and numbness and may impair bladder and bowel function. A person may feel a beltlike band of discomfort where the spinal cord is injured.

A computed tomography (CT) or magnetic resonance imaging (MRI) scan usually shows where the spinal cord is compressed and may indicate the cause. A myelogram may also be performed. With a myelogram, dye is injected around the spinal cord, and then x-rays are taken to determine where in the spinal cord the dye looks compressed or pinched off. This test is more complicated than a CT or MRI scan and is somewhat more uncomfortable, but it remains the gold standard when questions remain after a CT or MRI scan.

These tests may show a fracture, collapse, or dislocation of a vertebra; a ruptured disk; a bone growth; a pool of blood; an abscess; or a tumor. Additional tests are sometimes needed. For ex-

---

▲ see page 969

■ see box, page 324

Which Area of the Spinal Column is Damaged?

The spinal column is divided into four areas: cervical (neck), thoracic (chest), lumbar (lower back), and sacral (tailbone). Each area is referred to by a letter (C, T, L, or S). The vertebrae within each area of the spine are numbered beginning at the top. For example, the first vertebra within the cervical spine is labeled C1, the second within the cervical spine is C2, the second within the thoracic spine is T2, the fourth within the lumbar spine is L4, and so forth.

Nerves run from the spinal column to specific areas of the body. By noting where a person has weakness, paralysis, or other loss of function (and thus nerve damage), a neurologist can trace back and pinpoint where the spinal column is damaged.

Effects of Spinal Injury

Level of Injury	Effect*
C1 to C5	Paralysis of muscles used for breathing and of all arm and leg muscles; usually fatal.
C5 to C6	Legs paralyzed; slight ability to flex arms
C6 to C7	Paralysis of legs and part of wrists and hands; shoulder movement and elbow bending are relatively preserved
C8 to T1	Legs and trunk paralyzed; eyelids droop; loss of sweating on the forehead (Horner's syndrome); arms relatively normal; hands paralyzed
T2 to T4	Legs and trunk paralyzed; loss of feeling below the nipples
T5 to T8	Legs and lower trunk paralyzed; loss of feeling below the rib cage
T9 to T11	Legs paralyzed; loss of feeling below the umbilicus
T12 to L1	Paralysis and loss of feeling below the groin
L2 to L5	Different patterns of leg weakness and numbness
S1 to S2	Different patterns of leg weakness and numbness
S3 to S5	Loss of bladder and bowel control; numbness in the perineum

*Loss of bladder and bowel control can occur with severe injury anywhere along the spinal column

Dermatomes

Dermatomes are the areas of skin supplied with nerve fibers by a single spinal nerve root. There are 8 nerve roots for the 7 cervical vertebrae; otherwise, each of the 12 thoracic, 5 lumbar, and 5 sacral vertebrae has a single spinal nerve root that supplies specific areas of skin. The illustration shows how nerves supply the different areas. For example, the nerve coming from the fifth lumbar vertebra (L5) supplies nerve function to a strip of skin along the lower back, the outside of the thigh, the inside of the lower leg, and the heel.

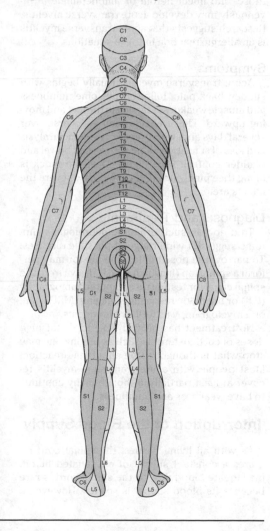

ample. If tests show an abnormal growth, a biopsy may be needed to determine if the growth is cancerous.

Treatment

The treatment of spinal cord compression depends on the cause, but when possible, the compression must be relieved immediately or the spinal cord may be permanently damaged. Relief often requires surgery, although radiation therapy may relieve compression caused by tumors. Corticosteroids such as dexamethasone are often given to help reduce swelling in or around the spinal cord that may be contributing to the compression.

Spinal cord compression caused by infection is treated immediately with antibiotics. The doctor, usually a neurosurgeon, drains the pus-filled area of infection (abscess); sometimes the doctor can drain an abscess by drawing out the pus through a syringe.

Cervical Spondylosis

Cervical spondylosis is a disease that affects middle-aged and older adults in whom the disks and vertebrae in the neck degenerate.

Symptoms

Cervical spondylosis narrows the spinal canal in the neck—the passageway that the spinal cord runs through—and compresses the spinal cord or spinal nerve roots, causing malfunction. Symptoms may reflect either spinal cord compression or nerve root damage. If the spinal cord is compressed, a change in gait is usually the first sign. Leg movements may become jerky (spastic), and walking becomes unsteady. The neck may be painful, especially when the nerve roots are affected. Weakness and loss of muscle in one or both arms may develop either before or after signs of spinal cord compression.

Diagnosis and Treatment

When a doctor suspects cervical spondylosis, magnetic resonance imaging (MRI) helps show where the spinal canal narrows, the degree of compression, and the distribution of nerve roots that may be involved.

Spinal cord malfunction from cervical spondylosis can improve or stabilize without treatment, or it can progress. Initially, the doctor may suggest treatment with a soft neck collar, neck traction, anti-inflammatory drugs, mild analgesics, and muscle relaxants to provide relief. However, when the disorder progresses or when an MRI scan shows severe compression, surgery is generally needed to stop symptoms from progressing. As a rule, surgery doesn't reverse changes that have already occurred because some of the nerves in the spinal cord are permanently damaged.

Spinal Cord and Brain Cysts

A syrinx is a fluid-filled sac (cyst) within the brain (syringobulbia) or spinal cord (syringomyelia).

Spinal cord and brain cysts are rare. About half the time, the cysts are present at birth, but for poorly understood reasons they enlarge during the teen or young adult years. Often, children who have cysts at birth also have other defects. Injury or tumors are the usual causes of cysts later in life.

Symptoms

Cysts that grow in the spinal cord press on it from within. Though most common in the neck, they can occur anywhere along the length of the spinal cord and often grow to involve a long segment of the cord. Usually, the nerves that detect pain and changes in temperature are most affected. Cuts and burns are common in people with this type of nerve damage because their fingers may not feel pain or heat. As the cysts extend further, they can cause spasms and weakness, beginning in the legs. Eventually, the muscles served by these nerves may begin to waste away.

Diagnosis and Treatment

A doctor may suspect a spinal cord cyst when a young child or teenager develops the symptoms described above. A magnetic resonance imaging (MRI) scan can outline the cyst (or a tumor if there is one). The doctor may be able to make the diagnosis from a myelogram, followed by a computed tomography (CT) scan if MRI isn't available.

A neurosurgeon may drain spinal cord cysts to prevent further deterioration, but surgery

doesn't always correct the problem. Severe deterioration of the nervous system may be irreversible, even if the surgery is successful.

Acute Transverse Myelitis

In acute transverse myelitis, nerve impulse transmission up and down the spinal cord is totally blocked at one or more points.

The cause of acute transverse myelitis isn't known for certain, but about 30 to 40 percent of the people affected develop the disorder after an otherwise minor viral illness. People with multiple sclerosis or certain bacterial infections or those who inject heroin or amphetamine intravenously may develop acute transverse myelitis. Research suggests that acute transverse myelitis is an allergic reaction in these situations.

Symptoms

Acute transverse myelitis usually begins with sudden back pain, followed by some numbness and muscle weakness starting in the feet and moving upward. These effects may get worse over several days and, when severe, result in paralysis and loss of sensation along with loss of bowel and bladder control. How high or low the block is along the spinal cord determines how severe the effects are.

Diagnosis and Treatment

To a doctor, such dramatic neurologic symptoms suggest a wide range of possible diseases. To narrow the possibilities, the doctor may perform a spinal tap (in which fluid is drawn from the spinal canal for testing), a computed tomography (CT) or magnetic resonance imaging (MRI) scan, or a myelogram,▲ as well as blood tests.

No treatment has proved beneficial, but high doses of corticosteroids such as prednisone may stop what is thought to be an allergic reaction. Most people with acute transverse myelitis recover at least partially, although many continue to have weakness and numbness.

Interruption of the Blood Supply

As with all living tissues, the spinal cord requires a constant supply of oxygenated blood. Inadequate blood flow to the spinal cord is rare because its blood supply is so rich. However, a

▲ see page 287

tumor, ruptured disk, or other, less common cause can compress the arteries and veins and interrupt the blood supply. In rare instances, the blood supply is blocked by atherosclerosis or a blood clot. The upper thoracic (chest) area is most vulnerable to an interruption of blood supply.

Symptoms

Interruption of the blood supply to the front of the spinal cord usually causes sudden back pain. This pain is followed by weakness and an inability to feel heat, cold, or pain in areas below the level where the blood supply has been interrupted. Symptoms are most noticeable during the first few days, and at least partial recovery may occur over time. If the blood supply to the back of the spinal cord isn't cut off as well, sensations carried in that portion—including touch, the ability to feel vibration, and the ability to sense where the feet and legs are without looking at them (position sense)—may remain intact.

Diagnosis and Treatment

To distinguish among the possible causes, a doctor orders a magnetic resonance imaging (MRI) scan or a myelogram. Along with the myelogram, or if the MRI scan is normal, a doctor may perform a spinal tap to check the spinal fluid's pressure or to check for an infection and for any abnormalities in the levels of protein and other substances. Unless a growth or ruptured disk is compressing the blood vessels and can be surgically removed, the blood supply can't be restored. If the blood supply is restored quickly, partial recovery is likely. Full recovery is rare.

Spinal Hematoma

A spinal hematoma results when leaking blood (hemorrhage) collects around the spinal cord and presses on it.

A hematoma may result from a back injury, from an abnormal blood vessel (arteriovenous malformation), or from bleeding in people who take anticoagulants or have a tendency to bleed.

Symptoms

A hematoma usually causes sudden pain and tenderness, followed by weakness and loss of sensation below the affected area of the spinal cord.▲

These effects may progress to complete paralysis in minutes or hours, although sometimes people recover spontaneously. Occasionally, blood flows upward into the brain, causing even more severe problems; coma and death are possible if a hematoma near the top of the spinal cord interferes with the ability to breathe.

Diagnosis and Treatment

The doctor makes a tentative diagnosis based on the symptoms and usually confirms it with a magnetic resonance imaging (MRI) scan, although a computed tomography (CT) scan or myelogram is sometimes used. Immediately removing the accumulated blood may prevent permanent injury to the spinal cord. Surgery using special techniques (microsurgery) can sometimes correct an arteriovenous malformation. People who take anticoagulants or have a bleeding disorder are given drugs to eliminate or reduce their tendency to bleed.

Nerve Root Disorders

Nerve roots project from the spinal cord, delivering signals to and receiving signals from almost all parts of the body. These nerve roots emerge from the spinal column through openings between vertebrae, and each nerve root supplies information or sensation to a particular area of the body.■ The nerve roots are organized in pairs: The motor nerves emerge from the front of the spinal cord and stimulate the muscles; the sensory nerves emerge from the back of the spinal cord and bring sensory information to the brain.

Causes

The most common cause of nerve root damage is a ruptured disk between the vertebrae.★ The collapse of a vertebra, which usually results when bones are weakened by cancer, osteoporosis, or severe injury, also can damage the nerve roots. Degenerative arthritis (osteoarthritis) is another common cause of nerve root damage; this disor-

---

▲ see box, page 324

■ see box, page 324

★ see page 328

der creates irregular projections of bone (bone spurs) that compress nerve roots. Narrowing of the space around the spinal cord (**spinal stenosis**) occurs in older people. Less commonly, spinal cord tumors or infections such as meningitis or herpes zoster (shingles) harm nerve roots.

Symptoms

Damage to a vertebra or to the disks between the vertebrae can put pressure on the nerve roots. The pressure causes pain, which often worsens when the person moves the back, coughs, sneezes, or strains (for example, while defecating). When nerve roots in the lower back are under pressure, pain may be felt only in the lower back, or the pain may travel along the sciatic nerve to the buttocks, thigh, calf, and foot (a pain called **sciatica**).

If the pressure is severe, the nerves can't carry signals to and from the muscles, leading to weakness and loss of feeling. Sometimes the ability to urinate and control bowel movements is impaired. When nerve roots in the neck are affected, pain may travel down the shoulder, arm, and hand or up the back of the head.

Diagnosis

Nerve root damage is a possibility when a person has pain, loss of sensation, or weakness at a specific level of the body supplied by a single nerve root. By noting where a person feels pain or has lost sensation, a doctor can deduce which nerve root is affected. During the physical examination, the doctor notes any tenderness the patient feels in that area of the spinal column. An x-ray can reveal whether the bones in the spinal column are thin, have been damaged, or are out of alignment. A computed tomography (CT) or magnetic resonance imaging (MRI) scan provides an even better picture of what is happening in and around the spinal cord. If MRI isn't available, a myelogram can be used to picture the defect. Other tests, especially one that measures electrical activity in nerves and muscles, may be needed.

Treatment

The treatment for nerve root disorders depends on the cause and severity. When the cause

is a collapsed vertebra resulting from osteoporosis, very little can be done other than bracing the back with a tight corset to limit motion. When a ruptured disk is the cause, treatment is available. An infection is immediately treated with antibiotics; if an abscess has formed, it is usually drained immediately. Spinal cord tumors are treated by surgical removal, radiation therapy, or both.

Analgesics may help relieve pain, regardless of the cause. Muscle relaxants are also used, but their effectiveness hasn't been proved. The side effects of muscle relaxants may overshadow their benefits, particularly in the elderly.

Ruptured Disk

The vertebrae of the spinal column are separated by disks made of cartilage. Each disk has a strong outer layer and a softer inner part that acts as a shock absorber to cushion the vertebrae during movement. If the disk degenerates, for example following an injury or with aging, the inner part of the disk can bulge or rupture through the outer layer (herniated disk). The ruptured inner part of the disk can compress or irritate a nerve root and may even injure it.

Symptoms

The location of the ruptured disk determines where a person will feel pain, lose sensation, or experience weakness.▲ How badly the nerve root is compressed or damaged determines how severe the pain or other symptoms will be.

Most ruptured disks are in the lower back (lumbar spine) and usually affect only one leg. Such a rupture can cause pain not only in the lower back but also down the sciatic nerve, which runs from the spinal column to the buttocks, leg, and heel (the pain is called sciatica). Ruptured disks in the lower back can also cause leg weakness, and a person may especially have difficulty lifting the front part of the foot (footdrop). A ruptured disk that is very large and centrally located in the spinal column can affect nerves that regulate bowel and bladder function, impairing the ability to defecate or urinate and making urgent medical attention necessary.

The pain of a ruptured disk is usually worse with movement and may be aggravated by coughing, laughing, urinating, or straining while defecating. Numbness and tingling of the legs, feet, and toes may occur. Symptoms may come on sud-

▲ see box, page 324

denly, spontaneously disappear, and return at intervals or may be constant and long-lasting.

The second most common place for a disk to rupture is the neck (cervical spine). Symptoms usually affect only one arm. When a disk in the cervical spine ruptures, the person usually has pain in the shoulder blade and armpit or in the upper ridge and tip of the shoulder, which travels down the arm to one or two fingers. The muscles in the arm can become weak; less often, finger movement is affected.

Diagnosis

The symptoms help a doctor make the diagnosis. During the physical examination, the doctor checks the spine for areas of tenderness and tests sensation, coordination, muscle strength, and reflexes (for example, the knee jerk). Using a procedure such as the straight leg test, in which the person lifts the leg without bending the knee, the doctor notes at what position the pain gets worse. The doctor assesses muscle tone in the rectum by inserting a finger into the rectum. Weakness of the muscles around the anus along with difficulty in urinating or controlling urination are particularly grave signs—treatment is urgent.

Spinal x-rays can show narrowing of the disk space, but computed tomography (CT) and magnetic resonance imaging (MRI) scans more clearly identify the problem. A myelogram can be useful, but this test has generally been replaced by MRI.

Treatment

Unless loss of nerve function is progressive and severe, most people with a ruptured disk in the lower back recover without surgery. Discomfort usually subsides with relaxation at home. In rare cases, people are confined to bed for a few days. Activities that put stress on the spine and cause pain—for example, lifting heavy objects, bending, or straining—should generally be avoided. For most people, traction isn't beneficial.

A firm, supportive mattress is helpful for sleeping. Many people benefit from simply adjusting their sleep posture—a pillow under the waist and another pillow under the shoulder may help people who sleep on their side; a pillow under the knees may help people who sleep on their back.

Aspirin and other nonsteroidal anti-inflammatory drugs usually help relieve pain; severe pain is treated with opioid analgesics.▲ Some people believe that muscle relaxants help, although their

A Ruptured Disk

When a disk in the spinal column ruptures, its soft inner material bulges out through a weak area in the hard outer layer. A ruptured disk causes pain and sometimes damages nerves.

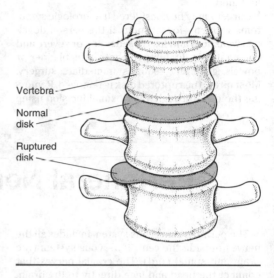

Vertebra

Normal disk

Ruptured disk

effectiveness is unproved. The elderly are especially likely to experience side effects from muscle relaxants.

Exercises are often recommended to reduce muscle spasms and pain and to hasten recovery. Normally, the spinal column in both the neck and lower back is curved forward. Flattening these curves or even reversing them by arching the back provides more space for the spinal nerves and relieves the pressure of the ruptured disk. Exercises that may be beneficial include flattening the back against a wall or the floor, lying down and pulling each knee alternately up to the chest or doing the same maneuver with both knees simultaneously, and doing sit-ups and deep knee bends. These exercises can be performed in sets of 10 about two or three times a day. A pamphlet illustrating the exercises may be available at the

▲ see box, page 292

doctor's office. Additionally, a physical therapist can demonstrate the exercises and prescribe a specific program to meet individual needs.

Adjusting the posture can promote beneficial changes in the back curvature. For example, when a person is sitting, the chair can be adjusted so that it leans forward, or a low foot stool can be used to keep the knees bent up and the spine flattened.

Surgery may be considered if neurologic symptoms worsen—for example, if the person develops weakness and loss of sensation or severe and constant pain. Inability to control the bladder or bowels generally requires immediate surgery. Most often, the ruptured disk is removed. Removing the disk through a very small incision using

microsurgery techniques is becoming more common. Dissolving a ruptured disk by injecting chemicals into it doesn't appear to be as effective as the other approaches and may be dangerous.

If the ruptured disk is in the cervical spine, traction and a supportive neck collar may help. Traction is a means of pulling on the spinal column to increase the space between vertebrae and relieve the pressure. It's generally applied at home using a mechanism that pulls upward on the neck and chin. To ensure that the equipment is used correctly, only a doctor or physical therapist should prescribe traction. Most symptoms are relieved by simple measures, but surgery may be required if pain and signs of nerve damage are severe and progressive.

CHAPTER 70

Peripheral Nerve Disorders

The peripheral nervous system includes all the nerves outside the central nervous system (the brain and spinal cord). The cranial nerves that connect the head and face directly to the brain, the nerves that connect the eyes and nose to the brain, and all the nerves that connect the spinal cord to the rest of the body are part of the peripheral nervous system.

The brain communicates with much of the body through the 31 pairs of spinal nerves that emerge from the spinal cord. Each pair of spinal nerves includes one nerve at the front of the spinal cord, which carries information from the brain to the muscles, and one nerve at the back, which carries sensory information to the brain. Spinal nerves connect to each other through plexuses in the neck, shoulder, and pelvis, then divide again to supply more distant parts of the body.

Peripheral nerves are actually bundles of nerve fibers. Some are very small (less than $1/64$ of an inch in diameter), and others are quite large (more than $1/4$ of an inch in diameter). Larger

fibers convey messages that activate muscles (motor nerve fibers) and the sensations of touch and position (sensory nerve fibers). Smaller sensory nerve fibers convey sensations of pain and temperature and control the automatic functions of the body, such as heart rate, blood pressure, and temperature (the autonomic nervous system). Schwann cells envelop each nerve fiber and generate multiple layers of a fatty insulation called the myelin sheath.

Dysfunction of peripheral nerves may result from damage to the nerve fiber itself, to the body of the nerve cell, to the Schwann cell, or to the myelin sheath. When the myelin sheath is damaged and myelin is lost (demyelination), nerves can't transmit impulses normally.▲ However, the myelin sheath can often regenerate rapidly, allowing complete recovery of nerve function. Unlike the myelin sheath, a nerve cell that is damaged repairs itself and regrows very slowly, if at all. Sometimes the regrowth may be misdirected, leading to abnormal nerve connections. For example, a nerve may connect to the wrong muscle, leading to a jerky or awkward movement, or a sensory nerve may grow abnormally, causing a person to misperceive where touch or pain is coming from.

▲ see box, page 319

Muscle-Brain Circuit

Nerves are connected and communicate their signals through synapses. Moving a muscle involves two complex nerve pathways: the sensory nerve pathway to the brain and the motor nerve pathway to the muscle. Twelve basic steps are pinpointed.

1. Sensory receptors in the skin detect sensations and transmit a signal to the brain.

2. The signal travels along a sensory nerve to the spinal cord.

3. A synapse in the spinal cord connects the sensory nerve to a spinal cord nerve.

4. The nerve crosses to the opposite side of the spinal cord.

5. The signal is sent up the spinal cord.

6. A synapse in the thalamus connects the spinal cord to nerve fibers that carry the signal to the sensory cortex.

7. The sensory cortex perceives the signal and triggers the motor cortex to generate a signal of movement.

8. The nerve carrying the signal crosses over at the base of the brain.

9. The signal is sent down the spinal cord.

10. A synapse connects the spinal cord to a motor nerve.

11. The signal follows the length of the motor nerve.

12. The signal reaches the motor end plate, where it stimulates muscle movement.

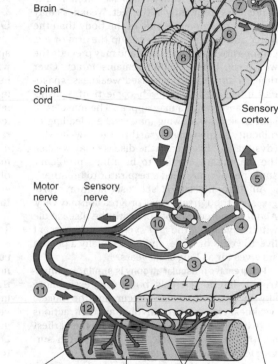

Disorders of Muscle Stimulation

The nerve route from the brain to the muscles is complex; dysfunction anywhere along the route can lead to muscle and movement problems. Without proper stimulation from nerves, muscles weaken, shrink (atrophy), and can become completely paralyzed even though the muscles themselves are normal. Muscle disorders that origi-

nate with nerve dysfunction include amyotrophic lateral sclerosis (Lou Gehrig's disease), progressive muscular atrophy, progressive bulbar palsy, primary lateral sclerosis, and progressive pseudobulbar palsy. In most instances, the cause is unknown. An inherited tendency to these disorders appears to be involved about 10 percent of the time.

These disorders have similarities—in all of them, nerves in the spinal cord or brain that stimulate muscle action (motor nerves) progressively deteriorate, causing muscle weakness that can end up as paralysis. However, each disorder affects a different part of the nervous system and a different set of muscles, so in each disorder a different part of the body is most affected. These disorders are more common in men than in women. Symptoms usually start when people are in their 50s.

Symptoms

Amyotrophic lateral sclerosis is a progressive disease that begins with weakness, often in the hands, less frequently in the feet. Weakness may progress more on one side of the body than the other and generally proceeds up the arm or leg. Cramps are common as well and may precede the weakness, but sensation remains intact. Over time, in addition to increased weakness, spasticity intervenes: Muscles become tight, spasms ensue, and tremors may appear. The muscles of speech and swallowing may weaken, leading to difficulty in speaking (dysarthria) and swallowing (dysphagia). Eventually the disease may weaken the diaphragm, leading to breathing problems; some people may need a respirator to breathe.

Amyotrophic lateral sclerosis is always progressive, though the rate of progression may vary. About 50 percent of people with the disease die within 3 years of the first symptoms, 10 percent live 10 years or more, and occasionally a person survives for as long as 30 years.

Progressive muscular atrophy is similar to amyotrophic lateral sclerosis, but it progresses more slowly, spasticity doesn't occur, and the muscle weakness is less severe. Involuntary contractions or twitching of muscle fibers may be the earliest symptoms. Many people with this disorder survive for 25 years or longer.

In **progressive bulbar palsy,** the nerves controlling the muscles of chewing, swallowing, and talking are affected so that these functions become increasingly difficult. People with progressive bulbar palsy also may develop odd emotional responses, switching from expressions of happiness to those of sadness quickly and without reason; inappropriate emotional outbursts are common. Swallowing difficulties often result in food

or saliva being inhaled (aspirated) into the lungs. Death usually occurs 1 to 3 years after onset of the disorder, often because of pneumonia.

Primary lateral sclerosis and **progressive pseudobulbar palsy** are rare, slowly progressive variants of amyotrophic lateral sclerosis. Primary lateral sclerosis affects primarily the arms and legs, and progressive pseudobulbar palsy affects the muscles of the face, jaw, and throat. In both disorders, severe muscle stiffness accompanies muscle weakness. Muscle twitches and atrophy do not develop; disability usually progresses over several years.

Diagnosis

Doctors suspect one of these disorders when an adult develops progressive muscle weakness without loss of sensation. Examinations and tests help rule out other causes of weakness. Electromyography, which measures electrical activity in muscles, can help determine whether the problem is in the nerves or muscles.▲ However, laboratory tests can't determine which of the possible nerve diseases is causing the problem. A doctor makes the diagnosis by considering which parts of the body are affected, when the disorder started, what symptoms appeared first, and how the symptoms changed over time.

Treatment

These disorders have no specific treatment or cure. Physical therapy helps the person maintain muscle strength and prevent the muscles from tightening (contractures). People with swallowing difficulties must be fed with great care to prevent their choking; some must be fed through a gastrostomy tube—a tube inserted through the abdominal wall into the stomach. Baclofen, a drug to reduce muscle spasms, sometimes relieves muscle cramps. Other drugs may decrease cramps and saliva formation.

Researchers are experimenting with certain substances that promote the growth of nerves (neurotrophic factors). Clinical studies to date have not proved their effectiveness.

Disorders of the Neuromuscular Junction

Nerves communicate with muscles at the neuromuscular junction. When a nerve stimulates a muscle at the neuromuscular junction, the mus-

▲ see page 287

cle contracts. Neuromuscular junction disorders include myasthenia gravis, Eaton-Lambert syndrome, and botulism.

MYASTHENIA GRAVIS

Myasthenia gravis is an autoimmune disease in which the neuromuscular junction functions abnormally, resulting in episodes of muscle weakness.

In myasthenia gravis, the immune system produces antibodies that attack the receptors that lie on the muscle side of the neuromuscular junction. The particular receptors damaged are those that receive the nerve signal by the action of acetylcholine, a chemical substance that transmits the nerve impulse across the junction (a neurotransmitter).

What causes the body to attack its own acetylcholine receptors isn't known, but genetic predisposition to the immune abnormality plays an essential part. The antibodies circulate in the blood, and mothers with myasthenia gravis may pass them through the placenta to their unborn children. This transfer of antibodies produces **neonatal myasthenia,** in which the baby has muscle weakness that disappears several days to a few weeks after birth.

Symptoms

The disease occurs more frequently in women than in men and usually begins between the ages of 20 and 40, although it may occur at any age. The most common symptoms are weakness of the eyelids (drooping eyelids); weak eye muscles, which causes double vision; and excessive, specific muscle fatigue after exercise. In 40 percent of the people with myasthenia gravis, the eye muscles are the first ones affected, but eventually 85 percent have this problem. Difficulty in speaking and swallowing and weakness of the arms and legs are common.

Characteristically, a muscle gets progressively weaker, so for example, a person who once could use a hammer well becomes too weak to use it repetitively. The degree of muscle weakness varies over the course of hours to days. The disease doesn't follow an even course; exacerbations are common. In severe bouts, people with myasthenia gravis may become virtually paralyzed but even then don't lose feeling. About 10 percent of the people develop a life-threatening weakness of the muscles needed for breathing (a condition called **myasthenic crisis**).

Diagnosis

Doctors suspect myasthenia gravis in anyone with general weakness, especially when the weakness involves the muscles of the eyes or face or increases with use of the affected muscles and recovers with rest. Because acetylcholine receptors are blocked, drugs that increase the amount of acetylcholine are beneficial, and a test using one of them can help confirm the diagnosis. Edrophonium is most commonly used as the test drug; when injected intravenously, it temporarily improves muscle strength in people with myasthenia gravis. Other diagnostic tests include measuring nerve and muscle function with an electromyogram and testing the blood for antibodies to acetylcholine.

Some people with myasthenia gravis have a tumor of the thymus gland (thymoma), which may be the cause of the immune system malfunction. A computed tomography (CT) scan of the chest can determine whether a thymoma exists.

Treatment

Drugs taken by mouth that increase the level of acetylcholine, such as pyridostigmine or neostigmine, may be given to treat the disease. A doctor may increase the dose during bouts of worsening symptoms. Long-acting capsules are available for nighttime use to help people who awaken in the morning with severe weakness or trouble swallowing. Other drugs may be needed to counteract the abdominal cramps and diarrhea that pyridostigmine and neostigmine often cause.

If the dose of an acetylcholine-supplementing drug is too high, the drug itself can cause weakness that is difficult for the doctor to differentiate from the myasthenia. Also, these drugs may lose effect with long-term use, so doctors must adjust the dose. Increasing weakness or decreasing drug effectiveness requires evaluation by a doctor with expertise in treating myasthenia gravis.

For people who don't respond fully to pyridostigmine or neostigmine, a doctor may prescribe corticosteroids such as prednisone or azathioprine. Corticosteroids may produce improvement within a few months. Current treatment programs use corticosteroids on alternate days to suppress the autoimmune response. Azathioprine, a drug that helps suppress antibody production, is also beneficial in some instances.

When drugs don't bring relief or when a person is in myasthenic crisis, plasmapheresis may be used.▲ Plasmapheresis is an expensive procedure that extracts toxic substances from the blood (in this case the abnormal antibody). Surgically removing the thymus gland helps about 80 percent of the people with generalized myasthenia gravis.

OTHER NEUROMUSCULAR JUNCTION DISORDERS

Eaton-Lambert syndrome is similar to myasthenia gravis in that it's also an autoimmune disease that causes weakness. However, Eaton-Lambert syndrome is caused by the inadequate release of acetylcholine rather than by abnormal antibodies to acetylcholine receptors. Eaton-Lambert syndrome can appear sporadically but usually occurs as a side effect of certain cancers, especially lung cancer.■

Botulism is a disorder caused by ingesting a food that contains a toxic substance produced by the bacterium *Clostridium botulinum*. The toxic substance paralyzes muscles by inhibiting the release of acetylcholine from nerves.★

Many drugs, certain insecticides (organophosphates), and the nerve gases used in chemical warfare can affect the neuromuscular junction. Some of these substances prevent the natural breakdown of acetylcholine after the nerve impulse has been transmitted to the muscle. Very high doses of some antibiotics can cause weakness in a similar way.

Plexus Disorders

A plexus distributes nerves in somewhat the way an electric junction box distributes wires to different parts of a house. Injury to nerves in the major plexuses, the nervous system's junction boxes, causes problems in the arms or legs that these nerves supply. Major plexuses in the body are the **brachial plexus,** located in the neck and distributing nerves throughout the arms, and the lumbosacral plexus, located in the lower back and distributing nerves to the pelvis and legs.

Causes

Often, a plexus is damaged when the body produces antibodies that attack its own tissues (an autoimmune reaction). An autoimmune reaction is probably responsible for **acute brachial neuritis,** a sudden malfunction of the brachial plexus. However, a plexus is more frequently damaged by physical injury or by a cancer. An accident that pulls the arm or severely bends the arm in its socket may damage the brachial plexus; similarly, a fall can injure the lumbosacral plexus. A cancer growing in the upper regions of the lung can invade and destroy the brachial plexus; a cancer of the intestine, bladder, or prostate can invade the lumbosacral plexus.

Symptoms and Diagnosis

A malfunction of the brachial plexus causes pain and weakness in an arm. The weakness may affect only a portion of the arm, such as the forearm or biceps, or the entire arm. When the cause is an autoimmune disorder, the arm loses strength within a day to a week and regains strength slowly over a few months. Recovery from an injury also tends to occur slowly, over several months, although some severe injuries may cause permanent weakness. Malfunction of the lumbosacral plexus causes pain in the lower back and leg and produces weakness of part or all of a leg. The weakness may be limited to movements of the foot or calf or may cause total leg paralysis. Recovery depends on the cause. Damage to the plexus from an autoimmune disease may resolve slowly over several months.

From the combined disturbances of feeling and motion, a doctor determines that a plexus is involved and, from the location, which plexus is affected. An electromyogram and nerve conduction studies can help locate the problem.● A computed tomography (CT) or magnetic resonance imaging (MRI) scan can help determine whether a cancer or other growth is causing the plexus disorder.

Treatment

The treatment depends on the cause of the plexus disorder. Cancer near the plexus may be treatable with radiation therapy or chemother-

---

▲ see box, page 741

■ see page 385

★ see page 516

● see page 287

apy. Occasionally, a tumor or a collection of blood that is harming the plexus must be removed surgically. Doctors sometimes prescribe corticosteroids for acute brachial neuritis and other plexus disorders in which an autoimmune cause is suspected, but they have no proven benefit. When physical injury causes a plexus disorder, time for healing may be all that is needed.

Thoracic Outlet Syndromes

Thoracic outlet syndromes are ill-defined disorders that are grouped together because they all cause pain and unusual sensations (paresthesias) in the hand, neck, shoulder, or arm.

Causes

Thoracic outlet syndromes are more common in women than in men and usually affect those between the ages of 35 and 55. The various causes of these disorders are often uncertain, but they may originate in the thoracic outlet, the passageway at the top of the rib cage (base of the neck) that allows the esophagus, major blood vessels, trachea, and other structures to pass between the neck and chest. This passageway is very crowded, and problems can occur when blood vessels or nerves to the arm become compressed between a rib and overlying muscle.

Symptoms and Diagnosis

The hands, arms, and shoulders may swell or take on a bluish tinge from lack of oxygen (a condition called cyanosis). No test can specifically identify a thoracic outlet syndrome. Rather, a doctor must rely on information obtained from the history, physical examination, and several tests.

Two tests may help the doctor determine whether the thoracic outlet passageway is so narrow that certain movements cut off blood flow to the arm. **Adson's test** is performed by determining whether the wrist pulse is reduced or obliterated when the person draws a deep breath and holds it while tipping the head back and turning it toward the opposite side. Elevating the arm and rotating it with the head turned to the unaffected side may also cut off the pulse (**Allen test**). A doctor may hear abnormal sounds through a stethoscope indicating abnormal blood flow in the affected artery. Angiography (x-rays taken after a special dye is injected into the bloodstream) may

Nerve Junction Boxes: The Plexuses

Much like the electrical junction box in a house, a nerve plexus is a network of interwoven nerves. Four nerve plexuses are located in the trunk of the body. The cervical plexus provides nerve connections to the head, neck, and shoulder; the brachial plexus, to the chest, shoulder, arm, forearm, and hand; the lumbar plexus, to the back, abdomen, groin, thigh, knee, and leg; and the sacral plexus, to the pelvis, buttocks, genitalia, thigh, leg, and foot. Because the lumbar and sacral plexuses are interconnected, they are sometimes referred to as the lumbosacral plexus. Intercostal nerves are located between the ribs.

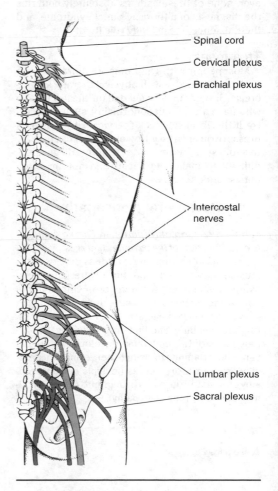

- Spinal cord
- Cervical plexus
- Brachial plexus
- Intercostal nerves
- Lumbar plexus
- Sacral plexus

When the Foot's Asleep

The foot falls asleep when the nerve supplying it is compressed. The compression interferes with the blood supply to the nerve, and the nerve gives off abnormal signals (tingling), called a paresthesia. Moving around removes the compression and restores the blood supply. As a result, nerve function resumes, and the paresthesia stops.

disclose abnormal blood flow to the arm.▲ However, none of these findings absolutely confirms the diagnosis of a thoracic outlet syndrome, and their absence doesn't fully rule it out.

Treatment

Most people with symptoms of a thoracic outlet syndrome improve with physical therapy and exercise. Surgery may be needed for the few people who have a clear-cut abnormality, such as an extra little rib in the neck (cervical rib) that puts pressure on an artery. However, most doctors try to avoid surgery because a definitive diagnosis is difficult to make and because symptoms often persist after surgery.

Peripheral Neuropathy

Peripheral neuropathy (peripheral nerve damage) is a malfunction of the peripheral nerves.

Peripheral neuropathy can disrupt sensation, muscle activity, or the function of internal organs. Symptoms may appear alone or in combination. For example, the muscles supplied by a damaged nerve can weaken and atrophy. Pain, numbness, tingling, swelling, and flushing (blushing) in various parts of the body may develop. The effects can follow damage to a single nerve **(mononeuropathy)**, two or more nerves **(multiple mononeuropathy)**, or many nerves throughout the body simultaneously **(polyneuropathy).**

▲ see page 287

MONONEUROPATHY

A mononeuropathy occurs when a single peripheral nerve is damaged.

Physical injury is the most common cause of a mononeuropathy. Often, the injury is caused by prolonged pressure on a nerve that runs close to the surface of the body near a bony prominence, such as an elbow, shoulder, wrist, or knee. Pressure during sound sleep may be prolonged enough to damage a nerve—especially in people who are under anesthesia or are drunk, in older persons restrained in bed, and in those who can't move or turn over because of paralysis. More unusual causes of prolonged pressure are a misfitting cast, improper use of crutches, and prolonged periods in cramped positions, as when gardening or when playing cards with elbows resting on the table. Nerves may also be damaged during strenuous activities, in an accident, by prolonged exposure to cold or heat, or by radiation given to treat cancer.

Infections may cause mononeuropathy by destroying a nerve. In some countries, leprosy is sometimes a cause of neuropathy.

Certain peripheral nerves are injured more often than others because they are in a vulnerable location. This is true of the median nerve in the wrist (resulting in carpal tunnel syndrome), the ulnar nerve in the elbow, the radial nerve in the upper arm, and the peroneal nerve in the calf.

Carpal tunnel syndrome: Carpal tunnel syndrome results from compression of the median nerve that travels through the wrist supplying the thumb side of the hand. This compression produces odd sensations, numbness, tingling, and pain in the first three fingers and the thumb side of the hand. Occasionally, it also produces pain and paresthesia (a burning or tingling sensation) in the arm and shoulder. The pain may be more severe while sleeping because of the way the hand is positioned. With time, the muscles in the hand on the thumb side can weaken and atrophy.

Carpal tunnel syndrome is common—especially in women—and may affect one or both hands. Particularly susceptible are people whose work requires repeated forceful movements with the wrist extended, such as using a screwdriver. Prolonged use of computer keyboards has also been claimed to cause carpal tunnel syndrome. Pregnant women and people who have diabetes or an underactive thyroid gland are at increased risk of developing carpal tunnel syndrome.

The disorder is best treated by avoiding positions that hyperextend the wrist or put extra pressure on the median nerve. Wrist splints and such measures as adjusting the angle of a computer keyboard may help. Injections of corticosteroids into the nerve occasionally bring temporary relief. If pain is severe or if the muscle atrophies or weakens, surgery is the best way to relieve pressure on the nerve. A surgeon releases the bands of fibrous tissue that place pressure on the median nerve. Before surgery, a doctor may first perform nerve conduction velocity tests to be certain that the problem is carpal tunnel syndrome.

Ulnar nerve palsy: The ulnar nerve passes close to the surface of the skin at the elbow and is easily damaged by repeatedly leaning on the elbow or sometimes by abnormal bone growth in the area. The result is ulnar nerve palsy, odd sensations and weakness in the hand. Severe, chronic ulnar nerve palsy can lead to muscle atrophy and a clawhand deformity. Nerve conduction studies can help locate the damaged nerve. Since surgical repair is often unsuccessful, the disorder is usually treated with physical therapy and by avoiding pressure over the elbow.

Radial nerve palsy: Prolonged compression of the radial nerve, which runs along the underside of the bone in the upper arm, results in radial nerve palsy. This disorder is sometimes called Saturday night palsy because it occurs in people who drink heavily and then sleep soundly with an arm draped over the back of a chair or under the head. The nerve damage weakens the wrist and fingers so the wrist may flop into a bent position with the fingers curved (wristdrop). Occasionally, the back of the hand may lose feeling. Usually, radial nerve palsy improves once the pressure is relieved.

Peroneal nerve palsy: Compression of the peroneal nerve, which lies close to the surface of the skin in the soft folds at the top of the calf behind the knee, results in peroneal nerve palsy. This weakens the muscles that lift the foot, causing footdrop. It's most common in thin people who are bedridden, people who are improperly strapped into a wheelchair, or people who habitually cross their legs for long periods of time.

Substances That May Cause Nerve Damage

Anti-infective drugs
- Emetine
- Chlorobutanol
- Sulfonamides
- Nitrofurantoin

Anticancer drugs
- Vinca alkaloids

Antiseizure drugs
- Phenytoin

Industrial poisons
- Heavy metals (such as lead or mercury)
- Carbon monoxide
- Triorthocresyl phosphate
- Orthodinitrophenol
- Many solvents

Sedatives
- Hexobarbital
- Barbital

POLYNEUROPATHY

Polyneuropathy is the simultaneous malfunction of many peripheral nerves throughout the body.

Causes

Polyneuropathy has many different causes. An infection can cause polyneuropathy, sometimes from a toxin produced by some bacteria (as in diphtheria) or from an autoimmune reaction (as in Guillain-Barré syndrome▲). Toxic agents can harm peripheral nerves and cause polyneuropathy or, more rarely, mononeuropathy. A cancer may cause polyneuropathy by directly invading or compressing the nerves or by producing toxic substances.

Nutritional deficiencies and metabolic disorders may cause polyneuropathy. For example, vitamin B deficiency affects peripheral nerves throughout the body. However, neuropathies related to nutritional deficiencies are uncommon in the United States.

▲ see page 338

Disorders that may cause **chronic polyneuropathy** include diabetes, kidney failure, and severe malnutrition. Chronic polyneuropathy tends to develop slowly, often over months or years, and usually begins in the feet or sometimes the hands. Poor control of blood sugar levels in diabetes causes several forms of polyneuropathy. The most common form of **diabetic neuropathy,** distal polyneuropathy, leads to a painful tingling or burning sensation in the hands and feet.▲ Diabetes can also cause mononeuropathy or multiple mononeuropathy that leads to weakness, typically of the eye and thigh muscles.

Symptoms

Tingling, numbness, burning pain, and an inability to sense vibration or the position of the arms, legs, and joints are prominent symptoms of chronic polyneuropathy. Pain is often worse at night and may be aggravated by touching the sensitive area or by temperature changes. Because they may not sense temperature and pain, people with chronic polyneuropathy often burn themselves and develop open sores (skin ulcers) from prolonged pressure or other injuries. Without pain as a warning of too much stress, joints are subject to injuries (Charcot's joints). An inability to sense the position of joints leads to unsteady walking and even standing. Eventually, muscles may weaken and atrophy.

Many people with peripheral neuropathy also develop abnormalities in the autonomic nervous system, which controls automatic functions in the body such as heartbeat, bowel function, bladder control, and blood pressure. When peripheral neuropathy affects the autonomic nerves, typical effects are diarrhea or constipation, inability to control the bowel or bladder, sexual impotence, and low or high blood pressure, most notably low blood pressure upon standing. The skin may become paler and drier, and sweating may be excessive.

Diagnosis

A doctor easily recognizes chronic polyneuropathy by its symptoms. A physical examination and special studies such as electromyography and nerve conduction velocity tests can provide additional information.■ However, a diagnosis of polyneuropathy is only the beginning; the cause must be sought. If the cause is a metabolic disorder rather than a physical injury, blood tests may reveal the underlying problem. For instance, blood tests may indicate pernicious anemia (vitamin B_{12} deficiency) or lead poisoning. Elevated blood sugar levels indicate poorly controlled diabetes, and elevated blood creatine levels suggest kidney failure. Urine tests may uncover heavy metal poisoning or multiple myeloma. Thyroid function tests or measurement of B vitamin levels may be appropriate in some people. Infrequently, a nerve biopsy is necessary.

Treatment and Prognosis

Both the treatment and outcome of chronic polyneuropathy depend on the cause. When neuropathy is related to diabetes, careful control of blood sugar levels may halt progression and improve symptoms, but recovery is slow. Treating multiple myeloma and kidney failure may also speed recovery. People with nerve damage from injury and compression may need surgical treatment. Physical therapy sometimes reduces the severity of muscle spasms or weakness.

Guillain-Barré Syndrome

Guillain-Barré syndrome (acute ascending polyneuritis) is a form of acute polyneuropathy that produces rapidly worsening muscle weakness, sometimes leading to paralysis.

The presumed cause is an autoimmune reaction—the body's immune system attacks the myelin sheath. In about 80 percent of the people, symptoms begin about 5 days to 3 weeks after a mild infection, surgery, or an immunization.

Symptoms

Guillain-Barré syndrome usually begins with weakness, tingling, and loss of sensation in both legs, then progresses upward to the arms. Weakness is the most prominent symptom. In 90 percent of the people who have Guillain-Barré syndrome, weakness is most severe within 2 to 3 weeks. In 5 to 10 percent, the muscles that support breathing become so weak that a respirator is needed. About 10 percent need to be fed intravenously or through a gastrostomy tube because the facial and swallowing muscles become weak.

▲ see page 720

■ see page 287

If the disease is very severe, the blood pressure may fluctuate, or the person may have an abnormal heart rhythm or other dysfunctions in the autonomic nervous system. One form of Guillain-Barré syndrome produces an unusual group of symptoms in which eye movements become paralyzed, walking is difficult, and normal reflexes disappear. Over all, about 5 percent of the people with Guillain-Barré syndrome die of the disease.

Diagnosis

Since laboratory tests can't specifically diagnose Guillain-Barré syndrome, doctors must recognize the disease from its pattern of symptoms. Analysis of cerebrospinal fluid from the spinal column (obtained by a spinal tap), electromyography, nerve conduction studies, and blood tests are performed mostly to exclude other possible causes of profound weakness.

Treatment

Guillain-Barré syndrome is a very serious disease that requires immediate hospitalization because it can worsen rapidly. Establishing the diagnosis is of the utmost importance because the sooner appropriate treatment is started, the better the chance that the outcome will be good. Patients are closely monitored so that breathing can be assisted with a respirator, if necessary. Nurses take precautions to prevent bedsores and injuries by providing soft mattresses and by turning the patient every 2 hours. Physical therapy is important to prevent tightening of muscles and to preserve joint and muscle function.

Once the diagnosis is made, plasmapheresis, in which toxic substances are filtered from the blood,▲ or infusion of autoimmune globulin is the treatment of choice. Corticosteroids are no longer recommended because they have no proven benefit and may actually worsen the disease.

People with Guillain-Barré syndrome can get better on their own, but convalescence without treatment can last a long time. People treated early can improve very quickly—in a matter of days to weeks. Otherwise, recovery takes several months, but most people recover almost completely. About 30 percent (and an even higher percentage of children with the disease) have residual weakness after 3 years. After initial improvement, about 10 percent of the people relapse and develop **chronic relapsing polyneuropathy.** Immune globulins and corticosteroids may be

helpful for this persistent form of Guillain-Barré syndrome. Plasmapheresis and drugs that suppress the immune system also help.

Hereditary Neuropathies

Hereditary neuropathies are nervous system disorders that are genetically passed from parents to children. The three main categories of hereditary neuropathies are hereditary motor neuropathies, which affect only motor nerves; hereditary sensory neuropathies, which affect only sensory nerves; and hereditary sensory-motor neuropathies, which affect both sensory and motor nerves. None of these neuropathies are common, but hereditary sensory neuropathies are especially rare.

Charcot-Marie-Tooth disease (also called **peroneal muscular atrophy**), the most common hereditary neuropathy, affects the peroneal nerve, causing muscle weakness and atrophy in the lower legs. This disease is inherited as an autosomal dominant trait.■

Symptoms of Charcot-Marie-Tooth disease depend on which form of the disease is inherited. Children with type 1 disease develop weakness in their lower legs during middle childhood, which causes footdrop and wasting of the calf muscles (stork leg deformity). Later, hand muscles begin to waste away. The children lose their ability to feel pain, heat, and cold in their hands and feet. The disease progresses slowly and doesn't affect life expectancy. People with type 2 disease, which progresses even more slowly, develop somewhat similar symptoms later in life.

Dejerine-Sottas disease (also called **hypertrophic interstitial neuropathy**) is rarer than Charcot-Marie-Tooth disease, starts in childhood, and is characterized by progressive weakness and loss of sensation in the legs. Muscle weakness progresses at a faster rate than in Charcot-Marie-Tooth disease.

The distribution of weakness, the age of onset, the family history, the presence of foot deformities (high arches and hammer toes), and the results of nerve conduction studies help doctors

---

▲ see box, page 741

■ see page 9

distinguish Charcot-Marie-Tooth disease from Dejerine-Sottas disease and other causes of neuropathy. No current treatment can keep the diseases from worsening. Wearing braces helps correct the footdrop, and sometimes orthopedic surgery is needed.

Spinal Muscular Atrophies

Spinal muscular atrophies are inherited diseases in which nerve cells in the spinal cord and brain stem degenerate, causing progressive muscle weakness and wasting.

Symptoms

Symptoms first appear in infancy and childhood. The muscle weakness of **acute spinal muscular atrophy (Werdnig-Hoffmann disease)** appears in babies 2 to 4 months old. The disease is inherited in an autosomal recessive pattern, which means that two nondominant genes are required, one from each parent.

Children with **intermediate spinal muscular atrophy** remain normal for a year or two and then develop weakness, worse in the legs than in the arms. They don't usually develop respiratory, cardiac, or cranial nerve problems. The disease progresses slowly.

Chronic spinal muscular atrophy (Wohlfart-Kugelberg-Welander disease) begins in children between 2 and 17 years of age and worsens slowly, so people with this disease live longer than those with other types of spinal muscular atrophy. Weakness and wasting of muscles begin in the legs and later spread to the arms.

Diagnosis and Treatment

Doctors test for these rare diseases when young children develop unexplained weakness and muscle wasting. Because these diseases are inherited, a family history may help make the diagnosis. The specific faulty gene has been found for some of the diseases. Electromyography helps the doctor make the diagnosis. Amniocentesis, a test that analyzes some of the mother's amniotic fluid during pregnancy, is of no help in diagnosing these diseases.

No specific treatments are available. Physical therapy, wearing braces, and special devices can sometimes help.

CHAPTER 71

Cranial Nerve Disorders

Twelve nerves—the cranial nerves—lead directly from the brain to various parts of the head. Except for cranial nerve VIII, which processes hearing and assists in maintaining equilibrium, cranial nerves III through XII control movements of the eyes, tongue, face, and throat. Cranial nerves V and IX receive sensations from the face, tongue, and throat. Cranial nerve I is the olfactory nerve, or the nerve of smell.▲ Cranial nerve II is the optic nerve, or the nerve of sight.■ A disorder of any of the cranial nerves can produce severe

loss of function, but three disorders—trigeminal neuralgia, glossopharyngeal neuralgia, and Bell's palsy—are the most common.

Trigeminal Neuralgia

*Also known as **tic douloureux,** trigeminal neuralgia involves a malfunction of the trigeminal nerve (cranial nerve V), which carries sensation from the face to the brain.*

Malfunction of the trigeminal nerve produces bouts of severe, piercing pain lasting seconds to minutes. Adults of any age can be affected by trigeminal neuralgia, but the disorder is more common in the elderly. The cause is unknown.

Symptoms

The pain can occur spontaneously but is often set off by touching a particular spot (trigger

▲ see page 342

■ see page 1051

point) or by an activity such as brushing the teeth or chewing. Repeated bursts of closely separated lightning-like flashes of excruciating pain can be felt in any part of the lower portion of the face. Most often the pain is felt in the cheek adjacent to the nose or in the jaw area. Recurring as often as 100 times a day, the pain can be totally incapacitating.

Diagnosis

Although no specific test exists for identifying trigeminal neuralgia, its characteristic pain makes it easy for a doctor to diagnose. Doctors also evaluate other possible causes of facial pain, such as diseases of the jaw, teeth, or sinuses or compression of the trigeminal nerve by a tumor or aneurysm.

Treatment

Since the bouts of pain are brief and recurrent, typical pain medications aren't usually helpful, but other drugs, especially certain antiseizure drugs (which stabilize nerve membranes), may be helpful. Carbamazepine is usually tried first, but phenytoin may be prescribed if carbamazepine doesn't work or produces severe side effects. Baclofen and several antidepressant drugs also help in some cases. Spontaneous remissions are common, but bouts of the disease often recur at wide intervals.

Trigeminal neuralgia sometimes results when an out-of-place artery compresses the nerve adjacent to the brain. In such cases an operation can separate the artery from the nerve and relieve the pain for at least a few years. For people with pain that can't be relieved by drugs and who may not be good candidates for surgery, a test can be done in which alcohol is injected into the nerve, temporarily blocking its function. If this relieves the pain, the nerve can be cut or permanently destroyed by injecting a drug into it. Such approaches often produce discomfort in the face and should be regarded as a last resort.

Glossopharyngeal Neuralgia

Glossopharyngeal neuralgia is a rare disorder in which a person has recurring attacks of severe pain in the back of the throat near the tonsils, sometimes affecting the ear on the same side.

Glossopharyngeal neuralgia usually begins after age 40 and occurs more often in men than in women. Its cause is unknown.

Bell's Palsy Paralyzes One Side of the Face

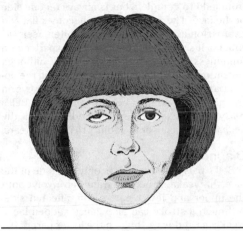

Symptoms

As in trigeminal neuralgia, attacks are intermittent and brief but cause excruciating pain and may be triggered by a particular action, such as chewing, swallowing, talking, or yawning. The pain may last several seconds to a few minutes and usually affects only one side.

Treatment

The same drugs used to treat trigeminal neuralgia—carbamazepine, phenytoin, baclofen, and antidepressants—may be helpful. When these measures fail, surgery may be needed to block or cut the glossopharyngeal nerve either in the neck or at the base of the brain.

Bell's Palsy

Bell's palsy is an abnormality of the facial nerve that leads to sudden weakness or paralysis of the muscles on one side of the face.

The facial nerve is the cranial nerve that stimulates the facial muscles. Although the cause of Bell's palsy is unknown, it may involve swelling of the facial nerve as a reaction to a viral infection, compression, or lack of blood supply.

Symptoms

Bell's palsy comes on suddenly. Several hours before developing weakness of the facial muscles, the person may have pain behind the ear. The ensuing facial weakness can range unpredictably from mild to complete but is always on one side of the face. The paralyzed side becomes flat and expressionless, but the person often feels as though it's twisted. Most people experience a numbness or heavy feeling in the face, although sensation actually remains normal. When the upper part of the face is involved, closing the eye on the affected side may be difficult. Rarely, Bell's palsy interferes with the production of saliva, the sensation of taste, or the ability to produce tears.

Diagnosis

Bell's palsy always affects only one side of the face; the weakness is sudden and can involve both the upper and lower part of the affected side. Although a stroke can also cause sudden facial weakness, it does so only in the lower part of the face. In addition, a stroke causes weakness of the arm and leg.▲

Other causes of facial nerve paralysis are rare and usually appear slowly. They include brain or other tumors that compress the nerve; destruction of the facial nerve by a viral infection such as herpes (Ramsay Hunt's syndrome); infections in the middle ear or mastoid sinuses; ■ Lyme disease; fractures of the bone at the base of the skull; and several other, even more rare, disorders. Usually, a doctor can exclude these disorders by taking the person's history and by noting the results of an x-ray, a computed tomography (CT) scan, or a magnetic resonance imaging (MRI) scan. A blood test for Lyme disease may be needed. No specific test exists for Bell's palsy.

Treatment

Bell's palsy has no specific treatment. Some doctors believe that corticosteroids such as prednisone should be given no later than 2 days after symptoms develop and continued for 1 to 2 weeks. Whether this treatment reduces pain and improves the chances for recovery has not been conclusively demonstrated.

If paralyzed facial muscles prevent the eye from closing completely, the eye must be protected from dryness. Lubricating eye drops, used every few hours, are often recommended. An eye patch may be needed. In people with severe paralysis, massaging the weakened muscles and stimulating the nerves may help prevent the facial muscles from tightening. If paralysis persists for 6 to 12 months or more, a surgeon may try to graft a healthy nerve (usually taken from the tongue) into the paralyzed facial muscle.

Prognosis

Complete recovery within 1 to 2 months is likely when the paralysis is partial. The outcome for people with total paralysis varies, although most recover completely. To help determine the likelihood of complete recovery, a doctor can test the facial nerve using electrical stimulation. Occasionally, as the facial nerve heals, it forms abnormal connections, resulting in unexpected movements of some facial muscles or spontaneous watering of the eyes.

CHAPTER 72

Smell and Taste Disorders

Since disorders of smell and taste are rarely life-threatening, they may not receive close medical attention. Yet, these disorders can be frustrating because they can affect a person's ability to enjoy food, drink, and pleasant aromas. They can also interfere with a person's ability to notice potentially harmful chemicals and gases, which could have serious consequences. Now and then, a disorder that impairs smell and taste can be serious.

▲ see page 352

■ see page 1006

How People Sense Flavors

The senses of taste and smell work together to enable people to recognize and appreciate flavors. The smell and taste center in the brain combines sensory information from both the tongue and nose.

Thousands of tiny taste buds cover most of the tongue's surface. When food is placed in the mouth, it stimulates receptors in the taste buds. The taste buds, in turn, send nerve impulses to the smell and taste center of the brain, which interprets them as taste. The taste buds on the tip of the tongue detect sweetness; those on the sides, saltiness and sourness; and those in the back, bitterness. Combinations of these four basic tastes produce a wide spectrum of flavors.

A small area on the mucous membrane that lines the nose (the olfactory epithelium) contains nerve endings that detect odor (olfactory nerves). When airborne molecules enter the nasal passage, they stimulate tiny hairlike projections (cilia) on these nerve cells. This stimulation sends nerve impulses through the swellings at the end of the nerves (olfactory bulbs), along the olfactory nerve, to the smell and taste center of

the brain. The center interprets these nerve impulses as a distinct odor. By this process, thousands of different odors can be distinguished.

To distinguish most flavors, the brain needs both taste and smell sensations. For example, to distinguish the flavor of a candy bar, the brain senses a sweet taste from the taste buds and the rich, full-bodied aroma of chocolate from the nose.

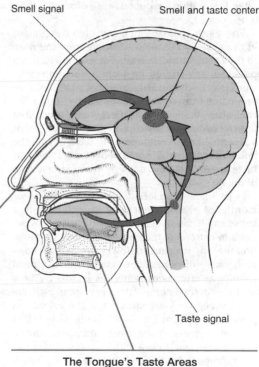

Smell signal

Smell and taste center

Taste signal

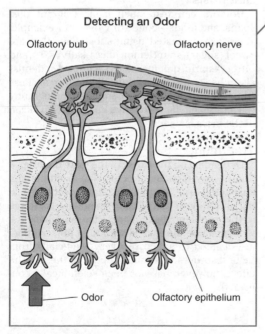

Detecting an Odor

Olfactory bulb

Olfactory nerve

Odor

Olfactory epithelium

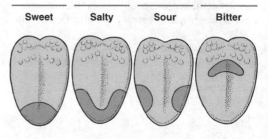

The Tongue's Taste Areas

Sweet	Salty	Sour	Bitter

Smell and taste are closely linked. The taste buds of the tongue identify taste; the nerves in the nose identify smell. Both sensations are communicated to the brain, which combines the information to recognize and appreciate flavors. While some tastes—such as salty, bitter, sweet, and sour—can be recognized without the sense of smell, more complex flavors (raspberry, for example) require both taste and smell sensations to be recognized.

A loss of or reduction in the ability to smell (anosmia) is the most common disorder of smell and taste. Because distinguishing one flavor from another is based in large part on smell, people often first notice a reduced sense of smell if their food seems tasteless.

The sense of smell can be affected by changes in the nose, in the nerves leading from the nose to the brain, or in the brain. For example, if nasal passages are stuffed up from a common cold, smell may be decreased simply because odors are prevented from reaching the smell receptors. Because the ability to smell affects taste, food often doesn't taste right to people with colds. Cells that sense smell can be temporarily damaged by the influenza (flu) virus; some people can't smell or taste for several days or even weeks after a bout of the flu.

Occasionally, the loss of smell or taste lasts for months or even becomes permanent. Cells that sense smell can be damaged or destroyed by serious infections of the nasal sinuses or by radiation therapy for cancer. However, the most common cause of permanent loss of smell is head trauma, as often occurs in a car accident. Fibers of the olfactory nerve—the nerve that contains smell receptors—are sheared at the cribriform plate—the bone at the skull base that separates the intracranial space from the nasal cavity. Rarely, a person is born without a sense of smell.

Oversensitivity to smell (hyperosmia) is much less common than anosmia. A distorted sense of smell that makes innocuous odors smell disagreeable (dysosmia) may result from infections in the sinuses or partial damage to the olfactory nerve. Dysosmia also may be caused by poor dental hygiene, which can result in mouth infections that smell bad and are sensed by the nose. Sometimes people with depression develop dysosmia. Some people who have seizures originating in the part of the brain where smell is perceived (the olfactory center) experience brief, vivid, unpleasant smell sensations (olfactory hallucinations).▲ These disagreeable smells are part of the seizure, not a misinterpretation of an odor.

A diminished or lost sense of taste (ageusia) is usually caused by conditions that affect the tongue. Examples are very dry mouth, heavy smoking (especially pipe smoking), radiation treatment to the head and neck, and side effects of drugs such as vincristine (a cancer drug) or amitriptyline (an antidepressant).

A distortion of taste (dysgeusia) may be caused by many of the same factors that result in loss of taste. Burns to the tongue may temporarily destroy taste buds, and Bell's palsy (a one-sided paralysis of the face caused by malfunction of the facial nerve)■ may dull the sense of taste on one side of the tongue. Dysgeusia may also be a symptom of depression.

Diagnosis

Doctors can test smell using fragrant oils, soaps, and foods—coffee or cloves, for example. Taste can be tested using substances that are sweet (sugar), sour (lemon juice), salty (salt), and bitter (aspirin, quinine, aloes). A doctor or dentist also checks the mouth for infection or dryness (too little saliva). Rarely, a computed tomography (CT) or magnetic resonance imaging (MRI) scan of the brain is needed.

Treatment

Depending on the cause of the taste disorder, a doctor may recommend changing or stopping a suspected drug, keeping the mouth wet by sucking on candy, or just waiting several weeks to see if the problem disappears. Zinc supplements, which can be purchased without a prescription, are claimed to speed recovery, especially from taste disorders that follow a bout of the flu. The effect, however, has not been scientifically confirmed.

▲ see page 347

■ see page 341

Seizure Disorders

A seizure is the response to an abnormal electrical discharge in the brain.

The term *seizure* describes various experiences and behaviors and isn't the same as *convulsion*, though the terms are sometimes used synonymously. Anything that irritates the brain can produce a seizure. Two thirds of people who experience a seizure never have another. One third go on to have recurring seizures (a condition called epilepsy).

Precisely what happens during a seizure depends on what part of the brain is affected by the abnormal electrical discharge. The discharge may involve a tiny area of the brain and lead only to the person noticing an odd smell or taste, or it may involve large areas and lead to a convul-

Causes of Seizures

High fever
- Heatstroke
- Infection

Brain infections
- AIDS
- Malaria
- Meningitis
- Rabies
- Syphilis
- Tetanus
- Toxoplasmosis
- Viral encephalitis

Metabolic disturbances
- Hypoparathyroidism
- High levels of sugar or sodium in the blood
- Low levels of sugar, calcium, magnesium, or sodium in the blood
- Kidney or liver failure
- Phenylketonuria

Insufficient oxygen to the brain
- Carbon monoxide poisoning
- Inadequate blood flow to the brain
- Near drowning
- Near suffocation
- Stroke

Destruction of brain tissue
- Brain tumor
- Head injury
- Intracranial hemorrhage
- Stroke

Other illnesses
- Eclampsia
- Hypertensive encephalopathy
- Lupus erythematosus

Exposure to toxic drugs or substances
- Alcohol (large amounts)
- Amphetamines
- Camphor
- Chloroquine
- Cocaine overdose
- Lead
- Pentylenetetrazol
- Strychnine

Withdrawal after heavy use
- Alcohol
- Sleep aids
- Tranquilizers

Adverse reactions to prescription drugs
- Ceftazidime
- Chlorpromazine
- Imipenem
- Indomethacin
- Meperidine
- Phenytoin
- Theophylline

Symptoms of Seizures Vary by Site

Site of Abnormal Electrical Discharge	Symptoms
Frontal lobe	Twitches in a specific muscle
Occipital lobe	Hallucinations of flashes of light
Parietal lobe	Numbness or tingling in a specific body part
Temporal lobe	Hallucinations of images and complicated repetitive behavior—for instance, walking in circles
Anterior temporal lobe	Chewing movements, lip smacking
Anterior deep temporal lobe	Intense hallucination of a smell, either pleasant or unpleasant

sion—jerking and spasms of muscles throughout the body. The person may also have brief attacks of altered consciousness; lose consciousness, muscle control, or bladder control; and become confused. Seizures are often preceded by auras—unusual sensations of smell, taste, or visions or an intense feeling that a seizure is about to begin. Sometimes these sensations are pleasant, and other times they are extremely unpleasant. About 20 percent of the people with epilepsy experience auras.

A seizure usually lasts for 2 to 5 minutes. When it stops, the person may have a headache, sore muscles, unusual sensations, confusion, and profound fatigue (called a postictal state). The person usually can't remember what happened during the seizure.

Infantile Spasms and Febrile Seizures

Two kinds of seizures occur almost exclusively in children. In **infantile spasms** (salaam seizures), a child lying on his back suddenly raises and bends the arms, bends the neck and upper body forward, and straightens the legs. Attacks last for only a few seconds but may recur many times a day. They generally occur in children under age 3; many typically evolve into other forms of seizure later in life. Most children with infantile spasms have associated intellectual impairment or neurodevelopmental delays; mental retardation usually continues into adulthood. The seizures are difficult to stop with antiepileptic drugs.

Febrile seizures result from fever in children from 3 months to 5 years old. They occur in about 4 percent of all children and tend to run in families. Most children who have a febrile seizure have only one, and most seizures last for less than 15 minutes. Children who have a febrile seizure are slightly more likely to develop epilepsy later in life.

Epilepsy

Epilepsy is a disorder characterized by the tendency to have recurring seizures.

Overall, 2 percent of the adult population has a seizure at some time. One third of that group has recurring seizures (epilepsy). In about 25 percent of adults with epilepsy, the cause is found when tests such as an electroencephalogram (EEG) reveal abnormal electrical activity or magnetic resonance imaging (MRI) reveals scarring in small areas of the brain. In some cases, these defects may be microscopic scars resulting from brain injury at birth or later. A few specific types of seizure disorders (such as juvenile myoclonic epilepsy) are inherited. In the remaining people with epilepsy, the disease is labeled *idiopathic*—that is, no evidence of damage is found in the brain, and the cause isn't known.

People with idiopathic epilepsy usually have their first seizure between the ages of 2 and 14. Seizures before age 2 are generally caused by brain defects, chemical imbalances, or high fevers. Seizures that begin after age 25 are more likely to result from brain trauma, a stroke, or a tumor or other disease.

Epileptic seizures may be triggered by repetitive sounds, flashing lights, video games, or even touching certain parts of the body. Even minor stimuli can trigger a seizure in people with epilepsy. Very strong stimuli—such as certain drugs, low levels of oxygen in the blood, or very low levels of sugar in the blood—can trigger a seizure even in people who don't have epilepsy.

Symptoms

Epileptic seizures are sometimes classified by their characteristics. **Simple partial seizures** begin with electrical discharges in a small area of the brain, and the discharges remain confined to that area. The person experiences abnormal sensations, movements, or psychic aberrations, depending on the part of the brain affected. For example, if an electrical discharge occurs in the part of the brain that controls the right arm's muscle movements, the right arm may begin to shake and jerk; if it occurs in the anterior deep temporal lobe (the part of the brain that senses smells),▲ the person may sense an intensely pleasant or unpleasant smell. A person who has a psychic aberration may experience, for example, a sense of déjà vu, in which unfamiliar surroundings inexplicably seem familiar.

In **jacksonian seizures,** symptoms begin in one isolated part of the body, such as the hand or foot, and then "march up" the limb as the electrical activity spreads in the brain. **Complex partial (psychomotor) seizures** begin with a 1- to 2-minute period during which the person loses touch with surroundings. The person may stagger, move the arms and legs in strange and purposeless ways, utter meaningless sounds, fail to understand what others say, and resist help. Confusion lasts for several more minutes, followed by full recovery.

Convulsive seizures (grand mal or tonic-clonic seizures) usually begin with an abnormal electrical discharge in a small area of the brain. The discharge quickly spreads to adjoining parts of the brain, causing the entire area to malfunction. In **primary generalized epilepsy,** abnormal discharges over a large area of the brain cause widespread malfunction from the beginning. In either case, a convulsion is the body's reaction to the abnormal discharges. In these convulsive seizures, a person experiences a temporary loss of consciousness, severe muscle spasms and jerking throughout the body, intense turning of the head to one side, clenching of teeth, and loss of bladder control. Afterward, the person may have a headache, be temporarily confused, and feel extremely tired. Usually, the person doesn't remember what happened during the seizure.

Petit mal (absence) seizures begin in childhood, usually before age 5. They don't produce the convulsions and other dramatic symptoms of grand mal seizures. Instead, a person has episodes of staring, fluttering eyelids, or twitching facial muscles that last 10 to 30 seconds. The person is unresponsive but doesn't fall down, collapse, or move jerkily.

In **status epilepticus,** the most serious seizure disorder, the seizure doesn't stop. *Status epilepticus is a medical emergency* because the person has convulsions with intense muscle contractions, is unable to breathe properly, and has widespread (diffuse) electrical discharges in the brain. Without rapid treatment, the heart and brain can become overtaxed and permanently damaged, and the person can die.

Diagnosis

A person who loses consciousness, has muscle spasms that shake the body, loses bladder control, or suddenly becomes confused and inattentive may be having a seizure. Yet true seizures are much less common than most people think—most episodes of brief unconsciousness or abnormal behavior aren't caused by abnormal electrical discharges in the brain.

An eyewitness report of the episode can be very helpful to doctors. The witness can describe exactly what happened, while the person who had the episode usually can't. An accurate description of the circumstances surrounding the episode is needed: how fast it started; whether it involved abnormal muscle movements, such as spasms of the head, neck, or facial muscles, tongue biting, or loss of bladder control; how long it lasted; and how quickly the person recovered. The doctor also needs to know what the person experienced. Did the person have a premonition or warning that something unusual was about to happen? Did anything happen that seemed to precipitate the episode, such as certain sounds or flashing lights?

Aside from noting a description of the episode, a doctor diagnoses a seizure disorder or epilepsy using an electroencephalogram (EEG), which measures electrical activity in the brain. The test is painless and poses no risk. Electrodes are

---

▲ see box, page 279

Brain Activity During a Seizure

An electroencephalogram (EEG) is a recording of the brain's electrical activity. The procedure is simple and painless: About 20 small electrodes are pasted to the scalp, and the brain's activity is recorded under normal conditions. Then the person is exposed to various stimuli, such as bright or flashing lights, to help provoke a seizure. During a seizure, electrical activity in the brain accelerates, producing a jagged waveform pattern. Such recordings of brain waves help identify epilepsy. Different types of seizures have different wave patterns.

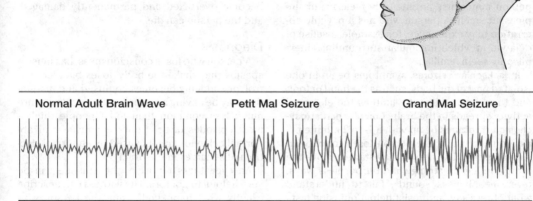

| Normal Adult Brain Wave | Petit Mal Seizure | Grand Mal Seizure |

pasted to the scalp to measure the electrical impulses within the brain. Because abnormal discharges are more likely to occur after too little sleep, EEGs are sometimes scheduled after a person has deliberately stayed awake for 18 to 24 hours.

Doctors examine the EEG recording for evidence of abnormal electrical discharges. Even if a seizure didn't occur during the EEG recording, abnormalities may be present. However, because the EEG is recorded for only a limited time, it can miss seizure activity and appear normal, even in a person who has epilepsy.

Once epilepsy is diagnosed, more tests are usually needed to seek a possibly treatable cause. Routine blood tests measure the levels of sugar, calcium, and sodium in the blood; determine whether the liver and kidneys are functioning

properly; and count the white blood cells, since a high number might indicate an infection. The doctor often orders an electrocardiogram▲ to see if an abnormal heart rhythm resulted in inadequate blood flow to the brain, which can cause a person to lose consciousness. The doctor generally orders a computed tomography (CT) or magnetic resonance imaging (MRI) scan to evaluate the brain for cancer and other tumors, previous strokes, small scars, and damage from injury. Sometimes a spinal tap (lumbar puncture)■ is needed to determine if the person has a brain infection.

Treatment

If a treatable cause such as a tumor, an infection, or abnormal blood sugar or sodium levels is identified, that condition is treated first. Once the medical condition is corrected, the seizures themselves may not need to be treated. When no cause is found or if the cause can't be completely cured or controlled, antiseizure drugs may be needed to prevent further seizures. Only time can tell if a

▲ see page 73

■ see box, page 374

person will have recurring seizures. About one third of the people do have recurring seizures, but the other two thirds ever have only one seizure. Medication is generally considered unnecessary for one-time seizures but necessary for recurring ones.

Seizures should be prevented for several reasons. Fierce, rapid muscle contractions can cause bodily harm and even result in broken bones. Sudden loss of consciousness can cause serious injury from falls and accidents. The turbulent electrical activity of a grand mal seizure can cause minor brain damage. However, most people who have epilepsy experience dozens or more seizures in their lives without suffering serious brain injury. Although individual seizures don't impair intelligence, recurring convulsive seizures may do so.

Antiseizure drugs can completely prevent grand mal seizures in more than half the people with epilepsy and greatly reduce the frequency of seizures in another third. Drugs are only slightly less effective for petit mal seizures. Half of the people who respond to drug treatment can eventually discontinue the treatment without having a relapse. No single drug can control all types of seizures. Some people can have their seizures controlled with a single drug, while others have to take several.

Because status epilepticus is an emergency, doctors must give the person large intravenous doses of an antiseizure drug as quickly as possible. Care is taken to prevent injuries during the prolonged seizure.

While antiseizure drugs are very effective, they may have side effects. Many cause drowsiness but, paradoxically, cause hyperactivity when given to children. Doctors order blood tests periodically to find out if the drug is affecting the kidneys, liver, or blood cells. People taking antiseizure drugs should be aware of possible side effects and should consult their doctor at the first sign of them.

The dose of an antiseizure drug is critical: It must be large enough to prevent seizures but not so large that side effects are a problem. The doctor adjusts the dose after asking about side effects and testing the level of drug in the blood. Antiseizure drugs should be taken just as prescribed. No other drugs should be taken at the same time without the doctor's permission because they might alter the amount of antiseizure drug in the blood. Anyone taking antiseizure drugs should

Drugs Used to Treat Seizures

Drug	Type of Seizure	Possible Side Effects
Carbamaze-pine	Generalized, partial	Low counts of white blood cells and red blood cells
Ethosuximide	Petit mal	Low counts of white blood cells and red blood cells
Gabapentin	Partial	Sedation
Lamotrigine	Generalized, partial	Rash
Pheno-barbital	Generalized, partial	Sedation
Phenytoin	Generalized, partial	Swollen gums
Primidone	Generalized, partial	Sedation
Valproate	Infantile spasms, petit mal	Weight gain, hair loss

see a doctor regularly for possible dose adjustment and should always wear a Medic Alert bracelet that names the seizure disorder and the drug being taken.

Most people who have epilepsy look and behave normally between seizures and can live normal lives. However, they may have to adjust some habits and behaviors. For example, people who are prone to seizures shouldn't drink alcoholic beverages. In addition, laws in most states forbid people with epilepsy to drive until they have been seizure-free for at least 1 year.

A family member or close friend should be trained to help if a seizure occurs. Although some people think they should attempt to protect the tongue, such efforts can do more harm than good. The teeth may be damaged, or the person may bite the helper unintentionally as the jaw muscles contract. The important steps are to protect the person from a fall, loosen clothing around the neck, and place a pillow under the head. A person who loses consciousness should be rolled onto one side to ease breathing. No one who has had a seizure should be left alone until he has awakened completely and can move about normally. Notifying the person's doctor is usually wise.

For about 10 to 20 percent of the people with epilepsy, drugs alone won't prevent seizures from recurring. If a defect in the brain can be identified as the cause and it's confined to a small area, surgically removing that area may solve the problem. Surgically removing the nerve fibers that connect the two sides of the brain (corpus callosum) may help people who have several sources for the seizures or who have seizures that spread to all parts of the brain very quickly. Brain surgery is considered only if all drugs have failed or their side effects can't be tolerated.

CHAPTER 74

Stroke and Related Disorders

When blood flow to the brain is disrupted, brain cells can die or be damaged from lack of oxygen. Brain cells can also be damaged if bleeding occurs in or around the brain. The resulting neurologic problems are called **cerebrovascular disorders** because of the brain (cerebrum) and blood vessel (vascular) involvement.

Insufficient blood supply to parts of the brain for brief periods causes **transient ischemic attacks,** temporary disturbances in brain function. Because the blood supply is restored quickly, brain tissue doesn't die, as it does in a **stroke.** A transient ischemic attack is often an early warning sign of a stroke.

In Western countries, strokes are the most common cause of disabling neurologic damage. High blood pressure and atherosclerosis—hardening of the arteries from fatty buildup—are the major risk factors for strokes. The incidence of strokes has declined in recent decades, mainly because people are more aware of the importance of controlling high blood pressure and high cholesterol levels.

How a stroke or transient ischemic attack affects the body depends on precisely where in the brain the blood supply was cut off or where bleeding occurred. Each area of the brain is served by specific blood vessels. For example, if a blood vessel in the area that controls the left leg's muscle movements becomes blocked, the leg will be weak or paralyzed. If the area that senses touch to the right arm is damaged, the right arm will lose feeling (sensation). The loss of function is greatest immediately after a stroke. However, some function is usually regained because, while some brain cells die, others are only injured and may recover.

Occasionally, a stroke or transient ischemic attack occurs when blood flow to the brain is normal but the blood doesn't contain enough oxygen. This can happen when a person has severe anemia, carbon monoxide poisoning, or a condition that produces abnormal blood cells or abnormal blood clotting, such as leukemia or polycythemia.

Transient Ischemic Attacks

A transient ischemic attack (TIA) is a disturbance in brain function resulting from a temporary deficiency in the brain's blood supply.

Causes
Small pieces of fatty material and calcium that build up on the wall of an artery (called atheromas)▲ can break off and lodge in the small blood vessels leading to the brain, temporarily blocking the blood supply and causing a TIA. Clumps of platelets or blood clots can also block a blood vessel, leading to a TIA. The risk of having a TIA is increased if a person has high blood pressure, atherosclerosis, heart disease (especially when the heart valves or the heart rhythm is abnormal), diabetes, or an excess of red blood cells (polycythemia). TIAs are more common in middle age

---

▲ see box, page 119

and are progressively more likely with advancing age. Occasionally, TIAs occur in young adults or in children who have heart disease or a blood disorder.

Symptoms

A TIA starts suddenly and usually lasts 2 to 30 minutes. Rarely does it last more than 1 to 2 hours. The symptoms vary, depending on which part of the brain is deprived of blood and oxygen. When the arteries that branch from the carotid artery are affected, blindness in one eye or sensation abnormalities and weakness are most common. When the arteries that branch from the vertebral arteries in the back of the brain are affected, dizziness, double vision, and general weakness are more common. Overall, however, many different symptoms can occur, such as the following:

• Loss of or abnormal sensations in an arm or leg or one side of the body
• Weakness or paralysis of an arm or leg or one side of the body
• Partial loss of vision or hearing
• Double vision
• Dizziness
• Slurred speech
• Difficulty in thinking of the appropriate word or saying it
• Inability to recognize parts of the body
• Unusual movements
• Loss of bladder control
• Imbalance and falling
• Fainting

While the symptoms are similar to those of a stroke, they are temporary and reversible. However, TIAs tend to recur. A person may have several in 1 day or only two or three in several years. About one third of the time, a TIA is followed by a stroke. Roughly half of such strokes occur within 1 year of the TIA.

Diagnosis

Sudden, temporary neurologic symptoms suggesting malfunction of a specific area of the brain are the doctor's first diagnostic clues. However, other disorders, including seizures, tumors, migraine headaches, or abnormal blood sugar levels, have similar symptoms, so further evaluation is needed. Since brain damage doesn't occur, a doctor can't make the diagnosis with a computed

Blood Route to the Brain

Blood is supplied to the brain through two pairs of large arteries: the carotid arteries and the vertebral arteries. The carotid arteries bring blood from the heart along the front of the neck, and the vertebral arteries bring blood from the heart along the back of the neck inside the spinal column. These large arteries empty into a circle of other arteries, from which smaller arteries branch off like roads from a traffic circle. The branches carry the blood to all parts of the brain.

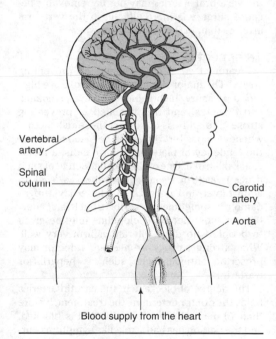

Vertebral artery

Spinal column

Carotid artery

Aorta

Blood supply from the heart

tomography (CT) or magnetic resonance imaging (MRI) scan, tests that can identify a stroke.

Doctors use several techniques to evaluate a possible blockage in one or both carotid arteries. The uneven flow of blood creates sounds, called bruits, that may be heard through a stethoscope. However, bruits can also be present without any significant blockage. The next step is usually an ultrasound scan and a Doppler flow study, two tests performed simultaneously to measure the size of the blockage and the amount of blood that can flow around it. If the carotid arteries are severely narrowed, the doctor may order an MRI scan of the arteries or perform cerebral angiography to determine the size and location of the blockage. In angiography, a fluid that can be seen on x-rays is injected into an artery while x-rays of the head and neck are taken.▲

Unlike the assessment of carotid arteries, ultrasound and Doppler studies are less helpful in assessing the vertebral arteries. MRI or angiography is the only sure way to verify that a vertebral artery is diseased. However, a blockage in the vertebral arteries may not be removable because surgery is more difficult in the vertebral arteries than in the carotid arteries.

Treatment

Treatment of TIAs is aimed at preventing stroke. The major risk factors for stroke are high blood pressure, high cholesterol level, smoking, and diabetes, and the first step in preventing stroke is to address or correct these risk factors whenever possible. Drugs can be taken to reduce the tendency of platelets to form clots, a major cause of stroke. One of the most effective of such drugs is aspirin, usually prescribed as $1/2$ of an adult tablet or 1 children's tablet a day. Dipyridamole is sometimes prescribed, but it isn't effective for most people. Ticlopidine may be given to people who don't tolerate aspirin very well. When stronger drugs are needed, a doctor may prescribe anticoagulants such as heparin or warfarin.

The degree of blockage in the carotid arteries helps the doctor determine the treatment. If more than 70 percent of the blood vessel is blocked, and the person has had strokelike symptoms during the previous 6 months, surgery to remove the blockage may be necessary to prevent a stroke. Smaller blockages are usually removed only when they have led to further TIAs or a stroke. In the usual operation—an endarterectomy—the surgeon removes fatty deposits (atheromas) in the carotid artery. However, this operation carries a

1 to 2 percent risk of causing a stroke. For small blockages that haven't produced any symptoms, the risks of surgery appear to be greater than doing nothing.

Stroke

A stroke (also called a cerebrovascular accident) is the death of brain tissue (cerebral infarction) resulting from lack of blood flow and insufficient oxygen to the brain.

A stroke can be either ischemic or hemorrhagic. In an ischemic stroke, the blood supply to part of the brain is cut off because either atherosclerosis or a blood clot has blocked a blood vessel. In a hemorrhagic stroke, a blood vessel bursts, preventing normal flow and allowing blood to leak into an area of the brain and destroy it.■

Causes

With an ischemic stroke, blockage can occur anywhere along the arterial pathways to the brain. For example, a large deposit of fatty material (atheroma)★ can develop in a carotid artery, reducing its blood flow to a trickle, like water through a clogged pipe. This condition is serious because each carotid artery normally supplies a large percentage of the brain's blood supply. Fatty material may also break off from the wall of the carotid artery, travel with the blood, and become stuck in a smaller artery, blocking it completely.

The carotid and vertebral arteries and their branches can become blocked in other ways. For example, a blood clot formed in the heart or on one of its valves can break loose (becoming an embolus), travel up through the arteries to the brain, and lodge there. The result is an embolic stroke **(cerebral embolism).** Such strokes are most common in people who have recently had heart surgery and in people who have defective heart valves or abnormal heart rhythms (especially atrial fibrillation). A **fat embolus** is a rare cause of stroke; many emboli can form if fat from the marrow of a broken bone is released into the bloodstream and eventually coalesces (consolidates) in an artery.

A stroke can occur if inflammation or an infection narrows blood vessels that lead to the brain. Drugs such as cocaine and amphetamines also can narrow the blood vessels in the brain and produce stroke.

▲ see page 287

■ see page 356

★ see box, page 119

A sudden drop in blood pressure can severely reduce blood flow to the brain, usually causing the person to faint. However, a stroke can result if the low blood pressure is severe and prolonged. This situation can occur when someone loses a lot of blood from an injury or during surgery, has a heart attack, or has an abnormal heart rate or rhythm.

Symptoms and Course

Most strokes begin suddenly, develop rapidly, and cause brain damage within minutes (**completed stroke**). Less commonly, strokes may continue to worsen for several hours to a day or two as a steadily enlarging area of brain tissue dies (**stroke in evolution**). The progression is usually, but not always, interrupted by somewhat stable periods during which the area temporarily stops enlarging or some improvement occurs.

Many different symptoms can occur, depending on which part of the brain is affected. Possible symptoms are the same as those for transient ischemic attacks. However, the neurologic dysfunction is more likely to be severe, widespread, associated with a coma or stupor, and permanent. In addition, strokes can cause depression or an inability to control emotions.

Strokes can cause edema or swelling in the brain. This swelling is particularly dangerous because the skull allows little room for expansion. The resulting pressure can damage brain tissue further, making neurologic problems worse even if the stroke itself doesn't enlarge.

Diagnosis

Doctors usually can diagnose a stroke from the history of events and from a physical examination. The physical examination helps a doctor pinpoint where the brain was damaged. A computed tomography (CT) or magnetic resonance imaging (MRI) scan is usually performed to confirm the diagnosis, but these tests may not reveal the stroke until several days later. A CT or MRI scan also helps rule out whether a hemorrhage or brain tumor caused the stroke. For the rare occasion when immediate surgery is being considered, the doctor may perform angiography.

Doctors try to determine the precise cause of the stroke. They are particularly interested in whether the stroke was caused by a traveling blood clot (embolism) that reached the brain or

Why Strokes Affect Only One Side of the Body

Strokes usually damage only one side of the brain. Because nerves in the brain cross over to the other side of the body, symptoms appear on the side of the body opposite the damaged side of the brain.

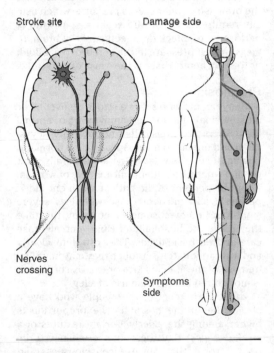

Stroke site

Damage side

Nerves crossing

Symptoms side

by blockage of a blood vessel from atherosclerosis (atherothrombosis).

When a blood clot or embolism is the cause, another stroke is very likely to follow unless the underlying problem is corrected. For example, if blood clots are forming in the heart because it's beating irregularly, treating the irregularity can prevent new clots from forming and causing another stroke. In this case, the doctor generally obtains an electrocardiogram (to look for abnormal heart rhythms) and may also recommend other tests of the heart. Such tests might include Holter monitoring, in which an electrocardiogram is taken continuously for 24 hours, and echocardiography, in which the chambers and valves of the heart are evaluated.▲

Other laboratory tests are of little help but are performed to be sure that the stroke wasn't caused by a deficiency of red blood cells (anemia), an excess of red blood cells (polycythemia), a cancer of the white blood cells (leukemia), or an infection. A spinal tap (lumbar puncture) is rarely necessary after a stroke. In fact, this test can be performed only if the doctor is sure that the brain isn't under excess pressure, which usually requires a CT or MRI scan. A spinal tap is performed to check for infection of the brain, to measure the pressure in the cerebrospinal fluid, or to see if hemorrhage is the cause of the stroke.

Prognosis

Many people who suffer a stroke recover all or most normal function and enjoy years of normal life. Others are physically and mentally devastated and unable to move, speak, or eat normally. During the first few days, doctors generally can't predict whether a patient will improve or worsen. About 50 percent of the patients with one-sided paralysis and most of those with less severe symptoms recover some function by the time they leave the hospital and can eventually take care of their basic needs. They can think clearly and walk adequately, although they may have limited use of the affected arm or leg. Use of an arm is more often limited than use of a leg.

About 20 percent of the people who have a stroke die in the hospital. The proportion is higher among the elderly. Certain features of a stroke suggest that the outcome is likely to be poor. Strokes that cause unconsciousness and those that impair breathing or heart function are particularly grave. Neurologic losses that remain after 6 months are likely to be permanent, although some people continue to improve slowly. Older people fare less well than younger people. People who already have other serious medical problems find it harder to recover.

Treatment

Symptoms that indicate a possible stroke require immediate medical attention; doctors can sometimes reduce the damage or prevent further

damage by acting quickly. Many effects of a stroke require medical care, especially during the first few hours. At first, doctors usually administer oxygen and insert an intravenous line to make sure the patient receives fluids and nourishment.

For a stroke in evolution, anticoagulants such as heparin may be given, but these drugs are useless once the stroke is completed. What's more, they aren't generally given to people with high blood pressure and are never given to people with a cerebral hemorrhage because they increase the risk of bleeding into the brain.

Recent research suggests that paralysis and other symptoms may be prevented or reversed if certain drugs that break up clots, such as streptokinase or tissue plasminogen activator, are given within 3 hours of a stroke's onset. An examination must be performed quickly to determine that the cause is a clot and not a hemorrhage, which can't be treated with clot-dissolving drugs. Other new measures, currently experimental, that may improve the chances of a favorable outcome involve blocking the receptors of certain neurotransmitters in the brain.

Once a stroke is completed, some brain tissue is dead, and reestablishing its blood supply can't restore its function. Therefore, surgery is usually of no benefit. However, removing blockages after a small stroke or a transient ischemic attack in someone whose carotid artery is more than 70 percent blocked may reduce the risk of future strokes.

To reduce the swelling and increased pressure on the brain in people with an acute stroke, drugs such as mannitol or, rarely, corticosteroids may be given. A person with a very severe stroke may be put on a respirator because of pneumonia or to maintain adequate breathing.

Measures are taken to prevent pressure sores on the skin, and close attention is given to bladder and bowel function. Often, accompanying problems such as heart failure, irregular heartbeats, high blood pressure, and lung infections must be treated. Because mood changes, especially depression, often follow a stroke, family or friends should inform the doctor if the person seems depressed.■ Depression can be treated with medication and psychotherapy.

Rehabilitation

Intensive rehabilitation can help many people learn to overcome disability despite the impairment of some brain tissue. Other parts of the

▲ see page 76

■ see page 403

brain can assume tasks previously performed by the damaged part.

Rehabilitation is started as soon as blood pressure, pulse, and breathing have stabilized. Doctors, therapists, and nurses combine their expertise to keep the patient's muscles strong, prevent muscular contractions and pressure sores (which can result from being in one position too long), and teach the patient to walk and talk again. Patience and perseverance are crucial.

After discharge from the hospital, many people benefit from continued rehabilitation in a hospital or nursing home, in scheduled visits to a rehabilitation center, or at home. Occupational and physical therapists can suggest ways to make life easier and the home safer for a person with disabilities.

Intracranial Hemorrhage

An intracranial hemorrhage is bleeding inside the skull.

Bleeding can occur within the brain or around it. Hemorrhages that occur inside the brain are **intracerebral hemorrhages,** those between the brain and the subarachnoid space are **subarachnoid hemorrhages,** those between the layers of the covering (meninges) of the brain are **subdural hemorrhages,** and those between the skull and covering of the brain are **epidural hemorrhages.** No matter where the bleeding occurs, brain cells are destroyed. Also, because the skull allows little room for tissue to expand, bleeding there quickly raises pressure dangerously.

Causes

Head injury is the most common cause of an intracranial hemorrhage in people under age 50.▲ Another cause is an **arteriovenous malformation,** an anatomical abnormality in the arteries or veins in or around the brain. An arteriovenous malformation may be present from birth, but it's only identified if symptoms develop. Bleeding from an arteriovenous malformation can cause sudden collapse and death and tends to strike teenagers and young adults.

Sometimes the wall of a blood vessel becomes weak and swells; such a weak blood vessel is called an **aneurysm.** The thin walls of an aneurysm could burst and cause the blood vessel to hemorrhage. An aneurysm in the brain is another cause of intracranial hemorrhage, leading to hemorrhagic stroke.

INTRACEREBRAL HEMORRHAGE

An intracerebral hemorrhage—a type of stroke—is caused by bleeding into brain tissue.

Symptoms and Diagnosis

An intracerebral hemorrhage begins abruptly with a headache, followed by signs of steadily increasing neurologic losses, such as weakness, inability to move (paralysis), numbness, loss of speech or vision, and confusion. Nausea, vomiting, seizures, and loss of consciousness are common and may occur within a few minutes.

Doctors can often diagnose intracerebral hemorrhages without ordering any tests, but computed tomography (CT) or magnetic resonance imaging (MRI) scans are generally performed when doctors suspect that a stroke has occurred. Both types of imaging can help doctors distinguish an ischemic stroke from a hemorrhagic stroke. The scans also can reveal how much brain tissue has been damaged and whether pressure is increased in other areas of the brain.

A lumbar puncture (spinal tap) isn't usually performed unless the doctor thinks the patient may have meningitis or some other infection, and brain imaging tests either aren't available or haven't revealed any problems.

Prognosis and Treatment

The treatment for a hemorrhagic stroke is similar to that for an ischemic stroke, with two important differences: Anticoagulants aren't given for the hemorrhage, and surgery may save the person's life but often leaves the person with severe neurologic disabilities. The goal of surgery in such cases is to remove blood that has accumulated in the brain and to relieve increased pressure.

Of all forms of stroke, intracerebral hemorrhage is most dangerous. The stroke is usually large and catastrophic, especially if the person has had chronic high blood pressure. More than half of the people who have large hemorrhages die within a few days. Those who do survive usually recover consciousness and some brain function as the body absorbs the leaked blood. Problems tend to remain, but many people with small hemorrhages recover to a remarkable degree.

▲ see page 357

Sites of Brain Hemorrhage

Cross Section of the Brain

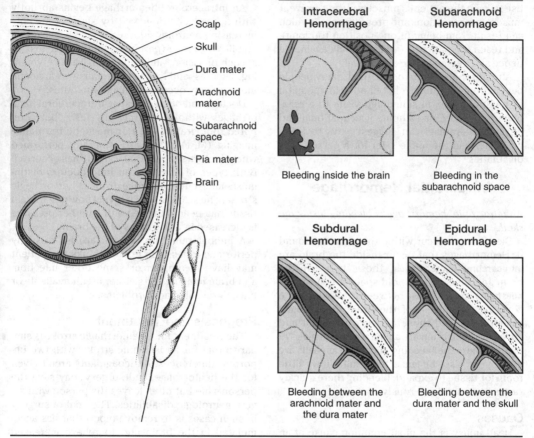

Scalp
Skull
Dura mater
Arachnoid mater
Subarachnoid space
Pia mater
Brain

Intracerebral Hemorrhage

Bleeding inside the brain

Subarachnoid Hemorrhage

Bleeding in the subarachnoid space

Subdural Hemorrhage

Bleeding between the arachnoid mater and the dura mater

Epidural Hemorrhage

Bleeding between the dura mater and the skull

SUBARACHNOID HEMORRHAGE

A subarachnoid hemorrhage is sudden bleeding into the space (the subarachnoid space) between the brain and its covering (meninges).▲

The usual source of the bleeding is a weak blood vessel (either an arteriovenous malformation or an aneurysm) that suddenly ruptures. Sometimes atherosclerosis or an infection damages a blood vessel, causing it to rupture. Ruptures can occur in people at any age but are most common between ages 25 and 50. Rarely, a subarachnoid hemorrhage can follow a head injury.

Symptoms

Aneurysms that cause subarachnoid hemorrhages usually produce no symptoms before rupturing. However, sometimes aneurysms press on a nerve or leak small amounts of blood before a major rupture, thereby producing warning signs, such as a headache, facial pain, double vision, or other visual problems. The warning signs can occur minutes to weeks before the rupture. Such symptoms should always be brought to a doctor's

▲ see box, page 279

attention quickly, because steps may be taken to prevent a massive hemorrhage.

A rupture usually produces a sudden, severe headache, often followed by a brief loss of consciousness. Some people remain in a coma, but more often they wake up, feeling confused and sleepy. Blood and cerebrospinal fluid around the brain irritate the surrounding membrane (meninges), producing headaches, vomiting, and dizziness. Frequent fluctuations in the heartbeat and breathing rate often occur as well, sometimes accompanied by seizures. Within hours or even minutes, the person may again become sleepy and confused. About 25 percent of the people have neurologic problems, usually paralysis on one side of the body.

Diagnosis

The diagnosis of a subarachnoid hemorrhage can usually be made with a computed tomography (CT) scan, which pinpoints the site of bleeding. Lumbar puncture, if necessary, can reveal any blood in the cerebrospinal fluid. Angiography is usually performed within 72 hours to confirm the diagnosis and guide any necessary surgery.

Prognosis

About one third of the people who have a subarachnoid hemorrhage die during the first episode because of extensive brain damage. Another 15 percent die within a few weeks from subse-

quent bleeding. Occasionally, a small bleeding site that has already sealed itself off doesn't show up on angiography, in which case the outlook is very good. Otherwise, without surgery for the aneurysm, people who survive after 6 months have a 5 percent chance every year of another episode of bleeding.

Many people recover most or all mental and physical function after a subarachnoid hemorrhage. However, neurologic problems sometimes linger.

Treatment

A person who may have had a subarachnoid hemorrhage is hospitalized immediately and instructed to avoid exertion. Analgesics are given to control the severe headaches. Occasionally, a drainage tube may be placed in the brain to relieve pressure.

Surgery that isolates, blocks off, or supports the walls of the weak artery reduces the risk of fatal bleeding later. This surgery is difficult, and regardless of the surgical procedure used, the death rate is high, especially in people who are in a stupor or coma. The best time for surgery is somewhat controversial and must be decided on the basis of individual factors. Most neurosurgeons recommend operating within 3 days of the start of symptoms. Delaying the operation 10 or more days reduces the risks of surgery but increases the chances of rebleeding in the interim.

CHAPTER 75

Head Injuries

The thick, hard bones of the skull help protect the brain. Despite having this natural helmet, the brain is susceptible to many kinds of injury. Head injuries kill and disable more people under age 50 than any other type of neurologic damage and, after gunshot wounds, are the second leading cause of death in men under age 35. Nearly half of those who suffer a severe head injury die.

The brain can be injured even if the skull isn't penetrated. Many injuries are caused by the sudden acceleration that follows a jolt, as may be delivered by a forceful blow to the head, or by the sudden deceleration that occurs when a moving

head strikes an immovable object. The brain can be damaged at the point of impact and on the opposite side. Acceleration-deceleration injuries are sometimes called *coup contrecoup* (French for hit-counterhit).

Severe head trauma can tear, shear, or rupture the nerves, blood vessels, and tissues in or around the brain. Nerve pathways can be disrupted, and bleeding or severe swelling can occur. Bleeding, swelling, and a buildup of fluid (edema) have an effect similar to that caused by a mass growing within the skull. Since the skull can't expand, increasing pressure can damage or destroy brain tissue. Because of the brain's position in the skull, pressure tends to push the brain downward. The upper part of the brain may be forced into the opening that connects it with the lower part (brain stem), a condition called **herniation**. A similar type of herniation can jam the cerebellum and brain stem through the opening at the base of the skull (foramen magnum) into the spinal cord. Herniations can be life-threatening because the brain stem controls such vital functions as heart rate and breathing.

Sometimes severe brain damage can occur with what appears to be a minor head injury. The elderly are particularly susceptible to bleeding around the brain (subdural hematoma) after a head injury. People taking drugs that prevent the blood from clotting (anticoagulants) are also at particular risk for bleeding around the brain after a head injury.

Brain damage often causes some degree of permanent dysfunction, which varies depending on whether the damage is limited to a specific area (localized) or more widespread (diffuse). Which functions are lost depend on which area of the brain is damaged. Specific, localized symptoms can help pinpoint the injured area. Changes may occur in movement, sensation, speech, sight, and hearing. Diffuse impairment of brain function can affect memory and sleep and can lead to confusion and coma.

Prognosis

The eventual consequences of a head injury range from complete recovery to death. The type and severity of disabilities depend on where and how badly the brain was injured. Many brain functions can be performed by more than one area, and uninjured areas of the brain sometimes take over functions that were lost when another area was damaged, permitting partial recovery. As people age, however, the brain becomes less able to shift functions from one area to another. For example, language skills are handled by several parts of the brain in young children but are concentrated on one side of the brain in adults. If the left hemisphere's language areas are severely damaged before the age of 8, the right hemisphere can assume near-normal language function. How-

ever, injury to language areas during adulthood is more likely to result in permanent deficits.

Some functions, such as vision and arm and leg movements (motor control), are controlled by unique regions on one side of the brain. Damage to any of those regions usually causes permanent deficits. Rehabilitation, however, can help people minimize the impact of these deficits on function.

People with a severe head injury sometimes develop amnesia and can't remember the events immediately before and after they lost consciousness.▲ Those who regain consciousness in the first week are most likely to recover their memory.

Some people with a head injury, even a minor one, develop postconcussion syndrome. They may continue to experience headaches and memory problems for a considerable time after the injury.

A **persistent** or **chronic vegetative state**—the most serious consequence of a nonfatal head injury—is a long-term state of total unconsciousness accompanied by nearly normal cycles of awakening and sleeping.■ It results when the upper parts of the brain, which control sophisticated mental functions, are destroyed but the thalamus and brain stem, which control sleep cycles, body temperature, breathing, and heart rate, are spared. If a vegetative state persists for more than a few months, recovery of consciousness is unlikely. Nevertheless, a person given skilled nursing care can live for years in this condition.

Diagnosis and Treatment

When a person with a head injury reaches the hospital, doctors and nurses first check vital signs: heart rate, blood pressure, and breathing. A ventilator may be needed for those who aren't breathing adequately on their own. Doctors immediately assess the person's state of consciousness and memory. They also test basic brain function by checking the size of the pupils and their reaction to light, evaluate the response to sensations such as heat or pinpricks, and test the ability to move the arms and legs. Computed tomography (CT) or magnetic resonance imaging (MRI) scans are ordered to evaluate possible brain injury. Standard x-rays can identify skull fractures but reveal nothing about brain injury.

Increasing sleepiness and confusion, a deepening coma, rising blood pressure, and a slowing pulse after a head injury are signs that the brain is swelling. Because the brain can be damaged quickly by the pressure of excess fluid, drugs are

---

▲ see page 362

■ see page 372

given to reduce the swelling. A small pressure gauge may be implanted in the skull to determine how well the treatment is working.

Specific Head Injuries

People suffer many kinds of head injury, including skull fractures, concussions, cerebral contusions and lacerations, and intracranial hematomas.

Skull Fractures

A skull fracture is a break in a skull bone.

Skull fractures can injure arteries and veins, which then bleed into spaces around the brain tissue. Fractures, especially at the base of the skull, can tear the meninges, the layers of tissue that line the brain. Cerebrospinal fluid, the fluid that circulates between the brain and the meninges, then can leak through the nose or ear. Bacteria occasionally enter the skull through such fractures, causing infection and severe damage to the brain.

Most skull fractures don't require surgery unless bone fragments are pressing against the brain or the skull bones have been jolted out of alignment.

Concussion

A concussion is a brief loss of consciousness and sometimes memory after an injury to the brain that doesn't cause obvious physical damage.

Concussions cause a malfunction of the brain but do not result in visible structural damage. They may occur after even a minor head injury, depending on how the brain is jarred within the skull. A concussion may leave the person somewhat confused, headachy, and abnormally sleepy; most people recover completely within a few hours or days.

Some people develop dizziness, difficulty in concentration, forgetfulness, depression, lack of feeling or emotion, and anxiety. These symptoms may last from a few days to several weeks but rarely longer. Meanwhile, the person may have trouble working, studying, and socializing. This condition is called **postconcussion syndrome.**

Postconcussion syndrome is puzzling; why these problems commonly occur after a *mild*

head injury is unknown. Experts disagree about whether the symptoms are caused by microscopic injuries or psychologic factors. Drug therapy and psychiatric treatment help some but not all people with postconcussion syndrome.

More worrisome than the postconcussion syndrome is the fact that more serious symptoms may develop hours or sometimes even days after the original injury. Worsening headaches, confusion, and increasing sleepiness indicate an urgent need for medical attention.

Generally, once a doctor has determined that more severe damage hasn't occurred, no treatment is needed. Yet, all people who have a head injury are told about the warning signs of worsening brain function. Parents of small children are told how to monitor the children for these changes during the hours after an injury. As long as symptoms don't get worse, acetaminophen may be used for pain. Aspirin may be used after the first 3 or 4 days if the injury isn't severe.

Cerebral Contusions and Lacerations

Cerebral contusions are bruises on the brain, usually caused by a direct, strong blow to the head. Cerebral lacerations are torn brain tissue, often accompanying visible head wounds and skull fractures.

Cerebral contusions and lacerations are more serious than concussions. Magnetic resonance imaging (MRI) scans show physical damage to the brain, which may be minimal or which may cause weakness on one side of the body along with confusion or even coma. If the brain swells, the brain tissue may be damaged further; very severe swelling may lead to herniation of the brain. As is often the case, treatment becomes more complex if severe brain injuries are accompanied by other injuries, especially chest injuries.

Intracranial Hematomas

Intracranial hematomas are collections of blood within the brain or between the brain and the skull.

Intracranial hematomas can occur from an injury or from a stroke.▲ Injury-related intracranial

---

▲ see page 352

hematomas usually form either inside the outer covering of the brain (subdural hematoma) or between the outer covering and the skull (epidural hematoma).▲ Both types of hematoma usually show up on computed tomography (CT) or magnetic resonance imaging (MRI) scans. Most hematomas develop rapidly and produce symptoms within minutes. Chronic hematomas, which are more common in the elderly, enlarge slowly, producing symptoms only after hours or days.

Large hematomas press on the brain, cause swelling, and eventually destroy brain tissue. They may also cause the upper part of the brain or the brain stem to herniate. A person with an intracranial hematoma may lose consciousness, fall into a coma, become paralyzed on one or both sides of the body, experience breathing difficulties or heart problems, or even die. Hematomas may also produce confusion and memory loss, especially in the elderly.

An epidural hematoma originates from bleeding from an artery that lies between the meninges (the tissue that lines and protects the brain) and the skull. Most epidural hematomas occur when an overlying skull fracture cuts the artery. Because blood is under more pressure in arteries than in veins, it spurts from arteries more rapidly. Symptoms sometimes begin immediately, usually as a severe headache, but they can be delayed for several hours. The headache sometimes disappears but returns several hours later, worse than before. Increasing confusion, sleepiness, paralysis, collapse, and a deep coma can quickly follow.

Early diagnosis is crucial and usually depends on an emergency CT scan. Epidural hematomas are treated as soon as they are recognized. A hole is drilled in the skull to drain the excess blood, and the surgeon seeks the source of the bleeding and stops it.

Subdural hematomas originate from bleeding from veins around the brain. Bleeding may start suddenly after a severe head injury or more slowly after a less serious one. Subdural hematomas that enlarge slowly are most common in elderly people, because their veins are fragile,

and in alcoholics, who may ignore mild to moderate head injuries. In both situations, the initial injury may seem minor: Symptoms may not be noticeable for several weeks. However, MRI or CT scans can detect the resulting pooled blood. A subdural hematoma in an infant can enlarge the head because the skull is soft and pliable; for cosmetic reasons at least, doctors usually drain the hematoma surgically.

Small subdural hematomas in adults often are absorbed spontaneously. Large subdural hematomas that cause neurologic symptoms are usually drained surgically. Indications for drainage include a persisting headache, fluctuating drowsiness, confusion, memory changes, and mild paralysis on the opposite side of the body.

Damage to Specific Brain Areas

Damage to the top layer of the brain (cerebral cortex) usually impairs a person's ability to think, govern emotions, and behave normally. Since specific areas of the cerebral cortex are generally responsible for specific kinds of behavior, the precise site and extent of injury determine the type of impairment.■

Frontal Lobe Damage

The frontal lobes of the cerebral cortex mainly control learned motor skills (for example, writing, playing musical instruments, or tying shoelaces). They also coordinate facial expressions and expressive gestures. Particular areas of the frontal lobes are responsible for specific skilled motor activities on the opposite side of the body.

The behavioral effects of frontal lobe damage vary according to the size and location of the physical defect. Small defects usually don't cause any noticeable behavioral changes if they affect only one side of the brain, although they sometimes cause seizures. Large defects toward the back of the frontal lobes may cause apathy, inattention, indifference, and sometimes incontinence. People with larger defects toward the front or side of the frontal lobes tend to be easily distracted, inappropriately euphoric, argumentative, vulgar, and rude; they may disregard the consequences of their behavior.

▲ see box, page 356

■ see page 278

Parietal Lobe Damage

The parietal lobes of the cerebral cortex combine impressions of form, texture, and weight into general perceptions. Mathematics and language skills stem somewhat from this area but more specifically from adjacent areas of the temporal lobes. The parietal lobes also help people orient themselves to space and sense the position of their body parts.

Small deficits in front parts of the parietal lobes cause numbness on the opposite side of the body. People with larger injuries can lose the ability to perform sequenced tasks (a condition called apraxia) and to display right-left orientation. Large deficits can affect a person's ability to recognize body parts or the space around his body or may even interfere with the memory of once well-known forms, such as clocks or cubes. As a result, a sudden injury to some parts of the parietal lobe can cause people to ignore the serious nature of their condition and to neglect or even deny paralysis that affects the side of the body opposite the brain injury. They may be confused or delirious and unable to dress themselves or perform other ordinary tasks.

Temporal Lobe Damage

The temporal lobes process immediate events into recent and long-term memory. They comprehend sounds and images, store and recall memory, and generate emotional pathways. Injury to the right temporal lobe tends to impair memory of sounds and shapes. Injury to the left temporal lobe drastically interferes with understanding language coming from external or internal sources and typically prevents the person from expressing language. People with a nondominant right temporal lobe injury may experience personality changes such as humorlessness, unusual degrees of religiosity, obsessiveness, and loss of libido.

Disorders Caused by Head Injury

Some of the specific disorders caused by a head injury include posttraumatic epilepsy, aphasia, apraxia, agnosia, and amnesia.

Posttraumatic Epilepsy

Posttraumatic epilepsy is a disorder in which seizures occur some time after the brain is injured by a blow to the head.

Seizures are the response to abnormal electrical discharges in the brain.▲ They develop in about 10 percent of the people who have severe head injuries but no penetrating wound of the brain and in 40 percent of those who do have a penetrating wound. Seizures may not appear until several years after an injury. The resulting symptoms often depend on where in the brain the seizure originates. Anticonvulsant drugs, such as phenytoin, carbamazepine, or valproate, usually can control posttraumatic epilepsy. In fact, some doctors prescribe such drugs after a serious head injury to prevent seizures, although most experts do not recommend the practice. Treatment is often continued for several years or indefinitely if seizures begin.

Aphasia

Aphasia is a loss of the ability to use language because of an injury to the language area of the brain.

People with aphasia are partly or entirely unable to understand or express words. In most people, the left temporal lobe and the nearby region of the frontal lobe control language function. Damage to any part of this small area by a stroke, tumor, head injury, or infection interferes with at least some aspect of language function.

Language problems take many forms. The variety of possible defects reflects the complex nature of language function. One person may lose only the ability to comprehend written words (**alexia**), while another may lose only the ability to recall or say the names of objects (**anomia**). Some people with anomia can't remember the right word at all; others may have a word in mind but be unable to say it. **Dysarthria** is the inability to articulate words properly. Though seemingly a language problem, dysarthria is caused by damage to the part of the brain that controls the mus-

▲ see page 345

Testing a Person With Aphasia

Broca's aphasia—answers to questions are given hesitantly but are sensible
Question: "What is this a picture of?" (dog barking)
Answer: "D—d—d—dg, eh, no...d-d ...damn...p-p-pet, yeah, yeah, pet, pet, pet...b—b—...makes noise."

Wernicke's aphasia—answers to questions are given fluently but are nonsensical
Question: "How are you today?"
Answer: "When? Easy for my river runs black boxes wizzel abata H on when boobles come."

cles used to make sounds or coordinate movements of the vocal apparatus.

People with **Wernicke's aphasia,** a condition that may follow temporal lobe damage, seem to speak fluently, but sentences come out as garbled, confused strings of words (sometimes referred to as a word salad). People with **Broca's aphasia** (expressive aphasia) largely grasp the meaning of words and know how they want to respond, but they have trouble saying the words. Their words are forced out slowly and with great effort, often interrupted by expletives.

Damage to both the left temporal and frontal lobes may initially make a person almost entirely mute. During recovery from such complete (global) aphasia, the person has impaired speech (dysphasia), writing (agraphia or dysgraphia), and verbal comprehension.

Speech therapists can often help people who develop aphasia after a stroke, head injury, or some other cause of language impairment. In general, treatment is started as soon as the person's medical condition permits.

Apraxia

Apraxia is the inability to perform tasks that require remembering patterns or sequences of movements.

Apraxia is an uncommon disability that is usually caused by damage to the parietal or frontal lobes. In apraxia, the memory of the sequence of movements needed to complete skilled or complex tasks seems to be erased; the arms or legs have no physical defect that explains why the task can't be performed. For example, buttoning a button actually consists of a series of steps. People with apraxia can't carry out such a sequence.

Some forms of apraxia affect only particular kinds of tasks. For instance, a person may lose the ability to draw a picture, write a note, button a jacket, tie a shoelace, pick up a telephone receiver, or play a musical instrument. Treatment is aimed at the underlying disorder that has caused the brain dysfunction.

Agnosia

Agnosia is a rare disorder in which a person can see and feel objects but can't associate them with their usual role or function.

People with certain forms of agnosia can't recognize familiar faces or common objects such as a spoon or a pencil, even though they can see and describe these things. Agnosia is caused by malfunctions in the parietal and temporal lobes of the brain, where memories of the uses and importance of familiar objects and sights are stored. Agnosia often comes on suddenly following a head injury or stroke. Some people with agnosia improve or recover spontaneously; others must learn to cope with their strange disability. No specific treatment exists.

Amnesia

Amnesia is the total or partial inability to recall recent or remote experiences.

The causes of amnesia are only partly understood. Injury to the brain can produce memory loss of events that occurred just before (retrograde amnesia) or just after (posttraumatic amnesia) the injury. Depending on the severity of the injury, most amnesias last for only minutes or hours and disappear without treatment. But with severe brain injury, the amnesia can be permanent.

Learning requires memory. Memories acquired during childhood are held more tightly than those acquired during adulthood, perhaps because young brains have special learning abilities. The brain's mechanisms for receiving information and recalling it from memory are located primarily in the occipital, parietal, and temporal lobes. Emotions originating from the brain's limbic system can influence both the laying down of memories and their retrieval. The limbic system is closely connected to areas responsible for alertness and awareness. Because memory involves many interwoven brain functions, virtually any type of brain damage can result in memory loss.

Transient global amnesia describes a sudden, severe, forgetful attack of confusion for time, place, and other people. Many people with transient global amnesia have no more than one attack in a lifetime; others may have repeated attacks. Attacks can last from 30 minutes to about 12 hours or so. Small arteries in the brain probably become intermittently blocked as a result of atherosclerosis. In young people, migraine headaches, which temporarily reduce blood flow to the brain, may bring about transient global amnesia. Heavy drinking or taking excessive amounts of tranquilizers, such as barbiturates and benzodiazepine drugs, can also cause brief attacks. The amnesia may totally disorient a person and block recall of events that happened during the previous few years. After an attack, the confusion usually clears quickly and total recovery is the rule.

Alcoholics and other malnourished people may develop an unusual form of amnesia called the **Wernicke-Korsakoff syndrome.** The syndrome consists of a combination of two disorders: an acute confusional state (a type of encephalopathy) and a longer lasting amnesia. Both disorders result from brain dysfunction caused by thiamine (vitamin B_1) deficiency. Drinking large amounts of alcohol without eating foods that contain thiamine decreases the brain's supply of this vitamin. Drinking large amounts of other liquids or receiving large amounts of fluid intravenously after surgery can also cause Wernicke's encephalopathy in a person who was previously poorly nourished.

People who develop acute Wernicke's encephalopathy tend to stagger, develop eye problems (such as paralysis of eye movements, double vision, or nystagmus), and become confused and drowsy. Their memory loss is severe. Thiamine given intravenously usually corrects the problem.

Types of Memory Affected by Amnesia

Immediate memory—recall of events that happened in the preceding few seconds

Intermediate memory—recall of events that happened a few seconds to a few days previously

Remote or long-term memory—recall of events from further back in time

Left untreated, acute Wernicke's encephalopathy can be fatal. For this reason, if an alcoholic develops unusual neurologic symptoms or becomes confused, thiamine treatment is usually started immediately.

Korsakoff's amnesia accompanies acute Wernicke's encephalopathy and may be permanent if it follows severe or repeated attacks of the encephalopathy or alcohol withdrawal. Severe memory loss often is accompanied by agitation and delirium. In chronic Korsakoff's amnesia, immediate memory is retained, but memory for recent and relatively long-term events is lost. Remote memory, however, sometimes survives. People with chronic Korsakoff's amnesia may be able to interact socially and hold a coherent conversation even though they're unable to remember anything that happened in the preceding few days, months, or years or even in the preceding few minutes. Bewildered by the lack of memory, they tend to make things up rather than admit that they can't remember.

Although Korsakoff's amnesia most commonly occurs with thiamine deficiency, a similar pattern of amnesia also can follow a severe head injury, cardiac arrest, or acute encephalitis. In alcoholics, administering lost thiamine corrects Wernicke's encephalopathy but doesn't always correct Korsakoff's amnesia. Sometimes the disorders gradually disappear on their own if alcohol is avoided and other contributing illnesses are treated.

Delirium and Dementia

Although delirium and dementia are often discussed together in medical books, they're really quite different. Delirium describes a sudden, usually reversible, change in mental state that is characterized by confusion and disorientation. Dementia is a chronic, slowly progressive illness resulting in loss of memory and a severe decline in all aspects of mental functioning; unlike delirium, dementia is usually irreversible.

Common Causes of Delirium

• Alcohol, street drugs, and poisons

• Toxic effects of medications

• Abnormal blood levels of electrolytes, salts, and minerals such as calcium, sodium, or magnesium resulting from medication, dehydration, or disease

• Acute infection with fever

• Normal-pressure hydrocephalus, a condition in which the fluid that cushions the brain fails to be properly reabsorbed and puts pressure on the brain

• Subdural hematoma, a collection of blood under the skull that can put pressure on the brain

• Meningitis, encephalitis, syphilis— infections affecting the brain

• Thiamine and vitamin B_{12} deficiencies

• Thyroid disease from either an underactive or overactive thyroid gland

• Brain tumors—some occasionally cause confusion and memory problems

• Fractures of the hip and long bones

• Poor heart or lung function resulting in low levels of oxygen or high levels of carbon dioxide in the blood

• Stroke

Delirium

Delirium is a potentially reversible condition that usually comes on suddenly; the person has diminished ability to pay attention and is confused, disoriented, and unable to think clearly.

Causes

Delirium is an abnormal mental state, not a disease, with a variety of symptoms that represent diminished mental functioning. Hundreds of conditions or disorders, ranging from simple dehydration to drug intoxication or life-threatening infections, can cause delirium. It most commonly affects the elderly and people whose brain is already impaired, including the very ill, people who take drugs that alter the mind or behavior, and people with dementia.

Symptoms

Delirium can begin in a number of ways, and a mild case may be difficult to recognize. The actions of delirious people vary but are roughly similar to those of a person who is getting progressively more intoxicated.

The hallmark of delirium is an inability to pay attention. Delirious people can't concentrate, so they have trouble processing new information and can't recall recent events. Almost all are disoriented to time and at least partially confused about where they are. They think in a confused way, ramble, and even become incoherent. In severe cases, they may not know who they are. They may be frightened by bizarre visual hallucinations, in which they see things or people that aren't there. Some may experience paranoia, believing that strange things are happening (delusions). Delirious people respond to their difficulties in various ways: Some become so quiet and withdrawn that those around them may not even realize that they are delirious; others become agitated and try to fight their hallucinations or delusions.

When drugs cause delirium, behavior is often altered in different ways, depending on the drug.

For example, people intoxicated from sleeping pills are likely to be very withdrawn, while those intoxicated from amphetamines may become aggressive and hyperactive.

Delirium can last hours, days, or even longer, depending on the severity and the medical circumstances. It often becomes worse at night (a phenomenon known as sundowning). Ultimately, a delirious person will fall into a restless sleep; depending on its cause, delirium may even progress to a coma.

Diagnosis

Doctors can easily recognize delirium that has passed the mild stage. Because delirium can be a sign of many serious illnesses—some of which are rapidly fatal—doctors try to determine the cause as quickly as possible. They first try to distinguish delirium from mental illness. In the elderly, doctors try to distinguish delirium from dementia by determining the person's usual mental function. However, people who have dementia can become delirious as well.

Doctors collect as much information about the person's medical history as possible. Friends, family, or other observers are asked how the confusion began, how quickly it progressed, and what they know about the person's physical and mental health, including use of medications, illicit drugs, and alcohol. Information may come from police, emergency medical personnel, or evidence such as pill bottles.

A full physical examination follows, and the doctor pays close attention to the person's neurologic responses. The doctor orders blood tests, x-rays, and often a spinal tap (lumbar puncture) to obtain cerebrospinal fluid for laboratory analysis.

Treatment

The treatment of delirium depends on its underlying cause. For example, doctors treat infections with antibiotics, fever with other drugs, and abnormal salt and mineral levels in the blood by regulating levels of fluids and salts.

People who are extremely agitated or who have hallucinations must be prevented from injuring themselves or their caregivers. Hospitals sometimes use padded restraints. Benzodiazepine drugs such as diazepam, triazolam, and temazepam can help relieve agitation. Antipsychotic drugs such as haloperidol, thioridazine, and chlorpromazine are usually given only to people

Is It Delirium or Psychosis?

Common Signs of Delirium (physical illness)	Common Signs of Psychosis (mental illness)
Confusion about current time, date, location, or identity	Usually aware of time, place, and identity
Difficulty paying attention	Able to pay attention
Loss of recent memory	Illogical thinking but retention of recent memory
Inability to think logically or perform simple calculations	Retained ability to calculate
Fever or other signs of infection	History of previous psychiatric disturbances
Preoccupations commonly inconsistent	Preoccupations often fixed and consistent
Hallucinations (if any) mostly visual	Hallucinations (if any) mostly auditory
Evidence of recent drug use	
Tremor	

who are aggressively paranoid or severely fearful, or to those who cannot be calmed with benzodiazepines. Hospitals use restraints with caution, and doctors are careful when prescribing drugs, particularly in the elderly, because restraints or drugs may cause more agitation or confusion and mask an underlying problem. However, if the delirium is induced by alcohol, doctors give benzodiazepines until agitation stops.

Dementia

Dementia is a decline in mental ability that usually progresses slowly, in which memory, thinking, judgment, and the ability to pay attention and learn are impaired, and personality may deteriorate.

Dementia can develop suddenly in young people when a severe injury, disease, or toxic sub-

Comparing Delirium and Dementia

Delirium	Dementia
Develops suddenly	Develops slowly
Lasts days to weeks	May be permanent
Associated with drug use or withdrawal, severe illness, problem with metabolism	May not be otherwise ill
Almost always worse at night	Often worse at night
Unable to pay attention	Attention wanders
Awareness fluctuates from lethargy to agitation	Awareness is often reduced but not subject to wide swings
Orientation to surroundings varies	Orientation to surroundings is impaired
Language is slow, often incoherent, and inappropriate	Sometimes has difficulty in finding the right word
Memory is jumbled, confused	Loss of memory, especially for recent events

stance (for example, carbon monoxide) destroys brain cells. However, dementia usually develops slowly and affects people over age 60. Nevertheless, dementia isn't a normal part of aging. As all people age, changes in the brain cause some memory loss—especially short-term memory— and some decline in learning ability. These normal changes don't affect the ability to function. Forgetfulness in older people is sometimes called **benign senescent forgetfulness,** and it's not necessarily a sign of dementia or early Alzheimer's disease. Dementia is a much more serious decline in mental ability, and one that gets worse with time. While people who are aging normally may forget details, people with dementia may forget entire recent events.

Causes

The most common cause of dementia is **Alzheimer's disease.** What causes Alzheimer's disease isn't known, but genetic factors play a role—the disease seems to run in some families and is caused or influenced by several specific gene abnormalities. In Alzheimer's disease, parts of the brain degenerate, destroying cells and reducing the responsiveness of the remaining ones to many of the chemicals that transmit signals in the brain. Abnormal tissues, called senile plaques and neurofibrillary tangles, and abnormal proteins appear in the brain and are recognizable by doctors during an autopsy. **Lewy body dementia** closely resembles Alzheimer's disease, although the microscopic changes found in the brain are different.

The second most common cause of dementia is **successive strokes.** The individual strokes are small, leaving little or no immediate weakness and seldom the kind of paralysis that results from larger strokes. These small strokes gradually destroy brain tissue; areas destroyed as a result of blocked blood supply are called infarcts. Since this type of dementia results from many small strokes, the condition is known as **multi-infarct dementia.** Most people with multi-infarct dementia have had high blood pressure or diabetes, both of which damage blood vessels in the brain.

Dementia can also follow a brain injury or an episode of cardiac arrest.

Other causes of dementia are uncommon. Pick's disease, a rare condition, is much like Alzheimer's disease except that it affects only a small area of the brain and progresses more slowly. About 15 to 20 percent of the people with Parkinson's disease sooner or later develop dementia. Dementia also occurs in people with AIDS and with Creutzfeldt-Jakob disease, a rare, rapidly progressive disease caused by an infection of the brain, probably by an infectious particle called a prion, which may be related to mad cow disease.

Normal-pressure hydrocephalus results when the fluid that normally surrounds the brain and protects it from injury fails to be properly reabsorbed, causing an unusual type of dementia. This hydrocephalus not only causes loss of mental function but also results in urinary incontinence and an unusual broad-based walking abnormality. Unlike many other causes of dementia, normal-pressure hydrocephalus sometimes can be reversed if treated early.

People who suffer repeated head injuries— boxers, for example—often develop **dementia pu-**

gilistica (chronic progressive traumatic encephalopathy); some of them also develop hydrocephalus.

Some older people who become depressed have **pseudodementia**—they only appear to have dementia. They eat and sleep little and complain bitterly about their memory loss, unlike those with true dementia, who often deny memory loss.

Symptoms

Dementia usually begins slowly and worsens over time, so the condition may not be identified at first. Memory, the ability to keep track of time, and the ability to recognize people, places, and objects all diminish. People with dementia have problems finding and using the right word and have difficulty with abstract thinking (such as working with numbers). Changes in personality are also common; often a particular personality trait is exaggerated.

Dementia resulting from Alzheimer's disease usually begins subtly. People whose disease develops while they are employed can't perform as well; in those who are retired, the changes may not be noticeable at first. The first sign may be forgetting recent events, although sometimes the disease begins with depression, fears, anxiety, decreased emotion, or other personality changes. Speech patterns may change slightly; the person may use simpler words, use words incorrectly, or be unable to find the appropriate word. An inability to interpret signals may make driving a car difficult. In time, the changes become more noticeable, and eventually the person can't function socially.

Unlike dementia caused by Alzheimer's disease, dementia caused by small strokes may follow a stair-step downward course, worsening suddenly but then improving somewhat, only to get worse again months or years later when another stroke occurs. Controlling high blood pressure and diabetes sometimes can prevent more strokes, and mild recovery sometimes occurs.

Some people with dementia hide their deficiencies well. They avoid complex activities such as balancing a checkbook, reading, and working. People who fail to modify their lives may become frustrated with the inability to perform daily tasks. They may forget to do important tasks or may perform them incorrectly; for example, they may fail to pay bills or become absentminded about turning off the lights or stove.

Dementia progresses at different rates in different people. Looking back at how fast it worsened over the previous year often gives an indication about the coming year. The dementia caused by AIDS generally begins subtly but progresses steadily over a few months or years. It rarely precedes other symptoms of AIDS. In contrast, Creutzfeldt-Jakob disease usually leads to severe dementia and often death within a year.

In its most advanced forms, dementia leads to a near complete destruction of the brain's ability to function. People with dementia become more withdrawn and less capable of controlling their behavior. They have noisy outbursts and mood swings, and they tend to wander. Eventually, they become unable to follow conversations and may lose the ability to speak.

Diagnosis

Forgetfulness is usually the first sign apparent to family members or a doctor. Doctors and other medical professionals usually can make the diagnosis by asking the person and the family a series of questions. Mental status testing is performed, in which doctors ask a set of simple questions and the person's answers are recorded and scored for correctness.▲ More sophisticated testing (neuropsychologic testing) may be needed to clarify the degree of impairment or to determine whether the person is experiencing true intellectual decline.

Doctors make the diagnosis of dementia based on the overall situation, taking into account the person's age, the family history, how the symptoms started and how they're progressing, and the presence of other diseases (such as high blood pressure or diabetes).

At the same time, doctors search for a treatable cause for the decreased mental function, such as thyroid disease, abnormal blood levels of electrolytes, infections, vitamin deficiencies, medication toxicity, or depression. Standard blood chemistry tests are always performed, and doctors review all of the person's prescription drugs to see if one or more of them may be at fault. The doctor may order a computed tomography (CT) or magnetic resonance imaging (MRI) scan to rule out a brain tumor, hydrocephalus, or a stroke.

▲ see box, page 283

Helping People With Dementia and Their Families

• Maintaining a familiar environment helps a person with dementia stay oriented. Moving to a new home or city, rearranging furniture, or even repainting can be disruptive. A large daily calendar, a night-light, a clock with large numbers, or a radio can also help orient the person.

• Hiding car keys and placing detectors on doors may help prevent accidents for those who wander. Identification bracelets may also be helpful.

• Establishing a regular routine for bathing, eating, sleeping, and other activities can give the person a sense of stability. Regular contact with familiar faces can also help.

• Scolding or punishing a person with dementia doesn't help, and it may make matters worse.

• Enlisting the aid of organizations that provide social and nursing services, often in the home, can be helpful. Transportation and meal services may be available. Full-time care can be very expensive, but many insurance plans cover some of the cost.

Doctors suspect Alzheimer's disease as the cause of dementia in an older person whose memory gradually deteriorates. Although a diagnosis made by examining a person can be correct about 85 percent of the time, the diagnosis of Alzheimer's disease is proved only by examining the brain during an autopsy. When an autopsy is performed, doctors find a loss of nerve cells. Tangles are seen within the remaining nerve cells, and plaques made up of amyloid, a type of abnormal protein, are scattered throughout the brain tissue. Tests on spinal fluid and special brain scans called positron emission tomography (PET) scans have been suggested as methods of diagnosing Alzheimer's disease, but such tests aren't yet reliable.

Treatment

Most dementias are incurable. The drug tacrine helps some people with Alzheimer's disease but produces serious side effects. It has generally been superseded by donepezil, which causes fewer side effects and may slow the progression of Alzheimer's disease for a year or more. Ibuprofen also may slow the course. The drugs work best during the early, mild stage of the disease.

The dementia caused by successive small strokes can't be treated, but its progression can be slowed or even stopped by treating the high blood pressure or diabetes associated with the strokes. Currently no treatment exists for dementia caused by either Creutzfeldt-Jakob disease or AIDS. Drugs used to treat Parkinson's disease don't help the accompanying dementia and some may aggravate the symptoms. When memory loss is caused by depression, antidepressant drugs and counseling may help, at least temporarily. If diagnosed early, dementia caused by normal-pressure hydrocephalus can sometimes be treated by removing the excess fluid within the brain through a drainage tube (shunting).

Doctors often use antipsychotic drugs, such as thioridazine and haloperidol, to control the agitation and outbursts that may accompany advanced dementia. Unfortunately, these drugs aren't very effective at controlling such behaviors, and they can cause serious side effects. Antipsychotic drugs work best in those who have paranoia or hallucinations.

A wide range of drugs, vitamins, and nutritional supplements have proved useless in treating dementia. Among them are lecithin, ergoloid mesylates, cyclandelate, and vitamin B_{12} (unless a B_{12} deficiency has been found). Many drugs, some of which can be purchased without a prescription (over the counter), worsen dementia. Sleep aids, cold remedies, antianxiety drugs, and some antidepressants are common offenders.

Even though dementia is chronic and intellectual function can't be restored, supportive measures can be remarkably helpful. For example, large clocks and calendars can help to orient people, and caregivers can make frequent comments that remind them of where they are and what's going on. A bright and cheerful environment, minimal new stimulation, and regular low-stress activities can be beneficial. If daily routines are simplified and the caregivers' expectations are reduced without a person sensing a total loss of dignity or self-esteem, some improvement may actually occur. Caregivers must provide appropriate direction but avoid treating the person like a child. Scolding a person with dementia for making mistakes or failing to learn or remember isn't helpful and can make situations worse.

Since dementia is usually progressive, planning for the future is essential. Such planning usually combines the efforts of a doctor, a social worker, nurses, and a lawyer. However, most responsibility falls on the family, and the stresses can be tremendous. Relief from the burdens of around-the-clock attention is often available, depending on the specific behavior and capabilities of the demented person and on the family and community resources. Social agencies, including the social service department of the local community hospital, can help locate appropriate sources of help. Options include day care programs, home nursing visits, part-time or full-time housekeeping assistance, and live-in assistance. As a person's condition deteriorates, a nursing home may provide the best care.

CHAPTER 77

Stupor and Coma

Activity levels in the normal brain vary constantly. The levels when a person is awake are very different from those when asleep. Brain activity while taking a difficult examination differs subtly from brain activity while relaxing quietly on a beach. These differing levels are all normal states, and the brain can switch quickly from one level of alertness to another. During abnormal states of alertness (altered levels of consciousness), the brain is not able to switch and function appropriately.

A part of the brain deep within the brain stem▲ controls arousal levels, rhythmically stimulating the brain into wakefulness and alertness. Conscious arousal normally receives visual input from the eyes, sounds from the ears, touch sensations from the skin, and input from every other sensory organ to adjust the appropriate level of alertness. When either the arousal system or its connections to other parts of the brain don't work properly, sensations can no longer influence the brain's levels of arousal and alertness appropriately. When this happens, a person's consciousness is impaired. Periods of impaired consciousness can be short or long and can range from mild confusion to complete unresponsiveness.

Several medical terms are used to describe abnormal levels of consciousness. In **delirium** and **confusional states,** a person may be fully awake but is disoriented; that is, the person may be confused by past and present events, may be agitated, and often is unable to interpret and understand properly.■ **Obtundation** is reduced arousal. **Hypersomnia** is excessively long or deep sleep from which a person can be awakened only by energetic stimulation.★ **Stupor** is deep unresponsiveness, during which a person can be aroused only briefly by being repeatedly shaken, spoken to loudly, pinched, stuck with a pin, or similarly stimulated. **Coma** is a state somewhat like anesthesia or deep sleep, from which a person cannot be aroused at all. A person in a deep coma lacks even the most primitive responses, such as avoiding pain.

Causes

Many serious illnesses, injuries, or abnormalities can affect the brain and cause stupor or coma. Brief unconsciousness can result from a minor head injury, a seizure, or reduced blood flow to the brain as may occur with a fainting spell or stroke. Prolonged unconsciousness can be caused by a more serious head injury, a severe illness such as encephalitis, a toxic reaction to medications, or the intentional ingestion of sed-

---

▲ see page 281

■ see page 364

★ see page 303

Conditions Associated With Impaired Consciousness

Condition	Possible Result
Stroke	A person can go into a coma after a stroke, either suddenly or gradually over several hours
Head injury (concussion, cuts, bruises), bleeding in or around the brain	A person can lapse into a coma immediately or slowly over several hours after a head injury. The cause of the coma can be direct injury to the brain or bleeding within the skull (hematoma)
Infection (meningitis, encephalitis, sepsis)	Infections of the brain or severe infections outside the brain that produce high fevers, toxic substances in the blood, and low blood pressure can alter brain function and lead to a coma
Lack of oxygen	The brain becomes irreversibly damaged after only a few minutes of complete oxygen deprivation. A lack of oxygen occurs most often with acute cardiac arrest, less often with severe lung disease
Inhaling high levels of carbon monoxide (for example, fumes from a car engine or from a home heating system)	Carbon monoxide attaches to the hemoglobin of the blood's red cells and blocks their capacity to carry oxygen. Severe carbon monoxide poisoning can cause a coma or irreversible brain damage because of oxygen deprivation
Epileptic seizure	Rarely, a coma follows a seizure, but the coma usually lasts only a few minutes
Toxic effects of prescription drugs, street drugs, or alcohol	Alcohol intoxication can make a person stuporous or produce a coma, especially when the blood alcohol level exceeds 0.2 percent. Many drugs, both prescribed and illicit, can cause a coma
Liver or kidney failure	A coma is a dreaded sign of liver failure, as occurs with acute hepatitis. Kidney failure rarely results in a coma because dialysis can cleanse the blood
Low or high blood sugar levels	An abnormally low blood sugar level (hypoglycemia) can cause a coma. Immediate treatment with intravenous glucose prevents permanent brain damage. An abnormally high blood sugar level (hyperglycemia) can also cause a coma but is much less common and less severe than that of hypoglycemia
Low or high body temperature	Very high fevers (above 108° F.) can damage the brain and cause a coma. A body temperature below 88° F. (hypothermia) slows the brain to a level of stupor or coma
Fainting (syncope)	A fainting-induced coma lasts only a few seconds unless the person suffers a head injury during the fall
Psychiatric disorders	Malingering (pretending to be ill or injured), hysteria, and catatonia (a schizophrenic condition during which a person appears to be in a stupor) may resemble loss of consciousness

ative drugs or other substances. The body's metabolism, which controls levels of salt, sugar, and other chemicals in the blood, can also affect brain function.

Diagnosis

Loss of consciousness may be a result of a minor health problem or a sign of serious illness; therefore, it always requires evaluation by a doctor. Unconsciousness may be a medical emergency, as when a person loses consciousness because choking has blocked the airway or because a high dose of insulin has dangerously lowered the blood sugar level. When treating an unconscious person, emergency personnel look first for the possibility of a life-threatening situation.

An unconscious person presents a challenge to doctors and emergency medical personnel. People with medical conditions that put them at risk of losing consciousness can help by carrying medical identification or wearing Medic Alert bands. Such people include those with diabetes, epilepsy, abnormal heart rhythms, asthma, and severe liver or kidney disease. Since an unconscious person can't communicate, family and friends must be honest with doctors about the person's use of drugs, alcohol, or other toxic substances. If a drug or a poisonous substance was ingested, the doctor will want to see a sample of that substance or its container.

First, emergency medical personnel or a doctor checks to be sure that the airway is open and that breathing, blood pressure, and pulse are normal. The doctor checks body temperature: A high temperature might be a sign of infection; an abnormally low temperature could mean the person was exposed to the cold for too long. The skin is examined for signs of injury, drug injections, or allergic reactions, and the scalp is checked for cuts and bruises. The doctor also performs as thorough a neurologic examination as is possible without the cooperation of the unconscious person.

The doctor examines the person for signs of brain damage. One indication of brain damage is Cheyne-Stokes breathing, an unusual pattern in which a person breathes rapidly, then more slowly, then not at all for several seconds. Unusual postures, especially decerebrate rigidity, in which the jaw is clenched and the neck, back, arms, and legs are still and extended, are also signs of significant brain damage. General limpness of the entire body is of even greater concern,

indicating total loss of activity in certain important parts of the central nervous system.

The eyes also provide important clues to the person's status. The position of the pupils, their ability to move, their size, their reaction to bright light, their ability to follow a moving object, and the appearance of the retina are all checked. Pupils of unequal size can be a sign of pressure somewhere in the brain. The doctor needs to know if the person's pupils are normally different sizes or if the person takes glaucoma medication, which can affect pupil size.

Laboratory tests give further clues about the possible reason for a person's stupor or coma. Blood tests measure blood sugar levels, red blood cell levels (for anemia), white blood cell levels (for infection), salt levels, alcohol levels (for intoxication), and blood levels of oxygen and carbon dioxide. Urine is tested for the presence of sugar and toxic chemicals.

Additional tests may include a computed tomography (CT) or magnetic resonance imaging (MRI) scan of the head to rule out the possibility of brain injury or bleeding. A doctor who even slightly suspects a brain infection performs a lumbar puncture (spinal tap) to remove and examine a sample of cerebrospinal fluid. In patients who may be in a coma from a brain tumor or brain hemorrhage, emergency CT or MRI brain imaging is performed before the lumbar puncture to be sure that the pressure on the brain is not elevated.

Treatment

The rapid development of an altered state of consciousness is a medical emergency requiring quick attention and treatment. Diagnosing what's wrong, a prerequisite for completely effective treatment, can't always be done quickly. Until specific test results are obtained (which can take hours or days), the person is admitted to a hospital intensive care unit, where nurses can monitor heart rate, blood pressure, temperature, and the amount of oxygen in the blood.

Oxygen is often given immediately, and an intravenous line is put in place so drugs can be given quickly. Glucose, a simple sugar, is usually given intravenously, even before the results of blood sugar tests are available. If doctors suspect that reduced consciousness was caused by a narcotic, the antidote naloxone may be given while they wait for blood and urine test results. If the unconscious person is suspected of having ingested something toxic, the doctor may pump the stomach to identify its contents and prevent more of the substance from being absorbed. Blood, fluids, and drugs may be administered to keep the heart beating and the blood pressure normal.

In the deepest stages of a coma, the brain may be so damaged that it can't carry out essential body functions, such as breathing. A respirator, a machine that helps the lungs to function, may be necessary.

Prognosis

The likelihood of recovery from a deep coma that lasts more than a few hours is difficult to predict. Recovery is more likely with some causes than with others. If the coma follows a head injury, substantial recovery may occur, even if the coma lasts several weeks (but not more than 3 months). Full recovery after the heart has stopped or the person is deprived of oxygen rarely occurs if the coma lasts as long as a month. For those who remain in a deep coma longer than a few weeks, the family needs to decide whether they want doctors to continue using a respirator, feeding tube, and drugs. The family should discuss these issues with the doctors and bring any advance medical directives, such as a living will or durable power of attorney for health care,▲ to the doctors' attention.

Occasionally, after a brain injury, lack of oxygen, or a severe brain-damaging illness, a person with severe brain damage may enter a **vegetative state.** A person in this state has relatively normal sleeping and waking patterns, breathes and swallows spontaneously, and may even show a startle reaction to loud noises but has temporarily or permanently lost all capacity for conscious thought and behavior. Most people in a vegetative state have prominent abnormal reflexes, including stiffening or jerking of the arms and legs.

The **locked-in state** is a rare condition in which a person is conscious and able to think but is so severely paralyzed that communication is possible only by opening and closing the eyes in response to questions. It can occur with severe peripheral nerve paralysis or with certain acute strokes.

The most severe loss of consciousness is **brain death.** In this condition, the brain has permanently lost all vital functions, including consciousness and the ability to maintain breathing. Without drugs and a respirator, death occurs quickly. Widely accepted legal definitions consider a person to be dead when the brain has ceased all functions, even though the heart continues to beat. As a rule, doctors can legally declare brain death 12 hours after they have corrected all treatable medical problems but the brain still doesn't respond (even to induced pain), the eyes don't react to light, and the person doesn't breathe without a respirator. When any doubt exists, an electroencephalogram (a recording of the electrical activity of the brain) will show no function. A brain-dead person who is on a respirator may have some reflexes if the spinal cord is still functioning.

CHAPTER 78

Infections of the Brain and Spinal Cord

The brain and spinal cord are remarkably resistant to infection, but when they do become infected the consequences are usually very serious. For example, meningitis, an inflammation of the covering of the brain and spinal cord (menin-ges), is usually caused by a bacterial or viral infection. Aseptic meningitis is a term sometimes used to describe an inflammation of the meninges that is usually caused by a virus but at times is an autoimmune reaction (as sometimes occurs in multiple sclerosis), is a side effect of a medication such as ibuprofen, or is caused by chemicals injected into the spinal canal. Encephalitis, inflammation of the brain itself, is usually caused by a

▲ see page 1368

viral infection but may also be caused by an autoimmune reaction. An abscess is a localized infection, much like a boil, that can form anywhere in the body, including the brain.

Bacteria and other infectious organisms can reach the meninges and other areas of the brain from distant sites in several ways. They can be carried by the bloodstream, or they can enter the brain by penetration—from an injury or surgery, for example. Abscesses can spread from infected structures adjoining the brain, such as the sinuses.

Bacterial Meningitis

Bacterial meningitis is an inflammation of the meninges caused by bacteria.

Causes

Three species of bacteria account for more than 80 percent of all cases of meningitis: *Neisseria meningitidis*, *Hemophilus influenzae*, and *Streptococcus pneumoniae*. All three are normally present in the external environment and may even reside in a person's nose and respiratory system without causing harm. Occasionally, these organisms infect the brain without an identifiable reason. In other cases, infection follows a head injury or results from an abnormality in the immune system. People most at risk of developing meningitis from one of these bacteria are those who abuse alcohol; who have had a splenectomy (removal of the spleen); or who have chronic ear and nose infections, pneumococcal pneumonia, or sickle cell disease.

Rarely, other types of bacteria such as *Escherichia coli* (found normally in the colon and feces) and *Klebsiella* cause meningitis. Infections with these bacteria usually follow a head injury, brain or spinal cord surgery, a widespread infection of the blood, or an infection acquired in a hospital; these infections are more common in people with an impaired immune system. People who have kidney failure or who are taking corticosteroids have a higher than normal risk of developing meningitis from *Listeria* bacteria.

Meningitis is most common in children between the ages of 1 month and 2 years. It's much less common in adults unless they have a special risk factor. However, small epidemics of meningococcal meningitis may occur in such environments as military training camps, a college dormitory, or other small groups of people in close contact.

Symptoms

A fever, headache, stiff neck, sore throat, and vomiting, often following a respiratory illness, are the major early symptoms of meningitis. A stiff neck isn't just soreness; trying to lower the chin to the chest causes pain or may be impossible. Adults may become desperately ill within 24 hours, and children even sooner. Older children and adults can become irritable, confused, and then increasingly drowsy. They can progress to stupor, coma, and finally death. The infection causes swelling of brain tissue and hampers blood flow, causing stroke symptoms that include paralysis.▲ Some people develop seizures. **Waterhouse-Friderichsen syndrome,** an overwhelming, rapidly progressive infection caused by *Neisseria meningitidis*, produces severe diarrhea, vomiting, seizures, internal bleeding, low blood pressure, shock, and often death.

In children up to age 2, meningitis usually causes a fever, feeding problems, vomiting, irritability, seizures, and high-pitched crying. The skin over the fontanelles (the soft spots between the skull bones) becomes taut, and the fontanelles may bulge. The flow of fluid around the brain may become blocked, causing the skull to enlarge (a condition called hydrocephalus). Unlike older children or adults, infants under 1 year of age may not develop a stiff neck.

Diagnosis

Since bacterial meningitis (especially when caused by *Neisseria meningitidis*) can lead to death within hours, urgent medical attention is needed. An unexplained fever in children up to age 2 warrants an immediate, complete evaluation by a doctor, especially if the child becomes increasingly irritable or unusually sleepy, refuses to eat, vomits, has seizures, or develops a stiff neck. If the doctor suspects bacterial meningitis, the child is generally given antibiotics even before test results are available.

▲ see page 351

Spinal Tap: How It's Performed

A small, hollow needle is inserted into the lower part of the spinal canal, usually between the third and fourth lumbar vertebrae, below the point where the spinal cord ends. Cerebrospinal fluid is allowed to drip into a test tube, and the sample is sent to a laboratory for examination.

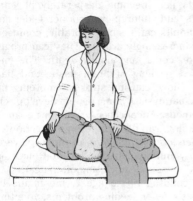

Cross Section of Spine

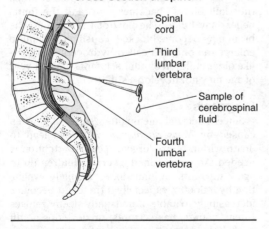

Spinal cord

Third lumbar vertebra

Sample of cerebrospinal fluid

Fourth lumbar vertebra

During the physical examination, the doctor looks for a skin rash (usually red and purple spots), cyanosis (a bluish skin color), neck stiffness, and other telltale signs of meningitis. One such sign is that the hips and knees may flex (pull up) when the child's head is pulled down toward the chest. Another is that the doctor may be unable to straighten the child's flexed knees when lifting the leg.

When doctors suspect meningitis, they must quickly determine if it's from a bacterial, viral, fungal, or other type of infection or from an irritation caused by something other than an infection (for example, a chemical). The possible causes are many, and the treatment differs for each.

The test usually used to diagnose meningitis and determine its cause is the spinal tap (lumbar puncture). A thin needle is inserted between two bones in the lower spinal column to withdraw a sample of cerebrospinal fluid from an area just below the spinal cord. The doctor then examines the fluid for bacteria under a microscope and sends a sample of it to the laboratory to be grown (cultured) and identified. The bacteria can be tested for susceptibility to treatment with different antibiotics. The sugar level, an increase in protein, and the number and type of white blood cells in the fluid also help determine the type of infection.

Besides performing a spinal tap, doctors may culture samples of blood, urine, nasal and throat mucus, and pus from skin infections to help make the diagnosis.

Treatment

Bacterial meningitis is treated immediately with intravenous antibiotics and with intravenous corticosteroids to suppress inflammation. Doctors may use one or more antibiotics to cover the most likely bacteria that might be causing the infection. Once the specific bacterium is identified (1 or 2 days later), the antibiotics may be changed to one that best treats the infection. Treatment also includes replacing fluids the person has lost because of fever, sweating, vomiting, and poor appetite.

The doctor watches for complications that may result from the brain infection. Bacterial meningitis (particularly if caused by *Neisseria meningitidis*) can lead to very low blood pressure, and the person needs additional fluids or medications to counteract this condition.

Prognosis

When treatment is started immediately, fewer than 10 percent of people with bacterial meningitis die. But when the diagnosis or treatment is delayed, permanent brain damage or death becomes more likely, especially in very young children and the elderly. Most people recover fully, but some develop seizures that require lifelong treatment. Permanent mental impairment and paralysis may also follow a bout of meningitis.

Prevention

A vaccine can help prevent meningitis caused by *Neisseria meningitidis*. The vaccine is used mainly in epidemics, in closed populations (such as on military bases) where an epidemic threatens, and with people who may be repeatedly exposed to the bacterium. Family members, medical personnel, and others in close contact with people with meningitis from *Neisseria meningitidis* may also be given an antibiotic such as rifampin or minocycline. All children should routinely be immunized with *Hemophilus influenzae* type b vaccine, which helps prevent the most common type of childhood meningitis.▲

Chronic Meningitis

Chronic meningitis is a brain infection that produces inflammation in the meninges lasting a month or longer.

Chronic meningitis usually affects people whose immune system is impaired because of AIDS, cancer, other severe diseases, anticancer drugs, or long-term use of prednisone.

Causes

Some infectious organisms may invade the brain and grow over a long time, gradually causing symptoms and damage. The most common are the fungus *Cryptococcus*, cytomegalovirus, the virus that causes AIDS, and the bacteria that cause tuberculosis, syphilis, and Lyme disease.

Some noninfectious diseases such as sarcoidosis and some cancers can irritate the meninges, producing chronic meningitis. Of the noninfectious causes, invasion of the meninges from lymphomas and leukemias is most common. Some drugs used to treat cancer, others used in organ transplants, and even such nonsteroidal anti-inflammatory drugs as ibuprofen also can inflame the meninges.

Symptoms

The symptoms of chronic meningitis are similar to those of bacterial meningitis, but the illness develops more slowly, generally over weeks rather than days. Fever is often less severe than in bacterial meningitis. Headache, confusion, and even backache and nerve abnormalities (such as weakness, tingling, numbness, and facial paralysis) are common.

Diagnosis

The diagnosis of chronic meningitis is suspected on the basis of its symptoms. However, bacterial meningitis that's been modified but not eliminated by a partial course of antibiotics and brain tumors or abscesses may be mistaken for chronic meningitis. To be sure of the diagnosis, doctors usually order a computed tomography (CT) or magnetic resonance imaging (MRI) scan of the head, followed by a spinal tap and an examination of the cerebrospinal fluid. The number of white blood cells in the fluid is higher than normal but usually is lower than in bacterial meningitis and contains a different population of white cells (lymphocytes rather than neutrophils). Infectious organisms may be visible under the microscope. The cerebrospinal fluid is always cultured to identify the specific organism. Additional tests may be ordered to check for tuberculosis or syphilis and for certain fungi and viruses.

Treatment

Chronic meningitis from certain noninfectious causes—sarcoidosis, for example—is usually treated with prednisone. Treatment of chronic infectious meningitis depends on the cause.

Chronic meningitis from a fungus is generally treated with intravenous antifungal drugs. Those most often used are amphotericin B, flucytosine, and fluconazole. When the infection is particularly difficult to cure, amphotericin B is sometimes given directly into the cerebrospinal fluid, either by repeated spinal taps or through an Ommaya reservoir—a device that's implanted under the scalp and delivers the drug to the ventricles of the brain through a small tube. For cryptococcal meningitis, amphotericin B is generally combined with flucytosine.

Recurrent herpes meningitis may be treated with acyclovir, and cytomegalovirus meningitis

---

▲ see box, page 1200

may be treated with ganciclovir. Most viral meningitides resolve on their own and require no specific treatment.

Viral Infections

Encephalitis *is an inflammation of the brain, usually caused by a virus and is referred to as viral encephalitis.* **Encephalomyelitis** *is an inflammation of both the brain and spinal cord, also caused by a virus.* **Aseptic meningitis** *is an inflammation of the meninges (the covering around the brain and spinal cord), usually caused by a virus.*

Several different viruses can infect the brain and spinal cord, including occasionally those that cause herpes and mumps. Some of these infections occur in epidemics, and some are spread by insects.

Some viruses don't primarily infect the brain and spinal cord but rather cause immune reactions that indirectly result in inflammation of these areas. This type of encephalitis (**parainfectious encephalitis** or **postinfectious encephalitis**) can follow measles, chickenpox, or rubella. The inflammation typically develops 5 to 10 days after a viral illness and can severely damage the nervous system.

Very rarely, a brain inflammation occurs weeks, months, or years after a viral infection. An example is **subacute sclerosing panencephalitis,** a brain inflammation that occasionally follows measles and usually occurs in children.▲

Symptoms

Viral brain infections can produce three different sets of symptoms. Some infections are mild, causing fever and a general feeling of illness, often without specific symptoms. Viral meningitis usually produces fever, headache, vomiting, weakness, and a stiff neck. Encephalitis disrupts normal brain function, causing personality changes, seizures, weakness of one or more parts of the body, confusion, sleepiness that can progress to coma, and the symptoms of meningitis.

Certain viruses produce additional symptoms. For example, the herpes simplex virus often induces repeated seizures in the early stages of encephalitis. The cerebrospinal fluid in herpes

simplex encephalitis contains red blood cells in addition to white blood cells—this is unusual in other milder types of viral infection. This virus also causes swelling in the temporal lobe of the brain, which can be diagnosed early by a magnetic resonance imaging (MRI) scan. A computed tomography (CT) scan begins to show changes only after severe damage has occurred.

Diagnosis

At first, doctors may have difficulty distinguishing viral or aseptic meningitis from bacterial meningitis, and encephalitis may closely resemble many other diseases that cause abnormal brain function. At the first sign of either of these conditions, doctors try to pinpoint the cause of the infection. They almost always perform a spinal tap to evaluate the cerebrospinal fluid. In viral infections, the number of white blood cells in the fluid is increased, but no bacteria are present. Culturing viruses from the fluid is difficult and takes many days.

Doctors also use immunologic tests that measure antibodies against viruses. Even with these tests, a specific virus is identified less than half the time. The doctor may order a CT or MRI scan to be sure the symptoms aren't being caused by a brain abscess, stroke, or structural problem, such as a hematoma, aneurysm, or tumor.

Prognosis and Treatment

Although infections that don't produce symptoms usually don't require treatment, antiviral drugs may help in more severe infections. Acyclovir is effective against herpes simplex but not against most other viruses.

Many people who have viral brain infections recover completely. The chances of survival and recovery depend largely on the type of virus. Herpes encephalitis causes severe brain damage but can be treated with acyclovir. To ensure a good recovery, treatment must be given before the person lapses into a coma. Infants are more likely to have permanent damage. Young children tend to recover over a long period, while adults tend to recover quickly. The drug zidovudine (AZT) may slow dementia caused by the AIDS virus. Progressive multifocal leukoencephalopathy is sometimes treated with cytarabine or vidarabine, but at best these drugs only slow progression of the infection.■

▲ see page 1267

■ see page 922

Causes of Chronic and Aseptic Meningitis

Infectious Causes

Viral diseases: Mumps, polio, lymphocytic choriomeningitis, herpes, chickenpox, eastern and western equine encephalitis, St. Louis encephalitis, infectious mononucleosis, AIDS, and infections by echovirus, coxsackievirus, or cytomegalovirus

Postinfectious causes (viral diseases that cause meningitis by an immune reaction after the main illness has cleared up): Measles, rubella (German measles), varicella (chickenpox)

Bacterial infections: Tuberculosis, syphilis, leptospirosis, mycoplasmosis, lymphogranuloma venereum, cat-scratch disease, brucellosis, cerebral Whipple's disease

Other infections: Rickettsiosis, toxoplasmosis, cryptococcosis, trichinosis, coccidioidomycosis, cysticercosis, malaria, amebiasis

Noninfectious Causes

Diseases that affect the brain: Brain tumors, stroke, multiple sclerosis, sarcoidosis, leukemia

Poison: Lead poisoning

Reaction to vaccines: Rabies and pertussis vaccines

Reaction to substances injected into the spinal column: Anticancer drugs (chemotherapy), antibiotics, dyes (for x-rays)

Drugs: Trimethoprim-sulfamethoxazole, azathioprine, carbamazepine, nonsteroidal anti-inflammatory drugs (ibuprofen, naproxen)

Brain Abscess

A brain abscess is a localized collection of pus in the brain.

Brain abscesses aren't common. They can result from the spread of an infection somewhere else in the head (such as in a tooth, the nose, or an ear), from a head wound that penetrates the brain, or from an infection somewhere else that's carried by the blood.

Symptoms

A brain abscess can cause many different symptoms, depending on its location. Symptoms include headaches, nausea, vomiting, sleepiness, seizures, personality changes, and other signs of brain dysfunction. These symptoms can develop over days or weeks. A person may have a fever and chills at first, but the symptoms may disappear as the body wards off the infection.

Diagnosis

The best test for a suspected brain abscess is generally a computed tomography (CT) or magnetic resonance imaging (MRI) scan. Although the CT or MRI scan usually shows the abscess, the collection of pus can resemble a brain tumor or stroke on the image. Additional tests may be needed so the doctor can rule out a tumor or stroke and determine which organism is causing the abscess. A biopsy of the abscess may be needed (a sample is removed for examination under a microscope and for culture).

Treatment

A brain abscess may be fatal unless treated with antibiotics. Those most commonly used are penicillin, metronidazole, nafcillin, and the cephalosporins, such as ceftizoxime. Antibiotics generally are continued for 4 to 6 weeks, and a CT or

MRI scan is repeated every 2 weeks. If the antibiotic doesn't cure the infection, a surgeon may have to drain the abscess.

Occasionally, a brain abscess causes increased pressure and swelling in the brain. This condition is very serious and can permanently damage the brain, so doctors treat it aggressively. They may give corticosteroids and drugs such as mannitol that reduce brain swelling and decrease the pressure.

Subdural Empyema

A subdural empyema is a collection of pus that develops between the brain and its surrounding tissue (the meninges), rather than in the brain itself.

Usually a subdural empyema is a complication of a sinus infection, but it can also result from a severe ear infection, head or brain injury, surgery, or a blood infection that follows a lung infection. The same kinds of bacteria that cause brain abscesses can cause subdural empyemas, and doctors treat these conditions the same way.

Like a brain abscess, a subdural empyema can cause headache, sleepiness, seizures, and other signs of brain dysfunction. The symptoms can evolve over several days, and without treatment they progress rapidly to a total loss of consciousness and death. CT and MRI scans are the best tests for helping the doctor make the diagnosis.

A spinal tap is of little help and may be dangerous. In infants, a needle can sometimes be inserted directly into the empyema through a fontanelle (a soft spot between the skull bones) to drain the pus, relieve pressure, and help with the diagnosis.

Parasitic Infections

In some parts of the world, worms can infect the brain. In the Western Hemisphere, **cysticercosis** is the most common of these infections. After a person eats food contaminated with *Cysticercus* eggs, stomach juices cause the eggs to hatch and form larvae. The larvae enter the bloodstream and are distributed to all parts of the body, including the brain. The larvae develop into cysts that can cause headaches and seizures. The cysts degenerate and the larvae die, triggering inflammation, swelling, and neurologic problems.

Schistosomiasis is a worm infection that can cause seizures, abnormal neurologic function, and increased pressure on the brain. **Echinococcosis** is an infection that can produce large cysts in the brain, causing many kinds of neurologic problems and seizures. **Coenurosis** is an infection that produces cysts, which can block the flow of fluid around the brain. Many of these infections can be controlled with drugs, such as praziquantel and albendazole, but sometimes the cysts must be removed surgically.

CHAPTER 79

Tumors of the Nervous System

A tumor is an abnormal mass anywhere in the body. Though technically a tumor can be a pocket of infection (an abscess) or inflammation, the term usually means an abnormal new growth (neoplasm) that can be either malignant (cancerous) or benign (noncancerous).

In most parts of the body, a benign tumor causes few or no problems, but any abnormal growth in the brain can cause considerable damage. A tumor can damage the brain in two ways: A growing tumor can directly destroy tissue or,

because the skull is hard and its contents can't expand, the pressure from a growing tumor on the brain can damage even areas far from the tumor. Tumors in the spinal cord also can cause damage by pressing on crucial nerve tissue. Neurofibromas, soft growths of abnormal nerve tissue, can damage peripheral nerves (those outside the brain and spinal cord) as well as nerve roots in the spine. And cancers elsewhere in the body sometimes affect the nervous system, resulting in paraneoplastic syndromes.

Brain Tumors That Originate in the Nervous System

Type of Tumor	Origin	Malignancy Status	Percentage of All Brain Tumors	People Affected
Chordoma	Nerve cells of the spinal column	Benign but invasive	Less than 1%	Adults
Germ cell tumors	Embryonic cells	Malignant or benign	1%	Children
Glioma (glioblastoma multiforme, astrocytoma, oligodendrocytoma)	Support cells of the brain, including astrocytes and oligodendrocytes	Malignant or relatively benign	65%	Children and adults (according to type)
Hemangioblastoma	Blood vessels	Benign	1 to 2%	Children and adults
Medulloblastoma	Embryonic cells	Malignant	Not applicable*	Children
Meningioma	Cells of the membrane covering the brain	Benign	20%	Adults
Osteoma	Bones of the skull	Benign	2%	Children and adults
Osteosarcoma	Bones of the skull	Malignant	Less than 1%	Children and adults
Pinealoma	Cells of the pineal gland	Benign	1%	Children
Pituitary adenoma	Pituitary epithelial cells	Benign	2%	Children and adults
Schwannoma	Schwann cells that wrap around nerves	Benign	3%	Adults

*Medulloblastoma is the major malignant brain tumor of childhood and rarely occurs in adults.

Brain Tumors

A **benign** brain tumor is an abnormal, but not cancerous, growth of tissue in the brain. A **malignant** brain tumor is any cancer in the brain that has the potential to invade and destroy neighboring tissue or that has spread (metastasized) to the brain from elsewhere through the bloodstream.

Several types of benign tumors can grow in the brain. They are named for the specific cells or tissues from which they originate: **Schwannomas** originate in the Schwann cells that form a wrapping around nerves; **ependymomas,** in cells that line the interior surface of the brain; **meningiomas,** in the meninges, the tissue that lines the outer surface of the brain; **adenomas,** in gland cells; **osteomas,** in the bony structures of the skull; and **hemangioblastomas,** in blood vessels. Certain benign brain tumors (such as craniopharyngiomas, chordomas, germinomas, teratomas, dermoid cysts, and angiomas) may even be present at birth.

Meningiomas are usually benign but may recur after they are removed. These tumors occur more often in women and usually appear between the ages of 40 and 60, but they can begin growing in childhood or later life as well. The symptoms and dangers inherent in these tumors depend on how big they are, how fast they grow, and where they are in the brain. If they become too large, they may cause mental deterioration much like dementia.

The most common malignant brain tumors are *metastases* from cancer that started in another part of the body. Cancers of the breast and lung, malignant melanoma, and blood cell cancers such as leukemia and lymphoma all can spread to the brain. Metastases may grow in a single area of the brain or in several different parts.

Primary brain tumors originate within the brain. Most often, primary brain tumors are **gliomas,** which grow from tissues that surround and support nerve cells. Several types of glioma are malignant; **glioblastoma multiforme** is the most common type. Others include the fast-growing **anaplastic astrocytomas,** the slower-growing **astrocytomas,** and **oligodendrogliomas. Medulloblastomas,** which are uncommon, usually affect children before puberty. **Sarcomas** and **adenocarcinomas** are rarer cancers that grow from structures other than nerve cells.

Brain tumors occur with equal frequency in men and women, but some types are more common in men and others are more common in women. For unknown reasons, lymphomas of the brain are appearing more often,▲ especially in people who have AIDS.

Symptoms

Symptoms result when brain tissue is destroyed or pressure builds on the brain; these symptoms occur whether a brain tumor is benign or malignant. However, when the brain tumor is a metastasis from a distant cancer, a person may also have symptoms related to that cancer. For example, lung cancer may produce coughing that brings up bloody mucus, or breast cancer may produce a lump in the breast.

The symptoms of a brain tumor depend on its size, its growth rate, and its location. Tumors in some parts of the brain can grow to considerable size before any symptoms are apparent; in other parts, even a small tumor can have devastating effects.

A headache is often the first symptom, although most headaches stem from causes other than a brain tumor.■ A brain tumor headache usually recurs frequently or is felt constantly without relief, is often severe, may start in someone who hasn't had headaches before, occurs at night, and is present upon awakening. Other common early symptoms of a brain tumor include poor balance and coordination, dizziness, and double vision. Later symptoms may include nausea and vomiting, intermittent fever, and abnormally fast or slow pulse and breathing rates. Just before death, extreme fluctuations in blood pressure may occur.

Some brain tumors cause seizures. Seizures are more common with benign brain tumors, meningiomas, and slow-growing cancers such as astrocytomas than with fast-growing cancers such as glioblastoma multiforme. A tumor can cause an arm or leg or one side of the body to become weak or paralyzed and can affect the ability to feel heat, cold, pressure, a light touch, or sharp objects. Tumors can also affect hearing, sight, and the sense of smell. Pressure on the brain can cause personality changes and can make a person feel drowsy, confused, and unable to think. Such symptoms are extremely serious and require immediate medical attention.

Diagnosis

A doctor suspects a brain tumor when a person has any of the characteristic symptoms. Though a doctor can often detect abnormal brain function by a physical examination, other procedures are undertaken to make the diagnosis.

Ordinary x-rays of the skull and brain provide little help in diagnosing brain tumors (with the occasional exception of a meningioma or pituitary adenoma). All types of brain tumors usually show up on a computed tomography (CT) or magnetic resonance imaging (MRI) scan, which can measure the tumor's size and exact position. When a brain tumor appears on a CT or MRI scan, more tests are done to determine the particular kind.

Pituitary tumors are generally discovered when they press on nerves that affect vision. Blood tests show abnormal levels of pituitary hormones, and the tumor can usually be diagnosed with a CT or MRI scan.

Some other tumors also cause abnormal levels of hormones in the blood, but most don't. A biopsy of the tumor must be performed (a sample

▲ see page 770

■ see box, page 295

Symptoms of Some Specific Brain Tumors

Astrocytomas and Oligodendrogliomas

Astroyctomas and oligodendrogliomas may be slow-growing tumors and may only cause seizures. When they are more malignant (anaplastic astrocytomas and anaplastic oligodendrogliomas), they can produce signs of abnormal brain function, such as weakness, loss of sensation, and an unsteady gait. The most malignant astrocytoma, **glioblastoma multiforme,** grows so fast that it increases pressure in the brain, producing headaches, slowed thinking, and if severe enough, sleepiness and coma.

Meningiomas

Benign tumors that originate in the covering (meninges) around the brain can cause different symptoms, depending on where they grow. They may cause weakness or numbness, seizures, an impaired sense of smell, bulging eyes, and changes in vision. In elderly people, they may cause memory loss and difficulty in thinking, similar to that found with Alzheimer's disease.

Pineal Tumors

The pineal gland, located in the middle of the brain, controls the body's biological clock, especially the normal cycling between wakefulness and sleep. Most common in childhood, atypical pineal tumors (germ cell tumors) often cause early puberty. They can obstruct drainage of the fluid around the brain, leading to enlargement of the brain and skull (hydrocephalus) and serious brain malfunction.

Pituitary Gland Tumors

The pituitary gland, located at the base of the skull, controls much of the body's endocrine system. Tumors of the pituitary gland usually are benign and secrete abnormally large amounts of pituitary hormones:

• An increased amount of growth hormone leads to extreme height (gigantism) or disproportionate enlargement of the head, face, hands, feet, and chest (acromegaly).
• An increased amount of corticotropin results in Cushing's syndrome.
• An increased amount of thyroid-stimulating hormone leads to hyperthyroidism.
• An increased amount of prolactin stops menstrual periods (amenorrhea), causes breast milk production in women who aren't breast-feeding (galactorrhea), and enlarges the breasts in men (gynecomastia).

Pituitary gland tumors can also destroy hormone-secreting tissues, eventually leading to insufficient levels of hormones in the body. Other symptoms may include headaches and a loss in the outer visual fields of both eyes.

---

is removed and examined under a microscope) to determine the type of tumor and whether it's malignant.

Sometimes microscopic examination of the cerebrospinal fluid, obtained through a spinal tap (lumbar puncture), shows cancer cells. A spinal tap can't be performed if there's any evidence of increased pressure within the skull, because the sudden change in pressure could cause **herniation,** one of the most dangerous potential complications of a brain tumor. With herniation, increased pressure within the skull forces brain tissue downward through the narrow opening at the base of the skull, thereby compressing the lower part of the brain (brain stem). As a result, the critical functions controlled by the brain stem—

breathing, heart rate, and blood pressure—begin to malfunction. If not diagnosed and treated early, herniation eventually results in coma and death.

A biopsy can usually be performed during surgery in which all or part of the tumor is removed. Sometimes tumors in deep parts of the brain are inaccessible and can't be approached safely and directly. In such cases, a biopsy may be performed using three-dimensional needle placement, a technique in which a special imaging device guides the placement of a needle and then cells from the tumor are drawn into the needle.

Treatment

The treatment of a brain tumor depends on its location and type. When possible, the tumor is

Benign Intracranial Hypertension or Brain Tumor?

Benign intracranial hypertension (also called **pseudotumor cerebri**) is a disorder in which the pressure around the brain increases without any evidence of a tumor, infection, blocked drainage of the fluid surrounding the brain, or other cause. The disorder is sometimes mistaken for a brain tumor. It's most common in women between the ages of 20 and 50, especially those who are overweight.

In most instances, neither the onset nor the eventual disappearance of benign intracranial hypertension can be traced to a particular event. In children, it sometimes follows the withdrawal of corticosteroids, or it occurs after a child has taken excessive amounts of vitamin A or the antibiotic tetracycline.

Benign intracranial hypertension usually begins with a headache that is often, but not always, mild. Late in the course of the disease, about 5 percent of the people temporarily lose their vision, either partially or completely, in one or both eyes. The doctor may also find swelling in the back of the eye, a condition called papilledema.

The doctor's first step in evaluating benign intracranial hypertension is to rule out any possible treatable cause of elevated pressure in the brain. The results of a computed tomography (CT) scan are usually normal, but the scan may show a slight compression of air and fluid spaces in the brain. A spinal tap usually shows elevated pressure of the cerebrospinal fluid, although chemically, the fluid seems normal.

Benign intracranial hypertension often disappears on its own within 6 months. No treatment is needed, but overweight people should lose weight. Aspirin or acetaminophen may relieve the headache. If the increased intracranial pressure isn't relieved within a few weeks, a doctor may prescribe the drug acetazolamide.

About 10 to 20 percent of the people with benign intracranial hypertension have recurrences, and a small percentage get progressively worse, eventually becoming blind. Once vision is lost, it may never return, even if the pressure in the skull is relieved. A surgically placed shunt may drain fluid from the brain in some people who have chronic benign intracranial hypertension.

---

removed surgically. Many brain tumors can be removed with little or no damage to the brain. However, some grow in an area that makes removal difficult or impossible without destroying essential structures. Surgery sometimes causes brain damage that can lead to partial paralysis, changes in sensation, weakness, and impaired intellect. Nevertheless, removing a tumor is essential if its growth threatens important brain structures. Even when surgical removal can't cure a cancer, surgery may be useful to reduce the tumor's size, relieve symptoms, and help the doctor determine the specific type of tumor and whether other treatments, such as radiation therapy, are warranted.

Some benign tumors must be surgically removed because their continued growth in a confined space can cause severe damage or death. Meningiomas are usually removed if at all possible, and the removal can generally be done safely and completely. However, very small meningiomas and those in elderly people may be left in place. Most other benign tumors, such as schwannomas and ependymomas, are treated similarly. Sometimes, radiation therapy is given after surgery to destroy any remaining tumor cells.

Most brain tumors, especially those that are malignant, are treated by some combination of surgery, radiation therapy, and chemotherapy. After as much of the tumor is removed as possible, radiation therapy is begun. Radiation rarely cures brain cancer but may shrink a tumor enough to keep it under control for many months or even years. Chemotherapy is used to treat some forms of brain cancer. Both metastatic and primary brain cancers may respond to chemotherapy.

Increased pressure on the brain is extremely serious and requires immediate medical attention. Drugs such as mannitol and corticosteroids are usually given by injection to reduce the pressure and prevent herniation. Sometimes, a small device is placed under the skull to measure the pressure on the brain so that treatment can be adjusted accordingly.

Treatment of metastases to the brain depends largely on where the cancer originated. Radiation therapy is often performed on the cancer growth in the brain. Surgical removal may benefit a person who has only a single metastasis. In addition to traditional treatments, some experimental treatments involving chemotherapy, radioactive implants in the tumor, and radiosurgery are being tried.

Prognosis

Despite treatment, only about 25 percent of the people with brain cancer are alive after 2 years. The outlook is slightly better with some types of tumors, such as astrocytomas and oligodendrogliomas, in which the cancer usually doesn't recur for 3 to 5 years after treatment. About 50 percent of all the people treated for medulloblastomas survive more than 5 years.

The treatment of brain cancer is more likely to be effective in people under age 45, in people with anaplastic astrocytoma rather than glioblastoma multiforme, and in those in whom most or all of the tumor can be surgically removed.

Spinal Cord Tumors

Spinal cord tumors are masses of new tissue growth, benign or malignant, in the spinal cord.

Tumors in the spinal cord can be either primary (originating in the spinal cord) or secondary (metastases of cancer that originated elsewhere in the body). Spinal cord tumors are much less common than brain tumors and are rare in children.

Only about 10 percent of primary spinal cord tumors originate in the nerve cells inside the spinal cord. Two thirds of them are **meningiomas** (originating in the cells of the meninges, which lines the brain and spinal cord) and **schwannomas** (originating in the Schwann cells, which form a wrapping around the nerves). Both meningiomas and schwannomas are benign (noncancerous) growths. Malignant (cancerous) growths include **gliomas,** which originate in other cells inside the spinal cord, and **sarcomas,** which originate in connective tissues in the spinal column. **Neurofibromas,** a type of schwannoma in which the Schwann cells develop into tumors, also may originate in the spinal cord as part of von Recklinghausen's disease.

Metastases spread to the spinal cord or its surrounding structures from cancers in other parts of the body, most commonly the lung, breast, prostate gland, kidney, or thyroid. Lymphomas also may spread to the spinal cord.

Symptoms

Spinal cord tumors usually cause symptoms by pressing on the nerves. Pressure on the nerve roots, the parts of the nerves that exit from the spinal column, ▲ can cause pain, numbness, tingling, and weakness. Pressure on the cord itself can cause spasticity, weakness, poor coordination, and decreased or abnormal sensations. The tumor may also cause difficulty with urination, loss of bladder control, or constipation.

Diagnosis

Doctors consider the possibility of a spinal cord tumor in people who have certain cancers in other parts of the body, who develop pain in a specific area of the spinal column, and who experience weakness, tingling, or poor coordination. Because of the way the nerves of the spinal cord are arranged, a doctor can locate the tumor by evaluating the parts of the body that aren't functioning normally.■

Doctors must rule out other disorders that can affect the function of the spinal cord, such as sore back muscles, bone bruises, an insufficient blood supply to the spinal cord, fractured vertebrae, and ruptured disks, as well as diseases such as syphilis, viral infections, multiple sclerosis, and amyotrophic lateral sclerosis.

Several procedures are used to help diagnose a spinal cord tumor. Although spinal x-rays can show changes in the bones, they usually don't show tumors that haven't yet affected the bone. Magnetic resonance imaging (MRI) is considered the best technique for examining all the structures of the spinal cord and column. A biopsy (removal of a sample of the tumor for examination under a microscope) is needed to diagnose the precise type of tumor.

▲ see page 327

■ see box, page 324

Treatment

Many tumors of the spinal cord and column can be removed surgically. Others can be treated with radiation therapy or with surgery followed by radiation therapy. When a tumor is compressing the spinal cord or its surrounding structures, corticosteroids may be given to reduce the swelling and preserve nerve function until the tumor can be removed.

Prognosis

Recovery generally depends on how much damage has already been done and how deep into the spinal cord the tumor has grown. Symptoms are reversed after treatment in about half of the people with spinal cord tumors. Removal of meningiomas, neurofibromas, and some primary tumors may be curative.

Neurofibromatosis

Neurofibromatosis **(von Recklinghausen's disease)** *is a genetically transmitted disease in which many soft, fleshy growths of abnormal nerve tissue (neurofibromas) appear in the skin and other parts of the body.*

Neurofibromas are growths of myelin-producing Schwann cells and other cells that surround and support peripheral nerves (those nerves located outside the brain and spinal cord). The growths usually start appearing after puberty and can be felt under the skin as small lumps.

Symptoms and Diagnosis

About one third of the people with neurofibromatosis notice no symptoms, and the disease is first diagnosed during a routine examination when a doctor finds lumps under the skin near nerves. In another third, the disease is first diagnosed when a person seeks help for a cosmetic problem. Many people have medium brown skin spots (café au lait spots) over the chest, back, pelvis, elbows, and knees. These spots may exist at birth or appear during infancy. Between ages 10 and 15, flesh-colored growths (neurofibromas) of varying size and shape begin appearing on the

---

▲ see page 327

■ see page 1012

skin. There may be fewer than 10 of these growths or thousands of them. In some people, the growths produce skeletal problems, such as abnormal curvature of the spine (kyphoscoliosis), rib deformities, enlarged long bones of the arms and legs, and bone defects of the skull and around the eye. In the remaining one third of the people with neurofibromatosis, the disease is diagnosed when they notice neurologic problems.

Neurofibromas may affect any nerve in the body but frequently grow on spinal nerve roots,▲ where they often cause few or no problems but can become a serious threat if they put pressure on the spinal cord. More commonly, neurofibromas put pressure on peripheral nerves, impairing their normal function. Neurofibromas that affect nerves in the head can cause blindness, dizziness, deafness, and incoordination. As the number of neurofibromas increases, more neurologic complications appear.

Besides having these problems, people with a rarer form of the disease, called type 2 neurofibromatosis, develop tumors **(acoustic neuromas)** in the inner ear.■ The tumors may cause hearing loss and sometimes dizziness, as early as age 20.

Treatment

No known treatment can stop the progression of neurofibromatosis or cure it, but individual growths can usually be removed surgically or shrunk with radiation therapy. When they have grown close to a nerve, surgical removal often requires removing the nerve as well. Because neurofibromatosis is an inherited disorder, genetic counseling is recommended when a person with this disorder is considering parenthood.

Paraneoplastic Syndromes

Paraneoplastic syndromes are the remote effects of cancer (most commonly lung and ovarian cancer) on many different functions of the body, often those of the nervous system.

Exactly how distant cancers affect the nervous system isn't completely understood. Some cancers release substances into the bloodstream that damage remote tissues by causing an autoimmune reaction. Other cancers secrete substances that directly interfere with the nervous system's function or actually destroy parts of the nervous system.

Paraneoplastic syndromes can produce a wide variety of neurologic symptoms, including dementia, mood swings, seizures, weakness (possibly progressive) of the limbs or the entire body, numbness, tingling, poor coordination, dizziness, double vision, and abnormal eye movements. The most common effect, **polyneuropathy,** is a dysfunction of peripheral nerves (those outside the brain and spinal cord).▲ A person feels weak, loses sensation, and has weak reflexes. Although polyneuropathy can't be directly treated, it's sometimes improved by treating the cancer.

A rare form of polyneuropathy, **subacute sensory neuropathy,** sometimes precedes the diagnosis of cancer. A person may have a disabling loss of sensation and poor coordination but little weakness. No treatment is available for subacute sensory neuropathy.

The substances produced by different cancers can have widely varying effects. Breast and ovarian cancers sometimes produce a substance that appears to induce an autoantibody that destroys the cerebellum, resulting in a disorder called **subacute cerebellar degeneration.** Symptoms of this disorder—unsteady gait, poor arm and leg coordination, difficulty in speaking, dizziness, double vision—may appear weeks, months, or even years before the cancer is discovered. Subacute cerebellar degeneration usually gets worse over weeks or months, often leaving the person severely disabled. The disorder isn't easy to diagnose before the cancer is found, although a computed tomography (CT) or magnetic resonance imaging (MRI) scan may show loss of brain tissue in the cerebellum. No effective treatment is available, but the disorder sometimes improves after the cancer is successfully treated.

Neuroblastoma, a childhood cancer, sometimes causes a rare combination of symptoms characterized by sudden, uncontrollable eye movements. The child also has poor coordination, along with rigidity, spasms, and muscle contractions in the body, arms, and legs. These symptoms are often relieved by treating the cancer and sometimes by taking corticosteroids such as prednisone.

In rare instances, Hodgkin's disease can indirectly affect the nerve cells of the spinal cord, weakening the arms and legs in a pattern similar to that of acute polyneuropathy. This condition usually improves with corticosteroids.

The **Eaton-Lambert syndrome** is a paraneoplastic syndrome similar to myasthenia gravis ■ that can occur in people with lung cancer. The syndrome involves antibodies that interfere with the substances that provide communication between nerves and muscles (neurotransmitters). Weakness develops before, during, or after the diagnosis of cancer. Occasionally, no cancer can be found. People with Eaton-Lambert syndrome may also develop fatigue, pain and tingling in the arms and legs, dry mouth, drooping eyelids, and impotence. Normal reflexes, such as the knee jerk reflex, are diminished or may even disappear.

The symptoms of Eaton-Lambert syndrome may subside when the underlying cancer is treated. Guanidine, a drug that triggers nerves to produce more of the substance that stimulates muscles, may relieve the weakness somewhat. Guanidine has serious side effects, however, including damage to the bone marrow and liver. Other treatments include plasmapheresis, a procedure in which toxic substances are removed from the blood,★ and administration of corticosteroids such as prednisone.

Cancers can also cause weakness by directly affecting muscles rather than nerves. The resulting disorders, **dermatomyositis** and **polymyositis,** weaken the strong muscles close to the trunk. People may develop a purplish rash on the nose and cheeks and swelling around the eyes (a heliotrope rash). Although dermatomyositis and polymyositis are most common in people over age 50 who have cancer, they occasionally affect people who don't have cancer. Treatment with corticosteroids such as prednisone is sometimes effective.

Radiation Damage to the Nervous System

Although doctors try to prevent radiation from damaging the nervous system during cancer treatments, such damage is sometimes unavoidable. Symptoms of injury from radiation can ap-

---

▲ see page 337

■ see page 333

★ see box, page 741

pear suddenly or slowly, can remain the same or get worse, and can be temporary or permanent. Sometimes symptoms don't appear until months or years after the radiation therapy is completed.

Exposing the brain to radiation can cause **acute encephalopathy,** with headaches, nausea and vomiting, sleepiness, confusion, and other neurologic symptoms. Acute encephalopathy usually begins shortly after the first or second dose of radiation is administered, but sometimes it begins 2 to 4 months after radiation therapy is completed. Symptoms usually diminish during the radiation treatments, and corticosteroids such as prednisone may help the person improve faster.

Sometimes, symptoms of brain damage appear many months or years after radiation therapy, a condition called **late-delayed radiation damage.** Symptoms can include progressively worsening dementia, memory loss, difficulty in thinking, mistaken perceptions, personality changes, and unsteadiness in walking.

Radiation therapy to the neck or chest may cause **radiation myelopathy,** in which a person may experience **Lhermitte's sign,** a sensation like an electric shock that begins in the neck or back, usually when the neck is bent forward, and shoots down to the legs. This type of radiation myelopathy usually improves without treatment. Another type of radiation myelopathy may develop many months or years after radiation therapy. This type causes weakness, loss of sensation, and sometimes the **Brown-Séquard syndrome,** with weakness on one side of the body and loss of pain and temperature sensation on the other. On the weak side of the body, the person may lose position sense (the ability to determine where the hands and feet are when not actually looking at them). This rare disorder usually doesn't subside and leaves many people paralyzed.

Nerves near the site of the radiation therapy may also become damaged. For example, radiation to the breast or lung may damage nerves in the arms, causing weakness or loss of feeling. Radiation to the groin may affect nerves in the legs, causing similar symptoms.

Mental Health Disorders

Overview of Mental Health Care

Mental health (psychiatric) disorders involve disturbances in thinking, emotion, and behavior. These disorders are caused by complex interactions between physical, psychologic, social, cultural, and hereditary influences.

Mental Illness in Society

A movement in recent decades to bring mentally ill patients out of institutions has been made possible by the development of effective antipsychotic drugs. With the deinstitutionalization movement, greater emphasis has been placed on viewing mentally ill people as members of families and communities.

Research has demonstrated that certain interactions between families and patients can improve or worsen mental illness. Therefore, family therapy techniques have been developed that dramatically prevent the chronically mentally ill from needing to be reinstitutionalized. Today the family of a mentally ill patient is more involved than ever as an ally in treatment. The family doctor also plays an important role in rehabilitating a patient into the community. In addition, mentally ill people who must be hospitalized are less likely to be isolated and restrained than in the past, and they are often discharged early into partial hospital programs and day treatment centers. These settings are less expensive because fewer staff are involved, the emphasis is on group therapy rather than individual therapy, and patients sleep at home or in halfway houses.

However, the deinstitutionalization movement has had its share of problems. Because mentally ill people who are not a danger to themselves or society can no longer be institutionalized or treated against their will, many have become homeless. Although these legal measures protect people's civil rights, they make it more difficult to provide needed treatment to many patients, some of whom may be extremely irrational. The homelessness also has an impact on society.

Everyone requires a social network to satisfy the human need to be cared for, accepted, and emotionally supported, particularly in times of stress. Research has demonstrated that strong social support may significantly improve recovery from both physical and mental illnesses. Societal changes have diminished the traditional support once offered by neighbors and families. As an alternative, self-help groups and mutual-aid groups have sprung up throughout the country.

Some self-help groups, such as Alcoholics Anonymous and Narcotics Anonymous, focus on addictive behavior. Others act as advocates for certain groups, such as the handicapped and the elderly. Still others, such as the National Alliance for the Mentally Ill, provide support for family members of people who have a severe illness.

Classification and Diagnosis of Mental Illness

In the field of medicine, the classification of diseases is constantly changing as knowledge changes. Similarly, in psychiatry, the knowledge of how the brain functions and is influenced by the environment and other factors is constantly becoming more sophisticated. Despite advances, knowledge of the intricate mechanisms involved in brain functioning is still in its infancy. However, because many research studies have shown that mental illnesses can be distinguished from one another with a high degree of reliability, a standardized approach to diagnosis is becoming more and more refined.

In 1952, the American Psychiatric Association first published the *Diagnostic and Statistical Manual of Mental Disorders* (DSM-I). The latest edition, DSM-IV, was published in 1994. This manual provides a classification system that attempts to separate mental illnesses into diagnostic categories based on descriptions of symptoms—what patients say and do as reflections of how they think and feel—and on the course of the illness.

The *International Classification of Disease, 9th Revision, Clinical Modification* (ICD-9-CM), a book published by the World Health Organization, uses diagnostic categories similar to those in the DSM-IV. This similarity suggests that diagnoses of specific mental illnesses are becoming more standard and consistent throughout the world.

Advances have been made in diagnostic methods. Several new brain imaging techniques have become available, including computed tomography (CT), magnetic resonance imaging (MRI), and positron emission tomography (PET), a type of scan that measures blood flow to specific areas of the brain.▲ These imaging techniques are being used to map brain structure and function in people with normal and abnormal behavior, giving scientists greater understanding of how the brain functions in people with and without mental illness. Research that has differentiated one psychiatric disorder from another has led to greater precision in diagnosis.

Treatment of Mental Illness

Most psychiatric treatment methods can be categorized as either somatic or psychotherapeutic. Somatic treatments include drug therapy and electroconvulsive therapy. Psychotherapeutic treatments include psychotherapy (individual, group, or family), behavioral therapy techniques (such as relaxation training and hypnosis), and hypnotherapy. Many psychiatric disorders require a combination of drug therapy and psychotherapy. Indeed, most studies suggest that for major psychiatric disorders, a treatment approach involving both drugs and psychotherapy is more effective than either treatment method used alone.

Drug Treatment

Over the last 40 years, a number of psychiatric drugs have been developed that are highly effective and widely used by psychiatrists and other doctors. These drugs are often categorized according to the disorder for which they are primarily prescribed. For example, **antidepressants,** including imipramine, fluoxetine, and bupropion, are used to treat depression. **Antipsychotic drugs,** such as chlorpromazine, haloperidol, and thiothixene, are helpful for people with psychotic disorders such as schizophrenia.■ New antipsychotic drugs, such as clozapine and risperidone, may be useful for some patients who have not responded to other antipsychotic drugs. **Antianxiety drugs,** such as clonazepam and diazepam, may be used to treat anxiety disorders such as panic disorder and phobias.★ **Mood stabilizers,** such as lithium and carbamazepine, have been used with some success in patients with manic-depressive illness.

Features of Psychotherapy

- Empathy and acceptance of the person's difficulties

- An explanation for the person's distress and a method for relieving it

- Information about the nature and source of the person's problems and the suggestion of possible alternatives for dealing with them

- A strengthening of the person's expectations of health through a trusting and confidential relationship with the therapist

- An increase in the person's emotional awareness that enables a change in attitude and behavior

Electroconvulsive Therapy

With electroconvulsive therapy, electrodes are attached to the head and a series of electric shocks are delivered to the brain to induce seizures. This therapy has consistently been shown to be the most effective treatment for severe depression. Contrary to its portrayal in the media, electroconvulsive therapy is safe and rarely causes any serious complications. The modern use of anesthetics and muscle relaxants has greatly reduced any risk to the patient.

Psychotherapy

In recent years, significant advances have been made in the field of psychotherapy. Psychotherapy is the treatment of a patient by a therapist using psychologic techniques and making systematic use of the patient-therapist relationship. Psychiatrists are not the only mental health professionals trained to practice psychotherapy. Others include clinical psychologists, social

▲ see page 287

■ see page 435

★ see box, page 397

workers, nurses, some pastoral counselors, and many paraprofessionals; however, psychiatrists are the only mental health professionals licensed to prescribe drugs.

Although individual psychotherapy is practiced in many different ways, most mental health professionals are affiliated with one of four schools of psychotherapy: dynamic, cognitive-behavioral, interpersonal, or behavioral. **Dynamic psychotherapy** is derived from psychoanalysis and is based on helping the patient understand unconscious conflicts and patterns that may be creating symptoms and difficulties with relationships. **Cognitive-behavioral therapy** focuses primarily on distortions in the patient's thinking. **Interpersonal therapy** focuses on how a loss or change in a relationship affects the patient. **Behavioral therapy** is geared toward helping patients unlearn conditioned ways of reacting to events around them. In practice, many psychotherapists combine techniques, depending on a patient's needs.

Psychotherapy is appropriate in a wide range of conditions. Even people who don't have a psychiatric disorder may find psychotherapy helpful in coping with such problems as employment difficulties, bereavement, or chronic illness in the family. **Group psychotherapy** and **family therapy** are also widely used.

Hypnosis and Hypnotherapy

Hypnosis and hypnotherapy are increasingly used to manage pain and treat physical disorders that have a psychologic component. These techniques may promote relaxation and thereby lower anxiety and reduce tension. For example, hypnosis and hypnotherapy can help people with cancer who have anxiety or depression in addition to pain.

CHAPTER 81

Psychosomatic Disorders

The term *psychosomatic disorder* has no precise definition. Most often, the term is applied to physical disorders thought to be caused by psychologic factors. However, no physical disorder is caused exclusively by psychologic factors. Rather, a physical disorder has a necessary biologic component—a factor essential for the disease to occur.

For example, to acquire tuberculosis, a person must be infected with the *Mycobacterium* bacterium, which causes tuberculosis. But many people infected with *Mycobacterium* have only a minor illness or no illness at all. Other factors are needed to produce the illness recognized as tuberculosis, possibly including a hereditary susceptibility; environmental factors, such as living in crowded conditions; the presence of malnutrition; and social or psychologic stress, such as the loss of a loved one, and the resulting emotional reaction, such as depression. Biologic, environmental, social, and psychologic factors combine to make someone infected with *Mycobacterium* ill with tuberculosis. The term psychosomatic covers the combination of factors.

Mind-Body Interaction

Social and psychologic stress can trigger or aggravate a wide variety of diseases, such as diabetes mellitus, systemic lupus erythematosus (lupus), leukemia, and multiple sclerosis. However, the relative importance of psychologic factors varies widely among different people with the same disorder.

Most people, on the basis of either intuition or personal experience, believe that emotional stress can precipitate or alter the course of even major physical diseases. How these stressors might do this isn't clear. Emotions obviously can affect certain body functions, such as heart rate, sweating, sleep patterns, and bowel movements, but other relationships are less obvious. For example, the pathways and mechanisms by which the brain and immune system interact still haven't been identified. Can the mind (brain) alter the activity of white blood cells and thus an immune response? If so, how does the brain communicate with the blood cells? After all, white blood cells travel through the body in blood or lymph vessels and aren't attached to nerves. Nevertheless, research has shown that such relationships do exist. For example, hives can be brought on by a physical allergy or a psychologic reaction. Depression can suppress the immune system, making a depressed person more susceptible to certain infections, such as those by the viruses that cause the common cold.

Stress, therefore, can cause physical symptoms even though no physical disease may be present. The body responds physiologically to emotional stress. For example, stress can cause anxiety, which then triggers the autonomic nervous system and hormones such as adrenaline to speed up the heart rate and to increase the blood pressure and amount of sweating. Stress can also cause muscle tension, leading to pain in the neck, back, head, or elsewhere. The emotional disturbance that triggered the symptoms may be overlooked when the patient and the doctor assume that they were caused by a physical disease. Many fruitless diagnostic tests may be done to uncover the cause of the fast heart rate, headaches, backaches, and so on.

Psychologic factors can also *indirectly* influence a disease's course. For example, some seriously ill people deny having a disease or deny its seriousness. Denial is a defense mechanism that helps reduce anxiety and makes a threatening situation more tolerable. If denial relieves anxiety, it may be beneficial. However, denial may prevent a person from complying with a treatment program, and this can have serious consequences. For example, a person with diabetes who denies the need for insulin injections and strict dietary management can have marked shifts in blood sugar levels and risks having complications such as diabetic coma. Similarly, a high percentage of people with high blood pressure (hypertension) or epilepsy fail to take their medications.

The mind-body interaction is a two-way street. Not only can psychologic factors contribute to the onset or aggravation of a wide variety of physical disorders, but also physical diseases can affect a person's thinking or mood. People with life-threatening, recurring, or chronic physical disorders commonly become depressed. Although depression under these circumstances may appear to be a normal reaction, the person's mental state still deserves attention. The depression may worsen the effects of the physical disease and add to the person's misery. Appropriate

---

Metaphors That Suggest Conversion Symptoms

"Oh, my aching back."

"I can't swallow that."

"The very idea makes me sick."

"I've been stabbed in the back."

"That makes me want to throw up."

---

treatment, including the use of antidepressants, often improves these situations.

A person who is anxious or depressed may instead express concerns about a physical problem. This phenomenon is most common in depressed people who seem unable to accept that their symptoms are primarily psychologic. The depression may lead to insomnia, lack of appetite, weight loss, and fatigue. Instead of saying "I'm so depressed," the person focuses on his symptoms in the belief that they are caused by a physical disorder. This is referred to as a "masked" depression. Some people are able to admit that they are depressed but then try to explain it as resulting from a physical disorder.

Conversion of Symptoms

A mechanism by which psychologic and social stress can suggest a physical disease is conversion. In conversion, the person unconsciously converts a psychologic conflict into a physical symptom. This diverts the person's focus away from a troublesome emotional issue to what may be a less frightening physical problem. Virtually any symptom imaginable may become a conversion symptom. Sometimes a conversion symptom is a metaphor for the person's psychologic problem. For example, a person with chest pain may be symbolically suffering from a broken heart after being rejected by a loved one, or a person with back pain may feel that his burdens are too difficult to carry.

A conversion symptom may also stem from identification with someone else who had the symptom. For example, a person may have chest pain, suggesting the possibility of a heart attack, after a parent, sibling, or coworker has had a heart attack. Or a man may develop chest pain as he approaches the age at which his father died of a heart attack.

Finally, the conversion symptom may be neither a metaphor nor the result of identifying with another person, but rather the reexperiencing of a symptom of a previous physical disorder. For example, a person who once had a painful bone fracture may reexperience that sort of bone pain as a conversion symptom. A person who has episodes of chest pain (angina) from coronary artery disease may sometimes have a similar pain as a conversion symptom (the pain is then called pseudoangina).

Conversion *symptoms* differ from conversion *disorder*, in which physical symptoms more often resemble those of a neurologic disease.▲ Conversion symptoms are milder and more transient and affect people who don't have a serious underlying psychiatric disease. Anyone can have conversion symptoms. The symptoms can be difficult for a doctor to diagnose, and a patient with these symptoms is likely to undergo various diagnostic tests to be certain there is no underlying physical disorder.

Most conversion symptoms disappear rather quickly after a medical evaluation and reassurance from a doctor. When conversion symptoms recur or fail to go away and become disabling, a somatoform disorder may be the cause.■

CHAPTER 82

Somatoform Disorders

Somatoform disorders encompass several psychiatric disorders in which people report physical symptoms but deny having psychiatric problems.

Somatoform disorders is a relatively new term for what many people refer to as psychosomatic disorder.★ In somatoform disorders, either the physical symptoms or their severity and duration can't be explained by any underlying physical disease. Somatoform disorders include somatization disorder, conversion disorder, and hypochondriasis.

Psychiatrists differ considerably in opinion as to the value and validity of using these diagnostic categories. However, categorizing the different somatoform disorders has given psychiatrists a way to describe the wide variety of symptoms seen in these patients and to differentiate the disorders based on these descriptions. Careful

descriptions may help psychiatrists sort out the different disorders that can be better studied scientifically.

Somatoform disorders have no generally accepted explanation. The individual patients who are diagnosed with a somatoform disorder vary greatly. Because there's no clear understanding of why or how people develop their symptoms, there are no generally agreed on, clear-cut modes of treatment.

Somatization Disorder

Somatization disorder is a chronic, severe illness characterized by many physical symptoms, particularly some combination of pain and gastrointestinal, sexual, and neurologic symptoms.

The causes of somatization disorder aren't known. It often runs in families. People with the disorder tend to also have personality disorders characterized by self-centeredness (narcissistic personality) and exaggerated dependence on others (dependent personality).●

Symptoms appear first in adolescence or early adulthood and are thought to occur predominantly in women. Male relatives of women with the disorder tend to have a high incidence of socially disapproved behavior and alcoholism.

▲ see page 394

■ see below

★ see page 390

● see page 426

Munchausen Syndrome: Faking Illness for Attention

Munchausen syndrome, also called malingering, isn't a somatoform disorder, but its features are somewhat similar in that psychiatric problems underlie a physical disorder. The key difference is that people with Munchausen syndrome consciously *fake* the symptoms of a physical disorder. They repeatedly fabricate illnesses and often wander from hospital to hospital for treatment.

However, Munchausen syndrome is more complex than simple dishonest fabrication and simulation of symptoms. The disorder is associated with severe emotional problems. People with the disorder are usually quite intelligent and resourceful; they not only know how to mimic diseases but also are sophisticated with regard to medical practices.

They can manipulate their care to be hospitalized and subjected to intense testing and treatment, including major operations. Their deceits are conscious, but their motivation and quest for attention are largely unconscious.

A bizarre variant of the syndrome is called **Munchausen by proxy.** In this disorder, a child is used as a surrogate patient, usually by a parent. The parent falsifies the child's medical history and may injure the child with drugs or add blood or bacterial contaminants to urine specimens, all in an effort to simulate disease. The motivation underlying such bizarre behavior appears to be a pathologic need for attention and for an intense relationship with the child.

Symptoms

A person with somatization disorder has many vague physical complaints. Although any part of the body may be affected, most often symptoms take the form of headaches, nausea and vomiting, abdominal pain, diarrhea or constipation, painful menstrual periods, fatigue, fainting, pain during intercourse, and loss of sexual desire. Although the symptoms are primarily physical, anxiety and depression also occur. People with somatization disorder are dramatic and emotional in describing their symptoms, often referring to them as "unbearable," "beyond description," or "the worst imaginable."

Extreme dependency emerges in the relationships of people with somatization disorder. They increasingly demand help and emotional support and may become enraged when they feel their needs aren't being met. They are often described as exhibitionistic and seductive. In an attempt to manipulate others, they may threaten or attempt suicide. Often dissatisfied with their medical care, they go from doctor to doctor.

The physical symptoms appear to be a way of communicating a plea for help and attention. The intensity and persistence of the symptoms reflect the person's intense desire to be cared for in every aspect of life. The symptoms also seem to serve other purposes, such as allowing the person to avoid the responsibilities of adulthood. The symptoms tend to be uncomfortable and prevent the person from engaging in many enjoyable pursuits, suggesting that the person also suffers feelings of unworthiness and guilt. The symptoms both prevent pleasure and act as punishment.

Diagnosis

People with somatization disorder aren't aware that their basic problem is psychologic, so they press their doctors for medical studies and treatments. The doctor is obliged to conduct many physical examinations and tests to determine whether the person has a physical disorder that adequately explains the symptoms. Referrals to specialists for consultations are common, even if the person has developed a reasonably satisfactory relationship with one doctor.

Once a doctor determines that the disorder is psychologic, somatization disorder can be distinguished from similar psychiatric disorders by its many symptoms and their tendency to persist over a period of years. Adding to the diagnosis are the dramatic nature of the complaints and the person's exhibitionistic, dependent, manipulative, and sometimes suicidal behavior.

Prognosis and Treatment

Somatization disorder tends to fluctuate in severity but persists throughout life. Complete relief of symptoms for any extended period is rare. Some people become more overtly depressed after many years, and their references to suicide become more ominous. Suicide is a definite risk.

Treatment is extremely difficult. People with somatization disorder tend to be frustrated and angered by any suggestion that their symptoms are psychologic. Therefore, doctors can't deal directly with the problem as a psychologic one, even when they recognize it. Drugs don't help much, and even if the person agrees to a psychiatric consultation, specific psychotherapy techniques aren't likely to be beneficial. Usually, the best treatment is a calm, firm, supportive relationship with a doctor who offers symptomatic relief and protects the person from very costly and possibly dangerous diagnostic or therapeutic procedures. However, the doctor must remain alert to the possibility that the person may develop a physical disease.

Conversion Disorder

In conversion disorder, physical symptoms that are caused by psychologic conflict resemble those of a neurologic disorder or other medical condition.

Symptoms of a conversion disorder are clearly caused by psychologic stress and conflict, which people unconsciously convert into physical symptoms. Although conversion disorders tend to occur during adolescence or early adulthood, they may first appear at any age. The condition is generally believed to be somewhat more common in women than in men.

Symptoms and Diagnosis

By definition, the symptoms of conversion disorder are limited to those that suggest a nervous system dysfunction—usually paralysis of an arm or leg or loss of sensation in a part of the body. Other symptoms include simulated convulsions and the loss of one of the special senses, such as vision or hearing.

Generally, the onset of symptoms is linked to some distressing social or psychologically stressful event. A person may have only a single episode or sporadic episodes, but usually the episodes are brief. If people with conversion symptoms are hospitalized, they generally improve within 2 weeks. However, 20 to 25 percent of the people have recurrences within a year.

The diagnosis tends to be difficult to make at first because the person believes that the symptoms stem from a physical problem and doesn't want to be seen by a psychiatrist. Doctors take great care to be certain no physical disorder is responsible for the symptoms.

Treatment

A trusting doctor-patient relationship is essential to treatment. As the doctor evaluates a possible physical disorder and reassures the person that the symptoms don't indicate a serious underlying disease, the person usually begins to feel better and the symptoms fade. When a psychologically distressing situation has preceded the onset of symptoms, psychotherapy can be particularly effective.

Occasionally, conversion symptoms recur frequently and even become chronic. Various treatment methods have been tried (and some may be helpful), although none has been uniformly effective. One method is hypnotherapy. The person is hypnotized, and psychologic issues that may be responsible for the symptoms are identified and discussed. Discussion continues after the hypnosis, when the person is fully alert. Other methods include narcoanalysis, a procedure similar to hypnosis except that the person is given a sedative to induce a state of semisleep. Behavior modification therapy, including relaxation training, has also been effective for some people.

Hypochondriasis

Hypochondriasis is a psychiatric disorder in which a person reports physical symptoms and is especially preoccupied with the certainty that these symptoms represent a serious disease.

Symptoms and Diagnosis

The person's concerns about having a serious disease are often based on a misinterpretation of normal bodily functions. For example, gurgling noises in the abdomen, and sometimes bloating and crampy discomfort, are normal as fluids move through the intestinal tract. People with hypochondriasis use such "symptoms" to explain their belief that they have a serious disease. Examination and reassurance by a doctor don't relieve their concerns; they tend to believe that the doctor has somehow failed to find the underlying disease.

Hypochondriasis is suspected when a healthy person with minor symptoms is preoccupied with the significance of those symptoms and doesn't respond to reassurance after careful evaluation. The diagnosis of hypochondriasis is confirmed when the situation persists for years and the person's symptoms can't be attributed to depression or another psychiatric disorder.

Treatment

The treatment is difficult because a person with hypochondriasis is convinced something inside the body is seriously wrong. Reassurance doesn't relieve these concerns. However, a trusting relationship with a caring doctor is beneficial, especially if regular visits with the doctor are followed by reassurance. If the person's symptoms aren't adequately relieved, the person may benefit from referral to a psychiatrist for further evaluation and treatment, along with continuation of the primary doctor's care.

CHAPTER 83

Anxiety Disorders

All people experience fear and anxiety. Fear is an emotional, physiologic, and behavioral response to a recognized external threat—for example, an intruder or a runaway car. Anxiety is an unpleasant emotional state that has a less clear source. Anxiety is often accompanied by physiologic and behavioral changes similar to those caused by fear. Because of these similarities, people often use the terms anxiety and fear interchangeably.

Anxiety is a response to stress, such as the breakup of an important relationship or exposure to a life-threatening disaster. One theory holds that anxiety may also be a reaction to a repressed sexual or aggressive impulse that's threatening to override the psychologic defenses that normally keep such drives in check. As such, anxiety indicates the presence of psychologic conflict.

Anxiety can arise suddenly, as in panic, or gradually over minutes, hours, or days. The anxiety itself can last for any length of time, from a few seconds to years. Anxiety ranges in intensity from barely noticeable qualms to full-blown panic.

Anxiety serves as one element in a wide range of flexible responses that are essential for people to survive in a dangerous world. A certain amount of anxiety introduces an appropriate element of caution in potentially dangerous situations. Most of the time, a person's level of anxiety makes appropriate and imperceptible shifts along a

spectrum of consciousness from sleep through alertness to anxiety and fear and back again. Sometimes, however, a person's anxiety response system operates improperly or is overwhelmed by events; in this case, an anxiety disorder can arise.

People react differently to situations. For example, some people find speaking before a group exhilarating, while others dread it. The ability to tolerate anxiety varies among people, and determining what constitutes abnormal anxiety can be difficult. However, when anxiety occurs at inappropriate times or is so intense and long-lasting that it interferes with a person's normal activities, then it is properly considered a disorder. Anxiety disorders can be so distressing and interfere so much with a person's life that they can lead to depression.▲ Some people have an anxiety disorder and depression at the same time. Others develop depression first and an anxiety disorder later.

Anxiety disorders are the most common type of psychiatric disorder. The diagnosis of an anxiety disorder is based largely on its symptoms. However, symptoms identical to those of an anxiety disorder can be caused by a medical condi-

▲ see page 403

How Anxiety Affects Performance

How anxiety affects performance can be shown on a curve. As the level of anxiety increases, performance efficiency increases proportionately, but only up to a point. As anxiety increases further, performance efficiency decreases. Before the peak of the curve, anxiety is adaptive, because it helps people prepare for a crisis and improve their functioning. Beyond the peak of the curve, anxiety is maladaptive and causes distress and dysfunction.

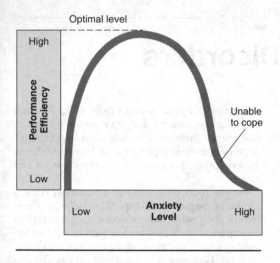

tion (for example, an overactive thyroid gland) or by the use of a prescribed or illicit drug (for example, corticosteroids or cocaine). A family history of an anxiety disorder may help the doctor make the diagnosis, since the predisposition to a specific anxiety disorder as well as a susceptibility to anxiety disorders in general often is hereditary.

Accurate diagnosis is important, since treatment varies from one disorder to another. Depending on the disorder, behavioral therapy, drugs, or psychotherapy, alone or in appropriate combinations, can significantly relieve the distress and dysfunction for most people.

▲ see page 447

■ see page 389

Generalized Anxiety Disorder

Generalized anxiety disorder consists of excessive, almost daily anxiety and worry (lasting 6 months or longer) about a variety of activities or events.

The anxiety and worry of generalized anxiety disorder are so extreme that they become difficult to control. In addition, the person experiences three or more of the following symptoms: restlessness, easy fatigue, difficulty concentrating, irritability, muscle tension, and disturbed sleep. Worries are general in nature; common worries include work responsibilities, money, health, safety, car repairs, and chores. The severity, frequency, or duration of the worries is disproportionately greater than the situation calls for.

Generalized anxiety disorder is common; about 3 to 5 percent of adults have it at some time during a given year. Women are twice as likely as men to have the disorder. It often begins in childhood or adolescence but may start at any age. For most people, the condition fluctuates, worsening at times (especially during times of stress), and persists over many years.

Treatment

Drugs are the primary treatment for generalized anxiety disorder. Antianxiety drugs such as benzodiazepines are usually prescribed; however, because long-term use of benzodiazepines can lead to physical dependence,▲ the drug must be tapered off slowly rather than stopped abruptly if discontinued. The relief that benzodiazepines bring usually outweighs any mild side effects.

Buspirone is another effective drug for many people with generalized anxiety disorder. Its use apparently doesn't lead to physical dependence. However, buspirone may take 2 weeks or longer to start working, in contrast to benzodiazepines, which begin to work within minutes.

Behavior therapy isn't usually beneficial because no clear-cut situations trigger the anxiety. Relaxation and biofeedback techniques may be of some help.

Generalized anxiety disorder may be associated with underlying psychologic conflicts. Such conflicts are frequently related to insecurities and self-critical attitudes that are self-defeating. For some people, psychotherapy may be effective in helping to understand and resolve internal psychologic conflicts.■

Antianxiety Drugs: Relief for Many Symptoms

Antianxiety drugs, also called anxiolytics, sedatives, and tranquilizers, target anxiety symptoms. Many relax muscles, reduce tension, help with sleeplessness, and thus provide temporary relief when anxiety limits a person's ability to cope with everyday life.

Different types of drugs are used to relieve anxiety, the most common of which are drugs called **benzodiazepines**. Benzodiazepines have general antianxiety effects; they promote mental and physical relaxation by reducing nerve activity in the brain. However, benzodiazepines can result in physical dependence, and they should be used cautiously by people who have or have had an alcohol dependency problem. Examples of benzodiazepines include alprazolam, chlordiazepoxide, diazepam, flurazepam, lorazepam, oxazepam, temazepam, and triazolam.

Before benzodiazepines were discovered, **barbiturates** were the drugs of choice for the treatment of anxiety. But the abuse potential of barbiturates is high, withdrawal problems are common, and barbiturates are more likely than benzodiazepines to be lethal if an overdose is accidentally or purposely taken. For these reasons, barbiturates are seldom prescribed for anxiety disorders.

An antianxiety drug called **buspirone** isn't chemically or pharmacologically related to the benzodiazepines or other antianxiety drugs.

It's not known how buspirone works, but it doesn't cause sedation or interact with alcohol. However, because its antianxiety effects may take 2 weeks or longer to become apparent, buspirone is useful only for people with generalized anxiety disorder rather than for those with intermittent, acute anxiety.

Antidepressant drugs are also sometimes prescribed for anxiety disorders. Different types of antidepressants can be used this way, including **selective serotonin reuptake inhibitors** (for example, fluoxetine, fluvoxamine, paroxetine, sertraline), **monoamine oxidase inhibitors** (for example, phenelzine, tranylcypromine), and **tricyclic antidepressants** (for example, amitriptyline, amoxapine, clomipramine, imipramine, nortriptyline, protriptyline). Antidepressants can help diminish core features of some disorders, for example, the obsessions and compulsions in obsessive-compulsive disorder or the panic in panic disorder. Although the antidepressants don't cause physical dependence, many have significant adverse effects. The selective serotonin reuptake inhibitors are particularly well tolerated.

Some antianxiety drugs can be taken once a day; others require several doses a day. Most people tolerate antianxiety drugs well. However, the choice of drug and its proper use require discussion between patient and doctor.

Anxiety Induced by Drugs or Medical Problems

Anxiety may result from a medical disorder or the use of a drug. Examples of medical disorders that may cause anxiety include neurologic disorders, such as a head injury, a brain infection, and inner ear disease; cardiovascular disorders, such as heart failure and arrhythmias; endocrine disorders, such as an overactive adrenal or thyroid gland; and respiratory disorders, such as asthma and chronic obstructive lung disease. Drugs that can induce anxiety include alcohol, stimulants, caffeine, cocaine, and many prescription drugs. Anxiety can also result when a drug is withdrawn.

Anxiety should subside after the medical condition is treated or the drug has been discontinued long enough for any withdrawal symptoms to abate. Any remaining anxiety can be treated with appropriate antianxiety drugs, behavior therapy, or psychotherapy.

Panic Attacks and Panic Disorder

Panic is acute and extreme anxiety with accompanying physiologic symptoms.

Panic *attacks* may occur in any anxiety disorder, usually in response to a specific situation tied to the main characteristic of the disorder. For example, a person with a phobia of snakes may panic when encountering a snake. However, these

Symptoms of a Panic Attack

A panic attack involves the sudden appearance of at least four of the following symptoms:

- Shortness of breath or sense of being smothered
- Dizziness, unsteadiness, or faintness
- Palpitations or accelerated heart rate
- Trembling or shaking
- Sweating
- Choking
- Nausea, stomachache, or diarrhea
- Feelings of unreality, strangeness, or detachment from the environment
- Numbness or tingling sensations
- Flushing or chills
- Chest pain or discomfort
- Fear of dying
- Fear of "going crazy" or losing control

situational panics differ from the spontaneous, unprovoked ones that define a person's problem as panic *disorder*.

Panic attacks are common, occurring in more than a third of adults each year. Women are two to three times more likely than men to have panic attacks. Panic disorder is uncommon and is diagnosed in slightly less than 1 percent of the population. Panic disorder usually begins in late adolescence and early adulthood.

Symptoms and Diagnosis

The symptoms of a panic attack—among others, shortness of breath, dizziness, increased heart rate, sweating, choking, and chest pain—peak within 10 minutes and usually dissipate within minutes, leaving little for a doctor to observe except the person's fear of another terrify-

▲ see page 399

■ see page 447

ing attack. Since panic attacks are often unexpected or occur for no apparent reason, people who have them frequently anticipate and worry about another attack—a condition called anticipatory anxiety—and avoid places where they have previously panicked. This avoidance of places is called agoraphobia.▲ If agoraphobia is severe enough, a person may become housebound.

Because symptoms of a panic attack involve many vital organs, people often worry that they have a dangerous medical problem involving the heart, lungs, or brain and seek help from a doctor or hospital emergency department. Although panic attacks are uncomfortable—at times extremely so—they aren't dangerous.

Treatment

Most people recover from panic attacks without treatment; a few develop panic disorder. Recovery without treatment is possible even for those who have recurring panic attacks or anticipatory anxiety, particularly if they are repeatedly exposed to the provocative stimulus or situation. People who don't recover on their own or who don't seek treatment continue to have panic attacks off and on indefinitely.

People respond better to treatment when they understand that panic disorder involves both biologic and psychologic processes. Drugs and behavioral therapy can generally control the symptoms. In addition, psychotherapy may help resolve any psychologic conflicts that might underlie the anxious feelings and behavior.

Drugs that are used to treat panic disorder include antidepressants and antianxiety drugs such as benzodiazepines. All types of antidepressants—tricyclics (such as imipramine), monoamine oxidase inhibitors (such as phenelzine), and selective serotonin reuptake inhibitors (SSRIs, such as fluoxetine)—have proved effective. Benzodiazepines work faster than antidepressants but can cause physical dependence■ and are probably more likely to cause certain adverse effects, such as sleepiness, impaired coordination, and slowed reaction time. SSRIs are preferred because they are effective and they have fewer side effects and cause less physical dependency than benzodiazepines.

When a drug is effective, it prevents or greatly reduces the number of panic attacks. A drug may have to be taken for long periods of time if panic attacks return once the drug is stopped.

Exposure therapy, a type of behavior therapy in which the person is exposed repeatedly to whatever triggers a panic attack, often helps to diminish the fear. Exposure therapy is practiced until the person develops a high level of comfort with the anxiety-provoking situation. In addition, people who are afraid they will faint during a panic attack can practice an exercise in which they spin in a chair or breathe quickly (hyperventilate) until they feel faint. This exercise teaches them that they won't actually faint during a panic attack. Practicing slow, shallow breathing (respiratory control) helps many people who tend to hyperventilate.

Psychotherapy with a view to gaining insight and better understanding of any underlying psychologic conflicts may also be useful. A psychiatrist assesses the person to determine whether this type of treatment is appropriate. Less intensive, supportive psychotherapy is always appropriate because a therapist can provide general information about the disorder, its treatment, realistic hope for improvement, and the support that comes from a trusting relationship with a doctor.

Phobic Disorders

Phobias involve persistent, unrealistic, intense anxiety in response to specific external situations, such as looking down from heights or coming near a small dog.

People who have a phobia avoid situations that trigger their anxiety, or they endure them with great distress. However, they recognize that their anxiety is excessive and therefore are aware that they have a problem.

AGORAPHOBIA

Although agoraphobia literally means fear of the marketplace or open spaces, the term more specifically describes the fear of being trapped without a graceful and easy way to leave if anxiety should strike. Typical situations that are difficult for people with agoraphobia include standing in line at a bank or supermarket, sitting in the middle of a long row in a theater or classroom, and riding on a bus or airplane. Some people develop agoraphobia after experiencing a panic attack in one of these situations. Other people simply feel uncomfortable in these settings and may never, or only later, develop panic attacks. Agoraphobia

often interferes with daily living, sometimes so drastically that it leaves the person housebound.

Agoraphobia is diagnosed in 3.8 percent of women and 1.8 percent of men during any 6-month period. The disorder most often begins in the early 20s; a first appearance after age 40 is unusual.

Treatment

The best treatment for agoraphobia is exposure therapy, a type of behavior therapy. With the help of a therapist, the person seeks out, confronts, and remains in contact with what he fears until his anxiety is slowly relieved by familiarity with the situation (a process called habituation). Exposure therapy helps more than 90 percent of the people who practice it faithfully.

If agoraphobia isn't treated, it usually waxes and wanes in severity and may even disappear without formal treatment, possibly because the person has conducted some personal form of behavior therapy.

People with agoraphobia who are deeply depressed may need to take an antidepressant. Substances that depress the central nervous system, such as alcohol or large doses of antianxiety drugs, may interfere with behavior therapy and are tapered off gradually before therapy is begun.

As with panic disorder, the anxiety in some people who have agoraphobia may have its roots in underlying psychologic conflicts. In such cases, psychotherapy (in which the person develops a better understanding of the underlying conflicts) may be helpful.

SPECIFIC PHOBIAS

Specific phobias are the most common of the anxiety disorders. About 7 percent of women and 4.3 percent of men have a specific phobia during any 6-month period.

Some specific phobias, such as the fear of large animals, the dark, or strangers, begin early in life. Many phobias stop as the person gets older. Other phobias, such as fear of rodents, insects, storms, water, heights, flying, or enclosed places, typically develop later in life. At least 5 percent of people are to some degree phobic about blood, injections, or injury, and these people can actually faint, which does not happen with other phobias and anxiety disorders. In contrast, many people with anxiety disorders hyperventilate, which can cause feelings of faintness, but they virtually never faint.

Treatment

A person can often cope with a specific phobia by avoiding the feared object or situation. For example, a city dweller who is afraid of snakes may have no trouble avoiding them. However, the city dweller who fears small, closed places such as elevators will have a problem working on an upper floor in a skyscraper.

Exposure therapy, a type of behavior therapy in which the person is gradually exposed to the feared object or situation, is the best treatment for a specific phobia. A therapist can help ensure that the therapy is carried out properly, although it can be done without a therapist. Even people with a phobia of blood or needles respond well to exposure therapy. For example, a person who faints while blood is drawn can have a needle brought close to a vein and then removed when the heart rate begins to slow down. Repeating this process allows the heart rate to return to normal. Eventually, the person can have blood drawn without fainting.

Drugs aren't very useful in helping people overcome specific phobias. However, benzodiazepines (antianxiety drugs) may give a person short-term control over a phobia, such as the fear of flying.

Psychotherapy, with a view toward gaining insight and understanding of internal conflicts,▲ may be helpful in identifying and treating the conflicts that may underlie a specific phobia.

SOCIAL PHOBIA

A person's ability to relate comfortably with others affects many aspects of life, including early family relationships, education, work, leisure, dating, and mating. Although some anxiety in social situations is normal, people with social phobia have so much anxiety that they either avoid social situations or endure them with great distress. Recent research shows that about 13 percent of people have a social phobia sometime in their lives.

Situations that commonly trigger anxiety among people with social phobia include public speaking; performing publicly, such as acting in a play or playing a musical instrument; eating in front of others; signing a document before wit-

nesses; and using a public bathroom. People with social phobia are concerned that their performance or actions will seem inappropriate. Often they worry that their anxiety will be obvious—that they'll sweat, blush, vomit, or tremble or that their voice will quiver; they'll lose their train of thought; or they won't be able to find the words to express themselves.

A more general type of social phobia is characterized by anxiety in almost all social situations. People with a general social phobia are usually concerned that if their performance falls short of expectations, they will feel humiliated and embarrassed.

Some people are shy by nature and show timidness early in life that later develops into social phobia. Others first experience anxiety in social situations at puberty. Social phobia often persists if left untreated, causing many people to avoid activities in which they would otherwise like to participate.

Treatment

Exposure therapy, a type of behavior therapy, works well for social phobia, but arranging for exposure to last long enough to permit habituation and comfort may not be easy. For example, a person who is afraid of speaking in front of his boss may not be able to arrange a series of speaking sessions in front of that boss. Substitute situations may help, such as joining Toastmasters (an organization for those who have anxiety about speaking in front of an audience) or reading a book to nursing home residents. Substitute sessions may or may not reduce anxiety during conversations with the boss.

Antidepressants, such as sertraline and phenelzine, and antianxiety drugs, such as clonazepam, can often help people with social phobia. Many people use alcohol as a social lubricant; in some cases, however, alcohol abuse and dependence can result.

Psychotherapy, which involves talking with a therapist to better understand underlying conflicts,■ may be particularly helpful for people who are capable of examining their own behavior and making changes in the way they think about and react to situations.

Obsessive-Compulsive Disorder

Obsessive-compulsive disorder is characterized by the presence of recurrent, unwanted, intrusive

---

▲ see page 389

■ see page 389

ideas, images, or impulses that seem silly, weird, nasty, or horrible (obsessions) and an urge or compulsion to do something that will relieve the discomfort caused by an obsession.

The pervading obsessional theme is harm, risk, or danger. Common obsessions include concerns about contamination, doubt, loss, and aggressiveness. Typically, people with obsessive-compulsive disorder feel compelled to perform rituals—repetitive, purposeful, intentional acts. Rituals used to control an obsession include washing or cleaning to be rid of contamination, checking to allay doubt, hoarding to prevent loss, and avoiding the people who might become objects of aggression. Most rituals, such as excessive hand washing or repeated checking to make sure a door has been locked, can be observed. Other rituals are mental, such as repetitive counting or making statements intended to diminish danger. Obsessive-compulsive disorder is different from obsessive-compulsive personality disorder.▲

People can become obsessional about anything, and their rituals aren't always logically connected to the discomfort that these rituals relieve. For example, a person who has been worried about contamination may have felt his discomfort decrease once when he happened to put his hand in his pocket. Since then, any time obsessions about contamination arise, he repeatedly puts his hand in his pocket.

Most people with obsessive-compulsive disorder are aware that their obsessions don't reflect actual risks. They realize that their physical and mental behavior is excessive to the point of being bizarre. Obsessive-compulsive disorder thus differs from psychotic disorders, in which people lose contact with reality.

Obsessive-compulsive disorder affects about 2.3 percent of adults and occurs about equally in men and women. Because people with this disorder are afraid they'll be embarrassed or stigmatized, they often perform their rituals secretly, even though the rituals may occupy several hours each day. About one third of the people with obsessive-compulsive disorder are depressed at the time the disorder is diagnosed. Altogether, two thirds become depressed at some point.

Treatment

Exposure therapy, a type of behavior therapy, often helps people with obsessive-compulsive disorder. In this type of therapy, the person is exposed to the situations or people that trigger obsessions, rituals, or discomfort. The person's discomfort or anxiety will gradually diminish if he prevents himself from performing the ritual during repeated exposure to the provocative stimulus. In this way, the person learns that the ritual isn't needed to decrease discomfort. The improvement usually persists for years, probably because those who have mastered this self-help approach continue to practice it as a way of life without much effort after formal treatment has ended.

Drugs can also help many people with obsessive-compulsive disorder. Three drugs (clomipramine, fluoxetine, and fluvoxamine) have been specifically approved for this use, and two others (paroxetine and sertraline) have also been demonstrated to be effective. Certain other antidepressant drugs are also used, but much less often.

Psychotherapy, with a view toward gaining insight and understanding of underlying conflicts,■ has generally not been effective for people with obsessive-compulsive disorder. Ordinarily, a combination of drugs and behavior therapy is the best treatment.

Posttraumatic Stress Disorder

Posttraumatic stress disorder is an anxiety disorder caused by exposure to an overwhelming, traumatic event, in which the person later repeatedly reexperiences the event.

Experiences that threaten death or serious injury can affect people long after the experience is over. Intense fear, helplessness, or horror can haunt a person. The traumatic situation is repeatedly reexperienced, usually in nightmares or flashbacks. The person persistently avoids things that are reminders of the trauma. Sometimes symptoms don't begin until many months or even years after the traumatic event took place. The person has a numbing of general responsiveness and symptoms of increased arousal (such as difficulty falling asleep or being easily startled). Symptoms of depression are common.

Posttraumatic stress disorder affects at least 1 percent of people sometime during their life. People at high risk, such as combat veterans and victims of rape or other violent acts, have a higher

▲ see page 428

■ see page 389

incidence. Chronic posttraumatic stress disorder doesn't disappear but often becomes less intense over time even without treatment. Nevertheless, some people remain severely handicapped by the disorder indefinitely.

Treatment

Treatment of posttraumatic stress disorder involves behavior therapy, drugs, and psychotherapy. In behavior therapy, the person is exposed to situations that may trigger memories of the painful experience. After some initial increase in discomfort, behavior therapy usually lessens a person's distress. Refraining from rituals, such as excessive washing to feel clean after a sexual assault, is also helpful.

Antidepressant and antianxiety drugs appear to provide some benefit. Because of the often intense anxiety associated with traumatic memories, supportive psychotherapy plays an especially important role. The therapist is openly empathic and sympathetic in recognizing the person's psychologic pain. The therapist reassures the person that his response is valid but encourages him to face his memories during behavioral desensitization therapy. The patient also is taught ways to control anxiety, which helps to modulate and integrate the painful memories into his personality.

People with posttraumatic stress disorder often feel guilty. For example, they may have behaved in ways that they believe were unacceptably aggressive and destructive during combat, or they may have survived a traumatic experience in which family members or friends died and experience survivor guilt. If so, insight-oriented psychotherapy can help people understand why they are punishing themselves and help rid them of guilt feelings. This psychotherapeutic technique may be needed to help the person retrieve key traumatic memories that had been repressed, so that the memories can be dealt with constructively.

Acute Stress Disorder

Acute stress disorder is similar to posttraumatic stress disorder, except that it begins within 4 weeks of the traumatic event and lasts only 2 to 4 weeks.

A person with acute stress disorder has been exposed to a terrifying event. The person mentally reexperiences the traumatic event, avoids things that remind him of it, and has increased anxiety. The person also has three or more of the following symptoms:
• A sense of numbing, detachment, or lack of emotional responsiveness
• Reduced awareness of surroundings (for example, being dazed)
• A feeling that things aren't real
• A feeling that he himself isn't real
• Inability to remember an important part of the traumatic event

Treatment

Many people recover from acute stress disorder once they are removed from the traumatic situation and given appropriate support in the form of understanding, empathy for their distress, and an opportunity to describe what happened and their reaction to it. Many people benefit from describing their experience several times. Sleep aids may be helpful, but other drugs can interfere with the natural healing process.

CHAPTER 84

Depression and Mania

Depression and mania represent the two major poles of mood disorders. Mood disorders are psychiatric illnesses in which emotional disturbances consist of prolonged periods of excessive depression or elation (mania). Mood disorders are also called affective disorders. *Affect* (emphasis on the first syllable) means *emotional state* as revealed through facial expressions and gestures.

Sadness and joy are part of the normal experience of everyday life and are different from the severe depression and mania that characterize mood disorders. Sadness is a natural response to loss, defeat, disappointment, trauma, or catastrophe. Sadness may be psychologically beneficial because it permits a person to withdraw from offensive or unpleasant situations, which may aid recovery.

Grief or bereavement is the most common of the normal reactions to a loss or separation, such as the death of a loved one, divorce, or romantic disappointment. Bereavement and loss don't generally cause persistent, incapacitating depression except in people predisposed to mood disorders.

Success and achievement normally incite feelings of elation. However, elation can sometimes be a defense against depression or a denial of the pain of loss. People who are dying sometimes have brief periods of elation and restless activity, and some recently bereaved people may even become elated rather than grieve normally. In people predisposed to mood disorders, these reactions may be the prelude to mania.

Although 25 to 30 percent of all people will experience some form of excessive mood disturbance during their life, only about 10 percent will have a disorder severe enough to require medical attention. Of these, a third have long-lasting (chronic) depression, and most of the remainder have recurring episodes of depression. Chronic and recurring depressions are termed **unipolar.** Nearly 2 percent of the population have a condition called **manic-depressive illness** or **bipolar disorder,** in which periods of depression alternate with periods of mania (or with periods of less severe mania known as hypomania).

Depression

Depression is a feeling of intense sadness; it may follow a recent loss or other sad event but is out of proportion to that event and persists beyond an appropriate length of time.

After anxiety, depression is the most common psychiatric disorder. An estimated 10 percent of the people who see their doctors for what they think is a physical problem are actually experiencing depression. Depression typically begins in the 20s, 30s, or 40s. People born in the latter part of the 20th century seem to have higher rates of depression than those of previous generations, in part because of higher rates of substance abuse.

An episode of depression typically lasts for 6 to 9 months, but in 15 to 20 percent of the people, it lasts for 2 years or more. Episodes generally tend to recur several times over a lifetime.

Causes

The causes of depression aren't fully understood. A number of factors may make a person more likely to experience depression, such as a family tendency (heredity), side effects of certain medications, an introverted personality, and emotionally upsetting events, particularly those involving a loss. Depression may also arise or worsen without any apparent or significant life stress.

Women are twice as likely as men to experience depression, though the reasons aren't entirely clear. Psychologic studies show that women tend to respond to adversity by withdrawing into themselves and blaming themselves. In contrast, men tend to deny adversity and throw themselves into activities. Of biologic factors, hormones are the ones most involved. Changes in hormone levels, which can create mood changes shortly before menstruation (premenstrual tension) and after childbirth (postpartum depression), might play some role in women. Similar hormonal changes may occur with the use of oral contraceptives in women who have experienced depression. Abnormal thyroid function, which is fairly common in women, may also be a factor.

Depression that follows a traumatic event, such as the death of a loved one, is called **situational depression.** Some people become temporarily depressed in reaction to certain holidays (holiday blues) or meaningful anniversaries, such as the anniversary of a loved one's death. Depression without an apparent precipitating event is called **endogenous depression.** These distinctions, however, aren't very important, since the effects and treatment of the depression are similar.

Depression may also occur with, or be caused by, a number of physical diseases or disorders. Physical disorders may cause a depression directly (such as when thyroid disease affects hormone levels, which can induce depression) or indirectly (such as when rheumatoid arthritis causes pain and disability, which can lead to depression). Often, depression that results from a physical disorder has both direct and indirect causes. For example, AIDS may cause depression directly if the human immunodeficiency virus (HIV), which causes AIDS, damages the brain; AIDS may cause depression indirectly by having an overall negative impact on the person's life.

Physical Disorders That Can Cause Depression

Side effects of drugs

Amphetamines (withdrawal from)

Antipsychotic drugs

Beta-blockers

Cimetidine

Contraceptives (oral)

Cycloserine

Indomethacin

Mercury

Methyldopa

Reserpine

Thallium

Vinblastine

Vincristine

Infections

AIDS

Influenza

Mononucleosis

Syphilis (late stage)

Tuberculosis

Viral hepatitis

Viral pneumonia

Hormonal disorders

Addison's disease

Cushing's disease

High levels of parathyroid hormone

Low and high levels of thyroid hormone

Low levels of pituitary hormones (hypopituitarism)

Connective tissue diseases

Rheumatoid arthritis

Systemic lupus erythematosus

Neurologic disorders

Brain tumors

Head injury

Multiple sclerosis

Parkinson's disease

Sleep apnea

Stroke

Temporal lobe epilepsy

Nutritional disorders

Pellagra (vitamin B_6 deficiency)

Pernicious anemia (vitamin B_{12} deficiency)

Cancers

Abdominal cancers (ovary, colon)

Cancer spreading in the entire body

Various prescription drugs, most notably drugs used to treat high blood pressure, can cause depression. For unknown reasons, corticosteroids often cause depression when they are produced in large amounts as part of a disease, as in Cushing's syndrome, but they tend to cause elation when they are given as medication.

A number of psychiatric conditions can predispose a person to depression, including certain anxiety disorders, alcoholism and other substance abuse disorders, schizophrenia, and the early phase of dementia.

Symptoms

Symptoms typically develop gradually over days or weeks. A person entering a depression may appear slow and sad or irritable and anxious. A person who tends to withdraw, speak little, stop eating, and sleep little is experiencing what is called a **vegetative depression.** A person who, in addition, is very restless—wringing the hands and talking continuously—is experiencing what is called an **agitated depression.**

Many people with depression can't experience emotions—including grief, joy, and pleasure—normally; in the extreme, the world appears to have become colorless, lifeless, and dead. Thinking, speech, and general activity may slow down so much that all voluntary activities stop. Depressed people may be preoccupied with intense feelings of guilt and self-denigrating ideas and may not be able to concentrate well. They are often indecisive and withdrawn, feel progressively helpless and hopeless, and think about death and suicide.

Most depressed people have difficulty falling asleep and awaken repeatedly, particularly early in the morning. A loss of sexual desire or pleasure in general is common. Poor appetite and weight loss sometimes lead to emaciation, and in women menstrual periods may stop. However, overeating and weight gain are common in milder depressions.

In about 20 percent of depressed people, the symptoms are milder but the illness lasts years, often decades. This **dysthymic variant** of depression often begins early in life and is associated with distinct changes in personality. People with this condition are gloomy, pessimistic, humorless, or incapable of having fun; passive and lethargic; introverted; skeptical, hypercritical, or constantly complaining; and self-critical and full of self-reproach. They are preoccupied with inadequacy, failure, and negative events, sometimes to the point of morbid enjoyment of their own failures.

Some depressed people complain of having a physical illness, with various aches and pains or fears of calamity or of becoming insane. Others think they have illnesses they believe to be incurable or shameful, such as cancer or sexually transmitted diseases, and that they are infecting other people.

About 15 percent of depressed people, most commonly those with severe depression, have delusions (false beliefs) or hallucinations, seeing or hearing things that aren't there. They may believe that they have committed unpardonable sins or crimes or may hear voices accusing them of various misdeeds or condemning them to death. In rare cases, they may imagine that they see coffins or deceased relatives. Feelings of insecurity and worthlessness may lead severely depressed people to believe that they are being watched and persecuted. These depressions with delusions are termed **psychotic depressions.**

Thoughts of death are among the most serious symptoms of depression. Many depressed people want to die or feel they are so worthless that they should die. As many as 15 percent of people with severe depression exhibit suicidal behavior. A suicide plan represents an emergency situation, and someone with such a plan should be hospitalized and kept under supervision until treatment reduces the risk of suicide.▲

Diagnosis

A doctor is usually able to diagnose depression from its signs and symptoms. A previous history of depression or a family history of depression helps to confirm the diagnosis.

Sometimes standardized questionnaires are used to help measure the degree of depression. Two such questionnaires are the Hamilton Depression Rating Scale, conducted verbally by an interviewer, and the Beck Depression Inventory, a self-administered questionnaire.

Laboratory tests, usually blood tests, may help a doctor determine the cause of some depressions. This is particularly useful for women, in whom hormonal factors could contribute to depression.

In cases that are difficult to diagnose, doctors may perform other tests to confirm the diagnosis of depression. For example, because sleep problems are such a prominent sign of depression, doctors who specialize in diagnosing and treating mood disorders may use a sleep electroencephalogram to measure the time it takes for rapid eye movement sleep (the period during which dreaming occurs) to begin after the person falls asleep.■ Normally, it takes about 90 minutes. In a person with depression, it usually takes less than 70 minutes.

▲ see page 411

■ see page 301

Prognosis and Treatment

An untreated depression may last 6 months or longer. Although mild symptoms persist in many people, functioning tends to return to normal. Nonetheless, most people with depression experience repeated episodes of depression, an average of four to five times over a lifetime.

Depression today is usually treated without hospitalization. However, sometimes a person should be hospitalized, especially if he is seriously contemplating suicide or has attempted it, is too frail because of weight loss, or is at risk for heart problems because of severe agitation.

Medications are the cornerstone of treatment for depression today. Other treatments include psychotherapy and electroconvulsive therapy. Sometimes a combination of these different therapies is used.

Drug Treatment

Several types of drugs—tricyclic antidepressants, selective serotonin reuptake inhibitors, monoamine oxidase inhibitors, and psychostimulants—are available, but they must be taken regularly for at least several weeks before they begin to work. The chances that any given antidepressant will work for a particular person are about 65 percent.

The adverse effects vary with each type of drug. The **tricyclic antidepressants** often cause sedation and lead to weight gain. They can also be associated with an increased heart rate, a decrease in blood pressure when the person stands, blurred vision, dry mouth, confusion, constipation, difficulty in starting to urinate, and delayed orgasm. These effects are called anticholinergic effects and are often more pronounced in the elderly.▲

Antidepressants that are similar to the tricyclic antidepressants have other adverse effects. Venlafaxine may slightly raise the blood pressure. Trazodone has been associated with painful erection (priapism). Maprotiline and bupropion taken in quickly escalating doses can induce seizures. However, bupropion doesn't cause sedation, doesn't affect sexual function, and is often useful in patients with depression and slowed thinking.

The **selective serotonin reuptake inhibitors (SSRIs)** represent a major improvement in the treatment of depression in that they tend to cause fewer adverse effects than the tricyclic antidepressants. Also they are generally quite safe in people who have depression and a coexisting physical disorder. Although they can cause nausea, diarrhea, and headache, these adverse effects are either mild or go away with continued use. For these reasons, doctors often select SSRIs first when treating depression. SSRIs are particularly useful in the treatment of dysthymia, which requires long-term drug therapy. Moreover, SSRIs are quite effective in obsessive-compulsive disorder, panic disorder, social phobia, and bulimia (an eating disorder), which often coexist with depression. The main disadvantage of SSRIs is that they commonly cause sexual dysfunction.

Monoamine oxidase inhibitors (MAOIs) represent another class of antidepressant drug. However, people who use MAOIs must adhere to a number of dietary restrictions and follow special precautions. For example, they should not eat foods or beverages that contain tyramine, such as beer on tap, red wines (including sherry), liqueurs, overripe foods, salami, aged cheeses, fava or broad beans, yeast extracts (marmite), and soy sauce. They must avoid drugs such as phenylpropanolamine and dextromethorphan, found in many over-the-counter cough and cold remedies, which cause the release of adrenaline and can cause a sudden and severe rise in blood pressure. Certain other drugs should also be avoided by people who take MAOIs, such as tricyclic antidepressants, selective serotonin reuptake inhibitors, and meperidine (a painkiller).

People taking MAOIs usually are instructed to carry an antidote, such as chlorpromazine or nifedipine, at all times. If a severe, throbbing headache occurs, they should take the antidote at once and go to the nearest emergency room. Because of the difficult dietary restrictions and necessary precautions, MAOIs are rarely prescribed except for depressed people who haven't improved with other antidepressants.

Psychostimulants, such as methylphenidate, are generally reserved for depressed people who are withdrawn, slowed, and fatigued or who haven't improved after using all other classes of antide-

---

▲ see box, page 41

pressants. Their abuse potential is high. Because psychostimulants tend to work quickly (within a day) and facilitate ambulation, they are sometimes prescribed for elderly depressed people who are convalescing from surgery or a protracted illness.

Psychotherapy

Psychotherapy used with antidepressants can greatly enhance the results of medication.▲ Individual or group psychotherapy can help the person gradually resume former responsibilities and adapt to the normal pressures of life, building on the improvement made by drug treatment. With interpersonal psychotherapy, the person receives supportive guidance for adjusting to changes in life roles. Cognitive therapy can help change a person's hopeless and negative thinking. Psychotherapy alone may be just as effective as drug therapy for milder depressions.

Electroconvulsive Therapy

Electroconvulsive therapy (ECT) is used to treat severe depression, particularly when the person is psychotic, is threatening to commit suicide, or is refusing to eat. This type of therapy is usually very effective and can relieve depression quickly, unlike most antidepressants, which can take up to several weeks. The speed with which electroconvulsive therapy takes effect can save lives.

With electroconvulsive therapy, electrodes are placed on the head and an electric current is applied to induce a seizure in the brain. For reasons that aren't understood, the seizure alleviates depression. Usually five to seven treatments, one treatment every other day, are given. Because the electric current can cause muscle contractions and pain, the person receives general anesthesia during treatments. Electroconvulsive therapy may cause some temporary (rarely permanent) loss of memory.

Mania

Mania is characterized by excessive physical activity and feelings of extreme elation that are grossly out of proportion to any positive event. Hypomania is a milder form of mania.

Types of Antidepressants

Tricyclic and similar antidepressants
Amitriptyline

Amoxapine

Bupropion

Clomipramine

Desipramine

Doxepin

Imipramine

Maprotiline

Nefazodone

Nortriptyline

Protriptyline

Trazodone

Trimipramine

Venlafaxine

Selective serotonin reuptake inhibitors
Fluoxetine

Fluvoxamine

Paroxetine

Sertraline

Monoamine oxidase inhibitors
Isocarboxazid

Pargyline

Phenelzine

Tranylcypromine

Psychostimulants
Dextroamphetamine

Methylphenidate

▲ see page 389

Physical Disorders That Can Cause Mania

Side effects of drugs

Amphetamines

Antidepressants (most)

Bromocriptine

Cocaine

Corticosteroids

Levodopa

Methylphenidate

Infections

AIDS

Encephalitis

Influenza

Syphilis (late stage)

Hormonal disorders

High levels of thyroid hormone

Connective tissue disease

Systemic lupus erythematosus

Neurologic disorders

Brain tumors

Head injury

Huntington's chorea

Multiple sclerosis

Stroke

Sydenham's chorea

Temporal lobe epilepsy

Although a person can have depression without manic episodes (unipolar disorder), mania most commonly occurs as a part of manic-depressive illness (bipolar disorder).▲ The few people who appear to experience only mania may

▲ see page 409

actually have mild or brief depressive episodes. Mania and hypomania are less common than depression, and they are also less easily recognized—while extreme and protracted sadness may prompt a visit to a doctor, elation much less commonly does (because people with mania are unaware that anything is wrong with their mental state or behavior). A doctor must rule out an underlying physical disease in a person who is experiencing mania for the first time, without a previous depressive episode.

Symptoms and Diagnosis

Manic symptoms typically develop rapidly over a few days. In the early (milder) stages of mania, the person feels better than normal and often appears brighter, younger, and more energetic.

A person who is manic is generally elated but may also be irritable, cantankerous, or frankly hostile. He typically believes he is quite well. A lack of insight into his condition, along with a huge capacity for activity, can make the person impatient, intrusive, meddlesome, and aggressively irritable when crossed. Mental activity speeds up (a condition called flight of ideas). The person is easily distracted and constantly shifts from one theme or endeavor to another. The person may have false convictions of personal wealth, power, inventiveness, and genius and may temporarily assume a grandiose identity, sometimes believing that he is God.

The person may believe he is being assisted or persecuted by others or have hallucinations, hearing and seeing things that aren't there. The need for sleep decreases. A manic person is inexhaustibly, excessively, and impulsively involved in various activities (such as risky business endeavors, gambling, or perilous sexual behavior) without recognizing the inherent social dangers. In extreme cases, mental and physical activity is so frenzied that any clear link between mood and behavior is lost in a kind of senseless agitation (delirious mania). Immediate treatment is then required, because the person may die of sheer physical exhaustion. In less severely overactive mania, hospitalization may be needed to protect the person and his family from ruinous financial or sexual behavior.

Mania is diagnosed by its symptoms, which are typically obvious to the observer. However, because people with mania are notorious for denying that there is anything wrong with them,

Symptoms of Mania

Mood

- Elation, irritability, or hostility
- Momentary tearfulness

Other psychologic symptoms

- Inflated self-esteem, boasting, grandiose behavior
- Racing thoughts, new thoughts triggered by word sounds rather than meaning, tendency to be distracted easily
- Heightened interest in new activities, increased involvement with people (who are often alienated because of the person's intrusive and meddlesome behavior), buying sprees, sexual indiscretions, foolish business investments

Psychotic symptoms

- Delusions of exceptional talent
- Delusions of exceptional physical fitness
- Delusions of wealth, aristocratic ancestry, or other grandiose identity
- Having visions or hearing voices (hallucinations)
- Paranoia

Physical symptoms

- Increased activity level
- Possible weight loss from increased activity and inattention to diet
- Decreased need for sleep
- Increased sexual desire

---

doctors usually have to obtain information from family members. Questionnaires aren't used as widely as in depression.

Treatment

Untreated episodes of mania end more abruptly than those of depression and are typically shorter, lasting from a few weeks to several months. Because mania is a medical and social emergency, a doctor makes all attempts to treat the patient in a hospital.

A drug called lithium can reduce the symptoms of mania. Because lithium takes 4 to 10 days to work, a drug that works rapidly, such as haloperidol, is often given at the same time to control excited thought and activity. However, haloperidol can cause muscle stiffness and unusual movements. Therefore, haloperidol is given in small doses, in combination with a benzodiazepine, such as lorazepam or clonazepam, which enhances haloperidol's antimanic effects while reducing its unpleasant side effects.

Manic-Depressive Illness

Manic-depressive illness, also called bipolar disorder, is a condition in which periods of depression alternate with periods of mania or lesser degrees of excitement.

Manic-depressive illness affects slightly less than 2 percent of the population to some degree. The illness is believed to be hereditary, although the exact genetic defect is still unknown. Manic-depressive illness is equally common in men and women and typically begins in the teens, 20s, or 30s.

Symptoms and Diagnosis

Manic-depressive illness usually begins with depression and includes at least one period of mania at some time during the illness. Episodes of depression typically last 3 to 6 months. In the most severe form of the illness, called **bipolar I disorder,** depression alternates with intense mania. In the less severe form, called **bipolar II disorder,** short depressive episodes alternate with hypomania. Symptoms of bipolar II disorder often recur in certain seasons, for example, depression occurs in the fall and winter, and brief excitement occurs in the spring or summer.

In an even milder form of manic-depressive illness, called **cyclothymic disorder,** periods of elation and depression are less severe, typically last for only a few days, and recur fairly often at irregular intervals. Although cyclothymic disorder may ultimately evolve into manic-depressive illness, in many people cyclothymic disorder never leads to major depression or mania. Having a cyclothymic disorder may contribute to a person's success in business, leadership, achievement, and artistic creativity. However, it may also cause uneven work and school records, frequent change of residence, repeated romantic breakups or marital failure, and alcohol and drug abuse. In about a third of people with cyclothymic disorder, these symptoms can lead to a mood disorder that requires treatment.

The diagnosis of manic-depressive illness is based on the distinctive pattern of symptoms. A doctor determines whether the person is experiencing a manic or depressive episode so that the correct treatment can be given. About one in three people with bipolar disorder experience manic (or hypomanic) and depressive symptoms *simultaneously*. This condition is known as a **mixed bipolar state.**

Prognosis and Treatment

Manic-depressive illness recurs in nearly all cases. Episodes may sometimes switch from depression to mania, or vice versa, without any period of normal mood in between. Some people cycle more rapidly through episodes than others. Up to 15 percent of the people with manic-depressive illness, mostly women, have four or more episodes a year. People who cycle rapidly are more difficult to treat.

Manic or hypomanic episodes in manic-depressive illness can be treated like acute mania. Depressive episodes are treated like depression. However, most antidepressants can cause swings from depression to hypomania or mania and sometimes cause rapid cycling between them. Therefore, these drugs are used for only short periods, and their effect on mood is closely monitored. At the first sign of a swing to hypomania or mania, the antidepressant is stopped. Antidepressants least likely to cause mood switching are bupropion and the monoamine oxidase inhibitors. Optimally, most people with manic-depressive disorder should be given mood-stabilizing drugs, such as lithium or an anticonvulsant.

Lithium has no effect on normal mood but reduces the tendency toward mood swings in about 70 percent of the people with manic-depressive illness. A doctor monitors the level of lithium in the blood with blood tests. Possible adverse effects of lithium include tremor, muscle twitching, nausea, vomiting, diarrhea, thirst, excessive urination, and weight gain. Lithium can make acne or psoriasis worse, can cause the blood levels of thyroid hormone to fall, and rarely can cause excessive urination. A very high level of lithium in the blood can cause a persistent headache, mental confusion, drowsiness, seizures, and abnormal heart rhythms. Adverse effects are more likely to occur in the elderly. Women who are trying to become pregnant must stop taking lithium, because lithium can (rarely) cause heart defects in a developing fetus.

Newer drug treatments have evolved over the past several years. These include the anticonvulsants **carbamazepine** and **divalproex.** However, carbamazepine can seriously reduce the number of red and white blood cells, and divalproex can cause liver damage (primarily in children). With careful monitoring by a doctor, these problems are rare, and carbamazepine and divalproex are useful alternatives to lithium, especially for people with the mixed or rapid cycling form of manic-depressive illness who haven't responded to other treatments.

Psychotherapy is often recommended for those taking mood stabilizing drugs, mostly to help them stay with the therapy. Some people taking lithium feel less alert, less creative, and less in control than normal. However, an actual decrease in creativity is uncommon, particularly since lithium allows people with manic-depressive illness to lead a steadier life, improving their overall work performance. Group therapy is often useful for helping people and their spouses or relatives understand the illness and better cope with it.

Phototherapy is sometimes used to treat people with manic-depressive illness, especially those who have milder and more seasonal depression: autumn-winter depression and spring-summer hypomania. With phototherapy, the person is placed in a closed room that is bathed in artificial light. The light is controlled to mimic the season that the therapist is trying to create: longer days for summer and shorter days for winter. If the dose of light is excessive, the person may switch to hypomania or, in some cases, eye damage can occur. Therefore, phototherapy should be supervised by a doctor who specializes in the treatment of mood disorders.

Suicidal Behavior

Suicidal behavior encompasses suicide gestures, suicide attempts, and completed suicide. Suicide plans and actions that appear unlikely to be fatal are called **suicide gestures.** Suicide actions that are intended to be fatal but that don't succeed are called **suicide attempts.** Some people who attempt suicide are discovered early and saved. Other people who attempt suicide are ambivalent about dying, and the attempt may fail because it is a plea for help combined with a strong wish to live. Finally, a **completed suicide** results in death. All suicidal thoughts and behaviors, whether gestures or attempts, must be taken seriously.

Self-destructive behavior may be direct or indirect. Suicide gestures, attempted suicide, and completed suicide are examples of direct self-destructive behavior. Indirect self-destructive behavior involves the undertaking, generally repeatedly, of dangerous activities without a conscious intention of dying. Examples of indirect self-destructive behavior include excessive drinking and drug use, heavy smoking, overeating, neglect of one's health, self-mutilation, reckless driving, and criminal behavior. People who engage in indirect self-destructive behavior are sometimes said to have a "death wish," but usually there are many reasons for the behavior.

Epidemiology

Because statistics on suicide are based mainly on death certificates and inquest reports, they almost certainly underestimate the true incidence. Even so, suicide is among the top 10 causes of death. Suicide accounts for 30 percent of the deaths among college students and for 10 percent of the deaths of people between ages 25 and 34. It is the second leading cause of death among adolescents.▲ However, more than 70 percent of the people who commit suicide are over age 40, and the frequency rises sharply in those over age 60, particularly for men. Suicide rates are higher in urban than in rural areas.

In contrast, suicide attempts are more common before middle age. Attempted suicide is particularly common among unmarried adolescent girls and unmarried men in their 30s. Although women attempt suicide three times more frequently than men, men complete suicide four times as often as women.

Married men and women are less likely to attempt or complete suicide than separated, divorced, or widowed men and women who live alone. Suicides are more common among family members of those who have attempted or completed suicide. The suicide rate among blacks has risen in recent years but is lower than that of whites. Although the rate has increased among black women, their overall rate remains low. Among Native Americans, the rate has risen in recent years, and in some tribes it is five times the national average, particularly among young men.

Many suicides take place in prisons, particularly by young men who haven't committed violent crimes. These men usually hang themselves, often during the first week of imprisonment. Group suicides, whether they involve large numbers or only two people (such as a pair of lovers or spouses), reflect an extreme form of identification with another person. Suicides in large groups tend to occur in highly emotional or fanatic religious settings that overpower the strong drive for self-preservation.

Suicide rates among lawyers, dentists, doctors (especially women doctors), and military personnel are higher than in the general population. Drug overdose is a common means of suicide among doctors, possibly because doctors can obtain drugs easily and know what constitutes a fatal dose.

Suicide occurs less often among practicing members of most religious groups (particularly Roman Catholics), who generally are supported by their beliefs, have close social bonds that protect against acts of self-destruction, and are forbidden by religious beliefs to commit suicide. However, religious affiliation and strong beliefs don't necessarily prevent impetuous, unplanned

---

▲ see page 1319

High Risk Factors for Completed Suicide

Personal and social factors

- Male
- Age over 60 years
- History of a previous suicide attempt
- History of suicide or mood disorder in family
- Recent separation, divorce, or widowhood
- Social isolation, with real or imagined unsympathetic attitude of relatives or friends
- Personally significant anniversaries, such as the anniversary of a loved one's death
- Unemployment or financial difficulties, particularly if they have caused a drastic fall in economic status
- Alcohol or drug abuse
- Detailed suicide planning and taking precautions against being discovered
- Recent humiliating life experience

Mental and physical factors

- Depression (especially manic-depressive illness)
- Agitation, restlessness, and anxiety
- Feelings of guilt, inadequacy, and hopelessness
- Self-denigrating talk or demeanor
- Impulsive, hostile personality
- Delusional conviction of having cancer, heart disease, or another serious disease
- Hallucinations in which a voice commands a suicide attempt
- Physical illness that is chronic, painful, or disabling, especially if the person has previously been healthy
- Use of drugs, such as reserpine, that can cause severe depression

suicidal acts that result from frustration, anger, and despair, especially when accompanied by feelings of guilt or unworthiness.

Suicide notes are left by about one in six people who complete suicide. The notes often refer to personal relationships and to events that will follow the person's death. Notes written by elderly people often express concern for those left behind, while notes written by younger people may be angry or vindictive. A note left by someone who attempts but doesn't complete suicide indicates that the attempt was premeditated; the risk of repeated attempts is, therefore, high.

Causes

Suicidal behavior usually results from the interaction of several factors:
- Mental disorders—primarily depression and substance abuse
- Social factors—disappointment, loss, and a lack of social support

▲ see page 403

- Personality disorders—impulsiveness and aggression
- An incurable physical illness

Well over half of the people who attempt suicide are depressed.▲ Marital problems, an ended or unhappy love affair, or a recent bereavement—particularly among the elderly—may precipitate the depression. Often one factor, such as a disruption in an important relationship, is seen as the last straw. Depression combined with a physical illness may lead to a suicide attempt. A physical disability, especially one that is chronic or painful, is more likely to end in a completed suicide. Physical illness, particularly one that is serious, chronic, and painful, plays an important role in about 20 percent of the suicides among elderly people.

Suicide is often the final act in a course of self-destructive behavior. Self-destructive behavior is significantly more common among people who have had traumatic childhood experiences, particularly those who suffered child abuse or neglect or the distresses of a single-parent home, perhaps because such people are more likely to have difficulties establishing secure, meaningful relationships. Attempted suicide is more likely among battered wives, many of whom were also abused as children.

Alcohol increases the risk of suicidal behavior by worsening feelings of depression and by diminishing self-control. About half of those who attempt suicide are intoxicated at the time of the attempt. Since alcoholism itself, particularly binge drinking, often causes deep feelings of remorse in the intervening periods, alcoholics are particularly suicide-prone even when sober.

Violent self-injury may occur during a deep but temporary depressive mood swing. Mood swings may be caused by drugs or a serious illness. A person who is experiencing a depressive mood swing is often only partially conscious and afterward may be only vaguely able to recall the suicide attempt. People who have epilepsy, especially those who have temporal lobe epilepsy, frequently experience brief but profound episodes of depression that, together with the availability of drugs prescribed for their condition, put them at a greater-than-normal risk of suicidal behavior.

In addition to depression, other mental disorders put people at risk for suicide. For example, people with schizophrenia, particularly those who are also depressed (a fairly common problem in schizophrenia), are more likely to attempt suicide than those who don't have the disorder.▲ The suicide method chosen by schizophrenics may be bizarre and is often violent. In schizophrenia, suicide attempts are usually successful. Suicide may occur early in the illness and may be the first obvious indication that the person had schizophrenia.

People with personality disorders are also at risk of attempted suicide, especially people who are emotionally immature, who tolerate frustration poorly, and who react to stress impetuously with violence and aggression.■ Such people may drink alcohol excessively, abuse drugs, or commit criminal acts. Suicidal behavior is sometimes precipitated by the stresses that inevitably result from the breakup of troubled relationships and the burdens of establishing new relationships and lifestyles. Another important aspect in attempted suicide is the element of Russian roulette, in which the person decides to let fate determine the outcome. Some unstable people find excitement in the perilousness of activities that involve flirting with death, such as reckless driving or dangerous sports.

Methods

The method a person chooses for committing suicide is often determined by availability and cultural factors. It may also reflect the seriousness of intent, since some methods, such as jumping from a tall building, make survival virtually impossible, while others, such as overdosing on a drug, make rescue possible. However, using a method that proves not to be fatal doesn't necessarily indicate that the person's intent was less serious.

Drug overdose is the method most frequently used in suicide attempts. Because doctors no longer prescribe barbiturates often, the number of overdoses with these drugs has decreased; however, the number of overdoses with other psychotropic drugs, such as antidepressants, is increasing. Aspirin overdose has dropped from more than 20 percent of the cases to about 10 percent. Two or more methods or a combination of drugs is used in about 20 percent of attempted suicides, which increases the risk of dying.

Of completed suicides, a gunshot is the method most frequently used in the United States. It is a method predominantly used by boys and men. Women are more likely to use nonviolent methods, such as poisoning (or drug overdose) and drowning, although the number of gunshot suicides among women has increased in recent years. Violent methods, such as gunshots or hanging, are uncommon among attempted suicides because they usually result in death.

A suicidal act often contains evidence of aggression toward others, as can be seen in murders followed by suicide and in the high incidence of suicide among prisoners serving terms for violent crimes.

Prevention

Any suicidal act or threat must be taken seriously. Because 20 percent of the people who at-

▲ see page 435

■ see page 426

Suicide Intervention: Crisis Hot Lines

A person threatening suicide is in crisis, and suicide prevention centers, located around the country, provide 24-hour hot lines to those in distress. Suicide prevention centers are staffed by specially trained volunteers.

When a potentially suicidal person calls a hot line, a volunteer seeks to establish a relationship with the suicidal person, reminding him of his identity (for instance, by using his name repeatedly). The volunteer may offer constructive help for the problem that brought on the crisis and encourage the person to take positive action to resolve it. The volunteer may remind the person that he

has family and friends who care and want to help. Finally, the volunteer may try to facilitate emergency face-to-face professional help for the suicidal person.

Sometimes a person may call a hot line to say that he has already committed a suicidal act (taken a drug overdose or turned on the gas) or is in the process of doing so. In this case, the volunteer tries to obtain the person's address. If that isn't possible, another volunteer contacts the police to trace the call and attempt a rescue. The person is kept talking on the telephone until the police arrive.

tempt suicide repeat the attempt within a year, all people who make suicide gestures or who attempt suicide need to be treated. About 10 percent of all attempted suicides are fatal.

Although sometimes a suicide or attempted suicide comes as a complete surprise or shock, even to close relatives, friends, and associates, in most cases warning signs were present. Because most people who commit suicide are depressed, having depression correctly diagnosed and treated is the most important practical step in preventing suicide. However, the risk of suicide actually increases near the start of treatment for depression, as the person becomes more active and decisive but still feels depressed.

Good psychiatric and social care after an attempted suicide is the best means of preventing further suicide attempts. Since many people who commit suicide have previously attempted suicide, a psychiatric assessment is carried out soon after a suicide attempt. The assessment helps a doctor identify problems that contributed to the act and plan appropriate treatment.

Treatment of Attempted Suicide

Many people who attempt suicide are admitted while unconscious to a hospital emergency department. When a person is known to have taken an overdose of a drug or poison, a doctor takes the following steps:

• Removes as much of the drug or poison as possible from the person's body by trying to prevent its absorption and speed its excretion

• Monitors vital signs and treats symptoms to keep the person alive
• Administers an antidote if the specific drug ingested is definitely known and if an antidote exists

Although most people are physically well enough to be discharged as soon as an injury is treated, they often are hospitalized for psychiatric assessment and treatment. During the psychiatric assessment, the person may deny having any problems. Fairly often, in fact, the severe depression that led to the suicidal act is followed by a short-lived mood elevation, so further suicide attempts are rare immediately after the initial attempt. Nevertheless, the risk of another suicide attempt is high unless the person's problems are resolved.

The length of hospital stay and the kind of treatment required vary. People who have a severe psychiatric illness are usually admitted to a psychiatric unit in the hospital for continued supervision until their suicide-inducing problems have been resolved or until the person can cope with them. Hospitalization may require involuntary commitment, a process by which a person can be held for care against his wishes because he is a danger to himself or others.

Impact of Suicide

A completed suicide has a powerful emotional impact on anyone involved. The person's family, friends, and doctor may feel guilt, shame, and remorse at having failed to prevent the suicide.

They may also feel anger toward the person. Eventually they realize that they couldn't be all-knowing or all-powerful and that the suicide in most cases couldn't have been prevented.

A suicide attempt has a similar impact. However, those who are close to the person have an opportunity to resolve their feelings by responding to the person's cry for help.

CHAPTER 86

Eating Disorders

Serious eating disorders are grouped into three categories: refusing to maintain a minimally normal body weight (anorexia nervosa), eating in binges and then purging (bulimia nervosa), and bingeing without purging (binge eating disorder). Bingeing is the rapid consumption of large amounts of food in a short period of time accompanied by a feeling of loss of control. Purging is self-induced vomiting or misuse of laxatives, diuretics, or enemas to rid the body of food.

Anorexia Nervosa

Anorexia nervosa is a disorder characterized by a distorted body image, an extreme fear of obesity, refusal to maintain a minimally normal body weight, and in women, the absence of menstrual periods.

About 95 percent of the people who have this disorder are females. It usually begins in adolescence, occasionally earlier, and less commonly in adulthood. Anorexia nervosa primarily affects people in middle and upper socioeconomic classes. In Western society, the number of people who have this disorder seems to be increasing.

Anorexia nervosa may be mild and transient or severe and long lasting. Death rates as high as 10 to 20 percent have been reported. However, because mild cases may not be diagnosed, no one knows exactly how many people have anorexia nervosa or what percentage die of it.

Its cause isn't known, but social factors appear to be important. The desire to be thin pervades Western society, and obesity is considered unattractive, unhealthy, and undesirable. Even before adolescence, children are aware of these attitudes, and two thirds of all adolescent girls diet or take other measures to control their weight.

Yet, only a small percentage of these girls develop anorexia nervosa.

Symptoms

Many women who later develop anorexia nervosa are meticulous and compulsive, with very high standards for achievement and success. The first indications of the impending disorder are increased concern with diet and concern about body weight, even among those who already are thin, as are most people who have anorexia nervosa. Preoccupation and anxiety about weight intensify as the person becomes thinner. Even when emaciated, the person claims to feel fat, denies that anything is wrong, doesn't complain about lack of appetite or weight loss, and usually resists treatment. The person usually doesn't see a doctor until brought by family members who are concerned.

Anorexia means "lack of appetite," but people who have anorexia nervosa are actually hungry and preoccupied with food. They study diets and calories; they hoard, conceal, and deliberately waste food; they collect recipes; and they prepare elaborate meals for others.

Half the people who have anorexia nervosa binge and then purge by vomiting or taking laxatives and diuretics. The other half simply restrict the amount of food they eat. Most also exercise excessively to control weight.

Women stop having menstrual periods, sometimes before losing much weight. Women and men may lose interest in sex. Typically, they have a low heart rate, low blood pressure, low body temperature, swelling of tissues caused by fluid accumulation (edema), and fine, soft hair or excessive body and facial hair. Anorectics who become very thin tend to remain active, even pursuing vigorous exercise programs. They don't have symptoms of nutritional deficiencies and are surprisingly free of infections. Depression is common, and people who have this disorder frequently lie about how much they have eaten and conceal their vomiting and their peculiar dietary habits.

Hormonal changes resulting from anorexia nervosa include markedly reduced levels of estrogen and thyroid hormone and increased levels of cortisol. If a person becomes seriously malnourished, every major organ system in the body is likely to be affected. Problems with the heart and with fluids and electrolytes (sodium, potassium, chloride) are the most dangerous. The heart gets weaker and pumps less blood through the body. The person may become dehydrated and prone to fainting. The blood may become acidic (metabolic acidosis), and potassium levels in the blood may decrease. Vomiting and taking laxatives and diuretics can worsen the situation. Sudden death, probably from abnormal heart rhythms, may occur.

Diagnosis and Treatment

Anorexia nervosa is usually diagnosed on the basis of severe weight loss and the characteristic psychologic symptoms. The typical anorectic is an adolescent girl who has lost at least 15 percent of her body weight, fears obesity, stops having menstrual periods, denies being sick, and otherwise appears healthy.

Usually, treatment consists of two steps. The first is restoring normal body weight. The second is psychotherapy, often supplemented with drugs.

When weight loss has been rapid or severe—for example, to more than 25 percent below the ideal body weight▲—restoring body weight is crucial; such weight losses can be life threatening. The initial treatment usually is carried out in a hospital where experienced staff members firmly but gently encourage the patient to eat. Rarely, the patient is fed intravenously or through a tube inserted in the nose and passed into the stomach.

When the person's nutritional status is acceptable, long-term treatment, which is best conducted by specialists in eating disorders, is

begun. This treatment may include individual, group, and family psychotherapy as well as drugs. When depression is diagnosed, antidepressants are prescribed.■ Treatment is aimed at establishing a calm, concerned, stable environment while encouraging the consumption of an adequate amount of food.

Bulimia Nervosa

Bulimia nervosa is a disorder characterized by repeated episodes of binge eating followed by purging (self-induced vomiting or taking laxatives, diuretics, or both), rigorous dieting, or excessive exercising to counteract the effects of bingeing.

As in anorexia nervosa, most people who have bulimia nervosa are female, are deeply concerned about body shape and weight, and belong to the middle or upper socioeconomic classes. Although bulimia nervosa has been portrayed as an epidemic, only about 2 percent of college women, believed to be those at highest risk, are true bulimics.

Symptoms

Bingeing (rapidly and quickly consuming relatively large amounts of food while feeling a loss of control) is followed by intense distress as well as by purging, rigorous dieting, and excessive exercising. The amount of food consumed in a binge may be quite large or no larger than a normal meal. Emotional stress often triggers bingeing, which usually is done in secret. A person must binge at least twice a week to be diagnosed as having bulimia nervosa but may binge more often. Although bulimics express concern about becoming obese and a few are obese, their body weight tends to fluctuate around normal.

Self-induced vomiting can erode tooth enamel, enlarge the salivary glands in the cheeks (parotid glands), and inflame the esophagus. Vomiting and purging can lower potassium levels in the blood, causing abnormal heart rhythms. Sudden death from repeatedly taking large quantities of ipecac to induce vomiting has been reported. Rarely, people who have this disorder eat so much during a binge that their stomach ruptures.

Compared with people who have anorexia nervosa, those who have bulimia nervosa tend to be more aware of their behavior and to feel remorseful or guilty about it. They are more likely to admit their concerns to a doctor or other confidant. Generally, bulimics are more outgoing.

▲ see box, page 647

■ see page 406

They also are more prone to impulsive behavior, drug or alcohol abuse, and obvious depression.

Diagnosis and Treatment

A doctor suspects bulimia nervosa if a person is overly concerned about weight gain and has wide fluctuations in weight, especially with evidence of excessive laxative use. Other clues include swollen salivary glands in the cheeks, scars on the knuckles from using the fingers to induce vomiting, erosion of tooth enamel from stomach acid, and a low level of potassium detected in a blood test. The diagnosis isn't confirmed until the person describes binge-purge behavior.

The two approaches to treatment are psychotherapy and drugs. Psychotherapy, generally best conducted by a therapist with experience in eating disorders, may be very effective. An antidepressant drug often can help control bulimia nervosa, even when a person is not obviously depressed, but the disorder may return after the drug is discontinued.

Binge Eating Disorder

Binge eating disorder is a disorder characterized by bingeing that isn't followed by purging.

In this disorder, bingeing contributes to excessive caloric intake. Unlike bulimia nervosa, binge eating disorder occurs most commonly in people who are obese and becomes more prevalent with increasing body weight. People who have binge eating disorder tend to be older than those who have anorexia nervosa or bulimia nervosa, and more (nearly half) are men.

Symptoms

People who have this disorder are distressed by it. About 50 percent of obese binge eaters are depressed, compared with only 5 percent of obese people who don't binge. Although this disorder doesn't result in the physical problems that can occur with bulimia nervosa, it is a problem for a person who is trying to lose weight.

Treatment

Because binge eating disorder has only recently been identified, no standard treatment programs have been developed for it. Most people who have it are treated in conventional weight-loss programs for obesity, which pay little attention to bingeing—even though 10 to 20 percent of the people in these programs have binge eating disorder. Most people who have the disorder accept this situation because they are more concerned about their obesity than their bingeing.

Specific treatments for binge eating are being developed, based on the treatment of bulimia nervosa; they include psychotherapy and drugs—antidepressants and appetite suppressants. Although both treatments are reasonably effective in controlling binge eating, psychotherapy appears to have longer-lasting effects.

CHAPTER 87

Sexuality and Psychosexual Disorders

Sexuality is a normal part of the human experience. However, the types of sexual behavior and attitudes about sexuality that are considered normal vary greatly within and among different cultures. For example, **masturbation,** which was once regarded as a perversion and even a cause of mental disease, is now recognized as a normal sexual activity throughout life. It is estimated that over 97 percent of males and 80 percent of females have masturbated. Although masturbation is normal and is often recommended as a "safe sex" option, it may cause guilt and psychologic suffering that stems from the disapproving attitudes of others. This can result in considerable distress and can even affect sexual performance.

Similarly, **homosexuality,** once considered abnormal by the medical profession, is no longer considered a disorder; it is widely recognized as a sexual orientation that is present from childhood. The prevalence of homosexuality is unknown, but it is estimated that about 6 to 10 percent of adults are involved exclusively in homosexual relationships throughout their lives. A much higher percentage of people have experimented with same-sex activities in adolescence but are heterosexually oriented as adults.

The causes of homosexuality aren't known, nor are the causes of heterosexuality. No particular hormonal, biologic, or psychologic influences have been identified as substantially contributing to a person's sexual orientation. Homosexuals discover that they are attracted to people of the same sex, just as heterosexuals discover that they are attracted to people of the opposite sex. The attraction appears to be the end result of biologic and environmental influences and isn't a matter of deliberate choice. Therefore, the popular term "sexual preference" makes little sense in matters of sexual orientation.

Most homosexuals adjust well to their sexual orientation, although they must overcome widespread societal disapproval and prejudice. That adjustment may take a long time and may be associated with substantial psychologic stress. Many homosexual men and women experience bigotry in social situations and in the workplace, adding to their stress.

For some heterosexuals and homosexuals, frequent sexual activity with different partners is a common practice throughout life. Such activity may indicate a low capacity for close emotional bonding. This may be a reason to seek professional counseling, especially since the transmission of certain diseases (for example, infection with the human immunodeficiency virus or AIDS, syphilis, gonorrhea, and cervical cancer) is linked to having many sexual partners.

Gender Identity Disorders

A gender identity disorder is the desire to be the opposite sex or the belief that one is "trapped" in a body of the wrong sex.

The difference between sex and gender can be simplified as the following: *sex* is biologic male-

ness or femaleness, and *gender* is how a person sees himself or herself, whether masculine or feminine. Gender role is the objective, public presentation in our culture as masculine or feminine. Sexual role is the public behavior associated with choosing a sexual partner (homosexual, heterosexual, or bisexual). For most people, gender identity (the private, inner sense of being masculine or feminine) is consistent with gender role (for example, a man feels and acts like a man).

Gender identity is generally established in early childhood (18 to 24 months of age). Boys come to know they're boys, and girls come to know they're girls. Even though a child may prefer activities sometimes considered to be more appropriate for the other sex, children with normal gender identity still see themselves as being a member of their own biologic sex. This means that a young girl who likes to play baseball and wrestle doesn't have a gender identity problem if she sees herself as, and is content with being, female. Similarly, a boy who plays with dolls and prefers cooking to sports doesn't have a gender identity problem unless he doesn't identify himself as male or isn't comfortable with being biologically male.

Although a child reared as a member of the opposite sex may be confused about gender, such confusion often clears up later in childhood. Children born with genitals that aren't clearly male or female▲ usually don't have a gender identity problem if they're decisively reared as one sex or the other, even if they are raised in the sex that is opposite from their chromosomal pattern.

Transsexualism

Transsexualism is a distinct gender identity disorder. People with this disorder believe that they are a victim of a biologic accident (that occurred before birth), cruelly imprisoned within a body incompatible with their real gender identity. A majority of transsexuals are biologic males who identify themselves as females, usually early in childhood, and regard their genitals and masculine features with repugnance. Transsexualism appears to be less common in biologic females.

Transsexuals may seek psychologic help, either to assist them in coping with the difficulties of living in a body that they don't feel comfortable with or to help them through a gender transition. Others may seek to change their appearance with the help of doctors who specialize in sex reas-

▲ see page 1237

signment surgery and plastic surgery. Some transsexuals may be satisfied with changing their gender role without major surgery by working, living, and dressing in society as members of the opposite sex. They change their outward appearance, may take hormone treatments, and obtain identification that confirms the change, but usually don't see a need for expensive, risky operations.

However, many transsexuals appear to be helped most by a combination of counseling, hormonal therapy, and genital surgery. In biologic males, sex transformation is accomplished through the use of female hormones (causing breast growth and other body changes) and surgery to remove the penis and testes and create an artificial vagina. In biologic females, sex transformation is accomplished through surgery to remove the breasts and the internal reproductive organs (uterus and ovaries), to close the vagina, and to create an artificial penis. The use of male hormones (testosterone) is important in female-to-male transformation and must precede surgery. With testosterone treatment, facial hair grows and the voice permanently deepens.

Although transsexuals who undergo sex reassignment surgery are unable to bear children, they are often able to have satisfactory sexual relations. The ability to achieve orgasm is often retained after surgery, and after receiving surgery, some report feeling comfortable sexually for the first time. However, few transsexuals endure the sex reassignment process for the sole purpose of being able to function sexually in the opposite sex. Confirmation of gender identity is the usual motivator.

Paraphilias

Paraphilias (deviant attractions) in extreme forms are socially unacceptable deviations from the traditionally held norms of sexual relationships.

The key features of a paraphilia include repetitive, intense, sexually arousing fantasies or behaviors that usually involve objects (shoes, underwear, leather or rubber products), the infliction of suffering or pain on oneself or one's partner, or having sex with nonconsenting persons (children, helpless persons, or in rape scenes). Once they are established, usually in late childhood or near puberty, these arousal patterns are usually lifelong.

Some degree of variety is very common in adult sexual relationships and fantasies. When people mutually agree to engage in them, noninjurious sexual behaviors of an unusual nature may be an intrinsic part of a loving and caring relationship. When taken to the extreme, however, such sexual behaviors are paraphilias, psychosexual disorders that seriously impair the capacity for affectionate, reciprocal sexual activity. Partners of people with a paraphilia may feel like an object or as if they are unimportant or unnecessary in the sexual relationship.

Paraphilias may take the form of fetishism, transvestism, pedophilia, exhibitionism, voyeurism, masochism, or sadism, among others. Most people with paraphilias are men, and many have more than one type of paraphilia.

Fetishism

In fetishism, sexual activity makes use of physical objects (the fetish), sometimes in preference to contact with humans. People with fetishes may become sexually stimulated and gratified by wearing another's undergarments, wearing rubber or leather, or holding, rubbing, or smelling objects, such as high-heeled shoes. People with this disorder may not be able to function sexually without their fetish.

Transvestism

In transvestism, a man occasionally prefers to wear women's clothing, or less commonly, a woman prefers to wear men's clothing. In neither case, however, does the person wish to change sex, as transsexuals do. Cross-dressing isn't always considered a mental disorder and may not adversely affect a couple's sexual relationship. Transvestism is a disorder only if it causes distress, results in impairment of some type, or involves "daredevil" behavior likely to lead to injury, loss of job, or imprisonment. Transvestites also cross-dress for reasons other than sexual stimulation, for example, to reduce anxiety, relax, or experiment with the feminine side of their otherwise male personalities.

Pedophilia

Pedophilia is a preference for sexual activity with young children. In Western societies, pedophilia is generally considered to be a desire to engage in sexual activity with children 13 years of age or younger. A person diagnosed with pedophilia is at least 16 years old and is generally at least 5 years older than the child victim.

Although state laws vary, the law generally considers a person to be committing statutory rape if the child is 16 years old or younger and the adult is over age 18. Statutory rape cases often do not meet the definition of pedophilia.

A person with pedophilia is severely distressed or preoccupied with sexual fantasies about children, even if no sexual activity actually takes place. Some pedophiles are attracted only to children, often of a specific age range, whereas other pedophiles are attracted to both children and adults. Both men and women can be pedophiles, and both boys and girls can be victims. Pedophiles may focus only on children within their families (incest), or they may prey on children in the community. Force or coercion may be used to engage children sexually, and threats may be invoked to prevent disclosure by the victim.

Pedophilia can be treated with psychotherapy and drugs that alter the sex drive. Such treatment may be sought voluntarily or only after criminal apprehension and legal action. Some pedophiles may respond to treatment; others don't. Incarceration, even long term, doesn't change pedophilic desires or fantasies.

Exhibitionism

In exhibitionism, a person (usually a man) exposes his genitals to unsuspecting strangers and becomes sexually excited when doing so. Masturbation may ensue after exposure. Further sexual contact is almost never sought, so exhibitionists rarely commit rape. Most exhibitionists who are apprehended are under 40 years old. Although women may exhibit their bodies in provocative ways, exhibitionism is rarely considered a psychosexual disorder in women.

Voyeurism

In voyeurism, a person becomes sexually aroused by watching someone who is disrobing, naked, or engaged in sexual activity. It is the act of "peeping" that is arousing, not sexual activity with the observed person. Some degree of voyeurism is particularly common among boys and men, and society often regards mild forms of this behavior as normal. As a disorder, however, voyeurism may become the preferred method of sexual activity and may consume countless hours of searching.

Most voyeurs are men. The amount and variety of sexually explicit materials and shows (for example, male strip shows) available to heterosexual women has increased significantly, but engaging in these activities lacks the element of secret observation that is the hallmark of voyeurism.

Masochism and Sadism

Masochism constitutes sexual enjoyment in being physically harmed, threatened, or abused. Sadism, the opposite of masochism, is the sexual enjoyment a person receives from inflicting actual physical or psychologic suffering on a sex partner. Some amount of sadism and masochism is commonly play-acted in healthy sexual relationships, and mutually compatible partners often seek one another out. For example, the use of silk handkerchiefs for simulated bondage and mild spanking during sexual activity are common practices between consenting partners and aren't considered sadomasochistic.

Masochism or sadism taken to the extreme, however, can result in severe bodily or psychologic harm, including death. The disorder of sexual masochism entails the need for real, not simulated, humiliation, beatings, or other submission to an aggressive, often sadistic, partner for the purpose of sexual arousal. For example, the deviant sexual activity may involve asphyxiophilia, whereby the person is partially choked or strangled (either by a partner or by the self-application of a noose around the neck). A temporary decrease in oxygen to the brain at the point of orgasm is sought as an enhancement to sexual release, but the practice may accidentally result in death.

Sexual sadism may exist solely in fantasy or may be needed for arousal or orgasm. Some sadists entrap unsuspecting and terrified "partners" who do not consent to the activity and are then raped. Other sadists specifically seek out sexual masochists through personal ads or other sources and fulfill their sadistic urges with a consenting masochist. Fantasies of total control and dominance are often important, and the sadist may bind and gag the partner in elaborate ways. In extreme cases, the sadist may torture, cut, stab, apply electrical shocks to, or kill the partner.

Disorders of Sexual Function

Normal sexual function in men and women involves both the mind (thoughts and emotions) and the body. The nervous, circulatory, and endocrine (hormonal) systems all interact to produce a sexual response, which has four stages: desire, arousal, orgasm, and resolution.

Desire is the wish to engage in sexual activity. It may be triggered by thoughts or verbal and visual cues.

Arousal is the state of sexual excitement. During arousal, blood flow to the genital area increases, leading to an erection in men and to enlargement of the clitoris, engorgement of the vaginal walls, and increased vaginal secretions in women.

Orgasm is the peak or climax of sexual excitement. In men, semen ejaculates from the penis. In women, the muscles surrounding the vagina contract rhythmically. At orgasm, both men and women experience increased muscle tension throughout the body and contractions of the pelvic muscles. Most people experience orgasm as highly pleasurable.

Resolution, a sense of well-being and general muscular relaxation, follows orgasm. During resolution, men are unable to have another erection for some time. The time between erections (refractory period) generally increases as men age. In contrast, many women are able to respond to additional stimulation almost immediately after orgasm.

A delicate and balanced interplay among all parts of the nervous system controls the sexual response. Part of the nervous system, called the parasympathetic nervous system, regulates the increased blood flow during arousal. Another part of the nervous system, the sympathetic nervous system, mainly controls orgasm. An abnormality in blood flow to the penis or vagina, physical damage to any of the genital organs, a hormonal imbalance, or the use of many drugs may interfere with the sexual response, even if the nervous system is functioning normally.

Sexual dysfunction may result from either physical or psychologic factors; many sexual problems result from a combination of both. For instance, a physical problem may lead to psychologic problems, such as anxiety, fear, or stress, and psychologic problems often aggravate a physical problem.

Premature Ejaculation

Premature ejaculation is ejaculation that occurs too early, usually before, upon, or shortly after penetration.

The problem is common among adolescent boys and may be intensified by feelings that sex is sinful. Fear of discovery, of making the partner pregnant, or of contracting a sexually transmitted disease, as well as anxiety about performance, may be contributing factors. Similar concerns may persist into adulthood and may be magnified by problems in a relationship. Although premature ejaculation rarely has a physical cause, inflammation of the prostate gland or a nervous system disorder may be involved.

Premature ejaculation can be a significant problem for couples. If the man ejaculates before his partner reaches orgasm, she may be left feeling unsatisfied and may become resentful.

Treatment

A therapist explains the mechanisms of premature ejaculation, provides reassurance, and offers simple advice. With one technique, the stop-and-start technique, the man learns to tolerate high levels of excitement without ejaculating. The technique involves stimulation of the penis, either manually or through intercourse, until the man feels that he will soon ejaculate unless stimulation stops. He signals his partner to stop stimulation, which is resumed after 20 to 30 seconds. The partners rehearse this technique at first with manual stimulation and later during intercourse. With practice, more than 95 percent of the men learn to control ejaculation for 5 to 10 minutes or even longer. The technique also helps reduce anxiety, which often aggravates the problem. Some men find that the use of condoms helps delay ejaculation.

Occasionally, premature ejaculation is caused by more serious psychologic problems, for which psychotherapy may be appropriate and helpful. When behavior therapy, such as the stop-and-

---

Psychologic Causes of Sexual Dysfunction

- Anger toward a partner

- Depression

- Fear of losing control, of dependence on another person, or of pregnancy

- Guilt

- Anxiety

- Ignorance or inhibitions about sexual behavior

- Previous traumatic sexual experiences (for example, rape, incest or sexual abuse, or sexual failure)

- Performance anxiety (worrying about performance during intercourse)

- Feeling like a spectator rather than a participant

- Discord or boredom with a partner

---

start technique, is inappropriate or rejected by the patient, or when it simply doesn't work, then drugs called selective serotonin reuptake inhibitors (such as fluoxetine, paroxetine, or sertraline) can be taken to delay ejaculation. This type of drug works by increasing the amount of serotonin in the body. They can be taken either daily or an hour or so before sexual intercourse.

Retarded Ejaculation

Retarded ejaculation is a condition in which an erection is maintained but ejaculation is delayed for a prolonged period.

Retarded ejaculation is rare. Yet as men get older, the time it takes to reach orgasm generally becomes longer. Some drugs, such as thioridazine, mesoridazine, and some blood pressure medications, can impair ejaculation. Impaired ejaculation can also be a side effect of certain antidepressant drugs, such as selective serotonin reuptake inhibitors. Diabetes can also impair ejaculation. Psychologic causes include fear of vaginal penetration and fear of ejaculating in the partner's presence.

The treatment involves behavioral therapy to reduce anxiety and learn techniques for timing ejaculation. The female partner first stimulates the man to ejaculate outside the vagina, then at the lips of the vagina, and finally inside the vagina. If this technique fails, other forms of psychotherapy may help.

Low Sexual Desire Disorder

Low sexual desire disorder is a persistent loss of sexual fantasy and little desire for sexual activity.

Low sexual desire occurs in both men and women. Some people lack interest in or desire for sexual activity all their lives. The disorder may be related to traumatic events in childhood or adolescence, suppression of sexual fantasies, or occasionally, abnormally low levels of the hormone testosterone (in either men or women). More commonly, the problem develops after years of normal sexual desire. Causes include boredom in a relationship, depression, a hormonal imbalance, and the use of sedatives, antianxiety drugs (tranquilizers), antidepressants, and certain drugs to treat high blood pressure.

Symptoms

A lack of interest in sex, even in ordinarily erotic situations, is the hallmark of this disorder. Sexual activity is usually infrequent and may cause discord between partners. Some people continue to have sexual relations fairly often because they want to please their partners or because they are urged or forced to do so. They may have no difficulty with performance but continually feel apathetic about sex. When boredom is the cause, the person may have little sexual desire for the usual partner but may have normal or even intense sexual desire for another.

Diagnosis and Treatment

A doctor or therapist asks the person about previous and current sexual interest and experience, tries to learn about the person's sexual maturation and any sexual trauma, and investigates the possibility of depression, discord between partners, and other related issues. Whenever possible, both partners are interviewed, first separately and then together. The doctor evaluates the person's medical condition and any drugs being taken that might be contributing to sexual problems. A blood test may be needed to measure testosterone and thyroid hormone levels in men and women.

Counseling or behavioral therapy, such as the sensate focus technique (an exercise in which partners learn to achieve an intimate sexual relationship), may improve communication between partners. For the few men who have a testosterone deficiency, injections of testosterone or testosterone patches may be helpful. If the use of a drug is responsible for low sexual desire, then decreasing the dose or switching to another drug may remedy the problem.

Sexual Aversion Disorder

Sexual aversion disorder is persistent, extreme aversion to virtually all sexual activity, characterized by fear and sometimes accompanied by panic attacks.

Sexual aversion disorder occasionally occurs in men but is much more common in women. The cause may be sexual trauma, such as incest, sexual abuse, or rape; a repressive family atmosphere, possibly linked to rigid religious training; or pain during first attempts at intercourse. Sexual activity may remind the person of pain even after intercourse is no longer physically painful.

Treatment

Couples counseling may help resolve discord in a relationship. Psychotherapy may be needed for people who have experienced sexual trauma. Behavioral therapy in which a person is gradually exposed to sexual activity, beginning with non-threatening activities and progressing to full sexual expression, may also be effective. Drugs may help relieve panic attacks associated with sexual activity.

Sexual Arousal Disorder in Women

Sexual arousal disorder is the persistent failure to attain or maintain sexual excitement despite adequate sexual stimulation. Sexual arousal disorder in women is similar to impotence in men;▲ both disorders have physical or psychologic causes.

The problem may be lifelong or, more frequently, occurs after a period of normal function. Psychologic factors such as marital discord, depression, and stressful situations are the predominant causes. A woman may associate sex with sinfulness and sexual pleasure with feelings of

Sex Therapy: The Sensate Focus Technique

The sensate focus technique is a method taught to couples who are having sexual difficulties as a result of psychologic rather than physical factors. The technique aims to make both partners aware of what each other finds pleasurable and to reduce anxiety about performance. It is often used in the treatment of low sexual desire disorder, sexual arousal disorder, inhibited orgasm, and impotence.

The technique has three steps. Both partners must achieve comfort at each level of intimacy before proceeding to the next step.

• The first step concentrates on caressing. Each partner gives the other as much pleasure as possible by touching and caressing parts of the body other than the breasts or genitals.

• The second step allows partners to touch the breasts, genitals, and other erogenous zones, but intercourse isn't permitted.

• The third step consists of sexual intercourse, concentrating on enjoyment rather than on orgasm.

guilt. Fear of intimacy may also play a part. Some women or their partners aren't aware of how the female genital organs function, especially the clitoris, and they may not know techniques of sexual arousal.

Many physical problems can cause sexual arousal disorder. Pain from endometriosis or an infection of the bladder (cystitis) or vagina (vaginitis) could affect a woman's ability to become sexually aroused. The estrogen deficiency that accompanies menopause or the surgical removal of the ovaries usually causes dryness and thinning of the vaginal walls and may result in sexual arousal disorder. A hysterectomy or mastectomy may affect a woman's sexual self-image.

▲ see page 1065

Other physical causes of sexual arousal disorder include an underactive thyroid gland; abnormal vaginal anatomy as a result of cancer, surgery, or radiation therapy; loss of sensation because of alcoholism, diabetes, or certain nervous system disorders such as multiple sclerosis; and the use of drugs to treat anxiety, depression, or hypertension.

Diagnosis and Treatment

A medical history and physical examination help the doctor determine if the cause is primarily psychologic or physical. Any physical problem is treated. For example, antibiotics may be prescribed for an infection of the bladder or vagina, and hormones can be taken to replace a deficiency. Counseling is often beneficial, as is learning the sensate focus technique.▲ Kegel exercises can strengthen the pelvic muscles and may help a woman feel more pleasure. In these exercises, the woman contracts her vaginal muscles hard (as if to stop her urinary stream) 10 to 15 times at least three times a day for 2 or 3 months.

Inhibited Orgasm

Inhibited orgasm is a disorder in which a woman either has no orgasms, has orgasms that are delayed much longer than she and her partner desire, or has orgasms that are difficult to achieve despite appropriate stimulation.

The disorder may be lifelong, may develop after a period of normal function, or may occur only in certain situations or with certain partners. About 10 percent of women never have an orgasm with any source of stimulation or in any situation. Most women can have an orgasm with stimulation of the clitoris, but probably more than half are often unable to have an orgasm during intercourse unless the clitoris is stimulated during vaginal penetration.

The causes of inhibited orgasm are similar to those of sexual arousal disorder. Intercourse may be consistently terminated by the partner before the woman reaches orgasm. Some women have no trouble developing adequate arousal but may be afraid to "let go," especially during intercourse. The reason may be feelings of guilt following a pleasurable experience or a fear of dependency on a partner. It may also represent a fear of losing control.

Treatment

Any physical causes identified by a doctor are treated appropriately. When psychologic causes predominate, individual or couples counseling may be helpful. The sensate focus technique is generally beneficial to women who are sexually inhibited.■ However, the technique is less beneficial to women who are able to have an orgasm from stimulation of the clitoris but aren't able to do so during intercourse.

A woman's knowledge of the function of her sex organs and of her responses is essential. She should know the best ways to stimulate her clitoris. Vaginal sensations may be enhanced by strengthening voluntary control of the muscles surrounding the vagina using Kegel exercises. In these exercises, the woman contracts her vaginal muscles hard (as if to stop her urinary stream) 10 to 15 times at least three times a day. Generally, after 2 or 3 months, muscle tone and sensitivity improve and the woman's sense of control increases.

Dyspareunia

Dyspareunia is genital or deep pelvic pain experienced during intercourse.

Dyspareunia can occur in men, although it isn't too common. Prostatitis, an inflammation of the prostate gland, or the use of certain antidepressant drugs, such as amoxapine, imipramine, and clomipramine, may cause a man to experience pain with orgasm.

Dyspareunia is more common in women. Pain during intercourse may develop during the first attempts at sexual intercourse or years later. The cause may be physical or psychologic.

In a woman who has never had intercourse, a membranous fold (hymen) may partially or completely cover the entrance to the vagina. Penile penetration during the first sexual encounter may tear the hymen, causing pain. Bruising of the genital area can also produce pain, as can inadequate vaginal lubrication, usually resulting from insufficient foreplay. The glands in the genital region (Bartholin's glands or Skene's glands) may become infected or inflamed, resulting in pain. An improperly fitting condom or diaphragm or an allergic reaction to contraceptive foams or jellies

---

▲ see box, page 423

■ see box, page 423

may irritate the vagina or cervix. A woman may have a congenital abnormality, such as a rigid hymen or an abnormal dividing wall in the vagina.

Estrogen deficiency, which usually occurs after menopause, causes drying and thinning of the vaginal walls, possibly resulting in pain during intercourse. Surgery to repair torn tissue after childbirth or other types of surgery that result in a narrowing of the vagina may produce subsequent pain during intercourse. Inflammation and infection of the vagina (vaginitis) are often painful. Other causes of dyspareunia include infections of the cervix, uterus, or fallopian tubes; endometriosis; pelvic tumors; and adhesions (fibrous tissue) that formed after a previous pelvic disease or surgery. Radiation therapy for a cancer may produce changes in the tissues that make intercourse painful.

A woman who has dyspareunia may develop anxiety and fear of sexual intercourse. Anger or repulsion toward a sexual partner are other possible problems that may need to be addressed.

Diagnosis and Treatment

The doctor tries to determine whether the cause is physical or psychologic (such as vaginismus) by taking a complete history and performing a pelvic examination. Abstaining from intercourse until the problem is resolved is important. However, sexual activity that doesn't involve vaginal penetration can continue.

Applying an anesthetic ointment reduces pain. Sitz baths may be helpful. Pain and muscle spasms may be prevented by liberally applying a lubricant before intercourse. However, water-based lubricants rather than petroleum jelly or other oil-based lubricants are preferable, as the oil-based products tend to dry the vagina and can also damage latex contraceptives such as condoms and diaphragms. Devoting more time to foreplay may increase vaginal secretions.

Women who have reached menopause may benefit from using a topical estrogen cream or taking oral estrogen to increase vaginal lubrication and counteract the effects of thinning vaginal walls. Sometimes a different position for intercourse, one involving less deep thrusting or one that gives the woman more control of penetration by being on top, reduces pain.

Inflammation and infection of the vagina are treated with appropriate drugs.▲ If the vulva is swollen and painful, applying wet dressings of alu-

minum acetate solution may help. Surgery may be needed to remove cysts or abscesses, open a rigid hymen, or repair an anatomic abnormality. A pessary, a device inserted into the vagina to support the uterus, helps some women. A poorly fitting diaphragm should be replaced with a different type, brand, or size, or a different method of birth control should be tried. Analgesics or sedatives may be needed in rare instances.

Vaginismus

Vaginismus is an involuntary contraction of the lower vaginal muscles that prevents the penis from penetrating the vagina.

Vaginismus results from a woman's unconscious desire to prevent penetration. A woman may develop vaginismus if intercourse has been painful in the past. She may not want to engage in intercourse for fear of becoming pregnant, of being controlled by the man, of losing control, or of being hurt during intercourse.

Diagnosis and Treatment

A medical history and physical examination often establish a physical problem or psychologic factor. Any physical problem can usually be corrected. If vaginismus persists, the woman is taught techniques to reduce the muscle spasms.

In the graduated dilation technique, the woman inserts lubricated dilators into her vagina. The dilators are very small at first, but progressively larger dilators are used as the level of comfort increases. Exercises to strengthen the pelvic muscles, such as Kegel exercises, while the dilators are in place are helpful. In these exercises, the muscles surrounding the vagina are squeezed hard and then relaxed, which allows the woman to develop a sense of control over them. The dilation technique can also be practiced regularly at home using the fingers.

Once the woman can tolerate having large dilators inserted without discomfort, she and her partner may try to have sexual intercourse again. Counseling for both the woman and her partner can ease this process and allay anxiety.

▲ see box, page 1083

Personality Disorders

Personality disorders are characterized by patterns of perceiving, reacting, and relating that are relatively fixed, inflexible, and socially maladaptive across a variety of situations.

Everyone has characteristic patterns of perceiving and relating to other people and events (**personality traits**). Put another way, all people tend to cope with stresses in an individual but repetitive style. For example, some people always respond to a troubling situation by seeking someone else's help. Others always assume that they can deal with problems on their own. Some people minimize problems; others exaggerate them.

Although people tend to always respond to a difficult situation in the same way, most are likely to try another approach if their first response is ineffective. In contrast, people with personality disorders are so rigid that they can't adapt to reality, which impairs their ability to function. Their maladaptive patterns of thinking and behaving become evident by early adulthood, often earlier, and tend to persist throughout life. They are likely to have trouble in their social and interpersonal relationships and at work.

People with personality disorders usually aren't aware that their behavior or thought patterns are inappropriate; on the contrary, they often believe their patterns are normal and right. Often, family members or social agencies send them for psychiatric help because their inappropriate behavior causes difficulty for others. In contrast, people with anxiety disorders trouble themselves but not others.▲ When people with personality disorders do seek help on their own—usually because of frustrations—they tend to believe their problems are caused by other people or a particularly difficult situation.

Personality disorders include the following types: paranoid, schizoid, schizotypal, histrionic, narcissistic, antisocial, borderline, avoidant, dependent, obsessive-compulsive, and passive-aggressive. Dissociative identity disorder, formerly called multiple personality disorder, is an entirely different disorder.■

Paranoid Personality

People with a paranoid personality project their own conflicts and hostilities onto others. They are generally cold and distant in their relationships. They tend to find hostile and malevolent intentions behind other people's trivial, innocent, or even positive acts and react with suspicion to changes in situations. Often, the suspiciousness leads to aggressive behaviors or rejection by others—results that seem to justify their original feelings.

Those who have a paranoid personality often take legal action against others, especially if they feel righteously indignant. They are unable to see their own roles in a conflict. Although they usually work in relative isolation, they may be highly efficient and conscientious.

Sometimes people who already feel alienated because of a defect or handicap (such as deafness) are more vulnerable to developing paranoid ideas.

Schizoid Personality

People with a schizoid personality are introverted, withdrawn, and solitary. They are emotionally cold and socially distant. They are most often absorbed with their own thoughts and feelings and are fearful of closeness and intimacy with others. They talk little, are given to daydreaming, and prefer theoretical speculation to practical action. Fantasy is a common coping mechanism.

Schizotypal Personality

People with a schizotypal personality, like those with a schizoid personality, are socially and emotionally detached. In addition, they display oddities of thinking, perceiving, and communicating. While these oddities are similar to those of people with schizophrenia,★ and while schizotypal personality is sometimes found in people with schizophrenia before they become ill, most adults with a schizotypal personality don't develop schizophrenia. Some people show signs of magical thinking—the idea that a particular

---

▲ see page 395

■ see page 432

★ see page 435

action can control something completely unrelated. For example, a person may believe that bad luck will really occur if he walks under a ladder or that he can cause harm to others by thinking angry thoughts. Those with a schizotypal personality may also have paranoid ideas.

Histrionic Personality

People with a histrionic (hysterical) personality conspicuously seek attention and behave dramatically. Their lively expressive manner results in easily established but often superficial relationships. Emotions often seem exaggerated, childish, and contrived to evoke sympathy or attention (often erotic or sexual) from others. People with a histrionic personality are prone to sexually provocative behavior or to sexualizing nonsexual relationships. They may not really want a sexual relationship; rather, their seductive behaviors often mask their wish to be dependent and protected. Some people with a histrionic personality also are hypochondriacal and exaggerate their physical problems to get the attention they need.

Narcissistic Personality

People with a narcissistic personality have a sense of superiority and an exaggerated belief in their own value or importance, which is what psychiatrists call "grandiosity." People with this personality type may be extremely sensitive to failure, defeat, or criticism and, when confronted by a failure to fulfill their high opinion of themselves, can easily become enraged or severely depressed. Because they believe themselves to be superior in their relationships with other people, they expect to be admired and often suspect that others envy them. They feel they're entitled to have their needs attended to without waiting, so they exploit others, whose needs or beliefs are deemed to be less important. Their behavior is usually offensive to others, who view them as being self-centered, arrogant, or selfish.

Antisocial Personality

People with an antisocial personality (previously called **psychopathic** or **sociopathic personality**), most of whom are male, show callous disregard for the rights and feelings of others. They exploit others for material gain or personal gratification (unlike narcissistic people who think they are better than others). Characteristically, such people act out their conflicts impulsively and irresponsibly. They tolerate frustration

---

Possible Consequences of Personality Disorders

- People with severe personality disorders are at high risk of behaviors that can lead to physical illness, such as alcohol or drug addiction; self-destructive behavior; reckless sexual behavior; hypochondriasis; and clashes with society's values.

- People with personality disorders are vulnerable to psychiatric breakdowns as a result of stress; the type of psychiatric disorder (for example anxiety, depression, or psychosis) depends in part on the type of personality disorder.

- People with personality disorders are less likely to follow a prescribed treatment regimen; even when the regimen is followed, they are likely to be less responsive than normal to medications.

- People with personality disorders often have a poor relationship with their doctors because they refuse to take responsibility for their behavior or feel overly distrustful, deserving, or needy. The doctor may then become blaming, distrusting, and ultimately rejecting of the person.

---

poorly, and sometimes they are hostile or violent. Despite the problems or harm they cause others by their antisocial behaviors, they typically don't feel remorse or guilt. Rather, they glibly rationalize their behavior or blame it on others. Dishonesty and deceit permeate their relationships. Frustration and punishment rarely cause them to modify their behaviors.

People with an antisocial personality are often prone to alcoholism, drug addiction, sexual deviation, promiscuity, and imprisonment. They are likely to fail at their jobs and move from one area to another. They often have a family history of antisocial behavior, substance abuse, divorce, and physical abuse. As children, they were usually emotionally neglected and often physically abused during their formative years. People with an antisocial personality have shorter life expectancies than average, but among those who survive, the condition tends to diminish or stabilize with age.

Borderline Personality

People with a borderline personality, most of whom are women, are unstable in their self-image, moods, behavior, and interpersonal relationships (which are often stormy and intense). Borderline personality becomes evident in early adulthood, but prevalence diminishes with age. People with a borderline personality have often been deprived of adequate care during childhood. Consequently they feel empty, angry, and deserving of nurturing.

When people with a borderline personality feel cared for, they appear lonely and waiflike, often needing help for depression, substance abuse, eating disorders, and past mistreatment. However, when they fear abandonment by a caring person, their mood shifts dramatically. They frequently show inappropriate and intense anger, accompanied by extreme changes in their view of the world, themselves, and others—shifting from black to white, hated to loved, or vice versa, but never to neutral. People with a borderline personality who feel abandoned and alone may wonder whether they actually exist (that is, they don't feel real). They can become desperately impulsive, engaging in reckless promiscuity or substance abuse. At times they're so out of touch with reality that they have brief episodes of psychotic thinking, paranoia, and hallucinations.

People with borderline personality disorder are commonly seen by primary care doctors; they tend to visit the doctor frequently with repeated crises or vague complaints but often don't comply with treatment recommendations. Borderline personality disorder is also the most common personality disorder treated by psychiatrists because people with the disorder relentlessly seek someone to care for them.

Avoidant Personality

People with an avoidant personality are oversensitive to rejection, and they fear starting relationships or anything else new because of the possibility of rejection or disappointment. People with an avoidant personality have a strong desire for affection and acceptance. They're openly distressed by their isolation and inability to relate comfortably to others. Unlike those with a borderline personality, people with an avoidant per-

---

▲ see page 400

sonality don't respond to rejection with anger; instead, they appear shy and timid. Avoidant personality disorder is similar to social phobia.▲

Dependent Personality

People with a dependent personality surrender major decisions and responsibilities to others and permit the needs of those they depend on to supersede their own. They lack self-confidence and feel intensely insecure about their ability to take care of themselves. They often protest that they can't make decisions and don't know what to do or how to do it. They are reluctant to express opinions even when they have them for fear of offending people they need. People with other personality disorders often have aspects of a dependent personality, but these traits are usually hidden by the more dominant ones of the other disorder. Sometimes adults with protracted illnesses develop dependent personalities.

Obsessive-Compulsive Personality

People with an obsessive-compulsive personality are reliable, dependable, orderly, and methodical but often can't adapt to change. They are cautious and analyze all aspects of a problem, which impairs decision making. Although these traits are in tune with Western cultural standards, people with an obsessive-compulsive personality take their responsibilities so seriously that they can't tolerate mistakes and pay so much attention to detail that they don't complete their tasks. Consequently, such people can become entangled with the means of accomplishing a task and forget its purpose. Their responsibilities make them anxious, and they rarely enjoy satisfaction from their achievements.

People with an obsessive-compulsive personality are often high achievers, especially in the sciences and other intellectually demanding fields in which order and attention to detail are desirable. However, they can feel detached from their feelings and uncomfortable with relationships or other situations in which they lack control, events are unpredictable, or they must rely on others.

Passive-Aggressive Personality

The behaviors of a person with a passive-aggressive (negativistic) personality are covertly designed to control or punish others. Passive-aggressive behavior is often displayed as procrastination, inefficiency, and sullenness. Fre-

Defense Mechanisms: Immature Ways to Cope

Defense Mechanism	Description	Result
Dissociation	Enables a person to numb current feelings	Causes a temporary but drastic experience of feeling separate from oneself, not existing, or being in an unreal world; can cause a dreamlike state (fugue or trance); may result in stimulus-seeking or self-destructive behaviors
Projection	Allows a person to attribute his own feelings or thoughts to others	Leads to prejudice, suspiciousness, and excessive worrying about external dangers
Fantasy	Provides escape from conflict and painful realities (for example, loneliness)	Allows imagination and private beliefs to take the place of involvement with the outside world and, most especially, with other people
Acting out	Allows a person to avoid thinking about a painful situation or experiencing a painful emotion	Leads to acts that are often irresponsible, reckless, and foolish
Splitting	Enables a person to use black-or-white, all-or-nothing perceptions to divide people into groups of idealized all-good saviors and vilified, all-bad evildoers	Avoids the discomfort of having both loving and angry feelings for the same person as well as feelings of uncertainty and helplessness

quently, people with a passive-aggressive personality agree to perform tasks that they really don't want to do and then proceed to subtly undermine completion of those tasks. Such behavior usually serves to express concealed hostility.

Diagnosis

A doctor bases the diagnosis of a personality disorder on a person's display of maladaptive thought or behavior patterns. These patterns tend to become apparent because the person stubbornly resists changing them despite their maladaptive consequences.

In addition, a doctor is likely to notice the person's inappropriate use of coping mechanisms, often called defense mechanisms. While everyone unconsciously uses defense mechanisms, people with personality disorders use them in inappropriate or immature ways.

Treatment

Although treatments differ according to the type of personality disorder, some general principles apply to all. Because most people with a per-

sonality disorder don't see a need for therapy, motivation often comes from someone else. Nevertheless, the person can usually respond to supportive but forceful confrontation about the maladaptive consequences of their thought and behavior patterns. This is usually most effective when it comes from peers or a psychotherapist.

A therapist repeatedly points out the undesirable consequences of the person's thought and behavior patterns, sometimes sets limits on behavior, and repeatedly confronts the person with reality. Involvement of the person's family is very helpful and often essential, since group pressure can be effective. Group and family treatment, group living in designated residential settings, and participation in therapeutic social clubs or self-help groups can all be valuable in treatment.

People with a personality disorder sometimes have anxiety and depression, which they hope can be relieved by drugs. However, the anxiety and depression that result from a personality disorder are rarely satisfactorily relieved by drugs, and such symptoms may be evidence that the person is undertaking some healthy self-examination. Moreover, drug therapy is frequently complicated by misuse of the drugs or by suicide attempts. If the person has another psychiatric disorder, such as major depression, phobia, or panic disorder, then drugs may be appropriate, although they will likely provide only limited relief.

Changing a personality takes a long time. No short-term treatment can successfully cure a personality disorder, but certain changes may be accomplished faster than others. Recklessness, social isolation, lack of assertiveness, or temper outbursts can respond to behavior modification therapy. However, long-term psychotherapy (talk therapy), aimed at helping the person understand the causes of his anxiety and recognize his maladaptive behavior, remains the cornerstone of most treatment. Some personality disorders, such as narcissistic or obsessive-compulsive types, may be best treated with psychoanalysis. Others, such as antisocial or paranoid types, are rarely amenable to any therapy.

CHAPTER 90

Dissociative Disorders

Dissociation is a psychologic defense mechanism in which one's identity, memories, ideas, feelings, or perceptions are separated from conscious awareness and can't be recalled or experienced voluntarily.

Everyone dissociates at times. For example, people often realize after driving home from work that they don't remember much of the trip because they were preoccupied with personal concerns or a program on the radio. During hypnosis, a person may dissociate feelings of physical pain. However, other forms of dissociation disrupt a person's sense of self and recollection of life's events.

Dissociative disorders include dissociative amnesia, dissociative fugue, dissociative identity disorder, depersonalization disorder, and a group of less well-defined conditions that psychiatrists refer to as dissociative disorder not otherwise specified. Dissociative disorders are usually precipitated by overwhelming stress. The stress may be caused by experiencing or witnessing a traumatic event, accident, or disaster. Or a person may experience inner conflict so intolerable that his mind is forced to separate incompatible or unacceptable information and feelings from conscious thought.

Dissociative Amnesia

Dissociative amnesia is an inability to recall important personal information, usually of a traumatic or stressful nature, which is too extensive to be explained by normal forgetfulness.

Usually the lost memory involves information that is normally part of routine conscious awareness or "autobiographical" memory—who one is; what one did; where one went; to whom one spoke; what was said, thought, and felt; and so on. Sometimes the information, though forgotten, continues to influence the person's behavior.

People with dissociative amnesia usually have one or more memory gaps spanning a few minutes to a few hours or days. However, memory gaps spanning years or even a person's entire life are well documented. Usually the boundaries around the memory gap are clear. Most people are aware that they have "lost some time," but some who have dissociative amnesia become aware of time loss only when they realize or are confronted with evidence that they have done things that they don't recall. Some people with amnesia forget some but not all events over a period of time; others can't recall their entire previous life or forget things as they occur.

The incidence of dissociative amnesia is unknown, but the disorder is most common in young adults. Amnesia is more common in people who have been involved in wars, accidents, or natural disasters. Many reports are made of people having amnesia for episodes of childhood sexual abuse, who later recalled the episodes in adulthood. Amnesia can occur after a traumatic event, and memory may return as a result of treatment, later events, or information the person receives. Nevertheless, whether such recovered memories reflect real events in the person's past remains unknown. Both accurate and inaccurate recovered memories have been demonstrated.

Causes

Dissociative amnesia appears to be caused by stress—traumatic experiences endured or witnessed, major life stresses, or tremendous internal conflicts. Episodes of amnesia may be preceded by abusive physical or sexual experiences and emotionally overwhelming situations in which there is a threat of injury or death—examples are rape, combat, or a natural disaster such as a fire or flood. Major life stresses typically include abandonment, the death of a loved one, and financial ruin. Turmoil over guilt-ridden impulses, apparently unresolvable difficulties with other people, or criminal behavior also may lead to amnesia. It is generally believed that some people, such as those who are easily hypnotized, are more likely to develop amnesia than others.

Symptoms and Diagnosis

The most common symptom of dissociative amnesia is the loss of memory. Shortly after becoming amnesic, a person may seem confused. Many amnesic persons are somewhat depressed. Some people are very distressed by their amnesia; others are not. Other symptoms and concerns depend on the importance of the forgotten information and its connection with the person's conflicts or on the consequences of forgotten behavior.

To make the diagnosis, the doctor performs physical and psychiatric examinations. The person's blood and urine are tested to determine whether a toxic substance such as an illicit drug could be causing the amnesia. An electroencephalogram may be performed to determine whether a seizure disorder is responsible.▲ Special psychologic tests can help the doctor characterize the person's dissociative experiences.

Treatment and Prognosis

A supportive environment in which the person feels secure is essential. This alone frequently leads to gradual spontaneous recovery of the missing memories.

If the memories aren't spontaneously recalled, or if the need to recall the memories is urgent, memory retrieval techniques are often success-

ful. Using hypnosis or drug-facilitated interviews, the doctor questions the amnesic person about his past. Great care is taken because the circumstances that stimulated the memory loss are likely to be recalled in the process and to be very upsetting. Memories recalled through such techniques can't be assumed to be accurate. Only external corroboration can determine their accuracy. However, filling in the memory gap to the greatest extent possible helps restore continuity to the person's identity and sense of self. Once the amnesia has disappeared, continued treatment helps the person understand the trauma or conflicts that caused the condition and find ways to resolve them.

Most people recover what appear to be their missing memories and resolve the conflicts that caused the amnesia. However, some people never break through the barriers that prevent them from reconstructing their missing past. The prognosis is determined in part by the person's life circumstances, particularly the stresses and conflicts that brought on the amnesia.

Dissociative Fugue

Dissociative fugue is a disorder in which a person has one or more episodes of sudden, unexpected, and purposeful travel from home during which he can't remember some or all of his past life and either has lost memory of who he is or has formed a new identity.

Dissociative fugue affects about 2 of every 1,000 people. It is much more common in people who have been in wars, accidents, and natural disasters.

Causes

The causes of dissociative fugue are similar to those of dissociative amnesia but with some additional factors. Often fugue occurs in circumstances under which malingering is suspected. Malingering is a state in which a person feigns illness, because it removes him from accountability for his actions, gives him an excuse to avoid responsibilities, or reduces his exposure to a known hazard, such as a dangerous job assignment. Furthermore, many fugues seem to represent disguised wish fulfillments (for example, an

▲ see box, page 348

escape from overwhelming stresses, such as divorce and financial ruin). Other fugues are related to feelings of rejection or separation, or they may protect the person from suicidal or homicidal impulses.

Symptoms and Diagnosis

A person in a fugue state, having lost his customary identity, usually disappears from his usual haunts, leaving his family and job. The person may travel far from home and begin a new job with a new identity, unaware of any change in his life. The fugue may last from hours to weeks or months, or occasionally even longer. The person may appear normal and attract no attention. However, at some point the person may become aware of the amnesia or confused about his identity. Sometimes the fugue can't be diagnosed until the person's previous identity returns, and the person is distressed to find himself in unfamiliar circumstances.

Often the person has no symptoms or is only mildly confused during the fugue. However, when the fugue ends, the person may experience depression, discomfort, grief, shame, intense conflict, and suicidal or aggressive impulses. In other words, the person suddenly may have to deal with the painful situation that the fugue allowed him to flee from. People might also feel confusion, distress, or even terror about having experienced a fugue state because they usually don't remember events that occurred during the fugue period.

A fugue is rarely recognized as it is occurring. A doctor may suspect fugue when a person seems confused about his identity or is puzzled about his past, or when confrontations challenge his new identity or absence of one. The diagnosis is usually made retroactively by a doctor reviewing the person's history and collecting information that documents the circumstances before the person left home, the travel itself, and the establishment of an alternate life. When dissociative fugues recur more than a few times, the person usually has dissociative identity disorder.

Treatment and Prognosis

Treatment for a fugue in progress entails having a doctor try to recover information about the person's true identity, to figure out why it was abandoned, and to help restore it. If the information can't be obtained directly from the person, assistance may be needed from law enforcement personnel and people working in social agencies.

Dissociative fugue is treated much the same as dissociative amnesia and may include the use of hypnosis or drug-facilitated interviews. However, often all efforts to restore the memory of the fugue period are unsuccessful. A psychiatrist may help the person to explore his patterns of handling the types of situations, conflicts, and moods that triggered (precipitated) the fugue episode.

Most fugues last hours or days and disappear on their own. Unless some behavior before or during the fugue has brought on its own complications, impairment is usually mild and short-lived. If the fugue was prolonged and the person's behavior before or during the fugue was problematic, the person may suffer considerable difficulties as a consequence. For example, a man may have abandoned his family and business responsibilities, committed a crime, or undertaken binding commitments in his fugue state.

Dissociative Identity Disorder

*Dissociative identity disorder, formerly called **multiple personality disorder**, is a condition in which two or more identities or personalities alternate in control of a person's behavior and in which there are episodes of amnesia.*

Dissociative identity disorder is a serious, chronic, and potentially disabling or fatal condition. An inability by some personalities to remember important personal information (amnesia) is mixed with simultaneous awareness of the information by other personalities. Some personalities appear to know and interact with one another in an elaborate inner world. For example, personality A may be aware of personality B and know what B does, as if observing B's behavior; personality B may or may not be aware of personality A. Other personalities may or may not be aware of personality B, and personality B may or may not be aware of them. People with this disorder frequently attempt suicide and are thought to be more likely to commit suicide than people with any other mental disorder.

Dissociative identity disorder appears to be a rather common mental disorder. It can be found in 3 to 4 percent of people hospitalized for other psychiatric problems and in a sizable minority of patients in drug abuse treatment facilities. Increased awareness of the disorder has led to it being diagnosed more often in recent years. Awareness of the consequences of child abuse and improved diagnostic methods have also led to more diagnoses of dissociative identity disorder. Although some authorities believe that increased reports of this disorder reflect the influence of doctors on suggestible patients, no evidence substantiates that view.

Causes

Dissociative identity disorder appears to be caused by the interaction of several factors:
• Overwhelming stress, such as emotional or physical abuse experienced during childhood
• An ability to separate one's memories, perceptions, or identity from conscious awareness (dissociative capacity)
• Abnormal development before a unified view of self and others can become strongly consolidated
• Insufficient protection and nurture during childhood

Human development requires that children be able to integrate complicated and different types of information and experiences. As children learn to achieve a cohesive, complex identity, they go through phases in which different perceptions and emotions are kept segregated. They may use these different perceptions to generate different selves, but not every child who suffers abuse or a major loss or trauma has the capacity to develop multiple personalities. Those who do have the capacity also have normal ways of coping, and most of these vulnerable children are sufficiently protected and soothed by adults, so dissociative identity disorder doesn't develop.

Symptoms

People with dissociative identity disorder often experience an array of symptoms that can resemble those of other psychiatric disorders. Symptoms may be similar to those of anxiety disorders, personality disorders, schizophrenic and mood disorders, or seizure disorders. Most people suffer symptoms of depression, anxiety (discomfort in breathing, rapid pulse, palpitations), phobias, panic attacks, sexual dysfunction, eating disorders, posttraumatic stress disorder, and symptoms simulating those of medical diseases. They may be preoccupied with suicide, and suicide attempts are common, as are episodes of self-mutilation. Many people with dissociative identity disorder abuse drugs or alcohol at some time in their lives.

The switching of personalities and the lack of awareness of one's behavior in the other personalities often make a person's life chaotic. Because

Dissociative Identity Disorder and Childhood Abuse: A Connection

Nearly all (97 to 98 percent) of the adults with dissociative identity disorder report having been abused during childhood. Abuse can be documented for 85 percent of the adults and 95 percent of the children and adolescents with dissociative identity disorder.

Although childhood abuse is a major cause of dissociative identity disorder, that doesn't mean all the specific abuses alleged by patients really happened. Some aspects of some reported experiences are clearly not accurate. Some patients were not abused but did suffer an important early loss, such as the death of a parent, a serious medical illness, or some other very stressful experience.

the personalities often interact with each other, people report hearing inner conversations and the voices of other personalities. This is a type of hallucination.

Several features are characteristic of dissociative personality disorder:
• Different symptoms that occur at different times
• A fluctuating ability to function, from managing well at work and home to becoming disabled
• Severe headaches or other physical pain
• Time distortions, time lapses, and amnesia
• Depersonalization and derealization—feeling detached from one's self and experiencing one's surroundings as unreal

People with dissociative identity disorder often hear from others about things they have done but don't remember doing. Others may also remark about changes in their behavior that they don't recall. They may discover objects, products, or handwriting that they can't account for or recognize. Often they refer to themselves as "we," "he," or "she." While most people can't recall much about the first 3 to 5 years of life, people with dissociative identity disorder in addition often can't remember much about childhood events that occurred between ages 6 and 11.

People with dissociative identity disorder typically have a history of three or more different previous psychiatric diagnoses and of not responding to treatment. They are very concerned with issues of control, both self-control and the control of others.

Diagnosis

To make the diagnosis of dissociative personality disorder, a doctor conducts a thorough medical and psychiatric interview, particularly inquiring about dissociative experiences. Special interviews have been developed to help doctors identify the disorder. Also, a doctor may interview the patient for prolonged periods, ask the patient to keep a journal between visits, and use hypnosis or drug-facilitated interviews to reach the personalities. These measures increase the likelihood that the person will shift from one personality to another during the evaluation.

Increasingly, doctors bring out various personalities by asking to speak to the part of the mind that was involved in a particular behavior. This behavior may be one that the patient either doesn't remember or had experienced as if he were watching it happen rather than living it (as if the experience were dreamlike or unreal).

Treatment and Prognosis

Dissociative identity disorder requires psychotherapy, usually facilitated by hypnosis. Symptoms may come and go spontaneously, but the disorder doesn't clear up on its own. Medication can relieve some specific symptoms but doesn't affect the disorder itself.

Treatment is often arduous and emotionally painful. The person may experience many emotional crises from the actions of the personalities and from the despair that may occur when traumatic memories are recalled during therapy. Several periods of psychiatric hospitalization are often necessary to help the person through difficult times and to come to grips with particularly painful memories. The doctor often uses hypnosis to help bring out (access) the personalities, facilitate communication between them, and stabilize and integrate them. Hypnosis is also used to reduce the painful impact of traumatic memories.

Generally, two or more psychotherapy sessions a week for at least 3 to 6 years are necessary. The sessions are aimed toward integrating the personalities into a single personality or toward achieving a harmonious interaction among the personalities that allows normal functioning without symptoms. Integration of personalities is ideal but not possible for all people with the disorder. Visits to the therapist are tapered off gradually but rarely terminated. Patients may come to rely on the therapist to help them deal with psychologic issues from time to time, just as they may periodically rely on their medical doctor.

The prognosis of people with dissociative identity disorder depends on the symptoms and features they experience. Some people have mainly dissociative symptoms and posttraumatic features; that is, in addition to their problems with identity and memory, they experience anxiety about traumatic events and the reliving and recalling of them. They generally function well and recover completely with treatment. Other people have additional serious psychiatric disorders, such as personality disorders, mood disorders, eating disorders, and drug abuse disorders. Their problems improve more slowly, and treatment may be either less successful or much longer and more crisis ridden. Finally, some people not only have other severe psychologic problems but also remain deeply involved with people who are alleged to have abused them. Treatment is often long and chaotic and is aimed at reducing and relieving symptoms rather than achieving integration. Sometimes even a patient with a poor prognosis will improve enough with therapy to work through the disorder and begin to make rapid strides toward recovery.

Depersonalization Disorder

Depersonalization disorder is characterized by persisting or recurring feelings of being detached from one's body or mental processes.

A person with depersonalization disorder usually feels as if he were an outside observer of his life. The person may experience himself and the world as unreal and dreamlike.

Depersonalization can be a symptom of other psychiatric disorders. In fact, depersonalization is the third most common psychiatric symptom (after anxiety and depression) and often occurs after a person experiences life-threatening danger, such as an accident, assault, or serious illness or injury. As a separate disorder, depersonalization disorder hasn't been studied widely, and its incidence and causes aren't known.

Symptoms and Diagnosis

People with depersonalization disorder have a distorted perception of their identity, body, and life, which makes them uncomfortable. Often the symptoms are temporary and appear at the same time as symptoms of anxiety, panic, or fear (phobia). However, symptoms can persist or recur for many years. People with the disorder often have a great deal of difficulty describing their symptoms and may fear or believe they are going crazy.

Depersonalization disorder can be a minor, passing disturbance with little noticeable effect on behavior. Some people can adjust to depersonalization disorder or even block its impact. Others are continually plagued with anxiety over their state of mind, worry that they are going crazy, or ruminate over the distorted perceptions of their body and their sense of estrangement from themselves and the world. Mental anguish may prevent them from focusing on work or routine activities of daily life, and they may become disabled.

The diagnosis of depersonalization disorder is based on the symptoms. A doctor evaluates the person to rule out physical disease (such as a seizure disorder), drug abuse, and the possibility of another psychiatric disorder. Special interview procedures may help the doctor recognize the problem.

Treatment and Prognosis

The feeling of depersonalization often disappears without treatment. Treatment is warranted only if the condition persists, recurs, or causes distress. Psychodynamic psychotherapy, behavior therapy, and hypnosis have been effective,▲ but no single type of treatment has proved effective for all people with depersonalization disorder. Tranquilizers and antidepressants help some people. Depersonalization is often associated with or precipitated by other mental disorders, which will need to be treated. Any stresses associated with the beginning (onset) of the depersonalization disorder must also be addressed.

Some degree of relief is usually achieved. Complete recovery is possible for many people, especially those whose symptoms occur in connection with stresses that can be addressed during treatment. A large number of people with depersonalization disorder don't respond well to treatment, although they may gradually improve on their own.

CHAPTER 91

Schizophrenia and Delusional Disorder

Schizophrenia and delusional disorder are distinct disorders that may share certain features, such as paranoia, suspiciousness, and unrealistic thinking. However, schizophrenia is a relatively common and serious mental disorder that is associated with psychosis—a loss of contact with reality—and a decline in general functioning. In contrast, delusional disorder is more rare and results in partial or more circumscribed disability.

Schizophrenia

Schizophrenia is a serious mental disorder characterized by loss of contact with reality (psychosis), hallucinations, delusions (false beliefs), abnormal thinking, and disrupted work and social functioning.

Schizophrenia is a major public health problem throughout the world. The prevalence of schizophrenia worldwide appears to be slightly less than 1 percent, although pockets of higher or lower prevalence have been identified. In the United States, people with schizophrenia occupy about one fourth of all hospital beds and account for about 20 percent of all Social Security disability days. Schizophrenia is more prevalent than Alzheimer's disease, diabetes, or multiple sclerosis.

▲ see page 389

A number of disorders share features of schizophrenia. Disorders that resemble schizophrenia, but in which symptoms have been present for less than 6 months, are called **schizophreniform disorders.** Disorders in which episodes of psychotic symptoms last at least 1 day but less than 1 month are called **brief psychotic disorders.** A disorder characterized by the presence of mood symptoms, such as depression or mania, along with more typical symptoms of schizophrenia is called **schizoaffective disorder.** A personality disorder that may share symptoms of schizophrenia, but in which the symptoms are generally not so severe as to meet the criteria for psychosis, is called **schizotypal personality disorder.**▲

Causes

Although the specific cause of schizophrenia is not known, the disorder clearly has a biologic basis. Many authorities accept a "vulnerability-stress" model, in which schizophrenia is viewed as occurring in people who are biologically vulnerable. What makes a person vulnerable to schizophrenia isn't known but may include genetic predisposition; problems that occurred before, during, or after birth; or a viral infection of the brain. Difficulty in processing information, an inability to pay attention, an impaired ability to behave in socially acceptable ways, and an inability to cope with problems in general may indicate vulnerability. In this model, environmental stresses, such as stressful life events or substance abuse problems, trigger the onset and recurrence of schizophrenia in vulnerable individuals.

Symptoms

The peak age for the onset of schizophrenia is between 18 and 25 for men and between 26 and 45 for women. However, onset in childhood or early adolescence■ or late in life is not uncommon. The onset may be sudden, over a period of days or weeks, or slow and insidious, over a period of years.

The severity and types of symptoms can vary significantly among different people with schizophrenia. Overall, the symptoms fall into three major groups: delusions and hallucinations; thought disorder and bizarre behavior; and deficit or negative symptoms. A person may have symptoms from one or all three groups. The symptoms are sufficiently severe as to interfere with the ability to work, interact with people, and care for oneself.

Delusions are false beliefs that usually involve a misinterpretation of perceptions or experiences. For example, people with schizophrenia may experience persecutory delusions, believing that they are being tormented, followed, tricked, or spied on. They may have delusions of reference, believing that passages from books, newspapers, or song lyrics are directed specifically at them. They may have delusions of thought withdrawal or thought insertion, believing that others can read their mind, that their thoughts are being transmitted to others, or that thoughts and impulses are being imposed on them by outside forces. **Hallucinations** of sound, sight, smell, taste, or touch may occur, although hallucinations of sound (auditory hallucinations) are by far the most common. A person may "hear" voices commenting on his behavior, conversing with one another, or making critical and abusive comments.

Thought disorder refers to disorganized thinking, which becomes apparent when speech is rambling, shifts from one topic to another, and loses its goal-directed quality. Speech may be mildly disorganized or completely incoherent and incomprehensible. **Bizarre behavior** may take the form of childlike silliness, agitation, or inappropriate appearance, hygiene, or conduct. Catatonic motor behavior is an extreme form of bizarre behavior in which a person may maintain a rigid posture and resist efforts to be moved or, in contrast, display purposeless and unstimulated motor activity.

Deficit or **negative symptoms** of schizophrenia include blunted affect, poverty of speech, anhedonia, and asociality. Blunted affect refers to a flattening of emotions. The person's face may appear immobile; he makes poor eye contact and lacks emotional expressiveness. Events that would normally make a person laugh or cry produce no response. Poverty of speech refers to a diminishment of thoughts reflected in a decreased amount of speech. Answers to questions may be terse, one or two words, creating the impression of an inner emptiness. Anhedonia refers to a diminished capacity to experience pleasure; the person may take little interest in previous activities and spend more time in purposeless ones. Asociality refers to a lack of interest in relation-

▲ see page 426

■ see page 1317

ships with other people. These negative symptoms are often associated with a general loss of motivation, sense of purpose, and goals.

Types of Schizophrenia

Some researchers believe schizophrenia is a single disorder, while others believe it is a syndrome (collection of symptoms) based on numerous underlying diseases. Subtypes of schizophrenia have been proposed in an effort to classify patients into more uniform groups. However, among individual patients, the subtype may change over time.

Paranoid schizophrenia is characterized by a preoccupation with delusions or auditory hallucinations; disorganized speech and inappropriate emotions are less prominent. **Hebephrenic or disorganized schizophrenia** is characterized by disorganized speech, disorganized behavior, and flat or inappropriate emotions. **Catatonic schizophrenia** is dominated by physical symptoms such as immobility, excessive motor activity, or the assumption of bizarre postures. **Undifferentiated schizophrenia** is often characterized by symptoms from all groups: delusions and hallucinations, thought disorder and bizarre behavior, and deficit or negative symptoms.

More recently, schizophrenia has been classified according to the presence and severity of negative or deficit symptoms. In people with the **negative or deficit subtype of schizophrenia,** negative symptoms, such as flattened emotions, lack of motivation, and diminished sense of purpose, are prominent. In people with **nondeficit or paranoid schizophrenia,** delusions and hallucinations are prominent, but relatively few negative symptoms are observed. Overall, people with nondeficit schizophrenia tend to be less severely disabled and more responsive to treatment.

Diagnosis

No definitive test exists to diagnose schizophrenia. A psychiatrist makes the diagnosis based on a comprehensive assessment of the person's history and symptoms. To establish the diagnosis of schizophrenia, symptoms must persist for at least 6 months and be associated with significant deterioration of work, school, or social functioning. Information from family, friends, or teachers is often important in establishing when the illness began.

The doctor will rule out the possibility that the patient's psychotic symptoms are caused by a mood disorder.▲ Laboratory tests are often performed to rule out substance abuse or an underlying medical, neurologic, or endocrine disorder that can have features of psychosis. Examples of such disorders include brain tumors, temporal lobe epilepsy, autoimmune diseases, Huntington's disease, liver disease, and adverse reactions to medications.

People with schizophrenia have brain abnormalities that may be seen on a computed tomography (CT) or magnetic resonance imaging (MRI) scan. However, the defects are insufficiently specific to be of help in diagnosing schizophrenia in individual patients.

Prognosis

Over a short time period (1 year), the prognosis of schizophrenia is closely related to how well a person follows a drug treatment plan. Without drug treatment, 70 to 80 percent of the people who have experienced a schizophrenic episode will relapse over the next 12 months and experience a subsequent episode. Drugs taken continuously can reduce the relapse rate to about 30 percent.

Over longer periods, the prognosis of schizophrenia varies. In general, one third of the people achieve significant and lasting improvement, one third achieve some improvement with intermittent relapses and residual disability, and one third experience severe and permanent incapacity. Factors associated with a good prognosis include sudden onset of illness, late age at onset, a good level of skills and accomplishments prior to becoming ill, and the paranoid or nondeficit subtype of illness. Factors associated with a poor prognosis include early age of onset, poor social and vocational functioning prior to becoming ill, a family history of schizophrenia, and the hebephrenic or deficit subtype of illness.

Schizophrenia is associated with about a 10 percent risk of suicide. On the average, schizophrenia reduces the life span of those affected by 10 years.

Treatment

The general goals of treatment are to reduce the severity of psychotic symptoms, prevent the recurrences of symptomatic episodes and the

▲ see page 402

Antipsychotic Drugs: How Do They Work?

Antipsychotic drugs appear to be most effective in treating hallucinations, delusions, disorganized thinking, and aggression. Although antipsychotic drugs are most commonly prescribed for schizophrenia, they appear to be effective in treating these symptoms whether they arise from mania, schizophrenia, dementia, or acute intoxication with a substance such as amphetamines.

The first effective antipsychotic drug, chlorpromazine, was marketed in 1955. Since then, more than a dozen similar antipsychotic drugs—fluphenazine, haloperidol, perphenazine, and thioridazine, to name a few—have been developed. Referred to as conventional antipsychotic drugs, they all work in essentially the same way: they block receptors of dopamine in the brain. Dopamine is a neurotransmitter, a chemical substance that helps carry electrical impulses along nerve pathways and between nerves. Excessive dopamine activity is associated with hallucinations and delusions. Blocking dopamine receptors can alleviate these symptoms.

Conventional antipsychotic drugs differ with regard to potency (high versus low), side effects (tendency toward sedation versus tendency toward muscle stiffness), and route of administration (oral versus injectable). Because all conventional antipsychotic drugs are equally effective in controlling the symptoms of schizophrenia, the selection of a particular drug is often based on its side effects and how well it is tolerated by an individual patient.

A relatively new class of antipsychotic drugs appears to work by blocking the receptors of both dopamine and serotonin (another neurotransmitter) in the brain. Clozapine is an example of such a drug. Clozapine has greater efficacy than conventional antipsychotic drugs in the treatment of schizophrenia symptoms. However, because it has very serious side effects, such as a dangerous drop in the white blood cell count, it is used only for people who don't respond to conventional drugs.

associated deterioration in functioning, and provide support to allow functioning at the highest level possible. Antipsychotic drugs, rehabilitation and community support activities, and psychotherapy represent the three major components of treatment.

Antipsychotic drugs can be effective in reducing or eliminating symptoms such as delusions, hallucinations, and disorganized thinking. After the acute symptoms have cleared, the continued use of antipsychotic drugs substantially reduces the probability of future episodes. Unfortunately, antipsychotic drugs have significant adverse effects that can include sedation, muscle stiffness, tremors, and weight gain. These drugs may also cause tardive dyskinesia, an involuntary movement disorder most often characterized by puckering of the lips and tongue or writhing of the arms or legs. Tardive dyskinesia may not go away even after the drug is discontinued. For those cases that persist, there is no effective treatment.

About 75 percent of the people with schizophrenia respond to conventional antipsychotic

drugs, such as chlorpromazine, fluphenazine, haloperidol, or thioridazine. Up to half of the remaining 25 percent may benefit from a relatively new antipsychotic drug called clozapine. Because clozapine can have severe side effects, such as seizures or potentially fatal bone marrow suppression, it is generally used only for patients who have not responded to other antipsychotic drugs. People who take clozapine must have their white blood cell counts measured weekly. Research is underway to identify other new drugs that don't have clozapine's potentially serious side effects. Risperidone is already available, and several other drugs are on the verge of FDA approval.

Rehabilitation and community support activities are directed at teaching the skills needed to survive in the community. These skills enable people with schizophrenia to work, shop, care for themselves, manage a household, and get along with others. Although hospitalization may be needed during severe relapses, and involuntary hospitalization may be necessary if the person poses a danger to himself or others, the general goal is to have people with schizophrenia live in the community. To achieve this goal, some people may need to live in a supervised apartment or group home where someone can ensure that drugs are taken as prescribed.

A small number of people with schizophrenia are unable to live independently, either because they have severe and unresponsive symptoms or because they lack the skills necessary to live in the community. They usually require full-time care in a safe and supportive setting.

Psychotherapy is another important aspect of treatment. Generally, the goal of psychotherapy is to establish a collaborative relationship between the patient, family, and doctor. That way the patient might learn to understand and manage his illness, to take antipsychotic drugs as prescribed, and to manage stresses that can aggravate the illness.

Delusional Disorder

Delusional disorder is characterized by the presence of one or more false beliefs that persist for at least 1 month.

In contrast to schizophrenia, delusional disorder is relatively uncommon and functioning is less impaired. The disorder generally first affects people in middle or late adult life.

The delusions in delusional disorder tend to be nonbizarre and involve situations that could conceivably occur in real life, such as being followed, poisoned, infected, loved at a distance, or deceived by one's spouse or lover. Several subtypes of delusional disorder are recognized.

In the **erotomanic subtype,** the central theme of the delusion is that another person is in love with the individual. Efforts to contact the object of the delusion through telephone calls, letters, or even surveillance and stalking may be common. Behavior related to the delusion may come in conflict with the law.

In the **grandiose subtype,** the person is convinced that he has some great talent or has made some important discovery.

In the **jealous subtype,** the person is convinced that a spouse or lover is unfaithful. This belief is based on incorrect inferences supported by dubious "evidence." Under such circumstances, physical assault may be a significant danger.

In the **persecutory subtype,** the person believes that he is being plotted against, spied on, maligned, or harassed. The person may repeatedly attempt to obtain justice by appealing to courts and other government agencies. Violence may be resorted to in retaliation for imagined persecution.

The **somatic subtype** involves a preoccupation with a bodily function or attribute, such as an imagined physical deformity, odor, or parasite.

Symptoms and Diagnosis

A delusional disorder may arise from a preexisting paranoid personality disorder.▲ Beginning in early adulthood, people with a paranoid personality disorder demonstrate a pervasive distrust and suspiciousness of others and their motives. Early symptoms may include feeling exploited, being preoccupied with the loyalty or trustworthiness of friends, reading threatening meanings into benign remarks or events, bearing grudges for a long time, and responding readily to perceived slights.

After ruling out other specific conditions that are associated with delusions, a doctor bases the diagnosis of delusional disorder largely on the person's history. It is particularly important for the doctor to assess the degree of dangerousness, particularly the extent to which the person is willing to act on his delusions.

Prognosis and Treatment

Delusional disorder does not generally lead to severe impairment or changes in personality. However, the person may become progressively involved with the delusion. Most people are able to remain employed.

A good doctor-patient relationship helps in the treatment of delusional disorder. Hospitalization may be needed if the doctor believes the patient is dangerous. Antipsychotic drugs aren't generally used but are sometimes effective in suppressing symptoms in some cases. A long-term treatment goal is to shift the person's focus away from the delusion to a more constructive and gratifying area, although this goal is frequently difficult to achieve.

▲ see page 426

Drug Dependence and Addiction

Addiction is the compulsive activity and overwhelming involvement with a specific activity. The activity may be gambling or may involve the use of almost any substance, such as a drug. Drugs can cause either psychologic dependence or both psychologic and physical dependence.

Psychologic dependence is based on a desire to continue taking a drug to induce pleasure or to relieve tension and avoid discomfort. Drugs that produce psychologic dependence usually act on the brain and have one or more of the following effects:

- Reduce anxiety and tension
- Cause elation, euphoria, or other pleasurable mood changes
- Produce feelings of increased mental and physical ability
- Alter sense perceptions

Psychologic dependence can be very powerful and difficult to overcome. It is particularly common with mood- and sensation-altering drugs that affect the central nervous system.

For addicts, drug-related activity becomes such a large part of daily life that an addiction generally interferes with the ability to work, study, or interact normally with family and friends. With severe dependence, the addict's thoughts and activities may be predominantly directed toward obtaining and taking the drug. An addict may manipulate, lie, and steal to pursue the addiction. Addicts have difficulty giving up drug use and often return to it following periods of abstinence.

Some drugs cause **physical dependence,** but physical dependence doesn't always accompany psychologic dependence. With drugs that cause physical dependence, the body adapts to the drug when it is used continually, leading to tolerance and to withdrawal symptoms when use stops. **Tolerance** is the need to progressively increase the dose of a drug to reproduce the effect originally achieved by smaller doses. **Withdrawal** symptoms occur when drug use is stopped or when the drug's effects are blocked by an antagonist. A person undergoing withdrawal feels sick and may develop many symptoms, such as headaches, diarrhea, or shaking (tremors). With-drawal can evoke a serious and even life-threatening illness.

Drug abuse involves more than a drug's physiologic actions. For example, people with cancer whose pain is treated for months or years with opioids such as morphine almost never become narcotic addicts, although they may become physically dependent. Rather, drug abuse is a concept defined mainly by behaviors that are dysfunctional and by societal disapproval. Almost every society throughout recorded history has sanctioned the use of some psychoactive drugs, even those known to be unhealthy. Mood-altering substances, such as alcohol and hallucinogenic mushrooms, play an important role in some religious rituals. Some societies accept substances that others don't permit. Societies may accept a substance and later reject it.

In the United States, the medical term *drug abuse* refers to dysfunction and maladaptation, but not dependence, brought on by the use of drugs. Colloquially, drug abuse often refers to the experimental and recreational use of illegal drugs, the use of legal drugs to relieve problems or symptoms in ways not prescribed by a doctor, and the use of drugs to the point of dependence. Drug abuse occurs in all socioeconomic groups and involves highly educated and professional people as well as those who are uneducated and unemployed.

Although abused drugs have powerful effects, the user's mood and the setting where a drug is taken significantly influence its effect. For example, a person who feels sad before drinking alcohol may become sadder as the alcohol takes effect. The same person might be cheered when drinking with friends who are happy when intoxicated. Predicting exactly what a drug will do for the same person each time it is used isn't always possible.

How drug dependence develops is complex and unclear. The process is influenced by the drug's chemical properties, the drug's effects, the drug user's personality, and other predisposing conditions, such as heredity and social pressures. In particular, the progression from experimentation to occasional use and then to tolerance and de-

Drugs That May Lead to Dependence

Drug	Psychologic Dependence	Physical Dependence
Depressants (downers)		
Alcohol	Yes	Yes
Narcotics	Yes	Yes
Sleep aids (hypnotics)	Yes	Yes
Benzodiazepines (antianxiety drugs)	Yes	Yes
Inhalants	Yes	Possibly
Volatile nitrites	Possibly	Probably not
Stimulants (uppers)		
Amphetamine	Yes	Yes
Methamphetamine (speed)	Yes	Yes
Methylenedioxymethamphetamine (MDMA, Ecstasy, Adam)	Yes	Yes
Cocaine	Yes	Yes
2-5-dimethoxy-4-methylamphetamine (DOM, STP)	Yes	Yes
Phencyclidine (PCP, angel dust)	Yes	Yes
Hallucinogens		
Lysergic acid diethylamide (LSD)	Yes	Possibly
Marijuana	Yes	Possibly
Mescaline	Yes	Possibly
Psilocybin	Yes	Possibly

pendence is poorly understood. People at high risk for addiction based on family history have not been proven to have biologic or physiologic differences in the way they respond to drugs, although some studies indicate that alcoholics may have a genetically diminished response to the effects of alcohol.

Much attention has been given to the so-called addictive personality. People who are addicted often have low self-esteem, are immature, are easily frustrated, and have difficulty solving personal problems and relating to people of the opposite sex. Addicts may try to escape reality and have been described as fearful, withdrawn, and depressed. Some have a history of frequent suicide attempts or self-inflicted injuries. Addicts have sometimes been described as having dependent personalities, grasping for support in their rela-

Effects of Alcohol in Nonalcoholics

Alcohol Level in the Blood	Effects
0.05 (50 mg/dL*)	Social high; tranquillity
0.08 (80 mg/dL)	Reduced coordination (reduced mental and physical abilities) Slowed reflexes (Both impair safe driving)
0.10 (100 mg/dL)	Noticeably impaired coordination
0.20 (200 mg/dL)	Confusion Reduced memory Severe impairment (unable to stand)
0.30 (300 mg/dL)	Loss of consciousness
0.40 (400 mg/dL and higher)	Coma, death

*Amount of alcohol in milligrams (mg) per deciliter (dL) of blood.

tionships and having difficulty taking care of themselves. Others exhibit overt and unconscious rage and uncontrolled sexual expression; they may use drugs to control their behavior. However, evidence suggests that most of these traits emerge as a result of long-term addiction and aren't necessarily an antecedent of drug abuse.

At times, family members or friends may behave in ways that allow an addict to continue to abuse drugs or alcohol; these people are considered codependents (also referred to as "enablers"). Codependents may call in sick for an addict or make excuses for the person's behavior. For example, a friend may say, "Pete didn't mean to put his fist through the wall; he was just a little upset because the bar ran out of his favorite beer." The codependent may plead with the addict to stop using drugs or alcohol but rarely does anything else to help the addict change his behavior.

▲ see page 1214

A family member or friend who cares should encourage the addict to stop abusing drugs and to enter a treatment program. If the addict refuses to seek help, the family member or friend may eventually have to threaten to pull back from regular contact. Such an approach seems harsh but can be coupled with a professionally guided intervention. This can be one way to convince an addict that behavioral changes must be made.

A pregnant addict exposes her fetus to the drugs she's using. Often, the pregnant addict doesn't admit to her doctors and nurses that she's abusing drugs or alcohol. The fetus may become physically dependent. Soon after delivery, the newborn can experience severe or even fatal withdrawal, ▲ particularly when the doctors and nurses haven't been informed of the mother's addiction. Babies who survive withdrawal may have many other problems.

Finally, a major concern with any illegal drug is that it isn't always what it is purported to be. Quality control with illegal drugs is nonexistent, and poor quality (widely varying degrees of potency or even misrepresentation of drug contents) represents yet another hazard of drug use.

Alcoholism

Alcoholism is a chronic disease characterized by a tendency to drink more than was intended, unsuccessful attempts at stopping drinking, and continued drinking despite adverse social and occupational consequences.

Alcoholism is common. Nearly 8 percent of adults in the United States have some problem with alcohol use. Men are four times more likely than women to become alcoholics. People of all ages are susceptible. Increasingly, children and adolescents have alcohol problems, with especially disastrous consequences.

Alcohol produces both psychologic and physical dependence. Alcoholism usually interferes with the ability to socialize and to work and leads to many other destructive behaviors. Alcoholics are frequently intoxicated, often daily. Drunkenness may disrupt family and social relationships; married couples often divorce. Extreme absenteeism from work can lead to unemployment. Alcoholics often can't manage their behavior, tend to drive while drunk, and suffer physical injury from falls, fights, or motor vehicle accidents. Some alcoholics may also become violent.

Causes

The cause of alcoholism is unknown, but alcohol use isn't the only factor. Of the people who drink alcohol, about 10 percent become alcoholics. Blood relatives of alcoholics have a higher incidence of alcoholism than people at random. Also, alcoholism is more likely to develop in the biologic children of alcoholics than in the adopted children, which suggests that alcoholism involves a genetic or biochemical defect. Some research suggests that people at risk for alcoholism are less easily intoxicated than nonalcoholics; that is, their brains are less sensitive to the effects of alcohol.

Aside from a possible genetic defect, certain background and personality traits may predispose a person to alcoholism. Alcoholics frequently come from broken homes, and relationships with their parents are often disturbed. Alcoholics tend to feel isolated, lonely, shy, depressed, or hostile. They may exhibit self-destructive behaviors, and they may be sexually immature. Nonetheless, alcohol abuse and dependency are so common that alcoholics can be identified among people of every personality type.

Biologic Effects

Alcohol is rapidly absorbed from the small intestine into the bloodstream. Because alcohol is absorbed faster than it's metabolized and eliminated from the body, alcohol levels in the blood rise rapidly. A small amount of alcohol in the blood is excreted unchanged in the urine, sweat, and exhaled air. The vast majority of alcohol is metabolized by the liver and yields about 210 calories for each ounce (7 cal/mL) of pure alcohol consumed.

Alcohol immediately depresses brain functions; how much so depends on its level in the blood—the higher the level, the greater the impairment. Levels of alcohol can be measured in the blood or estimated by measuring the amount in a sample of exhaled breath. State laws limit the level of blood alcohol a person can have while driving. Most states set the limit for driving at 0.1 (100 milligrams of alcohol per deciliter of blood), but other states (California, for example) set the limit at 0.08. Even a blood alcohol level of 0.08 can reduce a person's ability to drive a car safely.

Effects of Prolonged Alcohol Use

Type of Deficit	Effect
Nutritional	
Low folic acid levels	Anemia, birth defects
Low iron levels	Anemia
Low niacin levels	Pellagra (skin damage, diarrhea, depression)
Gastrointestinal	
Esophagus	Inflammation (esophagitis), cancer
Stomach	Inflammation (gastritis), ulcers
Liver	Inflammation (hepatitis), cirrhosis, cancer
Pancreas	Inflammation (pancreatitis), low blood sugar levels, cancer
Cardiovascular	
Heart	Abnormal heartbeat (arrhythmia), heart failure
Blood vessels	High blood pressure, atherosclerosis, stroke
Neurologic	
Brain	Confusion, reduced coordination, poor short-term memory (poor recall of recent events), psychosis
Nerve	Deterioration of nerves in arms and legs that control movements (reduced ability to walk)

Prolonged use of excessive amounts of alcohol damages many organs of the body, particularly the liver, brain, and heart. Like many other drugs, alcohol tends to induce tolerance, so that people who regularly have more than two drinks a day can drink more alcohol than nondrinkers without becoming intoxicated. Alcoholics also can become tolerant to other depressants; for example, those who take barbiturates or benzodiazepines usually need higher doses to achieve a therapeutic effect. Tolerance doesn't appear to alter the way alcohol is metabolized or excreted. Rather, alcohol induces the brain and other tissues to adapt to its presence.

If an alcoholic suddenly stops drinking, withdrawal symptoms are likely. **Alcohol withdrawal syndrome** usually begins 12 to 48 hours after a person stops drinking alcohol. Mild symptoms include tremor, weakness, sweating, and nausea. Some people develop seizures (called alcoholic epilepsy or rum fits). Heavy drinkers who stop drinking may develop alcoholic hallucinosis. They may have hallucinations and hear voices that seem accusatory and threatening, causing apprehension and terror. Alcoholic hallucinosis may last for days and can be controlled with antipsychotic drugs, such as chlorpromazine or thioridazine.

If left untreated, alcohol withdrawal may lead to a more serious set of symptoms called **delirium tremens** (DTs). Delirium tremens usually doesn't begin immediately; rather, it appears about 2 to 10 days after the drinking stops. In delirium tremens, the person is initially anxious and later develops increasing confusion, sleeplessness, nightmares, excessive sweating, and profound depression. The pulse rate tends to speed up. Fever may develop. The episode may escalate to include fleeting hallucinations, illusions that arouse fears and restlessness, and disorientation with visual hallucinations that may incite terror. Objects seen in dim light may be particularly terrifying. Eventually, the person becomes extremely confused and disoriented. A person with delirium tremens sometimes feels that the floor is moving, the walls are falling, or the room is rotating. As the delirium progresses, the hands develop a persistent tremor that sometimes extends to the head and body, and most people become severely uncoordinated. Delirium tremens can be fatal, particularly when untreated.

Other problems are directly related to the toxic effects of alcohol on the brain and liver. An alcohol-damaged liver is less able to rid the body of toxic substances that can cause **hepatic coma.** A

person developing hepatic coma becomes dull, sleepy, stuporous, and confused and usually develops an odd, flapping tremor of the hands. Hepatic coma is life threatening and needs to be treated immediately.

Korsakoff's syndrome (Korsakoff's amnesic psychosis)▲ usually occurs in people who regularly drink large amounts of alcohol, especially those who are malnourished and have a deficiency of B vitamins (particularly thiamine). A person with Korsakoff's syndrome loses his memory for recent events. Memory is so poor that a person often makes up stories to try to cover up the inability to remember. Korsakoff's syndrome sometimes follows a bout of delirium tremens. Some people with Korsakoff's syndrome also develop **Wernicke's encephalopathy;** symptoms include abnormal eye movements, confusion, uncoordinated movements, and abnormal nerve function. Korsakoff's syndrome can be fatal unless the thiamine deficiency is treated promptly.

In a pregnant woman, a history of chronic heavy alcohol use can be associated with severe birth defects in the developing fetus, including low birth weight, short length, small head size, heart damage, muscle damage, and low intelligence or mental retardation.■ Moderate social drinking (for example, two 4-ounce glasses of wine a day) isn't associated with these problems.

Treatment

Alcoholics who develop withdrawal symptoms generally treat themselves by drinking. Some people seek medical attention either because they don't want to continue drinking or because withdrawal symptoms are too severe. In either case, a doctor first checks for the possibility of an illness or head injury that could complicate the situation. The doctor then tries to characterize the type of withdrawal symptoms, determine how much the person usually drinks, and find out when the drinking ended.

Because vitamin deficiency causes potentially life-threatening withdrawal symptoms, doctors in emergency departments generally give large intravenous doses of vitamin C and B complex vitamins, especially thiamine. Intravenous fluids, magnesium, and glucose are often given to prevent some of the symptoms of alcohol withdrawal and to avoid dehydration.

Often, doctors prescribe a benzodiazepine drug for a few days to calm agitation and help prevent withdrawal symptoms. Antipsychotic

▲ see page 363

■ see page 1214

drugs are generally given to small numbers of people with alcoholic hallucinosis. Delirium tremens can be life threatening and is treated more aggressively to control the high fever and severe agitation. Usually intravenous fluids, drugs that lower fever (such as acetaminophen), sedatives, and close supervision are needed. With such treatment, delirium tremens generally begins to clear within 12 to 24 hours following onset.

After the urgent medical problems are resolved, a detoxification and rehabilitation program should be started. In the first phase of treatment, alcohol is completely withdrawn. Then an alcoholic has to modify his behavior. Staying sober is difficult. Without help, most people relapse within a few days or weeks. Group treatment is generally believed to be superior to one-on-one counseling; however, the treatment should be tailored to the individual. Enlisting the support of family members may be important as well.

Alcoholics Anonymous

No approach has benefited so many alcoholics as effectively as the help they can offer themselves by participating in Alcoholics Anonymous (AA). Alcoholics Anonymous operates within a religious context; alternative organizations exist for those seeking a more secular approach. An alcoholic must feel comfortable with the particular group—preferably joining one in which the members share interests aside from alcoholism. For example, some metropolitan areas have Alcoholics Anonymous groups for doctors and dentists or other professions and for people with certain hobbies, as well as for single people or homosexual men and women.

Alcoholics Anonymous provides a place where the recovering alcoholic can socialize away from the tavern with nondrinking friends who are always available for support when the urge to start drinking again becomes strong. The alcoholic hears other people confess—to the entire group—how they are struggling every day to avoid taking a drink. Finally, by providing a means to help others, Alcoholics Anonymous builds self-esteem and confidence formerly found only in drinking alcohol.

Drug Treatment

Sometimes an alcoholic can benefit from the use of a drug to avoid drinking alcohol. A drug called **disulfiram** (Antabuse) may be prescribed. This drug interferes with alcohol metabolism, causing acetaldehyde, a metabolite of alcohol, to build up in the bloodstream. Acetaldehyde is toxic and produces facial flushing, throbbing headache, rapid heart rate, rapid breathing, and sweating within 5 to 15 minutes after the person drinks alcohol. Nausea and vomiting may follow 30 to 60 minutes later. These uncomfortable and potentially dangerous reactions last 1 to 3 hours. The discomfort from drinking alcohol after taking disulfiram is so intense that few people risk taking alcohol—even the small amount in some over-the-counter cough and cold preparations or some foods.

A recovering alcoholic can't take disulfiram right after stopping drinking; the drug can be taken only after a few days of abstinence. Disulfiram can affect alcohol metabolism 3 to 7 days *after* the last dose of the drug. Because of the severe reaction to alcohol associated with the treatment, disulfiram should be given only to recovering alcoholics who really want help and are willing to cooperate with a doctor and treatment counselors. Pregnant women or people who have a serious illness shouldn't use disulfiram.

Another drug, **naltrexone**, can help people become less dependent on alcohol if it's used as part of a comprehensive treatment program that includes counseling. Naltrexone alters the effects of alcohol on certain endorphins in the brain, which may be associated with alcohol craving and consumption. A big advantage compared with disulfiram is that naltrexone doesn't make people sick. One disadvantage, however, is that a person taking naltrexone can continue to drink. Naltrexone shouldn't be taken by people who have hepatitis or liver disease.

Narcotic Addiction

Narcotic addiction is a strong psychologic and physical dependence—a compulsion to continue taking narcotics. Because tolerance develops, the dose must be continually increased to obtain the same effect, and continued use of the same or a similar narcotic is needed to prevent withdrawal.

Narcotics that have a legitimate medical use as powerful pain relievers are called opioids and include codeine (which has a low dependence potential), oxycodone (alone and in various combinations, such as oxycodone plus acetaminophen), meperidine, morphine, and hydromorphone.▲ Heroin, which is illegal in the United States, is one of the strongest narcotics.

Tolerance and mild withdrawal can develop within 2 to 3 days of continued use. Sometimes withdrawal symptoms occur when the drug is stopped. Most narcotics in equivalent doses can produce equivalent degrees of tolerance and physical dependence. Abusers may substitute one narcotic for another. People who have developed tolerance may show few signs of drug use and function normally in their usual activities as long as they have access to drugs. People who are given narcotics to treat serious pain have little risk of becoming addicted if they use the medication as prescribed.

Symptoms

Narcotics used to relieve pain may have other effects, such as constipation; flushed or warm skin and lowered blood pressure; itching; constricted pupils; drowsiness; slow, shallow breathing; a slow heart rate; and low body temperature. Narcotics may also produce euphoria, sometimes simply because a severe pain has finally been relieved.

Generally, symptoms of withdrawal are the opposite of the drug's effects: hyperactivity, a sense of heightened alertness, rapid breathing, agitation, an increased heart rate, and fever. The first sign of withdrawal is generally rapid breathing, usually accompanied by yawning, perspiration, crying, and a runny nose. Other symptoms include dilated pupils, gooseflesh, tremors, muscle twitching, hot and cold flashes, aching muscles, loss of appetite, gastrointestinal cramps, and diarrhea. Symptoms can appear as early as 4 to 6 hours after the narcotic use stops and generally peak within 36 to 72 hours. The withdrawal symptoms are worse in people who have used large doses for longer times. Because narcotics are eliminated from the body at different rates, the withdrawal symptoms differ for each drug.

▲ see box, page 292

■ see page 338

★ see page 1214

Complications

Many complications other than withdrawal arise from narcotic abuse, especially if the drugs are injected with shared, unsterilized needles. For example, viral hepatitis, which can spread through shared needles, causes liver damage. Bone infections (osteomyelitis)—particularly in the vertebrae—also can result from unsterile injections. Drug abuser's elbow (myositis ossificans) is caused by repeated, inept needle punctures; the muscle around the elbow is replaced with scar tissue. Many abusers begin with subcutaneous injections (skin popping), which can cause skin sores. As the addiction becomes stronger, the abusers may inject the drugs intravenously, returning to skin popping when their veins fill with scar tissue (tracks) and can't be injected.

Narcotic addicts develop lung problems, such as lung irritations from aspiration (inhaling saliva or vomit), pneumonia, abscesses, pulmonary emboli, and scarring, which develops from the talc in impure injections.

Problems with the immune system can develop. Addicts who inject drugs intravenously lose the ability to fight infections. Because the human immunodeficiency virus (HIV) can spread through shared needles, large numbers of people who inject narcotics also develop AIDS.

Narcotic addicts can develop neurologic problems, usually as the result of inadequate blood flow to the brain. Coma may result. Quinine, a common heroin contaminant, can cause double vision, paralysis, and other nerve injury symptoms, including Guillain-Barré syndrome.■ Infectious organisms from unsterile needles can sometimes infect the brain, causing meningitis and brain abscesses.

Other complications include skin abscesses, skin and lymph node infections, and blood clots.

Drug overdose presents a serious threat to life, particularly because narcotics can suppress respiration and can precipitate the filling of the lungs with fluid. Unanticipated high concentrations of heroin, injected or even inhaled, can lead to overdose and death.

Narcotic use during pregnancy is especially serious. Heroin and methadone easily cross the placenta into the fetus. An infant born to an addicted mother may quickly develop withdrawal symptoms, including tremors, high-pitched crying, jitters, seizures, and rapid breathing.★ A mother infected with HIV or hepatitis B may transmit the virus to her fetus.

Treatment

A narcotic overdose is a medical emergency that must be treated quickly to prevent death. The overdose may suppress breathing, and fluid may accumulate in the lungs (pulmonary edema) severely enough to require treatment with a ventilator. Doctors or emergency medical workers generally inject a drug called naloxone intravenously to block the narcotic's actions.

Few doctors have formal training or experience in treating narcotic addiction, and federal, state, and local laws limit what a doctor can do. Still, narcotic addicts should discuss their problems with a primary care doctor, who can recommend an addiction treatment center. Such centers can treat withdrawal symptoms while providing psychologic and social counseling.

Although withdrawal symptoms eventually abate, the acute withdrawal can be severe and last for several days. The unpleasant symptoms create a strong urge to start taking drugs again. The symptoms usually aren't life threatening and can be relieved with medication.

Substituting **methadone** for the narcotic is the preferred method of treating withdrawal. Methadone, itself a narcotic, is taken orally and alters brain function less than do other narcotics. Because methadone's effects last much longer than those of other narcotics, it can be taken less frequently, usually once a day. Maintaining addicts with large enough doses of methadone for months or years will enable them to be socially productive because their supply problems are met. For some, the treatment works. Others may not become socially rehabilitated.

Addicts must appear every day at a clinic, where methadone is dispensed in the smallest amount that prevents severe withdrawal symptoms from developing. Generally, 20 milligrams of methadone a day will block severe withdrawal symptoms; however, some addicts need higher doses. Once a methadone dose is established that lessens the intensity of the withdrawal reaction, the dose is usually reduced by about 20 percent a day. This leaves the person free of acute withdrawal symptoms but doesn't prevent a relapse to using heroin again.

Withdrawing from methadone maintenance can sometimes cause an uncomfortable reaction, such as deep muscle aches (bone pains). People withdrawing from methadone commonly feel upset and have trouble sleeping. Taking sleep aids for several nights may help. Many withdrawal reactions disappear after about 7 to 10 days, but weakness, insomnia, and severe anxiety may last for several months.

A few treatment centers may dispense L-alpha-acetylmethadol (LAAM), a longer-acting form of methadone. This eliminates the need to make daily clinic visits or take home medications. However, LAAM is still experimental, and the number of treatment facilities and the amount of research devoted to LAAM decreased when public funds for methadone maintenance were reduced.

Symptoms of narcotic withdrawal can also be relieved with a drug called **clonidine.** However, clonidine may cause some adverse effects, including low blood pressure, drowsiness, restlessness, insomnia, irritability, faster heartbeat, and headaches.

Naltrexone is a drug that blocks the effects of even very powerful intravenous doses of heroin. Depending on the dose, naltrexone's effects last from 24 to 72 hours. Because of this, an addict who has a stable social background can take this drug daily (or three times a week) to avoid the temptation of using heroin. A support group comprising the doctor, family, and friends is important to the treatment's success.

The **therapeutic community concept** emerged nearly 25 years ago in response to the problems of heroin addiction. Daytop Village and Phoenix House pioneered this nondrug approach. Treatment involves a communal, relatively long-term (usually 15-month) stay in a residential setting to help addicts build new lives through training, education, and redirection. These programs have helped many people, but precisely how well they've worked and how widely they should be applied remain unanswered.

The AIDS epidemic has motivated some people to suggest that sterile needles and syringes be provided to addicts who inject narcotics. Such distribution has been shown to reduce HIV transmission.

Addiction to Antianxiety Drugs and Sleep Aids

Prescription drugs used to treat anxiety and to induce sleep can cause both psychologic and physical dependence. Such drugs include benzodiazepines, barbiturates, glutethimide, chloral

Classifying the Abuse Potential of Prescription Drugs

Prescription drugs that can cause dependency are subject to restrictions dictated by United States government regulations. All prescription drugs regulated under the Controlled Substances Act are assigned a schedule or class number that determines how they may be prescribed. Substances in schedule I are considered to have a high abuse potential, no accepted medical use, and no acceptable safety data. Those in schedule II have a high abuse potential but have some appropriate medical uses. Schedule III drugs have less abuse potential; schedule IV and V drugs have the least abuse potential.

hydrate, and meprobamate. Each works in a different way and each has a different dependency and tolerance potential. Meprobamate, glutethimide, chloral hydrate, and barbiturates are prescribed less often than in the past, mainly because the benzodiazepines are safer.

Most people addicted to these drugs started out taking them for a medical reason. Sometimes a doctor may prescribe high doses for long periods to treat a severe problem, which promotes dependency. At other times, people may use more medication than is prescribed. In either case, dependency can develop within as little as 2 weeks of continual use.

Symptoms

Dependence on sleep aids and antianxiety drugs decreases alertness and results in slurred speech, poor coordination, confusion, and slowed breathing. These drugs may make a person alternately depressed and anxious. Some people experience memory losses, faulty judgment, shortened attention spans, and frightening shifts in their emotions. Older people may appear demented—they may speak slowly and have diffi-

▲ see page 301

■ see page 444

culty in thinking and in understanding others. Falls may occur that result in broken bones, especially hip fractures.

While these drugs cause sleepiness, they tend to reduce the amount of rapid eye movement (REM) sleep, the sleep stage in which dreaming takes place.▲ Interference with dreaming can make a person more irritable the next day. Sleep patterns may be seriously disturbed in people who discontinue the drug after developing both dependence and tolerance. The person may have more REM sleep than normal, more dreaming, and more frequent awakening. This sort of rebound reaction varies from person to person, but in general it is more severe and occurs more often in people who use higher drug doses for longer periods before withdrawal.

Abrupt withdrawal from any of these drugs can produce a severe, frightening, and potentially life-threatening reaction, much like alcohol withdrawal (delirium tremens).■ Serious withdrawal reactions are more common with barbiturates or glutethimide than with benzodiazepines. The person is hospitalized during the withdrawal process because of the possibility of a severe reaction.

Treatment

Stopping a severe withdrawal reaction is difficult, although treatment can relieve it. Within the first 12 to 20 hours, the person may become nervous, restless, and weak. The hands and legs may shake. By the second day, the tremors may be more severe and the person becomes even weaker. During the second and third days, most people who were taking daily doses that were eight or more times greater than the standard prescription dose have seizures, which are severe and can be fatal in the case of barbiturates and glutethimide. Occasionally, a seizure may occur even 1 to 3 weeks after withdrawal. Other effects that can occur during withdrawal include dehydration, delirium, insomnia, confusion, and visual and auditory hallucinations. Even with the best treatment, a person may not feel normal for a month or more.

Barbiturate withdrawal is generally worse than benzodiazepine withdrawal, although both can be very difficult. The time course of withdrawal reactions varies from drug to drug. Often, doctors treat withdrawal by restarting the problem drug at a lower dose and decreasing the dose over days or weeks.

Marijuana Abuse

Marijuana (cannabis) use is widespread. Surveys of high school students have periodically shown increases, decreases, and then increases in its use. In the United States, marijuana is commonly smoked in the form of cigarettes (joints) made from the stems, leaves, and flowering tops of the dried plant, almost always *Cannabis sativa*. Marijuana is also used as hashish, the pressed resin (tarry substance) of the plant. The active ingredient of marijuana is tetrahydrocannabinol (THC), which occurs in many variations, the most active being delta-9-THC. Delta-9-THC is made synthetically as a drug called dronabinol and is used in research and sometimes to treat the nausea and vomiting associated with cancer chemotherapy.

Some people become dependent on marijuana for psychologic reasons, and this dependence can have all the characteristics of severe addiction. Physical dependence on marijuana hasn't been demonstrated conclusively. As with the use of alcohol, marijuana can be used intermittently by many people without causing noticeable social or psychologic dysfunction or addiction.

Symptoms

Marijuana depresses brain activity, producing a dreamy state in which ideas seem disconnected and uncontrollable. Time, color, and spatial perceptions may be distorted and enhanced. Colors may seem brighter, sounds may seem louder, and appetite may be increased. Marijuana generally relieves tension and provides a sense of well-being. The sense of exaltation, excitement, and inner joyousness (a high) seems to be related to the setting in which the drug is taken—such as whether the smoker is alone or in a group and the prevailing mood.

Communicative and motor abilities decrease during marijuana use, so driving or operating heavy equipment is dangerous. People who use large quantities of marijuana may become confused and disoriented. They may develop a toxic psychosis, not knowing who they are, where they are, or what time it is. Schizophrenics are especially susceptible to these effects, and there is compelling evidence that schizophrenia may become worse with marijuana use. Occasionally, panic reactions occur, particularly in new users. Other effects include an increased heart rate, bloodshot eyes, and dry mouth.

Tolerance can develop in long-term marijuana users. Withdrawal reactions can include increased muscle activity (for example, jerkiness) and insomnia. However, because marijuana is eliminated from the body slowly over several weeks, a withdrawal reaction tends to be mild and is generally not perceptible to the moderate user.

Some studies have suggested that prolonged heavy use of marijuana in men may reduce the testosterone levels, the size of the testes, and the sperm count. Chronic use in women may lead to irregular menstrual cycles. However, these effects don't always occur, and the effects on fertility are uncertain. Pregnant women who use marijuana may have smaller babies than nonusers. In addition, delta-9-THC passes into the breast milk and may affect a breastfed infant in the same manner as the mother is affected.

Heavy, prolonged smoking of marijuana can have effects similar to those of cigarette smoking on the lungs. Bronchitis is common, and risk of lung cancer is probably increased.

Urine test results for marijuana generally remain positive for several days after use, even for casual users. For regular users, test results may remain positive longer while the drug is slowly released from body fat. The time is variable, depending on the percentage of THC and the frequency of use. Urine testing is an effective means of identifying marijuana use, but a positive urine test result means only that the person has used marijuana; it doesn't prove that the user is currently impaired (intoxicated). Sophisticated tests can determine up to a year later that marijuana has been ingested.

Amphetamine Abuse

Among the drugs classified as amphetamines are amphetamine, methamphetamine (speed), and methylenedioxymethamphetamine (MDMA, Ecstasy, or Adam).

Amphetamines may be chronically abused or used intermittently. Dependence is both psychologic and physical. Years back, amphetamine dependence may have started when the drugs were prescribed for weight loss, but most abuse now begins with illegal distribution of the drugs. Some amphetamines are not approved for medical use and some are manufactured and used illegally. Methamphetamine is the most commonly abused amphetamine in the United States. The abuse of MDMA, widespread in Europe for the past few years, has now reached the United States. Users often take this drug and go to "rave dances," where they dance and socialize in after-hours clubs. MDMA interferes with the reuptake of serotonin (one of the body's neurotransmitters) in the brain and is thought to be toxic to the nervous system.

Symptoms

Amphetamines increase alertness (reduce fatigue), heighten concentration, decrease the appetite, and enhance physical performance. They may induce a feeling of well-being or euphoria.

Many amphetamine abusers are depressed and use the mood-elevating effects of these stimulants to temporarily relieve the depression. Physical performance may, to some degree, temporarily improve. For example, in athletes running in a race, the difference between first and second place may be only a few tenths of a second, and amphetamines may produce that winning difference. Some people, such as long-distance truck drivers, may use amphetamines to help stay awake.

In addition to stimulating the brain, amphetamines increase the blood pressure and heart rate. Fatal heart attacks have occurred, even in healthy, young athletes. The blood pressure may become so high that a blood vessel in the brain ruptures, causing a stroke and possibly resulting in paralysis and death. Death is more likely when drugs such as MDMA are used in warm rooms with little ventilation, when the user is very active physically (for example, dancing fast), or when the user sweats heavily and doesn't drink enough water to restore lost fluids.

People who habitually use amphetamines several times a day rapidly develop tolerance. The amount used ultimately may exceed several *hundred* times the original dose. At such doses almost all abusers become psychotic, because amphetamines can cause severe anxiety, paranoia, and a distorted sense of reality. Psychotic reactions include auditory and visual hallucinations (hearing and seeing things that don't exist) and feelings of omnipotence. Although these effects can occur in any user, people with a psychiatric disorder, such as schizophrenia, are more vulnerable to them.

Treatment

Symptoms opposite to the drug's effects occur when an amphetamine is suddenly discontinued. The user will become tired or sleepy—an effect that may last for 2 or 3 days after stopping the drug. Some people are severely anxious and restless. Those abusers who were depressed when they started using amphetamines may become even more depressed when they stop. They may become suicidal but may lack the energy to attempt suicide for several days. Therefore, chronic users may need to be hospitalized during drug withdrawal.

A person experiencing delusions and hallucinations may be given an antipsychotic drug, such as chlorpromazine, which has a calming effect and alleviates distress. However, an antipsychotic drug may sharply lower the blood pressure. Usually, reassurance and a quiet, nonthreatening environment help a person to recover.

Cocaine Abuse

Cocaine produces effects similar to those of amphetamines but is a much more powerful stimulant. It may be taken orally, inhaled as a powder through the nose (snorted), or injected, usually directly into a vein (called mainlining). When boiled with sodium bicarbonate, cocaine is converted into a freebase form called crack cocaine, which can then be smoked. Crack cocaine acts almost as fast as cocaine injected intravenously. Cocaine produces a sense of extreme alertness, euphoria, and great power when injected intravenously or inhaled.

Symptoms

Cocaine increases the blood pressure and heart rate and can cause a fatal heart attack, even in healthy, young athletes. Other effects include constipation; intestinal damage; extreme nervousness; the feeling that something is moving under the skin (cocaine bugs), which is a sign of possible nerve damage; seizures (convulsions); hallucinations; sleeplessness; paranoid delusions; and violent behavior. The abuser may be dangerous to himself or others. Because cocaine's effects last only about 30 minutes, the abuser takes repeated doses. To reduce some of the extreme nervousness caused by cocaine, many addicts also abuse heroin or some other depressant, such as alcohol.

Women who become pregnant while addicted to cocaine are more likely than nonaddicts to miscarry. If the woman doesn't miscarry, the fetus may be damaged by the cocaine, which easily travels from the mother's blood into its blood-stream.▲ Babies born to addicts may have abnormal sleep patterns and poor coordination. Crawling, walking, and speech development may be delayed, but this may be the result of nutritional deficiencies, poor prenatal care, and maternal abuse of other drugs as well.

Tolerance to cocaine develops rapidly with frequent daily use. Withdrawal reactions include extreme fatigue and depression—the opposite of the drug's effects. Suicidal urges emerge when the abuser stops taking the drug. After several days, when mental and physical strength have returned, the abuser may attempt suicide.

As with intravenous heroin use, many infectious diseases, including hepatitis and AIDS, are transmitted when cocaine abusers share unsterile needles.

Diagnosis

Cocaine use is evident from the person's hyperactivity, dilated pupils, and increased heart rate. Anxiety and erratic, grandiose, and hypersexual behavior are evident with heavier use. Paranoia is often seen in those who are brought to the emergency department. Cocaine use can be confirmed by testing the urine and blood.

Treatment

Cocaine is a very short-acting drug, so treatment of a toxic reaction may not be necessary. Emergency medical staff watch the person closely to see if the dangerous (life-threatening) effects subside. Drugs may be given to lower the blood pressure or heart rate. Other drugs may be given to stop seizures. A very high fever may also require treatment.

Withdrawing from long-term cocaine abuse requires close supervision because the person may become depressed and suicidal. Entering a hospital or a drug treatment center may be necessary. The most effective methods of treating cocaine abuse are counseling and psychotherapy. Sometimes the psychologic disorders common to cocaine addicts, depression and manic-depression, are treated with antidepressants or lithium.

Hallucinogen Abuse

Hallucinogens include LSD (lysergic acid diethylamide), psilocybin (magic mushroom), mescaline (peyote), and 2,5-dimethoxy-4-methyl-amphetamine (DOM, STP), an amphetamine derivative.

These drugs generally don't produce true hallucinations; true hallucinations occur when a person believes that the abnormal things that he sees and hears are actually happening. In contrast, most hallucinogen users understand that the abnormal sensations aren't real and are caused by the drug. Therefore, these drugs are really pseudo or false hallucinogens.

Symptoms

Hallucinogens distort auditory and visual sensations. Additionally, sensations may cross over; for example, listening to music may cause colors to appear and move in time to the rhythm. The chief dangers of using these drugs are the psychologic effects and impaired judgment they produce, which can lead to dangerous decision making or accidents. For example, a user might think he can fly and may even jump out a window to prove it, resulting in severe injury or death.

Hallucinogens stimulate the brain. The actual effect can depend on the person's mood when the drug is taken and the setting in which he takes the drug. For example, users who were depressed before the drug was taken are likely to feel more sad when the drug takes effect.

The user's ability to cope with the visual and auditory distortions also affects the experience. An inexperienced, frightened user is less able to cope than someone who is more experienced and not afraid of the trip. A user under the influence of a hallucinogen, usually LSD, can develop extreme anxiety and begin to panic, resulting in a bad trip. The user may want to stop the trip, but that isn't possible. The trip is worse than a nightmare because a dreamer can wake up, ending the bad dream. A bad trip doesn't end quickly.

As the trip continues, the user begins to lose control and can temporarily become psychotic. Sometimes, a bad trip can be so severe or trigger such an innate vulnerability that the user remains psychotic for many days (or longer) after the drug's effects have worn off. A prolonged psychosis is more likely in a user with a preexisting psychologic disorder, which has become more obvious or worsened by the effects of the drug.

▲ see page 1214

Tolerance to LSD may develop; it can appear after about 72 hours of continual use. LSD users may also become tolerant to other hallucinogens. In general, people who have become tolerant to hallucinogens and abruptly stop taking them don't appear to suffer withdrawal symptoms.

Some people—especially chronic or repeated users of hallucinogens, particularly LSD—may experience flashbacks after they have discontinued abusing drugs. Flashbacks are similar to but generally less intense than the original experience. Flashbacks may be triggered by marijuana and possibly other drugs, including alcohol, or by stress or fatigue. They may also occur for no apparent reason. Generally, flashbacks disappear over a 6- to 12-month period but can recur as long as 5 years after the last use of LSD, especially when the user still suffers from an anxiety or other psychiatric disorder.

Diagnosis and Treatment

Episodes of panic and visual distortions, accompanied by various types of bizarre delusions, typify the acute use of hallucinogens. The pupils become dilated, but the heart rate isn't elevated to the same degree as with stimulants. Information from the user's friends is important to the diagnosis.

Most hallucinogen users never seek treatment. A quiet, dark room and calm, nonthreatening talk can help a user who is having a bad trip. The user needs reassurance that the effects are caused by the drug and will end. A person who experiences a prolonged psychosis may need psychiatric treatment.

Phencyclidine Abuse

Phencyclidine (PCP, angel dust), developed in the late 1950s as an anesthetic, strongly reduces pain perception. The legitimate medical use of PCP was discontinued in 1962 because patients who received it often developed severe anxiety and delusions; some became temporarily psychotic. PCP appeared as a street drug in 1967 and was often sold falsely as marijuana. All of the PCP now available on the street is synthesized illegally.

PCP is most often smoked after being sprinkled on plant material, such as parsley, mint leaves, tobacco, or marijuana. Occasionally PCP is taken orally or injected.

Symptoms

PCP depresses the brain, and abusers usually become confused and disoriented shortly after taking the drug. They may not know where they are, who they are, or what time or day it is. They may go into a trance as if hypnotized. Salivation and sweating may increase. PCP abusers can be combative, and because they don't feel pain, they may continue fighting even when hit hard. Blood pressure and heart rate also increase. Muscle tremors (shaking) are common.

Very high doses of PCP may cause high blood pressure, which can result in a stroke, auditory hallucinations (hearing voices), seizures (convulsions), a life-threatening high fever (hyperthermia), coma, and possibly death. Chronic PCP abuse may damage the brain, kidneys, and muscles. Abusers who are schizophrenic are more likely to become psychotic for days or weeks following PCP use.

Treatment

The treatment of an adverse reaction to PCP is directed at the specific effects. For example, drugs are given to lower high blood pressure or to stop seizures. When PCP abusers become agitated (as most do when brought for treatment), they are put in a quiet room and allowed to relax, although their blood pressure, heart rate, and respiration are monitored frequently. Soothing talk doesn't help; in fact, the person may become even more agitated. If quiet surroundings don't calm an agitated person, the doctor may give a tranquilizer such as diazepam. The stomach may be pumped and drugs given to hasten the excretion of PCP from the body.

Inhalant Abuse

Among teenagers, inhalants are abused more frequently than cocaine or LSD but less frequently than marijuana and alcohol. Abused inhalants are found in many common household products. These products are meant to be used only in a well-ventilated room, because many of the chemicals in them are powerful brain depressants. Even in a well-ventilated room, these chemicals have some depressant effects.

When the product's fumes are directly inhaled, the effects are stronger. The product may be sprayed into a plastic bag and inhaled (bagging, sniffing, or snorting), or a cloth soaked with the

Inhalants and Their Chemical Contents

Products	Chemicals
Adhesives	
Airplane glue	Toluene, ethyl acetate
Rubber cement	Hexane, toluene, methyl ethyl ketone, methyl butyl ketone
Polyvinyl chloride cement	Trichloroethylene
Aerosols	
Spray paint	Butane, propane, fluorocarbons, toluene, hydrocarbons
Hair spray	Butane, propane, fluorocarbons
Deodorant spray, air freshener	Butane, propane, fluorocarbons
Analgesic spray, asthma spray	Fluorocarbons
Solvents and gases	
Nail polish remover	Acetone, ethyl acetate
Paint remover	Toluene, methylene chloride, methanol acetone, ethyl acetate
Paint thinner	Petroleum distillates, esters, acetone
Typing correction fluid and thinner	Trichloroethylene, trichloroethane
Fuel gas	Propane
Cigarette lighter fluid	Butane
Gasoline	Mixed hydrocarbons
Cleaning agents	
Dry-cleaning fluid	Tetrachloroethylene, trichloroethane
Spot remover	Xylene, petroleum distillates, chlorohydrocarbons
Degreaser	Tetrachloroethylene, trichloroethane, trichloroethylene
Dessert topping sprays	
Whipped cream, whippets	Nitrous oxide (laughing gas)
Nitrite room deodorizers	
"Poppers" and "rush"	Alkyl nitrite, (iso)amyl nitrite, (iso)butyl nitrite, isopropyl nitrite, butyl nitrite

product may be placed next to the nose or in the mouth (huffing).

Symptoms

Users rapidly become intoxicated. Dizziness, drowsiness, confusion, slurred speech, and a reduced ability to stand and walk (unsteady gait) have been observed. These effects can last for minutes or more than an hour. The user may also become excited—not because the chemicals are stimulants, but because control is lost, as occurs with alcohol abuse. Death can occur, even the first time one of these products is directly inhaled, because of either severely depressed breathing or an irregular heartbeat (cardiac arrhythmia).

Some people, usually teenagers or even young children, ignite the inhaled fumes with matches, producing a fire that travels right through the nose and mouth into the lungs. The severe burns to the skin and internal organs can be fatal. Others have died of asphyxiation because the inhaled spray coated the lungs, preventing oxygen from entering the bloodstream.

Chronic abuse or exposure to these chemicals in the workplace can severely damage the brain, heart, kidneys, liver, and lungs. In addition, the bone marrow may be damaged, affecting red blood cell production and causing anemia. Although inhaling nitrous oxide (laughing gas) from whipped cream containers may seem to be harmless, prolonged exposure can cause numbness and weakness in the legs and arms, which can be permanent.

Glass vials of amyl nitrite have legitimate medical uses, for example, to relieve the chest pain caused by coronary artery disease. However, amyl nitrite can be abused, usually by homosexual men who seek to alter consciousness and enhance sexual pleasure. Amyl nitrite appears to enhance orgasm by affecting oxygen delivery to the brain. Although amyl nitrite is available through prescription or illegal synthesis, butyl nitrite and isobutyl nitrite are sold legally under a variety of names. Butyl nitrite and isobutyl nitrite briefly lower blood pressure, produce dizziness, and cause flushing, followed by a rapid heartbeat. For these reasons, they may be dangerous for people with heart conditions.

Treatment

Treating children and teenagers who abuse inhalants involves evaluating and managing any organ damage. It also involves education and counseling to address psychologic and sociologic problems. Recovery rates from inhalant abuse are among the poorest for any mood-altering substance.

Mouth and Dental Disorders

CHAPTER 93

Disorders of the Lips, Mouth, and Tongue

When healthy, the lining of the mouth (oral mucosa) is reddish pink, and the gums, which fit snugly around the teeth, are paler pink. The roof of the mouth (palate) is divided into two parts. The front part has ridges and is hard (hard palate); the back part is relatively smooth and soft (soft palate). The inside and outside surfaces of the lips are distinctly divided by a wet-dry border (the vermilion border); the outside surface is skin-like, and the inside surface is moist mucosa. The tongue is normally not smooth: Tiny projections (papillae), which contain taste buds, appear on the surface.

The mouth may be affected by local conditions (conditions affecting only a specific area of the body)—such as some infections and injuries.

Also, systemic diseases (diseases affecting the body generally)—such as diabetes, AIDS, and leukemia—can cause changes in the mouth. Sometimes, the first signs of these diseases appear in the mouth and are recognized by a dentist.

Mouth Disorders

Problems that may develop in the mouth include various sores and growths, such as canker sores and cancerous growths. Also, the lining of the mouth or the palate may undergo certain changes in color. Other problems include bad breath and salivary gland disorders.

Canker Sores

Canker sores are small, painful sores that appear inside the mouth.

The cause is unknown, but stress seems to play a role—for example, a college student may get canker sores during final exam week. A canker sore appears as a round white spot with a red border. The sore almost always forms on soft, loose tissue, particularly on the inside of the lip or cheek, on the tongue or soft palate, and sometimes in the throat. Small canker sores (less than one-half inch in diameter) often appear in groups of two or three; generally, they disappear by themselves within 10 days and don't leave scars. Larger canker sores are less common; they may be irregularly shaped, can take many weeks to heal, and frequently leave scars.

Symptoms

The main symptom of a canker sore is pain—usually far more pain than would be expected from something so small. The pain, which lasts 4 to 10 days, worsens if the tongue rubs the sore or if the person eats hot or spicy foods. Severe canker sores can cause fever, swollen neck glands, and a generally run-down feeling. Many people who get canker sores get them repeatedly—perhaps one or more times a year.

Diagnosis and Treatment

A doctor or dentist identifies a canker sore by its appearance and the pain it causes. However, sores caused by herpes simplex virus may resemble canker sores.

Treatment consists of relieving the pain until the sores heal by themselves. An anesthetic such as viscous lidocaine can be swabbed on canker sores or used as a mouth rinse. This anesthetic relieves the pain for several minutes and can make eating less painful though it may also impair a person's taste. A protective coating, carboxymethylcellulose, also may be applied to relieve the pain. If a person has many canker sores, a doctor or dentist may prescribe a tetracycline mouthwash. Also, a person who has repeated outbreaks of severe canker sores may use this mouthwash as soon as a new sore appears. Another treatment option, cauterization with silver nitrate, destroys the nerves under the canker sore. Occasionally, a doctor or dentist prescribes a corticosteroid ointment that's applied directly to severe canker sores. A dexamethasone mouth rinse or prednisone tablets can be prescribed for severe episodes.

Oral Herpes Infection

Primary oral herpes infection (primary herpetic gingivostomatitis) is an initial infection by the herpes simplex virus that can cause rapidly developing, painful sores on the gums and other parts of the mouth. Secondary herpes (recurrent herpes labialis) is a local reactivation of the virus that produces a cold sore.

Cause and Symptoms

Typically, an infant gets the herpes simplex virus from an adult who has a cold sore. The infant's first such infection (primary herpes) causes general gum inflammation and extensive mouth soreness. The child may have a fever, swollen lymph nodes in the neck, and general discomfort; thus, the child may be cranky. Most cases are mild and go unrecognized. Parents often mistake the problem for teething or another illness. Within 2 or 3 days, very small blisters (vesicles) form in the child's mouth. These may not be noticed because they rupture quickly, leaving the mouth raw and sore. The soreness may be anywhere in the mouth but always includes the gums. Though the child gets better in a week or so, the herpes simplex virus never leaves the body, and the infection commonly flares up later in life (secondary herpes). People who escape oral herpes in childhood but contract it as adults usually have more severe symptoms.

Unlike the original infection that causes widespread mouth soreness, the later flare-ups usually produce cold sores (fever blisters). These flare-ups are commonly triggered by sunburn on the lips, a cold, fever, food allergy, mouth injury, dental treatment, or anxiety. For a day or two before a blister appears, the person may feel tingling or discomfort (a prodrome) in the spot where the blister will erupt. This sensation is difficult to describe but is easily recognized by a person who has had herpes before. A raw, open sore may appear on the outer lip and then become crusty. Inside the mouth, a sore most commonly appears on the palate. Sores in the mouth start out as small blisters that quickly run together and form a painful, red sore.

Although merely a painful annoyance for most people, flare-ups of oral herpes simplex can be life-threatening in people with immune systems compromised by diseases (such as AIDS), chemotherapy, radiation therapy, or bone marrow transplants. In such people, large, persistent sores in the mouth can interfere with eating, and the spread of the virus to the brain can be fatal.

Treatment

The aim of treatment for **primary herpes** is to relieve the pain, so that the person can sleep, eat, and drink normally. The pain may keep a child from eating and drinking altogether, which, combined with a fever, can quickly lead to dehydration. Thus, a child should drink as much liquid as possible. An adult or older child can use a prescribed anesthetic mouthwash such as lidocaine to reduce pain. A mouth rinse containing baking soda may also be soothing.

Treatment for **secondary herpes** works best when started before the sore erupts—as soon as the person has the sensation that an attack is starting (prodrome). Taking vitamin C during the prodrome may make a cold sore clear up faster.

Protecting the lips from direct sunlight by wearing a brimmed hat or a lip balm containing sunscreen can reduce the chances of an outbreak of cold sores. Also, a person should avoid activities and foods that are known to cause flare-ups. Anyone who suffers frequent, severe flare-ups may benefit from taking lysine (available at health food stores) for long periods of time.

Acyclovir ointment may reduce the severity of an attack and clear up the sore more quickly. Lip balms like petroleum jelly may keep the lips from cracking and reduce the risk of spreading the virus to neighboring areas. Adults with severe sores should be given antibiotics to prevent bacterial infections, but antibiotics don't affect the virus. For severe cases and for people with immune system deficiencies, acyclovir capsules may be prescribed. Corticosteroids aren't used for herpes simplex because they may allow the infection to spread.

Other Mouth Sores and Growths

Any sore that lasts for 2 or more weeks should be examined by a dentist or a doctor, especially if it is *not* painful. Painful sores inside the lip or cheek usually have less serious causes; they can be canker sores or can result from biting the lip or cheek accidentally.

Sores inside the mouth are often white, sometimes with red borders. A mouth sore may form when a person keeps an aspirin between the cheek and gum in a misguided effort to relieve a toothache. Sores in the mouth can be a sign of Behçet's syndrome, which may also cause sores on the eyes and genitals.

A white, painless sore (chancre) that develops in the mouth or on the lips 1 to 13 weeks after a person has performed oral sex may be the first stage of syphilis. The sore usually goes away after several weeks. One to 4 months afterwards, a later sign of untreated syphilis—a white patch (mucous patch)—can also form on the lip or, more commonly, inside the mouth. Both the chancre and the mucous patch are so contagious that even kissing may spread the disease at these stages.

The floor of the mouth is a common area for cancer, particularly in middle-aged and elderly people who drink alcohol and smoke. Various types of cysts may also develop on the floor of the mouth. Often, these cysts are surgically removed because they annoy the person.

Large, fluid-filled blisters can form anywhere in the mouth. Commonly, they result from injury, but they may be related to diseases such as pemphigus. Some viral diseases, such as measles, can also cause temporary abnormalities inside the cheeks, especially in children.

Infections that spread from decayed lower teeth to the floor of the mouth can be serious. A very severe infection called Ludwig's angina can cause severe swelling in the floor of the mouth, even forcing the tongue upward, blocking the airway. When this occurs, emergency measures are needed to keep the person breathing.

When a person bites the inside of the cheek frequently, or repeatedly injures the inside of the mouth in some other way, an irritation fibroma may grow. This small, firm, painless bump can be removed surgically.

Warts can infect the mouth if a person sucks a wart growing on a finger. A different type of wart (condyloma acuminatum) may also be transmitted through oral sex. A doctor may treat a wart using several methods.

Palate

Necrotizing sialometaplasia is a sudden breakdown of the surface of the palate, creating a gaping sore in 1 or 2 days. Though the damage is often extensive and can be frightening, necrotizing sialometaplasia is painless. This disorder often follows injury to the area (during a dental procedure, for example) and clears up within 2 months.

A slow-growing projection of bone (torus) may form in the middle of the palate. This hard growth is both common and harmless. It appears during puberty and persists throughout life. Even a large growth can be left alone unless the mucosa over it gets scraped during eating or the person needs a denture that will cover the area.

Tumors on the palate, both cancerous and non-cancerous, occur most often in those between ages 40 and 60. In the early stages, there are few symptoms, though sometimes a person may notice a swelling in the palate or find that an upper denture has become unstable. Pain develops much later.

In late-stage syphilis, a hole (gumma) may appear in the palate.

Color Changes

If a person has anemia, the lining of the mouth may be pale instead of the normal healthy reddish pink. If the anemia is treated, the normal color will return.

Newly discolored areas in the mouth should be examined by a doctor or dentist because they may be a sign of an adrenal gland disease or cancer (melanoma). White areas can appear anywhere in the mouth and often are simply food debris that can be wiped away. But if the area is raw and painful and it bleeds after wiping, the problem may be a yeast infection (thrush).

White areas in the mouth may also be thickened layers of keratin; these areas are called leukoplakia. A tough protein, keratin normally protects the outermost layer of the skin but also is found in small quantities in the lining of the mouth. Sometimes keratin can build up in the mouth, particularly in people who smoke or use snuff or smokeless tobacco.

Reddened areas in the mouth (erythroplakia) may result when the lining of the mouth thins and blood vessels show through more than usual. White or red areas may be noncancerous (benign), precancerous, or cancerous (malignant). Such areas need to be checked by a dentist or doctor without delay.

A person with a fine, lacy network of white lines (lichen planus) inside the cheeks or on the side of the tongue may also have an itchy skin rash. Lichen planus can cause painful sores, but most of the time the condition causes no discomfort.

Spots that resemble tiny grains of white sand surrounded by a red ring (Koplik's spots), appearing on the inner cheeks opposite the back teeth, may be the first sign of measles.

Palate

Color changes in the palate can come from irritation or infection. The palate of a longtime pipe-smoker has a white, pebbly, hard appearance with many red spots (smoker's palate). If other sores last for more than 2 weeks, the person should see a doctor or dentist.

After a person has performed vigorous oral sex on a male partner, small pinhead-sized red spots from broken blood vessels (petechiae) may appear on the palate. These spots disappear within a few days. Such spots can also be a sign of a blood disorder or infectious mononucleosis. Red, overgrown areas on the palate most often result from poorly fitting dentures or dentures left in the mouth too long. Generally, all removable dental appliances, except for orthodontic retainers, should be taken out at bedtime, cleaned, and placed in a cup of water. In a person with AIDS, purplish patches caused by Kaposi's sarcoma may appear on the palate. To relieve discomfort and improve the palate's appearance, a doctor can treat these patches.

Bad Breath

Bad breath (halitosis) can be real or imagined. When real, it's most often caused by a combination of food lodged between the teeth and poor oral hygiene that results in gum disease and infection. Proper brushing and flossing can eliminate the problem.

Odors from foods that contain volatile oils, such as onions and garlic, pass from the bloodstream into the lungs and are breathed out. Oral hygiene can't remove these odors.

Certain diseases also produce bad breath. Liver failure gives the breath a mousy odor; kidney failure makes the breath smell like urine; and severe, uncontrolled diabetes makes the breath smell like nail polish remover (acetone). A lung abscess causes very severe halitosis.

Salivary Gland Problems

The largest pair of salivary glands lies just behind the angle of the jaw, in front of the ears. Two smaller pairs are deep in the floor of the mouth. Tiny salivary glands are distributed throughout the mouth.

When the flow of saliva is insufficient, the mouth feels dry. Because saliva offers some natural protection against tooth decay, less saliva can lead to more cavities. A dry mouth can result from drinking too little liquid, breathing through the mouth, or taking certain medications or from diseases that affect the salivary glands such as Sjögren's syndrome. The mouth also dries out somewhat as a person ages. A duct draining a salivary gland can be blocked by an accumulation of calcium called a stone. Such blockage makes saliva back up, causing the gland to swell. It also may become infected with bacteria. If swelling worsens just before mealtime or particularly when a person is eating a pickle, it surely results from a blocked duct. Here's why: Anticipating the sour pickle's taste stimulates saliva flow, but if the duct is blocked, the saliva has no place to go. Sometimes, a dentist can push the stone out by pressing on both sides of the duct. If that fails, a fine-wire–like instrument can be used to pull the stone out. As a last resort, the stone can be removed surgically.

An injury to the lower lip—for instance, from biting—may harm a tiny salivary gland and block the flow of saliva. As a result, the gland may swell and form a small, soft lump (mucocele) that appears bluish. Over a few weeks, the lump usually disappears by itself, but it can easily be removed by dental surgery if it becomes bothersome or frequently recurs.

Mumps, certain bacterial infections, and other diseases can cause the major salivary glands to swell. Swelling also can result from cancerous or noncancerous tumors in the salivary glands; this swelling is usually firmer than that caused by infection. If the tumor is cancerous, the gland may feel stone-hard.

Inflammation and infection of the salivary glands, often caused by a stone blocking the salivary duct, develop more frequently than tumors. Nevertheless, any salivary gland swelling warrants medical attention. To determine the cause of swelling, a dentist or doctor may obtain a sample (biopsy) of salivary gland tissue.

Locating the Major Salivary Glands

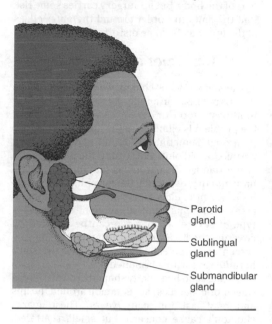

Parotid gland

Sublingual gland

Submandibular gland

Changes in the Lips

The lips may undergo changes in size, color, and surface. Some of these changes are harmless—for instance, as people age, their lips may grow thinner. Other changes may indicate medical problems.

Lip Size

An allergic reaction can make the lips swell. The reaction may be caused by sensitivity to certain foods, medications, cosmetics, or airborne irritants. But at least half the time, the cause remains a mystery.

Several other conditions can cause the lips to swell. One inherited condition, angioedema, causes recurrent bouts of swelling. Noninherited conditions—such as erythema multiforme, sunburn, or trauma—may also cause the lips to swell. Certain types of severe lip enlargement may be reduced with steroid injections. For other types, excess lip tissue may be removed surgically to improve appearance.

With age, the lips may grow thinner. They can be enlarged for cosmetic reasons using collagen injections or injections of fat taken from another part of the body. But lip surgery carries some risk that the smooth border around the outer edges of the lips may become distorted.

Lip Color and Surface

The sun's rays or cold, dry weather can make the lips peel. So can an allergic reaction to lipstick, toothpaste, food, or beverages. After the cause of the problem is eliminated, the lips usually return to normal. Sometimes, a doctor may prescribe a corticosteroid ointment to stop the peeling.

Sun damage in particular may make the lips hard and dry, especially the lower lip. Red speckles or a white, filmy look signals damage that increases the chance of subsequent cancer. This type of severe sun damage can be reduced by covering the lips with a lip balm containing sunscreen or by shielding the face from the sun's harmful rays with a brimmed hat.

Freckles and irregularly shaped brownish areas (melanotic macules) are common around the lips and may last for many years. These marks shouldn't cause concern, but small, scattered, brownish-black spots may be a sign of an inherited intestinal disease in which polyps form in the stomach and intestines (Peutz-Jeghers syndrome). Kawasaki syndrome can cause dryness and cracking of the lips and reddening of the lining of the mouth.

With inflammation of the lips (cheilitis), the corners of the mouth may become painful, irritated, red, cracked, and scaly. Fungus (thrush) may grow in the corners of the mouth, keeping them sore. Cheilitis may result from a lack of the B vitamin riboflavin in the diet, but this deficiency is rare in the United States.

Vertical skinfolds and irritated skin may develop in the corners of the mouth if complete dentures don't separate the jaws adequately. Treatment consists of adjusting or replacing the dentures.

A raised area or a sore with hard edges on the lip may be a form of skin cancer.

Changes in the Tongue

Injury is the most common cause of tongue discomfort. The tongue has many nerve endings for pain and touch and is far more sensitive to pain than most other parts of the body. The tongue is frequently bitten accidentally but heals quickly. A sharp, broken filling or tooth can do considerable damage to this delicate tissue.

An overgrowth of the normal projections on the tongue can give it a hairy appearance. These "hairs" may become discolored if a person smokes or chews tobacco, eats certain foods, or has colored bacteria growing on the tongue. The tongue may also appear hairy after fevers, after antibiotic treatment, or when peroxide mouthwash is used too often. The top of the tongue may look black if a person takes bismuth preparations for an upset stomach. Brushing the tongue with a toothbrush can get rid of such discoloration. A mesh of white lines or white curdlike material on the sides of the tongue that can be wiped away and leaves a bleeding surface may indicate thrush.

Redness of the tongue may be a sign of pernicious anemia or a vitamin deficiency. Iron deficiency anemia may also make the tongue look pale and smooth (because of a loss of its normal projections). The first sign of scarlet fever may be a change from the tongue's normal color to a strawberry, and then raspberry, color. Whitish patches, similar to those sometimes found inside the cheeks, may accompany fever, dehydration, the second stage of syphilis, thrush, lichen planus, leukoplakia, or mouth breathing. A smooth red tongue and painful mouth may indicate pellagra, a type of malnutrition caused by a deficiency of niacin in the diet. In geographic tongue, some areas of the tongue are white, and others are red and smooth. The areas of discoloration seem to move around over a period of years or a lifetime. The condition is usually painless, and no treatment is needed.

Although small bumps on both sides of the tongue are usually harmless, a bump on only one side may be cancerous. Unexplained red or white areas, sores, or lumps on the tongue—especially if painless—may be signs of cancer and should be examined by a doctor. Most mouth cancers grow on the sides of the tongue or on the floor of the mouth. Cancer almost never grows on the top of the tongue.

Sores on the tongue can be caused by herpes simplex virus, tuberculosis, bacterial infection, or early-stage syphilis. Sores can also be caused by allergies or by immune system diseases.

Glossitis is inflammation (redness, pain, swelling) of the tongue. Glossodynia is a burning or painful sensation of the tongue. Usually, it has no characteristic appearance or obvious cause; however, pressure exerted on the teeth by the tongue, an allergic reaction, or irritants such as alcohol, spices, or tobacco may cause this sensation.

Changing brands of toothpaste, mouthwash, or chewing gum may provide relief. Glossodynia is sometimes a sign of emotional upset or mental illness. Low doses of antianxiety medications can help. Regardless of cause, the condition often goes away with time.

CHAPTER 94

Tooth Disorders

To maintain healthy teeth, a person must remove plaque daily with a toothbrush and dental floss. Also, to reduce the risk of tooth decay, a person should limit the amount of sugar consumed. Fortunately, fluoridated water helps reduce this risk.

Limiting both tobacco and alcohol use keeps the mouth and teeth healthy, too. Tobacco—whether it's smoked, chewed, or dipped—makes gum disease worse. Tobacco, alcohol, and especially the combination of alcohol and tobacco cause mouth cancer.

Cavities

Cavities (dental caries) are decayed areas in the teeth, the result of a process that gradually dissolves a tooth's hard outer surface (enamel) and progresses toward the interior.

Along with the common cold and gum disease, cavities are among the most common human afflictions. If cavities aren't properly treated by a dentist, they continue growing. Ultimately, an untreated cavity can lead to tooth loss.

Cause

For tooth decay to develop, a tooth must be susceptible, acid-producing bacteria must be present, and food must be available for the bacteria to thrive. A susceptible tooth is one that has relatively little fluoride or has pronounced pits, grooves, or fissures that retain plaque (the collection of bacteria that accumulates on teeth). Although the mouth contains large numbers of bacteria, only certain types cause decay. The most common decay-causing bacterium is *Streptococcus mutans.*

Decay develops differently, depending on its location in the tooth. **Smooth surface decay,** the most preventable and reversible type, grows the slowest. In smooth surface decay, a cavity begins as a white spot where bacteria are dissolving the calcium of the enamel. Smooth surface decay between the teeth usually begins between ages 20 and 30.

Pit and fissure decay, which usually starts during the teen years in the permanent teeth, forms in the narrow grooves on the chewing surface and the cheek side of the back teeth; this decay progresses rapidly. Many people can't adequately clean these cavity-prone areas because the grooves are narrower than the bristles of a toothbrush.

Root decay begins on the bone-like tissue covering the root surface (cementum) that has been exposed by receding gums, usually in people past middle age.▲ This type of decay often results from difficulty cleaning the root areas and from a diet high in sugar. Root decay can be the most difficult type to prevent.

Decay in the enamel, the hard outer layer of the tooth, progresses slowly. After penetrating into the second layer of the tooth—the somewhat softer, less resistant dentin—decay spreads more rapidly and moves toward the pulp, the innermost part of the tooth, which contains the nerves and blood supply. Although a cavity may take 2 or 3 years to penetrate the enamel, it can travel from the dentin to the pulp—a much greater distance—in as little as a year. Thus, root decay that

▲ see page 467

How Cavities Develop

The illustration on the left shows a tooth with no cavities; the illustration on the right shows a tooth with the three types of cavities.

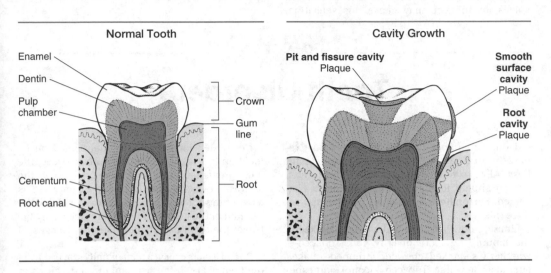

Normal Tooth

Enamel

Dentin

Pulp chamber

Crown

Gum line

Cementum

Root canal

Root

Cavity Growth

Pit and fissure cavity
Plaque

Smooth surface cavity
Plaque

Root cavity
Plaque

starts in the dentin can destroy a lot of tooth structure in a short time.

Symptoms

Not all tooth pain is caused by cavities. Toothaches may result from roots that are exposed but not decayed, excessively forceful chewing, or fractured teeth. Sinus congestion can make the upper teeth sensitive.

Usually, a cavity in the enamel causes no pain; the pain starts when the decay reaches the dentin. A person may feel pain only when drinking something cold or eating candy. This indicates that the pulp is still healthy. If the cavity is treated at this stage, the dentist can usually save the tooth, and most likely no further pain or chewing difficulties will develop.

A cavity that gets close to or actually reaches the pulp causes irreversible damage. Pain lingers even after a stimulus (cold water, for example) is removed. The tooth may even hurt without stimulation (spontaneous toothache).

When bacteria enter the pulp and the pulp dies, the pain may stop temporarily. But in a short time (hours to days), the tooth becomes sensitive when the person bites or when the tongue or a

finger presses on it because inflammation and infection spread out just beyond the end of the root, causing an abscess (a collection of pus). Pus accumulating around the tooth tends to push it out of its socket. Biting pushes it back in place, causing extreme pain. Pus can continue to accumulate and cause swelling in the adjacent gum or can spread more broadly through the jaw (cellulitis) and drain into the mouth or even through the skin near the jaw.

Diagnosis and Prevention

If a cavity is treated before it starts to hurt, the chance of damage to the pulp is reduced, and more of the tooth structure is saved. To detect cavities early, a dentist inquires about pain, examines the teeth, probes the teeth with dental instruments to test for sensitivity and softness, and may take x-rays. A person should have a dental examination every 6 months, though every examination will not include x-rays. Depending on the dentist's assessment of a person's teeth, x-rays may be taken anywhere from every 12 to 36 months.

Five general strategies are key to preventing cavities: good oral hygiene, proper diet, fluoride, sealants, and antibacterial therapy.

Oral Hygiene

Good oral hygiene, which involves brushing before or after breakfast and before bedtime and flossing daily to remove plaque, can effectively control smooth surface decay. Brushing prevents cavities from forming on the sides of the teeth, and flossing gets between the teeth where a brush can't reach. Food debris can be cleaned from beneath the gum margin and from the surfaces facing the lips, cheeks, tongue, and palate with a rubber-tipped gingival stimulator.

For a person with normal manual dexterity, proper brushing takes only about 3 minutes. Initially, plaque is quite soft, and removing it with a soft-bristled toothbrush and dental floss at least once every 24 hours makes decay unlikely. Once plaque becomes calcified, a process that begins after about 24 hours, removing it becomes more difficult.

Diet

Although all carbohydrates can cause tooth decay to some degree, the biggest culprits are sugars. All simple sugars have the same effect on the teeth, including table sugar (sucrose) and the sugars in honey (levulose and dextrose), fruits (fructose), and milk (lactose). Whenever sugar comes in contact with plaque, *Streptococcus mutans* bacteria in the plaque produce acid for about 20 minutes. *The amount of sugar eaten is irrelevant; the amount of time the sugar stays in contact with the teeth is the important issue.* Thus, sipping a sugary soft drink over an hour is more damaging than eating a candy bar in 5 minutes, even though the candy bar contains more sugar.

A person who tends to develop cavities should eat sweet snacks less often. Rinsing the mouth after eating a snack removes some of the sugar; brushing the teeth is more effective. Drinking artificially sweetened soft drinks also helps, though diet colas contain acid that can promote tooth decay. Drinking tea or coffee without sugar also can help people avoid cavities, particularly on exposed root surfaces.

Fluoride

Fluoride can make the teeth, particularly the enamel, more resistant to the acid that helps

The Language of Dentists

What most people call it	What dentists call it
Adult tooth	Permanent tooth
Baby tooth	Deciduous tooth
Back teeth	Molars
Bite	Occlusion
Braces	Orthodontic bands and wires, appliances
Cap	Crown
Cavities	Caries
Cleaning	Prophylaxis
Filling	Restoration
Front teeth	Incisors and canines
Gum	Gingiva
Gum disease	Periodontal disease, periodontitis
Harelip	Cleft lip
Laughing gas	Nitrous oxide
Lower jaw	Mandible
Plate	Complete or partial denture
Roof of the mouth	Palate
Side teeth	Bicuspids
Silver filling	Amalgam restoration
Tartar	Calculus
Uneven bite	Malocclusion
Upper jaw	Maxilla

Root Canal Treatment for a Badly Damaged Tooth

1. The tooth is anesthetized.

2. A rubber dam is placed around the tooth to isolate it from bacteria in the rest of the mouth.

3. An opening is drilled through the chewing surface of a back tooth or the tongue side of a front tooth.

4. Fine instruments are passed through the opening, into the pulp canal space, and all the remaining pulp is removed.

5. The canal is smoothed and tapered from the opening to the end of the root.

6. The canal is sealed with a filling.

cause cavities. Fluoride taken internally is particularly effective while the teeth are growing and hardening—until about age 11. Water fluoridation is the most efficient way to supply children with fluoride, and over half of the United States population now has drinking water with enough fluoride to reduce tooth decay. However, if a water supply has too much fluoride, the teeth can become spotted or discolored. If a child's water supply doesn't have enough fluoride, a doctor or dentist can prescribe sodium fluoride drops or tablets. A dentist may apply fluoride directly to the teeth of a person of any age who is prone to tooth decay. Toothpaste containing fluoride is also beneficial.

Sealants

Sealants may be used to protect hard-to-reach grooves on the back teeth. After thoroughly cleaning the area to be sealed, a dentist conditions the enamel and places a liquid plastic in and over the grooves of the teeth. When the liquid hardens, it forms such an effective barrier that any bacteria inside a groove stop producing acid because food can no longer reach them. A sealant lasts fairly long—about 90 percent remain after 1 year and 60 percent after 10 years—but may occasionally need repair or replacement.

Antibacterial Therapy

Some people have especially active, decay-causing bacteria in their mouth. A parent may pass these bacteria to a child, presumably by kissing. The bacteria flourish in the child's mouth after the first teeth come in and can then cause cavities. So a tendency toward tooth decay that runs in families doesn't necessarily reflect poor oral hygiene or bad eating habits.

For people who are very prone to decay, antibacterial therapy may be needed. The dentist first removes decayed areas and seals all pits and fissures in the teeth. Then the dentist prescribes a powerful mouth rinse (chlorhexidine) for several weeks to kill off the bacteria in any remaining plaque. The hope is that less harmful bacteria will replace the cavity-causing bacteria. To keep bacteria under control, the person may use daily home fluoride rinses and chew gum containing xylitol.

Treatment

If decay is halted before it reaches the dentin, the enamel can repair itself, and the white spot on the tooth disappears. Once decay reaches the dentin, the decayed part of the tooth must be removed and replaced with a filling (restoration). Treating the decay at an early stage helps maintain the strength of the tooth and limits the chance of damage to the pulp.

Fillings

Fillings are made of various materials and may be put inside the tooth or around it. Silver amalgam is most commonly used for fillings in back teeth, where strength is important and the silver color is relatively inconspicuous. Silver amalgam is relatively inexpensive and lasts an average of 14 years. Gold fillings (inlays) are more expensive, and at least two dental visits are required; however, they are stronger and can be used in very large cavities.

Composite resins and porcelain fillings are used in the front teeth, where silver would be conspicuous. Increasingly, these fillings are also being used in back teeth. Although they have the advantage of being the color of the teeth, they are more expensive than silver amalgam and may not last as long, particularly in the back teeth, which must take the full force of chewing.

Crowns, Bridges, and Implants

Damaged Tooth

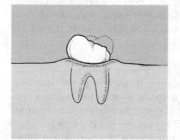

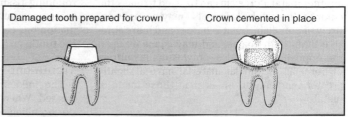

| Damaged tooth prepared for crown | Crown cemented in place |

To repair a damaged tooth, a dentist first prepares it by altering its shape. Then the dentist cements the crown onto the reshaped tooth.

Missing Tooth

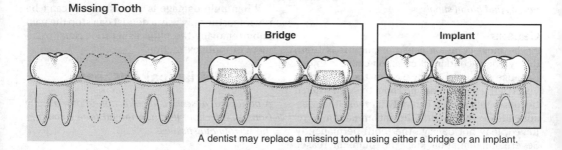

| Bridge | Implant |

A dentist may replace a missing tooth using either a bridge or an implant.

Glass ionomer, a tooth-colored filling, is formulated to release fluoride once in place, a benefit for people prone to decay at the gum line. Glass ionomer is also used to restore areas damaged by overzealous brushing.

Root Canal Treatment and Tooth Extraction

When decay advances far enough to permanently harm the pulp, the only way to eliminate the pain is to remove the pulp by root canal (endodontic) treatment or tooth extraction. Back teeth that have had root canal treatment are best protected by a crown, which replaces the entire chewing surface. The restoration method for front teeth that have had root canal treatment depends on the amount of tooth that remains.

Rarely, fever, headache, and swelling of the jaw, floor of the mouth, or throat may develop a week or two after root canal treatment. If such complications develop, the person should be examined by a dentist or doctor.

If the tooth is extracted, it should be replaced as soon as possible. Otherwise, neighboring teeth may change position and alter the person's bite. The replacement may be a bridge—a fixed partial denture in which teeth on either side of the missing tooth are covered with caps—or a removable denture. Also, implants may be used to replace missing teeth.

A crown is a restoration that fits over a tooth. Getting a properly shaped crown usually takes two visits to the dentist, though sometimes it takes several visits. On the first visit, the dentist prepares the tooth by tapering it slightly, takes an impression of the prepared tooth, and puts a temporary crown on it. A permanent crown is then fashioned in a dental prosthetics laboratory, using the impression. On the next visit, the temporary crown is removed, and the permanent crown is cemented onto the prepared tooth.

Usually, crowns are made of an alloy of gold or another metal. Porcelain can be used to mask the color of the metal. Crowns also may be made entirely of porcelain, but it is harder and more abrasive than tooth enamel and may cause wear on the opposing tooth. Also, crowns made entirely of porcelain or similar material have a slightly greater tendency to break than those made of metal.

Pulpitis

Pulpitis is painful inflammation of the tooth pulp, the innermost part of the tooth that contains the nerves and blood supply.

Causes

The most common cause of pulpitis is tooth decay; the second most common cause is injury. Because the pulp is encased in the unyielding walls of the tooth, it has no room to swell when it becomes inflamed. It can only increase the pressure inside the tooth. Mild inflammation, if relieved, may not damage the tooth permanently. Severe inflammation kills the pulp. Increased pressure may push the pulp out through the end of the root where it can injure the jawbone and surrounding tissues.

Symptoms and Diagnosis

Pulpitis causes intense tooth pain. To determine if the pulp is healthy enough to save, a dentist can perform certain tests. For example, a dentist can apply a cold stimulus. If the resulting pain from the stimulus stops within a few seconds after the cold stimulus is removed, the pulp is still healthy. The dentist can save it by removing the decayed part of the tooth and putting in a filling. However, if pain persists after the cold stimulus is removed or if pain occurs spontaneously, the pulp isn't healthy enough to save.

A dentist may also use an electric pulp tester, which indicates whether the pulp is alive but not whether it's healthy. If the person feels the small electrical charge delivered to the tooth, the pulp is alive. Sensitivity to tapping on a tooth often means that inflammation has spread to the surrounding tissue and bone. X-rays can confirm tooth decay and show whether spreading inflammation has caused bone loss around the root of the tooth.

Treatment

The inflammation stops when the cause is treated. When pulpitis is detected early, a temporary filling containing a sedative can eliminate the pain. This filling can be left in place for 6 to 8 weeks and then replaced with a permanent filling. Sometimes a permanent filling can be put in immediately.

When pulp damage is extensive and can't be reversed, the only way a dentist can stop the pain is by removing the pulp, using root canal treatment or tooth extraction.

Periapical Abscess

A periapical abscess is a collection of pus, usually from an infection, that has spread from a tooth to the surrounding tissues.

Cause

The body attacks infection with large numbers of white blood cells; pus is the accumulation of these white blood cells and dead tissue. Usually, pus from a tooth infection drains into the gums first, so the gums swell near the root of the tooth. Depending on the location of the tooth, the pus may then drain to the skin, mouth, throat, or skull.

Treatment

A dentist treats an abscess or cellulitis by eliminating the infection and draining the pus, which requires oral surgery or root canal treatment. Dentists often prescribe antibiotics to help eliminate the infection, but removing the diseased pulp and draining the pus are more important.

Periodontal Diseases

Periodontal diseases inflame and destroy the structures surrounding and supporting the teeth, primarily the gums, bone, and the outer layer of the tooth root.

Periodontal diseases are caused mainly by accumulation of bacteria. They can be affected by some general body conditions, such as diabetes mellitus, poor nutrition, leukemia, and AIDS as well as by smoking.

Gingivitis

Gingivitis is inflammation of the gums (gingiva).

Inflamed gums are red and swollen and bleed easily. Gingivitis, an extremely common condition, can develop any time after a person's teeth come in.

Causes and Symptoms

Gingivitis is almost always the result of inadequate brushing and flossing that allows plaque to remain along the gum line of the teeth. Plaque—a soft, sticky film made up primarily of bacteria—accumulates especially in faulty fillings and around the teeth next to poorly cleaned partial dentures, bridges, and orthodontic appliances. When plaque stays on the teeth for more than 72 hours, it hardens into tartar (calculus), which can't be completely removed by brushing and flossing. Although plaque is the main cause of gingivitis, other factors can make the inflammation worse, especially pregnancy, puberty, and birth control drugs.

Some **drugs** can cause an overgrowth of the gums, so that removing plaque becomes more difficult, and gingivitis often develops. Phenytoin (taken to control seizures), cyclosporine (taken by people who have had organ transplants), and calcium channel blockers such as nifedipine (taken to control blood pressure and heart rhythm disturbances) can cause such an overgrowth. Also, birth control pills or injections can aggravate gingivitis.

In **simple gingivitis,** the gums look red rather than pink. They swell and become movable instead of being firm and tight against the teeth. When the person brushes or eats, the gums often

bleed. If gingivitis is severe, the pillowcase may be bloodstained in the morning, particularly if the person breathes through the mouth while asleep.

In rare instances, **vitamin deficiencies** can cause gingivitis. Vitamin C deficiency (scurvy) can lead to inflamed, bleeding gums. Niacin deficiency (pellagra) also causes inflamed, bleeding gums and a predisposition to certain mouth infections.

Acute herpetic gingivostomatitis is a painful viral infection▲ of the gums and other parts of the mouth. The infection turns the gums bright red and causes many small, white or yellow sores inside the mouth.

Gingivitis of pregnancy, a worsening of mild gingivitis during pregnancy, is caused primarily by hormonal changes. However, some pregnant women may contribute to the problem by neglecting oral hygiene because they feel nauseated in the morning. During pregnancy, a minor irritation, often a buildup of tartar, may cause a lump-like overgrowth of gum tissue, called a pregnancy tumor. The bloated tissue bleeds easily if injured and may get in the way of eating.

Desquamative gingivitis is a poorly understood, painful condition that occurs most commonly in postmenopausal women. In this condition, the outer layers of the gums separate from the underlying tissue, exposing nerve endings. The gums become so loose that the outer layers can be rubbed away with a cotton swab or blown off with a dentist's air syringe.

Gingivitis of leukemia is the first sign of disease in about 25 percent of children with leukemia. An infiltration of leukemia cells into the gums causes the gingivitis, and reduced infection-fighting ability worsens it. The gums appear red and bleed easily. Often, the bleeding continues for several minutes or more because the blood doesn't clot normally in people with leukemia.

In **pericoronitis,** the gum swells over a tooth that hasn't fully emerged, usually a lower wisdom tooth. The flap of gum over the partially emerged tooth can trap fluids, bits of food, and bacteria. If the upper wisdom tooth emerges before the lower

▲ see page 456

one, it may bite on this flap, increasing the irritation. Infections can develop and spread to the throat or cheek.

Prevention and Treatment

Simple gingivitis can be prevented with good oral hygiene—the daily use of a toothbrush and dental floss. People who form a lot of tartar can use a tartar-control toothpaste that contains pyrophosphate. After tartar forms, only a professional cleaning (prophylaxis) can remove it. People with poor oral hygiene, medical conditions that can lead to gingivitis, or a tendency to produce plaque may need professional cleanings more often. Depending on how fast tartar forms, a person may need professional cleanings every 3 months to every year. Because of their excellent blood supply, the gums quickly become healthy again after tartar and plaque are removed as long as the person brushes and flosses carefully.

Medical conditions that might cause or worsen gingivitis should be treated or controlled. If a person must take a drug that causes gum tissue overgrowth, the excess gum tissue may need to be removed surgically. However, meticulous oral hygiene at home and frequent professional cleanings may slow the rate of overgrowth and eliminate the need for surgery.

Vitamin C and niacin deficiencies can be treated with the appropriate vitamin supplement and improved diet.

Acute herpetic gingivostomatitis usually gets better in 2 weeks without treatment. Intensive cleaning doesn't help, so a person should brush gently while the infection is still painful. A dentist may recommend an anesthetic mouth rinse to relieve discomfort during eating and drinking.

If a pregnant woman is neglecting oral hygiene because she becomes nauseated, a dentist can suggest ways to keep the teeth and gums clean without nausea. A woman may have a bothersome pregnancy tumor (a noncancerous gingival growth) surgically removed, but such tumors tend to recur until the pregnancy ends.

If desquamative gingivitis develops during menopause, hormone replacement therapy may help. Otherwise, a dentist may prescribe corticosteroid tablets or a corticosteroid paste that's applied directly to the gums.

To prevent bleeding, a person with gingivitis of leukemia should gently wipe the teeth and gums with a gauze pad or sponge instead of brushing and flossing. A dentist can prescribe chlorhexidine mouth rinse to control plaque and prevent mouth infections. When the leukemia is under control, good dental care can restore the gums to good health.

When a person has pericoronitis, a dentist may flush under the flap to rinse out the debris and bacteria. If x-rays show that a lower tooth is not likely to emerge completely, a dentist may remove the upper tooth and prescribe antibiotics for a few days before removing the lower one. Sometimes a dentist removes the lower tooth immediately.

Trench Mouth

Trench mouth (Vincent's infection, acute necrotizing ulcerative gingivitis) is a painful, noncontagious infection of the gums causing pain, fever, and fatigue.

The term trench mouth comes from World War I when many soldiers in the trenches developed the infection. Poor oral hygiene usually contributes to its development, as does physical or emotional stress, poor diet, or lack of sleep. The infection occurs most often in people who have simple gingivitis and experience a stressful event—for example, taking college exams or changing jobs. The condition is far more common among smokers than nonsmokers.

Symptoms

Usually, trench mouth begins abruptly with painful gums, an uneasy feeling, and fatigue. A foul breath odor also develops. The tips of the gums between the teeth erode and become covered with a gray layer of dead tissue. The gums bleed easily, and eating and swallowing cause pain. Often, the lymph nodes under the jaw swell, and a low-grade fever develops.

Treatment

Treatment begins with a gentle, thorough cleaning, during which the dentist removes all the dead gum tissue and tartar from the area. Because the cleaning can be painful, the dentist may use a local anesthetic. The patient may be told to rinse with hydrogen peroxide solution (3 percent hydrogen peroxide mixed half-and-half with water) several times a day instead of brushing for the first few days after the cleaning.

The patient visits the dentist every day or two for about 2 weeks. Professional cleanings continue until healing is well along. If the gums don't return to their normal shape and position, the dentist surgically reshapes them to prevent a recurrence or periodontitis. When trench mouth is severe or dental care isn't available, an antibiotic may be prescribed.

Periodontitis

Periodontitis (pyorrhea) occurs when gingivitis extends to the supporting structures of the tooth.

Periodontitis is one of the main causes of tooth loss in adults and is the main cause in older people.

Cause

Most periodontitis results from a long-term accumulation of plaque and tartar between the teeth and the gums. Pockets form between the teeth and gums and extend downward between the root of the tooth and the underlying bone. These pockets collect plaque in an oxygen-free environment, which promotes the growth of bacteria. If the condition continues, eventually so much jawbone near the pocket is destroyed that the tooth loosens.

The rate at which periodontitis develops differs considerably even among people with similar amounts of tartar. That's probably because their plaque contains different types and numbers of bacteria and because people have different responses to the bacteria. Periodontitis may produce bursts of destructive activity that last for months followed by periods when the disease apparently causes no further damage.

Many medical conditions—including diabetes mellitus, Down syndrome, Crohn's disease, a lack of white blood cells, and AIDS—can predispose a person to periodontitis. In people with AIDS, periodontitis progresses quickly.

Symptoms and Diagnosis

The early symptoms of periodontitis are bleeding, red gums, and bad breath (halitosis). Dentists measure the depth of the pockets in the gums with a thin probe, and x-rays show how much bone has been lost. As more and more bone is

Periodontitis: From Plaque to Tooth Loss

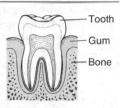

Healthy gums and bone hold the tooth firmly in place.
— Tooth
— Gum
— Bone

Plaque buildup irritates the gums, and they become inflamed. In time, the gums pull away from the tooth, creating a pocket that fills with more plaque.
— Plaque
— Pocket

The pockets get deeper, and the plaque hardens into tartar. More plaque accumulates on top.
— Tartar

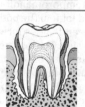

Plaque moves down to the root of the tooth and eventually destroys the bone supporting the tooth. Without this support, the tooth loosens and falls out.

lost, the teeth loosen and change position. Frequently, the front teeth tilt outward. Periodontitis usually doesn't cause pain until the teeth loosen enough to move while chewing or an abscess (collection of pus) forms.

Treatment

Unlike gingivitis, which usually disappears with good self-care, periodontitis requires professional care. A patient using good oral hygiene can clean only one twelfth of an inch below the gum line. A dentist can clean pockets up to one fifth of an inch deep using scaling and root planing, which thoroughly remove tartar and the diseased root surface. For pockets of one fourth of an inch or more, surgery is often required. A dentist or periodontist may also remove part of the separated gum so that the rest of the gum can reattach tightly to the teeth and the person can remove plaque at home.

A dentist may prescribe antibiotics, especially if an abscess has developed. A dentist may also insert antibiotic-impregnated filaments into deep pockets, so that high concentrations of the drug can reach the diseased area. Periodontal abscesses cause a burst of bone destruction, but immediate treatment with surgery and antibiotics may allow much of the damaged bone to grow back. When the mouth is sore after surgery, a 1-minute chlorhexidine mouth rinse twice a day may be temporarily substituted for brushing and flossing.

CHAPTER 96

Disorders of the Temporomandibular Joint

The temporomandibular joints are the two places—one on each side of the face, just in front of the ears—where the temporal bone of the skull connects to the lower jaw (mandible). Ligaments, tendons, and muscles support the joints and are responsible for jaw movement.

The temporomandibular joint is the most complicated joint in the body: It opens and closes like a hinge and slides forward, backward, and from side to side. During chewing, it sustains an enormous amount of pressure. The temporomandibular joint contains a piece of specialized cartilage called a disk that keeps the lower jawbone and skull from rubbing against each other.

Temporomandibular joint disorders, often called **TMJ**, include problems with the joints and the muscles surrounding them. Most often, the cause of temporomandibular joint disorder is a combination of muscle tension and anatomic problems within the joints. Sometimes, there's a psychological component as well. These disorders are most common in women between ages 20 and 50.

Symptoms include headaches, tenderness of the chewing muscles, and clicking or locking of the joints. Sometimes the pain seems to occur near the joint rather than in it. Temporomandibular joint disorder may be the reason for recurring

headaches that don't respond to usual medical treatment.

Dentists almost always diagnose temporomandibular joint disorder based simply on a person's medical history and a physical examination. Part of the examination involves pushing on the side of the face or placing the little finger in the person's ear and gently pressing forward while the person opens and closes the jaw. Also, the dentist gently palpates the muscles used for chewing to detect pain or tenderness and notes whether the jaw slides when the person bites.

Special x-ray techniques can help a dentist make the diagnosis. When a dentist suspects that the disk lies in front of its normal position (a condition called internal derangement), an x-ray in which dye is injected into the joint (an arthrogram) may be used. Though expensive, a computed tomography (CT) or magnetic resonance imaging (MRI) scan is used in rare instances to find out why a person isn't responding to treatment. Laboratory tests are rarely useful. Dentists occasionally use electromyography, which analyzes muscle activity, to monitor treatment and less commonly to make a diagnosis.

Eighty percent of people get better in 6 months without any treatment. From most to least common, temporomandibular joint disorders requiring treatment are muscle pain and tightness, in

An Inside Look at the Temporomandibular Joint

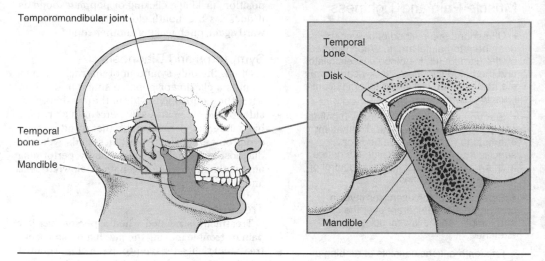

Temporomandibular joint

Temporal bone

Mandible

Temporal bone

Disk

Mandible

---

ternal derangement, arthritis, injury,▲ reduced or excessive mobility of the joint, and developmental (birth) abnormalities.

Muscle Pain and Tightness

Muscle pain and tightness around the jaw come mainly from muscle overuse, often brought on by psychological stress that causes a person to clench or grind the teeth (bruxism). Most people can place the tips of their index, middle, and ring fingers held vertically in the space between the upper and lower front teeth without forcing. When a person has problems with the muscles around the temporomandibular joint, this space usually is smaller.

Symptoms

People with muscle pain usually have very little pain in the joint itself. Rather, they feel pain and tightness on the sides of the face upon awakening or after stressful periods during the day. This pain and tightness result from muscle spasms brought on by repeated muscle or tooth clenching and tooth grinding. Clenching and grinding while asleep exert far more force than grinding while awake.

Treatment

People who realize that they clench or grind their teeth can take steps to break the habit. Usually, splint therapy is the main treatment. A thin plastic splint (nightguard) is made to fit over either the upper or lower set of teeth (usually the upper) and is adjusted to give the person an even bite. The splint reduces daytime and nighttime grinding, allowing the jaw muscles to rest and recover. The splint can also prevent damage to teeth that are under exceptional stress from the grinding.

A dentist may prescribe physical therapy, which can consist of ultrasound treatment, electromyographic biofeedback, spray and stretch exercises, or friction massage. Transcutaneous electrical nerve stimulation also may help. Stress management, sometimes along with electromyographic biofeedback, often brings dramatic improvement.

A dentist also may prescribe medication. For instance, a muscle-relaxing drug may be prescribed to ease tightness and pain, particularly while a patient waits for a splint to be made. How-

▲ see page 475

Physical Therapy for Jaw Muscle Pain and Tightness

• Ultrasound is a method of delivering deep heat to painful areas. When warmed by the ultrasound, the blood vessels dilate, and the blood can more quickly carry away the accumulated lactic acid that may cause muscle pain.

• Electromyographic biofeedback monitors muscle activity with a gauge. The patient attempts to relax the entire body or a specific muscle while watching the gauge. In this way, the patient learns to control or relax particular muscles.

• Spray and stretch exercises involve spraying a skin refrigerant over the cheek and temple, so the jaw muscles can be stretched.

• Friction massage consists of rubbing a rough towel over the cheek and temple to increase circulation and speed lactic acid removal.

• Transcutaneous electrical nerve stimulation involves using a device that stimulates the nerve fibers that do not transmit pain. The resulting impulses are thought to block the painful impulses the patient has been feeling.

ever, medications aren't a cure, generally aren't recommended for older people, and are prescribed for only a short time, usually for a month or less. Analgesics such as nonsteroidal antiinflammatory drugs (aspirin, for example) also relieve pain. Dentists avoid prescribing narcotics because they can be habit forming. Sleeping pills may be used occasionally to help people who have trouble sleeping because of the pain.

Internal Derangement

In internal derangement, the disk inside the joint lies in front of its normal position.

In internal derangement without reduction, the disk never slips back into its normal position, and jaw movement is limited. In internal derangement with reduction, which is more common, the disk lies in front of its normal position only when the mouth is closed. As the mouth opens and the jaw slides forward, the disk slips back into its normal position, making a clicking or popping sound as it does. As the mouth closes, the disk slips forward again, often making another sound.

Symptoms and Diagnosis

Often, the only symptom of internal derangement is a clicking or popping sound in the joint when the mouth opens wide or the jaw shifts from side to side. As many as 20 percent of all people have internal derangement that produces no symptoms except for these joint sounds. A dentist diagnoses internal derangement by performing an examination while the patient slowly opens and closes the mouth.

Treatment

Treatment is needed when a person has jaw pain or trouble moving the jaw. If a person seeks treatment right after symptoms develop, a dentist may be able to push the disk back into its normal position. If the person has had the condition for less than 3 months, the dentist may apply a splint that holds the lower jaw forward. This splint keeps the disk in position, permitting the supporting ligaments to tighten. Over 2 to 4 months, the dentist adjusts the splint to allow the jaw back to its normal position, with the expectation that the disk will remain in place.

A dentist instructs a person with internal derangement to avoid opening the mouth wide—for instance, when yawning or biting into a thick sandwich. People with this condition need to stifle yawns, cut food into small pieces, and eat food that's easy to chew.

If the condition can't be treated by nonsurgical means, an oral-maxillofacial surgeon may perform surgery to reshape the disk and sew it back into place. However, the need for surgery is relatively rare.

Often, people with internal derangement also have jaw muscle pain and tightness; after the muscle pain is treated, the other symptoms go away too. Dentists are more successful in treating muscle pain and tightness than in treating internal derangement.

Arthritis

Arthritis can affect the temporomandibular joints the same way it affects other joints. Osteoarthritis (degenerative joint disease), a type of arthritis in which the cartilage of the joints degenerates, is most common in older people. The cartilage in the temporomandibular joints isn't as strong as the cartilage in other joints. Because osteoarthritis occurs mainly when the disk is missing or has developed holes, the person feels a grating sensation in the joint when opening and closing the mouth. When osteoarthritis is severe, the top of the jawbone flattens out, and the person can't open the mouth wide. The jaw may also be shifted toward the affected side, and the person may be unable to move it back. Even without treatment, most of the symptoms improve after a few years, probably because the band of tissue behind the disk becomes scarred and functions like the original disk.

Rheumatoid arthritis affects the temporomandibular joint in only about 17 percent of people with this type of arthritis. When rheumatoid arthritis is severe, especially in young people, the top of the jawbone may degenerate and shorten. This damage can lead to sudden misalignment of many or all of the upper and lower teeth (malocclusion). If the damage is severe, the jawbone may eventually fuse to the skull (ankylosis), greatly limiting the ability to open the mouth. Rheumatoid arthritis usually affects both temporomandibular joints about equally, which is rarely the case in other types of temporomandibular joint disorders.

Arthritis in a temporomandibular joint also may result from injury, particularly injury that causes bleeding into the joint. Such injuries are fairly common in children who are struck on the side of the chin.

Treatment

A person with **osteoarthritis** in a temporomandibular joint needs to rest the jaw as much as possible, use a splint or other device to control muscle tightness, and take an analgesic for pain. The pain usually goes away in 6 months with or without treatment. Usually, jaw movement is sufficient for normal activities, though the jaw may not open as wide as it used to.

Rheumatoid arthritis of the temporomandibular joint is treated with the drugs used for rheumatoid arthritis of any joint; these may include an-

algesics, corticosteroids, methotrexate, and gold compounds. Maintaining joint mobility and preventing ankylosis (fusion of the joint) are particularly important. Usually, the best way to accomplish these goals is by exercising under a physical therapist's direction. To relieve symptoms, particularly muscle tightness, the person wears a splint at night that doesn't restrict jaw movement. If ankylosis freezes the jaw, the person may need surgery and, in rare cases, an artificial joint to restore jaw mobility.

Ankylosis

Ankylosis is loss of joint movement resulting from fusion of bones within the joint or calcification of the ligaments around it.

Typically, calcification of the ligaments around the joint isn't painful, but the mouth can open only about 1 inch or less. Fusion of bones within the joint causes pain and more severely limits jaw movement. Occasionally, stretching exercises help people with calcification, but people with calcification or bone fusion usually need surgery to restore jaw movement.

Hypermobility

Hypermobility (looseness of the jaw) results when the ligaments that hold the joint together become stretched.

In a person with hypermobility, the jaw may slip forward completely out of its socket (dislocation), causing pain and an inability to close the mouth. This can happen repeatedly. When it happens, a helper should stand in front of the person, place the thumbs on the gums next to the lower back teeth, and press first down and then back on the outer surface of the teeth. The jaw should snap back into position. The helper needs to keep the thumbs away from the chewing surfaces because the jaws close with considerable force.

Prevention consists of avoiding opening the mouth wide, so that the ligaments aren't excessively stressed. Thus, the person should stifle yawns and avoid large sandwiches and other foods that require opening the mouth wide. If dislocations occur frequently, surgery may be needed to reposition or shorten the ligaments and make the joint tighter.

Developmental Abnormalities

Abnormalities of the temporomandibular joint at birth are uncommon. Sometimes the top of the jawbone doesn't form or is smaller than normal. Other times, the top of the jawbone grows faster or for a longer time than normal. These abnormalities can cause facial deformities and misalignment of the upper and lower sets of teeth. Only surgery can correct these problems.

CHAPTER 97

Urgent Dental Problems

Certain dental problems require early treatment to relieve discomfort and minimize damage to the structures of the mouth. These problems include some toothaches; fractured, loosened, and knocked-out teeth; jaw fractures; and certain complications that develop after dental treatment. None of these problems is life threatening.

Toothaches

A toothache may result from a cavity,▲ an abscess,■ inflammation of the gum around the root of a tooth (pericoronitis),★ or sinus inflammation (sinusitis).●

If several upper teeth hurt when a person is chewing or is bending down (for instance, to tie a shoe), the cause is probably sinusitis—especially if the toothache develops while the person has a cold. Sinusitis can be diagnosed by a dentist or a doctor. Treatment is usually an antibiotic for the infection and a decongestant to help the infected sinuses drain. Inhaling steam for a day or two may also help.

Fractured, Loosened, and Knocked-Out Teeth

A person who has brief, sharp pain both while chewing and while eating something cold may have an incomplete (greenstick) fracture of a tooth. As long as the fracture is incomplete and part of the tooth hasn't split off, the dentist can correct the problem with a filling (restoration).

The upper front teeth, particularly protruding teeth (buck teeth), are prone to injury and fracture. If after an injury a tooth isn't sensitive to air, most likely only the hard outer surface (enamel) has been harmed. Even if the enamel has sustained a small chip, immediate treatment isn't required.

Fractures of the intermediate layer of the tooth (dentin) are usually painful when exposed to air and food, so people with such fractures seek dental help quickly. If the fracture affects the innermost part of the tooth (pulp), a red spot and often some blood will appear in the fracture. Root canal treatment may be needed to remove the remaining pulp before it dies and causes severe pain. If the patient is under age 12, root canal treatment may be postponed until the roots of the affected teeth are fully formed.◆

If an injury loosens a tooth in the socket or if the surrounding gum tissue bleeds a great deal, a person should see a dentist. Damaged baby (deciduous) teeth in the front of the mouth usually aren't a problem. If the damage is severe, the teeth can be removed without harming the permanent teeth or losing space for those that are yet to come. When the damaged deciduous teeth are in the back of the mouth, the dentist inserts a space-maintainer appliance, so that the permanent teeth won't be crowded out.

A knocked-out (avulsed) permanent tooth requires immediate treatment. The tooth should be wiped off with a clean tissue and placed back in its socket. If that isn't possible, the tooth should be placed in a glass of milk (the milk provides a

▲ see page 461

■ see page 466

★ see page 467

● see page 1016

◆ see page 465

good medium for sustaining the tooth). In either case, the patient and the tooth should be taken immediately to the nearest dentist. If a tooth is reimplanted within 30 minutes, the likelihood of long-term success is good. The longer the tooth is out of the socket, the worse the chances for long-term success. The dentist usually splints the tooth to the surrounding teeth for 7 to 10 days. Most reimplanted teeth eventually need root canal treatment. If the bone around the tooth also has been fractured, the tooth may have to be splinted for 6 to 10 weeks.

Jaw Fracture

A fractured jaw causes pain and usually changes the way the teeth fit together. Often, the mouth can't be opened wide or it shifts to one side when opening or closing. Most jaw fractures occur in the lower jaw (mandible). Fractures of the upper jaw (maxilla) may cause double vision (because the muscles of the eye attach nearby), numbness in the skin below the eye (because of injuries to nerves), or an irregularity in the cheekbone that can be felt when running a finger along it.

Any injury forceful enough to fracture the jaw may also injure the spine in the neck, so before a fractured jaw is treated, neck x-rays are often taken to rule out spinal damage. A blow powerful enough to fracture the jaw may also cause a concussion or bleeding within the skull. If a person suspects a jaw fracture, the jaw should be held in place with the teeth together and immobile. The jaw may be held with a hand or preferably with a bandage wrapped under the jaw and over the top of the head several times. The person wrapping the bandage must be careful not to cut off breathing. Medical help should be sought as soon as possible because fractures can cause internal bleeding and an airway obstruction.

At the hospital, the upper and lower jaws may be wired together; they remain wired for 6 weeks to allow the bone to heal. During this time, the person is able only to drink liquids through a straw. Many jaw fractures can be repaired surgically with a plate (a piece of metal that's screwed into the bone on each side of the fracture); the jaws are immobilized for only a few days, after which soft foods can be eaten for several weeks.

In children, some jaw fractures aren't immobilized. Instead, initial treatment allows restricted motion, and normal activity resumes in a few weeks. Antibiotics are usually given to a person with a compound fracture—one that extends through a tooth or its socket and opens to a contaminated area, such as the mouth.

Problems After Dental Treatment

Swelling is usual after certain dental procedures, particularly tooth extractions and periodontal surgery. Holding an ice pack—or better yet, a plastic bag of frozen peas or corn, which adapts to facial contours—to the cheek can prevent much of the swelling. When the person is awake during the first 18 hours, ice should be held on the cheek for 25-minute periods and then removed for 5-minute periods. If swelling persists or increases after 3 days or if pain is severe, an infection may have set in, and the patient should contact the dentist.

A **dry socket** (exposure of the bone in the socket causing delayed healing) may develop after a lower back tooth has been removed. Typically, discomfort improves for 2 or 3 days after the extraction and then suddenly worsens, usually accompanied by an earache. Although the condition goes away by itself after one to several weeks, a dentist can place an anesthetic dressing in the socket to eliminate the pain. The dentist replaces the dressing every day or two for about a week.

Bleeding after oral surgery is typical. Usually, it can be stopped by keeping steady pressure on the surgical site for the first hour, normally by having the person bite down on a piece of gauze. Bleeding in the mouth can be deceptive because a small amount of blood may mix with saliva and appear worse than it is. If bleeding continues, the area can be wiped clean, and another piece of gauze or a moistened tea bag can be held against the area with steady pressure. If bleeding continues for more than a few hours, the dentist should be notified. People who regularly take an anticoagulant or aspirin (even if they only take one aspirin every few days) should mention it to the dentist a week before surgery because these drugs increase the tendency to bleed. The dentist and the person's doctor may adjust the drug dosage or temporarily stop the drug.

Cancer and Other Growths of the Mouth

Oral cancers develop in 30,000 Americans and cause 8,000 deaths each year, mostly in people over age 40. This represents about 2.5 percent of cancer cases and 1.5 percent of all cancer-related deaths—a high rate considering the small size of the mouth in relation to the rest of the body. Along with cancers of the lungs and skin, cancers of the mouth are more preventable than most other cancers.

Noncancerous (benign) and cancerous (malignant) growths can originate in any type of tissue in and around the mouth, including bone, muscle, and nerve. Cancers that originate in the lining of the mouth or surface tissues are called carcinomas; cancers that originate in the deeper tissues are called sarcomas. Rarely, cancers found in the mouth region have spread there from other parts of the body—most commonly the lung, breast, and prostate.

Screening for oral cancer should be an integral part of medical and dental examinations because early detection is critical. Cancers less than a half inch across usually can be cured easily. Unfortunately, most oral cancers aren't diagnosed until they've spread to the lymph nodes of the jaw and neck. Because of delayed detection, 25 percent of oral cancers are fatal.

Risk Factors

People who use alcohol and tobacco are at greatest risk of developing oral cancer. The combination of alcohol and tobacco is more likely to cause cancer than either of them alone. About two thirds of oral cancers occur in men, but increased tobacco use among women over the past few decades is gradually closing the gender gap.

Cigarette smoking is more likely to cause oral cancer than cigar or pipe smoking. A brown, flat, freckle-like area (smoker's patch) may develop at the site where a cigarette or pipe is habitually held in the lips. Only a biopsy (removal of a tissue specimen and examination under a microscope) can determine whether the patch is cancerous.

Repeated irritation from the sharp edges of broken teeth, fillings, or dental prostheses (such as crowns and bridges) may add some risk for oral cancer. People who have had one oral cancer are at increased risk of developing another cancer.

Symptoms and Diagnosis

Oral cancers occur most commonly on the sides of the tongue, the floor of the mouth, and the back portion of the roof of the mouth (soft palate). Cancers on the tongue and floor of the mouth are usually squamous cell carcinomas. Kaposi's sarcoma is a cancer of the blood vessels near the skin. It occurs commonly in the mouth—usually on the roof of the mouth (palate)—of people with AIDS.

In those who use chewing tobacco and snuff, the insides of the cheeks and lips are common sites of cancer. These cancers are often slow-growing verrucous (warty) carcinomas.

Melanoma, a cancer that usually occurs on the skin, occurs less commonly in the mouth. An area in the mouth that has recently become brown or darkly discolored may be a melanoma and should be examined by a doctor or dentist. A melanoma must be distinguished from normal pigmented areas in the mouth, which occur in some families and are particularly common among dark-skinned and Mediterranean people.

Tongue

Tongue cancer is invariably painless in the early stage and is usually detected during a routine dental examination.

Cancer typically appears on the sides of the tongue. It almost never develops on the top of the tongue except in someone who has had untreated syphilis for many years. Squamous cell carcinomas of the tongue often look like open sores and tend to grow into the underlying structures.

A red area in the mouth (erythroplakia) is a predictor of cancer. Anyone with a red area on the sides of the tongue should see a doctor or dentist.

Floor of the Mouth

Cancer of the floor of the mouth is invariably painless in the early stage and is usually detected during a routine dental examination. As with cancer of the tongue, cancer of the floor of the mouth is usually squamous cell carcinoma, which looks like open sores and tends to grow into underlying structures.

Anyone with a red area (erythroplakia) on the floor of the mouth should see a doctor or dentist because it may indicate cancer.

Soft Palate

Cancer of the soft palate can be squamous cell carcinoma or cancer that begins in the small salivary glands in the soft palate. Squamous cell carcinoma often looks like an ulcer. Cancer beginning in the small salivary glands commonly appears as a small swelling.

Lining of the Mouth

When the moist inner lining of the mouth (oral mucosa) is irritated for a long period, a flat white spot that doesn't rub off (leukoplakia) may develop. The injured spot appears white because it's a thickened layer of keratin—the same material that covers the outermost part of the skin and normally is less abundant in the lining of the mouth. Unlike other white areas that develop in the mouth—usually from the buildup of food, bacteria, or fungi—leukoplakia can't be wiped off. Most leukoplakia results from the mouth's normal protective response against further injury. But in the process of forming this protective covering, some cells may become cancerous.

By contrast, a red area in the mouth (erythroplakia) results from a thinning of the lining of the mouth. The area appears red because the underlying capillaries are more visible. Erythroplakia is a much more ominous predictor of cancer than leukoplakia. A person with any red area in the mouth should see a doctor or dentist.

An ulcer is a hole that forms in the lining of the mouth when the top layer of cells breaks down, and the underlying tissue shows through. An ulcer appears white because of the dead cells inside the hole. Mouth ulcers frequently result from tissue injury or irritation—for instance, when the inside of the cheek is accidentally bitten or scraped. Other causes are canker sores and irritating substances, such as an aspirin, held against the gums. Noncancerous ulcers are invariably painful. An ulcer that doesn't hurt and lasts more than 10 days may be precancerous or cancerous and should be examined by a doctor or dentist.

A person who chews tobacco or uses snuff may develop white, ridged bumps on the insides of the cheeks. These bumps can develop into verrucous carcinoma.

Gums

A distinct lump or raised area on the gums (gingiva) isn't a cause for alarm. If such a lump isn't caused by a periodontal abscess or abscessed tooth, it may be a noncancerous growth caused by irritation. Noncancerous growths are relatively common and, if necessary, can be easily removed by surgery. In 10 to 40 percent of people, the noncancerous growths recur because the irritant remains. If the irritant is a poorly fitting denture, it should be adjusted or replaced.

Lips

The lips—most commonly the lower lip—are subject to sun damage (actinic cheilosis), which makes them cracked and red, white, or mixed red and white. A doctor or dentist may perform a biopsy to determine whether these rough spots on the lips are cancerous. Cancer on the outside of the lip is more common in sunny climates. Cancers of the lip and other parts of the mouth often feel rock hard and stick to the underlying tissue, while most noncancerous lumps in these areas are freely movable. Abnormalities in the upper lip are less common than those on the lower lip but are more likely to be cancerous and require medical attention.

A person who chews tobacco or uses snuff may develop white, ridged bumps on the inside of the lips. These bumps can develop into verrucous carcinoma.

Salivary Glands

Salivary gland tumors can be cancerous or noncancerous. They may occur in any of the three pairs of major salivary glands: parotid gland (on the side of the face in front of the ear), submandibular gland (under the side of the jaw), or sublingual gland (on the floor of the mouth in front of the tongue). Tumors can also occur in the minor salivary glands, which are scattered throughout most of the lining of the mouth. The early growth of salivary gland tumors may or may not be painful. Cancerous tumors tend to grow fast and feel hard.

Jaw

Many kinds of noncancerous cysts cause jaw pain and swelling. Often, they're next to an impacted wisdom tooth and, even though they're not cancerous, they can destroy considerable areas of the jawbone as they expand. Certain types of cysts are more likely to recur. Odontomas are noncancerous overgrowths of tooth-forming cells that look like small, misshapen extra teeth. Because they may take the place of normal teeth or get in the way of normal teeth coming in, they're often surgically removed.

Jaw cancer often causes pain and a numb or unusual sensation, somewhat like the feeling of a mouth anesthetic wearing off. X-rays can't always distinguish jaw cancers from cysts, noncancerous bone growths, or cancers that have spread from elsewhere in the body. However, x-rays usually show the irregular borders of jaw cancer and may show that the cancer has eaten away the roots of nearby teeth. Typically, a biopsy (removal of a tissue specimen and examination under a microscope) is needed to confirm a diagnosis of jaw cancer.

Prevention and Treatment

Staying out of the sun reduces the risk of lip cancer. Avoiding excessive alcohol and tobacco use can prevent most oral cancers. Smoothing rough edges from broken teeth or restorations is another preventive measure. Some evidence indicates that antioxidant vitamins, such as vitamins C and E, and beta-carotene may provide added protection, but further study is needed. If sun damage covers a large area of the lip, a lip shave in which all of the outer surface is removed, either by surgery or with a laser, may prevent a progression to cancer.

The success of treatment for oral and lip cancers depends largely on how far the cancer has progressed. Oral cancers rarely spread to distant sites in the body but tend to invade the head and neck. If the entire cancer and the surrounding normal tissue is removed before the cancer has spread to the lymph nodes, the cure rate is high. If the cancer has spread to the lymph nodes, cure is much less likely. During surgery, the nodes under and behind the jaw and along the neck as well as the cancer in the mouth are removed. Surgery for mouth cancers can be disfiguring and psychologically traumatic.

A person with mouth or throat cancer may receive radiation therapy and surgery or just radiation therapy. Radiation therapy often destroys the salivary glands and leaves the person's mouth dry, which can lead to cavities and other dental problems. Because jawbones exposed to radiation don't heal well, dental problems are treated before radiation is administered. Any teeth likely to become problems are removed, and time is allowed for healing. Good dental hygiene is important for people who have had radiation therapy for oral cancer. Such hygiene includes regular examinations and thorough home care, including daily home fluoride applications. If the person eventually has a tooth pulled, hyperbaric oxygen therapy may help the jaw heal better.

Chemotherapy has a limited therapeutic benefit for mouth cancers. The mainstays of treatment are surgery and radiation therapy.

Digestive Disorders

Biology of the Digestive System

The digestive system, which extends from the mouth to the anus, is responsible for receiving food, breaking it down into nutrients (a process called digestion), absorbing the nutrients into the bloodstream, and eliminating the undigestible parts of food from the body. The digestive tract consists of the mouth, throat, esophagus, stomach, small intestine, large intestine, rectum, and anus. The digestive system also includes organs that lie outside the digestive tract: the pancreas, the liver, and the gallbladder.

Mouth, Throat, and Esophagus

The mouth is the entrance to both the digestive and the respiratory systems. The inside of the mouth is lined with mucous membrane. Ducts from the salivary glands in the cheeks, under the tongue, and under the jaw all empty into the mouth. On the floor of the mouth lies the tongue, which is used to taste and mix food. Behind and below the mouth is the throat (pharynx).

Taste is sensed by taste buds on the surface of the tongue. Smell is sensed by olfactory receptors high in the nose. The sense of taste is relatively simple, distinguishing only sweet, sour, salty, and bitter. The sense of smell is much more complex, distinguishing many subtle variations.

Cutting with the front teeth (incisors) and chewing with the back teeth (molars) break down food into more easily digestible particles, while saliva from the salivary glands coats the particles with digestive enzymes and begins digestion. Between meals, the flow of saliva washes away bacteria that can cause tooth decay and other disorders. Saliva also contains antibodies and enzymes, such as lysozyme, that break down proteins and attack bacteria directly.

Swallowing begins voluntarily and continues automatically. A small muscular flap (epiglottis) closes to prevent food from going down the windpipe (trachea) toward the lungs, and the back portion of the roof of the mouth (soft palate) lifts to prevent food from going up the nose.

The esophagus—a thin-walled, muscular channel lined with mucous membrane—connects the throat with the stomach. Food is propelled through the esophagus not by gravity but by waves of rhythmic muscular contractions and relaxations, called peristalsis.

Stomach

The stomach is a large, bean-shaped, hollow, muscular organ consisting of three regions: the cardia, the body (fundus), and the antrum. Food enters the stomach from the esophagus by passing through a ring-shaped muscle (sphincter), which opens and closes. The sphincter normally prevents the contents of the stomach from flowing back into the esophagus.

The stomach serves as a storage area for food, contracting rhythmically and mixing the food with enzymes. The cells lining the stomach secrete three important substances: mucus, hydrochloric acid, and the precursor of pepsin (an enzyme that breaks down proteins). Mucus coats the cells of the stomach lining to protect them from being damaged by acid and enzymes. Any disruption of this layer of mucus—from infection by the bacterium *Helicobacter pylori*, for example, or from aspirin—can result in damage that leads to a stomach ulcer.

Hydrochloric acid provides the highly acidic environment needed for pepsin to break down proteins. The stomach's high acidity also serves as a barrier against infection by killing most bacteria. Acid secretion is stimulated by nerve impulses to the stomach, gastrin (a hormone released by the stomach), and histamine (a substance released by the stomach).

Pepsin is responsible for about 10 percent of protein breakdown. It's the only enzyme that digests collagen, which is a protein and a major constituent of meat.

Only a few substances, such as alcohol and aspirin, can be absorbed directly from the stomach and only in small amounts.

Small Intestine

The stomach releases food into the duodenum, the first segment of the small intestine. Food enters the duodenum through the pyloric sphincter in amounts that the small intestine can digest.

When full, the duodenum signals the stomach to stop emptying.

The duodenum receives pancreatic enzymes from the pancreas and bile from the liver. These fluids, which enter the duodenum through an opening called the sphincter of Oddi, are important in aiding digestion and absorption. Peristalsis also aids digestion and absorption by churning up food and mixing it with intestinal secretions.

The first few inches of the duodenal lining are smooth, but the rest of the lining has folds, small projections (villi), and even smaller projections (microvilli). These villi and microvilli increase the surface area of the duodenal lining, allowing for greater absorption of nutrients.

The rest of the small intestine, located below the duodenum, consists of the jejunum and the ileum. This part of the small intestine is largely responsible for the absorption of fats and other nutrients. Absorption is enhanced by the vast surface area made up of folds, villi, and microvilli. The intestinal wall is richly supplied with blood vessels that carry the absorbed nutrients to the liver through the portal vein. The intestinal wall releases mucus, which lubricates the intestinal contents, and water, which helps dissolve the digested fragments. Small amounts of enzymes that digest proteins, sugars, and fats are also released.

The consistency of the intestinal contents changes gradually as they travel through the small intestine. In the duodenum, water is pumped rapidly into the contents to dilute the stomach acidity. As the contents travel through the lower small intestine, they become more fluid with water, mucus, bile, and pancreatic enzymes being added.

Pancreas

The pancreas is an organ that contains two basic types of tissue: the acini, which produce digestive enzymes, and the islets, which produce hormones. The pancreas secretes digestive enzymes into the duodenum and hormones into the bloodstream.

The digestive enzymes are released from the cells of the acini and flow down various channels into the pancreatic duct. The pancreatic duct joins the common bile duct at the sphincter of Oddi, where both flow into the duodenum. The enzymes secreted by the pancreas digest proteins, carbohydrates, and fats. The proteolytic

enzymes, which break down proteins into a form that the body can use, are secreted in an inactive form. They're activated only when they reach the digestive tract. The pancreas also secretes large amounts of sodium bicarbonate, which protects the duodenum by neutralizing the acid that comes from the stomach.

The three hormones produced by the pancreas are insulin,▲ which lowers the level of sugar (glucose) in the blood; glucagon, which raises the level of sugar in the blood; and somatostatin, which prevents the other two hormones from being released.

Liver

The liver is a large organ with several functions, only some of which are related to digestion.

The nutrients of food are absorbed into the wall of the intestine, which is supplied with many tiny blood vessels (capillaries). These capillaries flow into veins that join larger veins and eventually enter the liver as the portal vein. This vein splits into tiny vessels inside the liver where the incoming blood can be processed.

Blood is processed in two ways: Bacteria and other foreign particles absorbed from the intestine are removed, and many nutrients absorbed from the intestine are further broken down so they can be used by the body. The liver performs the necessary processing at high speed and passes the blood, laden with nutrients, into general circulation.

The liver manufactures about half of the body's cholesterol; the rest comes from food. About 80 percent of the cholesterol made by the liver is used to make bile. The liver also secretes bile, which is stored in the gallbladder until it's needed.

Gallbladder and Biliary Tract

Bile flows out of the liver through the right and left hepatic ducts, which come together to form the common hepatic duct. This duct then joins with a duct coming from the gallbladder, called the cystic duct, to form the common bile duct. The pancreatic duct joins the common bile duct just where it empties into the duodenum.

▲ see page 717

Digestive System

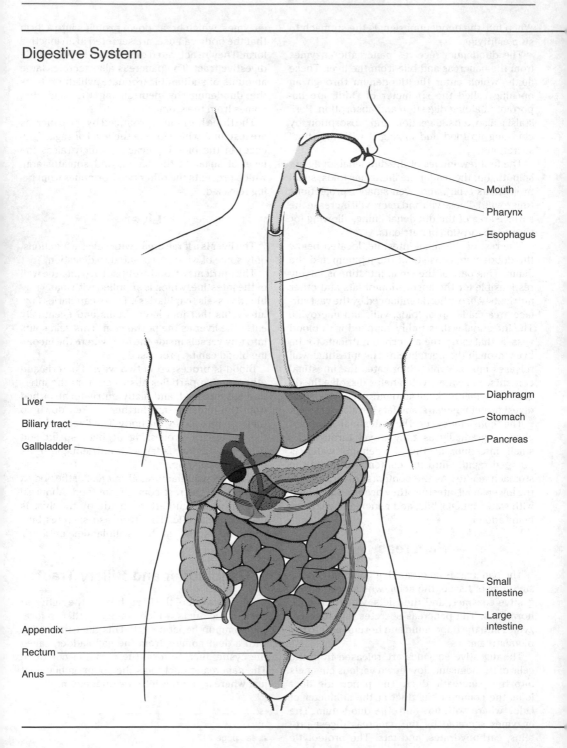

Mouth

Pharynx

Esophagus

Liver

Biliary tract

Gallbladder

Diaphragm

Stomach

Pancreas

Small intestine

Large intestine

Appendix

Rectum

Anus

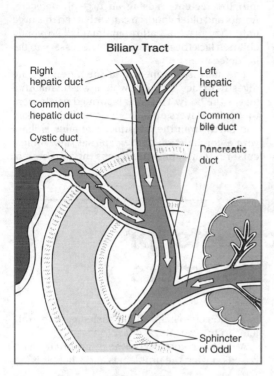

Biliary Tract

Right hepatic duct

Left hepatic duct

Common hepatic duct

Common bile duct

Cystic duct

Pancreatic duct

Sphincter of Oddi

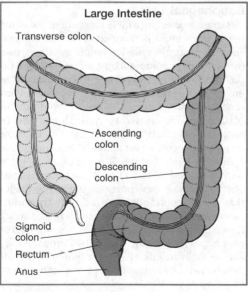

Large Intestine

Transverse colon

Ascending colon

Descending colon

Sigmoid colon

Rectum

Anus

Between meals, bile salts are concentrated in the gallbladder, and only a little bile flows from the liver. Food that enters the duodenum triggers a series of hormonal and nerve signals that cause the gallbladder to contract. As a result, bile flows into the duodenum and mixes with food contents. Bile has two important functions: It assists in the digestion and absorption of fats, and it's responsible for the elimination of certain waste products from the body—particularly hemoglobin from destroyed red blood cells and excess cholesterol. Specifically, bile is responsible for these actions:

• Bile salts increase the solubility of cholesterol, fats, and fat-soluble vitamins to aid in their absorption.

• Bile salts stimulate the secretion of water by the large intestine to help move the contents along.

• Bilirubin (the main pigment in bile) is excreted in bile as a waste product of destroyed red blood cells.

• Drugs and other waste products are excreted in bile and later eliminated from the body.

• Various proteins that play important roles in bile function are secreted in bile.

Bile salts are reabsorbed into the small intestine, extracted by the liver, and resecreted into bile. This recirculation of bile salts is known as the enterohepatic circulation. All the bile salts in the body circulate about 10 to 12 times a day. During each pass, small amounts of bile salts reach the colon, where bacteria break them down into various constituents. Some constituents are reabsorbed; the rest are excreted with the feces.

Large Intestine

The large intestine consists of the ascending (right) colon, the transverse colon, the descending (left) colon, and the sigmoid colon, which is connected to the rectum. The appendix is a small, finger-shaped tube projecting from the ascending (right) colon near the point where it joins the small intestine. The large intestine secretes mucus and is largely responsible for the absorption of water and electrolytes from the feces.

Intestinal contents are fluid when they reach the large intestine but are normally solid by the time they reach the rectum as feces. The many bacteria that inhabit the large intestine can further digest some material, aiding in the body's absorption of nutrients. Bacteria in the large intestine also make some important substances, such as vitamin K. These bacteria are necessary for healthy intestinal function, and some diseases and antibiotics can upset the balance among the different types of bacteria in the large intestine. The result is irritation that leads to the secretion of mucus and water, causing diarrhea.

Rectum and Anus

The rectum is a chamber that begins at the end of the large intestine, immediately following the sigmoid colon, and ends at the anus. Ordinarily, the rectum is empty because feces are stored

higher in the descending colon. Eventually, the descending colon becomes full, and feces pass into the rectum, causing an urge to defecate. Adults and older children can withstand this urge until they reach a bathroom. Infants and young children lack the muscle control necessary to delay defecation.

The anus is the opening at the far end of the digestive tract through which waste material leaves the body. The anus is formed partly from the surface layers of the body, including the skin, and partly from the intestine. The anus is lined with a continuation of the external skin. A muscular ring (anal sphincter) keeps the anus closed.

CHAPTER 100

Diagnostic Tests for Digestive Disorders

Tests performed on the digestive system make use of endoscopes (fiber-optic tubes that doctors use to view internal structures and to obtain tissue samples from inside the body), x-rays, ultrasound scans, radioactive tracers, and chemical measurements. These tests can help diagnose, locate, and sometimes treat a problem. Some tests require the digestive system to be cleared of stool (feces), some require 8 to 12 hours of fasting, and others don't require any preparation at all.

The first steps in diagnosing a problem are always a medical history and a physical examination. However, symptoms of digestive disorders are often vague, so doctors may have difficulty determining precisely what's wrong. Also, psychologic disorders such as anxiety and depression can affect the digestive system and contribute to the symptoms.

During a physical examination of a person with symptoms of a digestive problem, doctors examine the abdomen, anus, and rectum. They listen with a stethoscope for unusual sounds, feel for masses and enlarged organs, determine whether particular areas are sensitive to pressure, examine the anus and rectum by inserting a gloved finger, and obtain a small sample of stool to test for hidden (occult) blood. In women, a pelvic ex-

amination often helps distinguish digestive problems from gynecologic ones.

A doctor recommends the appropriate tests, based on what the problem is and where it is.

Esophageal Tests

Barium studies, in which the patient swallows barium, are often performed on the esophagus. For such a study (called a barium swallow), doctors tend to use fluoroscopy, a continuous x-ray technique that allows barium to be observed or filmed as it passes through the esophagus. Fluoroscopy allows a doctor to see the contractions of the esophagus as well as any anatomic defects, such as obstructions or ulcers. Often, these images are recorded on film or videotape.

Besides liquid barium, a patient may be given barium-coated food, so that a doctor can locate obstructions or view portions of the esophagus that aren't contracting normally. Both barium preparations taken together can show abnormalities such as esophageal webs (in which the esophagus is partially blocked by fibrous tissue), Zenker's diverticulum (an outpouching of the esophagus), esophageal erosions and ulcers, esophageal varices (esophageal varicose veins), and tumors.

Manometry is a test in which a tube with pressure gauges along its surface is placed in the esophagus. Using this device (called a manometer), a doctor can determine whether contractions of the esophagus can propel food normally.

An **esophageal pH test** (a test that measures acidity in the esophagus) can be performed during manometry. The test is used to determine if a person has acid reflux (reflux of stomach acid into the esophagus).▲ One or more measurements may be taken.

In the **Bernstein test** (esophageal acid perfusion test), a small amount of acid is placed in the esophagus through a nasogastric tube. This test, which is used to find out if chest pain is caused by acid irritation of the esophagus, is a good way to detect inflammation of the esophagus (esophagitis).

Intubation

Intubation is the process of passing a small, flexible plastic tube through the nose or mouth into the stomach or small intestine.

This procedure may be used for diagnostic or treatment purposes. Although intubation may cause gagging and nausea in some patients, it isn't painful. The tube size varies according to the purpose.

Nasogastric intubation (passage of a tube through the nose into the stomach) can be used to obtain a sample of stomach fluid. Doctors can then determine whether the stomach contains blood, or they can analyze the stomach's secretions for acidity, enzymes, and other characteristics. In poisoning victims, samples of the stomach fluid can be analyzed to identify the poison. In some cases, the tube is left in place, so that more samples can be obtained over several hours.

Nasogastric intubation may also be used to treat certain conditions. For example, cool water can be infused into the stomach to help stop bleeding, poisons can be pumped out or neutralized with activated charcoal, or liquid food can be administered to people who can't swallow.

Sometimes nasogastric intubation is used to continuously remove the contents of the stomach. The end of the tube is usually attached to a suction device, which removes gas and fluid from the stomach. This helps relieve pressure when the digestive system is blocked or otherwise not functioning properly.

In nasoenteric intubation, a longer tube is passed through the nose, through the stomach, and into the small intestine. This procedure can be used to sample intestinal contents, continuously remove fluids, or provide food. A tube with a small device at the end can be used to perform a biopsy (obtain a sample of the small intestine for examination). The tissue may be analyzed for enzyme activity, examined under a microscope, or evaluated in other ways. Because the stomach and small intestine don't feel pain, the procedure is painless.

Endoscopy

Endoscopy is an examination of internal structures using a fiber optic viewing tube (endoscope).

When passed through the mouth, an endoscope can be used to examine the esophagus (esophagoscopy), the stomach (gastroscopy), and the small intestine (upper gastrointestinal endoscopy). When passed through the anus, an endoscope can be used to examine the rectum and the lower portion of the large intestine (sigmoidoscopy) and the entire large intestine (colonoscopy).

Endoscopes range in diameter from about $\frac{1}{4}$ inch to about $\frac{1}{2}$ inch and range in length from about 1 foot to about 5 feet. Fiber-optic video systems allow the endoscope to be flexible while providing both a lighting source and a viewing system. Many endoscopes also are equipped with a small clipper to remove tissue samples and an electric probe to destroy abnormal tissue.

Doctors can get a good view of the lining of the digestive system with an endoscope. They can see areas of irritation, ulcers, inflammation, and abnormal tissue growth. Usually, they can obtain samples for examination. Endoscopes can also be used for treatment. A doctor can pass different types of instruments through a small channel in the endoscope. Electrocautery can be used to close off a blood vessel and stop bleeding or to remove small growths, and a needle can be used to inject drugs into esophageal varices and stop their bleeding.

Before having an endoscope passed through the mouth, a person usually must avoid food for several hours. Food in the stomach can obstruct the doctor's view and might be vomited up during

▲ see page 491

the procedure. Before having an endoscope passed into the rectum and colon, a person usually takes laxatives and is given enemas to clear out any stool.

Complications from endoscopy are relatively rare. Although endoscopes can injure or even perforate the digestive tract, they more commonly cause only irritation of the intestinal lining and a little bleeding.

Laparoscopy

Laparoscopy is an examination of the abdominal cavity using an endoscope.

Laparoscopy is usually done with the patient under general anesthesia. After the appropriate area of the skin is washed with an antiseptic, a small incision is made, usually in the navel. Then an endoscope is passed into the abdominal cavity. A doctor can look for tumors or other abnormalities, examine virtually any organ in the abdominal cavity, obtain samples, and even do reparative surgery.

X-ray Studies

X-rays often are used to evaluate digestive problems. **Plain abdominal x-rays,** the standard x-rays of the abdomen, don't require any preparation on the patient's part. The x-rays generally are used to show an obstruction or paralysis of the digestive tract or abnormal air patterns in the abdominal cavity. These standard x-rays can also show enlargement of organs such as the liver, kidneys, and spleen.

Barium studies often provide more information. After a person swallows barium, it looks white on x-rays and outlines the digestive tract, showing the contours and lining of the esophagus, stomach, and small intestine. The barium collects in abnormal areas, showing ulcers, tumors, erosions, and esophageal varices. X-rays may be taken at intervals to determine where the barium is. Or a fluoroscope may be used to observe the barium as it moves through the digestive tract. This process can also be filmed for later review. By observing the barium passing through the digestive tract, doctors can see how the esophagus and stomach function, determine if their contractions are normal, and tell whether food is getting blocked in the digestive system.

Barium also can be given in an enema to outline the lower part of the large intestine. Then, x-rays can show polyps, tumors, or other structural abnormalities. This procedure may cause crampy pain, producing slight to moderate discomfort.

Barium taken by mouth or given as an enema is eventually excreted in the stool, making the stool chalky white. Barium should be eliminated quickly after the studies because it can cause significant constipation. A gentle laxative can speed the elimination of barium.

Paracentesis

Paracentesis is the insertion of a needle into the abdominal cavity and the removal of fluid.

Normally, the abdominal cavity outside of the digestive tract contains only a small amount of fluid. However, fluid can accumulate in certain circumstances, such as when a person has a perforated stomach or intestine, liver disease, cancer, or a ruptured spleen. A doctor may use paracentesis to obtain a fluid sample for analysis or to remove excessive fluid.

Before paracentesis, a physical examination, sometimes accompanied by an ultrasound scan, is performed to confirm that the abdominal cavity contains excessive fluid. Next, an area of the skin, generally just below the navel, is washed with an antiseptic solution and numbed with a small amount of anesthetic. A doctor then pushes a needle attached to a syringe through the skin and muscles of the abdominal wall and into the area of fluid accumulation. A small amount may be removed for laboratory testing, or up to several quarts may be removed to relieve distention.

Abdominal Ultrasound Scan

Ultrasound scanning uses sound waves to produce pictures of internal organs. It can show the size and shape of many organs, such as the liver and pancreas, and can also show abnormal areas within them. Ultrasound scanning can also show the presence of fluid. It isn't a good method, however, for examining the lining of the digestive tract, so it isn't used to look for tumors and causes of bleeding in the stomach, small intestine, or large intestine.

An ultrasound scan is a painless procedure that poses no risk. The examiner (a doctor or technician) presses a small probe against the person's abdominal wall and directs sound waves to various parts of the abdomen by moving the probe. The pictures are then displayed on a video screen and recorded on video film.

Occult Blood Tests

Bleeding in the digestive system can be caused by something as insignificant as a little irritation or as serious as cancer. When bleeding is profuse, a person can vomit blood, pass bright red blood in the stool, or pass black, tarry stool (melena). Amounts of blood too small to be seen or to change the appearance of stool can be detected chemically, and the detection of such small amounts may provide early clues to the presence of ulcers, cancers, and other abnormalities.

During a rectal examination, the doctor obtains a small amount of stool on a gloved finger. This sample is placed on a piece of filter paper impregnated with chemicals. After another chemical is added, the color of the sample will change if blood is present. Alternatively, the person can take home a kit containing the impregnated filter papers. The person places samples of stool from about three different bowel movements on the filter papers, which are then mailed in special containers back to the doctor for testing. If blood is detected, further examinations are needed to determine the source.

CHAPTER 101

Disorders of the Esophagus

The esophagus is the channel that leads from the throat (pharynx) to the stomach. The walls of the esophagus propel food to the stomach with rhythmic waves of muscular contractions called peristalsis. Near the junction of the throat and the esophagus, there's a band of muscle called the upper esophageal sphincter. Slightly above the junction of the esophagus and the stomach, there's another band of muscle called the lower esophageal sphincter. When the esophagus isn't in use, these sphincters contract so that food and stomach acid don't flow up from the stomach to the mouth. During swallowing, the sphincters relax so food can pass to the stomach.

Two of the most common symptoms of esophageal disorders are dysphagia (an awareness of difficulty in swallowing) and chest or back pain.

Dysphagia is the sensation that food isn't progressing normally from the throat to the stomach or that it has become stuck on the way down. The sensation may be painful. The movement of liquids and solids may actually be impeded by physical abnormalities of the throat, esophagus, and nearby organs or by problems in the nervous system or muscles. Or the swallowing difficulty may be imagined.

Chest or back pain includes heartburn, pain during swallowing, and esophageal muscle pain.

Pain during swallowing may result from any of the following:

- Destruction of the esophageal lining (mucosa), as may result from inflammation caused by stomach acid reflux
- Bacterial, viral, or fungal infections of the throat
- Tumors, chemicals, or muscle disorders, such as achalasia and diffuse esophageal spasm

The pain may be perceived as a burning sensation or a tightness under the breastbone (sternum), which typically occurs as soon as the person swallows food or liquid. Severe, squeezing chest pain that occurs with difficulty swallowing hot or cold beverages is a typical symptom of esophageal muscle disorders.

Esophageal muscle pains may be difficult to distinguish from chest pain stemming from heart disease (angina). The pains occur when the esophageal muscles go into spasm.

Dysphagia Caused by Throat Disorders

A person can have trouble moving food from the upper part of the throat into the esophagus because of disorders affecting the throat. The problem occurs most often in people who have disorders of the voluntary (skeletal) muscles or the nerves that serve them. Examples include dermatomyositis, myasthenia gravis, muscular dystrophy, polio, pseudobulbar palsy, and disorders of the brain and spinal cord such as Parkinson's disease and amyotrophic lateral sclerosis (Lou Gehrig's disease). A person who takes a phenothiazine (an antipsychotic drug) may also have difficulty swallowing because the drug can affect the throat muscles. When any of these disorders causes difficulty in swallowing, the person often regurgitates food through the back of the nose or inhales it into the windpipe (trachea) and then coughs.

In **cricopharyngeal incoordination,** the upper esophageal sphincter (cricopharyngeal muscle) remains closed or it opens in an uncoordinated way. An abnormally functioning sphincter may allow food to repeatedly enter the windpipe and lungs, which may lead to chronic lung disease. A surgeon can correct the problem by cutting the sphincter so that it's permanently relaxed. If left untreated, the condition may lead to the formation of a diverticulum, a sac formed when the lining of the esophagus pushes outward and backward through the cricopharyngeal muscle.▲

Lower Esophageal Ring

Probably present at birth, a lower esophageal ring (Schatzki's ring) is a narrowing of the lower esophagus.

Normally, the lower esophagus has a diameter of $1\frac{1}{2}$ to 2 inches. If it's narrowed to about $\frac{1}{2}$ inch or less, the person may have trouble swallowing solids. This symptom can begin at any age, but usually it doesn't begin until after age 25. Rings more than $\frac{3}{4}$ of an inch in diameter usually produce no symptoms.

With a lower esophageal ring, difficulty in swallowing comes and goes. Often, barium x-rays■ are taken to detect the problem.

Chewing food thoroughly usually alleviates the problem. If this doesn't work, the constricting ring may be opened surgically. Alternatively, a doctor may use a dilator or may pass an endoscope (a flexible viewing tube with attach-

ments)★ through the mouth and throat to widen the passageway.

Esophageal Webs

Esophageal webs (Plummer-Vinson syndrome, sideropenic dysphagia) are thin membranes that grow across the inside of the esophagus from its surface lining (mucosa).

Although rare, webs occur most often in people who have untreated severe iron deficiency anemia. Webs in the upper esophagus usually make swallowing solids difficult. Taking x-ray movies (cineradiographs) as the patient swallows a barium drink (a test called a barium swallow) is usually the best procedure for diagnosing the problem.

Once the anemia has been treated successfully, the webs disappear. If not, a doctor can rupture them using a dilator or an endoscope.

Dysphagia Lusoria

Dysphagia lusoria is a swallowing difficulty caused by compression of the esophagus by a blood vessel.

This condition is a birth defect most commonly involving an abnormally placed right subclavian artery. The swallowing difficulty may occur in childhood or may develop later from atherosclerosis in the abnormal vessel.

Barium x-rays● can show the compressed esophagus. Arteriography (an x-ray of an artery taken after injection of a dye) is needed to confirm that the compression is caused by an artery. Surgery is only rarely needed.

Other Causes of Obstruction

In some people, narrowing (stricture) of the esophagus is congenital; in others, the problem results from damage caused by the repeated backflow of acid from the stomach (acid reflux). Narrowing also may be caused by compression against the outside of the esophagus. For example, compression can result from an enlarged left atrium of the heart, aortic aneurysm, abnormally formed subclavian artery, abnormal thyroid gland, a bony outgrowth from the spine, or a cancer—most commonly lung cancer. The most serious cause of blockage is esophageal cancer.◆ Because all these disorders decrease the diameter of the esophagus, they usually produce diffi-

---

▲ see page 492

■ see page 484

★ see page 485

● see page 484

◆ see page 549

culty in swallowing solid foods—particularly meat and bread—not liquids.

When the narrowing is caused by acid reflux, swallowing difficulty follows long-standing symptoms such as severe heartburn and periodic sharp pain behind the breastbone at night or when bending over; the swallowing difficulty gets progressively worse for years. With cancer of the esophagus, swallowing difficulty progresses rapidly in weeks or months.

An x-ray is usually taken to find the cause and location of an obstruction. Treatment and prognosis depend on the cause.

Diffuse Esophageal Spasm

Diffuse esophageal spasm (rosary bead or corkscrew esophagus) is a disorder of the propulsive movements (peristalsis) of the esophagus caused by malfunctioning nerves.

The normal propulsive contractions that move food through the esophagus are replaced periodically by nonpropulsive contractions. In 30 percent of people with this disorder, the lower esophageal sphincter opens and closes abnormally.

Symptoms

Muscle spasms throughout the esophagus typically are felt as chest pain under the breastbone coinciding with difficulty in swallowing liquids or solids. Pain also occurs at night and may be severe enough to awaken a person. Very hot or cold liquids may worsen the pain. Over many years, this disorder may evolve into achalasia.

Diffuse esophageal spasm also may produce severe pain without swallowing difficulty. This pain, often described as a squeezing pain under the breastbone, may accompany exercise or exertion, making it difficult to distinguish from angina (chest pain stemming from heart disease).

Diagnosis

X-rays taken while the person swallows a barium drink may show that food doesn't move normally down the esophagus and that contractions of the esophageal wall are disorganized. Esophageal scintigraphy (a sensitive imaging test that shows the movement of food labeled with a tiny amount of radioactive tracer) is used to detect abnormal movements of food through the esophagus. Pressure measurements (manometry) provide the most sensitive and detailed analysis of

How the Esophagus Works

As a person swallows, food moves from the mouth to throat, also called the pharynx (1). The upper esophageal sphincter opens (2), so food can enter the esophagus, where waves of muscular contractions, called peristalsis, (3) propel the food downward. The food then passes through the lower esophageal sphincter (4) and moves into the stomach (5).

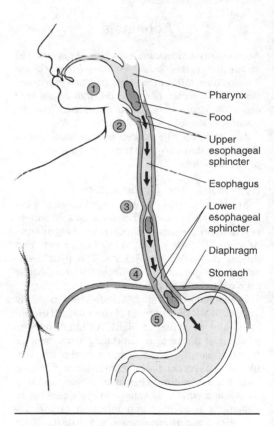

Pharynx
Food
Upper esophageal sphincter
Esophagus
Lower esophageal sphincter
Diaphragm
Stomach

the spasms. If these studies are inconclusive, manometry may be conducted after the person eats a meal or is given edrophonium to provoke the painful spasms.▲

▲ see page 485

Treatment

Often, diffuse esophageal spasm is difficult to treat. Nitroglycerin, long-acting nitrates, anticholinergics such as dicyclomine, or calcium channel blockers such as nifedipine may relieve the symptoms. Sometimes, potent analgesics are needed. Inflating a balloon inside the esophagus or passing bougies (progressively larger metal dilators) to dilate the esophagus may be helpful. A surgeon may have to cut the muscle layer along the full length of the esophagus if other less radical forms of treatment aren't effective.

Achalasia

Achalasia (cardiospasm, esophageal aperistalsis, megaesophagus) is a nerve-related disorder of unknown cause that can interfere with two processes: the rhythmic waves of contraction that propel food down the esophagus, called peristalsis, and the opening of the lower esophageal sphincter.

Achalasia may be caused by a malfunction of the nerves that surround the esophagus and supply its muscles.

Symptoms and Complications

Achalasia may occur at any age but usually begins, almost unnoticed, between ages 20 and 40 and then progresses gradually over many months or years. Difficulty swallowing both solids and liquids is the main symptom. The tight lower esophageal sphincter causes the esophagus above it to enlarge greatly.

Other symptoms may include chest pain, regurgitation of the contents of the enlarged esophagus, and coughing at night. Although uncommon, chest pain may occur during swallowing or for no apparent reason. About a third of the people who have achalasia regurgitate undigested food while sleeping. They may inhale food into their lungs, which can cause a lung abscess, bronchiectasis (widening and infection of the airways), or aspiration pneumonia. Achalasia also is a risk factor for esophageal cancer, though probably less than 5 percent of people with achalasia develop such cancer.

▲ see page 485

■ see page 485

Diagnosis and Prognosis

X-rays of the esophagus taken while the person is swallowing barium show an absence of peristalsis. The esophagus is widened, frequently to enormous proportions, but is narrow at the lower esophageal sphincter. Measurement of pressures inside the esophagus (manometry)▲ indicates a lack of contractions, increased closing pressure of the lower esophageal sphincter, and incomplete opening of the sphincter when the person swallows. Esophagoscopy■ (an examination of the esophagus through a flexible viewing tube with a video camera) shows widening but no obstruction.

Using an esophagoscope (flexible viewing tube), a doctor performs a biopsy (obtains tissue samples for examination under a microscope) to make sure the symptoms aren't caused by cancer at the lower end of the esophagus. The person is also examined to rule out scleroderma, a muscle disorder that can impair swallowing.

Often the cause of achalasia isn't serious and doesn't lead to any major illness. The prognosis isn't as good if stomach contents have been inhaled into the lungs because the lung complications are difficult to treat.

Treatment

The aim of treatment is to get the lower esophageal sphincter to open more easily. The first approach is to widen the sphincter mechanically—for example, by inflating a balloon inside it. The results of this procedure are satisfactory about 40 percent of the time, but repeated dilations may be needed. Nitrates (for example, nitroglycerin placed under the tongue before meals) or calcium channel blockers (for example, nifedipine) may delay the need for another dilation procedure by helping to relax the sphincter. In fewer than 1 percent of cases, the esophagus may rupture during the dilation procedure, leading to inflammation of the surrounding tissue (mediastinitis). Immediate surgery is needed to close the rupture in the wall of the esophagus.

As an alternative to mechanical dilation, a doctor may inject botulinum toxin into the lower esophageal sphincter. This newer therapy is as effective as mechanical dilation, but the long-term effects aren't yet known.

If dilation or botulinum toxin therapy doesn't work, surgery to cut the muscular fibers in the lower esophageal sphincter is usually performed. This surgery is successful about 85 percent of the time. However, about 15 percent of people experience episodic acid reflux after surgery.

Acid Reflux

Acid reflux (gastroesophageal reflux) is a backflow of stomach contents upward into the esophagus.

The lining of the stomach protects the stomach from the effects of its own acids. Because the esophagus lacks a similar protective lining, stomach acid that refluxes into it causes pain, inflammation (esophagitis), and damage.

Acid refluxes when the lower esophageal sphincter isn't functioning properly. The force of gravity contributes to reflux when the person is lying down. The degree of inflammation caused by reflux depends on the acidity of the stomach contents, the volume of the stomach acid in the esophagus, and the ability to clear the regurgitated fluid from the esophagus.

Symptoms and Complications

The most obvious symptom of acid reflux is heartburn, a burning pain behind the breastbone. The pain—which rises in the chest and may extend into the neck, throat, or even face—is caused by acid reflux from the stomach into the esophagus. It usually occurs after meals or while lying down. Heartburn may be accompanied by regurgitation of stomach contents into the mouth or excessive salivation. A high level of salivation that results when stomach acid irritates the inflamed lower esophagus is called water brash.

Complications of acid reflux include narrowing of an area of the esophagus (peptic esophageal stricture), esophageal ulcer, and precancerous changes in the lining of the esophagus (Barrett's syndrome). Inflammation of the esophagus may cause pain during swallowing and bleeding that's usually slight but can be massive. Narrowing makes swallowing solid foods increasingly more difficult. Peptic esophageal ulcers are painful open sores of the esophageal lining. The pain is usually behind the breastbone or just below it and can usually be relieved by antacids. Healing requires drugs that reduce stomach acid over a 4- to 12-week period. The ulcers heal slowly, tend to recur, and usually leave a narrowed esophagus after healing.

Diagnosis

The symptoms point to the diagnosis. X-ray studies, esophagoscopy (examination of the esophagus through a flexible viewing tube), pressure measurements (manometry) of the lower esophageal sphincter, esophageal pH (acidity) tests, and the Bernstein test (esophageal acid infusion test) are sometimes needed to help confirm the diagnosis and check for complications.▲ Proof that symptoms result from acid reflux is best provided by a biopsy (microscopic examination of a tissue specimen) or the Bernstein test, regardless of x-ray or esophagoscopic findings. A biopsy is also the only reliable way to detect Barrett's syndrome.

For the Bernstein test, an acid solution is placed in the lower esophagus. The test indicates that the problem is acid reflux if symptoms quickly appear and then disappear when a salt solution is placed in the lower esophagus.

Esophagoscopy can identify a number of possible causes and complications. Microscopic examination of a biopsy sample taken from the esophagus can accurately identify acid reflux, even when inflammation isn't seen during esophagoscopy.

X-rays taken after a person drinks a barium solution and then lies on an incline with the head lower than the feet may show reflux of the barium from the stomach into the esophagus. A doctor may press on the abdomen to increase the likelihood of reflux. The x-rays taken after the barium is swallowed also can reveal esophageal ulcers or a narrowed esophagus.

Pressure measurements at the lower esophageal sphincter indicate its strength and can distinguish a normal sphincter from a poorly functioning one.

Treatment

Several measures may be taken to relieve acid reflux. Raising the head of the bed about 6 inches can keep acid flowing away from the esophagus as a person sleeps. Avoiding coffee, alcohol, and other substances that strongly stimulate the stomach to produce acid also can help. Also, a person can take an antacid 1 hour after meals and

▲ see page 484

another at bedtime to neutralize stomach acid and possibly reduce leakage from the lower esophageal sphincter. Taking drugs such as cimetidine or ranitidine can reduce stomach acidity. A person also should avoid specific foods (for example, fats and chocolate), smoking, and certain drugs (for example, anticholinergics)—all of which increase the tendency of the lower esophageal sphincter to leak. A doctor may prescribe a cholinergic drug (for example, bethanechol, metoclopramide, or cisapride) to make the lower sphincter close more tightly.

Unless bleeding from esophagitis is massive, emergency surgery isn't needed. But bleeding may recur. Esophageal narrowing is treated with drug therapy and repeated dilation, which may be performed using balloons or bougies (progressively larger metal dilators). If dilation is successful, narrowing doesn't seriously limit what a person can eat. Omeprazole or lansoprazole therapy or surgery can alleviate severe inflammation, bleeding, stricture, ulcers, or symptoms that haven't responded to other treatments. Omeprazole and lansoprazole are the most effective drugs for rapidly healing esophageal inflammation caused by reflux. Barrett's syndrome, a precancerous condition, may or may not disappear when treatment relieves symptoms.

Injury From Corrosive Substances

Corrosive substances, such as cleaning solutions, can injure the esophagus if they're swallowed accidentally or deliberately, as in a suicide attempt.

Some drugs can cause severe irritation if they lodge temporarily in the esophagus. Pain during swallowing and, less commonly, narrowing of the esophagus may result.

Esophageal Pouches

Esophageal pouches (diverticula) are abnormal protrusions from the esophagus that rarely may cause swallowing difficulties.

There are three types of esophageal pouch: pharyngeal pouch or Zenker's diverticulum, mid-esophageal pouch or traction diverticulum, and epiphrenic pouch. Each has a different cause, but probably all are related to uncoordinated swallowing and muscle relaxation, as may occur in

disorders such as achalasia and diffuse esophageal spasm.

Symptoms, Diagnosis, and Treatment

A large pouch can fill with food that may be regurgitated later, when the person bends over or lies down. This may cause food to be inhaled into the lungs during sleep, resulting in aspiration pneumonia. Rarely, the pouch may enlarge and cause swallowing difficulty.

A video x-ray or cineradiograph (an x-ray that produces a moving image as a person swallows barium) is used to diagnose a pouch.

Treatment isn't usually needed, although surgery can remove the pouch if swallowing is impaired or aspiration into the lungs is likely.

Hiatal Hernia

Hiatal hernia is a protrusion of a portion of the stomach from its normal position in the abdomen through the diaphragm.

In a **sliding hiatal hernia,** the junction between the esophagus and the stomach and also a portion of the stomach, which are normally below the diaphragm, protrude above it.

In a **paraesophageal hiatal hernia,** the junction between the esophagus and stomach is in the normal place below the diaphragm, but a portion of the stomach is pushed above the diaphragm and lies beside the esophagus.

The cause of hiatal hernia is usually unknown; it may be a birth defect or the result of an injury.

Symptoms

More than 40 percent of people have a sliding hiatal hernia, but most have no symptoms. Symptoms that do occur usually are minor.

A paraesophageal hiatal hernia generally produces no symptoms. However, it may get trapped or pinched by the diaphragm and lose its blood supply. Such trapping is a serious and painful condition, called strangulation, that requires immediate surgery.

Rarely, microscopic or massive bleeding from the lining of the hernia may occur with either type of hiatal hernia.

Diagnosis and Treatment

Usually, x-rays clearly reveal a hiatal hernia, though a doctor may have to press vigorously on the abdomen to reveal a sliding hiatal hernia.

Understanding Hiatal Hernia

A hiatal hernia is an abnormal bulging of a portion of the stomach through the diaphragm.

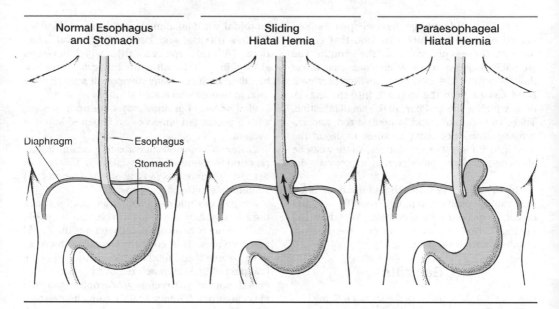

| Normal Esophagus and Stomach | Sliding Hiatal Hernia | Paraesophageal Hiatal Hernia |

Diaphragm — Esophagus

Stomach

A hiatal hernia usually requires no specific treatment, but any accompanying acid reflux is treated. A paraesophageal hernia may be corrected surgically to prevent strangulation.

Esophageal Laceration and Rupture

A laceration of the lower esophagus and the upper part of the stomach during forceful vomiting, retching, or hiccups is called Mallory-Weiss syndrome. The first symptom of the syndrome is usually bleeding from a ruptured artery. Mallory-Weiss syndrome is the cause of about 5 percent of bleeding episodes in the upper digestive (gastrointestinal) tract.

Diagnosis is made by esophagoscopy▲ or arteriography (an x-ray of an artery taken after injection of a dye). The laceration can't be detected on routine x-rays.

Most bleeding episodes stop by themselves, but sometimes a surgeon must tie off the bleeding artery. Bleeding may also be controlled by injecting vasopressin (a drug that constricts the artery) during arteriography.

The esophagus may be ruptured during endoscopy or other procedures in which instruments are inserted. With such ruptures, the risk of death is very high. Ruptures are usually caused by vomiting and rarely by heavy lifting or by straining during defecation. An esophageal rupture leads to tissue inflammation in the chest outside the esophagus and allows fluid to enter the space between the pleura covering the lungs, a condition called pleural effusion.■ Surgical repair of the esophagus and drainage of the area surrounding it are performed immediately.

▲ see page 485

■ see page 206

Disorders of the Stomach and Duodenum

The stomach is a large, bean-shaped, hollow, muscular organ that fills with food that comes through the esophagus from the mouth. The stomach secretes acid and enzymes that break down (digest) the food into smaller particles. Food passes from the stomach into the duodenum, which is the first part of the small intestine. There the stomach acid is neutralized, and enzymes in the duodenum continue to digest the food into still smaller substances, so they can be absorbed into the bloodstream to nourish the body.

The inside of the stomach and duodenum are remarkably resistant to injury from the acid and digestive enzymes they contain. Yet, they can become irritated, develop ulcers, become obstructed, and develop tumors.

Gastritis

Gastritis is inflammation of the stomach lining.

The lining of the stomach resists irritation and can usually withstand very strong acid. Nevertheless, the stomach lining can become irritated and inflamed for several reasons.

Bacterial gastritis commonly results from an infection by *Helicobacter pylori* organisms (bacteria that grow in the mucus-secreting cells of the stomach lining). No other bacteria are known to grow in the normally acidic stomach, but many types of bacteria may grow if the stomach doesn't produce acid. Such bacterial growth may cause temporary or persistent gastritis.

Acute stress gastritis, the most severe type of gastritis, is caused by a sudden severe illness or injury. The injury may not even be to the stomach. For example, extensive burns and injuries involving major bleeding are typical causes.

Chronic erosive gastritis can result from irritants such as drugs, especially aspirin and other non-

steroidal anti-inflammatory drugs (NSAIDs); Crohn's disease; and bacterial and viral infections. With this type of gastritis, which develops slowly in people who are otherwise healthy, bleeding or ulcers may develop. It's most common in people who abuse alcohol.

Viral or fungal gastritis may develop in people with a prolonged illness or an impaired immune system.

Eosinophilic gastritis may result from an allergic reaction to roundworm infestation. In this type of gastritis, eosinophils (a type of white blood cell) accumulate in the stomach wall.

Atrophic gastritis results when antibodies attack the stomach lining, causing it to become very thin and lose many or all of the cells that produce acid and enzymes. This condition usually affects elderly people. It also tends to occur in those who've had part of their stomach removed (a procedure called partial gastrectomy). Atrophic gastritis may cause pernicious anemia because it interferes with the absorption of vitamin B_{12} from food.▲

Ménétrier's disease is a form of gastritis whose cause isn't known. With this disease, the stomach walls develop thick, large folds; enlarged glands; and fluid-filled cysts. About 10 percent of people with Ménétrier's disease develop stomach cancer.

Plasma cell gastritis is another form of gastritis with an unknown cause. With this disease, plasma cells (a type of white blood cell) accumulate in the stomach wall and other organs.

Swallowing corrosives, such as cleaning fluids, or receiving high levels of radiation—for instance, during x-ray therapy—may also induce gastritis.

Symptoms

Symptoms vary, depending on the type of gastritis. In general, however, a person with gastritis has indigestion and discomfort in the upper abdomen.

In **acute stress gastritis,** the underlying illness, injury, or burn usually overshadows the stomach symptoms. However, the upper abdomen may

---

▲ see page 745

feel mildly uncomfortable. Shortly after the injury, small bruises may develop in the stomach lining. In a few hours, these bruises can change into ulcers. The ulcers and the gastritis may disappear if the person recovers quickly from the injury. If the person remains ill, however, the ulcers may enlarge and start to bleed, usually 2 to 5 days after the injury. The bleeding may turn the stools tarry black, turn the stomach fluid red, or if very severe, cause blood pressure to fall. The bleeding can be massive—and fatal.

Symptoms of **chronic erosive gastritis** include mild nausea and pain in the upper abdomen. However, many people, such as long-time aspirin users, have no pain. Some people may develop ulcerlike symptoms including pain when the stomach is empty. If the gastritis leads to bleeding stomach ulcers, symptoms may include passing tarry black stools (melena) or vomiting blood (hematemesis) or partially digested blood that looks like coffee grounds.

In **eosinophilic gastritis,** abdominal pain and vomiting may be caused by a narrowing or blockage of the stomach outlet to the duodenum.

In **Ménétrier's disease,** the most common symptom is stomach pain. Loss of appetite, nausea, vomiting, and weight loss are less common. Bleeding from the stomach is unusual. Fluid retention and tissue swelling (edema) may be caused by a loss of protein from the inflamed stomach lining. This lost protein mixes with the stomach contents and is eliminated from the body.

In **plasma cell gastritis,** abdominal pain and vomiting can occur along with a skin rash and diarrhea.

Gastritis from radiation therapy causes pain, nausea, and heartburn because of the inflammation and sometimes because of the development of stomach ulcers. Ulcers can perforate the stomach wall, spilling stomach contents into the abdominal cavity, causing peritonitis (inflammation of the abdominal lining) and excruciating pain. The resulting severe illness characterized by a rigid abdomen requires immediate surgery. In rare cases, after radiation therapy, scarring narrows the stomach outlet, causing abdominal pain and vomiting. Radiation can damage the protective stomach lining, so that bacteria can invade the stomach wall, causing a sudden, severe, extremely painful form of gastritis.

Diagnosis

Doctors suspect gastritis when a person has upper abdominal pain with nausea or heartburn. If the symptoms persist, tests often aren't needed, and treatment is started on the basis of the most likely cause.

If a doctor is uncertain about what the problem is, an examination of the stomach using an endoscope (a fiber-optic tube passed through the mouth)▲ may be needed. If necessary, a doctor can perform a biopsy (obtain a sample of the stomach lining for examination).

If the gastritis continues or recurs, a doctor looks for a cause, such as infection, and considers the person's diet, drugs, and drinking habits. Bacterial gastritis can be diagnosed by a biopsy. Many people with bacterial gastritis have antibodies to the bacterium causing it, and they can be detected by a blood test.

Treatment

Many doctors treat a *Helicobacter pylori* infection if it's causing symptoms. The infection can be controlled or eliminated with bismuth, antibiotics such as amoxicillin and clarithromycin, and the anti-ulcer drug omeprazole. At times, eliminating *Helicobacter pylori* from the stomach can be difficult.

Most people with acute stress gastritis recover fully when the underlying illness, injury, or bleeding is under control. However, 2 percent of the people in intensive care units have heavy bleeding from this condition, which is often fatal. Therefore, doctors try to prevent acute stress gastritis after a major illness, major injury, or severe burns. Antacids (which neutralize stomach acid) and potent antiulcer drugs (which reduce or halt stomach acid production) are commonly given after surgery and in most intensive care units to prevent and treat acute stress gastritis.

For people with heavy bleeding from stress gastritis, a wide variety of treatments have been used. Few, however, improve the prognosis: Such bleeding can be fatal. Blood transfusions may actually make bleeding worse. Bleeding points can be temporarily heat-sealed during endoscopy, but bleeding will start again if the underlying illness persists. If bleeding continues, clotting may

▲ see page 485

be induced in the appropriate blood vessel, or the entire stomach may have to be removed as a lifesaving measure.

Chronic erosive gastritis may be treated with antacids. The person should avoid certain drugs (for example, aspirin and other nonsteroidal anti-inflammatory drugs) and irritating foods. Coated aspirin tablets produce fewer ulcers than uncoated aspirin. Misoprostol probably reduces the risk of ulcers caused by nonsteroidal anti-inflammatory drugs.

For a person with eosinophilic gastritis, corticosteroids or surgery may be needed to relieve a blocked stomach outlet.

Atrophic gastritis can't be cured. Most people who have this disorder must take supplemental injections of vitamin B_{12}.

Ménétrier's disease may be cured by removing part or all of the stomach, but no drug treatment is effective.

Plasma cell gastritis may be treated with ulcer drugs that block the secretion of stomach acid.

Peptic Ulcer

A peptic ulcer is a well-defined round or oval sore where the lining of the stomach or duodenum has been eaten away by stomach acid and digestive juices. A shallow ulcer is called an erosion.

Pepsin is an enzyme that works together with the hydrochloric acid produced in the lining of the stomach to digest food, especially proteins. Peptic ulcers develop in the lining of the digestive tract that's exposed to acid and digestive enzymes—primarily the stomach and duodenum. The names of ulcers identify their anatomic locations or the circumstances under which they developed.

Duodenal ulcers, the most common type of peptic ulcer, occur in the duodenum, the first few inches of the small intestine just below the stomach. **Gastric ulcers,** which are less common, usually occur along the upper curve of the stomach. If part of the stomach is removed surgically, **marginal ulcers** can develop where the remaining stomach has been reconnected to the intestine. Repeated regurgitation of stomach acid into the lower part of the esophagus can cause inflammation (esophagitis) and **esophageal ulcers.** Ulcers occurring under the stress of severe illness, burns, or trauma are called **stress ulcers.**

Causes

An ulcer develops when the defense mechanisms protecting the duodenum or stomach from stomach acid break down—for example, when the amount of mucus production changes. The causes of such breakdowns aren't known.

Almost everyone produces stomach acid, but only 1 in 10 people develop ulcers. Different people generate different amounts of stomach acid, and each person's pattern of acid secretion tends to persist throughout life. In fact, infants can be identified as low, average, or high secretors. High secretors have a greater tendency to develop peptic ulcers than low secretors. However, most people who are high secretors never develop ulcers, and some people who are low secretors do develop them. Obviously, other factors besides acid secretion are involved.

Many people with **duodenal ulcers** have *Helicobacter pylori* bacteria in their stomach, and these bacteria are now considered a major cause of peptic ulcers. How the bacteria contribute to an ulcer is uncertain. They could interfere with the normal defenses against stomach acid, or they may produce a toxin that contributes to ulcer formation. Duodenal ulcers are almost never cancerous.

Gastric ulcers differ from duodenal ulcers in that they tend to develop later in life. Certain drugs—particularly aspirin, ibuprofen, and other nonsteroidal anti-inflammatory drugs—cause erosions and ulcers in the stomach, especially in the elderly. These erosions and ulcers tend to heal when the drugs are stopped and aren't likely to recur unless the person begins taking the drug again. Some cancerous (malignant) gastric ulcers also show healing, making them difficult to distinguish from noncancerous (benign) gastric ulcers, such as those caused by drugs.

Symptoms

The typical ulcer tends to heal and recur. Symptoms can vary with the location of the ulcer and the person's age. Children and the elderly may not have the usual symptoms or may have no symptoms at all. In these instances, ulcers are discovered only when complications develop.

Only about half the people with **duodenal ulcers** have typical symptoms: gnawing, burning, aching, soreness, an empty feeling, and hunger. The

Complications of Peptic Ulcers

Most ulcers can be cured without further complications. However, in some cases, peptic ulcers can develop potentially life-threatening complications such as penetration, perforation, bleeding, and obstruction.

Penetration

An ulcer can go through the muscular wall of the stomach or duodenum and continue into an adjacent solid organ, such as the liver or pancreas. This causes intense, piercing, persistent pain, which may be felt outside of the area involved—for example, the back may hurt when a duodenal ulcer penetrates the pancreas. The pain may intensify when the person changes position. If drugs don't heal the ulcer, surgery may be needed.

Perforation

Ulcers on the front surface of the duodenum, or less commonly the stomach, can go through the wall, creating an opening to the free space in the abdomen. The resulting pain is sudden, intense, and steady. It rapidly spreads throughout the abdomen. The person may feel pain in one or both shoulders, which may intensify with deep breathing. Changing position worsens the pain, so that the person often tries to lie very still. The abdomen is tender when touched, and the tenderness worsens if a doctor presses deeply and then suddenly releases the pressure. (Doctors called this symptom rebound tenderness.) Symptoms may be less intense in the elderly, in people taking corticosteroids, or in very ill people. A fever indicates an infection in the abdomen. If the condition isn't treated, shock can develop. This emergency situation requires immediate surgery and intravenous antibiotics.

Bleeding (hemorrhage)

Bleeding is a common complication of ulcers even when they aren't painful. Vomiting bright red blood or reddish-brown clumps of partially digested blood that look like coffee grounds and passing black or obviously bloody stools can be symptoms of a bleeding ulcer. Such bleeding may result from other gastrointestinal conditions as well, but doctors begin their investigation by looking for the source of bleeding in the stomach and duodenum. Unless bleeding is massive, a doctor performs an endoscopy (an examination using a flexible viewing tube). If a bleeding ulcer is seen, the endoscope can be used to cauterize it. If the source can't be found and the bleeding isn't severe, treatments include taking ulcer drugs, such as H_2 antagonists, and antacids. The person also receives intravenous fluids and takes nothing by mouth, so the gastrointestinal tract can rest. If the bleeding is massive or persistent, a doctor may use the endoscope to inject a material that causes clotting. If this measure fails, surgery is required.

Obstruction

Swelling of inflamed tissues around an ulcer or scarring from previous ulcer flare-ups can narrow the outlet from the stomach or narrow the duodenum. A person with this type of obstruction may vomit repeatedly—often regurgitating large volumes of food eaten hours before. A feeling of being unusually full after eating, bloating, and a lack of appetite are frequent symptoms of obstruction. Over time, vomiting can cause weight loss, dehydration, and an imbalance in body minerals. Treating the ulcers relieves the obstruction in most cases, but severe obstructions may require endoscopic or surgical correction.

pain tends to occur when the stomach is empty. The ulcer usually doesn't hurt on awakening, but pain develops by midmorning. The pain is steady and mild or moderately severe, and it's located in a definite area, almost always just below the breastbone. Drinking milk, eating, or taking antacids generally relieves the pain, but it usually returns 2 or 3 hours later. Pain that awakens the person at 1:00 or 2:00 A.M. is common. Frequently, the pain erupts once or more a day over a period of one to several weeks and then may disappear without treatment. However, pain usually recurs, often within the first 2 years and occasionally after several years. People generally develop patterns and often learn by experience when a recurrence is likely (commonly in spring and fall and during periods of stress).

The symptoms of **gastric ulcers** often don't follow the same pattern as those of duodenal ulcers; eating can cause pain rather than relieve it. Gastric ulcers are more likely to cause swelling of the tissues leading into the small intestine, which may prevent food from easily passing out of the stomach. This may cause bloating, nausea, or vomiting after eating.

With esophagitis or **esophageal ulcers,** the person usually feels pain while swallowing or lying down.

More severe symptoms appear when the complications of peptic ulcers, such as bleeding or perforation, occur.

Diagnosis

A doctor thinks of ulcers when someone has characteristic stomach pain. Tests may be needed to confirm the diagnosis because gastric cancer can cause similar symptoms. Also, when severe ulcers resist treatment, particularly if a person has several ulcers or they're in unusual places, a doctor may suspect other underlying conditions that cause the stomach to overproduce acid.

To help diagnose ulcers and identify their underlying cause, a doctor may use endoscopy, barium contrast x-rays, gastric analysis, and blood tests.▲

Endoscopy is an outpatient procedure in which a doctor inserts a long, flexible viewing tube (endoscope) through the mouth and looks directly into the stomach. Because ulcers are usually visible through an endoscope, many doctors use endoscopy as the first diagnostic procedure. Endoscopy is more reliable than x-rays for detecting ulcers in the duodenum and on the back wall of the stomach; endoscopy is also more reliable if the person has had stomach surgery. However, even a highly skilled endoscopist may miss 5 to 10 percent of gastric and duodenal ulcers. With an endoscope, a doctor can perform a biopsy

▲ see page 484

(obtain a tissue sample for examination) to determine if a gastric ulcer is cancerous. An endoscope also can be used to stop bleeding from an ulcer.

Barium contrast x-rays of the stomach and duodenum (also called a barium swallow or an upper gastrointestinal series) are useful when endoscopy doesn't reveal an ulcer. However, x-rays can miss up to 20 percent of peptic ulcers.

Gastric analysis is a procedure in which fluids are suctioned directly from the stomach and duodenum so the amount of acid can be measured. This procedure is done only if ulcers are severe or recurrent or if surgery is scheduled.

Blood tests can't detect an ulcer, but blood counts can detect anemia resulting from a bleeding ulcer. Other blood tests can detect the presence of *Helicobacter pylori.*

Treatment

One aspect of treating duodenal or gastric ulcers is neutralizing or decreasing stomach acidity. This process begins with eliminating possible stomach irritants, such as nonsteroidal antiinflammatory drugs, alcohol, and nicotine. Although bland diets may have a place in ulcer treatment, no strong evidence supports the belief that such diets speed healing or keep ulcers from recurring. Nevertheless, people should avoid foods that seem to make pain and bloating worse.

Antacids

Antacids relieve symptoms, promote healing, and decrease the number of recurrences of ulcers. Most antacids can be purchased without a doctor's prescription.

The capacity of an antacid for neutralizing stomach acid varies with the amount of antacid taken, with the person, and at different times for the same person. The taste of an antacid, its effect on bowel movements, its cost, and its effectiveness all determine a person's choice of antacids. Antacids are available as tablets or liquids. Tablets may be more convenient, but they aren't as effective as liquids.

Absorbable antacids rapidly and completely neutralize stomach acid. Sodium bicarbonate and calcium carbonate, the strongest antacids, may be taken from time to time for short-term relief. Because they're absorbed by the bloodstream, continual use may change the acid-alkaline balance in the blood, producing alkalosis (the milk-alkali syndrome). Therefore, these antacids generally shouldn't be used in large amounts for more than a few days. Symptoms of alkalosis include nausea, headache, and weakness, but these symptoms can result from many disorders.

Nonabsorbable antacids are preferred because they cause fewer side effects; in particular, they're unlikely to cause alkalosis. They combine with stomach acid to form compounds that stay in the stomach, reducing digestive juice activity and relieving ulcer symptoms without causing alkalosis. However, these antacids may interfere with the absorption of other drugs (such as tetracycline, digoxin, and iron) into the bloodstream.

Aluminum hydroxide is a relatively safe, commonly used antacid. However, aluminum may bind with phosphate in the gastrointestinal tract, reducing blood phosphate levels and causing a loss of appetite and weakness. The risk of these side effects is greater in alcoholics and people with kidney disease, including those receiving hemodialysis. Aluminum hydroxide may also cause constipation.

Magnesium hydroxide is a more effective antacid than aluminum hydroxide. Bowel movements will usually remain regular if only 4 doses of 1 to 2 tablespoons a day are taken; more than 4 doses may cause diarrhea. Because small amounts of magnesium are absorbed into the bloodstream, this drug should be taken in small doses by people with kidney damage. Many antacids contain both magnesium and aluminum hydroxide.

Ulcer Drugs

Ulcers are commonly treated for at least 6 weeks with drugs that reduce the output of acid in the stomach and duodenum. Any one of several ulcer drugs can neutralize or reduce gastric acid and relieve the symptoms, usually within a few days. If symptoms aren't completely relieved or if they return when the drug is stopped, additional testing is usually done.

Sucralfate may work by forming a protective coating in the base of an ulcer to promote healing. It works well on peptic ulcers and is a reasonable alternative to antacids. Sucralfate is taken three or four times a day and isn't absorbed into the bloodstream, so side effects are few. It may, however, cause constipation.

H_2 antagonists (cimetidine, ranitidine, famotidine, and nizatidine) promote ulcer healing by reducing the acid and digestive enzymes in the stomach and duodenum. These highly effective drugs are taken only once or twice a day. Most cause few serious side effects, and several are now available without a prescription. However, cimetidine may produce reversible breast enlargement in men. Less commonly, cimetidine may cause impotence in men who take high doses for prolonged periods. Mental changes (especially in the elderly), diarrhea, rash, fever, and muscle pains have been reported in less than 1 percent of the people treated with cimetidine. If a person who takes cimetidine suffers from any of these side effects, changing to another H_2 antagonist may solve the problem. Because cimetidine may interfere with the body's elimination of certain drugs—such as theophylline for asthma, warfarin for blood clotting, and phenytoin for seizures—people should make sure their doctor knows they're taking cimetidine.

Omeprazole and lansoprazole are very potent drugs that inhibit the production of the enzymes needed for the stomach to make acid. These drugs can completely inhibit acid secretion, and they have long-lasting effects. They promote healing in a greater percentage of people in a shorter period of time than do H_2 antagonists. They're particularly useful in treating people who have esophagitis with or without esophageal ulcers and people who have other conditions that affect gastric acid secretion, such as the Zollinger-Ellison syndrome.

Antibiotics increasingly are being used when the bacterium *Helicobacter pylori* is the major underlying cause of ulcers. The treatment consists of one or more antibiotics and a drug to reduce or neutralize stomach acid. Combinations of bismuth subsalicylate (a drug similar to sucralfate), tetracycline, and metronidazole or amoxicillin are most commonly used. Omeprazole and an antibiotic are also an effective combination. Such treatment may relieve ulcer symptoms even if ulcers have resisted previous treatment or have recurred repeatedly.

Misoprostol may be used to prevent gastric ulcers caused by nonsteroidal anti-inflammatory drugs. Doctors don't agree yet on all the specific circumstances in which misoprostol should be used. However, most agree that it's helpful in some people with arthritis who are taking high doses of nonsteroidal anti-inflammatory drugs. Misoprostol isn't used in all such patients because it produces diarrhea in about 30 percent of people, and only about 10 to 15 percent of people taking high doses of nonsteroidal anti-inflammatory drugs for arthritis develop peptic ulcers.

Surgery

Surgery for ulcers is seldom needed because drug therapy is so effective. Surgery is used primarily to deal with complications of a peptic ulcer such as a perforation, an obstruction that fails to respond to drug therapy or that recurs, two or more major episodes of bleeding ulcers, a gastric ulcer suspected of being cancerous, or severe and frequent recurrences of peptic ulcers. A number of different operations may be performed to treat these problems. However, ulcers may recur after surgery, and each procedure may cause problems of its own, such as weight loss, poor digestion, and anemia.

CHAPTER 103

Disorders of the Anus and Rectum

The anus is the opening at the end of the digestive tract where waste material (stool, feces) leaves the body. The rectum is the section of the digestive tract above the anus where stool is held before it passes out of the body through the anus.

The rectal lining consists of glistening, orange-tan tissue containing mucus glands—much like the rest of the intestinal lining. The anus is formed partly from the surface layers of the body, including the skin, and partly from the intestine. The lining of the rectum is relatively insensitive to pain, but the nerves from the anus and nearby external skin are very sensitive to pain. The veins from the anus drain into both the portal vein, which leads to the liver, and the general circulation. The lymph vessels of the rectum drain into the large intestine; those of the anus drain into the lymph nodes in the groin.

A muscular ring (anal sphincter) keeps the anus closed. This sphincter is controlled subconsciously by the autonomic nervous system; however, the lower part of it can be relaxed or tightened at will.

To diagnose disorders of the anus and rectum, a doctor inspects the skin around the anus for any abnormality. With gloved fingers, a doctor probes a man's rectum or a woman's rectum and vagina. Next, a doctor looks into the anus and rectum with a short, rigid viewing tube (anoscope). A 6- to 10-inch rigid viewing tube (proctoscope) also may be used. A sigmoidoscope, which is a longer flexible tube, may then be inserted so that the doctor can observe the large intestine as much as 2 feet from the anus. If the area in or around the anus is painful, a local, regional, or even general anesthetic may be given before sigmoidoscopy (examination with a sigmoidoscope). Sometimes a cleansing enema is given before sigmoidoscopy. Tissue samples and smears of secretions for microscopic examination and cultures may be obtained during sigmoidoscopy. A barium x-ray▲ also may be performed.

Hemorrhoids

Hemorrhoids are swollen tissues that contain veins and that are located in the wall of the rectum and anus.

Hemorrhoids may become inflamed, develop a blood clot (thrombus), bleed, or become enlarged and protrude. Hemorrhoids that remain in the anus are called internal hemorrhoids; those that protrude outside the anus are called external hemorrhoids.

Hemorrhoids may develop from repeated straining during bowel movements, and constipation may make straining worse. Liver disease increases the blood pressure in the portal vein, sometimes leading to the formation of hemorrhoids.

Symptoms and Diagnosis

Hemorrhoids can bleed, typically after a bowel movement, producing blood-streaked stool or toilet paper. The blood may turn water in the toilet bowl red. However, the amount of blood is usually small, and hemorrhoids rarely lead to severe blood loss or anemia.

▲ see page 486

Hemorrhoids that protrude from the anus may need to be pushed back gently with a finger, or they may go back by themselves. A hemorrhoid may swell and become painful if its surface is rubbed raw or if a blood clot forms in it. Less commonly, hemorrhoids may discharge mucus and create a feeling that the rectum isn't completely emptied. Itching in the anal region (pruritus ani) isn't a symptom of hemorrhoids, but it may develop because the painful area is difficult to keep clean.

A doctor can readily diagnose swollen, painful hemorrhoids by inspecting the anus and rectum. Anoscopy and sigmoidoscopy help a doctor determine if the person has a more serious condition, such as a tumor.

Treatment

Usually, hemorrhoids don't require treatment unless they cause symptoms. Taking stool softeners or psyllium may relieve constipation and the straining that accompanies it. Bleeding hemorrhoids can be treated with an injection of a substance that causes the veins to become obliterated with scar tissue; this procedure is called injection sclerotherapy.

Large internal hemorrhoids and those that don't respond to injection sclerotherapy are tied off with rubber bands. The procedure, called rubber band ligation, causes the hemorrhoid to wither and drop off painlessly. The treatment is applied to one hemorrhoid at a time at intervals of 2 weeks or longer. Three to six treatments may be needed. Hemorrhoids may also be destroyed using a laser (laser destruction), an infrared light (infrared photocoagulation), or an electric current (electrocoagulation). Surgery may be used if other treatments fail.

When a hemorrhoid with a blood clot causes pain, it's treated with warm sitz baths (baths in which the person sits in water), local anesthetic ointments, or witch hazel compresses. Pain and swelling usually diminish after a short while, and clots disappear over 4 to 6 weeks. Alternatively, a doctor may cut the vein and remove the clot in an attempt to relieve the pain rapidly.

Anal Fissure

An anal fissure (fissure in ano, anal ulcer) is a tear or ulcer in the lining of the anus.

Anal fissures are usually caused by an injury from a hard or large bowel movement. Fissures cause the sphincter to go into spasm, which may prevent healing.

Fissures cause pain and bleeding during or shortly after a bowel movement. The pain lasts for several minutes to several hours and then subsides until the next bowel movement. A doctor diagnoses a fissure by inspecting the anus.

Treatment

A stool softener or psyllium may reduce the injury caused by hard bowel movements, while lubricating and soothing the lower rectum. Lubricant suppositories also can be helpful. A warm sitz bath for 10 or 15 minutes after each bowel movement eases discomfort and helps increase blood flow, which promotes healing. When these simple measures fail, surgery generally is needed.

Anorectal Abscess

An anorectal abscess is a collection of pus caused by bacteria invading a space around the anus and rectum.

Abscesses just under the skin can be swollen, red, tender, and very painful. Often, a doctor can see an abscess in the skin around the anus. Using gloved fingers, a doctor can feel tender swelling in the rectum, even when no external swelling can be seen. Abscesses higher in the rectum may cause no rectal symptoms but may produce fever and pain in the lower abdomen.

Treatment

Antibiotics have limited value except in people who have a fever, diabetes, or an infection elsewhere in the body. Usually, treatment consists of injecting a local anesthetic, cutting into the abscess, and draining the pus. Occasionally, a person is hospitalized and given general anesthesia before a doctor cuts and drains an abscess. After all the pus has been drained, an abnormal channel to the skin (anorectal fistula) may develop.

Anorectal Fistula

An anorectal fistula (fistula in ano) is an abnormal channel from the anus or rectum usually to the skin near the anus but occasionally to another organ, such as the vagina.

Most fistulas begin in a deep gland in the wall of the anus or rectum. Sometimes fistulas result from drainage of an anorectal abscess, but often the cause can't be identified. Fistulas are more common among people who have Crohn's disease or tuberculosis. They also occur in those with diverticulitis, cancer, or an anal or rectal injury. A fistula in an infant is usually a birth defect; such fistulas are more common in boys than girls. Fistulas that connect the rectum and vagina may result from x-ray therapy, cancer, Crohn's disease, or an injury to the mother during childbirth.

Symptoms and Diagnosis

A fistula may be painful, or it may discharge pus. A doctor can usually see one or more openings of a fistula or can feel the fistula beneath the surface. A probe may be inserted to determine its depth and direction. Looking through an anoscope inserted into the rectum and exploring with the probe, a doctor may locate the internal opening. Inspection with a sigmoidoscope helps a doctor determine whether the problem is being caused by cancer, Crohn's disease, or another disorder.

Treatment

The only effective treatment is surgery (fistulotomy), during which the sphincter may be partially cut. If too much of the sphincter is cut, the person may have difficulty controlling bowel movements. If the person has diarrhea, active ulcerative colitis, or active Crohn's disease, all of which may delay wound healing, the operation usually isn't performed.

Proctitis

Proctitis is an inflammation of the lining of the rectum (rectal mucosa).

In ulcerative proctitis, a common form of proctitis, ulcers appear in the inflamed rectal lining. The condition may affect 1 to 4 inches of the lower rectum. Some cases readily respond to treatment; others persist or recur and require prolonged treatment. Some cases eventually evolve into ulcerative colitis.

Proctitis, which is becoming increasingly common, has several causes. It may result from Crohn's disease or ulcerative colitis. It also can result from a sexually transmitted disease (such as gonorrhea, syphilis, *Chlamydia trachomatis* in-

fection, herpes simplex, or cytomegalovirus infection), especially in homosexual men. Anyone whose immune system is impaired is also at increased risk of developing proctitis, particularly from infections caused by the herpes simplex virus or cytomegalovirus. Proctitis may be caused by a specific bacterium, such as *Salmonella*, or by the use of an antibiotic that destroys normal intestinal bacteria and allows other bacteria to grow in their place. Another cause of proctitis is radiation therapy directed at or near the rectum.

Symptoms and Diagnosis

Proctitis typically causes painless bleeding or the passage of mucus from the rectum. When the cause is gonorrhea, herpes simplex, or cytomegalovirus, the anus and rectum may be intensely painful.

To make the diagnosis, a doctor looks inside the rectum with a proctoscope or sigmoidoscope and takes a tissue sample of the rectal lining for examination. The laboratory then can identify bacteria, fungi, or viruses that may be causing the proctitis. A doctor also may examine other areas of the intestine using a colonoscope or barium x-rays.▲

Treatment

Antibiotics are the best treatment for proctitis caused by a specific bacterial infection. When proctitis is caused by using an antibiotic that destroys normal intestinal bacteria, metronidazole or vancomycin should destroy the harmful bacteria that have displaced the normal ones. When the cause is radiation therapy or isn't known, the person may get relief from a corticosteroid, such as hydrocortisone, and mesalamine, another anti-inflammatory drug. Both can be taken as an enema or as a suppository. Cortisone, a type of corticosteroid, comes in a foam that can be inserted with a cartridge and plunger. Sulfasalazine or a similar drug may be taken orally at the same time. If these forms of therapy don't relieve the inflammation, oral corticosteroids may help.

Pilonidal Disease

Pilonidal disease is an infection caused by a hair that injures the skin at the top of the cleft between the buttocks.

A pilonidal abscess is a collection of pus at the infection site; a pilonidal sinus is a chronic draining wound at the site.

▲ see page 486

Pilonidal disease usually occurs in young, hairy white men. To distinguish it from other infections, a doctor looks for pits—tiny holes in or next to the infected area. A pilonidal sinus can cause pain and swelling.

Generally, a pilonidal abscess must be cut and drained by a doctor. Usually, a pilonidal sinus must be removed surgically.

Rectal Prolapse

Rectal prolapse is a protrusion of the rectum through the anus.

Rectal prolapse causes the rectum to turn inside out, so that the rectal lining is visible as a dark red, moist, fingerlike projection from the anus.

A temporary prolapse of only the rectal lining (mucosa) often occurs in otherwise normal infants, probably when the infant strains during a bowel movement, and is rarely serious. In adults, prolapse of the rectal lining tends to persist and may worsen, so that more of the rectum protrudes.

Procidentia is a complete prolapse of the rectum. It occurs most often in women over age 60.

To determine the extent of a prolapse, a doctor examines the area while the person stands or squats and while the person strains. By feeling the anal sphincter with a gloved finger, a doctor often detects diminished muscle tone. A sigmoidoscopy and barium enema x-rays of the large intestine may reveal an underlying disease, such as disease in the nerves that supply the sphincter.

Treatment

In infants and children, a stool softener eliminates the urge to strain. Strapping the buttocks together between bowel movements usually helps the prolapse heal on its own.

In adults, surgery is needed to correct the problem. Surgery often cures procidentia. During one kind of abdominal operation, the rectum is lifted, pulled back, and attached to the sacral bone. In another, a segment of the rectum is removed.

For people who are too weak to undergo surgery because of old age or poor health, a wire or plastic loop can be inserted to encircle the sphincter; this technique is called the Thiersch procedure.

Anal Itching

Itchy skin around the anus (pruritus ani) can result from many causes:
- Skin disorders such as psoriasis and atopic dermatitis
- Allergic reactions such as contact dermatitis caused by anesthetic preparations applied to the skin, various ointments, or chemicals used in soap
- Certain foods such as spices, citrus fruits, coffee, beer, and cola as well as vitamin C tablets
- Microorganisms such as fungi and bacteria
- Infestation by parasites such as pinworms and, less commonly, scabies or lice infestation (pediculosis)
- Antibiotics, especially tetracycline
- Diseases such as diabetes or liver disease, anal disorders (for example, skin tags, cryptitis, draining fistulas), and cancers (for example, Bowen's disease)
- Poor hygiene that leaves irritating feces or excessive rubbing and use of soap
- Warmth and excessive sweating because of pantyhose, tight underwear (especially noncotton underwear), obesity, or hot weather
- Anxiety-itch-anxiety cycle

People with large external hemorrhoids may have itching because the area is difficult to keep clean.

Treatment

After bowel movements, the anal area should be cleaned with absorbent cotton, which may be moistened with plain warm water. Frequent dusting with baby powder or cornstarch may combat moisture. Corticosteroid creams, antifungal creams such as miconazole, or soothing suppositories may be used. Foods that can cause anal itching are avoided for a while to see if the condition improves. Clothing should be loose and bed linens light. If the condition doesn't improve and a doctor suspects cancer, a skin specimen may be obtained for examination.

Foreign Objects

Swallowed objects, such as toothpicks, chicken bones, or fish bones; gallstones; or a hard lump of feces may become lodged at the junction between the anus and rectum. Also, objects may be inserted intentionally. Enema tips, thermometers, and objects inserted for sexual stimulation may become lodged in the rectum. These larger objects usually become lodged in the midrectum.

Sudden, excruciating pain during bowel movements suggests that a foreign object, usually at the junction between the anus and rectum, is penetrating the lining of the rectum or anus. Other symptoms depend on the size and shape of the object, how long it has been there, and whether it has caused an infection or perforation.

A doctor can feel the object by probing with gloved fingers during an examination. An abdominal examination, sigmoidoscopy, and x-rays may be needed to make sure the wall of the large intestine hasn't been perforated.

Treatment

If a doctor can feel the object, a local anesthetic is usually injected under the skin and lining of the anus to numb the area. The anus can then be spread wider with a rectal retractor, and the object can be grasped and removed. Natural movements of the wall of the large intestine (peristalsis) generally bring the foreign object down, making the removal possible.

Occasionally, if a doctor can't feel the object or if the object can't be removed through the rectum, exploratory surgery is needed. The person is given regional or general anesthesia, so that the object can be gently moved toward the anus or the large intestine can be cut open to remove the object. After the object is removed, the doctor performs a sigmoidoscopy to determine whether the rectum has been perforated or otherwise injured.

CHAPTER 104

Disorders of the Pancreas

The pancreas is a leaf-shaped gland about 5 inches long. It's surrounded by the lower edge of the stomach and the wall of the duodenum (the first portion of the small intestine leading out of the stomach). The pancreas has two major functions: to secrete fluid containing digestive enzymes into the duodenum and to secrete the hormones insulin and glucagon,▲ which are needed to metabolize sugar, into the bloodstream.

The pancreas also secretes large quantities of sodium bicarbonate (the same chemical as baking soda) into the duodenum, which neutralizes the acid coming from the stomach. This sodium bicarbonate secretion flows through a collecting duct that runs along the center of the pancreas (pancreatic duct). This duct then joins with the common bile duct from the gallbladder and liver to form the ampulla of Vater, which joins the duodenum at the sphincter of Oddi.

Acute Pancreatitis

Acute pancreatitis is a sudden inflammation of the pancreas that may be mild or life threatening.

Normally, the pancreas secretes pancreatic juice through the pancreatic duct to the duodenum. This pancreatic juice contains digestive enzymes in an inactive form and an inhibitor that inactivates any enzymes that become activated on the way to the duodenum. Blockage of the pancreatic duct (for example, by a gallstone stuck in the sphincter of Oddi) stops the flow of the pancreatic juice. Usually, the blockage is temporary and causes limited damage, which is soon repaired. But if the blockage continues, activated enzymes accumulate in the pancreas, overwhelm the inhibitor, and begin to digest the cells of the pancreas, causing severe inflammation.

Damage to the pancreas may permit enzymes to ooze out and enter the bloodstream or the abdominal cavity, where they cause irritation and inflammation of the lining of the cavity (peritonitis) or of other organs. The part of the pancreas

---

▲ see page 717

that produces hormones, especially insulin, tends not to be damaged or affected.

Gallstones and alcoholism account for almost 80 percent of the hospital admissions for acute pancreatitis. One and a half times as many women as men experience acute pancreatitis caused by gallstones, whereas six times as many men as women experience acute pancreatitis caused by alcoholism. Gallstones that cause acute pancreatitis may become stuck in the sphincter of Oddi for a time, thus blocking the opening of the pancreatic duct; however, most gallstones pass into the intestinal tract. Drinking more than 4 ounces of alcohol a day for several years may cause the small ductules in the pancreas that drain into the pancreatic duct to clog, eventually causing acute pancreatitis. An attack of pancreatitis may be precipitated by an alcoholic binge or by an excessively large meal. Many other conditions can also cause acute pancreatitis.

Symptoms

Almost everyone with acute pancreatitis suffers severe abdominal pain in the upper midabdomen, below the breastbone (sternum). The pain often penetrates to the back. Rarely, the pain is felt first in the lower abdomen. Usually starting suddenly and reaching its maximum intensity in minutes, the pain is steady and severe, has a penetrating quality, and persists for days. Often, even large doses of an injected narcotic don't give complete relief. Coughing, vigorous movement, and deep breathing may make it worse; sitting upright and leaning forward may provide some relief. Most people feel nauseated and have to vomit, sometimes to the point of dry heaves—retching without producing any vomit.

Some people, especially those who develop acute pancreatitis because of alcoholism, may never develop any symptoms other than moderate pain. Others feel terrible. They look sick and sweaty, and they have a fast pulse (100 to 140 beats a minute) and shallow, rapid breathing. Inflammation of the lungs may contribute to the rapid breathing.

At first, body temperature may be normal, but it increases in a few hours to between 100° and 101° F. Blood pressure may be high or low, but it tends to fall when the person stands, causing

Locating the Pancreas

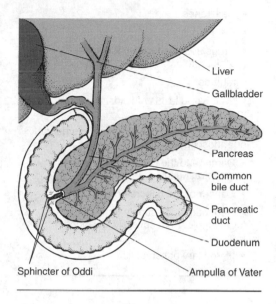

Liver
Gallbladder
Pancreas
Common bile duct
Pancreatic duct
Duodenum
Sphincter of Oddi
Ampulla of Vater

faintness. As the illness progresses, people tend to be less and less aware of their surroundings: Some are nearly unconscious. Occasionally, the whites of the eyes (sclera) become yellowish.

One in five people with acute pancreatitis develops some swelling in the upper abdomen. This swelling may occur because the movement of stomach and intestinal contents stops (a condition called gastrointestinal ileus) or because the inflamed pancreas enlarges and pushes the stomach forward. Fluid also may accumulate in the abdomen (a condition called ascites).

In severe acute pancreatitis (necrotizing pancreatitis), blood pressure may fall, possibly causing shock. Severe acute pancreatitis can be life threatening.

Diagnosis

Characteristic abdominal pain leads a doctor to suspect acute pancreatitis, especially in a person who has gallbladder disease or who is an alcoholic. On examination, a doctor often notes

---

Causes of Acute Pancreatitis

- Gallstones

- Alcoholism

- Drugs such as furosemide and azathioprine

- Mumps

- High blood levels of lipids, especially triglycerides

- Damage to the pancreas from surgery or endoscopy

- Damage to the pancreas from blunt or penetrating injuries

- Cancer of the pancreas

- Reduced blood supply to the pancreas, for example, from severely low blood pressure

- Hereditary pancreatitis

---

that the abdominal wall muscles are rigid. When listening to the abdomen with a stethoscope, a doctor may hear diminished bowel (intestinal) sounds.

No single blood test proves a diagnosis of acute pancreatitis, but certain tests corroborate the diagnosis. Blood levels of two enzymes produced by the pancreas, amylase and lipase, usually increase on the first day of the illness but return to normal in 3 to 7 days. Sometimes, however, these levels don't increase because so much of the pancreas has been destroyed during previous episodes of pancreatitis that few cells are left to release the enzymes. People with severe acute pancreatitis often have fewer red blood cells than normal because of bleeding into the pancreas and abdomen.

Standard x-rays of the abdomen may show dilated loops of intestine or rarely one or more gallstones. Ultrasound scanning may show gallstones in the gallbladder and sometimes in the common bile duct and also may detect swelling of the pancreas.

▲ see box, page 736

A computed tomography (CT) scan is particularly useful in detecting changes in the size of the pancreas and is used in severe cases and in cases with complications, such as extremely low blood pressure. Because the images are so clear, a CT scan helps a doctor make a precise diagnosis.

In severe acute pancreatitis, a CT scan helps determine the prognosis. If the scan indicates that the pancreas is only mildly swollen, the prognosis is excellent. If the scan shows large areas of destroyed pancreas, the prognosis is not so good.

Endoscopic retrograde cholangiopancreatography (an x-ray technique that shows the structure of the common bile duct and pancreatic duct) usually is done only when the suspected cause of pancreatitis is a gallstone in the common bile duct. A doctor passes an endoscope through the person's mouth and into the small intestine to the sphincter of Oddi. Then the doctor injects a radiopaque dye into the ducts. The dye is visible on the x-rays. If the x-rays show a gallstone, the doctor can use the endoscope to remove it.

Treatment

Most people with pancreatitis are hospitalized. A person who has mild acute pancreatitis must avoid all food and water because eating and drinking stimulate the pancreas to produce more enzymes. Fluids and nutrients are given intravenously. A tube is inserted through the nose and into the stomach to remove fluid and air, particularly if nausea and vomiting persist.

A person who has severe acute pancreatitis generally is admitted to an intensive care unit, where vital signs (pulse, blood pressure, and rate of breathing) are monitored closely. The output of urine is measured frequently. Also, blood samples are drawn to measure various components of the blood, including hematocrit, ▲ glucose levels, electrolyte levels, white blood cell count, and blood enzyme levels.

The person is fed intravenously and given nothing by mouth for at least 2 weeks and possibly for as long as 6 weeks. A tube is inserted through the nose and into the stomach to keep the stomach empty and often to give antacids to help prevent ulcers.

The blood volume is carefully maintained by giving intravenous fluids, and heart function is closely monitored. Oxygen is given through a face mask or nasal tubes to increase the amount in the bloodstream; if this therapy is inadequate, the person may be put on a respirator to assist breathing. Severe pain usually is treated with the drug meperidine.

Occasionally, surgery is needed during the first few days of severe acute pancreatitis. For instance, surgery may be used to alleviate pancreatitis that stems from an injury, or surgical exploration may be used to clarify an uncertain diagnosis. Sometimes, if a person's condition deteriorates after the first week of the illness, an operation is performed to remove infected, nonfunctioning pancreatic tissue.

Infection of an inflamed pancreas is a risk, particularly after the first week of illness. Sometimes, a doctor suspects an infection because the person's condition worsens, and a fever and high white blood cell counts develop after other symptoms start to subside. The diagnosis is made by culturing blood samples and performing computed tomography (CT) scans. A doctor may be able to withdraw a sample of infected material from the pancreas by inserting a needle through the skin and into the pancreas. Infections are treated with antibiotics and surgery.

Sometimes, a pseudocyst forms in the pancreas, filling with pancreatic enzymes, fluid, and tissue debris and expanding like a balloon. If a pseudocyst grows larger and causes pain or other symptoms, a doctor will decompress it. The need for decompression is particularly urgent if the pseudocyst expands rapidly, becomes infected, bleeds, or appears ready to rupture. Depending on the location of the pseudocyst, decompression is achieved either by inserting a catheter through the skin and allowing the pseudocyst to drain for several weeks or by performing a surgical procedure.

When acute pancreatitis results from gallstones, treatment depends on the severity. If the pancreatitis is mild, removal of the gallbladder can usually be delayed until symptoms subside. Severe pancreatitis caused by gallstones can be treated with endoscopy or surgery. The surgical procedure consists of removing the gallbladder and clearing out the ducts. In elderly people with other illness such as heart disease, endoscopy often is used first, but if this treatment fails, surgery should be performed.

Chronic Pancreatitis

Chronic pancreatitis is a long-standing inflammation of the pancreas.

In the United States, the most common cause of chronic pancreatitis is alcoholism. Other causes include a hereditary predisposition and an obstruction of the pancreatic duct resulting from duct narrowing or pancreatic cancer. Rarely, an episode of severe acute pancreatitis makes the pancreatic duct so narrow that chronic pancreatitis results. In many cases, the cause of chronic pancreatitis isn't known.

In tropical countries (for example, India, Indonesia, and Nigeria), chronic pancreatitis of unknown cause in children and young adults may give rise to diabetes and calcium deposits in the pancreas. The initial symptoms commonly result from the diabetes.

Symptoms

Symptoms of chronic pancreatitis generally fall into two patterns. In one, a person has persistent midabdominal pain that varies in intensity. In the other, a person has intermittent episodes of pancreatitis with symptoms similar to those of mild to moderate acute pancreatitis; the pain sometimes is severe and lasts for many hours or several days. With either pattern, as chronic pancreatitis progresses, cells that secrete the digestive enzymes are slowly destroyed, so eventually pain doesn't occur.

As the number of digestive enzymes decreases, food is inadequately absorbed, and the person may produce bulky, foul-smelling stools. The stool is light-colored and greasy and may even contain oil droplets. The malabsorption also leads to weight loss. Eventually, the insulin-secreting cells of the pancreas may be destroyed, gradually leading to diabetes.

Diagnosis

A doctor suspects chronic pancreatitis because of a person's symptoms or history of acute pancreatitis attacks. Blood tests are less useful in diagnosing chronic pancreatitis than in diagnosing acute pancreatitis, but they may indicate elevated levels of amylase and lipase. Also, blood tests can be used to check the level of glucose (a type of sugar) in the blood, which may be elevated.

Abdominal x-rays and ultrasound scans can show stones in the pancreas. Endoscopic retrograde pancreatography (an x-ray technique that shows the structure of the pancreatic duct) may reveal a dilated duct, narrowing of the duct, or stones in the duct. A computed tomography (CT) scan may show these abnormalities as well as the size, shape, and texture of the pancreas. And unlike endoscopic retrograde pancreatography, a CT scan doesn't require the use of an endoscope.

Treatment

During an attack, avoiding alcohol is essential. Avoiding all food and receiving only intravenous fluids can rest the pancreas and intestine and may relieve a painful flare-up. Often, however, narcotic analgesics still are needed to relieve the pain.

Later, eating four or five meals a day consisting of food low in fat and protein and high in carbohydrate may help reduce the frequency and intensity of the flare-ups. The person also must continue to avoid alcohol. If pain continues, a doctor searches for complications, such as an inflammatory mass in the head of the pancreas or a pseudocyst. An inflammatory mass may require surgery; a pancreatic pseudocyst that causes pain as it expands may have to be decompressed.

If the person has continuing pain and no complications, usually a doctor injects the nerves from the pancreas to block pain impulses from reaching the brain. If this procedure fails, surgery may be used. For instance, when the pancreatic duct is dilated, creating a bypass from the pancreas to the small intestine relieves the pain in about 70 to 80 percent of patients. When the duct isn't dilated, part of the pancreas may have to be removed. If most of the disease is in the tail of the pancreas (the part farthest from the duodenum), the tail can be removed. If the head of the pancreas is involved, it can be removed together with the duodenum. These operations may relieve pain in 60 to 80 percent of patients. Among recovering alcoholics, partial removal of the pancreas is used only for those who can manage the diabetes that will result after the surgery.

Taking tablets or capsules of pancreatic enzyme extracts with meals can make the stool less greasy and improve food absorption, but these problems are rarely eliminated. If necessary, a liquid antacid or an H_2 blocker may be taken with the pancreatic enzymes. With such treatment, the person usually gains some weight, has fewer daily bowel movements, has no more oil droplets in the stool, and generally feels better. If these measures are ineffective, the person can try decreasing fat intake. Supplements of the fat-soluble vitamins (A, D, and K) also may be required.

Adenocarcinoma of the Pancreas

Adenocarcinoma of the pancreas is a cancerous tumor that originates in the cells lining the pancreatic duct.

About 95 percent of cancerous tumors of the pancreas are adenocarcinomas. These tumors are nearly twice as common in men as in women and are slightly more common in blacks than in whites. Adenocarcinoma of the pancreas is two to three times more common in heavy smokers than in nonsmokers. And people with chronic pancreatitis have a higher risk of acquiring it.

The disease has become increasingly common in the United States as life expectancy has increased. It rarely develops before age 50; the average age at diagnosis is 55. Little is known about the cause.

Symptoms

Adenocarcinoma of the pancreas typically causes no symptoms until the tumor has grown large. Thus, at the time of diagnosis, the tumor has already spread (metastasized) beyond the pancreas to the neighboring lymph nodes or to the liver or lung in 80 percent of the cases.

Typically, the first symptoms are pain and weight loss. At the time of diagnosis, 90 percent of people have abdominal pain—usually severe pain in the upper abdomen that penetrates to the back—and weight loss of at least 10 percent of their ideal weight.

About 80 percent of these cancers occur in the head of the pancreas (the part nearest the duodenum and common bile duct). Therefore, jaundice caused by obstruction of the common bile duct is typically an early symptom. In people with jaundice, the yellow color affects not only the skin but also the whites of the eyes (sclera) and other tissues. The jaundice is accompanied by general itchiness.

Tumors in the body and tail of the pancreas (the middle part and the part farthest from the duodenum) may obstruct the vein draining the spleen, resulting in an enlargement of the spleen and varices (enlarged, tortuous, swollen varicose veins) around the stomach and esophagus. Severe bleeding may result, particularly from the esophagus, if these varicose veins rupture.

Diagnosis

Early diagnosis is difficult. When adenocarcinoma of the pancreas is suspected, the most commonly used diagnostic tests are ultrasound scans, computed tomography (CT), and endoscopic retrograde pancreatography (an x-ray technique that shows the structure of the pancreatic duct). To confirm the diagnosis, a doctor may obtain a sample of the pancreas for microscopic examination. The biopsy sample is obtained by inserting a needle through the skin while using a CT or ultrasound scan as a guide. A biopsy sample also may be taken from the liver to look for cancer that has spread. If a doctor strongly suspects adenocarcinoma of the pancreas, but the results of these tests are normal, the pancreas may be explored surgically.

Prognosis and Treatment

The prognosis is very poor. Fewer than 2 percent of the people with adenocarcinoma of the pancreas survive for 5 years after the diagnosis. The only hope of a cure is surgery, which is performed on patients whose cancer hasn't spread. Either the pancreas alone or the pancreas and the duodenum are removed. Even after such surgery, only 10 percent of patients live for 5 years, regardless of further treatment.

Mild pain may be relieved by aspirin or acetaminophen. Severe pain in the upper abdomen may be relieved by bending forward, tucking the head down, and bringing the knees up or by using medications such as oral codeine or morphine.▲ For 70 to 80 percent of those with severe pain, injections into nerves to block pain sensations may provide relief. The lack of pancreatic digestive enzymes can be treated with oral enzyme preparations. If diabetes develops, insulin treatment may be needed.

Cystadenocarcinoma

A rare type of pancreatic cancer, cystadenocarcinoma has a much better prognosis than adenocarcinoma. Only 20 percent of these cancers have spread by the time surgery is performed. If the cancer hasn't spread and the whole pancreas is removed surgically, the person has a 65 percent chance of surviving for at least 5 years.

Insulinoma

An insulinoma is a rare type of pancreatic tumor that secretes insulin, a hormone that lowers the levels of glucose in the blood.

Only 10 percent of insulinomas are cancerous.

Symptoms

The symptoms of an insulinoma result from low blood glucose levels. They occur when the person doesn't eat for many hours, most often in the morning after an all-night fast. The symptoms, which may mimic a variety of psychiatric and nerve disorders, include headache, confusion, vision abnormalities, muscle weakness, unsteadiness, and marked changes in personality. The low blood glucose levels may even lead to a loss of consciousness, convulsions, and coma. Symptoms that resemble those of anxiety or panic include faintness, weakness, trembling, awareness of the heartbeat (palpitations), sweating, hunger, and nervousness.

Diagnosis and Treatment

Diagnosing an insulinoma can be difficult. The person fasts for at least 24 hours, sometimes up to 72 hours, and is closely monitored, often in the hospital. After that time, the symptoms usually appear, and blood tests are performed to measure glucose and insulin levels. Very low glucose levels and high insulin levels indicate the presence of an insulinoma. The location must then be pinpointed. Imaging tests—such as computed tomography (CT) scanning and ultrasound scanning—can be used to locate the tumor, but sometimes exploratory surgery is needed.

The treatment for an insulinoma is surgical removal.

Gastrinoma

A gastrinoma is a pancreatic tumor that produces excessive levels of the hormone gastrin, which stimulates the stomach to secrete acid and enzymes, causing peptic ulcers.

▲ see page 291

Most people with this condition have several tumors clustered in or near the pancreas. About half of the tumors are cancerous.

Sometimes a gastrinoma occurs as part of a hereditary disorder, multiple endocrine neoplasia,▲ in which tumors arise from the cells of various endocrine glands, such as the insulin-producing cells of the pancreas.

Symptoms and Diagnosis

The excess gastrin secreted by the gastrinoma causes symptoms, called the Zollinger-Ellison syndrome. The syndrome includes mild to severe abdominal pain from peptic ulcers■ in the stomach, duodenum, and elsewhere in the intestine. Perforation, bleeding, and obstruction of the intestine can occur and are life threatening. However, for more than half the people with a gastrinoma, symptoms are no worse than those experienced by people with peptic ulcers from other causes. In 35 to 40 percent of patients, diarrhea is the first symptom.

A doctor suspects the diagnosis when a person has frequent or several peptic ulcers that don't respond to the usual ulcer treatments. Blood tests are then used to detect abnormally high gastrin levels. Also, samples of gastric juice—obtained by inserting a slender tube through the nose and into the stomach—show very high acid levels. Locating the tumors may be difficult because usually they're small and there are many of them. Doctors use several imaging techniques, such as computed tomography (CT), ultrasound scans, and arteriography.

Treatment

About 20 percent of those who don't have multiple endocrine neoplasia can be cured with surgery. For these patients before surgery and for the other patients, standard ulcer drugs—such as cimetidine, ranitidine, and famotidine—may relieve the symptoms. If they don't, omeprazole (which reduces acid secretion by other means) may be effective. If these treatments fail, an operation to remove the stomach (total gastrec-

tomy) may be necessary. This operation doesn't remove the tumor but the gastrin can no longer affect the stomach, so the symptoms disappear. If the stomach is removed, daily oral calcium supplements and monthly injections of vitamin B_{12} are required.

If malignant tumors have spread to other parts of the body, anticancer drugs (chemotherapy) may help reduce the number of tumor cells and the blood levels of gastrin. But such therapy doesn't cure the cancer, which is ultimately fatal.

Glucagonoma

A glucagonoma is a tumor that produces the hormone glucagon, which raises the level of glucose in the blood and produces a distinctive rash.

About 80 percent of these tumors are cancerous. However, they grow slowly, and many people survive for 15 years or more after the diagnosis. The average age at which symptoms begin is 50. About 80 percent of the people with glucagonomas are women.

Symptoms and Diagnosis

High levels of glucagon cause the symptoms of diabetes mellitus.★ Often, the person loses weight. Blood tests may reveal anemia and low levels of blood lipids, but in 90 percent of people, the most distinctive features are a scaling, reddish-brown skin rash (necrolytic migratory erythema) that starts in the groin and moves to the buttocks, forearms, and legs and a smooth, shiny, and bright red-orange tongue. The mouth also may have cracks at the corners.

The diagnosis is made by identifying high glucagon levels in the blood and then locating the tumor by angiography and exploratory abdominal surgery.

Treatment

Ideally, the tumor is surgically removed, eliminating all the symptoms. However, if removal isn't possible or the tumor has spread, anticancer drugs may reduce the levels of glucagon and lessen the symptoms. The drug octreotide also reduces glucagon levels, may clear up the rash, and may restore the appetite, facilitating weight gain. But octreotide may elevate blood glucose levels even more. Zinc ointment may be used to treat the skin rash. Sometimes the rash is treated with intravenous amino acids or fatty acids.

▲ see page 726

■ see page 496

★ see page 717

CHAPTER 105

Indigestion

Indigestion is an imprecise term that's used by different people to mean different things. Here the term is used to cover a wide range of digestive tract problems, including dyspepsia, nausea and vomiting, regurgitation, the sensation of having a lump in the throat (globus sensation), and bad breath (halitosis).

Dyspepsia

Dyspepsia is a pain or discomfort in the upper abdomen or chest that's often described as having gas, a feeling of fullness, or a gnawing or burning pain.

Dyspepsia has many causes. Some are serious disorders such as stomach ulcers, duodenal ulcers, stomach inflammation (gastritis), and stomach cancer. Anxiety can cause dyspepsia—possibly because an anxious person tends to sigh or gasp and swallow air, which can cause distention of the stomach or intestine as well as belching and flatulence. Also, anxiety can increase a person's perception of unpleasant sensations, so that minor discomfort becomes very distressing.

The bacterium *Helicobacter pylori*▲ can cause inflammation and ulcers of the stomach and duodenum, but whether the bacterium can cause mild dyspepsia in someone who doesn't have ulcers isn't clear.

Symptoms and Diagnosis

The pain or discomfort in the upper abdomen or chest may be accompanied by belching and loud intestinal sounds (borborygmi). For some people, eating makes the pain worse; for others, eating relieves the pain. Other symptoms include a poor appetite, nausea, constipation, diarrhea, and flatulence.

Often a person with dyspepsia is treated without having laboratory tests done. When tests are done, they fail to identify any abnormality in about 50 percent of those with dyspepsia. Even when abnormalities are found, they often don't account for all the symptoms.

Because dyspepsia can be an early warning of a serious disease, however, tests are done in certain cases. If dyspepsia continues for more than a few weeks, fails to respond to treatment, or is accompanied by weight loss or other unusual

Common Causes of Dyspepsia

- Swallowing air (aerophagia)
- Regurgitation (reflux) of acid from the stomach
- Stomach irritation (gastritis)
- Stomach or duodenal ulcer
- Stomach cancer
- Gallbladder inflammation (cholecystitis)
- Lactose intolerance (inability to digest milk and dairy products)
- Disorder of intestinal motility (for example, irritable bowel syndrome)
- Anxiety or depression

symptoms, the person undergoes tests. Laboratory tests usually include a complete blood cell count and a test for blood in the stool. Barium x-ray studies of the esophagus, stomach, or small intestine can be performed if the person is having trouble swallowing or is vomiting, losing weight, or experiencing pain that's either improved or worsened by eating. An endoscope (fiber-optic viewing tube)■ may be used to examine the inside of the esophagus, stomach, or intestine and to obtain a biopsy specimen of the stomach lining. The specimen then is examined microscopically to find out if it's infected by *Helicobacter pylori*. Other tests, such as those that measure the contractions of the esophagus or the response of the esophagus to acid, are sometimes helpful.

Treatment

If no underlying cause is found, a doctor treats the symptoms. An antacid or an H$_2$ blocker such as cimetidine, ranitidine, or famotidine can be

---

▲ see page 496

■ see page 485

tried for a short time. If the person has a *Helicobacter pylori* infection in the stomach lining, a doctor usually prescribes bismuth subsalicylate and an antibiotic such as amoxicillin or metronidazole.

Nausea and Vomiting

Nausea *is an unpleasant feeling in the abdomen that often ends with vomiting.* **Vomiting** *is the forceful expulsion of stomach contents through the mouth.*

Nausea and vomiting are caused by activation of the vomiting center in the brain. Vomiting is one of the more dramatic ways that the body eliminates harmful substances. It may be caused by eating or swallowing an irritating or poisonous substance or food that has spoiled.

Some people become nauseated and may vomit from the movement of a boat, car, or airplane. Vomiting may occur during pregnancy, particularly in the early weeks and especially in the morning; it can be severe. Many drugs, including anticancer (chemotherapy) drugs and opiate analgesics such as morphine, can cause nausea and vomiting. A mechanical obstruction of the intestine▲ eventually causes vomiting as food and fluid back up from the blockage. Also, irritation or inflammation of the stomach, intestine, or gallbladder can cause vomiting.

Psychologic problems also can cause nausea and vomiting (psychogenic vomiting). Such vomiting may be intentional—for instance, a person with bulimia vomits to lose weight. Or it may be unintentional—a conditioned response to achieve a benefit, such as to avoid going to school. Psychogenic vomiting also may result from a threatening or distasteful situation that causes anxiety. In some cases, psychologic factors that cause vomiting depend on a person's cultural background. For instance, most Americans would find eating chocolate-coated ants repulsive, but in other parts of the world they're considered a delicacy. Vomiting may be an expression of hostility, for instance when a child vomits during a temper tantrum. Or vomiting may be caused by intense psychologic conflict. For example, a woman who wants to have children

---

▲ see page 545

■ see page 491

may vomit on or near the anniversary of her hysterectomy (surgical removal of the uterus).

Symptoms, Diagnosis, and Treatment

Nausea, dry vomiting (retching), and considerable salivation often occur just before vomiting begins. Although the person generally feels unwell while vomiting, a feeling of relief often follows.

To identify the cause, a doctor first questions the person about other symptoms. Next, a doctor may perform simple tests such as a complete blood cell count and a urinalysis and then request more sophisticated blood tests and x-ray and ultrasound studies of the gallbladder, pancreas, stomach, and intestine.

If a physical cause of the vomiting can be found, it's treated. If the problem has a psychologic basis, treatment may consist of providing simple reassurance or prescribing medication. Regular visits may be needed to help resolve complex issues. To suppress the patient's nausea, a doctor may prescribe antiemetic drugs.

Regurgitation

Regurgitation is the spitting up of food from the esophagus or stomach without nausea or forceful abdominal muscle contractions.

Often, regurgitation is caused by acid coming up from the stomach (acid reflux).■ Regurgitation also may be caused by a narrowing (stricture) or a blockage of the esophagus. The blockage may result from one of several causes, including cancer of the esophagus. Blockage also may be caused by dysrhythmic nerve control of the esophagus and its sphincter at the opening to the stomach (lower esophageal sphincter).

Regurgitation without a physical cause is called rumination. Such regurgitation is common in infants but much less so in adults. Rumination in adults most often occurs in those who have emotional disorders, especially during periods of stress.

Symptoms, Diagnosis, and Treatment

Acid coming up from the stomach causes regurgitation of sour or bitter-tasting material. A narrowed or blocked esophagus causes tasteless fluid containing mucus or undigested food to be regurgitated.

In rumination, people regurgitate small amounts of food from the stomach, usually 15 to

30 minutes after eating. They then generally chew the material again and swallow it. The problem doesn't involve nausea, pain, or difficulty in swallowing.

A doctor looks for a physical cause of the regurgitation. Acid reflux is diagnosed by x-ray studies, measurements of pressure and acidity in the esophagus, and other tests. A diagnosis of narrowing or blockage of the esophagus requires x-rays or an examination with an endoscope (a fiber-optic viewing tube). ▲

Treatment of a narrowing or blockage of the esophagus depends on the cause.■ If no physical cause is found, the drug metoclopramide or cisapride, which stimulates the esophagus to contract normally, sometimes helps. Alternatively, relaxation therapy or biofeedback may bring relief.

Globus Sensation

Globus sensation (previously called globus hystericus) is the sensation of having a lump in the throat when there is no lump.

The sensation may result from abnormal muscle activity or sensitivity of the esophagus. It also may occur with frequent swallowing and drying of the throat brought on by anxiety, another strong emotion, or rapid breathing.

Globus sensation may make a person reluctant to eat. But the condition (which is similar to the normal reaction of feeling all choked up during events that trigger grief, anxiety, anger, pride, or happiness) is often relieved by eating, drinking, or crying.

Diagnosis and Treatment

To identify the cause of the sensation, a doctor asks the person questions and performs a physical examination. A doctor may order a complete blood cell count, a chest x-ray, a barium x-ray of the esophagus (barium swallow), and measurements of pressures in the esophagus.★ If the symptoms are typical, no physical abnormality is found, and social or psychologic stresses are apparent, a diagnosis of globus sensation is made.

Reassurance that there's no serious physical disorder may provide relief. No specific drug relieves globus sensation, but antianxiety or antidepressant drugs may help. If the problem is anxiety, depression, or some other psychosocial problem, it should be dealt with specifically, possibly with the help of a psychiatrist or psychologist.

Halitosis

Halitosis (bad breath) is an unpleasant odor in the breath.

Usually, bad breath is caused by certain foods or substances that have been swallowed or inhaled, by tooth or gum disease, or by the fermentation of food particles in the mouth. Bad breath can be a symptom of certain diseases that affect the entire body, such as liver disease, uncontrolled diabetes, or a disease in the lungs or mouth.

Bad breath usually isn't caused by problems in the intestine. Because the esophageal sphincter at the opening to the stomach (lower esophageal sphincter) is closed except during swallowing, odors can't rise from the stomach or further down the digestive system. However, a tumor in the esophagus or stomach may cause foul-smelling liquid or gas to be regurgitated into the mouth.

Psychogenic halitosis is the belief that one's breath smells bad when it actually doesn't. This problem may occur in people who tend to exaggerate normal body sensations. Sometimes psychogenic halitosis is caused by a serious mental disorder, such as schizophrenia. A person with obsessional thoughts may have an overwhelming sense of feeling dirty. A person who is paranoid may have the delusion that his organs are rotting. Both may believe their breath smells bad.

Treatment

Physical causes can be corrected or removed. For instance, people can stop eating garlic or improve their dental hygiene. Many deodorant mouthwashes and sprays are available; one of the best active ingredients is chlorophyll. Taking activated charcoal, which absorbs odors, is another remedy.

Some people with psychogenic halitosis may be helped by having a doctor assure them that they don't have bad breath. If the problem continues, a person may benefit from seeing a psychotherapist.

▲ see page 485

■ see page 487

★ see page 484

Gastroenteritis

Gastroenteritis is a general term for a group of conditions that are usually caused by infection and produce symptoms such as loss of appetite, nausea, vomiting, mild to severe diarrhea, cramps, and discomfort in the abdomen. Electrolytes, particularly sodium and potassium, are lost along with body fluids.▲ Merely inconvenient to a healthy adult, an electrolyte imbalance can cause life-threatening dehydration in the very ill, the very young, and the elderly.

Causes

Epidemics of diarrhea in infants, children, and adults are usually caused by microorganisms spread in water or food, generally after it's been contaminated by infected feces. Infections also can be transmitted from person to person, especially if someone with diarrhea doesn't thoroughly wash the hands after a bowel movement. Infections with one type of bacteria called *Salmonella* can be acquired by people who touch a reptile, such as a turtle or an iguana, and then put their fingers in their mouth.

Certain bacteria produce toxins that cause the cells in the intestinal wall to secrete electrolytes and water. One such toxin is responsible for the watery diarrhea that's a symptom of cholera.■ A toxin produced by the common bacterium *Escherichia coli* (*E. coli*) may cause traveler's diarrhea and some outbreaks of diarrhea in hospital nurseries.

Some bacteria, such as certain strains of *E. coli, Campylobacter, Shigella,* and *Salmonella* (including the type that causes typhoid fever), invade the lining of the intestine. They damage the underlying cells, causing tiny ulcerations that bleed and allow a considerable loss of fluid containing proteins, electrolytes, and water.★

Besides bacteria, several viruses, such as the Norwalk virus and the coxsackievirus, cause gastroenteritis. During the winter in temperate climates, rotaviruses cause most cases of diarrhea serious enough to send infants and toddlers to the hospital. Enterovirus and adenovirus infections can affect the lungs as well as the stomach and intestine.

Certain intestinal parasites, particularly *Giardia lamblia,* stick to or invade the lining of the intestine and cause nausea, vomiting, diarrhea, and a general sick feeling. The resulting illness, called giardiasis,● is more common in cold climates, such as in the Rocky Mountains, the northern United States, and northern Europe. If the disease becomes persistent (chronic), it can keep the body from absorbing nutrients, a condition called malabsorption syndrome.◆ Another intestinal parasite, called *Cryptosporidium,* causes watery diarrhea that is sometimes accompanied by abdominal cramps, nausea, and vomiting. In otherwise healthy people, the illness is usually mild, but in those with weakened immune systems, the infection may be severe or even fatal. Both *Giardia* and *Cryptosporidium* are most commonly acquired by drinking contaminated water.

Gastroenteritis may result from eating chemical toxins found in seafood, in plants such as mushrooms and potatoes, or in contaminated food. Also, lactose intolerance—the inability to digest and absorb milk sugar (lactose)—may cause gastroenteritis. The symptoms, which often occur after drinking milk, are sometimes mistakenly assumed to indicate a milk allergy. Accidentally ingesting heavy metals such as arsenic, lead, mercury, or cadmium in water or food may suddenly cause nausea, vomiting, and diarrhea. Many drugs, including antibiotics, can cause abdominal cramps and diarrhea.

Symptoms

The type and severity of the symptoms depend on the type and quantity of the microorganism or toxin ingested. Symptoms also vary according to the person's resistance to disease. Symptoms often begin suddenly—sometimes dramatically—with a loss of appetite, nausea, or vomiting. Audible rumbling of the intestine, abdominal

---

▲ see page 667

■ see page 869

★ see page 869

● see page 897

◆ see page 534

cramping, and diarrhea with or without visible blood and mucus may occur. Loops of intestine may be painfully distended with gas. The person may have a fever, feel generally sick, and experience aching muscles and extreme exhaustion.

Severe vomiting and diarrhea can lead to marked dehydration and a severe decrease in blood pressure (shock). Either excessive vomiting or diarrhea can cause a serious loss of potassium, resulting in low blood levels of potassium (hypokalemia). Low levels of sodium in the blood (hyponatremia) also may develop, particularly if the person replaces lost fluids by drinking liquids that contain little or no salt, such as water and tea. All of these imbalances are potentially serious.

Diagnosis

The diagnosis of gastroenteritis is usually obvious from the symptoms alone, but the cause often isn't. Sometimes other family members or coworkers have recently been ill with similar symptoms. Other times, the person can trace the illness to inadequately cooked, spoiled, or contaminated food, such as mayonnaise left out of the refrigerator too long or raw seafood. Recent travel, especially to certain foreign countries, may give clues as well.

If the symptoms are severe or last for more than 48 hours, stool samples may be examined in a laboratory for white blood cells and bacteria, viruses, or parasites. Laboratory tests on vomit, food, or blood also may help identify the cause.

If the symptoms persist beyond a few days, a doctor may need to examine the large intestine with a colonoscope (a flexible viewing tube) to find out whether the person has a disorder such as ulcerative colitis or amebic dysentery (amebiasis).

Treatment

Usually the only treatment needed for gastroenteritis is to drink adequate fluids. Even a person who is vomiting should drink small sips of fluids because fluids correct dehydration, which in turn may help stop the vomiting. If vomiting is prolonged or the person becomes severely dehydrated, intravenous fluids and electrolytes may be needed. Because children can become dehydrated more quickly, they should be given fluids with the appropriate mix of salts and sugars. Any

of the commercially available rehydration solutions are satisfactory. However, commonly used liquids such as carbonated beverages, teas, sports drinks, and fruit juices are not appropriate for children with diarrhea. If vomiting is severe, a doctor may give an injection or prescribe a suppository.

As the symptoms improve, the person may gradually add bland foods—such as cooked cereals, bananas, rice, applesauce, and toast—to the diet. If the modified diet doesn't eliminate the diarrhea after 12 to 24 hours and there's no blood in the stool to indicate a more serious bacterial infection, drugs such as diphenoxylate, loperamide, or bismuth subsalicylate may be given.

Because antibiotics can cause diarrhea and may encourage the growth of organisms resistant to antibiotics, they're rarely appropriate, even when a known bacterium is causing gastroenteritis. Antibiotics may be used, however, when certain bacteria such as *Campylobacter, Shigella,* and *Vibrio cholerae* are the cause.

Hemorrhagic Colitis

Hemorrhagic colitis is a type of gastroenteritis in which certain strains of the bacterium Escherichia coli (E. coli) *infect the large intestine and produce a toxin that causes sudden bloody diarrhea and sometimes other serious complications.*

In North America, the most common strain of *E. coli* that causes hemorrhagic colitis is called *E. coli* O157:H7. This strain appears in the intestines of healthy cattle. Outbreaks can be caused by eating undercooked beef, especially ground beef, or by drinking unpasteurized milk. The disease also can be transmitted from person to person, particularly among children in diapers. Hemorrhagic colitis can occur in people of all ages.

The *E. coli* toxins damage the lining of the large intestine. If they are absorbed into the bloodstream, they can also affect other organs, such as the kidney.

Symptoms

Severe abdominal cramps begin suddenly along with watery diarrhea that typically becomes bloody in 24 hours. The person's body temperature is usually normal or only slightly above normal, but occasionally it can reach more than 102° F. The diarrhea usually lasts 1 to 8 days.

About 5 percent of people infected with *E. coli* O157:H7 develop the hemolytic-uremic syndrome. Symptoms include anemia caused by the breakdown of red blood cells (hemolytic anemia), a low platelet count (thrombocytopenia), and sudden kidney failure. Some people also develop seizures, strokes, or other complications of nerve or brain damage. These complications typically develop in the second week of illness and may be preceded by a rising body temperature. Hemolytic-uremic syndrome is more likely to occur in children under age 5 and in the elderly. Even without these complications, hemorrhagic colitis may cause death in the elderly.

Diagnosis and Treatment

A doctor usually suspects hemorrhagic colitis when a person reports bloody diarrhea. To make the diagnosis, a doctor has stool specimens tested for *E. coli* O157:H7. These specimens should be obtained within a week of when symptoms start. Other tests, such as colonoscopy (an examination of the large intestine using a flexible viewing tube),▲ may be performed if a doctor suspects that other diseases may be causing the bloody diarrhea.

The most important aspects of treatment are drinking enough liquids to replace lost fluids and keeping to a bland diet. Antibiotics don't relieve the symptoms, eliminate the bacteria, or prevent complications. People who develop complications are likely to require intensive care in the hospital, including dialysis.

Staphylococcal Food Poisoning

Staphylococcal food poisoning is poisoning from eating food contaminated with the toxins of certain types of staphylococci, which are common bacteria; it generally results in diarrhea and vomiting.

The risk of an outbreak is high when food handlers with skin infections contaminate foods left at room temperature, allowing the bacteria to grow and produce their toxin in the food. The typical contaminated foods include custard, cream-filled pastry, milk, processed meats, and fish.

▲ see page 485

Symptoms and Diagnosis

Symptoms usually begin abruptly with severe nausea and vomiting starting about 2 to 8 hours after the contaminated food is eaten. Other symptoms may include abdominal cramping, diarrhea, and sometimes headache and fever. Severe fluid and electrolyte loss may cause weakness and very low blood pressure (shock). Symptoms usually last less than 12 hours, and recovery is usually complete. Occasionally, food poisoning is fatal, especially in the very young, the elderly, and people weakened by long-term illness.

The symptoms are usually all a doctor needs to make the diagnosis. Usually other people who ate the same food are similarly affected, and the disorder can be traced to a single source of contamination. To confirm the diagnosis, a laboratory must identify staphylococci in the suspected food. Microscopic specimens of vomit may also show staphylococci.

Prevention and Treatment

Careful food preparation can prevent staphylococcal food poisoning. Anyone who has a staphylococcal skin infection, such as boils or impetigo, shouldn't prepare food for others until the infection heals.

Treatment usually consists of little more than drinking adequate fluids. When the symptoms are severe, a doctor may give an injection or prescribe a suppository to help control nausea. Sometimes so much fluid is lost that fluids have to be given intravenously. Rapidly replacing fluids and electrolytes intravenously often brings dramatic relief.

Botulism

Botulism is an uncommon, life-threatening poisoning caused by the toxins produced by the bacterium Clostridium botulinum.

These toxins are the most potent poisons known and can severely damage nerves and muscles. (Because they cause nerve damage, they're called neurotoxins.) Doctors classify botulism as foodborne, wound, or infant botulism. As the terms imply, foodborne botulism results from ingesting contaminated food, and wound botulism results from a contaminated wound. Infant botulism, which also results from ingesting contaminated food, occurs in infants.

Causes

The bacterium *Clostridium botulinum* forms spores. Like seeds, spores can exist in a dormant state for many years, and they're highly resistant to destruction. When conditions are right—with moisture and nutrients present and oxygen absent—the spores start to grow and produce a toxin. Some toxins produced by *Clostridium botulinum* are highly poisonous proteins that resist destruction by the intestine's protective enzymes.

When contaminated food is eaten, the toxin enters the body through the digestive system, causing foodborne botulism. Home-canned foods are the most common sources of botulism, although commercially prepared foods have been responsible in about 10 percent of the outbreaks. Vegetables, fish, fruits, and condiments are the most common food sources. Beef, milk products, pork, poultry, and other foods have caused botulism as well.

Wound botulism occurs when a wound is contaminated with *Clostridium botulinum*. Inside the wound, the bacteria produce a toxin that is then absorbed into the bloodstream and produces symptoms.

Infant botulism occurs most frequently in babies who are 2 to 3 months old. Unlike foodborne botulism, infant botulism isn't caused by swallowing a previously formed toxin. It results from eating food containing spores, which then grow in the baby's intestine and produce a toxin. The cause of most cases isn't known, but some cases have been linked to the ingestion of honey. *Clostridium botulinum* is common in the environment, and many cases may result from the ingestion of small amounts of dust or soil.

Symptoms

Symptoms develop suddenly, usually 18 to 36 hours after the toxin enters the body, although symptoms can start as soon as 4 hours or as late as 8 days after the toxin enters. The more toxin that enters, the sooner the person becomes sick. Generally, people who become sick within 24 hours of eating contaminated food are the most severely affected.

The first symptoms commonly include dry mouth, double vision, drooping eyelids, and an inability to focus on nearby objects. The pupils of the eyes don't constrict normally when exposed to light during an eye examination; they may not constrict at all. In some people, nausea, vomiting, stomach cramps, and diarrhea are the first symptoms. Other people don't have these gastrointestinal symptoms at all, particularly those who have wound botulism.

The person has difficulty speaking and swallowing. Difficulty in swallowing can lead to inhalation of food and aspiration pneumonia.▲ The muscles of the arms and legs and the muscles involved in breathing become progressively weaker as symptoms gradually move down the body. The failure of the nerves to work properly affects muscle strength, although sensation is preserved. Despite such serious illness, the mind usually remains clear.

In about two thirds of the babies with infant botulism, constipation is the first symptom. Then paralysis of the nerves and muscles develops, beginning in the face and head and eventually reaching the arms, legs, and breathing muscles. The nerves on one side of the body may be damaged more than those on the other side. Problems range from mild lethargy and prolonged feeding time to severe loss of muscle tone and an inability to breathe properly.

Diagnosis

In foodborne botulism, the characteristic pattern of nerve and muscle impairment may lead a doctor to the diagnosis. However, often the symptoms are mistakenly thought to result from more common causes of paralysis, such as a stroke. A likely food source provides an additional clue. When botulism occurs in two or more people who ate the same food prepared in the same place, the diagnosis is easier. The diagnosis is confirmed when a laboratory test detects the toxin in the person's blood or a culture of a feces sample grows the bacterium. The toxin may also be identified in the suspected food. Electromyography (a test analyzing the electrical activity of muscles)■ shows abnormal muscle contractions after electrical stimulation in most but not all cases of botulism.

The diagnosis of wound botulism is confirmed when the toxin is found in the blood or when a culture of a wound tissue sample grows the bacterium.

▲ see page 200

■ see page 287

Finding the bacterium or its toxin in a sample of a baby's feces confirms the diagnosis of infant botulism.

Prevention and Treatment

The spores are highly resistant to heat and may survive boiling for several hours. The toxins, however, are readily destroyed by heat; therefore, cooking food at 176° F. for 30 minutes prevents foodborne botulism. Cooking food just before eating it almost always prevents foodborne botulism, but inadequately cooked foods can cause botulism if they're stored after cooking. The bacteria can produce some toxins at temperatures as low as 37.4° F., a typical refrigerator temperature.

Proper home and commercial canning and adequate heating of home-canned food before serving are essential. Canned foods showing any evidence of spoilage could be lethal and must be discarded. Also, cans that are swollen or leaking should be discarded promptly. Infants under 1 year of age shouldn't be fed honey because spores can be present.

Even minute amounts of a toxin entering the body by ingestion, inhalation, or absorption through the eye or a break in the skin can cause serious illness. Therefore, any food that may be contaminated should be disposed of carefully. A person should avoid skin contact as much as possible and should wash the hands immediately after handling the food.

A person who may have botulism should go immediately to the hospital. Treatment often can't wait for the results of laboratory tests, although they're done anyway to confirm the diagnosis. To rid the person's body of any unabsorbed toxin, a doctor may induce vomiting, wash out the stomach in a procedure called gastric lavage, and give the person a laxative to speed the passage of intestinal contents.

The greatest danger from botulism is a problem with breathing. Vital signs (pulse, breathing rate, blood pressure, and temperature) are measured regularly. If breathing problems begin, the person is transferred to an intensive care unit and may be temporarily placed on a respirator. Such intensive care has reduced the death rate from botulism from about 70 percent in the early 1900s to less than 10 percent today. Intravenous feeding may also be needed.

The antitoxin for botulism can't undo damage, but it may slow or stop further physical and mental deterioration, so the body can heal itself over a period of months. The antitoxin is given as soon as possible after botulism has been diagnosed. It's most likely to help if given within 72 hours of when symptoms begin. The antitoxin currently isn't recommended for infant botulism, but its effectiveness for this type of botulism is being studied.

Clostridium perfringens Food Poisoning

This type of gastroenteritis is caused by eating food contaminated by a toxin produced by the bacterium *Clostridium perfringens*. Some strains cause a mild to moderate disease that gets better without treatment; other strains cause a severe, often fatal, type of gastroenteritis. Some toxins can't be destroyed by boiling; others can. Contaminated meat is usually responsible for outbreaks of *Clostridium perfringens* food poisoning.

Symptoms, Diagnosis, and Treatment

The gastroenteritis is usually mild, although it can be a severe disorder with abdominal pain, abdominal distention from gas, severe diarrhea, dehydration, and shock. A doctor usually suspects the diagnosis when a local outbreak of the disease has occurred. The diagnosis is confirmed by testing contaminated food for *Clostridium perfringens*.

The person is given fluids and encouraged to rest. In severe cases, penicillin may help. If the disease destroys part of the small intestine, it may have to be removed surgically.

Traveler's Diarrhea

Traveler's diarrhea—also called intestinal flu, grippe, and turista—is a condition characterized by diarrhea, nausea, and vomiting that commonly occurs in travelers.

The organisms most likely to cause traveler's diarrhea are the types of *Escherichia coli* that produce certain toxins and some viruses such as the Norwalk virus.

Symptoms and Diagnosis

Nausea, vomiting, intestinal rumbling, abdominal cramping, and diarrhea can occur in any combination and with any degree of severity. Vomiting, headache, and muscle pain are particularly common in infections caused by the Norwalk virus. Most cases are mild and disappear without treatment. Tests are rarely needed.

Prevention and Treatment

Travelers should patronize restaurants with a reputation for safety and shouldn't eat food or drink beverages sold by street vendors. All food should be cooked and all fruit peeled. Travelers should drink only carbonated beverages or beverages made with water that has been boiled. Even ice cubes should be made with water that has been boiled. Salads containing uncooked vegetables should be avoided. Bismuth subsalicylate can provide some protection. The benefit of preventive antibiotics is controversial, but these drugs may be recommended for people who are particularly susceptible to the consequences of traveler's diarrhea, such as those whose immune system is impaired.

Treatment includes drinking plenty of fluids and eating a bland diet. Antibiotics aren't recommended for mild diarrhea unless the person has a fever or blood in the stool. These drugs can cause harm by eliminating bacteria that grow normally in the stool while encouraging the growth of bacteria that are resistant to the drugs.

Chemical Food Poisoning

Chemical food poisoning results from eating a plant or animal that contains a poison.

Mushroom (toadstool) poisoning can result from ingesting any of several species of mushroom. The potential for poisoning may vary within the same species, at different times of the growing season, and with cooking. In poisoning caused by many species of *Inocybe* and some species of *Clitocybe*, the dangerous substance is muscarine. Symptoms, which begin a few minutes to 2 hours after eating, may include increased tearing, salivation, constriction of the pupils, sweating, vomiting, stomach cramps, diarrhea, dizziness, confusion, coma, and occasionally convulsions. With appropriate treatment, the person usually recovers in 24 hours, although death can occur in a few hours.

In phalloidine poisoning, caused by eating *Amanita phalloides* and related species of mushroom,

symptoms start in 6 to 24 hours. People develop intestinal symptoms similar to those of muscarine poisoning, and kidney damage may cause reduced urination or none at all. Jaundice from liver damage is common and develops in 2 or 3 days. Sometimes the symptoms disappear on their own, but about half of the people who have phalloidine poisoning die in 5 to 8 days.

Plant and shrub poisoning can result from ingesting the leaves and fruits of many wild and domestic plants and shrubs. Green or sprouting underground roots that contain solanine may produce mild nausea, vomiting, diarrhea, and weakness. Fava beans may cause the breakdown of red blood cells (favism) in genetically susceptible people. Ergot poisoning results from eating grain contaminated by the fungus *Claviceps purpurea*. Fruit of the Koenig tree causes the vomiting sickness of Jamaica.

Seafood poisoning may be caused by bony fish or shellfish. Usually, poisoning by bony fish results from one of three toxins—ciguatera, tetraodon, or histamine. Ciguatera poisoning can occur after eating any of more than 400 species of fish from the tropical reefs of Florida, the West Indies, or the Pacific. The toxin is produced by certain dinoflagellates, microscopic sea organisms that the fish eat and that accumulate in their flesh. Larger, older fish are more toxic than younger, smaller ones. The flavor of the fish isn't affected. Current processing procedures can't destroy the toxin. Symptoms may begin 2 to 8 hours after the person eats the fish. Abdominal cramps, nausea, vomiting, and diarrhea last 6 to 17 hours. Later symptoms may include itchiness, a pins-and-needles sensation, headache, muscle aches, a reversal of hot and cold sensations, and facial pain. For months afterward, the unusual sensations may be disabling.

The symptoms of tetraodon poisoning from the puffer fish, which is found most commonly in the seas surrounding Japan, are similar to those of ciguatera poisoning. Death may result from paralysis of the muscles that regulate breathing.

Histamine poisoning from fish such as mackerel, tuna, and blue dolphin (mahimahi) occurs when the tissues of the fish break down after it has been caught, producing high levels of histamine. When ingested, histamine causes immediate facial flushing. It can also cause nausea, vom-

---

Chinese Restaurant Syndrome

What's popularly called the Chinese restaurant syndrome is not a type of chemical food poisoning. Rather it's a hypersensitivity reaction to monosodium glutamate (MSG), a flavor enhancer often used in Chinese cooking. In susceptible people, monosodium glutamate can produce facial pressure, chest pain, and burning sensations throughout the body. The amount of monosodium glutamate that can cause these symptoms varies considerably from person to person.

---

iting, stomach pain, and hives (urticaria) a few minutes after a person eats the fish. Symptoms usually last less than 24 hours.

From June to October, especially on the Pacific and New England coasts, shellfish such as mussels, clams, oysters, and scallops may ingest certain poisonous dinoflagellates. These dinoflagellates are found in such great numbers in the ocean at certain times that the water has a red cast, called the red tide. They produce a toxin that attacks nerves (such toxins are called neurotoxins). The toxin that produces **paralytic shellfish poisoning** persists even after the food has been cooked. The first symptom, a pins-and-needles sensation around the mouth, begins 5 to 30 minutes after eating. Nausea, vomiting, and abdominal cramps develop next. About 25 percent of people develop muscle weakness over the next few hours; occasionally, the weakness may progress to paralysis of the arms and legs. Occasionally, weakness of the muscles needed for breathing may be severe enough to cause death.

Contaminant poisoning may affect people who have ingested unwashed fruits and vegetables sprayed with arsenic, lead, or organic insecticides; acidic liquids served in lead-glazed pottery; or food stored in cadmium-lined containers.▲

▲ see page 1358

Treatment

Unless the person has experienced violent vomiting or diarrhea or the symptoms didn't appear until several hours after the food was eaten, attempts may be made to remove the poison using a procedure that washes out the stomach (gastric lavage). Drugs such as ipecac syrup may be used to induce vomiting, and a laxative may be given to empty the intestine. If nausea or vomiting continues, intravenous fluids containing salts and dextrose are given to correct dehydration and any acid or alkaline imbalance. Pain medications may be needed if stomach cramps are severe. A respirator and intensive nursing care may be required.

Anyone who becomes ill after eating an unidentified mushroom should try to vomit immediately and save the vomit for laboratory testing because different species are treated in different ways. Atropine is given for muscarine poisoning. In a person with phalloidine poisoning, a high-carbohydrate diet and intravenous dextrose and sodium chloride may help to correct the low level of sugar in the blood (hypoglycemia) caused by severe liver damage. Mannitol, a drug given intravenously, is sometimes used to treat severe ciguatera poisoning. Histamine blockers (antihistamines) may be effective in reducing the symptoms of histamine fish poisoning.

Adverse Effects of Drugs

Nausea, vomiting, and diarrhea are common side effects of many drugs. Common culprits include antacids containing magnesium as a major ingredient, antibiotics, anticancer drugs, colchicine (for gout), digitalis (usually used for heart failure), and laxatives. Laxative abuse can lead to weakness, vomiting, diarrhea, electrolyte loss, and other disturbances.

Recognizing that a drug is causing gastroenteritis can be difficult. In mild cases, a doctor can have a person stop taking the drug, then later start taking it again. If the symptoms subside when the person stops taking the drug, then start again when the drug is resumed, it may be the cause of the gastrointestinal symptoms. In severe cases of gastroenteritis, a doctor may instruct the person to stop taking the drug and never take it again.

Bowel Movement Disorders

Bowel (intestinal) function varies greatly not only from one person to another but also for any one person at different times. It can be affected by diet, stress, drugs, disease, and even social and cultural patterns. In most Western societies, the normal number of bowel movements ranges from two or three a week to as many as two or three a day. Changes in the frequency, consistency, or volume of bowel movements or the presence of blood, mucus, pus, or excess fatty material (oil, grease) in the stool may indicate a disease.

Constipation

Constipation is a condition in which a person has uncomfortable or infrequent bowel movements.

A person with constipation produces hard stools that may be difficult to pass. The person also may feel as though the rectum has not been completely emptied. Acute constipation begins suddenly and noticeably. Chronic constipation, on the other hand, may begin insidiously and persist for months or years.

Often the cause of acute constipation is nothing more than a recent change in diet or a decrease in physical activity, for example, when a person stays in bed for a day or two during an illness. Many drugs—for example, aluminum hydroxide (common in over-the-counter antacids), bismuth salts, iron salts, anticholinergics, antihypertensives, narcotics, and many tranquilizers and sedatives—can cause constipation. Acute constipation occasionally may be caused by serious problems such as an obstruction of the large intestine, poor blood supply to the large intestine, and nerve or spinal cord injury.

Too little physical activity and too little fiber in the diet are common causes of chronic constipation. Other causes include an underactive thyroid gland (hypothyroidism), high blood calcium levels (hypercalcemia), and Parkinson's disease. A decrease in the contractions in the large intestine (inactive colon) and discomfort during defecation also lead to chronic constipation. Psychologic factors are common causes of acute and chronic constipation.

Treatment

When a disease is causing constipation, the disease must be treated. Otherwise, constipation is best prevented and treated with a combination of adequate exercise, a high-fiber diet, and the occasional use of appropriate medications.

Vegetables, fruits, and bran are excellent sources of fiber. Many people find it convenient to sprinkle 2 or 3 teaspoons of unrefined miller's bran or high-fiber cereal on fruit two or three times a day. To work well, fiber must be consumed with plenty of fluids.

Laxatives

Many people use laxatives to relieve constipation. Some are safe for long-term use; others should be used only occasionally. Some are good for preventing constipation; others can be used to treat it.

Bulking agents (bran, psyllium, calcium polycarbophil, and methylcellulose) add bulk to the stool. The increased bulk stimulates the natural contractions of the intestine, and bulkier stools are softer and easier to pass. Bulking agents act slowly and gently and are among the safest ways to promote regular bowel movements. These agents generally are taken in small amounts at first. The dose is increased gradually until regularity is achieved. People who use bulking agents should always drink plenty of fluids.

Stool softeners, such as docusate, increase the amount of water that the stool can hold. Actually, these laxatives are detergents that decrease the surface tension of the stool, allowing water to penetrate the stool more easily and soften it. The increased bulk stimulates the natural contractions of the large intestine and helps the softened stools to move more easily out of the body.

Mineral oil softens the stool and facilitates its passage out of the body. However, mineral oil may decrease the absorption of certain fat-soluble vitamins. Also, if a person—for instance, someone who is debilitated—accidently inhales (aspirates) mineral oil, serious lung irritation can develop. Plus, mineral oil seeps from the rectum.

Osmotic agents pull large amounts of water into the large intestine, making the stool soft and loose. The excess fluid also stretches the walls of the large intestine, stimulating contractions. These laxatives consist of either salts—usually phosphate, magnesium, or sulfate—or sugars that are poorly absorbed—for example, lactulose and sorbitol. Some osmotic agents contain sodium. They may cause fluid retention in people with kidney disease or heart failure, especially when given in large or frequent doses. Osmotic agents containing magnesium and phosphate are partially absorbed into the bloodstream and can be harmful in people with kidney failure.▲ These laxatives, which generally work within 3 hours, are better for treating constipation than for preventing it. They're also used to clear stool from the intestine before x-rays of the digestive (gastrointestinal) tract are taken and before colonoscopy (an examination of the large intestine using a flexible viewing tube)■ is performed.

Stimulant laxatives directly stimulate the walls of the large intestine, causing it to contract and move the stool. These laxatives contain irritating substances such as senna, cascara, phenolphthalein, bisacodyl, or castor oil. They generally cause a semisolid bowel movement in 6 to 8 hours but often cause cramping as well. In suppositories, these laxatives often work in 15 to 60 minutes. Prolonged use of stimulant laxatives can damage the large intestine. Also, people can become addicted to stimulant laxatives, developing lazy bowel syndrome, which creates a dependency on the laxatives. Stimulant laxatives are often used to empty the large intestine before diagnostic procedures and to prevent or treat constipation caused by drugs that slow the contractions of the large intestine, such as narcotics.

PSYCHOGENIC CONSTIPATION

Many people believe they have constipation if they don't have a bowel movement every day. Other people think they have constipation if the appearance or consistency of their stool seems abnormal to them. However, daily bowel movements aren't necessarily normal, and less frequent bowel movements don't necessarily indicate a problem unless they represent a sub-

stantial change from previous patterns. The same is true of the color and consistency of stool; unless there's a substantial change in them, the person probably doesn't have constipation.

Such misconceptions about constipation can lead to overzealous treatment, especially the long-term use of stimulant laxatives, irritant suppositories, and enemas. Such treatment can severely damage the large intestine or induce lazy bowel syndrome and melanosis coli (abnormal changes in the lining of the large intestine caused by deposits of a pigment).

Before making a diagnosis of psychogenic constipation, a doctor first ensures that an underlying physical problem isn't causing irregular bowel movements. Diagnostic tests, such as a sigmoidoscopy (an examination of the sigmoid colon using a flexible viewing tube) or a barium enema,★ may be needed. If there's no underlying physical problem, the person needs to accept the existing pattern of bowel movements and not insist on a more regular pattern.

COLONIC INERTIA

Colonic inertia (inactive colon) is a decrease in contractions in the large intestine or an insensitivity of the rectum to the presence of stool, resulting in chronic constipation.

Colonic inertia often occurs in people who are elderly, debilitated, or bedridden, but it also occurs in otherwise healthy younger women. The large intestine stops responding to the stimuli that usually cause bowel movements: eating, a full stomach, a full large intestine, and stool in the rectum. Drugs used to treat medical conditions frequently cause or worsen the problem, especially narcotics (such as codeine) and drugs with anticholinergic properties (such as amitriptyline for depression or propantheline for diarrhea). Colonic inertia sometimes occurs in people who habitually delay defecation or who have used laxatives or enemas for a long time.

Symptoms

Constipation is a long-term, day-to-day problem; the person may or may not have abdominal discomfort. Often a doctor finds the rectum filled with soft stool, even though the person has no urge to defecate and can do so only with difficulty.

People with this condition may develop fecal impaction, in which the stool in the last part of the large intestine and rectum hardens and blocks the passage of other stool. This blockage leads to

---

▲ see page 593

■ see page 485

★ see page 486

cramps, rectal pain, and strong but futile efforts to defecate. Often, watery mucus material oozes around the blockage, sometimes giving the false impression of diarrhea.

Treatment

For colonic inertia, doctors sometimes recommend suppositories or enemas with 2 to 3 ounces of water, water and salts (saline enemas), or oils such as olive oil. For fecal impaction, laxatives—usually osmotic agents—are needed as well. Sometimes a doctor or nurse must remove hard impacted stool with a gloved finger or probe.

People who have colonic inertia should try to defecate daily, preferably 15 to 45 minutes after a meal because eating stimulates a bowel movement. Exercise often helps.

DYSCHEZIA

Dyschezia is difficulty in defecating caused by an inability to control the pelvic and anal muscles.

Having a normal bowel movement requires relaxation of the muscles in the pelvis and the circular muscles (sphincters) that keep the anus closed. Otherwise, efforts to defecate are futile, even with severe straining. People with dyschezia sense the need to have a bowel movement, but they can't have one. Even stool that isn't hard may be difficult to pass.

Conditions that can interfere with muscle movement include pelvic floor dyssynergia (a disturbance of muscle coordination), anismus (a condition in which the muscles fail to relax or paradoxically contract during defecation), a rectocele (hernia of the rectum into the vagina), enterocele (hernia of the small intestine into the rectum), rectal ulcer, and rectal prolapse.▲

Treatment with laxatives is generally unsatisfactory. Currently, relaxation exercises and biofeedback are being tested for pelvic floor dyssynergia and show much promise. Surgery may be needed to repair an enterocele or a large rectocele. Constipation can become so severe that stool must be removed by a doctor or nurse using a gloved finger or probe.

Diarrhea

Diarrhea is an increase in the volume, wateriness, or frequency of bowel movements.

A person with diarrhea caused by a significant medical problem usually has excessive volumes of stool, typically more than a pound of stool a day. People who eat large amounts of vegetable fiber normally may produce more than a pound, but it's well formed and not watery. Normally, stool is 60 to 90 percent water; diarrhea mainly results when the percentage exceeds 90.

Osmotic diarrhea occurs when certain substances that can't be absorbed into the bloodstream remain in the intestine. These substances cause excessive amounts of water to remain in the stool, leading to diarrhea. Certain foods (such as some fruits and beans) and hexitols, sorbitol, and mannitol (used as sugar substitutes in dietetic foods, candy, and chewing gum) can cause osmotic diarrhea. Also, lactase deficiency can lead to osmotic diarrhea. Lactase is an enzyme normally found in the small intestine that converts milk sugar (lactose) to glucose and galactose, so that it can be absorbed into the bloodstream. When people with a lactase deficiency drink milk or eat dairy products, lactose isn't converted.■ As it accumulates in the intestine, it causes osmotic diarrhea. The severity of osmotic diarrhea depends on how much of the osmotic substance is consumed. Diarrhea stops soon after the person stops eating or drinking the substance.

Secretory diarrhea occurs when the small and large intestines secrete salts (especially sodium chloride) and water into the stool. Certain toxins—such as the toxin produced in a cholera infection and those produced in other infectious diarrheas—can cause these secretions. The diarrhea can be massive—more than a quart an hour in cholera. Other substances that cause salt and water secretion include certain laxatives, such as castor oil, and bile acids (which may build up after surgery to remove part of the small intestine). Certain rare tumors—such as carcinoid, gastrinoma, and vipoma—also can cause secretory diarrhea.

Malabsorption syndromes★ can also lead to diarrhea. People with these syndromes can't digest foods normally. In generalized malabsorption, fats left in the large intestine because of malab-

---

▲ see page 503

■ see page 535

★ see page 534

Foods and Drugs That Can Cause Diarrhea

Foods and Drugs	Ingredient Causing Diarrhea
Apple juice, pear juice, sugar-free gums, mints	Hexitols, sorbitol, mannitol
Apple juice, pear juice, grapes, honey, dates, nuts, figs, soft drinks (especially fruit flavors)	Fructose
Table sugar	Sucrose
Milk, ice cream, frozen yogurt, yogurt, soft cheese, chocolate	Lactose
Antacids containing magnesium	Magnesium
Coffee, tea, cola drinks, over-the-counter headache remedies	Caffeine

sorption can cause secretory diarrhea, and carbohydrates may cause osmotic diarrhea. Malabsorption may be caused by such conditions as nontropical sprue, pancreatic insufficiency, surgical removal of part of the intestine, inadequate blood supply to the large intestine, a lack of certain enzymes in the small intestine, and liver disease.

Exudative diarrhea occurs when the lining of the large intestine becomes inflamed, ulcerated, or engorged, and it releases proteins, blood, mucus, and other fluids, which increase the bulk and fluid content of the stool. This type of diarrhea can be caused by many diseases, including ulcerative colitis, Crohn's disease (regional enteritis), tuberculosis, lymphoma, and cancer. When the lining of the rectum is affected, the person often feels an urgent need to defecate and has frequent bowel movements because the inflamed rectum is more sensitive to distention by stools.

Altered intestinal transit can cause diarrhea. For stool to have normal consistency, it must remain in the large intestine for a certain amount of time. Stool that leaves the large intestine too quickly is watery; stool that stays too long is hard and dry. Many conditions and treatments can decrease the amount of time that stool stays in the large intestine, including an overactive thyroid (hyperthyroidism); surgical removal of part of the small intestine, large intestine, or stomach; treatment for ulcers in which the vagus nerve is cut; surgical bypass of part of the intestine; and drugs such as antacids and laxatives containing magnesium, prostaglandins, serotonin, and even caffeine.

Bacterial overgrowth (the growth of normal intestinal bacteria in abnormally large numbers or the growth of bacteria normally not found in the intestines) can lead to diarrhea. Normal intestinal bacteria play an important role in digestion. Thus, any disruption of the intestinal bacteria can cause diarrhea.

Complications

Aside from discomfort, embarrassment, and the disruption of daily activities, severe diarrhea can lead to a loss of water (dehydration) and electrolytes such as sodium, potassium, magnesium, and chloride. If large amounts of fluid and electrolytes are lost, blood pressure can drop enough to cause fainting (syncope), heart rhythm abnormalities (arrhythmias), and other serious disorders. At particular risk are the very young, the elderly, the debilitated, and people with very severe diarrhea. Bicarbonate may be lost in the stool as well, leading to metabolic acidosis, a type of acid-base imbalance in the blood.

Diagnosis

A doctor first tries to establish whether the diarrhea appeared suddenly and for a short time or whether it's persistent. A doctor tries to determine whether changes in diet may be the cause; whether the person has other symptoms, such as a fever, pain, and rash; and whether the person has been exposed to others who have a similar condition. Based on the person's description and an examination of stool samples, the doctor and laboratory personnel determine if the stool is formed or watery, if it has an unusual odor, and if it contains fat, blood, or undigested materials. The volume of stool over a 24-hour period is also determined.

When diarrhea persists, often a sample of the stool must be examined microscopically for cells, mucus, fat, and other substances. The stool also can be tested for blood and substances that might produce osmotic diarrhea. Samples can be tested for infectious organisms, including certain bacteria, amebas, and *Giardia* organisms. If the person is surreptitiously taking a laxative, it also can be identified in the stool sample. A sigmoidoscopy (an examination of the sigmoid colon using a fiber-optic viewing tube) may be performed, so that a doctor can examine the lining of the anus and rectum.▲ Sometimes a biopsy (removal of a specimen of the rectal lining for microscopic examination) is performed.

Treatment

Diarrhea is a symptom, and its treatment depends on the cause. Most people with diarrhea only have to remove the cause, such as dietetic chewing gum or a certain drug, to suppress the diarrhea until the body heals itself. Sometimes chronic diarrhea is cured when the person stops drinking coffee or cola drinks containing caffeine. To help alleviate diarrhea, a doctor may prescribe a drug such as diphenoxylate, codeine, paregoric (tincture of opium), or loperamide. Sometimes even a bulking agent used for chronic constipation, such as psyllium or methylcellulose, helps relieve diarrhea. Kaolin, pectin, and activated attapulgite can help firm up the stool.

When severe diarrhea causes dehydration, hospitalization and fluid replacement with intravenous water and salts may be necessary. As long as the person isn't vomiting and doesn't feel nauseated, drinking liquids containing a balance of water, sugars, and salts can be very effective.

Fecal Incontinence

Fecal incontinence is the loss of control over bowel movements.

Fecal incontinence can occur briefly during bouts of diarrhea or when hard stool becomes lodged in the rectum (fecal impaction). People with injuries to the anus or spinal cord, rectal prolapse (protrusion of the rectal lining through the anus), dementia, neurologic injury from diabetes, tumors of the anus, or injuries to the pelvis during childbirth can develop persistent fecal incontinence.

A doctor examines the person for any structural or neurologic abnormality that may be causing fecal incontinence. This involves examining the anus and rectum, checking the extent of sensation around the anus, and usually performing a sigmoidoscopy (an examination of the sigmoid colon using a flexible viewing tube). Other tests, including an examination of the function of nerves and muscles lining the pelvis, may be needed.

The first step in correcting fecal incontinence is to try to establish a regular pattern of bowel movements that produce well-formed stool. Dietary changes, including the addition of a small amount of fiber, often help. If such changes don't help, a drug that slows bowel movements, such as loperamide, may succeed.

Exercising the anal muscles (sphincters) increases their tone and strength and helps prevent fecal incontinence from recurring. Using biofeedback, a person can retrain the sphincters and increase the sensitivity of the rectum to the presence of stools. About 70 percent of well-motivated people benefit from biofeedback.

If fecal incontinence persists, surgery may help in a small number of cases—for instance, when the cause is an injury to the anus or an anatomic defect in the anus. As a last resort, a colostomy (the surgical creation of an opening between the large intestine and the abdominal wall) may be performed. The anus is sewn shut, and the person defecates into a removable plastic bag attached to the opening in the abdominal wall.

Irritable Bowel Syndrome

Irritable bowel syndrome is a disorder of motility of the entire gastrointestinal tract that produces abdominal pain, constipation, or diarrhea.

Irritable bowel syndrome affects women three times more often than men. In this syndrome, the gastrointestinal tract is especially sensitive to many stimuli. Stress, diet, drugs, hormones, or minor irritants may cause the gastrointestinal tract to contract abnormally.

Periods of stress and emotional conflict that cause depression or anxiety frequently exacerbate episodes of irritable bowel syndrome. Some people with the syndrome appear to be much more aware of their symptoms, evaluate them more seriously, and experience greater disability than others. Other people with irritable bowel syndrome who experience similar stress and emotional conflicts either develop less severe gastrointestinal symptoms or react to them with less concern and disability.

During an episode, the contractions of the gastrointestinal tract become stronger and more frequent, and the resulting rapid transit of food and

▲ see page 485

feces through the small intestine often leads to diarrhea. Crampy pain seems to result from the strong contractions of the large intestine and increased sensitivity of the pain receptors in the large intestine. Episodes almost always occur when a person is awake; they rarely wake a person from sleep.

For some people, high-calorie meals or a high-fat diet may be to blame. For other people, wheat, dairy products, coffee, tea, or citrus fruits appear to aggravate the symptoms, but it's not clear that these foods are actually the cause.

Symptoms

There are two major types of irritable bowel syndrome. The spastic colon type, which is commonly triggered by eating, usually produces periodic constipation or diarrhea with pain. Sometimes constipation and diarrhea alternate. Mucus often appears in the stool. The pain may come in bouts of continuous dull aching or cramps, usually over the lower abdomen. The person may experience bloating, gas, nausea, headaches, fatigue, depression, anxiety, and difficulty concentrating. Having a bowel movement often relieves the pain.

The second type mainly produces painless diarrhea or relatively painless constipation. The diarrhea may begin very suddenly and with extreme urgency. Typically, the diarrhea follows soon after a meal, although it can sometimes occur immediately upon awakening. Sometimes the urgency is so strong that the person loses control and can't reach a bathroom in time. Diarrhea during the night is rare. Some people have bloating and constipation with relatively little pain.

Diagnosis

Most people with irritable bowel syndrome appear to be healthy. A physical examination generally doesn't reveal anything unusual except tenderness over the large intestine. Doctors generally perform some tests—for example, blood tests, a stool examination, and a sigmoidoscopy—to differentiate irritable bowel syndrome from inflammatory bowel disease▲ and the many other conditions that can cause abdominal pain and changes in bowel habits. These test results

are usually normal, although the stool may be watery. A sigmoidoscopy (an examination of the sigmoid colon using a flexible viewing tube)■ may cause spasms and pain, but the test results are otherwise normal. Sometimes other tests—such as abdominal ultrasound, x-rays of the intestines, or a colonoscopy (an examination of the large intestine using a flexible viewing tube)—are used.

Treatment

The treatment for irritable bowel syndrome differs from person to person. People who can identify particular foods or types of stress that bring on the problem should avoid them if possible. For most people, especially those who tend to be constipated, regular physical activity helps keep the gastrointestinal tract functioning normally.

In general, a normal diet is best. People with abdominal distention and increased gas (flatulence) should avoid beans, cabbage, and other foods that are difficult to digest. Sorbitol, an artificial sweetener used in dietetic foods and in some drugs and chewing gums, shouldn't be consumed in large amounts. Fructose (a common constituent of fruits, berries, and some plants) should be eaten only in small amounts. A low-fat diet helps some people. People who have both irritable bowel syndrome and lactase deficiency shouldn't eat dairy products.

Some people with irritable bowel syndrome can improve their condition by eating more fiber, especially if the main problem is constipation. They may take a tablespoon of raw bran with plenty of water and other fluids at each meal, or they can take psyllium mucilloid supplements with two glasses of water. Increasing the dietary fiber may aggravate some symptoms, such as flatulence and bloating.

Drugs that slow the function of the gastrointestinal tract and are considered to be antispasmodics, such as propantheline, haven't been proved effective, although they're frequently prescribed. Antidiarrheal drugs, such as diphenoxylate and loperamide, help people with diarrhea. Antidepressant drugs, mild tranquilizers, psychotherapy, hypnosis, and behavior modification techniques may help some people with irritable bowel syndrome.

▲ see page 527

■ see page 485

Flatulence

Flatulence is a feeling of an increased amount of gas in the gastrointestinal tract.

Air is a gas that can be swallowed with food. Swallowing small amounts of air is normal, but some people unconsciously swallow large amounts, especially when they feel anxious. Most swallowed air is later belched up, so only some passes from the stomach into the rest of the gastrointestinal system. Swallowing large amounts of air may make a person feel full, and the person may belch excessively or pass the air through the anus.

Other gases are produced in the gastrointestinal system by several means. Hydrogen, methane, and carbon dioxide are produced by bacterial metabolism of food in the intestine, especially after a person eats certain foods such as beans and cabbage. People who have deficiencies of the enzymes that break down certain sugars also tend to produce large amounts of gas when they eat foods containing the sugars. Lactase deficiency, tropical sprue, and pancreatic insufficiency all may lead to the production of large amounts of gas.

The body eliminates gas through belching, absorbing gas through the walls of the gastrointestinal tract into the blood and then excreting it through the lungs, and passing gas through the anus. Bacteria in the gastrointestinal system also metabolize some gases.

Symptoms

Flatulence is commonly thought to cause abdominal pain, bloating, belching, and excessive passing of gas through the anus; however, the exact relationship between flatulence and any of these symptoms isn't really known. Some people appear to be particularly sensitive to the effects of gas in the gastrointestinal system; others can tolerate large amounts without developing any symptoms.

Flatulence can produce repeated belching. People normally pass gas through the anus more than 10 times a day, but flatulence may cause a person to pass gas more often. Infants with crampy abdominal pain sometimes pass excessive amounts of gas. Whether these children actually produce more gas than others or are simply more sensitive to it isn't clear.

Treatment

Bloating and belching are difficult to relieve. If belching is the main problem, reducing the amount of air being swallowed can help. However, this can be difficult because people generally aren't aware of swallowing air. Avoiding chewing gum and eating more slowly in a relaxed atmosphere may help.

People who belch or pass gas excessively may need to change their diet by avoiding foods that are difficult to digest. Discovering which foods are causing the problem may require eliminating one food or one group of foods at a time. A person can start by eliminating milk and dairy products, then fresh fruits, and then certain vegetables and other foods. Belching may also result from drinking carbonated beverages or taking antacids such as baking soda.

Taking drugs sometimes helps people reduce their production of gas, although drugs generally aren't very effective. Simethicone, present in some antacids and also available separately, can provide a little relief. Sometimes other drugs—including other types of antacids, metoclopramide, and bethanechol—may help. Eating more fiber helps some people but worsens the symptoms in others.

CHAPTER 108

Inflammatory Bowel Diseases

Inflammatory bowel diseases are chronic disorders in which the intestine (bowel) becomes inflamed, often causing recurring abdominal cramps and diarrhea.

The two types of inflammatory bowel disease are Crohn's disease and ulcerative colitis, which have many similarities and sometimes are difficult to distinguish from each other. The cause of these diseases isn't known.

in about 45 percent, both the ileum and the large intestine are affected.

The cause of Crohn's disease isn't known. Research has focused on three main possibilities: a dysfunction of the immune system, infection, and diet.

Common Patterns of Crohn's Disease

Symptoms differ among people with Crohn's disease, but there are four common patterns:

- Inflammation with pain and tenderness in the right lower part of the abdomen

- Recurring acute intestinal obstructions that cause severe painful spasms of the intestinal wall, swelling of the abdomen, constipation, and vomiting

- Inflammation and chronic partial intestinal obstruction causing malnutrition and chronic debility

- Abnormal channels (fistulas) and pus-filled pockets of infection (abscesses) that often cause fever, painful masses in the abdomen, and severe weight loss

Crohn's Disease

Crohn's disease (regional enteritis, granulomatous ileitis, ileocolitis) is a chronic inflammation of the intestinal wall.

The disease typically affects the full thickness of the intestinal wall. Most commonly, it occurs in the lowest portion of the small intestine (ileum) and the large intestine, but it can occur in any part of the digestive tract from the mouth to the anus and even the skin around the anus.

In the past few decades, Crohn's disease has become more common both in Western and developing countries. It occurs about equally in both sexes, is more common among Jews, and tends to run in families that also have a history of ulcerative colitis. Most cases begin before age 30; the majority start between ages 14 and 24.

In each person, the disease affects specific areas of the intestine, sometimes with normal areas (skip areas) sandwiched between the affected zones. In about 35 percent of those with Crohn's disease, only the ileum is affected. In about 20 percent, only the large intestine is affected. And percent, only the large intestine is affected. And

Symptoms and Complications

The most common early symptoms of Crohn's disease are chronic diarrhea, crampy abdominal pain, fever, loss of appetite, and weight loss. A doctor may feel a lump or fullness in the lower part of the abdomen, most often on the right side.

Common complications of inflammation include the development of an intestinal obstruction, abnormal connecting channels (fistulas), and pus-filled pockets of infection (abscesses). Fistulas may develop that connect two different parts of the intestine. Fistulas also may connect the intestine and bladder or the intestine and the skin surface, especially around the anus. Perforation of the small intestine is a rare complication. When the large intestine is affected by Crohn's disease, rectal bleeding commonly occurs; after many years, the risk of cancer of the large intestine is increased. About a third of the people who develop Crohn's disease have problems around the anus, especially fistulas and cracks (fissures) in the lining of the mucus membrane of the anus.

Crohn's disease is associated with certain disorders affecting other parts of the body—such as gallstones, inadequate absorption of nutrients, and amyloid deposits (amyloidosis). When Crohn's disease causes a flare-up of gastrointestinal symptoms, the person may also experience inflammation of the joints (arthritis), inflammation of the whites of the eyes (episcleritis), mouth sores (aphthous stomatitis), inflamed skin nodules on the arms and legs (erythema nodosum), and blue-red skin sores containing pus (pyoderma gangrenosum). When Crohn's disease isn't causing a flare-up of gastrointestinal symptoms, the person still may experience inflammation of the spine (ankylosing spondylitis), inflammation of the pelvic joints (sacroiliitis), inflammation inside the eye (uveitis), and inflammation of the bile ducts (primary sclerosing cholangitis).

In children, gastrointestinal symptoms such as abdominal pain and diarrhea often aren't the main symptoms and may not appear at all. The main symptom may be joint inflammation, fever, anemia, or slow growth.

Some people recover completely after having a single attack affecting the small intestine. However, Crohn's disease usually flares up at irregular intervals throughout a person's life. Flare-ups can be mild or severe, brief or prolonged. Why the symptoms come and go and what triggers new episodes or determines their severity isn't known. The inflammation tends to recur in the same area of the intestine, but it may spread to other areas after a diseased area has been removed surgically.

Diagnosis

A doctor may suspect Crohn's disease in anyone with recurring, crampy abdominal pain and diarrhea, particularly if the person also has inflammation in the joints, eyes, and skin. No laboratory test specifically identifies Crohn's disease, but blood tests may show anemia, abnormally high numbers of white blood cells, low albumin levels, and other indications of inflammation.

Barium enema x-rays▲ can reveal the characteristic appearance of Crohn's disease in the large intestine. If the diagnosis is still in doubt, colonoscopy (an examination of the large intestine with a flexible viewing tube)■ and a biopsy (removal of a tissue specimen for microscopic examination) may help confirm the diagnosis. Although computed tomography (CT) can show the changes in the wall of the intestine and identify abscesses, it's not routinely used as an early diagnostic study.

Treatment and Prognosis

Crohn's disease has no known cure, but many treatments help reduce inflammation and relieve symptoms. Cramps and diarrhea may be relieved by anticholinergic drugs, diphenoxylate, loperamide, deodorized opium tincture, or codeine. These drugs are taken orally—preferably before meals. Taking methylcellulose or psyllium preparations sometimes helps prevent anal irritation by making the stool firmer.

Broad-spectrum antibiotics (antibiotics that are effective against many types of bacteria) are often prescribed. The antibiotic metronidazole may help relieve symptoms of Crohn's disease,

especially when it affects the large intestine or causes abscesses and fistulas around the anus. However, when used for a long time, metronidazole can damage nerves, resulting in pins-and-needles sensations in the arms and legs. This side effect usually disappears when the drug is stopped, but relapses of Crohn's disease after discontinuing metronidazole are common.

Sulfasalazine and chemically related drugs can suppress mild inflammation, especially in the large intestine. However, these drugs are less effective in sudden, severe flare-ups.

Corticosteroids such as prednisone may dramatically reduce fever and diarrhea, relieve abdominal pain and tenderness, and improve the appetite and sense of well-being. However, long-term corticosteroid therapy invariably results in serious side effects. Generally, high doses are taken to relieve major inflammation and symptoms; then the dose is reduced, and the drug is discontinued as soon as possible.

Drugs such as azathioprine and mercaptopurine, which modify the actions of the immune system, are effective for Crohn's disease that doesn't respond to other drugs and especially for maintaining long periods of remission. They significantly improve the person's overall condition, decrease the need for corticosteroids, and often heal fistulas. However, these drugs often don't produce benefits for 3 to 6 months and may have potentially serious side effects. Therefore, a doctor closely monitors the person for allergy, inflammation of the pancreas (pancreatitis), and a low white blood cell count.

Defined formula diets, in which each nutritional component is precisely measured, may improve the condition of intestinal obstructions or fistulas at least for a short time and also may help children grow more than they might otherwise. These diets may be tried before or in addition to surgery. Occasionally, patients need total parenteral nutrition or hyperalimentation, in which concentrated nutrients are given intravenously, to compensate for the poor absorption of nutrients that's typical of Crohn's disease.

▲ see page 486

■ see page 485

Ulcerative Proctitis

People who have ulcerative proctitis (inflammation and ulceration that's confined to the rectum) have the best prognosis. Severe complications are unlikely; however, in about 10 to 30 percent of the people, the disease eventually spreads to the large intestine (thus evolving into ulcerative colitis). Surgery is rarely needed, and life expectancy is normal. In some cases, though, the symptoms may prove exceptionally difficult to treat.

When the intestine is obstructed or when abscesses or fistulas won't heal, surgery may be needed. An operation to remove diseased sections of the intestine may relieve symptoms indefinitely, but it doesn't cure the disease. Inflammation tends to recur where the remaining intestine is rejoined. A second operation is needed in nearly half of the cases. Consequently, surgery is performed only if specific complications or the failure of drug therapy makes it necessary. Still, most people who have undergone surgery consider their quality of life to be better than it was before the operation.

Crohn's disease usually doesn't shorten a person's life. However, some people die of cancer of the digestive tract, which may develop in longstanding Crohn's disease.

Ulcerative Colitis

Ulcerative colitis is a chronic disease in which the large intestine becomes inflamed and ulcerated, leading to episodes of bloody diarrhea, abdominal cramps, and fever.

Ulcerative colitis may start at any age but usually begins between ages 15 and 30. A small group of people have their first attack between ages 50 and 70.

Unlike Crohn's disease, ulcerative colitis usually doesn't affect the full thickness of the intestine and never affects the small intestine. The disease usually begins in the rectum or the sigmoid colon (the lower end of the large intestine)

and eventually spreads partially or completely through the large intestine. In some people, most of the large intestine is affected early on.

About 10 percent of people who appear to have ulcerative colitis have only a single attack. However, some of those cases may actually be an undetected infection rather than true ulcerative colitis.

The cause of ulcerative colitis isn't known, but heredity and overactive immune responses in the intestine may be contributing factors.

Symptoms

An attack may be sudden and severe, producing violent diarrhea, high fever, abdominal pain, and peritonitis (inflammation of the lining of the abdomen). During such attacks, the person is profoundly ill. More often, an attack begins gradually, and the person has an urgency to defecate, mild cramps in the lower abdomen, and visible blood and mucus in the stool.

When the disease is limited to the rectum and the sigmoid colon, the stool may be normal or hard and dry; however, mucus containing large numbers of red and white blood cells is discharged from the rectum during or between bowel movements. General symptoms of illness, such as fever, are mild or absent.

If the disease extends farther up the large intestine, the stool is looser, and the person may have 10 to 20 bowel movements a day. Often, the person has severe abdominal cramps and distressing, painful rectal spasms that accompany the urge to defecate. There's no relief at night. The stool may be watery and contain pus, blood, and mucus. Frequently, it consists almost entirely of blood and pus. The person also may have a fever and a poor appetite and may lose weight.

Complications

Bleeding, the most common complication, often causes iron deficiency anemia. In nearly 10 percent of those with ulcerative colitis, a rapidly progressive first attack becomes very severe, with massive bleeding, perforation, or widespread infection.

In **toxic colitis,** a particularly severe complication, the entire thickness of the intestinal wall is damaged. The damage causes ileus—a condition in which the motion of the intestinal wall stops, so that the intestinal contents aren't propelled along their way. Abdominal distention develops. As toxic colitis worsens, the large intestine loses muscle tone, and within days—or even hours—it starts to dilate. X-rays of the abdomen show gas inside the paralyzed sections of intestine. When the large intestine becomes greatly distended, the condition is called toxic megacolon. The person is severely ill and may have a high fever. The person also has pain and tenderness in the abdomen and a high white blood cell count. However, of the people who receive prompt, effective treatment for their symptoms, fewer than 4 percent die. If the ulceration perforates the intestine, the risk of death is great.

The risk of **colon cancer** is higher in people with long-standing, extensive ulcerative colitis. The risk of colon cancer is highest when the entire large intestine is affected and the person has had ulcerative colitis for more than 10 years, regardless of how active the disease is. Colonoscopy (examination of the large intestine using a flexible viewing tube)▲ at regular intervals—preferably during symptom-free periods—is advised for people with a high risk of cancer. During colonoscopy, tissue samples are obtained throughout the large intestine for microscopic examination. As many as 1 in every 100 people with this disease may develop colon cancer each year. Most survive if the diagnosis of cancer is made during the cancer's early stages.

Like Crohn's disease, ulcerative colitis is associated with disorders affecting other parts of the body. When ulcerative colitis causes a flare-up of intestinal symptoms, the person also may experience inflammation of the joints (arthritis), inflammation of the whites of the eyes (episcleritis), inflamed skin nodules (erythema nodosum), and blue-red skin sores containing pus (pyoderma gangrenosum). When ulcerative colitis isn't causing intestinal symptoms, the person still may experience inflammation of the spine (ankylosing spondylitis), inflammation of the pelvic joints (sacroiliitis), and inflammation of the inside of the eye (uveitis).

Although people with ulcerative colitis commonly have minor liver dysfunction, only about 1 to 3 percent have symptoms of mild to severe liver disease. Severe disease can include liver inflammation (chronic active hepatitis); inflammation of the bile ducts (primary sclerosing cholangitis), which narrow and eventually close; and replacement of functional liver tissue with fibrous mate-

rial (cirrhosis). Inflammation of the bile ducts may appear many years before any intestinal symptoms of ulcerative colitis, and it increases the risk of cancer of the bile ducts.

Diagnosis

The patient's symptoms and a stool examination help establish the diagnosis. Blood tests reveal anemia, increased numbers of white blood cells, a low albumin level, and an elevated erythrocyte sedimentation rate. A sigmoidoscopy (an examination of the sigmoid colon using a flexible viewing tube)■ confirms the diagnosis and permits a doctor to directly observe the severity of the inflammation. Even during symptom-free intervals, the intestine rarely appears normal, and a tissue sample removed for microscopic examination shows chronic inflammation.

X-rays of the abdomen may indicate the severity and extent of the disease. Barium enema x-ray studies and colonoscopy (an examination of the entire large intestine using a flexible viewing tube) aren't usually done before treatment begins because they pose a risk of perforation when done during the active stages of the disease. At some point, however, the whole large intestine is usually evaluated by colonoscopy or by barium enema x-ray studies to determine the extent of the disease and to ensure that no cancer is present.

Inflammation of the large intestine has many causes other than ulcerative colitis. Thus, a doctor determines whether the inflammation is caused by an infection with bacteria or parasites. Stool samples obtained during sigmoidoscopy are examined under the microscope and cultured for bacteria. Blood samples are analyzed to determine whether the person may have acquired a parasitic infection, for example, during travel. Tissue samples are taken from the lining of the rectum and examined microscopically. A doctor also checks for sexually transmitted diseases of the rectum—such as gonorrhea, herpesvirus, or chlamydial infections★—especially if the patient is a homosexual male. In elderly people with atherosclerosis, inflammation may be caused by

---

▲ see page 485

■ see page 485

★ see page 937

poor blood supply to the large intestine. Colon cancer seldom produces a fever or a discharge of pus from the rectum, but a doctor must consider cancer as a possible cause of bloody diarrhea.

Treatment

Treatment aims to control the inflammation, reduce symptoms, and replace any lost fluids and nutrients. The person should avoid raw fruits and vegetables to reduce physical injury to the inflamed lining of the large intestine. A diet free of dairy products may decrease symptoms and is worth trying. Iron supplements may offset anemia caused by ongoing blood loss in the feces.

Anticholinergic drugs or small doses of loperamide or diphenoxylate are taken for relatively mild diarrhea. For more intense diarrhea, higher doses of diphenoxylate or deodorized opium tincture, loperamide, or codeine may be needed. In severe cases, a doctor closely monitors the patient taking these antidiarrheal drugs to avoid precipitating toxic megacolon.

Sulfasalazine, olsalazine, or mesalamine often is used to reduce the inflammation of ulcerative colitis and to prevent flare-ups of symptoms. These drugs usually are taken orally, but they can be given as an enema or a suppository.

People with moderately severe disease who aren't confined to bed usually take oral corticosteroids such as prednisone. Prednisone in fairly high doses frequently induces a dramatic remission. After prednisone controls the inflammation of ulcerative colitis, sulfasalazine, olsalazine, or mesalamine often is given as well. Gradually, the prednisone dosage is decreased, and ultimately, the prednisone is stopped. Prolonged corticosteroid treatment almost invariably produces side effects, although most subside when the drug is stopped. When mild or moderate ulcerative colitis is limited to the left side of the large intestine (descending colon) and the rectum, enemas with a corticosteroid or mesalamine may be given.

If the disease becomes severe, the person is hospitalized, and corticosteroids are given intravenously. People with heavy rectal bleeding may require blood transfusions and intravenous fluids.

Azathioprine and mercaptopurine have been used to maintain remissions in people with ulcerative colitis who would otherwise need long-term corticosteroid therapy. Cyclosporine has been given to some people who've suffered severe attacks and haven't responded to corticosteroid therapy, but about half of these people eventually require surgery.

Surgery

Toxic colitis is an emergency. As soon as a doctor detects it or suspects impending toxic megacolon, all antidiarrheal drugs are discontinued, the patient is given nothing to eat, a tube is inserted through the nose and into the stomach or small intestine and attached to intermittent suction, and all fluids, nutrition, and medication are given intravenously. The patient is monitored closely for indications of peritonitis or a perforation. If these measures fail to improve the person's condition in 24 to 48 hours, emergency surgery is needed: All or most of the large intestine is removed.

Surgery is performed on a nonemergency basis when cancer is diagnosed or precancerous changes are identified in the large intestine. Such surgery also may be performed because of narrowing of the large intestine or growth retardation in children. The most common reason for surgery is unremitting chronic disease that would otherwise make the person an invalid or chronically dependent on high doses of corticosteroids. In rare cases, severe colitis-related problems outside the intestine, such as pyoderma gangrenosum, may make surgery necessary.

Complete removal of the large intestine and rectum permanently cures ulcerative colitis. Living with a permanent ileostomy (a surgically created connection between the lowest portion of the small intestine and an opening in the abdominal wall) and an ileostomy bag has been the traditional price of this cure. However, various alternative procedures are available, the most common one being a procedure called ileo-anal anastomosis. In this procedure, the large intestine and most of the rectum are removed, and a small reservoir is created out of the small intestine and attached to the remaining rectum just above the anus. This procedure maintains continence, though some complications, such as inflammation of the reservoir, may occur.

Antibiotic-Associated Colitis

Antibiotic-associated colitis is inflammation of the large intestine resulting from the use of antibiotics.

Many antibiotics alter the balance among the types and quantity of bacteria in the intestine, thus allowing certain disease-causing bacteria to multiply.▲ The bacterium that most commonly causes problems is *Clostridium difficile,* which produces two toxins that can damage the protective lining of the large intestine.

The antibiotics that most often cause this disorder are clindamycin, ampicillin, and cephalosporins such as cephalothin. Other antibiotics that can cause the disorder include the penicillins, erythromycin, trimethoprim-sulfamethoxazole, chloramphenicol, and tetracycline. *Clostridium difficile* overgrowth can occur whether an antibiotic is taken by mouth or by injection. The risk increases with age, although young adults and children may be affected.

In mild cases, the lining of the intestine may become slightly inflamed. In severe colitis, the inflammation is extensive, and the lining is ulcerated.

Symptoms

Symptoms usually begin while the person is taking antibiotics. However, in a third of the patients, symptoms don't appear until 1 to 10 days after treatment has stopped, and in some people, symptoms don't appear for as long as 6 weeks afterward.

Typically, symptoms range from mild diarrhea to bloody diarrhea, abdominal pain, and fever. The most severe cases may involve life-threatening dehydration, low blood pressure, toxic megacolon,■ and perforation of the small intestine.

Diagnosis

A doctor diagnoses colitis by inspecting the inflamed large intestine, usually through a sigmoidoscope (a rigid or flexible viewing tube for examining the sigmoid colon).★ A colonoscope (a longer flexible viewing tube for examining the entire large intestine) may have to be used if the diseased section of intestine is higher than the reach of the sigmoidoscope.

The diagnosis of antibiotic-associated colitis is confirmed when *Clostridium difficile* is identified in a laboratory culture of a stool sample or its toxin is detected in the stool. The toxin can be detected in 20 percent of those with mild antibiotic-associated colitis and in more than 90 percent of those with severe antibiotic-associated colitis.

Laboratory tests may reveal an abnormally high number of white blood cells in the blood during severe attacks.

Treatment

If a person with antibiotic-associated colitis has severe diarrhea while taking antibiotics, the drugs are stopped immediately unless they're essential. Drugs that slow the movement of the intestine, such as diphenoxylate, generally are avoided because they may prolong the illness by keeping the disease-causing toxin in contact with the large intestine. Antibiotic-induced diarrhea without complications usually subsides on its own within 10 to 12 days after the antibiotic has been stopped. When it does, no other therapy is required. However, if mild symptoms persist, cholestyramine may be effective, probably because it binds itself to the toxin.

For most cases of severe antibiotic-associated colitis, the antibiotic metronidazole is effective against *Clostridium difficile.* The antibiotic vancomycin is reserved for the most severe or resistant cases.

Symptoms return in up to 20 percent of patients, and they need to be treated again. When diarrhea returns repeatedly, prolonged antibiotic therapy may be needed. Some patients are treated with preparations of lactobacillus given by mouth or bacteroides given rectally to restock the intestine with normal bacteria; however,

▲ see page 840

■ see page 531

★ see page 485

these treatments aren't used routinely. Rarely, antibiotic-associated colitis is acute and fulminating, and the person must be hospitalized to receive intravenous fluids, electrolytes, and blood transfusions. A temporary ileostomy (a surgically created connection between the small intestine and an opening in the abdominal wall that diverts stool from the large intestine and rectum) or surgical removal of the large intestine occasionally has been needed as a lifesaving measure.

CHAPTER 110

Malabsorption Syndromes

Malabsorption syndromes are disorders that develop because nutrients from food aren't being absorbed properly into the bloodstream from the small intestine.

Normally, foods are digested, and then nutrients are absorbed into the bloodstream mainly from the small intestine. Malabsorption may occur either because a disorder interferes with the digestion of food or because a disorder interferes directly with the absorption of nutrients.

Disorders that prevent adequate mixing of food with stomach acid and digestive enzymes may interfere with digestion. Such inadequate mixing may occur in a person who has had part of the stomach surgically removed. In some disorders, the body produces inadequate amounts or types of enzymes or bile, which are necessary for the breakdown of food. Such disorders include pancreatitis, cystic fibrosis, obstruction of the bile duct, and lactase deficiency. Too much acid in the stomach or too many of the wrong kinds of bacteria growing in the small intestine may also interfere with digestion.

Disorders that injure the intestinal lining may interfere with absorption. Infections, drugs such as neomycin and alcohol, celiac disease, and Crohn's disease all may injure the intestinal lining. The normal intestinal lining consists of folds, small projections called villi, and even smaller projections called microvilli. These projections create an enormous surface area for absorption. Anything that reduces this area may reduce absorption. Obviously, surgical removal of a section of the intestine reduces the surface area. Disorders that prevent substances from being passed into the bloodstream through the intestinal wall, such as blockage of the lymphatic vessels by lymphoma or poor blood supply to the intestine, also reduce absorption.

Symptoms

People with malabsorption usually lose weight. If fats aren't properly absorbed, the stool may be light-colored, soft, bulky, and foul smelling; such stool is called steatorrhea. The stool may stick to the side of the toilet bowl or may float and be difficult to flush away. Steatorrhea results from any condition that interferes with the absorption of fats, such as reduced bile flow, celiac disease, or tropical sprue.

Malabsorption can cause deficiencies of all nutrients or of proteins, fats, vitamins, or minerals selectively. The symptoms vary depending on the specific deficiencies. For example, people with a deficiency of the enzyme lactase may experience explosive diarrhea, abdominal bloating, and flatulence after drinking milk.

Other symptoms depend on the disorder that is causing the malabsorption. For example, an obstructed bile duct may cause jaundice; poor blood supply to the intestine may cause abdominal pain after meals.

Diagnosis

Doctors suspect malabsorption when a person loses weight and has diarrhea and nutritional deficiencies despite eating well. Weight loss alone can have other causes.

Laboratory tests can help confirm the diagnosis. Tests that directly measure fat in stool samples collected over 3 or 4 days are the most reliable ones for diagnosing malabsorption of fat. A finding of excess fat makes the diagnosis likely. Other laboratory tests can detect malabsorption of other specific substances, such as lactose or vitamin B_{12}.

Stool samples are examined with the unaided eye and under the microscope. Undigested food fragments may mean that food passes through the intestine too rapidly. Such fragments also can indicate an anatomically abnormal intestinal pathway, such as a direct connection between the stomach and the large intestine (gastrocolic fistula) that bypasses the small intestine. In a person with jaundice, stool with excess fat may be an indication of problems in the biliary system. A doctor looks especially for cancer of the pancreas or biliary tract in people with jaundice and excess fat in the stool. Fat globules and undigested meat fibers seen under the microscope indicate that the pancreas isn't functioning properly. A doctor also may see parasites or their eggs under the microscope—a finding that suggests malabsorption caused by parasitic infection.

X-rays of the abdomen rarely help with the diagnosis, though they sometimes indicate possible causes of the malabsorption. X-rays taken after the person drinks barium▲ may show an abnormal pattern of barium distribution in the small intestine that is characteristic of malabsorption, but these x-rays give no information about the cause.

A **biopsy** (removal of a tissue specimen for examination) may be needed to detect abnormalities of the small intestine. The specimen can be obtained by using an endoscope (a flexible viewing tube)■ or by using a thin tube with a small cutting instrument at the end. The specimen is examined under the microscope and may be tested for enzyme activity.

Pancreatic function tests are often performed because pancreatic malfunction is a common cause of malabsorption. In one test, the person receives a special diet; in another, the person receives an injection of the hormone secretin. In both tests, intestinal juices containing pancreatic secretions are then collected through a tube and measured.

Sugar Intolerance

The sugars lactose, sucrose, and maltose are broken down by the enzymes lactase, sucrase, and maltase, which are located in the lining of the small intestine. Normally, the enzymes break these sugars into simple sugars, such as glucose, which are then absorbed into the blood through the intestinal wall. If the necessary enzyme is lacking, the sugars aren't digested, and they can't be absorbed. Thus, they remain in the small intestine. The resulting high concentration of sugar draws fluid into the small intestine, causing diarrhea. The unabsorbed sugar is then fermented by

Symptoms of Nutrient Deficiencies

Nutrient	Symptoms
Iron	Anemia
Calcium	Bone thinning
Folic acid	Anemia
Vitamin B$_1$	Pins-and-needles sensation, especially in feet
Vitamin B$_2$	Sore tongue and cracks at edge of mouth
Vitamin B$_{12}$	Anemia, pins-and-needles sensation
Vitamin C	Weakness, bleeding gums
Vitamin D	Bone thinning
Vitamin K	Tendency to bruise and bleed
Protein	Tissue swelling (edema), usually in legs

bacteria in the large intestine, producing acidic stool and flatulence. Enzyme deficiency occurs in celiac disease, tropical sprue, and infections of the intestine. Enzyme deficiency also can be congenital, or it can be caused by antibiotics, especially neomycin.

Some degree of lactose intolerance occurs in about 75 percent of adults. It affects fewer than 20 percent of adults of northwestern European origin but 90 percent of Asians. Lactose intolerance is common among people from the Mediterranean area. About 75 percent of nonwhite North Americans gradually develop lactose intolerance between ages 10 and 20.

Symptoms

People with lactose intolerance usually can't tolerate milk and other dairy products, which contain lactose. Some people recognize this early

▲ see page 486

■ see page 485

in life and consciously or unconsciously avoid dairy products.

A child who can't tolerate lactose has diarrhea and doesn't gain weight when milk is part of the diet. An adult may have audible bowel sounds (borborygmi), abdominal bloating, flatulence, nausea, an urgent need to defecate, abdominal cramps, and diarrhea following a meal containing lactose. Severe diarrhea may prevent proper absorption of nutrients because they're expelled from the body too quickly. Similar symptoms can be caused by lack of the enzymes sucrase and maltase.

Diagnosis

A doctor suspects lactose intolerance when a person has symptoms after consuming dairy products. If a person has lactose intolerance, eating a test dose of lactose causes diarrhea, bloating, and a feeling of abdominal discomfort in 20 to 30 minutes. Because the test dose isn't broken down into glucose, levels of glucose in the blood don't rise as they normally would.

A biopsy of the small intestine may be performed. The specimen of the small intestine is viewed under the microscope and tested for lactase or other enzyme activity. This test can indicate other possible causes of the malabsorption.

Treatment

Lactose intolerance can be controlled by avoiding foods containing lactose—primarily dairy products. To prevent a calcium deficiency, people who must avoid dairy products may take calcium supplements. Alternatively, lactase can be added to milk; the lactase then breaks down the lactose in the milk before the person drinks it.

Celiac Disease

Celiac disease (nontropical sprue, gluten enteropathy, celiac sprue) is an inherited disorder in which an allergic intolerance to gluten, a protein, causes changes in the intestine that result in malabsorption.

About 1 in 300 people in southwestern Ireland and 1 in 5,000 or more in North America have celiac disease. This hereditary disorder is caused by sensitivity to gluten, a protein found in wheat and rye and to a lesser degree in barley and oats. In this disorder, part of the gluten molecule combines with antibodies in the small intestine, causing the normal brushlike lining of the intestine to flatten. The resulting smooth surface is much less able to digest and absorb foods. When foods containing gluten are avoided, the normal brushlike surface usually is restored, and normal intestinal function returns.

Symptoms

Celiac disease may begin at any age. In infants, no symptoms appear until foods containing gluten are first eaten. Celiac disease often doesn't cause diarrhea or fatty stools, and a child may have only mild symptoms, which are interpreted as those of a simple upset stomach. However, some children stop growing normally, suffer painful abdominal bloating, and begin passing pale, foul-smelling, bulky stools. Anemia develops from iron deficiency. If the level of protein in the blood falls low enough, the child retains fluid, and tissues may swell (edema). In some people, symptoms don't appear until adulthood.

The nutritional deficiencies resulting from malabsorption in celiac disease can cause additional symptoms. These symptoms include weight loss, bone pain, and a pins-and-needles sensation in the arms and legs. Some people who develop celiac disease in childhood may have abnormally bowed long bones. Depending on the severity and duration of the disorder, the person may have low blood levels of protein, calcium, potassium, or sodium. A deficiency of prothrombin, which is important in blood clotting, leads to easy bruising and prolonged bleeding after an injury. Girls with celiac disease may not have menstrual periods.

Diagnosis

Doctors suspect celiac disease when they see a pale child who has wasted buttocks and a potbelly despite eating an adequate diet—especially if there's a family history of the disease. Results of laboratory tests and x-rays may help a doctor make the diagnosis. A laboratory test that measures the absorption of xylose, a simple sugar, sometimes is useful. The diagnosis is confirmed by an examination of a biopsy specimen that reveals a flattened lining of the small intestine and by a subsequent improvement in the lining after the person stops eating gluten products.

Treatment

Eating even small amounts of gluten may cause symptoms, so all gluten must be excluded from the diet. Gluten is so widely used in food products that people with the disorder need detailed lists of foods to be avoided and expert advice from a dietitian. Gluten is found, for example, in commercial soups, sauces, ice creams, and hot dogs.

Sometimes children who are seriously ill when first diagnosed need a period of intravenous feeding. Such feedings are rarely needed for adults.

Some people respond poorly or not at all to gluten withdrawal. This can be either because the diagnosis is incorrect or because the disorder has entered an unresponsive phase. If the latter is true, corticosteroids may help.

Some people diagnosed with celiac disease who have avoided gluten for a long time can tolerate reintroducing it into their diet, possibly because the diagnosis was incorrect. Trying to reintroduce gluten may be reasonable, but if symptoms recur, gluten should be removed immediately from the diet.

Gluten-free diets substantially improve the prognosis for children and adults. However, celiac disease can be fatal—mainly for adults with a severe form. A small percentage of adults may develop lymphoma▲ (a type of cancer) in the intestine. Whether this risk is diminished by strictly adhering to a gluten-free diet isn't known.

Tropical Sprue

Tropical sprue is an acquired disorder in which abnormalities of the lining of the small intestine lead to malabsorption and deficiencies of many nutrients.

Tropical sprue occurs chiefly in the Caribbean, southern India, and Southeast Asia. Both natives and newcomers may be affected. Although the cause is unknown, possible causes include bacterial infection, viral infection, parasitic infection, vitamin deficiency (especially folic acid deficiency), and a toxin in spoiled foods (for instance, in rancid fats).

Symptoms and Diagnosis

Light-colored stool, diarrhea, and weight loss are typical symptoms of tropical sprue. So is a sore tongue from vitamin B_2 deficiency. Other symptoms of malabsorption also may develop. A deficiency of prothrombin, which is important in blood clotting, leads to easy bruising and prolonged bleeding after an injury. People with tropical sprue also may have symptoms of albumin, calcium, folic acid, vitamin B_{12}, and iron deficiencies. Typically, anemia develops from folic acid deficiency.■

Doctors consider a diagnosis of tropical sprue in anyone with anemia and symptoms of malabsorption who lives in or has lived in one of the endemic areas. X-rays of the small intestine may or may not be abnormal. Absorption of the simple sugar xylose can be easily measured; in 90 percent of those with tropical sprue, xylose isn't absorbed normally. A biopsy of the small intestine shows characteristic abnormalities.

Treatment

The best treatment for tropical sprue is an antibiotic, either tetracycline or oxytetracycline. Depending on how severe the disease is and how well it responds to treatment, the antibiotic may need to be taken for as long as 6 months. Nutritional supplements, especially folic acid, are given as needed.

Whipple's Disease

Whipple's disease (intestinal lipodystrophy) is a rare disorder that affects mainly men ages 30 to 60.

Whipple's disease is caused by an infection with the organism *Tropheryma whippelii*. The lining of the small intestine is always severely infected, but infection also may spread to other organs, such as the heart, lung, brain, joints, and eye.

Symptoms and Diagnosis

Symptoms of Whipple's disease include skin darkening, inflamed and painful joints, and diarrhea. Severe malabsorption causes weight loss and anemia. Other common symptoms are abdominal pain, cough, and pain when breathing caused by inflammation of the pleura (the membrane layers covering the lungs). Fluid may collect in the space between the pleural layers (a condition called pleural effusion),★ and the lymph nodes in the center of the chest may become enlarged. People with Whipple's disease may develop heart murmurs, which usually indicate that the infection has reached the heart, or liver enlargement, which usually indicates that it has reached the liver. Confusion, memory loss, or

---

▲ see page 770

■ see page 660

★ see page 206

uncontrolled eye movements indicate that the infection involves the brain. If left untreated, the disease is progressive and fatal.

The diagnosis of Whipple's disease is made by a biopsy of the small intestine or an enlarged lymph node that reveals characteristic microscopic abnormalities.

Treatment

Whipple's disease can be cured with antibiotics such as tetracycline, sulfasalazine, ampicillin, and penicillin. Symptoms improve rapidly, but complete tissue healing may take up to 2 years. The disease can recur.

Intestinal Lymphangiectasia

Intestinal lymphangiectasia (idiopathic hypoproteinemia) is a disorder of children and young adults in which the lymph vessels supplying the lining of the small intestine become enlarged.

Lymph vessel enlargement may be a birth defect. Or later in life, it may result from inflammation of the pancreas (pancreatitis) or stiffening of the sac around the heart (constrictive pericarditis),▲ which increases pressure on the lymphatic system.

Symptoms and Diagnosis

A person with lymphangiectasia has massive fluid retention (edema) because tissue fluid can't drain efficiently through the enlarged, obstructed lymph vessels. The swelling may affect different parts of the body unevenly, depending on which lymph vessels are involved. For example, fluid may accumulate in the abdominal and pleural cavities.

Nausea, vomiting, mild diarrhea, and abdominal pain also may develop. The number of lymphocytes in the blood may decrease. Protein is lost because lymph leaks from the swollen lymph vessels into the intestine and the feces; thus, the level of protein in the blood is low. This low protein level may cause further tissue swelling. Cholesterol levels in the blood may be abnormally low because cholesterol from food isn't absorbed well. Some people also have fatty stools.

To help diagnose this disorder, a doctor may use an intravenous injection of radioactive-labeled albumin. If abnormal amounts of the radioactive substance appear in the stool, the person has an excessive protein loss. A biopsy of the small intestine shows that the lymph vessels are enlarged.

Treatment

Intestinal lymphangiectasia is treated by correcting the cause of the lymph vessel enlargement. For instance, treating constrictive pericarditis may relieve pressure on the lymph vessels.

Some people improve by eating a low-fat diet and taking supplements of certain triglycerides, which are absorbed directly into the blood and not through the lymph vessels. If only a small part of the intestine is affected, it can be removed surgically.

CHAPTER 111

Diverticular Disease

A diverticulum is a saclike outpouching of any portion of the gastrointestinal (digestive) tract. By far, the most common site for diverticula is the large intestine. The presence of diverticula is called diverticulosis—a condition that tends to

develop after middle age. If diverticula become inflamed, the condition is called diverticulitis.

Diverticulosis

Diverticulosis is the presence of diverticula, usually in the large intestine.

Diverticula may appear anywhere in the large intestine but they're most common in the sigmoid colon, the last part of the large intestine just be-

▲ see page 104

fore the rectum.▲ A diverticulum bulges at a point of weakness, usually where an artery penetrates the muscle layer of the large intestine. Spasms are thought to increase pressure in the large intestine, thereby creating more diverticula and enlarging existing ones.

Diverticula vary in diameter from one tenth of an inch to more than an inch. They're uncommon before age 40, but they start becoming common after 40. Virtually anyone who reaches age 90 has many diverticula.

Giant diverticula are rare outpouchings that range from 1 to 6 inches in diameter. A person may have only a single giant diverticulum.

Symptoms

Most people with diverticulosis don't appear to have symptoms. However, some experts believe that when such people have unexplained painful cramps, diarrhea, and other bowel movement disturbances, the cause is actually diverticulosis. The opening of a diverticulum can bleed, sometimes heavily, into the intestine and out through the rectum. Such bleeding may result when feces wedge in the diverticulum and damage a blood vessel (usually the artery beside the diverticulum). Bleeding is more common when diverticula are in the ascending colon than when they're in the descending colon. Colonoscopy (an examination of the large intestine using a flexible viewing tube) can identify the source of bleeding.

Diverticula themselves aren't dangerous. Feces trapped in a diverticulum, however, may cause not only bleeding but also inflammation and infection, resulting in diverticulitis.

Treatment

The goal of treatment is usually to reduce intestinal spasms. Consuming a high-fiber diet (vegetables, fruits, and cereals) is the best way to reduce them. If a high-fiber diet alone isn't effective, a person may supplement it with millers' bran or may take a bulking agent, such as 3.5 grams of psyllium in 8 ounces of water once or twice daily. Methylcellulose also may help. Low-fiber diets should be avoided because more pressure may be needed to move the resulting intestinal contents.

Diverticulosis doesn't require surgery. However, giant diverticula do because they're more likely to become infected and to perforate.

Diverticulitis: Reasons for Elective Surgery

Condition	Reason
Two or more severe attacks of diverticulitis (or one severe attack in someone under age 50)	High risk of serious complications
Rapid progression of disease	High risk of serious complications
Persistent tender mass in the abdomen	May be cancer
X-ray showing suspicious changes in lower part of large intestine (sigmoid colon)	May be cancer
Pain when urinating—in men or in women who have had a hysterectomy	May be a warning of impending perforation into bladder
Sudden abdominal pain in people taking corticosteroids	Large intestine may have perforated into abdominal cavity

Diverticulitis

Diverticulitis is inflammation or infection of one or more diverticula.

Diverticulitis is less common in people under age 40 than in those over age 40. However, it can be severe in people of any age. Among people under age 50 who need surgery for diverticulitis, men outnumber women three to one; among those over age 70, women outnumber men three to one.

Symptoms and Diagnosis

Typically, the initial symptoms are pain, tenderness (usually in the lower left part of the abdomen), and fever.

▲ see box, page 483

Fistula: An Abnormal Connection

Most fistulas form between the sigmoid colon and the bladder, as shown.

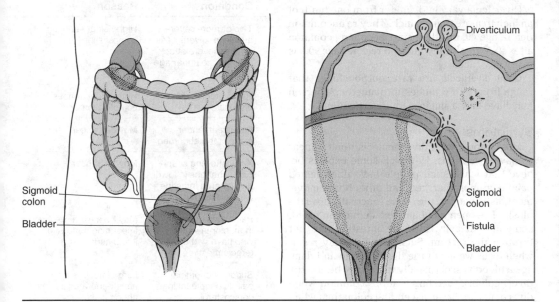

Diverticulum

Sigmoid colon

Bladder

Sigmoid colon

Fistula

Bladder

If a doctor knows that the person already has diverticulosis, a diagnosis of diverticulitis may be made almost entirely on the basis of the symptoms. A barium enema x-ray▲ study to confirm the diagnosis or evaluate the problem could damage or perforate an inflamed intestine, so this test is usually delayed for a few weeks.

Appendicitis and cancer of the large intestine or ovary are most often confused with diverticulitis. A computed tomography (CT) or ultrasound scan may be needed to make sure the problem isn't appendicitis or an abscess. To rule out cancer, a doctor may use colonoscopy, especially if there's bleeding. Exploratory surgery may be needed to confirm the diagnosis.

Complications

The inflammation occurring in diverticulitis can lead to abnormal connections (fistulas) between the large intestine and other organs. Most fistulas form between the sigmoid colon and the bladder. These fistulas are more common in men than in women, but a hysterectomy (removal of the uterus) increases a woman's risk. With such a fistula, intestinal contents, including normal bacteria, enter the bladder and cause urinary tract infections. Other fistulas may develop between the large intestine and the small intestine, uterus, vagina, abdominal wall, or even the thigh or chest.

Other possible complications of diverticulitis include inflammation of the surrounding structures, spreading inflammation of the intestinal wall, rupture of the wall of a diverticulum (perforation), abscess, infection of the abdomen (peritonitis), bleeding, and intestinal obstruction.■

▲ see page 486

■ see page 545

Treatment

Mild diverticulitis can be treated at home with rest, a liquid diet, and oral antibiotics. Symptoms usually disappear rapidly. After a few days, a person can begin a soft, low-fiber diet and take a daily psyllium seed preparation. After one month, a high-fiber diet can be resumed.

People with more severe symptoms—such as localized abdominal pain, fever, and other evidence of serious infection or complications—are generally admitted to the hospital. They're given intravenous fluids and antibiotics, and they stay in bed and take nothing by mouth until the symptoms subside.

If the condition doesn't improve, the person may need surgery, especially if pain, tenderness, and fever are increasing. Only about 20 percent of people who have diverticulitis require surgery because the condition doesn't improve; of those, about 70 percent have pain and inflammation, and the others have bleeding, fistulas, or an obstruction. Sometimes surgery for diverticulitis is recommended when a person has no evidence of inflammation, infection, or complications because the risk of developing a problem that will require surgery is high and because surgery before the problem develops will be simpler and safer.

Emergency surgery is necessary for patients who are hospitalized for intestinal pertoration and peritonitis. The surgeon generally removes the perforated segment and creates an opening between the large intestine and the skin surface, called a colostomy. The cut ends of the intestine are rejoined during a follow-up operation, and the colostomy is closed.

When massive bleeding occurs, the source can be identified by injecting a dye into the arteries that supply the large intestine and then taking an x-ray, a procedure called angiography. Injecting vasopressin (a drug that constricts arteries) may control the bleeding but can be dangerous, especially in the elderly. In some cases, bleeding starts again within a few days, requiring surgery. Removing the affected section of the intestine is possible only if the source of bleeding is known. Otherwise, much more of the intestine is removed in a procedure called subtotal colectomy. If bleeding stops (or slows significantly) without treatment, the best way to determine the cause of the bleeding is to perform a colonoscopy.

Treatment for a fistula involves removing the section of large intestine where the fistula begins and rejoining the cut ends.

CHAPTER 112

Gastrointestinal Emergencies

Certain gastrointestinal disorders can be life threatening and require emergency treatment—surgery, in some cases. These disorders include bleeding in the digestive tract, mechanical obstruction of the digestive tract, ileus (a temporary cessation of the tract's normal contractile movements), appendicitis (inflammation of the appendix), and peritonitis (inflammation of the lining of the abdominal cavity).

Gastrointestinal Bleeding

Bleeding may occur anywhere along the digestive (gastrointestinal) tract▲ from the mouth to the anus. It may appear as blood in the stool or vomit or may be hidden (occult) and detectable only by tests. Bleeding anywhere in the digestive tract may be worsened by another bleeding disorder.

Symptoms

Possible symptoms include vomiting blood (hematemesis), passing black tarry stools (melena), and passing visible blood from the rectum (hematochezia). Black tarry stools usually result from bleeding high up in the digestive tract—for example, the stomach or duodenum; the black color results from blood that has been exposed

▲ see box, page 482

The Wheres and Whys of Gastrointestinal Bleeding

Where	Why
Esophagus	• Torn tissue • Bleeding varicose veins • Cancer
Stomach	• Cancerous or noncancerous ulcer • Irritation (gastritis), as from aspirin or *Helicobacter pylori*
Small intestine	• Noncancerous duodenal ulcer • Cancerous or noncancerous tumor
Large intestine	• Cancer • Noncancerous polyp • Inflammatory bowel disease (Crohn's disease or ulcerative colitis) • Diverticular disease • Abnormal blood vessel in the intestinal wall (angiodysplasia)
Rectum	• Cancer • Noncancerous tumor
Anus	• Hemorrhoids • Tear of the anus (anal fissure)

to stomach acid and bacterial digestion for several hours before it exits the body. About 2 ounces of blood can produce a tarry stool. A single severe bleeding episode can produce tarry stools for as long as a week, so continuing tarry stools don't necessarily indicate persistent bleeding.

People with long-term bleeding may have symptoms of anemia, such as tiring easily, looking unnaturally pale, having chest pain, and feeling light-headed. In people who don't have such symptoms, a doctor may be able to detect an abnormal drop in blood pressure when a person sits up after lying down.

▲ see page 564

Symptoms indicating a serious blood loss include a rapid pulse rate, low blood pressure, and reduced urine production. A person may also have cold, clammy hands and feet. The reduced supply of blood to the brain caused by the blood loss may lead to confusion, disorientation, sleepiness, and even shock.

Symptoms of serious blood loss may differ, depending on whether the person has certain other diseases. For instance, a person with coronary artery disease may suddenly develop angina (chest pain) or symptoms of a heart attack. In a person who has serious gastrointestinal bleeding, the symptoms of other diseases—such as heart failure, high blood pressure, lung disease, and kidney failure—may worsen. In people with liver disease, bleeding into the intestine can cause a buildup of toxins that, in turn, results in symptoms such as changes in personality, awareness, and mental ability (liver encephalopathy).▲

Diagnosis

After a serious blood loss, a hematocrit measurement, a type of blood test, generally reveals a low concentration of red blood cells in the blood. Knowing about the symptoms that led up to a bleeding episode may help a doctor determine its cause. Pain in the abdomen that's relieved by food or antacids suggests a peptic ulcer; however, bleeding ulcers often aren't painful. Drugs that can damage the lining of the stomach, such as aspirin, may cause bleeding from the stomach that appears as blood in the stools.

Someone with gastrointestinal bleeding who has no appetite and has lost weight for no obvious reason is examined for the possibility of cancer. A person who has difficulty swallowing is examined for cancer of the esophagus or a narrowing in the esophagus. Very forceful vomiting and retching immediately before the bleeding suggests a torn esophagus, but about half of the people with such a tear don't vomit beforehand. Constipation or diarrhea along with bleeding or hidden blood in the stool may be caused by cancer or a polyp in the lower intestine, particularly in someone over age 45. Fresh blood on the surface of the stools may result from hemorrhoids or a problem within the rectum, such as cancer.

A doctor examines the patient for clues that may point to the source of the bleeding. For example, during a rectal examination, a doctor looks for hemorrhoids, rectal tears (fissures), and tumors. Then tests are chosen according to whether the doctor suspects that the bleeding is coming from the upper gastrointestinal tract (esophagus, stomach, and duodenum) or the lower gastrointestinal tract (lower small intestine, large intestine, rectum, and anus).

Suspected problems in the upper gastrointestinal tract usually are investigated first by inserting a tube through the nose and into the stomach and withdrawing fluid. Stomach fluid that resembles coffee grounds is created by the partial digestion of blood, indicating that bleeding is slow or has stopped. Continuous bright red blood indicates active, vigorous bleeding. Next, a doctor often uses a flexible endoscope (a viewing tube)▲ to examine the esophagus, stomach, and duodenum and find the source of the bleeding. If no gastritis or ulcer is found in the stomach or duodenum, a doctor may perform a biopsy (obtain a specimen for microscopic examination). A biopsy can determine if the bleeding results from an infection with *Helicobacter pylori*. Such an infection is treated and usually cured by antibiotic therapy.

A doctor looks for polyps and cancers in the lower gastrointestinal tract using x-rays after a barium enema■ has been administered or using an endoscope. A doctor may view the inside of the lower intestine directly with an anoscope, a flexible sigmoidoscope, or a colonoscope.

If these investigations don't reveal the source of bleeding, angiography (x-rays taken after an injection of a radiopaque substance) or scans taken after an injection of radioactive red blood cells may be used. These techniques are especially useful in revealing whether the cause of bleeding is a blood vessel malformation.

Treatment

In more than 80 percent of people with gastrointestinal bleeding, the body's defenses stop the bleeding. People who continue bleeding or who have symptoms of significant blood loss often are hospitalized and usually are admitted to an intensive care unit.

If a large amount of blood has been lost, a transfusion may be needed. Packed red blood cells may be used instead of whole blood to avoid overloading the blood circulation with fluid. After the blood volume has been restored, the person is observed closely for evidence of continued bleeding, such as an increased pulse rate, a drop in blood pressure, or a loss of blood from the mouth or anus.

Bleeding from varicose veins in the lower esophagus (esophageal varices) can be treated in several ways. One way involves inserting a catheter with a balloon through the mouth into the esophagus and inflating the balloon to press on the bleeding area. Another way is to inject the bleeding vessel with an irritating chemical that causes inflammation and scarring of the veins.

Bleeding in the stomach often can be stopped by procedures performed with an endoscope; these involve cauterizing the bleeding vessel with an electric current or injecting a material that causes clotting within blood vessels. If these procedures fail, surgery may be needed.

Bleeding of the lower intestine usually doesn't require emergency treatment. However, if necessary, an endoscopic procedure or abdominal surgery is performed. Sometimes, the bleeding can't be located precisely, so a segment of the intestine may be removed.

Bleeding Arteriovenous Malformations

Bleeding arteriovenous malformations are ruptures in abnormal blood vessels that connect arteries and veins.

Why arteriovenous malformations occur in the lining of the stomach and intestine is unknown. However, they're more common in people with disorders of the heart valves, kidneys, or liver; in people with connective tissue disease; and in people who have had radiation therapy of the intestine. These abnormal blood vessels range in diameter from the width of heavy fishing line to the width of a person's little finger. They're fragile and liable to bleed, sometimes heavily, especially in older people.

Symptoms and Diagnosis

Bleeding arteriovenous malformations of the stomach and intestine usually cause vomiting of blood or passing of black tarry stools. If the bleed-

▲ see page 485

■ see page 486

When Abdominal Pain Requires Surgery

Organ in Which Pain Originates	Conditions Requiring Immediate Surgery	Conditions Not Requiring Immediate Surgery
Esophagus	Perforation or rupture	Reflux of acid and esophagitis
Stomach	Perforated or bleeding ulcer, stomach cancer	Ulcer, gastritis, hiatal hernia
Small intestine	Perforated ulcer, obstruction	Uncomplicated ulcer, gastroenteritis, Crohn's disease
Appendix	Appendicitis	—
Large intestine and rectum	Diverticulitis with perforation or obstruction, cancer, obstructing polyp, ulcerative colitis, Crohn's disease (severe)	Crohn's disease (mild), uncomplicated diverticulitis
Liver	Cancer, abscess	Bruising, cyst
Biliary system	Gallstones with gallbladder inflammation or obstruction	Gallstones without inflammation or obstruction
Spleen	Rupture, abscess	—
Pancreas	Pancreatitis (severe)	Pancreatitis (mild)
Blood vessels	Bulging of an artery (aneurysm), blockage	—
Kidney	Stones	Infection
Bladder	Stones, cancer	Infection
Male genitals	Twisting of testicles	Infection of prostate or testicles
Female genitals	Ectopic pregnancy, abscess of ovary	Pelvic inflammatory disease
Peritoneum (lining of the abdominal cavity)	Peritonitis from perforation	Peritonitis from tuberculosis

ing is massive or prolonged, the person may develop anemia and other symptoms of blood loss. Episodes of bleeding usually start without warning and tend to recur.

The diagnosis usually is made by using an endoscope. However, arteriovenous malformations may be difficult to detect, especially when low blood volume or low output from the heart causes the blood vessels to partially collapse.

Treatment

Treatment of an underlying condition (for example, heart valve surgery or a kidney transplant) may eliminate the gastrointestinal bleeding. A doctor may be able to seal off the bleeding by cauterizing the blood vessel, using an endoscope, but new malformations can develop. The anemia caused by the loss of blood can be corrected with iron supplements.

Abdominal Pain

Abdominal pain can be caused by problems along the digestive tract or elsewhere in the abdomen. Such problems include a ruptured esophagus, a perforated ulcer, irritable bowel syndrome, appendicitis, pancreatitis, and gallstones. Some of these disorders are relatively minor; others may be life threatening. A doctor has to decide whether immediate treatment is needed or whether it can wait until diagnostic test results are available.

Diagnosis and Treatment

The nature of the pain and its timing in relation to eating or moving about may provide a doctor with clues to the diagnosis. If other family members have had an abdominal disorder, such as gallstones, the patient may have the same disorder.

The person's appearance can be an important clue. For instance, jaundice (apparent from a yellow tinge to the skin and whites of the eyes) suggests a disease of the liver, gallbladder, or bile ducts.

A doctor examines the abdomen, feeling for tenderness and any abnormal masses. When the wall of the abdomen is gently pressed, the person feels pain, and if the pressure is suddenly released, the pain may suddenly feel worse—a symptom called rebound tenderness. This symptom usually indicates inflammation of the lining of the abdominal cavity (peritonitis).

Diagnostic tests for abdominal pain include blood and urine analysis, x-rays, ultrasound scans, and computed tomography (CT).▲ Emergency exploratory surgery of the abdomen is often performed when the abdominal pain seems to result from an intestinal obstruction; a perforated or ruptured organ, such as the gallbladder, appendix, or intestine; or an abscess (an accumulation of pus).

Mechanical Obstruction of the Intestine

A mechanical obstruction of the intestine is a blockage that completely stops or seriously impairs the passage of intestinal contents.

An obstruction may occur anywhere along the intestine. The part of the intestine above the obstruction continues to function. As it fills with food, fluid, digestive secretions, and gas, it swells like a soft hose.

In newborns and infants, intestinal obstruction is commonly caused by a birth defect,■ a hard mass of intestinal contents (meconium), or a twisting of the intestine on itself (volvulus).

In adults, an obstruction of the duodenum may be caused by cancer of the pancreas; scarring from an ulcer, a previous operation, or Crohn's disease; or adhesions, in which a fibrous band of connective tissue traps the intestine. An obstruction also occurs when part of the intestine bulges through an abnormal opening (hernia), such as a weakness in the muscles of the abdomen, and becomes trapped. Rarely, a gallstone, a mass of undigested food, or a collection of worms may block the intestine.

In the large intestine, cancer is a common cause of obstruction. A twisted loop of intestine or a hard lump of feces (fecal impaction) also may cause a blockage.

If an obstruction cuts off the blood supply to the intestine, the condition is called strangulation. Strangulation occurs in nearly 25 percent of the cases of small-intestine obstruction. Usually strangulation results from the trapping of part of the intestine in an abnormal opening (strangulated hernia); the twisting of a loop of intestine (volvulus); or the telescoping of a loop of intestine into another loop (intussusception). Gangrene can develop in as little as 6 hours. With gangrene, the intestinal wall dies, usually causing perforation, which leads to inflammation of the lining of the abdominal cavity (peritonitis) and infection. Without treatment, the person may die.

Even without strangulation, the section of the intestine above the blockage enlarges. The intestinal lining becomes swollen and inflamed. If the condition isn't treated, the intestine can perforate, leaking its contents and causing inflammation and infection of the abdominal cavity.

Symptoms and Diagnosis

The symptoms of intestinal obstruction include cramping pain in the abdomen, accompanied by

▲ see page 484

■ see page 1231

What Causes Intestinal Strangulation

Strangulation (obstruction of the blood supply to the intestine) usually results from one of the three causes shown.

Strangulated Hernia	Volvulus	Intussusception

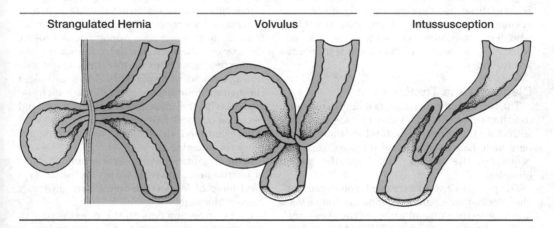

bloating. The pain may become severe and steady. Vomiting, which is common, begins later with large-intestinal obstruction than with small-intestinal obstruction. Complete obstruction causes severe constipation, while partial obstruction may cause diarrhea. A fever is common and is particularly likely if the intestinal wall is perforated. Perforation can rapidly lead to severe inflammation and infection, causing shock.

A doctor examines the abdomen for tenderness and abnormal swelling or masses. The normal sounds made by a functioning intestine (bowel sounds), which can be heard through a stethoscope, may be very loud and high pitched, or they may be absent. If perforation has caused peritonitis, the person will feel pain when the doctor presses on the abdomen; the pain increases when the doctor suddenly releases the pressure—a symptom called rebound tenderness.

X-rays may show dilated loops of intestine that indicate the location of the obstruction. The x-rays also may reveal air around the intestine in the abdomen, a sign of perforation.

Treatment

Anyone who may have an intestinal obstruction is hospitalized. Usually, a long, thin tube is passed through the nose and placed in the stomach or intestine. Suction is applied to the tube to remove the material that has accumulated above the blockage. Fluid and electrolytes (sodium and potassium) are given intravenously to replace water and salts lost from vomiting or diarrhea.

Sometimes an obstruction resolves itself without further treatment, especially if it results from adhesions. An endoscope advanced through the anus or a barium enema, which inflates the intestine, may be used to treat a few disorders, such as a twisted intestinal segment in the lower part of the large intestine. Most often, however, surgery is performed as soon as possible. During surgery, the blocked segment of intestine may be removed and the remaining parts joined.

Ileus

Ileus (paralytic ileus, adynamic ileus) is a condition in which the normal contractile movements of the intestinal wall temporarily stop.

Like a mechanical obstruction, ileus prevents the passage of intestinal contents. Unlike a mechanical obstruction, though, ileus rarely leads to perforation.

Ileus may be caused by an infection or a blood clot inside the abdomen, atherosclerosis that reduces the blood supply to the intestine, or an injury to an intestinal artery or vein. Ileus also may be caused by disorders outside the intestine, such as kidney failure or abnormal levels of blood electrolytes—low potassium or high calcium levels, for example. Other causes of ileus are certain drugs and an underactive thyroid gland. Ileus is common for 24 to 72 hours after abdominal surgery.

Symptoms and Diagnosis

The symptoms of ileus are abdominal bloating, vomiting, severe constipation, and cramps. A doctor hears few bowel sounds or none at all through a stethoscope. An x-ray of the abdomen shows bulging loops of intestine. Occasionally, a colonoscopy (an examination of the colon using a viewing tube)▲ is performed to evaluate the situation.

Treatment

The buildup of gas and liquid caused by ileus must be relieved. Sometimes a tube is passed into the large intestine through the anus to relieve the pressure. In addition, a tube is passed through the nose into the stomach or small intestine, and suction is applied to relieve pressure and distention. The person may not eat or drink anything until the crisis is over. Fluids and electrolytes are given intravenously.

Appendicitis

Appendicitis is inflammation of the appendix.

The appendix is a small, finger-shaped tube projecting from the large intestine near the point where it joins the small intestine. The appendix may have some immune function, but it isn't an essential organ.

Except for trapped hernias, appendicitis is the most common cause of sudden, severe abdominal pain and abdominal surgery in the United States. Appendicitis is most common between the ages of 10 and 30.

The cause of appendicitis isn't fully understood. In most cases, a blockage inside the appendix probably starts a process in which the appendix becomes inflamed and infected. If inflammation continues without treatment, the appendix can rupture. A ruptured appendix spills bacteria-laden intestinal contents into the abdomen, causing peritonitis, which may result in a life-threatening infection. A rupture also may cause an abscess to form. In a woman, the ovaries and fallopian tubes may become infected, and the resulting blockage of the tubes may cause infertility. A ruptured appendix also may allow bacteria to infect the bloodstream—a life-threatening condition called septicemia.

Symptoms

Less than half of the people with appendicitis have the combination of characteristic symptoms: nausea, vomiting, and excruciating pain in the lower right abdomen. Pain may begin suddenly in the upper abdomen or around the navel; then nausea and vomiting develop. After a few hours, the nausea passes, and the pain shifts to the right lower portion of the abdomen. When a doctor presses on this area, it's tender, and when the pressure is released, the pain may increase sharply—a symptom called rebound tenderness. A fever of 100° to 101° F. is common.

Pain, particularly in infants and children, may be general rather than confined to the right lower portion of the abdomen. In older people and in pregnant women, the pain is usually less severe, and the area is less tender.

If the appendix is ruptured, pain and fever may become severe. Worsening infection can lead to shock.

Diagnosis and Treatment

A blood test shows a moderate increase in the white blood cell count in response to the infection. Usually, in the early stages of appendicitis, most tests—including x-rays, ultrasound scanning, and computed tomography (CT)—are essentially useless.

Typically, a doctor bases the diagnosis on the physical examination findings. To avoid a rupture of the appendix, abscess formation, or inflammation of the lining of the abdominal cavity (peritonitis), a doctor performs surgery immediately.

In nearly 15 percent of the operations for appendicitis, the appendix is found to be normal. However, delaying surgery until a doctor is certain of the cause of the abdominal pain can be fatal: An infected appendix can rupture less than

▲ see page 485

24 hours after symptoms begin. Even when appendicitis isn't the cause, the appendix is usually removed. Then the surgeon examines the abdomen and tries to determine the true cause of the pain.

With an early operation, the chance of death from appendicitis is very low. The person can usually leave the hospital in 2 or 3 days, and convalescence is normally quick and complete.

For a ruptured appendix, the prognosis is more serious. Fifty years ago, a rupture often was fatal. Antibiotics have lowered the death rate to nearly zero, but repeated operations and a long convalescence may be necessary.

Peritonitis

Peritonitis is inflammation usually caused by an infection of the lining of the abdominal cavity (peritoneum).

The peritoneum is a thin, clear membrane that normally covers all abdominal organs and the inside walls of the abdomen. Peritonitis is usually caused by an infection spreading from an infected organ in the abdomen. Common sources are perforations of the stomach, intestine, gallbladder, or appendix. The peritoneum is remarkably resistant to infection. Unless contamination continues, peritonitis doesn't develop, and the peritoneum tends to heal with treatment.

Pelvic inflammatory disease in sexually active women is a common cause of peritonitis. An infection of the uterus and fallopian tubes—which may be caused by several types of bacteria, including the ones that cause gonorrhea and chlamydial infection—spreads into the abdominal cavity. In liver or heart failure, fluid may accumulate in the abdomen (ascites) and become infected.

Peritonitis can develop after surgery for several reasons. An injury to the gallbladder, ureter, bladder, or intestine during an operation can spill bacteria into the abdomen. Leakage also can occur during operations in which intestinal segments are joined.

Peritoneal dialysis (a treatment for kidney failure)▲ frequently results in peritonitis. The usual cause is an infection gaining access through the drains placed in the abdomen.

Peritonitis can also result from irritation without any infection. For example, inflammation of the pancreas (acute pancreatitis) can produce peritonitis. Also, talc or starch on a surgeon's gloves can cause peritonitis without infection.

Symptoms

The symptoms of peritonitis depend in part on the type and extent of the infection. Usually, the person vomits, has a high fever, and has a tender abdomen. One or more abscesses may form, and the infection can leave scarring in the form of bands of tissue (adhesions) that eventually may obstruct the intestine.

Unless peritonitis is treated promptly, complications develop rapidly. Peristalsis disappears, and fluid is retained in the small intestine and large intestine. Fluid also exudes from the bloodstream into the peritoneal cavity. Severe dehydration develops, and the bloodstream loses electrolytes. Major complications—such as lung, kidney, or liver failure and widespread clotting—follow.

Diagnosis

Rapid diagnosis is crucial. X-rays are taken with the patient lying down and standing. Free gas in the abdomen can be seen on x-rays and indicates a perforation. Occasionally, a needle is used to withdraw fluid from the abdominal cavity so that laboratory personnel can identify the infectious organism and test its sensitivity to various antibiotics. However, exploratory surgery is the most reliable means of diagnosis.

Treatment

Usually, the first measure is emergency exploratory surgery, particularly when appendicitis, a perforated peptic ulcer, or diverticulitis seems likely. For an episode of inflammation of the pancreas (acute pancreatitis) or pelvic inflammatory disease in women, emergency surgery usually isn't performed.

Antibiotics, often several at once, are given promptly. Also, a tube may be inserted through the nose and into the stomach or intestine to drain fluid and gas. Fluids and electrolytes may also be given intravenously to replace those that have been lost.

▲ see page 599

Cancer and Other Growths of the Digestive System

A wide variety of growths (tumors) can develop throughout the digestive (gastrointestinal) tract from the esophagus to the rectum. Some of these growths are cancerous (malignant), others are noncancerous (benign).

Esophagus

The most common noncancerous tumor of the esophagus is a leiomyoma, a tumor of the smooth muscle. The prognosis for most people with leiomyomas is excellent.

The most common esophageal cancer is carcinoma, either squamous cell carcinoma (also called epidermoid carcinoma) or adenocarcinoma. Other types of esophageal cancer include lymphoma (a cancer of lymphocytes), leiomyosarcoma (a cancer of the smooth muscle of the esophagus), and cancer that has spread (metastasized) from elsewhere in the body.

Cancer may occur anywhere in the esophagus. It may appear as a narrowing of the esophagus, a lump, or an abnormal flat area (plaque). Esophageal cancer is more common in people whose esophagus has narrowed because they once swallowed a strong alkali, such as lye used for cleaning. Esophageal cancer also is more common in those who have achalasia (a condition in which the lower esophageal sphincter fails to open properly),▲ esophageal blockages such as an esophageal web,■ or cancer of the head and neck. Smoking and alcohol abuse also increase the risk of esophageal cancer; in fact, they're the most important risk factors for squamous cell carcinoma. Changes in the lining of the esophagus appear to be a forerunner of cancer in some people. These changes take place after prolonged irritation of the esophagus from acid or bile backflow (reflux).

Symptoms and Diagnosis

Because cancer of the esophagus tends to obstruct the passage of food, the first symptom is usually difficulty in swallowing solids. Over several weeks, the problem progresses, and the person has difficulty swallowing soft foods and then liquids. The result is a marked weight loss.

Cancer of the esophagus is diagnosed by an x-ray procedure called a barium swallow.★ The person swallows a solution of barium that is radiopaque and therefore shows up on x-rays of the esophagus, outlining the obstruction. The abnormal area also should be examined with an endoscope (a flexible viewing tube).● An endoscope allows a doctor to collect a tissue specimen for microscopic examination (biopsy) and loose cells for microscopic examination (brush cytology).

Treatment and Prognosis

Fewer than 5 percent of people with cancer of the esophagus survive more than 5 years. Many die within a year of noticing the first symptoms.

Chemotherapy doesn't cure esophageal cancer, but when used either alone or with radiation therapy, it may reduce symptoms and prolong life. Surgery to remove the tumor, when it's possible, relieves symptoms for a time but seldom cures. Other measures that relieve symptoms include dilation of the narrowed area of the esophagus, insertion of a tube to keep the esophagus open, a bypass of the tumor using a loop of intestine, and laser therapy to destroy the cancer tissue obstructing the esophagus.

Stomach

Noncancerous tumors of the stomach are unlikely to cause symptoms or medical problems. Occasionally, however, some bleed or become cancerous.

About 99 percent of stomach cancers are adenocarcinomas. Other stomach cancers are leio-

---

▲ see page 490

■ see page 488

★ see page 484

● see page 485

myosarcomas (cancers of the smooth muscle) and lymphomas.

Stomach cancer is more common in older people. Less than 25 percent of such cancer occurs in people under age 50. Stomach cancer is extremely common in Japan, China, Chile, and Iceland. In the United States, it's more common in poor people, blacks, and people who live in the north. It's the seventh most common cause of death from cancer in the United States, occurring in about 8 of every 100,000 people. For unknown reasons, stomach cancer is becoming less common in the United States.

Causes

Stomach cancer often begins at a site where the stomach lining is inflamed. However, many experts believe that such inflammation is the result of stomach cancer rather than the cause of it. Some experts suggest that stomach ulcers can lead to cancer, but most people with ulcers and stomach cancer probably had an undetected cancer before the ulcers developed. *Helicobacter pylori*, the bacterium that plays a role in producing duodenal ulcers, also may play a role in some stomach cancers.

Stomach polyps, uncommon noncancerous round growths that project into the stomach cavity, are thought to be forerunners of cancer and therefore are removed. Cancer is particularly likely with certain types of polyp, a polyp larger than $^3/_4$ inch, or several polyps.

Certain dietary factors are thought to play a role in the development of stomach cancer. These factors include a high intake of salt, a high intake of carbohydrates, a high intake of preservatives called nitrates, and a low intake of green leafy vegetables and fruit. However, none of these factors have been proved to cause cancer.

Symptoms

In the early stages of stomach cancer, symptoms are vague and easily ignored. When symptoms do develop, they may help indicate where in the stomach the cancer is located. For instance, a feeling of fullness or discomfort after a meal may indicate cancer in the lower part of the stomach.

Weight loss or weakness usually results from difficulty in eating or from an inability to absorb some vitamins and minerals. Anemia may result from very gradual bleeding that causes no other symptoms. Uncommonly, a person may vomit large amounts of blood (hematemesis) or pass black tarry stools (melena). When stomach cancer is advanced, a doctor may be able to feel a mass through the abdominal wall.

Even in the early stages, a small stomach tumor may spread (metastasize) to distant sites. The spread of the tumor may cause liver enlargement, jaundice, fluid accumulation in the abdomen (ascites), and cancerous skin nodules. The spreading cancer also may weaken bone, leading to bone fractures.

Diagnosis

The symptoms of stomach cancer may be confused with those of a peptic ulcer.▲ If symptoms don't clear up after a person takes ulcer drugs or if the symptoms include weight loss, doctors suspect stomach cancer.

X-ray studies that use barium to outline changes in the surface of the stomach often are performed, but they rarely reveal small, early stomach cancers. Endoscopy (an examination using a flexible viewing tube) is the best diagnostic procedure because it allows a doctor to view the stomach directly; to check for *Helicobacter pylori*, the bacterium that may play a role in stomach cancer; and to obtain tissue samples for examination under a microscope.■

Treatment and Prognosis

Noncancerous stomach polyps are removed using endoscopy.

If carcinoma is confined to the stomach, surgery is usually performed to try to cure it. Most or all of the stomach and nearby lymph nodes are removed. The prognosis is good if the cancer hasn't penetrated the stomach wall too deeply. In the United States, the results of surgery are often poor because most people have extensive cancer by the time a diagnosis is made. In Japan, where cancers are detected earlier by mass screening using endoscopy, the results of surgery are better.

If carcinoma has spread beyond the stomach, the goal of treatment is to ease the symptoms and prolong life. Chemotherapy and radiation therapy may relieve symptoms. Sometimes surgery is used to relieve symptoms. For instance, if the passage of food is obstructed at the far end of the

▲ see page 496

■ see page 485

stomach, a bypass operation may relieve the symptoms. A connection is made between the stomach and the small intestine that allows food to pass. This connection relieves the symptoms of obstruction—pain and vomiting—at least for a while.

The results of chemotherapy and radiation therapy are better for gastric lymphomas than for carcinomas. Longer survival and even cure are possible.

Small Intestine

Most tumors of the small intestine are noncancerous. The less common cancerous tumors include carcinomas, lymphomas, and carcinoid tumors.

NONCANCEROUS TUMORS

Noncancerous tumors of the small intestine include abnormal growths of fat cells (lipomas), nerve cells (neurofibromas), connective tissue cells (fibromas), and muscle cells (leiomyomas). Most noncancerous tumors don't cause symptoms. However, larger ones may cause blood in the stool, a partial or complete intestinal obstruction, or intestinal strangulation if one part of the intestine telescopes into an adjacent part (a condition called intussusception).▲

When symptoms seem to indicate a tumor at the beginning or end of the small intestine, a doctor may use an endoscope (a flexible viewing tube) to observe the tumor and obtain a specimen for microscopic examination. A barium x-ray■ can show the entire small intestine and may be used to outline the tumor. Arteriography (an x-ray taken after a dye is injected into an artery) may be performed on an artery of the intestine, especially if the tumor is bleeding. Similarly, radioactive technetium can be injected into the artery and observed on x-rays as it leaks into the intestine; this procedure helps locate sites where the tumor is bleeding. The bleeding can then be corrected surgically.

Small growths may be destroyed through the endoscope by electrocautery, heat obliteration, or laser phototherapy. For large growths, surgery may be needed.

CANCEROUS TUMORS

Carcinoma in the small intestine is uncommon. However, people with Crohn's disease of the small intestine are more likely than others to develop

---

Kaposi's Sarcoma

An aggressive form of Kaposi's sarcoma occurs mainly in parts of Africa and in transplant recipients and people with AIDS. It may start anywhere in the intestine, but it usually begins in the stomach, small intestine, or far end of the large intestine. Although it usually causes no symptoms, a person may have protein and blood in the stool and diarrhea. A part of the intestine may telescope into an adjacent part (a condition called intussusception), which tends to obstruct the intestine and cut off its blood supply, creating an emergency. Kaposi's sarcoma also can appear as red-purple spots on the skin.

A doctor may suspect Kaposi's sarcoma when symptoms develop in a person who falls into one of the high-risk groups. Exploratory surgery is needed to confirm the diagnosis of Kaposi's sarcoma affecting the intestine.

Treatment is surgical removal of the sarcoma. If intussusception occurs, emergency surgery is necessary.

---

it. Lymphoma, a cancer that appears in the lymph system, may develop in the middle section of the small intestine (jejunum) or the lower section of the small intestine (ileum). Lymphoma may cause a segment of intestine to become rigid or elongated. This cancer is more common in people with celiac disease. The small intestine, particularly the ileum, is the second most common site (after the appendix) for carcinoid tumors.

The tumors may produce obstruction and bleeding into the intestine, which may cause symptoms such as blood in the stool, crampy abdominal pain, distention of the abdomen, and vomiting. Carcinoid tumors may secrete hormones that cause diarrhea and flushing of the skin.

A diagnosis of cancer of the small intestine is made by barium x-ray, endoscopy, or exploratory surgery. The best treatment is surgical removal of the tumor.

▲ see page 545

■ see page 486

Large Intestine and Rectum

Polyps in the large intestine and rectum are growths that usually are noncancerous. However, because some are precancerous, doctors generally recommend removing all polyps from the large intestine and rectum.

Cancer of the large intestine and rectum are common in Western countries.

POLYPS

A polyp is a growth of tissue from the intestinal wall that protrudes into the intestine and is usually noncancerous.

Polyps may grow with or without stalks and vary considerably in size. Most commonly, polyps develop in the rectum and lower part of the large intestine. They're less common higher up in the large intestine.

About 25 percent of the people with cancer of the large intestine also have polyps elsewhere in the large intestine. Strong evidence suggests that adenomatous polyps are likely to become cancerous if allowed to remain in the large intestine. The bigger the polyp, the greater the risk that it's cancerous.

Symptoms and Diagnosis

Most polyps don't cause symptoms, but the most common symptom is bleeding from the rectum. A large polyp may cause cramps, abdominal pain, or intestinal obstruction. Rarely, a polyp on a long stalk will drop down through the anus. Large polyps with fingerlike projections (villous adenomas) may excrete water and salts, causing profuse watery diarrhea that may result in low levels of potassium in the blood (hypokalemia). This type of polyp is more likely to be cancerous or to become cancerous.

A doctor may be able to feel polyps in the rectum with a gloved finger, but usually they're discovered during routine sigmoidoscopy (an examination of the rectum and lower part of the large intestine using a flexible viewing tube). When sigmoidoscopy reveals a polyp, colonoscopy (an examination of the large intestine using a flexible viewing tube)▲ is performed on the entire large intestine. This more complete and reliable examination is done because a person often

---

▲ see page 485

has more than one polyp and because one or more polyps may be cancerous. Colonoscopy also allows a doctor to take a biopsy specimen from any area that appears cancerous.

Treatment

First, the person is given laxatives and enemas to empty the intestine. Then the polyps are removed during colonoscopy using a cutting instrument or an electrified wire loop. If a polyp has no stalk or can't be removed during colonoscopy, abdominal surgery may be needed.

A pathologist examines polyps that have been removed. If a polyp is found to be cancerous, treatment depends on certain factors. For instance, the risk of the cancer spreading is higher when it has invaded the polyp's stalk or is nearer the cut end. The risk also may be considered high based on the pathologist's assessment of the polyp's microscopic appearance. If the risk is low, no further treatment is necessary. If the risk is high, the affected segment of the large intestine is removed surgically, and the cut ends of the intestine are rejoined.

When a person has a polyp removed, the entire large intestine is examined by colonoscopy a year later and then at intervals determined by the doctor. If such an examination is impossible because of a narrowing of the large intestine, a barium enema may be used. Any new polyps are removed.

FAMILIAL POLYPOSIS

Familial polyposis is a hereditary condition in which 100 or more precancerous, adenomatous polyps develop, carpeting the large intestine and rectum.

The polyps develop during childhood or adolescence. In nearly all untreated people, cancer of the large intestine (colon cancer) develops before age 40. Complete removal of the large intestine and rectum eliminates the risk of cancer. However, if the large intestine is removed and the rectum is joined to the small intestine, sometimes the rectal polyps disappear. Thus, many experts prefer the latter procedure. The remaining part of the rectum is inspected by sigmoidoscopy (an examination using a flexible viewing tube) every 3 to 6 months, so that new polyps can be removed. If new polyps appear too rapidly, the rectum must be removed, and the small intestine must empty through an opening in the abdominal wall. The surgically created connection between the small intestine and the abdominal wall is called an ileostomy.

Gardner's syndrome is a type of hereditary polyposis in which various types of noncancerous tumors occur elsewhere in the body as well as in the intestine. Like other types of familial polyposis, it carries a high risk of colon cancer.

Peutz-Jeghers syndrome is a hereditary condition in which many small lumps called juvenile polyps appear in the stomach, small intestine, and large intestine. People are born with these polyps, or they may develop during early childhood. People with the syndrome have brown skin and mucous membranes, especially of the lips and gums. The polyps don't increase the risk of cancer in the intestinal tract. However, people with Peutz-Jeghers syndrome are at increased risk for cancer of the pancreas, breast, lung, ovary, and uterus.

COLORECTAL CANCER

In Western countries, cancer of the large intestine and rectum (colorectal cancer) is the second most common type of cancer and the second leading cause of cancer death. The incidence of colorectal cancer begins to rise at age 40 and peaks between ages 60 and 75. Cancer of the large intestine (colon cancer) is more common in women; rectal cancer is more common in men. About 5 percent of the people with colon or rectal cancer have more than one cancer of the colorectum at the same time.

People with a family history of colon cancer have a higher risk of developing the cancer themselves. A family history of familial polyposis or a similar disease also increases the risk of colon cancer. People with ulcerative colitis or Crohn's disease have a higher risk of developing cancer. The risk is related to the person's age when the condition developed and the length of time the person has had the condition.

Diet plays some role in the risk of colon cancer, but exactly how it affects risk is unknown. Throughout the world, people at highest risk tend to live in cities and eat a diet typical of affluent Westerners. Such a diet is low in fiber and high in animal protein, fats, and refined carbohydrates such as sugar. Risk seems to be reduced by a diet high in calcium, vitamin D, and vegetables such as brussels sprouts, cabbage, and broccoli. Taking an aspirin every other day also seems to reduce the risk of colon cancer, but this measure

can't be recommended until more information is available.

Colon cancer usually begins as a buttonlike swelling on the surface of the intestinal lining or on a polyp. As the cancer grows, it begins to invade the intestinal wall. Nearby lymph nodes also may be invaded. Because blood from the intestinal wall is carried to the liver, colon cancer usually spreads (metastasizes) to the liver soon after spreading to nearby lymph nodes.

Symptoms and Diagnosis

Colorectal cancer grows slowly and takes a long time before it's extensive enough to cause symptoms. Symptoms depend on the type, location, and extent of the cancer. The right (ascending) colon has a large diameter and a thin wall. Because its contents are liquid, it doesn't become obstructed until late in the course of the cancer. A tumor in the ascending colon may enlarge so much that a doctor can feel it through the abdominal wall. Yet fatigue and weakness from severe anemia may be the person's only symptoms. The left (descending) colon has a smaller diameter and a thicker wall, and the feces are semisolid. Cancer tends to encircle this part of the colon, causing alternating constipation and frequent bowel movements. Because the descending colon is narrower and its wall thicker, the cancer is more likely to cause an obstruction earlier. The person may seek medical treatment because of crampy abdominal pain or severe abdominal pain and constipation. The feces may be streaked or mixed with blood, but often the blood can't be seen; a laboratory test is needed to detect it.

Most cancers bleed, usually slowly. In rectal cancer, the most common first symptom is bleeding during a bowel movement. Whenever the rectum bleeds, even if the person is known to have hemorrhoids or diverticular disease, doctors consider cancer. With rectal cancer, the person may have painful bowel movements and a feeling that the rectum hasn't been completely emptied. Sitting may be painful. However, the person usually feels no pain from the cancer itself unless it spreads to tissue outside the rectum.

As with other cancers, regular screening tests aid in the early detection of colorectal cancer. The stool can be tested for microscopic amounts of blood simply and inexpensively. To help ensure accurate test results, the person eats a high-fiber diet free of red meat for 3 days before providing

Spread of Cancer and Survival Rates

Spread of Cancer	5-Year Survival Rate
Cancer in intestinal lining (mucosa) only	90%
Cancer penetrating muscle layer of intestine	80%
Cancer spread to lymph nodes	30%

a stool sample. If this screening test indicates the possibility of cancer, further testing is required.

Before endoscopy, the intestine is emptied, often by using strong laxatives and several enemas. About 65 percent of colorectal cancers can be seen with a flexible, fiber-optic sigmoidoscope. If a polyp that may be cancerous is seen, the entire large intestine is examined with a colonoscope, which has a longer reach. Some growths that appear cancerous are removed using surgical instruments passed through the colonoscope; others must be removed during regular surgery.

Blood tests can be helpful in making the diagnosis. Levels of carcinoembryonic antigen in the blood are high in 70 percent of the people with colorectal cancer. If carcinoembryonic antigen levels are high before an operation to remove cancer, they may be low after it. If so, they can be measured at subsequent checkups. A rise in the level suggests that the cancer has recurred. Two other antigens, CA 19-9 and CA 125, are similar to carcinoembryonic antigen and may also be measured.

Treatment and Prognosis

The main treatment for colorectal cancer is surgical removal of a large segment of the affected intestine and the associated lymph nodes. About 70 percent of the people with colorectal cancer are good candidates for surgery. In the 30 percent who can't tolerate an operation because of poor health, some tumors can be removed by electro-coagulation. This procedure may relieve symptoms and prolong life, but cure is unlikely.

In most cases of colon cancer, the cancerous segment of the intestine is removed surgically, and the remaining ends are joined. For rectal cancer, the type of operation depends on how far the cancer is from the anus and how deeply it has grown into the rectal wall. The complete removal of the rectum and anus leaves the person with a permanent colostomy (a surgically created opening between the large intestine and the abdominal wall). With a colostomy, the contents of the large intestine empty through the abdominal wall into a bag, called a colostomy bag. If possible, only part of the rectum is removed, leaving a rectal stump and the anus intact. Then the rectal stump is rejoined to the end of the large intestine. Radiation therapy after surgical removal of visible rectal cancer may help control the growth of any residual tumors, delay a recurrence, and increase the chances of survival. People who have rectal cancer and one to four cancerous lymph nodes derive the most benefit from combined radiation and chemotherapy. In people with more than four cancerous lymph nodes, this treatment is less effective.

When colorectal cancer has spread and isn't likely to be cured by surgery alone, chemotherapy with fluorouracil and levamisole after surgery may prolong the person's life, but cure is still rare. When colorectal cancer has spread so much that all of it can't be removed, surgery to relieve the intestinal obstruction may ease symptoms. However, survival time is typically only about 7 months. When the cancer has spread only to the liver, chemotherapy drugs can be injected directly into the artery supplying the liver. A small pump inserted surgically beneath the skin or an external pump worn on a belt allows the person to be mobile during the treatment. Though expensive, this treatment may provide more benefit than ordinary chemotherapy; however, more research is needed. When cancer has spread beyond the liver, this approach has no advantage.

After colorectal cancer has been totally removed by surgery, most experts recommend two to five annual examinations of the remaining intestine, using colonoscopy. If these examinations don't detect any cancer, the person usually continues with follow-up examinations every 2 to 3 years thereafter.

Liver and Gallbladder Disorders

CHAPTER 114

Biology of the Liver and Gallbladder

Located in the upper right portion of the abdomen, the liver and gallbladder are connected by ducts known as the biliary tract. But despite this connection and the fact that the liver and the gallbladder participate in some of the same functions, they are very different. The wedge-shaped liver is the body's chemical factory. It is a complex organ that performs many vital functions, from regulating the levels of chemicals in the body to producing substances that make the blood clot during bleeding. The pear-shaped gallbladder, on the other hand, is simply a small storage tank for bile, a digestive fluid produced by the liver.

Liver

The liver is the largest—and in some ways the most complex—organ in the body. One of its major functions is to break down harmful substances absorbed from the intestine or manufactured elsewhere in the body, then excrete them as harmless by-products into the bile or the blood. By-products in the bile enter the intestine, then leave the body in the feces. By-products in the blood are filtered out by the kidneys, then leave the body in the urine.

View of the Liver and Gallbladder

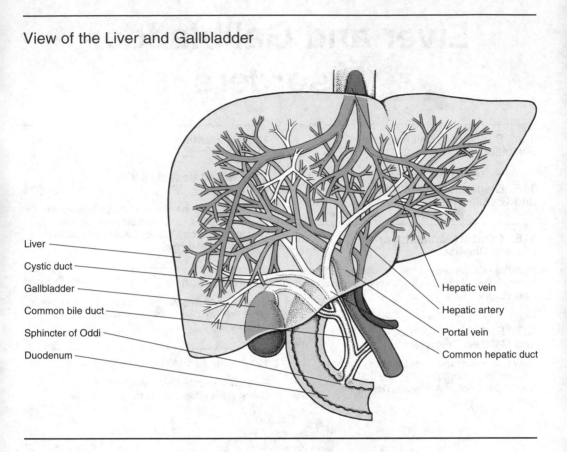

Liver

Cystic duct

Gallbladder

Common bile duct

Sphincter of Oddi

Duodenum

Hepatic vein

Hepatic artery

Portal vein

Common hepatic duct

The liver manufactures about half of the body's cholesterol; the rest comes from food. About 80 percent of the cholesterol made by the liver is used to make bile. Cholesterol is a vital part of every cell membrane and is needed to make certain hormones, including estrogen, testosterone, and the adrenal hormones.

The liver also converts substances in digested food into proteins, fats, and carbohydrates. Sugars are stored in the liver as glycogen and then broken down and released into the bloodstream as glucose when needed—for example, when blood sugar levels become too low.

Another function of the liver is to create (synthesize) many important compounds, especially proteins, that the body uses to carry out its functions. Among these are substances needed for the blood to clot when bleeding occurs. These substances are known as clotting factors.

The liver receives blood from both the intestine and the heart. Tiny capillaries in the intestinal wall drain into the portal vein, which enters the liver. The blood then flows through a latticework of tiny channels inside the liver, where digested nutrients and any harmful substances are processed. The hepatic artery brings blood to the liver from the heart. This blood carries oxygen for the liver tissue itself as well as cholesterol and other substances for processing. Blood from the intestine and heart then mix together and flow back to the heart through the hepatic vein.

Abnormalities of liver function can be divided broadly into two groups: those caused by a malfunction of the cells in the liver itself (such as cirrhosis or hepatitis), and those caused by an obstruction of bile flow from the liver through the biliary tract (such as bile stones or cancer).

Gallbladder and Biliary Tract

The gallbladder is a small, muscular storage sac that holds bile—the greenish-yellow, viscid digestive fluid produced by the liver. Bile flows out of the liver through the right and left hepatic ducts, which come together to form the common hepatic duct. This duct then joins with a duct coming from the gallbladder, called the cystic duct, to create the common bile duct. The common bile duct enters the upper intestine at the sphincter of Oddi, a few inches below the stomach.

About half the bile secreted between meals is diverted through the cystic duct and into the gallbladder. The rest of the bile flows directly through the common bile duct into the small intestine. When a person eats, the gallbladder contracts, emptying its bile into the intestine to help digest fats and certain vitamins.

Bile consists of bile salts; electrolytes; bile pigments, such as bilirubin; cholesterol; and other fats (lipids). It is responsible for the elimination of certain waste products from the body—particularly pigment from destroyed red blood cells and excess cholesterol—and it assists in the digestion and absorption of fats. Bile salts increase the solubility of cholesterol, fats, and fat-soluble vitamins to aid in their absorption from the intestine. Hemoglobin from destroyed red blood cells is converted into bilirubin (the main pigment in bile) and excreted in bile as a waste product. Also, various proteins that play important roles in bile function are secreted in bile.

Gallstones may obstruct the flow of bile from the gallbladder, causing pain (biliary colic) or gallbladder inflammation (cholecystitis). Stones may also migrate from the gallbladder to the bile duct, where they can cause jaundice by blocking normal bile flow to the intestine. The flow can also be blocked by tumors and other less common causes.

CHAPTER 115

Diagnostic Tests for Liver and Gallbladder Disorders

Laboratories can carry out a variety of tests that help doctors assess disorders of the liver, gallbladder, and biliary tract. Among the most important are a group of blood tests known as liver function tests. Depending on a patient's suspected problem, a doctor may also order certain imaging tests, such as an ultrasound scan, computed tomography, and magnetic resonance imaging. Also, a doctor may take a sample of liver tissue for examination under a microscope, a procedure called a liver biopsy.

Laboratory and Imaging Tests

Breath tests measure the ability of the liver to metabolize a variety of drugs. The drug, which is tagged with a radioactive tracer, may be given orally or intravenously. The amount of radioactivity in the person's breath is a measure of the amount of drug metabolized by the liver.

Ultrasound scanning uses sound waves to provide images of the liver, gallbladder, and biliary tract. The test is better for detecting structural abnormalities, such as tumors, than diffuse abnormalities, such as cirrhosis. It is the least expensive, safest, and most sensitive technique for creating images of the gallbladder and biliary tract.

Using ultrasound, a doctor can readily detect gallstones in the gallbladder. Ultrasound scanning easily distinguishes jaundice caused by bile duct obstruction from jaundice caused by liver cell malfunction. A type of ultrasound scanning, vascular Doppler ultrasound, can be used to show the blood flow in the blood vessels of the liver. A doctor also may use ultrasound scanning as a guide when inserting a needle to obtain a tissue sample for biopsy.

Liver Function Tests

Liver function tests are performed on blood samples. Most tests measure the levels of enzymes or other substances in the blood as a way of diagnosing liver problems. One test measures the time needed for blood to clot.

Test	What Is Measured	What the Test May Indicate
Alkaline phosphatase	An enzyme produced in the liver, bone, and placenta that is released into the blood during injury or during such normal activities as bone growth or pregnancy	Bile duct obstruction, liver injury, and some cancers
Alanine transaminase (ALT)	An enzyme produced in the liver that is released into the blood when liver cells are injured	Liver cell injury (as in hepatitis)
Aspartate transaminase (AST)	An enzyme released into the blood when the liver, heart, muscle, or brain is injured	Injury to liver, heart, muscles, or brain
Bilirubin	A component of the digestive juice (bile) produced by the liver	Obstruction to bile outflow, liver damage, excessive breakdown of red blood cells (from which bilirubin is made)
Gamma-glutamyl transpeptidase	An enzyme produced by the liver, pancreas, and kidneys and released into the blood when these organs are injured	Organ damage, drug toxicity, alcohol abuse, disease of the pancreas
Lactic dehydrogenase	An enzyme released into the blood when certain organs are injured	Damage to the liver, heart, lung, or brain and excessive breakdown of red blood cells
5'-nucleotidase	An enzyme contained only in the liver and released into the blood when the liver is injured	Bile duct obstruction or impaired bile flow
Albumin	A protein produced by the liver and normally released into the blood; one of albumin's functions is to hold fluid inside the blood vessels	Liver damage
Alpha-fetoprotein	A protein produced by the fetal liver and testes	Severe hepatitis or cancer of the liver or testes
Mitochondrial antibodies	Circulating antibodies against mitochondria, an inner component of cells	Primary biliary cirrhosis and certain autoimmune diseases, such as chronic active hepatitis
Prothrombin time	Time needed for blood to clot (clotting requires vitamin K and substances made by the liver)	Liver damage or poor absorption of vitamin K caused by a lack of bile

X-ray Techniques for Assessing the Biliary Tract

These three diagnostic techniques use a radiopaque contrast substance to outline the biliary tract on x-rays.

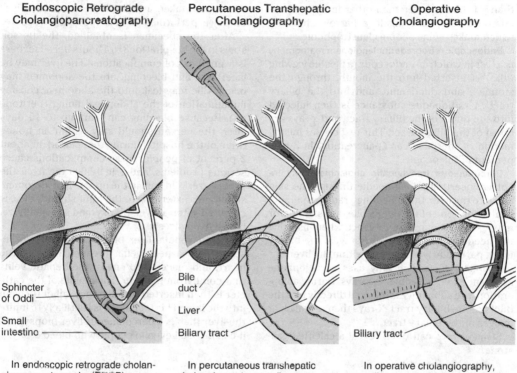

Endoscopic Retrograde Cholangiopancreatography	Percutaneous Transhepatic Cholangiography	Operative Cholangiography

Sphincter of Oddi

Small intestine

Bile duct

Liver

Biliary tract

Biliary tract

In endoscopic retrograde cholangiopancreatography (ERCP), a radiopaque contrast substance is introduced through an endoscope, which is inserted into the mouth and through the stomach into the duodenum (upper portion of the small intestine). The radiopaque substance is introduced past the sphincter of Oddi, and then flows back up the biliary system.

In percutaneous transhepatic cholangiography, a radiopaque contrast substance is injected through the skin directly into a small bile duct in the liver. The radiopaque substance then flows through the biliary tract.

In operative cholangiography, a radiopaque contrast substance is injected directly into the biliary tract during surgery.

Radionuclide (radioisotope) imaging uses a substance containing a radioactive tracer that is injected into the body and taken up by a particular organ. The radioactivity is detected by a gamma-ray camera attached to a computer that generates an image. **Liver scanning** is a type of radionuclide imaging that uses radioactive substances taken up by liver cells. **Cholescintigraphy,** another type of radionuclide imaging, uses radioactive substances excreted by the liver into the biliary tract, it is used to detect acute inflammation of the gallbladder (cholecystitis).

Computed tomography (CT) scanning can provide excellent liver images and is particularly useful in detecting tumors. It can detect diffuse disorders, such as fatty liver, and abnormally dense liver tissue caused by iron overload (hemochromatosis). However, because CT uses x-rays and is expensive, it is not as widely used as ultrasound.

Magnetic resonance imaging (MRI) provides excellent images, similar to those obtained with CT. However, it has drawbacks: It is more expensive than CT, takes longer than other imaging methods, and requires lying in a narrow chamber, which makes some people claustrophobic.

Endoscopic retrograde cholangiopancreatography is a test in which an endoscope (a flexible viewing tube) is inserted into the mouth, through the stomach and duodenum, and into the biliary tract. A radiopaque substance is then injected into the ducts of the biliary tract, and x-rays are taken of the biliary tract. This test causes inflammation of the pancreas (pancreatitis) in 3 to 5 percent of the people.

Percutaneous transhepatic cholangiography involves inserting a long needle through the skin and into the liver, then injecting a radiopaque substance into one of the liver's bile ducts. A doctor may use ultrasound for guidance when inserting the needle. The x-rays clearly reveal the biliary tract, particularly a blockage within the liver.

Operative cholangiography uses a radiopaque substance that is visible on x-rays. During an operation, the substance is injected directly into the ducts of the biliary tract. X-rays then reveal clear images of the biliary tract.

Simple x-rays can often reveal a calcified gallstone.

Liver Biopsy

A liver specimen can be obtained during exploratory surgery but is more often obtained by inserting a needle through the skin and into the liver. Before the procedure, the patient receives local anesthesia. Ultrasound or CT scans may be used to locate the abnormal area from which the specimen is taken. In most medical centers, a liver biopsy is performed as an outpatient procedure.

After the specimen is obtained, the person stays in the hospital for 3 to 4 hours because there is a small risk of complications. The liver may be lacerated, and bleeding into the abdomen may occur. Bile may leak into the abdomen, causing inflammation of the abdominal lining (peritonitis). Because bleeding can start up to 15 days later, the person should stay within an hour's drive of the hospital during that period. In about 2 percent of people, these complications cause serious problems, and 1 in 10,000 die from the procedure. Mild pain in the upper right abdomen, sometimes extending to the right shoulder tip, is common after a liver biopsy and is usually relieved by analgesics.

In transvenous liver biopsy, a catheter is inserted into a neck vein, threaded through the heart, and placed into one of the hepatic veins that come from the liver. The needle of the catheter is then inserted through the wall of the vein into the liver. This technique is less likely to injure the liver than is a percutaneous liver biopsy, and it can be used even in people who bleed easily.

CHAPTER 116

Clinical Manifestations of Liver Disease

Liver disease can manifest itself in many different ways. Manifestations of liver disease that are particularly important include jaundice, cholestasis, liver enlargement, portal hypertension, ascites, liver encephalopathy, and liver failure. When making the diagnosis of liver disease, a doctor considers a patient's description of his symptoms and conducts a physical examination.

Jaundice

Jaundice is a yellow discoloration of the skin and the whites of the eyes (sclerae) caused by abnor-

mally high levels of the bile pigment, bilirubin, in the bloodstream.

Old or damaged red blood cells are removed from the circulation mainly by the spleen. During the process, hemoglobin, the part of red blood cells that carries oxygen, is broken down into bilirubin. Bilirubin is carried to the liver and excreted into the intestine as a component of bile. If the excretion of bilirubin is hindered, excess bilirubin passes into the bloodstream, resulting in jaundice.

High levels of bilirubin in the blood may result when inflammation or other abnormalities of the liver cells hinder its excretion into bile. Alternatively, the bile ducts outside the liver may be blocked by a gallstone or a tumor. Less commonly, high levels of bilirubin may result from the breakdown of large numbers of red blood cells, as sometimes occurs in newborns with jaundice.▲

In Gilbert's syndrome, bilirubin levels are slightly increased, but usually not enough to cause jaundice. This sometimes hereditary condition is usually discovered during routine screening tests of liver function; it has no other symptoms and causes no problems.

Symptoms

In jaundice, the skin and the whites of the eyes appear yellow. The urine is often dark because bilirubin is excreted through the kidneys. Other symptoms appear depending on the underlying cause of the jaundice. For example, inflammation of the liver (hepatitis) may cause loss of appetite, nausea and vomiting, and fever. Blockage of bile may produce the symptoms of cholestasis.

Diagnosis and Treatment

A doctor uses laboratory tests and imaging studies to determine the cause of the jaundice.■ If the problem is a disease of the liver itself, for example, viral hepatitis, the jaundice will usually disappear as the condition of the liver improves. If the problem is blockage of a bile duct, then surgery or endoscopy (a procedure using a flexible viewing tube with surgical attachments) is usually performed as soon as possible to reopen the affected bile duct.

Cholestasis

Cholestasis is a reduction or stoppage of bile flow.

Bile flow may be impaired at any point between the liver cells and the duodenum (the upper por-

Major Clinical Features of Liver Disease

Jaundice

Enlarged liver

Fluid in the abdomen (ascites)

Confusion from encephalopathy

Gastrointestinal bleeding from varices

Portal hypertension

Skin
- Spiderlike blood vessels
- Red palms
- Florid complexion
- Itching

Blood
- Decreased number of red blood cells (anemia)
- Decreased number of white blood cells (leukopenia)
- Decreased number of platelets (thrombocytopenia)
- A tendency to bleed (coagulopathy)

Hormones
- High levels of insulin but poor response to it
- Cessation of menstrual periods and decreased fertility (in women)
- Impotence and feminization (in men)

Heart and blood vessels
- Increased heart rate and amount of blood pumped
- Low blood pressure (hypotension)

General
- Fatigue
- Weakness
- Weight loss
- Poor appetite
- Nausea
- Fever

tion of the small intestine). Even though bile isn't flowing, the liver continues to process bilirubin,

▲ see page 1212

■ see page 557

which escapes into the bloodstream. The bilirubin is then deposited in the skin and passed into the urine, causing jaundice.

For purposes of diagnosis and treatment, the causes of cholestasis are divided into two groups: those originating inside the liver and those originating outside of it. Causes within the liver include hepatitis, alcoholic liver disease, primary biliary cirrhosis, the effects of drugs, and the effects of hormonal changes during pregnancy (a condition called cholestasis of pregnancy). Causes outside the liver include a stone in a bile duct, a narrowing (stricture) of a bile duct, cancer of a bile duct, pancreatic cancer, and inflammation of the pancreas.

Symptoms

Jaundice and dark urine result from excessive bilirubin in the skin and urine, respectively. The stool is sometimes pale because of a lack of bilirubin in the intestine. The stool may also contain too much fat (a condition known as steatorrhea), because bile isn't available in the intestine to help digest dietary fat. The lack of bile in the intestine also means that calcium and vitamin D aren't properly absorbed. If the cholestasis persists, a lack of these nutrients can cause bone loss, which can result in bone pain and fractures. Substances needed for blood clotting are also poorly absorbed, creating a tendency to bleed easily.

Retention of bile products in the circulation may cause itching (with subsequent scratching and skin damage). Prolonged jaundice from cholestasis produces a muddy skin color and fatty yellow deposits in the skin. The underlying cause of cholestasis determines whether the person has other symptoms, such as abdominal pain, loss of appetite, vomiting, or fever.

Diagnosis

To determine whether the cause is within the liver, a doctor asks about symptoms of hepatitis, heavy alcohol intake, or recently used drugs that can cause cholestasis. Small, spiderlike blood vessels visible in the skin, an enlarged spleen, and fluid in the abdominal cavity (ascites) are signs that liver cells are diseased. If the cause is outside the liver, the person may experience chills, pain from the biliary tract or pancreas, and an enlarged gallbladder (which a doctor can feel or imaging studies can detect).

Typically, the blood levels of an enzyme called alkaline phosphatase are very high in people with cholestasis. A blood test that measures the level of bilirubin indicates the severity of the cholestasis but not its cause. Ultrasound, computed tomography (CT), or both are almost always done if blood test results are abnormal. This helps a doctor distinguish between liver disease and blockage of the bile ducts. If the cause appears to be within the liver, a liver biopsy (removal of a tissue specimen for microscopic examination) may be performed. A biopsy usually establishes the diagnosis. If the cause appears to be blockage of the bile ducts, an endoscopic procedure (using a flexible viewing tube) is often performed to clarify the nature of the blockage.

Treatment

A blockage outside the liver can usually be treated with surgery or therapeutic endoscopy (a procedure involving use of a flexible viewing tube with surgical attachments). A blockage inside the liver may be treated in various ways depending on the cause. If a drug is the suspected cause, the person stops taking it. If hepatitis is responsible for the blockage, then the cholestasis and jaundice usually disappear when the hepatitis has run its course.

Cholestyramine, taken orally, can be used to treat the itchiness. This drug binds with certain bile products in the intestine, so they can't be reabsorbed to irritate the skin. Unless the liver is severely damaged, taking vitamin K can improve blood clotting. Supplements of calcium and vitamin D are often taken if the cholestasis persists, but they aren't very effective in preventing bone disease. If too much fat is being excreted in the stool, the person may need to take triglyceride supplements.

Liver Enlargement

Liver enlargement (hepatomegaly) indicates liver disease. Even so, many people with liver disease have a normal-sized or even a shrunken liver. An enlarged liver usually causes no symptoms. However, if the enlargement is extreme, it may cause abdominal discomfort or a full feeling. If the enlargement occurs quickly, the liver may be tender to the touch. A doctor usually estimates the size of the liver by feeling it through the abdominal wall during a physical examination.

When feeling the liver, a doctor also notes its texture. The liver usually feels soft if it is enlarged because of acute hepatitis, fatty infiltration, congestion with blood, or early obstruction of the bile ducts. The liver feels firm and irregular if it is enlarged because of cirrhosis. Distinct lumps usually suggest cancer.

Portal Hypertension

Portal hypertension is abnormally high blood pressure in the portal vein, the large vein that brings blood from the intestine to the liver.

The portal vein receives blood drained from the entire intestine and from the spleen, pancreas, and gallbladder. After entering the liver, the blood divides into tiny channels that run through the liver. When blood leaves the liver, it drains back into the general circulation through the hepatic vein.▲

Two factors can increase blood pressure in the portal blood vessels: the volume of blood flowing through the vessels and increased resistance to the blood flow through the liver. In Western countries, the most common cause of portal hypertension is increased resistance to blood flow caused by cirrhosis.

Portal hypertension leads to the development of venous blood vessels (called collateral vessels) that connect the portal system to the general circulation, thus bypassing the liver. Because of this bypass, substances that are normally removed from the blood by the liver are able to pass into the general circulation. Collateral vessels develop at specific places, the most important of which is the lower end of the esophagus. Here the vessels become engorged and tortuous—that is, they become varicose veins (called **esophageal varices**). These engorged vessels are fragile and likely to bleed, sometimes seriously. Other collateral vessels may develop around the navel and at the rectum.

Symptoms and Diagnosis

Portal hypertension often enlarges the spleen. Fluid may leak out of the liver and distend the abdominal cavity, a condition called ascites. Varicose veins at the lower end of the esophagus and in the stomach lining bleed easily and sometimes massively. Varicose veins in the rectum may also bleed, though this is much less common.

A doctor can usually feel an enlarged spleen through the abdominal wall. Fluid in the abdomen can be detected by noting abdominal swelling and by listening for a dull sound when tapping (percussing) the abdomen. Ultrasound scans and x-rays provide considerable information about portal hypertension. Ultrasound may be used to examine the blood flow in the portal blood vessels and can detect the presence of fluid in the abdomen. Computed tomography (CT) scans can also be used to examine the enlarged veins. Pressure in the portal system may be measured directly using a needle inserted through the abdominal wall and into the liver or spleen.

Treatment

To reduce the risk of bleeding from esophageal varices, a doctor may try to reduce the pressure in the portal vein. One way is to give propranolol, a drug used to treat high blood pressure.

Bleeding from esophageal varices is a medical emergency. Drugs such as vasopressin or octreotide may be given intravenously to constrict the bleeding veins, and blood transfusions are given to replace lost blood. An endoscopic examination is usually done to confirm that the bleeding is from varices. The veins can then be blocked off with rubber bands or with chemical injections given through the endoscope. If the bleeding continues, a catheter with a balloon on the end can be passed through the person's nose and down the esophagus. Inflating the balloon compresses the varicose veins and usually stops the bleeding.

If the bleeding continues or recurs repeatedly, a surgical procedure may be done to create a bypass (called a shunt) between the portal venous system and the general (systemic) venous system. This lowers the pressure in the portal vein, because the pressure is much lower in the general venous system. There are various types of portal-

---

▲ see box, page 575

Causes of Ascites

Liver Disorders
- Cirrhosis, especially cirrhosis caused by alcoholism
- Alcoholic hepatitis without cirrhosis
- Chronic hepatitis
- Obstruction of the hepatic vein

Nonliver Disorders
- Heart failure
- Kidney failure, especially the nephrotic syndrome
- Constrictive pericarditis
- Carcinomatosis in which cancer spreads to sites in the abdominal cavity
- Tuberculosis affecting the lining of the abdominal cavity
- Reduced thyroid activity
- Inflammation of the pancreas

systemic shunt operations—including one that can be done under x-ray guidance in the radiology department using special tools. Shunt operations are usually successful in stopping the bleeding, but they are relatively dangerous. They also increase the risk of brain dysfunction from liver failure (liver encephalopathy).

Ascites

Ascites is the accumulation of fluid in the abdominal cavity.

Ascites tends to occur in long-standing (chronic) rather than in short-lived (acute) conditions. It occurs most commonly in cirrhosis, especially in cirrhosis caused by alcoholism. Ascites can also occur in nonliver diseases such as cancer, heart failure, kidney failure, and tuberculosis.

In people with liver disease, the fluid leaks from the surface of the liver and intestine. A combina-

▲ see page 486

tion of factors is responsible, including portal hypertension, decreased ability of the blood vessels to retain fluid, fluid retention by the kidneys, and alterations in various hormones and chemicals that regulate bodily fluids.

Symptoms and Diagnosis

Small amounts of fluid in the abdomen usually produce no symptoms, but massive amounts may cause abdominal distention and discomfort, as well as shortness of breath. When a doctor taps (percusses) the abdomen, the fluid makes a dull sound. When the abdomen contains large amounts of fluid, the abdomen is taut, and the navel (umbilicus) is flat or even pushed out. In some people with ascites, the ankles swell with excess fluid (edema).

If the presence or the cause of ascites isn't clear, ultrasound scanning may be used. Alternatively, a small sample of fluid can be withdrawn by inserting a needle through the abdominal wall—a procedure called diagnostic paracentesis.▲ Laboratory tests of the fluid can help determine the cause.

Treatment

The basic therapy for ascites is bed rest and a salt-restricted diet, usually combined with drugs called diuretics, which make the kidneys excrete more fluid in the urine. If the ascites makes breathing or eating difficult, the fluid may be removed through a needle—a procedure called therapeutic paracentesis. The fluid tends to reaccumulate in the abdomen unless the person also takes a diuretic drug. Often, large amounts of albumin (the major protein in plasma) are lost from the blood into the abdominal fluid, so albumin may be administered intravenously.

An infection occasionally develops in ascites fluid for no apparent reason, especially in people with alcoholic cirrhosis. This infection is called spontaneous bacterial peritonitis and is treated with antibiotics.

Liver Encephalopathy

Liver encephalopathy (also called portal-systemic encephalopathy, hepatic encephalopathy, or hepatic coma) is a disorder in which brain function deteriorates because toxic substances, which would normally be removed by the liver, build up in the blood.

Substances absorbed into the bloodstream from the intestines pass through the liver, where toxins are removed. In liver encephalopathy, toxins aren't removed because liver function is impaired. Also, because connections may have formed between the portal system and the general circulation (as a result of the liver disease), some toxins may bypass the liver altogether. A surgical bypass to correct portal hypertension (portal-systemic shunt) may have the same effect. Whatever the cause, the outcome is the same: Toxins can pass to the brain and affect its function. Exactly which substances are toxic to the brain isn't known; however, high blood levels of protein breakdown products, such as ammonia, appear to play a role.

In a person with long-standing liver disease, encephalopathy is usually triggered by an event such as an acute infection or an alcoholic binge, which increases liver damage. Or it may be triggered by eating too much protein, which increases the levels of protein breakdown products in the blood. Bleeding in the digestive tract, such as from esophageal varices, can also lead to a buildup of protein breakdown products, which may directly affect the brain. Certain drugs—especially some sedatives, analgesics, and diuretics—may also trigger encephalopathy. When such a precipitating cause is removed, the encephalopathy may disappear.

Symptoms and Diagnosis

The symptoms of liver encephalopathy are the result of decreased brain function, especially impaired consciousness. In the earliest stages, subtle changes appear in logical thinking, personality, and behavior. The person's mood may change, and judgment may be impaired. As the disorder progresses, the person usually becomes drowsy and confused, and movements and speech become sluggish. Disorientation is common. A person with encephalopathy may be agitated and excited, but this is uncommon. Seizures are also uncommon. Eventually, the person may lose consciousness and lapse into a coma.

Symptoms of impaired brain function in a person with liver disease provide a strong clue to the

diagnosis. The person may also have a sweet odor on the breath. When the person stretches out the arms, the hands can't be held steady, and the person displays a crude flapping motion.

An electroencephalogram (EEG) may help in diagnosing early encephalopathy. Even in mild cases, it shows abnormal brain waves. Blood tests usually show abnormally high levels of ammonia.

Treatment

A doctor looks for and tries to remove any precipitating cause, such as an infection or a drug that the person is taking. A doctor also tries to eliminate toxic substances from the intestines. Protein is eliminated from the diet, and oral or intravenous carbohydrates serve as the main source of calories. A synthetic sugar (lactulose), taken orally, has three beneficial effects: It alters the acidity of the intestines, thereby changing the type of bacteria present; it decreases the absorption of ammonia; and it acts as a laxative. (Cleansing enemas also may be given.) Occasionally, a person may take neomycin, an antibiotic, instead of lactulose. Neomycin reduces the quantity of intestinal bacteria that normally help digest protein.

With treatment, liver encephalopathy is frequently reversible. In fact, complete recovery is possible, especially if the encephalopathy was precipitated by a reversible cause. However, for a person in a severe coma as a result of acute liver inflammation, the condition is fatal up to 80 percent of the time despite intensive treatment.

Liver Failure

Liver failure is a severe deterioration in liver function.

Liver failure can result from any type of liver disorder, including viral hepatitis, cirrhosis, and liver damage from alcohol or drugs such as acetaminophen. A large portion of the liver must be damaged before liver failure occurs.

Symptoms and Diagnosis

A person with liver failure usually has jaundice, a tendency to bruise or bleed, ascites, impaired brain function (liver encephalopathy), and generally failing health. Other common symptoms include fatigue, weakness, nausea, and a loss of appetite.

The clinical manifestations alone provide strong evidence of liver failure. Blood tests usually show severely deranged liver function.

Prognosis and Treatment

Treatment depends on the cause and the specific clinical manifestations. The person is usually placed on a restricted diet. Protein consumption is carefully controlled: Too much protein can cause brain dysfunction; too little can cause weight loss. Sodium consumption is kept low to treat fluid accumulation in the abdomen (ascites).

Alcohol is completely avoided because it can worsen the liver damage.

Ultimately, liver failure is fatal if it isn't treated or if the liver disease is progressive. Even after treatment, it may be irreversible. In terminal cases, the person may die of kidney failure (hepatorenal syndrome) as the liver gives out. Liver transplantation, if performed soon enough, can restore a person to normal health, but it is suitable for only a small minority of patients with liver failure.

CHAPTER 117

Fatty Liver, Cirrhosis, and Related Disorders

Fatty liver, alcoholic liver disease, cirrhosis, primary biliary cirrhosis, primary sclerosing cholangitis, and alpha₁-antitrypsin deficiency are all disorders that appear to result from an injury to the liver. Many factors can injure the liver, but in some of these disorders, the nature of the injury is not known.

Fatty Liver

Fatty liver is an excessive accumulation of fat (lipid) inside the liver cells.

Sometimes the cause of fatty liver is not known, especially in newborns. In general, the known causes injure the liver in some way.

Fatty liver usually produces no symptoms. Rarely, it causes jaundice, nausea, vomiting, pain, and abdominal tenderness.

A physical examination that reveals an enlarged liver without any other symptoms suggests fatty liver. The diagnosis may be confirmed by performing a liver biopsy, in which a long hollow needle is used to obtain a small tissue sample for examination under a microscope.

The mere presence of excessive fat in the liver is not a serious problem. Treatment aims at eliminating the cause or treating the underlying disorder. Repeated liver injury from toxic substances such as alcohol may eventually progress from fatty liver to cirrhosis.

Alcoholic Liver Disease

Alcoholic liver disease is damage to the liver that results from excessive drinking of alcohol.

Alcoholic liver disease is a common, preventable health problem. In general, the amount of alcohol consumed (how much and how often) determines the risk and the degree of liver damage. Women are more vulnerable to liver damage than men. In women who drink over a period of years, the equivalent of as little as $\frac{2}{3}$ of an ounce of pure alcohol a day (6$\frac{1}{2}$ ounces of wine, 13 ounces of beer, or 2 ounces of whiskey) can cause liver damage. In men who drink over a period of years, the equivalent of as little as 2 ounces a day (20 ounces of wine, 40 ounces of beer, or 6 ounces of whiskey) can cause liver damage. However, the amount of alcohol that causes liver damage varies from person to person.

Alcohol may cause three types of liver damage: fat accumulation (fatty liver), inflammation (alcoholic hepatitis), and scarring (cirrhosis).

Alcohol also provides calories without essential nutrients, decreases the appetite, and causes poor absorption of nutrients because of its toxic effects on the intestine and pancreas. As a result, people who regularly drink alcohol without eating properly develop malnutrition.

Symptoms and Diagnosis

In general, symptoms depend on how long and how much a person has been drinking. Heavy drinkers usually first develop symptoms during their 30s and tend to develop severe problems by their 40s. In men, alcohol may produce effects similar to those produced by too much estrogen and too little testosterone—shrunken testes and breast enlargement.

People with liver damage from fat accumulation (fatty liver) usually have no symptoms. In a third of these people, the liver is enlarged and occasionally tender.

Inflammation of the liver induced by alcohol (alcoholic hepatitis) may produce a fever, jaundice, an increased white blood cell count, and a tender, painful, enlarged liver. The skin may develop spiderlike veins.

A person who has liver damage with scarring (cirrhosis) may have few symptoms or the features of alcoholic hepatitis. Such a person also may have complications of alcoholic cirrhosis: portal hypertension with spleen enlargement, ascites (fluid accumulation in the abdominal cavity), kidney failure from liver failure (hepatorenal syndrome), confusion (one of the main symptoms of liver encephalopathy), or liver cancer (hepatoma). To confirm the diagnosis of alcoholic liver disease in some cases, a doctor performs a liver biopsy. In this procedure, a hollow needle is inserted through the skin and a tiny piece of liver tissue is removed for examination under a microscope.▲

In people with alcoholic liver disease, the results of liver function tests may be normal or abnormal. However, blood levels of one liver enzyme, gamma-glutamyl transpeptidase,■ may be particularly high in people who abuse alcohol. Also, the person's red blood cells tend to be larger than normal, a telltale sign. Platelet levels in the blood may be low.

Prognosis and Treatment

If the person continues to drink alcohol, liver damage will progress and probably be fatal. If the person stops drinking, some of the liver damage (except that from scarring) may repair itself, and chances are good that the person will live longer.

Known Causes of Fatty Liver

- Obesity
- Diabetes
- Chemicals and drugs (such as alcohol, corticosteroids, tetracyclines, valproic acid, methotrexate, carbon tetrachloride, and yellow phosphorus)
- Malnutrition and a diet that is deficient in protein
- Pregnancy
- Vitamin A toxicity
- Bypass surgery of the small intestine
- Cystic fibrosis (most likely accompanied by malnutrition)
- Hereditary defects in glycogen, galactose, tyrosine, or homocystine metabolism
- Medium-chain aryldehydrogenase deficiency
- Cholesterol esterase deficiency
- Phytanic acid storage disease (Refsum's disease)
- Abetalipoproteinemia
- Reye's syndrome

The only treatment for alcoholic liver disease is to stop drinking alcohol. Doing so can be extremely difficult, and most people need to participate in a formal program to stop drinking, such as Alcoholics Anonymous.★

Cirrhosis

Cirrhosis is the destruction of normal liver tissue that leaves nonfunctioning scar tissue surrounding areas of functioning liver tissue.

Most of the common causes of liver injury result in cirrhosis. In the United States, the most

▲ see page 560

■ see box, page 558

★ see page 445

Causes of Cirrhosis

- Alcohol abuse
- Use of certain drugs
- Exposure to certain chemicals
- Infections (including hepatitis B and hepatitis C)
- Autoimmune diseases (including autoimmune chronic hepatitis)
- Bile duct obstruction
- Persistent obstruction to outflow of blood from the liver (such as occurs in the Budd-Chiari syndrome)
- Heart and blood vessel disturbances
- Alpha$_1$-antitrypsin deficiency
- High blood galactose levels
- High blood tyrosine levels at birth (congenital tyrosinosis)
- Glycogen storage disease
- Diabetes
- Malnutrition
- Hereditary accumulation of too much copper (Wilson's disease)
- Iron overload (hemochromatosis)

common cause of cirrhosis is alcohol abuse. Among people ages 45 to 65, cirrhosis is the third most common cause of death, after heart disease and cancer. In many parts of Asia and Africa, chronic hepatitis is a major cause of cirrhosis.▲

Symptoms

Many people with mild cirrhosis have no symptoms and appear to be well for years. Others are

▲ see page 573

■ see page 563

★ see page 564

● see box, page 558

weak, have a poor appetite, feel sick, and lose weight. If bile flow is chronically obstructed, the person has jaundice, itching, and small yellow skin nodules, especially around the eyelids. Malnutrition commonly results from a poor appetite and the impaired absorption of fats and fat-soluble vitamins caused by the reduced production of bile salts.

Occasionally, the person may cough up or vomit large amounts of blood because of bleeding from varicose veins at the lower end of the esophagus (esophageal varices). These enlarged blood vessels result from high blood pressure in the veins that run from the intestine to the liver. Such high blood pressure, called portal hypertension,■ along with poor liver function, may also lead to fluid accumulation in the abdomen (ascites).★ Kidney failure and liver encephalopathy also may develop.

Other symptoms of long-standing liver disease may develop, such as muscle wasting, redness of the palms (palmar erythema), a curling up of the fingers (Dupuytren's contracture of the palms), small spiderlike veins in the skin, breast enlargement in men (gynecomastia), salivary gland enlargement in the cheeks, hair loss, shrinking of the testes (testicular atrophy), and abnormal nerve function (peripheral neuropathy).

Diagnosis

An ultrasound scan may show that the liver is enlarged. A liver scan using a radioactive isotope creates an image showing which areas of the liver are functioning and which are scarred. Results of liver function tests● often are normal because only a small percentage of functioning liver cells are needed to carry out essential chemical functions. A definitive diagnosis is made by microscopic examination of a sample of liver tissue.

Prognosis and Treatment

Cirrhosis is usually progressive. If someone with early alcoholic cirrhosis stops drinking, the process of liver scarring usually stops, but scar tissue remains indefinitely. In general, the prognosis is poorer if serious complications—such as vomiting of blood, ascites, or abnormal brain function (encephalopathy)—have occurred.

Liver cancer (hepatocellular carcinoma) is more common in people with cirrhosis caused by chronic hepatitis B or hepatitis C infections, iron overload (hemochromatosis), and long-standing glycogen storage disease. Liver cancer can also occur in people with cirrhosis from alcohol abuse.

No cure exists for cirrhosis. The treatment includes withdrawing toxic agents such as alcohol, receiving proper nutrition including supplemental vitamins, and treating complications as they arise.

Liver transplantation may help a person with advanced cirrhosis. But if the person continues to abuse alcohol or if the underlying cause cannot be altered, a transplanted liver will also eventually develop cirrhosis.

Primary Biliary Cirrhosis

Primary biliary cirrhosis is inflammation and eventual scarring and obstruction of the bile ducts in the liver.

Primary biliary cirrhosis is most common among women ages 35 to 60, though it can occur in men and women of any age. The cause is not known, but the disease commonly occurs in people with autoimmune diseases, such as rheumatoid arthritis, scleroderma, or autoimmune thyroiditis.

Primary biliary cirrhosis begins with inflammation of the bile ducts in the liver. The inflammation blocks the flow of bile out of the liver; thus, bile remains in the liver cells or spills over into the bloodstream. As the inflammation spreads to the rest of the liver, a latticework of scar tissue develops throughout the liver.

Symptoms and Diagnosis

Usually, primary biliary cirrhosis starts gradually. Itching and sometimes fatigue are the first symptoms in about 50 percent of the people with primary biliary cirrhosis, and these symptoms can precede other symptoms by months or years. On physical examination, a doctor will feel an enlarged, firm liver in about 50 percent of people and an enlarged spleen in about 25 percent. About 15 percent have small yellow deposits in the skin (xanthoma) or eyelids (xanthelasma). Roughly 10 percent have increased skin pigmentation. Less than 10 percent have only jaundice. Other symptoms may include enlargement of the finger ends (clubbing) and abnormalities of the bone, nerves, and kidney. The stool may be pale and greasy and

have an offensive odor. Later, all the symptoms and complications of cirrhosis can develop.

At least 30 percent of people are diagnosed before symptoms develop because of abnormalities detected during routine blood testing. Antibodies against mitochondria (tiny structures contained within cells) are found in the blood of more than 90 percent of people with the disease.

When jaundice or liver test abnormalities are evident, one useful diagnostic tool is endoscopic retrograde cholangiopancreatography (ERCP). In this procedure, x-rays are taken after a radiopaque substance has been injected into the bile ducts through an endoscope.▲ This will show that no obstruction exists within the bile ducts, enabling the doctor to better identify the liver as the site of the problem. The diagnosis can be confirmed by a microscopic examination of a liver tissue specimen obtained using a hollow needle (liver biopsy).■

Prognosis and Treatment

The progression of primary biliary cirrhosis varies greatly. Initially, the disease may not diminish the quality of life, and a person with the disorder has a reasonably good prognosis. People with a slowly worsening disease seem to live longer. In some, the disease progresses relentlessly, culminating in severe cirrhosis in a few years. The prognosis is poor in people who have a rising blood level of bilirubin (jaundice). Metabolic bone disease (osteoporosis) develops in most.

No cure is known. Itching may be controlled by taking the drug cholestyramine. Supplements of calcium and vitamins A, D, and K may be needed because these nutrients are not properly absorbed when there is insufficient bile. The drug ursodiol (ursodeoxycholic acid) appears to somewhat lessen the progression of the disease and is generally well tolerated. Liver transplantation is the best treatment for those entering the final stages with complications. Prognosis for the transplanted liver is very good; less clear is whether primary biliary cirrhosis will recur in the transplanted liver.

▲ see box, page 559

■ see page 560

Primary Sclerosing Cholangitis

Primary sclerosing cholangitis is inflammation and eventual scarring and obstruction of the bile ducts inside and outside the liver.

In primary sclerosing cholangitis, the scarring narrows and eventually blocks the ducts, causing cirrhosis. The cause is not known but likely relates to abnormalities in the immune system. The disease most often affects young men. It commonly occurs in people with inflammatory bowel disease, especially ulcerative colitis.

Symptoms and Diagnosis

The disease usually begins gradually with worsening fatigue, itching, and jaundice. Attacks of upper abdominal pain and fever caused by inflammation of the bile ducts may occur, but they are uncommon. An affected person may have an enlarged liver and spleen or symptoms of cirrhosis. The person also may develop portal hypertension, ascites, and liver failure, which can be fatal.

The diagnosis usually is made using endoscopic retrograde cholangiopancreatography (ERCP) or percutaneous cholangiography.▲ In ERCP, x-rays are taken after a radiopaque substance is injected into the bile ducts through an endoscope. In percutaneous cholangiography, x-rays are taken after a direct injection of a radiopaque substance into the bile ducts. Microscopic examination of a liver tissue specimen obtained using a hollow needle (liver biopsy) may be necessary to confirm the diagnosis.

Prognosis and Treatment

Some people have no symptoms for as long as 10 years (the disease having been detected through routine liver function tests). Usually, primary sclerosing cholangitis gradually worsens.

Drugs such as corticosteroids, azathioprine, penicillamine, and methotrexate have not proven very effective and can cause severe adverse effects. The value of ursodiol remains unclear. Primary sclerosing cholangitis may require liver transplantation, which is the only known cure for this otherwise fatal disease.

Recurring infection of the bile ducts (bacterial cholangitis) is a complication of the disease and

requires treatment with antibiotics. Narrowed ducts can be dilated by an endoscopic or surgical procedure. Cancer of the bile ducts (cholangiocarcinoma) develops in 10 to 15 percent of the people with primary sclerosing cholangitis. The tumor is slow-growing, and treatment entails using an endoscopic procedure to place stents in the bile ducts to open up the diseased ducts. Occasionally, surgery is required.

Alpha$_1$-Antitrypsin Deficiency

Alpha$_1$-antitrypsin deficiency is a disorder in which a hereditary deficiency of alpha$_1$-antitrypsin may cause lung and liver disease.

Alpha$_1$-antitrypsin, an enzyme produced by the liver, is present in saliva, duodenal fluid, lung secretions, tears, nasal secretions, and cerebrospinal fluid. This enzyme inhibits the action of other enzymes that break down proteins. A lack of alpha$_1$-antitrypsin allows the other enzymes to damage tissue in the lungs. The deficiency in blood represents a failure of the liver to secrete the enzyme. Its retention inside liver cells may cause damage, fibrosis (scarring), and cirrhosis.

Symptoms and Prognosis

Up to 25 percent of children with alpha$_1$-antitrypsin deficiency develop cirrhosis and portal hypertension and die before age 12. About 25 percent die by age 20. Another 25 percent have only minor liver abnormalities and live into adulthood. The remaining 25 percent have no evidence of progressive disease.

Alpha$_1$-antitrypsin deficiency is uncommon in adults and, even if present, may not cause cirrhosis. More commonly, adults with the disorder develop emphysema, a lung disease that results in increasing shortness of breath. Liver cancer may eventually develop.

Treatment

Replacement therapy using synthetic alpha$_1$-antitrypsin has shown some promise, but liver transplantation remains the only successful treatment. Liver damage does not usually recur in the transplanted liver, which produces alpha$_1$-antitrypsin.

Treatment in adults is usually directed at the lung disease. Measures include preventing infection and getting a person who smokes to stop smoking.

▲ see box, page 559

Hepatitis

Hepatitis is inflammation of the liver from any cause.

Hepatitis commonly results from a virus, particularly one of five hepatitis viruses—A, B, C, D, or E. Less commonly, hepatitis results from other viral infections, such as infectious mononucleosis, yellow fever, and cytomegalovirus infection. The major nonviral causes of hepatitis are alcohol and drugs. Hepatitis can be acute (lasting less than 6 months) or chronic; it occurs commonly throughout the world.

Hepatitis A virus spreads primarily from the stool of one person to the mouth of another. Such transmission is usually the result of poor hygiene. Waterborne and foodborne epidemics are common, especially in developing countries. Eating contaminated raw shellfish is sometimes responsible. Isolated cases, usually arising from person-to-person contact, are also common. Most hepatitis A infections cause no symptoms and go unrecognized.

Hepatitis B virus is less easily transmitted than hepatitis A virus. One way it can be transmitted is through contaminated blood or blood products. However, because of precautions taken to ensure a safe blood supply, blood transfusions rarely are responsible for the transmission of the hepatitis B virus in the United States. Transmission commonly occurs among injecting drug users who share needles, as well as between sexual partners, both heterosexual and male homosexual. A pregnant woman infected with hepatitis B can transmit the virus to her baby during birth.

The risk of exposure to the hepatitis B virus is increased for patients undergoing kidney dialysis or in cancer units and for hospital personnel who have contact with blood. Also at risk are people in closed environments (such as prisons and institutions for the mentally retarded), where close personal contact exists.

Hepatitis B can be transmitted by healthy people who are chronic carriers of the virus. Whether insect bites can transmit this virus isn't clear. Many cases of hepatitis B have no known source. In areas of the world such as the Far East and parts of Africa, hepatitis B virus is responsible for many cases of chronic hepatitis, cirrhosis, and liver cancer.

Hepatitis C virus causes at least 80 percent of the hepatitis cases arising from blood transfusions, plus many scattered cases of acute hepatitis. It is most commonly transmitted by injecting drug users who share needles. Sexual transmission is uncommon. Hepatitis C virus is responsible for many cases of chronic hepatitis and some cases of cirrhosis and liver cancer. For unknown reasons, people with alcoholic liver disease often have hepatitis C as well; the combination of diseases sometimes produces a greater loss of liver function than would result from either disease alone. A small proportion of healthy people appear to be chronic carriers of the hepatitis C virus.

Hepatitis D virus occurs only as a co-infection with hepatitis B virus, and it makes the hepatitis B infection more severe. Drug addicts are at relatively high risk.

Hepatitis E virus causes occasional epidemics similar to those caused by hepatitis A virus. So far, these epidemics have occurred only in underdeveloped countries.

Acute Viral Hepatitis

Acute viral hepatitis is inflammation of the liver caused by infection with one of the five hepatitis viruses; for most people the inflammation begins suddenly and lasts only a few weeks.

Symptoms and Diagnosis

Symptoms of acute viral hepatitis usually begin suddenly. They include a poor appetite, a feeling of being ill, nausea, vomiting, and often a fever. In people who smoke, a distaste for cigarettes is a typical symptom. Occasionally, especially with hepatitis B infection, the person develops joint pains and wheals (itchy red hives on the skin).

After a few days, the urine becomes dark, and jaundice may develop. Most symptoms typically disappear at this point and the person feels better even though the jaundice is getting worse. Symptoms of cholestasis (a stoppage or reduction of bile flow)▲—such as pale stools and general itch-

▲ see page 561

ing—may develop. The jaundice usually peaks in 1 to 2 weeks, then fades over 2 to 4 weeks.

Acute viral hepatitis is diagnosed on the basis of the person's symptoms and the results of blood tests that evaluate liver function. In about half the people with this disease, a doctor will find the liver to be tender and somewhat enlarged.

Acute viral hepatitis must be distinguished from several other conditions that cause similar symptoms. For instance, the flulike symptoms early in the disease can mimic those of other viral diseases, such as influenza and infectious mononucleosis. Fever and jaundice are also symptoms of alcoholic hepatitis, which occurs in people who regularly drink significant amounts of alcohol.▲ The specific diagnosis of acute viral hepatitis can be made if blood tests reveal viral proteins or antibodies against hepatitis viruses.

Prognosis

Acute viral hepatitis can produce anything from a minor flulike illness to fatal liver failure. In general, hepatitis B is more serious than hepatitis A and is occasionally fatal, especially in elderly people. The course of hepatitis C is somewhat unpredictable: The acute illness is usually mild, but liver function may improve and then worsen repeatedly for several months.

A person with acute viral hepatitis usually recovers after 4 to 8 weeks, even without treatment. Hepatitis A rarely if ever becomes chronic. Hepatitis B becomes chronic in 5 to 10 percent of the infected people and can be mild or full-blown. Hepatitis C has the greatest likelihood of becoming chronic—about a 75 percent chance. Though usually mild and often without symptoms, hepatitis C is a serious problem because about 20 percent of the affected people eventually develop cirrhosis.

A person with acute viral hepatitis can become a chronic carrier of the virus. In the carrier state, the person has no symptoms but is still infected. This situation occurs only with hepatitis B and C viruses, not hepatitis A virus. A chronic carrier may eventually develop liver cancer.

▲ see page 566

Treatment

People with unusually severe acute hepatitis may require hospitalization, but in most cases treatment isn't necessary. After the first several days, appetite usually returns and the person doesn't need to stay in bed. Severe restrictions of diet or activity are unnecessary, and vitamin supplements are not required. Most people can safely return to work after the jaundice clears, even if their liver function test results aren't quite normal.

Prevention

Good hygiene helps prevent the spread of hepatitis A virus. Because the stool of people with hepatitis A is infectious, stool samples must be handled with special care by health practitioners. The same is true for the blood of people with any type of acute hepatitis. On the other hand, infected people don't require isolation—it does little to prevent the transmission of hepatitis A, and it won't prevent the transmission of hepatitis B or C.

Medical personnel reduce the chance of infection from blood transfusions by avoiding unnecessary transfusions, using blood donated by volunteers rather than paid donors, and screening all blood donors for hepatitis B and C. Because of screening, the number of cases of hepatitis B and C transmitted through a blood transfusion has been greatly reduced, though not eliminated.

Vaccination against hepatitis B stimulates the body's immune defenses and protects most people well. However, dialysis patients, people with cirrhosis, and people with an impaired immune system derive less protection from vaccination. Vaccination is especially important for people at risk of contracting hepatitis B, though it isn't effective once the disease is established. For these various reasons, universal vaccination of all people against hepatitis B is being increasingly recommended.

Hepatitis A vaccines are given to people at high risk of acquiring the infection, such as travelers to parts of the world where the disease is widespread. No vaccines are available against hepatitis C, D, and E viruses.

People who haven't been vaccinated and who are exposed to hepatitis may receive an antibody preparation (immune serum globulin) for protection. Antibodies are intended to give immediate protection against viral hepatitis, but the amount of protection varies greatly with different situations. For people who have been exposed—perhaps by an accidental needlestick—to blood infected with hepatitis B virus, hepatitis B immune globulin provides better protection than ordinary immune serum globulin. Infants born to mothers with hepatitis B are given hepatitis B immune globulin and are vaccinated. This combination prevents chronic hepatitis B in about 70 percent of those infants.

Chronic Hepatitis

Chronic hepatitis is inflammation of the liver that lasts at least 6 months.

Chronic hepatitis, though much less common than acute hepatitis, can persist for years, even decades. It is usually quite mild and doesn't produce any symptoms or significant liver damage. In some cases, though, continued inflammation slowly damages the liver, eventually producing cirrhosis and liver failure.

Causes

Hepatitis C virus is a common cause of chronic hepatitis; about 75 percent of acute hepatitis C cases become chronic. Hepatitis B virus, sometimes with hepatitis D virus, causes a smaller percentage of chronic infections. Hepatitis A and E viruses do not cause chronic hepatitis. Drugs such as methyldopa, isoniazid, nitrofurantoin, and possibly acetaminophen can also cause chronic hepatitis, particularly when they are taken for prolonged periods. Wilson's disease, a rare hereditary disease involving abnormal copper retention,▲ may cause chronic hepatitis in children and young adults.

No one knows exactly why the same viruses and drugs will cause chronic hepatitis in some people but not in others, or why the degree of severity varies. One possible explanation is that in people who develop chronic hepatitis, the immune system overreacts to the viral infection or drug.

In many people with chronic hepatitis, no obvious cause can be found. In some of these people, there appears to be an overactive immune system reaction that is responsible for the chronic inflammation. This condition, called **autoimmune hepatitis,** is more common among women than men.

Symptoms and Diagnosis

About a third of chronic hepatitis cases develop after a bout of acute viral hepatitis. The remainder develop gradually without any obvious previous illness.

Many people with chronic hepatitis have no symptoms at all. For those who do, the symptoms often include a feeling of illness, poor appetite, and fatigue. Sometimes the person also has a low fever and some upper abdominal discomfort. Jaundice may or may not develop. Features of chronic liver disease may eventually develop. These can include an enlarged spleen, spiderlike blood vessels in the skin, and fluid retention. Other features may occur, especially in young women with autoimmune hepatitis. These can involve virtually any body system and include acne, cessation of menstrual periods, joint pain, lung scarring, inflammation of the thyroid gland and kidneys, and anemia.

Although the person's symptoms and liver function test results provide helpful diagnostic information, a liver biopsy (removal of a tissue sample for examination under a microscope) ■ is essential for a definite diagnosis. Examining liver tissue under a microscope allows a doctor to determine the severity of the inflammation and whether any scarring or cirrhosis has developed. The biopsy may also reveal the underlying cause of the hepatitis.

Prognosis and Treatment

Many people have chronic hepatitis for years without developing progressive liver damage. For others, the disease gradually worsens. When this happens and the disease is the result of viral hepatitis B or C infection, the antiviral agent interferon-alpha may stop the inflammation. However, the drug is expensive, adverse effects are common, and hepatitis tends to recur once treatment is stopped. Therefore, such treatment is reserved for selected people with the infection. Ribavirin with interferon-alpha may be a better treatment.

Autoimmune hepatitis is usually treated with corticosteroids, sometimes together with azathioprine. These drugs suppress the inflammation, resolve the symptoms, and improve long-

▲ see page 662

■ see page 560

term survival. Nevertheless, scarring (fibrosis) in the liver may gradually worsen. Discontinuing therapy usually leads to a recurrence, so most people have to take the drugs indefinitely. Over a period of years, about 50 percent of the people with autoimmune hepatitis develop cirrhosis, liver failure, or both.

If a drug is suspected to cause the hepatitis, the person should stop taking it. Doing so may make the chronic hepatitis disappear.

Regardless of the cause or type of chronic hepatitis, any complications—such as ascites (fluid in the abdominal cavity)▲ or encephalopathy (abnormal brain function)■—require treatment.

CHAPTER 119

Blood Vessel Disorders of the Liver

The liver receives a quarter of its blood supply from the hepatic artery, which comes from the heart. The other three quarters of its blood supply comes from the portal vein, which drains the intestine. Blood draining from the intestine is filled with digested food substances for the liver to process.

Blood leaves the liver through the hepatic vein. This blood is a mixture of blood from the hepatic artery and blood from the portal vein. The hepatic vein drains into the vena cava—the largest vein in the body—which then empties into the heart.

Abnormalities of the Hepatic Artery

The hepatic artery provides the only blood supply to certain parts of the liver, particularly the supporting tissue and the walls of the bile ducts. Narrowing or blockage of the artery or its branches can cause considerable damage to these areas. Flow through the artery may be disrupted by an injury, such as a gunshot wound or surgical trauma, or by a blood clot. Blood clots generally are caused by inflammation of the arterial wall (arteritis), or by an infusion of anticancer drugs or other toxic or irritating substances into the artery.

Aneurysms can also affect the hepatic artery. Aneurysms are a bulge at a weak spot in an artery; an aneurysm in the hepatic artery is usually caused by infection, arteriosclerosis, injury, or polyarteritis nodosa. An aneurysm that presses on a nearby bile duct may narrow or even block it, and jaundice may develop because bile flow from the liver backs up. As many as three quarters of these aneurysms rupture, often causing massive bleeding. An aneurysm may be treated by inserting a catheter into the hepatic artery and injecting an irritating substance that causes a blockage. If this procedure (called embolization) fails, surgery is performed to repair the artery.

Veno-occlusive Disease

Veno-occlusive disease is blockage of the small veins in the liver.

Veno-occlusive disease may occur at any age, but children ages 1 to 3 are particularly vulnerable because they have smaller blood vessels. Blockage may be caused by drugs and other substances toxic to the liver, such as *Senecio* leaves (used in Jamaica to make herbal tea), dimethylnitrosamine, aflatoxin, and anticancer drugs such as azathioprine. Radiation therapy also can produce a blockage of the small veins, as can antibodies produced during rejection of a liver transplant.★

A blockage causes a backup of blood in the liver, reducing the liver's blood supply. The insufficient blood supply, in turn, damages the liver cells.

▲ see page 564

■ see page 564

★ see page 835

Blood Supply of the Liver

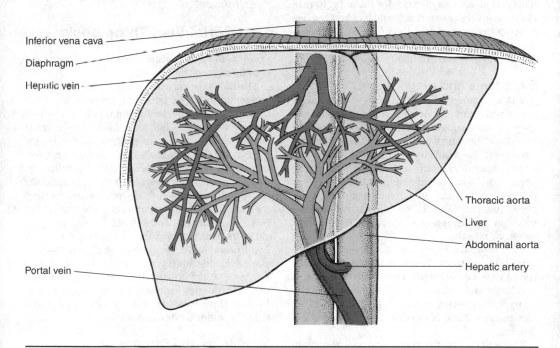

Inferior vena cava

Diaphragm

Hepatic vein

Thoracic aorta

Liver

Abdominal aorta

Hepatic artery

Portal vein

Symptoms, Prognosis, and Treatment

Blockage of the small veins causes the liver to swell with blood, making it tender to the touch. Fluid may leak from the surface of the swollen liver and accumulate in the abdomen, producing a condition called ascites.▲ The backup of blood in the liver also raises the pressure in the portal vein (a condition called portal hypertension) ■ and in the veins that empty into it. This higher pressure may cause varicose veins in the esophagus (esophageal varices), which may rupture and hemorrhage.

Typically, a blockage disappears quickly, and the person recovers with or without treatment. However, some people die of liver failure.★ In others, the pressure in the portal vein remains high and the injury leads to cirrhosis.● The only treatment is to stop taking the substance or drug causing the blockage. The exact course of the disease depends on the extent of damage and whether or not it recurs. A chronic course is more common, particularly when the blockage is caused by the consumption of herbal teas containing the toxic alkaloid.

Budd-Chiari Syndrome

Budd-Chiari syndrome is a rare disorder usually caused by blood clots that completely or partially block the large veins that drain the liver.

▲ see page 564

■ see page 563

★ see page 565

● see page 567

Usually the cause of Budd-Chiari syndrome is not known. Sometimes the person has a condition that increases the likelihood of blood clots—pregnancy or sickle cell disease, for instance. In rare cases, the veins are not actually blocked but are missing because of a birth defect. Fewer than a third of the people with Budd-Chiari syndrome survive for 1 year without effective treatment.

Symptoms and Diagnosis

The symptoms of Budd-Chiari syndrome may begin suddenly and be devastating, but usually they come on gradually. The liver swells with blood and becomes tender. Fluid leaks from the surface of the swollen liver into the abdominal cavity. Abdominal pain and mild jaundice may occur. The blood accumulation in the liver raises the pressure in the portal vein,▲ although the consequences, such as bleeding from varicose veins in the esophagus, may not develop for weeks or months.

After several months, jaundice, fever, and other symptoms of liver failure may appear. Sometimes the blood clots enlarge so much that they block the lower part of the largest vein entering the heart (the inferior vena cava). This blockage causes considerable swelling in the legs and abdomen.

The characteristic symptoms are the main clues to the diagnosis. X-rays of the veins taken after an injection of a radiopaque substance may reveal the precise location of the blockage. A magnetic resonance imaging (MRI) scan can also help in making the diagnosis. A liver biopsy (in which a sample of liver tissue is removed by needle for examination under a microscope) and ultrasound scans may help distinguish Budd-Chiari syndrome from similar diseases.

Treatment

If the vein is narrowed rather than blocked, anticoagulants (drugs that prevent clots) or thrombolytics (drugs that dissolve clots) may be used. In some cases, surgery may be performed to connect the portal vein to the vena cava, thus decompressing the portal vein through a bypass of the liver. Liver transplantation can be the most effective treatment.

Portal Vein Thrombosis

Portal vein thrombosis is a blockage of the portal vein by a blood clot.

The blockage may be caused by cirrhosis or by cancer of the liver, pancreas, or stomach. Or it may be caused by an inflammation of the bile ducts (cholangitis), inflammation of the pancreas (pancreatitis), or a liver abscess. In newborns, portal vein thrombosis may result from an infection of the navel (umbilicus). Portal vein thrombosis can occur in pregnant women, especially those with eclampsia (a disorder characterized by high blood pressure, protein in the urine, fluid retention, seizures, and sometimes coma).■

Portal vein thrombosis also can occur in any condition that backs up blood in the portal vein, such as Budd-Chiari syndrome, chronic heart failure, or chronic constrictive pericarditis. An abnormal tendency for blood to clot can cause portal vein thrombosis as well. The cause of portal vein thrombosis often cannot be found.

Symptoms and Diagnosis

Because the portal vein provides three quarters of the liver's blood supply, partial or complete blockage of the vein may damage liver cells, depending on where the clot is, how big it is, and how rapidly it develops. Blockage raises the pressure in the portal vein and the other veins that drain into it. The veins in the esophagus become enlarged. Often the first symptom of portal vein thrombosis is bleeding from varicose veins at the lower end of the esophagus (esophageal varices). The bleeding results in coughing up or vomiting of blood. The spleen typically enlarges, especially in children with this disorder. A doctor will then feel an enlarged spleen, which may be tender.

In about one third of the people with portal vein thrombosis, a blockage develops slowly, allowing other blood channels (collateral channels) to become established around the block, and eventually the portal vein reopens. Despite such reopening, portal hypertension may persist.

▲ see page 563

■ see page 1158

If the person has high pressure in the portal vein (portal hypertension), and microscopic examination of a liver tissue sample reveals that the cells are normal, portal vein thrombosis is the likely culprit. Ultrasound or computed tomography (CT) scans may show the blockage. The diagnosis is confirmed by angiography—an x-ray technique that creates images of the veins after a radiopaque substance is injected into the portal vein.

Treatment

Treatment is aimed at reducing the pressure in the portal vein and preventing bleeding from varicose veins in the esophagus. A doctor may first try to close the varicose veins by applying rubber bands or by injecting them with chemicals given through an endoscope (a flexible viewing tube with surgical attachments). Surgery may be necessary to create a connection (shunt) between the portal vein and the vena cava, causing blood flow to bypass the liver and reducing the pressure in the portal vein. However, the bypass operation increases the risk of liver encephalopathy (brain damage from liver disease).▲

Blood Vessel Disorders Resulting From Other Diseases

Severe heart failure can cause increased pressure in the veins leading from the liver. This increased pressure can lead to liver damage. Treating the heart failure often allows normal liver function to resume.

In sickle cell disease, abnormally shaped red blood cells block blood vessels inside the liver, causing liver damage.

Hereditary hemorrhagic telangiectasia (Rendu-Osler-Weber disease)■ is an inherited disorder that can affect the liver. When the liver is affected, small areas of abnormally wide blood vessels (telangiectasia) develop in the liver. These abnormal blood vessels create short circuits (shunts) between arteries and veins. The shunts can cause severe heart failure, which can further damage and enlarge the liver. The shunted blood flow also produces a continuous roaring noise (bruit) that can be heard through a stethoscope. Parts of the liver have scars (cirrhosis and fibrosis) and noncancerous tumors composed of blood vessels (hemangiomas).

CHAPTER 120

Liver Tumors

Liver tumors may be noncancerous (benign) or cancerous (malignant). Cancerous tumors may originate in the liver, or they may spread (metastasize) to the liver from other parts of the body. Cancer originating in the liver is called primary liver cancer; cancer originating elsewhere in the body is called metastatic cancer. The vast majority of liver cancers are metastatic.

Noncancerous liver tumors are relatively common but usually cause no symptoms. Most are detected when people have a scanning test—such as ultrasound, computed tomography (CT), or magnetic resonance imaging (MRI)—for an unrelated reason. However, some of these tumors cause the liver to enlarge or to bleed into the abdominal cavity. The liver usually functions normally, so blood tests show normal or only slightly elevated levels of liver enzymes.

Hepatocellular Adenoma

A hepatocellular adenoma is a common noncancerous tumor of the liver.

Hepatocellular adenomas occur mainly in women of childbearing age, probably because oral contraceptives increase the risk of this type of growth. These tumors usually cause no symptoms, so most remain undetected. Rarely, an adenoma suddenly ruptures and bleeds into the abdominal cavity, requiring emergency surgery. Adenomas caused by oral contraceptives often disappear when the woman stops taking the drug.

▲ see page 564

■ see page 754

In extremely rare cases, an adenoma may become cancerous.

Hemangioma

A hemangioma is a noncancerous tumor of the liver composed of a mass of abnormal blood vessels.

An estimated 1 to 5 percent of adults have small liver hemangiomas that cause no symptoms. These tumors are usually detected only if the person happens to undergo an ultrasound or computed tomography (CT) scan. They don't require treatment. In infants, large hemangiomas occasionally produce symptoms that lead to their detection, such as widespread clotting and heart failure. Surgery may be required.

Hepatoma

A hepatoma (hepatocellular carcinoma) is a cancer that begins in the liver cells.

Hepatomas are the most common type of cancer originating in the liver (primary liver cancer). In certain areas of Africa and Southeast Asia, hepatomas are even more common than metastatic liver cancer, and they are a prominent cause of death. In these areas, there is a high prevalence of chronic infection with the hepatitis B virus, which increases the risk of hepatomas more than 100-fold. Chronic infection with hepatitis C also increases the risk of hepatomas. Finally, certain cancer-causing substances (carcinogens) produce hepatomas. In subtropical regions where hepatomas are common, food is often contaminated by carcinogens called aflatoxins, substances that are produced by certain types of fungi.

In North America, Europe, and other areas of the world where hepatomas are less common, most people with hepatomas are alcoholics with long-standing liver cirrhosis. Additional types of cirrhosis are also associated with hepatomas, though the risk is lower with primary biliary cirrhosis than with other types.

Fibrolamellar carcinoma is a rare type of hepatoma that usually affects relatively young adults. It isn't caused by preexisting cirrhosis, hepatitis B or C infection, or other known risk factors.

─────────────────────

▲ see box, page 558

■ see page 560

Symptoms

Usually, the first symptoms of a hepatoma are abdominal pain, weight loss, and a large mass that can be felt in the upper right part of the abdomen. Alternatively, a person who has had cirrhosis for a long time may unexpectedly become much more ill. A fever is common. Occasionally, the first symptoms are acute abdominal pain and shock, caused by a rupture or bleeding of the tumor.

Diagnosis

In people with hepatomas, blood levels of alpha-fetoprotein typically are high.▲ Occasionally, blood tests reveal low levels of glucose or high levels of calcium, lipids, or red blood cells.

At first, the symptoms don't provide many clues to the diagnosis. However, once the liver enlarges enough to be felt, a doctor may suspect the diagnosis, especially if the person has long-standing cirrhosis. Occasionally, a doctor can hear rushing sounds (hepatic bruits) and scratchy sounds (friction rubs) when a stethoscope is placed over the liver.

Abdominal ultrasound and computed tomography (CT) scans sometimes detect cancers that haven't yet caused symptoms. In some countries where the hepatitis B virus is common, such as Japan, ultrasound scans are used to screen people with the infection for liver cancer. Hepatic arteriography (x-rays taken after a radiopaque substance is injected into the hepatic artery) may reveal hepatomas. Hepatic arteriography is particularly useful before surgical removal of the hepatoma because it shows the surgeon the precise location of the liver blood vessels.

A liver biopsy, in which a small sample of liver tissue is removed by needle for examination under a microscope,■ can confirm the diagnosis. The risk of bleeding or other injury during a liver biopsy generally is low.

Prognosis and Treatment

Usually, the prognosis for people with a hepatoma is poor because the tumor is detected too late. Occasionally, a person with a small tumor may do very well after the tumor is surgically removed.

Other Primary Liver Cancers

A **cholangiocarcinoma** is a cancer that originates in the lining of the bile channels in the liver or bile ducts. In the Orient, infestation with parasites called liver flukes may be partly responsible for this cancer. People with long-standing ulcerative colitis and sclerosing cholangitis occasionally develop cholangiocarcinoma.

A **hepatoblastoma** is one of the more common cancers in infants. Occasionally, it occurs in older children and may produce hormones called gonadotropins that result in early (precocious) puberty.▲ A hepatoblastoma is usually detected because of overall failing health and a large mass in the upper right part of the abdomen.

An **angiosarcoma** is a rare cancer originating in the blood vessels of the liver. An angiosarcoma may be caused by exposure to vinyl chloride in the workplace.

Diagnosis and Treatment

Cholangiocarcinomas, hepatoblastomas, and angiosarcomas can be diagnosed only by liver biopsy, in which a sample of liver tissue is removed by needle for examination under a microscope.■ Usually, treatment has little value, and most people die within a few months of when the tumor is detected. If the cancer is detected relatively early, however, the tumor may be surgically removed, offering the hope of long-term survival.

Metastatic Liver Cancers

Metastatic liver cancers are tumors that have spread to the liver from elsewhere in the body.

Metastatic liver cancer most commonly comes from the lung, breast, colon, pancreas, and stomach. Leukemia and other blood cell cancers, such as lymphomas, may involve the liver. Sometimes the discovery of a metastatic liver tumor is the first indication that a person has cancer.

Symptoms

Often, the first symptoms include weight loss and poor appetite. Typically, the liver is enlarged and hard and may be tender. Fever may be present. Occasionally the spleen is enlarged, especially if the cancer originated in the pancreas. The abdominal cavity may become distended with fluid, a condition called ascites.★ At first, jaundice is absent or mild, unless the cancer is blocking the bile ducts. In the weeks before the person dies, jaundice progressively worsens. Also, the person may become confused and drowsy as toxins accumulate in the brain, a condition called liver encephalopathy.●

Diagnosis

In the late stages of the disease, a doctor usually can diagnose metastatic liver cancer fairly easily, but the diagnosis is more difficult in the early stages. Ultrasound, computed tomography (CT), and magnetic resonance imaging (MRI) of the liver may reveal the cancer, but these scans can't always detect small tumors or distinguish a tumor from cirrhosis and other abnormalities. The tumors often cause liver malfunction, which can be detected by blood tests.

A liver biopsy, in which a sample of liver tissue is removed by needle for examination under a microscope, confirms the diagnosis in only about 75 percent of the cases. To improve the chances of obtaining cancerous tissue, ultrasound can be used to guide the insertion of the biopsy needle. Alternatively, a biopsy specimen may be obtained while a doctor looks at the liver through a laparoscope (a fiber-optic viewing tube that is inserted through the abdominal wall).

Leukemia usually is diagnosed based on the results of blood and bone marrow tests. Typically, a liver biopsy isn't needed.

Treatment

Depending on the type of cancer, anticancer drugs may temporarily shrink the tumor and prolong life, but they don't cure the cancer. Anticancer drugs may be injected into the hepatic artery, which then delivers a high concentration of the drugs directly to the cancer cells in the liver. This technique is more likely to shrink the tumor and to produce fewer side effects, but it hasn't been proved to prolong life. Radiation therapy to the liver can sometimes reduce severe pain, but it has little other benefit.

If only a single tumor is found in the liver, a surgeon may remove it, especially if it comes from cancer of the intestine. However, not all experts consider this surgery worthwhile. For most people with extensive cancer, all a doctor can do is relieve the symptoms.

▲ see page 1257

■ see page 560

★ see page 564

● see page 564

CHAPTER 121

Gallbladder Disorders

The gallbladder is a small, pear-shaped organ situated beneath the liver. The gallbladder stores bile, a greenish-yellow digestive fluid produced by the liver, until it is needed by the digestive system. Bile consists of bile salts, electrolytes, bilirubin, cholesterol, and other fats (lipids). Bile makes the cholesterol, fats, and vitamins in fatty foods more soluble, so they can be better absorbed by the body. Bile salts stimulate the large intestine to secrete water and other salts, which help move the intestinal contents along and out of the body. Bilirubin, a waste product consisting of the remains of worn-out red blood cells, is excreted in bile. The breakdown products of drugs and waste products processed by the liver are also excreted in bile.

Bile flows from the narrow collecting ducts inside the liver into the left and right hepatic ducts, then into the common hepatic duct, then into the larger common bile duct.▲ About half the bile secreted between meals flows directly through the common bile duct into the small intestine. The other half is diverted from the common bile duct through the cystic duct and into the gallbladder, where bile is stored. In the gallbladder, up to 90 percent of the water in the bile is absorbed into the bloodstream. What remains in the gallbladder is a concentrated solution of bile salts, biliary lipids, and sodium.

When food enters the small intestine, a series of hormonal and nerve signals trigger the gallbladder to contract and a sphincter (the sphincter of Oddi) to open. Bile then flows from the gallbladder into the small intestine to mix with food contents and perform its digestive functions.

A large proportion of the gallbladder's store of bile salts is released into the small intestine, and about 90 percent of the bile salts are reabsorbed into the bloodstream through the wall of the lower small intestine. The liver then extracts the bile salts from the blood and resecretes them back into the bile. The bile salts in the body go through this cycle about 10 to 12 times a day. Each time, small amounts of bile salts reach the large intestine, where they are broken down by bacteria. Some of the bile salts are reabsorbed in the large intestine; the rest are excreted in the stool.

Gallstones

Gallstones are collections of crystals in the gallbladder or the bile ducts (biliary tract). When gallstones are in the gallbladder, the condition is called **cholelithiasis;** *when gallstones are in the bile ducts, the condition is called* **choledocholithiasis.**

Gallstones are more common in women and in certain groups of people, such as Native Americans. The risk factors for gallstone formation include old age, obesity, a Western diet, and a genetic predisposition. In the United States, 20 percent of the people over age 65 have gallstones, but most never experience problems. Each year, more than half a million people have their gallbladder surgically removed—most of them doing so because gallstones have caused problems.

The major component of most gallstones is cholesterol, though some are made up of calcium salts. Bile contains large amounts of cholesterol that usually remains liquid. When bile becomes oversaturated with cholesterol, however, the cholesterol may become insoluble and precipitates out of the bile.

Most gallstones form in the gallbladder. Most gallstones in the bile ducts travel there from the gallbladder. Stones may form in a bile duct when bile backs up because a duct has narrowed abnormally or after the gallbladder has been removed.

Gallstones in the bile ducts can lead to a severe or life-threatening infection of the bile ducts (cholangitis), the pancreas (pancreatitis), or the liver. When the bile duct system is obstructed, bacteria can flourish and quickly establish infection in the ducts. The bacteria may spread to the bloodstream and cause infections elsewhere in the body.

Symptoms

Most gallstones don't cause any symptoms for long periods, if ever, particularly if they remain in the gallbladder. Rarely, however, large gallstones may gradually erode the gallbladder wall and en-

▲ see box, page 556

ter the small or large intestine, where they can cause an intestinal obstruction, called a gallstone ileus. Much more typically, gallstones pass from the gallbladder into the bile ducts. They may pass through these ducts and into the small intestine without incident, or they may remain in the ducts without obstructing the flow of bile or causing symptoms.

When gallstones partially or transiently obstruct a bile duct, a person experiences pain. The pain tends to come and go—a quality referred to as colic. Typically, this pain rises slowly to a plateau and then falls gradually. The pain may be sharp and intermittent, lasting up to several hours. The location of the pain varies. Most often, the pain is in the right upper part of the abdomen, which also may be tender. The pain may extend to the right shoulder blade. Often the person is nauseated and vomits; if an infection develops with duct obstruction, the person has a fever, chills, and jaundice. Usually, the obstruction is temporary and isn't complicated by an infection. Pain caused by duct obstruction may be indistinguishable from that caused by gallbladder obstruction.

A persistent obstruction that blocks the cystic duct causes the gallbladder to become inflamed (a condition called acute cholecystitis).▲ Gallstones that obstruct the pancreatic duct cause inflammation of the pancreas (pancreatitis) as well as pain, jaundice, and possibly infection. Sometimes, intermittent pain returns after the gallbladder has been removed; such pain may be caused by gallstones in the common bile duct.

Symptoms of indigestion and intolerance of fatty foods often are mistakenly blamed on gallstones. A person who experiences belching, bloating, a feeling of fullness, and nausea is just as likely to have peptic ulcer disease or indigestion as to have gallstones. Pain in the right upper part of the abdomen that occurs after eating fatty foods may result from gallstones. But indigestion after meals is common and only rarely indicates gallstones.

Diagnosis

Ultrasound scanning is the best method for diagnosing gallstones in the gallbladder. Cholecystography also is effective. With cholecystography, an x-ray shows the path of a radiopaque contrast substance as it is swallowed, absorbed

Rare Gallbladder Disorders

Cholesterol may be deposited in the lining of the gallbladder. The cholesterol deposits appear as small yellow specks that are highlighted against a red background (a condition called **strawberry gallbladder**). Eventually, noncancerous growths (polyps) may form inside the gallbladder. The disorder may occasionally cause pain and require surgical removal of the gallbladder.

Diverticulosis of the gallbladder, small fingerlike outpouchings of the gallbladder lining, may develop as a person ages. The diverticulosis may cause inflammation and require surgical removal of the gallbladder.

in the intestine, secreted into the bile, and stored in the gallbladder. If the gallbladder isn't functioning, the contrast material won't show up in the gallbladder. If the gallbladder is functioning, the outline of the gallstone is revealed in the x-rays by the contrast material. By using ultrasound and cholecystography together, a doctor can identify gallstones in the gallbladder 98 percent of the time. However, the tests may give false-positive results in a few people who don't have gallstones.

When a person has abdominal pain, jaundice, chills, and a fever, gallstones in the bile duct are a strong possibility. Blood test results usually show a pattern of abnormal liver function that suggests bile duct obstruction. Several tests can provide the additional information needed to make a firm diagnosis. These include ultrasound scans, computed tomography (CT), and various x-ray techniques using a radiopaque contrast substance to outline the bile ducts.■ Ultrasound scanning and CT can show whether the bile duct is dilated, but the ducts can be obstructed without being dilated. The x-ray techniques help detect an obstruction and, if present, whether it is caused by a gallstone.

▲ see page 582

■ see box, page 559

Which diagnostic x-ray technique is used depends on the situation. If the diagnosis is fairly certain, many doctors perform one of the x-ray techniques before deciding on surgery. If the diagnosis is uncertain, ultrasound scanning may be performed first.

Treatment

Most people who have "silent" gallstones in the gallbladder (that is, without symptoms) don't require treatment. People with intermittent pain can try avoiding or reducing their intake of fatty foods. Doing so may help prevent or reduce the number of pain episodes.

Gallstones in the Gallbladder

If gallstones in the gallbladder cause recurring attacks of pain despite dietary changes, a doctor may recommend gallbladder removal (cholecystectomy). Gallbladder removal doesn't cause nutritional deficiencies, and no dietary restrictions are required after surgery. About 1 to 5 people of every 1,000 who undergo this surgery die. During cholecystectomy, the doctor may investigate the possibility of stones in the bile ducts.

Laparoscopic cholecystectomy was introduced in 1990 and in an amazingly brief time has revolutionized surgical practice. About 90 percent of cholecystectomies are now performed laparoscopically. With laparoscopic cholecystectomy, the gallbladder is removed through tubes that are inserted through small incisions in the abdominal wall. The whole procedure is performed with the help of a camera (laparoscope), also placed in the abdomen through the incisions. Laparoscopic cholecystectomy has lessened postoperative discomfort, shortened the hospital stay, and reduced sick leave.

Other methods of eliminating gallstones introduced during the past decade include dissolution with methyl-*tert*-butyl ether and fragmentation with sonic shock waves (lithotripsy). An even earlier treatment involved dissolving gallstones with chronic bile acid therapy (chenodiol and ursodeoxycholic acid).

Gallstones in the Bile Ducts

Gallstones in the bile ducts can cause serious problems; therefore, they should be removed either by abdominal surgery or by a procedure called endoscopic retrograde cholangiopancreatography (ERCP). With ERCP, an endoscope (a flexible viewing tube with surgical attachments) is passed through the mouth, down the esophagus, through the stomach, and into the small intestine.▲ Radiopaque contrast material is passed into the bile duct through a tube in the sphincter of Oddi. In a procedure called a sphincterotomy, the muscle sphincter is opened wide enough to let the gallstones that were obstructing the bile duct pass through into the small intestine. ERCP and sphincterotomy are successful in 90 percent of cases. Fewer than 4 people in 1,000 die, and 3 to 7 people in 100 develop complications, making these procedures a safer option than abdominal surgery. Immediate complications include bleeding, inflammation of the pancreas (pancreatitis), and perforation or infection of the bile ducts. In 2 to 6 percent of the people, the ducts constrict again, and gallstones reappear. Gallstones located only in the gallbladder cannot be removed by ERCP.

Usually, ERCP alone is best for older people who have gallstones in their ducts and who have already had their gallbladder removed. For these people, the success rate is comparable to that of abdominal surgery. In most elderly people who have never had gallbladder problems, removing the gallbladder is unnecessary because only about 5 percent of elderly people have repeated symptoms of gallstones in the bile ducts.

People under age 60 with bouts of bile duct or gallbladder problems usually have their gallbladder removed electively after they have gone through ERCP and sphincterotomy. Otherwise, they are at some risk for developing acute gallbladder problems some time in later years. Most stones are removed from the bile duct during the ERCP procedure. If gallstones remain in the duct, they will often be passed subsequently through the permanent sphincterotomy. Any remaining gallstones can then be removed by endoscopy before the drain in the bile duct inserted during surgery is taken out.

Acute Cholecystitis

Acute cholecystitis is inflammation of the gallbladder wall, usually resulting from a gallstone in the cystic duct, that causes an attack of sudden, extreme pain.

▲ see box, page 559

At least 95 percent of the people with acute gallbladder inflammation have gallstones. Rarely, a bacterial infection causes inflammation.

Acute gallbladder inflammation without gallstones is a serious disease. It tends to occur after injuries, operations, burns, bodywide infections (sepsis), and critical illnesses—particularly in patients receiving prolonged intravenous feedings. The person usually has no previous signs of gallbladder disease before experiencing sudden, excruciating pain in the upper abdomen. Usually, the disease is very severe and can lead to gangrene or perforation of the gallbladder. Immediate surgery is necessary to remove the diseased gallbladder.

Symptoms

Pain, usually in the right upper part of the abdomen, is the first sign of gallbladder inflammation. The pain may worsen when the person breathes deeply and often extends to the lower part of the right shoulder blade. The pain may become excruciating; nausea and vomiting are usual.

The person typically feels a sharp pain when a doctor presses the upper right part of the abdomen. Within a few hours, the abdominal muscles on the right side may become rigid. At first, the person may have only a slight fever. Over time, it tends to become higher.

Typically, a gallbladder attack subsides in 2 or 3 days and completely disappears in a week. If it doesn't, the person may have serious complications. A high fever, shivering, a marked increase in the white blood cell count, and a cessation of the normal propulsive movement of the intestine (ileus) can indicate abscess formation, gangrene, or gallbladder perforation. Immediate surgery is needed for these conditions.

Other complications may occur. A gallbladder attack accompanied by jaundice or a backup of bile into the liver indicates that the common bile duct may be partially obstructed by a gallstone or by inflammation. If blood tests reveal an increased level of the enzyme amylase, the person may have inflammation of the pancreas (pancreatitis) caused by gallstone obstruction of the pancreatic duct.

Diagnosis

Doctors diagnose acute gallbladder inflammation based on the person's symptoms and the results of certain tests. Ultrasound scans often can help confirm the presence of gallstones in the gallbladder and can show thickening of the gallbladder wall. Hepatobiliary scintigraphy (an imaging technique used after a radioactive substance has been injected intravenously) provides the most accurate diagnosis. With this test, images are taken of the liver, the bile ducts, the gallbladder, and the upper part of the small intestine.

Treatment

A person with acute gallbladder inflammation generally is hospitalized, receives fluids and electrolytes intravenously, and is not allowed to eat or drink. A doctor may pass a tube through the nose and into the stomach, so that suctioning can be used to keep the stomach empty and thus reduce stimulation of the gallbladder. Usually, antibiotics are given as soon as acute gallbladder inflammation is suspected.

If the diagnosis is certain and the risk of surgery is small, the gallbladder usually is removed during the first day or two of the illness. However, if the person has another illness that increases the risk of surgery, then the operation may be delayed while that disease is treated. If the attack subsides, the gallbladder may be removed later—preferably after 6 weeks or more. If complications such as abscess formation, gangrene, or perforation of the gallbladder are suspected, immediate surgery generally is needed.

A small percentage of people have new or recurring episodes of pain that feel like gallbladder attacks even though they have no gallbladder. The cause of these episodes isn't known, but they may result from an abnormal function of the sphincter of Oddi, the opening that controls the release of bile into the small intestine. Pain is believed to result from increased pressure in the ducts caused by resistance to the flow of bile or pancreatic secretions. In some people, small gallstones remaining after surgery may cause pain. A doctor can use an endoscope (a viewing tube with surgical attachments) to widen the sphincter of Oddi. This procedure usually relieves symptoms in people who have a recognizable abnormality of the sphincter, but it won't help those who only have pain.

Chronic Cholecystitis

Chronic cholecystitis is long-standing inflammation of the gallbladder characterized by repeated attacks of severe, sharp abdominal pain.

Less Common Causes of Bile Duct Obstruction

Occasionally, a condition other than gallstones or tumors causes a bile duct obstruction. For instance, an injury during gallbladder surgery may cause an obstruction, or the duct may be narrowed as it passes through a chronically diseased pancreas. Rarer causes of obstruction include infection by the parasite *Ascaris lumbricoides* or *Clonorchis sinensis*.

A damaged gallbladder is thick-walled, contracted, and small. The walls consist largely of fibrous material. The lining inside the gallbladder may be ulcerated and scarred, and the gallbladder contains sludge or gallstones that often obstruct the cystic duct. This condition is probably caused by the damage and repeated repair of previous episodes of acute inflammation, often from gallstones.

Bile Duct Tumors

Aside from gallstones, cancer is the most common cause of bile duct obstruction. Most cancers originate in the head of the pancreas, which the common bile duct runs through. Less commonly, cancers originate in the biliary tract itself at the junction of the common bile duct and the pancreatic duct, in the gallbladder, or in the liver. Much less commonly, the bile ducts may be obstructed by cancer that has spread (metastasized) from

elsewhere in the body, or the bile ducts may be compressed by lymph nodes affected with lymphoma. Noncancerous (benign) tumors in bile ducts also cause obstruction.

Symptoms and Diagnosis

The symptoms of bile duct obstruction are jaundice, abdominal discomfort, loss of appetite, weight loss, and itching, usually without fever and chills. Symptoms gradually worsen. The diagnosis of cancer as the cause of the obstruction is made using ultrasound scanning, computed tomography (CT), or direct cholangiography (an x-ray taken after injection of radiopaque contrast material). To make a firm diagnosis, a doctor performs a biopsy (obtains a sample of tissue and examines it under a microscope).

Treatment

The treatment of bile duct tumors depends on the cause and circumstances. Surgery is the most direct way to determine the type of tumor, to find out if it can be removed, and to ensure that bile can flow around the obstruction. Most often, the cancer can't be completely removed, and most of these cancers don't respond well to radiation therapy. Chemotherapy may provide some relief from the symptoms.

Some people with bile duct obstruction from cancer experience pain, itching, and a buildup of pus caused by a bacterial infection. If they don't have surgery, then a doctor may insert a stent (a bypass tube) through a flexible endoscope to allow the bile and any pus to flow around the cancer. This procedure not only relieves the buildup of bile or pus but also helps control pain and relieve itching.

Kidney and Urinary Tract Disorders

Biology of the Kidneys and Urinary Tract

Normally, a person has two kidneys. Each kidney has a ureter, which drains urine from the kidney's central collecting area (renal pelvis) into the bladder. From the bladder, urine drains through the urethra, out of the body through the penis in males and the vulva in females.

The primary function of the kidneys is to filter metabolic waste products and excess sodium and water from the blood and help eliminate them from the body. The kidneys also help regulate blood pressure and red blood cell production.

Each kidney contains about a million filtering units (nephrons). A nephron begins as a hollow-walled, bowl-like structure (Bowman's capsule), which contains a tuft of blood vessels (the glomerulus). Collectively, these two structures are called a renal corpuscle.

Blood enters the glomerulus at high pressure. Much of the fluid part of blood is filtered through small pores in the walls of the blood vessels in the glomerulus and the inner layer of Bowman's capsule, leaving behind blood cells and most large molecules, such as proteins. The clear, filtered fluid (filtrate) enters Bowman's space (the area between the inner and outer layers of Bowman's capsule) and passes into the tube leading from Bowman's capsule. In the first part of the tube (proximal convoluted tubule), most of the sodium, water, glucose, and other filtered substances are reabsorbed and ultimately returned to the blood. The kidney also uses energy to selectively move a few large molecules, including drugs such as penicillin but not proteins, into the tubule. These molecules are excreted in the urine even though they're too big to pass through the pores of the glomerular filter. The next part of the nephron is the loop of Henle. As the fluid passes through the loop, sodium and several other electrolytes are pumped out and the remaining fluid becomes increasingly dilute. The dilute fluid passes up the next part of the nephron (distal convoluted tubule), where more sodium is pumped out in exchange for potassium.

Fluid from several nephrons passes into a collecting duct. In the collecting ducts, the fluid can continue through the kidney as dilute urine, or water can be absorbed from the urine and returned to the blood, making the urine more concentrated. Through hormones that affect kidney function, the body controls the concentration of urine according to its need for water.

Urine formed in the kidneys flows down the ureters into the bladder, but it doesn't flow passively like water through a pipe. The ureters are muscular tubes that push each small amount of urine along in waves of contraction. At the bladder, each ureter passes through a sphincter, a circular muscular structure that opens to let the urine through, then closes tightly like the aperture of a camera.

Urine accumulates in the bladder as it arrives regularly from each ureter. The bladder, which is expandable, gradually increases in size to accommodate the increasing volume of urine. When the bladder eventually fills, nerve signals are sent to the brain, conveying the need to urinate.

During urination, another sphincter, located between the bladder and urethra (at the bladder's outlet), opens, allowing urine to flow out. Simultaneously, the bladder wall contracts, creating pressure that forces the urine down the urethra. Tightening the muscles of the abdominal wall adds extra pressure. The sphincters through which the ureters enter the bladder remain tightly shut to prevent urine from flowing back up the ureters.

Symptoms of Kidney and Urinary Tract Disorders

Symptoms caused by kidney and urinary tract disorders vary according to the particular disorder and the part of the system affected.

Fever and a generally sick feeling (malaise) are common symptoms, although a bladder infection (cystitis) generally doesn't cause fever. A bacterial infection of the kidney (pyelonephritis) usually causes high fever. Kidney cancer occasionally causes fever.

Most people urinate about four to six times a day, mostly in the daytime. Frequent urination (frequency) without an increase in the total daily amount of urine is a symptom of a bladder infection or of something irritating the bladder, such as a foreign body, stone, or tumor. A tumor or other mass pressing on the bladder can also cause frequent urination. Bladder irritation can cause pain while urinating (dysuria) and a compelling need to urinate (urgency), which may feel like almost constant painful straining (tenesmus). The amount of urine is usually small, but bladder control may be lost if a person doesn't urinate immediately.

Frequent urination during the night (nocturia) may occur in the early stages of kidney disease, although the cause may simply be drinking a large amount of fluid, especially alcohol, coffee, or tea, in the late evening. A person may need to urinate frequently at night because the kidneys can't concentrate urine well. Frequent urination at night is also common in people who have heart failure, liver failure, or diabetes even though they don't have urinary tract disease. Frequent urination of very small amounts at night may result when urine backs up in the bladder because its outflow is obstructed; an enlarged prostate is the most common cause in older men.

Bed-wetting (enuresis) is normal during the first 2 or 3 years of life. After that, it may indicate a problem, such as delayed maturity of the muscles and nerves of the lower urinary tract, an infection or narrowing of the urethra, or inadequate control of the nerves of the bladder (neurogenic bladder). The problem is often genetic and occasionally psychologic.▲

A hesitating start when urinating, a need to strain, a weak and trickling stream of urine, and dribble at the end of urination are common symptoms of an obstructed urethra. In men, these symptoms are caused most commonly by an enlarged prostate and less often by a narrowing (stricture) of the urethra. Similar symptoms in a boy may mean that he was born with an abnormally narrow urethra or has a urethra with an abnormally narrow external opening. This opening may also be abnormally narrow in women.

An uncontrollable loss of urine (incontinence) can result from a variety of conditions. Urine may escape when a woman coughs, laughs, runs, or lifts because she has a cystocele (a herniation of the bladder into the vagina). A cystocele is generally caused by stretching and weakening of the pelvic muscles during childbirth or by changes that occur when estrogen levels decrease after menopause. Obstructed outflow from the bladder may cause incontinence whenever the pressure inside the bladder exceeds the force of the obstruction, although the bladder doesn't completely empty in this situation.

Passing gas in the urine, a rare symptom, usually indicates an abnormal connection (fistula) between the urinary tract and the intestine. A fistula may be a complication of diverticulitis, other types of intestinal inflammation, an abscess, or cancer. A fistula between the bladder and the vagina may also cause gas (air) to escape into the urine. Rarely, bacteria in the urine may produce gas.

Normally, adults pass about 3 cups to 2 quarts of urine daily. Many forms of kidney disease impair the kidney's ability to concentrate urine, in which case daily urine output can exceed $2\frac{1}{2}$ quarts. Very large amounts of urine are usually a response to a high blood glucose (sugar) concentration, a decreased concentration of antidiuretic hormone produced by the pituitary gland (diabetes insipidus),■ or the kidneys' lack of response to antidiuretic hormone (nephrogenic diabetes insipidus).★

Kidney disease or an obstruction of a ureter, the bladder, or the urethra may suddenly reduce the daily output of urine to less than 2 cups a day. The persistent output of less than about a cup of urine a day leads to the buildup of metabolic wastes in the blood (azotemia). Such low urine output may mean that the kidneys have suddenly failed or a chronic kidney problem has worsened.

Dilute urine can be nearly colorless. Concentrated urine is deep yellow. Food pigments can make the urine red, and drugs can produce a variety of colors: brown, black, blue, green, or red. Unless caused by food or drugs, colors other than yellow are abnormal. Brown urine may contain

▲ see pages 633 and 1249

■ see page 703

★ see page 615

Viewing the Urinary Tract

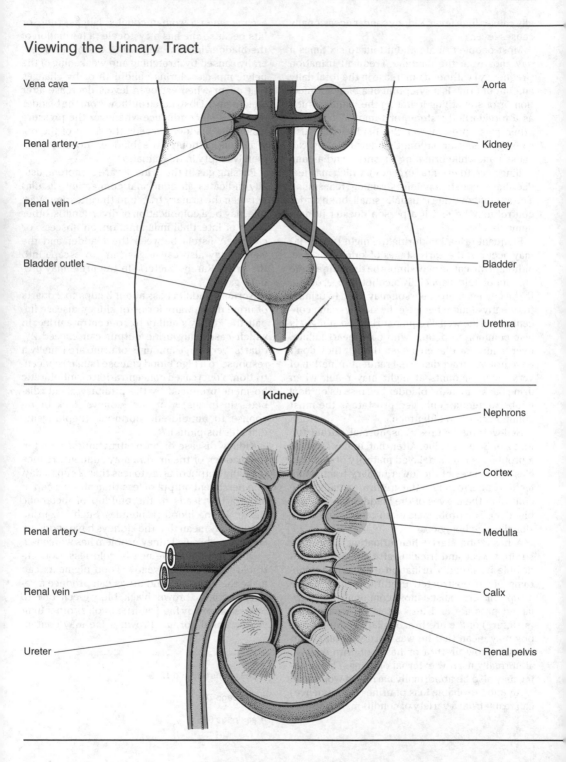

Vena cava

Renal artery

Renal vein

Bladder outlet

Aorta

Kidney

Ureter

Bladder

Urethra

Kidney

Renal artery

Renal vein

Ureter

Nephrons

Cortex

Medulla

Calix

Renal pelvis

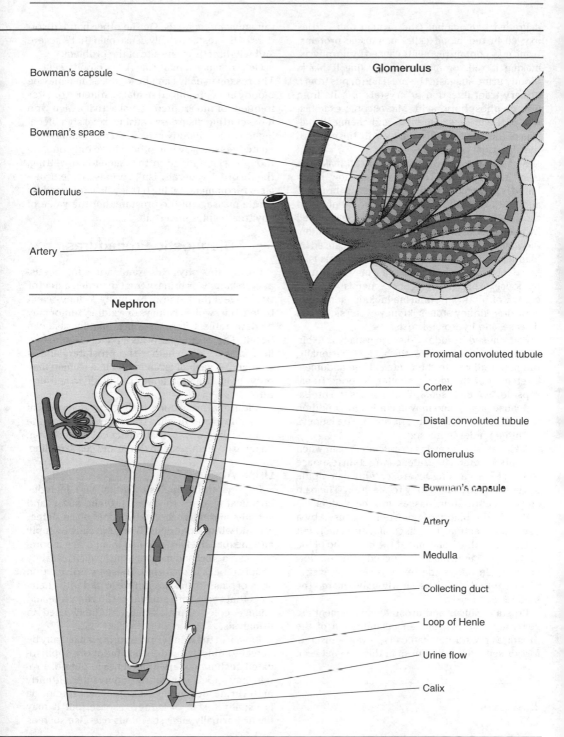

Bowman's capsule

Bowman's space

Glomerulus

Artery

Glomerulus

Nephron

Proximal convoluted tubule

Cortex

Distal convoluted tubule

Glomerulus

Bowman's capsule

Artery

Medulla

Collecting duct

Loop of Henle

Urine flow

Calix

degraded hemoglobin (the protein that carries oxygen in red blood cells) or muscle proteins. Urine may contain pigments caused by porphyria, making it red, or melanoma, making it black. Cloudy urine suggests the presence of pus from a urinary tract infection or crystals of salts from uric or phosphoric acid. Microscopic examination of the urine sediments▲ and chemical analysis of the urine usually can identify the cause of the abnormal color.

Blood in the urine (hematuria) can make the urine red to brown, depending on how much blood is present, how long it has been in the urine, and how acidic the urine is. An amount of blood too small to turn the urine red may be detected by chemical testing or microscopic examination. Blood in the urine without pain may be caused by bladder or kidney cancer. Such cancers usually bleed intermittently; the bleeding may stop spontaneously, though the cancer persists. Other causes of blood in the urine include glomerulonephritis, kidney stones, kidney cysts, sickle cell disease, and hydronephrosis.

Pain caused by kidney disease usually is felt in the side (flank) or small of the back. Occasionally, the pain radiates to the center of the abdomen. Stretching of the kidney's outer covering (renal capsule), which is sensitive to pain, is the probable cause of pain and may occur in any condition that makes the kidney tissue swell. The kidneys are often tender if pressed.

A kidney stone causes excruciating pain when it enters a ureter. The ureter contracts in response to the stone, causing severe, crampy pain in the lower back, often radiating to the groin. The pain stops once the stone passes into the bladder.

Pain in the bladder is most often caused by a bacterial infection. The discomfort is usually felt above the pubic bone and at the outer end of the urethra during urination. Blocked urine outflow causes pain above the pubic bone. However, a blockage that develops slowly may enlarge the bladder painlessly.

Prostate cancer and prostate enlargement are generally painless, but an inflammation of the prostate (prostatitis) can cause a vague discomfort or sensation of fullness in the area between

the anus and genitals. On the other hand, disorders of the testes usually cause pain that's severe and felt directly at the site of the problem.

Occasionally, a man ejaculates bloody semen. The reason usually can't be found. Semen may be bloody after prolonged sexual abstinence or after frequent or interrupted sexual activity. Men who have clotting disorders causing excessive bleeding may have bloody semen. Some men have repeated episodes, while others have only one. Although seeing blood in the semen is upsetting, the disorder generally isn't serious. Some urologists recommend taking tetracycline followed by gentle massage of the prostate, but the value of any treatment is uncertain.

Diagnostic Procedures

During the physical examination for a suspected kidney or urinary tract disorder, a doctor tries to feel the kidneys. Normally, kidneys can't be felt, but swollen kidneys or a kidney tumor may be detectable. Often, a swollen bladder also can be felt. The doctor performs a rectal examination in a man to feel whether the prostate gland is enlarged. A vaginal examination in a woman may provide information about the bladder and urethra.

Additional procedures to diagnose disorders of the kidneys and urinary tract may include urine analysis, blood tests that reflect kidney function, imaging procedures, and tissue and cell sampling.

Urine Analysis

Routine urine analysis (urinalysis) includes chemical analysis to detect protein, sugar, and ketones and microscopic examination to detect red and white blood cells. Tests that can be simply and inexpensively performed in an office laboratory can detect and measure the level of a variety of substances in the urine. These tests use a thin strip of plastic (dipstick) impregnated with chemicals that react with substances in the urine and change color. Dipsticks are routinely used in urinalysis.

Protein in the urine (proteinuria) can usually be detected quickly by dipstick, but more sophisticated techniques are sometimes required. Protein may appear constantly or only intermittently in the urine, depending on the cause. Proteinuria is usually a sign of kidney disease, but it may occur normally after strenuous exercise such as

▲ see page 591

marathon running. It can also occur in an uncommon, harmless genetic form called **orthostatic proteinuria,** in which protein isn't present in the urine after a person has been lying down, as when asleep, but appears after the person has been up for a while.

Glucose (sugar) in the urine (glucosuria) can be detected by dipstick, which is very accurate. The most common cause is diabetes. If glucose continues to appear in the urine after blood glucose levels are normal, a kidney abnormality is probably the problem.

Ketones in the urine (ketonuria) can be detected by dipstick. Ketones are formed when the body breaks down fat. Starvation, uncontrolled diabetes, and occasionally alcohol intoxication can produce ketones in the urine.

Blood in the urine (hematuria) is detectable by dipstick or examination under a microscope. Sometimes the urine contains enough blood to be visible, making the urine red or brown.

Nitrites in the urine (nitrituria) are also detectable by dipstick. Because nitrite levels increase when bacteria are present, this test is used to diagnose an infection quickly.

Leukocyte esterase (an enzyme found in certain white blood cells) in the urine can be detected by dipstick. Leukocyte esterase is a sign of inflammation, which is most commonly caused by a bacterial infection. The test may be falsely negative when the urine is very concentrated or contains glucose, bile salts, drugs such as the antibiotic rifampin, or a large amount of vitamin C.

The **acidity** of the urine is measured by dipstick. Certain foods may increase the acidity of urine.

The **concentration of urine** (osmolality, specific gravity) may be important in diagnosing abnormal kidney function. A doctor may analyze a random urine sample or may perform tests of the kidneys' ability to concentrate urine. In one such test, a person drinks no water or other fluids for 12 to 14 hours; in another, a person receives an injection of the hormone vasopressin. Afterward, urine concentration is measured. Normally, either test should make the urine highly concentrated. However, in certain kidney disorders, the urine is abnormally dilute.

Normally, urine contains a small number of cells and other debris shed from the inside of the urinary tract. A person who has urinary tract disease sheds more cells, which form a **sediment** if urine is centrifuged or allowed to settle. The sed-

Obtaining a Clean-Catch Urine Sample

1. The head of a man's penis or opening of a woman's urethra is washed.

2. The first few drops of urine are allowed to flow into the toilet, washing out the urethra.

3. Urination is resumed, and a sample is collected from the stream into a sterile cup.

iment can be examined under a microscope to provide information about the disease.

Urine cultures, in which bacteria are grown in a laboratory, are performed to diagnose a urinary tract infection. An uncontaminated sample of urine from the bladder is required and can be obtained by the clean-catch method. Other methods include passing a catheter through the urethra into the bladder or inserting a needle through the abdominal wall into the bladder (suprapubic needle aspiration).

Kidney Function Tests

Kidney function can be assessed by analyzing a blood sample as well as a urine sample. The kidney filtration rate can be estimated by measuring serum creatinine, a waste product. The level of blood urea nitrogen (BUN) can also indicate how well the kidneys are functioning, although many other factors can alter this level. Creatinine clearance—a more accurate test—can be approximated from a blood sample, using a formula that relates the serum creatinine level to a person's age, weight, and sex; determining it exactly requires a 24-hour urine collection.

Imaging Procedures

An **x-ray** of the abdomen can show the size and position of the kidneys, but an ultrasound scan is usually better for this purpose.

Intravenous urography is an x-ray technique used to display the kidneys and lower urinary tract. A radiopaque substance (often referred to as radiocontrast), which can be seen on x-rays, is given intravenously. The substance becomes concentrated in the kidneys, usually in less than 5 minutes. Then an x-ray film is taken. It provides a picture of the kidneys and the passage of the radiopaque substance through the ureters into the bladder. Intravenous urography doesn't work well in people with poorly functioning kidneys, which can't concentrate the radiopaque substance.

Sudden kidney failure occurs as an adverse effect in fewer than 1 out of 200 cases after a radiopaque substance has been injected for an x-ray procedure. The reason for kidney failure is unknown, but the risk is higher in those who are elderly or who have prior kidney insufficiency, diabetes mellitus, dehydration, or multiple myeloma. When an x-ray study using a radiopaque substance must be performed for a person at high risk, a doctor makes sure the person is given fluids intravenously beforehand. The doctor also uses a low dose of the radiopaque substance to reduce the risk as much as possible. Sometimes an alternative test, such as computed tomography, is used.

The **cystogram,** an x-ray image of the bladder, is obtained as part of the intravenous urography. However, a **retrograde cystogram,** produced when the radiopaque substance is introduced through the urethra, often provides more information about the bladder and ureters. X-ray films are taken before, during, and after urination.

In **retrograde urography,** radiopaque substances similar to those used in intravenous urography are inserted directly through a scope or catheter into a ureter. This technique provides good pictures of the bladder, ureters, and lower part of the kidneys when intravenous urography has been unsuccessful. Retrograde urography is also useful in investigating an obstruction of a ureter or in evaluating a person who is allergic to intravenous radiopaque substances. Disadvantages include the risk of infection and the need for anesthesia.

Ultrasound scanning uses sound waves to produce an image of anatomic structures. The technique is simple, painless, and safe. It can be used to study the kidneys, ureters, and bladder, with the added advantage that good pictures can be obtained even when the kidneys are functioning poorly. Ultrasound scans provide some indirect information about kidney function. Doctors use ultrasound scanning to measure the rate of urine production in a fetus older than 20 weeks by measuring how the bladder volume changes. This information helps a doctor determine how well the fetus' kidneys are functioning. For newborns, ultrasound scanning is the best way to investigate abdominal masses, urinary tract infections, and suspected birth defects of the urinary system, because the procedure is gentle and its results are highly accurate.

Ultrasound scanning is an excellent way to estimate kidney size and to diagnose a number of kidney abnormalities, including bleeding in the kidneys. Ultrasound scanning is used to locate the best place for a biopsy. It's the best diagnostic method for people who have advanced kidney failure, whose kidneys don't take up radiopaque substances, or who can't tolerate these substances.

A bladder filled with urine can be seen clearly on ultrasound scans. Although bladder tumors may be identified by ultrasound scanning, computed tomography is more reliable.

Computed tomography (CT) is more expensive than ultrasound scanning and intravenous urography but has some advantages. Because CT scans can distinguish solid structures from those that contain liquids, they're most useful in evaluating the type and extent of kidney tumors or other masses distorting the normal urinary tract. A radiopaque substance can be injected intravenously to obtain more information. CT scans can help determine how far a tumor has spread outside the kidney. A mixture of air and the radiopaque substance pumped into the bladder during CT can clearly reveal the outline of a bladder tumor.

Angiography, which involves injecting a radiopaque substance into an artery, is the most invasive of all kidney imaging procedures and is reserved for special situations, such as when a doctor must evaluate the blood supply to the kidneys. In many hospitals, conventional angiography is being replaced by spiral CT techniques. These techniques use computers to enhance the image produced when very small quantities of the radiopaque substance are used. Complications of angiography may include injury to the injected arteries and neighboring organs, reactions to the radiopaque substance, and bleeding.

Venography is x-ray imaging of veins using radiopaque substances. Complications are rare and are usually limited to leakage of blood and the radiopaque substance around the injection site.

Allergic reactions to the radiopaque substance can occur.

Magnetic resonance imaging (MRI) can provide information about kidney masses that can't be obtained by other techniques. For example, the shape of a tumor can be determined from the three-dimensional images produced by MRI. Solid kidney masses look different from hollow (cystic) ones, and the image of the fluid in a cyst helps a doctor distinguish bleeding from an infection. In addition, MRI produces excellent pictures of blood vessels and structures around the kidneys, so that a wide variety of diagnoses can be made. However, calcium deposits and stones in the kidney are unclear and better seen with CT.

Tissue and Cell Sampling

A **kidney biopsy,** in which a tissue sample is removed and examined under a microscope, may be performed so that a doctor can establish a diagnosis and observe the progress of treatment. A needle biopsy, in which the needle is inserted through the skin, is often part of the evaluation of kidney failure, and biopsies of a transplanted kidney are performed frequently to look for signs of rejection. For a biopsy of a person's own (native) kidney, the person lies face down, and a local anesthetic is injected into the skin and muscles of the back over the kidney. The biopsy needle is inserted and tissue is removed for microscopic examination. For a biopsy of a transplanted kidney, the needle is inserted directly through the abdominal wall. Ultrasound is used to help guide the needle to an abnormality.

Microscopic examination of the cells in the urine **(urine cytology)** is useful in diagnosing urinary tract cancers. For people at high risk—for example, smokers, petrochemical workers, and people with painless bleeding—urine cytology may be used to screen for cancer. For people who have had a bladder or kidney tumor removed, the technique may be used for follow-up evaluation. The results can be falsely positive, indicating cancer when none is present, because of another condition such as inflammation, or they can be falsely negative, failing to indicate cancer when it is present, possibly because of a low-grade cancer, in which the cells appear more normal.

CHAPTER 123

Kidney Failure

Kidney (renal) failure is abnormal kidney function in which the kidneys are unable to adequately excrete toxic substances from the body. Kidney failure has many possible causes, some of which lead to a rapid decline in kidney function (acute kidney failure), whereas others lead to a gradual decline in kidney function (chronic kidney failure).

Acute Kidney Failure

Acute kidney failure is a rapid decline in the kidneys' ability to clear the blood of toxic substances, leading to an accumulation of metabolic waste products, such as urea, in the blood.

Acute kidney failure can result from any condition that decreases the blood supply to the kidneys, obstructs the flow of urine after it has left the kidneys, or injures the kidneys themselves. Toxic substances may damage the kidneys. Such toxic substances include drugs, poisons, crystals precipitated in the urine, and antibodies that react against the kidneys.

Symptoms and Diagnosis

Symptoms depend on the severity of kidney failure, its rate of progression, and its underlying cause.

The condition that led to the kidney damage often produces serious symptoms unrelated to the kidneys. For example, high fever, shock, heart failure, and liver failure may occur before kidney failure and may be more serious than any of the symptoms of kidney failure. Some of the conditions that cause acute kidney failure also affect other parts of the body. For example, Wegener's granulomatosis, which damages blood vessels in

Major Causes of Acute Kidney Failure

Problem	Possible Causes
Insufficient blood supply to the kidneys	• Not enough blood because of blood loss, dehydration, or physical injury that blocks blood vessels • Heart pumping too weakly (heart failure) • Extremely low blood pressure (shock) • Liver failure (hepatorenal syndrome)
Obstructed urine flow	• Enlarged prostate • Tumor pressing on the urinary tract
Injuries within the kidneys	• Allergic reactions (for example, to radiopaque substances used for x-ray imaging) • Toxic substances • Conditions affecting the filtering units (nephrons) of the kidneys • Blocked arteries or veins within the kidneys • Crystals, protein, or other substances in the kidneys

the kidneys, may also damage blood vessels in the lungs, causing a person to cough up blood. Skin rashes are typical of some causes of acute kidney failure, including polyarteritis, systemic lupus erythematosus, and some toxic drugs.

Hydronephrosis▲ can cause acute kidney failure resulting from obstruction of urine flow. The backup of urine within the kidney causes the urine collecting area (renal pelvis) to stretch, producing crampy pain—ranging from mild to excruciating—usually in the side. About 10 percent of people have blood in the urine.

Doctors suspect acute kidney failure when urine output decreases. Blood tests that measure

▲ see page 625

■ see page 593

levels of creatinine and blood urea nitrogen (waste products in the blood that are normally cleared by the kidneys) help verify the diagnosis. A progressive rise in creatinine indicates acute kidney failure.

During a physical examination, the doctor assesses the kidneys to determine whether they are enlarged or tender. A narrowing of the main artery to a kidney may produce a rushing noise (bruit) that can be heard when a stethoscope is placed on the back over the kidneys.

If an enlarged bladder is detected, the doctor may insert a catheter to find out whether it's over-filled with urine. In older men especially, urine flow is usually obstructed at the bladder outlet (the opening into the urethra from the bladder). As a result, the bladder enlarges and urine backs up, damaging the kidneys. When an obstruction is suspected, rectal and vaginal examinations are also performed to find out whether a mass in either of those areas is causing the obstruction.

Laboratory tests can help pinpoint the cause and degree of kidney failure. First, the urine is thoroughly examined. If the kidney failure is caused by an inadequate blood supply or urinary obstruction, the urine typically appears normal. But if a problem within the kidney is causing failure, the urine may contain blood or clumps of red and white blood cells. The urine may also contain large amounts of protein or types of protein not normally present in urine.

Blood tests typically detect abnormally high urea and creatinine levels and metabolic imbalances, such as abnormal acidity (acidosis), a high potassium level (hyperkalemia), and a low sodium level (hyponatremia).

Imaging studies of the kidneys with ultrasound scanning or computed tomography (CT) are helpful. X-ray studies of the renal arteries or veins (angiography) may be performed if obstruction of blood vessels is the suspected cause. Magnetic resonance imaging (MRI) may be performed if the radiopaque substances used for x-ray studies are thought to be too dangerous. If these studies don't reveal the cause of kidney failure, a biopsy■ may be necessary.

Treatment

Acute kidney failure and its immediate complications can often be treated successfully. The survival rate ranges from less than 50 percent for people who have failure of several organs to about 90 percent for those who have decreased blood flow to the kidneys because body fluids have been lost through bleeding, vomiting, or diarrhea.

Often, simple but meticulous treatment is all that's required for the kidneys to heal themselves. Water intake is restricted to replacing the amount lost from the body. A person's weight is measured every day to monitor fluid intake. A weight gain from one day to the next indicates that too much fluid is being taken in. In addition to glucose or highly concentrated carbohydrate feedings, certain amino acids (the building blocks of protein) are given orally or intravenously to maintain adequate protein levels. The intake of all substances that are eliminated through the kidneys, including many drugs such as digoxin and some antibiotics, must be strictly limited. Because antacids that contain aluminum bind phosphorus in the intestines, they may be given to prevent the blood phosphorus level from rising too high. Sodium polystyrene sulfonate is sometimes given orally or rectally to treat a high blood level of potassium.

Kidney failure may be so severe that dialysis is needed to prevent serious harm to other organs and to control symptoms. In these cases, dialysis is started as soon as possible after diagnosis. Dialysis may be needed only to tide a person over until the kidneys recover their function, usually in several days to several weeks. On the other hand, if the kidneys are too badly damaged to recover, dialysis may be needed indefinitely, unless kidney transplantation▲ is performed.

Chronic Kidney Failure

Chronic kidney failure is a slowly progressive decline in kidney function that leads to the buildup of metabolic waste products in the blood (azotemia).

Injury to the kidneys by many diseases may lead to irreversible damage.

Symptoms

In chronic kidney failure, symptoms develop slowly. At first, a person has no symptoms; abnormal kidney function can be detected only by laboratory testing. A person with mild to moderate kidney failure may have only mild symptoms despite the increase in urea, a metabolic waste product, in the blood. At this stage, the person may need to urinate several times during the

---

Causes of Chronic Kidney Failure

- High blood pressure
- Urinary tract obstruction
- Glomerulonephritis
- Kidney abnormalities, such as polycystic kidney disease
- Diabetes mellitus
- Autoimmune disorders, such as systemic lupus erythematosus

---

night (nocturia), because the kidneys can't absorb water from the urine to concentrate it as they normally do during the night. As a result, urine volumes are larger. High blood pressure often develops in people who have kidney failure, because the kidneys can't eliminate excess salt and water. High blood pressure may lead to a stroke or heart failure.

As kidney failure progresses and toxic substances build up in the blood, the person may feel weary, tire easily, and become less mentally alert. As the buildup of toxic substances increases, nerve and muscle symptoms develop, including muscle twitches, muscle weakness, and cramps. The person may also feel a pins-and-needles sensation in the extremities and may lose sensation in certain areas. Convulsions (seizures) may result if high blood pressure or abnormalities in the blood chemistry cause the brain to malfunction. The buildup of toxic substances also affects the digestive tract, causing a loss of appetite, nausea, vomiting, inflammation of the lining of the mouth (stomatitis), and an unpleasant taste in the mouth. These symptoms may lead to malnutrition and weight loss. People who have advanced kidney failure commonly develop intestinal ulcers and bleeding. The skin may turn yellow-brown, and occasionally the concentration of urea is so high that it crystallizes

---

▲ see page 834

How Chronic Kidney Failure Affects the Blood

- Increased urea and creatinine concentrations
- Anemia
- Increased blood acidity (acidosis)
- Decreased calcium concentration
- Increased phosphate concentration
- Increased parathyroid hormone concentration
- Decreased vitamin D concentration
- Normal or slightly increased potassium concentration

from sweat, forming a white powder on the skin (uremic frost). Some people with chronic kidney failure have very uncomfortable generalized itching.

Diagnosis

Chronic kidney failure is diagnosed by blood tests. Typically, the blood becomes moderately acidic (acidosis). Two metabolic waste products, urea and creatinine, which are normally filtered out by the kidneys, build up in the blood. The calcium level decreases and the phosphate level increases. The blood potassium level is normal or only slightly increased but can become dangerously high. Urine volume tends to stay about the same—usually 2 to 8 pints a day—regardless of the amount of fluid consumed. Usually, the person has moderate anemia. Analysis of the urine may detect many abnormalities, including abnormal cells and concentrations of salts.

Prognosis and Treatment

Chronic kidney failure generally worsens regardless of treatment and is fatal if not treated. Dialysis or kidney transplantation may keep the person alive.

Conditions that cause or worsen kidney failure must be corrected as soon as possible. Such ac-

tions include correcting sodium, water, and acid-base imbalances; removing substances toxic to the kidneys; and treating heart failure, high blood pressure, infections, a high blood concentration of potassium or calcium (hypercalcemia), and any obstruction of urine flow.

Meticulous attention to diet helps control acidosis and increased concentrations of blood potassium and phosphate. A low-protein diet (0.2 to 0.4 grams per pound of ideal body weight) may slow the rate of progression from chronic kidney failure to end-stage kidney failure, when dialysis or kidney transplantation is necessary. People who have diabetes usually need one of these treatments at an earlier point than those who don't have diabetes. A vitamin supplement containing vitamins B and C is recommended when the diet is severely restricted or when dialysis is started.

A high concentration of blood triglycerides, which is common in people who have chronic kidney failure, increases the risk of complications, such as strokes and heart attacks. Drugs such as gemfibrozil may be taken to reduce the triglyceride level, although studies have not yet shown that these drugs reduce cardiovascular complications.

During kidney failure, changes in thirst usually determine how much water is consumed. Occasionally, water intake is restricted to prevent the sodium concentration in the blood from becoming too low. The intake of salt (sodium) usually isn't restricted unless fluid accumulates in the tissues (edema) or high blood pressure develops. Foods that are very high in potassium, such as salt substitutes, must be avoided, and foods that are high in potassium should not be consumed in excess. A high blood potassium level (hyperkalemia)▲ is dangerous because it increases the risk of abnormal heart rhythms and cardiac arrest. If the potassium level becomes too high, drugs such as sodium polystyrene sulfonate can adhere to potassium, causing it to be excreted in the stool; however, emergency dialysis may be required.

Bone formation may be impaired if certain conditions are present for a long time. These conditions include a low concentration of calcitriol (a derivative of vitamin D), poor intake and absorption of calcium, and high concentrations of blood phosphate and parathyroid hormone. The blood

▲ see page 670

phosphate concentration is controlled by restricting the intake of foods high in phosphorus, such as dairy products, liver, legumes, nuts, and most soft drinks. Drugs that bind phosphate, such as calcium carbonate, calcium acetate, and aluminum hydroxide (a common antacid), taken by mouth, may also help.

Anemia is caused by the kidneys' failure to produce sufficient amounts of erythropoietin (a hormone that stimulates red blood cell production). The anemia responds slowly to epoetin, a drug that can be injected. Blood transfusions are given only if the anemia is severe or is causing symptoms. Doctors also look for other causes of anemia, particularly dietary deficiencies of such nutrients as iron, folic acid (folate), and vitamin B_{12} or excesses of aluminum in the body.

A bleeding tendency in chronic kidney failure can be temporarily suppressed by transfusions of red blood cells or platelets or by such drugs as desmopressin or estrogens. Such treatment may be needed after an injury or before a surgical procedure or tooth extraction.

Symptoms of heart failure, which most commonly results from excessive sodium and water retention, improve if dietary sodium is reduced. Diuretics—furosemide, bumetanide, and torsemide—may also be effective, even when kidney function is poor. Moderate or severe increases in blood pressure are treated with standard blood pressure drugs to prevent heart and kidney function from being impaired.

When the initial treatments for kidney failure are no longer effective, long-term dialysis or transplantation is considered.

Dialysis

Dialysis is the process of removing waste products and excess water from the body.

There are two methods of dialysis: hemodialysis and peritoneal dialysis. In **hemodialysis,** blood is removed from the body and pumped into a machine that filters the toxic substances out of the blood and then returns the purified blood to the person. The total amount of fluid returned can be adjusted.

In **peritoneal dialysis,** fluid containing a special mixture of glucose and salts is infused into the abdominal cavity where it draws toxic substances from the tissues. The fluid is then drained out and discarded. The quantity of glucose can be adjusted to remove more or less fluid from the body.

Reasons for Dialysis

Doctors decide to begin dialysis when kidney failure is causing abnormal brain function (uremic encephalopathy), inflammation of the sac around the heart (pericarditis), high blood acidity (acidosis) that doesn't respond to other treatments, heart failure, or a very high blood potassium concentration (hyperkalemia). The symptoms of abnormal brain function caused by kidney failure are generally reversed by dialysis over several days or, rarely, in up to 2 weeks.

Many doctors use dialysis preventively in acute kidney failure when urine output is low, and they continue the treatments until blood tests indicate that kidney function is being restored. For chronic kidney failure, dialysis may be begun when tests indicate that the kidneys aren't removing waste products adequately or when a person can no longer perform normal daily activities.

The frequency of dialysis treatment varies according to the amount of kidney function remaining, but most people need dialysis three times a week. A successful dialysis program results in a reasonably normal life, a reasonable diet, an acceptable red blood cell count, normal blood pressure, and no progression of nerve damage. Dialysis may be used as long-term therapy for chronic kidney failure or as an interim measure before kidney transplantation. For acute kidney failure, dialysis may be needed for only a few days or weeks, until kidney function is restored.

Dialysis can also be used to remove certain drugs or poisons from the body. People often survive poisoning if given prompt assistance with breathing and heart function while the poison is being removed.

Problems

People undergoing dialysis need special diets and drugs. Because appetite is poor and protein is lost during peritoneal dialysis, these people generally need a diet relatively high in protein—roughly $\frac{1}{2}$ gram of protein per pound of ideal body weight a day. For those undergoing hemodialysis, consumption of sodium and potassium should be limited to 2 grams of each daily. Consumption of foods high in phosphorus also may have to be limited. Daily fluid intake is limited only for people who have a persistently low or a decreasing sodium concentration in the blood. Daily weighing is important, and excessive weight gain between hemodialysis treatments suggests consumption of too much fluid. For people undergoing peritoneal dialysis, restrictions on potassium (4 grams daily) and sodium (3 to 4 grams daily) are less severe.

Multivitamin and iron supplements are needed to replace the nutrients lost through dialysis. However, people undergoing dialysis who also receive many blood transfusions often get too much iron because blood contains large amounts of iron; therefore, they should not take iron supplements. Hormones, such as testosterone or erythropoietin, may be given to stimulate the production of red blood cells. Phosphate binders, such as calcium carbonate or calcium acetate, are used to remove excess phosphate.

A low blood calcium concentration or severe hyperparathyroid bone disease may be treated with calcitriol (a form of vitamin D) and supplemental calcium.

High blood pressure is common among people with kidney failure. It can be controlled in about half of these people simply by removing a sufficient amount of fluid during dialysis. The other half may need to take drugs to lower blood pressure.

For people undergoing chronic dialysis, the regular treatments keep them alive. However, dialysis often causes stress because the treatments are ongoing, several times a week for several hours.

People undergoing dialysis may experience losses in every aspect of their lives. The potential loss of independence can be especially distressing. These people are dependent on the treatment team. People undergoing hemodialysis need to arrange for transportation to and from dialysis centers on a regular basis because they must have uninterrupted access to this care. Dialysis sessions, often scheduled for the convenience of others, influence the person's work or school schedule and leisure activities. Regular employment may be impossible. People on dialysis may need help from the community to manage the high cost of treatments, drugs, special diets, and transpor-

tation. Older adults undergoing dialysis may become more dependent on their grown children or may not be able to continue living alone. Often, established family roles and responsibilities must be modified to fit the dialysis routine, creating stress and feelings of guilt and inadequacy.

People undergoing dialysis also face stressful losses and changes in body image and function. Children whose growth has been stunted may feel isolated and different from their peers. Young adults and adolescents coping with identity, independence, and body image issues may find these issues further complicated by dialysis.

As a result of these losses, many people undergoing dialysis become depressed and anxious. Nevertheless, most people do adjust to dialysis. How the people undergoing dialysis—and their treatment team—cope with these issues affects not only their social adjustment but also their long-term survival. Psychologic and social problems are generally reduced when dialysis programs encourage people to be independent and to resume pursuit of previous interests.

Psychologic and social counseling for depression, behavior problems, and issues involving losses or adjustments is often helpful to families as well as to those undergoing dialysis. These services are available from social workers, psychologists, and psychiatrists. Many dialysis centers provide psychologic and social support.

HEMODIALYSIS

Hemodialysis, a procedure in which the blood is removed from the body and circulated through a machine outside the body called a dialyzer, requires repeated access to the bloodstream. An artificial connection between an artery and a vein (an arteriovenous fistula) is made surgically to facilitate that access.

In hemodialysis, the person's blood flows through a tube connected to the arteriovenous (A-V) fistula and is pumped to the dialyzer. Heparin, a drug that prevents clotting, is used during dialysis to prevent blood from clotting in the dialyzer. Inside the dialyzer, a porous artificial membrane separates the blood from a fluid (the dialysate) that's similar in chemical composition to normal body fluids. Pressure in the dialysate compartment of the membrane unit is lower than that in the blood compartment, allowing fluid, waste products, and toxic substances in the blood to filter through the membrane into the dialysate. However, blood cells and large proteins are too large to filter through the small pores of the membrane. The dialyzed (purified) blood is returned to the person's body.

Dialyzers have different sizes and degrees of efficiency. Newer units are very efficient, allowing blood to flow faster and shortening dialysis time—for example, 2 to 3 hours, three times a week, compared with 3 to 5 hours, three times a week needed for an older unit. Most people who have chronic kidney failure need hemodialysis three times a week to remain healthy.

PERITONEAL DIALYSIS

In peritoneal dialysis, the peritoneum—a membrane that lines the abdomen and covers the abdominal organs—acts as a permeable filter. This membrane has a large surface area and a rich network of blood vessels. Substances from the blood can easily filter through the peritoneum into the abdominal cavity if conditions are right. Fluid is infused through a catheter inserted through the abdominal wall into the peritoneal space within the abdomen. The fluid must be left in the abdomen for a sufficient time to allow waste materials from the bloodstream to pass slowly into it. Then the fluid is drained out, discarded, and replaced with fresh fluid.

A soft silicone rubber or porous polyurethane catheter is usually used because it allows the fluid to flow smoothly and is unlikely to cause damage. A catheter can be put in place temporarily at the patient's bedside, or it may be put in place permanently in an operating room. One type of permanent catheter eventually forms a seal with the skin; it can be capped when not in use.

Various techniques are used for peritoneal dialysis. In the simplest technique, **manual intermittent peritoneal dialysis,** bags containing fluid are warmed to body temperature; the fluid is infused into the peritoneal cavity for 10 minutes, allowed to remain there for 60 to 90 minutes, and then drained in about 10 to 20 minutes. The entire treatment can take 12 hours. This technique is used chiefly to treat acute kidney failure.

Automated cycler intermittent peritoneal dialysis can be performed by people in their home, eliminating the need for constant nursing attention. A timed device automatically pumps fluid into and drains it from the peritoneal cavity. Usually, peo-

Possible Complications of Hemodialysis

Complication	Cause
Fever	Bacteria or fever causing substances (pyrogens) in the bloodstream Overheated dialysate
Life-threatening allergic reaction (anaphylaxis)	Allergy to a substance in the machine
Low blood pressure	Removal of too much fluid
Abnormal heart rhythms	Abnormal blood levels of potassium and other substances
Air embolus	Air entering blood in the machine
Bleeding in the intestine, brain, eyes, or abdomen	Heparin being used to prevent clotting in the machine

ple set the cycler at bedtime so the dialysis takes place while they're sleeping. These treatments need to be performed 6 or 7 nights a week.

In **continuous ambulatory peritoneal dialysis,** the fluid is kept in the abdomen for extremely long intervals. Typically, the fluid is drained and replenished four or five times a day. The fluids are packaged in collapsible polyvinyl chloride bags that can be folded when empty, tucked into a garment, and used for subsequent drainage without being disconnected from the catheter. People generally perform three of these fluid exchanges during the day, at intervals of 4 hours or longer. Each exchange takes 30 to 45 minutes. A longer exchange (8 to 12 hours) is performed at night, during sleep.

Another technique, **continuous cycler-assisted peritoneal dialysis,** uses an automated cycler to perform short exchanges at night during sleep, whereas longer exchanges are performed without the cycler during the day. This technique minimizes the number of exchanges during the day

Comparing Hemodialysis and Peritoneal Dialysis

When the kidneys fail, waste products and excess water can be removed from the blood by hemodialysis or peritoneal dialysis. In hemodialysis, blood is removed from the body and circulated through a machine called a dialyzer that filters the blood. In peritoneal dialysis, the peritoneum, a membrane in the abdomen, is used as the filter.

In hemodialysis, a connection between an artery and a vein (an arteriovenous fistula) is surgically created to facilitate the removal and return of blood. Blood flows through a tube connected to the fistula into the dialyzer. Inside the dialyzer, an artificial membrane separates the blood from a fluid (the dialysate) that's similar to normal body fluids. Fluid, waste products, and toxic substances in the blood filter through the membrane into the dialysate. The purified blood is returned to the person's body.

In peritoneal dialysis, a catheter is inserted through a small incision in the abdominal wall into the peritoneal space. The dialysate drains by gravity or is pumped through the catheter and left in the space long enough to allow waste products from the bloodstream to filter through the peritoneum into the dialysate. Then the dialysate is drained out, discarded, and replaced.

Hemodialysis

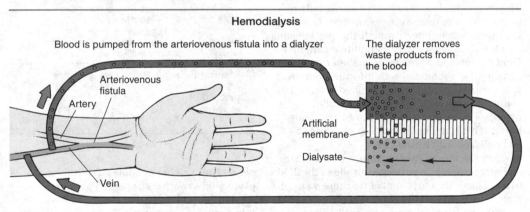

Blood is pumped from the arteriovenous fistula into a dialyzer

The dialyzer removes waste products from the blood

Arteriovenous fistula

Artery

Artificial membrane

Dialysate

Vein

Purified blood is pumped from the dialyzer into the arteriovenous fistula

Peritoneal Dialysis

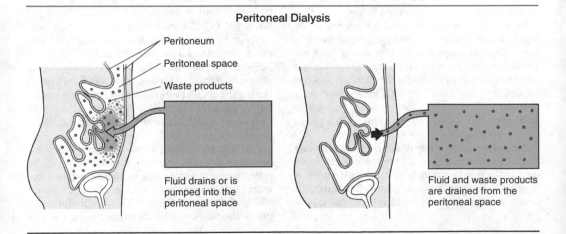

Peritoneum

Peritoneal space

Waste products

Fluid drains or is pumped into the peritoneal space

Fluid and waste products are drained from the peritoneal space

but prevents mobility at night because of cumbersome equipment.

Complications

Although many people undergo peritoneal dialysis for years without problems, complications can occur. Bleeding can occur at the site where the catheter leaves the body or within the abdomen, or an internal organ may be perforated during placement of the catheter. Fluid may leak around the catheter or into the abdominal wall. The flow of fluid may be obstructed by clots or other debris.

However, the most troublesome problem of peritoneal dialysis is infection. It can involve the peritoneum, the skin at the catheter site, or the area surrounding the catheter, causing an abscess. An infection usually occurs because of a lapse in sterile technique during some part of the dialysis procedure. Usually, antibiotics can clear up the infection; if not, the catheter may have to be removed until the infection clears up.

Other problems may be associated with dialysis. A low blood albumin level (hypoalbuminemia) is common. Rare complications include scarring of the peritoneum (peritoneal sclerosis) resulting in partial obstruction of the small intestine, subnormal levels of thyroid hormone (hypothyroidism), and seizures. A high blood sugar (glucose) level (hyperglycemia) is also rare, except in patients who have diabetes. Hernias of the abdomen and groin develop in about 10 percent of patients.

People undergoing peritoneal dialysis may be prone to constipation, which interferes with catheter drainage. Consequently, they may need to take laxatives or stool softeners.

Generally, peritoneal dialysis is not performed in people who have abdominal wall infections, abnormal connections between the chest and abdomen, a newly installed artificial blood vessel graft within the abdomen, or a recent abdominal wound.

CHAPTER 124

Nephritis

Nephritis is inflammation of the kidneys.

Inflammation of the kidneys generally is caused by an infection, as in pyelonephritis,▲ or an immune reaction that goes awry and injures the kidneys. An abnormal immune reaction can come about in two ways: (1) An antibody can attack either the kidney itself or an antigen (a substance that stimulates an immune reaction) attached to kidney cells, or (2) an antigen and antibody can combine somewhere else in the body and then become attached to cells in the kidney. Signs of nephritis, including blood and protein in the urine and impaired kidney function, depend on the type, location, and intensity of the immune reaction. Nonetheless, the many different conditions that injure the kidneys can produce similar types of damage, symptoms, and outcomes.

Generally, inflammation does not affect the entire kidney. The resulting disease depends on whether the inflammation affects primarily the glomeruli (the first part of the kidney's filtering apparatus), the tubules and the tissues that surround them (tubulointerstitial tissue), or the blood vessels within the kidneys, causing vasculitis.

Glomerulopathies

Kidney disorders in which inflammation affects mainly the glomeruli are called glomerulopathies. Although causes vary, glomerulopathies are similar because glomeruli respond to several types of injury in a similar way.

There are four major types of glomerulopathies. Acute nephritic syndrome starts suddenly and usually resolves quickly. Rapidly progressive nephritic syndrome starts suddenly and worsens rapidly. Nephrotic syndrome leads to the loss of

---

▲ see page 624

Inflammation in the Kidneys

Affected Area	Resulting Disease
Blood vessels	• Vasculitis
Glomeruli	• Acute nephritic syndrome • Rapidly progressive nephritic syndrome • Nephrotic syndrome • Chronic nephritic syndrome
Tubulointerstitial tissue	• Acute tubulointerstitial nephritis • Chronic tubulointerstitial nephritis

large amounts of protein in the urine. Chronic nephritic syndrome starts gradually and worsens very slowly, often over a period of years.

When the glomerulus is damaged, substances not normally filtered out of the bloodstream—such as proteins, blood, white blood cells, and debris—can pass through the glomerulus and enter the urine. Tiny blood clots (microthrombi) may form in the capillaries that supply the glomerulus; they, with other changes, may greatly reduce the amount of urine produced. In addition, the kidneys may become unable to concentrate urine, excrete acid from the body,▲ or balance the excretion of salts.■ At first, the glomerulus can partly compensate by growing bigger, but its increasing impairment causes urine production to fall and toxic metabolic waste products to build up in the blood.

Diagnosis

For all glomerulopathies, the precise diagnosis is made by performing a kidney biopsy. A small

---

▲ see page 676

■ see box, page 665

★ see box, page 741

specimen of the kidney is removed, usually by inserting a needle into the kidney through the skin. The specimen is examined under a microscope before and after it's been stained to visualize the type and location of immune reactions within the kidney.

An examination of a urine specimen (urinalysis) assists in the diagnosis, and simple blood tests indicate the extent of damage to kidney function. Measuring antibody levels in samples of blood can help track the progression of the disease by determining whether the levels are rising (the condition is worsening) or falling (the condition is improving).

Prognosis and Treatment

The course and prognosis of a glomerulopathy are highly variable and depend on the underlying cause. Although the immune reactions that cause many kidney diseases are now understood, in most instances treatment either isn't available or isn't specific to the immune disorder. Doctors try to modify the immune reaction by removing the antigen, the antibody, or the complex created by the combination of the two with procedures such as plasmapheresis, which removes harmful substances from the blood,★ or they try to suppress the immune reaction with anti-inflammatory and immunosuppressant drugs, such as corticosteroids, azathioprine, and cyclophosphamide. In some cases, drugs that prevent blood clotting are helpful. Whenever possible, specific treatment for the underlying disorder is given—for example, antibiotics for an infection.

Acute Nephritic Syndrome

Acute nephritic syndrome (acute glomerulonephritis; postinfectious glomerulonephritis) is an inflammation of the glomeruli that results in the sudden appearance of blood in the urine, with clumps of red blood cells (casts) and variable amounts of protein in the urine.

Acute nephritic syndrome may follow a streptococcal infection, such as strep throat. In such cases, the disorder is called poststreptococcal glomerulonephritis. The glomeruli are damaged by the accumulation of antigen from the dead streptococci clumped together with the antibodies that neutralized them. These clumps (immune complexes) coat the membranes of the glomeruli and interfere with their filtering function. Because the nephritis begins 1 to 6 weeks (average, 2 weeks) after the infection and the streptococci are already dead, antibiotics are ineffective. Poststreptococcal glomerulonephritis is most common in children over age 3 and in young adults. About 5 percent of cases occur after age 50.

Acute nephritic syndrome may also be caused by a reaction to other infections, such as infection of an artificial body part (prosthesis), bacterial endocarditis, pneumonia, abscesses of abdominal organs, chickenpox, infectious hepatitis, syphilis, and malaria. The last three infections may cause nephrotic syndrome rather than acute nephritic syndrome.

Symptoms and Diagnosis

About half the people with this syndrome have no symptoms. When symptoms do occur, the first to appear are fluid retention with tissue swelling (edema), low urine volume, and dark urine that contains blood. Edema may first appear as puffiness of the face and eyelids but later is prominent in the legs; it may become severe. High blood pressure and brain swelling may produce headaches, visual disturbances, and more serious disturbances of brain function. A laboratory analysis of the urine shows variable amounts of protein, and the concentration of urea and creatinine—two waste products—in the blood is often high.

Doctors investigate the possibility of poststreptococcal glomerulonephritis in people who develop such symptoms and whose laboratory test results indicate kidney dysfunction after a sore throat, impetigo, or—most convincing—a culture-proven streptococcal infection. Blood levels of antibodies against streptococci may be higher than normal. The nephrotic syndrome develops in about 30 percent of these people. Rarely, urine production stops completely as soon as poststreptococcal glomerulonephritis develops; blood volume increases suddenly, and the blood potassium level rises. Death may follow unless dialysis is started quickly.

Acute nephritic syndrome that follows an infection by organisms other than streptococci is usually easier to diagnose because its symptoms often begin while the infection is still obvious.

Prognosis and Treatment

Most people who have acute nephritic syndrome recover completely. However, if laboratory tests show large amounts of protein in the urine or a rapid decline in kidney function, kidney failure and lasting kidney damage are possible. In 1 percent of children and 10 percent of adults, the acute nephritic syndrome evolves into rapidly progressive nephritic syndrome. About 85 to 95 percent of children regain normal kidney function but may be at increased risk of developing high blood pressure later in life. About 40 percent of adults do not recover completely and continue to have kidney function abnormalities.

No treatment is available in most cases. Drugs that suppress the immune system (immunosuppressant drugs) and corticosteroids aren't effective; corticosteroids may even worsen the condition. If a bacterial infection is still present when acute nephritic syndrome is discovered, antibiotic therapy is started. When the condition results from an infected artificial body part, such as a heart valve, the prognosis remains good as long as the infection can be eradicated. Eradication often requires removal and replacement of the artificial part in addition to antibiotic therapy.

Following a diet that's low in protein and salt may be necessary until kidney function recovers. Diuretics may be given to help the kidneys excrete excess salt and water. High blood pressure may have to be treated with drugs. People who develop severe kidney failure may need dialysis.

Rapidly Progressive Nephritic Syndrome

Rapidly progressive nephritic syndrome (rapidly progressive glomerulonephritis) is an uncommon disorder in which most of the glomeruli are partly destroyed, resulting in severe kidney failure with protein, blood, and red blood cell clumps (casts) in the urine.

Rapidly progressive nephritic syndrome is part of a disorder that affects other organs as well as the kidneys in about 40 percent of the cases. Of the 60 percent of cases in which primarily the kidneys are affected, about one third appear to be caused by antibodies attacking the glomeruli, about one half have unknown causes, and the rest are caused by deposits of antibodies and antigens formed elsewhere in the body that are in the kidneys (immune complex disease).

What causes the body to produce antibodies against its own glomeruli is not known. The production of damaging antibodies may be related to viral infections or autoimmune disorders such as systemic lupus erythematosus. In some people who develop antibodies against their glomeruli, the antibodies also react with the small air sacs in the lungs, leading to Goodpasture's syndrome,▲ a condition in which the lungs and kidneys are damaged. Hydrocarbons, such as ethylene glycol, carbon tetrachloride, chloroform, and toluene, may damage the glomeruli, but they don't cause an immune reaction or the production of antibodies.

Symptoms and Diagnosis

Weakness, fatigue, and fever are the most obvious early symptoms. Nausea, loss of appetite, vomiting, joint pain, and abdominal pain are also common. About 50 percent of people had a flulike illness in the month before kidney failure started to develop. These people have puffiness (edema) caused by fluid retention and usually produce very little urine. High blood pressure is uncommon and rarely severe when it does occur. If the lungs are affected (Goodpasture's syndrome), the person coughs up blood and has difficulty breathing.

Blood is often visible in the urine, and clumps of red blood cells are always visible under a microscope. Blood tests detect anemia, sometimes severe, and usually detect an abnormally high number of white blood cells. Blood tests of kidney function detect some buildup of toxic metabolic waste products.

At first, the kidneys may appear enlarged on ultrasound scans or x-rays, but they gradually shrink. Often, a sample of kidney tissue is removed through a needle and sent to the laboratory for microscopic examination (biopsy) to confirm the diagnosis and to make sure the person doesn't have another condition that could be treated.

Prognosis

The prognosis depends on the severity of symptoms, which varies greatly. Because the early symptoms are subtle, many people who

---

▲ see page 189

have the disease aren't aware that they are sick and don't go to a doctor until kidney failure is severe. People who develop kidney failure will die within a few weeks unless they undergo dialysis.

The prognosis also depends on the cause and the affected person's age. When the cause is an autoimmune disease, in which the body forms antibodies against its own cells, treatment usually improves the situation. When the cause is unknown or the person is elderly, the prognosis is worse. Most people who are not treated develop kidney failure within 2 years.

Treatment

When doctors suspect rapidly progressive nephritic syndrome, a kidney biopsy is performed as soon as possible so that they can establish the diagnosis, estimate the prognosis, and plan treatment. Blood tests for antibodies and tests for infections are also performed.

When biopsy results show severe disease of the glomeruli, drugs are started promptly for maximum effectiveness. Corticosteroids are usually given intravenously at high doses for about a week and then by mouth. Cyclophosphamide or azathioprine, drugs that suppress the immune system, may also be given. In addition, a person may undergo plasmapheresis, in which blood is withdrawn from the person, filtered through a device that removes the antibodies, then returned to the person.

If the disease has progressed to a more advanced stage, dialysis may be the only useful treatment. The alternative is kidney transplantation, although the original disease can affect the transplanted kidney.

Nephrotic Syndrome

Nephrotic syndrome is a syndrome (a collection of symptoms) caused by many diseases that affect the kidneys, resulting in a severe, prolonged loss of protein into the urine, decreased blood levels of protein (especially albumin), retention of excess salt and water in the body, and increased levels of fats (lipids) in the blood.

Nephrotic syndrome can occur at any age. In children, it's most common between ages 18 months and 4 years, and more boys than girls are affected. In older people, the sexes are more equally affected.

Causes

Nephrotic syndrome can be caused by any of the glomerulopathies or a vast array of diseases. A number of drugs that are toxic to the kidneys can also cause nephrotic syndrome, as can intravenous heroin use. The syndrome may be associated with certain sensitivities. Some types of the syndrome are hereditary.

The nephrotic syndrome that's associated with human immunodeficiency virus (HIV) infection occurs mostly in black people who have the infection. The syndrome progresses to complete kidney failure in 3 or 4 months.

Symptoms

Early symptoms include loss of appetite, a generally sick feeling, puffy eyelids, abdominal pain, wasting of muscles, tissue swelling from excess salt and fluid retention, and frothy urine. The abdomen may be swollen because of a large accumulation of fluid there, and shortness of breath may be caused by fluid in the space surrounding the lungs (pleural effusion). Other symptoms may include swelling of the knees and, in men, the scrotum. Most often, the fluid causing tissue swelling moves around, accumulating in the eyelids in the morning and in the ankles after walking. Muscle wasting may be hidden by swelling.

A fall in blood pressure when standing up and generally low blood pressure, which may lead to shock, may develop in children. Adults may have low, normal, or high blood pressure. Urine output may decrease and kidney failure may develop because of the low blood volume and diminished blood supply to the kidney. Occasionally, kidney failure with low urine output occurs suddenly. When a person is first seen by a doctor, urine protein levels are usually high.

Nutritional deficiencies may result from the loss of nutrients, such as glucose, in the urine. Growth may be stunted. Calcium may be lost from bones. The hair and nails may become brittle and some hair may fall out. Horizontal white lines may develop in fingernail beds for unknown reasons.

The abdominal lining may become inflamed (peritonitis). Opportunistic infections—infections caused by normally harmless bacteria—are common. The high incidence of infection is thought to occur because the antibodies that normally fight infections are lost in the urine or not produced in normal amounts. Blood clotting becomes abnormal, significantly increasing the risk of clotting inside blood vessels (thrombosis), par-

What Can Cause Nephrotic Syndrome?

Diseases
- Amyloidosis
- Cancer
- Diabetes
- Glomerulopathies
- Human immunodeficiency virus (HIV) infection
- Leukemias
- Lymphomas
- Monoclonal gammopathy
- Multiple myeloma
- Systemic lupus erythematosus

Drugs
- Aspirin-like analgesics
- Gold
- Heroin taken intravenously
- Penicillamine

Allergies
- Insect bites
- Poison ivy
- Poison oak
- Sunlight

ticularly inside the main vein from the kidney. On the other hand, the blood may not clot, generally leading to excessive bleeding. High blood pressure accompanied by complications affecting the heart and brain is most likely to occur in people who have diabetes and those who have a connective tissue disease.▲

Diagnosis

The diagnosis of nephrotic syndrome is based on the symptoms and laboratory findings. Laboratory tests of urine detect high levels of protein with clumps of cells (casts). The blood concentration of albumin is low because this vital protein is lost in the urine and its synthesis is impaired. Urine levels of sodium are low and levels of potassium are high.

▲ see page 226

Blood lipid (fat) concentrations are high, sometimes up to or even exceeding 10 times normal. Urine lipid levels are also high. Anemia may be present. Blood clotting factors may be increased or decreased.

The doctor investigates possible causes of nephrotic syndrome, including drugs. Analysis of the urine and blood may reveal an underlying disorder. If the person has lost weight or is elderly, a search for cancer is undertaken. A kidney biopsy is especially useful in categorizing specific kidney tissue damage.

Prognosis

The prognosis varies depending on the cause of the nephrotic syndrome, the person's age, and the type of kidney damage as determined by microscopic examination of tissue in a biopsy. Symptoms may disappear completely if the nephrotic syndrome is caused by a treatable disorder, such as an infection or cancer, or by drugs. This situation occurs in about half the cases in children but less often in adults. The prognosis is generally good if the underlying disorder responds to corticosteroids. When the syndrome is caused by HIV infection, it usually progresses relentlessly. Children born with the nephrotic syndrome rarely live beyond their first birthday, although a few have survived by means of dialysis treatments or kidney transplantation.

Nephrotic syndrome has the best prognosis when it is caused by a mild type of glomerulonephritis, **minimal change disease;** 90 percent of children and nearly as many adults respond to treatment. The disease rarely progresses to kidney failure, although it's likely to recur. However, after a year of being free of the disease, a person is unlikely to have a recurrence.

Membranous glomerulonephritis, a more serious type of glomerulonephritis that causes nephrotic syndrome, is contracted mainly by adults and slowly progresses to kidney failure in 50 percent of those over 15 years of age. The remaining 50 percent are disease free or have persistent protein in the urine but adequate kidney function. In

the majority of children who have membranous glomerulonephritis, protein in the urine disappears completely and spontaneously within 5 years of being diagnosed.

Two other types, **familial nephrotic syndrome** and **membranoproliferative glomerulonephritis,** respond poorly to treatment, and the prognosis is less optimistic. More than half the people who have the familial type develop kidney failure within 10 years. In 20 percent, the prognosis is even worse: severe kidney disease develops within 2 years. The disease progresses more rapidly in adults than in children. Similarly, half the people with the membranoproliferative type progress to kidney failure within 10 years; the disease disappears in fewer than 5 percent. Another type, **mesangial proliferative glomerulonephritis,** virtually never responds to corticosteroids.

For nephrotic syndrome that results from systemic lupus erythematosus, amyloidosis, or diabetes, treatment is aimed mainly at suppressing symptoms rather than attempting a cure. Although newer treatments for systemic lupus erythematosus reduce symptoms and stabilize or improve abnormal test results, progressive kidney failure occurs in most people. In diabetic nephrotic syndrome, severe kidney disease usually develops in 3 to 5 years.

In cases of nephrotic syndrome resulting from conditions such as an infection, an allergy, or intravenous heroin use, the prognosis varies, depending on how early and effectively the underlying condition is treated.

Treatment

Treatment is aimed at the underlying cause. Treating an infection that causes nephrotic syndrome may cure the syndrome. If the syndrome is caused by a treatable disease, such as Hodgkin's disease or another kind of cancer, treating that disease can eliminate the kidney symptoms. If a heroin addict with the nephrotic syndrome stops using heroin in the early stages of the disease, symptoms may disappear. People who are sensitive to sunlight, poison oak, poison ivy, or insect bites should avoid these irritants. Allergy shots▲ (desensitization) may reverse the nephrotic syndrome associated with poison oak, poison ivy, or insect bites. If drugs are responsible

---

▲ see page 824

for the syndrome, stopping the drugs may eliminate the kidney problems.

If no cause can be found, the person is given corticosteroids and drugs that suppress the immune system, such as cyclophosphamide. However, such drugs cause problems for children because they can stunt growth and suppress sexual development.

General therapy includes a diet that contains normal amounts of protein and potassium but that is low in saturated fat and sodium. Eating too much protein raises protein levels in the urine. Angiotensin converting enzyme inhibitors, such as enalapril, captopril, and lisinopril, usually decrease protein excretion in the urine and lipid concentrations in the blood. However, these drugs may increase the blood potassium concentration in people who have moderate to severe kidney dysfunction.

If fluid accumulates in the abdomen, frequently eating small meals may help reduce symptoms. High blood pressure is usually treated with diuretics. Diuretics can also reduce fluid retention and tissue swelling but may increase the risk that blood clots will form. Anticoagulants may help control clot formation if it occurs. Infections can be life threatening and must be treated promptly.

Chronic Nephritic Syndrome

Chronic nephritic syndrome (chronic glomerulonephritis, slowly progressive glomerular disease) is a disorder occurring in several diseases in which the glomeruli are damaged and kidney function degenerates over a period of years.

The cause isn't known. In about 50 percent of people with chronic nephritic syndrome, there is evidence of an underlying glomerulopathy, although these people have no history of having symptoms.

Symptoms and Diagnosis

Because the syndrome causes no symptoms for years, it goes undetected in most people. It develops gradually, so a doctor may not be able to tell exactly when it began. It may be discovered during a routine medical examination of a person who is feeling well, has normal kidney function, and has no signs of a problem except the presence

of protein and possibly blood cells in the urine. In other cases, a person may have kidney failure, which causes nausea, vomiting, difficulty in breathing, itchiness, or fatigue. Fluid retention (edema) may occur. High blood pressure is common.

Because the symptoms of many kidney diseases are identical, a kidney biopsy is the most reliable method of distinguishing among them in the early stages of disease. A biopsy is rarely performed in advanced stages, when the kidneys are shrunken and scarred, because the chances of obtaining specific information about the cause would be small.

Prognosis and Treatment

Although many forms of therapy have been tried, none has prevented the disease from progressing. Taking drugs to reduce high blood pressure and restricting the intake of sodium are thought to help. Restricting the amount of protein eaten is modestly useful in reducing the rate of kidney deterioration. Kidney failure must be treated with dialysis or kidney transplantation.

Tubulointerstitial Nephritis

Tubulointerstitial nephritis may be acute or chronic. It may be caused by various diseases, drugs, or conditions that damage the kidneys.

Acute Tubulointerstitial Nephritis

Acute tubulointerstitial nephritis is kidney failure that begins suddenly, caused by damage to the kidney tubules and surrounding tissue.

The most common cause of acute tubulointerstitial nephritis is a drug, in which the person either has an allergy to it or suffers direct poisoning (a toxic reaction) from it. A toxic reaction may be caused by such drugs as amphotericin B and aminoglycosides. An allergic reaction may be triggered by such drugs as penicillin, the sulfonamides, diuretics, and nonsteroidal anti-inflammatory drugs, including aspirin.

Other causes include bacterial infection of the kidneys (pyelonephritis), cancers such as leukemia and lymphoma, and hereditary diseases.

The symptoms are highly variable. Some people develop the symptoms of a urinary tract infection: fever, painful urination, pus in the urine, and pain in the lower back or side (flank). Others have few symptoms, but laboratory tests detect signs of kidney failure. The amount of urine produced may be normal or less than normal.

The urine may be almost normal, with only a trace of protein or pus, but often the abnormalities are striking. The urine may contain protein at levels high enough to indicate nephrotic syndrome, microscopic or visible blood, or pus that includes eosinophils, a type of white blood cell. Eosinophils rarely appear in the urine, but when they do, a person almost certainly has acute tubulointerstitial nephritis caused by an allergic reaction.

When an allergic reaction is the cause, the kidneys usually are large because of inflammation caused by the allergy. The interval between the exposure to the allergen that caused the reaction and the development of the kidney abnormalities varies from 5 days to 5 weeks. Other symptoms of an allergic reaction include a fever, a rash, and an increased number of eosinophils in the blood.

A kidney biopsy is the only conclusive means of diagnosing this condition.

Some people must be treated for acute kidney failure.▲ Kidney function usually returns when the offending drug is stopped, although some kidney scarring is common. In some cases, the damage is irreversible. Corticosteroid therapy may speed the recovery of kidney function when the disorder is caused by an allergic reaction.

Chronic Tubulointerstitial Nephritis

Chronic tubulointerstitial nephritis is any chronic kidney disease in which damage of the tubules or surrounding tissue is more important than damage of the glomeruli or blood vessels.

This type of disorder is responsible for about a third of all cases of chronic kidney failure. About 20 percent of the cases of chronic tubulointerstitial nephritis result from taking a drug or toxin for a long time. The remainder may accompany a number of diseases.

Certain symptoms are common to all types of chronic tubulointerstitial nephritis. Puffiness or visible tissue swelling (edema) resulting from fluid retention usually is not present. Little protein is lost in the urine, and blood in the urine is uncommon. Blood pressure is normal or only slightly above normal in the early stages of the disease. If a large amount of protein or blood appears in the urine, glomerular disease is usually also present. If the kidney tubules aren't functioning normally, symptoms are similar to those of acute tubulointerstitial nephritis. Kidney stones form in some types of chronic tubulointerstitial nephritis.

CHAPTER 125

Blood Vessel Disorders of the Kidneys

The blood supply to the kidneys is vital for their proper function. Any interruption or reduction of the blood supply can cause problems, such as kidney damage, kidney dysfunction, and increased blood pressure.

Kidney Infarction

A kidney infarction is the death of an area of kidney tissue caused by a blockage of the renal artery, the main artery that carries blood to the kidney.

Blockage of the renal artery is rare, most frequently resulting when a particle that was floating in the bloodstream (embolus) lodges in the artery. The embolus may originate from a blood clot

▲ see page 593

(thrombus) in the heart or from the breakup of a cholesterol deposit (atheroma) in the aorta. Alternatively, the infarction may result from the formation of a blood clot (acute thrombosis) in the renal artery itself, resulting from injury to the artery. The injury may be caused by surgery, angiography, or angioplasty.▲ The clot may also result from severe atherosclerosis, arteritis (inflammation of arteries), sickle cell disease, or the rupture of a renal artery aneurysm—a bulge in the wall of the artery. A tear in the lining (acute dissection) of the renal artery causes blood flow in the artery to be blocked or the artery to rupture. Underlying causes of infarction include arteriosclerosis and fibrodysplasia (abnormal development of fibrous tissue in the wall of an artery).

A kidney infarction is occasionally produced intentionally (therapeutic infarction) to treat kidney tumors, massive loss of protein in the urine (proteinuria), or severe uncontrollable bleeding from the kidney. Blood flow to the kidney is blocked by passing a catheter into the artery that supplies the kidney.

Symptoms and Diagnosis

Small blockages of the renal artery often don't cause any symptoms. However, they may cause a steady aching pain in the lower back (flank pain) on the affected side. Fever, nausea, and vomiting may occur. Partial blockage of the artery may lead to high blood pressure.

Total blockage of both renal arteries—or of one renal artery in people who have only one kidney—completely stops urine production and shuts down the kidneys (acute kidney failure).

Blood tests usually show an abnormally high number of white blood cells. Protein and microscopic amounts of blood are present in the urine. Rarely, enough blood is present to be visible to the eye.

Imaging of the kidney is necessary to make the diagnosis, because none of the symptoms or laboratory tests can specifically identify a kidney infarction. During the first 2 weeks after a large infarction, the function of the affected kidney is poor. Intravenous urography or radionuclide imaging■ can show the poor kidney function because the kidney can't excrete normal amounts of the radiopaque substances (which are visible on x-rays) or radioactive tracers used in these tests. However, because poor kidney function can also be caused by conditions other than

---

Blood Vessel Disorders Affecting the Kidneys

- Inflammation of blood vessels (vasculitis), which can interfere with the blood supply

- Blockage of the renal artery, resulting in tissue death of the part of the kidney supplied by that vessel (kidney infarction)

- Blockage of small kidney (renal) blood vessels by small particles of fatty material broken off from blood vessel walls outside the kidney (atheroembolic kidney disease)

- Damage to all or part of the outer layer (cortex) of one or both kidneys (cortical necrosis)

- Damage to small blood vessels in the kidneys caused by high blood pressure (nephrosclerosis)

- Blockage of the renal vein (renal vein thrombosis)

---

infarction, an ultrasound scan or retrograde urography★ may be needed to distinguish among the possible causes. The best way to confirm the diagnosis and produce a clear picture of the problem is arteriography of the kidney, in which a radiopaque substance is injected into the renal artery. However, arteriography is performed only if the doctor is considering an attempt to relieve the obstruction. How well kidney function recovers may be evaluated by intravenous urography or radionuclide scanning repeated at 1-month intervals.

Treatment

The usual treatment is anticoagulants, which are given to prevent additional clots from blocking the renal artery. Drugs that dissolve clots (thrombolytics) are newer and may be more ef-

---

▲ see page 125

■ see page 609

★ see page 592

Kidney's Blood Supply

within $1\frac{1}{2}$ to 3 hours—the amount of time kidney tissue can tolerate the loss of its blood supply.

To remove the blockage, a doctor may thread a balloon catheter from the femoral artery in the groin to the renal artery. The balloon is then inflated to force open the obstructed area. This procedure is called percutaneous transluminal angioplasty.

The optimal treatment for kidney infarction is uncertain, but drug treatment is preferred. Although surgery can open obstructed blood vessels, it has greater risks of complications and death and does not improve kidney function more than anticoagulant or thrombolytic drugs alone. Surgery is the treatment of choice in one setting: when it is performed early (within 2 to 3 hours) to remove a blood clot in the renal artery resulting from an injury (traumatic renal artery thrombosis).

Although kidney function may improve with treatment, it usually isn't restored completely.

Atheroembolic Kidney Disease

Atheroembolic kidney disease is a condition in which numerous small pieces of fatty (atheromatous) material (emboli) clog the small renal arteries, causing the kidneys to fail.

Tiny pieces of fatty material lodged on a blood vessel wall break off, travel to the small renal arteries, and block the kidneys' blood supply. This condition may occur spontaneously or as a complication of surgery or procedures affecting the aorta, such as angiography, in which pieces of fatty material lining the aorta are unintentionally broken off. Atheroembolic kidney disease occurs most commonly in elderly people; the risk increases with age.

Symptoms

Atheroembolic disease usually proceeds gradually with progressive failure of the kidneys that causes no symptoms until the failure is advanced. If the blockage results from a procedure affecting the aorta, the time at which the blockage occurs is usually obvious, and the kidneys often fail suddenly. With complete kidney failure, a wide variety of symptoms appear, beginning with fatigue and a generally sick feeling (malaise). The symptoms aren't specifically caused by atheroembolic kidney disease, but they reflect disturbances in the muscles, nerves, heart, digestive tract, and skin that result from kidney failure.

Nephron

fective than other treatments. Drugs improve kidney function only when the artery is not completely blocked or when clots can be dissolved

Emboli are usually not limited to the renal arteries. They frequently obstruct the blood vessels of other organs, such as the pancreas and the intestine; common symptoms include abdominal pain, bloody stools, and diarrhea. If emboli travel to the extremities, such symptoms as a purplish netlike discoloration of the skin, painful muscle nodules, and even gangrene may result. Emboli that travel to an eye may cause sudden blindness.

Diagnosis and Treatment

Kidney failure is diagnosed easily with blood tests. Atheroembolic kidney disease is diagnosed by a kidney biopsy: Examination of a tissue sample obtained through a needle detects microscopic particles of fat blocking small arteries.

The only treatments for advanced kidney failure caused by atheroembolic kidney disease are kidney dialysis▲ and transplantation.■

Cortical Necrosis

Cortical necrosis is a rare form of kidney tissue death that affects some or all of the outer part of the kidneys (cortex) but not the inner part (medulla).

Cortical necrosis results from obstruction of the small arteries to the kidney cortex, which can be caused by many conditions.

Cortical necrosis can occur at any age. About 10 percent of the cases occur in infancy and childhood. More than half of the newborns with this condition had deliveries complicated by abrupt detachment of the placenta (abruptio placentae); the next most common cause is a bacterial infection of the bloodstream (bacterial sepsis). In children, cortical necrosis may follow an infection, dehydration, shock, or the hemolytic-uremic syndrome. In adults, bacterial sepsis causes a third of all cases of cortical necrosis. About 50 percent of reported cases occur in women who have complications of pregnancy, such as abrupt detachment of the placenta, abnormal position of the placenta (placenta previa), bleeding from the uterus, infections immediately after childbirth (puerperal sepsis), blockage of an artery (embolism) by amniotic fluid, death of the fetus within the uterus, and preeclampsia (high blood pressure with protein in the urine or fluid retention during pregnancy).

Other causes include rejection of a transplanted kidney, burns, inflammation of the pancreas (pancreatitis), injury, snakebite, and poisoning—for example, with phosphorus or arsenic.

Symptoms

Cortical necrosis may resemble other types of kidney failure. However, doctors suspect cortical necrosis when urine production decreases suddenly and radically without evidence of obstruction in the ureters or bladder and blood is found in the urine of a person who has a condition that may cause cortical necrosis. A fever is often present. Mild high blood pressure or even low blood pressure is common.

The small amount of urine that's produced contains protein and many red blood cells, along with white blood cells and casts (clumps of red and white blood cells and other debris). Levels of some enzymes, measurable in a blood sample, are abnormally high in the early stages of the disease.

Diagnosis and Treatment

The diagnosis can usually be established by ultrasound or computed tomography (CT) scanning. A kidney biopsy or arteriography can be performed, but it isn't needed in most cases. Calcium deposits seen on x-ray films suggest renal cortical necrosis, but they develop late in the disease as a result of healing and are found in only 20 to 50 percent of people.

Treatment is often complicated because the underlying condition must be treated. Kidney failure requires dialysis. Occasionally, people regain enough kidney function to discontinue dialysis after several months. About 20 to 40 percent partially recover kidney function. For the majority, however, kidney transplantation or lifelong dialysis is the only solution.

Malignant Nephrosclerosis

Malignant nephrosclerosis is a condition associated with severe high blood pressure (malignant hypertension) in which the smallest arteries (arterioles) in the kidneys are damaged and kidney failure progresses rapidly.

▲ see page 597

■ see page 834

Nephrosclerosis with malignant hypertension is most common in men during their 40s and 50s and in women during their 30s. It's more common among blacks than whites and uncommon among people who have high blood pressure.

Arteriosclerosis in the arteries of the kidney (benign nephrosclerosis) commonly accompanies aging and is associated with high blood pressure. Malignant nephrosclerosis is a much more severe condition that occurs with malignant hypertension. Malignant hypertension most commonly results from poorly controlled high blood pressure but may result from other conditions, such as glomerulonephritis, chronic kidney failure, narrowing of the renal artery (renal vascular hypertension), inflammation of kidney blood vessels (renal vasculitis), or, rarely, hormonal disorders such as pheochromocytoma, Conn's syndrome, or Cushing's syndrome.

Symptoms and Diagnosis

Symptoms are caused by injury to the brain, heart, and kidneys as a result of the severe high blood pressure; diastolic blood pressure is usually higher than 130 millimeters of mercury (mm Hg). Symptoms include restlessness, confusion, sleepiness, blurred vision, headache, nausea, and vomiting. By viewing the back of the eye with an ophthalmoscope, a doctor can see areas of bleeding, collections of fluid, and swelling of the optic nerve. The heart becomes enlarged, and heart failure is common. Coma may result from swelling (edema) of or bleeding within the brain.

Because the kidneys malfunction, protein can pass into the urine. Blood cells, detected by microscopic examination, appear in the urine, and casts of clumped red blood cells also may be seen. Anemia often results from the breakdown and impaired production of red blood cells. Widespread clotting within the blood vessels is also common. Blood levels of renin and aldosterone (substances produced by the kidneys that help regulate blood pressure) are extremely high.

Prognosis and Treatment

If the condition is not treated, about 50 percent of the people who have it die within 6 months, and most of the remainder die within a year. About

---

▲ see page 604

60 percent of the deaths result from kidney failure, 20 percent from heart failure, 20 percent from strokes, and 1 percent from heart attacks (myocardial infarctions). Lowering the blood pressure and treating the kidney failure significantly reduce the death rate, especially from heart and kidney failure and strokes.

People who have less severe kidney failure improve the most with treatment. For most people, the extraordinarily high blood pressure can be lowered satisfactorily with diet and drug therapy. Those who have progressive kidney failure can be kept alive by dialysis and occasionally improve enough that dialysis can be discontinued.

Renal Vein Thrombosis

Renal vein thrombosis is blockage of the renal vein, which carries blood away from the kidney.

The blockage may be acute (sudden) or chronic (gradual), producing a wide range of symptoms and usually resulting in the nephrotic syndrome,▲ in which large amounts of protein are lost in the urine.

In adults, this disorder usually occurs with other kidney disorders that cause loss of protein into the urine. It may be caused by kidney cancer or conditions that put pressure on the renal vein (for example, a tumor) or on the inferior vena cava, which the renal vein drains into. Other possible causes are oral contraceptive use, injury, or, rarely, thrombophlebitis migrans—a condition in which clotting occurs sequentially in different veins all over the body.

Symptoms and Diagnosis

People with renal vein thrombosis usually have no symptoms, and the disorder goes undetected. When it does cause symptoms, it follows one of two patterns, depending on whether the onset is gradual or sudden.

In adults, onset and progression are usually **gradual.** The urine contains protein, and urine volume diminishes. With **sudden** onset in adults, pain typically occurs in the side between the ribs and hips. The person has a fever, blood in the urine, scanty urine, retention of fluid and salt (sodium) causing tissue swelling (edema), an abnormally high number of white blood cells, and evidence of kidney failure on blood test results. Similar symptoms occur in children, but the disorder commonly starts with diarrhea, dehydration, and an increased tendency of the blood to clot. Massive destruction of the kidney occurs rarely.

Ultrasound scanning shows an enlarged kidney if the blockage developed suddenly or a shrunken kidney if the blockage developed gradually. Imaging tests such as intravenous urography and radionuclide scanning show poor kidney function. In these tests, a radiopaque substance is injected into a vein and its path tracked. X-ray films of the inferior vena cava or the renal vein (venography) may reveal the outline of the thrombosis. When additional information is needed, computed tomography (CT) or x-rays of the renal arteries may be performed.

Prognosis and Treatment

The outcome depends on the cause of the thrombosis, complications, and the degree of kidney damage. Death from this disorder is rare and usually results from a fatal underlying cause or from complications. One dangerous complication is pulmonary embolism, in which a clot becomes lodged in the lungs. Adequate kidney function depends on whether one or both kidneys are affected, whether blood flow is restored, and what the state of kidney function was before the thrombosis.

Rarely, surgery is performed to remove clots in the renal vein. A kidney is removed only if all of its tissue has died because its blood supply was blocked (total infarction). Anticoagulant drugs usually improve kidney function by preventing additional clot formation and can prevent pulmonary embolism. Using drugs that dissolve clots (thrombolytics) in addition to using anticoagulants is still experimental but promising.

CHAPTER 126

Metabolic and Congenital Kidney Disorders

Kidney abnormalities can be anatomic or metabolic in origin. Many are hereditary and present at birth (congenital).

Renal Tubular Acidosis

Renal tubular acidosis is a disorder in which the kidney tubules can't adequately remove acid from the blood to excrete into the urine.

Normally, the kidneys remove acid from the blood and excrete it into the urine. In renal tubular acidosis, the kidney tubules don't function properly, and insufficient amounts of acid are excreted into the urine. As a result, acid builds up in the blood, a condition called metabolic acidosis,▲ which leads to the following problems:
- Low potassium levels in the blood
- Calcium deposits in the kidney
- A tendency to become dehydrated
- Painful softening and bending of the bones (osteomalacia or rickets)

Renal tubular acidosis may be hereditary or may be caused by drugs, heavy metal poisoning, or an autoimmune disease, such as systemic lupus erythematosus or Sjögren's syndrome.

Symptoms and Diagnosis

Three types of renal tubular acidosis exist. Each type produces slightly different symptoms. When blood potassium levels are low, neurologic problems may develop, including muscle weakness, diminished reflexes, and even paralysis. Kidney stones may develop, causing damage to kidney cells and leading to chronic kidney failure.

A doctor considers the diagnosis of renal tubular acidosis when a person has certain characteristic symptoms or when routine blood tests reveal high acid levels and low potassium levels. Special tests help determine the type of renal tubular acidosis.

▲ see page 676

Types of Renal Tubular Acidosis

Type*	Cause	Underlying Abnormality	Resulting Symptoms and Metabolic Abnormalities
1	May be hereditary; may be triggered by an autoimmune disease or certain drugs; cause usually not known, especially in women	Inability to excrete acid into the urine	High blood acidity; mild dehydration; low blood potassium levels, leading to muscle weakness and paralysis; fragile bones; bone pain; kidney stones (calcium deposits); kidney failure
2	Usually caused by a hereditary disease such as Fanconi's syndrome, hereditary fructose intolerance, Wilson's disease, or Lowe's syndrome; may also be caused by heavy metal poisoning or certain drugs	Inability to reabsorb bicarbonate from the urine, so bicarbonate is lost	High blood acidity, mild dehydration, and low blood potassium levels
4	Not hereditary; caused by diabetes, an autoimmune disease, sickle cell disease, or an obstruction in the urinary tract	Deficiency of or inability to respond to aldosterone, a hormone that helps regulate potassium and sodium excretion in the kidneys	High blood acidity and high blood potassium levels that rarely cause symptoms, unless the potassium level is so high that irregular heartbeats and muscle paralysis develop

*Note: There is no type 3.

Treatment

Treatment depends on the type. Types 1 and 2 are treated by drinking a solution of bicarbonate (baking soda) every day to neutralize the acid in the blood. This treatment relieves the symptoms and prevents kidney failure and bone disease or keeps these problems from becoming worse. Other specially prepared solutions are available, and potassium supplements may also be required. In type 4, the acidosis is so mild that bicarbonate may not be needed. High potassium levels can be kept in check by drinking plenty of fluids and taking diuretics.

Renal Glycosuria

Renal glycosuria (glucosuria) is a condition in which glucose (sugar) is excreted into the urine, despite normal or low glucose levels in the blood.

The kidneys serve as a filter of the blood. When blood is filtered through the kidneys, glucose is removed along with many other substances. The filtered fluid passes through the network of tubules in the kidney, where wanted substances, including glucose, are reabsorbed and returned to the bloodstream and unwanted substances are excreted in urine. In most healthy people, glucose is completely reabsorbed back into the blood.

Normally, the body excretes glucose into the urine only when there is too much glucose in the blood. With renal glycosuria, glucose may be excreted into the urine despite normal glucose levels in the blood. This happens because the kidney tubules malfunction. Glycosuria may be an inherited condition.

Glycosuria has no symptoms or serious effects. A doctor makes the diagnosis when a routine urine test detects glucose in the urine even though blood glucose levels are normal. No treatment is needed, although occasionally a person with glycosuria develops diabetes.

Nephrogenic Diabetes Insipidus

Nephrogenic diabetes insipidus is a disorder in which the kidneys produce a large volume of dilute urine because they fail to respond to antidiuretic hormone and are unable to concentrate urine.

Both diabetes insipidus and the better-known type of diabetes, diabetes mellitus, ▲ result in the excretion of large volumes of urine. Otherwise, the two types of diabetes are very different.

Causes

Normally, the kidneys adjust the concentration of urine according to the body's needs. The kidneys make this adjustment in response to the level of antidiuretic hormone in the blood. Antidiuretic hormone, which is secreted by the pituitary gland, signals the kidneys to conserve water and concentrate the urine.

Two types of diabetes insipidus exist. In nephrogenic diabetes insipidus, the kidneys don't respond to antidiuretic hormone, so they continue to excrete a large amount of dilute urine. In the other type, the pituitary gland fails to secrete antidiuretic hormone.■

Nephrogenic diabetes insipidus may be hereditary. The gene that causes the disorder is recessive and carried on the X chromosome, so usually only males develop symptoms. However, females who carry the gene can transmit the disease to their sons.★ Other causes of nephrogenic diabetes insipidus include the use of certain drugs that can damage the kidneys. Such drugs include aminoglycoside antibiotics; demeclocycline, another antibiotic; and lithium, which is taken for manic-depressive disorder.

Symptoms and Diagnosis

When nephrogenic diabetes insipidus is hereditary, symptoms usually start soon after birth. The symptoms are excessive thirst (polydipsia) and the excretion of large volumes of dilute urine (polyuria). Because infants can't communicate thirst, they may become very dehydrated. They may develop a high fever accompanied by vomiting and convulsions.

If nephrogenic diabetes insipidus isn't quickly diagnosed and treated, the brain may be damaged, leaving the infant with permanent mental retardation. Frequent episodes of dehydration can also retard physical development. With treatment, however, an infant who has this disorder is likely to develop normally.

A doctor suspects nephrogenic diabetes insipidus based on the symptoms. Laboratory tests reveal high sodium levels in the blood and very dilute urine. Otherwise, kidney function seems normal. The diagnosis is confirmed by testing the kidney's response to antidiuretic hormone using the water deprivation test.●

Treatment

To prevent dehydration, people with nephrogenic diabetes insipidus must always drink adequate amounts of water as soon as they feel thirsty. Infants and young children must be given water frequently. People who drink enough water aren't likely to become dehydrated, but a prolonged period without water (generally more than 12 hours) can lead to serious dehydration. Certain drugs may help, such as thiazide diuretics (for example, hydrochlorothiazide) and nonsteroidal anti-inflammatory drugs (for example, indomethacin or tolmetin).

Cystinuria

Cystinuria is a rare disorder that results in excretion of the amino acid cystine into the urine, often causing cystine stones to form in the urinary tract.

Cystinuria is caused by an inherited defect of the kidney tubules. The gene that causes cystinuria is recessive, so people with the disorder must have inherited two abnormal genes, one from each parent.◆ People who carry the gene but don't have the disorder have one normal and one abnormal gene. These people may excrete larger than normal amounts of cystine into the urine, but seldom enough to form stones.

▲ see page 717

■ see page 703

★ see box, page 11

● see page 703

◆ see box, page 10

Symptoms and Diagnosis

Cystine stones form in the bladder, renal pelvis (area where urine collects and flows out of the kidney), or ureters (long narrow tubes that convey urine from the kidneys to the bladder). Symptoms usually start between ages 10 and 30. Usually, the first symptom is intense pain caused by a spasm of the ureter where a stone becomes lodged. Blockage of the urinary tract by stones may result in urinary tract infection and kidney failure.

A doctor tests for cystinuria when a person has recurring kidney stones. Cystine may form yellow-brown hexagonal crystals in the urine that are visible under a microscope. Excessive amounts of cystine in the urine can be detected and measured by several tests.

Treatment

Treatment consists of preventing cystine stones from forming by keeping the concentration of cystine in the urine low. To keep the cystine concentration low, a person with cystinuria must drink enough fluids to produce at least 8 pints of urine each day. During the night, however, when the person isn't drinking, less urine is produced and stone formation is more likely. This risk is reduced by drinking fluids before going to bed. Another treatment approach involves making the urine more alkaline by taking sodium bicarbonate and acetazolamide. Cystine dissolves more easily in alkaline urine than in acidic urine.

If stones continue to form despite these measures, a drug such as penicillamine may be tried. Penicillamine reacts with cystine to keep it dissolved. However, about half of all people who take penicillamine develop adverse effects, such as fever, rash, or joint pains.

Fanconi's Syndrome

Fanconi's syndrome is a rare disorder of tubule function that results in excess amounts of glucose, bicarbonate, phosphates, and certain amino acids in the urine.

Fanconi's syndrome may be hereditary or may be caused by the use of heavy metals or other chemical agents, vitamin D deficiency, kidney transplantation, multiple myeloma, or amyloidosis. Taking outdated tetracycline (an antibiotic) can also cause Fanconi's syndrome.

In hereditary Fanconi's syndrome, symptoms usually begin during infancy. A child may excrete a large amount of urine. Other symptoms include weakness and bone pain.

The symptoms and a blood test that shows high blood acidity may lead a doctor to suspect Fanconi's syndrome. The diagnosis is confirmed when urine tests detect high levels of glucose, phosphate, bicarbonate, uric acid, potassium, and sodium.

Fanconi's syndrome can't be cured. The high acidity of the blood (acidosis) may be neutralized by drinking sodium bicarbonate. Low blood potassium levels may require taking potassium supplements by mouth. Bone disease requires treatment with phosphates and vitamin D supplements given by mouth. Kidney transplantation may be lifesaving if a child with the disorder develops kidney failure.

Vitamin D–Resistant Rickets

Vitamin D–resistant rickets is a disorder in which the bones become painfully soft and bend easily because the blood contains low levels of phosphate and has inadequate amounts of the active form of vitamin D.

This very rare disorder is nearly always hereditary, passed as a dominant gene that is carried on the X chromosome.▲ The genetic defect causes a kidney abnormality that allows phosphate to be excreted into the urine, resulting in low blood phosphate levels. Because bone growth requires phosphate, this deficiency causes defective bones. Females with vitamin D–resistant rickets have less severe bone disease than males. In rare cases, the disorder develops as a result of certain cancers, such as giant cell tumors of bone, sarcomas, prostate cancer, and breast cancer. Vitamin D–resistant rickets isn't the same as rickets caused by vitamin D deficiency.■

Symptoms and Treatment

Vitamin D–resistant rickets usually begins in the first year of life. It ranges from so mild that it produces no noticeable symptoms to so severe that it produces bowing of the legs and other bone deformities, bone pain, and a short stature. Bony

▲ see page 9

■ see page 656

outgrowth where muscles attach to bones may limit movement at those joints. A baby's skull bones may close too soon, leading to convulsions. Laboratory tests show that blood calcium levels are normal, but phosphate levels are low.

The aim of treatment is to raise blood phosphate levels, which will promote normal bone formation. Phosphate can be taken by mouth and should be combined with calcitriol, the activated form of vitamin D. Taking vitamin D alone is not helpful. In some adults, rickets resulting from cancer has improved dramatically after the cancer was removed.

Hartnup Disease

Hartnup disease is a rare hereditary disorder that results in a skin rash and brain abnormalities because tryptophan and other amino acids aren't well absorbed from the intestine and excessive amounts of these substances are excreted into the urine.

Hartnup disease occurs when a person inherits two recessive genes for the disorder, one from each parent. The disorder affects how the body processes amino acids, which are the building blocks of proteins. People with the disorder aren't able to convert the amino acid tryptophan to the B vitamin niacinamide. Consequently, they can't absorb amino acids properly from the intestine and excrete excessive amounts of amino acids in the urine. The body is thus left with inadequate amounts of amino acids.

Symptoms
Symptoms may be triggered by sunlight, fever, drugs, or emotional or physical stress. A period of poor nutrition nearly always precedes an attack. The attacks usually become progressively less frequent with age. Most symptoms occur sporadically and are caused by a deficiency of niacinamide. A rash develops on parts of the body exposed to the sun. Mental retardation, a short stature, headaches, an unsteady gait, and collapsing or fainting are common. The person may become psychologically disturbed.

Diagnosis and Treatment
Laboratory tests performed on urine samples reveal the typical abnormal excretion pattern of amino acids and their breakdown products.

People with Hartnup disease can prevent attacks by maintaining good nutrition and supplementing their diet with niacinamide or niacin. A diet that's adequate in protein can overcome the deficiency caused by poor gastrointestinal absorption and excess excretion of amino acids into the urine.

Bartter's Syndrome

Bartter's syndrome is a disorder in which the kidneys overexcrete electrolytes (potassium, sodium, and chloride), resulting in low blood levels of potassium (hypokalemia) and high blood levels of the hormones aldosterone and renin.

Bartter's syndrome is usually hereditary and is caused by a recessive gene, thus a person with the disorder has inherited two recessive genes for the disorder, one from each parent.

Symptoms
Children with Bartter's syndrome grow slowly and appear malnourished. They may have muscle weakness and excessive thirst, may produce large amounts of urine, and may be mentally retarded.

The levels of sodium chloride and water in the blood become low. The body tries to compensate by producing more aldosterone and renin; these hormones reduce the levels of potassium in the blood.▲

Diagnosis and Treatment
A doctor suspects Bartter's syndrome based on the symptoms. Laboratory test results that reveal abnormal levels of potassium and hormones in the blood support the diagnosis.

Many of the consequences of Bartter's syndrome can be prevented by taking potassium supplements by mouth and a drug that reduces excretion of potassium into the urine, such as spironolactone (which also blocks the action of aldosterone), triamterene, amiloride, propranolol, or indomethacin. Drinking adequate amounts of fluids is necessary to compensate for the excessive fluid losses.

Liddle's Syndrome

Liddle's syndrome is a rare hereditary disorder in which the kidneys excrete potassium but retain too much sodium and water, leading to high blood pressure.

▲ see page 670

Polycystic Kidney Disease

In polycystic kidney disease, many cysts form in both kidneys. The cysts gradually enlarge, destroying some or most of the normal tissue in the kidneys.

Normal Kidney	Polycystic Kidney

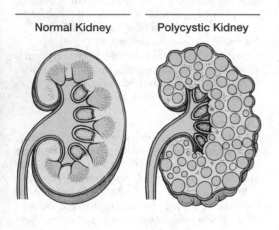

An abnormality in the kidneys causes Liddle's syndrome. Triamterene or amiloride, drugs that prevent potassium excretion, can be taken to increase the excretion of sodium and water and lower blood pressure.

Polycystic Kidney Disease

Polycystic kidney disease is a hereditary disorder in which many cysts form in both kidneys; the kidneys grow larger but have less functioning kidney tissue.

The genetic defect that causes polycystic kidney disease may be dominant or recessive. In other words, a person with the disease has inherited either a dominant gene from one parent or two recessive genes, one from each parent. Those with dominant gene inheritance usually have no symptoms until adulthood; those with recessive gene inheritance have severe illness in childhood.

▲ see page 356

■ see page 597

Symptoms

In children, polycystic kidney disease causes the kidneys to become very large and the abdomen to protrude. A severely affected newborn may die shortly after birth, because kidney failure in the fetus leads to poor development of the lungs. The liver is also affected, and at 5 to 10 years of age, a child with this disorder tends to develop high blood pressure in the blood vessel that connects the intestine and the liver (portal system). Eventually, liver failure and kidney failure occur.

In adults, polycystic kidney disease progresses slowly over many years. Typically, symptoms begin in early or middle adulthood, although occasionally the disease isn't discovered until after death at autopsy. Symptoms usually include back discomfort or pain, blood in the urine, infection, and intense crampy (colicky) pain from kidney stones. In other cases, fatigue, nausea, inadequate production of urine, and other consequences of kidney failure may result because the person has less functioning kidney tissue. Chronic infection, a frequent problem, can worsen the kidney failure. About half of those with polycystic kidney disease have high blood pressure at the time of diagnosis.

About a third of the people who have polycystic kidney disease also have cysts in the liver, but these cysts don't affect liver function. More than 20 percent of the people with the disease have dilated blood vessels in the skull, and 75 percent of these people ultimately have a brain hemorrhage (subarachnoid hemorrhage).▲

Diagnosis, Prognosis, and Treatment

A doctor suspects this disease on the basis of family history and symptoms. When the disease is advanced and the kidneys are very large, the diagnosis is obvious. Ultrasound scans and computed tomography (CT) reveal the characteristic moth-eaten appearance of the kidneys and liver caused by the cysts.

More than half of the people who have this disease develop kidney failure at some time in their life. Treating urine infections and high blood pressure may prolong life. Without dialysis■ or kidney transplantation, kidney failure is fatal.

Genetic counseling can help people with polycystic kidney disease understand the probability that their children will inherit the condition.

Medullary Cystic Disease

Medullary cystic disease is a disorder in which kidney failure develops along with cysts deep within the kidneys.

Medullary cystic disease is either hereditary or caused by a birth defect (congenital).

Symptoms usually begin before age 20, but symptoms vary greatly and a few people don't have any symptoms until much later. A person starts to produce excessive amounts of urine because the kidneys don't respond to antidiuretic hormone, which normally signals the kidneys to concentrate urine. This may cause an excessive amount of sodium to be excreted, so a large daily intake of fluids and salt (sodium) is needed. Retarded growth and evidence of bone disease are common in children. In many people, these problems develop slowly over several years, and the body compensates so well that the problems are not recognized until kidney failure is advanced.

Laboratory tests reveal poor kidney function. X-rays show that the kidneys are small. Ultrasound scans may detect cysts deep within the kidneys, although the cysts may be too small to be detected.

The disease progresses slowly but relentlessly. When kidney failure occurs, dialysis or kidney transplantation is needed.

Medullary Sponge Kidney

Medullary sponge kidney is a congenital disorder in which the urine-containing tubules of the kidneys are dilated, causing the kidney tissue to appear spongy.

Medullary sponge kidney causes no symptoms most of the time, but a person with the disorder is prone to painful kidney stones, blood in the urine, and kidney infections. Calcium deposits in the kidneys occur in more than half of the people with the disorder.

The symptoms lead a doctor to request x-rays of the kidneys, which reveal the calcium deposits. The diagnosis can be confirmed by an imaging technique in which a radiopaque substance, visible on x-rays, is injected intravenously and then observed on x-rays as it is excreted by the kidneys. Ultrasound scans may help but may not detect tiny cysts lying deep within the kidneys.

Treatment usually isn't necessary if medullary sponge kidney doesn't cause calcium deposits.

Taking thiazide diuretics, drinking a lot of fluids, and eating a low calcium diet may prevent stones from forming and obstructing the urinary tract. Surgery may be needed if the urinary tract becomes obstructed. Infections are treated with antibiotics.

Alport's Syndrome

Alport's syndrome (hereditary nephritis) is a hereditary disorder in which kidney function is poor, blood is present in the urine, and deafness and eye abnormalities sometimes occur.

Alport's syndrome is caused by a defective gene on the X chromosome,▲ but other factors influence how severe the disorder is in a person who has the gene. Women with the defective gene on one of their two X chromosomes usually don't have symptoms, although their kidneys may be somewhat less efficient than normal. Men with the defective gene (men don't have a second X chromosome to compensate for the defect) usually develop kidney failure between ages 20 and 30. Many people have no symptoms other than blood in the urine, but the urine may also contain varying amounts of protein, white blood cells, and casts (small clumps of material) of various types visible under a microscope.

Alport's syndrome can affect organs other than the kidneys. Hearing problems, usually an inability to hear sounds in the higher frequencies, are common. Cataracts can also occur, although less frequently than hearing loss. Abnormalities of the cornea, lens, or retina sometimes cause blindness. Other problems include abnormalities that affect several nerves (polyneuropathy) and a low blood platelet count (thrombocytopenia).■

People who develop kidney failure need to undergo dialysis or receive a kidney transplant. Genetic counseling is usually offered to people with Alport's syndrome who want to have children.

Nail-Patella Syndrome

The nail-patella syndrome is a rare hereditary disorder of the connective tissue that results in abnormalities of the kidneys, bones, joints, and fingernails.

▲ see page 10

■ see page 755

Most commonly, in people who have this syndrome, one or both kneecaps (patellas) are missing, one of the arm bones (the radius) is dislocated at the elbow, and the pelvic bone is abnormally shaped. They either have no fingernails or poorly developed ones, with pitting and ridges. The irises of the eyes may be variably colored.

The urine may contain proteins, usually in small amounts, and rarely blood, which may prompt the doctor to order kidney function tests. Kidney failure eventually develops in about 30

percent of the people with affected kidneys. The diagnosis is confirmed by bone x-rays and a biopsy of kidney tissue.

Most people don't need treatment. Those who develop kidney failure need dialysis or a kidney transplant. Genetic counseling is usually offered to people who want to have children. The gene that causes nail-patella syndrome is dominant, meaning that children of a person with the disorder have a 50 percent chance of inheriting the defective gene.

CHAPTER 127

Urinary Tract Infections

In healthy people, urine in the bladder is sterile: No bacteria or other infectious organisms are present. The urethra, the channel that carries urine from the bladder out of the body, contains either no infectious organisms or too few to cause infection. However, any part of the urinary tract can become infected. These infections are usually classified as lower or upper urinary tract infections; lower refers to infections of the urethra or bladder, and upper refers to infections of the kidneys or ureters.

The organisms that cause infection usually enter the urinary tract by one of two routes. The most common route by far is through the lower end of the urinary tract—the opening at the tip of a man's penis or the opening of a woman's urethra where it exits at the vulva. The result is an ascending infection that spreads up the urethra. The other possible route is through the bloodstream, usually directly to the kidneys.

Urinary tract infections may be caused by bacteria, viruses, fungi, or a variety of parasites.

Bacteria: Bacterial infections of the lower urinary tract—the bladder and urethra—are very common. They are more common in male than in

▲ see pages 916 and 946

■ see page 908

female newborns but become about 10 times more common in girls than in boys by age 1. Roughly 5 percent of adolescent girls develop urinary tract infections at some time, but adolescent boys rarely do. Among people between the ages of 20 and 50, urinary tract infections are about 50 times more common in women than in men. The infections become more common in both men and women, with less difference between the sexes, in later years.

More than 85 percent of urinary tract infections are caused by bacteria from a person's own intestine or vagina. Ordinarily, however, bacteria that enter the urinary tract are washed out by the flushing action of the bladder as it empties.

Viruses: Infections by the herpes simplex virus type 2 (HSV-2)▲ affect the penis in men and may affect the vulva, perineum, buttocks, cervix, or vagina in women. If the urethra is affected, urination may be painful and emptying the bladder may be difficult.

Fungi: Fungal infections ■ of the urinary tract are most commonly caused by *Candida* (yeast that causes candidiasis) in people who have a bladder catheter in place. Rarely, other types of fungus, including those that cause blastomycosis *(Blastomyces)* or coccidiomycosis *(Coccidioides),* can also infect the urinary tract. Fungi and bacteria often infect the kidneys at the same time.

Parasites: A number of parasites,▲ including worms, can cause urinary tract infections. **Malaria,** a disease caused by protozoan parasites carried by mosquitoes, can block the small blood vessels of the kidneys or can rapidly damage red blood cells (hemolysis), causing acute kidney failure. **Trichomoniasis,** also caused by a protozoan, is a sexually transmitted disease that can produce a copious greenish-yellow, frothy discharge from the vagina. Rarely, the bladder becomes infected. Trichomoniasis in men usually produces no symptoms, although it can cause inflammation of the prostate gland (prostatitis).

Schistosomiasis, a worm infection, can affect the kidneys, ureters, and bladder and is a common cause of severe kidney failure among people who live in Egypt and Brazil. The infection can cause persistent bladder infections that may eventually result in bladder cancer. **Filariasis,** a threadworm infection, obstructs lymphatic vessels, causing lymphatic fluid in the urine (chyluria). Filariasis can cause enormous swelling of tissues (elephantiasis), which may involve the scrotum and legs.

Urethritis

Urethritis is an infection of the urethra, the channel that carries urine from the bladder out of the body.

Urethritis may be caused by bacteria, fungi, or viruses. In women, the organisms generally travel to the urethra from the vagina. In most cases, the bacteria come from the lower intestine and reach the vagina from the anus. Men are much less likely to develop urethritis. Sexually transmitted organisms—such as *Neisseria gonorrhoeae,* which causes gonorrhea■—reach the vagina or penis during sexual intercourse with an infected partner and can spread to the urethra. When men do develop urethritis, the gonococcal organism is a very common cause. Although this organism may infect the urethra in women, the vagina, cervix, uterus, ovaries, and fallopian tubes are more likely to be infected. Chlamydia and the herpes simplex virus also can be transmitted sexually and can cause urethritis.

Symptoms

In men, urethritis usually begins with a discharge from the urethra. The discharge contains

Urinary Tract Infections

Organ	Infection
Urethra	Urethritis
Bladder	Cystitis
Ureters	Ureteritis
Kidneys	Pyelonephritis

pus when the gonococcal organism is involved or mucus when other organisms are involved. Other symptoms of urethritis include pain during urination and a frequent, urgent need to urinate. A vaginal infection may cause pain during urination as the urine, which is acidic, passes over the inflamed labia.

A gonorrheal infection of the urethra that isn't treated or is inadequately treated eventually can cause a narrowing (stricture) of the urethra. The stricture increases the risk of developing urethritis higher in the urethra and occasionally leads to the formation of an abscess★ around the urethra. The abscess can produce outpouchings from the urethral wall (urethral diverticula), which can also become infected. If the abscess perforates the skin, urine may flow through the newly created channel (urethral fistula).

Diagnosis and Treatment

The diagnosis of urethritis is usually apparent from the symptoms alone. A sample (urethral swab) of the discharge, if present, is collected and sent to a laboratory for analysis so that the infecting organism can be identified.

The treatment depends on the cause of the infection. Antibiotics are given for a bacterial infection. A herpes simplex infection may be treated with an antiviral drug, such as acyclovir.

▲ see page 895

■ see page 941

★ see page 856

Factors Contributing to Bacterial Urinary Tract Infections

Ascending Infections
• Blockage (for example, by stones) anywhere in the urinary tract
• Abnormal bladder function that prevents proper emptying, such as occurs in neurologic diseases
• Leaking of the valve between the ureter and the bladder, allowing urine and bacteria to flow backward from the bladder, possibly reaching the kidneys
• Insertion of a urinary catheter or an instrument by a doctor

Blood-borne Infections
• Infection in the bloodstream (septicemia)
• Infection of the heart valves (infective endocarditis)

Cystitis

Cystitis is an infection of the bladder.

Bladder infections are common in women, particularly during the reproductive years. Some women develop bladder infections repeatedly.

Bacteria in the vagina may travel to the urethra and into the bladder. Women often develop bladder infections after engaging in sexual intercourse, probably because the urethra was bruised during sex. Rarely, recurring bladder infections in women are caused by an abnormal connection between the bladder and the vagina (vesicovaginal fistula), which may cause no other symptoms.

Bladder infections are less common in men and generally start with an infection in the urethra that moves into the prostate, then into the bladder. Alternatively, a bladder infection can be caused by a catheter or an instrument used during surgery. The most common cause of recurring bladder infections in men is a persistent bacterial infection of the prostate.▲ Although antibiotics quickly clear bacteria from the urine in the bladder, most of these drugs can't penetrate well enough into the prostate to cure an infection there. Consequently, when drug therapy is stopped, the bacteria that remain in the prostate tend to reinfect the bladder.

Rarely, an abnormal connection between the bladder and the intestine (vesicoenteric fistula) develops, sometimes enabling bacteria that produce gas to enter and grow in the bladder. These infections can produce air bubbles in the urine (pneumaturia).

Symptoms

Bladder infections usually produce a frequent, urgent desire to urinate and a burning or painful sensation during urination. Pain is usually felt above the pubic bone and often in the lower back as well. Frequent urination during the night is another symptom. The urine is often cloudy and contains visible blood in about 30 percent of people. Symptoms may disappear without treatment. Sometimes a bladder infection produces no symptoms and is discovered when a urine examination (urinalysis) is performed for other reasons. Bladder infections without symptoms are particularly common in the elderly, who may develop urinary incontinence■ as a result.

A person whose nerve supply to the bladder is malfunctioning (neurogenic bladder) or a person who has had a catheter left continuously in the bladder may have a bladder infection with no symptoms until a kidney infection or an unexplained fever develops.

Diagnosis

A doctor can diagnose a bladder infection on the basis of its typical symptoms. A midstream (clean-catch) urine specimen★ is collected so that the urine isn't contaminated with bacteria from the vagina or the tip of the penis. The person begins to urinate into the toilet, stops, then urinates into a sterile container. The urine is examined under a microscope to see whether it contains red or white blood cells or other substances. Bacteria are counted, and the sample is cultured to identify the type of bacteria. If the person has an infection, one type of bacteria is usually present in large numbers.

▲ see page 1061

■ see page 631

★ see box, page 591

In men, a midstream urine specimen is usually sufficient for the diagnosis. In women, these specimens are sometimes contaminated by bacteria from the vagina. To ensure that the urine is not contaminated, a doctor often must obtain a specimen of a woman's urine directly from the bladder with a catheter.

Finding the cause of frequently recurring infections is important. Doctors may perform an x-ray study in which a radiopaque substance, visible on x-rays, is injected into a vein, then excreted into the urine by the kidneys.▲ The x-ray films provide images of the kidneys, ureters, and bladder. Performing voiding cystourethrography, which involves putting the radiopaque substance into the bladder and filming its exit, is a good way to investigate the backflow of urine from the bladder, particularly in children, and may also identify any narrowing of the urethra. A retrograde urethrogram, in which the radiopaque substance is inserted directly into the urethra, is useful for detecting a narrowing, outpouchings, or abnormal connections (fistulas) of the urethra in both men and women. Looking directly into the bladder with a fiber-optic scope (cystoscopy) may help diagnose the problem when a bladder infection doesn't improve with treatment.

Treatment

In the elderly, infection without symptoms generally requires no treatment.

As a first step, drinking plenty of fluids often eliminates a mild bladder infection. The flushing action of the urine washes many bacteria out of the body; the body's natural defenses eliminate the remainder.

Before prescribing antibiotics, the doctor determines whether the person has a condition that would make a bladder infection more severe, such as abnormalities of structure or nerve supply, diabetes, or a weakened immune system that reduces the person's ability to fight infection. Such conditions may require more aggressive treatment, particularly because the infection is likely to return as soon as the person stops taking antibiotics.

Taking an antibiotic by mouth for 3 days or even taking a single dose is usually effective if the infection hasn't led to any complications. For more stubborn infections, an antibiotic is usually taken for 7 to 10 days.

Antibiotics may be taken continually in low doses as prevention (prophylaxis) against infection by people who have more than two bladder infections a year. The yearly cost is only one fourth the cost of treating three or four infections a year. Typically, the antibiotic is taken daily, three times a week, or immediately after sexual intercourse.

A variety of drugs are used to relieve symptoms, especially frequent, insistent urges to urinate and painful urination. Certain drugs, such as atropine, may relieve muscle spasms. Other drugs, such as phenazopyridine, reduce the pain by soothing the inflamed tissues. Often, symptoms can be relieved by making the urine alkaline, which involves drinking baking soda dissolved in water.

Surgery may be necessary to relieve a physical obstruction to urine flow (obstructive uropathy) or to correct a structural abnormality that makes infection more likely, such as a drooping uterus and bladder. Draining urine from an obstructed area through a catheter helps control the infection. Usually, an antibiotic is given before surgery to reduce the risk of the infection spreading throughout the body.

Interstitial Cystitis

Interstitial cystitis is a painful inflammation of the bladder.

The cause of this inflammation is unknown because no infectious organisms are found in the urine. Typically, middle-aged women are affected. Symptoms include frequent, painful urination, and the urine often contains pus and blood detected by microscopic examination. Occasionally, blood is visible in the urine, and transfusions may be needed. The eventual result often is a shrunken bladder. The diagnosis is established by cystoscopy, which may detect small superficial areas of bleeding and ulcers. A number of treatments have been tried, but none is particularly satisfactory. When a patient has intolerable symptoms that don't respond to any treatment, the bladder may be surgically removed.

▲ see page 591

Ureteritis

Ureteritis is an infection of one or both ureters, the tubes that connect the kidneys to the bladder.

The spread of an infection from the kidneys or bladder is the most common cause. Another cause of ureteritis is a slowing of urine flow (urinary holdup) because of a defective nerve supply to part of the ureter.▲ The underlying kidney or bladder infection is treated. The sections of the ureter in which nerves are defective may be removed surgically.

Pyelonephritis

Pyelonephritis is a bacterial infection of one or both kidneys.

Escherichia coli, a bacterium that's normally found in the large intestine, causes about 90 percent of kidney infections among people who live in the community but only about 50 percent among hospitalized patients. Infections usually ascend from the genital area to the bladder. In a healthy urinary tract, the infection is usually prevented from moving up the ureters into the kidneys by the urine flow washing organisms out and by closure of the ureters at their entrance to the bladder. However, any physical obstruction to the flow of urine, such as a kidney stone or an enlargement of the prostate, or backflow of urine from the bladder into the ureters increases the likelihood of a kidney infection.

Infections can also be carried to the kidneys from another part of the body through the bloodstream. For instance, a staphylococcal skin infection can spread to the kidneys through the bloodstream.

Other conditions that increase the risk of a kidney infection include pregnancy, diabetes, and conditions that reduce the body's ability to fight infection.

Symptoms

Symptoms of a kidney infection usually begin suddenly with chills, fever, pain in the lower part of the back on either side, nausea, and vomiting.

▲ see page 629

■ see page 593

About a third of the people with kidney infections also have symptoms of a lower urinary tract infection, including frequent, painful urination. One or both kidneys may be enlarged and tender, with tenderness felt in the small of the back on the affected side. Sometimes the muscles of the abdomen are tightly contracted. A person may experience episodes of intense pain caused by spasms of one of the ureters (renal colic). The spasms may be caused by irritation from the infection or the passing of a kidney stone. In children, symptoms of a kidney infection often are slight and more difficult to recognize. In a long-standing infection (chronic pyelonephritis), the pain may be vague, and fever may come and go or not occur at all. Chronic pyelonephritis occurs only in people who have major underlying abnormalities, such as a urinary tract obstruction, large kidney stones that persist, or, most commonly, backflow of urine from the bladder into the ureters in young children. Chronic pyelonephritis can eventually damage the kidneys to such an extent that they can no longer function properly. The result is kidney failure.■

Diagnosis

The typical symptoms of a kidney infection lead a doctor to perform two common laboratory tests to determine whether the kidneys are infected: examining a urine specimen under a microscope and culturing bacteria in a urine specimen to determine which bacteria are present.

Additional tests are performed for people who have intense back pain from renal colic, those who don't respond to antibiotic treatment within 48 hours, those whose symptoms return shortly after antibiotic treatment is finished, and men, because they so rarely develop a kidney infection. Ultrasound or x-ray studies performed in these situations may reveal kidney stones, structural abnormalities, or other causes of urinary obstruction.

Treatment

Antibiotics are started as soon as the diagnosis of a kidney infection seems likely and the person's urine and blood samples have been taken for laboratory tests. The choice of drug or its dosage may be modified based on the laboratory test results. Antibiotic treatment to prevent recurrence of the infection usually continues for 2 weeks but may last as long as 6 weeks for men, in whom the infection commonly is more difficult to eradicate. A final urine sample is usually taken 4 to 6 weeks after the antibiotic treatment is finished to make sure the infection has been eradicated.

If tests reveal a predisposing condition, such as an obstruction, a structural abnormality, or a stone, surgery may be needed to correct the condition.

People who have frequent kidney infections or whose infections return after antibiotic treatment is finished may be advised to take a small dose of antibiotic every day as preventive therapy. The ideal duration of such therapy is unknown, but it's often stopped after a year. If the infection returns, therapy may be continued indefinitely.

CHAPTER 128

Urinary Tract Obstruction

An obstruction anywhere along the urinary tract—from the kidneys, where urine is produced, to the urethra, through which urine leaves the body—can increase pressure inside the urinary tract and slow the flow of urine. Urinary obstruction can distend the kidneys and also lead to urinary tract infections, stone formation, and the loss of kidney function. Infection may develop because bacteria that enter the urinary tract aren't flushed out when urine flow is obstructed.

Hydronephrosis

Hydronephrosis is distention (dilation) of the kidney with urine, caused by backward pressure on the kidney when the flow of urine is obstructed.

Normally, urine flows out of the kidneys at extremely low pressure. If the urine flow is obstructed, urine backs up in the small tubes of the kidney and the central collecting area (renal pelvis), distending the kidney and putting pressure on its delicate tissues. The pressure from prolonged and severe hydronephrosis ultimately damages the kidney's tissues so that kidney function is gradually lost.

Causes

Hydronephrosis commonly results from ureteropelvic junction obstruction (an obstruction located at the junction of the ureter and renal pelvis). Causes include the following:
• Structural abnormalities—for example, when the insertion of the ureter into the renal pelvis is too high

• Kinking in this junction resulting from a kidney shifting downward
• Stones in the renal pelvis
• Compression of the ureter by fibrous bands, an abnormally located artery or vein, or a tumor

Hydronephrosis can also result from an obstruction below the junction of the ureter and renal pelvis or from backflow of urine from the bladder. Causes include the following:
• Stones in the ureter
• Tumors in or near the ureter
• Narrowing of the ureter resulting from a birth defect, an injury, an infection, radiation therapy, or surgery
• Disorders of the muscles or nerves in the ureter or bladder
• Formation of fibrous tissue in or around the ureter resulting from surgery, x-rays, or drugs (especially methysergide)
• Ureterocele (bulging of the lower end of a ureter into the bladder)
• Cancers of the bladder, cervix, uterus, prostate, or other pelvic organs
• Obstruction that prevents urine flow from the bladder to the urethra, resulting from prostate enlargement, inflammation, or cancer
• Backflow of urine from the bladder resulting from a birth defect or an injury
• Severe urinary tract infection, temporarily preventing the ureter from contracting

Occasionally, hydronephrosis occurs during pregnancy if the enlarging uterus compresses the ureters. Hormonal changes during pregnancy

Hydronephrosis: A Distended Kidney

In hydronephrosis, the kidney is distended because urine flow is obstructed and urine backs up in the kidney's small tubes and central collecting area (renal pelvis).

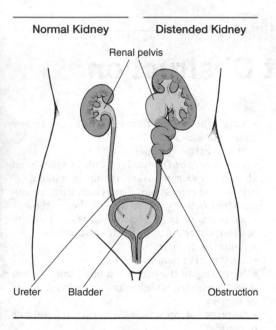

Normal Kidney   **Distended Kidney**

Renal pelvis

Ureter   Bladder   Obstruction

may aggravate the problem by reducing the muscular contractions of ureters that normally move urine to the bladder. This type of hydronephrosis usually ends when the pregnancy ends, although the renal pelvis and ureters may remain somewhat distended afterward.

Long-standing distention of the renal pelvis can inhibit the rhythmic muscular contractions that normally move urine down the ureters to the bladder. Nonfunctioning fibrous tissue may then replace the normal muscular tissue in the walls of the ureter, resulting in permanent damage.

Symptoms

Symptoms depend on the cause of the obstruction, its location, and its duration. When the ob-

struction begins quickly **(acute hydronephrosis)**, it usually produces renal colic—excruciating, intermittent pain in the flank (the area between the ribs and hip) on the affected side. When slowly progressive **(chronic hydronephrosis)**, it may produce either no symptoms or attacks of dull, aching discomfort in the flank on the affected side. A doctor may be able to feel a mass in the flank, particularly if the kidney is greatly distended in an infant or a child. Hydronephrosis may be intermittent and excruciatingly painful, resulting from temporary overfilling of the renal pelvis or temporary blockage of the ureter caused by a kidney that has shifted downward.

About 10 percent of people with hydronephrosis have blood in the urine. Urinary tract infections—with pus in the urine (usually identified by a laboratory test), fever, and discomfort in the area of the bladder or kidney—are fairly common. When urine flow is obstructed, stones (calculi) may form. Blood tests may detect a high urea level, which indicates that the kidneys aren't removing enough of this waste product from the blood. Hydronephrosis may cause vague intestinal symptoms, such as nausea, vomiting, and abdominal pain. These symptoms sometimes occur in children with hydronephrosis resulting from a birth defect in which the junction of the renal pelvis and ureter is too narrow. If untreated, hydronephrosis eventually damages the kidneys and can result in kidney failure.

Diagnosis

Several procedures are used to diagnose hydronephrosis. Ultrasound scanning can provide good images of the kidneys, ureters, and bladder and is particularly useful in children. In intravenous urography, the kidneys may be x-rayed after a radiopaque substance, which can be seen on x-rays, is injected into the bloodstream. X-ray images of the bladder and urethra can be produced after the injected radiopaque substance passes through the kidneys or after this substance is introduced into the urinary tract through the urethra in a procedure called retrograde urography. These tests can provide information about the flow of urine through the kidneys. Cystoscopy, in which a viewing tube containing a fiber-optic device is inserted into the urethra, is used to view the inside of the bladder directly.

Treatment and Prognosis

Urinary tract infections and kidney failure, if present, are treated promptly.

In **acute hydronephrosis,** urine that has accumulated above the obstruction in the kidney is drained as soon as possible—usually with a needle inserted through the skin—if kidney function has decreased, infection persists, or pain is severe. If the obstruction is complete, the infection is serious, or stones are present, a catheter to temporarily drain the urine may be inserted into the renal pelvis through the skin of the flank.

Chronic hydronephrosis is corrected by treating the cause and by relieving the urinary obstruction. A narrow or abnormal section of a ureter may be surgically removed and the cut ends joined together. Sometimes surgery to free the ureters from fibrous tissue is needed. If the junction of the ureters and bladder is obstructed, the ureters can be surgically detached, then attached to a different part of the bladder.

If the urethra is obstructed, treatment can include drugs such as hormone therapy for prostate cancer, surgery, or enlargement of the urethra with dilators. Other treatments may be needed for stones that block urine flow.

Surgery to correct acute hydronephrosis in one or both kidneys is usually successful when the infection can be controlled and the kidneys are functioning adequately. The prognosis is less certain for chronic hydronephrosis.

Stones in the Urinary Tract

Stones in the urinary tract (urinary calculi) are hard stonelike masses that form anywhere in the urinary tract and may cause pain, bleeding, obstruction of urine flow, or an infection.

Depending on where a stone forms, it may be called a kidney stone or bladder stone. The process of stone formation is called urolithiasis (renal lithiasis, nephrolithiasis).

Every year, about 1 out of 1,000 adults in the United States is hospitalized because of stones in the urinary tract. Stones may form because the urine becomes too saturated with salts that can form stones or because the urine lacks the normal inhibitors of stone formation. About 80 percent of the stones are composed of calcium; the remainder, of various substances, including uric acid, cystine, and struvite. Struvite stones—a mixture

of magnesium, ammonium, and phosphate—are also called infection stones, because they form only in infected urine.

Stones vary in size from too small to be seen with the eye alone to 1 inch or more in diameter. A large so-called staghorn calculus (stone) may be shaped by and may fill almost the entire renal pelvis and the tubes that drain into it (calices).

Symptoms

Stones, especially tiny ones, may not cause any symptoms. Stones in the bladder may cause pain in the lower abdomen. Stones that obstruct the ureter or renal pelvis or any of its drainage tubes may cause back pain or a severe colicky pain (renal colic). Renal colic is characterized by an excruciating intermittent pain, usually in the flank, that spreads across the abdomen, often to the genital area and inner thigh. Other symptoms include nausea and vomiting, abdominal distention, chills, fever, and blood in the urine. A person may need to urinate frequently, particularly as a stone passes down the ureter.

Stones may cause a urinary tract infection. When stones block the flow of urine, bacteria become trapped in urine that pools above the blockage, leading to an infection. When stones block the urinary tract for a long time, urine backs up in the tubes inside the kidney, producing pressure that can distend the kidney (hydronephrosis) and eventually damage it.

Diagnosis

Stones that cause no symptoms may be discovered by chance during a routine microscopic analysis of the urine (urinalysis). Stones that cause pain are generally diagnosed on the basis of the symptoms of renal colic, together with tenderness over the back and groin or pain in the genital area without an obvious cause. Microscopic analysis of the urine may disclose blood or pus in the urine as well as small stone crystals. Usually, no additional tests are needed, unless the pain persists for more than a few hours or the diagnosis is uncertain.

Additional tests that help make the diagnosis involve collecting 24-hour urine samples and blood samples, which are analyzed for levels of calcium, cystine, uric acid, and other substances known to produce stones.

Removing a Stone With Sound Waves

Kidney stones can sometimes be broken up by sound waves produced by a lithotriptor in a procedure called extracorporeal shock wave lithotripsy. After an ultrasound device or fluoroscope is used to locate the stone, the lithotriptor is placed against the back, and the sound waves are focused on the stone, shattering it. Then the patient drinks fluids to help flush the stone fragments out of the kidney, to be eliminated in the urine. Sometimes blood appears in the urine or the abdomen is bruised after the procedure, but serious problems are rare.

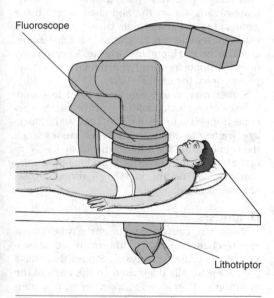

Fluoroscope

Lithotriptor

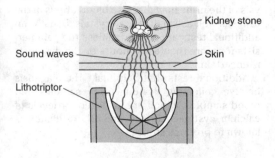

Fragmenting the Kidney Stone

Kidney stone

Sound waves

Skin

Lithotriptor

X-rays of the abdomen can show calcium and struvite stones. If needed, other procedures can be performed. In intravenous urography, a radiopaque substance, which is visible on x-rays, is injected into a vein and travels to the kidneys where it outlines uric acid stones so they can be seen on x-rays. In retrograde urography, the radiopaque substance is introduced into the urinary tract through the urethra.

Treatment

Small stones that aren't causing symptoms, obstruction, or an infection usually don't need to be treated. Drinking plenty of fluids increases urine production and helps wash out some stones; once a stone is passed, no other immediate treatment is needed. The pain of renal colic may be relieved with narcotic analgesics.

Often, a stone in the renal pelvis or uppermost part of the ureter that's $1/2$ inch or less in diameter can be broken up by ultrasound waves (extracorporeal shock wave lithotripsy). The pieces of stone are then passed in the urine. Sometimes, a stone is removed through a small incision in the skin (percutaneous nephrolithotomy), followed by ultrasound treatment. Small stones in the lower part of the ureter may be removed by an endoscope (a small, flexible tube) inserted into the urethra and through the bladder.

Uric acid stones are sometimes dissolved gradually by making the urine more alkaline (for example, with potassium citrate), but other types of stones can't be removed this way. Rarely, larger stones that are causing an obstruction may need to be removed surgically.

Prevention

Measures to prevent the formation of new stones vary, depending on the composition of the existing stones. These stones are analyzed, and urine levels of substances that can form stones are measured.

Most people with calcium stones have a condition called hypercalciuria, in which excess calcium is excreted in the urine. Thiazide diuretics such as trichlormethiazide reduce new stone formation in such people. Drinking large amounts of fluids—8 to 10 glasses a day—is recommended. Following a diet low in calcium and taking sodium cellulose phosphate, a resin, may help, but such measures can cause calcium levels to become too low. Potassium citrate may be given to increase a low urine level of citrate, a substance that inhibits calcium stone formation. A high level of oxalate in the urine, which contributes to calcium stone formation, may result from excess consumption of foods high in oxalate, such as rhubarb, spinach, cocoa, nuts, pepper, and tea, or from certain intestinal disorders. A change in diet may help, and the underlying disorder is treated.

Rarely, calcium stones result from another disorder, such as hyperparathyroidism, sarcoidosis, vitamin D toxicity, renal tubular acidosis, or cancer. In such cases, the underlying disorder is treated.

For stones that contain uric acid, a diet low in meat, fish, and poultry is recommended, because these foods increase the level of uric acid in the urine. Allopurinol may be given to reduce the production of uric acid. Potassium citrate may be given to make the urine alkaline, because uric acid stones form when urine acidity increases. Drinking large amounts of fluids also helps.

For struvite stones—which indicate a urinary tract infection—antibiotics are given.

CHAPTER 129

Neurogenic Bladder

A neurogenic bladder is the loss of normal bladder function caused by damage to part of the nervous system.

A neurogenic bladder may result from a disease, an injury, or a birth defect affecting the brain, spinal cord, or nerves leading to the bladder, its outlet (the opening into the urethra from the bladder), or both. A neurogenic bladder can be underactive, in which it is unable to contract (noncontractile) and unable to empty well, or it can be overactive (spastic), emptying by uncontrolled reflexes.

Causes

An underactive bladder usually results from interruption of local nerves supplying the bladder. The most common cause in children is a birth defect of the spinal cord, such as spina bifida or a myelomeningocele (a protrusion of the spinal cord through the vertebrae).▲

An overactive bladder usually results from an interruption of normal control of the bladder by the spinal cord and brain. A common cause is an injury or a disorder, such as multiple sclerosis, affecting the spinal cord, which may also result in paralysis of the legs (paraplegia) or the arms and legs (quadriplegia). Often, such an injury first causes the bladder to become flaccid for days,

weeks, or months (the shock phase). Later, it becomes overactive and empties without voluntary control.

Symptoms

The symptoms vary, according to whether the bladder is underactive or overactive.

Because an underactive bladder usually doesn't empty, it stretches until it becomes very large. This enlargement usually isn't painful because the bladder stretches slowly and has little or no local nerve supply. In some cases, the bladder remains large but constantly leaks small amounts of urine (overflow dribbling). Bladder infections are common in people who have an underactive bladder because the pool of residual urine in the bladder provides the conditions that encourage bacterial growth. Stones may form in the bladder, particularly if a person has a chronic bladder infection that requires the permanent placement of a catheter. Symptoms of a bladder infection may vary depending on the degree of nerve supply still functioning.

An overactive bladder may fill and empty without control and with varying degrees of warning,

---

▲ see box, page 1235

because it contracts and empties by reflex (involuntarily).

With an underactive or overactive bladder, the pressure and backflow of urine from the bladder up through the ureters may damage the kidneys. Among people who have a spinal cord injury, the contraction of the bladder and relaxation of the bladder outlet may not be coordinated, so that the pressure in the bladder stays elevated and does not allow the kidneys to drain.

Diagnosis

Often, a doctor can detect a large bladder by examining the lower abdomen. X-ray imaging studies using a radiopaque substance injected through a vein (intravenous urography) or through a catheter into the bladder (cystography) and urethra (urethrography) provide more information.▲ The x-rays can show the size of the ureters and bladder, and possibly stones and kidney damage, and give the doctor an indication of how the kidneys are functioning. Ultrasound imaging provides similar information. Cystoscopy is a procedure in which a doctor can look inside the bladder through a flexible scope that's inserted through the urethra usually painlessly.

The amount of urine left in the bladder after urination can be measured by inserting a catheter through the urethra to drain the bladder. Pressure within the bladder and urethra can be measured by connecting the catheter to a meter (cystometrography).

Treatment

When an **underactive bladder** is caused by a neurologic injury, a catheter may be inserted through the urethra to drain the bladder continuously or intermittently. The catheter is inserted as soon as possible after the injury to prevent the bladder muscle from becoming damaged by being overstretched and to prevent a bladder infection.

Permanent placement of a catheter causes fewer physical problems in women than in men. In a man, the catheter may cause inflammation of the urethra and surrounding tissue. However, for both men and women, use of a catheter that can be inserted by the patient periodically—four to

six times a day—and removed after the bladder is empty (intermittent self-catheterization) is preferred.

People who develop an **overactive bladder** may also need to have a catheter inserted for drainage if spasms of the bladder outlet prevent the bladder from emptying completely. For quadriplegic males who can't catheterize themselves, the sphincter (ringlike muscle that closes an opening) at the outlet may have to be cut to allow emptying, and an external collecting device can be worn. Electrical stimulation may be applied to the bladder, the nerves that control the bladder, or the spinal cord to induce the bladder to contract, but this type of treatment is still experimental.

Drug treatment may improve the bladder's storage of urine. Control of an overactive bladder can usually be improved with drugs that relax the bladder, such as anticholinergic drugs. However, these drugs commonly cause side effects, such as a dry mouth and constipation, and improving bladder emptying with drugs is difficult for people who have a neurogenic bladder.

Surgery to divert the urine to an external opening (ostomy) made in the abdominal wall or to increase the bladder size is sometimes recommended. Urine from the kidneys may be diverted to the body's surface by removing a short segment of the small intestine, connecting the ureters to it, and attaching it to the ostomy, allowing the urine to be collected in a bag. This procedure is called an ileal loop. The bladder can be enlarged with a segment of the intestine in a procedure called augmentation cystoplasty, and self-catheterization is performed. For infants, a connection is made between the bladder and an opening in the skin (vesicostomy) as a temporary measure until the child is old enough for definitive surgery.

Whether or not urine flow is diverted or catheters are used, extensive efforts are made to reduce the risk of having stones form in the urine. Kidney function is closely monitored. A kidney infection is treated promptly. Drinking at least eight glasses of fluids a day is recommended. A paralyzed person's position is changed frequently, and others are encouraged to walk as soon as possible. Although complete recovery is uncommon with any type of neurogenic bladder, some people recover considerably with treatment.

▲ see page 591

Urinary Incontinence

Urinary incontinence is the uncontrollable loss of urine.

Urinary incontinence can and does occur at any age, but the causes tend to be different among different age groups. The overall incidence of urinary incontinence increases progressively with age.

About 1 out of 3 older people has some problem with bladder control, and women are twice as likely as men to be affected. More than 50 percent of nursing home residents are incontinent. Urinary incontinence can be a reason for institutionalizing elderly people and contributes to the development of pressure sores, bladder and kidney infections, and depression. Urinary incontinence is also embarrassing and frustrating.

The kidneys constantly produce urine, which flows through two long tubes (the ureters) to the bladder, where urine is stored. The lowest part of the bladder (the neck) is encircled by a muscle (the urinary sphincter) that remains contracted to close off the channel that carries urine out of the body (the urethra), so that urine is retained in the bladder until it's full. At that point, messages travel along nerves from the bladder to the spinal cord, then are relayed to the brain, and a person becomes aware of the urge to urinate. The person can then consciously and voluntarily decide whether to release the urine from the bladder or to hold it for a while. When the decision is made to urinate, the sphincter muscle relaxes, allowing urine to flow out through the urethra, and the bladder wall muscles contract to push the urine out. That push can be augmented by contracting muscles in the abdominal wall and floor of the pelvis to increase the pressure on the bladder.

The entire process of holding and releasing (voiding) urine is complex, and the ability to control urination can be disrupted at various points in the process and by many abnormalities. The result of these disruptions is a loss of control—urinary incontinence.

Types of urinary incontinence are categorized by whether the incontinence started recently and suddenly or developed gradually and is persistent. Incontinence that starts suddenly often indicates a bladder problem. A bladder infection (cystitis) is the most common cause. Other causes include side effects of drugs, disorders that affect mobility or cause confusion, excess intake of caffeine-containing beverages or alcohol, and conditions that irritate the bladder or urethra, such as atrophic vaginitis and severe constipation. Persistent (chronic) incontinence may result from changes in the brain, changes in the bladder or urethra, or problems with the nerves to or from the bladder. These changes are particularly common in the elderly and in women after menopause.

Urinary incontinence is further categorized based on the pattern of symptoms as urge, stress, overflow, or total incontinence.

Causes and Types

Urge Incontinence is an urgent desire to urinate followed by uncontrolled loss of urine. Normally, people can hold urine for some time after first sensing that the bladder is full. In contrast, people with urge incontinence usually have little time to get to a bathroom. A woman may have this condition by itself or with varying degrees of stress incontinence (mixed incontinence). The most common sudden cause is a urinary tract infection. However, urge incontinence without infection is the most common type of incontinence in older people and often has no clear cause. Common causes of urge incontinence in older people are overactivity of the bladder and neurologic disorders, such as stroke and dementia, which interfere with the brain's ability to inhibit the bladder. Urge incontinence becomes a particular problem when an illness or injury prevents a person from getting to the bathroom quickly.

Stress incontinence is the uncontrolled loss of urine when coughing, straining, sneezing, lifting heavy objects, or performing any maneuver that suddenly increases pressure within the abdomen. Stress incontinence is the most common type of incontinence in women. It can be caused by weakness of the urinary sphincter. Sometimes the cause is changes in the urethra resulting from childbirth or pelvic surgery. In postmenopausal women, stress incontinence occurs because a

What Causes Incontinence?

Type	Description	Some Possible Causes
Urge incontinence	Inability to postpone urination more than a few minutes once the need to urinate is sensed	• Urinary tract infection • Overactivity of the bladder • Obstruction of urine flow • Bladder stones and tumors • Drugs, especially diuretics
Stress incontinence	Leakage of urine, usually in small bursts, caused by an increase in abdominal pressure that occurs when a person coughs, laughs, strains, sneezes, or lifts a heavy object	• Weakness of the urinary sphincter (the muscle that controls urine flow from the bladder) • In women, decreased resistance to urine flow through the urethra, usually caused by lack of estrogen • Anatomic changes caused by multiple childbirths or pelvic surgery • In men, removal of the prostate or injury to the upper part of the urethra or the bladder neck
Overflow incontinence	Buildup of urine in the bladder that becomes too great for the urinary sphincter to hold, so that urine leaks intermittently, often without bladder sensation	• Obstruction of urine flow, usually caused by enlargement or cancer of the prostate in men and by narrowing of the urethra (a birth defect) in children • Weakened bladder muscles • Nerve malfunction • Drugs
Total incontinence	Continual leakage because the urinary sphincter doesn't close	• Birth defect • Injury to the bladder neck—for example, during surgery
Psychogenic incontinence	Loss of control for psychologic reasons	• Emotional disturbances, such as depression
Mixed incontinence	Combination of the above problems (for example, many women have mixed stress and urge incontinence)	• Combination of the above causes

lack of the hormone estrogen contributes to a weakened urethra, thus reducing the resistance to urine flow through this channel. In men, stress incontinence may follow removal of the prostate (prostatectomy, transurethral resection of the prostate) when the upper part of the urethra or the bladder neck is injured.

Overflow incontinence is the uncontrolled leakage of small amounts of urine from a full bladder. The leakage occurs when the bladder becomes enlarged and insensitive because of chronic re-

tention of urine. Pressure in the bladder increases so much that small amounts of urine dribble out. During a physical examination, a doctor can often feel the full bladder.

The person ultimately may be unable to urinate because urine flow is blocked or because the muscles of the bladder wall can no longer contract. In children, blockage of the lower urinary tract may be caused by narrowing of the end of the urethra or of the bladder neck. In adults, blockage of the bladder outlet (the opening into the urethra from the bladder) is usually caused by benign prostate enlargement or prostate cancer in men. Less commonly, the blockage can be caused by narrowing of the bladder neck or the urethra (urethral stricture), which may occur after prostate surgery in men. Even constipation can cause overflow incontinence because when stool fills the rectum, pressure can be put on the bladder neck and urethra. A number of drugs that affect the brain or spinal cord or that interfere with nerve transmission, such as anticholinergic drugs and narcotics, may impair the bladder's ability to contract, resulting in a distended bladder and overflow incontinence.

Nerve malfunction resulting in a **neurogenic bladder**▲ can also cause overflow incontinence. A neurogenic bladder can result from many causes, including injury to the spinal cord and nerve damage from multiple sclerosis, diabetes, injury, alcoholism, or drug toxicity.

Total incontinence is the condition in which urine constantly drips from the urethra, day and night. It occurs when the urinary sphincter doesn't close adequately. Some children have this type of incontinence because of a birth defect in which the urethra didn't close off as a tube. In women with total incontinence, the cause is usually an injury to the bladder neck and urethra during childbirth. In men, the most common cause is an injury to the bladder neck and urethra resulting from surgery, particularly removal of the prostate because of cancer.

Psychogenic incontinence is incontinence resulting from emotional rather than physical causes. This type occurs occasionally in children and even in adults who have emotional problems. Persistent bed-wetting (enuresis) in children may be an example.■ A psychologic cause may be suspected when emotional distress or depression is evident and other causes of incontinence are ruled out.

Mixed types of incontinence sometimes occur. For example, a child may have incontinence resulting from both nerve malfunction and psychologic factors. A man may have overflow incontinence from prostate enlargement along with urge incontinence from a stroke. Older women often have a mixture of urge and stress incontinence.

Diagnosis

People commonly tend to live with incontinence without seeking professional help because they're too afraid or embarrassed to discuss the problem with their doctor or because they mistakenly believe that incontinence is a normal part of aging. Yet, many cases of incontinence can be cured or controlled, especially when treatment is started early.

Usually, the cause can be discovered and a plan for treatment can be developed after the doctor asks the person about the history of the problem and performs a physical examination. A urine analysis must be performed to determine whether an infection is present. The amount of urine left in the bladder after urination (residual urine) is often measured with the use of ultrasound scanning or urinary catheterization (placing a small tube called a catheter into the bladder). A large amount of residual urine indicates an obstruction or a problem with nerves or the bladder muscle.

Sometimes, special tests during urination (urodynamic evaluation) may be required. These tests measure the pressure in the bladder at rest and when filling and are particularly useful in chronic incontinence. A catheter is placed in the bladder. As the bladder is filled with water through the catheter, the pressure within the bladder is recorded. Normally, the pressure increases slowly. In some people, pressure builds in sudden spasms or rises too sharply before the bladder is completely filled. The pattern of pressure helps the doctor determine the mechanism of incontinence and the best treatment.

Another test measures the rate of urine flow. This test can help determine whether urine flow is obstructed and whether the bladder muscles can contract strongly enough to expel the urine.

Stress incontinence is diagnosed by reviewing the history of the problem, examining the vagina in women, and observing the loss of urine with coughing or straining. A pelvic examination also helps determine if the lining of the urethra or vagina is thinned because of lack of estrogen.

▲ see page 629

■ see page 1249

Treatment

Optimum treatment depends on careful analysis of the problem in each person and varies with the specific nature of the problem. The majority of people with urinary incontinence can be either cured or helped considerably.

Treatment often requires only taking some simple steps to change behavior. Many people can regain bladder control through behavioral modification techniques, such as urinating at regular intervals—every 2 to 3 hours—to keep the bladder relatively empty. Avoiding bladder irritants, such as caffeine-containing beverages, and drinking adequate amounts of fluids (six to eight 8-ounce glasses a day) to prevent the urine from becoming concentrated—which can irritate the bladder—can help. Drugs that affect bladder function adversely can often be stopped. Specific treatments, as outlined below, should be tried. If incontinence can't be fully controlled with specific treatments, specially designed incontinence pads and undergarments can protect the skin and enable people to remain dry, comfortable, and socially active. These items are unobtrusive and readily available.

Episodes of **urge incontinence** often can be prevented by urinating at regular intervals before the urge occurs. Bladder training techniques, which include pelvic muscle exercises and biofeedback, can be very helpful. Drugs that relax the bladder, such as propantheline, imipramine, hyoscyamine, oxybutynin, and dicyclomine, may help. Although many of the available drugs can be very helpful, each works somewhat differently and has potential adverse effects. For example, a drug that relaxes the bladder may reduce bladder irritability and strong urges to urinate, but it may cause dryness of the mouth or excessive retention of urine. Sometimes the drug's other effects can be used to advantage. For example, imipramine is an effective antidepressant and may be especially helpful to a person who is incontinent and also depressed. At times, combinations of drugs are useful. Drug therapy must be monitored and adjusted to each person's needs.

In many women with **stress incontinence,** applying estrogen cream to the vagina or taking estrogen tablets may relieve the problem. Estrogen in a skin patch has not been studied for the treatment of incontinence. Other drugs that help tighten the sphincter, such as phenylpropanolamine or pseudoephedrine, should be used with estrogen. For those with weak pelvic muscles, pelvic muscle (Kegel) exercises may help. Learning how to contract these muscles is not easily self-taught, so biofeedback is often used to help with training. Nurses or physical therapists can help teach these exercises. The exercises involve repeatedly contracting the muscles many times a day to build up strength and learning to use the muscles properly in situations that cause incontinence, such as coughing. Incontinence pads may be used to absorb the small amount of urine that usually leaks during stress.

More severe cases, which don't respond to nonsurgical treatments, can be corrected surgically using any of several procedures that lift up the bladder and strengthen the outflow passage. An injection of collagen around the urethra is effective in some cases.

For **overflow incontinence** caused by an enlarged prostate or other blockage, surgery is usually necessary. A variety of procedures are available to remove part or all of the prostate. The drug finasteride can often reduce the size of the prostate or stop its growth, so that surgery can be avoided or deferred. Drugs that relax the sphincter, such as terazosin, also often help.

When the cause is weak contraction of the bladder muscles, drugs that enhance bladder contraction, such as bethanechol, may be helpful. Gentle pressure applied by squeezing the lower abdomen with the hands just over the bladder may also be helpful, especially for people who can empty the bladder but have difficulty emptying it completely. In some cases, catheterization of the bladder is needed to drain the bladder and prevent complications, such as recurrent infections and kidney damage. The catheter may be put in place permanently, or it may be inserted and removed as needed.

Total urinary incontinence may be treated with various surgical procedures. For example, a urinary sphincter that doesn't close adequately may be replaced with an artificial one.

Treatment of **psychogenic incontinence** consists of psychotherapy, usually coordinated with behavioral modification and the use of devices that wake a child when bed-wetting starts or drugs that inhibit bladder contractions. A person who is incontinent and depressed may benefit from antidepressant drugs.

CHAPTER 131

Injury to the Urinary Tract

The urinary tract (kidneys, ureters, bladder, and urethra) may be injured by penetrating wounds, blunt force, radiation therapy, or surgery. The most common symptoms are blood in the urine, decreased urination, and pain. Such injuries may cause tenderness, swelling, bruising, and, if severe enough, dangerously low blood pressure (shock). Because metabolic wastes must be continuously filtered out of the blood by the kidneys and removed from the body through the urinary tract,▲ any injury that interferes with this process can be fatal. Preventing permanent damage to the urinary tract and even death may depend on prompt diagnosis and treatment.

Kidney Injuries

Blunt force is the usual cause of injury to the kidneys, occurring from motor vehicle accidents, falls, or sports injuries. Penetrating kidney injuries can result from gunshot or stab wounds. Damage varies widely. Minor injuries can result in small amounts of blood in the urine detectable only by microscopic examination, whereas major injuries are more likely to result in visible blood in the urine. If the kidney is severely injured (a condition called shattered kidney), bleeding may be severe and urine may leak into the surrounding tissues. If the kidney is torn from its stalk (renal pedicle), which contains the renal artery and vein, massive bleeding, shock, and death may result. Injury caused by extracorporeal shock wave lithotripsy (a common procedure used to break up kidney stones) may produce some transient blood in the urine, which usually is not significant, and the injury heals without treatment.

X-ray studies of the kidneys and urinary tract,■ such as intravenous urography with computed tomography (CT), can accurately determine the location and extent of the injury. Occasionally, more extensive imaging studies may be necessary.

Treatment begins with steps to control blood loss and prevent shock. Fluids are given intravenously to normalize blood pressure and stimulate urine production. When necessary, the appropriate x-ray study can be used to characterize the injury. For minor kidney injuries, such as those caused by extracorporeal shock wave lithotripsy, careful control of fluid intake and bed rest are often the only treatment needed. Major injuries that cause uncontrollable bleeding or leakage of large amounts of urine into the surrounding tissues often require surgical repair.

If the blood supply to the kidney is insufficient, normal kidney tissue, which must be supplied with blood to survive, may die and be replaced by scar tissue. Such injuries may lead to high blood pressure occurring weeks or months after a kidney injury. In general, if promptly diagnosed and treated, most kidney injuries have a good prognosis.

Ureteral Injuries

Most injuries to the ureters (the tubes leading from the kidneys to the bladder) occur during pelvic or abdominal operations, such as a hysterectomy, colon resection, or ureteroscopy (examination of the ureters with a fiber-optic tube). Frequently, such injuries aren't recognized until urination is reduced or urine leaks from the wound. Symptoms are generally nonspecific and may include pain or fever.

Other causes of ureteral injury include penetrating injuries, usually gunshot wounds. A ureteral injury from a blow to the body is uncommon. Rarely, blunt injuries, particularly those that cause the trunk to bend backward, can separate the upper part of the ureter from the kidney. Useful diagnostic tests include intravenous urography, computed tomography, and, when necessary, retrograde urography. In retrograde urography, x-rays are taken after a radiopaque substance, which is visible on x-rays, is injected directly into the ureter, outlining its entire course.

If a ureter is accidentally injured during surgery, another operation may be needed to repair it. A

▲ see page 586

■ see page 591

Kidney Injuries

The severity of kidney injuries varies widely. An injury may be minor, resulting in only bruising of the kidney. With a more severe injury, the kidney may be lacerated, and urine may leak into the surrounding tissue. If the kidney is torn from its stalk (renal pedicle), bleeding may be profuse, resulting in shock or death. Blood in the urine may or may not accompany any of these injuries.

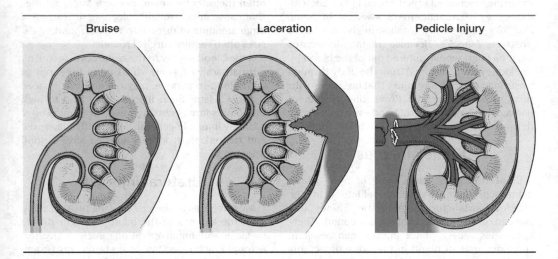

| Bruise | Laceration | Pedicle Injury |

urologic surgeon can reattach the ureter either to itself or to another part of the bladder. For lesser injuries, a catheter inserted into the ureter and kept there for 2 to 6 weeks may correct the problem, so that additional surgery can be avoided. Penetrating ureteral injuries, caused by gunshot or knife wounds, are best treated surgically.

Bladder Injuries

Crush injuries to the pelvis that result in fractures, often occurring in motor vehicle accidents, can cause the bladder to rupture. Penetrating wounds, usually from gunshots, also can injure the bladder. The main symptoms are blood in the urine or difficulty in urinating. The diagnosis is best established by cystography, a procedure in which a radiopaque substance, visible on x-rays, is injected into the bladder and x-rays are taken to look for leakage.

Minor tears (lacerations) may be treated by inserting a catheter into the urethra to drain urine for 7 to 10 days while the bladder heals itself. For more severe injuries, surgery is usually performed to determine the extent of the injury and repair any tears. The urine can then be more effectively drained from the bladder using two catheters, one inserted through the urethra (a transurethral catheter) and one inserted directly into the bladder through the lower abdomen (a suprapubic catheter). These catheters are removed in 7 to 10 days or once the bladder has healed satisfactorily.

Urethral Injuries

Common causes of significant injury to the urethra include pelvic fractures and straddle injuries (between the legs) in men. Surgical procedures directly on the urethra or during which instruments are passed into the urethra can also injure the urethra, but these injuries tend to be relatively minor. Symptoms include blood at the tip of the penis, bloody urine, and an inability to urinate. Rarely, urine leaks into the tissues of the abdominal wall, scrotum, or perineum (the area between the anus and vulva or scrotum). Narrowing (stricture) of the urethra at the injury site is a common complication that may develop later. These injuries can result in impotence, caused by damage to the arteries and nerves that supply the penis. The diagnosis of an injury is based on a retrograde urethrogram (an x-ray taken after a radiopaque substance is placed directly into the urethra).

For treatment of minor bruises to the urethra, a catheter is inserted through the urethra into the bladder for several days to drain the urine while the urethra heals itself. For all other injuries, urine must be diverted from the urethra using a catheter placed directly into the bladder. If a urethral stricture develops, it can be repaired surgically.

CHAPTER 132

Kidney and Urinary Tract Tumors and Cancers

Tumors of the kidney and urinary tract may occur in people of any age and either sex. Many of these tumors are cancerous.

Cancer of the Kidney

Cancer of the kidney (adenocarcinoma of the kidney; renal cell carcinoma; hypernephroma) accounts for about 2 percent of cancers in adults, affecting one and a half times as many men as women. Most solid kidney tumors are cancerous, but kidney cysts (hollow, fluid-filled growths) generally aren't.

Symptoms and Diagnosis

Blood in the urine is the most common first symptom, but the amount of blood may be so small that it's detected only under a microscope. On the other hand, the urine may be visibly red. The next most common symptoms are pain in the side and a fever. Sometimes a kidney tumor is first detected when a doctor feels an enlargement or lump in the abdomen, or a tumor may be discovered incidentally during evaluation of another problem, such as high blood pressure. Blood pressure may rise because an inadequate blood supply to part or all of the kidney triggers the release of chemical messengers that elevate blood pressure. The red blood cell count may also become abnormally high, resulting in secondary polycythemia,▲ because high levels of the hormone erythropoietin, produced by the diseased kidney, stimulate the bone marrow to increase red blood cell production.

If kidney cancer is suspected, intravenous urography, ultrasound scanning, or computed tomography (CT) may be used to visualize the tumor.■ Magnetic resonance imaging (MRI) may be used to provide even more information about how far the tumor has spread into nearby structures, including veins. If the tumor is hollow (a cyst), fluid may be withdrawn with a needle for analysis. X-ray studies, such as aortography and renal artery angiography, may be performed in preparation for surgery to provide more information about the tumor and the arteries supplying it.

Treatment and Prognosis

When the cancer hasn't spread beyond the kidney, surgically removing the affected kidney and lymph nodes provides a reasonable chance of cure. If the tumor has invaded the renal vein and

---

▲ see page 782

■ see page 592

even the vena cava (the large vein that carries blood to the heart) but hasn't spread (metastasized) to distant sites, surgery may still provide a chance for a cure. However, kidney cancer has a tendency to spread early, especially to the lungs. When it has spread to distant sites, it has a poor prognosis because it can't be cured by radiation, traditional anticancer drugs (chemotherapy), or hormones. Treating the cancer by enhancing the immune system's ability to destroy it causes some tumors to shrink and prolongs survival in some people.▲ One such treatment, interleukin-2, has been approved for treatment of kidney tumors, and various combinations of interleukin-2 and other biologic agents are being investigated. Rarely (in less than 1 percent of patients), removing the affected kidney causes tumors elsewhere in the body to shrink, but such regression in itself is not sufficient reason to remove a cancerous kidney when the cancer has already spread.

Cancers of the Renal Pelvis and Ureters

Cancer can occur in the cells lining the renal pelvis (transitional cell carcinoma of the renal pelvis) and the ureters. The renal pelvis is the part of the kidney that funnels urine into the ureters (the slender tubes that carry urine to the bladder).

Symptoms and Diagnosis

Blood in the urine is usually the first symptom. Crampy pain in the flank or lower abdomen may occur if urine flow is obstructed.

The diagnosis is made by intravenous urography or retrograde urography.■ CT scans can help a doctor distinguish a kidney stone from a tumor or blood clot and may help show how much the cancer has grown. Microscopic examination of a urine sample may detect cancer cells. A fiber-optic device—a ureteroscope or nephroscope— threaded up through the bladder or passed through the abdominal wall may be used to view, and occasionally even to treat, small tumors.

▲ see page 793

■ see page 591

★ see box, page 907

Treatment and Prognosis

If the cancer hasn't spread, the usual treatment is surgical removal of the kidney and ureter (nephroureterectomy) along with part of the bladder. However, in some situations—for example, when the kidneys aren't functioning well or a person has only one kidney—the kidney is usually not removed, because the person would then become dependent on dialysis. If the cancer has spread, chemotherapy is used, although this type of cancer doesn't respond quite as well to chemotherapy as does bladder cancer.

The prognosis is good when a cancer hasn't spead and can be completely removed surgically. Cystoscopies (insertions of a fiber-optic viewing tube to examine the inside of the bladder) are performed periodically after surgery, because people who have had this type of cancer are at risk of developing bladder cancer. If bladder cancer is detected at an early stage, it may be removed through the cystoscope or treated with anticancer drugs instilled into the bladder, just as any other bladder cancer is treated.

Cancer of the Bladder

An estimated 52,900 new cases of bladder cancer are diagnosed every year in the United States. About three times as many men as women develop bladder cancer. Certain chemicals become concentrated in the urine and cause cancer. Smoking is the strongest single risk factor and the underlying cause of at least half of all new cases. The chronic irritation that occurs with schistosomiasis★ (a parasitic infection) or bladder stones also predisposes people to bladder cancer, although irritation accounts for only a small proportion of all cases.

Symptoms and Diagnosis

Bladder cancer is often first suspected before any symptoms appear, when a routine microscopic examination of a urine specimen detects red blood cells. However, the urine may be visibly bloody. Later, symptoms may include pain and burning during urination and an urgent, frequent need to urinate. The symptoms of bladder cancer may be identical to those of a bladder infection (cystitis), and the two problems may occur together. Bladder cancer may be suspected if the symptoms don't disappear with treatment for an infection. Routine microscopic examination or other tests of urine may detect blood and pus cells, and special microscopic evaluation (cytology) frequently detects cancer cells.

Cystography or intravenous urography—x-ray films taken after injection of a radiopaque substance—may show an irregularity in the contour of the bladder wall, suggesting a possible tumor. Ultrasound scanning, CT, or MRI may also reveal an abnormality in the bladder, usually incidentally during evaluation of another problem. If any of these tests detects a growth, the doctor looks inside the bladder with a cystoscope passed through the urethra and removes samples of any suspicious areas for microscopic examination (biopsy). Sometimes the entire cancer is removed through the cystoscope.

Treatment and Prognosis

Cancers that remain on the bladder's inner surface or invade only the most superficial part of the muscle layer under the surface may be removed completely during cystoscopy. However, patients commonly develop new cancers later, sometimes in the same place or, more commonly, elsewhere in the bladder. The recurrence rate of superficial cancers, limited to the inner surface of the bladder, may be reduced by repeatedly instilling anticancer drugs or BCG (a substance that stimulates the body's immune system) into the bladder after all of the cancer has been removed during cystoscopy. These instillations may serve as treatment for a person with tumors that can't be removed during cystoscopy.

Cancers that have grown deep into or through the bladder wall can't be completely removed through a cystoscope. They are usually treated by total or partial removal of the bladder (cystectomy). Usually, the lymph nodes in the area are also removed to determine whether the cancer has spread. Radiation therapy alone or in combination with chemotherapy sometimes cures the cancer.

If the bladder is to be removed totally, a method of draining urine must be devised. Usually, urine is routed to an opening (stoma) made in the abdominal wall through a conduit made of intestine called an ileal loop. The urine is then collected in an external bag.

Several alternative methods of diverting urine are becoming increasingly common and are appropriate for some patients. These methods can be grouped into two categories: an orthotopic neobladder and a continent cutaneous diversion. In both, an internal reservoir is constructed from the intestine. For an orthotopic neobladder, the reservoir is connected to the urethra. The patient learns to empty this reservoir by relaxing the pelvic floor muscles and increasing pressure within the abdomen, so that urine passes through the urethra very much as it would naturally. Most patients are dry during the day, but some incontinence may occur at night. For a continent cutaneous urinary diversion, the reservoir is connected to a stoma in the abdominal wall. An external bag isn't needed, because the urine remains in the reservoir until the patient empties it by inserting a catheter through the stoma into the reservoir, which is emptied at regular intervals throughout the day.

Cancer that has metastasized requires chemotherapy. Several different combinations of drugs are active against this type of cancer, but only a relatively small proportion of people are cured.

Cancer of the Urethra

Cancer of the urethra is rare. It can occur in men and women. The first symptom is usually blood in the urine, which may be detectable only by examining a specimen under a microscope or which may color the urine red. Urine flow may become obstructed, making urination difficult or the stream of urine slow and thin. Fragile, bleeding growths at the external opening of a woman's urethra may be cancerous. A biopsy must be performed to positively identify a cancer. Radiation therapy, surgical removal, or a combination of both have been used to treat cancer of the urethra with variable results. The prognosis depends on the precise location in the urethra and the extent of the cancer.

A urethral caruncle is a more common small, red, painful, but noncancerous growth beside the external opening of a woman's urethra. It also causes bleeding into the urine. Surgical removal of the growth cures the problem.

Disorders of Nutrition and Metabolism

Overview of Nutrition

Nutrition is the process of consuming, absorbing, and using nutrients needed by the body for growth, development, and the maintenance of life; nutrients are chemical substances in foods that nourish the body.

Many nutrients can be synthesized in the body. Those that can't be synthesized in the body—called essential nutrients—must be consumed in the diet. They include amino acids (in proteins), certain fatty acids (in fats and oils), minerals, and vitamins. Nine of the 20 amino acids in proteins are essential nutrients.

If essential nutrients are not supplied in the quantities required, nutritional deficiency disorders may result. To determine whether a person is getting enough nutrients, a doctor asks about eating habits and diet, performs a physical examination to assess the composition (the amount of fat and muscle) and functioning of the body, and orders laboratory tests to measure the nutrient content of blood and tissues.

Generally, nutrients are divided into two classes: macronutrients and micronutrients. Macronutrients, which include proteins, fats, carbohydrates, and some minerals, are required daily in large quantities. They constitute the bulk of the diet and supply the energy and building blocks needed for growth, maintenance, and activity. Micronutrients are required in small quantities—milligrams (one thousandth of a gram) to micrograms (one millionth of a gram). They include vitamins and trace minerals that catalyze the utilization of macronutrients.

Other useful components of food aren't digested or metabolized to any appreciable extent. These components include some fibers, such as cellulose, pectins, and gums. Authorities recommend that 20 grams of fiber be consumed daily to improve movement in the gastrointestinal tract, moderate the changes in blood sugar and cholesterol that occur after meals, and increase the elimination of cancer-causing substances produced by the bacteria in the large intestine. Food additives such as preservatives, emulsifiers, antioxidants, and stabilizers improve the production, processing, storage, and packaging of foods.

Substances such as spices, flavors, odors, colors, phytochemicals (nonnutrients in plants, which have biologic activity in animals), and many other natural products improve the appearance, taste, and stability of food. Food in the daily diet contains as many as 100,000 substances, of which only 300 are nutrients and 45 are essential nutrients.

Macronutrients

The **organic macronutrients** are carbohydrates, fats, and proteins, which supply 90 percent of the dry weight of the diet and 100 percent of its energy. They are digested in the intestine and broken down into their basic units: sugars from carbohydrates, fatty acids and glycerol from fats, and amino acids from proteins. The energy content is 4 calories in a gram of protein or carbohydrate and 9 calories in a gram of fat (1 gram equals $^1/_{28}$ of an ounce). As sources of energy, carbohydrates, fats, and proteins are interchangeable in proportion to their energy content.

Energy intake varies markedly from about 1,000 to more than 4,000 calories a day depending on age, sex, and physical activity. Typically, sedentary women, young children, and older adults need about 1,600 calories a day; older children, active adult women, and sedentary men need about 2,000 calories; and active adolescent boys and young men need about 2,400 calories. About 55 percent of the calories commonly come from carbohydrates, about 30 percent from fats, and about 15 percent from proteins. If the energy intake is insufficient for the body's needs, weight loss occurs, and fat stored in the body—and to a lesser degree protein—is used to supply the energy needed. Total starvation causes death in 8 to 12 weeks.

The **essential fatty acids** make up about 7 percent of the fat consumed in a normal diet (which is 3 percent of the total calories or about 8 grams) and thus are considered macronutrients. They include linoleic acid, linolenic acid, arachidonic acid, eicosapentaenoic acid, and docosahexaenoic acid. Linoleic acid and linolenic acid are

Daily Food Pyramid: A Varied Diet for Good Health

General Guidelines

- Eat a variety of foods.

- Maintain a healthy weight.

- Choose a diet low in fat, especially saturated fats and cholesterol.

- Eat many vegetables, fruits, and grain products.

- Use sugar and salt (sodium) in moderation.

- Consume alcoholic beverages in moderation, if at all.

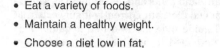

Fats
Oils
Sweets
Use sparingly

Milk
Yogurt
Cheese
2-3 Servings

Meat
Poultry
Fish
Dry beans
Eggs
Nuts
2-3 Servings

Fruits
2-4 Servings

Vegetables
3-5 Servings

Bread
Cereal
Rice
Pasta
6-11 Servings

found in vegetable oils; eicosapentaenoic acid and docosahexaenoic acid, which are essential for brain development, are found in fish oils. In the body, arachidonic acid can be formed from linoleic acid, and eicosapentaenoic and docosahexaenoic acid can be formed from linolenic acid, although fish oil is a more efficient source.

The **macrominerals** are calcium, phosphorus, sodium, chloride, potassium, and magnesium.▲ They are considered macronutrients because they are required in fairly large quantities (about 1 or 2 grams a day). Water, also a macronutrient, is required in amounts of 1 milliliter for each calorie of energy expended or about 2,500 milliliters (2.6 quarts) a day.

Micronutrients

Vitamins and trace minerals are micronutrients. Vitamins are classified as water soluble (vitamin C and eight members of the vitamin B complex) or fat soluble (vitamins A, D, E, and K).■

Essential trace minerals include iron, zinc, copper, manganese, molybdenum, selenium, iodide, and fluoride. Except for fluoride, all of these minerals activate enzymes required in metabolism.

▲ see box, page 653

■ see page 650

Fluoride forms a stable compound with calcium, helping stabilize the mineral content of bones and teeth and helping prevent tooth decay. Trace minerals such as arsenic, chromium, cobalt, nickel, silicon, and vanadium, which may be essential in animal nutrition, have not been established as requirements in human nutrition. All trace minerals are toxic at high levels, and some (arsenic, nickel, and chromium) have been identified as causes of cancer.

Nutritional Requirements

The objective of a proper diet is to achieve and maintain a desirable body composition and a large capacity for physical and mental work. The daily requirements for essential nutrients depend on a person's age, sex, height, weight, and metabolic and physical activity. After analyzing data from studies that have measured the requirements for the 45 essential nutrients in people on restricted diets, the Food and Nutrition Board of the National Academy of Sciences–National Research Council and the U.S. Department of Agriculture periodically publish recommended dietary allowances, computed to meet the needs of healthy people.

The U.S. Department of Agriculture originally proposed the basic four food groups (dairy products, meat and protein-rich vegetables, cereals and breads, and fruits and vegetables) as a guide to a balanced diet, but currently it suggests that the food guide pyramid is a better guide. This guide is intended to help people choose a diet that supplies essential nutrients as well as helps reduce the risk of such disorders as cancer, high blood pressure, coronary artery disease, and strokes. In this guide, the number of servings a day for each food group varies, depending on energy needs that range from 1,600 to more than 2,400 calories a day. For example, a person who consumes 1,600 calories a day could eat 6 servings from the bread group and 3 from the vegetable group, whereas a person who consumes 2,400 calories a day could eat 10 servings from the bread group and 5 from the vegetable group. In general, the consumption of fat should be reduced to about 30 percent of calories, and the consumption of fruits, vegetables, and cereals should be increased.

CHAPTER 134

Malnutrition

Malnutrition can result from either undernutrition or overnutrition. Both conditions are caused by an imbalance between the body's need for and the intake of essential nutrients.

Undernutrition, a deficiency of essential nutrients, can result from inadequate intake because of a poor diet or poor absorption from the intestine (malabsorption); abnormally high usage of nutrients by the body; or abnormal loss of nutrients through diarrhea, bleeding (hemorrhage), kidney failure, or excessive sweating. Overnutrition, an excess of essential nutrients, can result from overeating, excessive use of vitamins or other supplements, or underexercising.

Malnutrition develops in stages: First, changes occur in the levels of nutrients in blood and tissues, then changes occur in enzyme levels, next body organs and tissues malfunction, and then symptoms of illness and death occur.

The body needs more nutrients during certain stages of life, particularly in infancy, early childhood, and adolescence; during pregnancy; and while breastfeeding. In old age, nutritional needs are lower, but the ability to absorb nutrients is often reduced. Therefore, the risk of undernutrition is greater at these times of life, and even more so among people who are economically deprived.

Nutritional Assessment

To assess a person's nutritional status, a doctor asks about diet and medical problems, performs a physical examination, and orders certain laboratory tests. Blood levels of nutrients and substances that depend on nutrient levels (such as hemoglobin, thyroid hormones, and transferrin) are measured.

To determine a person's diet history, the doctor asks what foods were eaten in the previous 24 hours and what types of food are usually eaten. The person may be asked to keep a food diary, in which he lists everything he eats for 3 days. During the physical examination, the doctor observes the person's general appearance and behavior as well as the distribution of body fat and assesses the functioning of body organs.

Nutritional deficiencies can cause a number of medical problems. For example, gastrointestinal bleeding can cause iron deficiency anemia. A person being treated with high doses of vitamin A for acne may develop headaches and double vision as a result of vitamin A toxicity. Any body system can be affected by a nutritional disorder. For example, the nervous system is affected by niacin deficiency (pellagra), beriberi, vitamin B_6 (pyridoxine) deficiency or excess, and vitamin B_{12} deficiency. Taste and smell are affected by zinc deficiency. The cardiovascular system is affected by beriberi, obesity, a high-fat diet leading to hypercholesterolemia and coronary artery disease, and a high-salt diet leading to hypertension. The gastrointestinal tract is affected by pellagra, folic acid deficiency, and alcoholism. The mouth (lips, tongue, gums, and mucous membranes) is affected by a deficiency of B vitamins and scurvy. An enlarged thyroid gland may result from iodine deficiency. A tendency to bleed and skin symptoms such as rashes, dryness, and swelling from fluid retention (edema) can occur in scurvy, vitamin K deficiency, vitamin A deficiency, and beriberi. Bones and joints are affected by rickets, osteomalacia, osteoporosis, and scurvy.

A person's nutritional status can be determined in several ways. One is to measure height and weight and compare them with those in standardized tables. Another way is to calculate body mass index—the weight (in kilograms) divided by height (in meters squared). A body mass index of 20 to 25 is generally considered normal for men and women.

Still another way to assess nutritional status is by measuring skinfold thickness. A fold of skin on the back of the upper arm (the triceps skinfold) is pulled away from the arm so the layer of fat beneath the skin can be measured, usually with a caliper. Fat beneath the skin accounts for 50 per-

Who Is at Risk for Undernutrition?

- Infants and young children whose appetite is poor

- Adolescents experiencing rapid growth spurts

- Pregnant and breastfeeding women

- Elderly people

- People who have a chronic disease of the gastrointestinal tract, liver, or kidneys, particularly if they have recently lost 10 to 15 percent of their body weight.

- People on fad or crash diets for a long time

- Vegetarians

- People with alcohol or drug dependency who don't eat adequately

- People who have AIDS

- People taking drugs that interfere with appetite or with absorption or excretion of nutrients

- People who have anorexia nervosa

- People who have a prolonged fever, hyperthyroidism, burns, or cancer

cent of body fat. A skinfold measurement of about $1/2$ inch in men and about 1 inch in women is considered normal.

Nutritional status can also be assessed by measuring the circumference of the left upper arm to estimate the amount of skeletal muscle in the body (lean body mass).

X-rays can help determine bone density and the condition of the heart and lungs. They can also detect gastrointestinal disturbances caused by malnutrition.

When a doctor suspects severe malnutrition, he may order a complete blood cell count▲ and blood and urine tests to measure levels of vita-

▲ see box, page 736

Who Is at Risk for Overnutrition?

• Children and adults who have good appetites but don't exercise

• People who are more than 20 percent overweight

• People on high-fat, high-salt diets

• People who take high doses of nicotinic acid (niacin) for hypercholesterolemia

• Women who take high doses of vitamin B_6 (pyridoxine) for premenstrual syndrome

• People who take high doses of vitamin A for skin disorders

• People who take high doses of iron or other trace minerals without a prescription

mins, minerals, and waste products such as urea. Skin tests may also be ordered to assess certain types of immunity.

Risk Factors

Infants and children are at particular risk for undernutrition because they need a greater amount of calories and nutrients for growth and development.▲ They may develop deficiencies in iron, folic acid, vitamin C, and copper from inadequate diets. Insufficient intake of protein, calories, and other nutrients can lead to protein-energy malnutrition, a particularly severe form of undernutrition that retards growth and development. A bleeding tendency in newborns (hemorrhagic disease of the newborn) caused by a deficiency of vitamin K can be life threatening. As children approach adolescence, their nutritional requirements increase because their growth rate increases.

A woman who is pregnant or breastfeeding has an increased need for all nutrients to prevent malnutrition in herself and her baby. Folic acid supplements are recommended during pregnancy to

reduce the risk of brain or spinal defects (spina bifida) in the baby. Although women who have taken oral contraceptives are more likely to develop folic acid deficiency, there is no proof that the fetus will be deficient. The baby of an alcoholic woman may be physically and mentally impaired by fetal alcohol syndrome, because alcohol abuse and the resulting malnutrition affect fetal development.■ An infant who is breastfed exclusively can develop vitamin B_{12} deficiency if the mother is a vegetarian who eats no animal products (a vegan).

Elderly people may become malnourished because of loneliness, physical and mental handicaps, immobility, or chronic illness. In addition, their ability to absorb nutrients is reduced, possibly contributing to such problems as iron deficiency anemia, osteoporosis, and osteomalacia.

Aging is accompanied by a progressive loss of muscle that's unrelated to any disease or dietary deficiency. This loss averages about 22 pounds for men and 11 pounds for women. It accounts for the slowdown that occurs in metabolism, the decrease in total body weight, and the increase in body fat from about 20 to 30 percent in men and 27 to 40 percent in women. Because of these changes and a reduction in physical activity, older people need fewer calories and less protein than younger people do.

People who have a chronic disease that causes malabsorption tend to have trouble absorbing fat-soluble vitamins (A, D, E, and K), vitamin B_{12}, calcium, and iron. Liver disease impairs the storage of vitamins A and B_{12} and interferes with the metabolism of protein and glucose, a type of sugar. People who have kidney disease, including those on dialysis, are prone to deficiencies of protein, iron, and vitamin D.

Most vegetarians are ovo-lacto vegetarians: They don't eat meat and fish, but they do eat eggs and dairy products. Iron deficiency is the only risk from such a diet. Ovo-lacto vegetarians tend to live longer and develop fewer chronic disabling conditions than people who eat meat. However, their better health may also be a result of their abstention from alcohol and tobacco and their tendency to exercise regularly. Vegetarians who consume no animal products (vegans) are at risk of developing deficiencies of vitamin B_{12}. Oriental-style and other fermented foods, such as fish sauce, can provide vitamin B_{12}.

Many fad diets claim to enhance well-being or reduce weight. However, highly restrictive diets

▲ see page 1288

■ see page 1214

are nutritionally unsound: these diets have resulted in deficiencies of vitamins, minerals, and proteins; in disorders affecting the heart, kidneys, and metabolism; and even in some deaths. Very low calorie diets (fewer than 400 calories a day) can't sustain health for long.

Addiction to alcohol or drugs can disrupt a person's lifestyle to the point that adequate nourishment is neglected and the absorption and metabolism of nutrients are impaired. Alcoholism is the most common form of drug addiction, with serious effects on nutritional status. Consumed in large amounts, alcohol is a poison that damages tissue, particularly in the gastrointestinal tract, liver, pancreas, and nervous system (including the brain). People who drink beer and continue to consume food may gain weight, but people who consume a fifth of hard liquor daily tend to lose weight and become undernourished. Alcoholism is the most common cause of vitamin B_1 (thiamine) deficiency in the United States and may also lead to deficiencies of magnesium, zinc, and other vitamins.

Administration of Nutrients

When nutrients can't be given by mouth, they may be given through a tube (tube feeding) inserted into the gastrointestinal tract (enteral nutrition), or they may be given intravenously (parenteral nutrition). These methods may be used to feed people who are unwilling or unable to eat or who can't digest and absorb nutrients.

Tube Feeding

Tube feeding is used in various situations, including recovery from burns and inflammatory bowel disease. A thin plastic feeding tube (a nasogastric tube) is passed through the nose and gently down the throat until it reaches the stomach or small intestine. Although the insertion of this tube is mildly uncomfortable, most people have little discomfort once it's in place. If tube feeding must be used for a long time, the tube can be placed directly into the stomach or small intestine through a small incision in the abdominal wall.

The solutions used in tube feeding contain all the nutrients a person needs, including proteins, carbohydrates, fats, vitamins, and trace minerals. Fats supply 2 to 45 percent of the total calories.

Problems with tube feeding are uncommon and rarely serious. Some people have diarrhea and

Height-Weight Reference Chart for Adults*

| Height | Weight (pounds) | |
	Women	Men
4' 10"	92–121	—
4' 11"	95–124	—
5' 0"	98–127	—
5' 1"	101–130	105–134
5' 2"	104–134	108–137
5' 3"	107–138	111–141
5' 4"	110–142	114–145
5' 5"	114–146	117–149
5' 6"	118–150	121–154
5' 7"	122–154	125–159
5' 8"	126–159	129–163
5' 9"	130–164	133–167
5' 10"	134–169	137–172
5' 11"	—	141–177
6' 0"	—	145–182
6' 1"	—	149–187
6' 2"	—	153–192
6' 3"	—	157–197

*Height is without shoes; weight is without clothes.

abdominal discomfort. The esophagus can become irritated and inflamed by the nasogastric tube. Inhaling (aspirating) food into the lungs, a serious but rare complication, can be prevented by elevating the head of the bed to decrease regurgitation and by giving the solution slowly.

Intravenous Feeding

Intravenous feeding is used when people can't receive adequate nourishment through a nasogastric tube. For instance, people who are se-

How Starvation Affects Body Systems

System	Effects
Digestive system	• Low acid production by the stomach • Frequent, often fatal diarrhea
Cardiovascular system (heart and blood vessels)	• Reduced heart size, reduced amount of blood pumped, slow heart rate, and low blood pressure • Ultimately, heart failure
Respiratory system	• Slow breathing, reduced lung capacity • Ultimately, respiratory failure
Reproductive system	• Reduced size of ovaries in women and testes in men • Loss of sex drive (libido) • Cessation of menstrual periods
Nervous system	• Apathy and irritability, although intellect remains intact
Muscular system	• Low capacity for exercise or work because of reduced muscle size and strength
Hematologic system (blood)	• Anemia
Metabolic system	• Low body temperature (hypothermia), frequently contributing to death • Fluid accumulation in the skin, resulting mainly from disappearance of fat under the skin
Immune system	• Impaired ability to fight infections and repair wounds

verely malnourished and need to undergo surgery, radiation therapy, or chemotherapy or people who have severe burns, paralysis of the gastrointestinal tract, or persistent diarrhea or vomiting may be fed intravenously.

Intravenous feeding can supply part of a person's nutritional requirements or all of them (total parenteral nutrition). A number of solutions are available, and they can be modified for people who have kidney or liver disease. Total parenteral nutrition requires a larger intravenous tube (catheter) than those normally used for intravenous fluids. Consequently, a larger vein, such as the subclavian vein located approximately under the collarbone, is used.

A person receiving total parenteral nutrition is closely monitored for changes in weight and urine output and for signs of infection. If the blood levels of glucose become too high, insulin may be added to the solution. Infection is a constant risk because the catheter is usually left in place for a long time and the feeding solutions that pass through it have a high content of glucose—a substance in which bacteria can grow easily.

Total parenteral nutrition can cause other complications. The liver may enlarge if too many calories, particularly from fats, are consumed. The excess fat in the veins may also cause backaches, fever, chills, nausea, and a low platelet count. However, these problems occur in less than 3 percent of the people receiving total parenteral nutrition. Long-term total parenteral nutrition may produce bone pain.

Starvation

Starvation may result from fasting, famine, anorexia nervosa, severe gastrointestinal disease, stroke, or coma. The body resists starvation by breaking down its own tissues and using them as a source of calories—much like burning the furniture to keep a house warm. As a result, internal organs and muscle are progressively damaged, and body fat (adipose tissue) nearly disappears.

Adults can lose up to half of their body weight, and children can lose even more. Proportional weight loss is greatest in the liver and intestines, moderate in the heart and kidney, and least in the nervous system. The most obvious signs of emaciation are wasting in areas where the body normally stores fat, reduced muscle size, and protruding bones. The skin becomes thin, dry, inelastic, pale, and cold. The hair, which becomes dry and sparse, falls out easily. Most body systems are affected. Total starvation is fatal in 8 to 12 weeks.

Treatment

Restoring food intake to normal amounts requires a considerable amount of time, depending on how long a person has been without food and how severely the body is affected. The gastrointestinal tract shrinks during starvation and can't accommodate a normal diet all at once. Liquids such as juice, milk, broth, and clear soup are recommended for those who can take food by mouth. After a few days of liquids, a solid diet can be started and increased gradually to 5,000 or more calories a day. Usually, bland foods are recommended, given in small portions at frequent intervals to avoid diarrhea. A person should gain 3 to 4 pounds a week until a normal weight is reached. Some people need to be fed through a nasogastric tube at first. Intravenous feeding may be needed if malabsorption and diarrhea persist.

Protein-Energy Malnutrition

Between the extremes of starvation and adequate nutrition, there are various degrees of inadequate nutrition, such as protein-energy malnutrition, the leading cause of death in children of developing countries. Protein-energy malnutrition is caused by an inadequate consumption of calories, resulting in a deficiency of proteins and micronutrients (nutrients required in small quantities, such as vitamins and trace minerals). Rapid growth, an infection, an injury, or a chronic debilitating disease can increase the need for nutrients, particularly in infants and young children who are already malnourished.

Symptoms

There are three types of protein-energy malnutrition: dry (a person is thin and dehydrated), wet (a person is puffy because of fluid retention), and an intermediate type between the two extremes.

The dry type, called marasmus, results from almost total starvation. A child who has marasmus consumes very little food, often because the mother is unable to breastfeed, and is very thin from the loss of both muscle and body fat. Almost invariably, an infection develops. If the child is injured or if the infection becomes widespread, the prognosis is worse and the child's life is jeopardized.

The wet type is called kwashiorkor, an African word meaning "first child–second child." It comes from the observation that the first child develops kwashiorkor when the second child is born and replaces the first child at the mother's breast. The weaned first child is fed a thin gruel that's low in nutritional quality compared with mother's milk, so the child does not thrive. The protein defi-

ciency in kwashiorkor is usually more significant than the calorie (energy) deficiency, resulting in fluid retention (edema), skin disease, and discoloration of the hair. Because children develop kwashiorkor after they are weaned, they are usually older than those who have marasmus.

The intermediate type of protein-energy malnutrition is called marasmic kwashiorkor. Children with this type retain some fluid and have more body fat than those who have marasmus.

Kwashiorkor is less common than marasmus and usually occurs as marasmic kwashiorkor. It tends to be confined to parts of the world (rural Africa, the Caribbean, the Pacific islands, and Southeast Asia) where staples and foods used to wean babies—such as yams, cassava, rice, sweet potatoes, and green bananas—are protein-deficient and excessively starchy.

In marasmus, as in starvation, the body breaks down its own tissues to use as calories. Carbohydrates stored in the liver are depleted, proteins in muscle are broken down to synthesize new proteins, and stored fat is broken down to produce calories. As a result, the entire body shrinks.

In kwashiorkor, the body is less able to synthesize new proteins. Consequently, blood levels of proteins decrease, causing fluids to accumulate in the arms and legs as edema. Cholesterol levels also decrease and an enlarged fatty liver (excessive accumulation of fat inside the liver cells) develops.▲ The protein deficiency impairs body growth, immunity, the ability to repair damaged tissues, and the production of enzymes and hormones. In marasmus and kwashiorkor, diarrhea is common.

Behavioral development may be markedly slow in the severely malnourished child, and mental retardation may occur. Usually, an infant who has marasmus is affected more severely than an older child who has kwashiorkor.

Treatment

An infant who has protein-energy malnutrition is usually given intravenous feedings during the first 24 to 48 hours after hospitalization. Because such infants invariably have serious infections, an antibiotic is usually included in the intravenous fluids. A milk-based formula is given by mouth as soon as it can be tolerated. The amount

▲ see page 566

of calories given is gradually increased, so that an infant who weighed 13 to 17 pounds when admitted to the hospital gains about 7 pounds over 12 weeks.

Prognosis

Up to 40 percent of the children who have protein-energy malnutrition die. Death during the first days of treatment is usually caused by an electrolyte imbalance, an infection, an abnormally low body temperature (hypothermia), or heart failure. Stupor (semiconsciousness), jaundice, tiny skin hemorrhages, a low sodium level in the blood, and persistent diarrhea are ominous signs. The disap-

pearance of apathy, edema, and lack of appetite is a favorable sign. Recovery is more rapid from kwashiorkor than from marasmus.

The long-term effects of malnutrition in childhood are unknown. When children are adequately treated, the liver and immune system recover completely. However, in some children, the absorption of nutrients in the intestine remains impaired. The degree of mental impairment is related to how long a child was malnourished, how severe the malnutrition was, and at what age it began. A mild degree of mental retardation may persist into school age and possibly beyond.

CHAPTER 135

Vitamins and Minerals

Vitamins and minerals are a vital part of a healthy diet. If a person eats a variety of foods, the likelihood of developing a deficiency of these nutrients is very small. However, people who follow restrictive diets may not get enough of a particular vitamin or mineral. For example, strict vegetarians may become deficient in vitamin B_{12}, which is available only in animal products. On the other hand, consuming large amounts (megadoses) of vitamin and mineral supplements, without medical supervision, may have harmful (toxic) effects.

Vitamins

Vitamins are essential micronutrients, required by the body in small amounts. They are either fat soluble—A, D, E, and K—or water soluble—the B vitamins and vitamin C. The B vitamins include vitamins B_1 (thiamine), B_2 (riboflavin), and B_6 (pyridoxine), pantothenic acid, niacin, biotin, folic acid (folate), and vitamin B_{12} (cobalamin). The recommended daily allowance (RDA)—the amount an average person needs each day to remain healthy—has been determined for each vitamin. A person who consumes too little or too much of certain vitamins may develop a nutritional disorder.

When taken in daily doses that are more than 10 times the recommended daily allowance, vitamins A and D are toxic, but vitamins E and K (phylloquinone) are not. Niacin, vitamin B_6, and vitamin C are toxic when taken in high doses, but the other water-soluble vitamins are not.

Only two fat-soluble vitamins (A and E) are stored in the body to any extent. Vitamins D and K are stored in tiny amounts. Relative to requirements, vitamin C is stored in the smallest amounts, and vitamin B_{12} is stored in the largest amounts, requiring about 7 years to exhaust the body's reserves of 2 or 3 milligrams.

Vitamin A Deficiency

Vitamin A (retinol) is found mainly in fish liver oils, liver, egg yolk, butter, and cream. Green leafy and yellow vegetables contain carotenoids, such as beta-carotene, which the body slowly converts to vitamin A. Most of the body's vitamin A is stored in the liver. One form of vitamin A (retinal) is a component of the photoreceptors (nerve cells that are sensitive to light) in the eye's retina. Another form of vitamin A (retinoic acid) keeps the skin and the lining of the lungs, intestine, and urinary tract healthy. Drugs related to vitamin A (retinoids) are used to treat severe acne and are being investigated for the treatment of certain types of cancer.

Vitamins and Minerals

Nutrient	Principal Sources	Principal Importance	Effects of Deficiency and Excess	Daily Adult Requirement
Fat-soluble vitamins				
Vitamin A (retinol)	As vitamin A: Fish liver oils, beef liver, egg yolks, butter, cream As carotenoids (converted in the intestine to vitamin A): Dark green leafy vegetables, yellow vegetables and fruits, red palm oil	Normal vision, healthy skin and other surface tissues, defense against infections	*Deficiency:* Night blindness; thickening of skin around hair follicles; drying of the whites of the eyes and cornea—eventually progressing to bulging, ulceration, and rupture of the cornea with spillage of the eye's contents; blindness; spots on the whites of the eyes; risk of infections and death *Excess:* Headache, peeling of the skin, enlargement of the spleen and kidneys, bone thickening and joint pains	900 micrograms
Vitamin D	As vitamin D_2 (ergocalciferol): Irradiated yeast, fortified milk As vitamin D_3 (cholecalciferol): Fish liver oils, egg yolks, fortified milk; formed in the skin when exposed to sunlight (ultraviolet light)	Absorption of calcium and phosphorus from the intestine, bone mineralization, growth, and repair	*Deficiency:* Abnormal bone growth and repair, rickets in children, osteomalacia in adults, muscle spasms (occasionally) *Excess:* Poor appetite, nausea, vomiting, increased urination, weakness, nervousness, thirst, skin itching, kidney failure, calcium deposits throughout the body	10 micrograms
Vitamin E	Vegetable oil, wheat germ, leafy vegetables, egg yolks, margarine, legumes	Antioxidant	*Deficiency:* Rupture of red blood cells, nerve damage *Excess:* Increase in vitamin K requirement	10 milligrams
Vitamin K	Leafy vegetables, pork, liver, vegetable oils; produced by bacteria in the intestine	Formation of blood clotting factors, normal blood clotting	*Deficiency:* Bleeding	65 micrograms
Water-soluble vitamins				
Vitamin B_1 (thiamine)	Dried yeast, whole grains, meat (especially pork and liver), enriched cereals, nuts, legumes, potatoes	Carbohydrate metabolism, nerve and heart function	*Deficiency:* Beriberi in infants and adults, with heart failure and abnormal nerve and brain function	1.2 milligrams

(continued)

Vitamins and Minerals (Continued)

Nutrient	Principal Sources	Principal Importance	Effects of Deficiency and Excess	Daily Adult Requirement
Water-soluble vitamins (continued)				
Vitamin B$_2$ (riboflavin)	Milk, cheese, liver, meat, eggs, enriched cereal products	Carbohydrate metabolism, healthy mucous membranes	*Deficiency:* Fissures and scaling of the lips and corners of mouth, dermatitis	1.5 milligrams
Niacin (nicotinic acid)	Dried yeast, liver, meat, fish, legumes, whole-grain enriched cereal products	Chemical reactions in cells, carbohydrate metabolism	*Deficiency:* Pellagra (dermatosis, inflammation of the tongue, abnormal intestinal and brain function)	16 milligrams
Vitamin B$_6$ (pyridoxine)	Dried yeast, liver, organ meats, whole-grain cereals, fish, legumes	Amino acid and fatty acid metabolism, nervous system function, healthy skin	*Deficiency:* Convulsions in infants, anemias, nerve and skin disorders	2 milligrams
Biotin	Liver, kidneys, egg yolks, yeast, cauliflower, nuts, legumes	Carbohydrate and fatty acid metabolism	*Deficiency:* Inflammation of the skin and lips	60 micrograms
Vitamin B$_{12}$ (cobalamin)	Liver, meats (especially beef, pork, organ meats), eggs, milk and milk products	Maturation of red blood cells, nerve function, DNA synthesis	*Deficiency:* Pernicious anemia and other anemias (in strict vegetarians and people who have a fish tapeworm), some psychiatric disorders, poor vision	2 micrograms
Folic acid	Fresh leafy green vegetables, fruits, liver and other organ meats, dried yeast	Maturation of red blood cells, DNA and RNA synthesis	*Deficiency:* Decrease in the number of all types of blood cells (pancytopenia), large red blood cells (especially in pregnant women, infants, and people who have malabsorption disorders)	200 micrograms
Pantothenic acid	Liver, yeast, vegetables	Carbohydrate and fat metabolism	*Deficiency:* Neurologic disease, burning feet	6 milligrams
Vitamin C	Citrus fruits, tomatoes, potatoes, cabbage, green peppers	Bone and connective tissue growth and wound repair, function of blood vessels, antioxidant	*Deficiency:* Scurvy (bleeding, loose teeth, inflammation of the gums)	60 milligrams

(continued)

Vitamins and Minerals (Continued)

Nutrient	Principal Sources	Principal Importance	Effects of Deficiency and Excess	Daily Adult Requirement
Macrominerals				
Sodium	Salt, beef, pork, sardines, cheese, green olives, corn bread, potato chips, sauerkraut	Acid-base balance, nerve and muscle function	*Deficiency:* Low sodium levels in the blood, confusion, coma *Excess:* High sodium levels in the blood, confusion, coma	1 gram
Chloride	Same as for sodium	Electrolyte balance	*Deficiency:* Disturbance in acid-base balance	1.5 grams
Potassium	Whole and skim milk, bananas, prunes, raisins	Nerve and muscle function, acid-base and water balance	*Deficiency:* Low potassium levels in the blood, paralysis, heart disturbances *Excess:* High potassium levels in the blood, paralysis, heart disturbances	2 grams
Calcium	Milk and milk products, meat, fish, eggs, cereal products, beans, fruits, vegetables	Bone and tooth formation, blood clotting, nerve and muscle function, normal heart rhythm	*Deficiency:* Low calcium levels in the blood and muscle spasm *Excess:* High calcium levels in the blood, loss of intestinal tone, kidney failure, abnormal behavior (psychosis)	1 gram
Phosphorus	Milk, cheese, meat, poultry, fish, cereals, nuts, legumes	Bone and tooth formation, acid-base balance, component of nucleic acids, energy production	*Deficiency:* Irritability, weakness, blood cell disorders, abnormalities of the intestine and kidneys *Excess:* For people who have kidney failure, high phosphate levels in the blood	0.9 grams
Magnesium	Leafy green vegetables, nuts, cereal grains, seafood	Bone and tooth formation, nerve and muscle function, enzyme activation	*Deficiency:* Low magnesium levels in the blood, abnormal nerve function *Excess:* High magnesium levels in the blood, low blood pressure, respiratory failure, heart rhythm disturbances	0.3 grams

(continued)

Vitamins and Minerals (Continued)

Nutrient	Principal Sources	Principal Importance	Effects of Deficiency and Excess	Daily Adult Requirement
Microminerals				
Iron	Soybean flour, beef, kidneys, liver, beans, clams, peaches; however, less than 20% of iron in the diet is absorbed into the body	Formation of enzymes, which modify many chemical reactions in the body, and the main components of red blood cells and muscle cells	*Deficiency:* Anemia, difficulty in swallowing, spoon-shaped nails, intestinal abnormality, decreased work performance, impaired learning ability *Excess:* Iron deposits, liver damage (cirrhosis), diabetes mellitus, skin pigmentation	12 milligrams
Zinc	Organ meats, seafood; much of the zinc in the diet isn't absorbed	Component of enzymes and insulin, healthy skin, wound healing, growth	*Deficiency:* Slowed growth, delayed sexual maturation, diminished taste sensation	15 milligrams
Copper	Organ meats, oysters, nuts, dried legumes, whole-grain cereals	Enzyme component, formation of red blood cells, bone formation	*Deficiency:* Anemia in malnourished children *Excess:* Copper deposits in the brain, liver damage	2 milligrams
Manganese	Whole-grain cereals, dried fruits	Enzyme component	*Deficiency:* Weight loss, skin irritation, nausea and vomiting, changes in hair color, slowed hair growth *Excess:* Nerve damage	3.5 milligrams
Molybdenum	Dairy products, cereals	Enzyme activation	*Deficiency:* Acidosis, rapid heart rate, rapid breathing, blind spots, night blindness, irritability	150 micrograms
Selenium	Meats and other animal products; soil concentration influences plant content	Necessary for synthesis of an antioxidant enzyme	*Deficiency:* Muscle pain and weakness *Excess:* Loss of hair and nails, skin inflammation, possibly nerve abnormalities	60 micrograms
Iodine	Seafood, iodized salt, dairy products, drinking water in varying amounts (by region)	Formation of thyroid hormones, which regulate energy-control mechanisms	*Deficiency:* Enlargement of the thyroid gland (goiter), cretinism, deaf-mutism, abnormal fetal growth and brain development *Excess:* Occasionally causes high levels of thyroid hormone	150 micrograms

(continued)

Vitamins and Minerals (Continued)

Nutrient	Principal Sources	Principal Importance	Effects of Deficiency and Excess	Daily Adult Requirement
Microminerals (continued)				
Fluoride	Tea, coffee, fluoridated water	Bone and tooth formation	*Deficiency:* Increased risk of dental cavities, possibly bone thinning *Excess:* Fluorosis (excess accumulation of fluoride), mottling, pitting of permanent teeth, bony outgrowths of the spine	2.5 milligrams

Vitamin A deficiency is common in areas such as Southeast Asia, where polished rice—which lacks vitamin A—is the main source of food. Many diseases that affect the intestine's ability to absorb fats and therefore fat-soluble vitamins—such as celiac disease, cystic fibrosis, and obstruction of the bile ducts—increase the risk of vitamin A deficiency. Surgery of the intestine or pancreas may have the same effect.

Symptoms and Treatment

The first symptom of vitamin A deficiency is usually night blindness. Later, a foamy deposit (Bitot's spot) may appear in the white of the eye (sclera), and the cornea may harden and scar—a condition called xerophthalmia—which can lead to permanent blindness. In certain childhood diseases of malnutrition (marasmus and kwashiorkor), xerophthalmia is common not only because the diet lacks vitamin A but also because the deficiency of protein and energy (calories) inhibits the transport of vitamin A. The skin and the lining of the lungs, intestine, and urinary tract may harden. Vitamin A deficiency also produces inflammation of the skin (dermatitis) and increased susceptibility to infections. Some people have a mild anemia. In vitamin A deficiency, the blood level of vitamin A decreases to less than 15 micrograms per 100 milliliters (normal is 20 to 50).

This deficiency is treated by giving vitamin A supplements in a dose that's 20 times the recommended daily allowance for 3 days, followed by a dose that's three times the recommended daily allowance for 1 month. At this time, all symptoms should resolve. A person who is not free of symptoms after 2 months should be evaluated for malabsorption (the impaired absorption of nutrients in the intestine).

Vitamin A Excess

Excess vitamin A can cause toxicity, whether it's taken all at once (acute toxicity) or over a long period of time (chronic toxicity). Arctic explorers have developed drowsiness, irritability, headache, and vomiting within a few hours of eating polar bear or seal liver, both of which are rich in vitamin A. Tablets containing 20 times the recommended daily allowance of vitamin A, sold for the prevention and relief of skin disease, have occasionally caused similar symptoms, even when taken as directed.

Chronic toxicity in older children and adults usually results from taking large doses (10 times the recommended daily allowance) for months. Vitamin A toxicity may develop in infants within a few weeks. Early symptoms of chronic toxicity are sparse, coarse hair; partial loss of the eyebrows; cracked lips; and dry, rough skin. Severe headaches, increased pressure in the brain, and general weakness occur later. Bony outgrowths and joint pain are common, especially in children. The liver and spleen may enlarge. Babies of women who took isotretinoin (a vitamin A derivative used to treat skin conditions) during pregnancy may have birth defects.

The diagnosis of vitamin A toxicity is based on the symptoms and an abnormally high level of vitamin A in the blood. Symptoms disappear within 4 weeks after discontinuation of the vitamin A supplement.

Beta-carotene, found in vegetables such as carrots, is converted slowly to vitamin A in the body and can be consumed in large amounts without causing toxicity. Although the skin turns a deep yellow (carotenosis), especially on the palms and soles, no other adverse effects result.

Vitamin D Deficiency

Vitamin D exists in two forms. Vitamin D_2 (ergocalciferol) is found in yeast that's been exposed to ultraviolet light (irradiated), and vitamin D_3 (cholecalciferol) is found in fish liver oils and egg yolk. Vitamin D_3 is also produced in the skin when the skin is exposed to ultraviolet light, as occurs in sunlight. Milk may be fortified with either form of vitamin D. In the liver, vitamin D is converted to a form that can be transported in the blood. In the kidney, this form is further modified to produce vitamin D hormones, whose main function is to increase calcium absorption from the intestine and facilitate normal bone formation.

In vitamin D deficiency, the calcium and phosphate levels in the blood decrease, resulting in bone disease because not enough calcium and phosphate are available to maintain healthy bones. This condition is called rickets in children and osteomalacia in adults.

Vitamin D deficiency can be caused by either inadequate exposure to sunlight or a lack of vitamin D in the diet. Vitamin D deficiency during pregnancy may produce osteomalacia in the woman and rickets in her newborn. Because human milk doesn't contain large amounts of vitamin D, breastfed infants may develop rickets, even in the tropics if they are shielded from the sun. This deficiency may occur in elderly people because their skin produces less vitamin D when exposed to sunlight. Several rare forms of rickets caused by impaired metabolism of vitamin D are hereditary.

Symptoms, Diagnosis, and Treatment

Muscle spasms (tetany) caused by a low calcium level may be the first sign of rickets in infants. An older infant may be slow to sit and crawl, and the closing of the spaces between the skull bones (fontanelles) may be delayed. Children between the ages of 1 and 4 may have an abnormal curve in the spine, bowlegs, and knock-knees and may be slow to walk. For older children and adolescents, walking is painful. The flattening of the pelvic bones in adolescent girls may cause the birth canal to narrow. In adults, the loss of calcium from bones, particularly the spine, pelvis, and legs, causes weakness and may result in fractures.

The diagnosis of rickets or osteomalacia is based on the symptoms, the appearance of bones on x-ray films, and low blood levels of calcium, phosphate, and vitamin D by-products. Rickets and osteomalacia can be cured by giving vitamin D by mouth in daily doses five times the recommended daily allowance for 2 or 3 weeks. Certain hereditary forms of rickets usually improve when treated with vitamin D hormone.

Vitamin D Excess

Consuming 10 times the recommended daily allowance of vitamin D over several months can cause toxicity, which results in a high calcium level in the blood. The first symptoms of vitamin D toxicity are a loss of appetite, nausea, and vomiting, followed by excessive thirst, increased urination, weakness, nervousness, and high blood pressure. Calcium may be deposited throughout the body, particularly in the kidneys, where it may cause permanent damage. Kidney function becomes impaired, causing protein to pass into the urine and the blood level of urea, a waste product, to increase.

Treatment consists of discontinuing supplemental vitamin D and following a low-calcium diet to reduce the effects of a high calcium level in the body. Corticosteroids may be given to reduce the risk of tissue damage, and ammonium chloride may be given to keep the urine acidic, reducing the risk of calcium stones.

Vitamin E Deficiency

Vitamin E (alpha-tocopherol) is an antioxidant that protects the body's cells against damage by reactive chemical compounds known as free radicals. Vitamin E and selenium (an essential mineral that's a component of an antioxidant enzyme) have similar actions.

Premature infants have a very low vitamin E reserve and may become deficient if fed a formula high in unsaturated fats and low in vitamin E. Such fats are prooxidants (substances that are easily oxidized to form free radicals), are antagonistic to vitamin E, and may cause red blood cells to rupture (hemolysis). Disorders that interfere with fat absorption, such as celiac disease, cystic fibrosis, obstruction of the bile ducts, and Crohn's disease, can also reduce the absorption of vitamin E and increase the risk of a deficiency.

In premature infants, vitamin E deficiency may cause eye problems (retinopathy)▲ and bleeding within the brain—two problems that may result from exposure to the high oxygen level in incubators. In older children, the symptoms of vitamin E deficiency occur with intestinal malabsorption and resemble those of a neurologic disorder. They include reduced reflexes, difficulty in walking, double vision, loss of position sense, and muscle weakness.

A low blood level of vitamin E confirms the diagnosis. Taking large doses of supplemental vitamin E by mouth relieves most of the symptoms, but restoration of the nervous system may be delayed many months.

Vitamin E Excess

Large doses of vitamin E, which may be given to premature infants to reduce the risk of retinopathy, do not appear to have any significant adverse effects. In adults, high doses have very few visible adverse effects, except increasing the vitamin K requirement, which may cause bleeding in people taking anticoagulant drugs.

Vitamin K Deficiency

Vitamin K is a generic name for several related substances that are necessary for the normal clotting of blood. The principal form is vitamin K_1 (phylloquinone), found in plants, particularly green leafy vegetables. In addition, bacteria in the lower small intestine and the colon produce vitamin K_2 (menaquinone), which can be absorbed to a limited extent.

Hemorrhagic disease of the newborn, characterized by a tendency to bleed, is the principal form of vitamin K deficiency. It can develop because the placenta doesn't transmit fats and therefore the fat-soluble vitamin K very well; the newborn's liver is too immature to produce enough of the blood-clotting factors (proteins in blood that promote clotting and require vitamin K); no bacteria are in the intestine to produce vitamin K during the first few days of life; and breast milk is a poor source of vitamin K. A vitamin K injection should be given to newborns to protect them from this disease. Breastfed infants who haven't received this injection at birth are especially susceptible to vitamin K deficiency.

Because vitamin K is fat soluble, disorders that interfere with fat absorption, such as celiac disease and cystic fibrosis, can cause a vitamin K deficiency in children and adults. Taking excessive amounts of mineral oil may also prevent the absorption of vitamin K. This deficiency can also develop in people who take anticoagulant drugs to prevent blood clots.

Symptoms, Diagnosis, and Treatment

The main symptom is bleeding—into the skin, from the nose, from a wound, or in the stomach—accompanied by vomiting. Blood may be seen in the urine or stool. Most seriously, bleeding into the brain may occur in newborns.

When vitamin K deficiency is suspected, a blood test is performed to measure the level of prothrombin, one of the clotting factors that requires vitamin K. A low level (less than 50 percent of normal) suggests vitamin K deficiency. However, a low prothrombin level can also be caused by anticoagulant drugs or by liver damage. Usually, the diagnosis is confirmed if an injection of vitamin K increases the prothrombin level in a few hours and bleeding stops in 3 to 6 hours. If a person has severe liver disease, the liver may not be able to synthesize clotting factors despite injections of vitamin K. In such cases, plasma transfusions may be needed to replenish the clotting factors.■

Vitamin B_1 Deficiency

Vitamin B_1 (thiamine) is essential for a number of reactions involving enzymes, including the release of energy from glucose. Good sources of this vitamin are yeast, pork, legumes, and whole-grain cereals. Vitamin B_1 deficiency may develop when these foods are absent from the diet. When rice

---

▲ see page 1207

■ see page 738

is milled to remove the husk (polished), essentially all of the vitamins are lost. Asians are at risk for vitamin B_1 deficiency because their diet consists mainly of polished rice. However, boiling the rice before husking (parboiling) disperses the vitamin throughout the grain, preserving the vitamin and making it protective.

This deficiency may also result from reduced absorption caused by chronic diarrhea or an increased need for the vitamin caused by conditions such as hyperthyroidism, pregnancy, or a fever. People who have severe alcoholism substitute alcohol for food, thereby reducing the consumption of all vitamins including B_1. As a result, such people are at risk of developing nutritional deficiency disorders.

Symptoms and Treatment

Early symptoms are fatigue, irritability, memory impairment, loss of appetite, sleep disturbances, abdominal discomfort, and weight loss. Eventually, a severe vitamin B_1 deficiency (beriberi) may develop, characterized by nerve, brain, and heart abnormalities. In all forms of beriberi, red blood cell metabolism is altered, and vitamin B_1 levels in blood and urine are markedly reduced.

Nerve abnormalities (dry beriberi) begin as a prickling sensation (pins and needles) in the toes, a burning sensation in the feet that's particularly severe at night, muscle cramps in the calves, and pain in the legs and feet. If a person is also deficient in pantothenic acid, these symptoms may be worse. The calf muscles may become tender. Rising from a squatting position may become difficult, and the ability to feel vibration in the toes may be reduced. Eventually, the calf and thigh muscles may shrink (atrophy), and footdrop and toedrop (conditions in which the foot or toes hang limp and can't be raised) may occur because the nerves and the muscles aren't functioning properly. Wristdrop may also occur.

Brain abnormalities (Wernicke-Korsakoff syndrome,▲ cerebral beriberi) often result when a sudden severe vitamin B_1 deficiency, which can be caused by an alcoholic binge or severe vomiting in pregnancy, occurs and aggravates a chronic deficiency. Early symptoms of cerebral

---

▲ see page 363

■ see page 87

beriberi include mental confusion, laryngitis, and double vision. Later, a person may make up facts and experiences (confabulation) to fill in memory gaps. If Wernicke's encephalopathy (one part of the Wernicke-Korsakoff syndrome) isn't treated, symptoms may worsen, resulting in coma and even death. It's a medical emergency and should be treated with vitamin B_1 given intravenously at a dose of 100 times the recommended daily allowance for several days, followed by the vitamin given by mouth at 10 times the recommended daily allowance until the symptoms subside. Recovery is often incomplete because some brain damage may be permanent.

The heart abnormalities (wet beriberi) are characterized by a high output of blood from the heart, a fast heart rate, and dilation of blood vessels, causing the skin to be warm and moist. Because of the vitamin B_1 deficiency, the heart can't maintain this high output, and heart failure■ develops, with distended veins, shortness of breath, and fluid retention in the lungs and peripheral tissues. Treatment consists of giving vitamin B_1 intravenously at 20 times the recommended daily allowance for 2 or 3 days, followed by giving the vitamin by mouth.

Infantile beriberi occurs in infants who are breastfed by a mother who is deficient in vitamin B_1. It's characterized by heart failure, loss of voice, and damage to the peripheral nerves, typically between 2 and 4 months of life. Heart abnormalities usually resolve promptly and completely when treated with vitamin B_1.

Vitamin B_2 Deficiency

Vitamin B_2 (riboflavin) is important in many cell processes, particularly those leading to energy production and amino acid metabolism. Good sources of this vitamin are dairy products, meat, fish, and poultry. Vitamin B_2 deficiency is uncommon, except in areas where the diet consists mainly of polished rice. This deficiency may occur in people who have alcoholism, liver disease, or chronic diarrhea.

The most common symptoms are sores in the corners of the mouth, followed by cracks on the lips, which may leave scars. If thrush, a yeast infection, develops in these areas, grayish-white patches may appear. The tongue may turn magenta, and greasy (seborrheic) patches appear in the area between the nose and the lips. Occasionally, blood vessels grow into the cornea, causing discomfort in bright light. In males, the skin of the scrotum becomes inflamed. Symptoms resolve promptly when treated with supplemental vitamin B_2 at 10 times the recommended daily allowance.

Niacin Deficiency

Niacin (nicotinic acid) is found in many foods. Niacin is essential for the metabolism of many substances in the body.

Pellagra is the nutritional disorder caused by niacin deficiency. A deficiency of the amino acid tryptophan is also involved in the development of pellagra because tryptophan can be converted to niacin. People who live in areas where maize (Indian corn) is the major cereal are at risk of developing pellagra because maize is low in both tryptophan and niacin. Furthermore, the niacin in maize can't be absorbed in the intestine unless the maize is treated with alkali, as in the preparation of tortillas. Pellagra, a seasonal disorder, appears in the spring and lasts through the summer. It recurs in people on poor diets containing corn products.

Chronic alcoholics are at high risk for pellagra because of their poor diet. Pellagra develops in people who have Hartnup disease, a rare hereditary disorder in which tryptophan absorption in the intestine and kidneys is impaired. They need high doses of niacin to prevent symptoms.

Symptoms, Diagnosis, and Treatment

Pellagra is characterized by abnormalities of the skin, gastrointestinal tract, and brain. The first symptom is symmetric, reddened areas of skin that resemble a sunburn and become worse when exposed to sunlight (photosensitive). The skin changes don't disappear and may become brown and scaly.

The skin symptoms are usually followed by gastrointestinal disturbances, such as nausea, loss of appetite, and diarrhea, which is malodorous and sometimes bloody. The whole gastrointestinal tract is affected. The stomach may not produce enough acid (achlorhydria), and the tongue and mouth may become inflamed, turning bright scarlet. The vagina may also be affected.

Finally, mental changes occur, including fatigue, insomnia, and apathy; these symptoms usually precede a malfunctioning of the brain (en-

cephalopathy) characterized by confusion, disorientation, hallucinations, amnesia, and even manic-depressive psychosis.

The diagnosis is made on the basis of the diet history, symptoms, and low levels of niacin byproducts in the urine. Blood tests may also be useful. The treatment of pellagra consists of high doses (about 25 times the recommended daily allowance) of niacinamide, a form of niacin, plus high doses (10 times the recommended daily allowance) of other B vitamins. Vitamins B_1, B_2, and B_6 and pantothenic acid should be given because deficiencies of these vitamins produce some of the same symptoms as pellagra.

Niacin Excess

Niacin (but not niacinamide) in doses greater than 200 times the recommended daily allowance is prescribed for the control of high fat (lipid) levels in the blood. Such doses can cause severe flushing, itching, liver damage, skin disorders, gout, ulcers, and impaired glucose tolerance.

Vitamin B_6 Deficiency

Vitamin B_6 is a generic term for pyridoxine, pyridoxal, and pyridoxamine. These vitamins are important in catalyzing reactions involving amino acids in the cells of the blood, brain, and skin. This deficiency may result from poor absorption in the gastrointestinal tract or the use of drugs that deplete vitamin B_6 reserves in the body, including isoniazid, hydralazine, and penicillamine. The deficiency may also occur in hereditary disorders that inhibit the metabolism of vitamin B_6; these disorders can cause severe mental retardation, convulsions, and an anemia that's difficult to correct.

Vitamin B_6 deficiency can cause convulsions in infants and anemia, dermatitis, nerve damage (neuropathy), and confusion in adults. Other symptoms include a sore red tongue, cracks in the corners of the mouth, and numbness and a sensation of pins and needles in the hands and feet.

Blood tests can aid in the diagnosis. This deficiency is treated with high daily doses of vitamin B_6 (10 to 20 times the recommended daily allowance) until the symptoms resolve. Even higher doses may be needed when the deficiency is caused by a hereditary disorder.

Vitamin B₆ Excess

Taking high doses of vitamin B₆ (500 to 3,000 times the recommended daily allowance) prescribed for the carpal tunnel syndrome or premenstrual tension can severely damage nerves, destroying part of the spinal cord—which makes walking difficult. Recovery from this condition is slow, and some difficulty in walking may persist permanently after vitamin B₆ supplements are discontinued.

Biotin Deficiency

Biotin is a B vitamin that's necessary for the metabolism of fats and carbohydrates. Biotin is found in many foods. Good sources include liver, kidney, pancreas, eggs, milk, fish, and nuts. A deficiency is very unlikely in people who eat a balanced diet. However, eating raw egg whites for weeks can cause this deficiency because they contain a substance that binds with biotin in the body, preventing its absorption. Symptoms include sleepiness, weight loss, dermatitis, anxiety attacks, muscle pain, and certain nervous symptoms, such as exhaustion, insomnia, and hallucinations. This deficiency may also develop in people who are receiving long-term intravenous (parenteral) nutrition without biotin supplements. Laboratory tests detect a reduction in biotin levels in blood and urine.

Folic Acid and Vitamin B₁₂ Deficiencies

Folic acid (folate) and vitamin B₁₂ (cobalamin) function interdependently in the formation of normal red blood cells and in the production of an essential building block of DNA, thymidine. A deficiency of either of these vitamins results in a serious anemia (such as pernicious anemia), in which the red blood cells are few in number but large in size.▲ Symptoms include paleness, weakness, reduced acid secretion in the stomach, and nerve damage (neuropathy). Nerve damage occurs mainly in vitamin B₁₂ deficiency.

Pernicious anemia (vitamin B₁₂ deficiency anemia) is a condition in which vitamin B₁₂ can't be absorbed because the stomach doesn't produce

intrinsic factor, which combines with vitamin B₁₂ and transports it to the bloodstream. This anemia sometimes occurs because an overactive immune system attacks the stomach cells that produce intrinsic factor (an autoimmune reaction). Strict vegetarians—who lack vitamin B₁₂ because it's found only in animal products—and people who have hereditary disorders that block the transport or activity of this vitamin may develop other forms of vitamin B₁₂ deficiency.

Folic acid deficiency may occur in pregnant women on diets that lack green leafy vegetables and legumes, which contain folic acid. Infants can develop folic acid deficiency when the folic acid content of their formula is low.

The diagnosis of vitamin B₁₂ or folic acid deficiency is based on identifying an anemia with large red blood cells and detecting low levels of either or both vitamins in blood tests. A bone marrow sample showing large, immature red blood cell precursors confirms the diagnosis.

Treatment of pernicious anemia consists of monthly injections of vitamin B₁₂. Treatment of folic acid deficiency consists of folic acid taken by mouth.

Folic Acid Excess

Folic acid can be toxic under special conditions. In doses of 100 times the recommended daily allowance, it may increase the frequency of seizures in epileptics and worsen the neurologic damage in people who have vitamin B₁₂ deficiency.

Vitamin C Deficiency

Vitamin C (ascorbic acid) is found in citrus fruits, tomatoes, potatoes, cabbage, and green peppers. It's essential for the formation of connective tissue (the tissue that holds the body's structures together). It helps the body absorb iron and recover from burns and wounds. Like vitamin E, vitamin C is an antioxidant. Pregnancy, breastfeeding, overactivity of the thyroid gland (thyrotoxicosis), various kinds of inflammation, surgery, and burns all can significantly increase the body's requirements for vitamin C and the risk of a deficiency.

In infants, a lack of vitamin C in the formula and solid food may cause scurvy, a deficiency disease, between 6 and 12 months of life. Early symptoms include irritability, pain during movement, loss of

---

▲ see page 745

appetite, and failure to gain weight. The bones are thin and joints may be knobby. Bleeding beneath the tissue covering the bones (periosteum) and around the teeth is typical.

In adults, scurvy may occur when the diet is restricted, containing only dried meat and flour or tea, toast, and canned vegetables—typical foods eaten by elderly people who are disinterested in eating. After a few months on such a diet, bleeding occurs under the skin, particularly around hair follicles, under the fingernails, around the gums, and into the joints. A person may become depressed, tired, and weak. Blood pressure and heart rate fluctuate. Blood test results show a very low level of vitamin C.

In infants and adults, scurvy is treated with high doses of vitamin C for 1 week, followed by lower doses for 1 month.

Vitamin C Excess

High doses of vitamin C (500 to 10,000 milligrams) have been recommended by some to prevent the common cold, schizophrenia, cancer, hypercholesterolemia, and atherosclerosis. However, these recommendations have little or no scientific support. Doses higher than 1,000 milligrams a day cause diarrhea, kidney stones in susceptible people, and changes in the menstrual cycle. Some people who suddenly stop taking high doses develop rebound scurvy.

Minerals

Some minerals—sodium, chloride, potassium, calcium, phosphorus, and magnesium—are considered macronutrients because they're needed by the body in relatively large quantities; they're called macrominerals. Other minerals are micronutrients because they're needed by the body in small quantities; they're called microminerals or trace minerals. They include iron, zinc, copper, manganese, molybdenum, selenium, iodine, and fluoride. Deficiencies of minerals, except iron and iodine, are uncommon. Excesses of some minerals may cause toxicity.

Iron Deficiency

Iron is a component of many enzymes affecting important chemical reactions throughout the body. It's also a component of hemoglobin, which enables red blood cells to carry oxygen and deliver it to the body's tissues.

Food contains two types of iron—heme iron, which is found principally in animal products, and nonheme iron, which represents more than 85 percent of the iron in the average diet. Heme iron is absorbed much better than nonheme iron. However, the absorption of nonheme iron is increased when it's consumed with animal protein and vitamin C.

Iron deficiency is the most common nutritional deficiency in the world, producing anemia in men, women, and children. Bleeding (hemorrhage) results in loss of iron from the body, producing an iron deficiency that must be treated with iron supplements. Iron deficiency may also result from an inadequate diet. This deficiency is likely to occur during pregnancy because a large amount of iron must be supplied by the mother to the growing fetus. Because adolescent girls are growing and starting to menstruate, they are at risk of developing iron deficiency anemia if they follow diets that exclude meat.

When the iron reserves in the body are exhausted, anemia develops. Symptoms include paleness, spoon nails (a deformity in which the nails are thin and concave), weakness with impaired muscle performance, and changes in cognitive behavior.

The diagnosis of iron deficiency is made on the basis of the symptoms and blood test results showing anemia and low levels of iron and ferritin, a protein that stores iron. Iron deficiency is treated with high doses of iron once a day for several weeks. Treatment should be continued until red blood cells and iron reserves return to normal.

Iron Excess

Excess iron is toxic, causing vomiting, diarrhea, and damage to the intestine. Iron may accumulate in the body when a person is given iron therapy in excessive amounts or for too long, receives several blood transfusions, or has chronic alcoholism. Iron overload disease (hemochromatosis), a potentially fatal but easily treatable hereditary disorder in which too much iron is absorbed, affects over 1 million Americans. Usually, symptoms don't appear until middle age, developing insidiously. The skin becomes bronze-colored, and cirrhosis, liver cancer, diabetes, and heart failure develop, resulting in premature death.

Symptoms may include arthritis, impotence, infertility, hypothyroidism, and chronic fatigue. Blood tests can determine if a person has iron excess. All relatives of an affected person should be screened. Bloodletting is the treatment of choice. Early diagnosis and treatment permits a long, healthy life.

Zinc Deficiency

Zinc is widely distributed in the body because it's a component of more than 100 enzymes, including those responsible for RNA and DNA synthesis. The tissues that have the highest zinc content are the bones, liver, prostate, and testes. The level of zinc in the blood depends on the amount of zinc in the diet. Meat, liver, eggs, and seafood are rich sources of zinc, but cereals are not.

Whole-grain cereals contain substances, such as fiber and phosphates, that inhibit the absorption of zinc. Eating clay, which some people do habitually, inhibits the absorption of zinc and causes a zinc deficiency. Acrodermatitis enteropathica, a hereditary disorder in which zinc can't be absorbed, also produces zinc deficiency.

Symptoms include a loss of appetite, hair loss, dermatitis, night blindness, and impaired taste. The activity of the reproductive organs may be impaired, resulting in delayed sexual development and, in males, reduced sperm production. Growth may also be slowed. The body's immune system and ability to heal wounds may be impaired. In children, the first signs of this deficiency are slow growth, a loss of appetite, impaired taste, and the low zinc content of the hair.

The zinc level in blood is measured to help make the diagnosis. Treatment consists of taking zinc supplements.

Zinc Excess

Large amounts of zinc, usually acquired from consuming acidic foods or beverages placed in a zinc-coated (galvanized) container, can produce a metallic taste, vomiting, and stomach problems. Amounts of 1 gram or more may be fatal.

Copper Deficiency

Copper is a component of a variety of enzymes that are necessary for energy production, antioxidation, the synthesis of the hormone adrenaline, and the formation of connective tissue. A copper deficiency is rare in healthy people. It occurs most commonly in infants who are premature or recovering from severe malnutrition. People receiving long-term intravenous (parenteral) nutrition also are at risk of developing a copper deficiency.

Menkes' syndrome is a hereditary disorder causing copper deficiency. Symptoms include kinky hair, mental retardation, a low copper level in the blood, and a failure to synthesize the enzymes that require copper.

A copper deficiency produces fatigue and a low copper level in the blood. Decreases in the number of red blood cells (anemia), white blood cells (leukopenia), and one type of white blood cell called neutrophils (neutropenia) are common, as is decreased calcium in the bones (osteoporosis). Small, pinpoint hemorrhages in the skin and arterial aneurysms also occur.

Copper deficiency is treated with copper supplements for several weeks. However, people who have Menkes' syndrome do not respond well to these supplements.

Copper Excess

Any copper not bound to a protein is toxic. Consuming relatively small amounts of unbound copper may cause nausea and vomiting. Acidic food or beverages in prolonged contact with copper vessels, tubing, or valves can be contaminated with small amounts of copper. If larger amounts of copper salts, which are not bound to a protein, are inadvertently ingested or if compresses saturated with a solution of a copper salt are used to treat large areas of burned skin, enough copper may be absorbed to damage the kidneys, inhibit urine production, and cause anemia from the rupture of red blood cells (hemolysis).

Wilson's disease is a hereditary disorder in which copper accumulates in tissues and causes extensive damage. It affects 1 out of 30,000 people. In this disorder, the liver doesn't secrete copper into the blood or excrete copper into the bile. As a result, the copper level in the blood is low, but copper accumulates in the brain, eyes, and liver, causing cirrhosis. In the cornea of the eyes, the accumulated copper produces gold or greenish-gold rings. The first symptoms usually result from brain damage and include tremors, headaches, an inability to speak, incoordination, and even psychosis. Copper toxicity is treated with penicillamine, which binds copper and promotes its excretion—an example of chelation therapy. This treatment must be taken for life to preserve life.

Manganese Deficiency

Manganese is a component of several enzymes and is essential for normal bone structure. Rich sources include unrefined cereals and green leafy vegetables.

When the diet is deficient in manganese for a few weeks, the body seems to conserve this mineral effectively. The only symptom is a transient rash.

Hydralazine, an antihypertensive drug, can cause manganese deficiency and related side effects. These effects include pain radiating along a nerve (neuralgia), joint pain, a fever, a rash, enlarged lymph nodes, and an enlarged liver. Manganese salts are used to treat this condition.

Manganese Excess

Manganese toxicity is common only in people who mine and refine manganese ore. Prolonged exposure causes nerve damage, with symptoms resembling parkinsonism—tremors and difficulties in movement.

Molybdenum Deficiency

Molybdenum is necessary for the oxidation of sulfur, a component of proteins. It's found in milk, beans, breads, and cereals. A molybdenum deficiency caused by inadequate intake has not been observed in healthy people. However, the deficiency does occur under special conditions—for example, when a malnourished person who has Crohn's disease receives long-term total parenteral nutrition (all nutrients are given intravenously) without molybdenum supplements. Symptoms include a fast heart rate, shortness of breath, nausea, vomiting, disorientation, and finally coma. Treatment with molybdenum may result in a complete recovery.

Molybdenum Excess

People who consume large amounts of molybdenum may develop symptoms that resemble gout,▲ including a high uric acid level in the blood and joint pain. Miners exposed to molybdenum dust may develop nonspecific symptoms.

Selenium Deficiency

Selenium is necessary for the synthesis of one of the antioxidant enzymes. The symptoms of selenium deficiency, a rare condition, can be explained largely by a lack of antioxidants in the liver, heart, and muscles, resulting in tissue death and organ failure.

Premature infants and adults receiving total parenteral nutrition without selenium supplements are at risk of heart and muscle damage caused by a selenium deficiency. Treatment with selenium may result in a complete recovery.

Keshan disease, a disorder that is caused by a virus and damages heart muscle, can be prevented with selenium supplements. It affects about 1 percent of people who live in a part of China in which the selenium content of the soil and of plants grown in the soil is low.

Selenium Excess

Excess selenium can have harmful effects, which may result from taking nonprescription supplements of 5 to 50 milligrams a day. The symptoms are nausea and vomiting, the loss of hair and nails, a skin rash, and nerve damage.

Iodine Deficiency

Iodine is necessary for the synthesis of the thyroid hormones. Nearly 80 percent of the iodine in the body is found in the thyroid gland, most of it in the thyroid hormones. Seafood is a rich source of iodine. The amount of iodide, a form of iodine, in drinking water generally depends on the iodide content of local soil. Some 10 percent of the world population are at risk of developing iodine deficiency because they live at high altitudes where the drinking water is low in iodide. Iodide is added to some commercial table salt (iodized salt).

In iodine deficiency, the thyroid gland attempts to capture more iodide for the synthesis of thyroid hormones and enlarges. The iodide level in the blood and urine is very low. A pregnant

▲ see page 244

woman who is deficient in iodine may have a baby whose brain is improperly developed because of iodine deficiency—a condition called cretinism. Treatment consists of iodine in doses about 10 times the recommended daily allowance for several weeks.

Iodine Excess

Iodine toxicity is caused by consuming very large amounts of iodine daily (400 times the recommended daily allowance), sometimes as a result of living near the sea. Iodine excess can cause a goiter and sometimes hyperthyroidism.

Fluoride Deficiency

Fluoride, a form of fluorine, is an essential nutrient that strengthens bones and teeth. Sea fish and tea are rich in fluoride, but drinking water is the main source; its fluoride content varies from too little to too much in various parts of the world. A fluoride deficiency can lead to cavities in the teeth, which can be prevented by consuming enough fluoride in food and water. The addition of fluoride (fluoridation) to drinking water that's low in fluoride significantly reduces the risk of tooth decay.

Fluoride Excess

People in areas where the drinking water has a naturally high fluoride level may acquire too much of this element—a condition called fluorosis. Fluoride accumulates in the teeth, particularly permanent teeth, and in bones. Chalky white, irregular patches appear on the surface of the tooth enamel; they eventually turn yellow or brown, causing the enamel to appear mottled.

CHAPTER 136

Water Balance

Two thirds of body weight is water. A 150-pound person has about 10 gallons of body water. Of this, 6 to 7 gallons are inside the cells, 2 gallons are in the space surrounding the cells, and slightly less than 1 gallon, or about 8 percent of the total water, is in the bloodstream. This relatively small volume of water in the bloodstream is very important to body function and must be kept fairly constant. The water outside of the bloodstream acts as a reservoir that can either replenish or absorb excess water in the blood as needed.

Water enters the body primarily by absorption from the gastrointestinal tract. Water leaves the body primarily as urine excreted from the kidneys. The kidneys can excrete as much as several gallons of urine a day or can conserve water by excreting less than a pint a day. About $1\frac{1}{2}$ pints of water are also lost every day by evaporation from the skin and lungs. Profuse sweating, as occurs with vigorous exercise or in hot climates, can dramatically increase the amount of water lost

through evaporation. Normally, little water is lost from the gastrointestinal tract. However, as much as a gallon or more a day can be lost with protracted vomiting or severe diarrhea.

When water intake matches water loss, the body's water is in balance. To maintain water balance, healthy people with normal kidney function who are not sweating excessively should drink at least 1 quart of fluid a day. However, drinking $1\frac{1}{2}$ to 2 quarts a day is generally recommended for healthy adults to protect against dehydration as well as the development of kidney stones.▲

When the brain and kidneys are functioning properly, the body can cope with extreme changes in water intake. A person usually can drink enough water to compensate for excess water loss and thus maintain blood volume and the concentration of dissolved mineral salts (electrolytes) in the blood. However, a person may become dehydrated if unable to drink enough water to compensate for excessive water loss, as in protracted vomiting or severe diarrhea.

The amount of water in the body is closely linked to the amount of electrolytes. The blood sodium concentration (level) is a good indicator

▲ see page 627

of the amount of water in the body. The body works to keep total body water and thus the blood sodium level constant. When the sodium level is too high, the body retains water in order to dilute the excess sodium. Thirst develops and less urine is produced. When the sodium level drops too low, the kidneys excrete more water to bring the sodium level back into balance.▲

Dehydration

Dehydration is a deficiency of body water.

Dehydration occurs when the body's output of water is greater than its intake. The deficiency of water usually causes the sodium level in the bloodstream to rise. Vomiting, diarrhea, the use of diuretics (drugs that cause the kidneys to excrete excess amounts of water and salt), excessive heat, fever, and decreased water intake for any reason can lead to dehydration. Certain diseases such as diabetes mellitus, diabetes insipidus,■ and Addison's disease★ can lead to dehydration because excessive water is lost.

At first, dehydration stimulates the thirst centers of the brain, causing a person to drink more fluid. If water intake cannot keep up with water loss, dehydration becomes more severe. Sweating decreases, and less urine is produced. Water moves from the vast reservoir inside cells into the bloodstream. If dehydration continues unabated, the tissues of the body begin to dry out. The cells begin to shrivel and malfunction. Brain cells are among the most susceptible to dehydration so that one of the main signs of severe dehydration is mental confusion, which can progress to coma.

With the more common causes of dehydration, such as excessive sweating, vomiting, and diarrhea, electrolytes (especially sodium and potassium) are usually lost in addition to water.● Therefore, dehydration is often accompanied by a deficiency of electrolytes. When electrolytes are deficient, water doesn't move as readily from the large reservoir inside of cells into the blood. Thus, the amount of water circulating in the bloodstream is further reduced. Blood pressure can drop, causing light headedness or the sensation of impending blackout, particularly upon standing (orthostatic hypotension). If water and electrolyte losses continue, blood pressure can fall dangerously low, resulting in shock and severe damage to many internal organs, such as the kidneys, liver, and brain.

A Careful Balancing Act

Several mechanisms work together to maintain the balance of water in the body. One of the most important is the thirst mechanism. Nerve centers deep in the brain are stimulated when the body needs more water, resulting in the sensation of thirst. The sensation becomes stronger as the body's need for water increases, motivating a person to drink and replace the needed water.

Another mechanism for controlling the amount of water in the body involves the pituitary gland at the base of the brain. When the body is low in water, the pituitary gland secretes a substance into the bloodstream called antidiuretic hormone. Antidiuretic hormone stimulates the kidneys to retain as much water as possible.

When the body has insufficient water, the kidneys conserve water, while water automatically moves from the large reservoir in the cells to the bloodstream to maintain blood volume and blood pressure until the water can be replaced by increased intake. When the body has excess water, thirst is suppressed and the pituitary gland produces very little antidiuretic hormone, allowing the kidneys to excrete the excess water in the urine.

Treatment

For mild dehydration, drinking plain water may be all that is needed. However, when both water and electrolyte losses have occurred, salt (especially sodium and potassium) must also be replaced. Flavored commercial drinks, such as Gatorade, have been formulated to replace the salts (electrolytes) lost during vigorous exercise. These drinks can be used to prevent dehydration or treat mild dehydration. Drinking plenty of flu-

---

▲ see page 667

■ see page 703

★ see page 712

● see page 667

ids and consuming a little additional salt during or after exercise will work just as well. People with heart or kidney problems should consult their doctor about safely replacing fluids before engaging in exercise.

If blood pressure drops enough to cause shock or the threat of shock, medical personnel generally give solutions containing sodium chloride intravenously. Intravenous fluids are given rapidly at first and then more slowly as the person's physical condition improves.

The underlying cause of dehydration is always addressed. For example, if the person has diarrhea, then drugs to treat or stop the diarrhea may be necessary in addition to replacing fluids. If the kidneys are excreting too much water because the person has a deficiency of antidiuretic hormone, as can happen with diabetes insipidus, chronic treatment with synthetic antidiuretic hormone may be needed. Once the cause of dehydration has been treated, people recovering from dehydration are monitored to be sure that oral intake of fluids is once again sufficient to maintain hydration.

Overhydration

Overhydration is an excess of water in the body.

Overhydration occurs when the body's intake of water is greater than its output. The excess water in the body causes the sodium in the bloodstream to become overdiluted. Drinking excessive amounts of water doesn't usually cause overhydration if the pituitary gland, kidneys, and heart are functioning normally; an adult would have to drink more than 2 gallons of water a day to exceed the body's ability to excrete water.

Overhydration is much more common in people whose kidneys don't excrete water normally, such as those with heart, kidney, or liver disease. People with these problems may have to limit the amount of water they drink and the amount of salt they ingest.

As with dehydration, the organ most susceptible to overhydration is the brain. When overhydration occurs slowly, the brain cells have a chance to adapt, so very few symptoms occur. When overhydration occurs quickly, a person can develop mental confusion, seizures, and coma.

Doctors try to distinguish between overhydration and excess blood volume. With overhydration, excess water is found both within and around the cells and doesn't generally result in signs of fluid accumulation. With excess blood volume, the body also has too much sodium and therefore can't shift water into the reservoir within cells. In conditions of volume overload, such as heart failure and cirrhosis of the liver, fluid accumulates around cells in the chest, abdomen, and lower legs. Distinguishing between overhydration and excess blood volume is often quite complicated, as overhydration can occur by itself or along with excess blood volume.

Treatment

The treatment of overhydration depends to some degree on the underlying cause. However, regardless of the cause, fluid intake must be restricted. Drinking less than a quart of fluid a day usually improves overhydration over several days. Fluid should be restricted only at the advice of a doctor.

Sometimes doctors prescribe a diuretic to increase the excretion of water by the kidneys. In general, diuretics are more useful in the treatment of excess blood volume and therefore are most useful when overhydration is accompanied by excess blood volume.

CHAPTER 137

Salt Balance

Salts are simple chemical compounds made up of atoms that carry either a positive or a negative electrical charge. For example, table salt (sodium chloride) is made up of positively charged sodium and negatively charged chloride atoms. Sodium chloride forms crystals when it's dry but, like many other salts found in the body, readily dissolves in water.

When a salt dissolves in water, its components exist separately as charged particles called ions.

These dissolved, charged particles are collectively known as **electrolytes.** The level (concentration) of each electrolyte in a solution of dissolved salts can be measured and is generally expressed as the amount in milliequivalents (mEq) per volume of solution (usually per liter).

Electrolytes are dissolved in the three major compartments of body water▲: the fluid within the cells, the fluid in the space surrounding cells, and the blood (electrolytes are actually dissolved in the *serum,* or fluid part of blood). The normal concentrations of electrolytes in these fluids vary. Some electrolytes are found in high concentrations inside cells and in low concentrations outside them. Other electrolytes are found in low concentrations inside cells and in high concentrations outside them.

To function properly, the body must maintain the concentration of electrolytes in each of these compartments within very narrow limits. It does so by moving electrolytes into or out of cells. The kidneys filter the electrolytes in the blood and excrete enough of them in the urine to maintain a balance between daily intake and output.

Electrolyte concentrations can be measured in a sample of blood or urine by a laboratory. Doctors measure blood electrolyte concentrations to determine if an abnormality exists and, if so, to use the results to follow the response to treatment. Sodium, potassium, calcium, phosphate, and magnesium are the electrolytes most often involved in disorders of salt balance. Chloride and bicarbonate are also commonly measured; however, the blood chloride concentration usually parallels the blood sodium concentration, and bicarbonate is involved in disorders of acid-base balance.■

Regulation of Sodium

Most of the body's sodium is in the blood and the fluid that surrounds cells. Sodium is taken in through food and drink and lost through sweat and urine. Normal kidneys can adjust the amount of sodium excreted in the urine so that the total amount of sodium in the body varies little from day to day.

A disturbance in the balance between sodium intake and output affects the total amount of sodium in the body. Changes in the total amount of sodium are closely linked to changes in the volume of water in the blood. An overall loss of so-

Major Electrolytes in the Body

Positively Charged	Negatively Charged
Sodium (Na^+)	Chloride (Cl^-)
Potassium (K^+)	Phosphates ($HPO_4^=$ and $H_2PO_4^-$)
Calcium (Ca^{++})	
Magnesium (Mg^{++})	Bicarbonate (HCO_3^-)

dium from the body doesn't necessarily cause the blood sodium concentration to fall but rather may cause the blood volume to drop. When the blood volume drops, the blood pressure falls, the heart rate rises, and light-headedness and sometimes shock occur.

Conversely, the blood volume may rise when there's too much sodium in the body. The extra fluid accumulates in the space surrounding the cells and results in a condition called edema. One sign of edema is swelling of the feet, ankles, and lower legs. When both excess water and sodium are lost or gained by the body, both the blood volume and the blood sodium concentration can be affected.

The body continually monitors the blood sodium concentration and the blood volume. When the sodium concentration becomes too high, the brain senses thirst, prompting the person to drink water.★ Sensors in the blood vessels and kidneys detect when blood volume is becoming low and trigger a chain reaction that attempts to increase the volume of fluid in the blood. The adrenal gland secretes the hormone aldosterone, which causes the kidneys to retain sodium.● The pituitary gland secretes antidiuretic hormone, which causes the kidneys to conserve water. The retained sodium and water lead to decreased urine production, which eventually leads to an increase

---

▲ see page 664

■ see page 676

★ see box, page 665

● see page 712

What Causes the Syndrome of Inappropriate Antidiuretic Hormone?

Meningitis and encephalitis

Brain tumors

Psychosis

Lung diseases (including pneumonia and acute respiratory failure)

Cancer (especially of the lung or pancreas)

Drugs
• Chlorpropamide (a drug that lowers blood sugar levels)
• Carbamazepine (an antiseizure drug)
• Vincristine (an anticancer drug)
• Clofibrate (a drug that lowers cholesterol levels)
• Antipsychotic drugs
• Aspirin, ibuprofen, and many nonprescription analgesics
• Vasopressin and oxytocin (synthetic antidiuretic hormones)

in blood volume, and the blood pressure returns to normal. When sensors in the blood vessels and kidneys detect increased blood pressure and sensors in the heart detect increased blood volume, the kidneys are stimulated to excrete more sodium and urine, thus reducing blood volume.

Low Sodium Levels

Hyponatremia (low sodium blood level) is a blood sodium concentration below 136 milliequivalents (mEq) per liter of blood.

The sodium blood concentration falls too low when sodium has been overdiluted by too much water in the body. Sodium can be overdiluted in people who drink enormous amounts of water, as occasionally occurs in certain psychiatric disor-

---

▲ see page 712

■ see page 698

ders, and in hospitalized patients who receive large amounts of water intravenously. In either case, the amount of fluid taken in exceeds the kidneys' capacity to eliminate the excess. Smaller amounts of water intake—sometimes as little as 1 quart a day—can lead to hyponatremia in people whose kidneys aren't functioning properly, such as those with kidney failure. Hyponatremia also often occurs in people with heart failure and cirrhosis of the liver, in whom the blood volume is increased. In these conditions, the increased blood volume results in the sodium being overdiluted, although the total amount of sodium in the body is generally increased as well.

Hyponatremia occurs in people who have underactive adrenal glands (Addison's disease),▲ who excrete too much sodium. The wasting of sodium in the urine is caused by a deficiency of the adrenal hormone aldosterone.

People who have the syndrome of inappropriate secretion of antidiuretic hormone (SIADH) have low sodium concentrations for a different reason. In this disorder, the pituitary gland at the base of the brain secretes too much antidiuretic hormone.■ The antidiuretic hormone causes the body to retain water and dilute the amount of sodium in the blood.

Symptoms

The speed at which the blood sodium concentration falls partly determines the severity of symptoms. When the concentration falls slowly, symptoms tend to be less severe and don't begin until the concentration becomes extremely low. When the concentration falls quickly, symptoms are more severe and tend to occur with even minor decreases. The brain is particularly sensitive to changes in the blood sodium concentration. Therefore, lethargy and confusion are among the first symptoms of hyponatremia. As hyponatremia becomes more severe, muscles may twitch and seizures may occur. In the most severe cases, stupor, coma, and death may follow.

Treatment

Severe hyponatremia is an emergency that requires immediate and intensive treatment. After performing any necessary emergency measures, doctors slowly increase the blood sodium concentration with intravenous fluids; increasing the concentration too rapidly can result in permanent brain damage.

Fluid intake is restricted, and doctors attempt to identify and correct the underlying cause of the hyponatremia. In those with the syndrome of inappropriate secretion of antidiuretic hormone, potential causes are identified and treated if possible. Demeclocycline or thiazide diuretics, drugs that can decrease the effect of antidiuretic hormone on the kidneys, may be given if hyponatremia worsens or doesn't improve despite the restriction of fluid.

High Sodium Levels

Hypernatremia (high sodium blood level) is a blood sodium concentration above 145 milliequivalents (mEq) per liter of blood.

In hypernatremia, the body contains too little water relative to the amount of sodium. The blood sodium concentration generally rises abnormally high when water loss exceeds sodium loss, usually when a person drinks too little water. A high blood sodium concentration implies that a person either doesn't feel thirsty when he should, or he is thirsty but can't obtain enough water to drink. Hypernatremia may also be seen in people with abnormal kidney function, diarrhea, vomiting, fever, or excessive sweating.

Hypernatremia is most common among the elderly. Usually, the sense of thirst is slower to develop in the elderly and is less intense than in younger people. Elderly people who are bedridden or demented may be unable to obtain water to drink even if their sense of thirst is functioning. In addition, the kidneys are less able to concentrate the urine in advanced age, so the elderly can't conserve water as well. Older people who take diuretics, which force the kidneys to excrete more water, are particularly at risk for hypernatremia, especially when the weather is hot or they become ill and do not drink enough water. Hypernatremia is always serious but is especially so in the elderly. Nearly half of the older people hospitalized for this condition die. However, the death rate may be high because many of the victims have a severe underlying illness that allowed the hypernatremia to develop.

Hypernatremia can also result when the kidneys excrete excessive water, as in diabetes insipidus. In people with diabetes insipidus, either the pituitary gland secretes too little antidiuretic hormone (antidiuretic hormone causes the kidneys to retain water) or the kidneys don't respond

---

Major Causes of High Sodium Levels

- Head trauma or neurosurgery involving the pituitary
- Disorders of other electrolytes (high calcium levels and low potassium levels)
- Use of drugs such as lithium, demeclocycline, or diuretics
- Excess water losses (diarrhea, vomiting, fever, excessive sweating)
- Sickle cell disease
- Diabetes insipidus
- Limited access to water (especially in combination with any of the other causes)

---

appropriately to the hormone.▲ Despite the excess water loss from the kidneys, people with diabetes insipidus rarely develop hypernatremia if they have a normal thirst and access to water.

Symptoms

As with hyponatremia, the major symptoms of hypernatremia result from brain dysfunction. Severe hypernatremia can lead to confusion, muscle twitching, seizures, coma, and death.

Treatment

Hypernatremia is treated by replacing water. In all but the most mild cases, fluid is given intravenously. Blood tests are performed every few hours to help determine when enough fluid has been given. The blood sodium concentration is reduced very slowly, because correcting the condition too rapidly can cause permanent brain damage.

Doctors may perform additional blood or urine tests to determine why the sodium concentration is high. Once the underlying cause is identified, treatment can become more specific. For exam-

---

▲ see page 703

ple, if a person has diabetes insipidus, doctors can give antidiuretic hormone (vasopressin).

Regulation of Potassium

Potassium has major roles in cell metabolism and in nerve and muscle cell function. Unlike sodium, most of the body's potassium is located inside cells, not in the surrounding fluid or in the blood.

The concentration of potassium in the blood must be maintained within a narrow range. A potassium concentration that is too high or too low can have serious consequences, such as an abnormal heart rhythm or cardiac arrest. The potassium stored within the cells helps keep the potassium concentration in the blood constant.

As with other electrolytes, potassium balance is achieved by matching the amount of potassium taken in through food with the amount excreted. Although some potassium is lost through the gastrointestinal tract, most of the potassium leaves the body in the urine. Normally, the kidneys adjust the excretion of potassium to match changes in dietary intake. Some drugs and certain conditions cause potassium to move into or out of cells, also greatly affecting the potassium concentration in the blood.

Low Potassium Levels

Hypokalemia (low potassium blood level) is a blood potassium concentration below 3.8 milliequivalents (mEq) per liter of blood.

Normal kidneys are extremely good at conserving potassium. If the blood potassium concentration drops too low, usually it's because the kidneys aren't functioning normally or too much potassium has been lost through the gastrointestinal tract (because of vomiting, diarrhea, chronic laxative use, or colon polyps). Since many foods contain potassium, hypokalemia rarely is caused by too little intake.

Potassium may be lost in the urine for several reasons. By far the most common is the use of certain types of diuretics that cause the kidneys to excrete excess sodium, water, and potassium.

▲ see page 714

Other causes of hypokalemia are rare. In Cushing's syndrome, the adrenal glands produce excess amounts of corticosteroid hormones including aldosterone, a hormone that causes the kidneys to excrete large amounts of potassium.▲ The kidneys also excrete excessive potassium in people who eat large amounts of licorice or chew certain types of tobacco. People with Liddle's syndrome, Bartter's syndrome, and Fanconi's syndrome are born with rare defects in the kidneys' mechanism for conserving potassium.

Certain drugs, such as insulin and the asthma drugs albuterol, terbutaline, and theophylline, increase the movement of potassium into cells and can result in hypokalemia. However, use of these drugs is rarely the sole cause of hypokalemia.

Symptoms

Mild decreases in the blood potassium concentration usually cause no symptoms at all. A more severe deficiency (levels below 3.0 mEq per liter of blood) can cause muscle weakness, twitches, and even paralysis. The heart may develop abnormal rhythms, especially in people with heart disease. For this reason, hypokalemia is particularly dangerous in those taking the drug digoxin.

Treatment

Potassium usually can be replaced relatively easily by eating foods rich in potassium or by taking potassium salts (potassium chloride) orally. Because potassium can irritate the gastrointestinal tract, potassium supplements are given in small doses several times a day with food rather than in a single large dose.

Most people who take diuretics don't need to take potassium supplements. Nevertheless, doctors periodically check the blood potassium concentration so that the drug regimen can be altered if necessary.

When potassium deficiency is severe, potassium can be given intravenously. This is done cautiously, and generally only in the hospital, to avoid raising the blood potassium concentration too much.

High Potassium Levels

Hyperkalemia (high potassium blood level) is a blood potassium concentration higher than 5.0 milliequivalents (mEq) per liter of blood.

In general, a high blood potassium concentration is more dangerous than a low one. A potassium concentration above 5.5 mEq per liter of blood begins to affect the heart's electrical conducting system. If the blood concentration continues to rise, the heart rhythm becomes abnormal and the heart may stop beating.

Hyperkalemia usually results when the kidneys don't excrete enough potassium. Probably the most common cause of mild hyperkalemia is the use of drugs that block the kidneys' excretion of potassium, such as triamterene, spironolactone, and angiotensin converting enzyme inhibitors. Hyperkalemia can also be caused by Addison's disease, in which the adrenal glands don't produce sufficient amounts of the hormones that stimulate the kidneys to excrete potassium.▲ Addison's disease is becoming an increasingly common cause of hyperkalemia, as more people with AIDS develop problems with their adrenal glands.

Partial or complete kidney failure can result in severe hyperkalemia. Thus, people with poor kidney function generally must avoid foods high in potassium.

Hyperkalemia can also result when a large amount of potassium is suddenly released from the reservoir in cells. This might happen if a large amount of muscle tissue is destroyed (as in a crush injury), if a person has a severe burn, or if a person overdoses on crack cocaine. The rapid influx of potassium into the bloodstream can overwhelm the kidneys' ability to excrete it and result in life-threatening hyperkalemia.

Symptoms

Mild hyperkalemia causes few if any symptoms. Usually, hyperkalemia is first diagnosed in routine blood tests or when a doctor notices changes on an electrocardiogram. Occasionally, symptoms such as an irregular heartbeat occur; an irregular heartbeat may be experienced as palpitations.

Treatment

Immediate treatment is essential when the blood potassium concentration rises above 5 mEq per liter in someone with poor kidney function or above 6 mEq per liter in someone with normal kidney function. Potassium can be removed from the body through the gastrointestinal tract or the kidneys or by dialysis. Potassium can be removed by inducing diarrhea and by swallowing a preparation that contains a potassium-

---

Sources of Potassium

- Potassium supplements
- Salt substitutes (potassium chloride)
- Bananas
- Tomatoes
- Oranges
- Melons
- Potatoes and sweet potatoes
- Spinach, turnip greens, collard greens, kale, and other green leafy vegetables
- Most peas and beans

---

absorbing resin. This resin isn't absorbed from the gastrointestinal tract, so the potassium leaves the body in the stool. If the person's kidneys are functioning, a diuretic can be given to increase potassium excretion.

When treatment is needed even more rapidly, the person may be given an intravenous solution containing calcium, glucose, or insulin. Calcium helps protect the heart from the effects of high potassium, but this effect lasts only a few minutes. Glucose and insulin drive potassium from the blood into cells, thus lowering the blood potassium concentration. If these measures fail or if a person has kidney failure, dialysis may be necessary.

Regulation of Calcium

Calcium is essential for various body functions, including muscle contraction, nerve conduction, and the proper functioning of many enzymes. Most of the body's calcium is stored in the bones, but calcium is also found in cells and in the blood. The body controls precisely the amount of calcium in both cells and the blood.

Maintaining a normal calcium concentration in the blood depends on ingesting at least 500 to

---

▲ see page 712

Causes of Low Calcium Levels

Cause	Comments
Low levels of parathyroid hormone	Usually occurs after damage to or accidental removal of the parathyroid glands during surgery to remove the thyroid
Congenital lack of para-thyroid glands	A rare hereditary condition or one that occurs as part of DiGeorge syndrome
Pseudohypo-parathyroid-ism	An uncommon inherited disease; levels of parathyroid hormone are normal, but bone and kidney have a decreased response to the hormone
Vitamin D deficiency	Usually caused by poor nutri-tion, insufficient exposure to sunshine (vitamin D is activated when the skin is exposed to sunshine), liver disease, gastrointestinal disease that prevents absorp-tion of vitamin D, or the use of barbiturates and phenytoin, which decrease the effective-ness of vitamin D
Kidney damage	Interferes with vitamin D activation in the kidneys
Low magne-sium levels	Results in decreased para-thyroid hormone
Poor nutrition or malabsorp-tion	Occurs with or without vitamin D deficiency
Pancreatitis	Occurs when excess fatty acids in the blood from the injured pancreas combine with calcium
Low levels of albumin	Reduces amount of calcium bound to albumin but doesn't generally cause symptoms because the amount of free calcium remains normal

1,000 milligrams of calcium a day, absorbing an adequate amount of this calcium from the gastro-intestinal tract, and excreting excess calcium into the urine. Calcium moves out of the bones into the bloodstream as needed to maintain the blood calcium concentration. However, mobilizing too much calcium from the bones eventually weakens them and can lead to osteoporosis.

The calcium concentration in the blood is reg-ulated by two hormones: parathyroid hormone and calcitonin. **Parathyroid hormone** is produced by the four parathyroid glands located around the thyroid gland in the neck. When the calcium con-centration in the blood falls, the parathyroid glands produce more parathyroid hormone; when it rises, the parathyroid glands produce less hormone. Parathyroid hormone stimulates the gastrointestinal tract to absorb more calcium and causes the kidneys to activate vitamin D. Vitamin D further enhances the ability of the gastrointes-tinal tract to absorb calcium. Parathyroid hor-mone also stimulates the bones to release cal-cium into the blood and causes the kidneys to excrete less calcium into the urine. **Calcitonin,** a hormone produced by cells of the parathyroid, thyroid, and thymus glands, lowers the blood cal-cium concentration by stimulating the movement of calcium into the bones.

Low Calcium Levels

Hypocalcemia (low calcium blood level) is a blood calcium concentration below 8.8 milligrams (mg) per deciliter of blood.

The blood calcium concentration can be low as a result of several different problems. Hypocal-cemia is most common in disorders that result in chronic calcium loss from the urine or a failure to mobilize calcium from the bones. Since most of the calcium in the blood is carried by the protein albumin, too little albumin in the blood results in a low blood calcium concentration. However, hy-pocalcemia caused by too little albumin isn't usu-ally important, because only the calcium that isn't bound to albumin can prevent the symptoms of hypocalcemia.

Symptoms and Diagnosis

The blood calcium concentration can be ab-normally low without producing any symptoms. Over time, hypocalcemia can affect the brain and cause neurologic symptoms such as confusion, memory loss, delirium, depression, and halluci-nations. These symptoms are reversible if the cal-cium is restored. An extremely low calcium con-centration (below 7 mg per deciliter of blood) may cause muscle aches and tingling, often in the lips, tongue, fingers, and feet. Seizures and spasms of the muscles in the throat (leading to difficulty in breathing) as well as tetany (general stiffening and spasms of the muscles) can occur in severe cases. Changes in the heart's electrical conducting system occur and can be seen on an electrocardiogram.

An abnormal calcium concentration is usually first found during routine blood tests. Consequently, hypocalcemia is often diagnosed before symptoms become obvious. Once hypocalcemia is detected, a detailed history, complete physical examination, and other laboratory tests of blood and urine are required to establish the cause.

Treatment

The treatment varies, depending on the underlying cause. Calcium can be replaced either intravenously or orally. People who have chronic hypocalcemia may be able to correct the problem by taking oral calcium supplements. Once symptoms appear, the intravenous route is generally warranted. Taking vitamin D supplements as well helps to increase the absorption of calcium from the gastrointestinal tract.

High Calcium Levels

Hypercalcemia (high calcium blood level) is a blood calcium concentration above 10.5 milligrams (mg) per deciliter of blood.

Hypercalcemia can be caused by either increased gastrointestinal absorption or increased intake of calcium. People who ingest large amounts of calcium, as is occasionally done by those with peptic ulcers who drink a lot of milk and also take calcium-containing antacids, can develop hypercalcemia. An overdose of vitamin D similarly can affect the blood calcium concentration by greatly increasing the absorption of calcium from the gastrointestinal tract.

However, the most common cause of hypercalcemia is **hyperparathyroidism,** the excessive secretion of parathyroid hormone by one or more of the four parathyroid glands. Some 90 percent of people with primary hyperparathyroidism have a noncancerous tumor (adenoma) in one of these small glands. In the remaining 10 percent, the glands simply enlarge and produce too much hormone. In rare cases, cancers of the parathyroid glands cause hyperparathyroidism.

Hyperparathyroidism is more common in women than in men. It is more likely to develop in older people and in those who have previously received radiation therapy to the neck. Sometimes hyperparathyroidism occurs as part of the syndrome of multiple endocrine neoplasia, a rare hereditary disease.▲

People with cancer often have hypercalcemia. Cancers of the kidneys, lungs, or ovaries often secrete large amounts of a protein that has effects similar to those of parathyroid hormone—these effects are considered a paraneoplastic syndrome.■ Cancer also may spread (metastasize) to bone, destroying bone cells and releasing calcium into the blood. This occurs most commonly with cancers of the prostate, breast, and lung. Multiple myeloma (a cancer involving bone marrow) also can lead to the destruction of bone and result in hypercalcemia. Other cancers raise the blood calcium concentration by means not yet fully understood.

Diseases in which bone is destroyed or resorbed may also cause hypercalcemia. One such disease is Paget's disease. People who are immobilized, such as paraplegics, quadriplegics, or those on prolonged bed rest, can also develop hypercalcemia because bone tissue is resorbed.

Symptoms and Diagnosis

Because hypercalcemia often causes no symptoms at all, the condition is usually first discovered during routine blood tests. The underlying cause is often apparent from the person's history and recent activities (for example, drinking large amounts of milk and taking calcium-containing antacid tablets for indigestion), but usually laboratory tests or x-rays are needed to find a cause.

The earliest symptoms of hypercalcemia are usually constipation, loss of appetite, nausea and vomiting, and abdominal pain. The kidneys may produce abnormally large amounts of urine. As excess urine is produced, the fluid in the body decreases and symptoms of dehydration can occur.★ Very severe hypercalcemia often causes symptoms of brain dysfunction such as confusion, emotional disturbances, delirium, hallucinations, weakness, and coma. Abnormal heart rhythms and death can follow.

▲ see page 726

■ see page 797

★ see page 665

Kidney stones containing calcium may form in people with chronic hypercalcemia. If hypercalcemia is severe and prolonged, calcium-containing crystals may form in the kidneys, causing permanent damage.

Treatment

The treatment depends on how high and why the blood calcium concentration rose. If the calcium concentration is no higher than 11.5 mg per deciliter of blood, correcting the underlying cause is often sufficient. People who have normal kidney function and a tendency to develop hypercalcemia are usually advised to drink plenty of fluids, which stimulates the kidneys to excrete calcium and helps prevent dehydration.

If the calcium concentration is very high (higher than 15 mg per deciliter of blood) or if symptoms of brain dysfunction appear, fluids are given intravenously as long as the kidney function is normal. Diuretics such as furosemide increase the kidneys' excretion of calcium and are a mainstay of treatment. Dialysis is a highly effective, safe, reliable treatment but is usually reserved for those people with severe hypercalcemia not treatable by other methods.

Hyperparathyroidism is usually treated by surgically removing one or more of the parathyroid glands. For a successful result, the surgeon must remove all parathyroid tissue that's producing excessive amounts of hormone. Sometimes additional parathyroid tissue is located in places other than the parathyroid glands. In the hands of an experienced surgeon, surgery is successful in nearly 90 percent of cases.

Several other drugs can be used to treat hypercalcemia when other methods fail. They include plicamycin, gallium nitrate, calcitonin, bisphosphonates, and corticosteroids. The drugs work primarily by slowing the movement of calcium from bone.

Hypercalcemia caused by cancer is particularly difficult to treat. However, if the cancer can't be controlled, hypercalcemia usually returns despite the best treatment.

Regulation of Phosphate

The element phosphorus is present in the body almost exclusively in the form of phosphate (one phosphorus and four oxygen atoms). Most of the body's phosphate is contained in bone. The rest is primarily inside cells, where it's intimately involved in energy metabolism and is also used as a building block for such important molecules as DNA. Phosphate is excreted in the urine and stool.

Low Phosphate Levels

Hypophosphatemia (low phosphate blood level) is a blood phosphate concentration lower than 2.5 milligrams (mg) per deciliter of blood.

Chronic hypophosphatemia occurs in hyperparathyroidism, hypothyroidism (an underactive thyroid gland), poor kidney function, and long-term use of diuretics. Toxic amounts of the drug theophylline can reduce the amount of phosphate in the body. Taking large amounts of aluminum hydroxide antacids for a long time can also deplete the body's phosphate, especially in people undergoing kidney dialysis. Phosphate stores are depleted in people with severe malnutrition, diabetic ketoacidosis, severe alcohol intoxication, or severe burns. As people with these conditions recover, the blood phosphate concentration can quickly fall dangerously low because the body uses large amounts of phosphate.

Symptoms

A person may have hypophosphatemia without any illness. Symptoms occur only when the blood phosphate concentration drops very low. Initially the person may experience muscle weakness. Over time, bones can weaken, resulting in bone pain and fractures. An extremely low phosphate concentration (lower than 1.5 mg per deciliter of blood) can be very serious, leading to progressive muscle weakness, stupor, coma, and death.

Treatment

The treatment is determined by the severity of symptoms and the underlying cause. A person with no symptoms can take phosphate in an oral solution, but this usually causes diarrhea. One quart of low-fat or skim milk provides a large amount of phosphate and is generally easier to take. Intravenous phosphate may be given if hypophosphatemia is very severe or if phosphate can't be taken orally.

High Phosphate Levels

Hyperphosphatemia (high phosphate blood level) is a blood phosphate concentration higher than 4.5 milligrams (mg) per deciliter of blood.

Normal kidneys are so efficient at excreting excess phosphate that hyperphosphatemia rarely occurs except in people with severe kidney dysfunction. In people with kidney failure, hyperphosphatemia is a problem because dialysis is not very effective at removing phosphate.

Symptoms

There are few outward signs of hyperphosphatemia. When the blood phosphate concentration is elevated in dialysis patients, the blood calcium concentration becomes low. This stimulates the parathyroid glands to produce parathyroid hormone, which in turn raises the blood calcium concentration by mobilizing calcium from the bone. If this condition continues, progressive bone weakness can occur, resulting in pain and fractures from minimal trauma. Calcium and phosphate can crystallize in the walls of the blood vessels and heart, causing severe arteriosclerosis (hardening of the arteries) and leading to strokes, heart attacks, and poor circulation. Crystals can also form in the skin where they cause severe itching.

Treatment

Hyperphosphatemia in people with kidney damage is treated by decreasing phosphate intake and reducing the absorption of phosphate from the gastrointestinal tract. Foods high in phosphate should be avoided, and calcium-containing antacids should be taken with meals so that the calcium can bind to the phosphate in the intestines and not be absorbed.

Continuous stimulation of the parathyroid glands may cause hyperparathyroidism, requiring that the glands be surgically removed.

Regulation of Magnesium

A wide variety of enzymes in the body depend on magnesium to function properly. Most of the body's magnesium is found in bone; very little is in the blood. The amount of magnesium is maintained largely by eating a nutritious diet. Some magnesium is excreted in the urine; some is excreted in the stool.

Low Magnesium Levels

Hypomagnesemia (low magnesium blood level) is a blood magnesium concentration lower than 1.6 milliequivalents (mEq) per liter of blood.

Foods High in Phosphate

- Milk and dairy products
- Most peas and beans
- Spinach, turnip greens, collard greens, kale, and other green leafy vegetables
- Nuts
- Chocolate
- Dark-colored soft drinks (except root beer)

The disorders in which hypomagnesemia occurs are complex and usually are the result of metabolic and nutritional disturbances. The most common causes of hypomagnesemia are decreased intake associated with starvation or intestinal malabsorption and increased excretion by the kidneys. Hypomagnesemia also occurs frequently in people who consume large amounts of alcohol or who have protracted diarrhea. High levels of aldosterone, antidiuretic hormone, or thyroid hormone can cause hypomagnesemia by increasing the excretion of magnesium by the kidney. Treatment with diuretics, the antifungal drug amphotericin B, or the anticancer drug cisplatin can also cause hypomagnesemia.

Symptoms

Hypomagnesemia can lead to loss of appetite, nausea and vomiting, sleepiness, weakness, personality changes, muscle spasms, and tremors. If hypomagnesemia occurs in conjunction with hypocalcemia, the magnesium must be replaced before the calcium disorder can be treated successfully.

Treatment

Magnesium is replaced when the deficiency causes symptoms or when the magnesium concentration is very low (lower than 1 mEq per liter of blood). Magnesium can be taken orally or by injection into a muscle or vein.

High Magnesium Levels

Hypermagnesemia (high magnesium blood level) is a blood magnesium concentration higher than 2.1 milliequivalents (mEq) per liter of blood.

People almost never have hypermagnesemia unless they have kidney failure and are given magnesium salts or they take drugs that contain magnesium, such as some antacids or purgatives. Hypermagnesemia can lead to weakness, low blood pressure, and impaired breathing. The heart can stop beating if the magnesium concentration rises above 12 to 15 mEq per liter.

Treatment

The treatment of severe hypermagnesemia requires the administration of intravenous calcium gluconate and support of the circulatory and respiratory systems. Powerful intravenous diuretics can increase the kidneys' excretion of magnesium. If the kidneys aren't functioning well, dialysis may be needed.

CHAPTER 138

Acid-Base Balance

The degree of acidity is an important chemical property of blood and other bodily fluids. Acidity is expressed on the pH scale, in which 7.0 is neutral, above 7.0 is basic (alkaline), and below 7.0 is acidic. A strong acid has a very low pH (near 1.0), while a strong base has a very high pH (near 14.0). Blood is normally slightly alkaline, with a pH range of 7.35 to 7.45. The blood's acid-base balance is controlled precisely because even a minor deviation from the normal range can severely affect many organs.

The body uses three mechanisms to control the blood's acid-base balance. First, excess acid is excreted by the kidneys, largely in the form of ammonia. The kidneys have some ability to alter the amount of acid or base that is excreted, but this generally takes several days.

Second, the body uses pH buffers in the blood to guard against sudden changes in acidity. A pH buffer works chemically to minimize changes in the pH of a solution. The most important pH buffer in the blood uses bicarbonate. Bicarbonate, a basic compound, exists in equilibrium with carbon dioxide, an acidic compound. As more acid enters the bloodstream, more bicarbonate and less carbon dioxide are produced; as more base enters the bloodstream, more carbon dioxide and less bicarbonate are produced. In both cases, the effect on pH is minimized.

The third mechanism to control blood pH involves the excretion of carbon dioxide. Carbon dioxide is an important by-product of the metabolism of oxygen and, as such, is constantly produced by cells. The blood carries carbon dioxide to the lungs where it is exhaled. Respiratory control centers in the brain regulate the amount of carbon dioxide that is exhaled by controlling the speed and depth of breathing. When breathing is increased, the blood carbon dioxide level decreases and the blood becomes more basic. When breathing is decreased, the blood carbon dioxide level increases and the blood becomes more acidic. By adjusting the speed and depth of breathing, the respiratory control centers and lungs are able to regulate the blood pH minute by minute.

An abnormality in one or more of these pH control mechanisms can cause one of two major disturbances in acid-base balance: acidosis or alkalosis. **Acidosis** is a condition in which the blood has too much acid (or too little base), frequently resulting in a decrease in blood pH. **Alkalosis** is a condition in which the blood has too much base (or too little acid), occasionally resulting in an increase in blood pH. Acidosis and alkalosis are not diseases but rather are the results of a wide variety of disorders. The presence of acidosis or alkalosis provides an important clue to doctors that a serious metabolic problem exists.

Acidosis and alkalosis are categorized as metabolic or respiratory depending on their primary cause. Metabolic acidosis and metabolic alkalosis are caused by an imbalance in the production and excretion of acids or bases by the kidneys. Respiratory acidosis and respiratory alkalosis are caused primarily by lung or breathing disorders.

Metabolic Acidosis

Metabolic acidosis is excessive blood acidity characterized by an inappropriately low level of bicarbonate in the blood.

If an increase in acid overwhelms the body's pH buffering system, the blood can actually become acidic. As the blood pH drops, breathing becomes deeper and faster as the body attempts to rid the blood of excess acid by decreasing the amount of carbon dioxide. Eventually, the kidneys also try to compensate by excreting more acid in the urine. However, both mechanisms can be overwhelmed if the body continues to produce too much acid, leading to severe acidosis and eventually a coma.

Causes

The causes of metabolic acidosis can be grouped into three major categories.

First, the amount of acid in the body can be increased by ingesting an acid or a substance that is metabolized to acid. Most substances that cause acidosis when ingested are considered poisonous. Examples include wood alcohol (methanol) and antifreeze (ethylene glycol). However, even an overdose of aspirin (acetylsalicylic acid) can cause metabolic acidosis.

Second, the body can produce increased amounts of acid through metabolism. The body can produce excess acid as a result of several diseases; one of the most significant is type I diabetes mellitus. When diabetes is poorly controlled, the body breaks down fats and produces acids called ketones. The body also produces excess acid in the advanced stages of shock, when lactic acid is formed through the metabolism of sugar.

Third, metabolic acidosis may result when the kidneys aren't able to excrete enough acid. Even the production of normal amounts of acid may lead to acidosis when the kidneys aren't functioning normally. This type of kidney malfunction is called renal tubular acidosis and may occur in people with kidney failure or with abnormalities that affect the kidneys' ability to excrete acid.

Symptoms and Diagnosis

A person with mild metabolic acidosis may have no symptoms but usually has nausea, vomiting, and fatigue. Breathing becomes deeper or slightly faster, but most people don't even notice it. As the acidosis worsens, the person begins to feel extremely weak and sleepy and may feel confused and increasingly nauseated. If the acidosis worsens further, blood pressure can fall, leading to shock, coma, and death.

The diagnosis of acidosis generally requires the measurement of blood pH in a sample of arterial

Major Causes of Metabolic Acidosis and Alkalosis

Metabolic Acidosis

- Kidney failure
- Renal tubular acidosis (a form of kidney malformation)
- Diabetic ketoacidosis
- Lactic acidosis (buildup of lactic acid)
- Poisons such as ethylene glycol, salicylate (overdose), methanol, paraldehyde, acetazolamide, or ammonia chloride
- Loss of bases, such as bicarbonate, through the gastrointestinal tract from diarrhea, an ileostomy, or a colostomy

Metabolic Alkalosis

- Use of diuretics (thiazides, furosemide, ethacrynic acid)
- Loss of acid from vomiting or drainage of the stomach
- Overactive adrenal gland (Cushing's syndrome or use of corticosteroids)

blood, usually taken from the radial artery in the wrist. Arterial blood is used because venous blood is not an accurate measure of blood pH.

To learn more about the cause of the acidosis, doctors also measure the levels of carbon dioxide and bicarbonate in the blood. Additional blood tests may be performed to help determine the cause. For example, high blood sugar levels and ketones in the urine usually indicate uncontrolled diabetes. A toxic substance in the blood suggests that the metabolic acidosis is caused by poisoning or overdose. Sometimes the urine is examined microscopically, and its pH is also measured.

Treatment

The treatment of metabolic acidosis depends primarily on the cause. Whenever possible, doctors treat the underlying cause. For example, they may control diabetes with insulin or treat poisoning by removing the toxic substance from the blood. Occasionally dialysis is needed to treat severe overdoses and poisonings.

Metabolic acidosis may also be treated directly. If the acidosis is mild, intravenous fluids and treatment for the underlying disorder may be all that's needed. When acidosis is severe, bicarbonate may be given intravenously; however, bicarbonate provides only temporary relief and may cause harm.

Metabolic Alkalosis

Metabolic alkalosis is a condition in which the blood is alkaline because of an inappropriately high level of bicarbonate.

Metabolic alkalosis develops when the body loses too much acid. For example, a considerable amount of stomach acid is lost during periods of prolonged vomiting or when stomach acids are suctioned with a stomach tube (as is sometimes done in hospitals, particularly after abdominal surgery). In rare cases, metabolic alkalosis develops in a person who has ingested too much alkali from substances such as bicarbonate of soda. In addition, metabolic alkalosis can develop when excessive loss of sodium or potassium affects the kidneys' ability to control the blood's acid-base balance.

Symptoms and Diagnosis

Metabolic alkalosis may cause irritability, muscle twitching, and muscle cramps, or no symptoms at all. If the metabolic alkalosis is severe, prolonged contraction and spasms of muscles (tetany) can develop.

A sample of blood taken from an artery usually shows that the blood is alkaline. A sample of blood taken from a vein contains high levels of bicarbonate.

Treatment

Doctors usually treat metabolic alkalosis by replacing water and electrolytes (sodium and potassium) while treating the underlying cause. Occasionally when metabolic alkalosis is very severe, dilute acid in the form of ammonium chloride is given intravenously.

Respiratory Acidosis

Respiratory acidosis is excessive blood acidity caused by a buildup of carbon dioxide in the blood as a result of poor lung function or slow breathing.

The speed and depth of breathing control the amount of carbon dioxide in the blood. Normally when carbon dioxide builds up, the pH of the blood falls and the blood becomes acidic. High levels of carbon dioxide in the blood stimulate the parts of the brain that regulate breathing, which in turn stimulate faster and deeper breathing.

Causes

Respiratory acidosis develops when the lungs don't expel carbon dioxide adequately. This can happen in diseases that severely affect the lungs, such as emphysema, chronic bronchitis, severe pneumonia, pulmonary edema, and asthma. Respiratory acidosis can also develop when diseases of the nerves or muscles of the chest impair the mechanics of breathing. In addition, a person can develop respiratory acidosis if overly sedated from narcotics and strong sleeping medications that slow respiration.

Symptoms and Diagnosis

The first symptoms may be a headache and drowsiness. If respiratory acidosis worsens, drowsiness may progress to stupor and coma. Stupor and coma can develop within moments if breathing stops or is severely impaired or over hours if breathing is less dramatically impaired. The kidneys try to compensate for the acidosis by retaining bicarbonate, but this process takes many hours or days.

In general, the diagnosis of respiratory acidosis is readily apparent to doctors checking the results of blood pH and carbon dioxide measurements in samples of blood taken from an artery.

Treatment

The treatment of respiratory acidosis aims to improve the function of the lungs. Drugs to improve breathing may help people who have lung diseases such as asthma and emphysema. People who have severely impaired lung function, for whatever reason, may need artificial respiration with a mechanical ventilator.

Respiratory Alkalosis

Respiratory alkalosis is a condition in which the blood is alkaline because rapid or deep breathing results in a low blood carbon dioxide level.

Rapid, deep breathing, also called hyperventilation, causes too much carbon dioxide to be expelled from the bloodstream. The most common cause of hyperventilation, and thus respiratory alkalosis, is anxiety. Other causes of respiratory alkalosis include pain, cirrhosis of the liver, low oxygen levels in the blood, fever, and aspirin overdose.

Symptoms and Diagnosis

Respiratory alkalosis can make a person feel anxious and can cause a tingling sensation around the lips and face. If respiratory alkalosis worsens, muscles can go into spasm and the person can feel detached from reality.

Doctors usually can make the diagnosis of respiratory alkalosis by simply observing and talking to the person. When the diagnosis isn't obvious, a doctor can measure the level of carbon dioxide in a sample of blood taken from an artery. Frequently the blood pH is also elevated.

Treatment

Usually the only treatment needed is to slow down the rate of breathing. When respiratory alkalosis is caused by anxiety, a conscious effort to slow breathing may make the condition disappear. If pain is causing the person to breathe rapidly, relieving the pain usually suffices. Breathing into a paper (not a plastic) bag may help raise the blood carbon dioxide content as the person breathes carbon dioxide back in after breathing it out. Alternatively, the person can be taught to hold the breath as long as possible, then take a shallow breath and again hold it as long as possible, repeating this sequence 6 to 10 times.

As the carbon dioxide levels rise, the symptoms of hyperventilation improve, thus reducing the person's anxiety and stopping the attack.

CHAPTER 139

Disorders of Cholesterol and Other Fats

Fats, also called lipids, are energy-rich substances that serve as a major source of fuel for the body's metabolic processes. Fats are obtained from food or formed in the body, mostly in the liver, and can be stored in fat cells for future use. Fat cells also insulate the body from cold and help protect it from injury. Fats are essential components of cell membranes, of the myelin sheaths that surround nerve cells, and of bile.

The two major fats in the blood are cholesterol and triglyceride. The fats attach themselves to certain proteins so they can travel throughout the bloodstream; the combined fats and proteins are called lipoproteins. The major lipoproteins are chylomicrons, very low density lipoproteins (VLDL), low-density lipoproteins (LDL), and high-density lipoproteins (HDL).

Each type of lipoprotein serves a different purpose and is broken down and excreted in a slightly different way. For example, chylomicrons originate in the intestine and carry certain types of digested fat from the intestines into the bloodstream. A series of enzymes then remove the fat from the chylomicrons for use as energy or for storage in fat cells. Ultimately, the remaining chylomicron, stripped of much of its fat (triglyceride), is removed from the bloodstream by the liver.

The body regulates lipoprotein levels in several ways. One way is by reducing the synthesis of lipoproteins and their entry into the bloodstream. Another is by increasing or decreasing the rate at which lipoproteins are removed from the blood.

Abnormal levels of fats circulating in the bloodstream, especially cholesterol, can lead to long-term problems. The risk of having atherosclerosis and coronary artery or carotid artery disease (and therefore the risk of having a heart attack or stroke) increases as a person's total cholesterol level increases. Low cholesterol levels are therefore generally better than high ones, although extremely low cholesterol levels may not be healthy either. An ideal total cholesterol level is probably 140 to 200 milligrams of cholesterol per deciliter of blood (mg/dL) or less. The risk of a heart attack more than doubles when the total cholesterol level approaches 300 mg/dL.

Not all cholesterol increases the risk of heart disease. The cholesterol carried by LDL (the so-called bad cholesterol) increases the risk; the

Causes of High Fat Levels

Cholesterol

Diet high in saturated fats and cholesterol

Cirrhosis

Poorly controlled diabetes

Underactive thyroid gland

Overactive pituitary gland

Kidney failure

Porphyria

Heredity

Triglycerides

Excess calories in diet

Acute alcohol abuse

Severe uncontrolled diabetes

Kidney failure

Certain drugs
• Estrogens
• Oral contraceptives
• Corticosteroids
• Thiazide diuretics (to some extent)

Heredity

cholesterol carried by HDL (the so-called good cholesterol) lowers the risk and is beneficial. Ideally, LDL cholesterol levels should be below 130 mg/dL, and HDL cholesterol levels should be above 40 mg/dL. The HDL level should account for more than 25 percent of the total cholesterol. The total cholesterol level is less important as a risk factor for heart disease or strokes than the total cholesterol to HDL cholesterol ratio or the LDL to HDL ratio.

Whether high levels of triglycerides increase the risk of heart disease or strokes is uncertain. Blood levels of triglycerides above 250 mg/dL are considered abnormal, but high levels don't appear to uniformly increase the risk of atherosclerosis or coronary artery disease. However, extraordinarily high levels of triglycerides (above 800 mg/dL) may lead to pancreatitis.▲

Hyperlipidemia

Hyperlipidemia is abnormally high levels of fats (cholesterol, triglycerides, or both) in the blood.

Levels of lipoproteins, particularly LDL cholesterol, increase with age. Levels are normally higher in men than in women, but they start to rise in women after menopause. Other factors contributing to high levels of certain lipids (such

as VLDL and LDL) include a family history of hyperlipidemia, obesity, a high-fat diet, lack of exercise, moderate to high alcohol consumption, cigarette smoking, poorly controlled diabetes, and an underactive thyroid gland.

Most elevations in triglyceride and total cholesterol levels are temporary and not severe, mainly the result of eating fat. People's bodies clear fats from the blood at different rates. One person can eat large amounts of animal fats and never have the total cholesterol level rise above 200 mg/dL, while another person can follow a strict low-fat diet and never have the total cholesterol drop below 260 mg/dL. This difference seems in part to be genetically determined and largely relates to differences in the rate at which lipoproteins enter and are removed from the bloodstream.

Symptoms and Diagnosis

Usually, high fat levels cause no symptoms. Occasionally, when levels are particularly high, fat deposits form growths called xanthomas in tendons and in the skin. Extremely high levels of triglycerides (800 mg/dL and higher) may cause enlargement of the liver and spleen and symptoms of pancreatitis, such as severe abdominal pain.

A blood sample to measure the total cholesterol level can be taken at any time. However, blood samples to measure levels of HDL cholesterol, LDL cholesterol, and triglycerides are best taken after at least 12 hours of fasting.

▲ see page 504

Treatment

A diet low in cholesterol and saturated fats will reduce LDL levels. Exercise can help reduce the blood levels of LDL cholesterol and increase the blood levels of HDL cholesterol. Drinking a small amount of alcohol every day may raise the HDL cholesterol level and lower the LDL level, although having more than two drinks could have the opposite effect.

Generally, the best treatment for people who have high cholesterol or triglyceride levels is to lose weight if they're overweight, stop smoking, reduce the total amount of fat and cholesterol in their diet, increase exercise, and if necessary, take a lipid-lowering drug. However, when blood levels of fat are very high or don't respond to the usual treatments, the specific disorder should be identified with special blood tests so that specific treatment can be planned.

Hereditary Hyperlipidemias

Cholesterol and triglyceride levels are highest in people with hereditary hyperlipidemias, also called hyperlipoproteinemias, which interfere with the body's system for metabolizing and eliminating fats. Each of the five main types of hyperlipoproteinemia produces a different profile of blood fats and a different set of risks.

Type I hyperlipoproteinemia (familial hyperchylomicronemia) is a rare hereditary disorder, present at birth, in which the body is unable to clear chylomicrons from the blood. Children and young adults with type I hyperlipoproteinemia have recurrent bouts of abdominal pain. They have an enlarged liver and spleen and develop pinkish-yellow, fatty growths (eruptive xanthomas) on their skin. Blood tests show extremely high levels of triglycerides. This disorder doesn't lead to atherosclerosis but can cause pancreatitis, which can be fatal.▲ People who have the disorder must avoid eating fats of all types—saturated, unsaturated, and polyunsaturated.

Type II hyperlipoproteinemia (familial hypercholesterolemia) is a hereditary disorder that results in accelerated atherosclerosis and early death, usually from a heart attack. People with type II hyperlipoproteinemia have high levels of LDL cholesterol. Fat deposits form growths (xanthomas) in the tendons and skin. One in six men with this disorder has a heart attack by age 40, and two in three have a heart attack by age 60. Women with type II hyperlipoproteinemia are also at in-

Levels of Blood Fats

Laboratory Test	Ideal Range*
Total cholesterol	120 to 200 mg/dL
Chylomicrons	None (after 12 hours of fasting)
Very low density lipoproteins (VLDL)	1 to 30 mg/dL
Low-density lipoproteins (LDL)	60 to 160 mg/dL
High-density lipoproteins (HDL)	35 to 65 mg/dL
LDL to HDL ratio	Less than 3.5
Triglycerides	10 to 160 mg/dL

*mg/dL = milligrams per deciliter of blood.

creased risk, but the risk starts later—about one in two women with the disorder will have a heart attack by age 55. People who have two genes for this disorder (a rare occurrence) may have total cholesterol levels of 500 to 1,200 mg/dL and often die of coronary artery disease in childhood.

Treatment is aimed at avoiding risk factors such as smoking and obesity and at reducing the blood cholesterol levels with drugs; a diet that contains few or no fats, especially saturated fats and cholesterol; and exercise. Adding oat bran to the diet, which binds fats in the intestines, may be helpful. A lipid-lowering drug is often needed.

Type III hyperlipoproteinemia is an uncommon hereditary disorder that leads to high levels of VLDL cholesterol and triglycerides. In men with type III hyperlipoproteinemia, fatty growths appear in the skin by early adulthood; in women, fatty skin growths appear 10 to 15 years later. In both men and women, the growths will appear earlier if the person is overweight. Atherosclerosis often blocks arteries and reduces blood flow to the legs by middle age. Blood tests show high total cho-

▲ see page 504

Drugs Used to Lower Levels of Blood Fats

Type of Drug	Examples	How It Works
Bile acid absorber	• Cholestyramine • Colestipol	Binds bile acids in the intestine; enhances LDL removal from the bloodstream
Lipoprotein synthesis inhibitor	• Niacin	Reduces the rate of VLDL production (VLDL is the forerunner of LDL)
Coenzyme A reductase inhibitor	• Fluvastatin • Lovastatin • Pravastatin • Simvastatin	Blocks the synthesis of cholesterol; enhances the removal of LDL from the bloodstream
Fibric acid derivative	• Clofibrate • Fenofibrate • Gemfibrozil	Unknown, possibly increases the breakdown of fats

lesterol and triglyceride levels. The cholesterol consists mostly of VLDL. People with type III hyperlipoproteinemia often have mild diabetes and elevated blood levels of uric acid.

The treatment entails achieving and maintaining an ideal body weight and eating less cholesterol and saturated fats. Lipid-lowering drugs are usually needed. Blood fat levels can almost always be reduced to normal, slowing the rate of atherosclerosis.

Type IV hyperlipoproteinemia, a common disorder often affecting several members of a family, produces high levels of triglycerides. This disorder may increase a person's risk of developing atherosclerosis. People with type IV hyperlipoproteinemia are often overweight and have mild diabetes. Reducing weight, controlling diabetes, and avoiding alcohol are beneficial. Taking a lipid-lowering drug may also help.

Type V hyperlipoproteinemia is an uncommon disorder in which the body can't sufficiently metabolize and eliminate excess triglycerides. While sometimes hereditary, this disorder may be caused by abuse of alcohol, poorly controlled diabetes, kidney failure, or eating after a period of starvation. When inherited, the disorder usually first appears in early adulthood. People with type

V hyperlipoproteinemia may have large numbers of fatty growths (xanthomas) in the skin, an enlarged spleen and liver, and abdominal pain. Mild diabetes and high levels of uric acid are common. Many people are overweight. The major complication is pancreatitis, which is often brought on by eating fats and can be fatal. Treatment consists of avoiding fats in the diet, losing weight, and not drinking alcohol. Lipid-lowering drugs may be helpful.

Hypolipoproteinemia

Hypolipoproteinemia, low levels of fats in the blood, is rarely a problem but may indicate the presence of other diseases. For example, cholesterol levels may be low in someone with an overactive thyroid, anemia, malnutrition, or cancer, or whose absorption of foods from the gastrointestinal tract is faulty (malabsorption). Therefore, doctors may be concerned when total cholesterol levels fall below 120 mg/dL.

A few rare inherited disorders lower fat levels enough to have serious consequences. People with **hypobetalipoproteinemia** have extremely low levels of LDL cholesterol but usually have no symptoms and require no treatment. However, people with **abetalipoproteinemia** have no LDL cholesterol and can't make chylomicrons, resulting in the malabsorption of fat and fat-soluble vitamins, abnormal bowel movements, fatty stools (steatorrhea), odd-shaped red blood cells, and blindness from retinitis pigmentosa. Although abetalipoproteinemia can't be cured, taking massive doses of vitamin E and vitamin A may delay or slow damage to the nervous system. People with **Tangier disease** have extremely low HDL cholesterol levels, leading to abnormal nerve function and enlarged lymph nodes, tonsils, liver, and spleen.

Lipidoses

The lipidoses, diseases caused by abnormalities in the enzymes that break down (metabolize) fats, result in a toxic accumulation of fat by-products in tissues.

Groups of specific enzymes help the body break down each type of fat. Abnormalities in these enzymes can lead to the buildup of specific fatty substances that normally would have been broken down by the enzyme. Over time, accumulations of these substances can be harmful to many organs of the body.

GAUCHER'S DISEASE

Gaucher's disease is a hereditary disorder that leads to an accumulation of glucocerebrosides, a product of fat metabolism.

The genetic abnormality that causes Gaucher's disease is recessive; an affected person must inherit two abnormal genes to develop symptoms. This disease leads to enlargement of the liver and spleen and a brownish pigmentation of the skin. Accumulations of glucocerebrosides in the eyes cause yellow spots called pingueculae to appear. Accumulations in the bone marrow can cause pain.

Most people who have Gaucher's disease develop type 1, the adult chronic form, which results in an enlarged liver and spleen and bone abnormalities. Type 2, the infantile form, develops in infancy; infants with the disease have an enlarged spleen and severe nervous system abnormalities. Their neck and back may become rigidly arched because of muscle spasms. These infants usually die within a year. Type 3, the juvenile form, can begin at any time during childhood. Children with

the disease have an enlarged liver and spleen, bone abnormalities, and slowly progressive nervous system abnormalities. Children who survive to adolescence may live for many years.

Bone abnormalities may cause pain and swelling in the joints. Severely affected people may also develop anemia and an inability to produce white blood cells and platelets, resulting in pallor, weakness, susceptibility to infection, and excessive bleeding. When a doctor finds an enlarged liver or anemia and suspects Gaucher's disease, he usually performs a liver or bone marrow biopsy to confirm the diagnosis. A fetus can be diagnosed before birth by testing cells obtained by chorionic villus sampling or amniocentesis.▲

Many people with Gaucher's disease can be treated with enzyme replacement therapy, an expensive treatment in which enzymes are given intravenously, usually every 2 weeks. Enzyme replacement therapy is most effective for people who don't have nervous system complications. Blood transfusions may help relieve the anemia. The spleen may be surgically removed to treat anemia, low white blood cell counts, or low platelet counts or to relieve the discomfort of an enlarged spleen.

NIEMANN-PICK DISEASE

Niemann-Pick disease is a hereditary disorder in which the deficiency of a specific enzyme results in the accumulation of sphingomyelin (a product of fat metabolism) or there is an abnormal accumulation of cholesterol.

The gene responsible for Niemann-Pick disease is recessive, which means that a child with the disease has inherited a defective gene from both parents. The enzyme-deficiency type is most common in Jewish families.

Niemann-Pick disease has several forms, depending on the severity of the enzyme deficiency or of the cholesterol accumulation. In the severe juvenile form with enzyme deficiency, the enzyme is totally absent. Severe nervous system abnormalities develop because nerves can't use the sphingomyelin to produce myelin needed for the myelin sheath that normally surrounds many nerves.■ Children with the disease develop fatty

---

▲ see page 1134

■ see box, page 319

growths in the skin, areas of dark pigmentation, and an enlarged liver, spleen, and lymph nodes; they may be mentally retarded. These children commonly have anemia and low numbers of white blood cells and platelets, making them susceptible to infection and easy bruising.

Some forms of Niemann-Pick disease can be diagnosed in the fetus by chorionic villus sampling or amniocentesis. After birth, the diagnosis can be made by biopsy of the liver (a piece of liver tissue is removed and examined under a microscope). Niemann-Pick disease can't be cured, and children tend to die of infection or progressive dysfunction of the central nervous system.

FABRY'S DISEASE

Fabry's disease is a rare hereditary disorder that leads to an accumulation of glycolipid, a product of fat metabolism.

Because the defective gene is carried on the X chromosome, the full-blown disease occurs only in males, who have just one X chromosome. The accumulation of glycolipid causes angiokeratomas, noncancerous skin growths, to form over the lower part of the trunk. The corneas become cloudy, resulting in poor vision. A burning pain may develop in the arms and legs, and the person may have episodes of fever. Death typically is caused by kidney failure, heart disease, or stroke, any of which may result from high blood pressure.

Fabry's disease can be diagnosed in the fetus by chorionic villus sampling or amniocentesis. Treatment consists of taking analgesics to help relieve pain and fever. The disease can't be cured, but researchers are investigating a treatment in which the deficient enzyme is replaced by transfusion.

WOLMAN'S DISEASE

Wolman's disease is a hereditary disorder that results when specific types of cholesterol and glycerides accumulate in tissues.

This disease causes enlargement of the spleen and liver. Calcium deposits in the adrenal glands cause them to harden, and fatty diarrhea (steat-

---

▲ see box, page 741

orrhea) also occurs. Infants with Wolman's disease usually die by 6 months of age.

CEREBROTENDINOUS XANTHOMATOSIS

Cerebrotendinous xanthomatosis is a rare hereditary disease caused when cholestanol, a product of cholesterol metabolism, accumulates in tissues.

This disease eventually leads to uncoordinated movements, dementia, cataracts, and fatty growths (xanthomas) on tendons. The disabling symptoms often don't appear until a person is over 30. If started early, the drug chenodiol helps prevent progression of the disease, but it can't undo any damage already done.

SITOSTEROLEMIA

Sitosterolemia is a rare hereditary disease in which fats from fruits and vegetables accumulate in blood and tissues.

The buildup of fats leads to atherosclerosis, abnormal red blood cells, and fatty deposits on tendons (xanthomas). Treatment consists of reducing the intake of foods such as vegetable oils that are rich in plant fats and taking cholestyramine resin.

REFSUM'S DISEASE

Refsum's disease is a rare hereditary disorder in which phytanic acid, a product of fat metabolism, accumulates in tissues.

A buildup of phytanic acid leads to nerve and retinal damage, spastic movements, and changes in the bone and skin. Treatment involves avoiding eating green fruits and vegetables that contain chlorophyll. Plasmapheresis, in which phytanic acid is removed from the blood, may be helpful.▲

TAY-SACHS DISEASE

Tay-Sachs disease is a hereditary disorder in which gangliosides, products of fat metabolism, accumulate in tissues.

The disease is most common in families of Eastern European Jewish origin. At a very early age, children with this disease become progressively retarded and develop paralysis, dementia, blindness, and cherry-red spots in the retina. These children usually die by age 3 or 4. Tay-Sachs disease can be identified in the fetus by chorionic villus sampling or amniocentesis. It can't be treated or cured.

Obesity

Obesity is the accumulation of excessive body fat.

Except for those who are extremely muscular, people whose weight is 20 percent or more over the midpoint of their weight range on a standard height-weight table ▲ are considered obese. Obesity may be classified as mild (20 to 40 percent overweight), moderate (41 to 100 percent overweight), or severe (more than 100 percent overweight). Obesity is severe in only 0.5 percent of obese people.

Obesity in Adulthood

The prevalence of obesity in the United States is increasing—up 33 percent in the past decade alone. Overall, 31 percent of men and 35 percent of women are obese, but prevalence varies by age and race. Obesity is twice as common among older people as among younger people. The prevalence of obesity is about the same among black and white men, slightly higher among Hispanic men than among black and white men, and much higher among black and Hispanic women than among white women. For example, about 60 percent of middle-aged black women are obese compared with 33 percent of white women.

Causes

Obesity results from consuming more calories than the body uses. Genetic and environmental factors influence body weight, but precisely how they interact to determine a person's weight is still unclear. One proposed explanation is that body weight is regulated around a set point, similar to a thermostat setting. A higher-than-normal set point may explain why some people are obese and why losing weight and maintaining weight loss are difficult for them.

Genetic Factors: Recent research suggests that on the average, the genetic influence contributes to about 33 percent of body weight, but the contribution may be more or less in a particular person.

Socioeconomic Factors: Such factors strongly influence obesity, especially among women. In the United States, obesity is more than twice as common among women in lower socioeconomic groups as among women in higher ones. Why socioeconomic factors have such a strong influence on women's weight is not fully understood, but sanctions against obesity do increase with increasing social status. Women in higher socioeconomic groups have more time and resources for the dieting and exercise that enable them to conform to these social demands.

Psychologic Factors: Emotional disturbances, once considered an important cause of obesity, are now considered a reaction to the strong prejudice and discrimination against obese people. One type of emotional disturbance, a negative body image, is a serious problem for many young obese women. It leads to extreme self-consciousness and discomfort in social situations.

Two abnormal eating patterns that contribute to obesity in some people, binge eating disorder ■ and the night-eating syndrome, may be triggered by stress and emotional upset. Binge eating disorder is similar to bulimia nervosa except that the binges are not followed by self-induced vomiting. As a result, more calories are consumed. In the night-eating syndrome, a lack of appetite in the morning is followed by overeating, agitation, and insomnia in the evening.

Developmental Factors: An increase in the size or number of fat cells or both adds to the amount of fat stored in the body. Obese people, particularly those who became obese during childhood, may have up to five times more fat cells than people of normal weight. Because the number of cells can't be reduced, weight can be lost only by reducing the amount of fat in each cell.

Physical Activity: Reduced physical activity is probably one of the main reasons for the increase in obesity among people in affluent societies. In the United States, obesity is more than twice as common today as it was in 1900, even though the average number of calories consumed daily has

---

▲ see box, page 647

■ see page 417

decreased by 10 percent. Sedentary people need fewer calories. Increasing physical activity causes people of normal weight to eat more but may not cause obese people to eat more.

Hormones: Rarely, hormonal disorders cause obesity.

Brain Damage: Rarely, damage to the brain, particularly to the hypothalamus, can result in obesity.

Drugs: A number of commonly used drugs cause weight gain. They include corticosteroids such as prednisone and many antidepressants, as well as most other drugs used to treat psychiatric disorders.

Symptoms

Accumulation of excess fat below the diaphragm and in the chest wall may put pressure on the lungs, causing difficulty in breathing and shortness of breath, even with minimal exertion. The difficulty in breathing may seriously interfere with sleep, causing momentary cessation of breathing (sleep apnea), leading to daytime sleepiness and other complications.▲

Obesity may cause various orthopedic problems, including low back pain and worsening of osteoarthritis, particularly in the hips, knees, and ankles. Skin disorders are particularly common. Because obese people have relatively little body surface for their weight, they can't get rid of body heat efficiently and they sweat more than thinner people. Swelling of the feet and ankles, caused by accumulation of a small to moderate amount of fluid (edema), also is common.

Complications

Obese people have an increased risk of becoming ill or dying of most diseases, of injuries, and in accidents, and this risk further increases with increasing obesity. Risk is also affected by the location of excess fat. Fat tends to accumulate in the abdomen (abdominal obesity) of men and in the thighs and buttocks (lower-body obesity) of women. Abdominal obesity has been linked with a much higher risk of coronary artery disease and

with three of its major risk factors: high blood pressure, diabetes that starts in adulthood, and high levels of fats (lipids) in the blood. Why abdominal obesity increases these risks isn't known, but losing weight dramatically reduces them in people who have abdominal obesity. Losing weight lowers blood pressure in most people who have high blood pressure and allows over half the people who develop diabetes as adults to discontinue insulin or other drug treatment.

Certain cancers are more common in people who are obese than in those who aren't; they include cancer of the breast, uterus, and ovaries in women and cancer of the colon, rectum, and prostate in men. Menstrual disorders are also more common and gallbladder disease occurs three times more often in the obese.

Diagnosis and Treatment

Although obesity is self-evident, its extent is determined by measuring height and weight. Often, these measurements are converted to body mass index—the weight (in kilograms) divided by height (in meters squared). A value higher than 27 indicates mild obesity, and a value of 30 or higher indicates the need for treatment.

Paradoxically, women who have lower-body obesity, which has a far lower risk of health problems, seek treatment for obesity eight times more often than men. Untreated obesity tends to worsen, but the long-term effects of treatment are disappointing. Although considerable progress has been made in helping people lose weight, they usually regain it within 3 years. Concerns about whether regaining weight, called weight cycling, causes various health problems are unfounded, so such concerns should not prevent obese people from trying to lose weight.

To lose weight, obese people must consume fewer calories than they expend. Methods used to achieve this goal can be categorized into three groups: self-help, in which people, either on their own or in groups of like-minded people, use information from books or other sources; nonclinical programs provided by counselors who are not licensed health care practitioners; and clinical programs provided by licensed health care practitioners.

Most weight management programs are based on behavior modification. Dieting is usually considered less important than making permanent changes in eating and exercise habits. Reputable

---

▲ see page 304

programs teach people how to make safe, sensible, gradual changes in eating habits that increase the consumption of complex carbohydrates (fruits, vegetables, breads, and pasta) and decrease the consumption of fat. For mildly obese people, only a modest restriction of calories and dietary fat is recommended.

Programs that rely on very low calorie diets of 800 or even fewer calories per day have been developed for moderately obese people who want to lose weight more quickly. These diets are safe when medically supervised. However, enthusiasm for them has declined because they are expensive and people tend to regain weight after going off the diet.

Increasingly, doctors are prescribing drugs to reduce body weight. Generally, such a drug reduces weight by about 10 percent within 6 months and maintains the loss as long as the drug is continued. When it's discontinued, the weight is promptly regained.

The many serious complications of severe obesity (more than 100 percent overweight) make treatment important, and surgery is becoming the treatment of choice. Surgery, usually to reduce stomach size and therefore the amount of food that can be eaten at one time, can result in large weight losses, which commonly equal about half the person's excess weight, usually 80 to 150 pounds. Weight loss is rapid at first, then slows gradually over 2 years, and is often maintained. The loss usually relieves complications and improves the person's mood, self-esteem, body image, activity level, and ability to work and to relate to other people.

Surgery should be reserved for severely obese people and performed only within programs that specialize in this type of surgery and have demonstrated records of safety and efficacy. Within these programs, surgery is usually well tolerated: Less than 10 percent of these high-risk patients develop complications from surgery, and one percent or less die.

Obesity in Adolescence

The factors that influence obesity in adolescents are the same as those in adults. Often, a mildly obese adolescent gains weight rapidly and becomes substantially obese within a few years. Many obese adolescents have a poor self-image and become increasingly sedentary and socially isolated. Their parents often don't know how to help them.

Not many treatment choices for obese adolescents are available. Few commercial programs are designed for them, few doctors have experience in treating them, and experience with using drugs to help them is limited. Schools provide opportunities for education in nutrition and for physical activity, but these programs rarely do enough to enable adolescents to control obesity. Surgery is sometimes performed when obesity is severe.

Behavior modification can help adolescents control obesity. It consists of reducing caloric intake by establishing a well-balanced diet of ordinary foods, making permanent changes in eating habits, and increasing physical activity—such as walking, biking, swimming, and dancing. Summer camps for obese adolescents usually help them lose a significant amount of weight, but without continuing effort, the weight is usually regained. Counseling to help adolescents cope with their problems and poor self-esteem may be helpful.

CHAPTER 141

Porphyrias

Porphyrias are a group of disorders caused by deficiencies of enzymes involved in the synthesis of heme.

Heme, a chemical compound that carries oxygen and makes blood red, is a key component of hemoproteins, a type of protein found in all tissues. The largest amount of heme is synthesized in the bone marrow for manufacturing hemoglobin. The liver also produces large amounts of heme, and most is used as a component of cytochromes. Some cytochromes in the liver oxidize foreign chemicals, including drugs, so that they are more easily removed from the body.

Eight different enzymes drive the sequential steps in heme synthesis. When an enzyme in the pathway of heme production is deficient, chemical precursors of heme may accumulate in tissues (especially in the bone marrow or liver). These precursors, which include delta-aminolevulinic acid, porphobilinogen, and porphyrins, then appear in the blood and are excreted in the urine or stool.

Excess porphyrins cause photosensitivity, in which a person is overly sensitive to sunlight. This occurs because when exposed to light and oxygen, porphyrins generate a charged, unstable form of oxygen that can damage the skin. Nerve damage, leading to pain and even paralysis, occurs in some porphyrias, especially when delta-aminolevulinic acid and porphobilinogen accumulate.

The three most common porphyrias are porphyria cutanea tarda, acute intermittent porphyria, and erythropoietic protoporphyria. These disorders are very distinct. Their symptoms differ considerably, different tests are required for diagnosis, and different treatments are involved. Some features are shared with the other, less common porphyrias, which include delta-aminolevulinic acid dehydratase deficiency, congenital erythropoietic porphyria, hepatoerythropoietic porphyria, hereditary coproporphyria, and variegate porphyria.

All porphyrias except porphyria cutanea tarda are hereditary. All people with a particular hereditary porphyria have a deficiency of the same enzyme. However, unless they come from the same family, they are likely to have different mutations in the gene for that enzyme.

Porphyrias can be classified in several ways. Classification according to the specific enzyme deficiency is preferred. Another classification system distinguishes acute porphyrias, which cause neurologic symptoms, from cutaneous porphyrias, which cause skin photosensitivity. A third classification system is based on whether the excess precursors originate primarily in the liver, in which case the porphyria is hepatic, or primarily in the bone marrow, in which case the porphyria is erythropoietic.

A person who has symptoms of porphyria will have markedly abnormal laboratory test results.

But the tests must be properly selected and interpreted to confirm or exclude the presence of porphyria. In most cases, doctors measure the levels of delta-aminolevulinic acid and porphobilinogen in urine when they suspect an acute porphyria, and they measure the levels of porphyrin in the blood plasma when they suspect a cutaneous porphyria. Other tests, including red blood cell enzyme measurements, may be performed when the results of one of these screening tests are abnormal.

Porphyria Cutanea Tarda

Porphyria cutanea tarda, the most common form of porphyria, causes blistering of skin exposed to sunlight.

Porphyria cutanea tarda occurs throughout the world and is the only porphyria that isn't hereditary. This disorder, a hepatic porphyria, results when uroporphyrinogen decarboxylase, one of the enzymes in the liver necessary for heme synthesis, becomes inactivated. Contributing factors include iron, alcohol, estrogens, and infection with hepatitis C virus. Less commonly, porphyria cutanea tarda occurs in people infected with the human immunodeficiency virus (HIV). Although the disorder isn't hereditary, sometimes a partial deficiency of the uroporphyrinogen decarboxylase enzyme inherited from one parent makes a person susceptible to developing the disorder. In such cases, it is termed familial porphyria cutanea tarda.

Symptoms

Blisters occur on sun-exposed areas such as the backs of the hands, arms, and face. The skin, especially on the hands, is also sensitive to minor trauma. Crusting and scarring follow the blisters and take a long time to heal. Skin damage occurs because porphyrins produced in the liver are transported by the blood plasma to the skin. Hair growth on the face may increase. The liver is usually somewhat damaged, at times partly because of an infection with hepatitis C virus or the excessive use of alcohol. Cirrhosis of the liver and even liver cancer can develop over a long period of time.

Diagnosis

To diagnose porphyria cutanea tarda, a doctor tests the blood plasma, urine, and stool for porphyrins. Any porphyria that causes skin lesions is accompanied by a high level of porphyrins in the blood plasma. In porphyria cutanea tarda, the levels of porphyrins are also increased in the urine and stool.

Treatment

Porphyria cutanea tarda is the most readily treated porphyria. A procedure called a phlebotomy, in which a pint of blood is removed every 1 to 2 weeks, is most widely recommended. This makes the patient slightly iron deficient. The levels of porphyrins in the liver and blood plasma fall gradually, and the skin improves and eventually becomes completely normal. Usually only five to six phlebotomies are needed; anemia develops if too many are performed. Additional phlebotomies are needed only if the disorder recurs.

Taking very low doses of chloroquine or hydroxychloroquine is also effective. These drugs remove excess porphyrins from the liver. However, doses that are too high (even doses conventionally used in the treatment of other diseases) cause porphyrins to be removed too rapidly, resulting in a temporary worsening of the porphyria cutanea tarda and damage to the liver. Avoiding alcohol is also beneficial.

Acute Intermittent Porphyria

Acute intermittent porphyria, which causes neurologic symptoms, is the most common acute porphyria.

Acute intermittent porphyria, a hepatic porphyria, is caused by a deficiency of the enzyme porphobilinogen deaminase, also known as hydroxymethylbilane synthase. The enzyme deficiency is inherited from one parent, but most of those who inherit the trait never develop symptoms. Acute intermittent porphyria occurs in people of all races but is somewhat more common in Northern Europeans.

Other factors—drugs, hormones, or diet—are needed to activate the disorder and produce symptoms. Many drugs, including barbiturates, antiseizure drugs, and sulfonamide antibiotics, can bring on an attack. Hormones, such as progesterone and related steroids, can precipitate symptoms, as can low-calorie and low-carbohydrate diets or large amounts of alcohol. Stress as the result of an infection, another illness, surgery,

or a psychologic upset is also sometimes implicated. Usually a combination of factors is involved. Sometimes the factors that cause an attack can't be identified.

Symptoms

Symptoms occur in attacks lasting several days or longer. Attacks appear after puberty and are more common in women than in men. In some women, attacks develop during the second half of the menstrual cycle. Abdominal pain is the most common symptom. The pain can be so severe that the doctor may mistakenly think that abdominal surgery is needed. Gastrointestinal symptoms include nausea, vomiting, constipation or diarrhea, and abdominal bloating. The bladder may be affected, making urination difficult. A rapid heart rate, high blood pressure, sweating, and restlessness are also common during an attack.

All of these symptoms, including the gastrointestinal ones, result from effects on the nervous system. Nerves that control muscles can be damaged, leading to weakness, usually beginning in the shoulders and arms. The weakness can progress to virtually all the muscles, including those involved in breathing. Tremors and seizures may develop. High blood pressure can continue after the attack. Recovery may occur within a few days, although complete recovery from severe muscle weakness may take several months or years.

Diagnosis

The severe gastrointestinal and neurologic symptoms resemble those of many more common conditions. However, laboratory tests to measure the levels of two precursors of heme (delta-aminolevulinic acid and porphobilinogen) in the urine enable a doctor to make the diagnosis of acute intermittent porphyria. Levels of these precursors are very high during attacks of acute intermittent porphyria and remain high in people who have repeated attacks. The precursors can form porphyrins, which are reddish in color, and other substances that are brownish. Therefore, the urine may be discolored, especially after standing in light. Such changes in urine color may lead a doctor to suspect porphyria.

Treatment and Prevention

Severe attacks of acute intermittent porphyria are treated with heme, which must be given intravenously. Heme is available as hematin in the United States. Another product, heme arginate, has fewer side effects but is still investigational. Heme is taken up in the liver, where it compensates for the reduced synthesis of heme. Blood and urine levels of delta-aminolevulinic acid and porphobilinogen are promptly lowered and symptoms improve, usually within several days. If treatment is delayed, recovery takes longer and some nerve damage may be permanent.

Glucose given intravenously or a diet high in carbohydrates can also be beneficial, but these measures are less effective than heme. Pain can be controlled with drugs until the person responds to heme or glucose. The doctor will stop the person from taking any harmful drugs and, if possible, address other factors that may have contributed to the attack.

Attacks of acute intermittent porphyria can be prevented by maintaining good nutrition and avoiding the drugs that can provoke them. Crash diets to lose weight rapidly should be avoided. Heme can be used to prevent attacks, but there is no standard regimen. Premenstrual attacks in women can be prevented with one of the gonadotropin-releasing hormone analogues that are used to treat endometriosis, although this treatment is still investigational.

Erythropoietic Protoporphyria

Erythropoietic protoporphyria, in which protoporphyrin builds up in the bone marrow, red blood cells, and blood plasma, causes photosensitivity of the skin.

In this hereditary porphyria, the enzyme ferrochelatase is deficient. The enzyme deficiency, which is inherited from one parent, causes protoporphyrin to accumulate in the bone marrow and blood. Excess protoporphyrin passes through the liver into the bile and is eventually excreted in the stool.

Symptoms and Diagnosis

Symptoms usually start in childhood. Pain and swelling develop soon after the skin is exposed to sunlight. Because blistering and scarring are unusual, doctors don't always recognize the disease. Diagnosis is also difficult because protoporphyrin is very insoluble and isn't excreted in the urine. The diagnosis is therefore made when increased levels of protoporphyrin are detected in the plasma and red blood cells.

For unknown reasons, the severity of erythropoietic protoporphyria varies considerably from one person to another, even within a family. One person may be significantly affected by the disease, whereas a close relative with the same gene mutation may have little or no increase in porphyrins and no symptoms.

Treatment

Sunlight must be avoided. Beta-carotene, when taken in sufficient amounts to cause slight yellowing of the skin, is especially effective, as it makes many people more tolerant of sunlight. People with erythropoietic protoporphyria can develop gallstones that contain protoporphyrin; the gallstones may need to be surgically removed. A more severe complication is liver damage, which sometimes necessitates liver transplantation.

CHAPTER 142

Amyloidosis

Amyloidosis is a disease in which amyloid, an unusual protein that normally isn't present in the body, accumulates in various tissues.

Many forms of amyloidosis exist. In primary amyloidosis, the cause isn't known. However, the disease is associated with abnormalities of plasma cells, as is multiple myeloma, which may also be associated with amyloidosis. In second-

ary amyloidosis, the amyloidosis is secondary to another disease such as tuberculosis, infections of the bone, rheumatoid arthritis, familial Mediterranean fever, or granulomatous ileitis. A third form, hereditary amyloidosis, affects nerves and certain organs; it has been noted in people from Portugal, Sweden, Japan, and many other countries.

Another form of amyloidosis is associated with normal aging and particularly affects the heart. What causes amyloid to build up excessively usually isn't known. However, amyloidosis can be a response to various diseases that cause persistent infection or inflammation. Yet another form of amyloidosis is associated with Alzheimer's disease.

Symptoms

The accumulation of large amounts of amyloid can disturb the normal functioning of many organs. The symptoms of amyloidosis depend on where the amyloid builds up. Many people have few symptoms, while others develop severe, life-threatening disease.

In **primary amyloidosis,** typical sites of amyloid buildup are the heart, lungs, skin, tongue, thyroid gland, intestines, liver, kidney, and blood vessels. This accumulation can lead to heart failure, an irregular heartbeat, difficulty in breathing, a thickened tongue, an underactive thyroid gland, poor absorption of food, liver failure, kidney failure, and easy bruising or other abnormal bleeding because of its effect on blood clotting. Nerves may malfunction, leading to weakness and abnormal sensations. Carpal tunnel syndrome may develop. When amyloid affects the heart, death may occur as a result of severe heart failure or an irregular heartbeat.

In **secondary amyloidosis,** amyloid tends to build up in the spleen, liver, kidneys, adrenal glands, and lymph nodes. The spleen and liver tend to enlarge and to feel firm and rubbery to the doctor who examines them. Other organs and the blood vessels may also be affected, although the heart is rarely involved.

Diagnosis

Amyloidosis is sometimes difficult for doctors to recognize because it produces so many different problems. However, they may suspect amyloidosis when several organs fail or when a person bleeds easily for no apparent reason. The hereditary form is suspected when an inherited peripheral nerve disorder is discovered in a family.

The diagnosis is generally made by testing a small amount of abdominal fat obtained through a needle inserted near the navel. Alternatively, the doctor can take a sample of tissue for biopsy from the skin, rectum, gums, kidney, or liver. The amyloid shows up under the microscope with the use of special stains.

Treatment

Amyloidosis doesn't always require treatment. When amyloidosis is caused by another disease, treating the other disease usually slows or reverses the amyloidosis. However, amyloidosis caused by multiple myeloma has a bleak prognosis; most people who have both diseases die within 1 to 2 years.

Treatment for amyloidosis hasn't been very successful. People may find relief by taking prednisone and melphalan, sometimes with colchicine. Colchicine alone may help relieve amyloidosis that's triggered by familial Mediterranean fever. Accumulations of amyloid (amyloid tumors) in a specific area of the body can sometimes be removed surgically.

A person whose kidneys have been destroyed by amyloidosis may receive a kidney transplant. Someone with heart problems may receive a heart transplant. However, the transplanted organs may later become affected by the buildup of amyloid. In the hereditary form, the amyloid-producing defect occurs in the liver; therefore, a few people have had successful liver transplants to stop the disease's progression.

Hormonal Disorders

CHAPTER 143

Endocrine System and Hormones

The endocrine system consists of a group of organs (sometimes referred to as glands of internal secretion) whose main function is to produce and secrete hormones directly into the bloodstream. Hormones serve as messengers to coordinate activities of various parts of the body.

Endocrine Glands

The major organs of the endocrine system are the hypothalamus, the pituitary gland, the thyroid gland, the parathyroid glands, the islets of the pancreas, the adrenal glands, the testes, and the ovaries. During pregnancy, the placenta also acts as an endocrine gland in addition to its other functions.

The hypothalamus secretes several hormones that stimulate the pituitary: Some trigger the release of pituitary hormones; others suppress the release of pituitary hormones.

The pituitary gland is sometimes called the master gland because it coordinates many functions of the other endocrine glands.▲ Some pituitary hormones have direct effects; others simply control the rate at which other endocrine organs secrete their hormones. The pituitary controls the rate at which it secretes its own hormones through a feedback loop in which the blood levels of other endocrine hormones signal the pituitary

---

▲ see box, page 697

Major Endocrine Glands

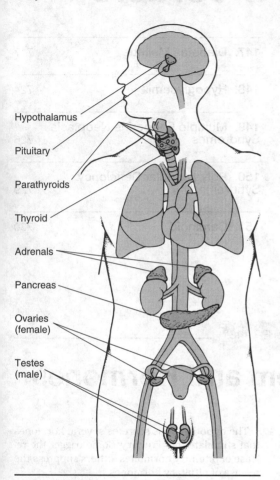

Hypothalamus

Pituitary

Parathyroids

Thyroid

Adrenals

Pancreas

Ovaries
(female)

Testes
(male)

of the endocrine system. Some of these organs produce substances that act only in the immediate vicinity of their release, while others don't secrete their products into the bloodstream. For example, the brain produces many hormones whose effects are confined mainly to the nervous system.

Hormones

Hormones are substances released into the bloodstream from a gland or organ that affect activity in cells at another site. Most hormones are proteins composed of amino acid chains of varying length. Others are steroids, fatty substances derived from cholesterol. Very small amounts of hormones can trigger very large responses in the body.

Hormones bind to receptors on a cell's surface or inside a cell. The binding of a hormone to a receptor speeds up, slows down, or in some other way alters the cell's function. Ultimately, hormones control the function of entire organs. They control growth and development, reproduction, and sexual characteristics. They influence the way the body uses and stores energy. Hormones also control the volume of fluid and the levels of salt and sugar in the blood. Some hormones affect only one or two organs, while others affect the whole body. For example, thyroid-stimulating hormone is produced in the pituitary gland and affects only the thyroid gland. In contrast, thyroid hormone is produced in the thyroid gland, but it affects cells throughout the body. Insulin, produced by the islet cells of the pancreas, affects the metabolism of glucose, protein, and fat throughout the body.

Endocrine Controls

When endocrine glands malfunction, hormone levels in the blood can become abnormally high or low, disrupting body functions. To control endocrine functions, the secretion of each hormone must be regulated within precise limits. The body needs to sense from moment to moment whether more or less of a given hormone is needed.

The hypothalamus and pituitary glands secrete their hormones when they sense that the blood level of another hormone that they control is too high or too low. Pituitary hormones then travel through the bloodstream to stimulate activity in their target glands. When the target hormone's

to slow down or speed up. Not all endocrine glands are under the pituitary's control; some respond directly or indirectly to concentrations of substances in the blood:
• The insulin-secreting cells of the pancreas respond to glucose and fatty acids.
• Parathyroid cells respond to calcium and phosphate.
• The adrenal medulla (part of the adrenal gland) responds to direct stimulation by the parasympathetic nervous system.

Many organs secrete hormones or hormonelike substances but aren't generally considered part

Major Hormones

Hormone	Where It Is Produced	Function
Aldosterone	Adrenal glands	Helps regulate salt and water balance by retaining salt and water and excreting potassium
Antidiuretic hormone (vasopressin)	Pituitary gland	Causes kidneys to retain water and, along with aldosterone, helps control blood pressure
Corticosteroid	Adrenal glands	Has widespread effects throughout the body; especially has anti-inflammatory action; maintains blood sugar level, blood pressure, and muscle strength; helps control salt and water balance
Corticotropin	Pituitary gland	Controls the production and secretion of hormones by the adrenal cortex
Erythropoietin	Kidneys	Stimulates red blood cell production
Estrogen	Ovaries	Controls the development of female sex characteristics and the reproductive system
Glucagon	Pancreas	Raises the blood sugar level
Growth hormone	Pituitary gland	Controls growth and development; promotes protein production
Insulin	Pancreas	Lowers the blood sugar level; affects the metabolism of glucose, protein, and fat throughout the body
Luteinizing hormone and follicle-stimulating hormone	Pituitary gland	Control reproductive functions, including the production of sperm and semen, egg maturation, and menstrual cycles; control male and female sexual characteristics (including hair distribution, muscle formation, skin texture and thickness, voice, and perhaps even personality traits)
Oxytocin	Pituitary gland	Causes muscles of the uterus and milk ducts in the breast to contract
Parathyroid hormone	Parathyroid glands	Controls bone formation and the excretion of calcium and phosphorus
Progesterone	Ovaries	Prepares the lining of the uterus for implantation of a fertilized egg and readies the mammary glands to secrete milk
Prolactin	Pituitary gland	Starts and maintains milk production in the mammary glands
Renin and angiotensin	Kidneys	Control blood pressure
Thyroid hormone	Thyroid gland	Regulates growth, maturation, and the speed of metabolism
Thyroid-stimulating hormone	Pituitary gland	Stimulates the production and secretion of hormones by the thyroid gland

The Function of Messengers

Although all cells respond to and most cells produce messengers, their effects are usually grouped into three major systems— the nervous, immune, and endocrine systems—essential for coordinating the body's activities. These three systems have much in common and cooperate closely. Their messengers are made up of proteins or derivatives of fat. Some messengers travel only a fraction of an inch; others travel a considerable distance through the bloodstream to reach their target.

The messengers attach themselves to their target cells using specific receptor proteins located either on the cell surface or within the cell. Some messengers alter the permeability of cell membranes to specific substances; for example, insulin alters the transport of glucose across cell membranes. Other messengers, such as epinephrine and glucagon, modify the activity of their receptors, causing them to produce other substances that act as second messengers. They affect the activity of the cell's genetic material, altering the cell's production of proteins or the activity of proteins already in the cell.

The effect of a given messenger depends on where it's secreted. For example, norepinephrine raises the blood pressure when the adrenal gland secretes it into the blood, but when norepinephrine is released within the nervous system, it stimulates the activity of only nearby nerve cells without affecting the blood pressure.

level in the blood is appropriate, the hypothalamus and pituitary gland recognize that no further stimulation is needed and they stop secreting hormones. This feedback system regulates all glands under pituitary control.

Certain hormones under pituitary control vary according to schedules. For example, a woman's menstrual cycle involves monthly fluctuations in the pituitary gland's secretion of luteinizing hormone and follicle-stimulating hormone. The ovarian hormones estrogen and progesterone also fluctuate monthly. Exactly how the hypothalamus and pituitary control these biorhythms isn't understood. However, the organs clearly respond to some sort of biologic clock.

Other factors also stimulate hormone production. Prolactin, a hormone secreted by the pituitary gland, causes milk glands in the breast to produce milk. A baby sucking on the nipple stimulates the pituitary gland to secrete more prolactin. The sucking also increases the secretion of oxytocin, which causes the milk ducts to contract, moving milk to the nipple for the hungry baby.

Glands such as the islets of the pancreas and the parathyroid glands, which aren't under pituitary control, have their own systems for sensing whether more or less hormone secretion is needed. For example, insulin levels increase shortly after eating because the body needs to process the sugars from the food. However, if insulin levels were to remain high, then blood sugar levels would fall dangerously low.

Other hormone levels vary for less obvious reasons. Corticosteroid and growth hormone levels are highest in the morning and lowest in midafternoon. Reasons for these daily variations aren't fully understood.

CHAPTER 144

Pituitary Gland Disorders

The pituitary is a pea-sized gland that sits in a bony structure (sella turcica) at the base of the brain. The sella turcica protects the pituitary but allows very little room for expansion. If the pituitary enlarges, it tends to push upward, often

pressing on the areas of the brain that carry signals from the eyes, possibly resulting in headaches or impaired vision.

The pituitary controls the function of most other endocrine glands and is, in turn, controlled

Pituitary: The Master Gland

The pituitary, a pea-sized gland at the base of the brain, produces a number of hormones, each of which affects a specific part of the body (a target organ). Because the pituitary controls the function of most other endocrine glands, it's often called the master gland.

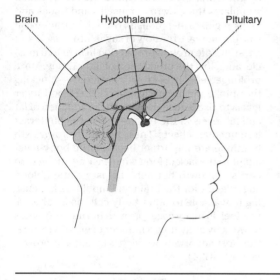

Brain   Hypothalamus   Pituitary

Hormone	Target Organ
Antidiuretic hormone	Kidney
Beta-melanocyte–stimulating hormone	Skin
Corticotropin	Adrenal glands
Endorphins	Brain
Enkephalins	Brain
Follicle-stimulating hormone	Ovaries or testes
Growth hormone	Muscles and bones
Luteinizing hormone	Ovaries or testes
Oxytocin	Uterus and mammary glands
Prolactin	Mammary glands
Thyroid-stimulating hormone	Thyroid gland

by the hypothalamus, a region of the brain that lies just above the pituitary. The pituitary gland has two distinct parts: the anterior (front) and the posterior (back) lobes. The hypothalamus controls the anterior lobe (adenohypophysis) by releasing factors, or hormonelike substances, through blood vessels that directly connect the two; it controls the posterior lobe (neurohypophysis) through nerve impulses.

The anterior lobe produces (secretes) hormones that ultimately control the function of the thyroid gland, adrenal glands, and reproductive organs (ovaries and testes); milk production (lactation) in the breasts; and overall body growth. It also produces hormones that cause the skin to darken and that inhibit pain sensations. The posterior lobe produces hormones that regulate water balance, stimulate the let-down of milk from the breasts in lactating women, and stimulate contractions of the uterus.

By detecting the levels of hormones produced by glands under the pituitary's control (target glands), the hypothalamus or the pituitary can determine how much stimulation or suppression the pituitary needs to adjust its target glands' activity.▲ The hormones produced by the pituitary (and the hypothalamus) are not all secreted continuously. Most are released in bursts every 1 to 3 hours with alternating periods of activity and inactivity. Some of the hormones—such as corticotropin, which controls the adrenal glands; growth hormone, which controls growth; and prolactin, which controls milk production—follow a circadian rhythm: The levels rise and fall predictably during the day, usually peaking just before awakening and dropping to their lowest levels

▲ see page 694

just before sleep. The levels of other hormones vary according to other factors. For example, in women, the levels of luteinizing hormone and follicle-stimulating hormone, which control reproductive functions, vary during the menstrual cycle.▲ Oversecretion or undersecretion of one or more of the pituitary hormones results in a wide variety of symptoms.

Anterior Pituitary Function

The anterior lobe of the pituitary gland accounts for 80 percent of the gland's weight. It releases hormones that either regulate normal growth and physical development or stimulate the activity of the adrenal glands, the thyroid gland, and the ovaries or testes. When the anterior lobe secretes too much or too little of its hormones, the other endocrine glands also overproduce or underproduce their hormones.

One of the hormones secreted by the anterior lobe is **corticotropin** (adrenocorticotropic hormone or ACTH), which stimulates the adrenal glands to secrete cortisol, the life-sustaining cortisonelike hormone, and several testosteronelike (androgenic) steroids. Without corticotropin, the adrenal glands shrink (atrophy) and stop secreting cortisol, which results in failure of the adrenal glands.■ Several other hormones are produced simultaneously with corticotropin. They include **beta-melanocyte–stimulating hormone,** which controls skin pigmentation, and **enkephalins** and **endorphins,** which control pain perception, mood, and alertness.

Thyroid-stimulating hormone, also produced by the anterior lobe, stimulates the thyroid gland to produce thyroid hormones.★ Very rarely, too much thyroid-stimulating hormone causes the thyroid to overproduce thyroid hormone, resulting in hyperthyroidism; too little causes the thyroid gland to underproduce thyroid hormone, resulting in hypothyroidism.

Two other hormones produced by the anterior lobe—**luteinizing hormone** and **follicle-stimulating**

▲ see page 1075

■ see page 712

★ see page 704

● see box, page 665

hormone, both gonadotropins—stimulate the ovaries and testes (gonads). In women, these two hormones stimulate the production of estrogen and progesterone and the monthly release of an egg (ovum) from the ovaries. In men, luteinizing hormone stimulates the testes to produce testosterone, and follicle-stimulating hormone stimulates them to produce sperm.

One of the most important hormones secreted by the anterior lobe is **growth hormone,** which stimulates the growth of muscles and bones and helps regulate metabolism. Growth hormone can sharply increase the flow of sugar into muscle and fat, stimulate protein production in liver and muscle, and slow the production of fatty tissue. More prolonged effects of growth hormone—blocking the uptake and use of sugars, causing blood sugar levels to rise, and increasing the production of fat and fat levels in the blood—seem to counteract its immediate effects. These two actions of growth hormone are important because the body must adapt to the lack of food when fasting. Along with cortisol, growth hormone helps maintain blood sugar levels for the brain and mobilizes fat, making it available to other body cells as an alternative fuel. In many cases, growth hormone appears to work by activating a number of growth factors, the most important of which is insulin-like growth factor I (IGF-I).

Posterior Pituitary Function

The posterior lobe of the pituitary gland secretes only two hormones: antidiuretic hormone and oxytocin. In reality, these hormones are produced by nerve cells within the hypothalamus; these nerve cells have projections (axons) that extend to the posterior pituitary, where the hormones are released. Unlike most pituitary hormones, antidiuretic hormone and oxytocin don't act by stimulating other endocrine glands; their excesses or deficiencies directly affect their target organs.

Antidiuretic hormone (also called vasopressin) promotes water conservation by the kidney. It helps the body retain the appropriate amount of water.● When a person is dehydrated, special receptors in the heart, lungs, brain, and aorta signal the pituitary gland to produce more antidiuretic hormone. Blood levels of electrolytes, such as sodium, chloride, and potassium, must be kept within a narrow range for cells to function normally. High levels of electrolytes, which are sensed by the brain, stimulate release of this hormone. Antidiuretic hormone release is also stimulated by pain, stress, exercise, low blood sugar levels, angiotensin, prostaglandins, and certain drugs, such as chlorpropamide, cholinergic drugs, and some drugs used to treat asthma and emphysema.

Alcohol, certain steroids, and a few other substances suppress the production of antidiuretic hormone. Lack of this hormone leads to diabetes insipidus, a condition in which the kidneys excrete too much water.▲ Antidiuretic hormone is sometimes produced in excess. Such is the case in the syndrome of inappropriate secretion of antidiuretic hormone, in which antidiuretic hormone levels are too high, causing the body to retain water and blood levels of some electrolytes, such as sodium, to fall. This syndrome occurs in people with heart failure and, in rare instances, in people with a diseased hypothalamus. Sometimes antidiuretic hormone is produced outside the pituitary, especially by some lung cancers. Thus, when doctors discover high levels of antidiuretic hormone, they check the function of the pituitary gland but also search for cancer.

Oxytocin causes the uterus to contract during childbirth and immediately after delivery to prevent excessive bleeding. Oxytocin also stimulates the contraction of certain cells in the breast that surround the mammary glands. Sucking on the nipple stimulates the pituitary gland to release oxytocin. The cells in the breast contract, moving milk from its site of production within the breast to the nipple.

Empty Sella Syndrome

In the empty sella syndrome, a characteristically enlarged sella turcica (a bony structure at the base of the brain) houses a normal-sized or small pituitary gland.

The empty sella syndrome is most common in women who are overweight or have high blood pressure. Some 10 percent of the people who have the syndrome develop high fluid pressure inside the skull,■ and about 10 percent have a chronically runny nose. Occasionally, a person has a small pituitary tumor, almost always benign, that secretes growth hormone, prolactin, or corticotropin. An ordinary x-ray of the skull or a computed tomography (CT) or magnetic resonance imaging (MRI) scan may reveal the enlarged sella turcica.

Usually, no treatment is needed for the empty sella syndrome. However, an enlarged sella turcica can also indicate an enlarged pituitary gland. A CT or MRI scan can help doctors distinguish the empty sella syndrome from other causes of an enlarged sella turcica. For example, a malignant or a benign tumor (adenoma) can enlarge the pituitary gland, affecting either it or the hypothalamus. An enlarged pituitary gland may produce symptoms such as headaches and, because the growing gland often presses on the optic nerve, a loss of vision. The vision loss is unique, initially affecting only the outermost fields of vision in both eyes.

Hypopituitarism

Hypopituitarism (an underactive pituitary gland) is a partial or complete loss of the anterior lobe's function.

Because hypopituitarism affects the function of endocrine glands that are stimulated by anterior pituitary hormones, the symptoms vary depending on which pituitary hormones are deficient. Although symptoms sometimes begin suddenly and dramatically, they usually begin gradually and may go unrecognized for a long time.

A deficiency of one, several, or all of the anterior pituitary hormones may develop. Deficiencies of gonadotropins (luteinizing hormone deficiency and follicle-stimulating hormone deficiency) in premenopausal women cause menstrual periods to stop (amenorrhea), infertility, vaginal dryness, and loss of some female sexual characteristics. In men, gonadotropin deficiencies result in impotence, shriveling (atrophy) of the testes, decreased sperm production and consequent infertility, and loss of some male sexual characteristics such as the growth of body and facial hair. Gonadotropin deficiencies also occur in Kallmann's syndrome. People with this syndrome may also have a cleft lip or palate, are colorblind, and are unable to sense smells.

Growth hormone deficiency usually produces few or no symptoms in adults but causes very slow growth, sometimes dwarfism, in children.★

▲ see page 703

■ see box, page 382

★ see page 1295

What Causes an Underactive Pituitary?

Causes affecting primarily the pituitary gland (primary hypopituitarism)
- Pituitary tumors
- Inadequate blood supply to the pituitary (from severe bleeding, blood clots, anemia, or other causes)
- Infections and inflammatory diseases
- Sarcoidosis or amyloidosis (unusual diseases)
- Irradiation
- Surgical removal of pituitary tissue
- Autoimmune disease

Causes affecting primarily the hypothalamus, which then affects the pituitary (secondary hypopituitarism)
- Tumors of the hypothalamus
- Inflammatory diseases
- Head injuries
- Surgical damage to the pituitary or to the blood vessels or nerves leading to it

Deficiency of thyroid-stimulating hormone leads to hypothyroidism, an underactive thyroid gland, which results in such symptoms as confusion, intolerance to cold, weight gain, constipation, and dry skin.▲ Corticotropin deficiency alone is rare; it leads to an underactive adrenal gland, which results in fatigue, low blood pressure, low blood sugar levels, and low tolerance for stress (for example, from major trauma, surgery, or infection).■

An isolated prolactin deficiency is a rare condition, but it may explain why some women can't produce breast milk after childbirth. Sheehan's syndrome is a rare complication, typically from excessive blood loss and shock during childbirth,

▲ see page 708

■ see page 712

★ see page 729

● see page 287

which results in partial destruction of the pituitary gland. Symptoms include fatigue, loss of pubic and underarm hair, and inability to produce breast milk.

Diagnosis

Because the pituitary gland stimulates other glands, a deficiency in pituitary hormones reduces the amount of hormones the other glands produce. Therefore, a doctor considers the possibility of pituitary malfunction when investigating a deficiency in another gland, such as the thyroid or adrenal gland. When symptoms suggest that several glands are underactive, a doctor immediately suspects hypopituitarism or a polyglandular deficiency syndrome.★

The pituitary gland is usually evaluated with a computed tomography (CT) or magnetic resonance imaging (MRI) scan to identify structural problems; blood tests are used to measure hormone levels. High-resolution CT or MRI scans help reveal individual (localized) areas of abnormal tissue growth as well as general enlargement or shrinkage of the pituitary gland. The blood vessels that supply the pituitary can be examined with angiography.● In the future, a positron emission tomography scan may provide even more information on pituitary gland function.

Growth hormone production by the pituitary is difficult to evaluate because no test reliably measures it. Because the body produces growth hormone in several bursts each day, with most bursts occurring during sleep, the blood level at any given moment doesn't indicate whether production is normal. Doctors often find it useful to measure the levels of insulin-like growth factor I (IGF-I) in the blood because the level of this hormone tends to change slowly in proportion to the overall amount of pituitary growth hormone secretion. Partial growth hormone deficiency is particularly difficult to evaluate. Furthermore, levels of growth hormone are usually low when thyroid or adrenal function is reduced.

Since the levels of luteinizing hormone and follicle-stimulating hormone fluctuate with the menstrual cycle, their measurement in women may be difficult to interpret. However, in postmenopausal women who aren't taking estrogen, luteinizing hormone and follicle-stimulating hormone levels are normally high. In men, the levels don't fluctuate greatly.

By temporarily inhibiting the pituitary gland's function, some conditions can resemble hypopituitarism. Prolonged starvation, as occurs in anorexia nervosa, is one cause of inhibited pituitary function. Men who develop cirrhosis of the liver after abusing alcohol for years develop symptoms resembling those of hypopituitarism, including enlarged breasts, atrophy of the testes, skin changes, and weight gain. A pituitary tumor that secretes prolactin is a common cause of luteinizing hormone and follicle-stimulating hormone deficiency. As the tumor grows, it may destroy the pituitary by pressure, causing loss of growth hormone, thyroid stimulating hormone, and corticotropin.

Treatment

The treatment focuses on replacing the deficient target hormones rather than on replacing the deficient pituitary hormones. For example, people deficient in thyroid-stimulating hormone are given thyroid hormone, those deficient in corticotropin are given adrenocortical hormones, and those deficient in luteinizing hormone and follicle-stimulating hormone are given estrogen, progesterone, or testosterone. Growth hormone may be given to children, but adults usually don't need growth hormone replacement.

A pituitary tumor that's responsible for hypopituitarism must be treated. If the tumor is small and not secreting prolactin, surgical removal through the nose is the treatment most experts favor. Tumors that produce prolactin can be treated with the drug bromocriptine. Supervoltage or proton beam irradiation of the pituitary gland can also be used to destroy the tumor. Large tumors and those that have extended beyond the sella turcica may be impossible to remove with surgery alone. If so, doctors use supervoltage irradiation after surgery to kill the remaining tumor cells. Irradiation of the pituitary tends to cause a slow loss of pituitary function. The loss may be partial or complete. Therefore, the function of the target glands is generally evaluated every 3 to 6 months for the first year and then yearly afterward.

Acromegaly

Acromegaly is excessive growth caused by oversecretion of growth hormone.

Oversecretion of growth hormone, which is almost always caused by a benign pituitary tumor (adenoma), produces changes in many tissues and organs. For example, many internal organs enlarge, including the heart, liver, kidneys, spleen, thyroid, parathyroid, and pancreas. Certain rare tumors of the pancreas and lung also can induce excessive production of growth hormonelike substances, with similar consequences.

Symptoms

In most cases, excessive secretion of growth hormone begins between the ages of 30 and 50, long after the end plates of the bones have closed. Therefore, the bones become deformed rather than elongated. A person's facial features become coarse, and the hands and feet swell. Larger rings, gloves, shoes, and hats are needed. Since changes occur slowly, they're usually not recognized for years. Coarse body hair increases as the skin thickens and frequently darkens. The sebaceous and sweat glands in the skin enlarge, producing excessive perspiration and often an offensive body odor.

Overgrowth of the jaw bone (mandible) can cause the jaw to protrude (prognathism). Cartilage in the voice box (larynx) may thicken, making the voice deep and husky. The tongue may enlarge and become more furrowed. The ribs may thicken, creating a barrel chest.

Joint pain is common; after many years, crippling degenerative arthritis may occur. The heart is usually enlarged, and its function may be so severely impaired that heart failure occurs. Sometimes a person feels disturbing sensations and weakness in the arms and legs as enlarging tissues compress the nerves. Nerves that carry messages from the eyes to the brain may also be compressed, causing loss of vision, particularly in the outer visual fields. The pituitary tumor may also cause severe headaches.

Nearly all women with acromegaly have irregular menstrual cycles. Some women produce breast milk even though they aren't breastfeeding (galactorrhea) because of either too much growth hormone or a related increase in prolactin. About a third of the men who have acromegaly become impotent.

In very rare instances, the oversecretion of growth hormone begins in childhood, before the end plates of the long bones have closed. Since bones continue to grow until their end plates close, this situation leads to exaggerated bone growth and abnormal height (**pituitary gigantism**). Although children have accelerated growth, their bones aren't deformed. However, the soft tissues around the bone are swollen, and some nerves may be enlarged. Puberty may be delayed, and the genitals may not develop fully.

Diagnosis

Because the changes induced by high levels of growth hormone occur slowly, acromegaly often isn't diagnosed until many years after the first symptoms appear. Serial photographs (those taken over many years) may help a doctor establish the diagnosis. An x-ray of the skull may show thickening of the bones, enlargement of the nasal sinuses, and enlargement or erosion of the sella turcica, the bony structure surrounding the pituitary gland. X-rays of the hands show thickening of the bones under the fingertips and swelling of the tissue around the bones. Many people with acromegaly develop high blood sugar levels.

The symptoms suggest the diagnosis of acromegaly, and a high level of growth hormone or insulin-like growth factor I (IGF-I) in a blood sample confirms it. If the blood test result is borderline, the person is given a large amount of sugar to see whether the level of growth hormone falls, as it should in a person who doesn't have acromegaly. Both blood sugar and growth hormone levels remain high in a person with acromegaly.

Treatment

To stop or reduce the overproduction of growth hormone, the tumor is removed or destroyed with surgery or radiation therapy. Radiation therapy involves the use of supervoltage irradiation, which is much less traumatic than surgery and generally doesn't affect the production of other pituitary hormones. However, this treatment may not return growth hormone levels to normal for several years. Doctors are trying other forms of radiation therapy in an effort to speed results.

Reducing the levels of growth hormone isn't easy, even with both surgery and radiation therapy. Injections of the drug octreotide can help block the production of growth hormone. Another drug, bromocriptine, may also help.

Galactorrhea

Galactorrhea is the production of breast milk in men or in women who aren't breastfeeding.

In both sexes, the most common cause of galactorrhea is a prolactin-producing tumor (prolactinoma) in the pituitary gland. Usually prolactinomas are very small when first diagnosed; however, they tend to be larger in men than in women. Oversecretion of prolactin and the development of galactorrhea may also be induced by drugs, including phenothiazines, certain drugs given for high blood pressure (especially methyldopa), and narcotics. Still another possible cause is hypothyroidism, an underactive thyroid gland.

Symptoms

Although breast milk production may be the only symptom of a prolactinoma, many women stop menstruating or develop abnormal menstrual periods. Women with prolactinomas also often develop hot flashes and vaginal dryness, which causes discomfort with sexual intercourse. Men with prolactinomas typically have headaches or lose their peripheral vision. About two thirds of the men lose interest in sex and become impotent.

Diagnosis

Finding the cause of abnormal breast milk production usually involves a combination of blood tests and a computed tomography (CT) or magnetic resonance imaging (MRI) scan. Signs of estrogen deficiency are obvious on physical examination. Doctors measure the blood levels of prolactin and other hormones, such as luteinizing hormone and follicle-stimulating hormone. High-resolution CT or MRI scans can reveal small prolactinomas. If a tumor is large, an ophthalmologist tests the person's visual fields for possible effects on vision.

Treatment

Prolactinomas are treated in different ways. When a person's prolactin levels aren't extraordinarily high, and a CT or MRI scan shows only a small pituitary tumor or none at all, a doctor may prescribe the drug bromocriptine or may not recommend treatment. In women, bromocriptine has the advantage of increasing estrogen levels— which are often low in women with high prolactin levels—thereby protecting them from developing osteoporosis. Bromocriptine also may enable women with prolactinomas to become pregnant and helps stop the embarrassing flow of breast milk. Estrogen or oral contraceptives that contain

estrogen may be given to women with small prolactinomas, as there is no evidence that estrogen
causes the small tumors to grow any more rapidly
than normal. Most experts recommend a CT or
MRI scan every year for at least 2 years to be sure
the tumor isn't enlarging substantially.

Doctors generally treat people who have larger
tumors (macroadenomas) with bromocriptine or
surgery after thoroughly testing the endocrine
system. Treatment is coordinated with an endo-
crinologist, a neurosurgeon, and a radiotherapist.
If bromocriptine reduces the prolactin levels and
symptoms disappear, surgery may not be necessary. When surgery is necessary, bromocriptine
may be prescribed to help shrink the tumor before the operation. Although surgery may initially
reduce the prolactin levels to normal, most prolactinomas eventually recur. Radiation therapy is
used only when the symptoms are worsening and
the tumor is enlarging despite treatment with
bromocriptine. The levels of other pituitary hormones may decrease for several years after radiation therapy.

Diabetes Insipidus

*Diabetes insipidus is a disorder in which insufficient
levels of antidiuretic hormone cause excessive
thirst (polydipsia) and excessive production of very
dilute urine (polyuria).*

Diabetes insipidus results from the decreased
production of antidiuretic hormone (vasopressin), the hormone that naturally restrains the
body from producing too much urine. Antidiuretic hormone is unique in that it's produced in
the hypothalamus, then stored and released into
the bloodstream by the posterior pituitary. Diabetes insipidus can also occur when antidiuretic
hormone levels are normal but the kidneys don't
respond normally to the hormone (a condition
called **nephrogenic diabetes insipidus**).▲

Causes

Diabetes insipidus may have several causes.
One possibility is that the hypothalamus may malfunction and produce too little antidiuretic hormone. Another is that the pituitary gland may fail
to release the hormone into the bloodstream.
Other causes include damage done during surgery on the hypothalamus or pituitary gland, a

brain injury—particularly a fracture of the base
of the skull—a tumor, sarcoidosis or tuberculosis,
an aneurysm or blockage in the arteries leading
to the brain, some forms of encephalitis or meningitis, and the rare disease histiocytosis X (Hand-
Schüller-Christian disease).

In rare cases, a person has psychologic symptoms of excessive thirst, resulting in a large intake
of fluid and excessive urination. These symptoms
resemble those of diabetes insipidus, except that
the person usually doesn't awaken during the
night to urinate. Over time, the excessive fluid
intake leads to diminished responsiveness to antidiuretic hormone.

Symptoms

Diabetes insipidus may begin gradually or suddenly at any age. Often the only symptoms are
excessive thirst and excessive urine production.
A person may drink huge amounts of fluid—4 to
40 quarts a day—to compensate for fluid lost in
urine. When compensation isn't possible, dehydration can quickly follow, resulting in low blood
pressure and shock. The person continues to urinate large quantities frequently during the night.

Diagnosis

Doctors suspect diabetes insipidus in people
who produce large amounts of urine. They first
test the urine for sugar to rule out the other type
of diabetes (diabetes mellitus). Blood tests show
abnormal levels of many electrolytes.

The water deprivation test is the simplest and
most reliable test for diabetes insipidus. Since the
person isn't allowed to drink liquids during the
test and severe dehydration may occur, the test
must be performed in a doctor's office or other
medical facility. Urine production, blood electrolyte (sodium) levels, and weight are measured
regularly for several hours. As soon as the blood
pressure falls or the heart rate increases, or more
than 5 percent of the body weight is lost, the test
is stopped and the person is given an injection of
antidiuretic hormone. The diagnosis of diabetes
insipidus is confirmed if, in response to the anti-

▲ see page 615

diuretic hormone, the person's excessive urination stops, the blood pressure rises, and the heart beats more normally.

Treatment

Whenever possible, the underlying cause of diabetes insipidus is treated. Vasopressin or desmopressin acetate, modified forms of antidiuretic hormone, may be taken as a nasal spray several times a day to maintain normal urine output. However, taking too much of these drugs can lead to fluid retention, swelling, and other problems. People with diabetes insipidus who are undergoing surgery or are unconscious are generally given injections of antidiuretic hormone.

Sometimes diabetes insipidus can be controlled with drugs that stimulate production of antidiuretic hormone, such as chlorpropamide, carbamazepine, clofibrate, and various diuretics (thiazides). These drugs are unlikely to relieve symptoms completely in people whose diabetes insipidus is severe.

CHAPTER 145

Thyroid Gland Disorders

The thyroid is a small gland, measuring about 2 inches across, that lies just under the skin below the Adam's apple in the neck. The two halves (lobes) of the gland are connected in the middle (called the isthmus), so the thyroid gland resembles the letter H or a bow tie. Normally, the thyroid gland can't be seen and can barely be felt, but if it becomes enlarged, a doctor can feel it easily

and a prominent bulge (goiter) may appear below or to the sides of the Adam's apple.

The thyroid gland secretes thyroid hormones, which control the speed at which the body's chemical functions proceed (metabolic rate). Thyroid hormones influence the metabolic rate in two ways: by stimulating almost every tissue in the body to produce proteins and by increasing the amount of oxygen that cells use. When the cells work harder, body organs work faster.

To produce thyroid hormones, the thyroid gland needs iodine, an element contained in food and water. The thyroid gland traps iodine and processes it into thyroid hormones. As thyroid hormones are used up, some of the iodine contained in the hormones returns to the thyroid gland and is recycled to produce more thyroid hormones.

The body has a complex mechanism for adjusting the level of thyroid hormones. First, the hypothalamus, located just above the pituitary gland in the brain, secretes **thyrotropin-releasing hormone,** which causes the pituitary gland to produce **thyroid-stimulating hormone.** Just as the name suggests, thyroid-stimulating hormone stimulates the thyroid gland to produce thyroid hormones. When the amount of thyroid hormones circulating in the blood reaches a certain level, the pituitary gland produces less thyroid-stimulating hormone; when the amount of thyroid hormones circulating in the blood decreases, the pituitary gland produces more thyroid-stimulating

Locating the Thyroid Gland

Thyroid cartilage

Thyroid

Trachea

Sternum

Clavicle

hormone—a negative feedback control mechanism.

Thyroid hormones are found in two forms. **Thyroxine (T₄)**, the form produced in the thyroid gland, has only a slight, if any, effect on speeding up the body's metabolic rate. Thyroxine is converted in the liver and other organs to the metabolically active form, **triiodothyronine (T₃)**. This conversion produces about 80 percent of the active form of the hormone; the remaining 20 percent is produced and secreted by the thyroid gland itself. Many factors control the conversion of T_4 to T_3 in the liver and other organs, including the body's needs from moment to moment. Most of the T_4 and T_3 is tightly bound to certain proteins in the blood and is active only when not bound to these proteins. In this remarkable way, the body maintains the correct amount of thyroid hormone needed to keep a steady metabolic rate.

For the thyroid gland to function normally, many factors must work well together: the hypothalamus, the pituitary gland, the thyroid hormone–binding proteins in the blood, and the conversion, in the liver and other tissues, of T_4 to T_3.

Laboratory Tests

To determine how well the thyroid gland is functioning, doctors use several laboratory tests. One of the most common is a test to measure the level of thyroid-stimulating hormone in the blood. Because this hormone stimulates the thyroid gland, blood levels are high when the thyroid gland is underactive (and thus needs more stimulation) and low when the thyroid gland is overactive (and thus needs less stimulation). If the pituitary gland isn't functioning normally (although this rarely happens), the level of thyroid-stimulating hormone alone won't accurately reflect thyroid gland function, and doctors then measure the level of free T_4.

Measuring the level of thyroid-stimulating hormone and the level of free T_4 circulating in the blood is usually all that is needed. However, doctors may also measure the level of a protein called thyroxine-binding globulin, because abnormal levels of this protein can lead to misinterpretation of a person's total thyroid hormone level. People who have kidney disease, some genetic disorders, or certain other diseases or who take anabolic steroids have lower levels of thyroxine-binding globulin. Conversely, levels of thyroxine-binding globulin may be increased in women who are pregnant or taking oral contraceptives or other forms of estrogen, in people in the early stages of hepatitis, and in people with some other diseases.

Some tests can be performed on the thyroid gland itself. For instance, if a doctor feels a growth in the thyroid gland, an ultrasound examination may be ordered; this procedure uses sound waves to determine whether the growth is solid or filled with fluid. A thyroid scan uses radioactive iodine or technetium and a device to produce a picture of the thyroid gland that will show any physical abnormalities. Thyroid scanning can also help the doctor determine whether the function of an area is normal, overactive, or underactive compared with the rest of the gland.

On rare occasions when a doctor isn't sure whether the problem lies in the thyroid gland or in the pituitary gland, functional stimulation tests may be ordered. One of these tests involves injecting thyrotropin-releasing hormone intravenously and then using blood tests to measure the pituitary gland's response.

Euthyroid Sick Syndrome

In the euthyroid sick syndrome, thyroid test results are abnormal even though the thyroid gland is functioning normally.

The euthyroid sick syndrome commonly occurs in people who have a severe illness other than thyroid disease. When people are sick, are malnourished, or have had surgery, the T_4 form of thyroid hormone isn't converted normally to the T_3 form. Large amounts of reverse T_3, an inactive form of thyroid hormone, accumulate. Despite this abnormal conversion, the thyroid gland continues to function and to control the body's metabolic rate normally. Because no problem exists with the thyroid gland, no treatment is needed. Laboratory tests show normal results once the underlying illness resolves.

Hyperthyroidism

Hyperthyroidism—a condition in which the thyroid gland is overactive—develops when the thyroid produces too much hormone.

Symptoms of Thyroid Disease

Hyperthyroidism (too much thyroid hormone)	Hypothyroidism (too little thyroid hormone)
Fast heartbeat	Slow pulse
High blood pressure	Hoarse voice
Moist skin and increased sweat	Slowed speech
	Puffy face
Shakiness and tremor	Loss of eyebrows
Nervousness	Drooping eyelids
Increased appetite with weight loss	Intolerance to cold
Sleep difficulties	Constipation
Frequent bowel movements and diarrhea	Weight gain
Weakness	Sparse, coarse, dry hair
Raised, thickened skin over shins	Dry, scaly, thick, coarse skin; raised, thickened skin over shins
Swollen, reddened, bulging eyes	Carpal tunnel syndrome
Sensitivity of eyes to light	Confusion
Constant stare	Depression
Confusion	Dementia

Hyperthyroidism has several causes, including immunologic reactions (believed to be the cause of Graves' disease). People with thyroiditis, an inflammation of the thyroid gland, typically go through a phase of hyperthyroidism. However, the inflammation may damage the thyroid gland, so that its initial overactivity is a prelude to either transient (more common) or permanent underactivity (hypothyroidism).

Toxic thyroid nodules (adenomas), areas of abnormal tissue growth within the thyroid gland, sometimes escape the mechanisms that normally control the thyroid gland and produce thyroid hormone in large quantities. A person may have one nodule or many. Toxic multinodular goiter (Plummer's disease), a disorder in which there

▲ see page 1034

are many nodules, is uncommon in adolescents and young adults and tends to increase with age.

In hyperthyroidism, regardless of the cause, the body's functions speed up. The heart pounds, beats more quickly, and may develop an abnormal rhythm, leading to an awareness of the heartbeat (palpitations). Blood pressure is likely to increase. Many people with hyperthyroidism feel warm even in a cool room. Their skin may become moist as they tend to sweat profusely, and their hands may develop a fine tremor. Many people feel nervous, tired, and weak, yet have an increased level of activity; have an increased appetite, yet lose weight; sleep poorly; and have frequent bowel movements, occasionally with diarrhea.

Older people with hyperthyroidism may not develop these characteristic symptoms but have what is sometimes called **apathetic** or **masked hyperthyroidism**. They simply become weak, sleepy, confused, withdrawn, and depressed. However, heart problems, especially abnormal heart rhythms, are seen more often in older people with hyperthyroidism.

Hyperthyroidism can cause changes in the eyes: puffiness around the eyes, increased tear formation, irritation, and unusual sensitivity to light. The person appears to stare. These eye symptoms disappear soon after the thyroid hormone secretion is controlled, except in people with Graves' disease, which causes special eye problems.

Hyperthyroidism may take the form of Graves' disease, toxic nodular goiter, or secondary hyperthyroidism.

GRAVES' DISEASE

Graves' disease (toxic diffuse goiter) is believed to be caused by an antibody that stimulates the thyroid to produce too much thyroid hormone. People with Graves' disease have the typical signs of hyperthyroidism and three distinctive additional symptoms. Since the entire gland is stimulated, it can become greatly enlarged, causing a bulge in the neck (goiter). People with Graves' disease may also have bulging eyes (exophthalmos)▲ and, less commonly, raised areas of skin over the shins.

The eyes bulge outward because of a substance that builds up in the orbit. This bulging occurs in addition to the intense stare and other eye changes of hyperthyroidism. The muscles that move the eyes become unable to function properly, making it difficult or impossible to move the eyes normally or to coordinate eye movements, resulting in double vision. The eyelids may not close completely, exposing the eyes to injury from foreign particles and dryness. These eye changes may begin years before any other symptoms of hyperthyroidism, providing an early clue to Graves' disease, or may not occur until other symptoms are noticed. Eye symptoms may even appear or worsen after the excessive thyroid hormone secretion has been treated and controlled.

Eye symptoms may be helped by elevating the head of the bed, by applying eyedrops, by sleeping with the eyelids taped shut, and occasionally by taking diuretics. The double vision may be helped by using eyeglass prisms. Finally, oral corticosteroid drugs, x-ray treatment to the orbits, or eye surgery may be needed.

In Graves' disease, a substance similar to the one deposited behind the eyes may be deposited in the skin, usually over the shins. The thickened area may be itchy and red and feels hard when pressed with a finger. As with deposits behind the eyes, this problem may begin before or after other symptoms of hyperthyroidism are noticed. Corticosteroid creams or ointments can help relieve the itching and hardness. Often the problem disappears without treatment for no apparent reason months or years later.

Toxic Nodular Goiter

In toxic nodular goiter, one or more nodules in the thyroid produce too much thyroid hormone and aren't under the control of thyroid-stimulating hormone. The nodules are true hyperfunctioning benign thyroid tumors and are not associated with the bulging eyes and skin problems of Graves' disease.

Secondary Hyperthyroidism

Hyperthyroidism may (rarely) be caused by a pituitary tumor that secretes too much thyroid-stimulating hormone, which in turn stimulates the thyroid to overproduce thyroid hormones. Another rare cause of hyperthyroidism is pituitary resistance to thyroid hormone, which results in the pituitary gland secreting too much thyroid-stimulating hormone.

Women with a hydatidiform mole▲ may also have hyperthyroidism because the thyroid gland is overstimulated by the high levels of human cho-

rionic gonadotropin in the blood. The hyperthyroidism disappears after the molar pregnancy is terminated and human chorionic gonadotropin vanishes from the blood.

Complications

Thyroid storm, sudden extreme overactivity of the thyroid gland, may produce fever, extreme weakness and loss of muscle, restlessness, mood swings, confusion, altered consciousness (even coma), and an enlarged liver with mild jaundice. *Thyroid storm is a life-threatening emergency requiring prompt treatment.* Severe strain on the heart can lead to a life-threatening irregular heartbeat (arrhythmia) and shock.

Thyroid storm is generally caused by untreated or inadequately treated hyperthyroidism and can be triggered by infection, trauma, surgery, poorly controlled diabetes, fear, pregnancy or labor, discontinuance of thyroid medication, or other stresses. It's rare in children.

Treatment

Hyperthyroidism can usually be treated with medication, but other options include surgically removing the thyroid gland or treating it with radioactive iodine. Each treatment has advantages and disadvantages.

The thyroid gland needs a small amount of iodine to work properly, but a large amount of iodine decreases the amount of hormone the gland makes and prevents the gland from releasing excess thyroid hormone. Therefore, doctors can use large doses of iodine to stop the gland from secreting excess thyroid hormone. Iodine treatment is particularly useful when doctors need to control hyperthyroidism quickly, as during thyroid storm or before emergency surgery. However, iodine isn't used for routine or long-term treatment of hyperthyroidism.

Propylthiouracil or methimazole, the drugs most commonly used to treat hyperthyroidism, slow thyroid function by decreasing the gland's production of thyroid hormone. Both drugs are taken orally, beginning with high doses that are later adjusted according to the results of thyroid hormone blood tests. These drugs can usually

---

▲ see page 1113

control thyroid function in 6 weeks to 3 months, but larger doses of the drugs may bring it under control faster—with an increased risk of adverse effects. These adverse effects include allergic reactions (most commonly, skin rashes), nausea, loss of taste, and on rare occasions, depressed synthesis of blood cells in the bone marrow. The bone marrow depression can deplete the number of white blood cells, creating a life-threatening situation in which the person is vulnerable to infection. While these two drugs are comparable in most ways, propylthiouracil may be safer than methimazole for use in pregnant women because less of it reaches the fetus. Carbimazole, a drug that is widely used in Europe, is converted into methimazole in the body.

Beta-blocking drugs such as propranolol help control some of the symptoms of hyperthyroidism. These drugs are effective in slowing down a fast heart rate, reducing shakiness (tremor), and controlling anxiety. Doctors therefore find beta-blockers particularly useful for people with thyroid storm and for people with bothersome or dangerous symptoms whose hyperthyroidism hasn't yet been brought under control by other treatments. However, beta-blockers don't control abnormal thyroid function.

Hyperthyroidism can also be treated with radioactive iodine, which destroys the thyroid gland. Radioactive iodine taken orally introduces very little radioactivity to the body as a whole but a great deal to the thyroid gland. Doctors try to adjust the dose of radioactive iodine to destroy only enough of the thyroid gland to bring its hormone production back to normal, without reducing thyroid function too much. However, most of the time, radioactive iodine treatment ultimately creates hypothyroidism (an underactive thyroid gland), a condition that requires thyroid hormone replacement therapy. People who need thyroid hormone replacement therapy take a thyroid hormone tablet daily for the rest of their lives to replace the natural hormone that's no longer being produced in sufficient quantities. About 25 percent of the people have hypothyroidism 1 year after radioactive iodine treatment, but the percentage increases steadily over the next 20 years or more. Concern that radioactive iodine may

cause cancer has never been confirmed. Radioactive iodine isn't given to pregnant women, since it crosses the placenta and may destroy the fetus' thyroid gland.

In a thyroidectomy, the thyroid gland is removed surgically. Surgery is an option especially for young people with hyperthyroidism. Surgery is also an option for people who have a very large goiter, as well as for people who are allergic to or who develop severe side effects from the drugs used to treat hyperthyroidism. Hyperthyroidism is permanently controlled in more than 90 percent of those who choose this option. Some degree of hypothyroidism occurs after surgery in some people, who then have to take replacement thyroid hormone for the rest of their lives. Rare complications include paralysis of the vocal cords and damage to the parathyroid glands (the tiny glands behind the thyroid gland that control calcium levels in the blood).

Hypothyroidism

Hypothyroidism is a condition in which the thyroid gland is underactive and produces too little thyroid hormone. Very severe hypothyroidism is called myxedema.

In Hashimoto's thyroiditis, the most common cause of hypothyroidism,▲ the thyroid gland is often enlarged, and hypothyroidism frequently results years later because the gland's functioning areas are gradually destroyed. The second most common cause of hypothyroidism is treatment of hyperthyroidism. Both radioactive iodine treatment and surgery tend to produce hypothyroidism.

A chronic lack of iodine in the diet produces an enlarged, underactive thyroid gland (goitrous hypothyroidism), the most common cause of hypothyroidism in many undeveloped countries. Since salt manufacturers began adding iodine to table salt and iodine-containing disinfectants are often used to sterilize cow's udders, this form of hypothyroidism has disappeared in the United States. Even rarer causes of hypothyroidism include some inherited disorders in which an abnormality of the enzymes in thyroid cells prevents the gland from making or secreting enough thyroid hormones. In other rare disorders, either the hypothalamus or the pituitary gland fails to secrete enough of the hormone needed to stimulate normal thyroid function.

▲ see page 709

Symptoms

Insufficient thyroid hormone causes bodily functions to slow down. In sharp contrast to hyperthyroidism, the symptoms of hypothyroidism are subtle and gradual and may be mistaken for depression. Facial expressions become dull, the voice is hoarse and speech is slow, eyelids droop, and the eyes and face become puffy and swollen. Many people with hypothyroidism gain weight, become constipated, and are unable to tolerate cold. The hair becomes sparse, coarse, and dry and the skin becomes coarse, dry, scaly, and thick. Many people develop carpal tunnel syndrome, which makes the hands tingle or hurt.▲ The pulse may slow, the palms and soles appear slightly orange (carotenemia), and the side part of the eyebrows slowly falls out. Some people, especially older people, may appear confused, forgetful, or demented—signs that can easily be mistaken for Alzheimer's disease or other forms of dementia.

If untreated, hypothyroidism can eventually cause anemia, a low body temperature, and heart failure. This situation may progress to confusion, stupor, or coma (myxedema coma), a life-threatening complication in which breathing slows, the person has seizures, and blood flow to the brain decreases. Myxedema coma can be triggered by exposure to the cold as well as by an infection, trauma, and drugs such as sedatives and tranquilizers that depress brain function.

Treatment

Hypothyroidism is treated by replacing the deficient thyroid hormone, using one of several different oral preparations. The preferred form is synthetic thyroid hormone, T_4. Another form, desiccated (dried) thyroid, is obtained from the thyroid glands of animals. In general, doctors find desiccated thyroid less satisfactory because the dose is harder to adjust and the tablets have variable amounts of T_3.

Treatment in an older person begins with small doses of thyroid hormone because too large a dose can cause serious side effects. The dose is gradually increased until the person's blood levels of thyroid-stimulating hormone return to normal. Medication is usually taken for life. In emergencies, such as myxedema coma, doctors may give thyroid hormone intravenously.

Thyroiditis

Thyroiditis, an inflammation of the thyroid gland, produces transient hyperthyroidism often followed by transient hypothyroidism or no change in thyroid function at all.

The three types of thyroiditis are Hashimoto's thyroiditis, subacute granulomatous thyroiditis, and silent lymphocytic thyroiditis.

HASHIMOTO'S THYROIDITIS

Hashimoto's thyroiditis (autoimmune thyroiditis) is the most common type of thyroiditis and the most common cause of hypothyroidism. For unknown reasons, the body turns against itself in an autoimmune reaction, creating antibodies that attack the thyroid gland.■ This type of thyroiditis is most common in elderly women and tends to run in families. The condition occurs eight times more often in women than in men and may occur in people with certain chromosomal abnormalities, including Turner's, Down, and Klinefelter's syndromes.

Hashimoto's thyroiditis often begins with a painless enlargement of the thyroid gland or a feeling of fullness in the neck. When doctors feel the gland, they usually find it enlarged, with a rubbery texture, but not tender; sometimes it feels lumpy. The thyroid gland is underactive in about 20 percent of the people when Hashimoto's thyroiditis is discovered; the rest have normal thyroid function. Many people with Hashimoto's thyroiditis have other endocrine disorders such as diabetes, an underactive adrenal gland, or underactive parathyroid glands, and other autoimmune diseases such as pernicious anemia, rheumatoid arthritis, Sjögren's syndrome, or systemic lupus erythematosus (lupus).

Doctors perform thyroid function tests on blood samples to determine whether the gland is functioning normally, but they base the diagnosis of Hashimoto's thyroiditis on the symptoms, a physical examination, and whether the person has antibodies that attack the gland (antithyroid

---

▲ see page 336

■ see page 816

antibodies), which can easily be measured in a blood test.

No specific treatment is available for Hashimoto's thyroiditis. Most people eventually develop hypothyroidism and must take thyroid hormone replacement therapy for the rest of their lives. Thyroid hormone may also be useful in decreasing the enlarged thyroid gland.

SUBACUTE GRANULOMATOUS THYROIDITIS

Subacute granulomatous (giant cell) thyroiditis, which is probably caused by a virus, begins much more suddenly than Hashimoto's thyroiditis. Subacute granulomatous thyroiditis often follows a viral illness and begins with what many people call a sore throat but actually proves to be neck pain localized to the thyroid. The thyroid gland becomes increasingly tender, and the person usually develops a low-grade fever (99° F. to 101° F.). The pain may shift from one side of the neck to the other, spread to the jaw and ears, and hurt more when the head is turned or when the person swallows. Subacute granulomatous thyroiditis is often mistaken at first for a dental problem or a throat or ear infection.

Inflammation usually causes the thyroid gland to release excessive thyroid hormones, resulting in hyperthyroidism, almost always followed by transient hypothyroidism. Many people with subacute granulomatous thyroiditis feel extremely tired.

Most people recover completely from this type of thyroiditis. Generally the condition goes away by itself within a few months, but sometimes it comes back or, more rarely, damages enough of the thyroid gland to cause permanent hypothyroidism.

Aspirin or other nonsteroidal anti-inflammatory drugs (such as ibuprofen) can relieve the pain and inflammation. In very severe cases, doctors may recommend corticosteroids such as prednisone, which should be tapered off over 6 to 8 weeks. When corticosteroids are stopped abruptly, symptoms often return in full force.

SILENT LYMPHOCYTIC THYROIDITIS

Silent lymphocytic thyroiditis occurs most often in women, typically just after childbirth, and causes the thyroid to become enlarged without becoming tender. For several weeks to several months, a person with silent lymphocytic thyroiditis has hyperthyroidism followed by hypo-

thyroidism before eventually recovering normal thyroid function. This condition requires no specific treatment, although the hyperthyroidism or hypothyroidism may require treatment for a few weeks. Often, a beta-blocker such as propranolol is the only drug needed to control the symptoms of hyperthyroidism. During the period of hypothyroidism, a person may need to take thyroid hormone, usually for no more than a few months. Hypothyroidism becomes permanent in about 10 percent of the people with silent lymphocytic thyroiditis.

Thyroid Cancer

Thyroid cancer is any one of four main types of malignancy of the thyroid: papillary, follicular, anaplastic, or medullary.

Thyroid cancer is more common in people who have been treated with radiation to the head, neck, or chest, most often for benign conditions (although radiation treatment for benign conditions is no longer carried out). Rather than causing the whole thyroid gland to enlarge, a cancer usually causes small growths (nodules) within the thyroid. Most thyroid nodules aren't cancerous, and thyroid cancers can generally be cured. Thyroid cancers often have a limited ability to take up iodine and produce thyroid hormone, but very rarely they produce enough hormone to cause hyperthyroidism. Nodules are more likely to be cancerous if only one nodule is found rather than several, if a thyroid scan shows that the nodule isn't functioning, if the nodule is solid rather than filled with fluid (cystic), if the nodule is hard, or if the nodule is growing quickly.

A painless lump in the neck is usually the first sign of thyroid cancer. When doctors find a nodule in the thyroid gland, they request several tests. A thyroid scan determines whether the nodule is functioning, since a nonfunctioning nodule is more likely to be cancerous than a functioning one. An ultrasound scan is less helpful but may be performed to determine whether the nodule is solid or filled with fluid. A sample of the nodule is usually taken by fine-needle biopsy for examination under a microscope—the best way to determine whether the nodule is cancerous.

PAPILLARY CANCER

Papillary cancer accounts for 60 to 70 percent of all thyroid cancers. Two to three times as many women as men have papillary cancer; however, since nodules are far more common in women, a nodule in a man is more suspicious for a cancer. Papillary cancer is more common in young people but grows and spreads more quickly in the elderly. People who have received radiation treatment to the neck, usually for a benign condition in infancy or childhood or for some other cancer in adulthood, are at greater risk of developing papillary cancer.

Surgery is the treatment for papillary cancer, which sometimes spreads to nearby lymph nodes. Nodules smaller than three quarters of an inch across are removed along with the thyroid tissue immediately surrounding them, although some experts recommend removing the entire thyroid gland. Surgery almost always cures these small cancers.

Since papillary cancer may respond to thyroid-stimulating hormone, thyroid hormone is taken in doses large enough to suppress secretion of thyroid-stimulating hormone and help prevent a recurrence. If a nodule is larger, most or all of the thyroid gland is usually removed, and radioactive iodine is often given in expectation that any remaining thyroid tissue or cancer that has spread away from the thyroid will take it up and be destroyed. Another dose of radioactive iodine may be needed to make sure the entire cancer has been destroyed. Papillary cancer is almost always cured.

FOLLICULAR CANCER

Follicular cancer accounts for about 15 percent of all thyroid cancers and is more common in the elderly. Follicular cancer is also more common in women than in men, but as with papillary cancer, a nodule in a man is more likely to be cancer. Much more aggressive than papillary cancer, follicular cancer tends to spread through the bloodstream, spreading cancerous cells to various parts of the body (metastases). Treatment for follicular cancer requires surgically removing as much of the thyroid gland as possible and destroying any remaining thyroid tissue, including the metastases, with radioactive iodine.

ANAPLASTIC CANCER

Anaplastic cancer accounts for less than 10 percent of thyroid cancers and occurs most commonly in elderly women. This cancer grows very quickly and usually causes a large growth in the neck. About 80 percent of the people with anaplastic cancer die within 1 year. Treatment with radioactive iodine is useless because anaplastic cancers don't take up radioactive iodine. However, treatment with anticancer drugs and radiation therapy before and after surgery has resulted in some cures.

MEDULLARY CANCER

In medullary cancer, the thyroid gland produces excessive amounts of calcitonin, a hormone produced by certain thyroid cells. Because medullary thyroid cancer can also produce other hormones, it can cause unusual symptoms. This cancer tends to spread (metastasize) through the lymphatic system to the lymph nodes and through the blood to the liver, lungs, and bones. Medullary cancer can develop along with other types of endocrine cancers in what is called multiple endocrine neoplasia syndrome.▲

Treatment requires removing the thyroid gland completely. Additional surgery may be needed so that doctors can determine whether the cancer has spread to the lymph nodes. More than two thirds of the people whose medullary thyroid cancer is part of multiple endocrine neoplasia syndrome live for at least 10 more years. When medullary thyroid cancer occurs alone, the chances of survival are not as good.

Because medullary thyroid cancer sometimes runs in families, close blood relatives of a person with this type of cancer should be screened for a genetic abnormality that can be easily detected in blood cells. If the screening test result is negative, the relative will almost certainly not develop medullary cancer. If the screening test result is positive, then the relative has or will develop medullary cancer, and thyroid surgery should be considered even before symptoms develop and the blood level of calcitonin rises. A high blood calcitonin level or an excessive rise in the level following stimulation tests also helps a doctor predict whether someone has or will develop medullary cancer. Finding an unusually high level of calcitonin will lead the doctor to suggest removing the thyroid gland, since early treatment provides the best chance of cure.

▲ see page 726

Adrenal Gland Disorders

The body has two adrenal glands, one near the top of each kidney. The inner part (medulla) of the adrenal glands secretes hormones such as adrenaline (epinephrine) that affect blood pressure, heart rate, sweating, and other activities also regulated by the sympathetic nervous system. The outer part (cortex) secretes many different hormones, including corticosteroids (cortisone-like hormones), androgens (male hormones), and mineralocorticoids, which control blood pressure and the levels of salt and potassium in the body.

The adrenal glands are part of a complex system that produces interacting hormones. The hypothalamus produces corticotropin-releasing hormone, triggering the pituitary gland to secrete corticotropin, which regulates the production of corticosteroids by the adrenal glands. Adrenal glands may stop functioning when either the pituitary or hypothalamus fails to produce sufficient amounts of the appropriate hormones. Underproduction or overproduction of any adrenal hormones can lead to serious illness.

Underactive Adrenal Glands

Addison's disease (adrenocortical insufficiency) results when underactive adrenal glands produce insufficient amounts of corticosteroids.

Addison's disease affects about 4 out of every 100,000 people. The disease can strike at any age and affects males and females about equally. In 30 percent of people with Addison's disease, the adrenal glands are destroyed by a cancer, amyloidosis, an infection such as tuberculosis, or another identifiable disease. In the other 70 percent, the cause isn't known for certain, but scientists strongly suspect the adrenal glands are destroyed by an autoimmune reaction.▲

The adrenal glands are also suppressed in people who take corticosteroids such as prednisone.

Ordinarily, the dose of corticosteroids is tapered slowly before the drug is stopped completely. When corticosteroids are stopped suddenly after being taken for a month or more, the adrenal glands may be unable to produce corticosteroids in sufficient amounts for several weeks or even months, depending on the dose of corticosteroids and the duration of treatment. Certain other drugs, such as ketoconazole taken to treat fungal infections, can also block the natural production of corticosteroids, resulting in a deficiency.

Corticosteroid deficiency can lead to many problems. For example, when corticosteroids are lacking, the body excretes large amounts of sodium and retains potassium, leading to low levels of sodium and high levels of potassium in the blood. The kidneys aren't able to concentrate urine, so when a person with a corticosteroid deficiency drinks too much water or loses too much sodium, the blood level of sodium falls. Inability to concentrate urine ultimately causes the person to urinate excessively and become dehydrated. Severe dehydration and a low sodium level reduce blood volume and can culminate in shock.

Corticosteroid deficiency also leads to an extreme sensitivity to insulin, a hormone normally present in the blood, so that the blood sugar levels may fall dangerously low. The deficiency prevents the body from manufacturing carbohydrates from protein, fighting infections, or healing wounds very well. Muscles weaken, and even the heart can become weak and unable to pump blood adequately.

To compensate for a deficiency of corticosteroids, the pituitary gland produces more corticotropin, the hormone that normally stimulates the adrenal glands. Since corticotropin also affects melanin production, people with Addison's disease often develop a dark pigmentation of the skin and the lining of the mouth. The excessive pigmentation usually occurs in patches. Even people with dark skin can develop excessive pigmentation, although the change may be hard to recognize. Excessive pigmentation doesn't occur

▲ see page 816

when adrenal insufficiency is caused by pituitary or hypothalamus insufficiency, conditions in which the basic problem is a deficiency of corticotropin.

Symptoms

Soon after developing Addison's disease, a person feels weak, tired, and dizzy when standing up after sitting or lying down. The skin becomes dark; this darkness may seem like tanning, but it appears on both sun-exposed and nonexposed areas. Black freckles may develop over the forehead, face, and shoulders; a bluish-black discoloration may develop around the nipples, lips, mouth, rectum, scrotum, or vagina. Most people lose weight, become dehydrated, have no appetite, and develop muscle aches, nausea, vomiting, and diarrhea. Many become unable to tolerate cold. Unless the disease is severe, symptoms tend to become apparent only during times of stress.

If the disease isn't treated, severe abdominal pains, profound weakness, extremely low blood pressure, kidney failure, and shock may occur, especially if the body is subjected to stress such as an injury, surgery, or severe infection. Death may quickly follow.

Diagnosis

Because the symptoms may start slowly and be subtle, and because no single laboratory test is definitive, doctors often don't suspect Addison's disease at the outset. Sometimes a major stress, such as an accident, operation, or serious illness, makes the symptoms more obvious and precipitates a crisis.

Blood tests may show a lack of corticosteroids, especially cortisol, as well as low sodium and high potassium levels. Measures of kidney function, such as tests for blood urea nitrogen and creatinine, usually indicate that the kidneys aren't working well. Corticosteroid levels, usually tested after an injection of corticotropin (a challenge test), can help the doctor distinguish adrenal gland insufficiency from pituitary gland insufficiency. When it is the latter, an injection of corticotropin-releasing hormone reveals whether the cause of the problem is hypothalamus insufficiency.

Treatment

Regardless of the cause, Addison's disease can be life-threatening and must be treated first with

A Close Look at the Adrenal Glands

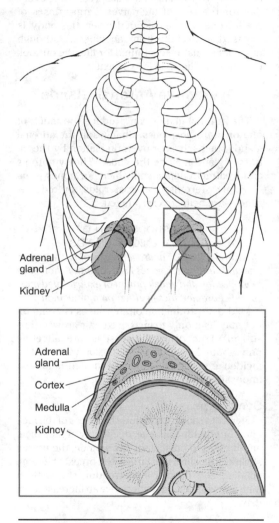

corticosteroids. Usually treatment can be started with prednisone taken orally. However, people who are severely ill may be given cortisol intravenously at first and then prednisone tablets. Most people with Addison's disease also need to take 1 or 2 tablets of fludrocortisone every day to help restore the body's normal excretion of sodium and potassium. Fludrocortisone can eventually be reduced or discontinued in some people; however, they will need to take prednisone every day for the rest of their lives. Larger doses of prednisone may be needed when the body is stressed, especially from an illness. Although treatment must be continued for life, the outlook for a normal life span is excellent.

Overactive Adrenal Glands

The adrenal glands can produce too much of one or more hormones. Changes in the adrenal glands themselves or overstimulation by the pituitary gland may be the cause. The symptoms and treatment depend on which hormones—androgenic steroids, corticosteroids, or aldosterone—are being overproduced.

OVERPRODUCTION OF ANDROGENIC STEROIDS

Overproduction of androgenic steroids (testosterone and similar hormones) is a condition that leads to virilization, the development of exaggerated masculine characteristics in either men or women.

Mild overproduction of androgens is common but may lead only to increased hair growth (hirsutism). True virilizing disease is rare, affecting only about 1 or 2 of every 100,000 women. The incidence of virilizing disease in men is almost impossible to guess.

Symptoms

Signs of virilization include hairiness of the face and body, baldness, acne, deepening of the voice, and increased muscularity. In women, the uterus shrinks, the clitoris enlarges, the breasts become smaller, and normal menstruation stops. Both men and women may experience an increased sex drive.

Diagnosis

The combination of body changes makes virilization relatively easy for a doctor to recognize. A test can determine the level of androgenic steroids in the urine. If the level is high, the dexamethasone suppression test can help determine whether the problem is a cancer, a noncancerous tumor (adenoma), or an enlargement of the hor-mone-producing portions of the adrenal cortex (adrenal hyperplasia). With this test, the corticosteroid dexamethasone is given orally. If the problem is adrenal hyperplasia, dexamethasone prevents the adrenal glands from producing androgenic steroids. If the problem is an adenoma or cancer of the adrenal glands, dexamethasone reduces androgenic steroid production only partially or not at all. The doctor may also order a computed tomography (CT) or magnetic resonance imaging (MRI) scan to obtain a view of the adrenal glands.

Treatment

Androgen-producing adenomas and adrenal cancers are usually treated by surgically removing the adrenal gland. For adrenal hyperplasia, small amounts of corticosteroids such as dexamethasone generally reduce the production of androgenic steroids, but these drugs may also cause symptoms of Cushing's syndrome if too large a dose is given.

OVERPRODUCTION OF CORTICOSTEROIDS

Overexposure to corticosteroids, whether from overproduction by the adrenal glands or from administration of excessive amounts by a doctor, results in Cushing's syndrome.

An abnormality in the pituitary gland, such as a tumor, can cause the pituitary to produce large amounts of corticotropin, the hormone that controls the adrenal glands. Pituitary tumors that overproduce corticotropin occur in about 6 in every 1 million people. Small-cell carcinoma in the lung and some other tumors outside the pituitary gland can produce corticotropin as well (a condition called ectopic corticotropin syndrome). This is the most common cause of excessive adrenal cortical function, found in at least 10 percent of people with small-cell carcinoma in the lung, a common type of tumor.

Sometimes the adrenal gland produces excessive corticosteroids even when corticotropin levels are low, usually when a benign tumor (adenoma) has developed in the adrenal gland. Benign tumors of the adrenal cortex are extremely common; half of all people have them by the age of 70. Only a small fraction of these benign tumors are active; the incidence of adenomas causing disease is about 2 in every 1 million people. Cancerous tumors of the adrenal cortex are equally common, but cancers causing endocrine disease are quite rare.

Symptoms

Because corticosteroids alter the amount and distribution of body fat, a person with Cushing's syndrome usually has a large, round face (moon face). Excessive fat develops throughout the torso and may be particularly noticeable at the top of the back (buffalo hump). Fingers, hands, and feet are usually slender in proportion to the thickened trunk. Muscles lose their bulk, leading to weakness. The skin becomes thin, bruises easily, and heals poorly when bruised or cut. Purple streaks that look like stretch marks may develop over the abdomen.

High corticosteroid levels over time raise the blood pressure, weaken bones (osteoporosis), and diminish resistance to infections. The risk of developing kidney stones and diabetes is increased, and mental disturbances, including depression and hallucinations, may occur. Women with Cushing's syndrome usually have an irregular menstrual cycle. Children who have the condition grow slowly and remain short. In some people, the adrenal glands also produce large amounts of androgenic steroids, leading to increased facial and body hair, balding, and an increased sex drive.

Diagnosis

Doctors who suspect Cushing's syndrome after observing the symptoms measure the blood level of cortisol, the main corticosteroid hormone. Normally, cortisol levels are high in the morning and decrease during the day. In people who have Cushing's syndrome, cortisol levels are very high in the morning and don't decrease late in the day as would be expected. Measuring cortisol in the urine can be useful because tests performed a few hours apart can indicate how much cortisol has been produced in that time.

If the cortisol levels are high, the doctor may recommend a dexamethasone suppression test. The test is based on the ability of dexamethasone to suppress the pituitary gland, thereby reducing adrenal gland stimulation. First a urine sample is tested for cortisol. Then dexamethasone is given, and cortisol levels are measured in another sample of urine. If the Cushing's syndrome is caused by pituitary stimulation, the level of cortisol will

fall; if the Cushing's syndrome is caused by stimulation from a nonpituitary source of corticotropin or an adrenal tumor, the urinary cortisol level will remain high.

Results of a dexamethasone suppression test may not be clear-cut. Other laboratory tests may be needed to help determine the precise cause of the syndrome. These tests may be followed by a computed tomography (CT) or magnetic resonance imaging (MRI) scan of the pituitary or adrenal glands and by a chest x-ray or CT scan of the lungs.

Treatment

Treatment is directed at the pituitary or adrenal gland, depending on the source of the problem. Surgery or radiation therapy may be needed to remove or destroy a pituitary tumor. Adenomas of the adrenal gland can often be removed surgically. Both adrenal glands may have to be removed if these treatments aren't effective or if no tumor is present. Any person who has had both adrenal glands removed, and many people who have had part of their adrenal glands removed, must take corticosteroids for life.

Some 5 to 10 percent of the people who have both adrenal glands removed develop **Nelson's syndrome**. In this condition, the pituitary gland enlarges, producing large amounts of corticotropin and other hormones such as beta-melanocyte–stimulating hormone, which darkens the skin. If necessary, Nelson's syndrome can be treated with radiation or surgical removal of the pituitary gland.

OVERPRODUCTION OF ALDOSTERONE

Overproduction of aldosterone (hyperaldosteronism) by the adrenal glands is a condition that affects the blood levels of sodium, potassium, bicarbonate, and chloride, leading to high blood pressure, weakness, and, rarely, periods of paralysis.

Aldosterone, a hormone produced and secreted by the adrenal glands, signals the kidney to excrete less sodium and more potassium. Aldosterone production is regulated partly by corticotropin in the pituitary and partly by a control mechanism in the kidneys (the renin-angiotensin-aldosterone system).▲ Renin, an enzyme pro-

---

▲ see box, page 114

duced in the kidneys, controls the activation of the hormone angiotensin, which stimulates the adrenal glands to produce aldosterone.

Hyperaldosteronism can be caused by a tumor (usually noncancerous) in the adrenal gland (a condition called Conn's syndrome). Sometimes hyperaldosteronism is a response to certain diseases. For example, the adrenal glands secrete large amounts of aldosterone if the blood pressure is very high or if the artery that carries blood to the kidneys is narrowed.

Symptoms

High levels of aldosterone can lead to low levels of potassium, causing weakness, tingling, muscle spasms, and paralysis. The nervous system may not function properly. Some people become extremely thirsty and urinate frequently, and some experience personality changes.

Symptoms of hyperaldosteronism are also associated with eating licorice, which contains a chemical very similar to aldosterone. In rare cases, people who eat a great deal of candy with real licorice flavoring may develop all the symptoms of hyperaldosteronism.

Diagnosis and Treatment

A doctor who suspects that high blood pressure or related symptoms are caused by hyperaldosteronism may measure the sodium and potassium levels in the blood. The doctor may also measure aldosterone levels and, if they're high, may prescribe spironolactone, a drug that blocks the action of aldosterone, to see if the levels return to normal. Other tests generally aren't needed.

When too much aldosterone is being produced, doctors examine the adrenal glands for an adenoma or cancer. While a computed tomography (CT) or magnetic resonance imaging (MRI) scan can be helpful, exploratory surgery is often necessary. If a growth is found, it can usually be removed. When a simple adenoma is removed, blood pressure returns to normal and other symptoms disappear about 70 percent of the time. If no tumor is found and the entire gland is overactive, partial removal of the adrenal glands may not control high blood pressure and complete removal will produce adrenal insufficiency,

requiring treatment for the rest of the person's life. However, spironolactone can usually control the symptoms, and drugs for high blood pressure are readily available. Rarely do both adrenal glands have to be removed.

Pheochromocytoma

A pheochromocytoma is a tumor that originates from the adrenal gland's chromaffin cells, causing overproduction of catecholamines, powerful hormones that induce high blood pressure and other symptoms.

With about 20 percent of pheochromocytomas, chromaffin cells grow outside their normal location in the adrenal glands. Only 5 percent of pheochromocytomas that grow within the adrenal glands are cancerous, but 30 percent of those outside the adrenal glands are cancerous. Pheochromocytomas occur in fewer than 1 in 1,000 people. They may occur in men or women at any age, but they're most common between ages 30 and 60.

Pheochromocytomas are usually very small. They rarely cause symptoms from pressure or obstruction and usually can't be felt by a doctor. However, even a small pheochromocytoma can produce a substantial amount of potent catecholamines, which causes many symptoms. The catecholamines include hormones such as adrenaline (epinephrine), norepinephrine, dopamine, and dopa, all of which stimulate high blood pressure. Catecholamines also trigger other symptoms usually associated with threatening situations that inspire panic attacks.

Some people who develop pheochromocytomas have a rare inherited condition, multiple endocrine neoplasia, that makes them prone to tumors in various endocrine glands, such as the thyroid, parathyroid, and adrenal glands.▲ Pheochromocytomas may also develop in people who have von Hippel-Lindau disease, in which blood vessels grow abnormally and form benign tumors (hemangiomas), and in those who have neurofibromatosis (von Recklinghausen's disease), in which fleshy tumors grow on nerves.

Symptoms

The most prominent symptom of a pheochromocytoma is high blood pressure, which may be very severe. In about 50 percent of the people, the high blood pressure is persistent. In the rest, the high blood pressure and other symptoms

▲ see page 726

come and go, sometimes triggered by pressure on the tumor, massage, medication (especially anesthesia and beta-blocking drugs), emotional trauma, and on rare occasions the simple act of urination. Other symptoms include any or all of the following: a fast and pounding heart rate, excessive sweating, light-headedness when standing, rapid breathing, flushing, cold and clammy skin, severe headaches, chest and stomach pain, nausea, vomiting, visual disturbances, tingling fingers, constipation, and an odd sense of impending doom. When these symptoms appear suddenly and forcefully, they can feel like a panic attack.

Diagnosis

A doctor may not suspect a pheochromocytoma because almost half the people have no symptoms other than persistent high blood pressure. However, when high blood pressure occurs in a young person, comes and goes, or accompanies other symptoms of pheochromocytoma, the doctor may request certain laboratory tests. For example, the level of certain catecholamines may be measured in urine samples.

Tests such as a computed tomography (CT) or magnetic resonance imaging (MRI) scan can help locate the pheochromocytoma. A test using injected radioactive chemicals that tend to accumulate in pheochromocytomas is also useful. A scan is then performed to see where the radioactive chemicals are.

Treatment

Usually the best treatment is to remove the pheochromocytoma. Surgery is often delayed, however, until a doctor can bring the tumor's secretion of catecholamines under control with medication, because having high levels of catecholamines can be dangerous during surgery. Phenoxybenzamine and propranolol are generally given together, and metyrosine or additional drugs are often needed to control blood pressure.

If the pheochromocytoma is a cancer that has spread, chemotherapy with cyclophosphamide, vincristine, and dacarbazine may help slow the tumor's growth. The dangerous effects of the excess catecholamines secreted by the tumor can often be blocked by continuing to take phenoxybenzamine and propranolol.

CHAPTER 147

Diabetes Mellitus

Diabetes mellitus is a disorder in which blood levels of glucose (a simple sugar) are abnormally high because the body doesn't release or use insulin adequately.

Doctors often use the full name *diabetes mellitus*, rather than *diabetes* alone, to distinguish this disorder from diabetes insipidus, a relatively rare disease.▲

Blood sugar (glucose) levels vary throughout the day, rising after a meal and returning to normal within 2 hours. Blood sugar levels are normally between 70 and 110 milligrams per deciliter (mg/dL) of blood in the morning after an overnight fast. They are usually lower than 120 to 140 mg/dL 2 hours after eating foods or drinking liq-

uids containing sugar or other carbohydrates. Normal levels tend to increase slightly but progressively after age 50, especially in people who are sedentary.

Insulin, a hormone released from the pancreas, is the primary substance responsible for maintaining appropriate blood sugar levels. Insulin allows glucose to be transported into cells so that they can produce energy or store the glucose until it's needed. The rise in blood sugar levels after eating or drinking stimulates the pancreas to pro-

---

▲ see page 703

duce insulin, preventing a greater rise in blood sugar levels and causing them to fall gradually. Because muscles use glucose for energy, blood sugar levels can also fall during physical activity.

Causes

Diabetes results when the body doesn't produce enough insulin to maintain normal blood sugar levels or when cells don't respond appropriately to insulin. People with **type I diabetes mellitus (insulin-dependent diabetes)** produce little or no insulin at all. Although about 6 percent of the United States population has some form of diabetes, only about 10 percent of all diabetics have type I disease. Most people who have type I diabetes developed the disease before age 30.

Scientists believe that an environmental factor—possibly a viral infection or a nutritional factor in childhood or early adulthood—causes the immune system to destroy the insulin-producing cells in the pancreas. Some genetic predisposition is most likely needed for this to happen. Whatever the cause, in type I diabetes more than 90 percent of the insulin-producing cells (beta cells) of the pancreas are permanently destroyed. The resulting insulin deficiency is severe, and to survive, a person with type I diabetes must regularly inject insulin.

In **type II diabetes mellitus (non–insulin-dependent diabetes),** the pancreas continues to manufacture insulin, sometimes even at higher than normal levels. However, the body develops resistance to its effects, resulting in a relative insulin deficiency. Type II diabetes may occur in children and adolescents but usually begins after age 30 and becomes progressively more common with age: About 15 percent of people over age 70 have type II diabetes. Obesity is a risk factor for type II diabetes; 80 to 90 percent of the people with this disease are obese. Certain racial and cultural groups are at increased risk: Blacks and Hispanics have a twofold to threefold increased risk of developing type II diabetes. Type II diabetes also tends to run in families.

▲ see page 1163

■ see page 676

Other less common causes of diabetes are abnormally high levels of corticosteroids, pregnancy (gestational diabetes),▲ drugs, and poisons that interfere with the production or effects of insulin, resulting in high blood sugar levels.

Symptoms

The first symptoms of diabetes are related to the direct effects of high blood sugar levels. When the blood sugar level rises above 160 to 180 mg/dL, glucose passes into the urine. When the level rises even higher, the kidneys excrete additional water to dilute the large amounts of glucose lost. Because the kidneys produce excessive urine, a person with diabetes urinates large volumes frequently (polyuria). The excessive urination creates abnormal thirst (polydipsia). Because excessive calories are lost in the urine, the person loses weight. To compensate, the person often feels excessively hungry (polyphagia). Other symptoms include blurred vision, drowsiness, nausea, and decreased endurance during exercise. In addition, people whose diabetes is poorly controlled are more susceptible to infections. Because of the severity of insulin deficiency, people with type I diabetes almost always lose weight before undergoing treatment. Most people with type II diabetes don't lose weight.

In people with type I diabetes, the symptoms begin abruptly and may progress rapidly to a condition called **diabetic ketoacidosis**. Despite high levels of sugar in the blood, most cells can't use sugar without insulin; thus, they turn to other sources of energy. Fat cells begin to break down, producing ketones, toxic chemical compounds that can make the blood acidic (ketoacidosis). The initial symptoms of diabetic ketoacidosis include excessive thirst and urination, weight loss, nausea, vomiting, fatigue, and—particularly in children—abdominal pain. Breathing tends to become deep and rapid as the body attempts to correct the blood's acidity.■ The person's breath smells like nail polish remover. Without treatment, diabetic ketoacidosis can progress to coma, sometimes within a few hours.

People with type I diabetes can develop ketoacidosis even after starting insulin treatment if they miss an insulin injection or become stressed by an infection, an accident, or a serious medical condition.

Long-term Complications of Diabetes

Tissue or Organ Affected	What Happens	Complication
Blood vessels	Atherosclerotic plaque builds up and blocks large or medium-sized arteries in the heart, brain, legs, and penis. The walls of small blood vessels are damaged so that the vessels do not transfer oxygen normally and may leak	Poor circulation causes wounds to heal poorly and can lead to heart disease, stroke, gangrene of the feet and hands, impotence, and infections
Eyes	The small blood vessels of the retina become damaged	Decreased vision and, ultimately, blindness
Kidney	Blood vessels in the kidney thicken; protein leaks into the urine; the blood isn't filtered normally	Poor kidney function; kidney failure
Nerves	Nerves are damaged because glucose isn't metabolized normally and because the blood supply is inadequate	Sudden or gradual weakness of a leg; reduced sensations, tingling, and pain in the hands and feet; chronic damage to nerves
Autonomic nervous system	The nerves that control blood pressure and digestive processes become damaged	Swings in blood pressure; swallowing difficulties and altered gastrointestinal function, with bouts of diarrhea
Skin	Poor blood flow to the skin and loss of feeling result in repeated injury	Sores, deep infections (diabetic ulcers); poor healing
Blood	White blood cell function is impaired	Increased susceptibility to infection, especially of the urinary tract and skin
Connective tissue	Glucose isn't metabolized normally, causing tissues to thicken or contract	Carpal tunnel syndrome; Dupuytren's contracture

People with type II diabetes may not have any symptoms for years or decades. When insulin deficiency progresses, symptoms may develop. Increased urination and thirst are mild at first and gradually worsen over weeks or months. Ketoacidosis is rare. If the blood sugar level becomes very high (often exceeding 1,000 mg/dL)—usually as the result of some superimposed stress such as an infection or drugs—the person may develop severe dehydration, which may lead to mental confusion, drowsiness, seizures, and a condition called **nonketotic hyperglycemic-hyperosmolar coma.**

Complications

Over time, elevated blood sugar levels damage blood vessels, nerves, and other internal structures. Complex sugar-based substances build up in the walls of small blood vessels, causing them to thicken and leak. As they thicken, they supply less and less blood, especially to the skin and nerves. Poorly controlled blood sugar levels also tend to cause the blood levels of fatty substances to rise, resulting in accelerated atherosclerosis (the buildup of plaque in blood vessels).▲ Atherosclerosis is between two and six times more common in diabetics than in nondiabetics and occurs in both men and women. Poor circulation through both the large and small blood vessels can harm the heart, brain, legs, eyes, kidneys, nerves, and skin and makes healing injuries slow.

▲ see page 118

For all of these reasons, people with diabetes may experience many serious long-term complications. Heart attacks and strokes are more common. Damage to the blood vessels of the eye can cause loss of vision (diabetic retinopathy). The kidneys can malfunction, resulting in kidney failure that requires dialysis. Damage to nerves can manifest in several ways. If a single nerve malfunctions (mononeuropathy), an arm or leg may suddenly become weak. If the nerves to the hands, legs, and feet become damaged (diabetic polyneuropathy), sensation may become abnormal and tingling or burning pain and weakness in the arms and legs may develop.▲ Damage to the nerves of the skin makes repeated injuries more likely because the person can't sense changes in pressure or temperature. Poor blood supply to the skin can also lead to ulcers, and all wounds heal slowly. Foot ulcers may become so deep and infected and heal so poorly that part of the leg may need to be amputated.

Recent evidence has shown that complications of diabetes can be prevented, delayed, or slowed by controlling blood sugar levels. Other unknown factors, including genetic ones, also determine the subsequent course of events.

Diagnosis

The diagnosis of diabetes is made when a person has abnormally high blood sugar levels. Blood sugar levels are often checked during a routine annual examination or a physical examination given before employment or participation in sports. A doctor may also check blood sugar levels to find the possible cause of such symptoms as increased thirst, urination, or hunger, or if the person has typical risk factors, such as a family history of diabetes, obesity, frequent infections, or any of the complications associated with diabetes.

To measure the blood sugar level, a blood sample is usually taken after the person has fasted for about 8 hours, but it may be taken after eating. Some elevation of blood sugar levels after eating is normal, but even then the levels shouldn't be very high. In people over 65 years old, the test is

best performed after fasting because older people have a greater increase in blood sugar levels after eating.

Another kind of blood test, an oral glucose tolerance test, may be performed in certain situations, such as when a doctor suspects that a pregnant woman has gestational diabetes.■ In this test, a person fasts, has a blood sample taken for the fasting blood sugar level, and then drinks a special solution containing a standard amount of glucose. More blood samples are then obtained over the next 2 to 3 hours.

Treatment

The main goal of diabetes treatment is to keep blood sugar levels within the normal range as much as possible. Completely normal levels are difficult to maintain, but the more closely they can be kept within the normal range, the less likely that temporary or long-term complications will develop. The main problem with trying to control blood sugar levels tightly is an increased chance of overshooting, resulting in low blood sugar levels (hypoglycemia).★

The treatment of diabetes requires attention to weight control, exercise, and diet. Many obese people with type II diabetes would not need medication if they lost weight and exercised regularly. However, weight reduction and increased exercise are difficult for most people with diabetes. Therefore, either insulin replacement therapy or an oral hypoglycemic medication is often needed. Exercise directly lowers blood sugar levels, often reducing the amount of insulin needed.

Diet management is very important. In general, people with diabetes shouldn't eat too much sweet food and should eat their meals on a regular schedule. However, eating a snack at bedtime or in the late afternoon often helps prevent hypoglycemia in people who inject themselves in the morning or evening with an intermediate-acting insulin. Since people with diabetes also have a tendency toward high cholesterol levels, dietitians usually recommend limiting the amount of saturated fat in the diet. Yet, the best way to reduce cholesterol levels is to control blood sugar levels and body weight.

Most people with diabetes benefit greatly from learning about their disease and what they can do to help control it. This education is best provided by a nurse trained in diabetes education. All diabetics must understand how diet and exercise affect their blood sugar levels and be aware

---

▲ see page 338

■ see page 1163

★ see page 724

of how to avoid complications, such as checking their skin for ulcerations. They must also take special care to avoid foot infections and can often benefit from having their toenails cut by a podiatrist. Yearly eye examinations are essential to check for changes in the blood vessels that can lead to blindness (diabetic retinopathy).

In case of injury or high or low blood sugar levels, people with diabetes should always carry a card or wear a Medic Alert bracelet identifying the disease. Alerting health care professionals to the presence of diabetes allows them to start life-saving treatment quickly.

Insulin Replacement Therapy

In type I diabetes, the pancreas can't produce insulin, so insulin must be replaced. Replacement can be accomplished only by injection; because insulin is destroyed in the stomach, it can't be taken by mouth. New forms of insulin, such as a nasal spray, are being tested. To date, these new forms haven't worked well because variability in the rate of absorption leads to problems in determining dose.

Insulin is injected under the skin into the fat layer, usually in the arm, thigh, or abdominal wall. Small syringes with very thin needles make the injections nearly painless. An air pump device that blows the insulin under the skin can be used for people who can't tolerate needles.

An insulin pen, which contains a cartridge that holds the insulin and closes like a large pen, is a convenient way to carry insulin, especially for those who take several injections a day outside the home. Another device is an insulin pump, which pumps insulin continuously from a reservoir through a small needle left in the skin. Additional doses of insulin can be programmed or triggered so that the pump more closely mimics the way the body normally produces insulin. For some people, the pump offers an added degree of control, while others find wearing the pump annoying or develop sores at the needle site.

Insulin is available in three basic forms, each with a different speed and duration of action. **Rapid-acting insulin,** such as regular insulin, is the fastest and shortest acting. This type of insulin often begins to lower blood sugar levels within 20 minutes, reaches maximum activity in 2 to 4 hours, and lasts for 6 to 8 hours. Rapid-acting insulin is often used by people who take several daily injections and is injected 15 to 20 minutes

before meals. **Intermediate-acting insulin,** such as insulin zinc suspension or isophane insulin suspension, starts to work in 1 to 3 hours, reaches its maximum activity in 6 to 10 hours, and works for 18 to 26 hours. This type of insulin may be used in the morning to provide coverage for the first part of the day or in the evening to provide coverage during the night. **Long-acting insulin,** such as extended insulin zinc suspension, has very little effect for about 6 hours but provides coverage for 28 to 36 hours. Insulin preparations are stable at room temperature for months, allowing them to be carried, brought to work, or taken on a trip.

Choosing which insulin to use may be complex. The decision is based on how tightly a person wishes to control his diabetes, how willing he is to monitor his blood sugar and adjust his dosage, how varied his daily activity is, how adept he is in learning about and understanding his disease, and how stable his blood sugar levels are during the day and from day to day.

The easiest regimen to follow is a single daily injection of one intermediate-acting insulin. However, such a regimen provides the least control over the blood sugar levels. Tighter control may be achieved by combining two insulins—a rapid-acting and an intermediate-acting insulin—in one morning dose. This requires more skill but offers more opportunity to adjust the blood sugar levels. A second injection may be taken at dinner or bedtime. Tightest control is usually achieved by injecting some rapid-acting and intermediate-acting insulin in the morning and evening along with several additional injections of rapid-acting insulin during the day.

Some people, especially older people, take the same amount of insulin every day; others adjust the insulin dose daily depending on their diet, exercise, and blood sugar patterns. The need for insulin varies with changes in food intake and amount of exercise. Thus, people who vary their diet and exercise very little usually need to make little change to their insulin dose. However, over time, insulin needs may change if the person experiences weight changes, emotional stress, or illness, especially infection. People who vary their diet and exercise patterns need to adjust their insulin accordingly.

Some people develop resistance to insulin. Because the insulin is not exactly like the insulin the body manufactures, the body can produce anti-

Characteristics of Oral Hypoglycemic Drugs

Drug	Duration of Action (hours)	Number of Daily Doses
Acarbose	About 4	3
Acetohexamide	12 to 18	1 to 2
Chlorpropamide	60	1
Glimepiride	Up to 24	1
Glipizide	Up to 24	1 to 2
Glyburide	Up to 24	1 to 2
Metformin	24 or more	2 to 3
Tolazamide	12 to 24	1 to 2
Tolbutamide	6 to 12	2 to 3

bodies to the insulin. These antibodies interfere with the insulin's activity, so a person with insulin resistance must take very large doses.

Insulin injections can affect the skin and underlying tissues at the injection site. An allergic reaction, which occurs rarely, produces pain and burning, followed by redness, itchiness, and swelling around the injection site for several hours. More commonly, the injections either cause fat deposits, making the skin look lumpy, or destroy fat, causing indentation of the skin. Changing the site of injection with each dose and switching the type of insulin generally prevent these complications. Insulin resistance and insulin allergy are uncommon with the use of synthetic human insulins, which are the insulins predominantly used today.

Oral Hypoglycemic Drugs

Oral hypoglycemic sulfonylurea drugs such as glipizide, glyburide, tolbutamide, and chlorpropamide can often lower blood sugar levels adequately in people with type II diabetes but aren't effective in type I diabetes. They lower the blood sugar levels by stimulating the pancreas to release insulin and by increasing its effectiveness. Another type of oral drug, metformin, does not affect the release of insulin but increases the body's response to its own insulin. A doctor may prescribe metformin alone or with a sulfonylurea drug. Yet another drug, acarbose, works by delaying absorption of glucose in the intestine.

Oral hypoglycemic drugs are usually prescribed for people with type II diabetes if diet and exercise fail to lower blood sugar levels adequately. The drugs can sometimes be taken only once a day, in the morning, although some people need two or three doses. If oral hypoglycemic drugs can't control blood sugar well enough, insulin injections alone or in combination with the oral drugs may be needed.

Monitoring Treatment

Monitoring blood sugar levels is an essential part of diabetes care. Although urine can also be tested for the presence of glucose, checking urine is not a good way to monitor treatment or adjust therapy. Fortunately, blood sugar levels can now be measured easily at home.

A drop of blood is obtained by pricking the tip of the finger with a small lancet. The lancet holds a tiny needle that can be jabbed into the finger or placed in a spring-loaded device that easily and quickly pierces the skin. Most diabetics find the pricking nearly painless. Then, a drop of blood is placed on a reagent strip. In response to sugar, the reagent strip changes color or undergoes some other chemical change. Some strips change color enough to read the blood sugar level when the color of the strip is compared to colors printed on a chart. A better and more accurate system is to use a machine that reads the changes in the test strip and reports the result on a digital display. Most of these machines time the reaction and read the result automatically. The machines are small, from the size of a pen to that of a pack of cigarettes.

People with diabetes should record their blood sugar levels and report them to their doctor or nurse for advice in adjusting the insulin or oral hypoglycemic drug dose. Some people can be taught to adjust the insulin dose on their own as necessary between visits to their doctor or nurse.

Doctors use a blood test called glycosylated hemoglobin, also called hemoglobin A_{1C}, to monitor treatment. When the blood sugar level is high, changes occur in hemoglobin, the chemical that carries oxygen in the blood. These changes are in direct proportion to the blood sugar level over an extended period. Thus, unlike the blood sugar measurement, which reveals the level at a particular moment, the glycosylated hemoglobin measurement demonstrates whether the blood sugar level has been controlled over the previous few weeks. The normal level for glycosylated hemoglobin is less than 7 percent. Diabetics rarely achieve such levels, but tight control aims to come close to it. Levels above 9 percent show poor control, and levels above 12 percent show very poor control. Most doctors who specialize in diabetes care recommend that glycosylated hemoglobin be measured every 3 to 6 months.

Treating Complications

Both insulin and oral drugs can lower blood sugar levels too much, causing **hypoglycemia.**▲ Hypoglycemia can also occur if a person with diabetes doesn't eat enough or on time or exercises strenuously without eating. When blood sugar levels are too low, the first organ affected is the brain. To protect the brain, the body immediately begins to manufacture glucose from glycogen stores in the liver. This process involves the release of epinephrine (adrenaline), which tends to induce hunger, anxiety, a sense of heightened awareness, and a shaky feeling. The lack of blood glucose to the brain can cause a headache.

Hypoglycemia must be treated quickly because within minutes it can become severe, leading to increasing confusion, coma, and rarely permanent brain injury. At the first sign of hypoglycemia, the person should eat some form of sugar. Therefore, people with diabetes should always carry candy, lumps of sugar, or glucose tablets to treat episodes of hypoglycemia. Other options are to drink a glass of milk (which contains lactose, a type of sugar), sugar water, or fruit juice or to eat a piece of cake, some fruit, or other sweet food. People with type I diabetes should always carry or have available glucagon (a hormone that raises blood sugar levels), which can be injected in case they aren't able to take any food containing sugar.

Diabetic ketoacidosis is a medical emergency. Without prompt and excellent treatment, diabetic ketoacidosis can cause a coma and death. Hos-

---

Symptoms of Low Blood Sugar Levels

- Sudden severe hunger
- Headache
- Sudden anxiety
- Tremulousness (shakiness)
- Sweating
- Confusion
- Unconsciousness, coma

---

pitalization, usually in an intensive care unit, is necessary. Large amounts of intravenous fluids are given along with electrolytes, such as sodium, potassium, chloride, and phosphate, to replace those lost through excessive urination. Insulin is generally given intravenously so that it works quickly and the dose can be adjusted frequently. Blood levels of glucose, ketones, and electrolytes are measured every few hours so that doctors can adjust the treatment. Doctors also take samples of arterial blood to measure its acidity. Sometimes additional treatments are needed to correct the acidity, although controlling blood sugar levels and replacing electrolytes usually allow the body to restore the normal acid-base balance.

The treatment of **nonketotic hyperglycemic-hyperosmolar coma** is similar to that of diabetic ketoacidosis. Fluid and electrolytes must be replaced. Blood sugar levels must be restored gradually to avoid sudden shifts of fluid into the brain. Blood sugar levels tend to be more easily controlled than in diabetic ketoacidosis, and blood acidity problems aren't severe.

Most of the long-term complications of diabetes are progressive unless the blood sugar level is tightly controlled. **Diabetic retinopathy,** however, can be directly treated. Laser surgery can seal the leaking eye blood vessels to prevent permanent damage to the retina. Early laser treatment can help prevent or substantially slow the loss of vision.

▲ see page 724

Hypoglycemia

Hypoglycemia is a condition in which blood sugar (glucose) levels are abnormally low.

Normally, the body maintains the level of blood sugar within a rather narrow range (about 70 to 110 milligrams per deciliter of blood). In diabetes, the blood sugar levels become too high; in hypoglycemia, the blood sugar levels become too low. Low blood sugar causes many organ systems in the body to malfunction. The brain is particularly sensitive to low blood sugar levels, because glucose is the brain's major energy source. The brain responds to low blood sugar levels and, through the nervous system, stimulates the adrenal glands to release epinephrine (adrenaline). This stimulates the liver to release sugar to adjust the level in the blood. If the level falls too low, the brain's function may be impaired.

Causes

Hypoglycemia has several different causes: excessive secretion of insulin from the pancreas, too high a dose of insulin or other medication given to a diabetic person to lower the blood sugar levels, an abnormality in the pituitary or adrenal glands, or an abnormality in the liver's storage of carbohydrate or production of glucose.

In general, hypoglycemia can be categorized as drug-related or non–drug-related. Most cases of hypoglycemia occur in diabetics and are drug-related. Non–drug-related hypoglycemia can be further divided into fasting hypoglycemia, in which hypoglycemia occurs after fasting, and reactive hypoglycemia, in which hypoglycemia occurs as a reaction to eating, usually of carbohydrates.

Most often, hypoglycemia is caused by insulin or other drugs (sulfonylureas) given to people with diabetes to lower the blood sugar levels. If the dose is too high for the amount of food eaten, the drug may lower the blood sugar levels too much. People with long-standing severe diabetes are particularly prone to severe hypoglycemia. This happens because their pancreatic islet cells don't produce glucagon normally and their adre-nal glands don't produce epinephrine normally—the major immediate mechanisms by which the body counteracts a low blood sugar level. Many drugs other than those for diabetes, most notably pentamidine used to treat a form of AIDS-related pneumonia, can cause hypoglycemia.

Hypoglycemia is sometimes seen in people with psychologic disturbances who surreptitiously administer insulin or hypoglycemic drugs to themselves. The people likely to do this are usually those who have access to the drugs, such as health care workers or relatives of diabetics.

Alcohol consumption, usually in people who drink heavily without eating for a long time (which depletes carbohydrates stored in the liver), can produce hypoglycemia severe enough to cause stupor. Hypoglycemia-induced stupor can even occur in a person whose blood alcohol level is below that legally allowed for driving. Police and emergency department personnel may not realize that a stuporous person whose breath smells of alcohol is hypoglycemic rather than just inebriated.

Prolonged strenuous exercise rarely induces hypoglycemia in otherwise healthy people. Prolonged fasting causes hypoglycemia only if a person has another disease, especially a disease of the pituitary or adrenal glands, or consumes large amounts of alcohol. The liver's carbohydrate stores may fall so low that the body can't maintain adequate blood sugar levels. In some people with a liver abnormality, just a few hours of fasting may cause hypoglycemia. Infants and children with an abnormality in any of the liver enzyme systems that metabolize sugars may develop hypoglycemia between meals.

Some people who have undergone certain types of stomach surgery develop hypoglycemia between meals (alimentary hypoglycemia, a type of reactive hypoglycemia). Hypoglycemia occurs because sugars are absorbed very quickly, stimulating excessive insulin production. The high level of insulin causes a rapid fall in the blood sugar level. Rarely, alimentary hypoglycemia occurs in people who haven't had surgery, in whom the condition is called idiopathic alimentary hypoglycemia.

In the past, doctors tended to diagnose reactive hypoglycemia in people who had symptoms resembling those of hypoglycemia 2 to 4 hours after a meal or to diagnose people with vague symptoms (mainly fatigue) as having hypoglycemia. However, measurement of blood sugar levels during an episode of symptoms doesn't reveal true hypoglycemia. Attempts have been made to reproduce reactive hypoglycemia with an oral glucose tolerance test, but this test doesn't accurately reflect what happens after a normal meal.

A type of reactive hypoglycemia that occurs in infants and children is caused by foods that contain the sugars fructose and galactose or the amino acid leucine. Fructose and galactose prevent the release of glucose from the liver; leucine stimulates overproduction of insulin from the pancreas. In either case, the result is a low blood sugar level some time after eating foods containing these nutrients. In adults, the ingestion of alcohol in combination with sugar, for example, as a gin and tonic, may precipitate reactive hypoglycemia.

Excessive insulin production also can cause hypoglycemia. Excessive production may result from a tumor of the pancreas' insulin-producing cells (an insulinoma) or, rarely, from a generalized proliferation of these cells. Infrequently, a tumor outside the pancreas causes hypoglycemia by producing an insulinlike hormone.

A rare cause of hypoglycemia is an autoimmune disease in which the body produces antibodies to insulin.▲ The levels of insulin in the blood fluctuate abnormally as the pancreas produces excessive insulin to cope with the antibodies. This condition may occur in people with or without diabetes.

Hypoglycemia can also result from kidney or heart failure, cancer, malnutrition, abnormal pituitary or adrenal function, shock, and severe infection. Extensive liver disease—for example from viral hepatitis, cirrhosis, or cancer—may also produce hypoglycemia.

Symptoms

The body first responds to a fall in blood sugar levels by releasing epinephrine (adrenaline) from the adrenal glands and certain nerve endings. Epi-

nephrine stimulates the release of sugar from body stores but also causes symptoms similar to those of an anxiety attack: sweating, nervousness, quivering, faintness, palpitations, and sometimes hunger. More severe hypoglycemia reduces the glucose supply to the brain, causing dizziness, confusion, fatigue, weakness, headaches, inappropriate behavior that can be mistaken for drunkenness, inability to concentrate, vision abnormalities, epilepsylike seizures, and coma. Prolonged hypoglycemia may permanently damage the brain. Both the anxietylike symptoms and impairment of brain function can begin slowly or suddenly, progressing from mild discomfort to severe confusion or panic within minutes. People who take insulin or oral hypoglycemic drugs for diabetes are most commonly affected.

In a person with an insulin-producing pancreatic tumor, symptoms are likely to occur early in the morning after an overnight fast, especially if the blood sugar stores are further depleted by exercise before breakfast. At first, people with a tumor usually have only occasional episodes of hypoglycemia, but over months or years, episodes become more frequent and severe.

Diagnosis

Doctors measure the blood sugar and then insulin levels when a nondiabetic and otherwise healthy person develops anxiety, drunkenlike behavior, or the other symptoms of impaired brain function described above. The symptoms of hypoglycemia rarely develop until the blood sugar level falls below 50 milligrams per deciliter of blood, although occasionally people develop symptoms at slightly higher levels, and some don't develop symptoms until their levels are much lower. Low blood sugar levels along with the symptoms of hypoglycemia confirm the diagnosis. If symptoms are relieved as the blood sugar level rises within a few minutes of ingesting sugar, the diagnosis is supported.

A doctor tests a person's blood sugar in the doctor's office. Blood sugar can be tested at home, using a drop of blood obtained by pricking the finger at the time symptoms occur and a device to monitor blood sugar levels, but home mon-

▲ see page 816

itoring of blood sugar is recommended only for diabetics. The oral glucose tolerance test, which is commonly used to help diagnose diabetes, is rarely used for diagnosing hypoglycemia because results are often misleading.

A doctor can almost always find the cause of hypoglycemia. The person's medical history, a physical examination, and simple laboratory tests are usually all that are needed to determine the cause. However, a few people may need to be hospitalized for more extensive testing. If the doctor suspects autoimmune hypoglycemia, the blood is tested for antibodies to insulin.

Measurements of insulin levels in the blood during fasting (sometimes up to 72 hours) may be needed to determine whether the person has an insulin-secreting tumor. Ideally, a tumor should be located before surgery. However, although some insulin-secreting tumors of the pancreas are visible on a computed tomography (CT) scan, magnetic resonance imaging (MRI) scan, or ultrasound imaging, tumors are usually so small that they can't be detected with these imaging devices. Frequently, exploratory surgery is needed to detect an insulin-secreting tumor.

Treatment

The symptoms of hypoglycemia are relieved within minutes of consuming sugar in any form, such as candy or glucose tablets, or of drinking a glass of fruit juice, a glass of water with several tablespoons of sugar, or a glass of milk (which contains lactose, a type of sugar). People with recurring episodes of hypoglycemia, especially diabetics, often prefer to carry glucose tablets because the tablets take effect quickly and provide a consistent amount of sugar. Both diabetic and nondiabetic people with hypoglycemia may benefit from consuming sugar followed by a food that provides longer-lasting carbohydrates (such as bread or crackers). When hypoglycemia is severe or prolonged and taking sugar by mouth isn't possible, doctors give glucose intravenously to prevent serious brain damage.

People who are known to be at risk for severe episodes of hypoglycemia may keep glucagon on hand for emergencies. Glucagon is a protein hormone secreted by the islet cells of the pancreas, which stimulates the liver to produce large amounts of glucose from its carbohydrate stores. It is given by injection and generally restores blood sugar within 5 to 15 minutes.

Insulin-secreting tumors should be removed surgically. However, since they are very small and difficult to locate, the surgery should be performed by a specialist experienced in dealing with this problem. Before surgery, the person may need a drug such as diazoxide to inhibit the tumor's insulin secretion. Sometimes more than one tumor is present, and if the surgeon doesn't find them all, a second operation may be necessary.

Nondiabetics who are prone to hypoglycemia often can avoid episodes by eating frequent small meals rather than the usual three meals a day. People prone to hypoglycemia should carry identification or a Medic Alert bracelet to inform emergency medical personnel of their condition.

CHAPTER 149

Multiple Endocrine Neoplasia Syndromes

Multiple endocrine neoplasias are rare inherited diseases in which benign or malignant (cancerous) tumors develop in several endocrine glands.

The tumors of multiple endocrine neoplasias can appear as early as infancy or as late as age 70. The abnormalities caused by multiple endocrine neoplasias result mostly from the excess hormones that the tumors produce.

Multiple endocrine neoplasias occur in three patterns, called types I, IIA, and IIB, although the types occasionally overlap.

Tumors of Multiple Endocrine Neoplasias

Tumor	Percentage of People With the Disease Who Have This Type of Tumor		
	Type I Disease	Type IIA Disease	Type IIB Disease
Noncancerous growths of the parathyroid glands	90% or more	25%	Less than 1%
Cancerous or noncancerous growths of the pancreas	80%	0%	0%
Noncancerous growths of the pituitary gland	65%	0%	0%
Cancerous growths (medullary carcinomas) of the thyroid gland	0%	More than 90%	More than 90%
Growths (usually noncancerous) of the adrenal gland (pheochromocytomas)	0%	50%	60%
Growths around nerves (neuromas)	0%	0%	100%

Type I Disease

People with multiple endocrine neoplasia type I develop tumors of the parathyroid glands (the small glands located next to the thyroid gland), the pancreas, the pituitary gland, or all three.

Almost all of the people with this disease have tumors of the parathyroid glands; the tumors cause the glands to produce too much parathyroid hormone (a condition called hyperparathyroidism).▲ The excess parathyroid hormone usually raises calcium levels in the blood, sometimes leading to kidney stones.

Most people with type I disease also develop tumors of the islet cells of the pancreas. About 40 percent of these tumors produce high levels of insulin and consequent low blood sugar levels (hypoglycemia), especially if the person hasn't eaten for several hours. More than half of islet cell tumors produce excessive gastrin, which signals the stomach to overproduce acid. People with these tumors generally develop peptic ulcers that often bleed, perforate and leak stomach contents into the abdomen, or obstruct the stomach. Diarrhea and fatty, smelly stools (steatorrhea) are common. The remaining islet cell tumors may produce other hormones, such as vasoactive intestinal polypeptide, which can cause severe diarrhea and lead to dehydration.

About one third of the time, the islet cell tumors are cancerous and sometimes spread (metastasize) to other areas of the body. But these cancers tend to grow more slowly than other types of pancreatic cancer.

About two thirds of the people with type I disease develop pituitary gland tumors. About 25 percent of these tumors produce the hormone prolactin, leading to menstrual abnormalities in women and impotence in men. Another 25 percent produce growth hormone, leading to acromegaly.■ A very small percentage of pituitary tumors produce corticotropin, leading to high levels of corticosteroid hormones and Cushing's syndrome.★ Nearly 25 percent appear to pro-

▲ see page 673

■ see page 701

★ see page 714

duce no hormones at all. Some pituitary tumors cause headaches, impaired vision, and decreased pituitary gland function.

Some people with type I disease develop thyroid and adrenal gland tumors. A very small percentage develop carcinoid tumors.▲ Some people also develop soft, noncancerous fatty growths just below the skin (lipomas).

Type IIA Disease

Multiple endocrine neoplasia type IIA can include a rare type of thyroid cancer (medullary carcinoma), pheochromocytoma (a type of adrenal gland tumor that is usually not cancerous), and overactive parathyroid glands.

Almost everyone with type IIA disease develops medullary thyroid cancer.■ About 50 percent develop pheochromocytomas, which usually raise blood pressure because of the epinephrine and other substances they produce.★ The high blood pressure may be intermittent or constant and is often very severe.

About 25 percent of the people with type IIA disease have overactive parathyroid glands and show symptoms of having increased blood calcium levels, which may lead to kidney stones and sometimes to kidney failure. In another 25 percent, the parathyroid glands increase in size without producing large amounts of parathyroid hormone, so the people don't have problems related to high calcium levels.

Type IIB Disease

Multiple endocrine neoplasia type IIB can consist of medullary thyroid cancer, pheochromocytoma, and neuromas (growths around the nerves). Some people with type IIB disease have no family history of it.

The medullary thyroid cancer that occurs in type IIB disease tends to develop at an early age

---

▲ see page 730

■ see page 711

★ see page 716

● see page 1306

and has been reported in infants as young as 3 months of age. The medullary thyroid cancers in type IIB also grow faster and spread more rapidly than those in type IIA disease.

Almost all the people with type IIB disease develop neuromas in their mucous membranes. The neuromas appear as glistening bumps around the lips, tongue, and lining of the mouth. Neuromas may also occur on the eyelids and glistening surfaces of the eyes, including the conjunctiva and cornea. The eyelids and lips may thicken.

Gastrointestinal tract abnormalities cause constipation and diarrhea. Occasionally, the colon develops large, dilated loops (megacolon). These abnormalities probably result from neuromas growing on the intestinal nerves.

People with type IIB disease often develop spinal abnormalities, especially curvature of the spine, as well as bony abnormalities of the feet and thighbones. Many people have long limbs and loose joints (a marfanoid habitus, so-called because the appearance is similar to that of someone with Marfan's syndrome).●

Treatment

No cure is known for any of the multiple endocrine neoplasias. Doctors treat each tumor individually, either by removing it or by correcting the hormone imbalance. Because medullary thyroid cancer is ultimately fatal if untreated, a doctor will most likely recommend surgically removing the thyroid gland if a person with type IIA disease has pheochromocytoma or hyperparathyroidism, even if the diagnosis of medullary thyroid cancer can't be established before the surgery. In type IIB disease, medullary thyroid cancer is particularly aggressive. A doctor will recommend removing the thyroid gland as soon as the diagnosis is established. This type of thyroid cancer can't be treated with radioactive iodine.

Screening

Since about half of the children of people with multiple endocrine neoplasia will inherit the disease, screening is important for early diagnosis and treatment. Tests for each type of tumor are currently available. Recently, the abnormal genes responsible for types IIA and IIB disease were identified. Tests for the abnormal gene will eventually be available, permitting earlier and more effective diagnosis and treatment.

CHAPTER 150

Polyglandular Deficiency Syndromes

Polyglandular deficiency syndromes are conditions in which several endocrine glands become underactive and produce lower than normal amounts of hormones.

People who develop a polyglandular deficiency syndrome probably have a genetic predisposition to it. Often, the activity of an endocrine gland is suppressed by an autoimmune reaction▲ that causes inflammation and destroys part or all of the gland. However, endocrine gland activity can also be suppressed by an infection, an inadequate blood supply to the gland, or a tumor. Frequently, after one gland is damaged, others also become damaged, causing many glands to slow or stop functioning (multiple endocrine gland failure).

Symptoms

The symptoms of polyglandular deficiency depend on which endocrine glands are malfunctioning. For example, hypothyroidism results when an underactive thyroid gland produces insufficient amounts of thyroid hormones;■ Addison's disease results when underactive adrenal glands produce insufficient amounts of corticosteroid hormones.★

Polyglandular deficiency syndromes are categorized into three types, according to whether symptoms develop in childhood or adulthood and which endocrine glands are involved.

Type 1 polyglandular deficiency syndrome usually develops in childhood. An underactive parathyroid gland (hypoparathyroidism) is the most common feature. The next most common are underactive adrenal glands (Addison's disease) and chronic yeast infections (chronic mucocutaneous candidiasis). The yeast infections probably occur because people with this syndrome have an inadequate immune response to common yeasts and don't react normally to fight infection. Rarely, underactive production of insulin in the pancreas causes diabetes. Additionally, people with type 1 polyglandular deficiency syndrome often have hepatitis, gallstones, difficulty in absorbing food, and premature balding.

Type 2 polyglandular deficiency syndrome generally develops in adults, usually around age 30. The adrenal glands always are underactive, and the thyroid gland frequently is. However, some people develop an overactive thyroid gland (hyperthyroidism). Underactive pancreatic function leads to insufficient amounts of insulin and, thus, diabetes. Neither hypoparathyroidism nor yeast infections are part of the type 2 syndrome.

Type 3 polyglandular deficiency syndrome develops in adults and may be considered a preliminary stage of the type 2 syndrome. People who have at least two of the following symptoms—an underactive thyroid gland, diabetes, pernicious anemia, loss of skin pigmentation (vitiligo), and hair loss (alopecia)—but no adrenal gland problems are categorized as having the type 3 syndrome. If adrenal gland failure develops, the syndrome becomes type 2.

Diagnosis

Blood tests are used to measure hormone production in the affected glands. Because one endocrine gland may be noticeably less active than others, a doctor may not notice until other symptoms develop that more than one endocrine gland is underactive. When additional tests show that several glands are underactive, the diagnosis of a polyglandular deficiency syndrome is confirmed.

Treatment

Although polyglandular deficiency syndromes can't be cured, doctors can prescribe hormone replacement therapy. A person with an underactive thyroid gland can be given thyroid hormone, a person with underactive adrenal glands can be given corticosteroids, and a person with diabetes can be given insulin. But hormone replacement therapy can't correct infertility or most other problems caused by underactive sex glands (gonads).

▲ see page 816

■ see page 708

★ see page 712

Carcinoid

Carcinoid is a cancer, usually occurring in the gastrointestinal tract, that can produce excessive amounts of several neuropeptides and amines, which have hormonelike effects. If the carcinoid spreads to the liver, it may cause episodes of flushing, bluish skin, abdominal cramps, diarrhea, heart damage, and other symptoms, which constitute the **carcinoid syndrome.**

Carcinoid tumors produce an excess of neuropeptides and amines (hormonelike substances) such as bradykinin, serotonin, histamine, and prostaglandins. Normally these substances control internal body functions. In excessive amounts, however, they can cause the symptoms of carcinoid syndrome.

Carcinoid tumors usually originate in hormone-producing cells that line the small intestine (enteroendocrine cells) or other cells of the gastrointestinal tract, pancreas, testes, ovaries, or lungs. What causes carcinoid tumors to form isn't known. On rare occasions, other cancers such as oat cell (small cell) carcinoma of the lung, islet cell carcinoma of the pancreas, and medullary carcinoma of the thyroid also produce substances that cause carcinoid syndrome.

When carcinoid tumors occur in the gastrointestinal tract, the hormonelike substances are released into the bloodstream and flow directly to the liver, where enzymes destroy them. Tumors that have spread (metastasized) to the liver release their hormonelike substances into the bloodstream without processing them first in the liver. Therefore, carcinoid tumors that originate in the gastrointestinal tract generally don't produce symptoms unless the tumors have spread to the liver. In this case, the hormonelike substances circulate throughout the body, causing symptoms of the carcinoid syndrome that vary, depending on which substances are produced. Carcinoid tumors in the lungs and ovaries also cause symptoms because the substances they produce bypass the liver and circulate widely in the bloodstream.

Symptoms

Fewer than 10 percent of the people with carcinoid tumors develop the carcinoid syndrome. Most people with carcinoid tumors have symptoms similar to those of other intestinal cancers, mainly cramping pain and changes in bowel movements as a result of obstruction.

The most common and often the earliest symptom of carcinoid syndrome is an uncomfortable flushing, typically of the head and neck. The flushing is thought to be caused by excess histamine and bradykinin, which dilate blood vessels. Flushing is often triggered by emotions, by eating, or by drinking alcohol or hot liquids. The skin can change color dramatically, from pale to red to a blue hue (cyanosis). Excess serotonin triggers the muscles around the intestines to contract, causing diarrhea, cramping, and malabsorption of foods. Malabsorption leads to malnutrition and produces fatty, very foul-smelling stools in some people.

Carcinoid syndrome can damage the heart and lungs. In many people, abnormal fibrous material develops in the heart (endocardial fibrosis), which damages the heart valves and impairs the heart's pumping ability. Because serotonin carried in the bloodstream is destroyed during passage through the lungs (before it reaches the left side of the heart), almost all heart problems occur in the right side. Whether serotonin is the only substance involved and how the body produces the fibrous material are both unknown. Some people with carcinoid syndrome develop asthmatic wheezing; others lose interest in sex and become impotent.

Diagnosis

Carcinoid tumors are diagnosed by x-ray, computed tomography (CT), magnetic resonance imaging (MRI), endoscopic studies, and chemical tests performed on urine.

When doctors suspect a carcinoid tumor, they confirm the diagnosis by measuring the amount of 5-hydroxyindoleacetic acid (5-HIAA)—one of the metabolites (chemical by-products) of serotonin—in the person's urine, which is collected over a 24-hour period. For at least 3 days before undergoing this test, the person should refrain from eating foods that are rich in serotonin—bananas, tomatoes, plums, avocados, pineapples, eggplants, and walnuts. Certain drugs, including guaifenesin (found in many cough syrups), methocarbamol (a muscle relaxant), and phenothiazines (tranquilizers), also interfere with test results.

To help make the diagnosis, a doctor sometimes gives drugs such as calcium gluconate, catecholamines, pentagastrin, or alcohol to provoke flushing. However, because provocative tests can cause uncomfortable and sometimes serious symptoms, they are done only under close observation in a hospital. A CT or MRI scan can help determine whether the tumor has spread to the liver. Extensive examination and sometimes exploratory surgery of the abdomen may be needed to locate the tumor (or tumors) and determine the extent of its growth.

Diagnostic arteriography and radionuclide scanning are important new techniques for both detecting a carcinoid tumor and determining its growth. A recent discovery shows that most carcinoids have receptors for the hormone somatostatin. Doctors can therefore inject a radioactive form of somatostatin into the blood and use nuclear scanning to detect carcinoids and metastases. About 90 percent of the tumors can be found using this technique.

Treatment

When the carcinoid tumor is restricted to a specific area, such as the lungs, appendix, small intestine, or rectum, surgical removal may cure the disease. If the tumor has spread to the liver, as can happen when a tumor originates outside the lungs, surgery rarely cures the disease but may help the doctor diagnose the problem and may relieve symptoms.

Neither radiation therapy nor chemotherapy is effective in curing carcinoid tumors. However, combinations of certain chemotherapy drugs (streptozocin with fluorouracil and sometimes doxorubicin) may relieve symptoms. A drug called octreotide can also relieve symptoms, and tamoxifen, interferon alfa, and eflornithine may reduce the tumor's growth. Phenothiazines, cimetidine, and phentolamine are used to control flushing. Prednisone is sometimes given to people with carcinoid tumors of the lung who have episodes of severe flushing. Diarrhea may be controlled with codeine, tincture of opium, diphenoxylate, cyproheptadine, or methysergide. High blood pressure may be treated with various antihypertensive drugs such as methyldopa and phenoxybenzamine.

Only surgical removal of carcinoid tumors that haven't metastasized can provide a cure. Nevertheless, the tumors grow so slowly that even people who have metastases often survive for 10 to 15 years.

Blood Disorders

Biology of Blood

Blood is a combination of liquid, cells, and cell-like particles that courses through the arteries, capillaries, and veins, delivering oxygen and essential nutrients to tissues and carrying away carbon dioxide and other waste products.

Liquid Components

More than half of the blood consists of a liquid (plasma), which is mostly water containing dissolved salts and proteins. The major protein in plasma is albumin. Others are antibodies (immunoglobulins) and clotting proteins. Plasma also contains hormones, electrolytes, fats, sugars, minerals, and vitamins.

Plasma does much more than transport blood cells. It provides a reservoir of water for the body, prevents blood vessels from collapsing and clogging, and helps maintain blood pressure and circulation throughout the body. Even more important, the antibodies in plasma actively defend the body against foreign substances such as viruses, bacteria, fungi, and cancer cells, while the clotting proteins control bleeding. Besides transporting hormones and regulating their effects, plasma cools and warms the body as needed.

Cellular Components

The cellular components of blood are red blood cells, white blood cells, and platelets, all of which are suspended in the plasma.

Red blood cells (erythrocytes), the most numerous of the three cellular components, normally make up almost half of the blood's volume. These cells are filled with hemoglobin, which enables them to carry oxygen from the lungs and deliver it to all body tissues. Oxygen is consumed to provide energy to cells, leaving carbon dioxide as a waste product, which the red blood cells carry away from the tissues and back to the lungs.

White blood cells (leukocytes) are fewer in number, with a ratio of about 1 white blood cell to

_____

▲ see page 811

■ see page 752

every 660 red blood cells. There are five main types of white blood cells that work together to provide the body's major mechanisms for fighting infections, including the production of antibodies.▲ **Neutrophils,** also called granulocytes because they contain enzyme-filled granules, are the most prevalent white blood cell type. They help protect the body against bacterial and fungal infections and ingest foreign debris. They consist of two types: band (immature) and segmented (mature) neutrophils. **Lymphocytes** consist of two main types: T lymphocytes, which help protect against viral infections and can detect and destroy some cancer cells, and B lymphocytes, which develop into cells that produce antibodies (plasma cells). **Monocytes** ingest dead or damaged cells and provide immunologic defenses against many infective organisms. **Eosinophils** kill parasites, destroy cancer cells, and are involved in allergic responses. **Basophils** also participate in allergic responses.

Platelets (thrombocytes) are cell-like particles smaller than red or white blood cells. As part of the blood's protective mechanism for stopping bleeding, they gather at a bleeding site, where they are activated. Once activated, they become sticky and clump together to form a plug that helps seal the blood vessel and stop the bleeding. At the same time, they release substances that help promote clotting.■

Red blood cells tend to flow smoothly through the bloodstream, but white blood cells do not. Many of them adhere to blood vessel walls or even penetrate the walls to enter other tissues. When white blood cells reach the site of an infection or other problem, they release substances that attract more white blood cells. The white cells function like an army, dispersed throughout the body but ready at a moment's notice to gather and fight off an invading organism.

Blood Cell Formation

Red blood cells, white blood cells, and platelets are produced in the bone marrow. In addition, lymphocytes are also produced in the lymph nodes and spleen, and T lymphocytes are produced and mature in the thymus, a small gland

How Blood Cells Develop

Stem cells divide and take different developmental pathways that result in the different types of blood cells and platelets. In this diagram, several intermediate forms are omitted.

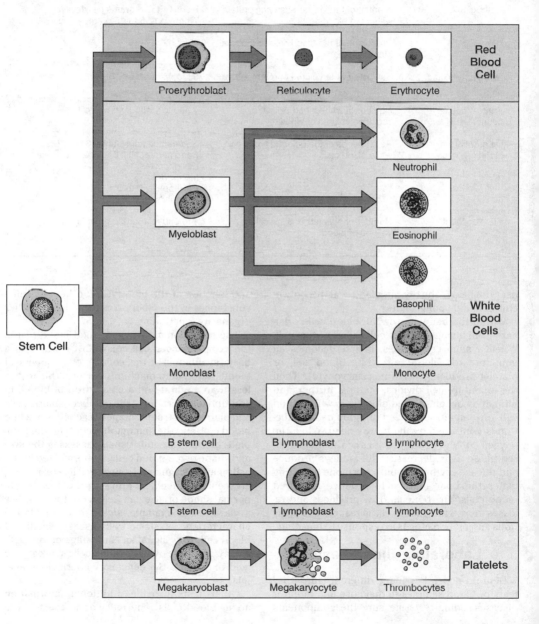

Complete Blood Cell Count

Test	What It Measures	Normal Values
Hemoglobin	Amount of this oxygen-carrying protein within red blood cells	Men: 14 to 16 grams per deciliter Women: 12.5 to 15 grams per deciliter
Hematocrit	Proportion of red blood cells to the total blood volume	Men: 42 to 50% Women: 38 to 47%
Mean corpuscular volume	Estimate of the volume of red blood cells	86 to 98 cubic micrometers
White blood cell count	Number of white blood cells in a specified volume of blood	4,500 to 10,500 per microliter
Differential white blood cell count	Percentages of the different types of white blood cells	Segmented neutrophils: 34 to 75% Band neutrophils: 0 to 8% Lymphocytes: 12 to 50% Monocytes: 15% Eosinophils: 0 to 5% Basophils: 0 to 3%
Platelet count	Number of platelets in a specified volume of blood	140,000 to 450,000 per microliter

near the heart. The thymus gland is active only in children and young adults.

Within the bone marrow, all blood cells originate from a single type of cell called a stem cell. When a stem cell divides, it first becomes an immature red blood cell, white blood cell, or platelet-producing cell (megakaryocyte). Then the immature cell divides, matures further, and ultimately becomes a red blood cell, white blood cell, or platelet. The speed of blood cell production is controlled by the body's need. When the oxygen content of body tissues or the number of red blood cells decreases, the kidneys produce and release erythropoietin, a hormone that stimulates the bone marrow to produce more red blood cells. The bone marrow produces and releases more white blood cells in response to infections and more platelets in response to bleeding.

Laboratory Blood Tests

Doctors depend on many different laboratory tests of blood samples to diagnose and monitor diseases. Some tests measure the components

and function of the blood itself; others examine substances in the blood to determine how other organs are functioning.

The most commonly performed blood test is the **complete blood cell count (CBC),** which is a basic evaluation of the cellular components of blood. Automated machines perform this test in less than a minute on a small drop of blood. In addition to determining the number of blood cells and platelets, the percentage of each type of white blood cell, and the hemoglobin content, the complete blood cell count usually assesses the size and shape of red blood cells. Abnormal red blood cells may be fragmented or shaped like teardrops, crescents, or needles. Knowing the specific abnormal shape or size can help a doctor diagnose a disease. For example, sickle-shaped cells are characteristic of sickle cell disease, small red blood cells may signal an early stage of iron deficiency, and large oval red blood cells suggest folic acid or vitamin B_{12} deficiency (pernicious anemia).

Other tests provide additional information about blood cells. The **reticulocyte count** is the number of newly formed (young) red blood cells (reticulocytes) in a specified volume of blood. Reticulocytes normally make up about 1 percent of the total number of red blood cells. When the body needs more red blood cells, as in anemia, the bone marrow normally responds by producing more reticulocytes. Thus, the reticulocyte count is a measure of bone marrow function. Tests to determine red blood cell fragility and membrane characteristics help doctors further evaluate the cause of the anemia.

White blood cells can be counted as a group (white blood cell count). When more detailed information is needed, a doctor requests a count of the specific types of white blood cells (differential white blood cell count).▲ Platelets also can be counted separately.

One of the most common tests performed on plasma is an analysis of electrolytes. Electrolytes include sodium, chloride, potassium, and bicarbonate, as well as less commonly measured substances such as calcium, magnesium, and phosphates. Other tests measure the amount of protein (usually albumin), sugar (glucose), and toxic waste products that the kidneys normally filter out (creatinine and blood urea nitrogen).

Most other blood tests help monitor the function of other organs. Because the blood carries so many substances essential to the body's functioning, blood tests can be used to find out what's happening in the body. In addition, testing blood is relatively easy. For example, thyroid function can be evaluated more easily by measuring the level of thyroid hormones in the blood than by directly sampling the thyroid. Likewise, measuring liver enzymes and proteins in the blood is easier than sampling the liver.

Bone Marrow Examination

Sometimes a sample of bone marrow must be examined to determine why blood cells are abnormal. A doctor can take two different types of bone marrow samples: a bone marrow aspirate and a bone marrow core biopsy. Both types are usually taken from the hipbone (iliac crest), although aspirates are sometimes taken from the breastbone (sternum). In young children, they are taken from a backbone (vertebra) or leg bone (tibia).

Taking a Bone Marrow Sample

Bone marrow samples are usually taken from the hipbone (iliac crest). The person may lie on one side, facing away from the doctor, with the knee of the top leg bent. After numbing the skin and tissue over the bone with a local anesthetic, the doctor inserts a needle into the bone and withdraws the marrow.

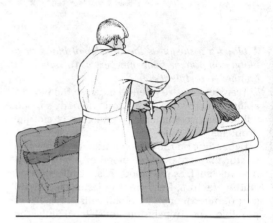

Both types of samples usually are taken at the same time. After the skin and tissue over the bone are numbed with a local anesthetic, the sharp needle of a syringe is inserted into the bone. For a bone marrow aspirate, the doctor pulls back on the plunger of the syringe and draws out a small amount of the soft bone marrow, which can be spread on a slide and examined under a microscope. Special tests, such as cultures for bacteria, fungi, or viruses and chromosomal analysis, can be performed on the sample. Although the aspirate often provides enough information to make a diagnosis, the process of drawing the marrow into the syringe breaks up the fragile bone marrow. As a result, determining the original arrangement of the cells is difficult.

▲ see page 761

When the exact anatomic relationships of cells must be determined and the structure of the tissues evaluated, the doctor also performs a core biopsy. A small core of intact bone marrow is removed with an internal coring device on the nee- dle. This core is preserved and sliced into thin sections that are examined under a microscope.

A bone marrow sampling generally involves only a slight jolt of pain, followed by minimal discomfort. The procedure takes only a few minutes.

CHAPTER 153

Blood Transfusion

A blood transfusion is the transfer of blood or a blood component from one person (a donor) to another (a recipient).

Transfusions are given to increase the blood's ability to carry oxygen, restore the body's blood volume, improve immunity, and correct clotting problems.

Depending on the reason for the transfusion, a doctor may order whole blood or a blood component—such as red blood cells, platelets, blood clotting factors, fresh frozen plasma (the liquid part of blood), or white blood cells.▲ Whenever possible, the transfusion consists of only the blood component that meets the patient's specific need, rather than whole blood. Giving a specific component is both safer and less wasteful.

In the United States, about 15 million transfusions are given every year. Thanks to better techniques for screening blood, transfusions today are safer than ever. But they still pose risks for the recipient, such as allergic reactions and infections. Even though the chance of contracting AIDS or hepatitis from transfusions is remote, doctors are well aware of these risks and order transfusions only when there seems to be no alternative.

Blood Collection and Classification

The Food and Drug Administration (FDA) strictly regulates the collection, storage, and transportation of blood and its components.

Many state and local health authorities, as well as the American Red Cross, the American Association of Blood Banks, and others, have their own additional standards.

Blood donors are screened for good health. Their pulse, blood pressure, and temperature are measured, and a blood sample is tested to check for anemia. They are asked whether they have or have had any condition that might disqualify them from donating blood. Conditions such as hepatitis, heart disease, cancer (except certain forms such as localized skin cancer), severe asthma, malaria, bleeding disorders, AIDS, and possible exposure to the AIDS virus can permanently disqualify a potential donor. Exposure to hepatitis, pregnancy, recent major surgery, poorly controlled high blood pressure, low blood pressure, anemia, or the use of certain drugs may temporarily disqualify a person from donating blood. These restrictions were developed to protect both the donor and the recipient. Generally, donors aren't allowed to give blood more than once every 2 months. The practice of paying donors for blood has almost disappeared; it encouraged needy people to present themselves as donors and deny having any conditions that would disqualify them.

For eligible donors, giving blood is very safe. The whole process takes about an hour; the actual donation takes only 10 minutes. There is usually a stinging sensation when the needle is inserted, but after that, the procedure is painless.

The standard unit of donated blood is about a pint. Freshly collected blood is sealed in plastic bags containing preservatives and an anticlotting compound. A small sample from each donation is

▲ see page 734

Testing Donated Blood for Infections

The transfusion of blood can transmit an infectious disease carried in the donor's blood. That's why health officials have stepped up their screening of blood donors and made blood testing more thorough. Today, all blood donations are tested for viral hepatitis, AIDS, syphilis, and selected other viruses.

Viral Hepatitis

Donated blood is tested for the types of viral hepatitis (types B and C) that are transmitted by blood transfusions. These tests can't identify all cases of infected blood, but with recent improvements in testing and donor screening, a transfusion poses almost no risk of transmitting hepatitis B. Hepatitis C remains the most common potentially serious infection transmitted by blood transfusions, with a current risk of about three infections for every 10,000 units of blood transfused.

AIDS

In the United States, donated blood is tested for the human immunodeficiency virus (HIV), the cause of AIDS. The test isn't 100 percent accurate, but potential donors are interviewed as part of the screening process. Interviewers ask about risk factors for AIDS— for instance, whether the potential donors or their sex partners have injected drugs or had sex with a male homosexual. Because of the blood test and the screening interview, the risk of contracting AIDS through a blood transfusion is extremely low—1 in 420,000, according to recent estimates.

Syphilis

Blood transfusions rarely transmit syphilis. Not only are blood donors screened and donations tested for syphilis, but the donated blood is also refrigerated at low temperatures, which kill the infectious organisms.

---

tested for infectious diseases such as AIDS, viral hepatitis, and syphilis. Refrigerated blood remains usable for 42 days. In special circumstances—for instance, to preserve a rare type of blood—red blood cells may be frozen and kept for up to 10 years.

Because transfusing blood that doesn't match the recipient's can be dangerous, donated blood is routinely classified by type as either A, B, AB, or O and as Rh-positive or Rh-negative. For example, a person's blood type may be O-positive or AB-negative. As a further precaution, before starting the transfusion, a technician mixes a drop of the donor's blood with the recipient's to make sure they're compatible; this is called cross-matching.

Blood and Blood Components

A person who needs a large amount of blood quickly—someone who is bleeding profusely, for example—may receive whole blood to help restore fluid volume and circulation. Whole blood also may be given when a needed blood component is unavailable separately.

The most commonly transfused blood component, packed red blood cells can restore the blood's oxygen-carrying capacity. This component may be given to a person who is bleeding or has severe anemia. Much more expensive than packed red blood cells, frozen-thawed red blood cells are usually reserved for transfusions of rare blood types.

Some people who need blood are allergic to it. If drugs don't prevent allergic reactions, a person may have to be given washed red blood cells. Washing the red blood cells removes from the donor's plasma almost all traces of substances that may cause allergic reactions.

Having too few platelets (thrombocytopenia) may result in severe and spontaneous bleeding. Transfusing platelets may restore the blood's clotting ability. Blood clotting factors are plasma proteins that normally work with platelets to help

Compatible Blood Types

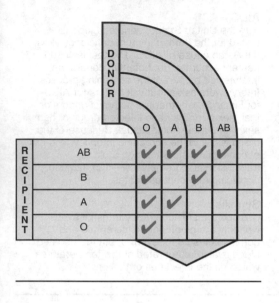

the blood clot. Without clotting, bleeding would not stop after an injury. Concentrated blood clotting factors can be given to people who have an inherited bleeding disorder, such as hemophilia or von Willebrand's disease.

Plasma is also a source of blood clotting factors. Fresh frozen plasma is used for bleeding disorders when it's not known which clotting factor is missing or when the replacement concentrate isn't available. Fresh frozen plasma also is used when bleeding is caused by insufficient production of clotting factor proteins resulting from liver failure.

Rarely, white blood cells are transfused to treat life-threatening infections in people whose white blood cell count is greatly reduced or whose white blood cells are functioning abnormally. Antibiotics are usually used in these situations. Antibodies (immunoglobulins), the disease-fighting components of blood, are sometimes given to build up immunity in people who have been exposed to an infectious disease such as chickenpox or hepatitis or who have low antibody levels.

Special Donation Procedures

In a traditional transfusion, one person donates whole blood and another person receives whole blood. However, the concept is broadening. Depending on the situation, people may receive only the cells from blood, only the clotting factors from blood, or only some other blood component. Transfusing only selected blood components allows the treatment to be specific, reduces the risks of side effects, and can efficiently use the different components from a single unit of blood to treat several people. In other situations, people may be given their own whole blood (autologous transfusion).

Apheresis

In apheresis, a donor gives only the specific blood component needed by a recipient rather than whole blood. If a recipient needs platelets, whole blood is drawn from the donor, and a machine that separates the blood into its components selectively removes the platelets and returns the rest of the blood to the donor. Because donors get most of their blood back, they can safely give 8 to 10 times as many platelets during one of these procedures as they would give in a single donation of whole blood.

Autologous Transfusion

The safest blood transfusion is one in which the donor is also the recipient because it eliminates the risk of incompatibility and blood-borne disease. Sometimes, when a patient is bleeding or undergoing surgery, the blood can be collected and given back. More commonly, people donate blood that will be given back later in a transfusion. For example, in the month before undergoing surgery, a person may donate several units of blood to be transfused if needed during or after the operation.

Directed or Designated Donation

Family members or friends can donate blood specifically for one another if the recipient's and donor's blood types and Rh factors are compatible. For some recipients, knowing who donated the blood is comforting, although a donation from a family member or friend isn't necessarily safer than one from an unrelated person. Blood from a

Treating Diseases With Blood Transfusion

Doctors use a type of blood transfusion called hemapheresis to treat certain diseases. Hemapheresis is a purification process. It consists of removing blood from a person, removing harmful substances or components from the blood, and returning the purified blood to the person.

The two most common types of hemapheresis are cytapheresis and plasmapheresis. **Cytapheresis** removes excess numbers of certain blood cells. It's used to treat polycythemia (an excess of red blood cells), certain types of leukemia (an excess of white blood cells), and thrombocytosis (an excess of platelets). **Plasmapheresis** (plasma exchange) removes harmful substances from plasma (the liquid part of blood). For example, it's used to treat myasthenia gravis and Guillain-Barré syndrome.

Difficult and expensive, hemapheresis is usually reserved for people with serious illnesses who haven't responded to conventional treatment. To be helpful, hemapheresis must remove the undesirable blood component faster than the body produces it. Hemapheresis should be repeated only as often as necessary, because the large fluid shifts between blood vessels and tissues that occur as blood is removed and returned may cause complications in people who are already ill. Hemapheresis can help control some diseases but is generally not a cure.

family member is treated with radiation to prevent graft-versus-host disease, which although rare, occurs more often when the recipient and donor are related.

Precautions and Reactions

To minimize the chance of a reaction during a transfusion, health care practitioners take several precautions. After double-checking that the blood about to be given is intended for the person about to receive it, they give the blood to the recipient slowly, generally over 2 hours or more for each unit of blood. Because most adverse reactions occur during the first 15 minutes of the transfusion, the recipient is closely observed at first. After that, a nurse may check on the recipient every 30 to 45 minutes and, if an adverse reaction occurs, stops the transfusion.

The vast majority of transfusions are safe and successful; however, mild reactions occur occasionally, and severe and even fatal reactions, rarely. The most common reactions are fever and allergic reactions (hypersensitivity), which occur in about 1 to 2 percent of transfusions. Symptoms include itchiness, rash, swelling, dizziness, fever, and headache. Less common are breathing difficulties, wheezing, and muscle spasms. Rarely is an allergic reaction severe enough to pose a danger. Treatments are available that allow transfusions to be given to people who previously had allergic reactions to them.

Despite careful typing and cross-matching of blood, mismatches can still occur that cause the transfused red blood cells to be destroyed shortly after the transfusion (a hemolytic reaction). Usually, this reaction starts as a general discomfort or anxiety during or immediately after the transfusion. Sometimes breathing difficulty, chest pressure, flushing, and severe back pain develop. Very rarely, the reactions become more severe and even fatal. A doctor can confirm that a hemolytic reaction is destroying red blood cells by checking to see whether hemoglobin released from these cells is in the patient's blood and urine.

Transfusion recipients can become overloaded with fluid. Recipients who have heart disease are most vulnerable, so their transfusions are given more slowly and they are monitored closely.

Graft-versus-host disease is an unusual complication that affects primarily people whose immune system is impaired by drugs or disease. In this disease, the recipient's (host's) tissues are attacked by the donated white blood cells (the graft). The symptoms include fever, rash, low blood pressure, tissue destruction, and shock.

Anemias

Anemias are conditions in which the number of red blood cells or amount of hemoglobin (the protein that carries oxygen) in them is below normal.

Red blood cells contain hemoglobin, which enables them to carry oxygen from the lungs and deliver it to all parts of the body. Because anemia reduces the number of red blood cells or the amount of hemoglobin in them, the blood can't carry an adequate supply of oxygen. Symptoms, caused by the inadequate oxygen supply, are varied. For example, anemia can cause fatigue, weakness, inability to exercise, and light-headedness. If the anemia becomes more severe, it can even lead to a stroke or heart attack.

Simple blood tests can identify anemia. The percentage of red blood cells in the total volume of blood (hematocrit) and the amount of hemoglobin in a blood sample can be determined. These tests are part of the complete blood cell count (CBC).▲

Anemia may be caused by excessive bleeding, decreased red blood cell production, or increased red blood cell destruction (hemolysis).

Excessive Bleeding

Excessive bleeding is the most common cause of anemia. When blood is lost, the body quickly pulls water from tissues outside the bloodstream in an attempt to keep the blood vessels filled. As a result, the blood is diluted and the percentage of red blood cells is reduced. Eventually, increased production of red blood cells corrects the anemia. However, the anemia may be severe at first, especially if it develops rapidly from a sudden loss of blood, such as from an accident, surgery, childbirth, or a ruptured blood vessel.

Losing large amounts of blood suddenly can create two problems: Blood pressure falls because the amount of fluid left in the blood vessels is insufficient, and the body's oxygen supply decreases because the number of oxygen-carrying red blood cells has diminished. Either problem may lead to a heart attack, stroke, or death.

Far more common than a sudden loss of blood is chronic (continuous or repeated) bleeding, which may occur in various parts of the body. Bleeding from recurrent nosebleeds and hemorrhoids is obvious. Chronic bleeding from other common sources—such as ulcers in the stomach and small intestine or polyps and cancers in the large intestine, especially colon cancer—may not be obvious because the amount of blood is small and doesn't appear as red blood in the stool; this type of blood loss is described as occult. Other sources of chronic bleeding include kidney or bladder tumors, which may cause blood to be lost in the urine, and heavy menstrual bleeding.

The anemia caused by bleeding ranges from mild to severe, and symptoms vary accordingly. The anemia may produce no symptoms, or it may produce faintness, dizziness, thirst, sweating, a weak and rapid pulse, and rapid breathing. Dizziness when a person sits or stands (orthostatic hypotension) is common. Anemia also can cause severe fatigue, shortness of breath, chest pain, and if severe enough, death.

How rapidly the blood is lost is a major determinant in whether symptoms will be mild or severe. When the blood loss is rapid—over several hours or less—loss of just a third of the body's blood volume can be fatal. When the blood loss is slower—over several days, weeks, or longer—loss of up to two thirds of the blood volume may cause only fatigue and weakness or no symptoms at all.

Treatment

Treatment depends on how rapidly blood is lost and how severe the anemia is. Transfusion of red blood cells is the only reliable treatment for rapid blood loss or severe anemia.■ Also, the source of bleeding must be found and the bleeding must be stopped. When blood loss is slower or the anemia less severe, the body may produce enough red blood cells to correct the anemia without transfusion. Because iron, which is required to produce red blood cells, is lost during bleeding, most people who have anemia need to take iron supplements, usually tablets.

▲ see box, page 736

■ see page 739

Common Causes of Anemia

Excessive Bleeding	Decreased Red Blood Cell Production	Increased Red Blood Cell Destruction
Sudden: • Accidents • Surgery • Childbirth • Ruptured blood vessel Chronic: • Nosebleeds • Hemorrhoids • Ulcers in the stomach or small intestine • Cancer or polyps in the gastrointestinal tract • Kidney or bladder tumors • Heavy menstrual bleeding	Iron deficiency Vitamin B_{12} deficiency Folic acid deficiency Vitamin C deficiency Chronic disease	Enlarged spleen Mechanical damage to red blood cells Autoimmune reactions against red blood cells Paroxysmal nocturnal hemoglobinuria Hereditary spherocytosis Hereditary elliptocytosis G6PD deficiency Sickle cell disease Hemoglobin C disease Hemoglobin S-C disease Hemoglobin E disease Thalassemia

Decreased Red Blood Cell Production

Many nutrients are needed for red blood cell production. The most critical are iron, vitamin B_{12}, and folic acid, but the body also needs trace quantities of vitamin C, riboflavin, and copper, as well as a proper balance of hormones, especially erythropoietin (a hormone that stimulates red blood cell production). Without these nutrients and hormones, red blood cell production is slow and inadequate, and the cells may be deformed and unable to carry oxygen adequately. Chronic disease also may lead to decreased red blood cell production.

Iron Deficiency Anemia

The body recycles iron: When red blood cells die, the iron in them is returned to the bone marrow to be used again in new red blood cells. The body loses large amounts of iron only when red blood cells are lost through bleeding, causing a deficiency of iron. Iron deficiency is one of the most common causes of anemia, and blood loss is virtually the only cause of iron deficiency in

adults. A diet low in iron may cause a deficiency in infants and small children, who need more iron because they are growing. In men and postmenopausal women, iron deficiency usually indicates bleeding in the gastrointestinal tract. Monthly menstrual bleeding may cause iron deficiency in premenopausal women.

Normal dietary iron intake usually can't compensate for iron loss from chronic bleeding, and the body has a very small iron reserve. Consequently, lost iron must be replaced with supplements. Because a developing fetus uses iron, pregnant women also take iron supplements.

In the United States, the average diet contains about 6 milligrams of iron for every 1,000 calories of food, so that the average person consumes about 10 to 12 milligrams of iron a day. Meat is the best source of iron, although some iron can be absorbed from other foods. Vegetable fibers, phosphates, bran, and antacids decrease the absorption of iron by binding with it. Vitamin C (ascorbic acid) is the only food element that can increase iron absorption. The body absorbs 1 to 2 milligrams of iron from food every day, which roughly equals the amount the body normally loses daily.

How Iron Deficiency Anemia Develops

Iron deficiency anemia usually develops gradually, in stages. Symptoms develop in the later stages.

Stage 1
Iron loss exceeds intake, depleting iron reserves, primarily in bone marrow. Blood levels of ferritin (a protein that stores iron) progressively decrease.

Stage 2
Because depleted iron reserves can't meet the needs of developing red blood cells, fewer red blood cells are produced.

Stage 3
Anemia begins to develop. Early in this stage, the red blood cells appear normal, but there are fewer of them. Hemoglobin levels and hematocrit are reduced.

Stage 4
The bone marrow tries to compensate for the lack of iron by speeding up cell division and producing very small (microcytic) red blood cells, which are typical of iron deficiency anemia.

Stage 5
As iron deficiency and anemia progress, the symptoms of iron deficiency may develop and symptoms of anemia worsen.

Symptoms

Anemia ultimately leads to fatigue, shortness of breath, an inability to exercise, and other symptoms. Iron deficiency may produce its own symptoms, such as pica (a craving for nonfoods such as ice, dirt, or pure starch), tongue irritation (glossitis), and cracks at the sides of the mouth (cheilosis) and in the fingernails, which have a spoonlike deformity (koilonychia).

Diagnosis

Blood tests are used to diagnose anemia. Usually, a person who has anemia is tested for iron

deficiency. Iron levels can be measured in the blood. Levels of iron and transferrin (the protein that carries iron when it isn't inside red blood cells) are measured and compared. If less than 10 percent of the transferrin is saturated with iron, iron deficiency is likely. However, the most sensitive test for iron deficiency is measuring the blood level of ferritin (a protein that stores iron). A low level of ferritin indicates iron deficiency. However, sometimes ferritin levels are normal or high despite iron deficiency because they can be artificially increased by liver damage, inflammation, infection, or cancer.

Occasionally, more sophisticated tests are needed to make the diagnosis. The most specific test is a bone marrow examination in which a sample of cells is examined under a microscope to determine their iron content.▲

Treatment

Because excessive bleeding is the most common cause of iron deficiency, the first step is to locate its source and stop the bleeding. Drugs or surgery may be needed to control excessive menstrual bleeding, repair a bleeding ulcer, remove a polyp in the colon, or treat bleeding from the kidneys.

Generally, treatment also includes replacing the lost iron. Most iron tablets contain ferrous iron sulfate, iron gluconate, or a polysaccharide. Iron tablets are absorbed best when taken 30 minutes before meals. In general, one iron tablet a day is sufficient, but occasionally two are needed. Because the intestine's ability to absorb iron is limited, larger doses are wasted and are likely to cause indigestion and constipation. Iron almost always turns stools black—a normal, harmless side effect.

Correcting iron deficiency anemia with iron supplements usually takes 3 to 6 weeks, even after the bleeding has stopped. Once the anemia is corrected, a person should continue to take iron supplements for 6 months to replenish the body's reserves. Blood tests are usually performed periodically to ensure that the person's iron supply is sufficient and that the bleeding has stopped.

Rarely, iron must be given by injection. Iron injections are reserved for people who can't tolerate iron tablets or who continue to lose large amounts of blood from ongoing bleeding. Whether iron is given by injections or tablets, recovery time from anemia is the same.

▲ see page 737

Vitamin Deficiencies

Besides iron, bone marrow needs both vitamin B_{12} and folic acid to produce red blood cells. If either is lacking, megaloblastic anemia can develop. In this type of anemia, the bone marrow produces large, abnormal red blood cells (megaloblasts). White blood cells and platelets also are usually abnormal.

Although megaloblastic anemia is most often caused by a lack of vitamin B_{12} or folic acid in the diet or an inability to absorb these vitamins, it is sometimes caused by drugs used to treat cancer, such as methotrexate, hydroxyurea, fluorouracil, and cytarabine.

VITAMIN B_{12} DEFICIENCY ANEMIA

Vitamin B_{12} deficiency anemia (pernicious anemia) is a megaloblastic anemia caused by a lack of vitamin B_{12}.

Inadequate absorption of vitamin B_{12} (cobalamin) causes pernicious anemia. This vitamin, available in meat, normally is readily absorbed in the ileum (the last part of the small intestine, leading to the large intestine). However, to be absorbed, the vitamin must combine with intrinsic factor, a protein produced in the stomach, which then carries the vitamin to the ileum, through its wall, and into the bloodstream. Without intrinsic factor, vitamin B_{12} remains in the intestine and is excreted in the stool. In pernicious anemia, the stomach doesn't produce intrinsic factor, vitamin B_{12} isn't absorbed, and anemia develops even if large amounts of the vitamin are taken in with food. But because the liver stores a large amount of vitamin B_{12}, anemia doesn't develop until 2 to 4 years after the body stops absorbing vitamin B_{12}.

Although lack of intrinsic factor is the most common cause of vitamin B_{12} deficiency, other possible causes include abnormal bacterial growth in the small intestine that prevents vitamin B_{12} absorption, certain diseases such as Crohn's disease, and surgery that removes the stomach or the part of the small intestine where vitamin B_{12} is absorbed. A strict vegetarian diet also may cause B_{12} deficiency.

Besides decreasing red blood cell production, vitamin B_{12} deficiency affects the nervous system, leading to tingling in the hands and feet, loss of sensation in the legs, feet, and hands, and spastic movements. Other symptoms may include a peculiar type of color blindness involving yellow and blue, a sore or burning tongue, weight loss, darkened skin, confusion, depression, and decreased intellectual function.

Diagnosis

Usually, vitamin B_{12} deficiency is diagnosed during routine blood tests for anemia. Megaloblasts (large red blood cells) are seen when a blood sample is examined under a microscope. Changes in white blood cells and platelets also can be detected, especially when a person has had anemia for a long time.

When this deficiency is suspected, the blood level of vitamin B_{12} is measured. If a deficiency is confirmed, tests to determine the cause may be performed. Generally, the tests focus on intrinsic factor. First, a blood sample is usually drawn to check for antibodies to intrinsic factor, which are found in about 60 to 90 percent of the people who have pernicious anemia. The second, more specific, test is a gastric analysis. A slender, flexible tube called a nasogastric tube is inserted through the nose, down the throat, and into the stomach. Then pentagastrin (a hormone that stimulates intrinsic factor secretion) is injected into a vein. A sample of the stomach contents is withdrawn and tested for intrinsic factor.

If still uncertain about the mechanism that produced the vitamin B_{12} deficiency, the doctor may order a Schilling test. First, a person is given a tiny amount of radioactive vitamin B_{12} by mouth, and its absorption is measured. Then intrinsic factor is given along with vitamin B_{12}, and its absorption is measured again. If vitamin B_{12} is absorbed with but not without intrinsic factor, the diagnosis of pernicious anemia is confirmed. Other tests are rarely needed.

Treatment

The treatment of vitamin B_{12} deficiency or pernicious anemia consists of replacing vitamin B_{12}. Because most people who have this deficiency can't absorb vitamin B_{12} taken by mouth, they must take it by injection. At first, injections are given daily or weekly for several weeks until the blood levels of vitamin B_{12} return to normal; then injections are given once a month. People who have this deficiency must take vitamin B_{12} supplements for life.

Folic Acid Deficiency Anemia

Folic acid (folate) deficiency anemia is a megaloblastic anemia caused by a lack of folic acid.

Folic acid is a vitamin found in raw vegetables, fresh fruit, and meat, but cooking usually destroys it. Because the body stores only a small amount in the liver, a diet lacking in folic acid leads to a deficiency within a few months.

Folic acid deficiency is more common in the Western world than vitamin B_{12} deficiency because many people don't eat enough raw leafy vegetables. People who have diseases of the small intestine, especially Crohn's disease and sprue, may have trouble absorbing folic acid. Certain antiseizure drugs and oral contraceptives also decrease absorption of this vitamin. Less commonly, pregnant and lactating women and people undergoing hemodialysis for kidney disease develop this deficiency because they have an increased need for folic acid. Because alcohol interferes with the absorption and metabolism of folic acid, those who drink large amounts of alcohol also develop this deficiency.

People who have folic acid deficiency develop anemia. Infants, but not adults, may have neurologic abnormalities, and this deficiency in a pregnant woman can cause spinal cord defects and other malformations in the fetus.

When doctors find megaloblasts (large red blood cells) in a person who has anemia, they measure the folic acid level in a blood sample. If folic acid deficiency is diagnosed, the treatment usually consists of taking one folic acid tablet daily. People who have trouble absorbing folic acid take supplements for life.

Vitamin C Deficiency Anemia

Vitamin C deficiency anemia is a rare type of anemia caused by a long-standing severe lack of vitamin C.

In this type of anemia, the bone marrow produces small red blood cells. This deficiency is diagnosed by measuring vitamin C levels in white blood cells. One vitamin C tablet daily corrects the deficiency and cures the anemia.

Chronic Disease

Chronic disease often leads to anemia, especially in the elderly. Conditions such as infections, inflammation, and cancer suppress red blood cell production in the bone marrow. Because iron stored in the bone can't be used by the developing red blood cells, this type of anemia is often called iron-reutilization anemia.

In all people, infections, even trivial ones, and inflammatory conditions such as arthritis and tendinitis inhibit the production of red blood cells in the bone marrow, resulting in fewer red blood cells. However, these conditions don't cause anemia unless they are severe or long lasting (chronic).

The more severe the disease, the more severe the resulting anemia, but anemia caused by chronic disease rarely becomes very severe. The hematocrit (percentage of red blood cells in the blood) rarely falls below 25 percent (normal is 45 to 52 percent in men and 37 to 48 percent in women), and the hemoglobin level (amount of this oxygen-carrying protein in red blood cells) rarely falls below 8 grams per deciliter of blood (normal is 13 to 18 grams per deciliter).

Because this type of anemia develops slowly and is generally mild, it usually produces no symptoms. When symptoms do occur, they usually result from the disease causing the anemia rather than from the anemia itself. Laboratory tests may indicate that chronic illness is the cause of anemia, but they can't confirm the diagnosis. Therefore, doctors first try to exclude other causes of anemia, such as excessive bleeding or iron deficiency.

Because no specific treatment exists for this type of anemia, doctors treat the disease causing it. Taking additional iron or vitamins doesn't help. On the rare occasion that the anemia becomes severe, transfusions or erythropoietin (a hormone that stimulates the bone marrow to produce red blood cells) may help.

Increased Red Blood Cell Destruction

Normally, red blood cells have a life span of about 120 days. When they get old, scavenger cells in the bone marrow, spleen, and liver detect and destroy them. If a disease destroys red blood cells prematurely (hemolysis), the bone marrow tries to compensate by producing new red blood cells faster—up to 10 times the normal rate. When destruction of red blood cells exceeds their production, hemolytic anemia results. Hemolytic anemias are relatively uncommon compared with the anemias caused by blood loss and decreased red blood cell production.

A number of factors can increase red blood cell destruction. The spleen may enlarge (splenomegaly). Obstacles in the bloodstream may break up the cells. Antibodies may bind to red blood cells and cause the immune system to destroy them in an autoimmune reaction. Sometimes red blood cells are destroyed because of abnormalities in the cells themselves—their shape and surface, their function, or their hemoglobin content. Red blood cell destruction can occur in disorders such as systemic lupus erythematosus and certain cancers, especially lymphomas. Various drugs such as methyldopa, dapsone, and sulfa drugs can also destroy red blood cells.

Symptoms of hemolytic anemia are similar to those of other anemias. Sometimes hemolysis is sudden and severe, resulting in a hemolytic crisis that includes chills, fever, back and stomach pain, light-headedness, and a significant drop in blood pressure. Jaundice and dark urine may result from the contents of the damaged red blood cells spilling into the blood. The spleen enlarges as it filters out many of the damaged red blood cells, sometimes causing abdominal pain. Continued hemolysis may produce pigmented gallstones, an unusual type of gallstone composed of the dark-colored contents of red blood cells.

Enlarged Spleen

Many disorders can cause the spleen to enlarge.▲ When it enlarges, it tends to trap and destroy red blood cells, creating a vicious circle: The more cells the spleen traps, the larger it grows, and the larger it grows, the more cells it traps.

Anemia caused by an enlarged spleen usually develops slowly, and symptoms tend to be mild. Often, the enlarged spleen also reduces the number of platelets and white blood cells in the bloodstream.

Treatment is usually aimed at the disorder that has caused the spleen to enlarge. Rarely, the anemia becomes severe enough to warrant surgical removal of the spleen (splenectomy).

Mechanical Damage to Red Blood Cells

Normally, red blood cells travel through blood vessels unharmed. However, they may be mechanically damaged by abnormalities in the blood vessels, such as an aneurysm (a pocket in a weakened blood vessel wall) or artificial heart valve, or by extremely high blood pressure. These abnormalities may break up normal red blood cells, causing their contents to spill into the blood. The kidneys eventually filter these substances out of the blood but may also be damaged by them.

When a number of red blood cells are damaged, **microangiopathic hemolytic anemia** develops. This disorder is diagnosed when fragments of the damaged red blood cells are seen in a blood sample examined under a microscope. The cause of the damage is then identified and, if possible, corrected.

Autoimmune Reactions

Sometimes the body's immune system malfunctions and destroys its own cells because it mistakenly identifies them as foreign substances (autoimmune reaction). When an autoimmune reaction is directed against red blood cells, the result is **autoimmune hemolytic anemia** (immune-mediated anemia). Autoimmune hemolytic anemia has many different causes, but in most people, the cause is unknown (idiopathic).

Autoimmune hemolytic anemia is diagnosed when laboratory tests identify antibodies (autoantibodies) in the blood that bind to and react against the body's own red blood cells.

Autoimmune hemolytic anemias are classified into two main types: warm-antibody hemolytic anemia, which is the most common type, and cold-antibody hemolytic anemia.

WARM-ANTIBODY HEMOLYTIC ANEMIA
Warm-antibody hemolytic anemia is a condition in which the body develops autoantibodies that react against red blood cells at body temperature.

These autoantibodies coat red blood cells, which are then identified as foreign and are destroyed by scavenger cells in the spleen or sometimes in the liver and bone marrow. This condition is more common in women than in men. About one third of the people who have this type of anemia have an underlying disease, such as a lymphoma, leukemia, or a connective tissue disease (especially systemic lupus erythematosus),

▲ see page 786

or have been exposed to certain drugs, primarily methyldopa.

Symptoms are often worse than would be expected from the severity of the anemia, probably because the anemia often develops rapidly. Because the spleen usually enlarges, the upper left part of the abdomen may be tender or uncomfortable.

Treatment depends on whether a cause is identified. Doctors first try to treat or eliminate the cause. If no cause is identified, a corticosteroid such as prednisone is often given in large doses, first intravenously, then orally. About one third of the people respond well to this drug, which is then tapered off and discontinued. The other two thirds may need to have the spleen surgically removed to stop it from destroying the autoantibody-coated red blood cells. Removal of the spleen controls the anemia in about half of the people. If these treatments fail, drugs that suppress the immune system such as cyclosporine and cyclophosphamide are tried.

Blood transfusions may cause problems for people who have autoimmune hemolytic anemia. The blood bank may be unable to find blood that doesn't react with the autoantibodies, and the transfusions themselves may stimulate production of more autoantibodies.

COLD-ANTIBODY HEMOLYTIC ANEMIA

Cold-antibody hemolytic anemia is a condition in which the body develops autoantibodies that react against red blood cells at room temperature or cold temperatures.

This type of anemia can be acute or chronic. The acute form often develops in people who have acute infections, especially certain pneumonias or infectious mononucleosis. The acute form usually doesn't last long, is relatively mild, and disappears without treatment. The chronic form is most common in women, particularly those over 40 who have rheumatism or arthritis.

Although the chronic form generally persists throughout life, the anemia is usually mild and produces few, if any, symptoms. But exposure to cold increases red blood cell destruction, may worsen joint aches, and may result in symptoms such as fatigue and blue discoloration of the arms and hands. As might be expected, people who have this disorder and live in cold climates have

substantially more symptoms than those who live in warm climates.

Cold-antibody hemolytic anemia is diagnosed by tests that detect antibodies on the red blood cell surface which are more active at temperatures below body temperature. No specific treatment exists, so treatment is aimed at relieving symptoms. The acute form associated with infections gets better on its own and rarely causes serious symptoms. Avoiding exposure to cold controls the chronic form.

Paroxysmal Nocturnal Hemoglobinuria

Paroxysmal nocturnal hemoglobinuria is a rare hemolytic anemia causing sudden, recurring bouts of red blood cell destruction by the immune system.

The sudden (paroxysmal) destruction of many red blood cells—which can occur at any time, not just at night (nocturnal)—causes hemoglobin to spill into the blood. The kidneys filter out the hemoglobin, which makes the urine dark (hemoglobinuria). This anemia is more common among young men but can appear at any age in either sex. Its cause isn't known.

Paroxysmal nocturnal hemoglobinuria can cause severe stomach cramps or back pain and clotting in the large veins of the abdomen and legs. The diagnosis is made by laboratory tests that can detect the abnormal red blood cells characteristic of this disorder.

Corticosteroids such as prednisone often help relieve symptoms, but no cure is available. People who develop blood clots may need to take an anticoagulant (a drug that reduces the blood's tendency to clot) such as warfarin. Bone marrow transplantation may be considered for people who have the most severe form of this anemia.

Red Blood Cell Abnormalities

Red blood cell destruction may occur because the red blood cells are deformed, have weak membranes that break easily, or lack the enzymes needed to function properly and maintain the flexibility that enables them to travel through narrow blood vessels. Such red blood cell abnormalities occur in certain inherited disorders.

Hereditary spherocytosis *is an inherited disorder in which the normally disk-shaped red blood cells become spherical.*

The misshapen, rigid red blood cells are trapped and destroyed in the spleen, resulting in anemia and an enlarged spleen. The anemia is usually mild but may be more severe if an infection develops. When the disorder is severe, jaundice and anemia may develop, the liver may enlarge, and gallstones may form. In young adults, this disorder may be mistaken for hepatitis. Bone abnormalities, such as a tower-shaped skull and extra fingers and toes, can occur. Treatment usually isn't needed, but severe anemia may require removal of the spleen. This procedure doesn't correct the shape of the red blood cells, but it reduces the number that are destroyed and thus corrects the anemia.

Hereditary elliptocytosis *is a rare disorder in which the red blood cells are oval or elliptical rather than disk-shaped.*

This disorder sometimes leads to mild anemia but requires no treatment. Removing the spleen may be helpful for severe anemia.

G6PD deficiency *is a disorder in which the enzyme G6PD (glucose-6-phosphate dehydrogenase) is missing from the red blood cell membrane.*

The G6PD enzyme helps process glucose, a simple sugar that is the main source of energy for red blood cells, and produce glutathione, which helps prevent the cells from breaking. This inherited disorder almost always affects males. It occurs in 10 percent of the black male population and a smaller percentage of white people from the Mediterranean area. Some people who have G6PD deficiency never develop anemia. Fever, viral or bacterial infections, diabetic crisis, and certain substances such as aspirin, vitamin K, and fava beans may trigger red blood cell destruction, resulting in anemia. Anemia can be prevented by avoiding the situations or substances that trigger it, but no treatment can cure G6PD deficiency.

Hemoglobin Abnormalities

Inherited abnormalities in hemoglobin may cause anemia. The red blood cells that contain abnormal hemoglobin may become misshapen or unable to carry or deliver an adequate supply of oxygen.

Red Blood Cell Shapes

Normal red blood cells are flexible and disk-shaped, thicker at the edges than in the middle. In several inherited disorders, red blood cells become spherical (hereditary spherocytosis), oval (hereditary elliptocytosis), or sickle-shaped (sickle cell disease).

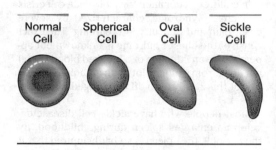

| Normal Cell | Spherical Cell | Oval Cell | Sickle Cell |

SICKLE CELL DISEASE

Sickle cell disease is an inherited condition characterized by sickle-shaped red blood cells and chronic hemolytic anemia.

Sickle cell disease affects blacks almost exclusively. About 10 percent of the blacks in the United States have one gene for sickle cell disease (they have sickle cell trait); they don't develop sickle cell disease. About 0.3 percent have two genes; they develop the disease.

In sickle cell disease, the red blood cells contain an abnormal form of hemoglobin (the protein that carries oxygen) that reduces the amount of oxygen in the cells, causing them to become crescent- or sickle-shaped. The sickle-shaped cells block and damage the smallest blood vessels in the spleen, kidneys, brain, bones, and other organs, reducing their oxygen supply. Because these deformed cells are fragile, they break up as they travel through blood vessels, causing severe anemia, blocked blood flow, organ damage, and possibly death.

Symptoms

People who have this disease always have some degree of anemia and mild jaundice, but they may have few other symptoms. However, anything that reduces the amount of oxygen in their blood, such as vigorous exercise, mountain climbing, flying at high altitudes without sufficient oxygen, or an illness, may bring on a sickle cell crisis—a sudden worsening of anemia, pain (often in the abdomen or long bones), fever, and sometimes shortness of breath. Abdominal pain may be severe, and vomiting may occur; symptoms may resemble those of appendicitis or an ovarian cyst.

In children, a common form of sickle cell crisis is a chest syndrome, characterized by severe chest pain and difficulty in breathing. The exact cause of the chest syndrome is unknown but appears to be an infection or a blocked blood vessel resulting from a blood clot or an embolus (a piece of clot that has broken off and lodged in a blood vessel).

Most people who have sickle cell disease develop an enlarged spleen during childhood. By the age of 9, the spleen is so badly injured that it shrinks and no longer functions. Because the spleen helps fight infection, these people are more likely to develop pneumococcal pneumonia and other infections. Viral infections particularly can decrease blood cell production, so anemia becomes more severe. The liver becomes progressively larger throughout life, and gallstones often form from the pigment of damaged red blood cells. The heart usually enlarges and heart murmurs are common.

Children who have sickle cell disease often have a relatively short torso but long arms, legs, fingers, and toes. Changes in the bones and bone marrow may cause bone pain, especially in their hands and feet. Episodes of joint pain with fever may occur, and the hip joint may become so damaged that it eventually needs to be replaced.

Poor circulation to the skin may cause sores on the legs, especially at the ankles. Damage to the nervous system may cause strokes. In older people, lung and kidney function may deteriorate. Young men may develop persistent, often painful erections (priapism).

Rarely, a person who has sickle cell trait has blood in the urine caused by bleeding from a kidney. If a doctor knows that this bleeding is related to the sickle cell trait, needless exploratory surgery can be avoided.

▲ see page 836

Diagnosis

Doctors recognize anemia, stomach and bone pain, and nausea in a young black person as signs of a sickle cell crisis. Sickle-shaped red blood cells and fragments of destroyed red blood cells can be seen in a blood sample examined under a microscope.

Electrophoresis, a blood test, can detect abnormal hemoglobin and indicate whether a person has sickle cell trait or sickle cell disease. Discovering the trait may be important for family planning, to determine the risk of having a child with sickle cell disease.

Treatment and Prevention

In the past, people who had sickle cell disease rarely lived beyond age 20, but today they usually live well past age 50. Rarely, a person who has sickle cell trait dies suddenly while undergoing very strenuous exercise that has caused severe dehydration, such as during military or athletic training.

Sickle cell disease can't be cured, so treatment is aimed at preventing crises, controlling the anemia, and relieving symptoms. People who have this disease should try to avoid activities that reduce the amount of oxygen in their blood and should promptly seek medical attention for even minor illnesses, such as viral infections. Because they are at increased risk of infection, they should be immunized with pneumococcal and *Hemophilus influenzae* vaccines.

Sickle cell crisis may require hospitalization. The person is given large amounts of fluid intravenously and drugs to relieve pain. Blood transfusions and oxygen may be given if a doctor suspects that anemia is severe enough to pose a risk of stroke, heart attack, or lung damage. Meanwhile, conditions that may have caused the crisis, such as an infection, are treated.

Drugs to control sickle cell disease, such as hydroxyurea, are being studied. Hydroxyurea increases the production of a form of hemoglobin found predominantly in fetuses, which decreases the number of red blood cells becoming sickle-shaped. Therefore, it reduces the frequency of sickle cell crises. Bone marrow from a family member or other donor who doesn't have the sickle cell gene may be transplanted in a person with the disease.▲ Although transplantation may be curative, it's risky, and recipients must take drugs that suppress the immune system for the rest of their lives. Gene therapy, a technique in which normal genes are implanted in precursor cells (cells that produce blood cells), is also under study.

HEMOGLOBIN C, S-C, AND E DISEASES

Hemoglobin C disease occurs in 2 to 3 percent of American blacks. Only people who have two genes for the disease develop anemia, which varies in severity. People who have this disease, particularly children, may have episodes of abdominal and joint pain, an enlarged spleen, and mild jaundice, but they don't have severe crises. In general, symptoms are few.

Hemoglobin S-C disease occurs in people who have one gene for sickle cell disease and one gene for hemoglobin C disease. It's much more common than hemoglobin C disease, and its symptoms are similar to those of sickle cell disease but much milder.

Hemoglobin E disease affects primarily blacks and people from Southeast Asia; it's rare in Chinese people. This disease produces anemia but none of the other symptoms that occur in sickle cell disease and hemoglobin C disease.

THALASSEMIAS

Thalassemias are a group of inherited disorders resulting from an imbalance in the production of one of the four chains of amino acids that make up hemoglobin.

Thalassemias are categorized according to the amino acid chain affected. The two main types are alpha-thalassemia (the alpha chain is affected) and beta-thalassemia (the beta chain is affected). Thalassemias are also categorized according to whether a person has one defective gene (thalassemia minor) or two defective genes (thalassemia major). Alpha-thalassemia is most common in blacks (25 percent carry at least one gene), and beta-thalassemia in people from the Mediterranean area and Southeast Asia.

One gene for beta-thalassemia produces mild to moderate anemia with no symptoms; two genes produce severe anemia with symptoms. About 10 percent of the people who have at least one gene for alpha-thalassemia also have a mild anemia.

All thalassemias have similar symptoms, but they vary in severity. Most people have a mild anemia. In more severe forms such as beta-thalassemia major, jaundice, skin ulcers, gallstones, and an enlarged spleen (sometimes huge) may develop. Overactive bone marrow may cause some bones, especially those in the head and face, to thicken and enlarge. The long bones may weaken and fracture easily. Children who have thalassemia may grow more slowly and reach puberty later than they normally would. Because iron absorption may be increased and frequent blood transfusions (providing more iron) are needed, excessive iron may accumulate and be deposited in the heart muscle, eventually causing heart failure.

Thalassemias are more difficult to diagnose than other hemoglobin disorders. Testing a drop of blood by electrophoresis is helpful but may be inconclusive, especially for alpha-thalassemia. Therefore, the diagnosis is usually based on hereditary patterns and special hemoglobin tests.

Most people who have a thalassemia don't need treatment, but people who have severe forms may need a bone marrow transplantation. Gene therapy is under study.

CHAPTER 155

Bleeding Disorders

Bleeding disorders, characterized by a tendency to bleed easily, may result from defects in the blood vessels or from abnormalities in the blood itself. The abnormalities may be in the blood clotting factors or the platelets.

Normally, blood is confined to the blood vessels—arteries, capillaries, and veins. When bleeding (hemorrhaging) occurs, blood spills from these vessels, inside or outside of the body. The body prevents or controls bleeding in several ways.

Hemostasis is the body's way of stopping injured blood vessels from bleeding. It involves three major processes: (1) constriction of the

Blood Clots: Plugging the Breaks

When an injury causes a blood vessel wall to break, platelets are activated: They change shape from round to spiny, stick to the broken vessel wall and each other, and begin to plug the break. They also interact with other components to form fibrin. Fibrin strands form a net that entraps more platelets and blood cells, producing a clot that plugs the break.

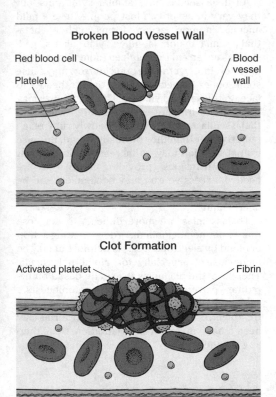

Broken Blood Vessel Wall

Red blood cell

Platelet

Blood vessel wall

Clot Formation

Activated platelet

Fibrin

blood vessels, (2) activity of the platelets (irregularly shaped cell-like particles in the blood that are involved in clotting), and (3) activity of the blood clotting factors (proteins dissolved in plasma, the liquid part of blood). Abnormalities in these processes can lead to either excessive bleeding or excessive clotting, both of which can be dangerous.

How the Body Prevents Bleeding

Blood vessel walls are the first barrier to blood loss. If a blood vessel is injured, it constricts so that blood flows out more slowly and clotting can start. At the same time, the accumulating pool of blood outside the blood vessel (a hematoma) presses against the vessel, helping prevent further bleeding.

As soon as the blood vessel wall breaks, a series of reactions activates the platelets so that they stick to the injured area. The "glue" that holds the platelets to the vessel walls is the von Willebrand factor, a plasma protein produced by the cells of the vessel walls. Collagen and other proteins, particularly thrombin, appear at the site of the injury, prompting the platelets to stick together. As platelets accumulate at the site, they form a mesh that plugs the injury; they change shape from round to spiny, and they release proteins and other chemicals that entrap more platelets and clotting proteins in the enlarging plug.

Thrombin converts fibrinogen, a soluble blood clotting factor, into long strands of insoluble fibrin that radiate from the clumped platelets and form a net that entraps more platelets and blood cells. The fibrin strands add bulk to the clot and help hold it in place to keep the vessel wall plugged. The series of reactions involves at least 10 blood clotting factors.

An abnormality in any part of the hemostatic process can cause problems. If blood vessels are frail, they can be injured easily or may not constrict. If the number of platelets is too low, if the platelets don't function normally, or if one of the clotting factors is abnormal or missing, clotting doesn't proceed normally. When clotting is abnormal, even a slight injury to a blood vessel may lead to major blood loss.

Because most clotting factors are produced in the liver, severe liver damage can cause a shortage of these factors in the blood. Vitamin K, found in green leafy vegetables, is necessary for production of the active forms of several clotting factors. Therefore, nutritional deficiencies or drugs that interfere with the normal function of vitamin K, such as warfarin, can cause bleeding. Abnormal bleeding can also occur when excessive clotting uses up large amounts of the clotting factors and platelets or when an autoimmune response (the body's immune system malfunctions and attacks the body) blocks the activity of clotting factors.

The reactions that result in the formation of a fibrin plug are balanced by other reactions that stop the clotting process and dissolve clots after the blood vessel has healed. Without this control system, minor blood vessel injuries could trigger widespread clotting throughout the body—which actually happens in some diseases. When clotting is uncontrolled, small blood vessels in critical places can become clogged. Clogged vessels in the brain cause strokes; clogged vessels leading to the heart cause heart attacks; and pieces of clots from veins in the legs, pelvis, or abdomen can travel through the bloodstream to the lungs and block major arteries there (pulmonary embolism).

Drugs That Affect Clotting

Certain types of drugs can help people who have conditions that put them at high risk of developing dangerous blood clots. In severe coronary artery disease, small accumulations of platelets may block an already narrowed coronary artery and cut off blood flow to the heart, resulting in a heart attack. Low doses of aspirin, as well as several other drugs, can reduce the stickiness of platelets so they won't clump together to block the artery.

Another type of drug, an anticoagulant, reduces the blood's tendency to clot by inhibiting the action of the clotting factors. Though often called blood thinners, anticoagulants don't really thin the blood. Commonly used anticoagulants are warfarin, given by mouth, and heparin, given by injection. People who have artificial heart valves or who are confined to bed for long periods are often given anticoagulants as a precaution against clot formation. People taking anticoagulants must be under close medical supervision. Doctors monitor the effects of these drugs with blood tests that measure clotting time, and they adjust the dose on the basis of test results. Doses that are too low may not prevent clots, while doses that are too high may cause severe bleeding.

Fibrinolytic drugs help dissolve clots that have already formed. Dissolving clots quickly may prevent the death of heart tissue deprived of its blood supply because of blocked blood vessels ▲ Three fibrinolytic drugs commonly used for dissolving clots in people who have had a heart attack are streptokinase, urokinase, and tissue plasminogen activator. These drugs may save lives when used during the first few hours after a heart

---

Bleeding Disorders: Why the Blood Doesn't Clot

Thrombocytopenia
The concentration of platelets in the blood is too low.

Von Willebrand's disease
Platelets don't stick to holes in blood vessel walls.

Hereditary platelet disorders
Platelets don't stick to each other to form a plug.

Hemophilia
Clotting factor VIII or clotting factor IX is missing.

Disseminated intravascular coagulation
Clotting factors are depleted because of excessive clotting

---

attack or when given for other clotting disorders, but they can also put people at risk of severe bleeding.

Easy Bruising

People may bruise easily because of fragile capillaries in the skin. Each time these small blood vessels break, a little blood leaks out, leaving tiny red dots in the skin (petechiae) and bluish-purple bruises (purpura). Women seem more prone than men to bruise from a minor injury, especially on the thighs, buttocks, and upper arms. Sometimes easy bruising runs in families. For most people, the condition isn't serious, but bruising easily may be a sign that something is wrong with the blood clotting elements, most likely the platelets. Blood tests can determine if such problems exist.

In older people, particularly those exposed to a great deal of sun, bruises commonly occur on the backs of the hands and the forearms (senile purpura). Older people are especially susceptible to easy bruising after bumps and falls because they have fragile blood vessels and a thinner layer

▲ see page 126

of fat under the skin, which normally serves as a cushion to help protect against injury. Blood leaks from damaged vessels, forming deep purple patches (hematomas). These bruises may persist for a long time, eventually becoming light green, yellow, or brown.

This condition is not a disease and no treatment is needed. Efforts to avoid injury can reduce the bruising.

Hereditary Hemorrhagic Telangiectasia

Hereditary hemorrhagic telangiectasia (Rendu-Osler-Weber disease) is a hereditary malformation of the blood vessels that makes them fragile and prone to bleeding.

Bleeding under the skin appears as small, red-to-violet discolorations, especially on the face, lips, lining of the mouth and nose, and tips of the fingers and toes. Similar small abnormalities may occur in the gastrointestinal tract. The fragile blood vessels may break, causing severe nosebleeds and bleeding from the gastrointestinal tract. Neurologic problems may also occur.

No specific treatment is available, but bleeding can be stopped by applying compresses or astringents. If bleeding recurs, a laser beam can be used to destroy the leaking blood vessel. Severe bleeding can be stopped by blocking the leaking artery with a pellet inserted through a catheter or by grafting normal tissue. Bleeding almost always recurs, resulting in iron deficiency anemia; consequently, people who have this disorder need to take iron supplements.

Connective Tissue Disorders

In certain hereditary diseases such as Ehlers-Danlos syndrome, collagen (a tough, fibrous protein in connective tissue) is abnormally weak and supple. Because collagen surrounds and supports the blood vessels that run through connective tissue,▲ abnormalities of collagen may make blood vessels unusually susceptible to breakage. No cure exists for these diseases; people who have them should try to avoid potentially injurious situations and control the bleeding when it occurs.

Allergic Purpura

Allergic purpura (Henoch-Schönlein purpura) is an inflammation of the small blood vessels that may be caused by an abnormal immune (autoimmune) reaction.

Allergic purpura, an uncommon disease, affects mainly young children but can affect older children and adults. Usually, it develops just after a respiratory tract infection, but it can be caused by drugs. The disease may develop suddenly and last a short time, or it may develop gradually and last a long time. Blood vessels in the skin, joints, gastrointestinal tract, or kidneys may become inflamed and leak.

Symptoms and Diagnosis

The disease may begin with the appearance of small areas of purplish spots (purpura)—most often on the feet, legs, arms, and buttocks—as blood leaks from vessels in the skin. Over several days, the purpuric spots may become raised and hard; crops of new spots may break out for several weeks after the first one appears. Swollen ankles, hips, knees, wrists, and elbows are common, usually accompanied by a fever and achy joints. Bleeding in the gastrointestinal tract may cause abdominal cramps and tenderness; nearly half the people who have allergic purpura have blood in the urine (hematuria). Most people recover completely within a month, but symptoms may appear and disappear several times. Sometimes the kidneys are permanently damaged.

The diagnosis is based on the symptoms. If blood or urine tests show changes in kidney function, a doctor may remove a small sample of tissue from the kidney with a needle for examination under a microscope (needle biopsy) to determine the extent of damage and to ensure that the cause is allergic purpura.

Prognosis and Treatment

If a doctor suspects that the allergic reaction is caused by a drug, the drug is discontinued immediately. Corticosteroids such as prednisone may help relieve swelling, joint pain, and abdominal pain, but they don't prevent kidney damage. Drugs that reduce the activity of the immune system (immunosuppressive drugs), such as azathioprine or cyclophosphamide, are sometimes used if kidney damage develops, but whether they help is not known.

▲ see page 4

Causes of Thrombocytopenia

Bone marrow doesn't produce enough platelets
- Leukemia
- Aplastic anemia
- Paroxysmal nocturnal hemoglobinuria
- Heavy alcohol consumption
- Megaloblastic anemias
- Some bone marrow disorders

Platelets become entrapped in an enlarged spleen
- Cirrhosis with congestive splenomegaly
- Myelofibrosis
- Gaucher's disease

Platelets become diluted
- Massive blood replacement or exchange transfusion (because platelets don't last long in stored blood)
- Cardiopulmonary bypass surgery

Use or destruction of platelets increases
- Idiopathic thrombocytopenic purpura
- HIV infection
- Purpura after blood transfusions
- Drugs such as heparin, quinidine, quinine, sulfa-containing antibiotics, some oral diabetes drugs, gold salts, and rifampin
- Chronic leukemia in newborns
- Lymphoma
- Systemic lupus erythematosus
- Conditions involving clotting within blood vessels, such as obstetric complications, cancer, blood poisoning (septicemia) from gram-negative bacteria, and traumatic brain damage
- Thrombotic thrombocytopenic purpura
- Hemolytic-uremic syndrome
- Adult respiratory distress syndrome
- Severe infections with blood poisoning

Thrombocytopenia

Thrombocytopenia is a deficiency of platelets (thrombocytes), which are involved in clotting.

The blood usually contains about 150,000 to 350,000 platelets per microliter. Abnormal bleeding can occur when the platelet count falls below 30,000 per microliter, although problems usually aren't apparent until it falls below 10,000 per microliter.

Many diseases can cause a low platelet count, but often no specific cause can be found. Four main reasons for a decrease in the number of platelets are that the bone marrow doesn't produce enough platelets, platelets become entrapped in an enlarged spleen,▲ use or destruction of platelets increases, and platelets become diluted.

Symptoms

Bleeding in the skin may be the first sign of a low platelet count. Many purple pinpoint bruises often appear on the lower legs, and minor injuries may cause small scattered bruises. The gums may bleed, and blood may be seen in the stool or urine. Menstrual periods may be unusually heavy. Sur-

gery and accidents can be dangerous because bleeding may be hard to stop.

Bleeding worsens as the number of platelets decreases. People who have very few platelets (usually fewer than 5,000 to 10,000 per microliter of blood) may lose large amounts of blood into the gastrointestinal tract or may develop life-threatening bleeding in the brain even though they haven't been injured.

Diagnosis

Doctors suspect thrombocytopenia in people who have abnormal bruising and bleeding. They often check platelet counts routinely in people who have disorders that cause thrombocytopenia. Sometimes they discover thrombocytopenia when blood tests are performed for other reasons in people who have no bleeding symptoms.

Determining the cause of thrombocytopenia is critical to treating the condition. The doctor must determine whether the person has a disorder that causes thrombocytopenia. If not, certain symp-

▲ see page 786

toms may help determine the cause. For example, people usually have a fever when thrombocytopenia results from an infection, an autoimmune disease such as systemic lupus erythematosus, or thrombotic thrombocytopenic purpura. But they usually don't have a fever when the cause is idiopathic thrombocytopenia or drugs. An enlarged spleen, which a doctor may be able to feel during a physical examination, suggests that the spleen is trapping platelets and that thrombocytopenia results from a disorder that causes the spleen to enlarge.

A sample of blood may be examined under a microscope, or the platelet count and volume may be measured with an electronic counter to determine the severity of thrombocytopenia and provide clues to its cause. A sample of bone marrow removed with the needle of a syringe (bone marrow aspiration) and examined under a microscope▲ may provide information about platelet production.

Treatment

Thrombocytopenia caused by a drug usually can be corrected by stopping the drug. People who have very low platelet counts are often treated in a hospital or advised to stay in bed to avoid accidental injury. When bleeding is severe, platelets may be transfused, particularly if the thrombocytopenia results from decreased platelet production.

IDIOPATHIC THROMBOCYTOPENIC PURPURA

Idiopathic thrombocytopenic purpura is a disorder in which a low platelet count with no discernible cause results in abnormal bleeding.

The cause of the platelet deficiency is unknown (idiopathic), but an abnormal immune reaction (autoimmune reaction), in which antibodies destroy a person's own platelets, appears to be involved. Although the bone marrow increases platelet production to compensate for the destruction, the supply cannot keep up with the demand.

In children, this disorder usually occurs after a viral infection and disappears without treatment after a few weeks or months.

Symptoms and Diagnosis

Symptoms may appear abruptly (acute form of the disorder) or develop more subtly (chronic form). Symptoms include red spots on the skin the size of a pinhead, unexplained bruises, bleeding from the gums and nose, and blood in the stool. Doctors make the diagnosis when they find a low platelet count and evidence of increased platelet destruction rather than decreased production in blood and bone marrow samples. No other causes of thrombocytopenia can be found.

Treatment

When treating adults, doctors first try to suppress the immune response with high doses of a corticosteroid such as prednisone. Corticosteroids almost always increase the platelet count, but the increase may be transient. Because continued use of a corticosteroid produces a number of undesired effects, the dose is tapered off as soon as possible. Drugs that suppress the immune system, such as azathioprine, are also sometimes used. When drugs aren't effective or the disorder recurs, removal of the spleen (splenectomy) cures the disorder in most people.

High doses of immune globulin or anti-Rh factor (for people who have Rh-positive blood) are given intravenously to treat people with acute life-threatening bleeding. They're also used for longer periods, especially in children, to keep platelet levels high enough to prevent bleeding.

THROMBOCYTOPENIA CAUSED BY DISEASE

Infection with the human immunodeficiency virus (HIV), the virus that causes AIDS, frequently results in thrombocytopenia. The cause appears to be antibodies that destroy platelets. The treatment is similar to that of idiopathic thrombocytopenic purpura. However, aggressive treatment may not be started until the platelet count is even lower because people who have AIDS seem to tolerate lower platelet counts before experiencing dangerous bleeding. The drug AZT (zidovudine), given to slow the replication of the AIDS virus, often increases the number of platelets.

Several other diseases can cause thrombocytopenia. Systemic lupus erythematosus decreases the number of platelets by producing antibodies. Disseminated intravascular coagulation causes tiny clots to form throughout the body, rapidly depleting platelets and clotting factors.

▲ see page 737

THROMBOTIC THROMBOCYTOPENIC PURPURA

Thrombotic thrombocytopenic purpura is a rare, life-threatening disorder in which small blood clots suddenly form throughout the body, leading to a sharp decrease in the number of platelets and red blood cells, fever, and widespread damage to many organs.

The cause of this disorder is unknown. The clotting can cut off the blood supply to parts of the brain, causing bizarre, fluctuating neurologic symptoms. Other symptoms include jaundice, blood and protein in the urine, kidney damage, abdominal pain, and abnormal heart rhythms. If not treated, the disorder is almost always fatal; with treatment, more than half the affected people survive.

Treatment

Repeated plasmapheresis (plasma exchange) or transfusions of large amounts of plasma (the liquid part of blood that remains after all the cells are removed) can stop the destruction of platelets and red blood cells. Corticosteroids and drugs that inhibit platelet function, such as aspirin and dipyridamole, may be used, but their effectiveness is uncertain. Although thrombotic thrombocytopenic purpura may occur as a single, isolated episode, people who have had the disorder should be monitored with blood tests and physical examinations for several years because sudden relapses requiring treatment are not unusual.

Hemolytic-Uremic Syndrome

Hemolytic-uremic syndrome is a disorder in which the number of platelets suddenly decreases, red blood cells are destroyed, and the kidney stops functioning.

This syndrome is most common in infants, small children, and women who are pregnant or have just given birth, although it can occur in older children, adults, and women who aren't pregnant. Sometimes a bacterial infection, anticancer drugs such as mitomycin, or potent immunosuppressive drugs seem to trigger the hemolytic-uremic syndrome, but usually the cause is unknown.

Symptoms and Diagnosis

The symptoms are those of a generalized bleeding disorder, similar to thrombotic thrombocytopenic purpura. However, few neurologic symptoms occur and kidney damage is always severe.

Treatment and Prognosis

Most infants and children recover, although they may need dialysis at intervals until their kidneys mend. Many adults, especially women who acquire the syndrome after giving birth, never recover full kidney function. For some people, plasmapheresis seems helpful. Most people who develop the syndrome while taking mitomycin die of complications within a few months.

Platelet Dysfunction

In some disorders, the number of platelets remains normal, but the platelets don't function normally; they are unable to prevent bleeding. The cause of such platelet dysfunction may be hereditary (for example, von Willebrand's disease) or acquired (for example, some drugs).

VON WILLEBRAND'S DISEASE

Von Willebrand's disease is a hereditary deficiency or abnormality of the von Willebrand factor in the blood, a protein that affects platelet function.

Von Willebrand's disease is the most common hereditary disorder of platelet function. The von Willebrand factor is found in plasma, platelets, and blood vessel walls. When the factor is missing or defective, the first step in plugging a blood vessel injury—platelets adhere to the vessel wall at the site of the injury—doesn't take place. As a result, bleeding doesn't stop as quickly as it should, although it usually stops eventually.

Symptoms and Diagnosis

Usually, a person with von Willebrand's disease has a parent who has a history of bleeding problems. Typically, a child bruises easily or bleeds excessively after a skin cut, tooth extraction, tonsillectomy, or other surgery. A woman may have increased menstrual bleeding. Bleeding may worsen at times. On the other hand, hormonal changes, stress, pregnancy, inflammation, and infections may stimulate the body to increase production of the von Willebrand factor and temporarily improve clot formation.

Aspirin and many of the drugs used for arthritis can aggravate bleeding because they interfere with platelet function. People who have von Wil-

Hereditary Platelet Disorders

Disorder	Frequency of Occurrence	Description	Severity of Bleeding
Von Willebrand's disease	Relatively common	Defective or missing von Willebrand factor, the protein that holds platelets to broken blood vessel walls, or deficient clotting factor VIII	Mild to moderate in most cases; may be severe in people who have very low levels of von Willebrand factor
Storage pool disease	Relatively uncommon	Defective platelet granules that impair platelet clumping	Mild
Chédiak-Higashi and Hermansky-Pudlak syndromes	Rare	Special forms of storage pool disease	Variable
Thromboxane A_2 dysfunction	Very rare	Impaired platelet response to stimuli for clumping	Mild
Thrombasthenia	Rare	Missing proteins on platelet surface that are needed for platelet clumping	Variable
Bernard-Soulier syndrome	Rare	Missing proteins on platelet surface and abnormally large platelets that don't stick to injured blood vessel walls	Variable

lebrand's disease can take acetaminophen for pain relief because it doesn't inhibit platelet function.

Laboratory tests may determine that the number of platelets is normal but bleeding time is abnormally long. Bleeding time is the amount of time elapsed before bleeding stops after a small cut is made on the forearm. To make the diagnosis, doctors may order tests that measure the amount of von Willebrand factor in the blood. Because the von Willebrand factor is the protein that carries factor VIII in the blood, the blood level of factor VIII may also be decreased.

▲ see page 740

Treatment

Many of the people who have von Willebrand's disease never need treatment. For excessive bleeding, a transfusion of concentrated blood clotting factors containing von Willebrand factor may be given.▲ For some mild forms of the disease, desmopressin may be given to increase the amount of the von Willebrand factor long enough for surgery or dental procedures to be performed without transfusions.

ACQUIRED PLATELET DYSFUNCTION

Several diseases and a variety of drugs can cause platelet dysfunction. Among the diseases are kidney failure, leukemia, multiple myeloma, cirrhosis of the liver, and systemic lupus erythematosus. The drugs include aspirin, ticlopidine, nonsteroidal anti-inflammatory drugs (used for arthritis, pain, and sprains), and penicillin in high doses. In most cases, the platelet dysfunction doesn't lead to severe bleeding.

Hemophilia

Hemophilia is a bleeding disorder caused by a deficiency in one of the blood clotting factors.

Hemophilia A (classic hemophilia), which accounts for about 80 percent of all cases, is a deficiency in clotting factor VIII. **Hemophilia B** (Christmas disease) is a deficiency in clotting factor IX. The bleeding patterns and consequences of these types of hemophilia are similar. Both are inherited through the mother (sex-linked inheritance) but affect male children almost exclusively.▲

Symptoms

Hemophilia is caused by several different gene abnormalities. The severity of the symptoms depends on how a particular gene abnormality affects the activity of factors VIII and IX. When the activity is less than 1 percent of normal, episodes of severe bleeding occur and recur for no apparent reason.

People whose clotting activity is 5 percent of normal may have only mild hemophilia. They rarely have unprovoked bleeding episodes, but surgery or injury may cause uncontrolled bleeding, which can be fatal. Milder hemophilia may not be diagnosed at all, although some people whose clotting activity is 10 to 25 percent of normal may bleed excessively after surgery, dental extractions, or a major injury.

Generally, the first bleeding episode occurs before 18 months of age, often after a minor injury. A child who has hemophilia bruises easily. Even an injection into a muscle can cause bleeding that results in a large bruise (hematoma). Recurring bleeding into the joints and muscles can ultimately lead to crippling deformities. Bleeding can swell the base of the tongue until it blocks the airway, making breathing difficult. A slight bump on the head can trigger substantial bleeding in the skull, causing brain damage and death.

Diagnosis

A doctor may suspect hemophilia in a young boy whose bleeding is unusual. A laboratory analysis of blood samples can determine whether the boy's clotting is abnormally slow. If it is, the doctor can confirm the diagnosis of hemophilia and can determine the type and severity by testing the activity of factors VIII and IX.

Treatment

People who have hemophilia should avoid situations that might provoke bleeding. They should be conscientious about dental care so they won't need to have teeth extracted. If people who have milder forms of hemophilia need to have dental or other surgery, the drug desmopressin may be given to improve clotting temporarily so that transfusions can be avoided. People who have hemophilia should also avoid certain drugs—aspirin, heparin, warfarin, and certain analgesics such as nonsteroidal anti-inflammatory drugs—that can aggravate bleeding problems.

Usually, treatment involves transfusions to replace the deficient clotting factor. These factors are found in plasma and, to a greater extent, in plasma concentrates. Some plasma concentrates are intended for home use and can be self-administered, either on a regular basis to prevent bleeding or at the first sign of bleeding. More often, they are administered three times a day, but both the dose and frequency depend on the severity of the bleeding problem. The dose is adjusted according to the results of periodic blood tests. During a bleeding episode, more clotting factors are needed, and treatment must be coordinated by a health care practitioner who is an expert in this disease.

In the past, the plasma concentrates carried the risk of transmitting blood-borne diseases such as hepatitis and AIDS. About 60 percent of the hemophiliacs who were treated with plasma concentrates in the early 1980s have been infected with HIV. However, the risk of transmitting HIV infection through plasma concentrates has been virtually eliminated by today's use of screened and processed blood■ and a genetically engineered factor VIII.

Some hemophiliacs develop antibodies to transfused factors VIII and IX. As a result, the transfusions are ineffective. If antibodies are detected in blood samples, the dosage of the plasma concentrates may be increased, or different types of clotting factors or drugs to reduce the antibody levels may be used.

▲ see box, page 11

■ see box, page 739

Disseminated Intravascular Coagulation

Disseminated intravascular coagulation (consumption coagulopathy) is a condition in which small blood clots disseminate through the bloodstream, blocking small blood vessels and depleting the clotting factors needed to control bleeding.

The condition begins with excessive clotting usually stimulated by a toxic substance in the blood. As the clotting factors are depleted, excessive bleeding occurs.

Symptoms and Diagnosis

Disseminated intravascular coagulation usually appears suddenly and may be very severe. If the condition follows surgery or childbirth, the surface of cut or torn tissues may bleed profusely and uncontrollably. Bleeding may persist at the site of an intravenous injection or puncture, and massive bleeding can occur in the brain, gastrointestinal tract, skin, muscles, and cavities of the body. At the same time, clots in small blood vessels can damage the kidneys—sometimes permanently—so that they can't produce urine.

Doctors order blood tests to monitor people at high risk for disseminated intravascular coagulation. These tests may show that the number of platelets in a blood sample has suddenly dropped and that the blood is taking a long time to clot. The diagnosis is confirmed if test results show diminished amounts of the clotting factors, unusually small clots, and large quantities of degradation products from the breakup of clots.

Treatment

The underlying cause of disseminated intravascular coagulation must be identified and corrected, whether it's an obstetric problem, an infection, or a cancer. The clotting problems may subside when the cause is corrected.

Because disseminated intravascular coagulation is life threatening, it's usually treated as an emergency until the underlying cause is corrected. Emergency treatment is complex because the person's condition fluctuates rapidly between bleeding excessively and clotting excessively. Platelets and clotting factors may be transfused to replace those depleted and to stop massive bleeding, but the benefits of platelet transfusions are short-lived. Sometimes heparin is used to slow the clotting.

Disorders of Circulating Anticoagulants

Circulating anticoagulants are substances in the blood that block an essential component of the blood clotting process. Usually, these anticoagulants are antibodies to a clotting factor such as factor VIII. In some diseases, the body produces these anticoagulants. Affected people develop symptoms of excessive bleeding similar to those of people taking anticoagulant drugs, such as heparin and warfarin.

People who have systemic lupus erythematosus often produce a circulating anticoagulant, which can be detected in laboratory tests that measure clotting. Paradoxically, this anticoagulant usually doesn't cause excessive bleeding; it sometimes causes excessive clotting. Women who have this anticoagulant seem prone to miscarriages.

White Blood Cell Disorders

White blood cells (leukocytes) are the body's defense against infective organisms and foreign substances. To defend the body adequately, a sufficient number of white blood cells must stimulate the right responses, get to where they are needed, and then kill and digest the harmful organisms and substances.▲

Like all blood cells, white blood cells are produced in the bone marrow. They develop from precursor (stem) cells that mature over time into one of the five major types of white blood cells—neutrophils, lymphocytes, monocytes, eosinophils, and basophils. Normally, a person produces about 100 billion white blood cells a day.

Usually, the number of white blood cells in a given volume of blood is determined automatically by a computerized cell-counting instrument. These instruments provide the total white blood cell count, expressed as cells per microliter of blood, as well as the proportion of each of the five major types of white blood cells. The total white blood cell count normally ranges between 4,000 and 10,000 cells per microliter.

Too few or too many white blood cells indicates a disorder. Leukopenia, a decrease in the number of white blood cells to fewer than 4,000 per microliter, makes a person more susceptible to infections. Leukocytosis, an increased number of white blood cells, may be a response to infections■ or foreign substances, or it can result from cancer, injury, stress, or certain drugs. Most white blood cell disorders involve neutrophils, lymphocytes, monocytes, and eosinophils. Disorders involving basophils are very rare.

Neutropenia

Neutropenia is an abnormally low number of neutrophils in the blood.

Neutrophils are the body's primary cellular defense system against bacteria and fungi. They also help heal wounds and ingest foreign debris, such as embedded splinters.

Neutrophils mature in the bone marrow in about 2 weeks. After entering the bloodstream, they circulate for about 6 hours, searching for infective organisms and other intruders. When they find one, they migrate into the tissues, attach themselves to the intruders, and produce toxic substances that kill and digest the intruders. This reaction may damage healthy tissue in the area of the infection. The entire process produces an inflammatory response in the infected area, which appears on the body's surface as redness, swelling, and heat.

Because neutrophils generally make up over 70 percent of the white blood cells, a decrease in the number of white blood cells usually means a decrease in the total number of neutrophils. When the neutrophil count falls below 1,000 cells per microliter, the risk of infections increases somewhat; when it falls below 500 cells per microliter, the risk of infections increases greatly. Without the key neutrophil defense, a person could die of an infection.

Causes

Neutropenia has a number of causes. The number of neutrophils can decrease because bone marrow production isn't adequate or because large numbers of white blood cells are destroyed in the circulation.

Aplastic anemia causes neutropenia as well as deficiencies in other types of blood cells. Certain rare hereditary diseases, such as infantile genetic agranulocytosis and familial neutropenia, also cause decreases in the number of white blood cells.

In cyclic neutropenia, a rare disorder, the number of neutrophils fluctuates between normal and low every 21 to 28 days; the neutrophil count may fall to almost zero and then spontaneously return to normal after 3 to 4 days. People who have cyclic neutropenia are prone to infections when the number of neutrophils is low.

Some people who have cancer, tuberculosis, myelofibrosis, vitamin B_{12} deficiency, or folic acid deficiency develop neutropenia. Certain drugs,

---

▲ see page 812

■ see page 841

Drugs That Can Cause Neutropenia

Antibiotics (penicillins, sulfonamides, and chloramphenicol)

Anticonvulsants

Antithyroid drugs

Cancer chemotherapy drugs

Gold salts

Phenothiazines

especially those used in cancer treatment (chemotherapy),▲ impair the bone marrow's ability to produce neutrophils.

Neutrophils are destroyed faster than they're produced in some bacterial infections, some allergic disorders, some autoimmune diseases, and some drug treatments. People with an enlarged spleen—for instance, those who have Felty's syndrome, malaria, or sarcoidosis—may have a low neutrophil count because the enlarged spleen traps and destroys neutrophils.■

Symptoms and Diagnosis

Neutropenia can develop suddenly over a few hours or days (acute neutropenia), or it can last for months or years (chronic neutropenia). Because neutropenia has no specific symptoms, it's likely to go unnoticed until an infection occurs. In acute neutropenia, a person can develop fever and painful sores (ulcers) around the mouth and anus. Bacterial pneumonia and other severe infections follow. In chronic neutropenia, the course may be less severe if the number of neutrophils isn't extremely low.

When a person has frequent or unusual infections, a doctor suspects neutropenia and orders a complete blood cell count to make the diagnosis. A low neutrophil count indicates neutropenia.

▲ see page 802

■ see page 786

★ see page 737

Next, the cause of the neutropenia is determined. A doctor usually takes a sample of bone marrow through a needle (bone marrow aspiration and biopsy).★ Although this procedure can be uncomfortable, it's usually not dangerous. The bone marrow sample is examined under a microscope to determine whether it looks normal, has a normal number of neutrophil precursor cells, and is producing a normal number of white blood cells. By determining whether the number of precursor cells is decreased and whether these cells are maturing normally, the doctor may be able to estimate the time needed for the neutrophil count to return to normal. If the number of precursor cells is decreased, new neutrophils will not appear in the bloodstream for 2 weeks or more; if the number is adequate and the cells are maturing normally, new neutrophils may appear in the bloodstream within days. Sometimes, bone marrow examination also reveals that other diseases, such as leukemia or other blood cell cancers, are affecting the bone marrow.

Treatment

The treatment of neutropenia depends on its cause and severity. Drugs that may cause neutropenia are discontinued whenever possible. Sometimes the bone marrow recovers by itself without treatment. People who have mild neutropenia (more than 500 neutrophils per microliter of blood) generally have no symptoms and may not need treatment.

People who have severe neutropenia (fewer than 500 cells per microliter) can rapidly succumb to infection because their bodies lack the means to fight the invading organisms. When these people develop infections, they are generally hospitalized and immediately given strong antibiotics, even before the cause and exact location of the infection are identified. Fever, the symptom that usually indicates infection in a person who has neutropenia, is an important sign that immediate medical attention is needed.

Growth factors that stimulate the production of white blood cells, particularly granulocyte colony-stimulating factor (G-CSF) and granulocyte-macrophage colony-stimulating factor (GM-CSF), are sometimes helpful. This form of treatment can eliminate neutropenic episodes in cyclic neutropenia. Corticosteroids may help if the neutropenia is caused by an allergic or autoimmune reaction. Antithymocyte globulin or some other type of immunosuppressive therapy (therapy that suppresses the activity of the immune system) may be used when an autoimmune disease—such as certain cases of aplastic anemia—is suspected. Removing an enlarged spleen may increase the neutrophil count if the spleen is trapping white blood cells.

People who have aplastic anemia may need to undergo bone marrow transplantation if immunosuppressive therapy fails.▲ Bone marrow transplantation can have significant toxic effects, requires a lengthy hospitalization, and can be performed only in certain situations. Generally, it isn't used to treat neutropenia alone.

Lymphocytopenia

Lymphocytopenia is an abnormally low lymphocyte count—below 1,500 cells per microliter of blood in adults or below 3,000 cells per microliter in children.

Normally, lymphocytes constitute 15 to 40 percent of all white blood cells in the bloodstream. Lymphocytes are central to the immune system: They protect the body against viral infection; they help other cells protect the body against bacterial and fungal infections; they develop into cells that produce antibodies (plasma cells); they fight cancer; and they help coordinate the activities of other cells in the immune system.■

Lymphocytopenia can be caused by a variety of diseases and conditions. The number of lymphocytes can decrease briefly during severe stress and during treatment involving corticosteroids such as prednisone, chemotherapy for cancer, and radiation therapy. People who have low T-lymphocyte counts usually have more severe lymphocytopenia and generally suffer more severe consequences than people who have low B-lymphocyte counts, but either deficiency can be fatal.

Symptoms and Diagnosis

Because lymphocytes make up a relatively small proportion of the white blood cells, a reduction in their number may not cause a significant decrease in the total number of white blood cells. Lymphocytopenia itself may cause no symptoms and is usually detected in a complete blood cell count that was ordered to diagnose other illnesses. Drastically reduced numbers of lymphocytes lead to infections with viruses, fungi, and parasites.

Lymphocytes: The Destroyer Cells

The two main types of lymphocytes are B lymphocytes, also called B cells, and T lymphocytes, also called T cells. B cells originate and mature in the bone marrow, whereas T cells originate in bone marrow but mature in the thymus gland. B cells develop into plasma cells, which produce antibodies. Antibodies help the body destroy abnormal cells and infective organisms such as bacteria, viruses, and fungi. T cells are divided into three groups, as follows:
- Killer T cells, which recognize and destroy abnormal or infected cells
- Helper T cells, which help other cells destroy infective organisms
- Suppressor T cells, which suppress the activity of other lymphocytes so they don't destroy normal tissue

---

With current laboratory technology, changes in numbers of specific types of lymphocytes can be detected. For instance, decreases in a type of T lymphocyte known as T4 cells are one way to measure the progression of AIDS.

Treatment

Treatment depends mainly on the cause. Lymphocytopenia caused by a drug usually resolves within days after a person stops taking the drug. When the cause is AIDS, generally little can be done to increase the number of lymphocytes, although certain drugs such as AZT (zidovudine) and ddI (didanosine) may increase the number of helper T cells.

When lymphocytopenia is a deficiency of B lymphocytes, the concentration of antibodies in the blood may fall below normal. In these cases, gamma globulin (a substance rich in antibodies) may be given to help prevent infections. If an infection does develop, specific antibiotic, antifungal, or antiviral drugs directed against the infective organism are given.

▲ see page 836

■ see page 810

Diseases That Cause Lymphocytopenia

Cancer (leukemias, lymphomas, Hodgkin's disease)

Rheumatoid arthritis

Systemic lupus erythematosus

Chronic infections

Rare hereditary disorders (certain agammaglobulinemias, DiGeorge syndrome, Wiskott-Aldrich syndrome, severe combined immunodeficiency syndrome, and ataxia-telangiectasia)

Acquired immunodeficiency syndrome (AIDS)

Some viral infections

Monocyte Disorders

Monocytes collaborate with other white blood cells to remove dead or damaged tissues, destroy cancer cells, and regulate immunity against foreign substances. Like other white blood cells, monocytes are produced in the bone marrow and then enter the bloodstream. Within a few hours, they migrate to tissues where they mature into macrophages, the scavenger cells (phagocytes) of the immune system. Macrophages are scattered throughout the body but accumulate in high concentrations in the lungs, liver, spleen, bone marrow, and linings of the major body cavities, where they survive for many months.

Certain types of infections (tuberculosis, for example), cancer, and disorders of the immune system increase the number of monocytes. In inherited diseases such as Gaucher's disease and Niemann-Pick disease, cellular debris accumulates in macrophages, causing dysfunction.

Eosinophilia

Eosinophilia is an abnormally high number of eosinophils in the blood.

Eosinophilia is not a disease, but it may be a response to a disease. An increased number of eosinophils in the blood usually indicates an appropriate response to abnormal cells, parasites, or substances that cause an allergic reaction (allergens).

Once produced in the bone marrow, eosinophils enter the bloodstream but stay there only a few hours before migrating to tissues throughout the body. When a foreign substance enters the body, it's detected by lymphocytes and neutrophils, which release substances that attract eosinophils to the area. Eosinophils then release toxic substances that can kill parasites and destroy abnormal human cells.

IDIOPATHIC HYPEREOSINOPHILIC SYNDROME

Idiopathic hypereosinophilic syndrome is a disorder in which the number of eosinophils increases to more than 1,500 cells per microliter of blood for more than 6 months without an obvious cause.

People of any age can develop idiopathic hypereosinophilic syndrome, but it's more common in men over 50 years old. The increased number of eosinophils can damage the heart, lungs, liver, skin, and nervous system. For example, the heart can become inflamed in a condition called Löffler's endocarditis, leading to formation of blood clots, heart failure, heart attacks, or malfunctioning heart valves.

The symptoms of this syndrome depend on which organs are damaged. They may include weight loss, fevers, night sweats, general fatigue, cough, chest pain, swelling, stomachache, skin rashes, pain, weakness, confusion, and coma. The syndrome is diagnosed when persistently increased numbers of eosinophils are found in people who have these symptoms. Before starting treatment, however, doctors must determine that the eosinophilia isn't being caused by a parasitic infection or an allergic reaction.

Without treatment, generally more than 80 percent of the people who have this syndrome die within 2 years; with treatment, more than 80 percent survive. Heart damage is the principal cause of death. Some people need no treatment other than close observation for 3 to 6 months, but most need drug treatment with prednisone or hydroxyurea. If this treatment fails, a variety of other drugs may be used, and they can be combined with a procedure to remove eosinophils from the blood (leukapheresis).

EOSINOPHILIA-MYALGIA SYNDROME

Eosinophilia-myalgia syndrome is a disorder in which eosinophilia is combined with muscle pain and tenderness, fatigue, swelling, joint pain, cough, shortness of breath, rashes, and neurologic abnormalities.

Usually rare, this syndrome appeared in the early 1990s in people who took large amounts of tryptophan, a popular health food store product sometimes recommended by doctors to enhance

sleep. An impurity in the product, rather than tryptophan itself, probably caused the syndrome.

This syndrome can last weeks to months after tryptophan is discontinued and can cause permanent neurologic damage and, in rare cases, death. No cure is known; physical rehabilitation is generally recommended.

CHAPTER 157

Leukemias

Leukemias are cancers of the blood cells.

Leukemias usually affect the white blood cells. The cause of most types of leukemia isn't known. Viruses cause some leukemias in animals, such as cats. A virus known as HTLV-I (human T-cell lymphotropic virus type I), which is similar to the virus that causes AIDS, is strongly suspected to be the cause of a rare type of leukemia in people, adult T-cell leukemia. Exposure to radiation and certain chemicals, such as benzene, and use of some anticancer drugs increase the risk of developing leukemia. Also, people who have certain genetic disorders, such as Down syndrome and Fanconi's syndrome, are more likely to develop leukemia.

White blood cells develop from stem cells in the bone marrow.▲ Leukemia results when the process of maturation from stem cell to white blood cell goes awry and produces a cancerous change. The change often involves a rearrangement of pieces of chromosomes—the cell's complex genetic material. Because the chromosomal rearrangements (chromosomal translocation) disturb the normal control of cell division, the affected cells multiply without restraint, becoming cancerous. They ultimately occupy the bone marrow, replacing the cells that produce normal blood cells. These leukemic (cancer) cells may also invade other organs, including the liver, spleen, lymph nodes, kidneys, and brain.

There are four major types of leukemia, named for how quickly they progress and which kind of white blood cell they affect. Acute leukemias progress rapidly; chronic leukemias progress slowly.

Lymphocytic leukemias affect lymphocytes; myeloid (myelocytic) leukemias affect myelocytes. Myelocytes develop into granulocytes, another term for neutrophils.

Acute Lymphocytic Leukemia

Acute lymphocytic (lymphoblastic) leukemia is a life-threatening disease in which the cells that normally develop into lymphocytes become cancerous and rapidly replace normal cells in the bone marrow.

Acute lymphocytic leukemia, the most common cancer in children, accounts for 25 percent of all cancers in children under age 15. It most often affects children between the ages of 3 and 5 but can also affect adolescents and, less commonly, adults.

Very immature cells that normally develop into lymphocytes become cancerous. These leukemic cells accumulate in the bone marrow, destroying and replacing cells that produce normal blood cells. They're released into the bloodstream and transported to the liver, spleen, lymph nodes, brain, kidneys, and reproductive organs, where they continue to grow and divide. They can irritate the lining of the brain, causing meningitis, and can cause anemia, liver and kidney failure, and other organ damage.

▲ see box, page 735

Major Types of Leukemia

Type	Progression	White Blood Cell Affected	Number of Cases Diagnosed Yearly in the United States
Acute lymphocytic (lymphoblastic) leukemia	Rapid	Lymphocytes	5,200
Acute myeloid (myelocytic, myelogenous, myeloblastic, myelomonocytic) leukemia	Rapid	Myelocytes	7,000
Chronic lymphocytic leukemia, including Sézary syndrome and hairy cell leukemia	Slow	Lymphocytes	8,500
Chronic myelocytic (myeloid, myelogenous, granulocytic) leukemia	Slow	Myelocytes	5,800

Symptoms

The first symptoms usually occur because the bone marrow fails to produce enough normal blood cells. These symptoms include weakness and shortness of breath, resulting from too few red blood cells (anemia); infection and fever, resulting from too few normal white blood cells; and bleeding, resulting from too few platelets. In some people, a severe infection is the first problem, but in others, the onset is more subtle, with progressive weakness, fatigue, and paleness. Bleeding may occur in the form of nosebleeds, gums that bleed easily, purple skin blotches, or easy bruising. Leukemic cells in the brain may cause headaches, vomiting, and irritability, and those in the bone marrow may cause bone and joint pain.

Diagnosis

Common blood tests, such as the complete blood cell count,▲ can provide the first evidence that a person has leukemia. The total number of white blood cells may be decreased, normal, or increased, but the number of red blood cells and platelets is almost always decreased. More important, very immature white blood cells (blasts) are seen in blood samples examined under a microscope. Since blasts aren't normally seen in the blood, their presence may be all that is needed to diagnose leukemia. However, a bone marrow biopsy■ is almost always performed to confirm the diagnosis and determine the type of leukemia.

Prognosis and Treatment

Before treatment was available, most people who had acute leukemia died within 4 months of diagnosis. Now, many people are cured. For more than 90 percent of people who have acute lymphocytic leukemia (usually children), the first course of chemotherapy brings the disease under control (remission). The disease returns in many, but 50 percent of children show no signs of the leukemia 5 years after treatment. Children between the ages of 3 and 7 have the best prognosis; people over age 20 fare less well. Children or adults whose initial white blood cell counts are lower than 25,000 cells per microliter of blood tend to have a better prognosis than those whose white blood cell counts are initially higher.

The goal of treatment is to achieve complete remission by destroying leukemic cells so that normal cells can once again grow in the bone marrow. A person receiving chemotherapy may need to stay in the hospital for a few days or weeks, depending on how quickly the bone marrow recovers. Before normal bone marrow function returns, the person may need to have red blood cell transfusions to treat anemia, platelet transfusions to treat bleeding, and antibiotics to treat infections.

▲ see page 736

■ see page 737

Several combinations of chemotherapy drugs are commonly used, and doses are repeated for several days or weeks. One combination consists of prednisone taken by mouth and weekly doses of vincristine with either anthracycline or asparaginase given intravenously. Other drugs are being investigated.

For treatment of leukemic cells in the brain, methotrexate is usually injected directly into the spinal fluid, and radiation therapy is applied to the brain. Even when a doctor has little evidence that the cancer has spread to the brain, some type of treatment is usually applied there.

A few weeks or months after the initial, intensive treatment aimed at destroying leukemic cells, additional treatment (consolidation chemotherapy) is given to destroy any remaining leukemic cells. Treatment may last 2 to 3 years, although some courses are somewhat shorter.

Leukemic cells may begin to appear again (relapse), often in the bone marrow, brain, or testes. The reappearance of leukemic cells in the bone marrow is particularly serious. Chemotherapy must be given again, and although most people respond to treatment, the disease has a strong tendency to come back. Bone marrow transplantation offers these people the best chance of cure, but this procedure can be performed only if bone marrow can be obtained from a person who has a compatible tissue type (HLA-matched)—almost always a close relative.▲ When leukemic cells reappear in the brain, chemotherapy drugs are injected into the spinal fluid one or two times a week. Treatment of relapse involving the testes consists of chemotherapy along with radiation therapy.

Acute Myeloid Leukemia

Acute myeloid (myelocytic, myelogenous, myeloblastic, myelomonocytic) leukemia is a life-threatening disease in which myelocytes (the cells that normally develop into granulocytes) become cancerous and rapidly replace normal cells in the bone marrow.

This type of leukemia affects people of all ages but mostly adults. Exposure to large doses of radiation and use of some cancer chemotherapy drugs increase the likelihood of developing acute myeloid leukemia.

The leukemic cells accumulate in the bone marrow, destroying and replacing cells that produce normal blood cells. They're released into the bloodstream and transported to other organs, where they continue to grow and divide. They can form small tumors (chloromas) in or just under the skin and can cause meningitis, anemia, liver and kidney failure, and other organ damage.

Symptoms and Diagnosis

The first symptoms usually occur because the bone marrow fails to produce enough normal blood cells. These symptoms include weakness, shortness of breath, infection, fever, and bleeding. Other symptoms may include headaches, vomiting, irritability, and bone and joint pain.

A complete blood cell count can provide the first evidence that a person has leukemia. Very immature white blood cells (blasts) are seen in blood samples examined under a microscope. Also, a bone marrow biopsy is almost always performed to confirm the diagnosis and determine the type of leukemia.

Prognosis and Treatment

Between 50 and 85 percent of people who have acute myeloid leukemia respond to treatment. Between 20 and 40 percent of people show no signs of the disease 5 years after treatment; bone marrow transplantation has increased that success rate to between 40 and 50 percent. People over age 50 and those who develop acute myeloid leukemia after undergoing chemotherapy and radiation therapy for other diseases have the poorest prognosis.

Treatment is aimed at bringing about prompt remission—the destruction of all leukemic cells. However, acute myeloid leukemia responds to fewer drugs than other types of leukemia do, and treatment often makes patients sicker before they get better. Patients get sicker because the treatment suppresses bone marrow activity, resulting in fewer white blood cells (particularly granulocytes), and having too few granulocytes makes infection likely. The hospital staff takes meticulous care to prevent infections and promptly treats any that occur with antibiotics. Red blood cell transfusions and platelet transfusions may also be needed.

The first course of chemotherapy generally includes cytarabine for 7 days and daunorubicin for 3 days. Sometimes, additional drugs such as

---

▲ see page 836

thioguanine or vincristine and prednisone are given, but their role is limited.

People whose disease is in remission usually receive additional chemotherapy (consolidation chemotherapy) a few weeks or months after the initial treatment to help ensure that as many leukemic cells as possible are destroyed.

Treatment to the brain usually isn't needed, and long-term treatment hasn't been shown to improve survival. Bone marrow transplantation may be performed in people who haven't responded to treatment and in younger people who have responded to a first course of treatment, to eradicate any remaining leukemic cells.

Chronic Lymphocytic Leukemia

Chronic lymphocytic leukemia is characterized by a large number of cancerous mature lymphocytes (a type of white blood cell) and enlarged lymph nodes.

More than three fourths of the people who have this type of leukemia are over age 60; it affects men two to three times more often than women. This type of leukemia is rare in Japan and China and remains uncommon in Japanese people who have moved to the United States—a clue that genetics plays some role in its development.

The number of cancerous mature lymphocytes increases first in the lymph nodes. They then spread to the liver and spleen, both of which begin to enlarge. As these lymphocytes invade the bone marrow, they crowd out normal cells, resulting in anemia and a decreased number of normal white blood cells and platelets in the blood. The level and activity of antibodies, the proteins that help fight infections, also decrease. The immune system, which defends the body against foreign substances, often becomes misguided, reacting to and destroying normal body tissues. This misguided activity can result in the destruction of red blood cells and platelets, inflammation of blood vessels, inflammation of joints (rheumatoid arthritis), and inflammation of the thyroid gland (thyroiditis).

Some types of chronic lymphocytic leukemia are classified by the type of lymphocyte involved. B-cell leukemia (leukemia of B lymphocytes▲) is

---

▲ see page 810

■ see page 778

the most common type, accounting for nearly three fourths of all cases of chronic lymphocytic leukemia. T-cell leukemia (leukemia of T lymphocytes) is much less common. Other types include Sézary syndrome (the leukemic phase of mycosis fungoides■) and hairy cell leukemia, a rare type of leukemia that produces a large number of abnormal white blood cells with distinctive projections that are visible under a microscope.

Symptoms and Diagnosis

In early stages of the disease, most people have no symptoms except enlarged lymph nodes. Symptoms may include fatigue, loss of appetite, weight loss, shortness of breath when exercising, and a sense of abdominal fullness resulting from an enlarged spleen. The T-cell leukemias may invade the skin early in the course of the disease, resulting in an unusual skin rash as seen in Sézary syndrome. As the disease progresses, people may appear pale and bruise easily. Bacterial, viral, and fungal infections generally don't occur until late in the course of the disease.

Sometimes the disease is discovered accidentally when blood counts ordered for some other reason show an increased number of lymphocytes—more than 5,000 cells per microliter. In these situations, a bone marrow biopsy is usually performed. If the person has chronic lymphocytic leukemia, an abnormally large number of lymphocytes are seen in the bone marrow. Blood tests also may show that the person has anemia, a reduced number of platelets, and a decreased level of antibodies.

Prognosis

Most types of chronic lymphocytic leukemia progress slowly. A doctor determines how far the disease has progressed (staging) to predict the patient's prospects for recovery. Staging is based on factors such as the number of lymphocytes in the blood and bone marrow, size of the spleen and liver, presence or absence of anemia, and platelet count. People who have B-cell leukemia often survive 10 to 20 years after the diagnosis is made and usually don't need treatment in the early stages. People who are severely anemic and have fewer than 100,000 platelets per microliter of blood are more likely to die within a few years than those who are not severely anemic and have more normal platelet counts. Usually, death occurs because the bone marrow can no longer produce a sufficient number of normal cells to carry oxygen, fight infections, and prevent bleeding. The prognosis for people who have T-cell leukemia is somewhat worse.

For reasons probably related to changes in the immune system, people who have chronic lymphocytic leukemia are more likely to develop other cancers.

Treatment

Because chronic lymphocytic leukemia progresses slowly, many people don't need treatment for years—until the number of lymphocytes begins to increase, lymph nodes begin to enlarge, or the number of red blood cells or platelets decreases. Anemia is treated with blood transfusions and injections of erythropoietin (a drug that stimulates red blood cell formation). Low platelet counts are treated with platelet transfusions, and infections with antibiotics. Radiation therapy is used to shrink enlarged lymph nodes, liver, or spleen when the enlargement is causing discomfort.

Drugs used to treat the leukemia itself don't cure the disease or prolong survival and may cause severe side effects. *Overtreatment is more dangerous than undertreatment.* A doctor may prescribe anticancer drugs alone or with corticosteroids when the number of lymphocytes becomes very large. Prednisone and other corticosteroids may produce striking and rapid improvement in people who have advanced leukemia. However, the response is usually brief, and corticosteroids have many adverse effects after long-term use, including an increased risk of severe infections. For B-cell leukemia, drug treatment includes alkylating agents, which kill cancer cells by interacting with their DNA. For hairy cell leukemia, interferon alfa and pentostatin are highly effective.

Chronic Myelocytic Leukemia

Chronic myelocytic (myeloid, myelogenous, granulocytic) leukemia is a disease in which a cell in the bone marrow becomes cancerous and produces a large number of abnormal granulocytes (a type of white blood cell).

This disease may affect people of any age and of either sex but is uncommon in children under 10 years old.

Most of the leukemic granulocytes are produced in the bone marrow, but some are produced in the spleen and liver. These cells range from very immature to mature forms, whereas only immature forms are seen in acute myeloid leukemia. Leukemic granulocytes tend to crowd out normal cells in the bone marrow, often leading to the formation of large amounts of fibrous tissue that replaces the normal bone marrow. During the course of the disease, more and more immature granulocytes enter the bloodstream and bone marrow (accelerated phase). During this phase, anemia and thrombocytopenia (a decreased number of platelets) develop, and the proportion of immature white blood cells (blasts) increases dramatically.

Sometimes the leukemic granulocytes undergo more changes, and the disease progresses to blast crisis. In blast crisis, the cancerous stem cells begin to produce only immature granulocytes, a sign that the disease has become much worse. At this time, chloromas (tumors composed of rapidly reproducing granulocytes) can grow in the skin, bones, brain, and lymph nodes.

Symptoms

In its early stages, chronic myelocytic leukemia may produce no symptoms. However, some people become fatigued and weak, lose their appetite, lose weight, develop a fever or night sweats, and notice a sensation of being full—which is usually caused by an enlarged spleen. Lymph nodes may also enlarge. Over time, people who have this type of leukemia become very sick as the number of red blood cells and platelets decreases, leading to paleness, bruising, and bleeding. Fever, lymph node enlargement, and formation of skin nodules filled with leukemic granulocytes (chloromas) are particularly worrisome signs.

Diagnosis

Chronic myelocytic leukemia is often diagnosed from a simple blood test. The test may show an abnormally high white blood cell count, anywhere from 50,000 to 1,000,000 white blood cells per microliter (normal is fewer than 11,000). In blood samples examined under a microscope, immature white blood cells, normally found only in bone marrow, are seen in many stages of maturation (differentiation). The number of other types of white blood cells, such as eosinophils and basophils, also increases, and immature forms of red blood cells may be present.

Tests that analyze chromosomes or portions of chromosomes are needed to establish a diagnosis. Chromosomal analysis of the leukemic white blood cells almost always shows a rearrangement of chromosomes. The leukemic cells often have a Philadelphia chromosome (a chromosome that has a specific piece of another chromosome attached to it), as well as other abnormal chromosomal arrangements.

Treatment and Prognosis

Although most treatments don't cure the disease, they do slow its progress. About 20 to 30 percent of people who have chronic myelocytic leukemia die within 2 years of the diagnosis, and about 25 percent die each year after that. However, many people who have this type of leukemia survive 4 years or more after diagnosis, ultimately dying during the accelerated phase or blast crisis. Treatment for a blast crisis is similar to that for acute lymphocytic leukemia. The average survival time after a blast crisis is only 2 months, but chemotherapy can sometimes extend survival to 8 to 12 months.

Treatment is considered successful if the white blood cell count is reduced to fewer than 50,000 cells per microliter. Even the best treatment available can't destroy all of the leukemic cells. The only chance for cure is a bone marrow transplantation.▲ The transplantation of bone marrow—which must come from a donor who has a compatible tissue type, almost always a close relative—is most effective during the early stages of the disease and is considerably less effective during the accelerated phase or blast crisis. More recently, the drug interferon alfa has been shown to normalize the bone marrow and bring about remission, but its long-term benefit is not yet known.

Hydroxyurea, which can be taken by mouth, is the most widely used chemotherapy drug for this disease. Busulfan also is helpful, but because of serious toxic effects, it generally is used for shorter periods than is hydroxyurea.

Besides drugs, radiation therapy to the spleen is sometimes given to help reduce the number of leukemic cells. Sometimes the spleen must be surgically removed (splenectomy) to alleviate abdominal discomfort, increase the number of platelets, and decrease the need for transfusions.

CHAPTER 158

Lymphomas

Lymphomas are cancers (malignancies) of the lymphatic system.

The lymphatic system carries a specialized type of white blood cells called lymphocytes through a network of tubular channels (lymph vessels) to all parts of the body, including the bone marrow.■ Scattered throughout this network are collections of lymphocytes in lymph nodes (commonly but incorrectly called lymph glands). Cancerous lymphocytes (lymphoma cells) can be confined to a single lymph node or can spread throughout the body to almost any organ.

The two major types of lymphoma are Hodgkin's lymphoma, more commonly known as Hodgkin's disease, and non-Hodgkin's lymphoma. Non-Hodgkin's lymphoma has several subtypes that include Burkitt's lymphoma and mycosis fungoides.

Hodgkin's Disease

Hodgkin's disease (Hodgkin's lymphoma) is a type of lymphoma distinguished by a particular kind of cancer cell called a Reed-Sternberg cell that has a distinctive appearance under a microscope.

Reed-Sternberg cells are large cancerous lymphocytes that have more than one nucleus. They can be seen when a biopsy specimen of lymph node tissue is examined under a microscope.

Hodgkin's disease is classified into four types on the basis of characteristics of tissue seen under a microscope.

▲ see page 836

■ see box, page 809

Four Types of Hodgkin's Disease

Type	Microscopic Appearance	Incidence	Progression
Lymphocyte predominance	Very few Reed-Sternberg cells but many lymphocytes	3% of cases	Slow
Nodular sclerosis	A small number of Reed-Sternberg cells and a mixture of other types of white blood cells; areas of fibrous connective tissue	67% of cases	Moderate
Mixed cellularity	A moderate number of Reed-Sternberg cells and a mixture of other types of white blood cells	25% of cases	Somewhat rapid
Lymphocyte depletion	Numerous Reed-Sternberg cells and few lymphocytes; extensive strands of fibrous connective tissue	5% of cases	Rapid

Cause

In the United States, 6,000 to 7,000 new cases of Hodgkin's disease occur every year. The disease is more common in males than in females—about three men are affected for every two women. People can develop Hodgkin's disease at any age, but it rarely occurs before age 10. It's most common in people between ages 15 and 34 and in those over 60. The cause is unknown, although some authorities suspect a virus, such as the Epstein-Barr virus. However, the disease doesn't appear to be contagious.

Symptoms

Hodgkin's disease usually is discovered when a person has an enlarged lymph node, most often in the neck but sometimes in the armpit or groin. Although usually painless, the enlarged node may be painful for a few hours after a person drinks large amounts of alcohol. Sometimes enlarged lymph nodes deep within the chest or abdomen, which are usually painless, are found unexpectedly on a chest x-ray or computed tomography (CT) scan performed for other reasons.

Along with enlarged lymph nodes, Hodgkin's disease sometimes produces additional symptoms such as fever, night sweats, and weight loss. For reasons not known, the skin may itch intensely. Some people have Pel-Ebstein fever, an unusual pattern of high temperature for several days alternating with normal or below-normal temperature for days or weeks. Other symptoms may develop, depending on where the lymphoma cells are growing. A person may have no symptoms or only a few of these symptoms.

Diagnosis

In Hodgkin's disease, lymph nodes usually enlarge slowly and painlessly, with no apparent infection. A rapid enlargement of lymph nodes—which may occur when a person has a cold or infection—isn't typical of Hodgkin's disease. If the lymph nodes remain enlarged for more than a week, a doctor may suspect Hodgkin's disease, especially when a person also has a fever, night sweats, and weight loss.

Abnormalities in blood cell counts and other blood tests may provide supportive evidence, but to make the diagnosis, a doctor must perform a biopsy of the affected lymph node to see if Reed-Sternberg cells are present. The type of biopsy depends on which node is enlarged and how much tissue is needed to be certain of the diagnosis. A doctor must remove enough tissue to be able to distinguish Hodgkin's disease from other diseases that can cause lymph node enlargement —including non-Hodgkin's lymphoma, other cancers with similar symptoms, infectious mono-

Symptoms of Hodgkin's Disease

Symptoms	Cause
Decreased number of red blood cells (resulting in anemia), white blood cells, and platelets; possibly bone pain	Lymphoma is invading bone marrow
Loss of muscle strength; hoarseness	Enlarged lymph nodes are compressing nerves in the spinal cord or nerves to the vocal cords
Jaundice	Lymphoma is blocking flow of bile from the liver
Swelling of the face, neck, and upper extremities (superior vena cava syndrome)	Enlarged lymph nodes are blocking flow of blood from the head to the heart
Swelling of legs and feet	Lymphoma is blocking lymphatic flow from the legs
Illness similar to pneumonia	Lymphoma is invading the lungs
Decreased ability to fight infection and increased susceptibility to fungal and viral infections	Disease is continuing to spread

nucleosis, toxoplasmosis, cytomegalovirus disease, leukemia, sarcoidosis, tuberculosis, and AIDS.

When the enlarged node is near the surface of the neck, a needle biopsy may be performed. In this procedure, an area of skin is anesthetized and a small piece of the node is removed with a needle and syringe. If this type of biopsy doesn't provide enough tissue to diagnose and classify Hodgkin's disease, a small incision must be made and a larger piece of the lymph node is removed. When the enlarged lymph node is not near the surface—for example, when it is deep within the chest—surgery may be more complex.

Staging Hodgkin's Disease

Before treatment is started, doctors must determine how extensively the lymphoma has spread—the stage of the disease. A superficial examination may detect only a single enlarged lymph node, but staging procedures may detect considerably more disease that's hidden (occult). The disease is classified into four stages based on the extent of its spread and symptoms. Choice of treatment and the prognosis are based on the stage. The chance that treatment will completely cure the disease is excellent for people who have stage I, II, or III disease and better than 50 percent for people who have stage IV disease.

The four stages are subdivided, based on the absence (A) or presence (B) of one or more of the following symptoms: unexplained fever (more than 100° F. for 3 consecutive days), night sweats, and unexplained loss of more than 10 percent of body weight in the preceding 6 months. For example, a stage may be described as IIA or IIB.

Several procedures are used to stage or evaluate Hodgkin's disease. A chest x-ray helps detect enlarged nodes near the heart. Lymphangiograms are x-rays taken after a small dose of dye that can be seen on x-rays (radiopaque dye) is injected into lymph vessels in the foot. The dye travels to and outlines lymph nodes deep in the abdomen and pelvis. This procedure has largely been replaced by CT scanning of the abdomen and pelvis. Faster and more comfortable than lymphangiography, CT is quite accurate in detecting enlarged lymph nodes or spread of the lymphoma to the liver and other organs.

Gallium scanning is another procedure that can be used for staging and following the effects of treatment. A small dose of radioactive gallium is injected into the bloodstream, and 2 to 4 days later, a body scan is performed with a device that detects the radioactivity and then produces an image of the internal organs.

Sometimes surgery to examine the abdomen (laparotomy) is needed to determine whether the lymphoma has spread there. During this procedure, surgeons often remove the spleen (splenectomy) and perform a liver biopsy to determine whether the lymphoma has spread to these organs. A laparotomy is performed only when its results are likely to affect the choice of treatment—for example, when a doctor needs to know whether to use radiation therapy or chemotherapy or both.

Treatment

Two effective treatments are radiation therapy and chemotherapy. With one or both of these treatments, most people who have Hodgkin's disease can be cured.

Radiation therapy alone cures about 90 percent of people who have stage I or II disease. Treatments are usually given on an outpatient basis over the course of about 4 or 5 weeks. Radiation is beamed at the affected areas and at the surrounding lymph nodes. Greatly enlarged lymph nodes in the chest are treated with radiation therapy that is usually preceded or followed by chemotherapy. With this dual approach, 85 percent of the people are cured.

Treatment for stage III disease varies with the situation. When a person has no symptoms, sometimes radiation therapy alone is sufficient. However, only 65 to 75 percent of such people are cured. The addition of chemotherapy increases the likelihood of cure to 75 to 80 percent. When a person has symptoms in addition to enlarged lymph nodes, chemotherapy is used with or without radiation therapy. For such people, cure rates range from 70 to 80 percent.

In stage IV disease, a combination of chemotherapy drugs is used. Two common (traditional) combination chemotherapy regimens are MOPP (mechlorethamine, vincristine [Oncovin], procarbazine, and prednisone) and ABVD (doxorubicin [Adriamycin], bleomycin, vinblastine, and dacarbazine). Each cycle of chemotherapy lasts for 1 month, with total treatment time being 6 or more months. Alternative treatments include other combinations of chemotherapy drugs. Even at this advanced stage of the disease, treatment cures more than 50 percent of the people.

The decision to use chemotherapy in treating Hodgkin's disease is difficult for both patients and doctors. Although chemotherapy greatly improves a person's chances for a cure, side effects can be serious. The drugs may cause temporary or permanent sterility, an increased risk of infection, and reversible hair loss. Leukemia and other cancers develop in some people in 5 to 10 years or even longer after treatment with either chemotherapy or radiation therapy and in even more people who have been treated with both.

A person who doesn't improve after radiation therapy or chemotherapy or who improves but then relapses within 6 to 9 months has less of a chance for long-term survival than a person who

Staging and Prognosis of Hodgkin's Disease

Stage	Extent of Spread	Likelihood of Cure*
I	Limited to the lymph nodes of only one part of the body (for example, the right side of the neck)	More than 95%
II	Involves lymph nodes in two or more areas on the same side of the diaphragm, either above or below it (for example, some enlarged nodes in the neck and some in the armpit)	90%
III	Involves lymph nodes both above and below the diaphragm (for example, some enlarged nodes in the neck and some in the groin)	80%
IV	Involves lymph nodes and other parts of the body (such as the bone marrow, lungs, or liver)	60 to 70%

*Survival for 15 years with no further disease

relapses 1 year or more after the initial treatment. Further chemotherapy combined with large doses of radiation therapy and bone marrow or blood stem-cell transplantation▲ may still be helpful in certain people. Large doses of chemotherapy combined with bone marrow transplantation has a high risk of overwhelming infection, which may be fatal; however, about 20 to 40 percent of people who undergo bone marrow transplantation remain free of Hodgkin's disease for 3

▲ see page 836

Combination Chemotherapy Regimens for Hodgkin's Disease

Regimen	Drugs	Comments
MOPP	Mechlorethamine (nitrogen mustard) Vincristine (Oncovin) Procarbazine Prednisone	Original regimen, developed in 1968; occasionally used today
ABVD	Doxorubicin (Adriamycin) Bleomycin Vinblastine Dacarbazine	Developed to reduce side effects of MOPP such as permanent sterility and leukemia. Produces side effects such as heart and lung toxicity. Cure rate is similar to that of MOPP; more commonly used than MOPP
ChlVPP	Chlorambucil Vinblastine Procarbazine Prednisone	Hair loss is minimal compared with that in MOPP and ABVD
MOPP/ ABVD	Alternating cycles of MOPP and ABVD	Developed to improve overall cure rate but not yet proved to do so. Relapse-free survival rate is improved compared with that in other regimens
MOPP/ABV hybrid	MOPP, alternating with Doxorubicin (Adriamycin) Bleomycin Vinblastine	Developed to improve overall cure rate and decrease toxicity compared with that in MOPP/ABVD. Undergoing evaluation

years or more and may be cured. The best results are achieved in people who are under 55 years old and in otherwise good health.

Non-Hodgkin's Lymphoma

Non-Hodgkin's lymphomas are a group of related cancers (malignancies) that originate in the lymphatic system and usually spread throughout the body.

Some of these lymphomas progress very slowly—over years—while others spread rapidly—over months. Non-Hodgkin's lymphoma is more common than Hodgkin's disease. In the United States, about 50,000 new cases are diagnosed every year, and the number of new cases is increasing, especially among older people and those who have HIV infection (AIDS).

Although the cause of non-Hodgkin's lymphoma isn't known, evidence suggests a link to a still unidentified virus. However, the disease doesn't appear to be contagious. A rare type of rapidly progressive non-Hodgkin's lymphoma is related to infection caused by HTLV-I (human T-cell lymphotropic virus type I), a retrovirus similar in function to the human immunodeficiency virus (HIV), which causes AIDS. Non-Hodgkin's lymphoma can also be a complication of AIDS, accounting for some of the increase in new cases.

Symptoms

The first noticeable symptom is often enlarged lymph nodes in a single area, such as the neck or groin, or throughout the body. The lymph nodes enlarge slowly and are usually painless. Occasionally, enlarged lymph nodes in the tonsils cause difficulty in swallowing. Enlarged lymph nodes deep within the chest or abdomen may press against various organs, causing difficulty in breathing, loss of appetite, severe constipation,

Symptoms of Non-Hodgkin's Lymphoma

Symptoms	Cause	Probability of Developing Symptom
Difficulty in breathing Swelling of the face	Enlarged lymph nodes in the chest	20 to 30%
Loss of appetite Severe constipation Abdominal pain or distention	Enlarged lymph nodes in the abdomen	30 to 40%
Progressive swelling of the legs	Blocked lymph vessels in the groin or abdomen	10%
Weight loss Diarrhea Malabsorption (interference with digestion and passage of nutrients into the blood)	Invasion of the small intestine	10%
Fluid accumulation around the lungs (pleural effusion)	Blocked lymph vessels in the chest	20 to 30%
Thickened, dark, itchy areas of skin	Infiltration of the skin	10 to 20%
Weight loss Fever Night sweats	Spread of the disease throughout the body	50 to 60%
Anemia (an insufficient number of red blood cells)	Bleeding into the gastrointestinal tract Destruction of red blood cells by an enlarged and overactive spleen Destruction of red blood cells by abnormal antibodies (hemolytic anemia) Destruction of bone marrow because of invasion by the lymphoma Inability of the bone marrow to produce sufficient numbers of red blood cells because of drugs or radiation therapy	30%; eventually almost 100%
Susceptibility to severe bacterial infections	Invasion of the bone marrow and lymph nodes, causing decreased antibody production	20 to 30%

abdominal pain, or progressive swelling of the legs. If the lymphoma invades the bloodstream, leukemia may develop. Lymphomas and leukemias have many similar characteristics.▲ Non-Hodgkin's lymphomas are more likely to invade the bone marrow, gastrointestinal tract, and skin than Hodgkin's disease.

In children, the first symptoms of non-Hodgkin's lymphoma are likely to be infiltrations of lymphoma cells into the bone marrow, blood, skin, intestine, brain, and spinal cord, rather than

enlarged lymph nodes. The infiltrations cause anemia, rashes, and neurologic symptoms, such as weakness and abnormal sensation. The lymph nodes that do become enlarged are usually deep ones, leading to accumulation of fluid around the lungs, which causes difficulty in breathing; pressure on the intestine, which causes loss of appe-

▲ see page 765

tite or vomiting; and blocked lymph vessels, which causes fluid retention.

Diagnosis and Staging

A biopsy of the lymph node must be taken to diagnose non-Hodgkin's lymphoma and distinguish it from Hodgkin's disease and others that cause enlarged lymph nodes.

Non-Hodgkin's lymphoma may be classified according to the microscopic appearance of the biopsied lymph node cells and the type of lymphocyte (B or T lymphocyte)▲ from which the lymphoma cells originated. Although various classification systems have been devised, one that is currently used relates cell type to prognosis. It categorizes lymphomas as low grade, having a favorable prognosis; intermediate grade, having an intermediate prognosis; and high grade, having an unfavorable prognosis. Because these categories are based on prognosis without treatment, they are slightly misleading: Many low-grade lymphomas become fatal after years or decades, and many intermediate- and high-grade lymphomas can now be completely cured.

Non-Hodgkin's lymphoma usually has spread widely by the time it's diagnosed; in only 10 to 30 percent of the people, the disease is localized (in just one part of the body). To determine how far the disease has spread and how much lymphoma tissue is present (staging), computed tomography (CT) scans of the abdomen and pelvis are usually performed; gallium scanning may also be useful. Staging rarely requires surgery. In most cases, a bone marrow biopsy is also performed. Staging for non-Hodgkin's lymphoma is similar to that for Hodgkin's disease but is not as accurate in making a prognosis. New staging systems that can make a more accurate prognosis are being devised on the basis of the results of certain blood tests and the person's overall condition.

Treatment

For some people, complete cure is possible; for others, treatment extends life and relieves symptoms for many years. The likelihood of cure or

---

▲ see box, page 763

long-term survival depends on the type of non-Hodgkin's lymphoma and the stage the disease has reached when treatment starts. Generally, the types that originate from T lymphocytes don't respond to therapy as well as those that originate from B lymphocytes. Cure is less likely for people who are over age 60, those in whom the lymphoma has spread throughout the body, those who have large tumors (accumulations of lymphoma cells), and those whose functioning is limited by severe fatigue and immobility.

People in **early stages** of the disease (stages I and II) are often treated with radiation limited to the site of the lymphoma and adjacent areas. Although radiation therapy usually doesn't cure people who have low-grade lymphomas, it may extend their survival, usually by 5 to 8 years. With radiation therapy, people who have intermediate-grade lymphomas generally survive 2 to 5 years, but people who have high-grade lymphomas survive only 6 months to a year. However, combination chemotherapy with or without radiation therapy can cure over half of the people who have intermediate- and high-grade lymphomas if started early in the course of the disease.

Most people are already in **late stages** of the disease (stages III and IV) when the diagnosis is made. Those who have low-grade lymphomas may not need immediate treatment, but frequent checkups are necessary to make sure the disease isn't causing potentially serious complications. Chemotherapy is indicated for people who have intermediate-grade lymphomas. Those who have high-grade lymphomas need immediate intensive chemotherapy because these lymphomas grow rapidly.

Many potentially effective chemotherapy regimens are available. Chemotherapy drugs may be given one at a time for low-grade lymphomas or together as combination therapy for intermediate- or high-grade lymphomas. Advances in combination chemotherapy have improved the likelihood of complete cure to between 50 and 60 percent for people who have advanced disease. Researchers are investigating the use of intensive chemotherapy regimens with growth factors and bone marrow transplantation.

New therapies being studied include toxin-conjugated monoclonal antibodies, which are

Combination Chemotherapy Regimens for Non-Hodgkin's Lymphomas

Regimen	Drugs	Comments
Single agents	Chlorambucil or Cyclophosphamide	Used for low-grade lymphomas to decrease size of lymph nodes and relieve symptoms
CVP (COP)	Cyclophosphamide Vincristine (Oncovin) Prednisone	Used for low-grade and some intermediate-grade lymphomas to decrease size of lymph nodes and relieve symptoms; produces a faster response than single agents
CHOP	Cyclophosphamide Doxorubicin (Adriamycin) Vincristine (Oncovin) Prednisone	Considered standard of care for most intermediate-grade and some high-grade lymphomas; very high doses are being investigated in high-risk patients
C-MOPP	Cyclophosphamide Vincristine (Oncovin) Procarbazine Prednisone	Older regimen, used for intermediate-grade and some high-grade lymphomas; also used in people who have heart problems and can't tolerate doxorubicin
M-BACOD	Methotrexate Bleomycin Doxorubicin (Adriamycin) Cyclophosphamide Vincristine (Oncovin) Dexamethasone	Has more toxic effects than CHOP and requires close monitoring of lung and kidney function; overall benefits similar to CHOP
ProMACE/CytaBOM	Procarbazine Methotrexate Doxorubicin (Adriamycin) Cyclophosphamide Etoposide alternating with Cytarabine Bleomycin Vincristine (Oncovin) Methotrexate	ProMACE regimen alternates with CytaBOM; overall benefits similar to CHOP
MACOP-B	Methotrexate Doxorubicin (Adriamycin) Cyclophosphamide Vincristine (Oncovin) Prednisone Bleomycin	Main advantage is therapy duration (only 12 weeks), but weekly treatments are required (most other regimens are given every 3 to 4 weeks for 6 cycles); overall benefits similar to CHOP

antibodies (immunoglobulins) that have toxic substances, such as radioactive compounds or plant proteins called ricins, attached to them. These tailor-made antibodies attach specifically to lymphoma cells and release the toxic substance, which kills the lymphoma cells.

Standard chemotherapy is of limited value when relapse occurs. New salvage drug regimens are being tested that are more dangerous than other treatments but offer a better chance of curing the lymphoma.

In bone marrow transplantation,▲ bone marrow is removed from the patient (and purged of

▲ see page 836

lymphoma cells) or from a compatible donor and transplanted into the patient. This procedure enables blood cell counts, reduced by high-dose chemotherapy, to recover more quickly. Bone marrow transplantation is most successful in people under 55 years old. Although it cures 30 to 50 percent of the patients who were not cured by standard chemotherapy, it has some risks. About 5 percent (or less) of the patients die of infection during the early critical weeks after the transplant, before the bone marrow recovers and can produce enough white blood cells to fight infection. Bone marrow transplantation is also being evaluated in people who respond well to initial chemotherapy but are at high risk of relapsing.

BURKITT'S LYMPHOMA
Burkitt's lymphoma is a very high grade non-Hodgkin's lymphoma that originates from a B lymphocyte and tends to spread to areas outside the lymphatic system, such as the bone marrow, blood, central nervous system, and spinal fluid.

Although Burkitt's lymphoma can develop at any age, it's most common in children and young adults, particularly males. It may develop in people who have AIDS.

Unlike other lymphomas, Burkitt's lymphoma has a specific geographic distribution: It's most common in central Africa and rare in the United States. It's caused by the Epstein-Barr virus, which causes infectious mononucleosis in people who live in the United States; however, people who have Burkitt's lymphoma can't spread the disease to others. Why the same virus causes lymphoma in central Africa but mononucleosis in the United States isn't clear.

Symptoms
Large numbers of lymphoma cells may accumulate in the lymph nodes and organs of the abdomen, causing it to swell. Lymphoma cells may invade the small intestine, resulting in blockage or bleeding. The neck and jaw may swell, sometimes painfully.

Diagnosis and Treatment
To make the diagnosis, a doctor performs a biopsy of the abnormal tissue and orders procedures to determine how far the disease has spread (staging). Rarely is the disease confined to one area (localized). If the lymphoma has spread to the bone marrow, blood, or central nervous system at the time of diagnosis, the prognosis is poor.

Without treatment, Burkitt's lymphoma progresses rapidly and is fatal. Surgery may be needed to remove affected parts of the intestine, which otherwise may bleed, become blocked, or rupture. Chemotherapy is intensive. Drugs include combinations of cyclophosphamide, methotrexate, vincristine, doxorubicin, and cytarabine. Chemotherapy can cure about 80 percent of those who have localized disease and 70 percent of those who have moderately advanced disease. For disease that has spread widely (disseminated), the usual cure rate is 50 to 60 percent, but it decreases to 20 to 40 percent if the lymphoma has invaded the central nervous system or bone marrow.

MYCOSIS FUNGOIDES
Mycosis fungoides is a rare, persistent, slow-growing type of non-Hodgkin's lymphoma that originates from a mature T lymphocyte and affects the skin; it may progress to the lymph nodes and internal organs.

Mycosis fungoides starts so subtly and grows so slowly that it may not be noticed at first. It becomes a long-lasting, itchy rash—sometimes a small area of thickened, itchy skin that later develops nodules and slowly spreads.

In some people, mycosis fungoides develops into leukemia (Sézary syndrome), in which abnormal lymphocytes appear in the bloodstream. The skin itches intensely, becomes dry and red, and peels.

Diagnosis and Treatment
Even with a biopsy, doctors have trouble diagnosing this disease in its early stages. However, later in the course of the disease, a biopsy shows lymphoma cells in the skin. Most people are over age 50 by the time mycosis fungoides is diagnosed. Even without treatment, they can expect to live another 7 to 10 years.

The thickened areas of skin are treated with a form of radiation called beta rays or with sunlight and cortisone-like steroid drugs. Nitrogen mustard applied directly to the skin can help reduce the itching and size of the affected areas. Interferon drugs can also reduce symptoms. If the disease spreads to lymph nodes and other organs, chemotherapy may be needed.

Plasma Cell Disorders

Plasma cell disorders (plasma cell dyscrasias, monoclonal gammopathies) are conditions in which one group (clone) of plasma cells multiplies excessively and produces a large quantity of abnormal antibodies.

Plasma cells develop from lymphocytes, a type of white blood cell, and normally produce antibodies to help the body fight infection. There are thousands of different types of plasma cells, found mainly in bone marrow and lymph nodes. Each plasma cell divides and multiplies to form a clone, composed of many identical cells. The cells of a clone produce only one specific type of antibody (immunoglobulin).▲

In plasma cell disorders, one clone of plasma cells grows excessively and overproduces one type of antibody-like molecule. Because these cells and the antibodies they produce aren't normal, they don't help protect the body against infections. In addition, normal antibody production often decreases, making a person more susceptible to infections. The ever-increasing number of abnormal plasma cells invades and damages various tissues and organs.

In **monoclonal gammopathies of undetermined significance,** plasma cells are abnormal but not cancerous. They produce a large quantity of abnormal antibodies but usually don't cause significant problems. These disorders often remain stable for years—as long as 25 years in some people— and don't require treatment. They're more common in older people. For unknown reasons, these disorders progress to multiple myeloma, a plasma cell cancer, in 20 to 30 percent of people. Multiple myeloma may appear abruptly and usually requires treatment. Macroglobulinemia, another plasma cell disorder, also can develop in people who have monoclonal gammopathies of undetermined significance.

Multiple Myeloma

Multiple myeloma is a plasma cell cancer in which a clone of abnormal plasma cells multiplies, forms tumors in the bone marrow, and produces a large quantity of abnormal antibodies that accumulate in the blood or urine.

In the United States, multiple myeloma accounts for about 1 percent of all cancers; about 12,500 new cases are diagnosed every year. This uncommon cancer affects men and women equally and usually is seen in people over 40 years old. Its cause is unknown.

Plasma cell tumors (plasmacytomas) are most common in the pelvic bones, spine, ribs, and skull. Occasionally, they develop in areas other than bones, particularly in the lungs and reproductive organs.

The abnormal plasma cells almost always produce a large quantity of abnormal antibodies, and the production of normal antibodies is reduced. As a result, people who have multiple myeloma are especially susceptible to infections.

Pieces of the abnormal antibodies frequently end up in the kidneys, damaging them and sometimes causing kidney failure. Deposits of antibody pieces in the kidneys or other organs can lead to amyloidosis,■ another serious disorder. Abnormal antibody pieces in the urine are called Bence Jones proteins.

Symptoms and Diagnosis

Sometimes multiple myeloma is diagnosed before a person has any symptoms—for instance, when an x-ray performed for other reasons reveals punched-out areas in the bones that are typical of this disorder.

Multiple myeloma often causes bone pain, especially in the spine or ribs, and weakens bones, which may fracture easily. Although bone pain is usually the first symptom, occasionally the disorder is diagnosed only after anemia (too few red

---

▲ see page 811

■ see page 690

blood cells), recurring bacterial infections, or kidney failure develops. Anemia results when the abnormal plasma cells crowd out the normal cells that produce red blood cells in the bone marrow. Bacterial infections result because abnormal antibodies are ineffective against infections. Kidney failure results when pieces of the abnormal antibodies (Bence Jones proteins) damage the kidneys.

In rare instances, multiple myeloma interferes with blood flow to the skin, fingers, toes, and nose because the blood thickens (hyperviscosity syndrome). Inadequate flow of blood to the brain can result in neurologic symptoms, such as confusion, visual problems, and headaches.

Several blood tests may help a doctor diagnose this disorder. A complete blood cell count may detect anemia and abnormal red blood cells. Usually, the erythrocyte sedimentation rate, a test that measures how quickly red blood cells (erythrocytes) settle to the bottom of a test tube, is abnormally high. Calcium levels are abnormally high▲ in one third of the people who have this disorder because changes in the bone result in calcium leaking into the bloodstream. However, the key diagnostic tests are serum protein electrophoresis and immunoelectrophoresis, blood tests that detect and identify the abnormal antibody that's the telltale sign of multiple myeloma. This antibody is found in about 85 percent of the people who have this disorder. Also, urine electrophoresis and immunoelectrophoresis can detect Bence Jones proteins, which are found in 30 to 40 percent of the people who have multiple myeloma.

Often, x-rays show loss of bone density (osteoporosis) and punched-out areas of bone destruction. A bone marrow biopsy,■ in which a sample of marrow is obtained with a needle and syringe and examined under a microscope, shows a large number of plasma cells abnormally arranged in sheets and clusters; the cells also may appear abnormal.

▲ see page 673

■ see page 737

★ see page 836

Treatment

Treatment is aimed at preventing or relieving symptoms and complications, destroying abnormal plasma cells, and slowing progression of the disorder.

Strong analgesics and radiation therapy directed at the affected bones can help relieve bone pain, which can be severe. People who have multiple myeloma, especially with Bence Jones proteins in the urine, need to drink plenty of fluids to dilute the urine and help prevent dehydration, which can make kidney failure more likely. Staying active is important; prolonged bed rest tends to accelerate osteoporosis and make the bones more vulnerable to fractures. However, running and heavy lifting should be avoided because the bones are weakened.

People who have signs of infection—fever, chills, or reddened areas of the skin—should see a doctor promptly because they may need antibiotics. Those who have severe anemia may need red blood cell transfusions, although for some, erythropoietin—a drug that stimulates red blood cell formation—may adequately treat the anemia. High calcium levels in the blood can be treated with prednisone and intravenous fluids and sometimes with diphosphonates, drugs that lower calcium levels. People who have high levels of uric acid in the blood may benefit from allopurinol.

Chemotherapy slows the progression of multiple myeloma by killing the abnormal plasma cells. The drugs most frequently used are melphalan and cyclophosphamide. Because chemotherapy kills normal cells as well as abnormal ones, the blood cells are monitored and the dose is adjusted if the number of normal white blood cells and platelets decreases too much. Corticosteroids such as prednisone or dexamethasone are also given as part of the chemotherapy. For those who have a good response to chemotherapy, the drug interferon may enable the response to last longer.

High-dose chemotherapy combined with radiation therapy is still experimental. Because this combination is so toxic, stem cells must be collected from a person's blood or bone marrow before treatment; these cells are then returned (transplanted)★ to the person after treatment.

Generally, this procedure is reserved for people who are under 50 years old.

Currently, no cure is available for multiple myeloma. However, treatment slows its progress in more than 60 percent of its victims. Those who respond to chemotherapy can expect to live for 2 to 3 years after the disorder is diagnosed, sometimes much longer. Occasionally, people who survive for many years after successful treatment of multiple myeloma develop leukemia or fibrous tissue (scarring) in the bone marrow. These late complications may result from chemotherapy and often lead to severe anemia and an increased susceptibility to infections.

Macroglobulinemia

Macroglobulinemia (Waldenström's macroglobulinemia) is a disorder in which plasma cells produce an excessive quantity of macroglobulins (large antibodies) that accumulate in the blood.

Macroglobulinemia results from a group (clone) of abnormal, cancerous lymphocytes and plasma cells. Men are affected more often than women, and the average age at which the disorder appears is 65 years. Its cause is unknown.

Symptoms and Diagnosis

Many people who have macroglobulinemia have no symptoms. Others, whose blood has thickened (hyperviscosity syndrome) because of the large quantity of macroglobulins, have reduced blood flow to the skin, fingers, toes, and nose as well as a variety of other symptoms. These symptoms include abnormal bleeding from the skin and mucous membranes (such as the lining of the mouth, nose, and intestinal tract), fatigue, weakness, headache, dizziness, and even coma. The thickened blood also may aggravate heart conditions and cause increased pressure in the brain. Tiny blood vessels in the back of the eyes can become engorged and may bleed, resulting in damage to the retina and impaired eyesight.

People who have macroglobulinemia may also have swollen lymph nodes, rashes, an enlarged liver and spleen, recurring bacterial infections, and anemia.

Macroglobulinemia often produces cryoglobulinemia, a condition characterized by cryoglobulins, which are abnormal antibodies that precipitate (form solid particles) in the blood when cooled below body temperature and dissolve when warmed. People who have cryoglobulinemia may become very sensitive to cold or develop Raynaud's phenomenon, in which the hands and feet become very painful and turn white when they're exposed to cold.

Blood tests detect abnormalities in people who have macroglobulinemia. The number of red and white blood cells and platelets may be abnormally low, and the erythrocyte sedimentation rate, which measures how quickly red blood cells (erythrocytes) settle to the bottom of a test tube, usually is abnormally high. Blood clotting test results may be abnormal, and other tests may detect cryoglobulins. Bence Jones proteins (pieces of abnormal antibodies) may be found in the urine. But the most useful diagnostic tests are serum protein electrophoresis and immunoelectrophoresis, which detect the large quantity of abnormal macroglobulins in a blood sample.

X-rays may show a loss of bone density (osteoporosis). A bone marrow biopsy, in which a sample of marrow is obtained with a needle and syringe and examined under a microscope, may reveal an increased number of lymphocytes and plasma cells, which helps confirm the diagnosis.

Prognosis and Treatment

The course of the disorder varies from person to person. Even without treatment, many people survive for 5 years or more.

A person whose blood is thickened must be treated promptly with plasmapheresis, a procedure in which blood is withdrawn, the abnormal antibodies are removed from it, and the red blood cells are returned to the person. Chemotherapy, usually with chlorambucil, can slow the growth of abnormal plasma cells but doesn't cure macroglobulinemia. Alternatively, melphalan or cyclophosphamide may be used as well as various other drugs, alone or in combinations.

CHAPTER 160

Myeloproliferative Disorders

Myeloproliferative disorders are conditions in which the cells that produce blood cells (precursor cells) develop and reproduce abnormally in the bone marrow or are crowded out by overgrowth of fibrous tissue.

The four major myeloproliferative disorders are polycythemia vera, myelofibrosis, thrombocythemia, and chronic myelocytic leukemia.▲ Myelofibrosis differs from the other three disorders in that fibroblasts (cells that produce fibrous or connective tissue), which aren't precursor cells, are involved. However, the fibroblasts appear to be stimulated by abnormal precursor cells, possibly megakaryocytes (cells that produce platelets).

Polycythemia Vera

Polycythemia vera is a disorder of blood cell precursors, resulting in an excess of red blood cells.

This disorder is rare; only five people out of every million have it. The average age at which the disorder is diagnosed is 60 years, but it can develop at an earlier age.

Symptoms

The excess of red blood cells increases the volume of blood and makes it thicker so that it flows less easily through small blood vessels (hyperviscosity). However, the number of red blood cells may be increased for a long time before symptoms appear.

Often, the earliest symptoms are weakness, fatigue, headache, light-headedness, and shortness of breath. Vision may be distorted, and a person may have blind spots or may see flashes of light. Bleeding from the gums and small cuts is common, and the skin, especially the face, may look red. A person may itch all over, particularly after a hot bath. Burning sensations in the hands and feet or, more rarely, bone pain may be felt. As the disorder progresses, the liver and spleen may enlarge, causing a dull, intermittent ache in the abdomen.

The excess of red blood cells may be associated with other complications, including stomach ulcers, kidney stones, and clotting in veins and arteries, which can cause heart attacks and strokes and can block blood flow to the arms and legs. Rarely, polycythemia vera progresses to leukemia; certain treatments increase the likelihood of this progression.

Diagnosis

Polycythemia vera may be diagnosed by routine blood tests■ performed for other reasons, even before a person has any symptoms. Hemoglobin (the protein that carries oxygen in red blood cells) levels and hematocrit (the percentage of red blood cells in the total blood volume) are abnormally high. A hematocrit reading higher than 54 percent in a man or 49 percent in a woman may indicate polycythemia, but the diagnosis can't be made on the basis of an abnormal hematocrit alone. A test that uses radioactively labeled red blood cells to determine the total number of red blood cells in the body can help make the diagnosis. Rarely, a bone marrow biopsy (removal of a sample for examination under a microscope) is needed.★

A high hematocrit reading also may indicate **relative polycythemia,** a condition in which the number of red blood cells is normal but the amount of fluid in the blood is low.

An excess of red blood cells caused by conditions other than polycythemia vera is called **secondary polycythemia.** For example, low levels of oxygen in the blood stimulate the bone marrow to produce more red blood cells. Therefore, people who have chronic lung disease or heart disease, those who smoke, and those who live at high altitudes may have an increased number of red blood cells. To distinguish polycythemia vera from some forms of secondary polycythemia, a doctor measures the oxygen levels in a sample of blood taken from an artery. If the oxygen levels are abnormally low, secondary polycythemia is likely.

▲ see page 769

■ see page 736

★ see page 737

Major Myeloproliferative Disorders

Disorder	Bone Marrow Characteristics	Blood Characteristics
Polycythemia vera	Increased number of erythroid (red blood cell) precursors	Increased number of red blood cells
Myelofibrosis	Excess fibrous tissue	Increased number of immature red and white blood cells and misshapen red blood cells
Thrombocythemia	Increased number of megakaryocytes (cells that produce platelets)	Increased number of platelets
Chronic myelocytic leukemia	Increased number of myelocytes (precursors of granulocytes, a type of white blood cell)	Increased number of mature and immature granulocytes

Blood levels of erythropoietin, a hormone that stimulates the bone marrow to produce red blood cells, also may be measured. Levels of erythropoietin are extremely low in polycythemia vera but are normal or high in secondary polycythemia. Rarely, cysts in the liver or kidneys and tumors in the kidneys or brain produce erythropoietin; people with these conditions have high levels of erythropoietin and may develop secondary polycythemia.

Prognosis and Treatment

Without treatment, about half the people who have polycythemia vera with symptoms die in less than 2 years. With treatment, they live an average of 15 to 20 years.

The aim of treatment is to slow down production and decrease the number of red blood cells. Usually, blood is removed from the body in a procedure called a phlebotomy. A pint of blood is removed every other day until the hematocrit begins to decrease. When the hematocrit reaches a normal level, blood is removed every few months, as needed.

In some people, the abnormal production of blood cells in the bone marrow accelerates, increasing the number of platelets (cell-like particles involved in clotting) in the bloodstream or greatly enlarging the liver or spleen. Because phlebotomy also increases the number of platelets and doesn't reduce the size of body organs, these people need chemotherapy to suppress blood cell production. Hydroxyurea is the anticancer drug usually given.

Other drugs can help control some of the symptoms. For example, antihistamines can help relieve itching, and aspirin can relieve burning sensations in the hands and feet as well as bone pain.

Myelofibrosis

Myelofibrosis is a disorder in which fibrous tissue may replace the precursor cells that produce normal blood cells in the bone marrow, resulting in abnormally shaped red blood cells, anemia, and an enlarged spleen.

In the bone marrow, cells called fibroblasts produce fibrous (connective) tissue that forms a lattice supporting the blood-producing cells. In myelofibrosis, an abnormal precursor cell stimulates the fibroblasts to produce too much fibrous tissue, which crowds out the blood-producing cells. With diminished red blood cell production, fewer red blood cells are released into the bloodstream, and anemia develops. Many of these red blood cells are immature or misshapen. White blood cells and platelets also may be misshapen, and there may be too many or too few of them.

Eventually, fibrous tissue replaces so much of the bone marrow that production of all blood cells is reduced. When this happens, the anemia becomes severe, the reduced number of white blood cells can't fight infections, and the reduced number of platelets can't prevent bleeding.

The body produces blood cells outside the bone marrow, mainly in the liver and spleen, which may enlarge; this condition is called agnogenic myeloid metaplasia.

Myelofibrosis sometimes accompanies leukemia, polycythemia vera, multiple myeloma, lymphoma, tuberculosis, or infections of the bone, but its cause is unknown. People who have been exposed to certain toxic substances, such as benzene and radiation, are at increased risk of developing myelofibrosis. It's most common in people between 50 and 70 years old. Because the disorder generally progresses slowly, people who have it usually live for 10 years or longer. Occasionally, the disorder progresses rapidly. This form, called malignant myelofibrosis or acute myelofibrosis, is a type of leukemia.

Symptoms and Diagnosis

Often, myelofibrosis produces no symptoms for years. Eventually, the anemia makes people weak and tired; they don't feel well and lose weight. The enlarged spleen and liver may cause pain in the abdomen.

The misshapen, immature red blood cells, seen in blood samples viewed under a microscope, and anemia suggest myelofibrosis, but a bone marrow biopsy (removal of a sample for examination under a microscope) is needed to confirm the diagnosis.

Treatment

No available treatment can effectively reverse or permanently slow the progression of this disorder, although the anticancer drug hydroxyurea may decrease the size of the liver or spleen.

Treatment is aimed at delaying complications. Bone marrow transplantation may offer hope in selected cases. In some people, red blood cell production can be stimulated with erythropoietin, but in others, blood transfusions are needed to treat the anemia. Rarely, the spleen becomes extremely large and painful and may have to be removed. Infections are treated with antibiotics.

Thrombocythemia

Thrombocythemia is a disorder in which an excess of platelets is produced, leading to abnormal blood clotting.

Platelets, also called thrombocytes, are normally produced in the bone marrow by cells called megakaryocytes. In thrombocythemia, megakaryocytes become abnormal and produce too many platelets.

This disorder usually occurs in people over 50 years old. It's called primary thrombocythemia when the cause isn't known and secondary thrombocythemia when the cause is another condition, such as bleeding, removal of the spleen, infections, rheumatoid arthritis, certain cancers, or sarcoidosis.

Symptoms

An excess of platelets, which are essential to blood clotting, can cause clots to form spontaneously, blocking the flow of blood through vessels. Symptoms include tingling and other abnormal sensations in the hands and feet, cold fingertips, headaches, weakness, and dizziness. Bleeding, usually mild, may occur, often consisting of nosebleeds, easy bruising, slight oozing from the gums, or bleeding in the gastrointestinal tract. The spleen and liver may enlarge.

Diagnosis

Symptoms suggest the diagnosis of thrombocythemia, and blood tests can confirm it. The platelet count is higher than 500,000 per microliter of blood—about twice the normal number—and often above 1,000,000 per microliter. Viewed under a microscope, a blood sample has abnormally large platelets, clumps of platelets, and fragments of megakaryocytes.

To distinguish between primary and secondary thrombocythemia, a doctor looks for signs of other conditions that could increase the platelet count. Sometimes a bone marrow biopsy (removal of a sample for examination under a microscope) is helpful.

Treatment

If another condition accounts for the increased platelet count (secondary thrombocythemia), treatment is aimed at that condition. If the treatment is successful, the platelet count usually returns to normal levels.

If no cause for the increased platelet count is found (primary thrombocythemia), a drug that slows platelet production is usually given. Usually, treatment is started when the platelet count exceeds 750,000 per microliter of blood or when bleeding or clotting complications develop. The drug is continued until the platelet count falls below 600,000 per microliter. Usually, the anticancer drug hydroxyurea is used, although sometimes the anticlotting drug anagrelide is used. Because hydroxyurea also can slow production of white and red blood cells, the dose must be adjusted to maintain an adequate number of these cells. Small doses of aspirin, which makes platelets less sticky and impairs clotting, may delay the need for these drugs.

If drug treatment doesn't slow platelet production quickly enough, a person may be treated with plateletpheresis. In this procedure, blood is withdrawn, platelets are removed from it, and the platelet-depleted blood is returned to the person. This procedure usually is combined with drug treatment.

CHAPTER 161

Spleen Disorders

The spleen produces, monitors, stores, and destroys blood cells. It is a spongy, soft, purplish organ about as big as a person's fist and is located in the upper part of the abdominal cavity, just under the rib cage on the left side.

The spleen functions as two organs. The white pulp is part of the infection-fighting (immune) system, and the red pulp removes unwanted material, such as defective red blood cells, from the blood.

Certain white blood cells (lymphocytes) produce protective antibodies and play an important role in fighting infection. Lymphocytes can be produced and reach maturity in the white pulp.

The red pulp contains other white blood cells (phagocytes) that ingest unwanted material, such as bacteria or defective cells, from the circulating blood. The red pulp monitors red blood cells, determines which ones are abnormal or too old or damaged to function properly, and destroys them. Consequently, the red pulp is sometimes called the red blood cell graveyard.

The red pulp also serves as a reservoir for blood elements, especially white blood cells and platelets (cell-like particles involved in clotting). In many animals, the red pulp releases these blood elements into the circulating blood when the body needs them; however, in humans, releasing these elements is not an important function of the spleen.

If the spleen is removed surgically (splenectomy), the body loses some of its ability to produce protective antibodies and to remove un-

Viewing the Spleen

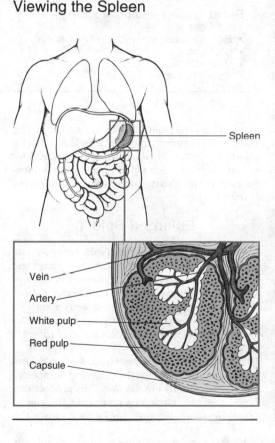

Spleen

Vein

Artery

White pulp

Red pulp

Capsule

Causes of an Enlarged Spleen

Infections
- Hepatitis
- Infectious mononucleosis
- Psittacosis
- Subacute bacterial endocarditis
- Brucellosis
- Kala-azar
- Malaria
- Syphilis
- Tuberculosis

Anemias
- Hereditary elliptocytosis
- Hereditary spherocytosis
- Sickle cell anemia (mainly in children)
- Thalassemia

Blood cancers and proliferative disorders
- Hodgkin's disease and other lymphomas
- Leukemia
- Myelofibrosis
- Polycythemia vera

Inflammatory diseases
- Amyloidosis
- Felty's syndrome
- Sarcoidosis
- Systemic lupus erythematosus

Liver diseases
- Cirrhosis of the liver

Storage diseases
- Gaucher's disease
- Hand-Schüller-Christian disease
- Letterer-Siwe disease
- Niemann-Pick disease

Other causes
- Cysts in the spleen
- External pressure on veins from the spleen or to the liver
- Blood clot in a vein from the spleen or to the liver

wanted bacteria from the blood. As a result, the body's ability to fight infection is reduced. After a short time, other organs (primarily the liver) increase their infection-fighting ability to compensate for this loss, so the increased risk of infection is not lifelong.

Enlarged Spleen

When the spleen enlarges (splenomegaly), its ability to trap and store blood cells increases. Splenomegaly can reduce the number of red and white blood cells and platelets in the circulation.

Many diseases can make the spleen enlarge. To pinpoint the cause, a doctor must consider disorders ranging from blood cancers to chronic infections.

When the enlarged spleen traps large numbers of abnormal blood cells, the cells clog the spleen, interfering with its functioning. This process can begin a vicious circle: the more cells the spleen traps, the larger it grows; the larger it grows, the more cells it traps.

When the spleen removes too many blood cells from the circulation (hypersplenism), a variety of

problems may develop, including anemia (too few red blood cells), frequent infections (because of too few white blood cells), and bleeding problems (because of too few platelets). Eventually, the greatly enlarged spleen also traps normal blood cells, destroying them along with the abnormal ones.

Symptoms

An enlarged spleen doesn't cause many symptoms, and none of them reveals the specific cause of enlargement. Because the enlarged spleen lies next to the stomach and may press against it, a person may feel full after eating a small snack or even without eating. A person may also have abdominal or back pain in the area of the spleen; the pain may spread to the left shoulder, especially if parts of the spleen don't get enough blood and start to die.

Diagnosis

Usually, a doctor can feel an enlarged spleen during a physical examination. An x-ray of the abdomen may also show that the spleen is enlarged. In some cases, computed tomography (CT) scans are needed to determine how large the spleen is and whether it is pressing on other organs. A magnetic resonance imaging (MRI) scan provides similar information and also traces blood flow through the spleen. Other specialized scanning devices use mildly radioactive particles to assess the spleen's size and function and to determine whether it is accumulating or destroying large numbers of blood cells.

Blood tests show decreased numbers of red blood cells, white blood cells, and platelets. When blood cells are examined under a microscope, their shape and size may provide clues to the cause of the spleen enlargement. An examination of bone marrow▲ may detect cancer of the blood cells (such as leukemia or lymphoma) or an accumulation of unwanted substances (such as storage diseases). These disorders can cause an enlarged spleen.

Blood protein measurement can help rule out such conditions as multiple myeloma, amyloidosis, malaria, kala-azar, brucellosis, tuberculosis, and sarcoidosis. Levels of uric acid (a waste product found in blood and urine) and of leukocyte alkaline phosphatase (an enzyme found in some blood cells) are measured to determine whether certain leukemias and lymphomas are present. Liver function tests help determine whether the liver is damaged along with the spleen.

Treatment

When possible, a doctor treats the underlying disease that caused the enlarged spleen. Surgical removal of the spleen is rarely necessary and can cause problems, including susceptibility to serious infection. However, these risks are worth taking in certain critical situations: when the spleen destroys red blood cells so rapidly that severe anemia develops; when it so depletes stores of white blood cells and platelets that infection and bleeding are likely; when it is so large that it causes pain or puts pressure on other organs; or when it is so large that parts of it bleed or die. As an alternative to surgery, radiation therapy can sometimes be used to shrink the spleen.

Ruptured Spleen

Because the spleen lies in the upper left part of the abdomen, a severe blow to the stomach area can rupture the spleen, tearing its covering and the tissue inside. A ruptured spleen is the most common serious complication of abdominal injury from car accidents, athletic mishaps, or beatings.

When the spleen ruptures, a large volume of blood may pour out into the abdomen. The spleen's tough outer capsule may contain the bleeding temporarily, but surgery is needed immediately to prevent life-threatening blood loss.

Symptoms

A ruptured spleen makes the abdomen painful and tender. Blood in the abdomen acts as an irritant and causes pain; the abdominal muscles contract reflexively and feel rigid. If the blood leaks out gradually, no symptoms may occur until the body's blood supply is so depleted that blood pressure falls or oxygen can't be transported to the brain and heart. Such a situation is an emergency requiring immediate blood transfusions to maintain adequate circulation and surgery to stop the leak; without these actions, the person could go into shock and die.

Diagnosis and Treatment

X-rays of the abdomen are taken to determine if the symptoms may be caused by something other than a ruptured spleen. Scanning procedures using radioactive material to trace blood flow and find leaks may be performed, or fluid in the abdomen may be withdrawn by a needle and sampled to see if it's bloody. When doctors strongly suspect that the spleen has ruptured, the person is rushed to surgery to stop the potentially fatal loss of blood. Usually the entire spleen is removed, but sometimes surgeons are able to close off a small rupture and save the spleen.

Before and after removal of the spleen, certain precautions are needed to prevent infections. For example, vaccinations against pneumococcus are given before a splenectomy whenever possible, and yearly vaccinations against influenza are recommended after a splenectomy. Many doctors also recommend prophylactic antibiotics.

▲ see page 737

Cancer

CHAPTER 162

Causes and Risks of Cancer

A cancer is a cell that has lost its normal control mechanisms and thus has unregulated growth.

Cancer can develop from any tissue within any organ. As cancer cells grow and multiply, they form a mass of cancerous tissue that invades adjacent tissues and can spread (metastasize) around the body.

How Cancer Develops

Cancer cells develop from normal cells in a complex process called transformation. The first step in the process is **initiation,** in which a change in the cell's genetic material primes the cell to become cancerous. The change in the cell's genetic material is brought about by an agent called a carcinogen—such as a chemical, virus, radiation, or sunlight. However, not all cells are equally susceptible to carcinogens. A genetic flaw in the cell or another agent, called a promoter, may make it more susceptible. Even chronic physical irritation may make cells more susceptible to becoming cancerous. In the next step, **promotion,** a cell that has been initiated becomes cancerous.

Promotion has no effect on noninitiated cells. Thus, several factors, often the combination of a susceptible cell and a carcinogen, are needed to cause cancer.

In the process by which a normal cell becomes a cancerous cell, ultimately its DNA undergoes change. Changes in a cell's genetic material are often hard to detect, but sometimes a change in the size or shape of one specific chromosome indicates a certain type of cancer. For example, an abnormal chromosome called the Philadelphia chromosome is found in about 80 percent of the people with chronic myelocytic leukemia.▲ Genetic changes have also been identified in brain tumors and cancers of the colon, breast, lung, and bone.

A series of chromosomal changes may be needed for some cancers to develop. Studies of familial polyposis of the colon (a hereditary intestinal disorder in which polyps develop and be-

▲ see page 769

Carcinogens: Chemicals That Can Cause Cancer

Chemical	Type of Cancer
Environmental and industrial	
Arsenic	Lung
Asbestos	Lung, pleura
Aromatic amines	Bladder
Benzene	Leukemia
Chromates	Lung
Nickel	Lung, nasal sinuses
Vinyl chloride	Liver
Associated with lifestyle	
Alcohol	Esophagus, mouth, throat
Betel nuts	Mouth, throat
Tobacco	Head, neck, lungs, esophagus, bladder
Used in medicine	
Alkylating agents	Leukemia, bladder
Diethylstilbestrol	Liver, vagina (if exposed before birth)
Oxymetholone	Liver
Thorotrast	Blood vessels

come cancerous) have suggested how this might work in colon cancer: The normal lining of the colon begins to grow more actively (hyperproliferate) because the cells no longer have a suppressor gene on chromosome 5 that normally controls the growth of the lining. A slight change in DNA then promotes changes to form an adenoma (a benign tumor). Another gene (the RAS oncogene) makes the adenoma grow more ac-

▲ see page 792

tively. The subsequent loss of a suppressor gene on chromosome 18 further stimulates the adenoma, and finally the loss of a gene on chromosome 17 converts the benign adenoma to cancer. Additional changes may make the cancer metastasize.

Even when a cell becomes cancerous, the immune system can often destroy it before it replicates and becomes established as a cancer.▲ Cancer is more likely to develop when the immune system isn't functioning normally, as in people with AIDS, those receiving immunosuppressive drugs, and those with certain autoimmune diseases. However, the immune system is not foolproof; cancer can escape the immune system's protective surveillance even when it's functioning normally.

Risk Factors

A host of genetic and environmental factors increases the risk of developing cancer.

Family history is one important factor. Some families have a significantly higher risk of developing certain cancers than other families. For example, a woman's risk of developing breast cancer increases 1.5 to 3 times if her mother or sister had breast cancer. Some breast cancers are linked to a specific gene mutation, more common in some ethnic groups and families. Women with this gene mutation have an 80 to 90 percent chance of developing breast cancer and a 40 to 50 percent chance of developing ovarian cancer. Researchers have found that 1 percent of Ashkenazi Jewish women have this gene mutation. Many other cancers, including some skin cancers and colon cancers, tend to run in families as well.

People with chromosomal abnormalities have an increased risk of cancer. For example, people with Down syndrome, who have three instead of the usual two chromosomes numbered 21, have a 12 to 20 times higher risk of developing acute leukemia.

A number of environmental factors increase the risk of cancer. One of the most important is cigarette smoking. Smoking cigarettes substantially increases the risk of developing cancers of the lung, mouth, larynx, and bladder.

Extended exposure to ultraviolet radiation, primarily from sunlight, causes skin cancer. Ionizing radiation, which is particularly carcinogenic, is used in x-rays, produced in nuclear power plants and atomic bomb explosions, and reaches the earth from space. For example, survivors of the atomic bombs dropped on Hiroshima and Nagasaki during World War II have an increased risk of developing leukemia. Exposure to uranium in mine workers has been linked to the development of lung cancer 15 to 20 years later; the risk is greatly increased if the mine workers also smoked cigarettes. Long-term exposure to ionizing radiation predisposes people to develop cancer of the blood cells, including acute leukemia.

Diet is another important risk factor for cancer, particularly cancers of the gastrointestinal system. A high-fiber diet reduces the likelihood of developing colon cancer. A diet high in smoked and pickled foods increases the chance of developing stomach cancer. Current evidence suggests that following a diet in which less than 30 percent of the total calories comes from fat reduces the risk of colon, breast, and possibly prostate cancer. People who drink large amounts of alcohol are at much higher risk of esophageal cancer.

Many chemicals are known to cause cancer and many others are suspected of causing cancer. Exposure to certain common chemicals can greatly increase a person's chance of developing cancer, often years later. For example, asbestos exposure may cause lung cancer and mesothelioma (cancer of the pleura).▲ Cancer is even more prevalent in cigarette smokers who were exposed to asbestos.

The risk of cancer also varies according to where people live. The risk of colon and breast cancers is low in Japan, yet in Japanese immigrants to the United States, the risk increases and eventually equals that of the rest of the American population. The Japanese have extremely high rates of stomach cancer. However, for Japanese born in the United States, the incidence is lower. This geographic variation in cancer risk is probably multifactorial: a combination of genetics, diet, and environment.

Several viruses are known to cause cancer in humans and several others are suspected of causing cancer. The papillomavirus that causes genital warts is probably one cause of cervical cancer in women. Cytomegalovirus causes Kaposi's sarcoma. Hepatitis B virus can cause liver cancer, although whether it's a carcinogen or a promoter isn't known. In Africa, the Epstein-Barr virus causes Burkitt's lymphoma; in China, it causes cancers of the nose and pharynx. Obviously, some additional factor, either environmental or genetic, is needed for the Epstein-Barr virus to cause cancer. Some human retroviruses, such as the human immunodeficiency virus,■ cause lymphomas and other cancers of the blood system.

Infection with the parasite *Schistosoma* (*Bilharzia*) may cause bladder cancer by chronically irritating the bladder. Yet, other causes of chronic bladder irritation don't cause cancer. Infection with *Clonorchis*, found mainly in the Far East, can lead to cancer of the pancreas and bile ducts.

Cancer Epidemiology

Cancer risk has changed over time. Some once common cancers have become rare. For example, cancer of the stomach was four times more prevalent in the United States in 1930 than it is today, probably because people today consume much less smoked, pickled, and spoiled food. On the other hand, lung cancer occurrence in the United States increased from 5 people per 100,000 in 1930 to 114 people per 100,000 in 1990, and the rate of lung cancer in women has skyrocketed. These changes are almost certainly the result of increased cigarette smoking. Cigarette smoking has also led to an increase in cancers of the mouth.

Age is an important factor in the development of cancer. Some cancers, such as Wilms' tumor, acute lymphocytic leukemia, and Burkitt's lymphoma, occur almost exclusively in young people. Why these cancers occur in the young is not well understood, but genetic predisposition is one factor. However, most cancers are more common in older people. Many cancers, including those of the prostate, stomach, and colon, are most likely to occur after age 60. Over 60 percent of the cancers diagnosed in the United States are in people over 65 years of age. Overall, the risk of developing cancer in the United States doubles every 5 years after age 25. The increased cancer rate is probably a combination of increased and prolonged exposure to carcinogens and weakening of the body's immune system, all associated with a longer life span.

▲ see page 209

■ see box, page 927

Cancer and the Immune System

The body's immune system attacks and eliminates not only bacteria and other foreign substances but also cancer cells. A cancer cell is not a foreign cell; rather, it is a cell whose biologic function has been altered in such a way that it doesn't respond to the body's normal mechanisms for controlling cell growth and reproduction. The abnormal cells can continue to grow, resulting in cancer.

Much of the body's protection against cancer is carried out directly by cells of the immune system rather than by antibodies circulating in the bloodstream.▲ For example, the presence of tumor antigens on cancer cells can activate certain white blood cells (lymphocytes and, to a lesser degree, monocytes), which carry out an immunologic surveillance, looking for cancer cells and destroying them.

The immune system's critical role in controlling cancer cell development is exemplified by an astounding statistic: Cancer is 100 times more likely to occur in people who take drugs that suppress the immune system (for example, because of an organ transplant or a rheumatic disease) than in people with normal immune systems. In addition, sometimes a transplanted organ has a cancer that wasn't diagnosed before the transplantation. The cancer may have been growing slowly or not at all in the organ donor. However, the cancer starts growing and spreading rapidly in the recipient, whose immune system is suppressed by drugs to protect the transplant. Typically, when the immunosuppressive drugs are stopped, the transplanted organ is rejected and the transplanted cancer is destroyed as well.

Tumor Antigens

An antigen is a foreign substance recognized and targeted for destruction by the body's immune system.■ Antigens are found on the surface of all cells, but normally a person's immune system doesn't react to his own cells. When a cell

becomes cancerous, new antigens—unfamiliar to the immune system—appear on the cell's surface. The immune system may regard these new antigens, called tumor antigens, as foreign and may be able to contain or destroy the cancer cells. However, even a fully functioning immune system can't always destroy all cancer cells.

Tumor antigens have been identified in several types of cancer, including malignant melanoma, bone cancer (osteosarcoma), and some gastrointestinal cancers. People with these cancers may have antibodies against the tumor antigens. The antigens generally don't elicit an immune response adequate to control the cancer. The antibodies seem unable to destroy the cancer and sometimes even seem to *stimulate* its growth.

Certain tumor antigens can be used to advantage, however. Antigens released into the bloodstream by some cancers can be detected with blood tests. These antigens are sometimes called **tumor markers.** Great interest has focused on whether tumor markers can be used as screening tests in people who have no symptoms of cancer. Because the tests are expensive and not very specific, for the most part their use in routine screening is currently inadvisable. Instead, tumor markers are much more valuable in both the diagnosis and treatment of cancer. For example, blood tests can help determine if a cancer treatment is effective. If the tumor marker no longer appears in the blood sample, the treatment has probably been successful. If the marker disappears and later reappears, the cancer has probably returned.

Carcinoembryonic antigen (CEA) is a tumor antigen found in the blood of people with cancer of the colon, breast, pancreas, bladder, ovary, or cervix. High levels of this antigen may also be found in people who are heavy cigarette smokers and in those who have cirrhosis of the liver or ulcerative colitis. Therefore, having a high carcinoembryonic antigen level doesn't always mean that a person has cancer. Measuring the carcinoembryonic antigen level in people who have been treated for cancer helps doctors detect a recurrence.

Alpha-fetoprotein (AFP), which is normally produced by fetal liver cells, is found in the blood of people with liver cancer (hepatoma). In addition,

▲ see page 811

■ see page 813

alpha-fetoprotein is often found in people with certain cancers of the ovary or testis and in children and young adults with pineal gland tumors.

Beta–human chorionic gonadotropin (β–HCG), a hormone produced during pregnancy that serves as the basis for pregnancy tests, also occurs in women who have a cancer originating in the placenta and in men with various types of testicular cancer. Beta–human chorionic gonadotropin is a very sensitive tumor marker. Its use in monitoring the effects of treatment has helped improve the cure rates for these cancers to well over 95 percent.

Prostate-specific antigen (PSA) levels are high in men with noncancerous (benign) enlargement of the prostate and considerably higher in men with prostate cancer. What constitutes a meaningfully abnormal level is somewhat uncertain, but men with an elevated prostate-specific antigen level should be evaluated further for prostate cancer.▲ Monitoring the blood level of prostate-specific antigen after treatment for cancer can indicate whether the cancer has recurred.

Blood levels of **CA-125**, another antigen, are measurably increased in women with a variety of ovarian diseases, including cancer. Since ovarian cancer is often difficult to diagnose, some cancer experts advocate screening for CA-125 in women over 40 years old. However, its lack of sensitivity and specificity mean that it isn't yet a reliable screening test.

Elevated levels of **CA 15-3** occur in breast cancer, **CA 19-5** in pancreatic cancer, **β₂-microglobulin** in multiple myeloma, and **lactate dehydrogenase** in testicular cancer, but none of them can be recommended for cancer screening. However, they are useful in monitoring the response to treatment of a person already diagnosed with cancer.

Immunotherapy

To improve the immune system's ability to find and destroy cancer, researchers have developed **biologic response modifiers**. These substances are used for the following functions:
• To stimulate the body's antitumor response by increasing the number of tumor-killing cells or producing one or more chemical messengers (mediators)
• To serve directly as tumor-killing agents or chemical messengers
• To decrease the body's normal mechanisms for suppressing the immune response

• To alter tumor cells to increase their likelihood of triggering an immune response or make them more likely to be damaged by the immune system
• To improve the body's tolerance to radiation therapy or the chemicals used in chemotherapy

Interferon is the best-known and most widely used biologic response modifier. Almost all human cells produce interferon naturally, but it can also be made by recombinant molecular biologic techniques. Although its mechanisms of action are not totally clear, interferon has a role in the treatment of several cancers. Excellent responses (including some cures) have occurred in about 30 percent of people with Kaposi's sarcoma, 20 percent of young people with chronic myelogenous leukemia, and 15 percent of people with renal cell carcinoma. In addition, interferon prolongs the expected disease-free period in people who are in remission from multiple myeloma and some forms of lymphoma.

In **killer cell therapy**, some of a cancer patient's own lymphocytes (a type of white blood cell) are removed from a blood sample. In the laboratory, the lymphocytes are exposed to a substance called interleukin-2 (a T-cell growth factor) to create lymphokine-activated killer cells, which are injected back into the person intravenously. These cells are more capable than the body's natural cells of detecting and destroying cancer cells. Although about 25 to 50 percent of the people who have malignant melanoma or kidney cancer respond well to lymphokine-activated killer cell therapy, this form of therapy is still experimental.

Humoral (antibody) therapy boosts the body's production of antibodies. Substances such as extracts of weakened (attenuated) tuberculosis bacteria, which are known to boost the immune response, have been tried with some cancers. Injecting the tuberculosis bacteria directly into a melanoma almost always causes the cancer there to recede. Occasionally, the effect extends to tumors that have spread to other parts of the body (metastases). Doctors have also successfully used tuberculosis bacteria to control bladder cancer that has not invaded the bladder wall.

Another experimental approach involves linking tumor-specific antibodies with anticancer drugs. The antibodies, which are synthesized in

▲ see page 1060

the laboratory and injected into a person, guide the drugs to cancer cells.

Alternatively, other antibodies created in the laboratory can adhere to both the cancer cell and a killer lymphocyte, bringing the two cells together so the killer lymphocyte can destroy the cancer cell. So far, such research hasn't resulted in any widely applicable cancer therapies.

Recent research offers hope for new treatments. Some of them use pieces of oncogenes, which are important in cell regulation and growth.

CHAPTER 164

Diagnosis of Cancer

An evaluation of cancer begins with a history and physical examination. Together, they help a doctor assess a person's risk of cancer and decide which tests are necessary. In general, as part of a routine physical examination, a cancer-related checkup should be performed to check for cancers of the thyroid, testes, mouth, ovaries, skin, and lymph nodes.

Screening tests try to identify cancer before it causes symptoms. If a screening test gives a positive result, further tests are needed to be certain of the diagnosis. A diagnosis of cancer must always be made with absolute certainty, a process that usually requires a biopsy. Determining the specific type of cancer is also absolutely essential. When cancer is found, staging tests help determine its exact location and whether it has spread. Staging also helps doctors plan appropriate treatment and determine prognosis.

Screening for Cancer

Cancer screening tests serve to detect the *possibility* that a cancer is present. They can reduce the number of cancer deaths: When cancer is detected in its earliest stages, it can usually be treated before it spreads. Screening tests usually aren't definitive; results are confirmed or disproved with further examinations and tests.

Although screening tests can help save lives, they can also be costly and sometimes have psychologic or physical repercussions. Generally, screening tests produce a relatively high number of **false-positive results**—results that suggest a cancer may be present when it actually isn't. Screening tests can also produce **false-negative results**—results that show no hint of a cancer that is actually present. False-positive results can cre-

ate undue psychologic stress and can lead to other tests that are expensive and risky. False-negative results can lull people into a false sense of security. For these reasons, health care practitioners carefully consider whether or not to perform such tests.

Two of the most widely used screening tests in women are the Papanicolaou (Pap) test to detect cervical cancer and mammography to detect breast cancer. Both screening tests have been successful in reducing the death rates from these cancers.

Measuring the blood level of prostate-specific antigen is a common screening test in men. Levels of prostate-specific antigen are high in men with prostate cancer, but levels are also elevated in men with benign enlargement of the prostate. Whether prostate-specific antigen should be used to screen for prostate cancer is still unresolved. Drawbacks to its use as a screening test include its cost and the incidence of false-positive results.

Another common screening test involves checking the stool for occult blood. Occult blood can't be seen by the eye alone; the stool sample must be tested. Finding occult blood in the stool is an indication that something is wrong in the colon. The problem may be cancer, although many other disorders can also cause small amounts of blood to leak into the stool.

Some screening tests can be done at home. For example, monthly breast self-examinations are exceedingly valuable in helping women detect breast cancer. Periodically examining the testes can help men detect testicular cancer, one of the most curable forms of cancer when diagnosed early. Periodically checking the mouth for sores can help detect mouth cancer in an early stage.

Cancer Screening Recommendations

Procedure	Frequency
Lung cancer	
Chest x-ray Sputum cytology	Not recommended on a routine basis
Rectal and colon cancer	
Stool examination for occult blood	Yearly after age 50
Rectal examination	Yearly after age 40
Sigmoidoscopic examination	Every 3 to 5 years after age 50
Prostate cancer	
Rectal examination and blood test for prostate-specific antigen	Yearly after age 50
Cervical, uterine, and ovarian cancers	
Pelvic examination	Every 1 to 3 years between ages 18 and 40, then yearly

Procedure	Frequency
Cervical cancer	
Papanicolaou (Pap) test	Yearly between ages 18 and 65. After 3 or more consecutive normal exams, a Pap test may be performed less often at the doctor's discretion. Most women over 65 need Pap tests less often
Breast cancer	
Breast self-examination	Monthly after age 18
Breast physical examination	Every 3 years between ages 18 and 40, then yearly
Mammography	Initial baseline exam between ages 35 and 40, every 1 to 2 years from age 40 to 49, and yearly after age 50

Modified from American Cancer Society publications #2070-LE and 92-10M-No. 3402; used with permission.

Diagnosing Cancer

Since many different types of cancer exist and their treatments vary, diagnosing the presence of cancer and determining the specific type of cancer are absolutely essential. This virtually always requires obtaining a sample of the suspected tumor for examination under a microscope. A variety of special tests on that sample may be required to further characterize the cancer. Knowing the type of cancer helps the doctor determine what tests to perform, because each cancer tends to follow a pattern of growth and spread.

In up to 7 percent of cancer patients, tests identify metastases before the original cancer is distinguished. Sometimes the original cancer cannot be discovered. However, doctors can usually identify the type of primary tumor by performing a biopsy of the metastasis and examining the tissue under a microscope. Nonetheless, identification is not always easy or certain. To what extent doctors search for a primary tumor is determined from the tissue diagnosis. In general, doctors seek the primary tumor if treating it will significantly affect survival (for example, breast cancer). If identifying the primary tumor will not change the program of therapy or the projected survival, extensive testing to locate it has no value.

Staging Cancer

When cancer is found, staging tests help doctors plan appropriate treatment and determine prognosis. A variety of tests are used to determine the tumor's location, its size, its growth into nearby structures, and its spread to other parts of the body. Staging is critical to determine if cure is likely. People with cancer sometimes become impatient and anxious during staging tests, wishing for a prompt attack on the tumor. However,

Tests for Staging Cancers

Cancer Site	Type of Biopsy Performed	Other Tests Performed
Breast	Needle or whole-lump biopsy	Mammogram Liver and bone scans Brain CT scan Estrogen- and progesterone-receptor testing on the biopsy sample
Gastrointestinal tract	Tissue for biopsy taken by endoscopy or with a needle (usually guided by a CT scan) through the skin for liver, pancreas, or other organs	Chest x-ray Barium x-ray Ultrasound scan CT scan Liver scan Blood tests for liver enzymes
Lung	Biopsy of the lung and possibly the sac around the lung (pleura) Mediastinoscopy	Chest x-ray CT scan Sputum cytology
Lymphatic system	Lymph node biopsy Bone marrow biopsy	Chest x-ray Blood cell counts Ultrasound scan CT scan Radioisotope scan Exploratory surgery Splenectomy
Prostate	Needle biopsy	Blood tests for acid phosphatase and prostate-specific antigen (PSA) Ultrasound scan
Testes	Testis removed for biopsy	Chest x-ray CT scan
Uterus, cervix, ovaries	Tissue for biopsy taken during exploratory surgery	Pelvic examination under anesthesia Ultrasound scan CT scan Barium enema examination

staging allows doctors to determine an intelligent, planned course of attack.

Staging may use scans, such as liver and bone scans, dye studies, or computed tomography (CT) or magnetic resonance imaging (MRI) to determine whether the cancer has spread. Mediastinoscopy, in which the center of the chest (the mediastinum) is viewed with a fiber-optic instrument,▲ is used to determine whether cancer, usu-

ally lung cancer, has spread to nearby lymph nodes. A bone marrow biopsy, in which tissue is taken from the center of a bone and examined under a microscope, can help determine whether a cancer has spread to the bone marrow.■

Sometimes surgery may be needed to determine the cancer's stage. For example, a laparotomy (an abdominal operation) allows the surgeon to remove or treat colon cancer while determining whether the cancer has spread to nearby lymph nodes, from which it could travel to the liver. An analysis of lymph nodes removed from the armpit during a mastectomy helps determine how far breast cancer has spread and whether

▲ see page 163

■ see page 737

postsurgical therapy is needed. An operation to remove the spleen (splenectomy) helps in staging Hodgkin's disease.

Ultrasound scanning is a painless, noninvasive procedure that uses sound waves to show the structure of internal organs. It's helpful for identifying and determining the size of certain cancers, particularly of the kidneys, liver, pelvis, and prostate. Doctors also use ultrasound to guide the removal of tissue samples during a needle biopsy.

Computed tomography (CT) scanning is used to detect cancer in the brain, lungs, and abdominal organs, including the adrenal glands, lymph nodes, liver, and spleen. A lymphangiogram is a test in which dye is injected into the feet and followed with x-rays as it flows upward. The test helps identify abnormalities in the abdominal lymph nodes. Although uncommonly done since the advent of CT imaging, lymphangiograms continue to have value in staging Hodgkin's disease and testicular cancer.

Magnetic resonance imaging (MRI) is an alternative to CT scans. With this procedure, a very powerful magnetic field generates exquisitely detailed anatomical images. It is of particular value in detecting cancers of the brain, bone, and spinal cord. No x-rays are involved, and MRI is extremely safe.

CHAPTER 165

Complications of Cancer

Cancers and their satellite tumors (metastases) can invade and thereby alter the function of an organ or put pressure on surrounding tissues; either may result in a wide variety of symptoms and medical problems. In people with metastatic cancer, pain can result from the cancer growing inside nonexpandable bone, from pressure on nerves, or from pressure on other tissues.

Many cancers produce substances such as hormones, cytokines, and proteins that can affect the function of other tissues and organs, resulting in a variety of symptoms termed paraneoplastic syndromes. Sometimes the problems caused by cancer are so severe that they must be treated as an emergency.

Paraneoplastic Syndromes

Paraneoplastic syndromes are collections of symptoms caused not by the tumor itself but by products of the cancer.

Some of the substances that a tumor can produce are hormones, cytokines, and a variety of other proteins. These products affect organs or tissues by their chemical effect, thus the term *paraneoplastic.* Exactly how cancers affect distant sites isn't completely understood. Some cancers release substances into the bloodstream that damage remote tissues by causing an autoimmune reaction. Other cancers secrete substances that directly interfere with the function of different organs or actually destroy tissues.

Symptoms such as low blood sugar, diarrhea, and high blood pressure can result. Often paraneoplastic syndromes affect the nervous system.▲ Although some of the symptoms can be treated directly, treating a paraneoplastic syndrome usually requires controlling the underlying cancer.

Cancer Emergencies

Cancer emergencies include cardiac tamponade, pleural effusion, superior vena cava syndrome, spinal cord compression, and hypercalcemic syndrome.

Cardiac tamponade is the accumulation of fluid in the baglike structure surrounding the heart (pericardium or pericardial sac), which puts pressure on the heart and interferes with its ability to pump blood. Fluid can accumulate when a cancer invades the pericardium and irritates it. The cancers most likely to invade the pericardium are lung cancer, breast cancer, and lymphoma.

Cardiac tamponade occurs suddenly when so much fluid accumulates that the heart can't beat

---

▲ see page 384

Some Effects of Paraneoplastic Syndromes

Area Affected	Effects	Cancer Responsible
Brain, nerves, and muscles	Neurologic deficits, muscle pain, weakness	Lung cancer
Blood and blood-forming tissues	Anemia, high blood platelet count, high white blood cell count, widespread clotting within the blood vessels, low platelet count, easy bruising	All cancers
Kidneys	Membranous glomerulitis resulting from antibodies in the bloodstream	Colon or ovarian cancer, lymphoma, Hodgkin's disease, leukemia
Bones	Enlarged fingertips (clubbing)	Lung cancer or lung metastases from a variety of cancers
Skin	A variety of skin lesions, often pigmented; for instance, acanthosis nigricans, an eruption of velvety, warty, benign growths and dark pigmentation in the armpit, in the neck, and around the genitals	Gastrointestinal or liver cancer, lymphoma, melanoma
Entire body	Fever	Leukemia, lymphoma, Hodgkin's disease, kidney or liver cancer

normally. Before the onset of tamponade, the person usually feels a vague pain or pressure in the chest that worsens upon lying down and gets better upon sitting up. Once the tamponade develops, the person has severe difficulty in breathing; the neck veins swell during inhalation.

Doctors diagnose cardiac tamponade with chest x-rays, electrocardiograms, and echocardiograms. To relieve the pressure, a doctor inserts a needle into the pericardial sac and draws the fluid into a syringe (pericardiocentesis). A sample of the fluid is examined under a microscope to see whether it contains cancer cells. Subsequently, the doctor cuts an opening in the pericardium (pericardial window) or strips the pericardium to prevent tamponade from recurring. Additional treatment depends on the type of cancer present.

▲ see page 210

Pleural effusion—fluid in the baglike structure around the lungs (pleural sac)—can cause breathlessness. Fluid can accumulate in the pleural sac for many reasons, one of which is cancer. A doctor drains the fluid by inserting a syringe needle between the ribs into the pleural sac. If fluid starts to accumulate again rapidly after this procedure, the doctor inserts a drainage tube through the chest wall and leaves it in the pleural sac until the person's condition improves. Special chemicals may be inserted into the pleural sac to irritate its walls, inducing them to fuse together. This eliminates the space where fluid can enter and reduces the likelihood of a recurrence.

Superior vena cava syndrome occurs when the cancer partially or completely blocks the veins (superior vena cava) that drain blood from the upper part of the body into the heart. Blockage of the superior vena cava causes the veins in the upper part of the chest and neck to swell, resulting in swelling of the face, neck, and upper part of the chest.▲

Spinal cord compression syndrome occurs when cancer compresses the spinal cord or the spinal cord nerves, resulting in pain and loss of function.▲ The longer a person has a neurologic deficit, the less likely normal nerve function will return. In general, treatment is best begun within 12 to 24 hours after the onset of symptoms. A doctor gives corticosteroids such as prednisone intravenously (to reduce the swelling) and radiation therapy. Rarely, when the cause of the spinal cord compression isn't known, surgery may help pinpoint the diagnosis and treat the problem by allowing the surgeon to decompress the spinal cord.■

Hypercalcemic syndrome occurs when the cancer produces a hormone that raises the blood calcium level or directly invades bone. The person develops confusion, which can progress to coma and cause death. Various drugs can promptly reduce the calcium levels.★

CHAPTER 166

Cancer Treatment

Successful cancer treatment focuses not only on the primary tumor but also on tumors that may have spread to other parts of the body (metastases). Surgery or radiation therapy to specific areas of the body is therefore often combined with chemotherapy for the whole body. Even when a cure is impossible, symptoms can often be relieved with palliative therapy, improving the quality and length of life.

Response to Treatment

While being treated for cancer, people are assessed to see how the cancer is responding to therapy. The most successful treatment produces a cure. A cure is defined as a complete remission in which all evidence of cancer disappears (complete response). Researchers sometimes estimate cures in terms of the 5-year or 10-year disease-free survival rates, in which the cancer completely disappears and doesn't recur within a defined period, often 5 or 10 years. With a partial response, the size of one or more tumors is reduced by more than half; this response can reduce symptoms and may prolong life, although the cancer eventually grows back. The least successful treatment produces no response.

Sometimes a cancer completely disappears but returns later; the interval between these two events is called the disease-free survival time. The interval from complete response to the time of death is the total survival time. In people who have a partial response, the duration of response is measured from the time of the partial response to the time when the cancer begins to enlarge or spread again.

Some cancers respond well to chemotherapy. Others improve but aren't cured. Some cancers (melanoma, kidney cell cancer, pancreatic cancer, brain cancer) respond poorly to chemotherapy and are termed resistant. Other cancers (breast cancer, small-cell lung cancer, leukemia) may have excellent initial responses to chemotherapy but after repeated treatment may develop resistance to the drugs. Because multidrug-resistant genes are found in both normal cells and cancer cells, exposure to one drug can make a tumor resistant to unrelated cancer drugs. Presumably these genes exist to provide cells with the means to escape destruction by a noxious material. As a result, the cell may pump out the drug in self-defense, making the therapy ineffective. Researchers are trying to determine how to suppress the activity of these genes.

▲ see page 383

■ see page 323

★ see page 673

Percentage of People With Cancer Who Are Disease-Free After 5 Years

Cancer Site	People With Cancer at Any Stage	People With Localized Cancer	People With Regional Metastases	People With Distant Metastases
Bladder	80	92	48	8
Breast (in women)	80	94	73	18
Cervix	67	90	51	12
Colon-rectum	59	91	60	6
Kidney	56	87	57	9
Lung	13	47	15	2
Mouth	52	79	42	19
Ovary	42	90	41	21
Pancreas	3	9	4	2
Prostate	80	94	85	29
Skin (melanoma)	85	93	57	15
Uterus	83	94	67	27

Acute lymphoblastic leukemia and acute myelogenous leukemia are two potentially curable cancers. Hodgkin's disease and many of the non-Hodgkin's lymphomas (diffuse large-cell lymphoma, Burkitt's lymphoma, and lymphoblastic lymphoma) are cured in about 80 percent of children and adults. Chemotherapy cures more than 90 percent of men who have advanced testicular cancer, and about 98 percent of women with choriocarcinoma (a cancer of the uterus).

Surgery

Surgery is one of the oldest forms of cancer therapy. Of the 1 million Americans who developed cancer in 1988, 64 percent had surgery and 62 percent of that group were cured. Treatment and outlook (prognosis) are determined largely by judging the severity and spread of the cancer through a process called staging.▲ Since some cancers can often be cured with surgery alone when treated in their early stages, seeing a doctor as soon as possible is vitally important.

Radiation Therapy

Radiation preferentially destroys cells that divide rapidly. Usually this means cancer, but radiation can also damage normal tissues, especially tissues in which cells normally reproduce rapidly such as skin; hair follicles; the lining of the intestines, ovary, or testis; and the bone marrow. Accurately targeting the radiation therapy protects normal cells as much as possible.

Cells that have an adequate oxygen supply are more susceptible to the damaging effects of radiation. Cells closer to the center of a large tumor often have a poor blood supply and low oxygen levels. As the tumor shrinks, the surviving cells

▲ see page 795

Early-Stage Cancers That May Be Cured With Surgery Alone

Cancer	Percentage of People Disease-Free After 5 Years
Bladder	81
Breast (in women)	82
Cervix	94
Colon	81
Kidney	67
Larynx	76
Lung (non–small-cell)	37 to 70
Mouth	67 to 76
Ovary	72
Prostate	80
Testis	65
Uterus	74

Early-Stage Cancers That May Be Cured With Radiation Therapy Alone

Cancer	Percentage of People Disease-Free After 5 Years
Breast (in women)	29
Cervix	60
Hodgkin's disease	71 to 88
Lung	9
Nasal sinuses	35
Nasopharynx	35
Non-Hodgkin's lymphoma	60 to 90
Prostate	67 to 80
Testis (seminoma)	84
Throat	10

appear to obtain an improved blood supply, which may make them more vulnerable to the next dose of radiation. Dividing the radiation into a series of doses over a prolonged period increases the lethal effects on tumor cells and decreases the toxic effects on normal cells. Cells have the capacity to repair themselves after being exposed to radiation; the treatment plan aims for maximum repairs of normal cells and tissues.

Radiation therapy is usually performed with equipment called a linear accelerator. The rays are directed very closely to the tumor. How the rays will adversely affect normal tissues depends on how large an area is being irradiated and its proximity to the tissues. For example, radiation to tumors of the head and neck often causes inflammation of the mucous membranes in the nose and mouth, resulting in soreness and ulcerations. Radiation to the stomach or abdomen often causes inflammation of the stomach (gastritis) and of the lower intestine (enteritis), resulting in diarrhea.▲

Radiation therapy plays a key role in curing many cancers, including Hodgkin's disease, early-stage non-Hodgkin's lymphoma, squamous cell cancer of the head and neck, seminoma (a testicular cancer), prostate cancer, early-stage breast cancer, early-stage non–small-cell lung cancer, and medulloblastoma (a brain or spinal cord tumor). For early cancers of the larynx and prostate, the rate of cure is essentially the same with radiation therapy as with surgery.

Radiation therapy can reduce symptoms when a cure isn't possible, as in multiple myeloma and advanced lung, esophageal, head and neck, and stomach cancers. Radiation therapy can also relieve symptoms caused by metastases to the bones or brain.

▲ see page 1342

Cancers That May Be Cured With Chemotherapy Alone

Cancer	Percentage of People Disease-Free After 5 Years
Burkitt's lymphoma	44 to 74
Choriocarcinoma	98
Diffuse large-cell lymphoma	64
Hodgkin's disease	74
Leukemia (acute non-lymphocytic leukemia)	
• Children	54
• Adults under 40 years	40
• Adults over 40 years	16
Lung (small-cell)	25
Lymphoblastic lymphoma	50
Testis (nonseminomatous)	88

Chemotherapy

Although an ideal anticancer drug would destroy cancer cells without harming normal cells, no such drug exists. Despite the narrow margin between benefit and harm, however, many people with cancer can be treated with anticancer drugs (chemotherapy) and some can be cured. Today the side effects of chemotherapy can be minimized.

Anticancer drugs are grouped into several categories: alkylating agents, antimetabolites, plant alkaloids, antitumor antibiotics, enzymes, hormones, and biologic response modifiers. Often, two or more drugs are used in combination. The rationale to combination chemotherapy is to use drugs that work at different parts of the cell's metabolic processes, thereby increasing the likelihood that more cancer cells will be killed. In addition, the toxic side effects of chemotherapy may be reduced when drugs with different toxicities are combined, each at a lower dose than would be needed if one drug were used alone. Finally, drugs with very different properties are sometimes combined. For example, drugs that kill tumor cells may be combined with drugs that stimulate the body's immune system against cancer (biologic response modifiers). ▲

Mustard gas, used as a weapon in World War I, is an example of an alkylating agent. Alkylating agents interfere with the DNA molecule, altering its structure or function so that it can't replicate, which then prevents the cell from multiplying. The difference between a beneficial dose and a harmful dose, however, is small. Side effects include nausea; vomiting; hair loss; bladder irritation (cystitis) with blood in the urine; low white blood cell, red blood cell, and platelet counts; low sperm count in men (and possible permanent sterility); and an increased risk of leukemia.

Antimetabolites are a broad group of drugs that interfere with steps in the synthesis of DNA or RNA, preventing cell replication. Besides causing the same side effects as alkylating agents, certain antimetabolites cause a skin rash, darkening of the skin (increased pigmentation), or kidney failure.

Plant alkaloids are drugs that can stop cell division as it happens, preventing the formation of new cells. Side effects are similar to those of the alkylating agents.

Antitumor antibiotics also injure DNA, preventing cell replication. Side effects are similar to those of the alkylating agents.

A person with acute lymphoblastic leukemia may be given asparaginase, an enzyme that depletes the blood of the amino acid asparagine, which the leukemia needs for continued growth. Side effects include life-threatening allergic reactions, loss of appetite, nausea, vomiting, fever, and high blood sugar levels.

Hormone therapies raise or lower levels of certain hormones to limit the growth of cancers that either depend on those hormones or are inhibited by them. For instance, some breast cancers need estrogen to grow. The antiestrogen drug tamoxifen blocks the effects of estrogen and may shrink the cancer. Similarly, prostate cancer may be inhibited by estrogen or antitestosterone drugs.

▲ see page 793

Where and How Chemotherapy Is Administered

Where	How	How Frequently
Hospital	Directly to the blood vessels that supply the area of tumor growth	Varies, depending on the cancer: several drugs in one day, one dose every day for several days, continuously over several days, doses once a week, one dose or a few days of medication once a month
Outpatient clinic		
Doctor's office	Intravenous drip (from a bag or bottle of intravenous solution for several minutes to several hours)	
Less commonly, in the operating room to apply drug close to the tumor		
At home (by nurse, self, or family member)	Intravenous push (directly into a vein, central venous catheter, or implanted port for several minutes)	Treatments can be given for several weeks to several years
	Orally (capsules, tablets, or liquid)	A course of treatment may be given only once, or several courses of treatment may be given, with intervals between treatment courses

Side effects vary, depending on the hormone taken. Giving estrogen to a man may have feminizing effects, such as breast enlargement. Giving antiestrogen drugs to a woman may cause hot flashes and irregular menstrual periods.

Interferon, the first effective biologic response modifier, is now commonly used to treat Kaposi's sarcoma and multiple myeloma.▲ Another type of immunotherapy uses immune-stimulated cells (lymphokine-activated killer cells) to specifically attack tumors, such as melanoma and kidney cell cancer. A treatment that uses antibodies to tumor cells, which are labeled with either a radioactive material or a toxin, has demonstrated effectiveness in treating some lymphomas.

Combination Therapy

For some cancers, the best therapy is a combination of surgery, radiation, and chemotherapy. Surgery or radiation therapy treats cancer that is confined locally, while chemotherapy kills cancer cells that have escaped beyond the local region. Sometimes radiation or chemotherapy is given before surgery to shrink a tumor, or after surgery to destroy any remaining cancer cells. Chemotherapy combined with surgery improves the chances of survival for people with colon cancer, breast cancer, or bladder cancer that has spread

to regional lymph nodes. Surgery and chemotherapy can sometimes cure advanced ovarian cancer.

Cancer of the rectum has been successfully treated with chemotherapy and radiation therapy. In advanced colon cancer, chemotherapy administered after surgery can prolong the disease-free survival. About 20 to 40 percent of head and neck cancers are cured with chemotherapy followed by radiation therapy or surgery. For those who aren't cured, these treatments can relieve symptoms (palliative therapy).

Surgery, radiation therapy, and chemotherapy play definite roles in treating Wilms' tumor and embryonal rhabdomyosarcomas. In Wilms' tumor, a childhood kidney cancer, the goal of surgery is to remove the primary cancer, even if tumor cells have spread to places in the body far from the kidney. Chemotherapy is started at the time of surgery, and radiation therapy is given later to treat local areas of residual disease.

Unfortunately, some tumors (such as those in the stomach, pancreas, or kidney) respond only partially to radiation therapy, chemotherapy, or a combination of the two. Nevertheless, these

▲ see page 793

Effectiveness of Combination Therapies

Type of Therapy	Type of Cancer	Percentage of People Disease-Free After 5 Years
Surgery and radiation	Bladder	54
	Endometrium	62
	Hypopharynx	33
	Lung	32
	Mouth	36
Surgery and chemotherapy	Breast	62
	Ovary (carcinoma)	28 to 40
	Prostate	50 to 68
	Stomach	54
Radiation and chemotherapy	Central nervous system (medulloblastoma)	71 to 80
	Ewing's sarcoma	70
	Lung (small-cell)	16 to 20
	Rectum (squamous cell carcinoma)	40
Surgery, radiation, and chemotherapy	Embryonal rhabdomyosarcoma	80
	Kidney (Wilms' tumor)	80
	Lung	32
	Oral cavity, hypopharynx	20 to 40

therapies can relieve pain from pressure or symptoms that result when the tumor infiltrates the surrounding tissues. Some resistant tumors (for example, non–small-cell lung cancer, esophageal cancer, pancreatic cancer, kidney cancer) can be treated to increase survival time. Progress in cancer therapy has come with better combinations of drugs, altered dosages, and better coordination with radiation therapy.

Side Effects of Treatment

Almost everyone who receives chemotherapy or radiation therapy experiences certain side effects, most commonly nausea or vomiting and low blood cell counts. People treated with chemotherapy often lose their hair. Relieving side effects is an important aspect of therapy.

Nausea and Vomiting

Nausea and vomiting can usually be prevented or relieved with drugs (antiemetics). Nausea may be reduced without using drugs by eating small meals frequently and avoiding foods that are high in fiber, that produce gas, or that are very hot or very cold.

Low Blood Cell Counts

Cytopenia, a deficiency of one or more types of blood cell, can develop during cancer therapy.

For example, a person may develop abnormally low numbers of red blood cells (anemia), white blood cells (neutropenia or leukopenia), or platelets (thrombocytopenia).▲ In general, cytopenia does not need to be treated. However, if anemia is severe, packed red blood cells can be transfused. Similarly, if thrombocytopenia is severe, platelets can be transfused to lower the risk of bleeding.

A person with neutropenia (abnormally low numbers of neutrophils, a type of white blood cell) is at increased risk of developing an infection. That's why a fever higher than 100.4° F. in a person with neutropenia is treated as an emergency. The person is evaluated for infection and may require antibiotics and even hospitalization. White blood cells are rarely transfused because they survive only a few hours and produce many side effects. Instead, certain substances (such as granulocyte-stimulating factor) can be administered to stimulate white blood cell production.

Other Common Side Effects

Radiation therapy or chemotherapy can cause inflammation or even ulcers of the mucous membranes, such as the lining of the mouth. Mouth ulcers are painful and can make eating difficult. A variety of oral solutions (usually containing an antacid, an antihistamine, and a local anesthetic) can reduce the discomfort. On rare occasions, nutritional support must be given by a feeding tube that's placed directly into the stomach or small intestine or even by vein. A variety of drugs can reduce the diarrhea caused by radiation therapy to the abdomen.

Newer Approaches and Investigational Treatments

One new approach to treating cancer is called dose-intensity chemotherapy, which uses especially high doses of drugs. This therapy is used for tumors that have recurred even though they had a good response when first treated with drugs. Such tumors have already demonstrated sensitivity to the drug; the strategy is to markedly increase the drug dose to kill more cancer cells and thus prolong survival.

However, dose-intensity chemotherapy can cause life-threatening injury to the bone marrow. Therefore, dose-intensity chemotherapy is commonly combined with rescue therapy, in which bone marrow is harvested before the chemotherapy is administered. After the treatment, the marrow is returned to the patient. Blood stem cells can be isolated from a blood sample and used instead of bone marrow in some cases. Although still investigational, these treatments have been tried for breast cancer, lymphoma, Hodgkin's disease, and myeloma.

A true bone marrow transplant from a tissue-matched donor (usually a sibling) can be performed after dose-intensity chemotherapy in people with acute leukemia. Complications include graft-versus-host disease, in which the transplanted tissue destroys the host's tissue.■

New techniques of radiation therapy, such as proton or neutron beam radiation, can effectively treat certain tumors. Radiation-activated dyes and photodynamic therapy show great promise.

Immunotherapy uses techniques such as biologic response modifiers, killer cell therapy, and humoral (antibody) therapy to stimulate the body's immune system against cancer.★ These techniques have been used to treat a number of different cancers such as melanoma, kidney cancer, Kaposi's sarcoma, and leukemia.

Finally, one of the most important potential therapeutic approaches is to find drugs that help prevent cancer. Retinoids (vitamin A derivatives) have been effective in reducing the recurrence rate of some cancers, especially those of the mouth, larynx, and lungs. Unfortunately, other agents, such as beta-carotene and related antioxidants, have not been shown to prevent cancer.

▲ see page 734

■ see page 836

★ see page 793

Immune Disorders

CHAPTER 167

Biology of the Immune System

Just as the human mind allows a person to develop a concept of intellectual self, the immune system provides a concept of biologic self. The function of the immune system is to defend the body against invaders. Microbes (germs or microorganisms), cancer cells, and transplanted tissues or organs are all interpreted by the immune system as nonself against which the body must be defended.

Although the immune system is intricate, its basic strategy is simple: to recognize the enemy, mobilize forces, and attack. Understanding the anatomy and components of the immune system makes it possible to see how this strategy works.

Anatomy

The immune system maintains its own system of circulation—the lymphatic vessels—which permeates every organ in the body except the brain. The lymphatic vessels contain a pale, thick fluid (lymph) consisting of a fat-laden liquid and white blood cells.

Along the lymphatic vessels are special areas—the lymph nodes, tonsils, bone marrow, spleen, liver, lungs, and intestines—where lymphocytes can be recruited, mobilized, and deployed to appropriate sites as part of the immune response. The ingenious design of this system ensures the ready availability and quick assembly of an immune response anywhere it is needed. This system can be seen at work when a wound or an infection in a fingertip leads to an enlarged lymph node at the elbow, or when a throat infection causes the lymph nodes under the jaw to swell. The lymph nodes swell because the lymphatic vessels drain the infection by carrying it to the nearest area where an immune response can be organized.

Understanding the Immune System

Antibody: A protein, made by B lymphocytes, that reacts with a specific antigen; also called an immunoglobulin.

Antigen: Any molecule capable of stimulating an immune response.

Cell: The smallest living unit of tissue, composed of a nucleus and cytoplasm surrounded by a membrane. The nucleus houses DNA, and the cytoplasm contains structures (organelles) that carry out the cell's functions.

Chemotaxis: A process of attracting and recruiting cells in which a cell moves toward a higher concentration of a chemical substance.

Complement: A group of proteins that helps to attack antigens.

Cytokines: Soluble proteins, secreted by cells of the immune system, that act as messengers to help regulate an immune response.

Endocytosis: The process by which a cell engulfs (ingests) certain antigens.

Histocompatibility: Literally means compatible tissue. Used to determine whether a transplanted tissue or organ (for example, bone marrow or a kidney transplant) will be accepted by the recipient. Histocompatibility is determined by the major histocompatibility complex molecules.

Human leukocyte antigens (HLA): A synonym for human major histocompatibility complex.

Immune response: The response to an antigen by components of the immune system, either cells or antibodies.

Immunoglobulin: A synonym for antibody.

Interleukin: A type of cytokine that influences a variety of cells.

Leukocyte: A white blood cell. Lymphocytes and neutrophils, among others, are leukocytes.

Lymphocyte: The main cell of the lymphatic system, further categorized as B lymphocytes (which produce antibodies) and T lymphocytes (which help the body distinguish self from nonself).

Macrophage: A large cell that engulfs (ingests) microbes after they have been targeted for destruction by the immune system.

Major histocompatibility complex (MHC): A group of molecules important in helping the body distinguish self from nonself.

Molecule: A group (aggregation) of atoms chemically combined to form a unique chemical substance.

Natural killer cell: A type of lymphocyte that can kill certain microbes and cancer cells.

Neutrophil: A large white blood cell (leukocyte) that ingests antigens and other substances.

Peptide: Two or more amino acids chemically bonded to form a single molecule.

Protein: A large number of amino acids chemically bonded in a chain. Proteins are large peptides.

Receptor: A molecule on the cell surface or in the cytoplasm that fits another molecule like a lock and key.

Components of the Immune System

The immune system is composed of cells and soluble substances. The major cells of the immune system are the white blood cells. Macrophages, neutrophils, and lymphocytes are all types of white blood cells. Soluble substances are molecules that are not contained in cells but are dissolved in a liquid, such as plasma.▲ The major soluble substances are antibodies, complement

▲ see page 734

Lymphatic System: Defending Against Infection

The lymphatic system is a network of lymph nodes connected by lymphatic vessels. Lymph nodes contain a mesh of tissue in which lymphocytes are tightly packed. This mesh of lymphocytes filters, attacks, and destroys harmful organisms that cause infections. Lymph nodes are often clustered in areas where the lymphatic vessels branch off, such as the neck, armpits, and groin.

Lymph, a fluid rich in white blood cells, flows through the lymphatic vessels. Lymph helps return water, proteins, and other substances from the body's tissues to the bloodstream. All substances absorbed by the lymph pass through at least one lymph node and its filtering mesh of lymphocytes.

Other bodily organs and tissues—the thymus, liver, spleen, appendix, bone marrow, and small collections of lymphatic tissue such as the tonsils in the throat and Peyer's patch in the small intestine—are also part of the lymphatic system. They too help the body fight infection.

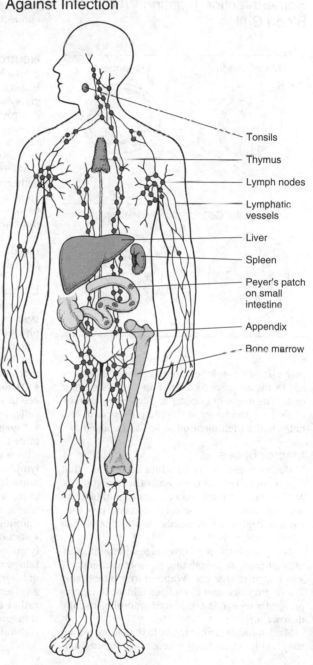

Tonsils

Thymus

Lymph nodes

Lymphatic vessels

Liver

Spleen

Peyer's patch on small intestine

Appendix

Bone marrow

Some Infection-Fighting White Blood Cells

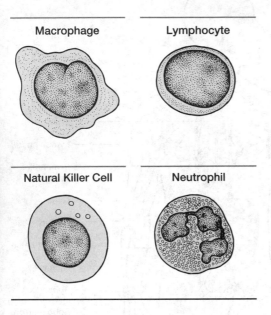

Macrophage

Lymphocyte

Natural Killer Cell

Neutrophil

proteins, and cytokines. Some soluble substances act as messengers to attract and activate other cells. The major histocompatibility complex molecule is at the heart of the immune system and helps in the identification of self and nonself.

Macrophages

Macrophages are large white blood cells that ingest microbes, antigens, and other substances. An antigen is any substance that can stimulate an immune response. Bacteria, viruses, proteins, carbohydrates, cancer cells, and toxins all can serve as antigens.

The cytoplasm of macrophages contains granules, or packets, consisting of several chemicals and enzymes that are wrapped in a membrane. These enzymes and chemicals allow the macrophage to digest the ingested microbe, usually destroying it.

Macrophages are not found in the blood; rather, they reside strategically where body organs inter-

face with the bloodstream or the outside world. For example, macrophages are found where the lungs receive outside air and where liver cells connect with blood vessels. Similar cells in the blood are called monocytes.

Neutrophils

Like macrophages, neutrophils are large white blood cells that ingest microbes and other antigens and have granules that contain enzymes to destroy ingested antigens. However, unlike macrophages, neutrophils circulate in the blood; they need a specific stimulus to exit from the blood and enter tissues.

Macrophages and neutrophils often work together: Macrophages initiate an immune response and send signals to mobilize neutrophils to join them at a trouble spot. When the neutrophils arrive, they destroy the invaders by digesting them. The accumulation of neutrophils and the killing and digesting of microbes lead to the formation of pus.

Lymphocytes

Lymphocytes, the main cells of the lymphatic system, are relatively small compared to macrophages and neutrophils. Unlike neutrophils, which live no more than 7 to 10 days, lymphocytes can live for years or even decades. Most lymphocytes fall into three major categories:

• B lymphocytes are derived from a parent (stem) cell in the bone marrow and mature into plasma cells, which secrete antibodies.

• T lymphocytes are formed when stem cells migrate from the bone marrow to the thymus gland, where they undergo division and maturation. T lymphocytes learn how to differentiate self from nonself in the thymus gland. Mature T lymphocytes leave the thymus gland and enter the lymphatic system, where they function as part of the immune surveillance system.

• Natural killer cells, slightly larger than T and B lymphocytes, are so named because they kill certain microbes and cancer cells. The "natural" part of their name indicates that they are ready to kill a variety of target cells as soon as they are formed rather than requiring the maturation and education process that B and T lymphocytes need. Natural killer cells also produce some cytokines,

Basic Y Structure of Antibodies

All antibody molecules have a basic Y-shaped structure in which the various pieces are held together by chemical structures called disulfide bonds. An antibody molecule is divided into variable and constant regions. The variable region determines which antigen the antibody will bind to. The constant region determines the antibody's class—IgG, IgM, IgD, IgE, or IgA.

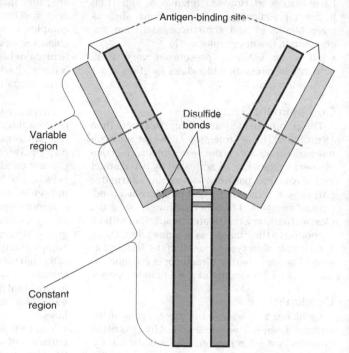

Antigen-binding site

Disulfide bonds

Variable region

Constant region

messenger substances that regulate some of the functions of T lymphocytes, B lymphocytes, and macrophages.

Antibodies

When stimulated by an antigen, B lymphocytes mature into cells that make antibodies. Antibodies are proteins that interact with the antigen that initially stimulated the B lymphocytes. Antibodies are also called immunoglobulins.

Each antibody molecule has a unique part that binds to a specific antigen and a part whose structure determines the antibody class. There are five classes of antibodies: IgM, IgG, IgA, IgE, and IgD.

• **IgM** is the antibody that is produced upon initial exposure to an antigen. For example, when a child receives his first tetanus vaccination, antitetanus antibodies of the IgM class are produced 10 to 14 days later (the primary antibody response). IgM is abundant in the blood but is not normally present in organs or tissues.

• **IgG**, the most prevalent type of antibody, is produced upon subsequent exposure to an antigen. For example, after receiving a second tetanus shot (booster), a child produces IgG antibodies in 5 to 7 days. This secondary antibody response is faster and more abundant than the primary antibody response. IgG is present in both the blood and the tissues. It is the only antibody that is transferred across the placenta from the mother to the fetus. The mother's IgG protects the fetus and newborn until the infant's immune system can produce its own antibodies.

• **IgA** is the antibody that plays an important role in the body's defenses against the invasion of microorganisms through mucous membrane–lined surfaces, including the nose, eyes, lungs, and intestines. IgA is found in the blood and in secretions such as those in the gastrointestinal tract and in the nose, eyes, lungs, and breast milk.

• **IgE** is the antibody that causes acute (immediate) allergic reactions. In this regard, IgE is the only class of antibody that seemingly does more harm than good. However, IgE may be important in fighting against parasitic infections, such as river blindness and schistosomiasis, that are common in the developing world.

• **IgD** is an antibody present in very small amounts in circulating blood. Its function is not well understood.

Complement System

The complement system comprises more than 18 proteins. These proteins act in a cascade, with one protein activating the next protein. The complement system can be activated by two distinct pathways. One pathway, called the alternative pathway, is activated by certain microbial products or antigens. The other pathway, called the classical pathway, is activated by specific antibodies bound to their antigens (immune complexes). The complement system functions to destroy foreign substances, either directly or in conjunction with other components of the immune system.

Cytokines

Cytokines function as the messengers of the immune system. They are secreted by cells of the immune system in response to stimulation. Cytokines amplify (or help) some aspects of the immune system and inhibit (or suppress) others. Many cytokines have been identified, and the list continues to grow.

Some cytokines can be given by injection as treatment of certain diseases. For example, **interferon alfa** is effective in treating certain cancers, such as hairy cell leukemia. Another cytokine, **interferon beta,** may be helpful in treating multiple sclerosis. A third cytokine, **interleukin-2,** may be beneficial in treating malignant melanoma and kidney cancer, although its use has adverse effects. Yet another cytokine, **granulocyte colony-stimulating factor,** which stimulates the production of neutrophils, can be given to cancer patients who have low numbers of neutrophils because of chemotherapy.

▲ see page 816

Major Histocompatibility Complex

All cells have molecules on their surface that are unique to a specific person. These molecules are called major histocompatibility complex molecules. Through its major histocompatibility complex molecules, the body is able to distinguish self from nonself. Any cell expressing identical major histocompatibility complex molecules is ignored; any cell expressing nonidentical major histocompatibility complex molecules is rejected.

There are two types of major histocompatibility complex molecule (also called human leukocyte antigens or HLA): class I and class II. Class I major histocompatibility complex molecules are present on all cells in the body except red blood cells. Class II major histocompatibility complex molecules are present on the surfaces only of macrophages and B lymphocytes and on T lymphocytes that have been stimulated by an antigen. A person's class I and class II major histocompatibility complex molecules are unique. Although identical twins have identical major histocompatibility molecules, the chance is low (one in four) that nonidentical twins will have identical molecules and extraordinarily low for nonsiblings.

The cells of the immune system learn to differentiate self from nonself in the thymus gland. When the immune system starts developing in the fetus, stem cells migrate to the thymus, where they divide and develop into T lymphocytes. While developing in the thymus gland, any T lymphocyte that reacts to the thymus' major histocompatibility complex molecules is eliminated. Any T lymphocyte that tolerates the thymus' major histocompatibility complex and learns to cooperate with cells expressing the body's unique major histocompatibility complex molecules is allowed to mature and leave the thymus.

The result is that mature T lymphocytes tolerate the body's own cells and organs and can cooperate with the body's other cells when called on to defend the body. If T lymphocytes were not made tolerant of the body's own major histocompatibility complex molecules, they could attack the body. However, sometimes T lymphocytes lose the ability to differentiate self from nonself, resulting in the development of autoimmune diseases such as systemic lupus erythematosus (lupus) or multiple sclerosis.▲

Immunity and the Immune Response

The immune system has evolved an intricate network of checks and balances that can be categorized as innate and learned immunity.

Everyone is born with **innate immunity**. The components of the immune system involved in innate immunity—macrophages, neutrophils, and complement—react similarly to all foreign substances, and the recognition of antigens does not vary from person to person.

As its name indicates, **learned immunity** is acquired. At birth, a person's immune system has not yet encountered the outside world or started to develop its memory files. The immune system learns to respond to every new antigen encountered. Learned immunity is, therefore, specific to the antigens encountered during a person's lifetime. The hallmark of specific immunity is its ability to learn, to adapt, and to remember.

The immune system carries a record or memory of every antigen a person encounters, whether through the lungs (by breathing), the intestine (by eating), or the skin. This is possible because lymphocytes are long-lived. When lymphocytes encounter an antigen for the second time, they mount a quick, vigorous, specific response to that antigen. This specific immune response is why people do not contract chickenpox or measles more than once and what makes vaccination successful in preventing disease. For example, to prevent polio, a person is given a vaccine made from a weakened form of the poliovirus. If the person is later exposed to the poliovirus, the immune system searches its memory files, finds the blueprint for poliovirus, and quickly activates the appropriate defenses. The result is that the poliovirus is eliminated by specific antibodies that neutralize the virus before it has a chance to multiply and invade the nervous system.

Innate immunity and learned immunity are not independent of each other. Each system interacts and influences the other, either directly or through the induction of cytokines (messengers). Rarely does a stimulus trigger a single response. Instead, several responses occur, some of which may act together or occasionally may conflict with each other. Yet all responses revolve around the three basic principles of recognition, mobilization, and attack.

Recognition

Before the immune system can respond to an antigen, it must be able to recognize the antigen. It is able to do so through a process called antigen processing. Macrophages are the major antigen-processing cells, but other cells, including B lymphocytes, can also process antigens.

Antigen-processing cells ingest an antigen and chop it into small fragments. The fragments are then packaged within the major histocompatibility complex molecules and shuttled to the surface of the cell membrane. The area of the major histocompatibility complex that has the antigen fragment then binds (attaches) to a special molecule on the surface of the T lymphocyte called the T-cell receptor. The T-cell receptor is designed to fit—like a key in a lock—the part of the major histocompatibility complex bearing an antigen fragment.

T lymphocytes have two major subsets that differ in their ability to bind (attach) to one of the two classes of major histocompatibility complex molecules. The T-lymphocyte subset with a CD8 molecule on its surface can bind to class I major histocompatibility complex molecules. The T-lymphocyte subset with a CD4 molecule on its surface can bind to class II major histocompatibility complex molecules.

Mobilization

Once an antigen has been recognized by an antigen-processing cell and T lymphocyte, a series of events to mobilize the immune system follows. When an antigen-processing cell ingests an antigen, it releases cytokines—for example, interleukin-1, interleukin-8, or interleukin-12—that act on certain other cells. Interleukin-1 mobilizes other T lymphocytes; interleukin-12 stimulates natural killer cells to become more potent killers and to secrete interferon; interleukin-8 acts as a beacon, guiding neutrophils to the site where the antigen was spotted. This process of attracting and recruiting cells is called chemotaxis.

When T lymphocytes are triggered through their T-cell receptors, they produce several cytokines that help to recruit other lymphocytes, thus amplifying the immune response. Cytokines can also activate the nonspecific (innate) immune defenses. Cytokines therefore bridge innate and learned immunity.

How T Lymphocytes Recognize Antigens

T lymphocytes are part of the immune surveillance system. They help identify antigens, which are substances foreign to the body. However, to be recognized by a T lymphocyte, an antigen must be processed and "presented" to the lymphocyte in a form it can identify, as shown here.

1. An antigen circulating in the body has a structure that a T lymphocyte cannot recognize.
2. An antigen-processing cell, such as a macrophage, engulfs the antigen.

3. Enzymes in the antigen-processing cell break the antigen into fragments.
4. Some antigen fragments become linked with major histocompatibility complex molecules and are then shuttled to the surface of the cell membrane.
5. A T-cell receptor, located on the surface of a T lymphocyte, recognizes the antigen fragment linked with a major histocompatibility complex molecule and binds to it.

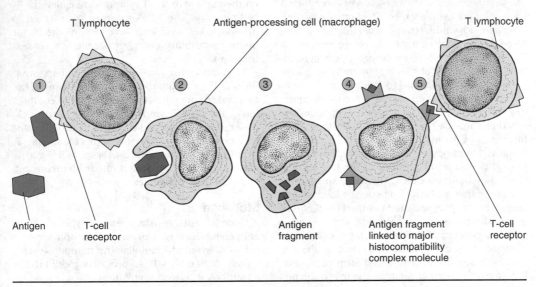

T lymphocyte   Antigen-processing cell (macrophage)   T lymphocyte

Antigen   T-cell receptor   Antigen fragment   Antigen fragment linked to major histocompatibility complex molecule   T-cell receptor

Attack

Much of the immune system's machinery is geared toward killing or eliminating invading microbes once they have been recognized. Macrophages, neutrophils, and natural killer cells are able to eliminate many foreign invaders.

If an invader cannot be eliminated completely, walls can be built to imprison it. The prison wall is made of special cells and is called a granuloma. Tuberculosis is an example of an infection that is not totally eliminated; the bacteria that cause tuberculosis are imprisoned within a granuloma. Most healthy people who are exposed to these bacteria fend off the tuberculosis infection, but

some bacteria survive indefinitely, usually in the lung, surrounded by a granuloma. If the immune system is weakened (even 50 or 60 years later), the prison walls crumble and the bacteria that cause tuberculosis start to multiply.

The body does not fight all invaders the same way. Invaders that stay outside the body's cells (extracellular organisms) are relatively easy to fight; the immune system mobilizes defenses to facilitate their ingestion by macrophages and other cells. How the immune system goes about this depends on whether the invaders are encapsulated (have a thick capsule around them) or are nonencapsulated. Invaders that gain access to the inside of cells (intracellular organisms) and remain viable (alive) and functional are fought in a different way altogether.

Encapsulated Extracellular Organisms

Some bacteria have a capsule that shields their cell wall, preventing macrophages from recognizing them. A common example of encapsulated bacteria are streptococci, which cause strep throat. The immune response is to have B lymphocytes produce antibodies against the capsule. Antibodies also neutralize the toxins that certain bacteria produce.

Once created, antibodies attach themselves to the capsules. The bacterium-antibody unit is called an **immune complex**. The immune complex attaches itself to a receptor on a macrophage. This engagement facilitates the ingestion of the whole complex by the macrophage, where the bacteria are digested. Immune complexes also activate the complement cascade. Attachment of products of the complement cascade to the immune complex makes it very easy for macrophages to identify immune complexes to ingest.

Nonencapsulated Extracellular Organisms

Some bacteria have only a cell wall; they do not have a capsule and are considered nonencapsulated. *Escherichia coli*, a common cause of food poisoning and urinary tract infections, is an example of a nonencapsulated bacterium. When nonencapsulated bacteria invade the body, macrophages, natural killer cells, cytokines, and the complement cascade spring into action.

Macrophages have sensors that recognize molecules on the surface of nonencapsulated bacteria. When these molecules and sensors are engaged, the bacterium is engulfed by the macrophage in a process called phagocytosis. Phagocytosis stimulates the macrophage to release several cytokines that attract neutrophils. The neutrophils then engulf and kill even more bacteria. Some of the cytokines released by the macrophages activate natural killer cells, which can then kill some of the bacteria directly or can help the neutrophils and macrophages kill more efficiently.

Nonencapsulated bacteria also activate the complement cascade. Complement helps destroy the bacteria and releases a product that serves as a signal to attract neutrophils, which then destroy the remaining bacteria.

Intracellular Organisms

Some microorganisms, such as tuberculosis bacteria, survive best inside a cell. Because these organisms must enter a cell to live, they have no particular defenses against being ingested. While being ingested, these organisms are sequestered within the cell in a protective structure called a vesicle or vacuole. The vesicles can fuse with other vesicles inside the cytoplasm, such as vesicles that assemble and package class II major histocompatibility complex molecules.

As these vesicles fuse, the major histocompatibility complex picks up some of the fragments of the bacteria. When the major histocompatibility complex is shuttled to the cell surface, it contains these foreign fragments. Major histocompatibility complex molecules are recognized by T lymphocytes, which respond to the antigen fragment by releasing cytokines. The cytokines activate macrophages. This activation results in the production of new chemicals within the cell. These chemicals now allow the macrophage to kill organisms inside the cell.

Some cytokines promote the production of antibodies. Antibodies are helpful in the defense against organisms outside the cell; however, they are ineffective against infections inside it.

Viruses are an example of another organism that must enter a cell in order to survive. However, viruses are processed not in vesicles but in special structures called proteosomes. Proteosomes break the virus into fragments that are transported to another structure within the cell, called the rough endoplasmic reticulum—the cell's factory for making proteins. Class I major histocompatibility complex molecules are also assembled within the rough endoplasmic reticulum. As the class I major histocompatibility complex molecules are assembled, they pick up virus fragments and take them along when they are shuttled to the cell surface.

Certain T lymphocytes recognize the class I molecules, which now contain the virus fragments, and bind to them. When the connection is completed, a signal sent through the cell membrane triggers the activation of antigen-specific T lymphocytes, most of which evolve into killer T cells. Unlike natural killer cells, however, killer T cells kill only the cells infected with the particular virus that stimulated their activation. For example, killer T cells help fight the influenza virus. The reason why most people need 7 to 10 days to recover from influenza is because that is how much time is needed to generate killer T cells that are specifically designed to fight the influenza virus.

Autoimmune Reactions

Sometimes the immune system malfunctions, misinterprets the body's tissues as foreign, and attacks them, resulting in an autoimmune reaction. Autoimmune reactions can be triggered in several ways:

• A substance in the body that is normally strictly contained in a specific area (and thus is hidden from the immune system) is released into the general circulation. For example, the fluid in the eyeball is normally contained within the eyeball's chambers. If a blow to the eye releases this fluid into the bloodstream, the immune system may react against it.

• A normal body substance is altered. For example, viruses, drugs, sunlight, or radiation may change a protein's structure in a way that makes it seem foreign.

• The immune system responds to a foreign substance that is similar in appearance to a natural body substance and inadvertently targets the body substance as well as the foreign substance.

• Something malfunctions in the cells that control antibody production. For example, cancerous B lymphocytes may produce abnormal antibodies that attack red blood cells.

The results of an autoimmune reaction vary. Fever is common. Various tissues may be destroyed, such as blood vessels, cartilage, and skin. Virtually any organ can be attacked by the immune system, including the kidneys, lungs, heart, and brain. The resulting inflammation and tissue damage can cause kidney failure, breathing problems, abnormal heart function, pain, deformity, delirium, and death.

A large number of disorders almost certainly have an autoimmune cause, including lupus (systemic lupus erythematosus), myasthenia gravis, Graves' disease, Hashimoto's thyroiditis, pemphigus, rheumatoid arthritis, scleroderma, Sjögren's syndrome, and pernicious anemia.

CHAPTER 168

Immunodeficiency Disorders

Immunodeficiency disorders are a group of diverse conditions in which the immune system doesn't function adequately, so infections are more common, recur more frequently, are unusually severe, and last longer than usual.

Frequent and severe infections—whether in a newborn, a child, or an adult—that don't respond readily to antibiotics suggest a problem with the immune system. Some problems with the immune system also lead to rare cancers or unusual infections with viruses, fungi, and bacteria.

Causes

Immunodeficiency may be present from birth (**congenital immunodeficiency**) or may develop later in life. Immunodeficiency disorders that are

present from birth are usually hereditary. Although rare, more than 70 different hereditary immunodeficiency disorders are known. In some disorders, the number of white blood cells decreases; in others, the number of cells is normal but they malfunction. In still others, the white blood cells aren't affected, but other components of the immune system are abnormal or missing.

Immunodeficiency that occurs later in life (**acquired immunodeficiency**) is usually caused by disease. Acquired immunodeficiency is much more common than congenital immunodeficiency. Some diseases cause only a minor impairment of the immune system, while others may destroy the body's ability to fight infection. Human immunodeficiency virus (HIV) infection, which results in acquired immunodeficiency syndrome (AIDS), is well known.▲ The virus attacks and destroys the white blood cells that normally fight viral and fungal infections. However, many different condi-

▲ see page 926

tions can impair the immune system. In fact, nearly every prolonged serious illness affects the immune system to some degree.

People who have spleen problems often have some degree of immunodeficiency. Not only does the spleen help trap and destroy bacteria and other infective organisms that enter the bloodstream, but also it is one of the places in the body where antibodies are produced. The immune system is affected if the spleen is surgically removed or destroyed by a disease, such as sickle cell disease. People without a spleen, especially infants, are particularly susceptible to certain bacterial infections, such as those caused by *Hemophilus influenzae, Escherichia coli,* and *Streptococcus.* Children without a spleen should be given pneumococcal and meningococcal vaccines in addition to the usual childhood vaccines. Young children without a spleen take antibiotics continuously for at least the first 5 years of life. All people with a spleen deficiency should take antibiotics at the first sign of an infection with fever.

Malnutrition can also seriously impair the immune system. The malnutrition may involve a deficiency of all nutrients, or it may involve primarily proteins and certain vitamins and minerals (especially vitamin A, iron, and zinc). When malnutrition results in a weight that is less than 80 percent of the ideal weight, the immune system is usually somewhat impaired. When the weight is reduced to less than 70 percent of ideal weight, the immune system is usually severely impaired. Infections, which are common in people with impaired immune systems, both depress the appetite and increase the body's metabolic demands, resulting in a vicious circle of worsening malnutrition.

How severely the immune system is impaired depends on the degree and duration of the malnutrition and on the presence or absence of an underlying disease, such as cancer. When good nutrition is restored, the immune system quickly returns to normal.

Symptoms

Most healthy infants have six or more minor respiratory tract infections a year, particularly when exposed to other children. In contrast, infants with impaired immunity usually develop severe bacterial infections that persist, recur, or lead to complications. For example, sinus infections, chronic ear infections, and chronic bronchitis commonly follow sore throats and head

Some Causes of Acquired Immunodeficiency

Hereditary and metabolic diseases
- Diabetes
- Down syndrome
- Kidney failure
- Malnutrition
- Sickle cell anemia

Chemicals and treatments that suppress the immune system
- Cancer chemotherapy
- Corticosteroids
- Immunosuppressive drugs
- Radiation therapy

Infections
- Chickenpox
- Cytomegalovirus infection
- German measles (congenital rubella)
- Human immunodeficiency virus infection (AIDS)
- Infectious mononucleosis
- Measles
- Severe bacterial infection
- Severe fungal infection
- Severe tuberculosis

Blood diseases and cancer
- Agranulocytosis
- All cancers
- Aplastic anemia
- Histiocytosis
- Leukemia
- Lymphoma
- Myelofibrosis
- Myeloma

Surgery and trauma
- Burns
- Removal of the spleen

Miscellaneous
- Alcoholic cirrhosis
- Chronic hepatitis
- Normal aging
- Sarcoidosis
- Systemic lupus erythematosus

colds in these infants. The bronchitis may progress to pneumonia.

The skin and mucous membranes lining the mouth, eyes, and genitals are susceptible to infection. Thrush, a fungal infection of the mouth,

Signs of Chronic Infection

• Pale, thin appearance

• Skin rash

• Pustules

• Eczema

• Broken blood vessels

• Hair loss

• Purple blotches

• Redness of the lining of the eye (conjunctivitis)

• Enlarged lymph nodes, such as those in the neck, armpits, and groin

• Scarred and perforated eardrums

• Crusted nostrils (from discharge)

• Enlarged liver and spleen

• In infants, redness around the anus from chronic diarrhea

along with mouth sores (ulcers) and inflammation of the gums, may be an early sign of impaired immunity. Inflammation of the eyes (conjunctivitis), hair loss, severe eczema, and areas of enlarged, broken capillaries under the skin are also signs of a possible immunodeficiency disorder. Infections in the gastrointestinal tract may lead to diarrhea, extreme gassiness, and weight loss.

Diagnosis

At first, a hereditary problem with the immune system may be difficult to diagnose. When severe or rare infections occur repeatedly, in either young children or adults, a doctor suspects an immunodeficiency disorder. Since immunodeficiency disorders in very young children are often hereditary, the presence of recurring infections in other children in the family is an important clue. Infections with common organisms that normally don't make people sick, such as *Pneumocystis* or cytomegalovirus, suggest a problem with the immune system.

In older children and adults, the doctor reviews the medical history to determine if a drug, an

exposure to a toxic substance, a previous surgery (such as a tonsillectomy or adenoidectomy), or another medical condition might be the cause. A sexual history is also important, since human immunodeficiency virus (HIV) infection, a common cause of immune dysfunction in adults, is often acquired through sexual contact. Newborns can be infected with HIV if their mothers are infected; older children can be infected through sexual abuse.

The type of infection gives the doctor clues to the type of immunodeficiency. For example, when infections are caused by certain bacteria such as *Streptococcus*, the problem is likely to be that the B lymphocytes don't produce enough antibodies. Severe infections from viruses, fungi, and unusual organisms such as *Pneumocystis* usually result from T-lymphocyte problems. Infections with the bacteria *Staphylococcus* and *Escherichia coli* usually indicate that phagocytic white blood cells (cells that kill and ingest invading microorganisms) aren't moving properly or aren't effectively killing the invaders. Infections with the bacterium *Neisseria* are often a sign of problems in the complement system, proteins in the blood that help rid the body of infection.

The age at which problems begin is also important. Infections in infants under 6 months of age usually indicate T-lymphocyte abnormalities; infections in older children usually indicate problems with antibody production and B lymphocytes. Immunodeficiency that begins in adulthood is rarely hereditary; a much more likely cause is AIDS or other conditions such as diabetes, malnutrition, kidney failure, and cancer.

Defining the exact nature of the immunodeficiency disorder requires laboratory testing, usually of the blood. First, a doctor determines the total number of white blood cells and the number of specific types of white blood cells. The white blood cells are examined under a microscope for abnormalities in appearance. Antibody (immunoglobulin) levels are checked, as are the numbers of red blood cells and platelets. The levels of complement can also be measured.

If any test results are abnormal, additional tests are generally needed. For example, if the number of lymphocytes (a type of white blood cell) is low, the doctor may measure the levels of T lymphocytes and B lymphocytes. Laboratory tests can even determine which type of T or B lymphocyte is affected. In AIDS, for example, the number of

CD4 T lymphocytes is decreased in comparison to the number of CD8 T lymphocytes.

Another useful laboratory test helps determine whether white blood cells are functioning normally by measuring their ability to grow and divide in response to certain chemical stimuli called mitogens. Their ability to destroy foreign cells and organisms can also be tested.

The function of T lymphocytes can be tested by using a skin test to analyze the body's ability to react to foreign substances. In this test, small amounts of protein from common infectious organisms such as yeast are injected under the skin. Normally, the body reacts by sending T lymphocytes to the area, causing the area to become slightly swollen, red, and warm. This test is not used until a child is 2 years old.

Prevention and Treatment

Some of the diseases that impair the immune system later in life can be prevented or treated. For example, close control of blood sugar levels in people with diabetes helps improve the ability of white blood cells to prevent infections. Successfully treating cancer is likely to restore the function of the immune system. Safe sex practices help prevent the spread of HIV (the virus that causes AIDS). Attention to diet can prevent immune disorders that arise from malnutrition.

People who have immunodeficiency disorders should maintain excellent nutrition, have good personal hygiene, and avoid eating undercooked food and being in contact with people who have infectious diseases. Some people must drink only bottled water. They should avoid smoking, inhaling secondhand cigarette smoke, and using illegal drugs. Fastidious dental care helps prevent infections in the mouth. Those who are able to produce antibodies are vaccinated, but only killed viral and bacterial vaccines rather than live vaccines (such as oral polio vaccine, measles-mumps-rubella vaccine, and BCG vaccine) are used in people with a B-lymphocyte or T-lymphocyte deficiency.

Antibiotics are given at the first sign of an infection. An infection that's rapidly worsening requires prompt medical attention. Some people, particularly those with Wiskott-Aldrich syndrome and those without a spleen, are given preventive antibiotics as a prophylactic measure before infections occur. Trimethoprim-sulfamethoxazole is often used to prevent pneumonia.

Drugs that enhance the immune system, such as levamisole, inosiplex, and thymic hormones, haven't been successful in treating people who have low numbers of or poorly functioning white blood cells. Low antibody levels can be raised with infusions or injections of immune globulin, usually given monthly. Injections of interferon gamma are beneficial in treating chronic granulomatous disease.

Experimental procedures, such as transplantation of fetal thymic cells and fetal liver cells, have occasionally been helpful, particularly for people with the DiGeorge anomaly. In severe combined immunodeficiency disease with adenosine deaminase deficiency, enzyme replacement is sometimes possible. Gene therapy shows promise for this and a few other congenital immunodeficiency disorders in which the genetic defect has been identified.

A bone marrow transplant sometimes corrects a severe, congenital immune system defect. This procedure is generally reserved for the most severe disorders, such as severe combined immunodeficiency disease.

Most people who have abnormal white blood cells aren't given blood transfusions unless the donated blood has first been irradiated, because white blood cells in the donated blood may attack those in the recipient's blood, creating a serious, even fatal, illness (graft-versus-host disease).▲

People whose families are known to carry the genes for inherited immunodeficiencies may seek counseling to avoid having children with the disorders. Agammaglobulinemia, the Wiskott-Aldrich syndrome, severe combined immunodeficiency disease, and chronic granulomatous disease are some disorders that can be diagnosed in the fetus by testing a sample of fetal blood or amniotic fluid. For many of these disorders, the parents or siblings can be tested to determine if they carry the defective gene.

X-linked Agammaglobulinemia

X-linked agammaglobulinemia (Bruton's agammaglobulinemia), which affects only boys, results in decreased numbers or absence of B lymphocytes and very low levels of antibodies because

▲ see page 741

of a defect in the X chromosome. Infants with X-linked agammaglobulinemia develop infections of the lungs, sinuses, and bones, usually from bacteria such as *Hemophilus* and *Streptococcus*, and they may develop some unusual viral infections of the brain. However, infections generally don't occur until sometime after 6 months of age because protective antibodies from the mother remain in the infant's bloodstream until that time. Children with X-linked agammaglobulinemia can develop polio if they are given live polio vaccine (the oral vaccine). They may also develop arthritis.

Injections or infusions of immune globulin are given throughout life to provide antibodies and help prevent infections. Antibiotics are needed whenever bacterial infections occur. Despite these measures, many boys with X-linked agammaglobulinemia develop chronic sinus and lung infections and have a tendency to develop cancer as well.

Common Variable Immunodeficiency

Common variable immunodeficiency, which occurs in males and females of any age but generally doesn't develop until age 10 to 20, results in very low antibody levels despite normal numbers of B lymphocytes. T lymphocytes function normally in some people but not in others.

Autoimmune disorders, including failure of the adrenal glands (Addison's disease), thyroiditis, and rheumatoid arthritis, often develop.▲ A tendency to develop diarrhea is common, and food may not be absorbed well from the gastrointestinal tract. Injections or intravenous infusions of immune globulin are given throughout life, and antibiotics are given whenever infections occur.

Selective Antibody Deficiency

With selective antibody deficiency, the total level of antibodies is normal, but a specific class of antibody is deficient. The most common deficiency is that of immunoglobulin A (IgA). Selective IgA deficiency is sometimes familial but more often occurs without an apparent cause. The disorder can also result from using phenytoin, an antiseizure drug.

Most people with selective IgA deficiency have little or no noticeable problem, but others can develop chronic respiratory infections and allergies. Some people with IgA deficiency produce anti-IgA antibodies if they're given transfusions of IgA-containing blood, plasma, or immune globulin, which may result in a severe allergic reaction the next time they receive a dose of plasma or immune globulin. Wearing a Medic Alert bracelet can alert doctors to take precautions against reactions. Usually, no treatment for IgA deficiency is needed. Antibiotics are given to those who have repeated infections.

Severe Combined Immunodeficiency Disease

Severe combined immunodeficiency disease is the most serious of the immunodeficiency disorders. In this disorder, B lymphocytes and antibodies are deficient, and the T lymphocytes are deficient or nonfunctioning and therefore unable to adequately fight infections. Several different defects of the immune system result in severe combined immunodeficiency disease, including deficiency of the enzyme adenosine deaminase. Most infants with severe combined immunodeficiency disease first develop pneumonia and thrush (a fungal infection of the mouth); diarrhea usually develops by 3 months of age. More serious infections, including pneumocystis pneumonia, can also develop. If not treated, these children generally die before age 2. Antibiotics and immune globulin are helpful but not curative. The best treatment is a bone marrow or umbilical cord blood transplantation.

Wiskott-Aldrich Syndrome

The Wiskott-Aldrich syndrome affects only boys and causes eczema, a low number of platelets, and a combined deficiency of B and T lymphocytes that leads to repeated infections. Because the platelet number is low, bleeding problems, such as bloody diarrhea, may be the first symptom. The B and T lymphocyte deficiency makes the children susceptible to infections with bacteria, viruses, and fungi. Respiratory tract infections are common. Children who survive past age 10 are likely to develop cancers such as lymphoma and leukemia.

▲ see page 816

Surgically removing the spleen often helps relieve the bleeding problems, because people with Wiskott-Aldrich syndrome have low numbers of platelets and platelets are destroyed in the spleen.▲ Antibiotics and infusions of immune globulin may be helpful, but a bone marrow transplantation offers the best hope.

Ataxia-Telangiectasia

Ataxia-telangiectasia is an inherited disorder that affects both the immune and nervous systems. Abnormalities in the cerebellum, a part of the brain that controls coordination, lead to uncoordinated movements (ataxia). The abnormal movements usually develop just when the child begins to walk but may be delayed until age 4. Slurred speech, muscle weakness, and sometimes mental retardation develop. Telangiectasia, in which capillaries in the skin and eyes are prominent, develops between ages 1 and 6, usually most obviously on the eyes, ears, sides of the nose, and arms.

Pneumonia, bronchial infections, and sinus infections develop frequently and may lead to chronic lung problems. Problems with the endocrine system can result in small testes, infertility, and diabetes. Many children with ataxia-telangiectasia develop cancers, especially leukemia, brain tumors, and stomach cancer.

Antibiotics and injections or infusions of immune globulin help somewhat in preventing infections but don't cure the neurologic problems. Ataxia-telangiectasia generally progresses to worsening muscle weakness, paralysis, dementia, and death.

Hyper-IgE Syndrome

Hyper-IgE syndrome, also called Job-Buckley syndrome, is an immunodeficiency disorder characterized by very high levels of IgE antibodies and repeated infections with the *Staphylococcus* bacterium. The infections may involve the skin, lungs, joints, or other organs. Many people with this disorder have weak bones and therefore suffer recurrent fractures. Some have signs of allergy, such as eczema, nasal stuffiness, and asthma. The treatment consists of taking antibiotics continually or intermittently for the staphylococcal infections. The antibiotic trimethoprim-sulfamethoxazole is often used as a preventive measure.

Chronic Granulomatous Disease

Chronic granulomatous disease, which affects mostly boys, is caused by an inherited defect in white blood cells that destroys their ability to kill certain bacteria and fungi. The white blood cells don't produce hydrogen peroxide, superoxide, and other chemicals that help fight these infections. Symptoms of the disease usually appear in early childhood but may not start until the early teens. Chronic infections occur in the skin, lungs, lymph nodes, mouth, nose, and intestines. Abscesses can develop around the anus and in the bones and brain. The lymph nodes tend to enlarge and drain, the liver and spleen enlarge, and the child may grow slowly. Antibiotics help treat the infections. Weekly injections of interferon gamma have been shown to decrease infections. Bone marrow transplantation has been successful in curing the disease in a few instances.

Transient Hypogammaglobulinemia of Infancy

In transient hypogammaglobulinemia of infancy, infants develop low antibody levels beginning at about 3 to 6 months of age. The condition is more common in premature infants, since they receive fewer maternal antibodies during gestation. The condition isn't hereditary and affects boys and girls equally. It generally lasts 6 to 18 months. Since most infants manufacture some antibodies and don't have a problem with infections, they need no treatment.

However, some infants with transient hypogammaglobulinemia—particularly those born prematurely—develop infections frequently. Treatment with immune globulin is very effective at preventing and helping treat infections and is usually given for about 3 to 6 months. Antibiotics are used as needed.

DiGeorge Anomaly

The DiGeorge anomaly occurs because of abnormal fetal development. The condition usually isn't hereditary and can occur in both boys and

▲ see page 785

Congenital Immunodeficiency Disorders

Disorders in which antibody levels are low
- Common variable immunodeficiency
- Selective antibody deficiency (for example, IgA deficiency)
- Transient hypogammaglobulinemia of infancy
- X-linked agammaglobulinemia

Disorders in which the function of white blood cells is impaired

T-lymphocyte problems
- Chronic mucocutaneous candidiasis
- DiGeorge anomaly

T-lymphocyte and B-lymphocyte problems
- Ataxia-telangiectasia
- Severe combined immunodeficiency disease
- Wiskott-Aldrich syndrome
- X-linked lymphoproliferative syndrome

Disorders in which the killing function of white blood cells is abnormal
- Chédiak-Higashi syndrome
- Chronic granulomatous disease
- Leukocyte glucose-6-phosphate dehydrogenase deficiency
- Myeloperoxidase deficiency

Disorders in which white blood cell movement is abnormal
- Hyperimmunoglobulinemia E
- Leukocyte adhesion defect

Disorders in which the complement system is abnormal
- Complement component 3 (C3) deficiency
- Complement component 6 (C6) deficiency
- Complement component 7 (C7) deficiency
- Complement component 8 (C8) deficiency

girls. Children born with this condition don't have a thymus gland, an important gland for normal T-lymphocyte development. Without T lymphocytes they can't fight infections well. Recurring infections begin soon after birth, and the degree of immune impairment varies considerably. Sometimes the defect is only partial, and T-lymphocyte function improves on its own.

Children with DiGeorge anomaly typically have heart problems and unusual facial features, including low-set ears, a small receding jawbone, and wide-spaced eyes. Because they also have no parathyroid glands, their blood calcium levels are low and they often develop seizures shortly after birth.

For children with severe immunodeficiency, bone marrow transplantation may help. Transplanting a fetal or newborn thymus gland (from an aborted or miscarried fetus) into a child with DiGeorge anomaly may also help. Sometimes the heart problems are worse than the immunologic ones and may require surgery to prevent severe heart failure or death. Treatment of the low calcium levels is also important.

Chronic Mucocutaneous Candidiasis

Chronic mucocutaneous candidiasis results from poorly functioning white blood cells, which allow infections with the fungus *Candida* to develop and persist in infants or young adults. The fungus may cause mouth infections (thrush), as well as infections of the scalp, skin, and nails. Chronic mucocutaneous candidiasis is somewhat more common in girls than in boys, and its severity varies. Some people develop hepatitis and chronic lung disease. Many have endocrine problems, such as underactive parathyroid glands.

Internal infections with *Candida* are rare. Generally, the infections can be treated with the antifungal drug nystatin or clotrimazole. More severe infections require a more powerful antifungal drug, such as ketoconazole given orally or amphotericin B given intravenously. Although the disease is generally incurable, bone marrow transplantation was successful in a single case.

Allergic Reactions

Allergic reactions, also called **hypersensitivity reactions,** are reactions of the immune system in which normal body tissue is injured. The mechanisms by which the immune system defends the body and by which a hypersensitivity reaction can injure it are similar. Thus, antibodies, lymphocytes, and other cells, which are normal protective components of the immune system,▲ are involved in allergic reactions as well as in blood transfusion reactions, autoimmune disease, and organ transplant rejection.

When most people use the term *allergic reaction,* they are referring to reactions that involve antibodies of the immunoglobulin E (IgE) class. IgE antibodies bind to special cells, including basophils in the circulation and mast cells in tissues. When IgE antibodies that are bound to those cells encounter antigens, in this case called **allergens,** the cells are prompted to release chemicals that injure surrounding tissues. An allergen can be almost anything—a dust particle, plant pollen, a drug, or food—that acts as an antigen to stimulate an immune response.

Sometimes the term *atopic disease* is used to describe a group of often inherited IgE-mediated diseases, such as allergic rhinitis and allergic asthma. Atopic diseases are noted by their tendency to produce IgE antibodies to harmless inhalants, such as pollens, molds, animal danders, and dust mites. Eczema (atopic dermatitis) is also an atopic disease, although the role of IgE antibodies in this disorder is less clear.■ A person with an atopic disease, however, is not at increased risk for developing IgE antibodies to injected allergens, such as drugs or insect venoms.

Allergic reactions range from mild to severe. Most reactions consist of just the annoyance of watery, itchy eyes and some sneezing. At the other extreme, allergic reactions can be life threatening if they involve sudden difficulty in breathing, heart malfunction, and very low blood pressure, leading to shock. This type of reaction, called **anaphylaxis,** may occur in sensitive people in a variety of situations, such as soon after eating certain foods, taking certain drugs, or being stung by a bee.

Diagnosis

Because each allergic reaction is triggered by a specific allergen, identifying that allergen is the main goal of diagnosis. The allergen may be a seasonal plant or plant product, such as grass or ragweed pollen, or a substance such as cat dander, drugs, or foods. The allergen may cause an allergic reaction when it lands on the skin or in the eye, is inhaled, is eaten, or is injected. Often, the allergen can be identified through careful detective work by both the doctor and the patient.

Tests may help determine if the symptoms are allergy-related and identify the allergen involved. A blood sample may show many eosinophils, a type of white blood cell that often increases in number during allergic reactions. The radioallergosorbent test (RAST) measures blood levels of IgE antibodies specific to individual allergens, which may help to diagnose an allergic skin reaction, seasonal allergic rhinitis, or allergic asthma.

Skin tests are most useful for identifying particular allergens. For skin testing, dilute solutions made from extracts of trees, grasses, weeds, pollens, dust, animal dander, insect venom, foods, and some drugs are individually injected into a person's skin in tiny amounts. If the person is allergic to one or more of these substances, the site at which the relevant solution was injected develops an edematous wheal (a hivelike swelling with surrounding redness) within 15 to 20 minutes. The radioallergosorbent test can be used when a skin test can't be done or wouldn't be safe. Both tests are highly specific and accurate, although the skin test is generally a bit more accurate and often cheaper and the results are available immediately.

Treatment

Avoiding an allergen is better than trying to treat an allergic reaction. Avoiding the substance

---

▲ see page 808

■ see page 961

may entail stopping use of a particular drug, installing air conditioners with filters, banning a pet from the house, or not consuming a particular kind of food. Sometimes a person allergic to a substance associated with a certain job may have to change jobs. People with strong seasonal allergies may consider moving to a region where the allergen doesn't exist.

Other measures involve reducing exposure to an allergen. For instance, someone with an allergy to house dust may remove dust-collecting furniture, carpets, and draperies; cover mattresses and pillows with plastic protectors; dust and wet-mop rooms frequently; use air conditioning to reduce the high indoor humidity that favors the breeding of dust mites; and install high-efficiency air filters.

Because some allergens, especially airborne allergens, can't be avoided, doctors often use methods to block the allergic response and prescribe drugs to relieve the symptoms.

Allergen Immunotherapy

When an allergen can't be avoided, allergen immunotherapy (allergy injections) may provide an alternative solution. With immunotherapy, tiny amounts of the allergen are injected under the skin in gradually increasing doses until a maintenance level is reached. This treatment stimulates the body to produce blocking or neutralizing antibodies that may act to prevent an allergic reaction. Eventually, the blood level of IgE antibodies, which react with the antigen, also may fall. Immunotherapy must be carried out carefully, however, because exposure too soon to a high dose of the allergen can itself produce an allergic reaction.

Although many people undergo allergen immunotherapy, and studies show that it helps, its cost-effectiveness and risk-to-benefit ratio aren't always favorable. Some people and some allergies tend to respond better than others. Immunotherapy is used most often for people allergic to pollens, house dust mites, insect venoms, and animal dander. Immunotherapy for people allergic to foods is generally not advised because of the danger of anaphylaxis.

The procedure is most effective when maintenance injections are continued throughout the year. Treatments are usually given once a week at first; most people can later get by with maintenance injections every 4 to 6 weeks.

Because adverse reactions can follow an immunotherapy injection, doctors usually insist that the patient remain in the office for at least 20 minutes after an injection. Sneezing, coughing, flushing, tingling sensations, itching, chest tightness, wheezing, and hives are all possible symptoms of an allergic reaction. If mild symptoms occur, medication (typically one of the antihistamines, such as diphenhydramine or chlorpheniramine) may help block the allergic reaction. More severe reactions require an injection of epinephrine (adrenaline).

Antihistamines

Antihistamines are the drugs most commonly used for treating allergies (they're not used for treating asthma). There are two types of histamine receptors in the body: histamine$_1$ (H$_1$) and histamine$_2$ (H$_2$). The term *antihistamines* generally refers to drugs that block the histamine$_1$ receptor; stimulation of this receptor by histamine results in injury to target tissues. Histamine$_1$ blockers shouldn't be confused with drugs that block the histamine$_2$ receptor (H$_2$ blockers), which are used to treat peptic ulcers and heartburn.

Many unpleasant but relatively minor effects of an allergic reaction—itchy eyes, runny nose, and itchy skin—are caused by the release of histamine. Other effects of histamine, such as shortness of breath, low blood pressure, and swelling in the throat that can cut off air flow, are more dangerous.

All antihistamines have similar desired effects; they differ mostly in their undesired or adverse effects. Both the desired and the generally undesired effects vary considerably with the specific antihistamine and the person using it. For example, some antihistamines have a greater sedative effect than others, although susceptibility to this effect varies. Sometimes generally undesired effects can be used to advantage. For example, because some antihistamines have what is called anticholinergic effects that dry mucous membranes, they can be used to relieve the runny nose caused by a cold.

Some antihistamines are available without a prescription (over the counter), come in short-acting and extended-release forms, and may be combined with decongestants, which constrict blood vessels and help reduce nasal stuffiness.▲ Other antihistamines require a prescription and a doctor's supervision.

Most antihistamines tend to cause drowsiness. In fact, because of their potent sedative effect, antihistamines are the active ingredient in many over-the-counter sleep aids. Most antihistamines also have strong anticholinergic effects, which can cause confusion, light-headedness, dry mouth, constipation, difficulty with urination, and blurred vision, especially in the elderly.■ However, most people don't experience adverse effects and can use over-the-counter drugs, which cost much less than the nonsedating prescription antihistamines. Drowsiness and other side effects may also be minimized by starting with a small dose and gradually increasing to a dose that is effective in controlling symptoms. A group of non-sedating antihistamines that also does not cause anticholinergic side effects is now available. This group includes astemizole, cetirizine, loratadine, and fexofenadine.

Some Prescription and Nonprescription Antihistamines

Prescription	Nonprescription
Astemizole	Brompheniramine
Azatadine	Chlorpheniramine
Cetirizine	Clemastine
Cyproheptadine	Dexbrompheniramine
Dexchlorpheniramine	Diphenhydramine
Fexofenadine	Phenindamine
Loratadine	Pyrilamine
Methdilazine	Triprolidine
Promethazine	
Trimeprazine	
Tripelennamine	

Types of Allergic Reactions

The different types of allergic reactions are generally categorized by what causes them, the part of the body most affected, and other features.

Allergic rhinitis is a common type of allergic reaction. It is an allergy to airborne particles—usually pollens and grasses but sometimes molds, dusts, and animal danders—that causes sneezing; an itchy, runny, or stuffy nose; itching; and irritated eyes. Allergic rhinitis may be seasonal or perennial (year-round).

Seasonal Allergic Rhinitis

Seasonal allergic rhinitis is an allergy to airborne pollens, commonly referred to as **hay fever** *or* **pollinosis**.

Pollen seasons vary considerably in different parts of the country. In the eastern, southern, and midwestern United States, the pollens that cause hay fever in the spring usually come from trees such as oak, elm, maple, alder, birch, juniper, and olive; in the early summer, from grasses such as bluegrasses, timothy, redtop, and orchard grass;

and in the late summer, from ragweed. In the western United States, the grasses pollinate for much longer, and there are other fall weeds. Occasionally, seasonal allergy is caused by mold spores.

Symptoms and Diagnosis

Once the pollen season starts, the nose, roof of the mouth, back of the throat, and eyes itch gradually or abruptly. Watery eyes, sneezing, and a clear watery discharge from the nose usually follow. Some people develop headaches, coughing, and wheezing; become irritable and depressed; lose their appetite; and have trouble sleeping. The inner eyelids and whites of the eyes may become inflamed (conjunctivitis). The lining of the nose may become swollen and bluish-red, leading to a runny nose and stuffiness.

Seasonal allergic rhinitis is usually easy to recognize. Skin tests and the person's history of symptoms can help the doctor determine which pollen is causing the problem.

▲ see page 59

■ see box, page 41

Treatment

Antihistamines are the usual initial treatment for seasonal allergic rhinitis. Sometimes a decongestant such as pseudoephedrine or phenylpropanolamine is taken orally along with the antihistamine to help relieve the stuffy, runny nose. However, people with high blood pressure should avoid decongestants unless their use is recommended and monitored by a doctor.

Cromolyn sodium, a nasal spray, is another drug that may be useful. Cromolyn requires a prescription and is more expensive than common antihistamines; its effects are generally limited to the areas where it's applied, such as the nose and the back of the throat. When antihistamines and cromolyn can't control uncomfortable allergy symptoms, corticosteroid sprays may be prescribed by a doctor. Corticosteroid sprays are remarkably effective, and the newer ones have essentially no adverse effects. When these measures fail, oral corticosteroids may be necessary for a short time (usually less than 10 days) to bring a difficult situation under control.

People who have severe adverse effects from taking drugs, who often have to take oral corticosteroids, or who develop asthma should consider allergen immunotherapy, a series of injections that may help prevent symptoms of allergy.▲ Allergen immunotherapy for seasonal allergic rhinitis should begin some months before the pollen season.

Perennial Allergic Rhinitis

Perennial (year-round) allergic rhinitis causes symptoms similar to those of seasonal allergic rhinitis, but the symptoms vary in severity, often unpredictably, throughout the year.

The allergen in a year-round allergy may be house dust mites, feathers, animal dander, or molds. Conjunctivitis isn't common. Nasal congestion, which is common, may block the eustachian tubes in the ears, causing hearing problems, particularly in children. A doctor must

---

▲ see page 824

■ see page 1015

★ see page 1015

---

distinguish perennial allergic rhinitis from recurring sinus infections (sinusitis) and growths inside the nose (nasal polyps).■ Sinusitis and nasal polyps could be complications of the allergic rhinitis.

Some people who have chronic nasal inflammation, sinusitis, nasal polyps, negative skin test results, and large numbers of eosinophils (a type of white blood cell) in their nasal secretions are prone to a severe reaction to aspirin or other nonsteroidal anti-inflammatory drugs. The adverse reaction in these people is usually manifested as a severe asthma attack that's not easily treated. People who tend to have this reaction should avoid using nonsteroidal anti-inflammatory drugs.

People who have a chronically stuffy and runny nose but no sinusitis, nasal polyps, or any demonstrable allergy may have a different condition—vasomotor rhinitis—which is not caused by allergy.★

Treatment

If specific allergens are identified, the treatment for perennial allergic rhinitis is very similar to that for seasonal allergic rhinitis. Although the use of oral corticosteroids is generally not advised, prescription corticosteroid nasal sprays can be very helpful. Nonprescription decongestant nose drops or sprays shouldn't be used for more than a few days at a time, because using them continually for a week or more may result in a rebound effect that can worsen or prolong nasal inflammation. Sometimes surgery is needed to remove nasal polyps or treat a sinus infection.

Allergic Conjunctivitis

Allergic conjunctivitis is an allergic inflammation of the conjunctiva, the delicate membrane that covers the inner eyelid and the external surface of the eye.

In most people, allergic conjunctivitis is part of a larger allergy syndrome, such as seasonal allergic rhinitis. However, allergic conjunctivitis can occur alone in some people who have direct contact with airborne substances such as pollens, fungal spores, dust, and animal dander. The whites of the eyes become red and swollen, and the eyes itch and may water a great deal. The eyelids may become swollen and red.

Sensitization, exposure to an antigen that results in a hypersensitivity reaction, can also occur with medications placed in the eye, cosmetics such as eyeliner and face powder, or chemicals that are conveyed to the eyes by fingers (as can happen in working with chemicals). These reactions, usually involving the skin on the eyelid and around the eye, are examples of contact dermatitis.

Treatment

Oral antihistamines are the main treatment for allergic conjunctivitis. Antihistamines can also be taken in eye drops, in which they're usually combined with vasoconstrictors to reduce the redness. However, the antihistamine itself, or something else in the solution, sometimes makes the allergic reaction worse, so taking oral antihistamines is generally preferable. Cromolyn, which is also available as eye drops, mainly prevents allergy symptoms when a person expects to come into contact with an allergen. Eye drops containing corticosteroids may be used in very severe cases but can cause complications, such as glaucoma. An ophthalmologist has to check the eye pressure regularly when a person is being treated with corticosteroids applied directly to the eyes.

Bathing the eyes with bland eyewashes such as artificial tears can help reduce irritation. Any substance that may be causing the allergic reaction should be avoided. Contact lenses shouldn't be worn during episodes of conjunctivitis. Allergen immunotherapy may be recommended when other treatments don't produce satisfactory results.

Food Allergy and Intolerance

A food allergy is an allergic reaction to a particular food. A much more common condition, food intolerance, isn't an allergic reaction but is any other undesirable effect of eating a particular food.

Many people can't tolerate certain foods for various reasons other than food allergy; for example, they may lack an enzyme necessary for digesting the food. If a person's digestive system can't tolerate certain foods, the result can be gastrointestinal distress, gas, nausea, diarrhea, or other problems. In general, allergic reactions aren't responsible for these symptoms. Many controversial claims are made about "food allergy," in which foods are blamed for ailments ranging from hyperactivity in children to chronic fatigue. Other unsubstantiated claims blame food allergy

for arthritis, poor athletic performance, depression, and other problems.

Symptoms

A common problem, which may be a manifestation of food allergy, starts in infancy and is most likely to arise when atopic diseases (such as allergic rhinitis or allergic asthma) run in the family. The first indication of an allergic predisposition may be a skin rash such as eczema (atopic dermatitis). The rash may or may not be accompanied by gastrointestinal symptoms such as nausea, vomiting, and diarrhea and may or may not be triggered by a food allergy. By the child's first birthday, the eczema is often less of a problem. Children with food allergies are likely to develop other atopic diseases as they get older, including allergic asthma and seasonal allergic rhinitis. However, in adults and in children over age 10, the food is unlikely to be responsible for respiratory symptoms, even though skin test results remain positive.

A few people develop very severe allergic reactions to specific potent allergens in foods, especially nuts, legumes, seeds, and shellfish. People with these food allergies may react violently to eating even a tiny amount of the offending food. They may break out all over in a rash, feel their throat swell and close up, and have trouble breathing. A sudden drop in blood pressure can lead to dizziness and collapse. This life-threatening emergency is called anaphylaxis.▲ Some people develop anaphylaxis only if they exercise immediately after eating the offending food.■

Food additives can cause symptoms as the result of either an allergy or an intolerance. Some foods contain toxins or chemicals (for example, histamine) that are responsible for nonallergic adverse reactions. Compounds such as monosodium glutamate (MSG) don't cause allergies. Sulfites (for example, metabisulfite, which is found in many food products as a preservative) and dyes (for example, tartrazine, a yellow dye found in candies, soft drinks, and many commercially prepared foods) have been reported to trigger asthma and hives in people sensitive to the substance. Some people develop migraine headaches after eating certain foods.

▲ see page 828

■ see page 832

Common Food Allergies

Milk

Eggs

Shellfish

Nuts

Wheat

Peanuts

Soybeans

Chocolate

Food allergies and intolerances are usually fairly obvious, although distinguishing a true allergy from an intolerance isn't always easy. Digestion apparently prevents allergic responses to many orally ingested allergens in adults. An example is **bakers' asthma,** in which bakery workers wheeze when they breathe in flour dust or other grains, yet can eat the grains without having an allergic reaction.

Diagnosis

Skin tests are sometimes useful in helping diagnose a food allergy; a positive test result doesn't necessarily mean a person is sensitive to a particular food, but a negative test result makes sensitivity to that food unlikely. After a positive test result, an allergist may need to perform an oral challenge test for definitive diagnosis. In an oral challenge test, the suspected food is hidden in a carrier substance such as milk or applesauce and fed to the patient. If no symptoms develop, the patient isn't allergic to that food. The best challenge tests are blinded; that is, sometimes the suspected food is in the carrier substance and sometimes not. In these tests, the doctor can determine with certainty that the patient has a sensitivity to the offending food.

An elimination diet may help identify the cause of an allergy. The person stops eating foods that might conceivably be causing the symptoms. Foods are later reintroduced one at a time. The

doctor may provide a starting diet, which must be followed strictly, using pure products. Following this diet isn't easy, because many food products are hidden as ingredients of other foods. For example, ordinary rye bread contains some wheat flour. No foods or fluids may be consumed other than those specified in the starting diet. Eating in restaurants isn't advisable, since the person (and doctor) must know every ingredient of every meal eaten.

Treatment

No specific treatment is available for food allergies except to stop eating the foods that trigger them. Anyone who is seriously allergic and who develops rashes, swelling (hives) of the lips and throat, or shortness of breath must be very careful to avoid the offending foods.

Desensitization by eating small amounts of a food or placing drops of food extracts under the tongue hasn't proved effective. Antihistamines are of little practical value as preventive agents but can be useful for acute general reactions with hives (urticaria) and giant hives (angioedema).

Anaphylaxis

Anaphylaxis is an acute, generalized, potentially severe and life-threatening allergic reaction in a person who was previously sensitized by prior exposure to an allergen and who comes into contact with the same allergen again.

Anaphylaxis can be caused by any allergen. The most common ones are drugs, insect stings, certain foods, and allergen immunotherapy injections. Anaphylaxis can't occur on the first exposure to an allergen. For example, a person's first exposure to penicillin or first bee sting doesn't trigger anaphylaxis, but subsequent exposure may. However, many people don't recall a first exposure.

An anaphylactic reaction begins when the allergen enters the bloodstream and reacts with an antibody of the immunoglobulin E (IgE) class. This reaction stimulates cells to release histamine and other substances involved in immune inflammatory reactions. In response, the airways in the lungs may constrict, causing wheezing; blood vessels may dilate, causing blood pressure to drop; and the walls of blood vessels may leak fluid, causing swelling and hives. The heart may malfunction, beat erratically, and pump blood inadequately. The person may go into shock.▲

▲ see page 111

Anaphylac*toid* reactions resemble anaphylac*tic* reactions but may occur after the *first* injection of certain drugs (for example, polymyxin, pentamidine, opioids, or contrast media used in x-ray studies). The mechanism doesn't involve IgE antibodies, so it isn't an allergic reaction. Aspirin and other nonsteroidal anti-inflammatory drugs can cause anaphylactoid reactions in some people, particularly those with perennial allergic rhinitis and nasal polyps.

Symptoms

Symptoms begin immediately or nearly always within 2 hours after exposure to the offending substance. The person may feel uneasy, become agitated, and develop palpitations, tingling, itchy and flushed skin, throbbing in the ears, coughing, sneezing, hives, swellings, or increased difficulty in breathing because of asthma or a closing off of the windpipe. Cardiovascular collapse can occur without respiratory symptoms. Usually an episode involves either respiratory or cardiovascular symptoms, not both, and the person has the same pattern of symptoms in subsequent episodes. However, anaphylaxis may progress so rapidly that it may lead to collapse, convulsions, loss of bladder control, unconsciousness, or stroke within 1 to 2 minutes. Anaphylaxis may prove fatal unless emergency treatment is given immediately.

Prevention

A person who has had anaphylaxis from a bee sting is very likely to have a repeat experience if stung again. The same is true for repeated exposure to any other allergen, such as a drug. Testing a person's skin reaction isn't practical every time a drug is administered. However, people who have a history of allergy to animal serum (for example, horse-derived tetanus antitoxin) or penicillin are tested before receiving these products.

Long-term allergen immunotherapy will prevent anaphylaxis in people who are known to be allergic to such unavoidable allergens as insect stings. Immunotherapy isn't used when the offending substance can be avoided, such as penicillin and other drugs. However, if a person needs a particular drug (such as penicillin or an antitoxin derived from horse serum), desensitization can be done rapidly with careful monitoring in the doctor's office or hospital.

Some people have a history of anaphylactoid reactions to dyes (contrast media) injected for certain x-ray studies. Although doctors try to avoid using these dyes in such patients, some disorders can't be diagnosed without them. Special contrast media can then be used, which reduce the incidence of reactions. In addition, drugs that block anaphylactic reactions, such as prednisone, diphenhydramine, or ephedrine, may be useful when given before the dye is injected.

Treatment

The first treatment for anaphylaxis is an epinephrine injection. People who are allergic to insect stings or certain foods, especially people who have had an attack of anaphylaxis, should always carry a self-injecting syringe of epinephrine for fast emergency treatment.

Usually this treatment stops an anaphylactic reaction. However, anyone having an anaphylactic reaction should go to a hospital emergency department as soon as possible, because careful monitoring of the cardiovascular and respiratory systems may be needed, with the availability of rapid, sophisticated treatment.

Hives

Hives, also called **urticaria,** *is a reaction in the skin characterized by small, pale or reddened swellings (wheals).*

Related to and sometimes coexisting with hives is a condition known as **angioedema,** which involves larger areas and deeper tissues beneath the skin. Hives and angioedema are anaphylactic-type reactions that are limited to the skin and underlying tissues. They may be triggered by allergens or other agents or their cause may be unknown. Common allergens are drugs, insect stings or bites, allergy shots, and certain foods, particularly eggs, shellfish, nuts, and fruits. Sometimes hives erupt suddenly after the person has eaten even an extremely tiny amount of a food. Other times hives occur only after eating large amounts of a food (for example, strawberries). Also, hives sometimes follow viral infections such as hepatitis, infectious mononucleosis, and German measles.

Hives that recur over weeks or months are often difficult to explain; a specific cause may never be found. An allergy is rarely the cause, although the unwitting long-term use of a food additive, a drug, or other chemical may be responsible. Examples include preservatives, dyes, and other food additives; minute traces of penicillin in milk (used by farmers to treat infections in cows); and some nonprescription drugs. A concurrent chronic disease (systemic lupus erythematosus, polycythemia vera, lymphoma, hyperthyroidism, or an infection) is uncommonly associated with hives. Although psychologic factors are often suspected, they're rarely identified.

Certain drugs, such as aspirin, may aggravate symptoms. A person whose hives are caused by aspirin may react similarly to other nonsteroidal anti-inflammatory drugs, such as ibuprofen, or to tartrazine, a yellow dye used to color some foods and drugs. Angioedema that recurs with no sign of ordinary hives may be a disorder called hereditary angioedema.▲

Symptoms and Diagnosis

Itching is usually the first symptom of hives, quickly followed by wheals—smooth, slightly elevated areas that are redder or paler than the surrounding skin and usually remain small (less than $\frac{1}{2}$ inch across). When the wheals are larger (up to 8 inches across), the center areas may be clear, forming rings. Ordinarily, crops of hives come and go; one spot may remain for several hours, then disappear, only to reappear elsewhere.

With angioedema, the swelling often covers large areas and extends deep beneath the skin. It may involve part or all of the hands, feet, eyelids, lips, or genitals or even the lining of the mouth, throat, and airways, making breathing difficult.

When hives appear suddenly and disappear quickly without a recurrence, a medical examination usually isn't needed; it rarely reveals a cause other than whatever was obvious to begin with. But when angioedema or hives recur without explanation, a medical evaluation is usually advisable.

Treatment

Hives that appear suddenly generally disappear without any treatment within days and sometimes within minutes. If the cause isn't obvious, the person should stop taking all nonessential drugs until the reaction subsides. Taking antihistamines such as diphenhydramine, chlor-

pheniramine, or hydroxyzine partially relieves the itching and reduces the swelling. Taking prednisone, a corticosteroid, for several days may reduce very severe swelling and itching.

Anyone who collapses or has difficulty swallowing or breathing must receive emergency treatment. An epinephrine (adrenaline) injection is given along with antihistamines as quickly as possible. Treatment is best continued in a hospital emergency department where the person's treatment can be carefully monitored and adjusted as needed.

Chronic hives may also be relieved by antihistamines. The antidepressant doxepin is effective for some adults. Because corticosteroids taken for more than 3 to 4 weeks cause many adverse effects, they are prescribed only for serious symptoms when all other treatments have failed and are given for as short a time as possible. About half the time, untreated chronic hives disappear within 2 years. Controlling stress often helps reduce the frequency and severity of attacks.

Hereditary Angioedema

Hereditary angioedema is a genetic disorder associated with a deficiency of C1 inhibitor, a protein in the blood.

C1 inhibitor is part of the complement system, a group of proteins involved in some immune and allergic reactions. Deficiency or subnormal activity of C1 inhibitor causes episodes of swelling in local areas of skin and the tissue beneath it or in the mucous membranes that line body openings such as the mouth, throat, and gastrointestinal tract. Injury or viral illness often precipitates attacks, which can be aggravated by emotional stress. Attacks typically produce areas of swelling that are painful rather than itchy and are unaccompanied by hives. Many people have nausea, vomiting, and cramps. The most serious complication is swelling of the upper airways, which can interfere with breathing. Blood tests that measure C1 inhibitor levels or activity establish the diagnosis.

Treatment

A drug called aminocaproic acid can sometimes end an attack of hereditary angioedema. Epinephrine, antihistamines, and corticosteroids are often given, although there's no proof that

▲ see below

these drugs are effective. Breathing can quickly become obstructed, and a breathing tube may need to be placed in the person's windpipe during an acute attack.

Certain treatments may help prevent an attack. For example, before undergoing minor surgery or dental procedures, a person with hereditary angioedema may be given a transfusion of fresh plasma to raise levels of C1 inhibitor in the blood. Administering purified C1 inhibitor can prevent attacks of hereditary angioedema, but it isn't yet available for general use. For long-term prevention, oral anabolic steroids (androgens) such as stanozolol or danazol can stimulate the body to produce more C1 inhibitor. Because these drugs can have masculinizing side effects, the doses are carefully evaluated and monitored when given to women.

Mastocytosis

Mastocytosis is a disorder in which mast cells, histamine-producing cells involved in immune reactions, accumulate in skin tissues and sometimes in various other parts of the body.

The most common form of mastocytosis may be limited to the skin, especially in children, or may involve other organs, such as the stomach, intestines, liver, spleen, lymph nodes, and bones. Rarer forms of mastocytosis may be associated with a serious blood disorder (such as acute leukemia, lymphoma, chronic neutropenia, or a myeloproliferative disorder) or with the very serious diseases called mast cell leukemia and aggressive mastocytosis. Some 90 percent of people with common mastocytosis and less than 50 percent of people with other forms of mastocytosis have urticaria pigmentosa—small, reddish-brown spots scattered over the body, which often produce hives and redness when rubbed or scratched.

The cause of mastocytosis isn't known. More and more mast cells accumulate over a period of years, resulting in a gradual increase in symptoms, but the symptoms can usually be controlled for decades with medication. Some people with mastocytosis have joint and bone pain and are prone to severe allergic reactions, including symptoms similar to those of anaphylaxis. They may also develop peptic ulcers and chronic diarrhea because their stomach produces too much histamine.

Treatment

Treatment of mastocytosis requires two types of antihistamine: histamine$_1$ receptor blockers, the kind taken for allergies, and histamine$_2$ receptor blockers, the kind taken for peptic ulcers. If the mastocytosis is associated with a serious underlying disorder, treatment is much more complex.

Physical Allergy

Physical allergy is a condition in which allergic symptoms develop in response to a physical stimulus, such as cold, sunlight, heat, or a minor injury.

Itching, skin blotches, and hives are the most common symptoms of physical allergy. In some people, the airways to the lungs tighten and breathing becomes difficult. A strong reaction to sunlight (photosensitivity) can produce both hives and unusual skin blotches.▲ Photosensitivity also may result from concurrent use of certain drugs or substances applied to the skin.

People who are especially sensitive to heat may develop a condition called cholinergic urticaria: small, intensely itchy, individual hives, each surrounded by a ring of redness. Cholinergic urticaria is also brought on by exercise, emotional stress, or any activity that causes sweating. People who are particularly sensitive to cold may develop hives, skin puffiness, asthma, or runny nose and nasal stuffiness when exposed to cold.

Treatment

The best way to deal with any physical allergy is to prevent it by avoiding whatever tends to cause it. People with allergy symptoms should stop using cosmetics and skin creams, lotions, and oils for a while to see if one of these substances may be aggravating the allergy. An antihistamine such as diphenhydramine, cyproheptadine, or hydroxyzine can usually relieve itching. Cyproheptadine tends to work best for hives caused by cold, and hydroxyzine for hives caused by stress. People who are very sensitive to sunlight should use sunscreens and minimize sun exposure.

▲ see page 987

Exercise-Induced Allergic Reactions

In some people, exercise can result in an episode of asthma or an acute anaphylactic reaction.

Asthma is one type of abnormal exercise-induced reaction. Exercise-induced asthma frequently occurs in people who ordinarily have asthma, but some people have asthma only with exercise. A sensation of tightness in the chest, associated with wheezing and difficulty in breathing, occurs after 5 to 10 minutes of vigorous exercise, typically beginning after the exercise has stopped. Exercise-induced asthma is more likely to occur when the air is cold and dry.

A much rarer condition is exercise-induced anaphylaxis, which can occur after vigorous exercise. In some people it occurs only after eating a specific food before exercising.

Treatment

For exercise-induced asthma, the goal of treatment is to make exercise possible without bringing on symptoms. The goal can usually be achieved by inhaling a beta-adrenergic drug about 15 minutes before starting to exercise. Cromolyn is effective in some people. For people who ordinarily have asthma, controlling the asthma by usual means often prevents the exercise-induced form.▲

People who have exercise-induced anaphylaxis should avoid either the exercise or the food known to trigger symptoms when combined with exercise. Some people find that gradually increasing the degree and duration of exercise makes them more tolerant of exercise. A self-injecting syringe of epinephrine should always be carried for prompt emergency treatment.

CHAPTER 170

Transplantation

Transplantation is the transfer of living cells, tissues, or organs from one person (the donor) to another (the recipient) or from one part of the body to another (for example, skin grafts) with the goal of restoring a missing function.

Transplantation can be of enormous benefit to people with a variety of otherwise incurable problems. Blood transfusions, which affect millions of people every year, are the most common type of transplantation. Transplantation of other organs usually entails finding a compatible donor as well as accepting the risks involved in undergoing major surgery, using powerful immunosuppressant drugs, facing possible rejection of the organ transplant, and dealing with serious complications or death. However, for people whose vital organs—such as the heart, lungs, liver, kidneys, or bone marrow—stop working properly and can't be restored to normal function, transplantation of a functional replacement organ may offer the only chance for survival.

Donated tissues or organs may come from a living person or from someone who has recently died. Tissues and organs from a living donor are preferable because they're more likely to be transplanted successfully. However, organs such as the heart, liver, lungs, and eye components (the cornea and lens) can come only from someone who has recently died, usually as the result of an accident rather than a disease.

Living donors are usually family members. Bone marrow and kidneys are the organs most often donated by a living donor. Because the body has two kidneys and can function well with only one, often a family member can safely donate a kidney. Portions of liver and lung tissue have also been transplanted from some living donors. An organ from a living donor is transplanted within minutes of being removed.

The national system overseeing organ donation is far from perfect. In many states, people may indicate the desire to donate organs when they register with their state's department of motor vehicles; this wish is recorded on their driver's license. So that organ transplantation can be performed without delay, a computerized database

▲ see page 176

tracks information on people who need a particular organ and their tissue type (in order to match compatibility).

Some organs survive for only a few hours outside the body; others can be kept cold for transplantation up to several days. Sometimes several people can benefit from transplantation of organs from one body. For example, one donor might theoretically provide two people with corneas, two with new kidneys, one with a liver, two with lungs, and another with a heart.

Tissue Matching

Transplanting tissues and organs from one person to another is a complex process. The immune system normally attacks and destroys foreign tissue (a problem known as graft rejection). Donated tissue must match the recipient's tissue as closely as possible in order to reduce the severity of rejection.

To match tissues as closely as possible, doctors determine both the donor's and the recipient's tissue type. **Antigens** (substances capable of stimulating an immune response) are present on the surface of every cell of the body; when a person receives transplanted tissue, the antigens on the transplanted tissue alert the recipient's body that the tissue is foreign. Three specific antigens on the surface of red blood cells—the **A, B, and Rh antigens**—determine whether a blood transfusion will be accepted or rejected.▲ That's why blood is typed according to these three antigens. Other tissues carry a greater variety of antigens, making possible more extensive matching. A group of antigens called the **human leukocyte antigens (HLA)**■ is most important when transplanting tissues other than red blood cells. The better the match of the HLA antigens, the more likely the transplantation will be successful. However, experts are still debating how much benefit results from matching, especially for liver transplants.

Generally, before any organ is transplanted, tissues from both the donor and recipient are examined for HLA type. In identical twins, the HLA antigens are exactly the same. In parents and in most siblings, several of the HLA antigens are the same but some differ. One in four pairs of siblings share HLA antigens and are quite compatible. In people from different families, few HLA antigens are the same.

Why Corneal Transplants Usually Work

Corneal transplants are a common and highly successful type of transplantation. A scarred or cloudy cornea can be replaced with a clear, healthy one using a microscopic surgical procedure that takes about an hour. Donor corneas come from people who have recently died.

A cornea is rarely rejected because it doesn't have its own blood supply—it receives oxygen and other nutrients from nearby tissues and fluid. Since antibodies (proteins produced in response to antigens, in this case, foreign tissue) and cells of the immune system, which circulate in the blood, don't reach the transplanted cornea, rejection of a corneal transplant is less likely than rejection of tissue with a rich blood supply.

Suppression of the Immune System

Even if HLA types are closely matched, transplanted organs are usually rejected unless the recipient's immune system is kept under control. Rejection, when it occurs, usually begins soon after the transplantation is performed but can become evident weeks or even months later. Rejection can be minor and easily suppressed, or it can be major and progress despite treatment. Rejection not only can destroy the transplanted tissue or organ but also can cause fever, chills, nausea, fatigue, and sudden changes in blood pressure.

The discovery that certain drugs can suppress the immune system has greatly increased the success rate of transplantation. But immunosuppressant drugs carry risks. While they suppress the immune system's reaction to the transplanted organ, they also keep the immune system from fighting infections and destroying other foreign material.

▲ see box, page 740

■ see page 812

One-Year Success Rates of Organ Transplants

Organ	Success Rates in 1980	Success Rates in 1995
Kidney	60%	90%
Heart	60%	90%
Liver	30%	80%
Pancreas	20%	70%
Lung and heart-lung	*	70%

*Data aren't available because lung and heart-lung transplants have been performed in large numbers of people for less than 10 years.

Intensive suppression of the immune system is usually necessary only during the first few weeks after a transplant or when a transplanted organ appears to be undergoing rejection. After that, smaller doses of drugs, which must be taken indefinitely, will usually suppress the immune system just enough to control rejection.

Many different types of drugs can act as immunosuppressants. Corticosteroids such as prednisone are frequently used. They may be given intravenously at first, then continued orally after surgery. Azathioprine has long been a mainstay of immunosuppressive treatment, and several other drugs, including tacrolimus and (most recently) mycophenolate mofetil, have been approved for this purpose. Cyclosporine is another commonly used immunosuppressant. Others include cyclophosphamide, used primarily in bone marrow transplantation; antilymphocyte globulin and antithymocyte globulin; and monoclonal antibodies against T lymphocytes.

Kidney Transplantation

For people whose kidneys don't function, kidney transplantation provides a lifesaving alternative to dialysis and is successfully performed in people of all ages. In the United States, about 11,000 kidneys are transplanted each year. About 90 percent of kidneys from living donors function

well a year after being transplanted. During each year that follows, 3 to 5 percent of those kidneys fail. The results are almost as good with kidneys transplanted from someone who has just died: 85 to 90 percent function after 1 year, and 5 to 8 percent fail during each successive year. Transplanted kidneys sometimes function for more than 30 years. People with successful kidney transplants usually lead normal, active lives.

Transplantation is a major operation because the donated kidney must be attached to the recipient's blood vessels and urinary tract. More than two thirds of all transplanted kidneys are transplanted after the death of the donor, usually a healthy person who died in an accident. The kidneys are removed, cooled, and transported quickly to a medical center for transplantation to a person who has a compatible tissue type and whose blood serum doesn't contain antibodies to the tissue.

Despite the use of drugs to suppress the immune system, one or more episodes of rejection typically occur shortly after transplant surgery. Rejection may cause weight gain from fluid retention, fever, and tenderness and swelling over the area where the kidney was implanted. Blood tests can reveal deteriorating kidney function. If doctors aren't sure whether rejection is taking place, they can perform a needle biopsy (remove a small piece of kidney tissue through a needle and examine it under a microscope).

Rejection can usually be reversed by increasing the dosage or number of immunosuppressant drugs. If the rejection can't be reversed, the transplantation fails. The rejected kidney may be left in place unless the fever persists, the area over the transplant remains tender, blood appears in the urine, or blood pressure remains high. When transplantation fails, dialysis must be started again. A second attempt at transplantation with another kidney can often be made after the person has recovered from the first; the chances for success are almost as good as for first transplants.

Most rejection episodes and other complications occur within 3 to 4 months of the transplantation. After that, unless the immunosuppressant drugs cause adverse effects or a severe infection intervenes, the recipient continues to take immunosuppressant drugs, because stopping them even briefly could allow the body to reject the new kidney. Rejection that takes place over many weeks or months is rare. If it occurs, the recipient's blood pressure may increase, kidney function deteriorates, and the transplant slowly fails.

The incidence of cancers appearing in kidney transplant recipients is 10 to 15 times greater than in the general population. The risk of developing cancer of the lymph system (lymphoma) is about 30 times greater than normal, probably because the immune system is being suppressed.▲

Liver Transplantation

While dialysis is an option for people with kidney disease, no similar treatment is available for people with severe liver disease. Liver transplantation is the only option when the liver can no longer function. Some people who might have benefited from liver transplantation die before a suitable liver becomes available.

Although the success rate of liver transplantation is somewhat lower than that of kidney transplantation, 70 to 80 percent of the recipients survive for at least 1 year. Most of these survivors are recipients whose liver was destroyed by primary biliary cirrhosis, hepatitis, or the use of a medication toxic to the liver. Liver transplantation as treatment of liver cancer is rarely successful. The cancer usually returns in the transplanted liver or elsewhere; fewer than 20 percent of recipients survive for even a year.

Surprisingly, liver transplants are rejected less vigorously than transplants of other organs, such as the kidney and heart. Nonetheless, immunosuppressant drugs must be taken after surgery. If the recipient has an enlarged liver, nausea, pain, fever, jaundice, or abnormal liver function as shown by blood test results, the doctor may perform a needle biopsy (remove a small piece of liver tissue through a needle and examine it under a microscope). The biopsy results help determine whether the liver is being rejected and whether the dosage of immunosuppressant drugs should be increased.

Heart Transplantation

Unthinkable just a few decades ago, heart transplantation is now a reality. Some 95 percent of heart transplant recipients are substantially better able to exercise and perform daily chores than they were before the transplant. More than 70 percent of heart transplant recipients return to work.

Heart transplantation is reserved for people who have the most serious types of heart disease and can't be treated with drugs or other forms of surgery. In some medical centers, mechanical heart machines can keep patients alive for weeks or months until a suitable donor heart can be found. However, many such patients die while waiting.

People who have heart transplants need immunosuppressant drugs after surgery. Rejection of the heart usually causes fever, weakness, and rapid or otherwise abnormal heartbeats. Poor heart function leads to low blood pressure, swelling (edema), and a buildup of fluid in the lungs. Very mild rejection may cause no symptoms at all, but an electrocardiogram (ECG) may show changes. If doctors suspect rejection, they usually perform a biopsy. In this procedure, a catheter with a small knife at the end is threaded through a vein in the neck to the heart, and a small piece of heart tissue is removed. The tissue is then examined under a microscope. If doctors find evidence of rejection, they modify the doses of immunosuppressant drugs.

Infections cause nearly half of all deaths that occur after heart transplantation. Another complication is atherosclerosis (clogged arteries), which develops in the coronary arteries of about one fourth of heart transplant recipients.

Lung and Heart-Lung Transplantation

Lung transplantation has improved considerably in recent years. Usually a single lung is transplanted, but both lungs are sometimes replaced. When lung disease has also damaged the heart, lung transplantation is sometimes combined with heart transplantation. Procuring lungs is a problem because preserving a lung for transplantation is difficult. Therefore, transplantation must be performed as soon as possible after a lung has been obtained.

Lung transplants can come from a living donor or from someone who has recently died. Not more than one entire lung can be taken from a living donor, and usually only one lobe is donated. Both lungs or the heart and lungs can be taken from a person who has died.

▲ see page 792

Some 80 to 85 percent of the people who receive lung transplants survive for at least 1 year, and about 70 percent survive for 5 years. Several complications can threaten the survival of lung and heart-lung transplant recipients. The risk of infection is high because the lungs are continually exposed to air, which isn't sterile. One of the most common complications is poor healing at the site where the airway is attached. In some people who receive lung transplants, the airways become partially blocked with scar tissue, which requires additional treatment.

Rejection of a lung transplant can be difficult to detect, evaluate, and treat. In more than 80 percent of the recipients, some evidence of rejection occurs within a month of the operation. Rejection produces fever, shortness of breath, and weakness; the weakness occurs because of insufficient oxygen in the blood. As with other transplanted organs, lung transplant rejection may be controlled by a change in the type or dosage of immunosuppressant drugs. A later complication of lung transplantation is closure of the small airways, which may represent gradual rejection.

Pancreatic Transplantation

Transplantation of the pancreas is performed only for certain people with diabetes.▲ Unlike transplantation of other organs, it's not a last resort to save a life but rather is intended to prevent the complications of diabetes and especially to control blood sugar more effectively than can be done by injecting insulin several times a day. Experimental studies suggest that pancreatic transplantation can slow or eliminate the complications of diabetes. Nevertheless, pancreatic transplantation isn't appropriate for most diabetics; it is generally reserved for those whose blood sugar is most difficult to control and who have not developed serious complications.

More than half the people who undergo pancreatic transplantation for diabetes have normal levels of blood sugar afterward, often without using insulin. However, the recipient of a new pancreas must take immunosuppressant drugs, which increases the risk of infection and other complica-

tions. Therefore, the risk of taking insulin and having less than ideal control of diabetes is traded for the risk of being immunosuppressed and having better control of diabetes. Because of the risk of immunosuppression, most pancreatic transplants have been performed on diabetic people who also needed a kidney transplant because of kidney failure.

Researchers are investigating the possibility of transplanting only the pancreatic cells that produce insulin (the islet cells) rather than the entire pancreas. While the results so far are encouraging, this procedure is still experimental.

Bone Marrow Transplantation

Bone marrow transplantation was first used as part of the treatment of leukemia, certain types of lymphoma, and aplastic anemia. As the techniques and success rates improve, bone marrow transplantation is gaining wider use. For example, some women with breast cancer and children with certain genetic diseases now receive bone marrow transplants. When cancer patients have chemotherapy or radiation therapy, normal blood-producing cells in the bone marrow can be destroyed along with the cancerous cells. But sometimes the patient's bone marrow can be removed and then reinjected after the patient has received high doses of chemotherapy. Thus, a cancer patient may be able to receive very high doses of radiation therapy and chemotherapy to destroy all cancer cells.

When bone marrow is transplanted from a donor, the recipient's HLA type must closely match the donor's HLA type; therefore, the most likely donors are close family members. The transplantation procedure itself is simple. Usually while the donor is under general anesthesia, a doctor removes marrow from the hip bone with a syringe and prepares it for transplantation. The doctor then injects the marrow into the recipient's vein. The donor's bone marrow migrates to and takes root in the recipient's bones, and the cells begin to divide. Ultimately, if all goes well, the recipient's bone marrow is entirely replaced.

Nevertheless, the procedure is risky because the recipient's white blood cells have been destroyed by radiation therapy and chemotherapy. It takes about 2 to 3 weeks for the transplanted bone marrow to produce enough white blood

_____

▲ see page 717

cells to protect against infections. As a result, the risk of serious infection is higher during this interval. Another problem is that the new bone marrow may produce immunologically active cells that attack the host's cells (graft-versus-host disease).▲ And despite a bone marrow transplant, cancer may recur.

Transplantation of Other Organs

People who have had extensive burns or other massive skin loss can receive **skin grafts.** Skin grafting is best performed by removing healthy skin from one part of the body and grafting it to another. When such grafting isn't possible, skin from a donor or even from animals (such as pigs) can provide temporary protection until normal skin grows to replace it. Efforts are also being made to increase the amount of skin available for grafting by growing small pieces of the person's skin in a tissue culture.

Cartilage is sometimes transplanted in children, usually to repair defects in the ears or nose. Transplanted cartilage is rarely attacked by the body's immune system. **Bone grafting** generally consists of taking bone material from one part of the body to replace missing bone in another part. Bone transplanted from one person to another doesn't survive, but it stimulates new bone growth and serves as a good scaffold for bridging and stabilizing defects until new bone can form.

Transplantation of the **small intestine** is experimental and may be attempted for people whose intestines have been destroyed by disease or do not function well enough to sustain life. Most of these transplants haven't lasted for long periods, but success rates are improving.

▲ see page 741

Infections

CHAPTER 171

Biology of Infectious Disease

Microorganisms are everywhere: in the soil, in freshwater and seawater, below the ocean floor, and in the air. Every day, we eat, drink, and breathe them. Yet, despite their seemingly overwhelming presence, organisms rarely invade, multiply, and produce infection in humans. And even when they do, the infection is sometimes so mild that it doesn't cause symptoms.

Relatively few microorganisms are actually capable of causing disease. Many microorganisms live on the skin, in the mouth, in the airways, in the intestine, and in the genitals (particularly the vagina). Whether a microorganism remains as a harmless companion to its human host or invades and causes disease depends on the nature of the microorganism and on the human body's defenses.

Resident Flora

A healthy person lives in harmony with normal microbial flora, which establishes itself on (colonizes) particular body sites. The normal microbial flora that usually occupies a site is called the resident flora. Rather than causing disease, resident flora usually protects the body against disease-causing organisms. If disturbed, resident flora promptly reestablishes itself. Microorganisms that colonize the host for hours to weeks but don't establish themselves permanently are called transient flora.

Environmental factors—such as diet, sanitary conditions, air pollution, and hygienic habits—influence which species make up a person's resident flora. For example, lactobacilli are organisms that commonly live in the intestine in people who consume a lot of dairy products. *Hemophilus influenzae* is a bacterium that colonizes the airways of people who have chronic obstructive pulmonary disease.

Under certain conditions, organisms that are part of a person's resident flora may cause disease. For instance, *Streptococcus pyogenes* may inhabit the throat without causing harm, but if the body's defenses are weakened or if the streptococci are a particularly dangerous strain, it may cause streptococcal pharyngitis (throat infection). Similarly, other organisms that are part of the resident flora can become invasive, causing disease in people whose defense barriers are disrupted. For instance, people with colon cancer are vulnerable to invasion by microorganisms that normally live in the intestine; these microorganisms can travel through the blood and infect the heart valves. Exposure to massive doses of radiation can also cause these microorganisms to invade and cause overwhelming infection.

How Infection Develops

Most infectious diseases are caused by microorganisms that invade the body and multiply. Invasion by most microorganisms begins when they adhere to a person's cells. Adherence is a very specific process, involving "lock-and-key" connections between the human cell and the microorganism.▲ Whether the microorganism remains near the invasion site or spreads to distant sites depends on such factors as whether it produces toxins, enzymes, or other substances.

Some microorganisms that invade the body produce toxins, which are poisons that affect nearby or distant cells. Most toxins contain components that bind specifically with molecules on certain cells (target cells), where they cause disease. Diseases in which toxins play a central role include tetanus, toxic shock syndrome, and cholera. A few infectious diseases are caused by toxins produced by microorganisms outside the body. Food poisoning caused by staphylococci is one example.

After invasion, the microorganisms must multiply to produce infection. Then one of three things can happen. First, the microorganisms can continue to multiply and overwhelm the body's defenses. This process can cause enough damage to kill the person. Second, a state of balance can be achieved, producing a chronic infection. Neither the microorganisms nor the person wins this fight. Third, the person, with or without medical treatment, can eradicate the invading microorganism. This process restores health and often provides lasting immunity against another infection by the same microorganism.

Many disease-causing organisms have properties that increase the severity of disease (virulence) and resist the body's defense mechanisms. For instance, some bacteria produce enzymes that break down tissue, allowing the infection to spread faster.

Some microorganisms have ways of blocking the body's defense mechanisms. For example, a microorganism may be able to interfere with the body's production of antibodies or the development of T cells (a type of white blood cell) specifically armed to attack them. Others have outer coats (capsules) that resist being ingested by white blood cells. The fungus *Cryptococcus* actually develops a thicker capsule after it enters the lungs. The reason: Its capsule grows thicker when it is surrounded by carbon dioxide, and there is more carbon dioxide in the lungs than in the soil, where the fungus normally lives. The body's defense mechanisms are thus not as effective when *Cryptococcus* infects the lungs. Some bacteria resist being split open (lysed) by substances circulating in the bloodstream. Some even produce chemicals that counter the effects of antibiotics.

What Type of Relationship Exists?

Three types of relationships can occur between a microorganism and its human host:
- Symbiotic, in which the microorganism and the host both benefit
- Commensal, in which the microorganism gains but the host suffers no harm
- Parasitic, in which the microorganism gains and the host is harmed

Bacteria and fungi account for most microorganisms that have symbiotic and commensal relationships.

How Infection Affects the Body

Certain infections cause changes in the blood, heart, lungs, brain, kidneys, liver, or intestines. By identifying these changes, a doctor can determine that a person has an infection.

Blood Changes

As part of the body's defenses against infection, the white blood cell count commonly is increased. The increase can occur within several hours, largely as a result of the release of white blood cells from stores in the bone marrow. The number of neutrophils, one type of white blood cell, increases first. If an infection persists, the number of monocytes, another type of white blood cell, increases. The number of yet another type of white blood cell, the eosinophil, increases with allergic reactions and parasitic infestations, but usually not with bacterial infections.

Certain infections, such as typhoid fever, actually decrease the white blood cell count. This decrease may occur because the infection is so overwhelming that the bone marrow can't produce white blood cells fast enough to replace the ones lost fighting the invasion.

Anemia may develop from bleeding caused by the infection, by destruction of red blood cells, or

▲ see box, page 814

Infection From Medical Devices

Usually, people think of infection as occurring when microorganisms invade the body and adhere to specific cells. But microorganisms can also adhere to medical devices placed in the body—such as catheters, artificial joints, and artificial heart valves—and begin to form colonies. When the medical device is inserted into the body, the microorganisms can spread, causing infection.

by inhibition of the bone marrow. Severe infection may result in widespread clotting in the blood vessels, a condition called disseminated intravascular coagulation.▲ The best way to reverse this condition is to treat the underlying disease, in this case, the infection. A fall in blood platelet levels without any other changes may also indicate underlying infection.

Heart, Lung, and Brain Changes

Possible heart changes during an infection include an increased heart rate and either an increased or a decreased output of blood. Although most infections increase the pulse rate, some infections, such as typhoid fever, cause a slower pulse rate than would be expected for the severity of the fever. Blood pressure may fall. In an overwhelming infection, blood vessel dilation may lead to a severe drop in blood pressure (septic shock).■

Infection and fever generally make a person breathe faster (increase the respiratory rate), which means more carbon dioxide is transferred from the blood and exhaled, making the blood more acidic. Lung stiffness may increase, which can interfere with breathing and lead to a condition called acute respiratory distress syndrome.★ The breathing muscles in the chest may also become fatigued.

Abnormalities of brain function may occur in severe infection, whether or not a microorganism directly invades the brain. The elderly are particularly prone to confusion. A high fever can cause seizures.

Kidney, Liver, and Intestinal Changes

Kidney changes may range from a small loss of protein in the urine to acute kidney failure. Heart weakening, including the fall in blood pressure, or the direct effects of the microorganism on the kidney may cause these changes.

Many infections may alter liver function, even though the microorganism doesn't directly attack the liver. A common problem is jaundice caused by a backup of bile (cholestatic jaundice).● Jaundice is a worrisome sign when it results from infection.

A serious infection may cause stress ulcers in the upper intestine, leading to bleeding. Usually, only a small blood loss occurs, but in a small percentage of people, a major blood loss may occur.

Body's Defenses Against Infection

The body's defenses against infection include natural barriers, such as the skin; nonspecific mechanisms, such as certain types of white blood cells and fever; and specific mechanisms, such as antibodies. Usually, if an organism gets through the body's natural barriers, the nonspecific and specific defense mechanisms destroy it before it multiplies.

Natural Barriers

Usually, the skin prevents invasion by many microorganisms unless it is physically damaged, for example, by injury, insect bite, or burns. Yet exceptions occur, such as infection with the human papillomavirus, which causes warts.

Other effective natural barriers are the mucous membranes, such as the linings of the airways and the intestine. Typically, mucous membranes are coated with secretions that fight microorganisms.

▲ see page 760

■ see page 859

★ see page 164

● see page 560

For instance, the mucous membranes of the eyes are bathed in tears, which contain an enzyme called lysozyme. This enzyme attacks bacteria and helps protect the eyes from infection.

The airways effectively filter particles in the incoming air. The tortuous passages through the nose, with their walls coated in mucus, tend to remove much of the incoming matter. If an organism reaches the lower airways, the coordinated beating of tiny hairlike processes (cilia) coated with mucus transport it away from the lung. Coughing further helps remove the organism.

The gastrointestinal tract has a series of effective barriers, including acid in the stomach and the antibacterial activity of pancreatic enzymes, bile, and intestinal secretions. The contractions of the intestine (peristalsis) and the normal shedding of cells lining the intestine help remove harmful microorganisms.

The genitourinary tract of a man is protected by the length of the urethra (about 8 inches). Because of this protective mechanism, bacteria seldom enter a man's urethra, unless they are unintentionally placed there by surgical instruments. Women are protected by the acidic environment of the vagina. The flushing effect as the bladder empties is another defense mechanism in both sexes.

People with impaired defense mechanisms are more vulnerable to certain infections.▲ For instance, those whose stomach secretes no acid are particularly vulnerable to tuberculosis and infection with *Salmonella* bacteria. The balance among the different types of organisms in the intestinal resident flora is also important in maintaining the body's defenses. Sometimes, an antibiotic taken for an infection elsewhere in the body can disrupt the balance among resident flora, allowing the number of disease-causing organisms to increase.

Nonspecific Defense Mechanisms

Any injury, including an invasion by bacteria, causes inflammation. Inflammation partly serves to direct certain defense mechanisms to the site of injury or infection. With inflammation, the blood supply increases, and white blood cells can pass out of the blood vessels into the inflamed area more easily. The number of white blood cells in the bloodstream also increases; the bone marrow releases large numbers from storage, then begins to make new ones.

The first type of white blood cells on the scene are neutrophils, which start engulfing the invading organisms and attempt to contain the infection in a small space.■ If the infection continues, monocytes, another type of white blood cell with even greater ability to engulf organisms, arrive in increasing quantities. However, these nonspecific defense mechanisms can be overwhelmed by large numbers of organisms or by other factors that reduce the body's defenses, such as air pollutants (including tobacco smoke).

Fever

Fever, an elevation of body temperature above 100° F. (as measured by an oral thermometer), is actually a protective response to infection and injury. The elevated body temperature enhances the body's defense mechanisms while causing relatively minor discomfort for the person.

Normally, body temperature goes up and down each day. It is lowest at about 6:00 A.M. and highest at about 4:00 to 6:00 P.M. Although normal body temperature is usually said to be 98.6° F., the maximum normal at 6:00 A.M. is 98.9° F., and the maximum normal at 4:00 P.M. is 99.9° F.

The part of the brain called the hypothalamus controls body temperature, and a fever results from an actual resetting of the hypothalamus' thermostat. The body raises its temperature to the new higher thermostat level by moving (shunting) blood from the skin surface to the interior of the body, thus reducing heat loss. Shivering may occur to increase heat production by muscle contraction. The body's efforts to conserve and produce heat continue until blood reaches the hypothalamus at the new higher temperature. Then that temperature is maintained in the normal manner. Later, when the thermostat is reset to its normal level, the body eliminates excess heat through sweating and shunting of blood to the skin. Chills may result when the temperature is lowered.

Fever may follow a pattern in which temperature peaks each day and then returns to normal. Alternatively, fever may be remittent, in which the temperature varies but doesn't return to normal.

▲ see page 933

■ see page 810

Selected Causes of Fever

• Infection, such as bacterial or viral infection

• Cancer

• An allergic reaction

• Hormone disorders, such as pheochromocytoma or hyperthyroidism

• Autoimmune diseases, such as rheumatoid arthritis

• Excessive exercise, especially in hot weather

• Excessive exposure to the sun

• Certain drugs, including anesthetics, antipsychotics, and anticholinergics as well as an overdose of aspirin

• Damage to the hypothalamus (the part of the brain that controls temperature), such as by a brain injury or tumor

Certain people, for example, alcoholics, the very old, and the very young, may have a *drop* in temperature as a response to severe infection.

Substances that cause fever are called pyrogens. Pyrogens may come from inside or outside the body. Examples of pyrogens formed outside the body are microorganisms and the substances they produce, such as toxins. Pyrogens from outside the body actually cause fever by stimulating the body to release its own pyrogens. Pyrogens formed inside the body are usually produced by a type of white blood cell called a monocyte. However, infection isn't the sole cause of fever; fever also may result from inflammation, cancer, or an allergic reaction.

Determining the Cause of Fever

Usually, fever has an obvious cause, such as influenza or pneumonia. But sometimes the cause is subtle, such as infection of the lining of the

▲ see page 1279

heart (bacterial endocarditis). When a person has a fever of at least 101° F. and extensive investigation fails to reveal a cause, a doctor may refer to it as a fever of unknown origin.▲ The potential causes of such a fever include any disorder that raises the body temperature, but the common causes in adults are infections, diseases caused by antibodies against the person's own tissues (autoimmune diseases), and an undiscovered cancer (especially leukemia or lymphoma).

To determine the cause, a doctor begins by asking the patient about present and previous symptoms and diseases, current medications, exposure to infections, recent travel, and so on. The pattern of the fever usually doesn't help with the diagnosis. However, there are some exceptions. For example, a fever that occurs every other day or every third day is typical of malaria.

Recent travel, especially overseas, or exposure to certain materials or animals may give clues to the cause. The southwestern United States is a source of coccidioidomycosis, and the Ohio and Mississippi River valleys are sources of histoplasmosis. A person who has drunk contaminated water (or who has used ice made from contaminated water) may have typhoid fever. Someone working in a meatpacking plant may have brucellosis.

After asking such questions, the doctor performs a thorough physical examination to find a source of infection or evidence of disease. Depending on the severity of the fever and the condition of the patient, the examination may be conducted in the doctor's office or in the hospital.

Blood tests can be used to detect antibodies against an organism, to grow the organism in a culture, and to determine the number of white blood cells. Increased levels of a specific antibody may be noted, which can help identify the invading organism. Increases in the white blood cell count usually indicate infection. The differential count (the proportion of different types of white blood cells) gives further clues. An increase in neutrophils, for instance, suggests an acute bacterial infection. An increase in eosinophils suggests a parasitic infestation—for example, by tapeworm or roundworm.

Ultrasound, computed tomography (CT), and magnetic resonance imaging (MRI) scans can help in diagnosis. Labeled white blood cell scanning can be used to identify areas of infection or inflammation. For such a test, the person receives an injection of white blood cells containing a radioactive marker. Because white blood cells are drawn to areas of infection and because the injected white blood cells have a radioactive marker, the scan can detect an area of infection. If these test results are negative, the doctor may need to obtain a biopsy specimen from the liver, bone marrow, or another suspected site. The specimen is then examined under a microscope.

Treating Fever

Because of the potential benefits of fever, there is some debate as to whether it should be treated routinely. However, a child who has had a seizure resulting from fever (febrile seizure) should be treated. Similarly, an adult with a heart or lung problem usually receives treatment because fever can increase the need for oxygen. Oxygen requirements increase 7 percent for every 1° F. increase in body temperature over 98.6° F. Fever can also cause changes in brain function.

Drugs used to lower body temperature are called antipyretics. The most widely used and effective antipyretics are acetaminophen and the nonsteroidal anti-inflammatory drugs, such as aspirin. However, aspirin isn't given to children and teenagers to treat a fever because it increases the risk of Reye's syndrome,▲ which can be fatal.

Specific Defense Mechanisms

Once an infection develops, the full power of the immune system comes into action.■ The immune system produces several substances that specifically attack the invading organism. For example, antibodies attach to invading organisms and help immobilize them. The antibodies may directly kill the organisms or may make it easier for the white blood cells to target and kill them. Also, the immune system may send cells known as killer T cells (yet another type of white blood cell) to specifically attack the invading organism.

Anti-infective drugs, such as antibiotic, antifungal, or antiviral agents, can aid the body's natural defenses. However, if the immune system is severely impaired, these drugs often aren't effective.

CHAPTER 172

Immunizations to Prevent Infection

Vaccines contain noninfectious parts of bacteria or viruses or whole bacteria or viruses that have been altered so that they can't cause infection. The body responds to a vaccine by creating immune defenses (such as antibodies and white blood cells).★ These defenses then prevent disease when the person is exposed to the infective bacteria and viruses.

Vaccines available today are highly reliable, and most people tolerate them well. However, they don't work in everyone, and they occasionally cause adverse effects.

Some vaccines are given almost routinely—for example, the tetanus toxoid is preferably given to adults every 10 years. Others are given mainly to specific groups of people—the influenza vaccine, for instance, is given to elderly people in nursing homes and to others at high risk for developing the viral infection and its complications. A series of vaccinations are routinely given to children.● Other vaccines are given after exposure to a specific disease—for instance, the rabies vaccine may be given to a person who has been bitten by a dog.

Adults who acquire an infection before they can be vaccinated or whose immune systems don't

---

▲ see page 1280

■ see page 812

★ see page 808

● see box, page 1200

Protecting Against Disease

In the United States, vaccines are available for the following diseases:

- Adenovirus (available only to the United States Armed Forces)
- Anthrax
- Cholera
- Diphtheria
- *Hemophilus influenzae* type b infections (meningitis)
- Hepatitis A
- Hepatitis B
- Influenza
- Japanese encephalitis
- Measles
- Meningococcal meningitis
- Mumps
- Pertussis (whooping cough)
- Plague
- Pneumococcal infection (meningitis, pneumonia)
- Polio
- Rabies
- Rotavirus infection
- Rubella (German measles)
- Tetanus
- Tuberculosis
- Typhoid
- Varicella (chickenpox)
- Yellow fever

respond adequately to an infection may be given immunoglobulin, which consists of a mixture of antibodies.

Common Adult Vaccinations

Depending on their circumstances, adults may be advised to receive vaccines against measles, mumps, rubella, tetanus, hepatitis B, influenza, and pneumococcal infections (especially pneumococcal pneumonia).

Measles, Mumps, and Rubella

Anyone born after 1956 who has never had measles, mumps, or rubella and who has not been immunized with two doses of the vaccine—but who is likely to be exposed to these diseases—should be vaccinated. For example, people beginning college should be vaccinated. Pregnant women and people who are allergic to eggs or the antibiotic neomycin shouldn't be vaccinated.

A person can receive an individual vaccine for measles, mumps, or rubella. However, the combined vaccine is better because anyone who needs protection against one of these infections usually also needs protection against the other two.

Tetanus

Because tetanus infections often are fatal, vaccination is important. A primary series of three injections over a 6-month period should be administered in childhood or to an adult who has not already received the primary series in childhood. A booster dose of the vaccine should be given to adults every 10 years. The tetanus vaccine is available alone or in combination with a diphtheria vaccine administered in a single injection.

Hepatitis B

Anyone who is at high risk for contracting the hepatitis B virus should receive the hepatitis B vaccine. People at high risk include doctors and other health care workers, mortuary workers, people receiving frequent blood transfusions or hemodialysis, injecting drug users, sexually active people, sex partners of known carriers of hepatitis B, and anyone who is exposed to the virus.

Normally, the vaccine is given to a person only once, in a series of three or four injections. However, if a person who has been vaccinated is exposed to the virus, that person's antibody levels should be measured. If these are low, the person may need another vaccination. People with a history of a severe allergic reaction to baker's yeast should not receive the vaccine.

Influenza

People at high risk for developing influenza or its complications should be vaccinated. These people include residents of nursing homes, those over age 65, doctors, and other health care workers. Others at risk include people with chronic heart or lung disease, disorders of metabolism (for example, diabetes), kidney failure, abnormal hemoglobins (for example, sickle cell disease), an impaired immune system, and human immunodeficiency virus (HIV) infection.

Influenza epidemics usually begin in late December or midwinter. Therefore, the best time to obtain the vaccine is during September or October.

Pneumococcal Infection

The vaccine for pneumococcal infection should be given to people who are at high risk for developing influenza, those whose spleen has been removed or doesn't function, those with cancer of the blood cells, those with spinal fluid leakage, and alcoholics.

The vaccine is effective in about two out of three adults, although it is less effective in the elderly. Although the vaccine probably provides lifetime protection, people at high risk are advised to receive the vaccine every 6 years.

Vaccination Before Foreign Travel

Residents of the United States may be required to obtain specific vaccines before traveling to areas that have infectious diseases not normally found in the United States. The Centers for Disease Control and Prevention (CDC), located in Atlanta, Georgia, provides the most up-to-date information on vaccination requirements in their Travelers' Health Section.▲

CHAPTER 173

Anti-infective Drugs

Anti-infective drugs (drugs that combat infection) include antibacterial, antiviral, and antifungal drugs. These drugs are made to be as toxic as possible to the infecting organism and as safe as possible for human cells—that is, they are made to have selective toxicity. Producing drugs with selective toxicity to combat bacteria and fungi is relatively easy, because bacterial and fungal cells are so different from human cells. However, producing a drug that will harm a virus without harming the infected human cell is very difficult, because viruses lose their identity inside a human cell, reprogramming the cell to make virus particles.

Antibiotics

Antibiotics are drugs used to treat bacterial infections. Unfortunately, an increasing number of bacteria are developing resistance to currently available antibiotics. This resistance develops in part because of the overuse of the antibiotics. Therefore, new antibiotics are constantly being developed to combat the increasingly resistant

bacteria. Eventually though, the bacteria will also become resistant to the newer antibiotics.

Antibiotics are classified on the basis of their strength. Bactericidal antibiotics actually kill bacteria; bacteriostatic antibiotics merely prevent them from multiplying, allowing the body to eliminate the remaining bacteria. For most infections, the two types of antibiotic seem equally effective, but if the immune system is impaired or the person has a severe infection, such as bacterial endocarditis or meningitis, a bactericidal antibiotic usually is more effective.

Selecting an Antibiotic

Doctors may choose an antibiotic to treat a particular infection based on their best guess as to which bacterium is responsible. In addition, the laboratory routinely identifies the infecting bacterium, thus helping the doctor choose an anti-

▲ see page 1402

Anti-infective Drugs: Uses and Side Effects

Drug	Common Uses	Side Effects
Antibiotics		
Aminoglycosides Amikacin Gentamicin Kanamycin Neomycin Streptomycin Tobramycin	Infections caused by gram-negative bacteria, such as *Escherichia coli* and *Klebsiella*	• Hearing loss, vertigo, and kidney damage
Cephalosporins Cefaclor Cefadroxil Cefazolin Cefixime Cefoperazone Cefotaxime Cefotetan Cefoxitin Ceftazidime Ceftriaxone Cefuroxime Cephalexin Cephalothin Loracarbef	Wide range of infections	• Gastrointestinal upset and diarrhea • Nausea (if alcohol taken concurrently) • Allergic reactions
Macrolides Azithromycin Clarithromycin Erythromycin Troleandomycin	Streptococcal infections, syphilis, respiratory infections, mycoplasmal infections, Lyme disease	• Nausea, vomiting, and diarrhea (especially at higher doses) • Jaundice
Penicillins Amoxicillin Ampicillin Azlocillin Carbenicillin Cloxacillin Mezlocillin Nafcillin Penicillin Piperacillin Ticarcillin	Wide range of infections Penicillin used for streptococcal infections, syphilis, and Lyme disease	• Gastrointestinal upset and diarrhea • Allergy with serious anaphylactic reactions • Brain and kidney damage (rare)
Polypeptides Bacitracin Colistin Polymyxin B	Ear, eye, or bladder infections Usually applied directly to the eye or inhaled into the lungs; rarely given by injection	• Kidney and nerve damage (when given by injection)
Quinolones Ciprofloxacin Enoxacin Norfloxacin Ofloxacin	Urinary tract infections, bacterial prostatitis, bacterial diarrhea, gonorrhea	• Nausea (rare)

Anti-infective Drugs: Uses and Side Effects (Continued)

Drug	Common Uses	Side Effects
Antibiotics (continued)		
Sulfonamides Mafenide Sulfacetamide Sulfamethizole Sulfamethoxazole Sulfasalazine Sulfisoxazole Trimethoprim- sulfamethoxazole	Urinary tract infections (except sulfacetamide and mafenide); mafenide is used topically for burns	• Nausea, vomiting, and diarrhea • Allergy (including skin rashes) • Crystals in urine • Kidney failure • Decrease in white blood cell count • Sensitivity to sunlight
Tetracyclines Doxycycline Minocycline Tetracycline	Syphilis, chlamydial infections, Lyme disease, mycoplasmal infections, rickettsial infections	• Gastrointestinal upset • Sensitivity to sunlight • Staining of teeth • Potential toxicity to mother and fetus during pregnancy
Miscellaneous antibiotics		
Aztreonam	Infections caused by gram-negative bacteria	• Allergic reactions
Chloramphenicol	Typhoid and other *Salmonella* infections, meningitis	• Severe decrease in white blood cell count (rare)
Clindamycin	Streptococcal infections, respiratory infections, lung abscess	• Severe diarrhea
Ethambutol	Tuberculosis	• Eye damage (reversible if stopped early)
Imipenem	Extremely wide range of infections	• Temporary low blood pressure, seizures
Isoniazid	Tuberculosis	• Serious but reversible liver damage • Allergy
Lincomycin	Streptococcal infections, respiratory infections	• Severe diarrhea
Metronidazole	Vaginitis caused by *Trichomonas* or *Gardnerella*, pelvic and abdominal infections	• Nausea • Headache • Metallic taste • Dark urine
Nitrofurantoin	Urinary tract infections	• Nausea and vomiting • Allergy
Pyrazinamide	Tuberculosis	• Elevated uric acid levels in blood

(continued)

Anti-infective Drugs: Uses and Side Effects (Continued)

Drug	Common Uses	Side Effects
Antibiotics (continued)		
Miscellaneous antibiotics (continued)		
Rifampin	Tuberculosis and leprosy	• Rash • Hepatitis • Red-orange saliva, sweat, tears, and urine
Spectinomycin	Gonorrhea	• Allergy • Fever
Vancomycin	Serious infections resistant to other antibiotics	• Chills and fever (when given intravenously)
Antiviral drugs		
Acyclovir	Herpes simplex, herpes zoster, and chickenpox	• Confusion, seizures, or coma (with intravenous infusion) • Side effects are few when drug is used topically
Amantadine	Influenza (prevention)	• Nervousness • Light-headedness • Slurred speech • Unsteadiness
Didanosine (ddI)	Human immunodeficiency virus infection	• Peripheral nerve damage, inflammation of the pancreas
Foscarnet	Cytomegalovirus, herpes simplex infections	• Kidney damage • Seizures
Ganciclovir	Herpes zoster, herpes simplex, and cytomegalovirus infections	• Toxic to bone marrow precursors of blood cells, resulting in anemia and clotting problems
Idoxuridine	Herpes simplex sores on skin or eyes	• Irritation, pain, and swelling (when applied to eyes or eyelids)
Indinavir	Human immunodeficiency virus infection	• Kidney stones
Interferon-alfa	Hairy cell leukemia, Kaposi's sarcoma, genital warts	• Flulike symptoms (fever, muscle aches, headache, tiredness) • Nausea and diarrhea
Lamivudine (3TC)	Human immunodeficiency virus infection	• Peripheral nerve damage, hair loss
Ribavirin	Respiratory syncytial virus infection	• Breakdown of red blood cells, causing anemia

(continued)

Anti-infective Drugs: Uses and Side Effects (Continued)

Drug	Common Uses	Side Effects
Antiviral drugs (continued)		
Rimantadine	Influenza (prevention)	• Fewer side effects than amantadine
Ritonavir	Human immunodeficiency virus infection	• Nausea, vomiting, diarrhea
Saquinavir	Human immunodeficiency virus infection	—
Stavudine (d4T)	Human immunodeficiency virus infection	• Peripheral nerve damage
Trifluridine	Herpes simplex of the eye	• Stinging of eyes • Swelling of eyelids
Vidarabine	Herpes simplex and herpes zoster Eye infection: Direct application Brain infection: Intravenous infusion	• Nausea and vomiting • Tremor (intravenous infusion) • Liver and bone marrow damage • Side effects are few when drug is used topically
Zalcitabine (ddC)	Human immunodeficiency virus infection	• Peripheral nerve damage
Zidovudine (AZT)	Human immunodeficiency virus infection	• Toxic to bone marrow precursors of blood cells, resulting in anemia and clotting problems
Antifungal drugs		
Amphotericin B	Wide variety of fungal infections	• Chills, fever, headache, and vomiting • Lowered blood potassium levels • Kidney damage
Fluconazole	*Candida* and other fungal infections	• Less liver toxicity than ketoconazole
Flucytosine	*Candida* and *Cryptococcus* infections	• Bone marrow and kidney damage
Griseofulvin	Fungal infections of the skin, hair, and nails	• Rash
Itraconazole	*Candida* and other fungal infections	• Less liver toxicity than ketoconazole
Ketoconazole	*Candida* and other fungal infections	• Blocks production of testosterone and cortisol • Liver toxicity

biotic. However, these tests generally take a day or two to produce results and thus can't be used to guide the initial choice.

Even when a bacterium has been identified and its sensitivity to antibiotics has been determined in the laboratory, the choice of an antibiotic isn't simple. Sensitivities in the laboratory aren't always the same as those in an infected person. The effectiveness of the treatment depends on such factors as how well the drug is absorbed by the bloodstream, how much drug reaches different body fluids, and how quickly the body eliminates the drug. Also, drug selection takes into account the nature and seriousness of the illness, the side effects of the drug, the possibility of allergies or other serious reactions to the drug, and the cost of the drug.

Combinations of antibiotics are sometimes needed to treat severe infections, particularly when the sensitivities of the bacteria to antibiotics aren't yet known. Combinations also are important for certain infections, such as tuberculosis, in which bacteria rapidly develop resistance to a single antibiotic. Sometimes, two antibiotics have a more powerful effect than just one, and such combinations may be used to treat infections caused by bacteria that are difficult to eradicate, such as *Pseudomonas*.

Taking Antibiotics

For severe bacterial infections, antibiotics usually are first given by injection—typically an intravenous injection. When the infection is under control, antibiotics can be taken orally. Antibiotics must be taken until the infecting organism is eliminated from the body, which may be days after the symptoms disappear. Stopping treatment too soon may result in a relapse or may encourage the development of resistant bacteria. For this reason, the antibiotic is usually taken for several days after all evidence of the infection is gone.

Certain antibiotics are used to treat infections with rickettsiae—microorganisms that are similar to both bacteria and viruses.▲ Rickettsiae are smaller than bacteria but larger than viruses. Like viruses, rickettsiae can survive only inside the

cells of another organism, but like bacteria, rickettsiae are vulnerable to antibiotics. Specifically, chloramphenicol and the tetracyclines are the most effective against rickettsial infections.

Antibiotics are used not only to treat infections but also to prevent them. To be effective and to avoid the development of resistance in bacteria, preventive antibiotic therapy must be used for only a short time, and the antibiotic must be potent against the particular bacterium. One example of preventive therapy is taking antibiotics while traveling to prevent traveler's diarrhea. Also, preventive antibiotics are often used in people exposed to someone with meningitis caused by meningococcus because of the risk of infection.

People with abnormal heart valves routinely take preventive antibiotics before surgery, including dental surgery. These people have an increased risk of heart valve infection (endocarditis) from bacteria normally found in the mouth and other parts of the body. Such bacteria may enter the bloodstream during surgery and travel to the damaged heart valves. Preventive antibiotics also may be taken by people whose immune system isn't fully functional, such as people with leukemia, people receiving chemotherapy for cancer, or people with AIDS. Otherwise healthy people undergoing surgery that has a high risk of infection (such as major orthopedic or intestinal surgery) may also take preventive antibiotics.

Unfortunately, antibiotics are often used without a good reason. For instance, they are commonly misused to treat viral illnesses, such as colds and flu.

Side Effects

An antibiotic may cause an allergic reaction, as commonly occurs with penicillin, or may trigger other side effects. For example, aminoglycosides can harm the kidneys and inner ear.

Antibiotic treatment may be continued despite side effects, especially if the antibiotic is the only one effective against the person's infection. A doctor weighs the seriousness of the side effect against the seriousness of the infection.

Antiviral Drugs

Antiviral drugs may work by interfering with any of the processes that a virus goes through to

▲ see page 893

replicate (reproduce): attachment to the cell, uptake into the cell, removal of its viral coat to release its genetic material, and manufacture of new virus particles by the cell.

Because viruses can only replicate inside cells and they use the same metabolic pathways that healthy cells use, antiviral drugs often are more toxic to human cells than are antibiotics. Another problem with antiviral drugs is that viruses may rapidly develop resistance to them.

Antifungal Drugs

Antifungal drugs may be applied directly to a fungal infection of the skin or other surface, such as the vagina or the inside of the mouth. Antifungal drugs may also be taken orally or injected.

Generally, antifungal drugs cause more side effects than do antibiotics. Antifungal drugs also are generally less effective, so fungal infections are difficult to treat and often become long-lasting (chronic). Antifungal therapy often lasts for weeks and must be repeated.

CHAPTER 174

Infections of the Skin and Underlying Tissue

Infections of the skin and the underlying tissue include cellulitis, necrotizing fasciitis, skin gangrene, lymphadenitis, acute lymphangitis, and skin abscesses. Most of these are bacterial infections. Many other skin infections exist, including those caused by fungi,▲ parasites,■ viruses,★ and other bacteria.●

Cellulitis

Cellulitis is a spreading bacterial infection in the skin and the tissues just beneath the skin.

Cellulitis may be caused by many different bacteria; the most common is *Streptococcus*. Streptococci spread rapidly over a wide area because they produce enzymes that prevent tissues from confining the infection. Staphylococci, another type of bacteria, also can cause cellulitis, but it is usually limited to a smaller area. Other bacteria cause cellulitis after certain types of injuries, such as animal bites or skin injuries that occur in freshwater or salt water.

Cellulitis most commonly develops in the legs. Usually the infection appears after the skin has been damaged by an injury, ulceration, athlete's foot, or dermatitis. Areas of the skin that become swollen with fluid (edema) are most vulnerable. Cellulitis tends to recur in or near scars from surgery (for example, surgery for varicose veins).

However, cellulitis also can occur in skin that hasn't been injured.

The infection can spread quickly and can enter the lymph vessels and bloodstream. When this happens, infection can spread throughout the body.

Symptoms and Complications

The first symptoms are redness and tenderness over a small area of skin. The infected skin becomes hot and swollen, and it may look like an orange peel (a condition called peau d'orange). In one form of cellulitis, called erysipelas, the edges of the infected area are raised. Small red spots (petechiae) commonly appear; larger spots caused by bleeding in the skin (ecchymoses) rarely appear. Small fluid-filled blisters (vesicles) or large fluid-filled blisters (bullae) may appear on the infected skin and may rupture.

As the infection spreads to a larger area, nearby lymph nodes may become enlarged and tender.

▲ see page 979

■ see page 982

★ see page 984

● see page 976

Lymph nodes in the groin may be affected by leg infections; lymph nodes in the armpit may be affected by arm infections. Red streaks running between the infection and the nearby lymph nodes may appear on the skin.

A person with cellulitis may have a fever, chills, a rapid heart rate, headache, and low blood pressure and may become confused. Sometimes these symptoms start several hours before any symptoms appear on the skin, but in many cases they don't occur at all.

Occasionally, abscesses may form as a result of cellulitis. Rare but serious complications include the spread of the infection under the skin resulting in tissue death (as in streptococcal gangrene and necrotizing fasciitis) and the spread of the infection through the bloodstream (bacteremia)▲ to other parts of the body. When cellulitis affects the same site repeatedly, nearby lymph vessels may be damaged, causing permanent swelling of the affected tissue.

Diagnosis

The bacteria that cause cellulitis are difficult to identify even when blood sample analysis and skin biopsies (microscopic examination of a tissue sample) are used. However, analysis of samples taken from pus or an open wound may help identify the bacteria. Sometimes, doctors need to perform tests to differentiate cellulitis from a blood clot in the deep veins of the leg (deep vein thrombosis),■ because the symptoms of these disorders are similar.

Treatment

The person starts taking an antibiotic as soon as a doctor diagnoses cellulitis. Also, the affected part of the body is kept immobile and elevated to help reduce swelling. Cool, wet dressings applied to the infected area may relieve discomfort.

For cellulitis caused by streptococci, usually an oral penicillin is prescribed. In severe cases, penicillin may be given intravenously, and clindamycin may be added to the treatment program. People who are allergic to penicillin may take

---

▲ see page 859

■ see page 141

★ see page 882

erythromycin for mild cases or clindamycin for severe cases. For cellulitis caused by staphylococci, a doctor may prescribe dicloxacillin; for severe infections, a doctor may prescribe oxacillin or nafcillin.

Symptoms of cellulitis usually disappear after a few days of antibiotic therapy. However, symptoms often get worse before they get better, probably because with the abrupt death of the bacteria, enzymes that cause tissue damage are released.

If cellulitis recurs repeatedly in the legs, treating skin problems may help. For instance, athlete's foot, which can cause cellulitis, may be treated with antifungal medications. A person with recurring cellulitis also may receive monthly penicillin injections or may take oral penicillin for 1 week each month.

Necrotizing Fasciitis

Necrotizing fasciitis is an extremely severe form of cellulitis that destroys infected tissue under the skin.

A particularly nasty strain of *Streptococcus* causes this infection. It's contracted in the same way as any other cellulitis, but it proceeds to destroy tissue at a rapid pace (some call it "flesh-eating disease"). The skin takes on a violet color, and large fluid-filled blisters (bullae) and gangrene may develop. The person usually feels very ill and has a fever, a rapid heart rate, and mental deterioration ranging from confusion to unconsciousness. Blood pressure may fall because large amounts of fluid are excreted into the infected area.

The treatment for necrotizing fasciitis is antibiotic therapy and surgical removal of the dead tissue. In some cases, an affected arm or leg may have to be amputated. The death rate is about 30 percent. Elderly people, those who have other medical problems, and those in whom the disease has reached an advanced stage have a poor prognosis.

Skin Gangrene

Gangrene is the death of tissue, usually associated with loss of blood supply to the affected area, followed by bacterial invasion.

Gangrene results from an infection caused by clostridia and sometimes by other bacteria. Clostridia are a type of bacteria called anaerobic bacteria, which grow only in the absence of oxygen.★

Clostridia produce gas as they grow, so the infection is sometimes called gas gangrene.

Major injuries—for example, a crushed leg—can interrupt the supply of blood and oxygen to an injured area, creating a situation that allows clostridia to grow. Infection develops within hours or days after the injury. Gangrene also may develop in a surgical wound, particularly when the blood supply to the wound is poor. People with poor circulation are particularly at risk.

Symptoms

The skin may look pale at first, but it becomes red or bronze and finally green. Infection with clostridia also makes the skin warm and swollen. The infection may spread extensively under the skin, often producing large fluid-filled blisters (bullae). The fluid from these blisters looks brown and smells foul. The gas produced by the clostridia often bubbles in the fluid, and the bubbles may make the skin feel crackly when touched.

Within several days, the infection can progress from very mild cellulitis to extensive gangrene that causes shock, kidney failure, delirium, and death. The infection may even progress dramatically within hours, destroying large amounts of skin and muscle.

Diagnosis

Often the symptoms are enough to make a doctor suspect gangrene. X-rays may show gas under the skin. Computed tomography (CT) scans and magnetic resonance imaging (MRI) can help determine the amount of gas and the extent of the tissue destruction. Fluid may be taken from the wound and cultured in the laboratory to confirm that the organism causing the infection is *Clostridium*. However, surgery to remove dead tissue or to amputate a limb is often needed before a doctor can be certain which organism is causing the infection.

Treatment and Prognosis

When gangrene is suspected, an antibiotic is usually given as soon as fluid samples have been taken from the wound but before the test results are available. Antibiotics that destroy a wide spectrum of bacteria are usually chosen, although penicillin is all that is needed to eliminate clostridia.

In addition to prescribing antibiotics, a doctor surgically removes destroyed tissue. Sometimes,

especially when circulation is poor, part or all of a limb must be amputated to prevent the spread of the infection.

High-pressure (hyperbaric) oxygen therapy may also be used to treat extensive skin gangrene. With this treatment, the person is placed in a chamber containing high-pressure oxygen, which helps to kill clostridia.

Despite treatment, about one out of five people with skin gangrene dies.

Lymphadenitis

Lymphadenitis is inflammation of one or more lymph nodes.

An infection from any type of organism—bacteria, viruses, protozoa, rickettsiae, or fungi—can cause lymphadenitis. Typically, the infection spreads to a lymph node from a skin, ear, nose, or eye infection.

Symptoms and Diagnosis

Infected lymph nodes enlarge and are usually tender and painful. Sometimes the skin over the infected nodes looks red and feels warm.

Usually, the cause of lymphadenitis is an obvious nearby infection. When the cause can't be found easily, a biopsy (removal and microscopic examination of a tissue sample) may be needed.

Treatment and Prognosis

Treatment depends on the organism causing the infection. For a bacterial infection, an antibiotic usually is given intravenously or orally. Warm compresses may help relieve the pain in inflamed lymph nodes. Usually, once the infection has been treated, the lymph nodes slowly shrink, and the pain subsides. Sometimes, the enlarged nodes remain firm but no longer feel tender.

Acute Lymphangitis

Acute lymphangitis is inflammation of one or more lymphatic vessels and is usually caused by a streptococcal infection.

The lymphatic vessels are small channels that carry lymph from tissue to the lymph nodes and throughout the body.▲ Streptococci bacteria usually enter these vessels from a scrape, a wound,

---

▲ see box, page 809

or an infection (typically cellulitis) in an arm or leg. Red, irregular, warm, tender streaks develop under the skin in the affected arm or leg. The streaks usually stretch from the infected area toward a group of lymph nodes, such as those in the groin or armpit. The lymph nodes become enlarged and feel tender.

The person commonly experiences a fever, chills, rapid heart rate, and headache. Sometimes these symptoms occur before the skin changes appear. The spread of the infection from the lymph system into the bloodstream can cause infection throughout the body, often with startling speed. Ulcers may form in the skin over the infected lymph vessel.

A blood test may show that the number of white blood cells has increased to fight the infection. The organisms causing the infection usually can't be sampled and cultured in the laboratory unless they have spread through the bloodstream or can be taken from pus or an open wound.

Most people are cured quickly with antibiotics that kill staphylococci and streptococci, such as dicloxacillin, nafcillin, or oxacillin.

Skin Abscesses

Skin abscesses (cutaneous abscesses) are collections of pus caused by a bacterial infection.

Abscesses usually form when a minor skin injury allows bacteria normally present on the skin to penetrate and cause an infection.▲ A skin abscess appears as a swollen, painful, tender area that may feel as though it is filled with thick fluid.

Bacteria may spread from the abscess to infect the surrounding tissue, causing cellulitis. Bacteria also may infect nearby lymph vessels and the lymph nodes into which they drain, causing the nodes to swell. The person may have a fever.

Treatment

A doctor may treat an abscess by cutting it open and draining the pus. For this procedure, a doctor uses a local anesthetic, such as lidocaine. After draining the abscess, the doctor probes it to make sure all of the pockets of pus have been drained. Any remaining pus is washed out with a salt solution. Sometimes the drained abscess is packed with gauze, which is removed 24 to 48 hours later. Applying mild heat and elevating the affected area may speed healing.

If the abscess is completely drained, antibiotics usually aren't needed. They are needed, however, if the infection has spread or if the abscess is on the middle or upper part of the face because of the high risk that the infection will spread to the brain. Antibiotics that kill staphylococci and streptococci—such as nafcillin, dicloxacillin, and oxacillin—may be used.

CHAPTER 175

Abscesses

An abscess is an accumulation of pus, usually caused by a bacterial infection.

When bacteria invade healthy tissue, the infection spreads through the area. Some cells die and disintegrate, leaving spaces where fluid and infected cells accumulate. White blood cells, the body's defenders against infection, move into these spaces, and after engulfing bacteria, they die. The dead white blood cells accumulate as

▲ see below

pus, a creamy substance that fills the area. As pus collects, healthy tissue is pushed aside. Tissue eventually grows around the abscess and walls it off; this is the body's attempt to prevent the further spread of infection. If an abscess ruptures internally, the infection may spread either inside the body or under the skin surface, depending on the location of the abscess.

A bacterial infection may lead to an abscess in several ways. For example, a puncture wound from a dirty needle may force bacteria under the skin. Or bacteria may spread from an infection elsewhere in the body. Also, bacteria that normally live on the body but cause no harm can sometimes cause an abscess. The chances of an abscess forming increase if there is dirt or a foreign body in the infected area; if the area of bacterial invasion has a poor blood supply, as occurs in diabetes; or if the person's immune system is impaired, as occurs in AIDS.

Abscesses can develop anywhere in the body, including the lungs,▲ mouth,■ rectum,★ and muscles. They are fairly common in or just below the skin, especially on the face.

Symptoms and Diagnosis

Where an abscess is located and whether it interferes with the function of an organ or a nerve determine its symptoms. Symptoms can include pain, tenderness, heat, swelling, redness, and possibly a fever. An abscess that forms just under the skin usually appears as a visible bump. When an abscess is about to rupture, it develops a whitish center as the overlying skin grows thinner. An abscess deep inside the body often grows quite large before it causes symptoms. Unnoticed, a deep abscess is likely to spread infection throughout the body.

Doctors can easily recognize an abscess on or just beneath the skin but often miss a deep abscess. When a person has such an abscess, blood tests often reveal an abnormally large number of white blood cells. X-rays, ultrasound scanning, computed tomography (CT), or magnetic resonance imaging (MRI) can be used to determine the size and position of an abscess. Because abscesses and tumors often cause the same symptoms and produce similar images, a definitive diagnosis sometimes requires that a doctor obtain a sample of the pus or surgically remove the abscess for examination under a microscope.

Treatment

Often an abscess heals without treatment by rupturing and discharging its contents. Occasionally, the abscess disappears slowly without rupturing as the body destroys the infection and absorbs the debris. The abscess may leave a hard lump.

An abscess can be pierced and drained to relieve pain and promote healing. To drain a large abscess, a doctor must probe it to break down the walls and release all the pus. When drained, large abscesses leave a large empty space (dead space), which a doctor may temporarily pack with gauze. Sometimes, inserting temporary artificial drains (usually thin plastic tubes) is necessary.

Because an abscess doesn't have a blood supply, antibiotics usually aren't helpful. After an abscess has been drained, antibiotics may be prescribed to prevent a recurrence. Antibiotics also are taken when an abscess spreads infection to other parts of the body. A laboratory analysis of bacteria from the pus helps a doctor select the most effective antibiotic.

Abdominal Abscesses

Abscesses may form below the diaphragm, in the middle of the abdomen, in the pelvis, or behind the abdominal cavity. Abscesses also may form in or around any abdominal organ, such as the kidneys, spleen, pancreas, or liver, or in the prostate gland. Often, abdominal abscesses are caused by injury, infection or perforation of the intestine, or infection of another abdominal organ.

An **abscess below the diaphragm** may form when infected fluid, for example, from a ruptured appendix, is moved upward by the pressure of abdominal organs and by the suction created when the diaphragm moves during breathing. Symptoms may include a cough, painful breathing, and pain in one shoulder—an example of referred pain that occurs because the shoulder and the diaphragm share the same nerves and the brain incorrectly interprets the source of the pain.

Abscesses in the midabdomen may result from a ruptured appendix, a perforated large intestine, inflammatory bowel disease, or diverticular disease. The abdomen is usually painful in the area of the abscess.

Pelvic abscesses result from the same disorders that cause abscesses in the midabdomen and from gynecologic infections. Symptoms may include abdominal pain, diarrhea from intestinal irritation, and an urgent or frequent need to urinate caused by bladder irritation.

Abscesses behind the abdominal cavity (called retroperitoneal abscesses) lie behind the perito-

---

▲ see page 200

■ see page 466

★ see page 501

neum, the membrane that lines the abdominal cavity and organs. The causes, which are similar to those of other abscesses in the abdomen, include inflammation of the appendix (appendicitis) and of the pancreas (pancreatitis). Pain, usually in the lower back, worsens when the person moves the leg at the hip.

Abscesses in the kidneys are caused either by bacteria from an infection traveling to the kidneys through the bloodstream or by a urinary tract infection traveling to the kidney and then spreading to the kidney tissue. Abscesses on the surface of the kidneys (perinephric abscesses) are nearly always caused by the rupture of an abscess inside the kidney, which spreads the infection to the surface and the surrounding tissue. Symptoms of a kidney abscess include a fever, chills, and pain in the lower back. Urination may be painful, and sometimes the urine is bloody.

Abscesses in the spleen are caused by an infection traveling through the bloodstream to the spleen, by an injury to the spleen, or by the spread of an infection from a nearby abscess, such as one below the diaphragm. Pain may occur in the left side of the abdomen, the back, or the left shoulder.

Abscesses inside the pancreas typically form after an attack of acute pancreatitis. Symptoms such as fever, abdominal pain, nausea, and vomiting often begin a week or more after a person recovers from pancreatitis.

Liver abscesses may be caused by bacteria or by amebas (single-celled parasites). Amebas from an intestinal infection reach the liver through the lymphatic vessels. Bacteria can reach the liver from an infected gallbladder; a penetrating or blunt wound; an infection in the abdomen, such as a nearby abscess; or an infection carried by the bloodstream from elsewhere in the body. Symptoms of liver abscesses include loss of appetite, nausea, and a fever. A person may or may not have abdominal pain.

Prostate abscesses usually result from a urinary tract infection that leads to a prostate gland infection (prostatitis). These abscesses most com-

monly occur in men between ages 40 and 60. Typically, a man with a prostate abscess experiences painful, frequent, or difficult urination. Less commonly, he feels internal pain at the base of the penis and notices pus or blood in his urine.

Diagnosis and Treatment

In nearly all cases of abdominal abscesses, the pus must be drained, either by surgery or by a needle inserted through the skin. To guide the placement of the needle, a doctor uses computed tomography (CT) or ultrasound scanning. Laboratory analysis of the pus identifies the infecting organism so that the most effective antibiotic can be selected.

Head and Neck Abscesses

Abscesses commonly develop in the head and neck, particularly behind the throat and in the salivary glands of the cheeks (parotid glands). Abscesses can also develop in the brain.▲

Abscesses behind and to the side of the throat (pharyngomaxillary abscesses) usually result from throat infections, including infections of the tonsils or adenoids.■ Children are more likely than adults to develop a throat abscess.★ An abscess can also form within a lymph node located beside the throat (a parapharyngeal abscess).● Less commonly, these abscesses come from a nearby infection, such as a tooth abscess or a salivary gland infection. Along with having a fever and sore throat, the person feels ill. Opening the mouth may be difficult. The infection may spread, causing neck swelling. If the abscess damages the carotid arteries in the neck, clotting or massive bleeding can result.

An abscess also may form at the outlet of one of the parotid glands. The abscess is usually caused by an infection spreading from the mouth. This type of abscess typically occurs in elderly or chronically ill people who have a dry mouth resulting from a low fluid intake or from certain drugs, such as antihistamines. Symptoms include pain and swelling in one cheek, fever, and chills that begin suddenly.

Muscle Abscesses

Abscesses occasionally form deep in muscles. These abscesses may be caused by bacteria spreading from a nearby infection in a bone or

▲ see page 377

■ see page 1018

★ see page 1265

● see page 1019

other tissue or spreading through the bloodstream from a distant part of the body.

Pyomyositis is a disorder in which muscle becomes infected by pus-producing bacteria that often cause abscesses to form. Pyomyositis is more common among people in the tropics and occurs in people with impaired immune systems. The muscles most commonly affected are those in the thighs, buttocks, and upper arms and those around the shoulders. Symptoms include cramping pain followed by swelling, mild fever, and increasing discomfort, especially when the infected muscle is moved.

Hand Abscesses

Abscesses in the hands are fairly common and usually result from injury. An abscess in the soft

pad at the tip of a finger nearly always results from a minor injury, such as a splinter or needle prick. Severe pain, warmth, and redness develop over the abscess, often with swelling of nearby lymph nodes in the arm. Infection of the bone underneath the abscess may cause more pain.

Abscesses may occur around the tendons that run along the inside of the fingers. This type of abscess is caused by an injury that penetrates one of the creases on the palm side of a finger. Infection and pus form around the tendon and rapidly destroy tissue. The gliding mechanism of the tendon becomes damaged, so the finger can barely move. Symptoms include swelling and inflammation of the finger, tenderness over the tendon sheath, and extreme pain when trying to move the finger. Swollen lymph nodes near the abscess and fever are common.

CHAPTER 176

Bacteremia and Septic Shock

Bacteremia, the presence of bacteria in the bloodstream, is common and usually causes no symptoms. Most bacteria that enter the bloodstream are rapidly removed by white blood cells.▲ Sometimes, however, there are too many bacteria to be removed easily, and an infection called sepsis develops, causing severe symptoms. In some cases, sepsis leads to a life-threatening condition called septic shock.

Bacteremia and Sepsis

Bacteremia is the presence of bacteria in the bloodstream. Sepsis is an infection in the bloodstream.

Very mild, temporary bacteremia may occur when a person clenches his jaw, because bacteria living on the gums around the teeth are forced into the bloodstream. Bacteria often enter the bloodstream from the intestine, but they are rapidly removed as the blood passes through the liver.

Sepsis becomes more likely when there is an infection in the body, such as in the lungs, abdomen, urinary tract, or skin. Sepsis can also result when surgery is performed on an infected area or on a part of the body where bacteria normally

grow, such as the intestine. The insertion of any foreign object—such as an intravenous catheter, a urinary catheter, or drainage tube—may also cause sepsis. The likelihood of sepsis increases the longer the object is left in place. Sepsis commonly occurs in injecting drug users. It is also more likely to occur in a person whose immune system isn't functioning properly—for example, a person receiving anticancer drugs.

Symptoms

Because the body can usually clear small numbers of bacteria quickly, temporary bacteremia rarely causes symptoms. However, once sepsis becomes established, symptoms include shaking, chills, fever, weakness, nausea, vomiting, and diarrhea.

Sepsis may cause infections in sites throughout the body (called metastatic infection) if not treated quickly. Infections may settle in the lining of the brain (meningitis), in the sac around the heart (pericarditis), in the inside lining of the

▲ see page 810

heart (endocarditis), in bones (osteomyelitis), and in the large joints. An abscess (a collection of pus)▲ may occur almost anywhere.

Diagnosis

Sepsis is the likely diagnosis when a person with an infection anywhere in the body suddenly develops a high fever. If the person has sepsis, usually the number of white cells in the blood is greatly increased. Blood cultures are used to grow and identify the infecting organism. However, bacteria may not grow in a blood culture, particularly if the person is taking antibiotics. Samples for culture are also taken from material coughed up from the lungs (sputum), from urine, from wounds, and from sites where catheters enter the body.

Treatment and Prognosis

Bacteremia caused by surgery or by the insertion of a catheter into the urinary tract usually requires no treatment, as long as the catheter is removed quickly. However, before undergoing such procedures, people at risk of developing serious infections—those with heart valve disease or immune system deficiencies, for example—generally are given antibiotics to prevent sepsis.

Sepsis is very serious, and the risk of death is high. A doctor must begin treatment with antibiotics immediately, even before laboratory culture results that identify the type of bacteria causing the infection are available. A delay in starting antibiotic treatment greatly decreases the chances of survival. Initially, a doctor bases the choice of antibiotic on which bacteria are most likely to be present. This depends on where the infection started—the urinary tract, mouth, lungs, intestine, or another site. Often, two antibiotics are given together to increase the chances of killing the bacteria. Later, when the culture results are available, the doctor can substitute the antibiotic that is most effective against the specific bacteria causing the infection. In some cases, surgery may

---

▲ see page 856

■ see page 1217

★ see page 812

● see page 812

be needed to eliminate the source of the infection, such as an abscess.

Septic Shock

Septic shock is a condition in which blood pressure falls to life-threateningly low levels as a result of sepsis.

Septic shock occurs most often in newborns,■ people over age 50, and people with a compromised immune system. Septic shock is more of a risk when white blood cell counts are low, as occurs in people who have cancer, who are taking anticancer drugs, or who have chronic diseases, such as diabetes or cirrhosis.

Septic shock is caused by toxins produced by certain bacteria★ and by cytokines, which are substances made by the immune system to fight an infection.● Blood vessels widen (dilate), causing the blood pressure to fall despite increases in both the heart rate and the volume of blood pumped. The blood vessels also may become leaky, allowing fluid to escape from the bloodstream into tissues and cause swelling. Blood flow to the vital organs, particularly the kidneys and brain, is reduced. Later, the blood vessels constrict in an attempt to raise blood pressure, but the heart's output of blood decreases, so that blood pressure remains very low.

Symptoms and Diagnosis

Often the first indications of septic shock, even 24 hours or more before blood pressure falls, are reduced mental alertness and confusion. These symptoms are caused by reduced blood flow to the brain. The output of blood from the heart increases, but the blood vessels dilate, thus lowering the blood pressure. Often, the person breathes very fast, so that the lungs blow off excess carbon dioxide, and the level of carbon dioxide in the blood decreases. Early symptoms may include a shaking chill; a rapid rise in temperature; warm, flushed skin; a bounding pulse; and blood pressure that rises and falls. Urinary flow decreases despite the increased output of blood by the heart. In later stages, the body temperature often falls below normal. As shock worsens, several organs may fail, including the kidneys (causing low urine output), the lungs (causing breathing difficulties and low levels of oxygen in the blood), and the heart (causing fluid retention and swelling). Blood clots may form inside blood vessels.

Blood tests show high or low levels of white blood cells, and the number of platelets may decrease. Levels of metabolic waste products (such as urea nitrogen)—measured easily in the blood—keep rising if the kidneys fail. An electrocardiogram (ECG) may show irregularities in heart rhythm, indicating inadequate blood supply to the heart muscle. Blood cultures are taken to identify the infecting bacteria.

Treatment and Prognosis

As soon as symptoms of septic shock are apparent, the person is admitted to an intensive care unit for treatment. Large amounts of fluid are given intravenously to raise the blood pressure, which is monitored carefully. Dopamine or norepinephrine may be given to constrict blood vessels, so that blood pressure is raised and blood flow to the brain and heart is increased. If lung failure develops, the person may need a mechanical ventilator.

High doses of intravenous antibiotics are given as soon as blood specimens have been taken for laboratory cultures. Until the laboratory identifies the infecting bacteria, two antibiotics usually are given together to increase the chances of killing the bacteria.

Any abscesses are drained, and any catheters that may have started the infection are removed. Surgery may be performed to remove any dead tissue, such as gangrenous tissue of the intestine. Despite all efforts, more than one fourth of the people with septic shock die.

CHAPTER 177

Bacillary Infections

Bacilli are a type of bacteria classified according to their distinctive rod-like shape. Bacteria are either spherical (coccal), rod-like (bacillary), or spiral/helical (spirochetal) in shape. The exact shape is dictated by the bacterium's cell wall, a rigid, complex, layered structure.

Although bacteria are classified in part by their distinctive shape, most bacteria—including bacilli—also are classified as either gram-positive or gram-negative depending on their color after a stain, called the Gram's stain, is applied during laboratory testing. Bacteria that stain blue are gram-positive, whereas those that stain pink are gram-negative. However, the classification of bacteria as gram-negative or gram-positive also corresponds to certain characteristics of the bacteria's outer wall, the kind of infections produced by the bacteria, and the types of antibiotics that are likely to kill the bacteria.

Gram-Positive Bacillary Infections

In the bacterial world, gram-positive bacteria are a minority. They are generally susceptible to penicillin and are usually slow to develop resistance to this antibiotic. Some gram-positive bacteria (such as certain streptococci) can penetrate deep into the tissue, whereas others inflict harm by producing extremely poisonous substances (for example, the toxins produced by *Clostridium botulinum*). Three infections caused by gram-positive bacilli are erysipelothricosis, listeriosis, and anthrax.

Erysipelothricosis

Erysipelothricosis is a slowly developing skin infection that is caused by the bacterium Erysipelothrix rhusiopathiae.

Although *Erysipelothrix rhusiopathiae* grows primarily on dead or decaying matter, it can also infect insects, shellfish, fish, birds, and mammals. People usually become infected after an occupational injury, typically a penetrating wound that occurs while handling animal matter (such as meat, poultry, fish, shellfish, bones, or shells).

Symptoms and Diagnosis

Within a week of becoming infected with *Erysipelothrix rhusiopathiae*, a raised, purplish-red, hard area appears on the skin at the site of injury. Other symptoms include itching, burning, and swelling around the affected area. The hand is the

Shapes of Bacteria

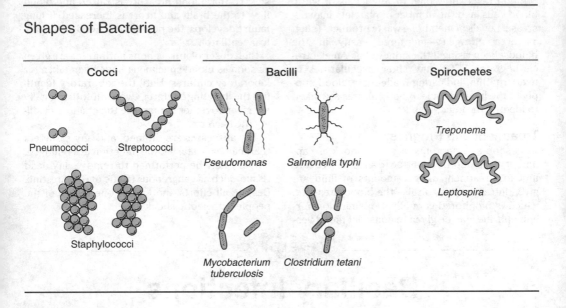

| Cocci | Bacilli | Spirochetes |

Cocci: Pneumococci, Streptococci, Staphylococci

Bacilli: Pseudomonas, Salmonella typhi, Mycobacterium tuberculosis, Clostridium tetani

Spirochetes: Treponema, Leptospira

most common site of infection, and swelling may limit its use. The affected area may slowly enlarge. Although the infection generally resolves even without treatment, pain and disability may remain for 2 to 3 weeks. In rare cases, the infection can spread to the bloodstream and affect either the joints or the heart valves.

A doctor bases the diagnosis on the symptoms and the circumstances that caused the infection. The diagnosis may be confirmed by sending a sample of skin scraped from the outer edge of the affected area for culture.

Treatment

A single dose of injected penicillin or a 1-week course of oral erythromycin cures the infection. If the joints or heart valves are infected, longer treatment with intravenous antibiotics is required.

Listeriosis

Listeriosis, a disease caused by Listeria monocytogenes, *varies in symptoms according to the site of infection and the age of the infected person.*

▲ see page 373

Listeria bacteria are found worldwide in the environment and in the intestines of birds, spiders, crustaceans, and nonhuman mammals. In humans, listeriosis may affect almost any organ of the body. Newborns, people over age 70, and those with a suppressed or impaired immune system are most susceptible to listeriosis. Most infections occur between July and August. Listeriosis is usually acquired by consuming contaminated dairy products or raw vegetables.

Symptoms and Diagnosis

In adults, the most common form of listeriosis is meningitis, an infection of the membranes covering the brain and spinal cord (meninges).▲ Brain abscesses may form in up to 20 percent of these cases. Meningitis produces fever and a stiff neck; if the person isn't treated, confusion, coma, and death can occur.

Listeria can sometimes infect the eyes, making them red and painful. The infection then can spread to the lymph nodes, blood, and meninges. In rare instances, *Listeria* infection of the heart valves can produce heart failure.

A doctor may suspect listeriosis based on the person's symptoms. To make a definite diagnosis, a sample of tissue or body fluid is taken and sent to a laboratory for culture. Antibodies against *Listeria* can also be measured in a blood sample.

Treatment

Penicillin generally cures listeriosis. If the infection has affected the heart valves, a second antibiotic, such as tobramycin, may also be given. Eye infections can be treated with oral erythromycin.

Anthrax

Anthrax is a disease caused by the bacterium Bacillus anthracis, *which can infect the skin, lungs, and gastrointestinal tract.*

Anthrax is a highly contagious and potentially fatal disease. It usually spreads to people from animals, especially cows, goats, and sheep. Dormant bacteria (spores) can live in the soil and in animal products (such as wool) for decades. Although infection in people is usually through the skin, it can also occur from eating contaminated meat or inhaling spores or bacteria.

Symptoms and Diagnosis

Symptoms may appear 12 hours to 5 days after exposure to the bacteria. A skin infection begins as a red-brown bump that enlarges, with considerable swelling at the edges. The bump blisters and hardens, then the center breaks open and oozes a clear fluid before forming a black scab (eschar). Lymph nodes in the affected area may swell, and the person may feel ill, sometimes experiencing muscle aches, headache, fever, nausea, and vomiting.

Pulmonary anthrax (woolsorter's disease) results from inhaling the spores of the anthrax bacterium. The spores multiply in the lymph nodes near the lung. The lymph nodes then start to break down and bleed, spreading the infection to nearby structures in the chest. Infected fluid builds up in the lungs and in the space between the lungs and the chest wall. At first, the symptoms are vague and similar to those of influenza. However, the fever worsens, and in a few days severe breathing difficulties develop, followed by shock and coma. Infection of the brain and its meninges (meningoencephalitis) may also occur. Even with early treatment, this form of anthrax is almost always fatal.

Gastrointestinal anthrax is rare. The bacteria can grow into the wall of the intestine and release a toxin that causes extensive bleeding and tissue death. The infection can be fatal if it spreads into the bloodstream.

Knowing that a person has had contact with animals helps a doctor make the diagnosis. To diagnose a pulmonary infection, a doctor may obtain a sputum sample for culture; however, the laboratory isn't always able to identify the bacteria. Sometimes treatment is started when anthrax is suspected but laboratory confirmation isn't yet available.

Prevention and Treatment

People at high risk of contracting anthrax—such as veterinarians, laboratory technicians, and employees of textile mills that process animal hair—can be vaccinated.

An anthrax skin infection is treated with penicillin injections or with oral tetracycline or erythromycin. Lung infections require intravenous penicillin. Other antibiotics also may be given. Corticosteroids may also be used to reduce lung inflammation. If treatment is delayed (usually because the diagnosis isn't made promptly), death is likely.

Gram-Negative Bacillary Infections

The distinctive feature of gram-negative bacteria is the presence of a double membrane surrounding each bacterial cell. Although all bacteria have an inner cell membrane, gram-negative bacteria have a unique outer membrane. This outer membrane excludes certain drugs and antibiotics from penetrating the cell, partially accounting for why gram-negative bacteria are generally more resistant to antibiotics than are gram-positive bacteria.

The outer membrane of gram-negative bacteria is rich in a molecule called lipopolysaccharide. If gram-negative bacteria enter the bloodstream, lipopolysaccharide can trigger a cascade of events, including high fever and a drop in blood pressure. For this reason, lipopolysaccharide is often referred to as an endotoxin.

Gram-negative bacteria have a great facility for exchanging genetic material (DNA) among strains of the same species and even among different species. This means that if a gram-negative bacterium either undergoes a genetic change (mutation) or acquires genetic material that confers resistance to an antibiotic, the bacterium may later share its

Some Examples of Gram-Negative Bacilli

Bartonella	Proteus
Brucella	Providencia
Campylobacter	Pseudomonas
Enterobacter	Salmonella
Escherichia	Serratia
Francisella	Shigella
Hemophilus	Vibrio
Klebsiella	Yersinia
Morganella	

DNA with another strain of bacteria and the second strain can become resistant as well.

Hemophilus Infections

Hemophilus *infections are infections caused by* Hemophilus *bacteria.*

Hemophilus bacteria grow in the upper airways of children and adults but rarely cause disease. The strain that most commonly causes disease is *Hemophilus influenzae.* It can cause meningitis (infection of the lining of the brain and spinal cord), bacteremia (a bloodstream infection), septic arthritis (infected joints), pneumonia, bronchitis, otitis media (middle ear infection), conjunctivitis (eye infection), sinusitis, and acute epiglottitis (infection of the area just above the voice box). Although these infections may occur in adults, they are more common in children.

Other *Hemophilus* bacteria may cause respiratory tract infections, infections of the heart (endocarditis), and brain abscesses. *Hemophilus ducreyi* causes chancroid, a sexually transmitted disease.▲

▲ see page 942

■ see box, page 1200

Children are routinely immunized with a vaccine against *Hemophilus influenzae* type b to prevent meningitis caused by that organism.■

Brucellosis

Brucellosis (undulant, Malta, Mediterranean, or Gibraltar fever) is an infection caused by Brucella *bacteria.*

Brucellosis can be contracted by having direct contact with the secretions and excretions of infected animals; by drinking the unpasteurized milk of cows, sheep, or goats; or by eating dairy products (such as butter and cheese) that contain living *Brucella* organisms. Transmission from person to person is rare. The disease is most prevalent in rural areas and is an occupational illness of meat packers, veterinarians, farmers, and livestock producers.

Symptoms and Complications

Symptoms begin 5 days to several months—usually 2 weeks—after infection with the bacteria and vary, especially in the early stages. The disease can start suddenly with chills and fever, severe headache, pains, an ill feeling, and occasionally diarrhea. The disease also can start insidiously with a mild sick feeling, muscle pain, headache, and pain in the back of the neck. As the disease progresses, a fever of 104° to 105° F. occurs in the evening; the temperature subsides gradually, becoming normal or nearly normal each morning, when profuse sweating develops.

Typically, this intermittent fever lasts 1 to 5 weeks and is followed by a 2- to 14-day period in which symptoms are greatly diminished or absent. Then the fever returns. This pattern may occur only once, but some people develop chronic brucellosis and experience repeated waves of fever and remission over months or years.

After the initial phase, the symptoms usually include severe constipation, appetite loss, weight loss, abdominal pain, joint pain, headache, backache, weakness, irritability, insomnia, depression, and emotional instability. Later, the lymph nodes, spleen, and liver may enlarge.

People with uncomplicated brucellosis usually recover in 2 to 3 weeks. Complications are rare but may include infections of the heart, brain, and lining of the brain, as well as inflammation of the nerves, testes, gallbladder, liver, and bone. Persistent cases usually lead to prolonged ill health, but the disease is rarely fatal.

Diagnosis

A doctor may suspect brucellosis in a person who has been exposed to infected animals or animal products, such as unpasteurized milk. The diagnosis may be based on taking a sample of blood—or less often, a sample of cerebrospinal fluid, urine, or tissue—from an infected person and sending it to a laboratory for culture. Blood tests also may reveal high levels of antibodies to the infecting bacteria.

Prevention and Treatment

Avoiding unpasteurized milk and cheese that hasn't been aged helps prevent *Brucella* infections. People handling animals or animal carcasses should wear goggles or glasses and rubber gloves and should cover any cuts in the skin. Eliminating infected animals and vaccinating young healthy animals can help prevent the spread of infection.

Relapses are common when only a single antibiotic is used, so a combination of antibiotics is often prescribed. Doxycycline or tetracycline and daily injections of streptomycin lower the risk of a relapse. Children under age 8 can be given trimethoprim-sulfamethoxazole and either streptomycin or rifampin, because tetracycline might cause tooth damage. In severe cases, corticosteroids such as prednisone also are used. A person with severe muscle pains may need a strong pain reliever, such as codeine.

Tularemia

Tularemia (rabbit fever, deer fly fever) is a bacterial infection caused by the organism Francisella tularensis.

People become infected with *Francisella tularensis* by eating or touching infected animals. The bacterium can penetrate unbroken skin. The disease is also transmitted when bacteria in animal tissues become airborne and are inhaled, as well as by infected ticks and similar blood-sucking pests.

Types of Tularemia

There are four types of tularemia. In the most common type **(ulceroglandular type)**, ulcers develop on the hands and fingers, and lymph nodes on the same side as the infection swell. The second type **(oculoglandular type)** infects the eye, causing redness and swelling along with swollen lymph nodes; this type probably results from touching the eye with an infected finger. In the third type **(glandular type)**, lymph nodes swell but no ulcers develop, suggesting that the source is ingested bacteria. The fourth type **(typhoidal type)** leads to a high fever, abdominal pain, and exhaustion. If tularemia reaches the lung, pneumonia can result.

Hunters, butchers, farmers, fur handlers, and laboratory workers are most commonly infected. In the winter, most cases result from contact with wild rabbits (especially while skinning them). In the summer, infection usually results from handling infected animals or being bitten by infected ticks or similar pests. Rarely, tularemia may be caused by eating undercooked meat or drinking contaminated water. Person-to-person transmission hasn't been reported.

Symptoms

The symptoms start suddenly 1 to 10 days—usually 2 to 4 days—after contact with the bacterium. Initial symptoms include headaches, chills, nausea, vomiting, a fever of up to 104° F., and severe exhaustion. Extreme weakness, recurring chills, and profuse drenching sweats develop. In 24 to 48 hours, an inflamed blister appears at the infection site—usually the finger, arm, eye, or roof of the mouth—except in the glandular and typhoidal types of tularemia. The blister rapidly fills with pus and opens to form an ulcer. Single ulcers commonly appear on the arms or legs, but many ulcers usually appear in the mouth or eye. Typically, only one eye is affected. Lymph nodes around the ulcer enlarge and may produce pus, which later drains.

People with tularemic pneumonia may become delirious. However, the pneumonia may cause only mild symptoms, such as a dry cough that causes a burning sensation in the middle of the chest. A rash may appear at any time during the course of the disease.

Diagnosis

A doctor suspects tularemia in a person who develops the sudden symptoms and characteristic ulcers of the infection after having been exposed to ticks or having had even slight contact with a wild mammal, especially a rabbit. Infections acquired by laboratory workers frequently affect only the lymph nodes or lungs and are difficult to diagnose. A diagnosis can be confirmed by growing bacteria in samples of the ulcers, lymph nodes, blood, or sputum.

Treatment

Tularemia is treated with antibiotics, which are injected or taken orally for 5 to 7 days. Moist bandages are placed on the ulcers and changed frequently. These bandages help prevent the spread of infection and swelling of the lymph nodes. In rare cases, large abscesses need to be drained. Applying warm compresses to an affected eye and wearing dark glasses give some relief. People with intense headaches are usually treated with pain relievers, such as codeine.

People who are treated almost always survive. About 6 percent of untreated people die. Death usually results from overwhelming infection, pneumonia, infection of the lining around the brain (meningitis),▲ or infection of the lining of the abdominal cavity (peritonitis).■ Relapses are uncommon but can occur if treatment is inadequate. A person who has had tularemia develops immunity to reinfection.

Plague

Plague (Black Death) is a severe infection that is caused by the bacterium Yersinia pestis.

The bacteria that cause plague infect primarily wild rodents, such as rats, mice, squirrels, and prairie dogs. In the past, massive plague epidemics, such as the Black Death of the Middle Ages, killed large numbers of people. More recent outbreaks have been limited to an occasional single person or small clusters of people. More than 90 percent of the human plague infections in the United States occur in the southwestern states, particularly Arizona, California, Colorado, and New Mexico.

Plague usually is transmitted from infected animals to people by fleas. A cough or sneeze, which disperses bacteria in droplets, can spread the infection from one person to another. Transmission from household pets, especially cats, can also occur through fleabites or the inhalation of infected droplets.

Symptoms and Diagnosis

Plague can take one of several forms—bubonic, pneumonic, septicemic, or pestis minor. The symptoms vary depending on the form of plague.

Bubonic plague symptoms usually appear 2 to 5 days after exposure to the bacterium, but can appear any time from a few hours to 12 days later. Symptoms start suddenly with chills and a fever of up to 106° F. The heartbeat becomes rapid and weak, and the blood pressure may drop. Swollen lymph nodes (buboes) appear with or shortly before the fever. Typically, the nodes are extremely tender to the touch, firm, and surrounded by swollen tissue. The overlying skin is smooth and red but not warm. The person is likely to become restless, delirious, confused, and uncoordinated. The liver and spleen may swell substantially and can easily be felt during examination by a doctor. Lymph nodes may fill with pus and drain during the second week. More than 60 percent of untreated people die. Most deaths occur between the third and fifth day.

Pneumonic plague is an infection of the lungs with the plague bacteria. Symptoms, which begin abruptly 2 or 3 days after exposure to the bacteria, include a high fever, chills, rapid heartbeat, and often a severe headache. A cough develops in 24 hours. The sputum is clear at first, but rapidly becomes flecked with blood, and then becomes uniformly pink or bright red (resembling raspberry syrup) and foamy. Rapid and labored breathing is common. Most untreated people die within 48 hours of the start of symptoms.

▲ see page 373

■ see page 548

Septicemic plague, another form of plague, is an infection in which the bubonic form spreads into the blood. It may cause death even before other symptoms of bubonic or pneumonic plague appear.

Pestis minor is a mild form of plague that usually occurs only in a geographic area where the disease is prevalent (endemic). Its symptoms—swollen lymph nodes, fever, headache, and exhaustion—subside within a week.

Plague is diagnosed by analyzing laboratory cultures of bacteria grown from samples of blood, sputum, or lymph nodes.

Prevention and Treatment

Prevention is based on controlling rodents and using repellents to avoid fleabites. Vaccination is available, but it isn't necessary for most people traveling to areas where plague cases have been reported. Travelers who are at risk of exposure may take preventive doses of tetracycline.

When a person is thought to have plague, a doctor begins treatment immediately. In septicemic or pneumonic plague, treatment must start within 24 hours. Prompt treatment reduces the chance of death to less than 5 percent. Many antibiotics are effective.

Unlike those with bubonic plague, people with pneumonic plague must be isolated. Anyone who has been in contact with a person with pneumonic plague must be observed closely for signs of infection or treated.

Cat-Scratch Disease

Cat-scratch disease is an infection at the site of a cat scratch caused by the bacterium Bartonella henselae.

After a person is scratched by a cat infected with *Bartonella henselae*, the bacteria tend to infect the walls of the blood vessels. The cat usually shows no signs of illness.

Symptoms

Within 3 to 10 days of getting a minor scratch, the person usually develops a red, crusted blister up to $2\frac{1}{2}$ inches in diameter. Rarely, a blister containing pus (pustule) appears. Lymph nodes in the area swell, become firm, and are tender when touched. Later, they fill with pus and may drain through the skin. The person may feel ill, have a lack of appetite, and have a fever or headache.

About 10 percent of the infected people have other symptoms, such as eye problems, which cause visual changes, or brain swelling, which causes a headache or stupor.

In almost all infected people, the skin clears up and the swelling in the lymph nodes disappears within 2 to 5 months. Recovery is complete. A severe form of cat-scratch disease can occur in people with AIDS.

Diagnosis and Treatment

The diagnosis of cat-scratch disease seems likely if a person has swollen lymph nodes for more than 3 weeks after being scratched by a cat. In uncertain cases, a blood sample may be tested for antibodies to *Bartonella henselae*.

Treatment consists of applying heat and taking pain relievers. A fluid-filled lymph node that is painful can usually be drained with a needle to alleviate the pain. Antibiotics may be given to help eradicate the bacteria, especially in people with AIDS.

Pseudomonas Infections

Pseudomonas infections are infections caused by Pseudomonas *bacteria, especially* Pseudomonas aeruginosa.

Pseudomonas is the main cause of two common, minor infections that can affect otherwise normal, healthy people: swimmer's ear and hot-tub folliculitis. **Swimmer's ear (otitis externa)** is an infection of the external ear canal resulting from prolonged exposure to freshwater.▲ It can be treated with antibiotic eardrops. **Hot-tub folliculitis** is a skin rash consisting of tiny pimples, some of which may contain a drop of pus in their center. Treatment consists of keeping the skin dry and occasionally applying an antibiotic ointment.

Serious *Pseudomonas* infections most frequently occur in hospitals, and the organism is commonly found in moist areas, such as sinks and urine receptacles. Surprisingly, this organism is even found in certain antiseptic solutions. The most serious infections from *Pseudomonas* occur in debilitated people whose immune system is impaired by medications, other treatments, or disease.

▲ see page 1002

Pseudomonas can infect the blood, skin, bones, ears, eyes, urinary tract, heart valves, and lungs. Burns can become severely infected with *Pseudomonas,* leading to a blood infection that often proves fatal.

Symptoms

The symptoms depend on the site of the infection, but *Pseudomonas* infections tend to be severe. Malignant external otitis, an ear infection, can cause severe ear pain and nerve damage and is most common in people with diabetes. *Pseudomonas* organisms can cause ulcers in the eye after gaining entry through an eye injury, a contaminated contact lens, or contaminated lens fluid. *Pseudomonas* infection may be found in deep puncture wounds, especially puncture wounds of the foot in children.

Pseudomonas can cause severe pneumonia in hospitalized patients, especially those in intensive care. This type of bacteria also is a common cause of urinary tract infections, usually in people who have had urologic procedures or those who have an obstruction of the urinary tract.

The bacteria often invade the blood of people with burns and those who have cancer. Without treatment, an overwhelming infection can lead to shock and death. The infection often causes a rash of purple-black areas about $\frac{3}{8}$ inch in diameter; these areas have a sore at the center surrounded by redness and swelling. The rash often occurs in the underarm and groin.

Rarely, *Pseudomonas* infects heart valves. People who have received an artificial heart valve are more vulnerable; however, natural heart valves can be infected, especially among injecting drug users.

Treatment

When the infection is restricted to an external area, such as the skin, a doctor will surgically remove dead tissue and large abscesses and then irrigate the site with an antibiotic solution. Malignant external otitis, internal infections, and blood infections require days or weeks of intravenous antibiotic therapy. Sometimes an infected heart valve can be cured with antibiotics, but often open heart surgery is needed to replace the valve.

Campylobacter Infections

Campylobacter *infections are infections of the gastrointestinal tract or blood caused by* Campylobacter *bacteria.*

The most common form of *Campylobacter* infection is gastroenteritis,▲ which may be acquired by drinking contaminated water, eating undercooked poultry or meat, or having contact with infected animals. *Campylobacter* bacteria are also a cause of diarrhea among travelers to developing countries. *Campylobacter* bacteria may also cause a bloodstream infection (bacteremia), most often in people with an existing disease such as diabetes or cancer. An organism that causes stomach ulcers was once called *Campylobacter pylori* but has been renamed *Helicobacter pylori.*■

Symptoms

The gastroenteritis caused by *Campylobacter* bacteria includes diarrhea, abdominal pain, and cramps, which may be severe. The diarrhea may be bloody, and a fever ranging from 100° to 104° F. may occur.

A fever that comes and goes may be the only symptom of a *Campylobacter* infection outside the gastrointestinal tract. Additional symptoms of a body-wide (systemic) *Campylobacter* infection may include a joint that becomes painful, red, and swollen; abdominal pain; and enlargement of the liver or the spleen. Rarely, the infection can involve the heart valves (endocarditis)★ or the brain and spinal cord (meningitis).●

Diagnosis and Treatment

A doctor diagnoses *Campylobacter* infections by obtaining a laboratory analysis of samples of blood, stool, or other body fluids.

Various antibiotics are used alone or in combination to treat these infections. Ciprofloxacin, tetracycline, or erythromycin usually clears the *Campylobacter* bacteria and cures the diarrhea. Bloodstream infections usually require treatment with intravenous antibiotics.

▲ see page 514

■ see page 494

★ see page 101

● see page 373

Cholera

Cholera is an infection of the small intestine caused by the bacterium Vibrio cholerae.

Cholera bacteria produce a toxin that causes the small intestine to secrete immense amounts of fluid rich in salts and minerals. Because the bacteria are sensitive to stomach acid, people with a deficiency of acid are more susceptible to the disease. People living in areas in which cholera is common (endemic) gradually develop some natural immunity.

Cholera is spread by ingesting water, seafood, or other foods contaminated by the excrement of infected people. Cholera occurs in parts of Asia, the Middle East, Africa, and Latin America. In these areas, outbreaks usually occur during the warm months, and the incidence is highest among children. In other areas, epidemics may occur in any season, and people of all ages are equally susceptible.

Other species of *Vibrio* bacteria also can infect humans. The diarrhea produced is usually much less severe than that of cholera.

Symptoms and Diagnosis

Symptoms, which begin 1 to 3 days after infection with the bacterium, range from a mild, uncomplicated episode of diarrhea to a severe, potentially fatal disease. Some infected people have no symptoms.

The disease usually starts with sudden, painless, watery diarrhea and vomiting. In severe cases, the diarrhea causes a loss of more than 1 quart of fluid an hour, but the usual loss is much less. In severe cases, the resulting critical water and salt depletion leads to severe dehydration with intense thirst, muscle cramps, weakness, and minimal urine production. Severe loss of fluid from tissues causes the eyes to become sunken and the skin on the fingers to become severely wrinkled. If the infection isn't treated, the resulting severe imbalances in blood volume and the increased concentration of salts can lead to kidney failure, shock, and coma.

Symptoms usually subside in 3 to 6 days. Most people are free of the organism in 2 weeks, but a few become long-term carriers.

The diagnosis of cholera is confirmed by recovering the bacteria from rectal swabs or fresh stool samples. Because the *Vibrio cholerae* bacterium does not grow in routine stool cultures, a doctor must request a special culture for *Vibrio* organisms.

Prevention and Treatment

Purification of water supplies and proper disposal of human excrement are essential for controlling cholera. Other precautions include using boiled water and avoiding uncooked vegetables or inadequately cooked fish or shellfish. The vaccine for cholera provides only partial protection and therefore generally isn't recommended. Prompt treatment with the antibiotic tetracycline can help prevent the disease in people sharing the same household as a person infected with cholera.

Rapid replacement of lost body fluids, salts, and minerals is central to treatment. For severely dehydrated people who can't drink, fluid is given intravenously. In epidemics, people sometimes receive fluids via a tube inserted through the nose into the stomach. Once dehydration is corrected, the general goal of treatment is to replace the exact amount of fluid lost in bowel movements and vomit. Solid foods can be eaten after vomiting stops and the appetite returns.

Early treatment with tetracycline or another antibiotic kills the bacteria and usually stops the diarrhea in 48 hours.

More than 50 percent of untreated people with severe cholera die. Fewer than 1 percent of those who receive prompt, adequate fluid replacement die.

Enterobacteriaceae Infections

Enterobacteriaceae are a group of bacteria that can cause infections of the gastrointestinal tract or other organs of the body. Many of these organisms normally inhabit the gastrointestinal tract. The group includes *Salmonella, Shigella, Escherichia, Klebsiella, Enterobacter, Serratia, Proteus, Morganella, Providencia,* and *Yersinia.*

Although *Escherichia coli (E. coli)* normally inhabits the gastrointestinal tract, certain strains of *E. coli* can cause bloody, watery, or inflammatory diarrhea (traveler's diarrhea). In children, diarrhea caused by enterohemorrhagic *E. coli* may produce the hemolytic-uremic syndrome,▲ a disease that destroys red blood cells and causes

---

▲ see page 757

kidney failure. *E. coli* also is a common cause of urinary tract infections and can infect the bloodstream, gallbladder, lungs, and skin. *E. coli* bacteremia and meningitis occur in newborns, particularly premature newborns. Antibiotics usually are started immediately and later changed if culture results show that another antibiotic would be more effective. For a simple urinary tract infection, a sulfa drug may be taken orally. Intravenous antibiotics are required for severe infections.

Klebsiella, Enterobacter, and *Serratia* infections usually are acquired in the hospital, mainly by patients who have a reduced ability to fight infections. These bacteria often infect the same sites of the body as *E. coli. Klebsiella* pneumonia is a rare but severe lung infection that is most common in diabetics and alcoholics. The person may cough up dark brown or dark red phlegm. The pneumonia may cause abscesses in the lung and collections of pus to form in the lung's lining (empyema). If treated early enough, *Klebsiella* pneumonia can be cured with intravenous antibiotics, usually cephalosporins or quinolones.

Proteus comprises a group of bacteria normally found in soil, water, and feces. They also can cause deep infections, particularly in the abdominal cavity, urinary tract, and bladder.

TYPHOID FEVER

Typhoid fever is an infection caused by the bacterium Salmonella typhi.

Typhoid bacteria are shed in the feces and urine of infected people. Inadequate hand washing after defecation or urination may spread *Salmonella typhi* to food or water supplies. Flies may spread the bacteria directly from feces to food. Rarely, hospital workers who haven't taken adequate precautions may develop typhoid fever by handling the soiled bed linens of infected people.

The bacteria enter the gastrointestinal tract and gain access to the bloodstream. Inflammation of the small and large intestine follows. In severe cases, which can be life threatening, the affected tissue develops bleeding sores and may perforate.

About 3 percent of the people who are infected with *Salmonella typhi* and haven't received treat-

ment shed bacteria in their stool for more than a year. Some of these carriers never have symptoms of typhoid fever. Most of the estimated 2,000 carriers in the United States are elderly women with chronic gallbladder disease.

Symptoms and Diagnosis

Usually, symptoms begin gradually 8 to 14 days after infection. They include a fever, headache, joint pain, sore throat, constipation, loss of appetite, and abdominal pain and tenderness. Less commonly, painful urination, cough, and nosebleeds develop.

If treatment isn't started, the body temperature slowly rises over 2 to 3 days, remains at 103° to 104° F. for 10 to 14 days, begins to fall gradually at the end of the third week, and reaches normal levels during the fourth week. This sustained fever often is accompanied by a slow heartbeat and extreme exhaustion. Delirium, stupor, or a coma may occur in severe cases. In about 10 percent of the people, clusters of small, pink spots appear on the chest and abdomen during the second week of the illness and last for 2 to 5 days. Sometimes the infection causes pneumonia-like symptoms, only a fever, or symptoms similar to those of a urinary tract infection.

Although the symptoms and the history of the person's illness can suggest typhoid fever, the diagnosis must be confirmed by identifying the bacteria in cultures of blood, stool, urine, or other body tissues.

Complications

Although most people recover fully, complications can occur, primarily in those who aren't treated or in whom treatment is delayed. Intestinal bleeding occurs in many people; about 2 percent of them have severe bleeding. Usually, bleeding occurs during the third week of the illness. Intestinal perforation occurs in 1 to 2 percent of people and produces severe abdominal pain as the contents of the intestine infect the abdominal cavity, a condition called peritonitis.▲

Pneumonia may develop during the second or third week and usually results from a pneumococcal infection, although the typhoid bacteria can also cause pneumonia. Infection of the gallbladder and liver also may occur. A blood infection (bacteremia) occasionally leads to infection of bones (osteomyelitis), heart valves (endocarditis), the lining of the brain (meningitis), the kid-

▲ see page 548

neys (glomerulitis), or the genital or urinary tract. A muscle infection can lead to abscesses.

In about 10 percent of untreated cases, symptoms of the initial infection recur 2 weeks after the fever breaks. For unknown reasons, antibiotics taken during the initial illness increase the recurrence rate to 15 to 20 percent. If antibiotics are given for the relapse, the fever dissipates much more quickly than it did in the original illness, but occasionally another relapse occurs.

Prevention and Treatment

The oral vaccine against typhoid fever offers 70 percent protection. It is given only to people who have been exposed to the organism and to those who are at high risk of exposure, including laboratory workers studying the organism and people traveling to areas where the disease is common. Travelers to such areas should avoid eating raw leafy vegetables and other foods served or stored at room temperature. Recently prepared foods served hot or chilled, bottled carbonated beverages, and raw foods that can be peeled are generally safe. Unless water is known to be safe, it should be boiled or chlorinated before drinking.

With prompt antibiotic therapy, more than 99 percent of typhoid fever cases are cured. Typically, people who die are malnourished, very young, or very old. Stupor, coma, and shock are signs of severe infection and a poor prognosis.

Convalescence may last several months, but antibiotics decrease the severity and complications of typhoid fever as well as the duration of the symptoms. The antibiotic chloramphenicol is used worldwide, but increasing resistance to it has prompted the use of other drugs. If the person is delirious, comatose, or in shock, corticosteroids may be used to reduce brain inflammation.

Frequent feedings are needed because of gastrointestinal bleeding or other gastrointestinal disruption. Sometimes intravenous feedings are given until the person can digest food. People with intestinal perforation need antibiotics that kill a broad range of bacteria (because many different types of bacteria will spill into the peritoneal cavity) and perhaps surgery to repair or remove the perforated section of intestine.

Relapses are treated the same way as the initial illness, but antibiotics are usually needed for only 5 days.

What Increases the Risk of *Salmonella* Infection?

- Removal of part of the stomach
- Lack of stomach acids
- Long-term antacid use
- Sickle cell anemia
- Lack of a spleen
- Louse-borne relapsing fever
- Malaria
- Bartonellosis
- Cirrhosis
- Leukemia
- Lymphoma
- Human immunodeficiency virus infection (including AIDS)

Carriers (people who don't have symptoms but who shed the bacteria in their stool) must report to the local health department and are prohibited from working with food. The bacteria can be completely eradicated in many carriers after 4 to 6 weeks of antibiotic therapy.

NONTYPHOIDAL *SALMONELLA* INFECTIONS

About 2,200 types of *Salmonella* are known, including the type that causes typhoid fever. Each type can produce gastrointestinal upset, enteric fever, and specific localized infections. Infected meat, poultry, raw milk, eggs, and egg products are common sources of *Salmonella*. Other sources include infected pet reptiles, carmine red dye, and contaminated marijuana. *Salmonella* infections remain a significant public health problem in the United States.

Symptoms and Diagnosis

Salmonella infections may cause gastrointestinal upset or enteric fever; sometimes the infection affects a specific site. Some infected people have no symptoms but are carriers.

Gastrointestinal upset usually starts 12 to 48 hours after ingesting *Salmonella* bacteria. Symptoms begin with nausea and crampy abdominal pain soon followed by diarrhea, fever, and sometimes vomiting. Usually the diarrhea is watery, although a person may produce pasty, semisolid stool. The upset is usually mild and lasts 1 to 4 days, but it may last much longer. Diagnosis is confirmed in a laboratory by culturing a sample of stool or rectal swab taken from an infected person.

Enteric fever occurs when *Salmonella* bacteria enter the blood. The fever produces extreme exhaustion (prostration). Typhoid fever is the prototype of this illness. A less severe form can be caused by other *Salmonella* strains.

A specific site may be infected by *Salmonella.* For example, the bacteria can lodge and multiply in the digestive tract, blood vessels, heart valves, lining of the brain or spinal cord, lungs, joints, bones, urinary tract, muscles, or other organs. Occasionally, a tumor may become infected, developing an abscess that provides a source for continued blood infection.

Carriers don't have symptoms but continue to shed the bacteria in their stool. Fewer than 1 percent of the people with nontyphoidal *Salmonella* infections continue to shed bacteria in their stool for a year or more.

Treatment

Gastrointestinal upset is treated with fluids and a bland diet. Antibiotics prolong the excretion of bacteria in the stool and therefore aren't recommended for people who have only gastrointestinal upset. However, infants, people in nursing homes, and those with human immunodeficiency virus (HIV) infection are treated with antibiotics because they are at higher risk for complications. In carriers who don't have symptoms, the infection usually resolves on its own; antibiotic treatment is rarely needed.

When an antibiotic is needed, ampicillin, amoxicillin, or ciprofloxacin generally is effective; however, resistance to these antibiotics is common. Antibiotics are taken for 3 to 5 days, but people with HIV infection generally require longer treatment to prevent relapses. People with *Salmonella* bacteria in their blood must take antibiotics for 4 to 6 weeks. Abscesses are treated by surgical drainage and 4 weeks of antibiotic therapy. People with infected blood vessels, heart valves, or other sites generally require surgery and prolonged antibiotic therapy.

SHIGELLOSIS

Shigellosis (bacillary dysentery), an intestinal infection that results in severe diarrhea, is caused by Shigella *bacteria.*

Shigella bacteria cause dysentery throughout the world and are responsible for 5 to 10 percent of diarrheal illnesses in many areas. The infection is spread by contact with the feces of infected people. A person may contract the disease from oral-to-anal contact or from contaminated food, water, objects, or flies. Epidemics are most frequent in overcrowded populations with inadequate sanitation. Children usually have more severe symptoms.

Symptoms

Shigella bacteria cause disease by penetrating the lining of the intestine, resulting in swelling and sometimes shallow sores. Symptoms start 1 to 4 days after infection. In young children, the illness starts suddenly with a fever, irritability or drowsiness, loss of appetite, nausea and vomiting, diarrhea, abdominal pain and bloating, and pain during defecation. Within 3 days, pus, blood, and mucus appear in the stool. The number of bowel movements generally increases rapidly—up to more than 20 a day. Weight loss and dehydration become severe.

Adults, however, may not develop a fever, and often the stool doesn't have blood or mucus initially. The illness may begin with episodes of abdominal pain, the urge to defecate, and the passing of formed stool, which temporarily relieves the pain. These episodes recur with increasing severity and frequency. Diarrhea becomes severe, and soft or liquid stool contains mucus, pus, and often blood.

Rarely, the illness begins suddenly with clear or cloudy stools; occasionally, it begins suddenly with bloody stools. Vomiting is common and can rapidly result in dehydration. Severe dehydration, which can lead to shock and death, is limited mainly to chronically ill adults and children under age 2.

A tentative diagnosis may be based on the symptoms of a person who lives in an area where *Shigella* is common. However, the diagnosis is confirmed by culturing a fresh stool sample.

Complications

Shigellosis may cause delirium, convulsions, and coma but little or no diarrhea. This infection may be fatal within 12 to 24 hours.

Other bacterial infections can accompany shigellosis, especially in debilitated and dehydrated patients. Ulcers in the intestine resulting from shigellosis can lead to severe blood loss.

Uncommon complications include damage to nerves, joints, or the heart, and, rarely, perforation of the intestine. Severe straining during bowel movements may cause rectal prolapse, in which part of the rectum is pushed out of the body. Permanent loss of bowel control can result.

Treatment

In most cases, the disease resolves within 4 to 8 days. Severe cases may last 3 to 6 weeks.

Treatment consists mainly of replacing fluids and salts lost because of diarrhea. Antibiotics are indicated when the patient is very young, when the disease is severe, or when the spread of infection to other people is likely. The severity of the symptoms and length of time the stool contains *Shigella* bacteria can be reduced with antibiotics, such as trimethoprim-sulfamethoxazole, norfloxacin, ciprofloxacin, and furazolidone.

CHAPTER 178

Coccal Infections

Bacteria can be classified in several ways, including by their shape. Bacteria that have a spherical shape are called cocci.▲ Cocci that can cause infection in humans include staphylococci, streptococci, pneumococci, and meningococci.

Staphylococcal Infections

Staphylococcal infections are those caused by staphylococci, which are common gram-positive bacteria.

Normally found in the nose and on the skin of 20 to 30 percent of healthy adults (and less commonly in the mouth, mammary glands, and genitourinary, intestinal, and upper respiratory tracts), staphylococci do no harm most of the time. However, a break in the skin or another injury may allow the bacteria to penetrate the body's defenses and cause infection.

People prone to staphylococcal infections include newborns, breastfeeding women, people with chronic diseases (especially lung disease, diabetes, and cancer), those with skin conditions and surgical incisions, and those whose immune systems are suppressed by corticosteroids, radiation therapy, immunosuppressive drugs, or anticancer medications.

Symptoms

Staphylococci can infect any site in the body, and the symptoms depend on the location of the infection. The infection may be mild or life threatening. Commonly, staphylococcal infections produce pus-filled pockets, such as abscesses and boils (furuncles and carbuncles). Staphylococci can travel through the blood and cause abscesses in internal organs, such as the lungs, as well as infections of bones (osteomyelitis) and the inner lining of the heart and its valves (endocarditis).

Staphylococci tend to infect the skin. Staphylococcal abscesses on the skin appear as warm, pus-filled pockets below the surface. They usually rupture like a large pimple and ooze pus onto the skin, where further infection can occur if the pus isn't cleaned off. Staphylococci can also cause cellulitis, a spreading infection under the skin.■ Usually, boils also are caused by staphylococci. Two particularly serious staphylococcal skin infections are toxic epidermal necrolysis★ and the

---

▲ see box, page 862

■ see page 977

★ see page 965

scalded skin syndrome,▲ both of which lead to large-scale peeling of skin.

Newborns may develop staphylococcal infections, usually within 6 weeks after birth. The most common symptom is large blisters filled with clear fluid or pus that appear in the armpit, groin, or neck skinfolds. More severe staphylococcal infections can cause many skin abscesses, sloughing of the skin in large patches, blood infection, infection of the membranes covering the brain and spinal cord (meningitis), and pneumonia.

Breastfeeding mothers may develop staphylococcal breast infections (mastitis) and abscesses 1 to 4 weeks after delivery. Such infections often are contracted by the infant in the hospital nursery and transferred to the mother's breast during feeding.

Staphylococcal pneumonia is a severe infection.■ People with chronic lung diseases (such as chronic bronchitis and emphysema) and those with influenza are particularly at risk. Staphylococcal pneumonia often causes a high fever and severe lung symptoms, such as shortness of breath, rapid breathing, and cough productive of sputum that may be tinged with blood. In newborns—and sometimes adults—staphylococcal pneumonia may cause lung abscesses and an infection of the pleura (the membrane layers surrounding the lungs). The infection, called thoracic empyema, worsens the difficulties in breathing caused by the pneumonia.

Although a staphylococcal infection of the blood (staphylococcal bacteremia) often develops from a staphylococcal infection elsewhere in the body, it usually comes from an infected intravenous device, such as a catheter, which gives staphylococci direct access to the bloodstream. Staphylococcal bacteremia is a common cause of death in severely burned people. Typically, the bacteremia causes a persistent, high fever and sometimes shock.

Staphylococci in the bloodstream can lead to an infection of the inner lining of the heart and its valves (endocarditis),★ especially in injecting drug users. The infection can quickly damage the valves, leading to heart failure and death.

Bone infections (osteomyelitis) predominantly affect children, although they also affect the elderly, especially those with deep skin ulcers (bedsores). Bone infections cause chills, fever, and bone pain. Redness and swelling appear over the infected bone, and fluid may build up in joints near the areas invaded by the bacteria. The site of infection may be painful, and the person usually has a fever. Sometimes x-rays and other radiologic scans can identify an area of infection, but they generally don't help the doctor make an early diagnosis.

A staphylococcal infection of the intestine often causes a fever, abdominal bloating and distention, a temporary halting of the intestine's normal contractile movements (ileus), and diarrhea. The infection is most common in hospitalized patients, especially those who have undergone abdominal surgery or received antibiotic treatment.

Surgery increases the risk of staphylococcal infection. The infection may produce abscesses at the stitches or may cause extensive destruction of the incision site. Such infections usually appear a few days to several weeks after an operation but may develop more slowly if the person received antibiotics at the time of surgery. A postoperative staphylococcal infection may worsen and progress to toxic shock syndrome.

Treatment

For most skin infections, oral antibiotics, such as cloxacillin, dicloxacillin, and erythromycin, are adequate. More severe infections, especially blood infections, require intravenous antibiotic therapy, often for up to 6 weeks.

The choice of an antibiotic depends on the site of infection, the severity of the illness, and which of the antibiotics most effectively kills the particular bacteria. Methicillin-resistant *Staphylococcus aureus* is resistant to most commonly used antibiotics and is a major concern because the bacterium is increasingly common in big city and university hospitals. Among the few antibiotics that are usually effective against methicillin-resistant *Staphylococcus aureus* are vancomycin and trimethoprim-sulfamethoxazole. Vancomycin kills the bacteria, whereas trimethoprim-sulfamethoxazole acts by inhibiting their ability to multiply.

▲ see page 978

■ see page 196

★ see page 101

An abscess that develops must be drained. Draining an abscess on the skin is relatively simple. A doctor makes a small cut in the area and applies pressure to clean out the infected material. Abscesses deeper in the body may require surgery.

Toxic Shock Syndrome

Toxic shock syndrome is an infection usually caused by staphylococci, which may rapidly worsen to severe, untreatable shock.

In 1978, toxic shock syndrome was first recognized as a distinct syndrome in several children between 8 and 17 years of age. In 1980, a large number of cases appeared, mainly in young women—almost always those who were using tampons. About 700 cases were reported in the United States in 1980. By 1981, after widespread publicity and the removal of the "superabsorbent" varieties of tampons from the market, the incidence of toxic shock syndrome fell dramatically. Cases still occur in some women who don't use tampons and in some who have just had surgery or given birth. About 15 percent of the cases occur in men who have undergone surgery. Mild cases are fairly common.

Although the strain of *Staphylococcus* that causes most cases of toxic shock syndrome is known, the event that triggers the syndrome isn't. The presence of a tampon may encourage the bacteria to produce a toxin that enters the blood through small cuts in the vaginal lining or through the uterus into the abdominal cavity. This toxin appears to cause the symptoms.

Symptoms and Diagnosis

Symptoms start suddenly with a fever of 102° to 105° F. A severe headache, sore throat, red eyes, extreme tiredness, confusion, vomiting, profuse watery diarrhea, and a sunburn-like rash all over the body quickly develop. Within 48 hours, the person also may experience fainting and develop shock. Between the third and seventh days, the skin peels, particularly on the palms and soles.

The syndrome causes anemia. Kidney, liver, and muscle damage is very common, especially during the first week. Heart and lung problems may also develop. Most organs recover fully after the symptoms disappear.

The diagnosis is usually based on the person's symptoms. Although there is no laboratory test available that specifically identifies toxic shock syndrome, blood tests usually are performed to exclude other possible causes of the symptoms.

Prevention, Treatment, and Prognosis

Precise recommendations for preventing toxic shock syndrome are hard to formulate. Generally, women should avoid constant tampon use during menstruation. Superabsorbent tampons, which are more likely to cause toxic shock syndrome, shouldn't be used.

A person who is suspected of having toxic shock syndrome should be hospitalized immediately. Treatment is started by removing a tampon, diaphragm, or other foreign objects, and antibiotics are given as soon as possible.

About 8 to 15 percent of people with full-blown toxic shock syndrome die. Recurring episodes are common in women who continue to use tampons in the 4 months after an episode of toxic shock syndrome, unless antibiotic treatment has eliminated the staphylococci.

Streptococcal Infections

Streptococcal infections are caused by gram-positive bacteria called streptococci.

The various disease-causing strains of streptococci are grouped by their behavior, chemistry, and appearance. Each group tends to produce specific types of infections and symptoms.

• **Group A** streptococci are the most virulent species for humans, who are their natural host. These streptococci can cause strep throat (a streptococcal infection of the throat), tonsillitis, wound and skin infections, blood infections (septicemia), scarlet fever, pneumonia, rheumatic fever, Sydenham's chorea (St. Vitus' dance),▲ and kidney inflammation (glomerulonephritis).

• **Group B** streptococci most commonly cause dangerous infections in newborns (neonatal sepsis)■ and infections in the joints (septic arthritis) and heart (endocarditis).

• **Groups C and G** streptococci often are carried by animals but also grow in the human throat,

---

▲ see page 313

■ see page 1217

intestine, vagina, and skin. These streptococci can cause severe infections, including strep throat, pneumonia, skin infections, wound infections, postpartum and neonatal sepsis, endocarditis, and septic arthritis. After an infection with one of these bacteria, kidney inflammation may develop.

• **Group D** streptococci and enterococci grow normally in the lower digestive tract, vagina, and surrounding skin. They can also cause infections in wounds and in the heart valves, bladder, abdomen, and blood.

Infections with certain types of streptococci can cause an autoimmune reaction in which the body attacks its own tissues.▲ Such reactions may occur after an infection such as strep throat and may lead to rheumatic fever, chorea, and kidney damage (glomerulonephritis).

Symptoms

Streptococci may live in the respiratory tract, intestine, vagina, or elsewhere in the body without causing problems. Occasionally, such bacteria are found in an inflamed area (such as the throat or vagina) of a person who is a carrier, and the streptococci are incorrectly identified as the cause of the infection.

The most common type of streptococcal infection is a throat infection (strep throat). Typically, symptoms appear suddenly and include sore throat, a general feeling of illness (malaise), chills, fever, headache, nausea, vomiting, and a rapid heartbeat. The throat is beefy red, the tonsils are swollen, and lymph nodes in the neck may be enlarged and tender. Children may have convulsions. In children under age 4, the only symptom may be a runny nose. A cough, an inflammation of the larynx (laryngitis), and a stuffy nose are uncommon in streptococcal infections; these symptoms suggest another cause, such as a cold or allergy.

Scarlet fever is caused by streptococcal toxins that lead to a widespread, pink-red rash. The rash is most obvious on the abdomen, on the sides of

the chest, and in the skinfolds. Other symptoms include a pale area around the mouth, a flushed face, an inflamed red tongue, and dark red lines in the skinfolds. The outer layer of reddened skin often peels after the fever subsides.

Streptococci also cause several types of skin infection but rarely produce abscesses. Rather, the infections tend to spread in the deep layers under the skin, producing cellulitis and sometimes hot, red eruptions called erysipelas (St. Anthony's fire). Streptococci, alone or with staphylococci, also can spread along the top layers of the skin, producing scabby, crusted eruptions (impetigo).■

Certain strains of streptococci may cause a rapidly spreading and destructive infection under the skin (necrotizing fasciitis).★ For unknown reasons, outbreaks of this infection have become more common recently.

Diagnosis

Although symptoms may suggest a streptococcal infection, the diagnosis must be confirmed by tests. The best way to be certain of a streptococcal infection is to culture a sample from the infected area. After overnight growth, a culture shows characteristic bacterial colonies.

To diagnose strep throat, a culture is taken by rubbing a sterile swab over the back of the throat. The sample then is placed in a Petri dish and allowed to grow overnight. Alternatively, Group A streptococci may be detected by special, rapid tests that can produce results within a few hours. If the result of a rapid test is positive, the slower overnight culture is not needed. Because both methods can detect streptococci in people who do not need treatment, examination by a doctor is necessary.

Treatment

People with strep throat and scarlet fever generally get better in 2 weeks, even without treatment. Nonetheless, antibiotics can shorten the duration of symptoms in young children and prevent serious complications, such as rheumatic fever. They also help prevent the spread of the infection to the middle ear, sinuses, and mastoid bone as well as to other people. An antibiotic, usually oral penicillin V, should be started promptly after the appearance of symptoms.

▲ see page 816

■ see page 976

★ see page 854

Diseases Caused by Pneumococci

Pneumonia
• Perhaps the most serious infection caused by pneumococci
• Usually affects only one lobe of the lung at a time but may spread to other lobes

Thoracic empyema (infection of the pleura surrounding the lungs)
• Pneumococci are the most common cause of this pus-forming infection
• May require surgical drainage

Otitis media (middle ear infection)
• Pneumococci cause about half the cases in infants and children
• If not treated, infection can spread to the sinuses, mastoid bones, and membranes covering the brain and spinal cord, causing meningitis

Bacterial meningitis (infection of the membranes covering the brain and spinal cord)
• Pneumococci are among the most common causes in all age groups
• May spread from a blood or lung infection, an ear or sinus infection, an infection of the skull bones (such as mastoiditis), or a skull fracture

Bacteremia (blood infection)
• May start from pneumonia or meningitis and spread to heart valves

Pneumococcal endocarditis (infection of the heart valves)
• Can be especially dangerous because bacteria and debris accumulate on heart valves—particularly injured, deformed, or artificial valves—causing damage
• In severe cases, damaged heart valves can rupture, leading to rapidly progressive heart failure

Peritonitis (infection of the abdominal cavity)
• Usually occurs in young girls from an infection that spreads upward from the vagina through the fallopian tubes into the abdominal cavity
• May occur in people with cirrhosis

Pneumococcal arthritis
• Rare cause of joint infection
• Usually occurs with endocarditis or meningitis

Other streptococcal infections, such as cellulitis, necrotizing fasciitis, and endocarditis, are very serious and require intravenous penicillin, sometimes together with other antibiotics. Group A streptococci are usually eliminated by penicillin. Some Group D streptococci, and especially enterococci, are resistant to penicillin and most antibiotics; there is no reliable antibiotic therapy available for many enterococcal strains.

Symptoms such as a fever, headache, and sore throat can be treated with drugs that reduce pain (analgesics) and fever (antipyretics), such as acetaminophen. Neither bed rest nor isolation is necessary; however, family members or friends who have similar symptoms or who have had complications from a streptococcal infection may be at risk for infection.

Pneumococcal Infections

Pneumococcal infections are infections caused by the gram-positive bacterium Streptococcus pneumoniae.

Pneumococci commonly inhabit the upper respiratory tract of humans, their natural host, particularly during the winter and early spring. Despite their location, pneumococci only occasionally cause pneumonia. Because pneumococcal pneumonia▲ rarely spreads from one person to another, people with the disease need not avoid contact with others. Pneumococci also

---

▲ see page 195

may cause infections in the brain, ear, and other organs.

People especially at risk of developing pneumococcal pneumonia include those with chronic illnesses and compromised immune systems—for example, people with Hodgkin's disease, lymphoma, multiple myeloma, malnutrition, and sickle cell disease. Because antibodies produced in the spleen normally help prevent pneumococcal infection, people who have had their spleen removed or who have a nonfunctioning spleen are also at risk. Pneumococcal pneumonia also may develop after chronic bronchitis or if a common respiratory virus, notably the influenza virus, damages the lining of the respiratory tract.

Prevention and Treatment

A highly effective pneumococcal vaccine is available for people over age 2. The vaccine protects against the most common strains of pneumococci and reduces the chances of developing pneumococcal pneumonia and bacteremia by 80 percent and the chances of dying of them by 40 percent. The vaccine is recommended for the elderly and for people with chronic heart and lung disease, diabetes, Hodgkin's disease, infection

with human immunodeficiency virus, or disorders of metabolism. It may also be helpful for children with sickle cell disease and for people who have had their spleen removed or who have a nonfunctioning spleen.

Penicillin is the preferred treatment for most pneumococcal infections. It is taken orally for ear and sinus infections and given intravenously for more severe infections.

Neisserial Infections

Neisseria meningitidis (meningococci) is a gram-negative coccal bacterium for which humans are the natural host. Meningococci may cause infection of the layers covering the brain and spinal cord (meningitis),▲ blood infection, and other severe infections in children and adults. *Neisseria gonorrhoeae,* also gram-negative cocci for which humans are the natural host, cause gonorrhea, a sexually transmitted disease that can infect the urethra, vagina, and anus and can spread to the joints.■ Many other species of *Neisseria* normally inhabit the throat and mouth, vagina, and intestine, but they rarely cause disease.

CHAPTER 179

Spirochetal Infections

Spirochetes are corkscrew-shaped bacteria★ that tend to move with an undulating and propeller-like motion. The main strains (species) of spirochetes include *Treponema, Borrelia, Leptospira,* and *Spirillum.*

Treponematoses

Treponematoses are nonvenereal infections caused by a spirochete that is indistinguishable from Trep-

onema pallidum, *which is the bacterium that causes syphilis.*

Treponematoses include persistent infections that are found in specific geographic areas, such as endemic syphilis, yaws, and pinta. Endemic syphilis occurs mainly in the arid countries of the eastern Mediterranean region and West Africa. Yaws occurs in humid equatorial countries. Pinta is common among the Indians of Mexico, Central America, and South America.

Symptoms

Endemic syphilis (bejel) begins in childhood with a slimy patch on the inside of the cheek followed by blisters on the trunk, arms, and legs. The leg bones commonly are involved. In later stages of the disease, soft, gummy lumps develop in the nose and on the roof of the mouth (soft palate).

▲ see page 373

■ see page 941

★ see box, page 862

Yaws (frambesia) begins several weeks after exposure to *Treponema* bacteria as a slightly raised sore at the site of infection, usually on a leg. The sore heals, but soft tumor-like nodules of tissue (granulomas) then erupt on the face, arms, legs, and buttocks. These granulomas heal slowly and may recur. Painful open sores may develop on the soles of the feet (crab yaws). Later, areas of the shinbones may be destroyed, and many other disfiguring growths, especially around the nose (gangosa), may occur.

Pinta begins as flat, reddened areas on the hands, feet, legs, arms, face, and neck. After several months, slate-blue patches develop in the same areas on both sides of the body and over bony places, such as the elbow. Later, the patches lose their pigmentation. Thickened skin may develop in the patches on the palms and soles.

Diagnosis and Treatment

A doctor makes the diagnosis based on the typical symptoms of a person who has lived in an area where such diseases are common. People with treponematoses will test positive for venereal disease; however, the tests can't distinguish between nonvenereal infections and syphilis.

The lesions are destructive and leave scars. However, a single injection of penicillin kills the bacteria, so the skin can heal. Public health measures are in place to locate and treat people who are infected and those with whom they have been in contact.

Relapsing Fever

Relapsing fever (tick fever, recurrent fever, or famine fever) is a disease caused by several strains of Borrelia *bacteria.*

Depending on the geographic location, relapsing fever is spread by body lice or soft ticks. Louse-borne relapsing fever occurs only in parts of Africa and South America, whereas tick-borne relapsing fever occurs in North and South America, Africa, Asia, and Europe. In the United States, the disease is generally confined to the western states, where it most commonly occurs between May and September.

Body lice become infected with these spirochete bacteria when they feed on an infected person; the infection can be transmitted to another person when the louse changes hosts. When the louse is crushed, the bacteria are released and enter skin that has been scraped or bitten. Ticks become infected by feeding on rodents, which harbor the bacteria naturally. The infection is transmitted to humans through a tick bite.

Symptoms and Diagnosis

People exposed to the bacteria may not show symptoms for 3 to 11 days—typically, 6 days. The initial symptoms include sudden chills followed by a high fever, rapid heartbeat, severe headache, vomiting, muscle and joint pain, and often delirium. In the early stages, a reddish rash may appear over the trunk, arms, and legs. A doctor may see broken blood vessels in the membrane covering the eyeball and in the skin and mucous membranes. As the disease progresses, fever, jaundice, an enlarged liver and spleen, heart inflammation, and heart failure may occur, especially with the louse-borne infection. The fever remains high for 3 to 5 days, and then it and other symptoms clear abruptly.

After 7 to 10 days, the fever and symptoms reappear suddenly, often accompanied by pain in the joints. Jaundice is more common during a relapse. Louse-borne relapsing fever is usually associated with a single relapse, whereas multiple relapses (2 to 10 times at 1- to 2-week intervals) are common with the tick-borne disease. The episodes gradually become less severe, and the person eventually recovers as immunity develops.

Relapsing fever may be confused with many diseases, including malaria and Lyme disease. The pattern of recurring fever is the clue to diagnosing the disease. The diagnosis is confirmed when the spirochete bacteria are found in a blood sample taken during an episode of fever. Because ticks feed briefly and painlessly at night, a person may not be able to recall having been bitten by a tick.

Prognosis, Prevention, and Treatment

Fewer than 5 percent of people with relapsing fever die; however, those who are very young, very old, malnourished, or debilitated are at greater risk. Complications of the disease include eye inflammation, asthma flare ups, and the eruption of a red rash (erythema multiforme) all over the body. The brain, the spinal cord, and the iris of the eye may also become inflamed. A pregnant woman may miscarry.

Dusting undergarments and the inside of clothing with malathion or lindane powder, where available, protects against relapsing fever caused by body lice. Tick bites are more difficult to prevent, because most insecticides and repellents aren't effective against ticks. However, those containing diethyltoluamide (deet) for the skin and permethrin for clothing may help protect against tick bites.

Antibiotic treatment with tetracycline, erythromycin, or doxycycline cures the infection. Although the drug usually is taken orally, it may be given intravenously if severe vomiting makes swallowing impractical.

Optimally, treatment is started either early in a fever stage or during a symptomless interval. Starting therapy near the end of a fever may induce the Jarisch-Herxheimer reaction, in which a high fever and a rise and subsequent fall (sometimes to dangerously low levels) in blood pressure may occur. This reaction is typical and sometimes fatal in people with the louse-borne disease.

Dehydration is treated with fluids given intravenously. Severe headache is treated with pain relievers such as codeine. Dimenhydrinate or prochlorperazine may be given for nausea.

Lyme Disease

Lyme disease is caused by the spirochete Borrelia burgdorferi, *which is usually transmitted by tiny deer ticks.*

The disease was recognized and named in 1975 when a cluster of cases occurred in the small community of Lyme, Connecticut. Since then, Lyme disease has appeared in 47 states, including those along the northeastern coast from Massachusetts to Maryland as well as Wisconsin, Minnesota, California, and Oregon. The disease is well recognized in Europe and has been reported in the former Soviet Union and in China, Japan, and Australia. Lyme disease usually occurs in the summer and early fall, most often in children and young adults who live in wooded areas.

Borrelia burgdorferi bacteria enter the skin at the site of a tick bite. After 3 to 32 days, the bacteria migrate outward in the skin and spread in the lymph or through the blood to other organs or skin sites.

Symptoms

The disease typically begins in the skin as a large red spot, usually on the thigh, buttock, trunk, or armpit. The spot expands to a diameter of 6 inches (15 centimeters), often with a central clearing. At least 75 percent of the infected people have this early sign. Nearly half of the people develop more, usually smaller, red areas soon after the large red spot appears.

Many people with Lyme disease feel ill and have such symptoms as fatigue, chills and fever, headaches, stiff neck, and muscle and joint aches. Less common symptoms include backache, nausea and vomiting, sore throat, swollen lymph nodes, and an enlarged spleen. Although most symptoms may come and go, the ill feeling and fatigue may persist for weeks.

Several weeks or months after the first symptoms appear, abnormalities of nerve function develop in about 15 percent of people; these last for several months and usually disappear completely. The most common problem is an infection of the lining of the brain (meningitis),▲ which causes a stiff neck, headache, inflammation of facial nerves, and weakness on one side of the face (palsy). Other areas of weakness also may develop. In 8 percent of people, heart disorders—including irregular heartbeats (arrhythmias) and inflammation of the sac around the heart (pericarditis)—develop. Pericarditis can cause chest pain.

Additionally, weeks to months after symptoms begin, arthritis develops in about half the people. In some cases, arthritis appears as late as 2 years after the first symptoms. Episodes of swelling and pain in a few large joints, especially the knee, typically recur for several years. The affected knees are commonly more swollen than painful, often hot when touched, and, in rare instances, red. Cysts may develop behind the knee and rupture, suddenly worsening the pain. About 10 percent of people with Lyme arthritis develop persistent knee problems.

Diagnosis

Borrelia burgdorferi bacteria are very difficult to culture in the laboratory, and no single test can

▲ see page 373

reliably diagnose Lyme disease. Therefore, the diagnosis is usually based on the typical symptoms of Lyme disease occurring in a person who has been exposed to conditions where tick infestation is likely, together with results of several tests. The most commonly used test is a measurement of the level of antibodies to the bacterium in the blood.

Treatment

Although all stages of Lyme disease respond to antibiotics, early treatment best helps prevent any complications. An antibiotic such as doxycycline, amoxicillin, penicillin, or erythromycin may be taken orally during the early stages of the disease. Antibiotics are given intravenously for late, severe, or persistent disease.

Antibiotics also help to relieve arthritis, although treatment may be needed for up to 3 weeks. Aspirin or other nonsteroidal anti-inflammatory drugs relieve the pain of swollen joints. Fluid that collects in affected joints may be drained, and the use of crutches may be helpful.

Leptospirosis

Leptospirosis is a group of infections—including Weil's syndrome, infectious (spirochetal) jaundice, and canicola fever—that are caused by Leptospira *bacteria.*

Leptospirosis occurs in many wild and domestic animals. Some animals act as carriers and shed the bacteria in their urine; others become ill and die. People acquire these infections through contact with the animal or its urine.

Although leptospirosis is an occupational disease of farmers and sewer and slaughterhouse workers, most people become infected during such activities as swimming in contaminated water. The 40 to 100 cases reported each year in the United States occur mainly in late summer and early fall. Because leptospirosis typically causes vague flulike symptoms, many cases probably go unreported.

Symptoms and Diagnosis

People usually develop symptoms within 2 to 20 days of becoming infected with the *Leptospira* bacteria. The disease usually starts abruptly with a fever, headache, severe muscle aches, and chills. Symptoms involving the lungs (including the coughing up of blood) occur in 10 to 15 per-

cent of infected people. Episodes of chills and fever, which often reaches 102° F., continue for 4 to 9 days. Pinkeye appears on the third or fourth day.

The fever clears for a few days, but reappears together with other symptoms between the sixth and twelfth day. At this time, inflammation of the lining of the brain (meningitis)▲ usually occurs, causing a stiff neck, headache, and sometimes stupor and coma. These symptoms don't result from infection of the brain lining, however, but rather from inflammation caused by the toxic effects of the body's attempts to destroy the bacteria. A pregnant woman who becomes infected with leptospirosis may miscarry.

Weil's syndrome is a severe form of leptospirosis that causes a continuous fever, stupor, and a reduced ability of the blood to clot, which leads to bleeding within tissues. This syndrome begins as the less severe forms of leptospirosis do. Blood tests reveal anemia, and by the third to sixth day, signs of kidney damage and liver injury appear. Kidney abnormalities may cause painful urination or blood in the urine. Liver injury tends to be mild and usually heals completely.

A doctor can confirm the diagnosis of leptospirosis by identifying the bacteria in cultures of blood, urine, or cerebrospinal fluid samples or, more commonly, by detecting antibodies against the bacteria in the blood.

Prognosis and Treatment

Infected people who don't develop jaundice usually recover. Jaundice indicates liver damage and increases the death rate to 10 percent or higher in people over age 60.

The antibiotic doxycycline can prevent the disease during an outbreak. Penicillin, ampicillin, or similar antibiotics are given to treat the disease. In severe cases, antibiotics may be given intravenously. People with the disease don't have to be isolated, but care must be taken when handling and disposing of their urine.

Rat-Bite Fever

Rat-bite fever is an infection caused by one of two different bacteria transmitted by a rodent bite.

▲ see page 373

Up to 10 percent of rat bites result in rat-bite fever. It is mainly a disease of ghetto dwellers, the homeless, and biomedical laboratory personnel.

Streptobacillus moniliformis, a bacterium that lives in the mouth and throat of healthy rats, is the most common cause of rat-bite fever in the United States. It is not a spirochete. Outbreaks of infection have been linked to people drinking unpasteurized, contaminated milk; when the bacterium is transmitted in this way, the disease is called Haverhill fever. Usually, however, infection follows a bite by an infected wild rat or mouse. Occasionally, the infection is transmitted by weasels and other rodents.

The initial wound usually heals promptly. However, 1 to 22 days after the bite (usually fewer than 10 days), chills, fever, vomiting, headache, and back and joint pains develop abruptly. A rash of small red spots appears on the person's hands and feet after 3 days. In many people, joint swelling and pain follow within a week and may continue for several days or months if treatment is not given. Rare but serious complications include infection of the heart valves and abscesses of the brain or other tissues. A doctor makes the diagnosis by identifying the bacteria in cultures grown from a sample of blood or joint fluid. Treatment consists of penicillin given either orally or intravenously; however, erythromycin can be substituted for people who are allergic to penicillin.

Another type of rat-bite fever (called sodoku) is caused by the spirochete *Spirillum minus*. This infection is common in Asia but rare in the United States. It is also acquired through a rat bite or occasionally a mouse bite. The wound usually heals promptly, but inflammation recurs at the site between 4 and 28 days after the bite (usually more than 10 days). The inflammation is accompanied by a fever that comes and goes and swollen lymph nodes in the affected area. A red rash sometimes appears. Other symptoms include an ill feeling, headache, and fatigue during episodes of the fever. If treatment is not given, the fever typically reappears every 2 to 4 days for up to 8 weeks, and sometimes for up to a year.

A doctor makes the diagnosis by identifying the bacteria in a sample of blood. Alternatively, a sample of tissue from the rash or from a lymph node may be taken. A person with this form of rat-bite fever is usually treated with penicillin, given either orally or intravenously; tetracycline is given to those who are allergic to penicillin.

CHAPTER 180

Anaerobic Bacterial Infections

Anaerobic bacteria differ from other bacteria in several ways. They thrive in areas of the body that have low levels of oxygen (such as the intestine) and in decaying tissue, particularly deep and dirty wounds, where other bacteria can't live and where the body's defenses can't easily reach. Anaerobic bacteria don't need oxygen to exist; in fact, some can't survive in its presence. They tend to cause infections that form collections of pus (abscesses).▲

Hundreds of species of anaerobic bacteria live normally and harmlessly on the skin and mucous membranes, such as the lining of the mouth, intestine, and vagina; several hundred billion bacteria may exist in a cubic inch of stool. If the normal environment of certain species of anaerobic bacteria is disrupted by surgery, poor blood supply, or other tissue damage, they can invade the host's tissues, causing serious—even deadly—infections.

Disease-causing anaerobic bacteria include clostridia—which live in dust, soil, vegetation, and the intestinal tract of humans and animals— and peptococci and peptostreptococci—which are part of the normal bacterial population (flora) of the mouth, upper respiratory tract, and large intestine. Other anaerobic bacteria include *Bacteroides fragilis*, which is part of the normal flora of the large intestine, and *Prevotella melaninogenica* and *Fusobacterium,* which are part of the normal flora of the mouth.

▲ see page 856

Symptoms and Diagnosis

The symptoms of anaerobic infections depend on the site of the infection. Infections include dental abscesses, jawbone infections, periodontal disease, chronic sinusitis and middle ear infection, and abscesses in the brain, spinal cord, lung, abdominal cavity, liver, uterus, genitals, skin, and blood vessels.

To diagnose an anaerobic infection, a doctor usually obtains a sample of pus or body fluid and sends it to the laboratory for a culture. The sample must be handled carefully because exposure to air can kill the anaerobic bacteria, thus making the culture worthless.

Prevention and Treatment

A severe anaerobic bacterial infection usually can be prevented by treating an infection that is limited to a specific area before it spreads. Cleaning wounds thoroughly, removing foreign objects, and starting antibiotic treatment early are helpful preventive measures. Intravenous antibiotics are used before, during, and after abdominal surgery to prevent infection.

Deep wound infections tend to be caused by anaerobic bacteria; such infections are treated primarily by drainage of the abscess and surgical removal (debridement) of dead tissue. Because anaerobic bacteria are difficult to grow in the laboratory, a doctor usually starts giving antibiotics before knowing the results of a laboratory culture. Deep wound infections often contain more than one type of bacteria, so several intravenous antibiotics may be given at the same time. Penicillin is used for infections caused by a mixture of bacteria in the mouth or throat. Because infections originating in the intestine usually include *Bacteroides fragilis*, which is resistant to penicillin, other antibiotics are used.

Clostridial Infections

Many anaerobic infections are caused by clostridia, which produce various toxins that damage tissue or the nervous system.

The most common clostridial infections are short-lived and relatively mild food poisonings.▲ In addition, clostridia may cause inflammation that sometimes destroys the walls of the large and small intestine, a condition called necrotizing enteritis. Although this infection can occur as an isolated case, it may also occur in outbreaks caused by eating contaminated meat.

Diseases Caused by Clostridia

Disease	Bacteria
Tetanus	*Clostridium tetani*
Botulism and infant botulism	*Clostridium botulinum, Clostridium baratii*
Food poisoning	*Clostridium perfringens*
Antibiotic-associated colitis	*Clostridium difficile*
Necrotizing enteritis	*Clostridium perfringens*
Uterine and wound infections	*Clostridium perfringens* and others

Clostridia also infect wounds. Lethal clostridial infections, including skin gangrene■ and tetanus, are relatively rare but may occur if a person is injured or is an injecting drug user. Botulism occurs from eating food contaminated with a toxin produced by some clostridia.★

Severe illness often results from clostridial infections, which can be complicated by deep tissue destruction. The risk of death is high, especially in people with cancer and the elderly.

TETANUS

Tetanus (lockjaw) is a disease caused by a toxin produced by the bacterium Clostridium tetani.

Spasm of the jaw muscles accounts for the name lockjaw. Although it is becoming rare in the United States, tetanus occurs in many parts of the world, especially in developing countries.

Spores of *Clostridium tetani* can live for years in soil and animal feces. Once the tetanus bacteria gain entry into a person's body, infection can develop in both superficial wounds and deep, contaminated wounds. In the United States, people with burns or surgical wounds and injecting drug

▲ see page 518

■ see page 854

★ see page 516

users are particularly at risk of developing a tetanus infection. After childbirth, an infection of the woman's uterus and the umbilical stump of the newborn (tetanus neonatorum) can occur.

Tetanus bacteria produce a toxin as they grow. It is the toxin, not the bacteria themselves, that causes the symptoms of infection.

Symptoms

Symptoms usually appear 5 to 10 days after infection with the bacteria, but they can appear as soon as 2 days or as late as 50 days. The most common symptom is jaw stiffness. Other symptoms include restlessness, difficulty in swallowing, irritability, headache, fever, sore throat, chills, muscle spasms, and stiffness in the neck, arms, and legs. As the disease progresses, a person may have difficulty in opening the jaw (trismus). Spasm of the facial muscles produces a facial expression of a fixed smile and raised eyebrows. Rigidity or spasm of abdominal, neck, and back muscles can cause a distinctive posture with the head and heels pulled back and the body arched forward. Spasms of muscular sphincters in the lower abdomen can lead to constipation and retention of urine.

Minor disturbances—such as noise, a draft, or the bed being jarred—can trigger painful muscle spasms and profuse sweating. During full-body spasms, a person can't cry out or speak because of rigid chest muscles or throat spasm. This condition also prevents normal breathing, causing oxygen deprivation or fatal suffocation.

The person usually has no fever. Breathing and the heart rate usually increase, and reflexes may be exaggerated.

Tetanus also can be limited to a group of muscles near the wound. Spasms near the wound may persist for weeks.

Diagnosis and Prognosis

A doctor suspects tetanus when muscle stiffness or a spasm occurs after a person has suffered a wound. Although *Clostridium tetani* can sometimes be cultured from a swab sample taken from the wound, negative culture results don't exclude a diagnosis of tetanus.

Tetanus has a worldwide mortality rate of 50 percent. Death is most likely in the very young and very old and in injecting drug users. The prognosis is grave if symptoms worsen rapidly or treatment is delayed.

Prevention and Treatment

Preventing tetanus by vaccination is far better than treating tetanus once it develops. In young children, the tetanus vaccine is given as part of the series that includes the diphtheria and pertussis (whooping cough) vaccines.▲ Adults should receive tetanus boosters every 5 to 10 years.

A person who suffers a wound and who has had a tetanus booster in the past 5 years doesn't need any further vaccination. However, a person who hasn't had a booster dose in the past 5 years receives one as soon as possible after an injury. A person who has never been vaccinated or didn't receive the complete series of vaccinations is given an injection of tetanus immunoglobulin and the first of three monthly vaccinations.

Wound care includes prompt, thorough cleaning—especially in deep puncture wounds—because dirt and dead tissue promote the growth of *Clostridium tetani*. Antibiotics such as penicillin or tetracyclines also may be given but aren't substitutes for the surgical removal of damaged tissue.

Tetanus immunoglobulin is given to neutralize the toxin. Antibiotics such as penicillin and tetracycline are given to prevent further toxin production. Other drugs provide sedation, control seizures, and relax the muscles.

The person is usually hospitalized and kept in a quiet room. For people with moderate to severe infections, a ventilator may be required to assist breathing. Nourishment is given intravenously or via a tube inserted through the nose and into the stomach. Bladder and rectal catheterization are often needed to remove body waste. The patient is frequently turned over in bed and forced to cough to help prevent pneumonia. Codeine is given to reduce pain. Other drugs may be given to control the blood pressure and heart rate.

Because a tetanus infection doesn't make the body immune to subsequent infections, the full series of vaccinations must be given after the person recovers.

▲ see box, page 1200

Actinomycosis

Actinomycosis is a chronic infection caused mainly by Actinomyces israelii, *a bacterium that may be present on the gums, teeth, and tonsils.*

This infection causes abscesses to develop at several sites. It occurs in four forms and most often affects adult men. Actinomycosis occasionally occurs in women who use an intrauterine device (IUD) for contraception.

The **abdominal form** is caused by swallowing mouth secretions contaminated with the bacteria. The infection affects the intestines and the lining of the abdominal cavity (peritoneum). Pain, fever, vomiting, diarrhea or constipation, and severe weight loss are common symptoms. A mass develops in the abdomen, and pus may drain to the skin through channels connecting the mass to the abdominal wall.

The **cervicofacial form** (called lumpy jaw) usually begins as a small, flat, hard swelling in the mouth, on the skin of the neck, or below the jaw. The swelling may sometimes cause pain. Subsequently, soft areas develop that discharge a fluid containing small, round, yellowish sulfur granules. The infection may then extend to the cheek, tongue, throat, salivary glands, skull bones, or brain and its lining (meninges).

The **thoracic form** causes chest pain, fever, and a cough that brings up sputum. These symptoms, however, may not appear until the lungs are severely infected. Tracts may even perforate the chest wall, allowing pus to drain through the skin.

In the **generalized form**, infection carried in the blood reaches the skin, spinal vertebrae, brain, liver, kidneys, ureters, and, in women, the uterus and ovaries.

Diagnosis

The symptoms, x-ray findings, and isolation of the *Actinomyces israelii* bacterium in samples of pus, sputum, or tissue help a doctor make the diagnosis. With some intestinal infections, a sample can't be obtained, and surgery is needed to make the diagnosis.

Prognosis and Treatment

Lumpy jaw is the most easily treated form of actinomycosis. The prognosis is worse for the thoracic, abdominal, and generalized forms. The prognosis is the worst when the brain and spinal cord are affected: More than 50 percent of people with these infections have neurologic damage, and more than 25 percent die.

Most people get better slowly with treatment, but months of antibiotic therapy and repeated surgical procedures often are needed. Surgical drainage of large abscesses and antibiotic treatment with penicillin or tetracycline may be continued for several weeks after the symptoms clear up.

CHAPTER 181

Tuberculosis

Tuberculosis is a contagious, potentially fatal infection caused by the airborne bacterium Mycobacterium tuberculosis, M. bovis, *or* M. africanum.

Tuberculosis refers to disease most commonly caused by *Mycobacterium tuberculosis*, but occasionally caused by *M. bovis* or *M. africanum*. Although other mycobacteria cause diseases that mimic tuberculosis, those infections are not contagious, and most respond poorly to drugs that are very effective against tuberculosis.

People have been contracting tuberculosis since ancient times. Tuberculosis became a major scourge in Europe during the Industrial Revolution, when overcrowding in cities was common, accounting for more than 30 percent of all deaths. With the development of the antibiotics streptomycin in the 1940s, isoniazid in the 1950s, ethambutol in the 1960s, and rifampin in the 1970s, the battle against tuberculosis seemed to be won. However, in the mid-1980s, the number of cases

Diseases Resembling Tuberculosis

Many types of mycobacteria exist. Some of these mycobacteria are similar to the ones that cause tuberculosis; they can cause infections with many of the same symptoms as tuberculosis. Although these mycobacteria are common, they generally cause infection only in people with an impaired immune system. The bacteria infect primarily the lungs but may also attack the lymph nodes, bones, skin, and other tissues.

The most common are a group of mycobacteria known as *Mycobacterium avium* complex (MAC). These mycobacteria are highly resistant to most antibiotics, including those used to treat tuberculosis. Infections caused by these bacteria are not contagious.

Lung infection caused by *Mycobacterium avium* complex may occur in middle-aged men whose lungs have been damaged by prolonged smoking, an old tuberculosis infection, bronchitis, emphysema, or other diseases. Infection with this mycobacterium is most common, however, in people with AIDS.

The infection usually develops slowly. The first symptoms include coughing and spitting up mucus. As the infection progresses, the person may regularly spit up blood and have trouble breathing. A chest x-ray may reveal an infection. However, a laboratory analysis of sputum taken from an infected person usually is needed to distinguish the infection from tuberculosis. Treatment with antibiotics is often not effective, even when several drugs are used in combination. However, newer drugs will soon become available that may delay the progression of such infections in older people. Mild cases in people without AIDS may clear up without treatment.

In people with AIDS or other diseases that impair the immune system, *Mycobacterium avium* complex can spread throughout the body. Symptoms include a fever, anemia, blood disorders, diarrhea, and stomach pain. Although antibiotics may temporarily relieve symptoms, the infection is often fatal unless the body's immune response improves.

Lymph node infection caused by *Mycobacterium avium* complex may occur in children, generally those between 1 and 5 years of age. The infection is usually caused by eating soil or drinking water that is contaminated with the mycobacteria. Antibiotics do not usually cure the infection, but the infected lymph nodes may be removed by surgery.

Other mycobacteria grow in swimming pools and even in home aquariums and can cause skin disorders. These infections may clear up without treatment. However, people with chronic infections usually need treatment with tetracycline or another antibiotic for 3 to 6 months. Another type of mycobacteria, *Mycobacterium fortuitum,* can infect wounds and artificial body parts, such as a mechanical heart valve or breast implant. Antibiotics and surgical removal of the infected areas usually cure the infection.

---

in the United States began to rise again. AIDS, combined with overcrowding and unsanitary conditions in many urban areas, homeless shelters, and prisons, has again made tuberculosis a serious public health problem. The problem is especially worrisome because some strains of tuberculosis bacteria have become resistant to the antibiotics used to treat the disease. Nonetheless, in the United States, tuberculosis is starting again to decline as an epidemic.

Tuberculosis is more common among the elderly. Of almost 23,000 cases reported in the United States in 1995, about 28 percent involved persons over age 65. There are three basic reasons why there are more cases in the elderly: (1) Many older persons became infected when tuberculosis was more common; (2) aging may reduce the effectiveness of the body's immune system, which can allow dormant bacteria to become reactivated; and (3) elderly people in chronic care facilities are likely to be in close contact with other elderly people at risk of contracting tuberculosis.

The disease is also more common in blacks than in whites, partly because blacks are more likely to live in poverty and partly because of how tuberculosis has evolved. For thousands of years, tuberculosis exacted a heavy toll in Europe, which was populated primarily by whites; those who happened to be more resistant to the disease were favored for survival and reproduction. These people thus passed on their tuberculosis-resistance genes to subsequent generations. In contrast, ancestors of American blacks first encountered tuberculosis after arrival in America, allowing much less time for them to develop tuberculosis-resistance genes to pass on to their progeny.

How Infection Develops

In the United States today, tuberculosis is solely transmitted by inhaling indoor air contaminated with *Mycobacterium tuberculosis*. For the air to become contaminated, a person with active tuberculosis must cough out the bacteria, which may remain in the air for several hours. However, a fetus may acquire tuberculosis from its mother before or during birth by breathing in or swallowing infected amniotic fluid, and an infant may acquire tuberculosis after birth by breathing in air containing infected droplets.▲ In developing countries, children may become infected with another mycobacterium that causes tuberculosis. This organism, called *Mycobacterium bovis*, may be transmitted in unpasteurized milk.

The immune system of a person infected with tuberculosis usually destroys the bacteria or seals them off at the site of infection. In fact, about 90 to 95 percent of all tuberculosis infections heal without ever being noticed. However, sometimes the bacteria aren't destroyed but remain dormant inside the scavenger white blood cells (called macrophages) for many years. About 80 percent of tuberculosis infections are caused by activation of dormant bacteria. Bacteria living in scars left by the initial infection—usually in the top of one or both lungs—may begin to multiply. Activation of dormant bacteria can occur when the person's immune system becomes impaired—for example, from AIDS, the use of corticosteroids, or very advanced age—in which case the infection can be life threatening.

Usually, a person infected with tuberculosis has a 5 percent chance of developing an active infec-

tion within 1 to 2 years. The progression of tuberculosis varies greatly among people, depending on such factors as race. For example, tuberculosis often progresses more rapidly in blacks and Native Americans than in whites. However, the rate of progression depends, in particular, on the strength of a person's immune system. For example, progression to an active infection is many times more likely and much faster in people with AIDS. A person with AIDS who becomes infected with tuberculosis has a 50 percent chance of developing active tuberculosis within 2 months. If the infecting bacteria happen to be resistant to antibiotics, a person with AIDS and tuberculosis has a 50 percent chance of *dying* within 2 months.

Active tuberculosis usually begins in the lungs (pulmonary tuberculosis). Tuberculosis that affects other parts of the body (extrapulmonary tuberculosis) usually comes from pulmonary tuberculosis that has spread through the blood. As in the lung, the infection may not cause disease, but the bacteria may remain dormant in a small scar.

Symptoms and Complications

At first, an infected person may simply feel unwell or have a cough that is blamed on smoking or a recent episode of flu. The cough may produce a small amount of green or yellow sputum in the morning. The amount of sputum usually increases as the disease progresses. Eventually, the sputum may be streaked with blood, although large amounts of blood are rare.

One of the most common symptoms is awakening in the night drenched with a cold sweat so profuse that the person has to change nightclothes or even the bedsheets. Such a sweat is caused by the subsiding of a low-grade fever that is not apparent to the person.

Shortness of breath may signal the presence of air (pneumothorax) or fluid (pleural effusion) in the pleural space.■ About a third of infections that become manifest do so as a pleural effusion. About 95 percent of pleural effusions in young

---

▲ see page 1222

■ see page 205

Tuberculosis: A Disease of Many Organs

Site of Infection	Symptoms or Complications
Abdominal cavity	Fatigue, slight tenderness, appendicitis-like pain
Bladder	Painful urination
Brain	Fever, headache, nausea, drowsiness, brain damage leading to coma
Pericardium (the membranous sac around the heart)	Fever, enlarged neck veins, shortness of breath
Joints	Arthritis-like symptoms
Kidney	Kidney damage, infection around the kidney
Reproductive organs Men Women	Lump in scrotum Sterility
Spine	Pain, leading to collapsed vertebrae and leg paralysis

adults are caused by a recent infection with *Mycobacterium tuberculosis*. The diagnosis is usually difficult to make, but experienced doctors know the condition must be treated as tuberculosis or else about half of the infections will progress to full-blown tuberculosis in the lung or another organ.

In a new tuberculosis infection, the bacteria travel from the lesion in the lung to the lymph nodes that drain the lung. If the body's natural defenses can control the infection, it goes no further and the bacteria become dormant. However, in children the lymph nodes may become large and compress the bronchial tubes, causing a brassy cough and possibly even resulting in a collapsed lung. Occasionally, bacteria spread up the lymph channels to form a cluster of lymph nodes in the neck. An infection in these lymph nodes may break through the skin and discharge pus.

Tuberculosis can affect organs of the body other than the lung, a condition called extrapulmonary tuberculosis. The kidney and bones are probably the most common sites for extrapulmonary tuberculosis. Tuberculosis in the kidneys may produce few symptoms, but the infection may destroy part of the kidney. Tuberculosis can then spread to the bladder, but unlike other bladder infections, it may cause few symptoms.

In men, the infection may also spread to the prostate, seminal vesicles, and epididymis, producing a lump in the scrotum. In women, tuberculosis can scar the ovaries and fallopian tubes, causing sterility. From the ovaries, the infection may spread to the peritoneum (the membrane lining the abdominal cavity). Symptoms of this condition, called tuberculous peritonitis, may vary from fatigue and vague stomach pain with slight tenderness to excruciating pain that resembles that of appendicitis.

The infection may spread to a joint, causing tuberculous arthritis. The joint becomes inflamed and painful. The most commonly affected joints are the weight-bearing ones (the hips and knees), but the bones of the wrist, hand, and elbow may also be affected.

Tuberculosis can infect the skin, bowel, and adrenal glands. The infection has even been reported in the wall of the aorta (the main artery of the body), causing it to rupture. When tuberculosis spreads to the pericardium (the membranous sac around the heart), the pericardium becomes distended with fluid, a condition called tuberculous pericarditis. The fluid may impair the heart's ability to pump blood. Symptoms include fever, enlargement of the neck veins, and shortness of breath.

A tuberculosis infection that breaks out in the base of the brain (tuberculous meningitis) is extremely dangerous. In the United States and other developed countries, tuberculous meningitis is now most common among the elderly. In developing countries, it is most common among children from birth to age 5. Symptoms of tuberculous meningitis include fever, constant headache, nausea, and drowsiness that can lead to coma. The neck is often so stiff that the chin can't touch the chest. The longer treatment is delayed, the more likely irreparable brain damage will occur. Sometimes, as a person with tuberculous meningitis gets better, a tumor-like mass called a tuberculoma remains in the brain. The tuberculoma may cause symptoms such as muscle weakness, much as a stroke does, and may need to be surgically removed.

In children, the bacteria may infect the spine (vertebrae) and the ends of the long bones of the arms and legs. Pain occurs if the vertebrae are infected. Because x-rays of the person's spine may appear normal, other diagnostic techniques, such as computed tomography (CT) or magnetic resonance imaging (MRI), may be required. If the condition isn't treated, one or two vertebrae may collapse and lead to leg paralysis.

In developing countries, tuberculosis bacteria may be transmitted through contaminated milk and settle in the lymph nodes of the neck or in the small intestine. Because the mucous membrane of the digestive tract is resistant to the bacteria, infection results only if a large number of bacteria remain in the small intestine for a long time or if the immune system is impaired. Intestinal tuberculosis may not produce any symptoms but may result in an abnormal growth of tissue at the infected area, which may be mistaken for cancer.

Diagnosis

Often, the first indication of tuberculosis is an abnormal chest x-ray, taken as part of a diagnostic evaluation for a vague illness. On the x-ray, the disease shows up as irregular white areas against the normally dark background, although other infections and cancer can produce the same x-ray results. The x-ray may reveal pleural effusion or even an enlarged heart (pericarditis).

The diagnosis depends on results of the tuberculin skin test and examination of sputum for *Mycobacterium tuberculosis*. Although a tuberculin skin test is one of the most useful tests for diagnosing tuberculosis, it indicates only that an infection by the bacteria has occurred some time in the past. It doesn't reveal if the infection is currently active, only that live tuberculosis bacteria are present somewhere in the body.

A tuberculin skin test is performed by injecting a small amount of protein derived from tuberculosis bacteria between the layers of the skin, usually on the forearm. A control substance is

---

What is Miliary Tuberculosis?

A potentially life-threatening type of tuberculosis may result when a large number of the bacteria spread throughout the body by way of the bloodstream. This infection is called miliary tuberculosis because the millions of tiny lesions are the size of millet, the small round seeds in wild bird food.

Symptoms of miliary tuberculosis can be very vague and difficult to identify; they include weight loss, fever, chills, weakness, general discomfort, and difficulty in breathing. Involvement of the bone marrow may cause severe anemia and other blood abnormalities, suggesting leukemia. An intermittent release of bacteria into the bloodstream from a hidden lesion may cause a fever that comes and goes, with gradual wasting of the body.

---

sometimes injected at another site. The control substance is made from something that most people react to—yeast or fungi, for example. About 2 days later, the injection site is checked: Swelling and redness indicate a positive result. A person with no reaction to the control substance may have an immune system that isn't functioning properly. In this case, a negative tuberculin test result could be inaccurate. People with severe tuberculosis and a defective immune system also may have falsely negative test results.

To be sure of the diagnosis, a doctor has to obtain a sample of sputum, infected fluid, or tissue for laboratory analysis. A needle may be used to obtain a sample of fluid from the chest, the abdomen, a joint, or around the heart. A minor surgical procedure called a biopsy may be necessary to obtain a small piece of infected tissue. Sputum may provide an adequate sample from the lung; alternatively, a doctor may use an instrument called a bronchoscope to inspect the bronchial tubes and obtain samples of mucus or lung tissue.

A spinal tap to obtain a sample of spinal cord fluid (cerebrospinal fluid) may be needed to look for evidence of tuberculous meningitis, an infection of the membranes covering the brain and spinal cord. The fluid sample is sent to a laboratory equipped to perform a test called polymerase chain reaction (PCR). Although test results are available quickly, a doctor generally begins antibiotic therapy on the mere *suspicion* of tuberculous meningitis in order to prevent death and minimize brain damage.

Evaluating the kidneys for tuberculosis is considerably more difficult than evaluating the lungs. A sample of the person's urine can be used for a PCR test, but other tests may also be needed to determine what damage the disease has already caused. For example, a doctor may use an x-ray technique in which a dye is injected. The dye outlines the kidneys on the x-rays and reveals any abnormal masses or cavities that may be caused by tuberculosis. Occasionally, the doctor will use a needle to obtain a tissue sample of a mass. The sample is examined under a microscope to help distinguish between cancer and tuberculosis.

To confirm tuberculosis of the female reproductive organs, a doctor may examine the pelvis through a tube with a light on the end (laparoscope). Sometimes the disease may be found by microscopic examination of scrapings taken from inside the uterus.

In some cases, a sample of tissue from the liver, a lymph node, or the bone marrow is required. Although such samples usually can be obtained using a needle, surgery may be necessary to obtain them.

Treatment

Antibiotics can usually cure even the most advanced cases of tuberculosis. There are five antibiotics that can be used, each of which can kill all but one in a million of the bacteria. Because an infection of active pulmonary tuberculosis often contains a billion or more bacteria, any drug given alone would leave behind a thousand organisms totally resistant to it. Therefore, at least two drugs with different mechanisms of action are always given, which together can kill off virtually all the bacteria. Treatment must be continued long after the patient feels completely well, because it takes that long to kill all the slow-growing bacteria and reduce the chance of a relapse to near zero.

The most commonly used antibiotics are isoniazid, rifampin, pyrazinamide, streptomycin,

and ethambutol. The first three drugs may be contained in the same capsule. This reduces the number of pills the person has to take each day and also ensures that the person takes the appropriate drugs.

Isoniazid, rifampin, and pyrazinamide can cause nausea and vomiting, as a result of their effects on the liver. When nausea and vomiting occur, the drugs must be stopped until liver function tests can be performed. If test results show a reaction to one of the drugs, a satisfactory substitute can usually be found to complete treatment.

Ethambutol is started in a relatively large dose to help reduce the number of bacteria quickly. The dose is reduced after 2 months to avoid harmful side effects to the eyes. Streptomycin was the first drug found to be effective against tuberculosis but must be given by injection. Although streptomycin is still a very effective drug for advanced infections, it can affect a person's balance and hearing if it is given in large doses or is continued beyond 3 months.

Surgery to remove a portion of the lung is almost never needed today if the person faithfully follows the drug treatment plan. However, sometimes surgery is needed to drain pus from wherever it has accumulated and occasionally to correct a deformity of the spine caused by tuberculosis.

Prevention

There are several ways to prevent tuberculosis. For example, a germicidal ultraviolet light can be used in places where people with a variety of sicknesses may have to sit together for several hours, such as hospital and emergency room waiting areas. Such a light kills the bacteria in the air.

The drug isoniazid is very effective when given to people at greatest risk for developing tuberculosis. Such people include those who have been in close contact with someone with the disease, such as health care workers whose tuberculin skin test result has changed from negative to positive and whose chest x-ray shows no disease. The latter signifies a recent infection that is not fully developed; it can be cured by taking isoniazid daily for 6 to 9 months. Studies have shown that about 10 percent of people with recent infections develop tuberculosis if treatment is not given, *regardless of their age.*

The benefit of preventive therapy is obvious in people under age 25 who react to the tuberculin skin test, because there is a good chance that the infection is recent and can be cured easily before it takes hold. Benefits of preventive treatment in adults over age 25 is difficult to show. The risk of toxicity from the antibiotics may be greater than the risk of developing tuberculosis, except when the reaction is the likely result of a recent infection.

A person who has tested positive with the tuberculin skin test and becomes infected by the human immunodeficiency virus (HIV, the virus that causes AIDS) is at very high risk of developing active infection; isoniazid is therefore given for as long as feasible to prevent the development of tuberculosis. People with HIV infection who do not react to the tuberculin skin test, but who are at considerable risk of contact with persons with active tuberculosis, may also be given isoniazid.

This preventive treatment is effective in eliminating tuberculosis bacteria before they become established.

People with pulmonary tuberculosis who are undergoing treatment do not need to be isolated for more than a few days, because the drugs work quickly to reduce infectiousness. However, those who cough and who fail to take their medication properly may need to be isolated longer, so that they don't spread the disease. A person usually is not contagious after 10 to 14 days of drug treatment. However, if a person works with people who are at high risk, such as those with AIDS or young children, a doctor may require repeated analysis of a sputum sample to determine when there is no danger of transmission of the infection.

In developing countries, a vaccine called BCG is in wide use to prevent infection by *Mycobacterium tuberculosis.* Its value is controversial, and it is used only in those countries where the likelihood of contracting tuberculosis is very high.

CHAPTER 182

Leprosy

Leprosy (Hansen's disease) is a chronic infection, caused by the bacterium Mycobacterium leprae, *that results in damage primarily to the peripheral nerves (nerves outside the brain and spinal cord), skin, mucous membrane of the nose, testes, and eyes.*

The mode of transmission of leprosy is uncertain. When an untreated, severely ill person sneezes, the *Mycobacterium leprae* bacteria are dispersed in the air. About half the people with leprosy probably contracted it through close contact with an infected person. Infection with *Mycobacterium leprae* can also probably come from soil, contact with armadillos, and possibly even contact with bedbugs and mosquitoes.

About 95 percent of people who are exposed to *Mycobacterium leprae* don't develop leprosy because their immune system fights off the infection. In those who do develop the disease, the infection can range from mild (tuberculoid lep-

rosy) to severe (lepromatous leprosy). The mild, tuberculoid form of leprosy isn't contagious.

More than 5 million people worldwide are infected with *Mycobacterium leprae.* Leprosy is most common in Asia, Africa, Latin America, and the islands of the Pacific Ocean. About 5,000 people in the United States are infected: Most of them are in California, Hawaii, and Texas. Almost all cases of leprosy in the United States involve people who have emigrated from developing countries. The infection can start at any age, most commonly beginning in people in their 20s and 30s. The severe, lepromatous form of leprosy is twice as common in men as in women, whereas the mild, tuberculoid form is equally common in both sexes.

Symptoms

Because the bacteria that cause leprosy multiply very slowly, symptoms usually do not begin until at least 1 year after a person has been infected, on average appearing 5 to 7 years subsequently, and often many years later. The signs and symptoms of leprosy depend on the individual person's immune response. The type of leprosy that results determines the long-term prognosis, likely complications, and the need for antibiotic treatment.

In **tuberculoid leprosy,** a rash appears, consisting of one or a few flat, whitish areas. Such areas are numb to the touch because the mycobacteria have damaged the nerves.

In **lepromatous leprosy,** small bumps or larger elevated rashes of variable size and shape appear on the skin. Body hair, including eyebrows and eyelashes, disappears.

Borderline leprosy is an unstable condition that shares features of both forms of leprosy. For people with borderline leprosy, their condition may either improve, in which case it comes to resemble the tuberculoid form, or worsen, in which case it becomes more like the lepromatous form.

During the course of untreated or even treated leprosy, certain immune reactions may occur, sometimes resulting in fever and inflammation of the skin, peripheral nerves, and less commonly the lymph nodes, joints, testes, kidneys, liver, and eyes. Depending on the type of reaction and its severity, treatment with corticosteroids or thalidomide may be effective.

Mycobacterium leprae is the only bacterium that invades peripheral nerves, and almost all of its complications are a direct consequence of that invasion. The brain and spinal cord are not affected. Because the ability to sense touch, pain, and hot and cold decreases, people with peripheral nerve damage may unknowingly burn, cut, or otherwise harm themselves. Also, damage to peripheral nerves may cause muscle weakness, at times resulting in clawing of the fingers and a "drop foot" deformity. Hence, people with leprosy may become disfigured.

People with leprosy also may develop sores on the soles of the feet. Damage to the nasal passages can result in a chronically stuffy nose. Eye damage may lead to blindness. Men with lepromatous leprosy may become impotent and infertile, because the infection can reduce both the amount of testosterone and the amount of sperm produced by the testes.

Diagnosis

The symptoms, such as distinctive skin rashes that don't disappear, a loss of the sense of touch, and particular deformities that result from muscle weakness, provide strong clues to the diagnosis of leprosy. Microscopic examination of a sample of infected skin tissue confirms the diagnosis. For diagnostic purposes, neither blood tests nor cultures are useful.

Prevention and Treatment

In the past, the deformities caused by leprosy led to ostracism, and people with the disease often were isolated in institutions or colonies. In some countries, this practice is still common. Although early treatment can prevent or correct most major deformities, people with leprosy are likely to suffer psychologic and social problems.

Isolation, however, is unnecessary. Leprosy is contagious only in the untreated lepromatous form, and even then it isn't easily transmitted to others. Furthermore, most people are naturally immune to leprosy, and only those in a household with an infected person for an extended time are at risk of developing an infection. Doctors and nurses who treat people with leprosy do not appear to be at increased risk.

Antibiotics can arrest the progression of leprosy or even cure the disease. Because some of the mycobacteria may be resistant to certain antibiotics, a doctor may prescribe more than one drug, particularly for people with lepromatous leprosy. Dapsone, the antibiotic most commonly used to treat leprosy, is relatively inexpensive and generally safe to use; it only occasionally causes allergic skin rashes and anemia. Rifampin, which is more expensive, is even stronger than dapsone; its most serious side effects are damage to the liver and flulike symptoms. Other antibiotics that may be given to people with leprosy include clofazimine, ethionamide, minocycline, clarithromycin, and ofloxacin.

Antibiotic therapy must be continued for a long time, because the bacteria are difficult to eradicate. Depending on the severity of infection and the doctor's judgment, treatment may continue from 6 months to many years. Many people who have lepromatous leprosy take dapsone for the rest of their lives.

Rickettsial Infections

Rickettsiae are microorganisms that share features of both bacteria and viruses. Like bacteria, rickettsiae have enzymes and cell walls, use oxygen, and can be controlled or destroyed by antibiotics. Like viruses, rickettsiae can live and multiply only inside cells. Ehrlichieae are similar to rickettsiae and cause similar disease.

Rickettsiae and Ehrlichieae normally live in ticks, mites, fleas, and lice, and they can be spread to humans by the bites of these bloodsucking insects. In people, rickettsiae usually live inside the cells lining small blood vessels, causing the blood vessels to become inflamed or blocked or to bleed into the surrounding tissue.

Symptoms and Diagnosis

A rickettsial infection may cause a fever, a skin rash, and a feeling of illness (malaise). Because the characteristic rash often doesn't appear for several days, an early diagnosis is difficult. Flea or lice infestation or a prior tick bite, particularly in a geographic area where a rickettsial disease is common (endemic), is a helpful clue in making the diagnosis.

The diagnosis of a rickettsial infection can be confirmed by identifying the organism in special cultures of blood or tissue specimens, by identifying the organism under a microscope using certain stains, or by identifying antibodies to the organism in a blood sample.

Treatment

A rickettsial infection responds promptly to early treatment with the antibiotic chloramphenicol or tetracycline, both of which are taken by mouth. Noticeable improvement usually takes 24 to 36 hours, and fever usually disappears in 2 to 3 days. When treatment begins late, improvement is slower and the fever lasts longer. Antibiotics are continued for at least 24 hours after the fever disappears.

Antibiotics may be taken intravenously by people who are too ill to take them orally. If a person is severely ill and in a late stage of disease, a corticosteroid may be taken for a few days in addition to the antibiotic to relieve serious toxic symptoms and help relieve the inflammation of blood vessels.

Murine Typhus

Murine typhus (rat flea typhus, urban typhus of Malaya) is caused by Rickettsia typhi *and produces a fever and rash.*

Rickettsia typhi lives in fleas that infest rats, mice, and other rodents. Rat fleas transmit the rickettsiae to humans. The disease occurs worldwide, often in outbreaks, particularly in congested urban areas where rats are common.

Symptoms and Treatment

Symptoms appear 6 to 18 days after infection. Usually, the first symptoms are shaking chills, headache, and fever. The fever lasts about 12 days. About 80 percent of patients with the infection develop a faint, slightly raised, pink rash after 4 to 5 days. At first, the rash covers only a small part of the body and is difficult to see. After 4 to 8 days, it gradually fades.

The disease is treated with antibiotics, as are other rickettsial infections. Most patients with murine typhus recover fully. However, death may occur in the elderly and in debilitated persons, especially those with an impaired immune system.

Rocky Mountain Spotted Fever

Rocky Mountain spotted fever (spotted fever, tick fever, tick typhus) is caused by Rickettsia rickettsii *and is transmitted by ixodid ticks.*

Rickettsia rickettsii is unique to the Western Hemisphere. Although the organism was first detected in the Rocky Mountain states, it is found in all of the United States except Maine, Hawaii, and Alaska. It is especially common on the Atlantic seaboard. The disease occurs mainly from May to September, when adult ticks are active and people are likely to be in tick-infested areas. In the southern states, cases occur throughout the year. People who spend a lot of time outdoors in tick-infested areas—such as children under age 15—have an increased risk of infection. Infected ticks transmit the rickettsiae to rabbits, squirrels, deer, bears, dogs, and humans. The disease is not transmitted directly from person to person.

Some Other Rickettsial Infections

Disease	Infecting Organism	Where the Infection Is Found	Features of the Infection
Epidemic typhus	*Rickettsia prowazekii*, transmitted by lice	Throughout the world	After an incubation of 7 to 14 days, onset is sudden, with fever, headache, and extreme fatigue (prostration). A rash appears on the 4th to 6th day. Untreated, the infection may be fatal, especially in those over age 50 years.
Scrub typhus	*Rickettsia tsutsugamu-shi*, transmitted by mites	Asiatic-Pacific area, bounded by Japan, India, Australia, and Thailand	After an incubation of 6 to 21 days, onset is sudden, with fever, chills, and headache. A rash appears on the 5th to 8th day.
Ehrlichiosis	*Ehrlichia canis* or a closely related species, transmitted by the brown dog tick	Throughout the world	Resembles Rocky Mountain spotted fever, but without the rash. Untreated, the infection is often fatal.
Rickettsialpox	*Rickettsia akari*, transmitted by mites	First observed in New York City, has also occurred in other areas in the United States and in Russia, Korea, and Africa	About 1 week before the onset of fever, a small buttonlike ulcer (sore) with a black center appears on the skin; fever comes and goes, lasts about a week, and is accompanied by chills, profuse sweating, headache, sensitivity to the sun, and muscle pains.
Q fever	*Coxiella burnetii (Rickettsia burnetii)*, transmitted by inhaling infected droplets containing the rickettsiae or by consuming infected raw milk	Throughout the world	After an incubation of 9 to 28 days, onset is sudden, with fever, severe headache, chills, extreme weakness, muscle aches, chest pain, and pneumonitis, but no rash.
Trench fever	*Bartonella quintana*, transmitted by lice	Mexico, Tunisia, Eritrea, Poland, and Russia	After a 14- to 30-day incubation, onset is sudden, with fever, weakness, dizziness, headache, and severe back and leg pain; the illness may be prolonged and debilitating.

The rickettsiae live and multiply in the cells lining blood vessels. Commonly infected are blood vessels in and under the skin and those in the brain, lungs, heart, kidneys, liver, and spleen. The blood vessels may become blocked by blood clots.

Symptoms

Symptoms begin suddenly 3 to 12 days after a tick bite. The sooner after infection the symptoms appear (that is, the shorter the incubation period), the more severe the symptoms. A severe headache, chills, extreme exhaustion (prostration), and muscle pains occur. A fever of 103° to 104° F. develops within several days and, in severe cases, remains high for 15 to 20 days. The fever may be temporarily absent in the morning. A hacking, dry cough develops.

On about the fourth day of the fever, a rash appears on the wrists, ankles, palms, soles, and forearms and rapidly extends to the neck, face, armpits, buttocks, and trunk. At first, the rash is flat and pink, but later it becomes slightly raised and darker. Warm water—for example, from a warm bath—makes the rash more evident. In about 4 days, small purplish areas (petechiae) develop because of bleeding in the skin. An ulcer may form when such areas merge.

Involvement of blood vessels in the brain can cause headache, restlessness, an inability to sleep, delirium, and coma. The liver may enlarge; liver inflammation may cause jaundice, although this is rare. Inflammation of the airways (pneumonitis) may develop. Also, pneumonia and brain and heart damage may develop. Although uncommon, low blood pressure and even sudden death occur in severe cases.

Prevention and Treatment

No vaccine against Rocky Mountain spotted fever is available. Tick repellents such as deet (diethyltoluamide) should be applied to the skin and clothing of anyone who works in tick-infested areas. These repellents are effective but occasionally cause toxic reactions, especially in children. Body hygiene and frequent searches for ticks are important to prevent infection. Ticks should be removed carefully, because rickettsiae may be transmitted if an infected tick that is swollen with blood is crushed between the fingers.

There are no practical means of ridding entire outdoor areas of ticks. However, controlling populations of small animals helps reduce the number of ticks. Insecticides are also helpful.

Rocky Mountain spotted fever can cause serious illness or death. Therefore, when a doctor suspects Rocky Mountain spotted fever, an antibiotic is given immediately, before laboratory test results become available. Similarly, any person who lives in a wooded area and who has a fever, headache, or illness should be treated with an antibiotic before the laboratory test results are known—even if a tick bite has not been detected. Antibiotic therapy has significantly reduced the death rate from about 20 to 7 percent. Death usually occurs when treatment is delayed.

Severely ill patients with Rocky Mountain spotted fever often have inadequate blood circulation, which can lead to kidney failure, anemia, tissue swelling, and coma. They also may have considerable leakage from infected blood vessels. For this reason, if intravenous fluids are needed, they are given cautiously to avoid increasing fluid accumulation in the lungs or brain, particularly during the later stages of illness.

CHAPTER 184

Parasitic Infections

A parasite is an organism, such as a single-celled animal (protozoan) or worm, that survives by living inside another, usually much larger, organism (the host).

Parasitic infections are common in rural Africa, Asia, and South America but are rare in developed countries. However, people from developed countries who visit developing countries can be infected by parasites and unknowingly return home with the infection, which may not be readily diagnosed because it is so uncommon.

Worms most commonly enter the body through the mouth, although some enter through the skin. Those that infect the intestine may stay there or may burrow through the intestinal wall and infect other organs. Worms that penetrate the skin often bore through the soles of the feet or enter the skin from infected water while a person is swimming.

If a doctor suspects that a person may have a parasitic infection, samples of blood, stool, or urine may be obtained for laboratory analysis. A doctor may also draw a sample of fluid from an organ or tissue that may be infected. Repeated examinations usually are necessary to find the parasites in these samples.

Parasites often reproduce in the host they infect, so their eggs are sometimes found in the host. If parasites reproduce in the digestive tract, the eggs may be found in the person's stool. To make the diagnosis of a parasitic infection, a doctor will usually collect three samples of stool at 1- or 2-day intervals. Sometimes stool samples are obtained with a sigmoidoscope (a flexible viewing tube used to examine the lower portion of the large intestine).▲ The person providing a stool sample shouldn't take antibiotics, laxatives, or antacids, because these drugs can reduce the number of parasites and make their detection in the laboratory more difficult.

Alternatively, to make the diagnosis, sometimes fluid is withdrawn from the duodenum (upper part of the small intestine), or a sample of the intestinal contents is obtained using a nylon string passed through the mouth.

Amebiasis

Amebiasis is an infection of the large intestine caused by Entamoeba histolytica, *a single-celled parasite.*

Entamoeba histolytica exists in two forms during its life cycle: the active parasite (trophozoite) and the dormant parasite (cyst). Trophozoites live among the intestinal contents and feed on bacteria or on the wall of the intestine. When infection begins, the trophozoites may cause diarrhea, which expels them from the body. Outside the body, the fragile trophozoites die. When the person doesn't have diarrhea, the trophozoites usually become cysts before leaving the intestine. The cysts are very hardy and may spread either directly from person to person or indirectly through food or water.

Direct transmission, the more common route in the United States, occurs through contact with infected stool. Amebiasis is more likely to spread among institutionalized people with poor sanitation practices than among noninstitutionalized people and by sexual contact, particularly among male homosexuals, rather than by casual contact.

Indirect transmission of the cysts is more common in areas where sanitation is poor, such as in migrant labor camps. Fruits and vegetables may be contaminated when grown in soil fertilized by human stool, washed in polluted water, or prepared by someone who is infected.

Symptoms

Most people who are infected, particularly those who live in temperate climates, have no symptoms. Sometimes, the symptoms are so vague that they are barely noticed. Symptoms may include intermittent diarrhea and constipation, increased gas (flatulence), and cramping abdominal pain. The abdomen may be tender when touched, and the stool may contain mucus and blood. The person may have a slight fever. Between attacks, symptoms diminish to recurring cramps and loose or very soft stools. Wasting of the body (emaciation) and anemia are common.

Invasion of the intestinal wall by trophozoites may cause a large lump (ameboma) to form. The ameboma may obstruct the intestine and be mistaken for cancer. Occasionally, trophozoites perforate the intestinal wall. The release of intestinal contents into the abdominal cavity causes severe abdominal pain and an abdominal infection (peritonitis), which requires immediate medical attention.

Trophozoite invasion of the appendix and the surrounding intestine may cause a mild form of appendicitis. Surgery for appendicitis can spread the trophozoites around the abdomen. Therefore, surgery may be delayed for 48 to 72 hours while drugs are given to kill the trophozoites.

An abscess filled with trophozoites may form in the liver. Symptoms include pain or discomfort in the area over the liver, an intermittent fever, sweats, chills, nausea, vomiting, weakness, weight loss, and, occasionally, mild jaundice.

Occasionally, the trophozoites spread through the bloodstream, causing infection in the lungs, brain, and other organs. The skin may also become infected, especially around the buttocks and genitals, as may wounds caused by surgery or injury.

Diagnosis

Amebiasis is diagnosed in a laboratory by examining samples of stool obtained from an infected person; three to six samples may be

▲ see page 485

needed to make the diagnosis. A proctoscope (a flexible viewing tube) may be used to look inside the rectum and to obtain a tissue sample of any ulcers found there.

People with a liver abscess almost always have high levels of antibodies against the parasite in their blood. However, because these antibodies may remain in the bloodstream for months or years, high antibody levels don't necessarily indicate a current abscess. Therefore, if a doctor thinks a liver abscess has formed, a drug that kills amebae (an amebicide) may be prescribed. If the drug is effective, amebiasis is assumed to be the correct diagnosis.

Treatment

Several amebicide drugs taken orally—such as iodoquinol, paromomycin, and diloxanide—kill the parasites in the intestine. Metronidazole or dehydroemetine is taken for severe disease and for disease outside the intestine. Stool samples are reexamined 1, 3, and 6 months after treatment to make sure the person is cured.

Giardiasis

Giardiasis is an infection of the small intestine caused by Giardia lamblia, *a single-celled parasite.*

Giardiasis occurs worldwide and is especially common among children and in places where sanitation is poor. In the United States, giardiasis is one of the most common parasitic infections of the intestine. It is more common in male homosexuals and in people who have traveled to developing countries. It is also more common in people who have low stomach acidity, have had their stomach removed surgically, have chronic pancreatitis,▲ or have an impaired immune system.

The parasite is transmitted from one person to another by cysts passed in the stool. Transmission may occur directly between children or sex partners or indirectly through contaminated food or water.

Symptoms and Diagnosis

The symptoms, which are usually mild, include intermittent nausea, belching, increased gas (flatulence), abdominal discomfort, bulky and foul-smelling stools, and diarrhea. If the infection is severe, the person may fail to absorb important nutrients from food, resulting in significant weight loss. The reason giardiasis interferes with nutrient absorption isn't known.

Giardia lamblia: An Intestinal Parasite

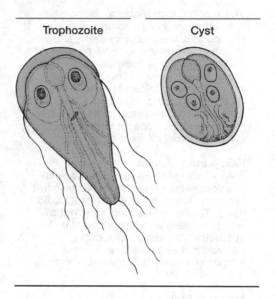

Trophozoite   Cyst

The symptoms suggest the diagnosis to the doctor. Laboratory test results that reveal the parasite in the person's stool or in secretions taken from the duodenum confirm the diagnosis. Because people who have been infected for a long time tend to excrete the parasites at unpredictable intervals, repeated stool examinations may be needed.

Treatment

Taken orally, the drug quinacrine is very effective against giardiasis. However, it may cause gastrointestinal upset, and rarely it leads to extremely abnormal behavior (toxic psychosis). Metronidazole also is effective and produces fewer side effects, but it isn't currently approved for treatment of giardiasis by the Food and Drug Administration. Furazolidone is less effective than either quinacrine or metronidazole, but be-

▲ see page 507

Symptoms and Patterns of Malaria

Vivax and Ovale Malaria

An attack may begin abruptly with a shaking chill, followed by sweating and a fever that comes and goes. Within a week, the typical pattern of intermittent attacks is established. A period of headache or of feeling ill may be followed by a shaking chill. The fever lasts 1 to 8 hours. After the fever subsides, the person feels well until the next chill. New attacks tend to occur every 48 hours in vivax malaria.

Falciparum Malaria

An attack may begin as chills. The person's temperature rises gradually, then falls suddenly. The attack may last for 20 to 36 hours. The person may feel more ill than with vivax malaria and have a severe headache. Between attacks, during intervals that vary from 36 to 72 hours, the person usually feels miserable and has a mild fever.

Malariae Malaria

An attack often begins abruptly. The attack is similar to that of vivax malaria but recurs every 72 hours.

cause it is available in a liquid, it can be given to children. A pregnant woman may be treated with paromomycin, but only if her symptoms are severe.

People who live with an infected person or who have had sexual contact with such a person should see a doctor for testing and, if necessary, treatment.

Malaria

Malaria is an infection of red blood cells caused by Plasmodium, *a single-celled organism.*

Malaria is spread by the bite of an infected female *Anopheles* mosquito, a transfusion with contaminated blood, or an injection with a needle that was previously used by a person with the infection. Four species of parasites—*Plasmodium vivax, Plasmodium ovale, Plasmodium falciparum,* and *Plasmodium malariae*—can infect humans and cause malaria.

Drugs and insecticides have made malaria rare in the United States and in most developed countries, but the infection remains common in the tropics. Visitors from the tropics or travelers returning from those areas sometimes bring the infection with them, possibly causing a small outbreak.

The life cycle of the malarial parasite begins when a female mosquito bites a person with malaria. The mosquito ingests blood containing malarial parasites, which move to the mosquito's salivary glands. When the mosquito bites another person, the parasites are injected along with the mosquito's saliva. Inside the person, the parasites move to the liver, where they multiply. They mature over an average of 2 to 4 weeks, then leave the liver and invade the person's red blood cells. The parasites multiply inside the red blood cells, eventually causing the infected cells to rupture.

Plasmodium vivax and *Plasmodium ovale* may remain in the liver cells while periodically releasing mature parasites into the bloodstream, causing attacks of malarial symptoms. *Plasmodium falciparum* and *Plasmodium malariae* don't remain in the liver. However, if the infection is untreated or inadequately treated, the mature form of *Plasmodium falciparum* may persist in the bloodstream for months, and the mature form of *Plasmodium malariae* may remain in the bloodstream for years, causing repeated attacks of malarial symptoms.

Symptoms and Complications

Symptoms usually begin 10 to 35 days after a mosquito injects the parasite into a person. Often, the first symptoms are a mild fever that comes and goes, headache, muscle aches, and chills, together with a general feeling of illness (malaise). Sometimes symptoms begin with shaking chills followed by fever. These symptoms last 2 or 3 days and are frequently thought to be symptoms of the flu. Subsequent symptoms and patterns of disease vary among the four types of malaria.

In falciparum malaria, abnormal brain function may occur, a complication called cerebral malaria. Symptoms include a fever of at least 104° F., severe headache, drowsiness, delirium, and confusion. Cerebral malaria can be fatal. It most commonly occurs in infants, pregnant women, and travelers to high-risk areas. In vivax malaria, delirium may occur when the fever is high, but otherwise brain symptoms are uncommon.

In all types of malaria, the total white blood cell count is usually normal, but the numbers of lymphocytes and monocytes, two specific types of white blood cells, increase.▲ Usually, mild jaundice develops if malaria is untreated, and the spleen and liver become enlarged. Low levels of blood sugar (glucose) are common and may be severe in people who have high levels of parasites. Blood sugar levels may drop even lower in people being treated with quinine.

Sometimes malaria persists when low levels of parasites remain in the blood. Symptoms include apathy, periodic headaches, a feeling of illness, poor appetite, fatigue, and attacks of chills and fever. The symptoms are considerably milder, and the attacks don't last as long as the first attack.

If the person is untreated, the symptoms of vivax, ovale, or malariae malaria subside spontaneously in 10 to 30 days but may recur at variable intervals. Untreated falciparum malaria is fatal in up to 20 percent of people.

Blackwater fever is a rare complication of malaria caused by the rupture of large numbers of red blood cells. The rupture releases red pigment (hemoglobin) into the bloodstream. The hemoglobin, which is then excreted in the urine, turns the urine dark. Blackwater fever occurs almost exclusively in people with chronic falciparum malaria, especially those who have taken quinine for treatment.

Diagnosis

A doctor suspects malaria when a person has periodic attacks of chills and fever with no apparent cause. The suspicion is greater if within the previous year the person had visited an area where malaria is prevalent and if the spleen is enlarged. Identifying the parasite in a blood sample confirms the diagnosis. More than one sample may be needed to make the diagnosis because the level of parasites in the blood varies over time. The laboratory report identifies the species of *Plasmodium* found in the sample, because the treatment, complications, and prognosis vary depending on the species involved.

Some Reminders About Malaria

- Drugs taken for prevention are not 100 percent effective

- Symptoms can begin a month or more after the infecting mosquito bite

- Early symptoms are nonspecific and often are mistaken for those of influenza

- Rapid diagnosis and early treatment are important, particularly for falciparum malaria, which is fatal in up to 20 percent of infected people

Prevention and Treatment

People who live in malaria-infested areas or who travel to them can take precautions. They can use long-lasting insecticide sprays in homes and outbuildings, place screens on doors and windows, use mosquito netting over their beds, and apply mosquito repellents on their skin. They also can wear enough clothing, particularly after sundown, to protect as much of the skin as possible against mosquito bites.

Drugs can be taken to prevent malaria during travel to a malaria-infested area. The drug is started a week beforehand, continued throughout the stay, and extended for a month after leaving. The most commonly used drug is chloroquine. However, many areas of the world have strains of *Plasmodium falciparum* that are resistant to this drug. Other drugs include mefloquine and doxycycline. However, doxycycline can't be taken by children under age 8 or by pregnant women.

No drug therapy is completely effective in preventing the infection. Travelers who develop a fever while in a malaria-infested area should be examined by a doctor immediately. Pyrimethamine-sulfadoxine, a combination of drugs, may be used for self-treatment until medical help is available.

Treatment depends on which type of malaria the person has and on whether the geographic

▲ see page 810

Toxoplasmosis: Symptoms and Problems

The symptoms of toxoplasmosis can vary, depending on what form the infection takes.

Mild lymphatic toxoplasmosis may resemble infectious mononucleosis. Symptoms can include enlarged lymph nodes in the neck and armpits that usually aren't tender, a feeling of illness, muscle pain, and a fluctuating low fever that can last for weeks or months but that eventually disappears. The person also may have mild anemia, low blood pressure, a low white blood cell count, an increased number of blood lymphocytes, and slightly abnormal results of liver function tests. Commonly, however, infected people have only enlarged, painless lymph nodes in the neck.

Chronic toxoplasmosis produces inflammation inside the eye. Often, the other symptoms are vague.

Acute disseminated toxoplasmosis can cause a rash, high fever, chills, and extreme exhaustion. This type of toxoplasmosis occurs primarily in people with an impaired immune system. In some people, infection causes inflammation of the brain and its lining (meningoencephalitis), liver (hepatitis), lungs (pneumonitis), or heart (myocarditis).

Toxoplasmosis in people with AIDS can spread throughout the body. Most often, brain inflammation (encephalitis) occurs, which may paralyze half the body, diminish sensation in specific areas, and cause convulsions, trembling, headache, confusion, or coma.

---

area has strains of the parasite that are resistant to chloroquine. For an acute attack of falciparum malaria in an area known to have chloroquine-resistant strains, a person may take quinine or receive quinidine intravenously. For the other types of malaria, resistance to chloroquine is less common, and therefore a person usually takes chloroquine followed by primaquine.

Toxoplasmosis

Toxoplasmosis is an infection caused by Toxoplasma gondii, *a single-celled parasite.*

Sexual reproduction by this parasite occurs only in the cells lining the intestine of cats. Eggs (oocysts) are shed in a cat's stool. People become infected by eating raw or undercooked meat containing the dormant form (cysts) of the parasite or by being exposed to soil containing oocysts from cat feces. If a pregnant woman becomes infected, the infection can be transferred to her fetus through the placenta. The woman may then have a miscarriage, or the baby may be stillborn or born with congenital toxoplasmosis.▲

▲ see page 1220

Symptoms

For children born with congenital toxoplasmosis, symptoms may be severe and rapidly fatal, or no symptoms may appear. Symptoms can include inflammation of the eyes, leading to blindness; severe jaundice; easy bruising; convulsions; a large or small head; and severe mental retardation. Very mild symptoms may appear shortly after birth, but more often they appear months or several years later.

Toxoplasmosis acquired after birth seldom causes symptoms and is usually diagnosed when a blood test reveals antibodies against the parasite. However, symptoms sometimes do appear. These vary, depending on whether the person has mild lymphatic toxoplasmosis, chronic toxoplasmosis, or acute disseminated toxoplasmosis. Toxoplasmosis in people with AIDS presents a different array of problems.

Diagnosis

The diagnosis of toxoplasmosis is usually made by a blood test that reveals antibodies against the parasite. However, if a person's immune system is impaired, a doctor may instead depend on computed tomography (CT) and magnetic resonance imaging (MRI) of the brain to make the diagnosis.

Treatment and Prognosis

Toxoplasmosis in newborns and in people who have an impaired immune system is treated with spiramycin or sulfadiazine plus pyrimethamine. Toxoplasmosis in people with AIDS tends to recur so frequently that treatment is usually continued indefinitely. Treatment during pregnancy is controversial because the drug could potentially harm the fetus. Because the disease disappears on its own in most adults with a normal immune system, pregnant women usually aren't treated with drugs unless a vital organ—such as the eye, brain, or heart—is infected or the symptoms are severe and persist throughout the body.

The prognosis for people with toxoplasmosis acquired after birth is good—except in those with an impaired immune system, such as people with AIDS, in whom toxoplasmosis is often fatal.

Babesiosis

Babesiosis is an infection of red blood cells caused by Babesia *parasites.*

Hard-bodied ticks—the same deer ticks that transmit Lyme disease—transmit *Babesia* parasites. Although infection in animals is common, people are rarely infected. Symptoms include fever and anemia caused by the breakdown of red blood cells.

In people whose spleen has been removed, the risk of death is high. In these people, the infection closely resembles falciparum malaria; it produces a high fever, anemia, hemoglobin in the urine, jaundice, and kidney failure. A person with a functioning spleen has a milder illness that usually disappears on its own within weeks or months. Most cases of babesiosis in the United States (which are acquired on the offshore islands of New York and Massachusetts) are mild.

The diagnosis is made by identifying the parasites, which resemble those that cause malaria. Treatment consists of taking the drug clindamycin.

Trichuriasis

Trichuriasis is an infection caused by Trichuris trichiura, *an intestinal roundworm.*

This parasite occurs mainly in the subtropics and tropics, where poor sanitation and a warm, moist climate provide the conditions needed for the eggs to incubate in the soil.

Infection results when a person swallows food containing eggs that have incubated in the soil for 2 to 3 weeks. The larvae hatch in the small intestine, migrate to the large intestine, and embed their heads in the intestinal lining. Each larva grows to about $4\frac{1}{2}$ inches. Mature females produce about 5,000 eggs a day, which are passed in the stool.

Symptoms and Diagnosis

Only a heavy infection causes the symptoms of abdominal pain and diarrhea. Very heavy infections may cause bleeding from the intestine, anemia, weight loss, and appendicitis. Occasionally, the rectum may fall through the anus (a condition called rectal prolapse), especially in a child or a woman in labor.

The barrel-shaped eggs are usually visible in stool samples examined under a microscope.

Prevention and Treatment

Prevention depends on using sanitary toilet facilities, maintaining good personal hygiene, and avoiding uncleaned vegetables. No treatment is needed for light infections. When treatment is needed, mebendazole is the preferred drug, but it can't be used in pregnant women because of its potentially harmful effects on the fetus.

Ascariasis

Ascariasis is an infection caused by Ascaris lumbricoides, *an intestinal roundworm.*

The infection occurs worldwide but is more common in warm areas with poor sanitation, where it persists largely because of indiscriminate defecation by children.

The life cycle of the *Ascaris* parasite resembles that of the parasite that causes trichuriasis, except that the larvae also migrate through the lungs. Once a larva hatches, it migrates through the wall of the small intestine and is carried by the lymphatic vessels and the bloodstream to the lungs. There it passes into the air sacs (alveoli), ascends the respiratory tract, and is swallowed. The larva matures in the small intestine, where it remains as an adult worm. Adult worms range from 6 to 20 inches in length and from $\frac{1}{10}$ to $\frac{2}{10}$ inch in diameter. Symptoms may be caused by the migration of the larva through the lung and by the presence of the adult worm in the intestine.

Symptoms and Diagnosis

The migration of larvae through the lungs can cause fever, coughing, and wheezing. A heavy intestinal infection may cause abdominal cramps and, occasionally, intestinal obstruction. Poor absorption of nutrients may be caused by a heavy concentration of worms. Adult worms occasionally obstruct the appendix, the biliary tract, or the pancreatic duct.

Infection with the adult worm is usually diagnosed by identifying eggs in a sample of stool. Occasionally, laboratory tests reveal adult worms in the stool or vomit or larvae in the sputum. In the blood, the number of eosinophils, a type of white blood cell, may increase. Signs of the migration may be seen on a chest x-ray.

Prevention and Treatment

Prevention requires using adequate sanitation and avoiding uncleaned vegetables. Treatment consists of taking pyrantel pamoate or mebendazole. However, mebendazole can't be taken by pregnant women because of its potentially harmful effects on the fetus.

Hookworm Infection

Hookworm infection is caused by an intestinal roundworm, either Ancylostoma duodenale *or* Necator americanus.

About one fourth of the world's population is infected with hookworms. Infection is most common in warm, moist places where sanitation is poor. *Ancylostoma duodenale* is found in the Mediterranean area, India, China, and Japan; *Necator americanus* is found in the tropical areas of Africa, Asia, and the Americas. These hookworms are now rarely transmitted in the southern part of the United States.

In the life cycle of either hookworm, eggs are discharged in stool and hatch in the soil after incubating for 1 to 2 days. In a few days, larvae are released and live in the soil. A person can become infected by walking barefoot through a field contaminated by human feces because the larvae can penetrate the skin. The larvae reach the lungs through the lymphatic vessels and bloodstream. Then they climb the respiratory tract and are swallowed. About a week after penetrating the skin, they reach the intestine. The larvae attach themselves by their mouths to the lining of the upper small intestine and suck blood.

Symptoms and Diagnosis

An itchy, flat, raised rash (ground itch) may develop where the larvae penetrated the skin. A fever, coughing, and wheezing may be caused by the migration of the larvae through the lungs. Adult worms often cause pain in the upper abdomen. Iron deficiency anemia and low levels of protein in the blood can result from intestinal bleeding. In children, slow growth, heart failure, and widespread tissue swelling may result from prolonged, severe blood loss.

If the infection produces symptoms, the eggs usually are visible in a sample of stool. If the stool isn't examined for several hours, the eggs may hatch and release larvae.

Treatment

A doctor's first priority is to correct the anemia, which usually improves with oral iron supplements but may require iron injections. In severe cases, a blood transfusion may be needed. When the person's condition is stable, an oral drug such as pyrantel pamoate or mebendazole is taken for 1 to 3 days to kill the hookworm. These drugs can't be taken by pregnant women.

Trichinosis

Trichinosis is a parasitic infection caused by Trichinella spiralis.

Trichinosis occurs in most parts of the world but is rare or absent in regions where pigs are fed root vegetables, as in France. In the United States, it has become rare.

Infection results from eating raw or inadequately cooked or processed pork or pork products. In rare cases, infection can result from eating the meat of bears, boars, and some marine mammals. Any of these animals may contain a cyst form of the larvae (trichinae). When the cyst wall is digested in the stomach or duodenum, it releases larvae that penetrate the wall of the small intestine. Within 2 days, the larvae mature and mate. The male worms play no further role in causing infections. The females burrow into the intestinal wall and by the seventh day begin to discharge living larvae.

Each female may produce more than 1,000 larvae. Production continues for about 4 to 6 weeks, after which the female worm dies and is digested. The tiny larvae are carried around the body by

Life Cycle of the Hookworm

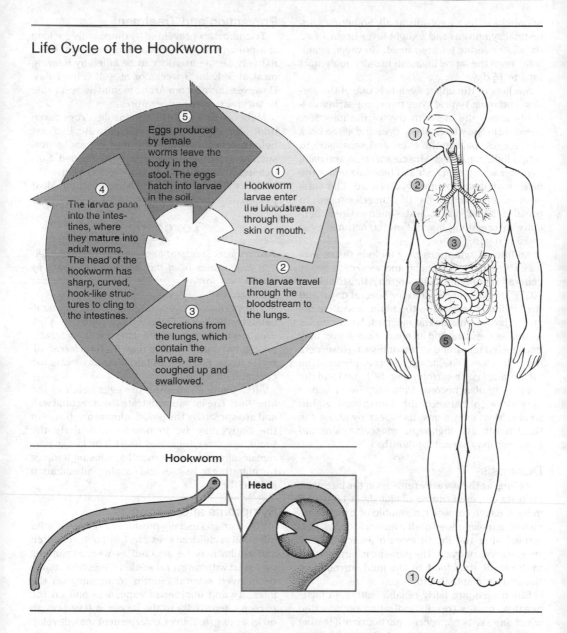

⑤ Eggs produced by female worms leave the body in the stool. The eggs hatch into larvae in the soil.

① Hookworm larvae enter the bloodstream through the skin or mouth.

④ The larvae pass into the intestines, where they mature into adult worms. The head of the hookworm has sharp, curved, hook-like structures to cling to the intestines.

② The larvae travel through the bloodstream to the lungs.

③ Secretions from the lungs, which contain the larvae, are coughed up and swallowed.

Hookworm

Head

the lymphatic vessels and bloodstream. Only larvae that reach skeletal muscles survive. They penetrate the muscles, causing inflammation. By the end of the third month, they form cysts.

Certain muscles, such as the tongue, the muscles of the eye, and the muscles between the ribs, are particularly likely to be infected. Larvae that reach the heart muscle are killed by the intense inflammatory reaction that they provoke.

Symptoms

The symptoms vary, depending on the number of invading larvae, the tissues invaded, and the general physical condition of the person. Many people have no symptoms at all. Sometimes, intestinal symptoms and a slight fever begin 1 to 2 days after eating infected meat. However, symptoms from the larval invasion usually don't start for 7 to 15 days.

Swelling of the upper eyelids is one of the earliest and most typical symptoms, appearing suddenly about the eleventh day of the infection. Bleeding in the whites of the eyes and at the back of the eyes, pain in the eyes, and sensitivity to bright light come next. Muscle soreness and pain, together with a skin rash and bleeding under the nails, may develop shortly afterward. The soreness is pronounced in the muscles used to breathe, speak, chew, and swallow. Great difficulty in breathing may follow, sometimes even causing death.

Additional symptoms may include thirst, profuse sweating, fever, chills, and weakness. Fever generally comes and goes—often rising to at least 102° F., remaining elevated for several days, and then falling gradually. As the immune system destroys larvae outside the muscles, lymph nodes as well as the brain and its membrane linings may become inflamed, and vision or hearing disorders may develop. The lungs or the pleura (the membrane layers surrounding the lungs) and the heart may also become inflamed. Heart failure may develop between the fourth and eighth weeks. Most symptoms disappear by about the third month, although vague muscular pains and tiredness may persist for months.

Diagnosis

As long as the parasite remains in the intestine, no tests can confirm the diagnosis. A biopsy of muscle tissue (in which a sample of tissue is removed and examined under a microscope), performed after the fourth week of infection, may reveal larvae or cysts. The parasite is rarely found in the stool, the blood, or the fluid surrounding the brain and spinal cord.

Blood tests are fairly reliable, although false-negative results (results indicating no infection when one exists) can occur, particularly if testing is done within 2 weeks of the start of the disease. Levels of eosinophils (a type of white blood cell) usually begin increasing about the second week, reach their maximum about the third or fourth week, and then gradually decline. Skin tests are unreliable.

Prevention and Treatment

Trichinosis is prevented by thoroughly cooking raw pork, pork products, and other meats. Alternatively, larvae usually can be killed by freezing meat at 5° F. for 3 weeks or at −4° F. for 1 day. However, larvae from Arctic mammals seem able to survive colder temperatures.

Mebendazole and thiabendazole, drugs taken orally, are effective against the parasite. Bed rest helps relieve muscular pain; however, analgesics, such as aspirin or codeine, may be needed. Corticosteroids, such as prednisone, may be used to reduce inflammation of the heart or brain. Most people with trichinosis recover fully.

Toxocariasis

Toxocariasis (visceral larva migrans) is an infection that results from the invasion of organs by roundworm larvae, such as Toxocara canis *and* Toxocara cati.

The parasite's eggs develop in soil contaminated by the feces of infected dogs and cats. Children's sandboxes, where cats often defecate, pose a hazard. The eggs may be transferred directly to the mouth if a child plays in or eats the contaminated sand.

After being swallowed, the eggs hatch in the intestine. The larvae penetrate the intestinal wall and are spread by the blood. Almost any tissue of the body may be involved—particularly the brain, eye, liver, lung, and heart. The larvae may remain alive for many months, causing damage by migrating to tissues and causing inflammation around them.

Symptoms and Diagnosis

Toxocariasis usually produces a relatively mild infection in children ages 2 to 4, but older children and adults may be affected as well. Symptoms may start within several weeks of infection or may be delayed several months, depending on the intensity and number of exposures and on the person's sensitivity to the larvae. A fever, cough or wheezing, and liver enlargement may develop first. Some people have a skin rash, spleen enlargement, and recurring pneumonia. Older children tend to have no or mild symptoms, but they may develop an eye lesion that impairs vision and that may be confused with a malignant tumor of the eye.

A doctor may suspect toxocariasis in a person who has high levels of eosinophils (a type of white blood cell), an enlarged liver, inflammation of the lungs, a fever, and high levels of antibodies in the blood. Examination of liver tissue obtained by biopsy may reveal evidence of larvae or of inflammation resulting from their presence.

Prevention and Treatment

Infected dogs and cats, particularly those under 6 months old, should be dewormed regularly, starting before they are 4 weeks old. Covering sandboxes when not in use prevents animals from defecating in them.

The infection in humans usually goes away without treatment in 6 to 18 months. The effectiveness of any treatment is uncertain. Mebendazole is probably the best treatment, and diethylcarbamazine may be helpful. Prednisone sometimes is taken to control the symptoms.

Beef Tapeworm Infection

Beef tapeworm infection is an intestinal infection caused by the tapeworm (cestode) Taenia saginata.

The infection is particularly common in Africa, the Middle East, Eastern Europe, Mexico, and South America. Although uncommon in the United States, the infection does occur in many states.

The adult worm lives in the human intestine and may grow 15 to 30 feet in length. Egg-bearing sections of the worm (proglottids) are passed in the stool and are eaten by cattle. The eggs hatch in the cattle and invade the intestinal wall. They are then carried in the bloodstream to skeletal muscle, where they form cysts (cysticerci). People are infected by eating the cysts in raw or undercooked beef.

Symptoms and Diagnosis

Although infection usually causes no symptoms, some people have upper abdominal pain, diarrhea, and weight loss. Occasionally, an infected person may feel a piece of the worm move out through the anus.

The diagnosis usually is made when a piece of the worm is found in the stool. A doctor may press the sticky side of cellophane tape against the area around the anus, place the tape on a glass slide, and examine it under a microscope for the parasite's eggs.

A Beef Tapeworm

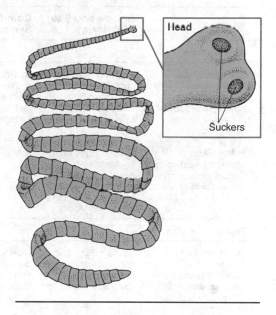

Prevention and Treatment

Beef tapeworm infection may be prevented by cooking beef at a minimum temperature of 133° F. for at least 5 minutes.

An infected person is treated with niclosamide or praziquantel taken orally. The stool is rechecked after 3 months and 6 months to ensure that the infection is cured.

Pork Tapeworm Infection

Pork tapeworm infection is an intestinal infection caused by the adult tapeworm Taenia solium. Infection with the larval stage of the worm causes cysticercosis.

Pork tapeworm infections are common in Asia, the former Soviet Union, Eastern Europe, and Latin America. Infection in the United States is rare, except among immigrants and travelers from high-risk areas.

The adult tapeworm measures 8 to 10 feet in length. It consists of a head armed with several small hooks and a body composed of 1,000 egg-

Other Worm Infections

Infection	Source and Site of Entry	Common Symptoms	Diagnostic Clues	Treatment
Roundworms				
Strongyloidiasis (threadworm) Occurs in moist tropics; infrequently in the southern United States	*Source:* Fecal contamination of soil (larvae) *Entry site:* Skin, usually feet	Radiating pain in pit of stomach, diarrhea, hives or rash in a linear pattern	Larvae in stool or duodenum	Thiabendazole
Enterobiasis (pinworm, seatworm) Occurs worldwide, especially in children	*Source:* Eggs from contaminated articles, spread by contact from anus to fingers to mouth *Entry site:* Mouth	Itching around anus	Eggs found near anus; adult worms near anus	Pyrantel pamoate Mebendazole
Tapeworms				
Dwarf tapeworm infection Occurs worldwide; in the southern United States, in children	*Source:* Eggs that contaminate the environment *Entry site:* Mouth	Diarrhea, abdominal discomfort in children with a massive infection	Eggs in stool	Praziquantel Niclosamide
Echinococcosis Occurs in sheep-raising areas of the world and in Alaska, Utah, Arizona, and Nevada	*Source:* Dog feces *Entry site:* Mouth	Abdominal mass, pain, cough, coughing up blood	Living in area where infection is present, liver or lung cyst, antibodies to tapeworm, spot on chest x-ray	Mebendazole Surgical removal
Flukes				
Intestinal flukes In the United States, occurs only as infections imported from the Far East or tropics	*Source:* Vegetation or freshwater fish *Entry site:* Mouth	Usually no symptoms; sometimes, abdominal pain, diarrhea, intestinal obstruction	Eggs in stool	Praziquantel
Sheep liver flukes Occurs worldwide in sheep-raising countries	*Source:* Watercress that contains cysts *Entry site:* Mouth	Acute abdominal pain, inflammation of the gallbladder	Immature eggs in stool or bile	Praziquantel Bithionol
Fish flukes (clonorchiasis) Occurs in the Far East	*Source:* Freshwater fish *Entry site:* Mouth	Abdominal pain, jaundice, diarrhea	Eggs in stool and intestinal contents	Praziquantel

(continued)

Other Worm Infections (Continued)

Infection	Source and Site of Entry	Common Symptoms	Diagnostic Clues	Treatment
Flukes (continued)				
Lung flukes Occurs extensively in Africa, the Far East, and Latin America; rarely, in the United States and Canada	*Source:* Crabs and crayfish containing cysts *Entry site:* Mouth	Difficulty in breathing, coughing up blood	Immature eggs in stool or sputum, positive blood test results	Praziquantel
Blood flukes (schistosomiasis) Occurs in the Far East, Africa, Latin America, and the Near East	*Source:* Infested water containing fork-tailed cercariae from snail hosts *Entry site:* Skin	Severe diarrhea, scarring of intestinal or bladder walls or liver, blood in urine	Developing eggs in stool or urine	Praziquantel Oxamniquine Metrifonate

containing sections (proglottids). Its life cycle resembles that of the beef tapeworm, except that pigs, rather than cattle, serve as the intermediate host. People also may act as intermediate hosts; the eggs reach the stomach either when a person swallows them or when proglottids are regurgitated from the intestine to the stomach. The embryos are released inside the stomach. They then penetrate the intestinal wall and travel to muscles, internal organs, the brain, and tissue under the skin, where they form cysts. Live cysts cause only a mild tissue reaction, whereas dead ones invoke a vigorous reaction.

Symptoms and Diagnosis

Infection with the adult worm usually doesn't cause any symptoms. Heavy infection with cysts may cause muscle pain, weakness, and fever. If the infection reaches the brain and its membrane linings, they may become inflamed. Seizures can occur as well.

In adult worm infections, eggs may be seen around the anus or in the stool. The proglottid or the head of the worm must be found in the stool and examined under a microscope to distinguish the pork tapeworm from other tapeworms. Live cysts in such tissues as the brain are best seen by computed tomography (CT) or magnetic resonance imaging (MRI). Sometimes cysts can be found by microscopic examination of a sample of tissue taken from a skin nodule. Blood tests for antibodies against the parasite also are available.

Prevention and Treatment

Thoroughly cooking pork prevents infection. The infection is treated with niclosamide or praziquantel taken orally.

Fish Tapeworm Infection

Fish tapeworm infection (diphyllobothriasis) is an intestinal infection caused by the adult tapeworm Diphyllobothrium latum.

Fish tapeworm infection occurs in Europe (particularly Scandinavia), Japan, Africa, South America, Canada, and the United States (especially Alaska and the Great Lakes region). Infection often is caused by eating raw or undercooked freshwater fish.

The adult worm has several thousand egg-containing sections (proglottids) and is 15 to 30 feet long. Eggs are released from proglottids inside the intestine and are expelled in the stool. The egg hatches in freshwater and releases the embryo, which is eaten by small crustaceans. Crustaceans in turn are eaten by fish. People are infected when they eat raw or undercooked infected freshwater fish.

Symptoms and Diagnosis

The infection usually produces no symptoms, although some people may experience mild intestinal upset. In rare cases, the tapeworm causes anemia by depriving the person of vitamin B_{12}. Eggs are found in the stool.

Prevention and Treatment

Thoroughly cooking freshwater fish or freezing them at 14° F. for 48 hours prevents infection. The infection is treated with niclosamide or praziquantel taken orally.

CHAPTER 185

Fungal Infections

A type of plant, fungi include molds and mushrooms. Spores of many fungi are everywhere in the environment. Often these spores float in the air. Of the wide variety of spores that land on the skin or are inhaled into the lungs, some can cause minor infections, which only rarely spread to other parts of the body. A few types of fungi, such as the *Candida* strains, can live normally on body surfaces or in the intestines. These normal body inhabitants only occasionally cause local infections of the skin, vagina, or mouth, but seldom do more harm. Occasionally, however, certain strains of fungi can produce severe infections of the lungs, the liver, and the rest of the body.

Fungi have a special tendency to cause infections in people with a compromised immune system. For example, people with AIDS or those undergoing treatment for cancer are more likely to develop serious fungal infections. Sometimes, people with impaired immunity develop infections caused by types of fungi that seldom, if ever, inflict harm in people whose immune systems are functioning normally. Such infections include mucormycosis and aspergillosis.▲

Some fungal infections are more common in certain geographic areas. For example, in the United States, coccidioidomycosis occurs almost exclusively in the Southwest, whereas histoplasmosis is common in the East and Midwest, especially in the Ohio and Mississippi River valleys. Blastomycosis occurs only in North America and Africa.

Because many fungal infections develop slowly, months or years may pass before a person realizes medical attention is needed. These infections may be difficult to treat, and treatment usually takes a long time. A variety of antifungal drugs are available.■

Histoplasmosis

Histoplasmosis is an infection caused by the fungus Histoplasma capsulatum *that occurs mainly in the lungs but can sometimes spread to all parts of the body.*

The spores of *Histoplasma* are present in the soil, particularly in certain eastern and midwestern states of the United States. Farmers and others working with infected soil are most likely to inhale the spores. Severe disease may result when large numbers of spores are inhaled. People with human immunodeficiency virus (HIV) infection are more likely to develop histoplasmosis, especially the form that spreads throughout the body.

Symptoms and Prognosis

Most people who are infected don't have any symptoms. However, in those who show signs of infection, histoplasmosis occurs in one of three forms: the acute form, the progressive disseminated form, or the chronic cavitary form.

In the **acute form,** symptoms usually appear 3 to 21 days after a person inhales the fungal spores. The person may feel sick and have a fever and a cough. Symptoms usually disappear without treatment in 2 weeks and rarely last longer than 6 weeks. This form of histoplasmosis is seldom fatal.

▲ see page 935

■ see box, page 851

The **progressive disseminated form** doesn't normally affect healthy adults. It usually occurs in infants and in people who have an impaired immune system (such as those with AIDS). Symptoms may worsen either very slowly or extremely rapidly. The liver, spleen, and lymph nodes may enlarge. Less commonly, the infection causes ulcers in the mouth and intestines. In rare cases, the adrenal glands may be damaged, causing Addison's disease.▲ Without treatment, the progressive disseminated form of histoplasmosis is fatal in 90 percent of people. Even with treatment, death may occur rapidly in people with AIDS.

The **chronic cavitary form** is a lung infection that develops gradually over several weeks, producing a cough and increased difficulty in breathing. Symptoms include weight loss, a feeling of illness (malaise), and a mild fever. Most people recover without treatment within 2 to 6 months. However, breathing difficulties may gradually worsen, and some people may cough up blood, sometimes in large amounts. Lung damage or bacterial invasion of the lungs eventually may cause death.

Diagnosis and Treatment

To make the diagnosis, a doctor obtains samples from an infected person's sputum, lymph nodes, bone marrow, liver, mouth ulcers, urine, or blood. These samples are then sent to a laboratory for culture and analysis.

People with the acute form of histoplasmosis rarely require drug treatment. Those with the progressive disseminated form, however, often respond well to treatment with amphotericin B given intravenously or to itraconazole given orally. In the chronic cavitary form, itraconazole or amphotericin B may eliminate the fungus, although the destruction caused by the infection leaves behind scar tissue. Breathing problems similar to those caused by chronic obstructive pulmonary disease usually remain. Therefore, treatment should begin as soon as possible to limit lung damage.

Coccidioidomycosis

Coccidioidomycosis (San Joaquin fever, valley fever) is an infection caused by the fungus Coccidioides immitis that usually affects the lungs.

Risk Factors for Developing Fungal Infections

Therapy that suppresses the immune system
- Anticancer drugs (chemotherapy)
- Corticosteroids and other immunosuppressant drugs

Diseases and conditions
- AIDS
- Kidney failure
- Diabetes
- Lung disease, such as emphysema
- Hodgkin's disease or other lymphomas
- Leukemia
- Extensive burns

Coccidioidomycosis occurs either as a mild lung infection that disappears without treatment (the acute primary form) or as a severe, progressive infection that spreads throughout the body and is often fatal (the progressive form). The progressive form is often a sign that the person has a compromised immune system, usually because of AIDS.

The spores of *Coccidioides* occur in soil in certain areas of North America, Central America, and South America. Farmers and others who work with soil are most likely to inhale the spores and become infected. People who become infected while traveling may not develop symptoms of the disease until after they leave the area.

Symptoms

Most people with the acute primary form of coccidioidomycosis have no symptoms. If symptoms develop, they appear 1 to 3 weeks after the person becomes infected. The symptoms are mild in most people and may include a fever, chest pain, and chills. The person also may cough up sputum and occasionally blood. Some people de-

---

▲ see page 712

velop desert rheumatism—a condition consisting of inflammation of the surface of the eye (conjunctivitis) and joints (arthritis) and the formation of skin nodules (erythema nodosum).

The progressive form of the disease is unusual and may develop weeks, months, or even years after the acute primary infection or after living in an area where the disease is common. Symptoms include a mild fever and losses of appetite, weight, and strength. The lung infection may worsen, causing increased shortness of breath. The infection also may spread from the lungs to the bones, joints, liver, spleen, kidneys, and the brain and its lining.

Diagnosis

A doctor may suspect coccidioidomycosis if a person who lives in or has recently traveled through an infected area develops these symptoms. Samples of sputum or pus are taken from the infected person and sent to a laboratory for analysis. Blood tests may reveal the presence of antibodies against the fungus. Such antibodies appear early but disappear in the acute primary form of disease; the antibodies persist in the progressive form.

Prognosis and Treatment

The acute form of coccidioidomycosis usually clears up without treatment, and recovery usually is complete. However, people with the progressive form are treated with intravenous amphotericin B or oral fluconazole. Alternatively, the doctor may treat the infection with itraconazole or ketoconazole. Although drug treatment can be effective in localized infections, such as those in skin, bones, or joints, relapses often occur after treatment is stopped. The most serious types of progressive disseminated coccidioidomycosis are often fatal, especially meningitis (infection of the membranes of the brain and spinal cord). If a person develops meningitis, fluconazole is used; alternatively, amphotericin B may be injected into the spinal fluid. Treatment must be continued for years, often for the rest of the patient's life. Untreated meningitis is always fatal.

Blastomycosis

Blastomycosis (North American blastomycosis, Gilchrist's disease) is an infection caused by the fungus Blastomyces dermatitidis.

Blastomycosis is primarily a lung infection, but occasionally it spreads through the bloodstream. Spores of *Blastomyces* probably enter the body through the respiratory tract when they are inhaled. It is not known where in the environment the spores originate, but beaver huts were linked to one outbreak. Most infections occur in the United States, chiefly in the Southeast and the Mississippi River valley. Infections have also occurred in widely scattered areas of Africa. Men between the ages of 20 and 40 are most commonly infected. The disease is rare in people with AIDS.

Symptoms and Diagnosis

Blastomycosis of the lungs begins gradually with a fever, chills, and drenching sweats. A cough that may or may not bring up sputum, chest pain, and difficulty in breathing may develop. Although the lung infection usually worsens slowly, it sometimes gets better without treatment.

The disseminated form of blastomycosis may affect many areas of the body. A skin infection may begin as small, raised bumps (papules), which may contain pus (papulopustules). The papules and papulopustules last for a short time and spread slowly. Raised, warty patches then develop, surrounded by tiny, painless abscesses—some that are the size of a pinpoint. Bones may develop painful swellings. In men, painful swelling of the epididymis (a cordlike structure attached to the testes) or deep discomfort from an infection of the prostate gland (prostatitis) may occur.

A doctor can make the diagnosis by examining a sample of sputum or infected tissue, such as skin, under the microscope. If fungi are seen, the sample can be cultured and analyzed in a laboratory to verify the diagnosis.

Treatment

Blastomycosis may be treated with intravenous amphotericin B or oral itraconazole. With treatment, the person begins to feel better in a week, and the fungus disappears rapidly. Without treatment, the infection slowly worsens and leads to death.

Candidiasis

Candidiasis (candidosis, moniliasis) is an infection caused by strains of Candida, *especially* Candida albicans.

Infection of the mucous membranes, as occurs in the mouth or vagina, is common in people with a normal immune system.▲ However, these infections are more common or persistent in people with diabetes or AIDS and in pregnant women.

People with an impaired immune system commonly develop candidiasis that spreads throughout the body. People at risk of developing an infection in the bloodstream (candidemia) include those with a low white blood cell count—which can be caused by leukemia or by treatment for other cancers—and those who have a catheter placed in a blood vessel. An infection of the heart valves (endocarditis) may result from surgery or other invasive procedures involving the heart and blood vessels.

Symptoms and Diagnosis

Symptoms of candidiasis vary, depending on which tissue is infected. For example, infection of the mouth (thrush) causes creamy, white, painful patches to form inside the mouth. Patches in the esophagus can make it difficult for a person to swallow or eat. An infection of the heart valves can cause a fever, a heart murmur, and enlargement of the spleen. An infection of the retina (the light-sensitive membrane on the inner surface of the back of the eye) can cause blindness. An infection of the blood (candidemia) or kidney can cause a fever, very low blood pressure (shock), and a decrease in urine production.

Many candidal infections are apparent from the symptoms alone. For a definite diagnosis, a doctor must be able to see the fungi in a skin sample under a microscope. Samples of blood or spinal fluid that have been cultured may also reveal the presence of the *Candida* fungi.

Prognosis and Treatment

When candidiasis occurs only in the mouth or vagina, antifungal drugs may be applied directly to the area, or fluconazole can be taken orally. Candidiasis that has spread throughout the body is a severe, progressive, and potentially fatal disease that usually is treated with intravenous amphotericin B, although fluconazole is effective for some people.

Certain medical conditions, such as diabetes, can worsen candidiasis and must be controlled to help eradicate the infection.

Sporotrichosis

Sporotrichosis is an infection caused by the fungus Sporothrix schenckii.

Sporothrix is typically found on rosebushes, barberry bushes, sphagnum moss, and other mulches. Most often, farmers, gardeners, and horticulturists are infected.

Sporotrichosis usually affects the skin and nearby lymph vessels. Occasionally, the lungs or other tissues may be infected.

Symptoms and Diagnosis

An infection of the skin and nearby lymph vessels typically starts on a finger as a small, nontender nodule that slowly enlarges and then forms a sore. Over the next several days or weeks, the infection spreads through the lymph vessels that lead from the finger through the hand and arm to the lymph nodes, forming nodules and sores along the way. Usually, the person has no other symptoms.

An infection of the lungs may cause pneumonia, with a slight chest pain and cough, usually in people who have some other lung disease, such as emphysema. Less commonly, an infection may occur in other parts of the body, such as the bones, joints, muscles, or eyes. Very rarely, an infection occurs in the spleen, liver, kidney, genitals, or brain.

The characteristic nodules and sores may lead a doctor to suspect sporotrichosis. The diagnosis is confirmed by culturing and identifying *Sporothrix* from samples of infected tissue.

Treatment

Sporotrichosis that affects the skin usually spreads very slowly and is seldom fatal. The skin infection is treated with itraconazole taken orally. Oral potassium iodide may be prescribed instead, but it is not as effective and causes side effects in most people, such as rash, runny nose, and inflammation of the eyes, mouth, and throat. For life-threatening, body-wide infection, amphotericin B is given intravenously, but oral itraconazole may prove to be as good or better as it is tested in more and more cases.

▲ see pages 946 and 980

Viral Infections

A virus is a small infectious organism—much smaller than a fungus or bacterium—that needs a living cell in order to reproduce. The virus attaches to a cell, often a specific type of cell. Once inside a cell, the virus releases its DNA or RNA (which contains the information needed to create new virus particles) and takes control of some aspects of the cell's metabolism. The components of the virus are then manufactured inside the cell and must be properly assembled for the virus to be released and remain infectious.

What happens to the cell depends on the type of virus. Some viruses kill the cells they infect. Others alter the cell function so that the cell loses control over normal cell division and becomes cancerous. Some viruses incorporate a part or all of their genetic information into the host cell DNA, but they remain silent (or latent) until the cell is disturbed in a way that permits the virus to emerge again.

Most viruses have a preferred host. Some, such as the influenza virus, can infect humans and a variety of other animals. However, some strains of influenza have adapted in a way that allows them to infect one species of animal more efficiently than others. Most viruses commonly found in people are transmitted from person to person. Some viruses, such as the rabies virus or encephalitis viruses, infect animals primarily and humans only occasionally.

The body has a number of specific and nonspecific defenses against viruses. Physical barriers, such as the skin and mucous membranes, discourage easy entry. Infected cells also make interferon(s), a family of glycoproteins that can make noninfected cells more resistant to infection by many viruses.

If a virus does enter the body, various types of white blood cells, such as lymphocytes, are able to attack and destroy infected cells.▲ The two main types of lymphocytes are B lymphocytes and T lymphocytes. When exposed to a viral attack, T lymphocytes increase in number and mature into either helper cells, which aid antibody-producing B lymphocytes, or cytotoxic (killer) cells, which can attack cells infected by a specific virus. T lymphocytes also produce chemicals (called cytokines) that speed this maturation process.■ The cytokines from helper cells can help B lymphocytes and their derivatives, the plasma cells, to produce antibodies that target specific viruses and make them noninfectious before they can infect another cell.

Immunity can be produced by receiving a vaccine. Vaccines are made to resemble a specific virus, such as the virus that causes influenza or measles, which can be given to people without causing the disease. In response to a vaccine, the body increases the number of T and B lymphocytes that are able to recognize the specific virus. In this way, vaccines can produce immunity to a specific virus. Many vaccines are available to prevent common and severe infections, including influenza, measles, mumps, polio, chickenpox (varicella), rabies, German measles (rubella), hepatitis A and B, Japanese encephalitis, and yellow fever.★ However, sometimes a virus changes (mutates) to evade the vaccine antibody, and revaccination becomes necessary.

Immediate protection against a viral infection can be achieved by receiving an injection or infusion of immunoglobulin. Immunoglobulin contains antibodies that were produced by another person or by an animal. For instance, a person traveling to an area where hepatitis A is prevalent may be given an injection of hepatitis A immunoglobulin. However, immunoglobulin can make some vaccines, such as measles or polio, less effective if given at the same time as the vaccine.

Drugs that combat a viral infection are called antiviral drugs.● There are far fewer antiviral drugs than there are antibacterial drugs (antibi-

▲ see page 810

■ see page 812

★ see page 845

● see page 852

otics) Compared with most antibiotics, antiviral drugs are generally more difficult to design, more specific for their targeted organism, and generally more toxic. Antibiotics are not effective for viral infections, but if a person has a bacterial infection as well as a viral infection, an antibiotic is often necessary.

Respiratory Viral Infections

Probably the most common viral infections are those of the lungs and airways. These illnesses include the common cold, influenza, throat infection (pharyngitis or laryngitis), croup in small children,▲ and inflammation of the windpipe (tracheitis) or other airways (bronchiolitis, bronchitis).■

Common Cold

The common cold is a viral infection of the lining of the nose, sinuses, throat, and large airways.

Many different viruses cause colds. Picornaviruses, such as the rhinoviruses, cause most spring, summer, and fall colds. Influenza viruses and respiratory syncytial viruses, which appear regularly in the late fall and winter, cause a spectrum of illnesses, including colds. Influenza viruses spread easily from person to person in infected droplets that are coughed or sneezed into the air. Rhinoviruses and respiratory syncytial viruses also are spread this way, but perhaps mainly by direct contact with infected secretions carried on the fingers.

Why a person is more likely to become infected at one time than another isn't entirely known. Becoming chilled doesn't by itself cause colds or increase a person's susceptibility to infection by a respiratory virus. A person's general health or eating habits don't seem to make any difference either. Neither does having an abnormality of the nose or throat, such as enlarged tonsils or adenoids. However, people who are fatigued or emotionally distressed, those who have allergies of the nose or throat, and women who are halfway between menstrual periods may be more likely to notice the symptoms of a cold.

Symptoms and Complications

Symptoms of the common cold start 1 to 3 days after infection. Usually, the first symptoms are discomfort in the nose or throat. Later the person starts sneezing, has a runny nose, and feels mildly ill. Usually, fever does not develop, but sometimes a slight fever appears when symptoms are beginning. Secretions from the nose are watery and clear and can be annoyingly plentiful during the first day or two. Later the secretions become thicker, opaque, yellow-green, and less abundant. Many people also develop a cough. Symptoms usually disappear in 4 to 10 days, although a cough with or without sputum often lasts into the second week.

Complications may prolong the symptoms. Infection of the windpipe (trachea) along with some tightness in the chest and a burning discomfort are more likely in some people and with some viruses. People with persistent bronchitis or asthma may have more difficulty breathing during and after a cold. A bacterial infection of the ears, the sinuses, or the windpipe and airways (tracheobronchial infection) may follow the cold and requires treatment with antibiotics.

Diagnosis

Most colds can be readily diagnosed based on the typical symptoms. However, bacterial infections, allergies, and other disorders can cause similar symptoms. The same viruses that cause colds also can cause symptoms similar to those of influenza. A high fever suggests that the infection is not a simple cold. Tests to diagnose a cold usually aren't needed unless complications develop.

Treatment

A person with a cold should stay warm and comfortable and try to avoid spreading the infection to others. This is often most readily done in the earliest stages of infection. Anyone with a fever or severe symptoms should probably rest at home. Drinking fluids helps to keep secretions loose and easier to expel.

Cold remedies are popular, but most of their benefits are doubtful.★ Aspirin may even in-

---

▲ see page 1273

■ see page 1274

★ see page 56

Preventing the Common Cold

Because so many different viruses cause colds and because the number of antibodies produced against a cold virus declines over time, most people continue to get colds throughout their lives. An effective vaccine for every respiratory virus has not been devised, but a vaccine for influenza is updated annually for new influenza strains, and vaccines are being developed for other viruses, such as respiratory syncytial virus and parainfluenza virus.

The best preventive measures involve good hygiene. Because many cold viruses are spread by contact with infected secretions, frequently washing the hands, carefully disposing of used tissues, and cleaning items and surfaces can help to reduce their spread.

Many treatments to prevent colds have been proposed and tested, but none has been shown to be reliably effective. Large doses of vitamin C (up to 2,000 milligrams a day) have not been shown to reduce the risk of acquiring colds or the amount of virus shed from an infected person.

When sprayed into the nose, interferon, a drug that enhances the ability of cells to resist infection, may prevent infection by some types of cold viruses (particularly rhinoviruses). However, it does not work after infection is established, may cause inflammation and nosebleeds, and has limited effect against certain viruses, such as influenza and parainfluenza viruses.

crease virus shedding, while improving symptoms only slightly. If a drug is needed to relieve pain or fever in a child or adolescent, acetaminophen or ibuprofen is preferred, because aspirin is associated with an increased risk of Reye's syndrome, a potentially fatal condition.▲

A nasal decongestant provides only temporary, limited relief. Antihistamines may help dry up a

▲ see page 1280

runny nose, but they have been shown to do so only in people with a history of allergy and they cause drowsiness and other side effects, particularly in the elderly. Inhaling steam or mist from a vaporizer is a method some find useful to loosen secretions and reduce chest tightness, and washing the nasal passages with an isotonic salt solution can help to remove tenacious secretions. Because coughing may be the only way to clear secretions and debris from the airways during a viral infection, it is preferable to leave a cough untreated unless it interferes with sleep or causes great discomfort. A severe cough may be treated with a cough suppressant. Antibiotics aren't effective against a cold; they should be used only if a bacterial infection also develops.

Influenza

Influenza (flu) is a viral infection that causes a fever, runny nose, cough, headache, a feeling of illness (malaise), and inflammation of the lining of the nose and airways.

Every year, widespread outbreaks of respiratory illness caused by influenza occur during late fall or early winter. The illness occurs throughout the world. Although many respiratory viruses can cause the symptoms of influenza, the influenza A or influenza B virus is usually responsible for the epidemics in the late fall or winter.

The virus is spread by inhaling infected droplets that have been coughed or sneezed out by an infected person or by having direct contact with an infected person's secretions. Handling infected household articles may sometimes be responsible.

Symptoms

Influenza differs from the common cold. Symptoms start 24 to 48 hours after infection and can begin suddenly. Chills or a chilly sensation may be the initial indication of influenza. Fever is common during the first few days, and the temperature may rise to 102° to 103° F. Many people feel sufficiently ill to remain in bed; they have aches and pains throughout the body, most pronounced in the back and legs. Headache is often severe, with aching around and behind the eyes. Bright light may make the headache worse.

At first, the respiratory symptoms may be relatively mild, with a scratchy sore throat, a burning sensation in the chest, a dry cough, and a runny nose. Later, the cough can become severe and bring up sputum. The skin may be warm and flushed, especially on the face. The mouth and throat may redden, the eyes may water, and the whites of the eyes may be mildly inflamed. The ill person, especially a child, may have nausea and vomiting.

After 2 or 3 days, most symptoms disappear rapidly, and the fever usually ends, although fever sometimes lasts up to 5 days. However, bronchitis and coughing may persist for 10 days or longer, and changes in the airways may take 6 to 8 weeks to completely resolve. Weakness and fatigue may persist for several days or occasionally for weeks.

Diagnosis

Because most people are familiar with the symptoms of influenza, and because influenza occurs in epidemics, influenza is often correctly diagnosed by the person who has it or by family members. The severity of the illness and the presence of a high fever distinguish influenza from the common cold. Although not always necessary or available, a blood test can identify an influenza infection. Even better at establishing the diagnosis of influenza is the recovery of the virus in a culture of respiratory secretions.

Prevention

A person exposed to an influenza virus produces antibodies, which protect against reinfection by that particular virus. Vaccination against influenza every year, however, is the best way to avoid contracting influenza. Influenza vaccines contain inactivated (or "killed") influenza virus strains or viral particles. A vaccine may be monovalent (one strain) or polyvalent (usually three strains). A monovalent vaccine permits a larger dose against a new virus strain, and a polyvalent vaccine boosts resistance against more than one strain. A different vaccine is introduced every year based on predictions of which strains are most likely to cause influenza. The predictions take into account the strain of virus that predominated during the previous flu season and the strain causing disease in other parts of the world in the current preseason.

Vaccination is particularly important for those who are likely to become very ill if infected. In the United States, vaccination should take place during the fall, so that levels of antibodies will be

Complications of Influenza

Although influenza is a serious illness in anyone, most healthy people feel well again in 7 to 10 days. Complications of influenza can make the illness more serious. The very young, the very old, and people with heart, lung, or nervous system disease have a particularly high risk of complications and death.

Rare cases of influenza result in severe inflammation of the airways with bloody secretions (hemorrhagic bronchitis). Viral pneumonia is the most severe complication; it can progress rapidly and cause death in as early as 48 hours. It is uncertain what determines whether pneumonia will occur, but it is most likely to occur during an epidemic caused by a strain of influenza A for which few people have immunity and strikes people at highest risk. Bacterial pneumonia may also complicate influenza because the lungs' ability to eliminate or control bacteria in the respiratory tract is affected.

The influenza virus very rarely has been associated with inflammation of the brain (encephalitis), heart (myocarditis), or muscle (myositis). Encephalitis may make the person drowsy, confused, or even comatose. Myocarditis may cause heart murmurs or heart failure.

Reye's syndrome is a serious and potentially fatal complication that occurs most commonly in children during epidemics of influenza B, particularly if they have received aspirin or a drug containing aspirin.

highest during the peak influenza months—November through March. For most people, about 2 weeks are needed for the vaccination to provide protection. However, children or other people who have never been exposed to an influenza virus need to receive two doses of vaccine, separated by 1 month, for adequate immunity.

Amantadine or rimantadine, two antiviral drugs, can protect against influenza A but not influenza B. They are used during epidemics of influenza A to protect those in close contact with infected people and others at high risk who have not been vaccinated. The drug may be discontinued 2 to 3 weeks after a person is vaccinated. If a vaccine can't be given, amantadine or rimantadine is taken throughout the epidemic, usually for 6 to 8 weeks. These drugs can cause nervousness, sleeplessness, and other side effects, especially in the elderly and in those with brain or kidney disease. Rimantadine tends to cause fewer side effects than amantadine.

Treatment

The main treatment for influenza is to stay in bed or rest adequately, to maintain hydration by drinking plenty of fluids, and to avoid exertion, ideally from the time the symptoms begin until 24 to 48 hours after the body temperature returns to normal. People with severe symptoms but without complications may take acetaminophen, aspirin, ibuprofen, or naproxen. Because of the danger of Reye's syndrome, children should not be given aspirin. Acetaminophen is, however, acceptable for use in children if needed. Other measures as listed for the common cold, such as nasal decongestants and steam inhalation, may relieve symptoms.

If taken early in the course of uncomplicated influenza A infection, amantadine or rimantadine helps to reduce the duration and severity of fever and respiratory symptoms. Neither reduces the severity of viral pneumonia, but either may be given to try to improve the likelihood of recovery. Ribavirin, which can be inhaled as an aerosol or taken orally, has been demonstrated to shorten the duration of the fever and affect the virus' ability to reproduce, but its use is still experimental. Ribavirin may, however, be given to relieve the symptoms of viral pneumonia.

A secondary bacterial infection is treated with antibiotics. Bacterial pneumonia caused by one type of bacteria, the pneumococcus, may be prevented with a polyvalent vaccine containing the common types of pneumococci.▲ However, the vaccine isn't given to someone who already has influenza.

Herpesvirus Infections

The two main types of herpesvirus that cause infections involving blisters on the skin are herpes simplex and herpes zoster. Another herpesvirus, Epstein-Barr virus, causes infectious mononucleosis. Cytomegalovirus, another of the herpesviruses, can produce an illness indistinguishable from infectious mononucleosis. A more recently identified herpesvirus (herpesvirus 6) causes a childhood illness known as roseola infantum. Human herpesvirus 7 has not been definitely linked with any illness at this time. In some studies, herpesvirus 8 has been interpreted to be the cause of Kaposi's sarcoma in people with AIDS.

Herpes Simplex

Herpes simplex infection produces recurring episodes of small, painful, fluid-filled blisters on the skin or mucous membranes.

Herpes simplex produces an eruption on the skin or mucous membranes. The eruption subsides, although the virus remains in an inactive (latent) state inside the ganglia (a group of nerve cell bodies) that supply the sensory nerves to the infected area. Periodically, the virus is reactivated and begins replicating, often causing skin eruptions of blisters in the same location as the earlier infection. However, the virus may be present in the skin without causing an obvious blister; the virus in this state can serve as a source for infecting other people. Eruptions may be triggered by overexposure to sunlight, a fever, physical or emotional stress, suppression of the immune system, or certain foods and drugs, but often the inciting factors are unknown.

The two types of herpes simplex virus that infect the skin are HSV-1 and HSV-2. HSV-1 is the usual cause of cold sores on the lips (herpes labialis)■ and sores on the cornea of the eye (herpes simplex keratitis) ★; it is usually transmitted by contact with secretions from or around the mouth. HSV-2 usually causes genital herpes and is transmitted primarily by direct contact with the sores, most often during sexual contact.●

▲ see page 195

■ see page 456

★ see page 1041

● see page 946

Symptoms and Complications

A recurrence of herpes simplex is heralded by tingling, discomfort, or itching, which precedes the blisters by several hours to 2 to 3 days. Blisters surrounded by a reddish rim may appear anywhere on the skin or mucous membranes, but they occur most often in and around the mouth, on the lips, and on the genitals. The blisters (which can be painful) tend to form in clusters, which join together into a larger single site. After a few days, the blisters begin to dry, forming a thin, yellowish crust and shallow ulcers. Healing typically begins within 1 to 2 weeks after the appearance and is usually completed by 21 days. Blisters in moist body areas, however, are sometimes slower to heal. Some scarring may occur if eruptions keep developing in the same place or if a secondary bacterial infection occurs.

The first herpes infection in infants or young children may cause painful sores and inflammation in the mouth and gums (gingivostomatitis) or painful inflammation of the vulva and vagina (vulvovaginitis). These conditions also cause irritability, loss of appetite, and fever. In infants and less often in older children, the infection may spread by way of the blood to involve internal organs, including the brain—an infection that can be fatal.

A woman who has had an HSV-2 infection can transmit the infection to her fetus, especially if an episode occurred in the last 3 months of pregnancy.▲ Herpes simplex virus in a fetus may cause a mild inflammation of the membrane surrounding the brain (meningitis) or occasionally severe brain inflammation (encephalitis).

If infants or adults with a skin condition called atopic eczema become infected with herpes simplex virus, they can develop a potentially fatal illness called eczema herpeticum.■ *Therefore, people with atopic eczema should avoid being near anyone with an active herpes infection.* In people with AIDS, herpes infections of the skin may be particularly severe and persistent. Inflammation of the esophagus and intestine, ulcers around the anus, pneumonia, or nerve abnormalities also occur more frequently in people with AIDS.

A swollen, painful, red fingertip caused by herpes simplex virus entering through a break in the skin is called **herpetic whitlow.** It most often occurs in health care workers who have not had herpes simplex and who touch body fluids containing herpes simplex virus.

Diagnosis

Herpes simplex is sometimes difficult for a doctor to recognize. It can be confused with an allergic reaction, other viral infections, or even a skin reaction to certain drugs. The location of the blisters on the body can sometimes be helpful in making the diagnosis.

A doctor who suspects herpes simplex can examine scrapings from the blisters under a microscope. If the person has herpes simplex infection, these scrapings will show large infected cells. Cultures for the virus, blood tests for increased antibody levels, and biopsy techniques can confirm the diagnosis. These tests are rarely needed, however. A diagnosis may be possible at a very early stage, using newer techniques such as the polymerase chain reaction, which can be used to identify the DNA from the herpes simplex virus in a body tissue or fluid.

Treatment

For most people, the only treatment needed for herpes labialis is to keep the infected area clean by gentle washing with soap and water. The area should then be carefully dried; allowing the blisters to stay moist may worsen the inflammation, delay healing, and possibly promote a bacterial infection. To prevent or treat a bacterial infection, an antibiotic ointment such as neomycin-bacitracin may be applied to the skin. If a bacterial infection appears to be progressing or is causing additional symptoms, the doctor may prescribe antibiotics taken orally or by injection.

Antiviral creams such as idoxuridine, trifluridine, and acyclovir are sometimes effective when placed directly on the blisters. Acyclovir or vidarabine, taken orally, may be used for severe bodywide herpes infections. Taking acyclovir daily is sometimes needed to suppress repeated eruptions, particularly when the genitals are involved. Specific treatment measures may be needed for herpes simplex keratitis★ or genital herpes.●

▲ see page 1219

■ see page 961

★ see page 1041

● see page 946

What is Postherpetic Neuralgia?

Pain in areas of skin supplied by the infected nerves is called postherpetic neuralgia. This pain may persist for months or years after an episode of shingles. It does not indicate that the virus continues to be actively replicating. The pain of postherpetic neuralgia may be constant or intermittent, and it may worsen at night or in response to heat or cold. Sometimes the pain is incapacitating.

Postherpetic neuralgia occurs most often in older people: 25 to 50 percent of those over age 50 who have shingles also have some postherpetic neuralgia. However, only about 10 percent of all people with shingles develop postherpetic neuralgia. Few have severe pain.

In most instances, the pain subsides within 1 to 3 months, but in 10 to 20 percent of cases, the pain may persist for more than 1 year, and has rarely lasted for more than 10 years.

Although a number of treatments for postherpetic neuralgia have been tried, no treatment has been found to be routinely successful. In most instances, pain is mild and requires no specific treatment.

Shingles

Shingles (herpes zoster) is an infection that produces a severely painful skin eruption of fluid-filled blisters.

Shingles is caused by the same herpesvirus, varicella-zoster virus, that causes chickenpox.▲ The initial infection with varicella-zoster virus, which may be in the form of chickenpox, ends with the virus entering the nerves in the ganglia (a group of nerve cell bodies) of spinal or cranial nerves and remaining latent there. Shingles always is limited to the skin distribution of the nerve root(s) involved (dermatomes).■

▲ see page 1270

■ see box, page 325

The herpes zoster virus may never cause symptoms again, or it may be reactivated many years later. Shingles occurs when the virus is reactivated. Sometimes, reactivation occurs when the body's immunity is reduced by another disorder, such as AIDS or Hodgkin's disease, or by drugs that impair the immune system. Most often, the reason for reactivation is unknown. The occurrence of shingles does not usually mean that a significant disease process is underway. Shingles may occur at any age but is most common after age 50.

Symptoms and Complications

Some people feel unwell and have chills, a fever, nausea, diarrhea, or difficulties with urination in the 3 or 4 days before shingles develops. Others experience pain or only a tingling sensation or itching in an area of skin. Clusters of small fluid-filled blisters surrounded by a small red area develop. The blisters occupy only a limited area of skin supplied by the affected nerves. Most often, blisters appear on the trunk and usually on only one side. However, a few blisters may appear elsewhere as well. The involved area of the body is usually sensitive to any stimulus, including very light touch, and may be severely painful.

The blisters begin to dry and scab about 5 days after they appear. Until scabbing occurs, the blisters contain herpes zoster virus, which can cause chickenpox if transmitted to susceptible persons. Blisters that cover large areas of skin or that persist for more than 2 weeks usually indicate that the immune system isn't functioning properly.

One attack of shingles usually gives a person lifelong immunity from further attacks; fewer than 4 percent of people have further attacks. Most people recover without any lasting effects. However, scarring of the skin, which can be extensive, may occur even if the person doesn't develop a secondary bacterial infection. Involvement of the branch of the facial nerve to the eye can be quite serious.

Diagnosis

A doctor may have trouble diagnosing shingles before the blisters appear, but the location of the initial pain in a vague band on one side of the body can be a useful clue. Depending on the nerves involved, the pain may resemble that caused by appendicitis, a kidney stone or gall-stone, or inflammation of the large intestine. The blisters produced by shingles may be nearly identical to those produced by herpes simplex. However, blisters from herpes simplex tend to occur in a different, more restricted pattern on the skin; tend to be fewer; and may recur repeatedly in the same location. If necessary, laboratory tests may be used to confirm the diagnosis.

Treatment

The best treatment for herpes zoster still isn't certain. Neither corticosteroids nor an antiserum with high levels of antibodies to varicella-zoster virus have an effect on shingles once it begins. No drug can eliminate the virus. However, antiviral drugs such as acyclovir or famciclovir may be given to shorten the duration of the skin eruption, particularly in people who have an impaired immune system. Keeping the skin clean is important to prevent secondary bacterial infections.

Aspirin or codeine may relieve pain temporarily and can be useful if pain prevents activities or sleep. Aspirin should be avoided in children because of the risk of Reye's syndrome.

Infectious Mononucleosis

Infectious mononucleosis is a disease characterized by fever, sore throat, and enlarged lymph nodes, which is caused by Epstein-Barr virus—one of the herpesviruses.

After first invading the cells lining the nose and throat, Epstein-Barr virus spreads to the B lymphocytes (the white blood cells responsible for producing antibodies). Epstein-Barr virus infection is very common, affecting children, adolescents, and adults alike. About 50 percent of all American children have had an Epstein-Barr virus infection before age 5. However, the virus isn't very contagious. Teenagers and young adults usually catch infectious mononucleosis by kissing or having other intimate contact with someone infected with the Epstein-Barr virus.

The Epstein-Barr virus is associated with Burkitt's lymphoma, a type of cancer that occurs mainly in tropical Africa. The virus also may play a role in certain tumors of B lymphocytes in people with impaired immune systems, such as those with organ transplants or AIDS, and in some cancers of the nose and throat. Although the precise role the Epstein-Barr virus plays in these cancers isn't known, it is thought that specific parts of the virus' genetic material alter the growth cycle of infected cells.

Symptoms and Complications

In most children under age 5, the infection produces no symptoms. In adolescents and adults, it may or may not produce symptoms. The usual time between infection and the appearance of symptoms (incubation period) is thought to be 30 to 50 days.

The four major symptoms are fatigue, a fever, sore throat, and swelling of the lymph nodes. Not everyone has all four symptoms. Usually, the infection begins with a feeling of illness that lasts several days to a week. Then comes a fever, sore throat, and enlarged lymph nodes. The fever usually peaks at around 103° F. in the afternoon or early evening. The throat may be very sore, and pus-like material may be produced at the back of the throat. Any lymph node may be enlarged, but those in the neck are most commonly enlarged. Fatigue is usually most pronounced in the first 2 to 3 weeks.

In more than 50 percent of the people with infectious mononucleosis, the spleen enlarges. The liver may enlarge slightly. Less commonly, jaundice and swelling around the eyes may occur. Skin rashes occur infrequently, but in one study nearly everyone infected with Epstein-Barr virus who received the antibiotic ampicillin developed a rash. Other complications include inflammation of the brain (encephalitis), seizures, various nerve abnormalities, inflammation of the brain lining (meningitis), and behavioral abnormalities.

The spleen may be more susceptible to injury, and rupture of the spleen is a possible but uncommon complication. If it occurs, emergency surgery to remove the spleen may be required. The number of white blood cells is usually elevated, but the number of white blood cells, blood platelets, and red blood cells may fall. They usually return to normal without treatment. Rarely, enlarged lymph nodes in the neck may press on the airway. Congestion in the lungs may develop but often doesn't cause symptoms.

Diagnosis

A doctor diagnoses infectious mononucleosis based on the symptoms. However, the symptoms of infectious mononucleosis are not specific and

---

Chronic Fatigue Syndrome

Chronic fatigue syndrome is an illness that occurs mainly among adults aged 20 to 40 years. Twice as many women as men develop chronic fatigue syndrome. Symptoms include debilitating fatigue, interference with the ability to concentrate, and, in some cases, a low-grade fever and swelling of the lymph nodes.

The Epstein-Barr virus was initially suspected as a possible cause, but little evidence supports this theory.

---

may resemble those of other infections. For example, cytomegalovirus infection causes a syndrome that is difficult to distinguish from infectious mononucleosis. Other viruses and toxoplasmosis can also produce symptoms similar to those of infectious mononucleosis, as can the side effects of some drugs and some noninfectious diseases.

A blood test can confirm the diagnosis of infectious mononucleosis. With the test, a doctor can detect antibodies to the Epstein-Barr virus. The body also produces new B lymphocytes to eliminate the infected ones. These lymphocytes have a characteristic appearance under the microscope and occur in large numbers in the blood of people with infectious mononucleosis. Streptococcal infection of the throat, which might resemble infectious mononucleosis, can be identified by a throat culture and requires antibiotic treatment to prevent abscesses and reduce the likelihood of rheumatic fever.

Prognosis and Treatment

Most people with infectious mononucleosis recover fully. The length of the illness varies. The acute phase lasts about 2 weeks, after which most people are able to resume their usual activities. However, fatigue may persist for several more weeks and, occasionally, for months.

Rarely (in less than 1 percent of infections), death can occur. Death is most often caused by complications, such as brain inflammation, rupture of the spleen, or airway obstruction, or is particularly likely in a person whose immune system is impaired.

People with infectious mononucleosis are encouraged to rest until the fever, sore throat, and feeling of illness disappear. Because of the risk of rupturing the spleen, heavy lifting and contact sports should be avoided for 6 to 8 weeks, even if the spleen isn't noticeably enlarged.

Acetaminophen or aspirin can be used for fever and pain. However, aspirin should be avoided in children because of the slight possibility of Reye's syndrome, which can be fatal. Some complications, such as severe swelling of the airway, may be treated with corticosteroids. Although acyclovir reduces the production of the Epstein-Barr virus, it has little effect on the symptoms of infectious mononucleosis.

Central Nervous System Viral Infections

Central nervous system viral infections are caused by a variety of viruses that affect primarily the brain and spinal cord and sometimes their surrounding membranes (meninges).

Rabies

Rabies is a viral infection of the brain that causes irritation and inflammation of the brain and spinal cord.

The rabies virus is present in the saliva of infected animals. An animal with rabies transmits the infection to other animals or humans by biting and sometimes licking. The virus travels from the site of initial inoculation along the nerves to the spinal cord and the brain, where it multiplies. It subsequently travels down nerves to the salivary glands and into the saliva.

Many different animals can transmit rabies to people. Although dogs are frequently the source of infection for people, cats, bats, raccoons, skunks, foxes, and others may be responsible. It is unusual for mice, rats, or other small mammals to be rabid, partly because the bite of another animal is usually fatal for them. In the United States, vaccination has largely eliminated rabies in dogs. However, rabies in dogs is still fairly common in most countries of Latin America, Africa, and Asia, where pets aren't always vaccinated against the disease. Infected animals may have either "furious" rabies or "dumb" rabies. In furious rabies, the animal is agitated and vicious, then later becomes paralyzed and dies. In dumb rabies, the localized or generalized paralysis is prominent from the beginning.

In the United States, most cases of human rabies during the last 30 years have been caused by bites of infected wild animals. Rabid wild animals may show furious behavior, but less obvious changes in behavior are more likely. Nocturnal animals (bats, skunks, raccoons, and foxes) infected with rabies may come out during the day and may not show normal fear of humans.

Though extremely rare, rabies may be acquired by breathing infected air. Two cases occurred when explorers breathed the air of a bat-infested cave.

Symptoms

Symptoms usually begin 30 to 50 days after infection, but the incubation period varies from 10 days to more than a year. The incubation period is usually shortest in people who were bitten on the head or trunk or who received many bites.

In 20 percent of people, rabies starts with paralysis in the lower legs that moves up through the body. However, the disease commonly starts with a short period of mental depression, restlessness, a sick feeling, and a fever. Restlessness increases to uncontrollable excitement, and the person produces a lot of saliva. Spasms of the muscles of the throat and voice box can be excruciatingly painful. These spasms are caused by irritability of the area in the brain responsible for swallowing and breathing. A slight breeze or an attempt to drink water can induce these spasms. Thus, a person with rabies can't drink. For this reason, the disease is sometimes called hydrophobia (fear of water).

Diagnosis

When a person is bitten by a sick or wild animal, the biggest concern is rabies. Determining whether an animal has rabies usually requires an examination of a brain tissue sample. The animal should be captured and observed. Typically, the animal must be killed to examine the brain. If a dog or cat without symptoms bites a person, however, a veterinarian may confine and observe the animal for 10 days. If the animal remains healthy, the veterinarian can safely conclude that the animal didn't have rabies at the time of the bite.

If a person who has been bitten by an animal develops symptoms of progressive brain inflammation (encephalitis), rabies is the likely cause. Viral testing of the person isn't helpful until symptoms appear. A skin biopsy, in which a sample of skin is taken (usually from the neck) for examination under a microscope, can reveal the virus.

Prevention and Treatment

Steps to prevent rabies can be taken before exposure to the rabies virus or immediately after exposure. For example, a vaccine can be administered to people at high risk for exposure to the virus. These people include veterinarians, laboratory workers who handle potentially infected animals, people who live or stay more than 30 days in developing countries where rabies in dogs is widespread, and people who explore bat caves. Vaccination gives most people some degree of protection for the rest of their lives. However, antibody levels fall with time, and people at high risk of further exposure should receive a booster dose of vaccine every 2 years.

People who have been bitten by a rabid animal rarely develop rabies if appropriate preventive steps are taken immediately. People bitten by rabbits and rodents (including squirrels, chipmunks, rats, and mice) require no further treatment unless there is definite suspicion of rabies; these animals are rarely infected. However, people bitten by wild animals such as skunks, raccoons, foxes, and bats need further treatment unless the biting animal can be captured and proved to be free of rabies.

Treating a bite wound immediately may be the most valuable preventive measure. The contaminated area is cleaned thoroughly with soap. Deep puncture wounds are flushed out with soapy water. Once the wound has been cleaned, people not previously immunized with rabies vaccine are given an injection of rabies immunoglobulin, with half of the dose given at the location of the bite. For people who have not been previously immunized, rabies vaccine injections are given on the day of exposure and on days 3, 7, 14, and 28. Pain and swelling at the injection site are usually minor. Serious allergic reactions are rare during the series of five injections; fewer than 1 percent of people develop a fever when they receive the vaccine.

If a person who is bitten has already been vaccinated, the risk of acquiring rabies is reduced, but the wound still needs to be cleaned promptly and two doses of vaccine must be given (on days 0 and 2).

Before current therapy was available, death usually occurred in 3 to 10 days. Most people died of blocked airways (asphyxia), convulsions, exhaustion, or widespread paralysis. Although death from rabies was once considered inevitable, a few people did survive. Survival in those instances can be attributed to intensive care to control symptoms affecting the lungs, heart, and brain. Administration of neither vaccine nor rabies immunoglobulin appears to be helpful once a person develops symptoms.

Creutzfeldt-Jakob Disease

Creutzfeldt-Jakob disease (subacute spongiform encephalopathy) is a progressive, inevitably fatal infection that produces muscle spasms and progressive loss of mental function.

Creutzfeldt-Jakob disease occurs throughout the world. Little is known about how it is usually spread. A few people have acquired it from receiving contaminated corneal or possibly other tissue transplants from infected donors or from contaminated instruments used during brain surgery. Growth hormone prepared from a cadaver's pituitary gland can also be the source of infection. (Synthetic growth hormone is now available.) The risk of the disease is slightly increased in people who have undergone brain surgery. A few pathologists have acquired Creutzfeldt-Jakob disease, presumably from cadavers.

Creutzfeldt-Jakob disease primarily affects adults, particularly those in their late 50s. The causative organism has been difficult to identify because no foreign RNA or DNA has been discovered in association with the disease. However, evidence indicates the presence of a specific protein, called a prion, in those with the disease.

A disease similar to Creutzfeldt-Jakob disease occurs in sheep **(scrapie)** and cattle **(mad-cow disease)**. The infection is transmitted to offspring, and there is speculation that it can be acquired by eating infected tissues. Transmission across species of animals is uncertain, but it is suspected that the incidence of mad-cow disease increased when cattle were fed sheep entrails, and human cases may have occurred when people ate affected beef.

Symptoms

For months or years after exposure, no symptoms occur. Slowly, brain damage increases and loss of intellectual ability (dementia) becomes apparent. At first, the symptoms may resemble those of other dementias ▲—neglect of personal hygiene, apathy, irritability, forgetfulness, and confusion. Some people tire easily, are sleepy, are unable to fall asleep, or suffer from other sleep disorders. Then the symptoms accelerate, usually much more rapidly than in Alzheimer's disease, until the person is profoundly demented.

Muscle twitching usually appears in the first 6 months after symptoms begin. Trembling, clumsiness, and peculiar body movements also may develop. Vision may become blurry or dim. Most people die, often of pneumonia, after about 3 to 12 months of illness. About 5 to 10 percent of people survive for 2 years or more.

Diagnosis

A doctor considers the diagnosis of Creutzfeldt-Jakob disease when evaluating a person with dementia. In most people with dementia, Creutzfeldt-Jakob disease is an unlikely cause, unless mental function is deteriorating quickly or is accompanied by muscle twitching. The diagnosis of Creutzfeldt-Jakob disease usually is not confirmed while the person is alive, since it requires taking a piece of brain tissue for specific testing. Such testing is safe but is done only when Creutzfeldt-Jakob disease seems a likely possibility.

Prevention and Treatment

Creutzfeldt-Jakob disease can't be cured, and its progress can't be slowed. A doctor tries to make the person comfortable and treats the symptoms. Because the disease is transmissible, people must avoid transplantation or ingestion of infected human or animal tissues.

Progressive Multifocal Leukoencephalopathy

Progressive multifocal leukoencephalopathy is a rare manifestation of polyomavirus infection of the

---

▲ see page 367

brain that often progresses rapidly once it produces symptoms.

The disease affects the brain and spinal cord and is caused by the JC virus, which is a polyomavirus. It has become most common in people with impaired T-lymphocyte (immunologic) function, such as those with leukemia, lymphoma, or AIDS. Men are more frequently affected than women.

Symptoms and Diagnosis

Many people are infected with JC virus with no apparent symptoms. As with herpesviruses, the JC virus appears to remain latent until something (such as an impaired immune system) causes it to reactivate. Therefore, progressive multifocal leukoencephalopathy usually appears only years after the initial infection.

The symptoms may begin either gradually or suddenly. Once they start, the symptoms usually worsen rapidly and vary depending on the part of the brain infected. Paralysis affecting half the body is common. Headaches and seizures occur in rare instances. A progressive loss of intellectual ability (dementia) affects about two out of three people. Increasing difficulty in speaking and partial blindness may also occur. Death is very common within 1 to 6 months of when symptoms start, but some people have survived.

A doctor bases the diagnosis on the progressively worsening symptoms. Noninvasive techniques, such as computed tomography (CT) and magnetic resonance imaging (MRI), can help to make the diagnosis. However, a definite diagnosis often can't be made until after the person has died, when the brain tissue can be examined.

Treatment

There is no proven treatment for progressive multifocal leukoencephalopathy. In those who have survived, researchers suspect that certain immune system functions may have been responsible for stopping the infection or for destruction of brain tissue.

Tropical Spastic Paraparesis

Tropical spastic paraparesis is a slowly progressive viral infection of the spinal cord that causes weakness in the legs.

The infection is caused by the human T-cell lymphotropic virus type I (HTLV-I). This virus, a retrovirus, also can cause a type of leukemia. Tropical spastic paraparesis may be spread by sexual contact or by contaminated needles. It can also be transmitted from mother to child either across the placenta or in breast milk.

The symptoms may begin years after the initial infection. In the process of responding to infection with HTLV-I, the immune system may injure nerve tissue, causing the symptoms. Weakness and muscle stiffness in both legs begin gradually and worsen slowly. Some sensation in the feet may be lost.

Although no cure is available, marked improvement has occurred in people treated with corticosteroids, which may suppress the immune response. Plasmapheresis has also produced temporary improvement.

Arbovirus Infections

Arbovirus is a term used for a virus that is spread to humans by bites from insects, such as ticks and mosquitoes, which become infected from infected animals, including domestic animals and birds.

Arbovirus Encephalitis

Arbovirus encephalitis is a severe infection of the brain caused by one of several viruses.

The most common types of viral encephalitis transmitted by insect bites in the United States are western equine encephalitis, eastern equine encephalitis, St. Louis encephalitis, and California encephalitis. The virus responsible for each of these infections is spread by a specific mosquito type found in a particular geographic area. The diseases are endemic zoonoses in the region, but outbreaks occur periodically when the population of infected animals increases. Infections in humans are incidental and do not enhance the spread of the virus.

Western equine encephalitis occurs throughout the United States in all age groups, but it particularly affects children under 1 year of age. Eastern equine encephalitis occurs predominantly in the eastern United States, mainly in young children and people over age 55, and is more likely to be fatal than the western type. Both types tend to be severe in children under 1 year of age, causing permanent nerve or brain damage. Outbreaks of St. Louis encephalitis have occurred throughout the United States, particularly in Texas and some midwestern states; the risk of death is greatest in older people. There are several related viruses in the California group of viruses, including the California virus (most common in the western United States), the La Crosse virus (most common in the midwestern United States), and the Jamestown Canyon virus (most common from New York westward). All of the viruses in the California group affect mainly children.

Symptoms and Treatment

The usual first symptoms include headache, drowsiness, and fever. Vomiting and a stiff neck are less common signs of an infection of the brain and spinal cord. Muscle trembling, mental confusion, convulsions, and coma may develop rapidly. Occasionally, the arms and legs become paralyzed.

Unlike the encephalitis caused by herpes simplex virus, there is no specific treatment. Care is generally supportive. A doctor tries to maintain the person's heart and lung function while the infection runs its course.

Other Arbovirus Infections

In other parts of the world, different but related arboviruses that cause encephalitis are transmitted periodically from nature to man. Such diseases include Venezuelan equine encephalitis, Japanese encephalitis, Russian spring-summer encephalitis, and other types of encephalitis named for the geographic area in which they occur.

One of the most recognized and historically important arbovirus infections is the one designated as **yellow fever.** Yellow fever, a viral disease transmitted by mosquitoes, results in fever, bleeding, and jaundice. It can be fatal. The disease is most common in Central Africa and Central and South America.

Dengue fever is one of the most prevalent arbovirus infections that occurs worldwide in the tropics and subtropics. The infection, transmitted by mosquitoes, results in fever, lymph node swelling, and bleeding. It causes severe joint and muscle pains and is sometimes called breakbone fever. It can be fatal. It occurs most often in children under age 10, and recurrent infections with variant types of virus(es) are common in subsequent years.

Arenavirus Infections

Arenaviruses and some viruses related to the arboviruses are viruses that can spread to humans by exposure to rodents or aerosols originating from their droppings.

Lymphocytic Choriomeningitis

Lymphocytic choriomeningitis is an arenavirus disease that usually produces an influenza-like illness.

The arenavirus that causes lymphocytic choriomeningitis is common in rodents, especially the gray house mouse and the hamster. These animals are usually infected by the virus for life and excrete it in urine, feces, semen, and nasal secretions. Exposure to contaminated dust or food is usually responsible for infection in people. The disease generally occurs in the winter when wild rodents seek shelter indoors.

Symptoms

An influenza-like illness develops 1 to 3 weeks after infection. In most of those who develop symptoms, a fever of 101° to 104° F. occurs and may include shaking (rigors). Other symptoms include a sick feeling, nausea, light-headedness, weakness, muscle pains, a headache behind the eyes made worse by bright light, and a poor appetite. Sore throat, painful joints, and vomiting may occur. The illness may include swollen finger joints and inflammation of the testes. Hair from the scalp may be lost as well.

Often, the disease occurs in two phases, with inflammation of the membrane covering the brain (meningitis) developing 1 to 2 weeks after the influenza-like illness. People who develop meningitis have a headache and stiff neck. They usually recover completely. Occasionally, people develop inflammation of the brain (encephalitis) with a headache and drowsiness. Permanent nerve damage is unusual but can occur.

Diagnosis and Treatment

During the first week of the illness, the symptoms resemble those of influenza or a similar viral infection, so tests usually aren't performed. If they are, a chest x-ray may show some lung inflammation, and blood tests reveal low levels of white blood cells and platelets. If the symptoms suggest meningitis, a spinal tap is performed to remove a sample of the fluid surrounding the brain and spinal cord (cerebrospinal fluid). If the person has lymphocytic choriomeningitis, the cerebrospinal fluid usually contains many white blood cells, principally lymphocytes. The disease is diagnosed by identifying the virus in the cerebrospinal fluid or by detecting rising blood levels of the antibody against the virus.

No specific treatment is available. A doctor tries to relieve the symptoms until the infection subsides.

Hemorrhagic Fevers

In several parts of the world, infections typically found in animals (zoonoses) are prevalent in humans. These infections are related to the local habitat and the viruses' vectors for transmission. Some viruses cause a severe, usually fatal infection, characterized by hemorrhagic fever, widespread bleeding, and failure of many organs. These infections include Bolivian and Argentinian hemorrhagic fever and Lassa fever.

Lassa fever is an arenavirus infection transmitted from rodents to humans or from human to human, which results in fever, vomiting, and bleeding. It is highly fatal and requires strict isolation of cases. It occurs mainly in West Africa.

Hantavirus Infection

Hantavirus infection is a viral disease that is spread from rodents to humans and causes severe infections of the lungs and kidneys.

Hantaviruses are bunyaviruses distantly related to the California group of encephalitis viruses. Hantaviruses are present throughout the world in the urine, feces, and saliva of various rodents, including field and laboratory mice and rats. People acquire the infection by having contact with rodents or their droppings, or possibly by inhaling virus particles in the air. No evidence of human-to-human spread has been found. Re-

---

Ebola and Marburg Viruses

Ebola and Marburg are two complex viruses of Africa classified as filoviruses. They cause severe hemorrhagic fevers in humans.

The Ebola virus probably originates in monkeys. It is often transmitted among humans by exposure to blood or infected body tissues. The infection results in fever, diarrhea, bleeding, and loss of consciousness. It is often fatal, but less virulent strains of the virus may exist. It occurs mainly in East, South, and Central Africa.

The Marburg virus is acquired from exposure to infected primate tissues. The virus is highly infectious, causing severe disease that affects many organs. Death is almost always inevitable. The reservoir for the virus seems to reside only in Central Africa.

---

cent outbreaks of hantavirus infection involving the lungs have occurred in the southwestern United States. However, the same or related viruses have been found elsewhere in the United States, and they may be expected to exist wherever the appropriate animal host(s) lives.

Symptoms

Hantavirus infection of the lungs begins with a fever and muscle pain. Abdominal pain, diarrhea, or vomiting also may develop. After 4 to 5 days, the person may develop a cough and shortness of breath, which may become severe within hours. A drastic, life-threatening fall in blood pressure (shock) may result from a loss of fluid into the lungs. Death almost invariably follows shock. Infection involving the lungs is fatal in a large majority of recognized cases. Those who survive may recover completely.

Kidney infection may be mild or severe. The mild form of kidney infection begins suddenly with a high fever, headache, backache, and abdominal pain. On the third or fourth day, small bruise-like patches appear on the whites of the eyes and the roof of the mouth along with a rash on the abdomen. About 20 percent of people become very ill and somewhat drowsy. Kidney function deteriorates, so toxic substances build up in the blood, leading to nausea, loss of appetite, and fatigue. The rash disappears in about 3 days. Urine output rises above normal, and the person recovers over several weeks.

The severe form of kidney infection begins similarly, but the fever is highest on the third or fourth day. A typical early symptom is a widespread reddening of the face, resembling sunburn. Pressing lightly on the skin produces a persistent red mark. Pinpoint bleeding (petechiae) develops on the third to fifth days, at first on the roof of the mouth and then on any area of the skin subjected to pressure. Bleeding beneath the whites of the eyes occurs at about the same time. On about the fifth day, blood pressure may fall sharply, and shock may develop. About the eighth day, blood pressure returns to normal, but urine production falls. Urine production increases again around the eleventh day. At this time, bleeding, particularly in the brain, may cause death. Hantavirus infection of the kidney is fatal in about 5 percent of people. Some who survive have permanent kidney damage.

Treatment

Generally, a doctor provides supportive care. The antiviral drug ribavirin may help if given early enough. For a lung infection, providing oxygen and monitoring the blood pressure appear to be most critical to recovery from illness. For a kidney infection, dialysis may be needed and can be lifesaving.

CHAPTER 187

Human Immunodeficiency Virus Infection

Human immunodeficiency virus (HIV) infection is an infection by one of two viruses that progressively destroys white blood cells called lymphocytes, causing acquired immunodeficiency syndrome (AIDS) and other diseases that result from the impaired immunity.

In the early 1980s, epidemiologists (people who study the factors that affect the frequency and distribution of diseases) recognized a sudden increase in two conditions among American homosexual men. One was Kaposi's sarcoma, a rare cancer; the other was pneumocystis pneumonia, a form of pneumonia that occurs only in people with a compromised immune system. The failure of the immune system that allowed the growth of rare cancers and the development of rare infections came to be known as AIDS. Immune system failure was found also in injecting drug users, hemophiliacs, and recipients of blood transfusions as well as in bisexual men. Some time later, the syndrome began to occur in heterosexuals who weren't drug users, hemophiliacs, or recipients of blood transfusions.

Researchers soon discovered that a virus was causing AIDS. The two AIDS-producing viruses are HIV-1 and HIV-2. HIV-1 is most common in the Western Hemisphere, in Europe, in Asia, and in Central, South, and East Africa. HIV-2 is the main AIDS-producing virus in West Africa, although many people there are infected by the HIV-1 strain.

AIDS has reached epidemic proportions, with more than 500,000 cases and 300,000 deaths reported in the United States through October 1995. The World Health Organization estimates that in 1996 20 million people worldwide were infected with HIV and that the number will climb to 30 to 40 million by the year 2000. More than a million people in the United States are thought to be currently infected with HIV.

Pathogenesis

In order to establish infection in a person, the virus must enter cells such as lymphocytes, a type of white blood cell. The genetic material of the virus is incorporated into the DNA of an infected cell. The virus reproduces itself inside the cell, eventually destroying the cell and releasing new virus particles. The new virus particles then infect other lymphocytes and can destroy them as well.

The virus attaches to lymphocytes that have a receptor protein, called CD4, in their outer membrane. Cells with CD4 receptors are usually called CD4-positive (CD4+) cells or helper T lymphocytes. Helper T lymphocytes serve to activate and coordinate other cells of the immune system, such as B lymphocytes (which produce antibodies), macrophages, and cytotoxic (CD8+) T lymphocytes, all of which help to destroy cancerous cells and invading organisms.▲ Because HIV infection destroys helper T lymphocytes, it weakens the body's system for protecting itself from infection and cancer.

People infected with HIV lose helper T lymphocytes (CD4+ cells) in three phases over months or years. A healthy person has a CD4+ lymphocyte count of roughly 800 to 1,300 cells per microliter of blood. In the first few months after HIV infection, this count may decrease by 40 to 50 percent. During these early months, the person can transmit HIV to other people because many virus particles are circulating in the blood. Although the body fights the virus, it is unable to clear up the infection.

After about 6 months, the number of virus particles in the blood reaches a steady level, which varies from person to person. Enough remain, however, to continue to destroy CD4+ lymphocytes and to transmit the disease to other people. Many years may pass during which the HIV-infected person has a slowly declining, below-normal count of CD4+ lymphocytes. High levels of virus particles and low levels of CD4+ lymphocytes help the doctor identify people at the highest risk of developing AIDS.

In the 1 to 2 years before recognizable AIDS develops, the count of CD4+ lymphocytes usually drops more rapidly. The person's vulnerability to infection increases as the CD4+ lymphocyte count falls below 200 cells per microliter of blood.

HIV infection also disrupts the function of B lymphocytes, the part of the immune system that produces antibodies, often causing them to produce excess antibodies.■ These antibodies are

What is a Retrovirus?

The human immunodeficiency virus (HIV) is a retrovirus, a type of virus that stores genetic information as RNA rather than as DNA. When the virus enters a targeted host cell, it releases its RNA and an enzyme (reverse transcriptase), and then makes DNA using the viral RNA as a pattern. The viral DNA then is incorporated into the host cell DNA.

Each time a host cell divides, it also makes a new copy of the integrated viral DNA along with its own genes. The viral DNA can take over the functions of the cell (become activated), causing the cell to produce new virus particles. These new viruses are released from the infected cell to invade other cells.

directed mainly against HIV itself and those infections with which the person had previous contact, but the antibodies are not very helpful against many of the opportunistic infections of AIDS. At the same time, destruction of CD4+ lymphocytes by the virus reduces the immune system's ability to recognize new invaders and target them for attack.

Transmission of Infection

The transmission of HIV requires contact with a body fluid that contains infected cells or virus particles; such fluids include blood, semen, vaginal secretions, cerebrospinal fluid, and breast milk. HIV also is present in tears, urine, and saliva, but in much lower concentrations.

HIV is transmitted in the following ways:
• Sexual relations with an infected person, during which the mucous membrane lining the mouth, vagina, or rectum is exposed to contaminated body fluids
• Injection or infusion of contaminated blood, as occurs with blood transfusions, the sharing of

▲ see page 812

■ see page 811

Simplified Life Cycle of the Human Immunodeficiency Virus

Like all viruses, human immunodeficiency virus (HIV) reproduces using the genetic machinery of its host cell, usually a CD4 lymphocyte. Currently licensed drugs inhibit two critical viral enzymes—reverse transcriptase and protease, which the virus uses to reproduce—and drugs targeting a third enzyme, integrase, are being developed.

1. The HIV virus first attaches to and penetrates its target cell.
2. The HIV's RNA, the genetic code of the virus, is released into the cell. To reproduce, the RNA must be converted into DNA. The enzyme that performs the conversion is called reverse transcriptase. The HIV virus mutates easily at this point because reverse transcriptase is prone to errors during conversion of viral RNA to DNA.
3. The viral DNA then enters the cell's nucleus.
4. With the help of an enzyme called integrase, the viral DNA becomes integrated with the cell's DNA.

5. The DNA now replicates and reproduces RNA and proteins. The proteins are in the form of a long chain that must be cut into pieces after the virus leaves the cell.
6. A new virus is assembled from RNA and short pieces of protein.
7. The virus buds through the cell membrane of the cell, wrapping itself in a fragment of the cell membrane (envelope).
8. To become infectious for other cells, another viral enzyme (HIV protease) must cut structural proteins within the budded virus, causing them to rearrange into the mature form of HIV.

Key

〜 Viral RNA   〰 Viral DNA   〰 Cell DNA

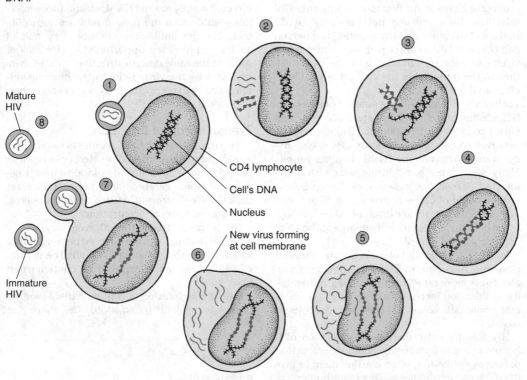

Mature HIV

Immature HIV

CD4 lymphocyte

Cell's DNA

Nucleus

New virus forming at cell membrane

needles, or an accidental prick from an HIV-contaminated needle
• Transfer of the virus from an infected mother to a child before or during birth or through the mother's milk

Susceptibility to HIV infection increases when the skin or a mucous membrane is torn or damaged, as can happen during vigorous vaginal or anal intercourse. Many studies have shown that sexual transmission of HIV is more likely if either sex partner has herpes, syphilis, or other sexually transmitted diseases▲ that may cause breaks in the skin. However, HIV can be transmitted by an infected person to a noninfected person by vaginal or anal intercourse even if neither has other sexually transmitted diseases or obvious breaks in the skin. HIV transmission also can occur during oral sex, although it is less common than during intercourse.

In the United States and Europe, the transmission of HIV among homosexual men and injecting drug users has been more common than transmission among heterosexuals. However, the rate of transmission among heterosexuals is rapidly increasing. In the United States, more than 10 percent of the people with AIDS are women, and HIV infection is increasing at a faster rate among women than among men. HIV transmission in Africa, the Caribbean, and Asia is primarily heterosexual, and HIV infection occurs equally among men and women.

Before 1992, most American women with HIV were infected by injecting drugs with contaminated needles. However, the number of cases resulting from sexual transmission has slowly surpassed the number attributed to drug abuse.

A health care worker who is accidentally pricked with an HIV-contaminated needle has a 1 in 300 chance of contracting HIV. The risk of HIV infection increases if the needle penetrates deeply or if contaminated blood is injected. Taking an antiretroviral drug such as AZT (zidovudine) appears to reduce the likelihood of becoming infected after a needlestick, but does not eliminate the risk.

AIDS is now the leading cause of death among people with hemophilia, who require frequent infusions of whole blood or other plasma products. Before 1985, many people in the United States with hemophilia received blood products infected with HIV. Since then, all blood collected is

tested for HIV, and plasma products are now treated with heat to eliminate the risk of HIV infection.

HIV infection in a large number of women of childbearing age has led to HIV infection in children.■ The virus can be transmitted to the fetus early in pregnancy through the placenta or at birth during passage through the birth canal. Children who are breastfed can contract HIV infection through breast milk. A few children contract HIV infection through sexual abuse.

HIV isn't transmitted by casual contact or even by close, nonsexual contact at work, school, or home. No case of HIV transmission has been traced to the coughing or sneezing of an infected person or to a mosquito bite. Transmission from an infected doctor or dentist to a patient is extremely rare.

Symptoms

Some people develop symptoms similar to those of infectious mononucleosis a few weeks after first contracting HIV infection. A fever, rashes, swollen lymph nodes, and general discomfort can last 3 to 14 days. Most symptoms then disappear, although the lymph nodes may stay enlarged. Additional symptoms may not appear for years. However, large amounts of the virus circulate in the blood and other body fluids immediately, so a person becomes contagious soon after becoming infected. Within several months of contracting HIV, people may repeatedly experience mild symptoms that don't yet fit the definition of full-blown AIDS.

A person may have symptoms of HIV infection for years before developing the distinctive infections or tumors that define AIDS. These symptoms include swollen lymph nodes, weight loss, a fever that comes and goes, an unwell feeling, fatigue, recurring diarrhea, anemia, and thrush—a fungal infection of the mouth. Weight loss (wasting) is a particularly troublesome problem.

By definition, AIDS begins with a low CD4+ lymphocyte count (less than 200 cells per microliter of blood) or the development of opportunistic infections (infections by organisms that don't

---

▲ see page 937

■ see page 1275

cause disease in people with a healthy immune system). Cancers such as Kaposi's sarcoma and non-Hodgkin's lymphoma may also develop.

Both the HIV infection itself and the opportunistic infections and cancers produce the symptoms of AIDS. For example, HIV can infect the brain and cause dementia, with loss of memory, difficulty in concentration, and a reduced speed of information processing. However, only a few people with AIDS die from the direct effects of HIV infection. Usually, death is caused by the cumulative effects of many opportunistic infections or tumors. Organisms and diseases that normally pose little threat to healthy people can rapidly lead to death in those with AIDS, especially when the CD4+ lymphocyte count drops below 50 cells per microliter of blood.

Several opportunistic infections and cancers are typical of the onset of AIDS. Thrush, an overgrowth of the yeast *Candida* in the mouth, vagina, or esophagus, may be the first infection to appear.▲ The earliest symptom of HIV infection in a woman may be frequent vaginal yeast infections that aren't easily cured. However, recurring vaginal yeast infections are commonly seen in otherwise healthy women and may be caused by other factors, such as oral contraceptives, antibiotics, and hormonal changes.

Pneumonia caused by the fungus *Pneumocystis carinii* is a common and recurring opportunistic infection in people with AIDS. Pneumocystis pneumonia■ is often the first serious opportunistic infection to develop; it was the most common cause of death among HIV-infected people before methods to treat and prevent the pneumonia were improved.

Chronic infection with *Toxoplasma* (toxoplasmosis)★ persisting since childhood is common, but causes symptoms in only a minority of people with AIDS. When it reactivates in patients with

AIDS, *Toxoplasma* causes severe infection primarily in the brain.

Tuberculosis is more frequent and more deadly in people who have HIV infection● than in those who do not and is difficult to treat if the strains of the tuberculosis bacterium are resistant to several antibiotics. Another mycobacterium, *Mycobacterium avium* complex,◆ is a common cause of fever, weight loss, and diarrhea in people with advanced disease. It can be both treated and prevented with recently developed drugs.

Gastrointestinal infections also are common with AIDS. *Cryptosporidium,* a parasite that may be acquired from contaminated food or water, causes severe diarrhea, abdominal pain, and weight loss.

Progressive multifocal leukoencephalopathy (PML), a viral infection of the brain, can affect neurologic function.♥ The first symptoms are usually a loss of strength in an arm or leg and loss of coordination or balance. Within days or weeks, the person may be unable to walk and stand, and death usually occurs within a few months.

Cytomegalovirus commonly infects people with AIDS. Reinfection tends to occur in people with advanced disease, often in the retina of the eyes, causing blindness. Treatment with antiviral drugs can control cytomegalovirus. People with AIDS are also highly susceptible to many other bacterial, fungal, and viral infections.

Kaposi's sarcoma, a tumor that appears as painless, red to purple, raised patches on the skin,✚ affects people with AIDS, especially homosexual men. People with AIDS also can develop tumors of the immune system (lymphomas), which may first appear in the brain or other internal organs. Women are prone to developing cancers of the cervix. Homosexual men are prone to developing cancer of the rectum.

Diagnosis

A relatively simple, highly accurate blood test (called the ELISA test) can be used to screen people for HIV infection. With this test, HIV antibodies can be detected in a blood sample; the results of the test are routinely confirmed by even more accurate tests. However, several weeks or longer may lapse after infection with the virus before the antibody test is positive. Highly sensitive tests (P24 antigen) may detect the virus at this time and are currently used to screen blood donated for transfusions.

▲ see page 946

■ see page 199

★ see box, page 901

● see page 885

◆ see box, page 886

♥ see page 922

✚ see page 994

Within several weeks after infection, most people develop antibodies against HIV. A small number of infected people don't produce measurable amounts of antibodies for several months or longer. Eventually, the ELISA test detects the antibodies in virtually all infected people. Almost all people with antibodies to HIV are both infected and contagious.

If the ELISA test result indicates an HIV infection, the test is repeated on the same blood sample to confirm the findings. If the results are again HIV positive, the next step is to confirm them with a more accurate and expensive blood test, such as a Western blot test. This test also identifies antibodies to HIV, but is more specific than the ELISA test. In other words, if the Western blot test result is positive, the person almost certainly is infected with HIV.

Prognosis

Exposure to HIV doesn't always lead to infection, and some people who have been repeatedly exposed over years remain uninfected. Moreover, many infected people have remained well for over a decade. Without benefit of current drug treatments, a person infected with HIV had a 1 to 2 percent chance of developing AIDS in the first several years after infection; the chance continued at about 5 percent each year thereafter. The risk of developing AIDS within 10 to 11 years of contracting the infection was about 50 percent. An estimated 95 to 100 percent of infected people will eventually develop AIDS, but the long-term effects of newly developed drugs used in combination may improve this outlook.

The first drugs used to treat HIV, such as AZT (zidovudine) and ddI (didanosine), have reduced the numbers of opportunistic infections and increased the life expectancy of people with AIDS, and combinations of these drugs produce even better results. Newer nucleoside drugs, such as d4T (stavudine) and 3TC (lamivudine), and HIV protease inhibitors, such as saquinavir, ritonavir, and indinavir, are even more potent. In some, combination therapy reduces the amount of virus in the blood to undetectable levels. Cures, however, have not been proven.

Techniques for measuring the amount of HIV virus (plasma RNA) in the blood (for example, polymerase chain reaction [PCR] and branched deoxyribonucleic acid [bDNA] tests) help a doctor monitor the effects of these drugs. These levels vary widely from less than a few hundred

---

Strategies for Preventing the Transmission of HIV

For uninfected people
- Abstinence
- Safe (protected) sex

For HIV-positive people
- Abstinence
- Safe (protected) sex
- No blood or organ donation
- Avoiding pregnancy
- Notification of previous and prospective partners

For drug abusers
- Halting the practice of sharing or reusing needles
- Entering drug treatment programs

For medical and dental professionals
- Wearing of latex gloves whenever there is a possibility of contact with body fluids
- Proper use and disposal of hollow needles

---

to over a million RNA-containing viruses per milliliter of plasma and best predict the patient's prognosis. Powerful drugs often lower the level by 10-fold to 100-fold. The ability of the new drug combinations and monitoring techniques to improve survival is promising, but has not yet been fully assessed.

Early in the AIDS epidemic, many people with AIDS had a rapid decline in their quality of life after their first hospitalization, often spending a large portion of their remaining time in the hospital. Most people died within 2 years of developing AIDS.

With the development of new antiviral drugs and improved methods to treat and prevent opportunistic infections, many people retain their physical and mental abilities for years after the diagnosis of AIDS. Thus, AIDS has become a treatable, if not yet curable, disease.

Prevention

Programs for preventing the spread of HIV have focused mainly on educating the public about the transmission of the virus, in an attempt to modify the behavior of people most at risk. Educational and motivational programs have met with mixed success because many people have difficulty changing their addictive or sexual behaviors. Advocating the use of condoms, which is one of the best means of preventing the spread of HIV, remains a controversial issue for some Americans. Making clean needles available to drug addicts, another proven method of reducing the spread of AIDS, has also met with public resistance.

Vaccines to prevent infection by HIV or to slow the progression in those already infected have so far proved elusive. Dozens of vaccines are being tested and many have failed, but research continues.

Hospitals and clinics generally don't isolate HIV-positive patients unless they have contagious infections, such as tuberculosis. HIV-contaminated surfaces can easily be cleaned and disinfected because HIV is inactivated by heat and with common disinfectants such as hydrogen peroxide and alcohol. Hospitals have strict procedures for handling samples of blood and other body fluids to prevent the transmission of HIV and other contagious organisms. These universal precautions apply to all samples from all patients, not just those known to come from a person infected with HIV.

Treatment

Many drugs are now available to treat HIV infection, including the nucleoside reverse transcriptase inhibitors, such as AZT (zidovudine), ddI (didanosine), ddC (zalcitabine), d4T (stavudine), 3TC (lamivudine), and abacavir; the nonnucleoside reverse transcriptase inhibitors, such as nevirapine, delavirdine, and efavirenz; and the protease inhibitors, such as saquinavir, ritonavir, indinavir, and nelfinavir. All prevent the virus from reproducing and thereby slow the progression of the disease. HIV usually develops resistance to all these drugs when they are used alone after periods of a few days to a few years, depending on the drug and the person.

Treatment appears to be most effective when at least two of the drugs are given in combination. Drug combinations may delay the onset of AIDS in HIV-positive people and extend life compared with the use of single drugs. Doctors aren't certain how soon after infection these drugs should be started, but people with high levels of HIV in

their blood, even people with high CD4+ counts and no symptoms, should be treated. Previous studies that appeared to show no advantage to starting treatment early are not necessarily relevant now that many other drugs and combinations have been developed. However, the cost and side effects of two or three drug treatments may be too great for some people in the United States and for many people in less developed countries.

AZT, ddI, d4T, and ddC may cause side effects such as abdominal pain, nausea, and headaches (especially AZT). Extended use of AZT can damage the bone marrow, causing anemia. ddI, ddC, and d4T can damage the peripheral nerves, and ddI may damage the pancreas. Among the nucleosides, 3TC appears to be associated with the fewest side effects.

All protease inhibitors may cause several side effects, including nausea and vomiting, diarrhea, and abdominal discomfort. Indinavir causes a mild, reversible increase in liver enzymes that does not produce any symptoms and can also cause severe back pain (renal colic) similar to that caused by kidney stones. Ritonavir has the disadvantage of raising and lowering the levels of many other drugs through its effect on the liver. Metabolic changes (such as elevated blood sugar and fat levels) and obvious redistribution of body fat ("protease paunch") occur in many patients taking any protease inhibitor and less frequently with other HIV drugs.

People with AIDS usually are prescribed many drugs to prevent infections. To prevent pneumocystis pneumonia, when the CD4+ lymphocyte count drops below 200 cells per microliter of blood, the combination of sulfamethoxazole and trimethoprim is highly effective. This combination of drugs also prevents toxoplasmic brain infections. For people with CD4+ lymphocyte counts less than 75 to 100 cells per microliter of blood, azithromycin taken weekly or clarithromycin or rifabutin taken daily may prevent *Mycobacterium avium* infections. People recovering from cryptococcal meningitis or those experiencing repeated bouts of thrush (infections of the mouth, esophagus, or vagina with the *Candida* fungus) may be given fluconazole, an antifungal drug, for prolonged periods. People with recurrent episodes of herpes simplex infections of the mouth, lips, genitals, or rectum may require prolonged treatment with the antiviral drug acyclovir to prevent relapses.

Infections in People With Impaired Defenses

Both physical barriers and the immune system defend the body against organisms that can cause infection. Physical barriers include the skin, teardrops, earwax, mucus (for example, in the nose), and stomach acid. Also, the normal flow of urine washes out organisms that ascend the urinary tract. The immune system, which is complex and sophisticated, is made up of, among other components, white blood cells and antibodies that identify and eliminate organisms.▲

A wide variety of diseases, drugs, and other treatments can cause a breakdown in the body's natural defenses. Such a breakdown may result in infections, which may be caused by organisms that normally live harmlessly on or in the body.■

Risk Factors

People with extensive burns have an increased risk of infection because the damaged skin opens up the body to invasion by harmful organisms. Similarly, people undergoing procedures that reduce their physical defenses have an increased risk of infection. Such procedures include the insertion of a catheter into the urinary tract or a blood vessel or the insertion of a tube into the lungs. Many drugs can suppress the immune system, including anticancer drugs (chemotherapy), drugs used to prevent organ rejection after a transplant (for example, azathioprine, methotrexate, or cyclosporine), and corticosteroid drugs (for example, prednisone).

People with AIDS have a dramatic decrease in their ability to fight certain kinds of infections, particularly late in the disease. These people are at risk for opportunistic infections—that is, infections by organisms that generally don't infect people whose immune systems are functioning normally. They also become more severely ill from many common infections, such as herpes.

Infections are more likely and usually more severe in the elderly than in younger adults, probably because aging reduces the effectiveness of the body's immune system. Many long term

(chronic) disorders that are common in the elderly—such as chronic obstructive pulmonary disease, cancer, and diabetes—also increase the risk of infection. In addition, the elderly are more likely to be in a hospital or a nursing home, where the risk of acquiring a serious infection is greater. In hospitals, the widespread use of antibiotics allows antibiotic-resistant organisms to thrive, and infections with these organisms often are more severe and more difficult to treat than infections acquired at home.

Antibiotics taken to eradicate disease-causing organisms may actually increase the person's risk of developing an infection. Sometimes, antibiotics kill not only the harmful bacteria but also the harmless ones that normally live on the skin or the helpful ones that live in the intestine. When this happens, fungi or antibiotic-resistant bacteria can multiply and cause a second infection, called a superinfection. Superinfections are more likely in the very young and the very old and in people with chronic or incapacitating diseases. Superinfections may also occur in people taking several antibiotics or antibiotics that kill a wide range of organisms (broad-spectrum antibiotics).

Prevention and Treatment

A number of steps can be taken to protect people who have an increased risk of infection. Hand washing is the most effective way of preventing the transmission of infection from one person to another. A susceptible person also can be isolated in a private hospital room with a closed door. To further reduce the risk of infection, visitors may be asked to don clean gowns and masks and to wash their hands and put on gloves before entering the patient's room.

Despite the chance that antibiotics may increase the risk of infection by suppressing some

---

▲ see page 808

■ see page 840

What Suppresses the Immune System?

Any of the following conditions or therapies can suppress a person's immune system, making infection more likely.

- Abnormalities of white blood cells, particularly neutrophils or T or B lymphocytes
- Abnormal antibody production
- Cancers (for example, leukemia, Hodgkin's disease, myeloma)
- AIDS (infection with human immunodeficiency virus)
- Failure of blood cell production (aplastic anemia)
- Diabetes
- Overproduction of corticosteroids (Cushing's disease)
- Chemotherapy (anticancer drugs)
- Radiation therapy (for cancer)
- Immunosuppressive drugs (for autoimmune diseases)
- Corticosteroids (for asthma, allergies, autoimmune diseases)

bacteria and allowing others to grow faster, these drugs can greatly reduce the risk of infection when used properly. This is called the prophylactic use of antibiotics. Antibiotics are given prophylactically before many types of surgery, particularly abdominal operations and organ transplants.

Vaccination also can prevent infections.▲ People who are at increased risk for developing infections, especially the elderly and people with AIDS, should receive all the vaccinations necessary to reduce this risk. In active immunization, a vaccine

▲ see page 845

is injected or taken orally, causing the body to produce antibodies (proteins designed explicitly to eliminate specific disease-carrying organisms). Vaccines are given to prevent or reduce the severity of such diseases as influenza, pneumococcal infections, chickenpox, shingles, hepatitis A, hepatitis B, measles, and rubella. In passive immunization, antibodies are injected, providing immediate but temporary protection. Passive immunization is particularly useful when the immune system is unable to produce enough antibodies to protect an infected person or when immediate protection is needed, for example, after exposure to the hepatitis virus.

Because superinfections and opportunistic infections often are resistant to most antibiotics, they can be very difficult to treat. Long-term treatment may be needed. Samples of an infected person's blood or other tissues or fluids are taken and sent to a laboratory for analysis; identification of the infecting organism helps the doctor determine which drugs will be most effective. Until the most effective antibiotic has been identified, a doctor makes a best guess and begins antibiotic treatment. For serious infections, combinations of antibiotics often are used. In rare cases, a person with a very low level of white blood cells may be given transfusions of white blood cells.

Specific Infections

People with impaired defenses are at risk for a number of infections, including but not limited to nocardiosis, aspergillosis, mucormycosis, and cytomegalovirus infection.

Nocardiosis

Nocardiosis is an infection caused by the bacterium Nocardia asteroides *that usually starts in the lungs and can spread to the skin and brain.*

Nocardia asteroides usually lives on decaying matter in the soil. The bacteria are carried by air contaminated with soil dust and are breathed into the lungs. In rare cases, the bacteria enter the body by being swallowed or by passing through the skin. Chronically ill people and those receiving drugs that suppress the immune system are at increased risk for nocardiosis. However, about half of the people with nocardiosis, usually the elderly, have no preexisting disease. At present, nocardiosis is an uncommon complication of AIDS.

Symptoms

Nocardiosis often begins as a lung infection, such as pneumonia. It can spread through the bloodstream, causing pockets of pus (abscesses) in many areas of the body, including the brain and, less frequently, the kidney. Abscesses develop in or beneath the skin in about a third of the cases.

With pneumonia caused by *Nocardia*, the most common symptoms are a cough, general weakness, chills, chest pain, shortness of breath, fever, loss of appetite, and weight loss. Fluid may collect in the pleural space (the space between the membrane layers covering the lungs). These symptoms are similar to those of tuberculosis or other types of bacterial pneumonia.

About a third of people with nocardiosis develop brain abscesses and experience severe headaches and altered sensations or weakness. The part of the body that becomes weakened depends on where in the brain the abscess is located.

Diagnosis and Treatment

The diagnosis of nocardiosis is based on identifying *Nocardia asteroides* in samples of body fluid or tissue taken from an infected person.

With or without treatment, nocardiosis can be fatal. The prognosis is better if the infection is only in the lungs than if it has spread to other parts of the body, for example, to the brain. The prognosis is worse for people receiving immunosuppressive therapy.

Penicillin is effective in only about 40 percent of the cases. Sulfadiazine may be effective but must be taken for several months. For some people, only amikacin is effective.

Aspergillosis

Aspergillosis, caused by the fungus Aspergillus, *is an infection primarily affecting the lungs.*

The *Aspergillus* fungus is commonly found in compost heaps, around the house, on food, and on the body. Some people experience an allergic reaction to the *Aspergillus* present on their body surfaces even though it hasn't invaded tissues to cause an infection.▲

Aspergillosis occurs when the *Aspergillus* organisms on a body surface invade the deeper tissues, such as the ear canals or the lungs, particularly in a person who has had tuberculosis or bronchitis. A fungus ball (aspergilloma) can grow in the lungs. The ball is composed of a tangled mass of fungus fibers, blood clotting fibers, and white blood cells. It gradually enlarges, destroying lung tissue in the process. In people with suppressed body defenses, such as those who have had a heart or liver transplant, aspergillosis can spread through the bloodstream to the brain and kidneys. It is a recognized but uncommon infection in people with AIDS.

Symptoms

Aspergillosis of the ear canal causes itching and occasionally pain. Fluid draining overnight from the ear may leave a stain on the pillow.

The fungus ball in the lungs may cause no symptoms and be discovered only by a chest x-ray. It may, however, cause repeated coughing up of blood, and rarely severe, even fatal, bleeding.

Infection of the deeper tissues makes a person very ill. Symptoms include fever, chills, shock, delirium, and blood clots. The person may develop kidney failure, liver failure (causing jaundice), and breathing difficulties. Death can occur quickly.

Diagnosis and Treatment

The symptoms alone provide strong clues for making the diagnosis. If possible, a sample of infected material is taken and sent to a laboratory for culture. It may take a few days for the fungus to grow enough to be identified, but treatment must be started immediately, because this disease can kill quickly.

Aluminum acetate (Burow's solution) is used to bathe an infected ear canal. The fungus ball in the lung is usually removed surgically. An antifungal drug, such as amphotericin B, usually is infused intravenously. Ketoconazole and itraconazole are alternative drugs that are taken orally for an infection of the deeper tissues. Some strains of *Aspergillus,* however, are resistant to these drugs.

▲ see page 188

Mucormycosis

Mucormycosis (phycomycosis) is an infection caused by a fungus belonging to a large group of organisms called Mucorales.

Mucormycosis under the skin (subcutaneous mucormycosis) is a form of infection that occurs in Southeast Asia and Africa. Usually, it heals without treatment; however, it can cause grotesque swellings under the skin of the neck and chest.

Mucormycosis of the nose and brain (rhinocerebral mucormycosis) occurs in the United States and is a severe and usually fatal infection. This form of mucormycosis typically affects people whose body defenses are weakened by disease, such as uncontrolled diabetes. The symptoms include pain, fever, and an infection of the eye socket (orbital cellulitis) with a bulging of the affected eye (proptosis). Pus is discharged from the nose. The divider between the nostrils (septum), the roof of the mouth (palate), or the facial bones surrounding the eye socket or sinuses may be destroyed. A brain infection may cause convulsions, an inability to speak properly, and partial paralysis.

Diagnosis and Treatment

Because the symptoms of mucormycosis can resemble those of other infections, a doctor may not be able to diagnose it immediately. Taking samples of infected body tissues for a culture may not be helpful, because the fungus is difficult to grow in a laboratory. A doctor may make the diagnosis by noting the person's symptoms and condition, including a poor immunologic status or uncontrolled diabetes.

A person with mucormycosis generally is treated with amphotericin B given intravenously or injected directly into the spinal fluid. Infected tissue may be removed by surgery. If the person also has diabetes, blood sugar (glucose) levels are brought down to within the normal range.

Cytomegalovirus Infection

Cytomegalovirus infection is a viral infection that may be acquired before birth or at any age after birth.

The cytomegalovirus is everywhere. Actively infected people may shed the virus in their urine or saliva for months. The virus is also excreted in cervical mucus, semen, stool, and breast milk. Children in institutions such as schools and day care centers often spread the virus to each other. The virus also is commonly spread by male homosexuals who have unprotected sex. Cytomegalovirus infection may develop in people who receive infected blood or an infected transplanted organ, such as a kidney.

When the cytomegalovirus enters the body, it may or may not cause an active disease. Once in the body, the virus may be dormant for years but become active and cause disease at any time. Between 60 and 90 percent of adults have had a cytomegalovirus infection at some time, although they usually have no symptoms. A serious infection generally occurs only in people with an impaired immune system—for example, those who have received a bone marrow transplantation or those with AIDS.

Symptoms

Cytomegalovirus infection before birth may cause a miscarriage, stillbirth, or the death of the newborn. Death is caused by bleeding, anemia, or extensive liver or brain damage.▲

The vast majority of people who acquire the infection after birth and harbor the virus have no symptoms. However, a healthy person who is infected may feel ill and have a fever. If a person receives a transfusion of blood containing the cytomegalovirus, symptoms may begin 2 to 4 weeks later. These symptoms include a fever lasting 2 to 3 weeks and sometimes inflammation of the liver (hepatitis), possibly with jaundice. The number of lymphocytes, a type of white blood cell, may increase. Occasionally, a rash develops.

A person whose immune system is impaired and who is infected with cytomegalovirus is particularly likely to develop a severe infection; such a person may become very ill and die. In people with AIDS, cytomegalovirus often infects the retina of the eye, causing blindness. Infection of the brain (encephalitis) or ulcers of the intestine or esophagus may also develop. People who receive an organ transplant infected with cytomegalovirus are at high risk of dying, because as part of the transplantation process they receive drugs to suppress their immune system.

▲ see page 1220

Diagnosis and Treatment

Cytomegalovirus infection may develop gradually and not be recognized immediately. Clues that are helpful in making the diagnosis are the person's symptoms and impaired immune system. Once cytomegalovirus infection is suspected, tests are conducted to detect the virus in the urine and in other body fluids or tissues. Because the virus can be shed for months or years after an infection has disappeared, the discovery of cytomegalovirus does not prove that the virus is causing an active infection. An increase in antibody levels against the virus, as measured by blood tests taken several days apart, strongly indicates that the virus is causing the infection. In a person with an eye infection of the back of the eye or retina (retinitis), a doctor can see abnormalities using an ophthalmoscope (an instrument that allows viewing of the internal eye structures). In newborns, the diagnosis usually is made by culturing the urine during the first 3 weeks of life.

Mild cytomegalovirus infection usually is not treated but subsides by itself. When the infection threatens a person's life or eyesight, the antiviral drug ganciclovir or foscarnet may be taken. However, these drugs have serious side effects. Also, they may not cure the infection. However, ongoing treatment often slows the disease's progression.

CHAPTER 189

Sexually Transmitted Diseases

Sexually transmitted (venereal) diseases are infections that are often, if not always, passed from person to person through sexual contact.

Because sexual activity provides an easy opportunity for organisms to find new hosts, a wide variety of infectious microorganisms can be spread by sexual contact. These range from microscopic viruses (for example, the human immunodeficiency virus) to visible insects (for example, the crab or pubic louse). Transmission of some sexually transmitted diseases does not require genital penetration. Although sexually transmitted diseases usually result from having vaginal, oral, or anal sex with an infected partner, occasionally they may be transmitted by kissing or by close body contact. Agents of some sexually transmitted diseases may be transmitted through food and water or blood transfusions, contaminated medical instruments, or needles used by injecting drug users.

Incidence

Sexually transmitted diseases are among the most common infectious diseases in the world. In Western countries, the numbers of people with these diseases increased steadily from the 1950s through the 1970s but generally stabilized in the 1980s. At the end of the 1980s, however, the numbers began increasing again in many countries, including the United States, particularly for syphilis and gonorrhea.

More than 250 million people throughout the world—almost 3 million in the United States—are infected with gonorrhea every year. For syphilis, the figures are 50 million people worldwide and 400,000 in the United States. Other sexually transmitted diseases, such as trichomoniasis and genital herpes, are probably more common, but because doctors aren't required to report them, the numbers are less reliable.

Today, treatments can rapidly cure most sexually transmitted diseases and prevent them from spreading. However, a number of new or drug-resistant variants of older organisms have spread widely, in part because of air travel. Such mobility was partly responsible for the rapid spread of the human immunodeficiency virus (HIV), which causes AIDS.

Controlling sexually transmitted diseases depends on promoting safe sex practices and providing good medical facilities for diagnosis and treatment. Educating people about how to prevent the spread of sexually transmitted diseases—especially encouraging condom use—is critical.

Diseases That May Be Sexually Transmitted

Earliest recognized sexually transmitted diseases
- Chancroid
- Gonorrhea
- Granuloma inguinale
- Lymphogranuloma venereum
- Syphilis

More recently recognized sexually transmitted diseases
- Chlamydial cervicitis
- Crabs (lice, pediculosis pubis)
- Genital candidiasis (usually not sexually transmitted)
- Genital herpes
- Genital warts
- HIV infection and AIDS
- Molluscum contagiosum
- Nongonococcal urethritis (often a chlamydial or mycoplasmal infection)
- Scabies
- Trichomoniasis

Diseases sometimes transmitted sexually
- Amebiasis
- Campylobacteriosis
- Cytomegalovirus infection
- Giardiasis
- Hepatitis A and B
- Salmonellosis
- Shigellosis

Another aspect of control of some diseases is contact tracing. Health care workers try to trace and treat all sexual contacts of an infected person.

▲ see page 571

■ see page 985

★ see page 982

● see page 982

◆ see page 926

♥ see page 1221

People who have been treated are reexamined to make sure they are cured.

Classification

Traditionally, five diseases have been classified as sexually transmitted diseases: syphilis, gonorrhea, chancroid, lymphogranuloma venereum, and granuloma inguinale. However, many other diseases are sexually transmitted, including genital herpes, hepatitis,▲ molluscum contagiosum,■ pubic lice,★ scabies,● and HIV infection, which causes AIDS.◆ Other infections, including salmonellosis and amebiasis, are sometimes transmitted during sexual activity but aren't usually thought of as sexually transmitted diseases.

Sexually transmitted diseases are sometimes grouped by the symptoms and signs they cause. Syphilis, genital herpes, and chancroid all cause ulcers (sores) on the skin or membranes lining the vagina or mouth. Both gonorrhea and chlamydial infections cause urethritis (inflammation and discharge of the urethra) in men; cervicitis (inflammation and discharge of the cervix) in women; pelvic infections in women; and eye infections in newborns.

Syphilis

Syphilis is a sexually transmitted disease caused by the bacterium Treponema pallidum.

The *Treponema pallidum* bacterium enters the body through mucous membranes, such as those of the vagina or mouth, or through the skin. Within hours, the bacterium reaches nearby lymph nodes, then spreads throughout the body via the blood. Syphilis may also infect a fetus during pregnancy,♥ causing birth defects and other problems.

The number of people with syphilis peaked during World War II, then fell dramatically until about 1960, when rates began increasing again. During this period, a large number of syphilis cases occurred in homosexual men. The numbers remained relatively stable until about the mid-1980s when, because of the AIDS epidemic and the resulting practice of safe sex, the incidence of syphilis among homosexual men fell. Consequently, the overall number of people with syphilis fell. This reduction was followed, however, by a rapid increase in new cases of syphilis among crack cocaine users—primarily among women or their newborns. Recently, focused programs of control have again reduced the incidence of syphilis in most areas in the United States.

A person who has been cured of syphilis doesn't become immune and can become infected with syphilis again.

Symptoms

Symptoms of syphilis usually begin 1 to 13 weeks after infection; the average is 3 to 4 weeks. Infection with *Treponema pallidum* progresses through several stages: the primary, secondary, latent, and tertiary stages. Infection may persist for many years and uncommonly causes heart damage, brain damage, and death.

Primary Stage

In the primary stage, a painless sore or ulcer (chancre) appears at the infection site—often on the penis, vulva, or vagina. The chancre also may appear on the anus, rectum, lips, tongue, throat, cervix, fingers, or, rarely, other parts of the body. Usually, a person has only one sore, but occasionally several sores develop.

The chancre begins as a small, red, raised area, which soon turns into an open sore (ulcer), but remains painless. The sore doesn't bleed, but when rubbed it leaks a clear fluid that is highly infectious. Nearby lymph nodes usually become enlarged, but they are also painless. Because the sore causes so few symptoms, it is often ignored. About half of the infected women and a third of the infected men are unaware of the sore. The sore usually heals in 3 to 12 weeks, after which the person appears to be entirely well.

Secondary Stage

The secondary stage usually begins with a skin rash, which typically appears 6 to 12 weeks after infection. About 25 percent of the infected people still have a healing sore at this time. The skin rash may be short-lived or may last for months. Even if a person isn't treated, the rash usually clears up. New rashes, however, may appear weeks or months later.

In the secondary stage, mouth sores are common, affecting more than 80 percent of people. About 50 percent have enlarged lymph nodes throughout the body, and about 10 percent have inflammation of the eyes. The eye inflammation usually causes no symptoms, although occasion-

ally the optic nerve swells, which may cause some blurring of vision. About 10 percent of people have inflamed bones and joints that ache painfully. Kidney inflammation may cause protein to leak into the urine. Jaundice may result from inflammation of the liver. A small number of people develop an inflammation of the lining of the brain (acute syphilitic meningitis), which causes headaches, neck stiffness, and sometimes deafness.

Raised areas (condylomata lata) may develop where the skin adjoins mucous membrane—for example, at the inner edges of the lips and vulva—and in moist areas of the skin. These extremely infectious areas may flatten and turn a dull pink or gray. The hair often falls out in patches, leaving a moth-eaten appearance. Other symptoms include a feeling of illness (malaise), loss of appetite, nausea, fatigue, fever, and anemia.

Latent Stage

After the person has recovered from the secondary stage, the disease enters a latent stage, in which no symptoms occur. This stage may last for years or decades—or for the rest of the person's life. During the early part of the latent stage, infectious sores sometimes recur.

Tertiary Stage

During the third (tertiary) stage of syphilis, a person isn't contagious. Symptoms range from mild to devastating. Three main types of symptoms may occur: benign tertiary syphilis, cardiovascular syphilis, and neurosyphilis.

Benign tertiary syphilis is rare today. Lumps called gummas appear in various organs, grow slowly, heal gradually, and leave scars. These lumps may occur almost anywhere in the body, but they are most common on the leg just below the knee, upper trunk, face, and scalp. The bones may be affected, resulting in a deep, penetrating pain that is usually worse at night.

Cardiovascular syphilis usually appears 10 to 25 years after the initial infection. A person may develop an aneurysm (weakening and dilation) of the aorta (the main artery leaving the heart) or leakage of the aortic valve. These changes may lead to chest pain, heart failure, or death.

Neurosyphilis (syphilis of the nervous system) affects about 5 percent of all people with untreated syphilis. The three major types are meningovascular neurosyphilis, paretic neurosyphilis, and tabetic neurosyphilis.

Syphilis of the Nervous System

About 5 percent of all people with untreated syphilis develop neurosyphilis, or syphilis of the nervous system, but cases are rare in developed countries. Symptoms vary with the three major types of neurosyphilis.

Meningovascular neurosyphilis is a chronic form of meningitis. The type of symptoms depend on whether the brain is primarily affected or whether both the brain and spinal cord are affected. When the brain is primarily affected, the symptoms include headache, dizziness, poor concentration, tiredness and lack of energy, difficulty sleeping, stiff neck, blurred vision, mental confusion, seizures, swelling of the optic nerve (papilledema), abnormalities of the pupils, difficulty speaking (aphasia), and paralysis of a limb or of half the body. When both the brain and spinal cord are affected, the symptoms include increasing difficulty in chewing, swallowing, and talking; weakness and wasting of shoulder and arm muscles; a slowly progressive paralysis with muscle spasms (spastic paralysis); an inability to empty the bladder; and an inflammation of a section of the spinal cord, resulting in the loss of bladder control and sudden paralysis while the muscles remain relaxed (flaccid paralysis).

Paretic neurosyphilis (also called general paralysis of the insane) begins gradually as behavioral changes in people who are in their 40s or 50s. These people slowly become demented. Symptoms may include convulsions, difficulty in speaking, temporary paralysis of half the body, irritability, difficulty in concentrating, memory loss, defective judgment, headaches, difficulty in sleeping, fatigue, lethargy, deterioration in personal hygiene and grooming habits, mood swings, loss of strength and energy, depression, delusions of grandeur, and lack of insight.

Tabetic neurosyphilis (tabes dorsalis) is a progressive disease of the spinal cord that begins gradually. Typically, the first symptom is an intense, stabbing pain in the legs that comes and goes irregularly. The person becomes unsteady while walking, especially in the dark, and may walk with the feet wide apart, sometimes stamping the feet. Because the person can't sense when the bladder is full, urine builds up, causing a loss of bladder control and repeated urinary tract infections. Impotence is common. The person may have tremors of the mouth, the tongue, the hands, and the whole body. Handwriting is usually shaky and illegible.

Most people with tabetic neurosyphilis are thin and have sad-looking faces. They have spasms of pain in various organs, especially the stomach. These stomach spasms can cause vomiting. Similar painful spasms may affect the rectum, bladder, and larynx (voice box). Because of the lack of sensation in the feet, open sores may develop on the soles. These sores may penetrate deeply and even reach the underlying bone. Because the person loses sensation of pain, the joints may become injured.

Diagnosis

A doctor suspects syphilis based on the person's symptoms. A definitive diagnosis is based on the results of laboratory tests and a physical examination.

Two types of blood test are used. The first is a screening test, such as the Venereal Disease Research Laboratory (VDRL) or the rapid plasma reagin (RPR) test. Screening tests are easy to perform and inexpensive. They sometimes give false-positive results but have the advantage of becoming negative when repeated after successful treatment. A doctor may need to repeat a screening test because the results can be negative in the first few weeks of primary syphilis. The second type of blood test, which is more accurate, detects antibodies to the bacterium that causes syphilis; however, once a positive result is obtained, subsequent results will always be positive, even after successful treatment. One such test, the fluorescent treponemal antibody absorption (FTA-ABS) test, is used to confirm that a positive screening test is caused by syphilis.

In the primary or secondary stages, syphilis may be diagnosed by obtaining fluid from a skin or mouth sore and identifying the bacteria under a microscope. The screening antibody test on a sample of blood can also be used. For neurosyphilis, a lumbar puncture is needed to obtain spinal fluid for antibody testing. In the latent stage, syphilis is diagnosed only by antibody tests of the blood and spinal fluid. In the tertiary stage, syphilis is diagnosed from the symptoms and with an antibody test.

Treatment and Prognosis

Because people with primary- or secondary-stage syphilis are infectious, they must avoid sexual contact until they and their sex partners have completed treatment. With primary-stage syphilis, all partners for the previous 3 months are in danger. With secondary-stage syphilis, all partners for the previous year are in danger. Such partners need to be screened with an antibody test performed on a blood sample and, if the result is positive, need to be treated.

Penicillin, usually the best antibiotic for all stages of syphilis, is typically given by injection. For primary-stage syphilis, penicillin is injected into each buttock only once. For secondary-stage syphilis, two additional injections at 1-week intervals are usually given. Penicillin is also given for latent-stage syphilis and for all forms of tertiary-stage syphilis, although more frequent or longer treatment given intravenously may be needed. People who are allergic to penicillin may receive doxycycline or tetracycline orally for 2 to 4 weeks.

More than half of the people with syphilis in its early stages, especially those with secondary-stage syphilis, develop a reaction (called the Jarisch-Herxheimer reaction) 2 to 12 hours after the first treatment. This reaction is believed to result from the sudden death of millions of bacteria. Symptoms of the reaction include a feeling of overall illness, a fever, headache, sweating, shaking chills, and temporary worsening of the syphilitic sores. Rarely, people with neurosyphilis may experience seizures or paralysis.

People with latent- or tertiary-stage syphilis are examined at regular intervals after treatment. Results of antibody tests usually remain positive for many years—sometimes for a lifetime. These results don't indicate a new infection. Other blood tests are used to check for new infections.

After treatment, the prognosis for primary-, secondary-, and latent-stage syphilis is excellent. The prognosis is poor for tertiary-stage syphilis of the brain or heart, because existing damage usually can't be reversed.

Gonorrhea

Gonorrhea is a sexually transmitted disease caused by the bacterium Neisseria gonorrhoeae *that infects the inner lining of the urethra, cervix, rectum, and throat or the whites (conjunctivae) of the eyes.*

Gonorrhea may spread through the bloodstream to other parts of the body, especially the skin and joints. In women, it may ascend the genital tract to infect the membranes inside the pelvis, causing pelvic pain and reproductive problems.

Symptoms

In men, the first symptoms usually appear 2 to 7 days after infection. Symptoms start with mild discomfort in the urethra, followed a few hours later by mild to severe pain during urination and discharge of pus from the penis. The man has a frequent and urgent need to urinate, and the urge worsens as the disease spreads to the upper part of the urethra. The penile opening may become red and swollen.

In women, the first symptoms may appear 7 to 21 days after infection. Often, infected women have no symptoms for weeks or months, and the disease is discovered only after the woman's male partner is diagnosed and she is examined as a contact. If symptoms occur, they are usually mild. However, some women have severe symptoms, such as a frequent need to urinate, pain while urinating, a discharge from the vagina, and fever. The cervix, uterus, fallopian tubes, ovaries, urethra, and rectum may be infected, causing deep pelvic pain or tenderness during intercourse. Pus, which appears to come from the vagina, may be coming from the cervix, the urethra, or the glands near the vaginal opening.

Women and homosexual men who engage in anal sex may contract gonorrhea of the rectum. The disease may cause discomfort around the anus and a discharge from the rectum. The area around the anus may become red and raw, and the stool may be coated with mucus and pus. When a doctor examines the rectum with an anoscope (a viewing tube), mucus and pus may be visible on the wall of the rectum.

Complications of Gonorrhea

In a rare complication of gonorrhea, the infection spreads through the bloodstream to one or a few joints, which become swollen, tender, and extremely painful, limiting movement. Bloodstream infection may also cause red pus-filled spots on the skin, fever, a general feeling of illness, or pain in many joints that moves from joint to joint (arthritis-dermatitis syndrome).

The interior of the heart may be infected (endocarditis). Infection of the covering of the liver (perihepatitis) causes pain similar to that of gallbladder disease. These infections are treatable and rarely fatal, but recovery from arthritis or endocarditis may be slow.

Oral sex with an infected partner may result in gonorrhea of the throat (gonococcal pharyngitis). Usually, the infection produces no symptoms, but sometimes it causes a sore throat and discomfort during swallowing.

If infected fluids come into contact with the eyes, an external eye infection may develop (gonorrheal conjunctivitis).▲ Newborns may be infected with gonorrhea by the mother during birth, causing swelling of both eyelids and a discharge of pus from the eyes.■ In adults, the same symptoms may occur, but often only one eye is affected. Blindness may result if the infection isn't treated.

Vaginal infection in infant and young girls is usually the result of sexual abuse by adults, but uncommonly results from handling infected household articles. Symptoms may include irritation, redness, and swelling of the vulva, with a discharge of pus from the vagina. The girl may be sore in the vaginal area or have pain during urination. The rectum also may be inflamed. The underpants may be stained with discharge.

▲ see page 1038

■ see page 1216

Diagnosis

A doctor can make a diagnosis almost immediately by identifying the bacterium (gonococcus) under a microscope. In more than 90 percent of infected men, such a diagnosis can be made using a sample of discharge from the penis. However, such a diagnosis can be made in only about 60 percent of infected women using a sample of the discharge from the cervix. If no bacteria are seen under the microscope, the discharge is sent to the laboratory for culture.

If a doctor suspects an infection of the throat or rectum, samples from these areas are sent for culture. Although a blood test for gonorrhea isn't available, a doctor may take a sample of blood to determine whether the person also has syphilis or human immunodeficiency virus (HIV) infection. Some people have more than one sexually transmitted disease.

Treatment

Doctors usually treat gonorrhea with a single injection of ceftriaxone into a muscle or with a weeklong course of oral antibiotics (usually doxycycline). If gonorrhea has spread through the bloodstream, the person usually is treated in the hospital, often with intravenous antibiotics. Because infection with *Chlamydia* is common in both men and women with gonorrhea but is difficult to diagnose, patients are given a weeklong course of doxycycline or tetracycline or a single dose of azithromycin, another long-acting antibiotic.

If symptoms recur or persist at the end of treatment, doctors may obtain specimens for culture to make sure the person is cured. In men, symptoms of urethritis may recur, a condition called postgonococcal urethritis. Postgonococcal urethritis, most commonly caused by *Chlamydia* and other organisms that don't respond to treatment with ceftriaxone, occurs particularly in people who do not follow the treatment plan as prescribed.

Chancroid

Chancroid is a sexually transmitted disease caused by Hemophilus ducreyi *bacteria that produces painful, persistent genital sores (ulcers).*

Once rare in North America, the number of chancroid cases has recently increased. A person who has a chancroid ulcer is more likely to become infected with human immunodeficiency virus (HIV) if exposed to the virus.

Symptoms and Diagnosis

Symptoms begin 3 to 7 days after infection. Small, painful blisters on the genitals and around the anus rapidly rupture to form shallow ulcers. These sores may enlarge and join together. The lymph nodes in the groin may become tender, enlarged, and matted together, forming an abscess (an accumulation of pus). The skin over the abscess may become red and shiny and may break down, so that pus is discharged onto the skin.

The diagnosis of chancroid is based on its appearance and on the results of tests for other causes of ulcers. Taking a sample of pus from an ulcer and growing the bacterium in the laboratory, which is technically difficult, can help the doctor make the diagnosis.

Treatment

An antibiotic, either ceftriaxone or erythromycin, is injected every 6 hours for at least 7 days. Pus may be removed from a swollen lymph node with a syringe.

A person with chancroid is monitored by a doctor for at least 3 months to make sure the infection is cured. If possible, all sex partners are traced, so they can be examined and treated as necessary.

Lymphogranuloma Venereum

Lymphogranuloma venereum is a sexually transmitted disease caused by Chlamydia trachomatis, *a bacterium that grows only within cells.*

Lymphogranuloma venereum is caused by types of *Chlamydia trachomatis* other than those that cause inflammation of the urethra (urethritis) and cervix (cervicitis). Lymphogranuloma venereum occurs mostly in tropical and subtropical areas and is uncommon in the United States.

Symptoms and Diagnosis

Symptoms begin 3 to 12 days or more after infection. A small, painless, fluid-filled blister develops usually on the penis or in the vagina. Typically, the blister becomes an ulcer that quickly heals—often going unnoticed. Next, lymph nodes in the groin on one or both sides may become enlarged and tender. The skin covering the infected area becomes warm and red, and if untreated, openings (sinuses) may appear in the skin over the lymph nodes. These openings discharge pus or bloody fluid and usually heal, but they may leave a scar and may recur. Other symptoms include fever, a feeling of illness (malaise), headache, joint pain, poor appetite, vomiting, backache, and an infection of the rectum that results in a discharge of blood-stained pus.

With prolonged or repeated episodes, the lymphatic vessels may become obstructed, causing tissue to swell. Rectal infection may cause scarring, which may result in a narrowing of the rectum.

A doctor suspects lymphogranuloma venereum based on its characteristic symptoms. The diagnosis can be confirmed by a blood test that identifies antibodies against *Chlamydia trachomatis.*

Treatment

If given early in the disease, treatment with oral doxycycline, erythromycin, or tetracycline for 3 weeks results in rapid healing. After treatment, a doctor should regularly check that the infection is cured. Attempts are made to identify all sexual contacts of the infected person so they can also be examined and treated.

Granuloma Inguinale

Granuloma inguinale is a sexually transmitted disease caused by the bacterium Calymmatobacterium granulomatis *that leads to chronic inflammation of the genitals.*

Granuloma inguinale is rare in temperate climates, such as the northern United States, but common in some tropical and subtropical areas.

Symptoms and Diagnosis

Symptoms begin about 1 to 12 weeks after infection. The first symptom is a painless, red nodule that slowly grows into a round, raised lump. Sites of infection include the penis, scrotum, groin, and thighs in men and the vulva, vagina, and surrounding skin areas in women. In both men and women, the anus, buttocks, and face may be infected. Eventually, the raised lumps may cover the genitals. Healing is slow, and scar tissue forms. Commonly, the nodules become infected with other organisms. If granuloma inguinale is left untreated, the infection may spread throughout the body to the bones, joints, or liver, causing severe weight loss, fever, and anemia.

A doctor diagnoses granuloma inguinale from the characteristic bright red lumps. Microscopic examination of specimens from the edge of the lumps can confirm the diagnosis.

Treatment

Any of several antibiotics may be taken, including streptomycin, tetracycline, erythromycin, chloramphenicol, and trimethoprim-sulfamethoxazole. For 6 months after treatment, the patient should be monitored by a doctor to make sure the infection has been cured.

Nongonococcal Urethritis and Chlamydial Cervicitis

Nongonococcal urethritis and chlamydial cervicitis are sexually transmitted diseases usually caused by Chlamydia trachomatis *or (in men)* Ureaplasma urealyticum *but occasionally by* Trichomonas vaginalis *or herpes simplex virus.*

These infections are called "nongonococcal" to indicate that they aren't caused by *Neisseria gonorrhoeae,* the bacterium that causes gonorrhea.▲ *Chlamydia trachomatis* causes about 50 percent of the urethral infections in men not caused by gonorrhea and most of the pus-forming infections of the cervix in women not caused by gonorrhea. Most of the remaining cases of urethritis are caused by *Ureaplasma urealyticum,* a mycoplasma-like bacterium.

Chlamydiae are small bacteria that can reproduce only inside cells. Ureaplasmas are very small bacteria that lack a rigid cell wall but that can reproduce outside cells.

Symptoms and Diagnosis

Usually between 4 and 28 days after intercourse with an infected person, an infected man feels a

mild burning sensation in his urethra while urinating. A discharge from the penis usually develops. The discharge may be clear or cloudy, but it is generally less thick than with gonorrhea. Early in the morning, the opening of the penis is often red and stuck together with dried secretions. Occasionally, the disease begins more dramatically. The man finds urinating painful, needs to urinate frequently, and has discharges of pus from the urethra.

Although most women infected with *Chlamydia* have no symptoms, some have a frequent urge to urinate, pain while urinating, pain in the lower abdomen, pain during sexual intercourse, and secretions of yellow mucus and pus from the vagina.

Anal or oral sex with an infected partner can lead to infection of the rectum or throat. These infections may cause pain and a yellow discharge of pus and mucus.

In most cases, an infection with *Chlamydia trachomatis* can be diagnosed by examining discharge from the penis or cervix in a laboratory. *Ureaplasma urealyticum* infections are not diagnosed specifically in routine medical settings. Because culturing is difficult and other techniques for diagnosis are expensive, the diagnosis of *Chlamydia* or *Ureaplasma* infection often is presumed on the basis of the characteristic symptoms along with evidence against the presence of gonorrhea.

Complications and Prognosis

If an infection caused by *Chlamydia trachomatis* isn't treated, symptoms disappear in 4 weeks in about 60 to 70 percent of the people. However, a chlamydial infection may cause a number of complications. Whether *Ureaplasma* has a role in these complications is unclear.

If untreated, a chlamydial infection in women often ascends to the fallopian tubes, where inflammation may cause pain, and scarring may cause infertility and ectopic pregnancy.■ These latter complications may occur in the absence of prior symptoms and result in considerable suffering and medical costs. In men, *Chlamydia* may cause epididymitis, which produces painful swelling of the scrotum on one or both sides.★

Treatment

Chlamydial and ureaplasmal infections are usually treated with tetracycline or doxycycline taken orally for at least 7 days or with a single dose of azithromycin. Pregnant women should

▲ see page 941

■ see page 1153

★ see page 1063

not take tetracycline. In about 20 percent of the people, the infection returns after treatment. Treatment is then repeated for a longer period.

Infected people who have sexual intercourse before completing treatment may infect their partners. Thus, sex partners are treated simultaneously if possible.

Trichomoniasis

Trichomoniasis is a sexually transmitted disease of the vagina or urethra caused by Trichomonas vaginalis, *a single-celled organism with a whiplike tail.*

Although *Trichomonas vaginalis* can infect the genitourinary tract of either men or women, symptoms are more common in women. About 20 percent of women experience trichomoniasis of the vagina during their reproductive years.

In men, the organism infects the urethra, prostate, and bladder, but it only rarely causes symptoms. In some populations, *Trichomonas* may account for 5 to 10 percent of all cases of nongonococcal urethritis. The organism is more difficult to detect in men than in women.

Symptoms

In women, the disease usually starts with a greenish-yellow, frothy vaginal discharge. In some women, the discharge may be slight. The vulva (the external female genital organs) may be irritated and sore, and sexual intercourse may be painful. In severe cases, the vulva and surrounding skin may be inflamed and the labia swollen. Pain on urination or frequency of urination may occur, resembling the symptoms of a bladder infection.

Men with trichomoniasis generally have no symptoms but can infect their sex partners. Some men have a temporary frothy or pus-like discharge from the urethra, pain during urination, and a need to urinate frequently. These symptoms usually occur early in the morning. The urethra may be mildly irritated, and occasionally moisture appears at the opening of the penis. Infection of the epididymis, causing pain in the testes, occurs rarely. The prostate also may become infected, but the role of *Trichomonas* is unclear. These infections are the only known complications of trichomoniasis in men.

Complications of Chlamydial and Ureaplasmal Infections

Complication	Possible Effect
In men	
Infection of the epididymis	Pain in the testis
Narrowing (stricture) of the urethra	Obstructed urine flow
In women	
Infection of the fallopian tubes	Pain, ectopic pregnancy, and infertility
Infection of the covering of the liver and the area surrounding the liver	Upper abdominal pain
In men and women	
Infection of the whites of the eyes (conjunctivitis)	Eye pain and discharge
In newborns	
Conjunctivitis	Eye pain and discharge
Pneumonia	Fever and cough

Diagnosis

In women, the diagnosis can usually be made within minutes by examining a sample of vaginal secretions under a microscope. Tests for other sexually transmitted diseases are usually performed as well.

In men, secretions from the end of the penis should be obtained in the morning before urination. The secretions are examined under a microscope, and a sample of the secretions is sent to the laboratory for culture. A urine culture may also be helpful, because this is more likely to detect *Trichomonas* missed by microscopic examination.

Treatment

A single oral dose of metronidazole cures up to 95 percent of infected women, provided their sex partners are treated simultaneously. Because it's not known whether a single-dose treatment is effective in men, men are usually treated for 7 days.

If taken with alcohol, metronidazole may cause nausea and flushing of the skin. The drug also may cause a decrease in white blood cells and, in women, an increased susceptibility to vaginal yeast infections (genital candidiasis). Metronidazole is probably best avoided during pregnancy, at least during the first 3 months. Infected people who have sexual intercourse before the infection is cured are likely to infect their partners.

Genital Candidiasis

*Genital candidiasis is a yeast (fungus) infection of the vagina or penis, commonly referred to as **thrush,** caused by* Candida albicans.

The *Candida* yeast normally resides on the skin or in the intestines. From these areas, it can spread to the genitals. *Candida* isn't usually transmitted sexually.

Candidiasis is a very common cause of vaginitis. Genital candidiasis has become more common mainly because of the increasing use of antibiotics, oral contraceptives, and other drugs that change the environment in the vagina in a way that favors the growth of *Candida*. Candidiasis is more common in women who are pregnant or menstruating and in diabetics. Less commonly, the use of drugs (such as corticosteroids or cancer chemotherapy) and diseases that suppress the immune system (such as AIDS) can facilitate the infection.

Symptoms and Diagnosis

Women with genital candidiasis usually develop itching or irritation of the vagina and vulva and may have a vaginal discharge. Frequently, the irritation is severe, but the discharge is light. The vulva may be reddish and swollen. The skin may be raw and may crack. The vaginal wall is usually covered with a white cheese-like material, but it may look normal.

Men often have no symptoms, but the end of the penis (the glans) and the foreskin (in uncircumcised men) may be sore and irritated, especially after sexual intercourse. Occasionally, men may notice a slight discharge from the penis. The end of the penis and the foreskin may be reddish,

may have small crusted blisters or sores, and may be covered with white cheese-like material.

Immediate diagnosis can be made by taking specimens from the vagina or the penis and examining them under a microscope. Specimens also may be sent to the laboratory for culture.

Treatment

In women, candidiasis can be treated by washing the vagina with soap and water, drying it with a clean towel, and then applying an antifungal cream containing clotrimazole, miconazole, butoconazole, or tioconazole and terconazole. Alternatively, ketoconazole, fluconazole, or itraconazole can be taken orally. In men, the penis (and foreskin in uncircumcised men) should be washed and dried before an antifungal cream (containing, for example, nystatin) is applied.

Occasionally, women who take oral contraceptives must stop using them for several months during treatment for vaginal candidiasis because they can make the infection worse. Women who are at unavoidable risk of vaginal candidiasis, such as those who have an impaired immune system or who are taking antibiotics for a long period of time, may need an antifungal drug or other preventive therapy.

Genital Herpes

Genital herpes is a sexually transmitted disease of the genital area, the skin around the rectum, or adjacent areas caused by herpes simplex virus.

There are two types of herpes simplex virus, called HSV-1 and HSV-2. HSV-2 is usually transmitted sexually, whereas HSV-1 usually infects the mouth. Both herpes simplex virus types may infect the genitals, the skin around the rectum, or the hands (especially the nail beds) and may be transmitted to other parts of the body (such as the surface of the eyes). Herpes sores don't usually become infected with bacteria, but some people with herpes also have other sexually transmitted organisms, such as syphilis or chancroid, in the same ulcers.

Symptoms

Symptoms of the initial (primary) outbreak begin 4 to 7 days after infection. The first symptoms are usually itching, tingling, and soreness. Then comes a small patch of redness, followed by a group of small, painful blisters. The blisters break and fuse to form circular sores. The sores, which are usually painful, usually become crusted after a few days. Urinating may be difficult, and walking may be painful. The sores heal in about 10 days but may leave scars. Lymph nodes in the groin are usually slightly enlarged and tender. The first outbreak is more painful, prolonged, and widespread than subsequent ones and may be associated with fever and feeling ill.

In men, the blisters and sores may develop anywhere on the penis, including the foreskin if the penis is uncircumcised. In women, the blisters and sores may develop on the vulva, in and around the vagina, and on the cervix. Those who have anal intercourse may develop blisters and sores around the anus or in the rectum.

In people with impaired immune systems, such as those with human immunodeficiency virus (HIV) infection, herpes sores may be severe, spread to other areas of the body, persist for weeks or longer, and, uncommonly, become resistant to treatment with acyclovir.

The symptoms tend to recur in the same or adjacent areas, because the virus persists in nearby pelvic nerves and reactivates to reinfect the skin. HSV-2 is better able to reactivate in the pelvic nerves. HSV-1 reactivates more effectively in the facial nerves, where it causes fever blisters or herpes labialis (herpes of the lips). Nonetheless, either virus can cause disease in either area. Prior infection with either virus provides partial immunity to the other, making symptoms of the second virus less severe.

Diagnosis

A doctor suspects herpes based on the person's symptoms. A diagnosis can be made immediately by examining samples from the sores under a microscope. To confirm the diagnosis, swabs from a sore are sent to special laboratories for culture. The results may be available in as little as 48 hours. Blood tests may show evidence of past infections or suggest a recent one if antibody levels are rising.

Treatment

No treatment can cure genital herpes, but treatment may shorten an outbreak. The number of outbreaks can be reduced by continuous low-

---

Complications of Genital Herpes

About 3 to 12 days after the blisters first appear in the genital area, the herpes virus may spread to other body parts. Serious complications, however, are rare. The covering of the brain (meninges) may become infected, causing vomiting, a headache, and neck stiffness. The spinal cord may become infected, causing weakness in the legs. The nerves in the pelvic area also may be affected, causing temporary pain, constipation, inability to urinate, and in men, impotence. Although rare, the virus may spread through the bloodstream to the skin, joints, liver, or lungs—particularly in newborns or people with an impaired immune system.

The most common complication of genital herpes is repeated return of the blisters and sores, which are usually confined to one side of the body and milder than the initial outbreak. A person may feel sick and have itching, tingling, or pain in the affected area before each attack. The risk of recurrence in the genital area is greater with HSV-2 than with HSV-1. However, the rate of recurrence varies greatly. In some people, the outbreaks recur frequently for many years. Sores may recur beyond the genital area to the buttocks, groin, or thighs.

---

dose therapy with antiviral drugs. Treatment is most effective if started early, usually within 2 days of the start of symptoms. Acyclovir or related antiviral drugs can be taken orally or applied in a cream directly on the sores. These drugs reduce the shedding of the live virus from the sores, thus reducing the risk of transmission. The drug can also lessen the severity of symptoms during the initial outbreak. However, even early treatment of the first attack doesn't prevent recurrences.

Patients with a history of herpes may be infectious to their sexual partners even when they are not aware of an outbreak.

Genital Warts

Genital warts (condylomata acuminata) are warts in or around the vagina, penis, or rectum caused by sexually transmitted papillomaviruses.

Genital warts are common and cause concern because they are unsightly, may become infected with bacteria, and may indicate an impaired immune system. In women, papillomavirus types 16 and 18, which occur in the cervix but do not cause warts on the external genitals, may cause cervical cancer.▲ These types and other papillomaviruses may cause cervical intraepithelial neoplasm (indicated by an abnormal Pap test result) or cancer of the vagina, vulva, anus, penis, mouth, throat, or esophagus.

Symptoms and Diagnosis

Genital warts occur most often on warm, moist surfaces of the body. In men, the usual areas are on the end and shaft of the penis and below the foreskin (if the penis is uncircumcised). In women, genital warts occur on the vulva, the vaginal wall, the cervix, and the skin surrounding the vaginal area. Genital warts may develop in the area around the anus and in the rectum, especially in homosexual men and in women who engage in anal sex.

The warts usually appear 1 to 6 months after infection, beginning as tiny soft, moist, pink or red swellings. They grow rapidly and may develop stalks. Multiple warts often grow in the same area, and their rough surfaces give them the appearance of a small cauliflower. The warts may grow very rapidly in pregnant women, in people with an impaired immune system (for example, from AIDS or treatment with immunosuppressive drugs), and in those who have inflammation of the skin.

Genital warts usually can be diagnosed from their appearance. However, they may be mistaken

---

▲ see page 1109

for sores found in the secondary stage of syphilis. Unusual looking or persistent warts may be removed surgically and examined under a microscope to make sure that they aren't cancerous. Women who have warts on the cervix should undergo regular Pap tests.

Treatment

No treatment is completely satisfactory. External genital warts may be removed by laser, cryotherapy (freezing), or surgery using local anesthetics. Chemical treatments, such as podophyllum resin or purified toxin or trichloroacetic acid, can be applied directly to the warts. This approach, however, requires many applications over weeks to months, may burn the surrounding skin, and frequently fails.

Warts in the urethra may be treated with anticancer drugs, such as thiotepa or fluorouracil. Alternatively, the warts may be removed from the urethra by endoscopic surgery (a procedure in which a flexible viewing tube with surgical attachments is used). Interferon-alfa injections into the wart are under study as a possible treatment, but their usefulness isn't yet known.

Genital warts return frequently and require repeated treatment. In men, circumcision may help to prevent recurrence. All sex partners should be examined and treated, if necessary.

Sexually Transmitted Intestinal Infections

Various bacteria *(Shigella, Campylobacter,* and *Salmonella)*, viruses (hepatitis A), and parasites *(Giardia* and other amebas) that cause intestinal infections may be transmitted sexually—particularly by activities in which the mouth comes into contact with the genitals or anus. Symptoms are typically those of the specific organism transmitted and may involve combinations of diarrhea, fever, bloating, nausea and vomiting, abdominal pain, and jaundice. Infections recur frequently, especially in homosexual men with many sex partners. Some infections cause no symptoms.

Skin Disorders

Biology of the Skin

The skin isn't just a protective wrapping. It's an organ system that regulates body temperature, senses painful and pleasant stimuli, keeps substances from entering the body, and provides a shield from the sun's harmful effects. Skin color, texture, and folds help mark people as individuals. Anything that goes wrong with skin function or appearance can have important consequences for physical and mental health.

Each layer of skin performs specific tasks. The top layer, the epidermis, is actually thinner over most of the body than plastic wrap. The top portion of the epidermis, the stratum corneum, contains keratin, which is formed from the remains of dead cells and protects the skin from harmful substances. At the bottom of the epidermis are the melanocytes, the cells that produce melanin—the dark-colored pigment of skin.

Below the epidermis lies the dermis, which contains pain and touch receptors, whose tentacles reach up to the skin surface, and many of the functional glands of the skin: sweat glands, which produce sweat; sebaceous glands, which produce oil; and hair follicles, which produce hair. Also within the dermis lie blood vessels that provide nutrition to the skin and make it feel warm and nerves that branch throughout the layers of the skin.

Below the dermis lies a layer of fat that helps insulate the body from heat and cold.

Over different parts of the body, the thickness and color of the skin and the number of sweat glands, sebaceous glands, hair follicles, and nerves vary. The top of the head has many hair follicles; the soles of the feet have none. The soles and the palms have much thicker epidermis and keratin layers. The fingertips and toes contain many nerves and are extremely sensitive to touch.

The skin tends to change throughout a person's lifetime. A baby's skin has a much thicker fat layer and a much thinner layer of protective keratin. As people age, they lose much of the underlying fat, the dermis and epidermis become thinner, the elastic fibers in the dermis become fragmented, and the skin becomes more wrinkled. The flow of blood in the skin also decreases with age, so dam-

What's Under the Skin?

This cross-sectional view shows the skin layers and structures beneath the surface.

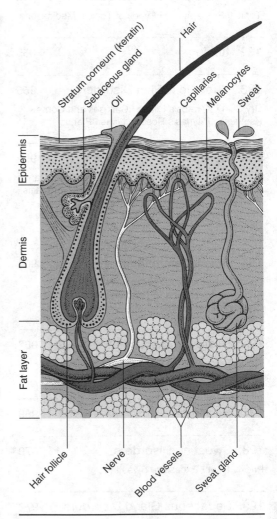

Medical Names for Marks and Growths on the Skin

Atrophic skin: Paper-thin, wrinkled skin.

Crust (scab): Dried blood, pus, or skin fluids on the surface of the skin. A crust can form wherever the skin has been damaged.

Erosion: Loss of part or all of the top surface of the skin. Erosions occur when infection, pressure, irritation, or temperature has damaged the skin.

Excoriation: A hollowed-out or linear crusted area, caused by scratching, rubbing, or picking at the skin.

Lichenification: Thickened skin that has deep grooves and wrinkles.

Macule: A flat, discolored spot of any shape, less than 0.4 of an inch in diameter. Freckles, flat moles, port-wine stains, and many rashes are macules. A **patch** is like a macule, but larger.

Nodule: A solid bump, 0.2 to 0.4 of an inch in diameter, that may be raised. A nodule sometimes appears to form below the surface of the skin and press upward.

Papule: A solid bump less than 0.4 of an inch in diameter. Warts, insect bites, skin tags, and some skin cancers are papules. A **plaque** is a larger papule.

Pustule: A blister containing pus (a collection of white blood cells).

Scales: Areas of heaped-up, dead epidermal cells, producing a flaky, dry patch. Scales occur with psoriasis, seborrheic dermatitis, and many other conditions.

Scar: An area where normal skin has been replaced by fibrous (scar-forming) tissue. Scars form after destruction of some part of the dermis.

Telangiectasia: Dilated blood vessels within the skin that have a tortuous appearance.

Ulcer: Like an erosion, only deeper, penetrating at least part of the dermis. The causes are the same as for erosions.

Vesicle: A small, fluid-filled spot less than 0.2 of an inch in diameter. A **blister** (bulla) is a larger vesicle. Insect bites, herpes zoster (shingles), chickenpox, burns, and irritations form vesicles and blisters.

Wheal (hive): Swelling in the skin that produces an elevated, soft, spongy area that appears relatively suddenly and then disappears. Wheals are common allergic reactions to drugs, insect bites, or something that touched the skin.

aged skin heals more slowly in older people. Older skin also makes less protective oil, so the skin dries out more easily.

Diagnosing Skin Conditions

Doctors can identify many skin conditions simply by looking at them. Revealing characteristics include size, shape, color, and location of the abnormality, as well as the presence or absence of other signs or symptoms. Sometimes, a doctor has to remove a small piece of skin for examination under a microscope, a procedure called a biopsy. For this simple procedure, the doctor generally numbs a small area of skin with a local anesthetic and, using a small knife (scalpel) or round cutter (biopsy punch), removes a piece of skin about one-eighth inch in diameter. Often, the doctor uses a stitch to close the site and stop the bleeding.

When doctors think the skin may be infected, they scrape off some material from the skin, send it to a laboratory, and have the specimen placed in a culture medium. If the specimen contains bacteria, fungi, or viruses, they grow in the culture and can be identified.

Other laboratory tests also help doctors diagnose skin infections. In a Wood's light examination, a certain frequency of ultraviolet (black) light makes some fungi visible and may make some pigmentation abnormalities more visible. The Tzanck test helps diagnose viral skin infections such as herpes. With a small scalpel, the doctor scrapes the surface of the inflamed skin and examines it under a microscope. Recognizable enlarged or grouped cells indicate a viral infection. The skin sample also can be sent to a laboratory for a viral culture.

Many problems that appear on the skin are limited to the skin. Sometimes, however, the skin reveals a medical condition of the entire body. For example, people who have systemic lupus erythematosus develop an unusual reddish rash on their cheeks, usually after sun exposure. Consequently, doctors often must consider many possible causes when evaluating skin problems. Examining the entire skin surface and looking for certain patterns of a rash can help them identify any possible medical illness. To check the distribution of a skin problem, the doctor may ask a patient to undress completely, even though the patient only noticed an abnormality on a small area of skin. Doctors may also order blood tests or other laboratory tests even if a person seems to have a problem limited only to the skin.

CHAPTER 191

Topical Skin Medications

Virtually all skin medications are either topical or systemic. Topical medications are applied directly to the affected area of the skin. Systemic medications are taken by mouth or injected and are distributed throughout the body. Rarely, when a high concentration of a medication is needed at the affected area, a doctor may inject a medication just under the skin; this is called an intradermal injection.

Some skin medications require a prescription; others can be purchased without one. Although generally considered safer than prescription drugs, over-the-counter drugs must be used with caution. Applying the wrong medication may worsen a skin condition or may mask symptoms, making the diagnosis difficult for a doctor.

Topical Preparations

The active ingredients (medications) in a topical preparation are mixed with (suspended in) a vehicle (an inert carrier for the medications). Thus, the formulation and consistency vary among topical preparations. The vehicle determines the consistency of the product and whether the active ingredients remain on the surface or penetrate the skin—whether the preparation is thick and greasy or light and watery. Depending on the vehicle used, the preparation will be an ointment, cream, lotion, solution, powder, or gel.

Ointments, which contain a lot of thick oil and very little water, feel greasy and are difficult to wash off. Ointments are most appropriate when the skin needs lubrication or moisture. Although messier to use than water-based cream preparations, ointments are usually better at delivering active ingredients into the skin.

Creams, the most commonly used preparations, are emulsions of oil in water. They're easy to apply and appear to vanish when rubbed into the skin.

Lotions are similar to creams but contain more water. They're actually suspensions of finely dispersed powdered material in a base of water or oil and water. Lotions are easy to apply and are particularly useful for cooling or drying the skin.

Solutions are liquids in which a drug is dissolved. Solutions tend to dry rather than moisturize the skin. The most commonly used liquids are alcohol, propylene glycol, polyethylene glycol, and plain water.

Powders are dried forms of substances that are used to protect areas where skin rubs against skin—for instance, between the toes or buttocks, in the armpits or groin, or under the breasts. Powders dry skin that's macerated (softened and damaged by moisture) and reduce friction by absorbing moisture. Powders may be incorporated into protective creams, lotions, and ointments.

Gels are water-based substances thickened without oil or fat. The skin doesn't absorb gels as well as it absorbs preparations containing oil or fat.

Types of Topical Medications

Topical medications can be divided into seven often overlapping categories: cleansing agents, protective agents, anti-infective agents, moisturizing agents, drying agents, symptom-relieving agents, and anti-inflammatory agents.

Cleansing Agents

The principal cleansing agents are soaps, detergents, and solvents. Soap is the most popular cleanser, but synthetic detergents are used as well. Certain soaps dry the skin; others have a creamy base that doesn't dry it. Some liquid soaps moisturize the skin; others dry it.

Because baby shampoos are excellent cleansing agents and are usually gentle to the skin, they're good for cleansing wounds, cuts, and abrasions. Also, people with psoriasis, eczema, and other scaling diseases can use baby shampoos to wash away dead skin. Oozing (weeping) lesions, however, should generally be cleaned only with water because even gentle soaps and detergents can irritate the area.

Many chemicals are added to cleansing agents. For example, antidandruff shampoos and lotions may contain zinc dipyrithione, selenium sulfide, or tar extracts to help treat flaking skin. Cleansing compounds may also contain small amounts of acetic acid, aluminum acetate, and magnesium sulfate (as in Epsom salts).

Protective Agents

Many different kinds of preparations help protect the skin. Oils and ointments supply an oil-based barrier that can help protect scraped or irritated skin and retain moisture. Powders may protect skin that rubs against skin or clothing. Synthetic hydrocolloid dressings protect bedsores (pressure ulcers) and other areas of raw skin. Sunscreens filter out harmful ultraviolet light.

Anti-infective Agents

Viruses, bacteria, and fungi can all infect the skin. By far, the best way to prevent such infections is by carefully washing the skin with soap and water. Other agents can disinfect more strongly or treat established infections. Most disinfecting agents are used only by nurses and doctors to sterilize their skin and their patients' skin before surgery. However, certain medications are commonly used to treat fungal and bacterial infections. For instance, antibiotics are applied to the skin for acne and superficial skin infections. Clotrimazole and miconazole are commonly applied to the skin to treat fungal infections. Both

are available without a prescription. Other antifungal agents such as ketoconazole creams are available by prescription only. Medications such as gamma benzene hexachloride (lindane) help treat infections such as scabies.

Moisturizing Agents

Moisturizers don't actually add moisture to the skin; they help the skin hold its natural moisture. Most moisturizers are creams or lotions containing oil. Putting a thin film of oil on the skin helps prevent water in the skin from evaporating. The best time to apply these agents is when the skin is already moistened—immediately after a bath or shower, for instance. Some stronger moisturizers contain compounds such as urea.

Drying Agents

Excessive moisture in the skin can cause maceration—a problem that usually occurs where skin rubs skin, trapping moisture, especially on hot, humid days. The areas most commonly affected are between the toes or buttocks, in the armpits or groin, and under the breasts. These moist areas also provide fertile breeding grounds for infections, especially with fungi and bacteria.

Talcum powder is the most commonly used drying agent. Talc absorbs moisture from the skin surface. Most of the many talc preparations vary only in their scents and packaging. Cornstarch, another good drying agent, has the disadvantage of encouraging the growth of fungi. For this reason, talc is generally better.

Solutions containing aluminum salts are useful when the skin is damaged from excessive wetness. These solutions are often used in hospitals and nursing homes.

Symptom-Relieving Agents

Skin disease is often accompanied by itching. Sometimes one medication is applied to relieve the itching, while another is used to treat the disease. Itching and mild pain can sometimes be controlled with soothing agents such as chamomile, eucalyptus, camphor, menthol, zinc oxide, talc, glycerin, and calamine. Antihistamines such as diphenhydramine are sometimes included in topical preparations to relieve the itching associated with allergic reactions. Although antihistamines block certain types of allergic reactions, they probably relieve itching by their sedative effects.

Strengths of Selected Topical Corticosteroids

Potency	Medication	Formulation
Low	Hydrocortisone	Cream, ointment, or lotion 2.5% or 1.0%
Medium	Betamethasone valerate	Cream 0.1%
	Fluocinolone acetonide	Cream or ointment 0.025%
	Hydrocortisone valerate	Cream or ointment 0.2%
	Triamcinolone acetonide	Cream, ointment, or lotion 0.1% or 0.025%
High	Betamethasone dipropionate	Cream or ointment 0.05%
	Betamethasone valerate	Ointment 0.1%
	Fluocinolone acetonide	Cream 0.2%
	Halcinonide	Cream or ointment 0.1%
Very High	Clobetasol propionate	Cream or ointment 0.05%
	Halobetasol propionate	Cream or ointment 0.05%

However, antihistamines can sensitize a person and cause an allergic reaction. To control certain forms of itching, a person should use oral antihistamines rather than topical antihistamines.

Anti-inflammatory Agents

Topical or oral corticosteroids (cortisone-like drugs) can help reduce inflammation (swelling, itching, and redness). Corticosteroids are most effective for rashes caused by allergic or inflammatory reactions to poison ivy, metals, cloth, or other substances. Because they lower resistance to bacterial and fungal infections, they usually shouldn't be used on infected areas or wounds. However, corticosteroids are sometimes mixed with antifungal agents to help reduce itching caused by a fungus. Combinations of corticosteroids and antibiotics are seldom used because they're generally no more effective than the corticosteroids alone. Also, antibiotics (especially neomycin) increase the risk of an allergic reaction that can complicate the problem.

Topical corticosteroids are sold as lotions, creams, and ointments. Creams are most effective if rubbed in gently until they vanish. In general, the ointments are the most potent. The type and concentration of corticosteroid in the preparation determines the overall strength. Hydrocortisone is available in concentrations of up to 1 percent without a prescription; concentrations of 0.5 percent or less offer little benefit. Stronger corticosteroid preparations require a prescription. Doctors usually prescribe potent corticosteroids first, then less potent corticosteroids as the skin heals. Generally, topical corticosteroids are applied two to three times a day in small amounts. Where the skin is already thin, such as on the face, they should be used sparingly and never for more than a few days.

When a stronger dose is needed, a doctor may inject a corticosteroid just under the skin. Another way to deliver a strong dose is to apply a nonporous occlusive dressing over a topical corticosteroid to increase the drug's absorption and effectiveness. For example, a polyethylene film (household plastic wrap) may be applied over cream or ointment preparations and left on overnight. With this method, creams and ointments are less irritating than lotions. Occlusive dressings increase the risk of adverse reactions to the corticosteroids, so they're generally reserved for conditions such as psoriasis and severe eczema.

Itching

Itching (pruritus) is a sensation that instinctively demands scratching.

Persistent scratching may cause redness and deep cuts in the skin. In fact, scratching can so irritate the skin that it leads to more itching, creating a vicious circle. Prolonged scratching and rubbing can thicken and scar the skin.

Causes

Itching may be caused by a skin condition or a systemic disease (a disease that affects the body generally). Skin conditions that cause severe itching include infestations with parasites (scabies, pediculosis), insect bites, hives, atopic dermatitis, and allergic and contact dermatitis. Often, contact with wool clothing or irritants such as solvents or cosmetics causes itching. Dry skin, especially in the elderly, causes severe, widespread itching.

Systemic diseases that can cause itching include liver disease (especially jaundice), kidney failure, lymphomas, leukemias, and other blood disorders. Sometimes people with thyroid disease, diabetes, or cancer develop itching. Itching is common during the later months of pregnancy.

Usually, it doesn't indicate any abnormality, but it can result from mild liver problems. Many drugs can cause itching, including barbiturates and aspirin as well as any drug to which a particular person has an allergy.

Treatment

Doctors treat itching by determining the cause and trying to eliminate it. Especially while the skin is inflamed, a doctor may encourage a patient to use a nonprescription, gentle, moisturizing cream or lotion without scents or colors. Additives that provide color or scent may irritate the skin and may even cause itching. Soothing compounds such as menthol, camphor, chamomile, eucalyptus, and calamine also can help. Corticosteroid creams, which help decrease inflammation and control itching, should be used only when itching is limited to a small area.

Taking antihistamines such as hydroxyzine and diphenhydramine by mouth may help, but they usually cause sleepiness. Generally, antihistamines shouldn't be applied to the skin because they can cause allergic reactions.

CHAPTER 193

Superficial Skin Disorders

The uppermost layer of the skin, called the stratum corneum or the keratin layer, consists of many layers of flattened, dead cells and acts as a barrier to protect the underlying tissue from injury and infection. By slowing evaporation, oils in this skin layer help hold moisture in the deeper layers, maintaining the skin's soft, pliable texture.▲

The stratum corneum is only a part of the epidermis, which is a thin layer of skin over most of the body. In some places, such as the palms of the hands and the soles of the feet, the epidermis is naturally thick, with the stratum corneum providing extra protection from impacts and abrasions. The epidermis may also be thick and hard in excessively dry areas.

Disorders of the superficial skin layers involve the stratum corneum and deeper layers of the epidermis and range from those causing temporary discomfort to those causing chronic disabilities.

▲ see box, page 950

Dry Skin

Dry skin is common, especially in people past middle age. Common causes are cold weather and frequent bathing. Bathing washes away surface oils, allowing the skin to dry out. Dry skin may become irritated and often itches—sometimes it sloughs off in small flakes and scales. Scaling most often affects the lower legs.

Sometimes, severe dry skin (ichthyosis) results from an inherited scaling disease, such as ichthyosis vulgaris or epidermolytic hyperkeratosis. A person with ichthyosis vulgaris has fine scales and no blisters; someone with epidermolytic hyperkeratosis has thick, warty scales and painful, foul-smelling blisters. Ichthyosis also results from nonhereditary disorders, such as leprosy, underactive thyroid, lymphoma, AIDS, and sarcoidosis.

Treatment

The key to treating simple dry skin is keeping the skin moist. Taking fewer baths allows protective oils to remain on the skin. Ointments or creams such as petroleum jelly (Vaseline), mineral oil, or unscented moisturizers also can hold water in the skin. Harsh soaps, detergents, and the perfumes in some moisturizers irritate the skin and may further dry it out. Rubbing or scratching dry skin can lead to infection and scarring.

When scaling is a problem, solutions or creams containing salicylic acid may help remove the scales. For adults, a doctor may recommend wrapping the skin with a barrier bandage made of plastic film or cellophane after applying these treatments. *For children, however, such bandages should not be used.*

For some forms of severe ichthyosis, creams containing vitamin A (tretinoin) are effective. Vitamin A compounds help the skin shed excessive scales. Etretinate, a drug related to vitamin A, is prescribed for some forms of ichthyosis. For epidermolytic hyperkeratosis, antibiotics and a strong disinfecting soap such as chlorhexidine may be used.

Keratosis Pilaris

Keratosis pilaris is a common disorder in which dead cells shed from the upper layer of skin and form plugs that fill the openings of hair follicles.

The plugs cause small, pointed pimples to break out, most commonly on the upper arms, thighs, and buttocks. The face may break out as well, particularly in children. People with keratosis pilaris are more likely to break out in cold weather, but the pimples tend to clear up by themselves in the summer.

The cause isn't known, though keratosis pilaris tends to run in families, so heredity probably plays a role. Generally, the pimples cause only cosmetic problems.

Treatment

Keratosis pilaris tends to clear up by itself. Petroleum jelly mixed with either water, cold cream, or salicylic acid may help flatten the bumps. Stronger salicylic acid preparations or tretinoin cream can also be used.

Calluses and Corns

A callus is an area on the uppermost layer of skin, the stratum corneum or keratin layer, that becomes abnormally thick and forms a protective pad in response to repeated rubbing.

Calluses can form anywhere on the body but usually develop over a bony spot on the hands, feet, and elbows or on other areas that take repeated wear or abuse, as on a violinist's jaw.

A corn is a pea-sized, thickened area of keratin that occurs on the feet.

Hard corns appear over the joints of the toes; corns between the toes are usually soft. Unlike most calluses, corns can be painful because the thickened skin transfers pressure to the underlying bone.

Diagnosis

Generally, calluses and corns are easy to recognize. Sometimes, corns are confused with plantar warts, which also contain a thickened keratin layer. However, warts are very sensitive when squeezed from the sides, while corns are more sensitive to direct pressure downward or inward against the bone.

Treatment

Corns and calluses are easier to prevent than to treat. Calluses may be avoided by removing the source of irritation or, if this isn't possible, by wearing a glove, pad, or other protective device. Most pharmacies sell protective pads and rings of suitable shapes for this purpose. Most often caused by ill-fitting shoes, corns may go away if better-fitting shoes are worn. Using a keratin-dissolving medication may get rid of corns more quickly. These medications—called keratolytic agents—often contain salicylic acid. They may be applied as a paste that dries on contact, or a pad containing the medication may be placed on the area. However, if keratolytic agents aren't applied carefully, the acid can damage adjacent normal tissue. Corns and calluses can also be thinned with a pumice stone during bathing or shaved with a scalpel by a doctor or nurse.

In a person with diabetes and poor circulation, corns and calluses may heal slowly, especially if they're on the feet. Doctors recommend that people with diabetes take special care of their feet.

Psoriasis

Psoriasis is a chronic, recurring disease recognizable by silvery scaling bumps and various-sized plaques (raised patches).

An abnormally high rate of growth and turnover of skin cells causes the scaling. The reason for the rapid cell growth is unknown, but immune mechanisms are thought to play a role. The condition often runs in families. Psoriasis is common, affecting 2 to 4 percent of whites; blacks are less likely to get the disease. Psoriasis begins most often in people ages 10 to 40, although people in all age groups are susceptible.

Symptoms

Psoriasis usually starts as one or more small psoriatic plaques that become excessively flaky. Small bumps may develop around the area. Although the first plaques may clear up by themselves, others may soon follow. Some plaques may remain thumbnail-sized, but others may grow to cover large areas of the body, sometimes in striking ring-shaped or spiral patterns.

Psoriasis typically involves the scalp, elbows, knees, back, and buttocks. The flaking may be mistaken for severe dandruff, but the patchy nature of psoriasis, with flaking areas interspersed among completely normal ones, distinguishes the disease from dandruff. Psoriasis can also break out around and under the nails, making them thick and deformed. The eyebrows, armpits, navel, and groin may also be affected.

Usually, psoriasis produces only flaking. Even itching is uncommon. When flaking areas heal, the skin takes on a completely normal appearance,

and hair growth is unchanged. Most people with limited psoriasis suffer few problems beyond the flaking, although the skin's appearance may be embarrassing.

Some people, however, have extensive psoriasis or experience serious effects from psoriasis. Psoriatic arthritis produces symptoms very similar to those of rheumatoid arthritis. Very rarely, psoriasis covers the entire body and produces exfoliative psoriatic dermatitis, in which the entire skin becomes inflamed. This form of psoriasis is serious because, like a burn, it keeps the skin from serving as a protective barrier against injury and infection. In another uncommon form of psoriasis, pustular psoriasis, large and small pus-filled pimples (pustules) form on the palms of the hands and soles of the feet. Sometimes, these pustules are scattered on the body.

Psoriasis may flare up for no apparent reason, or a flare-up may result from severe sunburn, skin irritation, antimalaria drugs, lithium, beta-blocker drugs (such as propranolol and metoprolol), or almost any medicated ointment or cream. Streptococcal infections (especially in children), bruises, and scratches can also stimulate the formation of new plaques.

Diagnosis

Psoriasis may be misdiagnosed at first because many other disorders can produce similar plaques and flaking. As psoriasis develops, the characteristic scaling pattern is usually easy for doctors to recognize, so diagnostic tests usually aren't needed. However, to confirm a diagnosis, a doctor may perform a skin biopsy (removal of a skin specimen and examination under a microscope).

Treatment

When a person has only a few small plaques, psoriasis responds quickly to treatment. Using ointments and creams that lubricate the skin (emollients) once or twice a day can keep the skin moist. Ointments containing corticosteroids are effective, and their effectiveness can be enhanced by applying them and then wrapping the area in cellophane. Vitamin D cream is also effective in many patients.

Ointments and creams containing salicylic acid or coal tar are also used to treat psoriasis. Most of these medications are applied twice a day to the affected area. Stronger medications like anthralin are used sometimes, but they can irritate the skin and stain sheets and clothing. When the scalp is affected, shampoos containing these active ingredients are often used.

Ultraviolet light also can help clear up psoriasis. In fact, during summer months, exposed regions of affected skin may clear up spontaneously. Sunbathing often helps to clear up the plaques on larger areas of the body; exposure to ultraviolet light under controlled conditions is another common therapy. For extensive psoriasis, such light therapy may be supplemented by psoralens, drugs that make the skin extra sensitive to the effects of ultraviolet light. The combination of psoralens and ultraviolet light (PUVA) is usually effective and may clear up the skin for several months. However, PUVA treatment can increase the risk of skin cancer from ultraviolet light; therefore, the treatment must be closely supervised by a doctor.

For serious forms of psoriasis and widespread psoriasis, a doctor may give methotrexate. Used to treat some forms of cancer, this drug interferes with the growth and multiplication of skin cells. Doctors use methotrexate for people who don't respond to other forms of therapy. It can be effective in extreme cases but may cause adverse effects on the bone marrow, kidneys, and liver. Another effective medication, cyclosporine, also has serious side effects.

The two most effective medications for treating pustular psoriasis are etretinate and isotretinoin, which are also used to treat severe acne.

Pityriasis Rosea

Pityriasis rosea is a mild disease that causes scaly, rose-colored, inflamed skin.

Pityriasis rosea is possibly caused by an infectious agent, although none has been identified. It can develop at any age but is most common in young adults. It usually appears during spring and autumn.

Symptoms

Pityriasis rosea begins as a rose red or light tan area that doctors call a herald or mother patch. This round or oval area usually develops on the torso. In 5 to 10 days, many similar but smaller patches appear on other parts of the body. These secondary patches are most common on the torso, especially along and radiating from the spine. Most people with pityriasis rosea have few symptoms, and the rash usually isn't very itchy.

However, fatigue, headaches, and occasionally troublesome itching may occur.

Treatment

Usually the rash goes away in 4 to 5 weeks without treatment, although sometimes it lasts for 2 months or more. Both artificial and natural sunlight may clear up pityriasis rosea faster and relieve the itching. A cream containing menthol can relieve the itching. Rarely, oral corticosteroids are prescribed for severe itching.

Lichen Planus

Lichen planus, a recurring itchy disease, starts as a rash of small discrete bumps that then combine and become rough, scaly plaques (raised patches).

About half of those who get lichen planus also develop mouth sores. The cause of lichen planus isn't known. An identical rash sometimes breaks out in people exposed to drugs containing gold, bismuth, arsenic, quinine, quinidine, or quinacrine and to certain chemicals used to develop color photographs. Thus, lichen planus may be the body's response to some external chemical or other agent.

Symptoms

The first episode may begin gradually or suddenly and persist for weeks or months. Although lichen planus usually clears up by itself, patches often come back, and the episodes may recur for years. The rash almost always itches—sometimes severely. The bumps are usually violet and have angular borders; when light is directed at them from the side, the bumps display a distinctive sheen. New bumps may form wherever scratching or a mild skin injury occurs. Sometimes a dark discoloration remains after the rash heals.

Usually, the rash is distributed symmetrically—most commonly in the mouth, on the torso, on the inner surfaces of the wrists, on the legs, on the head of the penis, and in the vagina. The face is seldom affected. On the legs, the rash may become especially large and scaly. The rash sometimes results in patchy baldness on the scalp.

Lichen planus mouth sores are particularly vexing; they are usually bluish-white and may form in a line. Often mouth sores appear before the skin rash, and although mouth sores usually don't hurt, they sometimes cause deeper sores that may be painful. Cycles of outbreaks followed by healing are common. Though unusual, long-standing sores may result in mouth cancer.

Diagnosis

Diagnosis may be difficult because many conditions resemble lichen planus. A dermatologist can usually recognize it by its appearance and pattern of recurrence, but a skin biopsy (removal of a specimen and examination under a microscope) may be needed to confirm the diagnosis.

Treatment

Drugs or chemicals that may be causing lichen planus should be avoided. For people who suffer from itching, an antihistamine such as diphenhydramine, hydroxyzine, or chlorpheniramine may be prescribed, although it may cause sleepiness. Corticosteroids may be injected into the bumps, applied to the skin, or given orally, sometimes with other medications, such as tretinoin. For painful mouth sores, a mouthwash containing lidocaine may be used before meals to form a pain-killing coating.

Lichen planus may disappear and then recur after several years. Prolonged treatment may be needed during outbreaks of the disease; between outbreaks, no treatment is needed.

CHAPTER 194

Dermatitis

Dermatitis (eczema) is an inflammation of the upper layers of the skin, causing blisters, redness, swelling, oozing, scabbing, scaling, and usually itching.

Continuous scratching and rubbing may eventually lead to thickening and hardening of the skin. Some types of dermatitis affect only specific parts of the body.

Contact Dermatitis

Contact dermatitis is inflammation caused by contact with a particular substance; the rash is confined to a specific area and often has clearly defined boundaries.

Substances can cause skin inflammation by one of two mechanisms—irritation (irritant contact dermatitis) or allergic reaction (allergic contact dermatitis). Even very mild soaps, detergents, and certain metals may irritate the skin after frequent contact. Sometimes repeated exposure, even to water, may dry out and irritate the skin. Strong irritants, such as acids, alkalis (such as drain cleaners), and some organic solvents (such as acetone in nail polish remover), may cause skin changes in a few minutes.

With an allergic reaction, the first exposure to a particular substance (or in some cases, the first several exposures) doesn't cause a reaction, but the next exposure may cause itching and derma-

Common Causes of Allergic Contact Dermatitis

Cosmetics: hair-removing chemicals, nail polish, nail polish remover, deodorants, moisturizers, aftershave lotions, perfumes, sunscreens

Metal compound (in jewelry): nickel

Plants: poison ivy, poison oak, poison sumac, ragweed, primrose

Drugs in skin creams: antibiotics (penicillin, sulfonamides, neomycin), antihistamines (diphenhydramine, promethazine), anesthetics (benzocaine), antiseptics (thimerosal), stabilizers

Chemicals used in clothing manufacturing: tanning agents in shoes; rubber accelerators and antioxidants in gloves, shoes, undergarments, other apparel

titis within 4 to 24 hours. People may use (or be exposed to) substances for years without a problem, then suddenly develop an allergic reaction. Even ointments, creams, and lotions used to treat dermatitis can cause such a reaction. About 10 percent of women are allergic to nickel, the most common cause of dermatitis from jewelry. People may also develop dermatitis from any of the materials they touch while at work (occupational dermatitis).

When dermatitis results after a person touches certain substances and then exposes the skin to sunlight, the condition is called photoallergic or phototoxic contact dermatitis. Such substances include sunscreens, aftershave lotions, certain perfumes, antibiotics, coal tar, and oils.

Symptoms

The effects of contact dermatitis range from a mild, short-lived redness to severe swelling and blisters. Often, the rash contains tiny, itching blisters (vesicles). At first, the rash is limited to the contact site, but later it may spread. The rash area may be very small (for example, the earlobes if earrings cause dermatitis), or it may cover a large area of the body (for example, if a body lotion causes dermatitis).

If the substance causing the rash is removed, the redness usually disappears in a few days. Blisters may ooze and form crusts, but they soon dry. Residual scaling, itching, and temporary thickening of the skin may last for days or weeks.

Diagnosis

Determining the cause of contact dermatitis isn't always easy because the possibilities are endless. Also, most people aren't aware of all the substances that touch their skin. Often, the location of the initial rash is an important clue.

If a doctor suspects contact dermatitis but a careful process of elimination doesn't pinpoint the cause, patch testing can be performed. For this test, small patches containing substances that commonly cause dermatitis are placed on the skin for 2 days to see if a rash develops beneath one of them.

Although useful, patch testing is complicated. A doctor must decide which substances to test, how much of each substance to apply, and when the tests should be done. Also, the results of patch testing can be hard to interpret. Tests may be falsely positive or negative. Most people can discover the source of their dermatitis without patch testing by systematically eliminating possible causes. However, patch testing can provide important clues in identifying the cause.

Treatment

Treatment consists of removing or avoiding whatever is causing the contact dermatitis. To prevent infection and avoid irritation, a person should clean the area regularly with water and gentle soap. Blisters should not be cut open. Dry bandages may also help prevent infection.

Corticosteroid creams or ointments usually relieve the symptoms of mild contact dermatitis, unless the person has a lot of blistering, as is common with poison ivy. Corticosteroid tablets (such as prednisone) are sometimes prescribed for severe cases of contact dermatitis. Although antihistamines relieve itching in some situations, they are not particularly helpful in most cases of contact dermatitis.

Chronic Dermatitis of the Hands and Feet

Chronic dermatitis of the hands and feet includes a group of disorders in which the hands and feet are frequently inflamed and irritated.

Chronic dermatitis of the hands results from repetitive tasks and contact with chemicals; chronic dermatitis of the feet results from the warm, moist conditions in socks and shoes. Chronic dermatitis may make the skin of the hands and feet itch or hurt.

Contact dermatitis, one type of chronic dermatitis of the hands, usually results from irritation by chemicals (such as soaps) or by rubber gloves.

Pompholyx, a long-lasting condition that produces itchy blisters on the palms and sides of the fingers, can also appear on the soles of the feet. The blisters are often scaly, red, and oozing. Pompholyx is sometimes called dyshidrosis, which means "abnormal sweating," but the condition has nothing to do with sweating.

Fungal infection is a common cause of an eruption on the feet, especially tiny blisters or deep red rashes. Sometimes, a person who has a chronic fungal infection on the feet develops dermatitis on the hands because of an allergic reaction to the fungus.

Treatment

Treatment of chronic dermatitis depends on the cause. Most often, the best treatment is to remove the chemical that is irritating the skin. Corticosteroid creams can be applied to treat the inflammation. Bacterial infections that may develop in open skin sores are treated with antibiotics. When a fungus is causing the symptoms, an antifungal drug is used.

Atopic Dermatitis

Atopic dermatitis is a chronic, itchy inflammation of the upper layers of the skin that often develops in people who have hay fever or asthma and in people who have family members with these conditions.

People with atopic dermatitis usually have many other allergic disorders. The relationship between the dermatitis and these disorders isn't clear; some people may have an inherited tendency to produce excessive antibodies, such as immunoglobulin E, in response to a number of different stimuli.▲

Many conditions can make atopic dermatitis worse, including emotional stress, changes in temperature or humidity, bacterial skin infections, and contact with irritating clothing (especially wool). In some infants, food allergies may provoke atopic dermatitis.

Symptoms

Atopic dermatitis sometimes appears in the first few months after birth. Infants may develop red, oozing, crusted rashes on the face, scalp, diaper area, hands, arms, feet, or legs. Often, the dermatitis clears up by age 3 or 4, although it commonly recurs. In older children and adults, the rash often occurs (and recurs) in only one or a few spots, especially on the upper arms, in front of the elbows, or behind the knees.

Although the color, intensity, and location of the rash vary, the rash always itches. The itching often leads to uncontrollable scratching, triggering a cycle of itching-scratching-rash-itching that makes the problem worse. Scratching and rubbing can also tear the skin, leaving an opening for bacteria to enter and cause infections.

For unknown reasons, people with long-term atopic dermatitis sometimes develop cataracts while in their 20s or 30s. In people with atopic dermatitis, herpes simplex, which usually affects a small area and is mild, may produce a serious illness with eczema and high fever (eczema herpeticum).

Diagnosis

Several visits to a doctor may be needed to establish the diagnosis. No test for atopic dermatitis exists. A doctor makes the diagnosis based on the typical pattern of the rash and often on whether other family members have allergies. Though atopic dermatitis may closely resemble seborrheic dermatitis in infants, doctors try to distinguish between them because their complications and treatments are different.

Treatment

No cure exists, but certain measures can help. Avoiding contact with substances known to irritate the skin can prevent a rash.

Corticosteroid creams or ointments can relieve a rash and control itching. However, powerful corticosteroid creams applied over large areas or for a long time can cause serious medical problems, especially in infants, because these drugs are absorbed into the bloodstream. If a corticosteroid cream or ointment appears to be losing its effectiveness, it may be replaced with petroleum jelly for a week or more at a time. Applying petroleum jelly or vegetable oil to the skin can help keep it soft and lubricated. When the corticosteroid is restarted after a brief break, it is more likely to be effective.

Some people with atopic dermatitis find that bathing worsens their rash; soap and water and even drying the skin, especially rubbing with a towel, may be irritating. For these people, bathing less often, lightly blotting the skin with a towel, and applying oils or unscented lubricants like moisturizing skin creams to the moist skin are helpful.

An antihistamine (diphenhydramine, hydroxyzine) can sometimes control the itching, partly by acting as a sedative. Because these drugs may cause sleepiness, they're most useful at bedtime.

Keeping fingernails short may help reduce skin damage from scratching and decrease the chance of infection. Learning to recognize the signs of atopic dermatitis skin infection (increased redness, swelling, red streaks, and fever) and seeking medical help as soon as possible are important. Such infections are treated with oral antibiotics.

Because corticosteroid tablets and capsules can produce serious side effects, doctors use them only as a last resort for people with stubborn cases. These oral drugs can stunt growth, weaken bones, suppress the adrenal glands, and

---

▲ see page 811

cause many other problems, especially in children. Also, their helpful effects are only short-lived.

For unknown reasons, ultraviolet light treatments plus oral doses of psoralen, a drug that intensifies the effects of ultraviolet light on the skin, may help adults. This treatment is rarely recommended for children because of its potential long-term side effects, including skin cancer and cataracts.

Seborrheic Dermatitis

Seborrheic dermatitis is an inflammation of the upper layers of the skin, causing scales on the scalp, face, and occasionally on other areas.

Seborrheic dermatitis often runs in families, and cold weather usually makes it worse.

Symptoms

Seborrheic dermatitis usually begins gradually, causing dry or greasy scaling of the scalp (dandruff), sometimes with itching but without hair loss. In more severe cases, yellowish to reddish scaly pimples appear along the hairline, behind the ears, in the ear canal, on the eyebrows, on the bridge of the nose, around the nose, and on the chest. In newborns less than one month old, seborrheic dermatitis may produce a thick, yellow, crusted scalp rash (cradle cap) and sometimes yellow scaling behind the ears and red pimples on the face. Frequently, a stubborn diaper rash accompanies the scalp rash. Older children may develop a thick, tenacious, scaly rash with large flakes of skin.

Treatment

In **adults,** the scalp can be treated with shampoos containing pyrithione zinc, selenium sulfide, salicylic acid and sulfur, or tar. The person usually uses these shampoos every other day until the dandruff is controlled and then twice weekly. Often, treatment must be continued for many months; if the dermatitis returns after the treatment is stopped, it can be restarted. Lotions that contain corticosteroids are also used on the head and other affected areas. On the face, only weak corticosteroid lotions, such as 1 percent hydrocortisone, should be used. Even weak corticosteroids must be used cautiously because long-term use can thin the skin and cause other problems. If corticosteroid therapy doesn't eliminate the rash, ketoconazole cream is sometimes used.

In **young children** who have a thick scaly rash on the scalp, salicylic acid in mineral oil may be rubbed gently into the rash with a soft toothbrush at bedtime. The scalp is also shampooed daily until the thick scale is gone.

In **infants,** the scalp is washed with mild baby shampoo, and hydrocortisone cream is rubbed into the scalp.

Nummular Dermatitis

Nummular dermatitis is a persistent, usually itchy rash and inflammation characterized by coin-shaped spots with tiny blisters, scabs, and scales.

The cause isn't known. Nummular dermatitis usually affects middle-aged people, occurs along with dry skin, and is most common in winter. However, the rash may come and go without any apparent reason.

The round spots start as itchy patches of pimples and blisters that later ooze and form crusts. The rash may be widespread. Often, spots are more obvious on the backs of the arms or legs and on the buttocks, but they also appear on the torso.

Many different treatments have been used, but none is effective in everyone. Treatments include oral antibiotics, corticosteroid creams and injections, other drugs, and ultraviolet light therapy.

Generalized Exfoliative Dermatitis

Generalized exfoliative dermatitis is a severe inflammation that affects the entire skin surface and leads to extreme redness and scaling.

Certain drugs (especially penicillins, sulfonamides, isoniazid, phenytoin, and barbiturates) may cause this condition. In some cases, it's a complication of other skin diseases, such as atopic dermatitis, psoriasis, and contact dermatitis. Certain lymphomas (cancers of the lymph nodes) may also cause generalized exfoliative dermatitis. In many cases, no cause can be found.

Symptoms

Exfoliative dermatitis may start rapidly or slowly. The entire skin surface becomes red, scaly, thickened, and sometimes crusted. Some people have itching and swollen lymph nodes. Although many people have a fever, they may feel cold because so much heat is lost through the damaged skin. Large amounts of fluid and protein may seep out, and the damaged skin is a poor barrier against infection.

Treatment

Early diagnosis and treatment are important to prevent infection and fluid and protein loss from becoming life threatening.

Any drug or chemical that could be causing the dermatitis should be eliminated. If lymphoma is causing the dermatitis, treating the lymphoma helps clear up the dermatitis. People with severe exfoliative dermatitis often need to be hospitalized and given antibiotics (for infection), intravenous fluids (to replace the fluids lost through the skin), and nutritional supplements. Care may include medications and heated blankets to control body temperature. Cool baths followed by applications of petroleum jelly and gauze may help protect the skin. Corticosteroids (such as prednisone) given orally or intravenously are used only when other measures are unsuccessful or the disease worsens.

Stasis Dermatitis

Stasis dermatitis is a chronic redness, scaling, warmth, and swelling (inflammation) on the lower legs, often culminating in dark brown skin.

Stasis dermatitis results from pooling of blood and fluid under the skin, so it tends to occur in people who have varicose veins and swelling (edema).

Symptoms

Stasis dermatitis usually occurs on the ankles. At first, the skin becomes reddened and mildly scaly. Over several weeks or months, the skin turns dark brown. The underlying pooling of blood often is ignored for long periods, during which the swelling increases as does the possibility of infection and eventual severe skin damage (ulceration).

Treatment

Long-term treatment is aimed at reducing the chances of blood pooling in the veins around the ankles. Keeping the legs above the level of the heart stops blood from pooling in the veins and fluid from accumulating in the skin. Properly fitted support hose can help prevent serious skin damage by preventing fluid accumulation in the lower legs. Additional treatment usually isn't necessary.

For dermatitis of recent onset, soothing compresses, such as gauze pads soaked in tap water, may make the skin feel better and can help prevent infection by keeping the skin clean. If the condition worsens—increased warmth, redness, small ulcers, or pus—a more absorbent dressing can be used. Corticosteroid creams are also helpful and are often combined with zinc oxide paste and applied in a thin layer.

When a person has large or extensive ulcers, more substantial dressings are needed. Zinc oxide paste has been used traditionally, but newer types of bandages with built-in absorbing materials are more effective. Antibiotics are used only when the skin is already infected. Sometimes, skin from elsewhere on the body may be grafted to cover very large ulcers.

Some people may need an Unna's boot, a cast-like device filled with a gelatin paste that contains zinc. The boot helps protect the skin from irritation, and the paste helps heal the skin. If the boot is uncomfortable or unmanageable, the same type of paste can be used under bandages held by elastic supports.

In stasis dermatitis, the skin is easily irritated; antibiotic creams, first-aid (anesthetic) creams, alcohol, witch hazel, lanolin, or other chemicals should not be used because they can make the condition worse.

Localized Scratch Dermatitis

Localized scratch dermatitis (lichen simplex chronicus, neurodermatitis) is a chronic, itchy inflammation of the top layer of the skin. It causes dryness, scaling, and dark, thickened patches that have oval, irregular, or angular shapes.

The cause is unknown, but psychologic factors may play a role. The condition doesn't seem to be allergic. More women than men have localized scratch dermatitis, and it's common among Asians and Native Americans. It usually develops between ages 20 and 50.

Symptoms and Diagnosis

Localized scratch dermatitis can occur anywhere on the body, including the anus (pruritus ani) and the vagina (pruritus vulvae). In the early stages the skin looks normal, but it itches. Later, dryness, scaling, and dark patches develop as a result of the scratching and rubbing.

Doctors try to discover the possible psychologic stress or underlying allergies or diseases that may be causing the initial itching. When the condition occurs around the anus or vagina, the doctor may investigate the possibility of pinworms, trichomoniasis, hemorrhoids, local discharges, fungal infections, warts, contact dermatitis, or psoriasis as the cause.

Treatment

For the condition to clear up, the person must stop the scratching and rubbing that's irritating the skin. To help control the itching, doctors prescribe antihistamines to be taken by mouth and corticosteroid creams to be rubbed gently on the affected area. Surgical tape saturated with a corticosteroid provides a therapeutic drug and prevents the person from scratching. The doctor may inject longer-acting corticosteroids under the skin to control the itching. Other medications to control itching, such as hydroxyzine or doxepin, may also help some people.

When this condition develops around the anus or vagina, the best treatment is corticosteroid cream. Zinc oxide paste may be applied over the cream to protect the area; the paste can be removed with mineral oil. Hard rubbing with toilet paper after a bowel movement can aggravate the condition.

CHAPTER 195

Skin Inflammation

The skin can break out in a variety of rashes, sores, and blisters (skin eruptions). Sometimes the skin quickly returns to normal, but some skin eruptions are long lasting and even life threatening. Many times the cause is never discovered. Commonly, drugs taken internally cause various skin reactions.

Drug Rashes

Drug rashes are side effects of medications.▲

Drugs cause rashes in several ways. Most drug rashes are allergic reactions to medications. After taking the first (or any subsequent) dose of a particular drug, a person may become sensitized to the drug. Later exposure to the drug may trigger an allergic reaction. Usually within minutes, though sometimes hours or days later, the skin breaks out in a rash. Other allergic symptoms—including a runny nose, watery eyes, or an asthma attack—may occur along with the rash.

Drugs also produce rashes directly without involving an allergic reaction. For example, corticosteroids (cortisone-like drugs) may produce acne and cause skin to become thin, and anticoagulants (blood thinners) may cause bruising when blood leaks under the skin.

Certain drugs make the skin particularly sensitive to the effects of sunlight (photosensitivity). These drugs include certain antipsychotic medications, tetracycline, antibiotics that contain sulfa, chlorothiazide, and some artificial sweeteners. No rash appears when the drug is taken, but later exposure to the sun produces an area of red, sometimes itchy, skin or gray-blue discoloration.

Drugs can cause almost any type of rash, but among the most important rashes that may result from drugs are hives (urticaria),■ toxic epidermal necrolysis, erythema multiforme, Stevens-Johnson syndrome, and erythema nodosum.

Symptoms

Drug rashes vary in severity from mild redness with pimples over a small area to peeling of the entire skin. Rashes may appear suddenly after a person takes a drug (for example, hives may erupt after taking penicillin), or they may be delayed for hours or days. Rarely, drug rashes show up years later; for example, arsenic may cause the skin to flake, change color, and even become cancerous years after ingestion.

▲ see page 42

■ see page 829

Common Rashes That Can Be Caused by Drugs

Rash	Description	Examples of Drugs That Can Cause the Rash
Fixed drug eruption	A dark red or purple rash that re-appears at the same spot each time a particular drug is taken. The rash most often appears in the mouth or on the genitals.	Usually antibiotics (tetracyclines and antibiotics containing sulfa), phenol-phthalein (which is used in some laxatives)
Purpuric eruptions	Purple blotches on the skin. The blotches most often appear on the legs.	Diuretics, some anticoagulants
Acne	An eruption of pimples and red blotches scattered mainly over the face, shoulders, and upper chest.	Corticosteroids, iodides, bromides, phenytoin, anabolic steroids
Hives (urticaria)	Raised, firm red and white bumps that signify an allergic reaction.	Penicillin, aspirin, certain dyes used in drug manufacturing
Morbilliform or maculopapu-lar rash	Flat, red, ill-defined rash, sometimes also with bumps or pimples; resem-bles measles.	Almost any drug, but especially barbiturates, ampicillin, sulfa drugs, other antibiotics
Stevens-Johnson syndrome or less severe rashes affect-ing the mucous membranes	Small blisters or a hive-like rash on the lining of the mouth or the vagina or on the tip of the penis.	Penicillins, antibiotics containing sulfa, barbiturates, some drugs for high blood pressure and diabetes
Exfoliative dermatitis	Thickened, red, and scaly skin over the entire body.	Penicillins, antibiotics containing sulfa

Diagnosis

Rashes have many possible causes, and cur-rently no laboratory tests confirm that a rash re-sults from a drug. Figuring out whether a drug is responsible may be difficult because a rash can result from only a minute amount of a drug, it can erupt long after a person has taken a drug, and it can persist for weeks or months after a person has stopped taking a drug. Every drug a person has taken is suspect, including those bought with-out a prescription; even eyedrops, nose drops, and suppositories are possible causes. Some-times the only way to determine which drug is causing a rash is to have the person stop taking all but life-sustaining drugs. Whenever possible, chemically unrelated drugs are substituted. If there are no such substitutes, the person starts taking the drugs again one at a time to see which one causes the reaction. However, this method

can be hazardous if the person had a severe aller-gic reaction to the drug.

Treatment

Most drug reactions disappear when the re-sponsible drug is stopped. When the skin rash is dry or itchy, a corticosteroid ointment may help relieve symptoms. Although most cases of hives clear up quickly without treatment, oral antihis-tamines or oral corticosteroids may be needed; very serious eruptions are treated with an injec-tion of epinephrine or a corticosteroid.

Toxic Epidermal Necrolysis

Toxic epidermal necrolysis is a life-threatening skin disease in which the top layer of the skin peels off in sheets.

A third of the cases are caused by a reaction to a drug, most often penicillin, antibiotics containing sulfa, barbiturates, anticonvulsants, nonsteroidal anti-inflammatory drugs, or allopurinol. In another third of the cases, toxic epidermal necrolysis appears along with some other serious disease, complicating the diagnosis. In the remaining third of the cases, no cause can be found. The condition is uncommon in children.

Symptoms

Toxic epidermal necrolysis typically begins with a painful red area that quickly spreads. Blisters may develop, or the top layer of skin may simply peel off without blistering. Often, just a gentle touch or pull peels off large sheets of skin. This makes the affected area look as if it's been scalded. (A similar-looking condition, staphylococcal scalded skin syndrome, results from a staphylococcal infection in infants, young children, and adults whose immune systems are abnormal.) As toxic epidermal necrolysis progresses, the person usually experiences discomfort, chills, and fever. Within 3 days, enormous areas of skin may peel off, and the condition often spreads to the mucous membranes of the eyes, mouth, and genitals.

As with severe burns, the skin loss is life threatening. Huge amounts of fluids and salts can seep from the large, raw, damaged areas. A person who has this condition is very susceptible to infection at the sites of damaged, exposed tissues; such infections are the most common cause of death in those with this condition.

Treatment

People with toxic epidermal necrolysis are hospitalized and immediately taken off drugs suspected of causing the condition. When possible, these people are treated in the burn unit and given scrupulous care to avoid infection. Hospital personnel wash their hands before touching the patient, keep the patient isolated from other hospital patients, and cover the patient's skin with protective bandages. Fluids and salts, which are lost through the damaged skin, are replaced intravenously. Using corticosteroids to treat the condition is controversial: Some doctors believe that giving large doses within the first few days is beneficial; others believe that corticosteroids should not be used. These drugs suppress the immune system, which increases the potential for serious infection. If an infection develops, doctors give antibiotics immediately.

Erythema Multiforme

Erythema multiforme is a disorder characterized by patches of red, raised skin that often look like targets and usually are distributed symmetrically over the body.

Probably more than half the cases are caused by herpes simplex. This viral infection may be obvious before the erythema multiforme appears. In the rest of the cases, possible causes include virtually any drug (most often penicillins, antibiotics containing sulfa, and barbiturates) and other infectious diseases (for example, coxsackievirus or echovirus infection, mycoplasmal pneumonia, psittacosis, and histoplasmosis). Rarely, certain vaccines cause erythema multiforme. Doctors are unsure how herpes simplex and certain drugs cause this condition, but a type of allergic reaction is suspected.

Symptoms

Usually, erythema multiforme appears suddenly, with reddened patches and blisters erupting most often on the palms of the hands or soles of the feet and on the face. Blisters on the lips and on the lining of the mouth can ooze blood. Erythema multiforme produces flat, round, red marks distributed equally on both sides of the body; these red areas may develop dark concentric rings with purple-gray centers (target or iris lesions). The reddened areas sometimes itch. A person with erythema multiforme may have cold sores (or have had them before), feel tired, and have pain in the joints and a fever. Attacks of erythema multiforme may last 2 to 4 weeks and may recur in the fall and spring for several years.

Stevens-Johnson syndrome—in which blisters break out on the lining of the mouth, throat, anus, genital region, and eyes—is a very severe form of erythema multiforme. Reddened areas may develop on the rest of the skin. The damage to the lining of the mouth makes eating difficult, and closing the mouth may be painful, so the person may drool. The eyes may become very painful, swell, and become so filled with pus that they seal shut. The corneas can become scarred. The opening through which urine passes may also be affected, making urination difficult and painful.

Treatment

Erythema multiforme usually heals on its own, but Stevens-Johnson syndrome can be fatal. Doctors try to treat any infectious cause or eliminate any drugs that are suspected causes. When the cause of erythema multiforme is thought to be herpes simplex, oral acyclovir is usually given.

Blisters or sores on the skin usually are covered with tap water compresses. Oral corticosteroids may be used in severe or persistent, recurring cases, but their use is controversial.

At the slightest indication of infection, antibiotics are prescribed. When erythema multiforme makes eating or drinking impossible, nutrition and fluids are given intravenously.

Erythema Nodosum

Erythema nodosum is an inflammatory disorder that produces tender red bumps (nodules) under the skin, most often over the shins but occasionally on the arms and other areas.

Quite often, erythema nodosum isn't a separate disease but a sign of some other disease or of sensitivity to a drug. Young adults are most prone to the condition, which may recur for months or years. In children, erythema nodosum most commonly follows a cold or sore throat, especially one caused by streptococci. In adults, streptococcal infection and sarcoidosis are the most common causes. Other causes include leprosy, coccidioidomycosis, histoplasmosis, tuberculosis, psittacosis, lymphogranuloma venereum, and ulcerative colitis. This disorder can also be a reaction to drugs—especially antibiotics containing sulfa, iodides, bromides, and oral contraceptives.

Symptoms and Diagnosis

Usually appearing on the shins, erythema nodosum nodules resemble raised bruises that gradually change from pink to bluish-brown. Fever and joint pain are common; lymph nodes in the chest occasionally become enlarged.

The painful nodules are usually the telltale sign for the doctor. Biopsy of a nodule (removal of a specimen and examination under a microscope) can help in making a diagnosis. There's no specific laboratory test for identifying the underlying cause.

Treatment

Drugs that might be causing erythema nodosum are stopped, and any underlying infections are treated. If the disorder is caused by a streptococcal infection, a person may have to take antibiotics for a year or more.

Bed rest may help relieve the pain caused by the nodules. If no infection or drug cause can be found, the doctor may recommend aspirin, which can be very effective. Individual nodules may be treated by injecting them with a corticosteroid; when a person has many nodules, corticosteroid tablets sometimes are prescribed.

Granuloma Annulare

Granuloma annulare is a chronic skin condition of unknown cause in which small, firm, raised bumps (nodules) form a ring with normal or slightly sunken skin in the center.

The nodules are either yellowish or the color of the surrounding skin; a person may have one ring or several. The nodules usually cause no pain or itching; they most often form on the feet, legs, hands, or fingers of children and adults. In a small percentage of people with this condition, clusters of granuloma annulare nodules erupt when the skin is exposed to the sun.

Most often, granuloma annulare heals without any treatment. Corticosteroid creams under waterproof bandages, corticosteroid-containing tape, or injected corticosteroids may help clear up the rash.

CHAPTER 196

Blistering Diseases

Many diseases and injuries can cause blistering, but three autoimmune diseases—pemphigus, bullous pemphigoid, and dermatitis herpetiformis—are among the most serious. In an autoimmune disease, the immune system, which normally attacks foreign invaders of the body—such as infectious agents—is wrongly activated against a normal component of the body—in this case, a component of skin.

Pemphigus

Pemphigus is an uncommon, sometimes fatal, disease in which blisters (bullae) of varying sizes break out on the skin, the lining of the mouth, the vagina, the thin covering of the penis, and other mucous membranes.

Pemphigus develops most often in middle-aged or elderly people. It rarely develops in children. The disease is caused by an autoimmune attack against the structures on epidermal cell surfaces that maintain cell-to-cell contact and tissue texture.

Symptoms

The hallmarks of pemphigus are clear, usually soft, fluid-filled blisters of various sizes; in some forms of pemphigus, scaling patches appear. Slight pinching or rubbing may easily detach the surface of the skin from the lower layers.

The blisters often first appear in the mouth and soon rupture, forming painful ulcers. More blistering and ulceration may follow until the entire lining of the mouth is affected. A similar pattern holds for the skin: Blisters first form on apparently normal skin, then rupture, leaving raw, crusted wounds. Blisters may be widespread, and once ruptured, they may become infected.

Diagnosis and Treatment

Routine microscopic examination and immune testing of a skin specimen for antibody deposits provide a doctor with a definitive diagnosis of this disease.

The first goal of treatment is to stop new blisters from forming. Partial suppression of the immune system with a corticosteroid drug like prednisone taken orally is likely to achieve this goal, but at the cost of making the body more susceptible to infections. Usually for the first 7 to 10 days, the corticosteroid drug is given at a high dose; then the dose is slowly reduced. To keep the disease in check, a person may need to take the drug for several months or even years.

Other drugs that suppress the immune system—such as methotrexate, cyclophosphamide,

azathioprine, and gold salts—may also be prescribed, so that the dose of the corticosteroid drug can be lowered. These powerful drugs have their own side effects, however. Immunosuppressant drugs may also be used along with plasmapheresis, a process in which antibodies are filtered from the blood.

The raw skin surfaces require extraordinary care, similar to the care given to burn patients. Antibiotics and other drugs may be needed to treat infections in ruptured blisters. Dressings impregnated with petroleum jelly or other types of dressings can protect raw, oozing areas.

Bullous Pemphigoid

Bullous pemphigoid is an autoimmune disease that causes blistering.

Although not as dangerous as pemphigus, bullous pemphigoid may persist for a long time. This disease tends to afflict older people.

The blisters are hard and tight, and the skin between blisters is red and may be swollen. Unlike with pemphigus, blisters usually don't form in the mouth. Bullous pemphigoid usually itches; early on, itching and hive-like areas may be the only symptoms.

Diagnosis and Treatment

Routine microscopic examination and immune testing of a skin specimen for antibody deposits provide a doctor with a definitive diagnosis of this disease.

Usually, a corticosteroid drug taken orally is used to suppress the immune system and control the disease. Initially, a high dose is given; over several weeks, the dose is tapered.

Dermatitis Herpetiformis

Dermatitis herpetiformis is an autoimmune disease in which clusters of intensely itchy, small blisters and hive-like swellings break out and persist.

The disease mainly affects adults between 15 and 60; it rarely affects blacks or Asians. In people with the disease, glutens (proteins) in wheat, rye, barley, and oat products activate the immune system, which attacks parts of the skin and somehow causes the rash and itching. People who suffer from dermatitis herpetiformis almost invariably have signs of intestinal disease (celiac disease).▲ These people also have a tendency to develop thyroid disease.

▲ see page 536

Small blisters usually develop gradually, mostly on the elbows, knees, buttocks, lower back, and the back of the head. Sometimes they break out on the face and neck. Itching and burning are likely to be severe.

Diagnosis and Treatment

The diagnosis is based on an examination of fresh skin specimens to locate antibodies in the skin structures.

Treatment may not be needed if a person adheres strictly to a diet free of wheat, rye, barley, and oats. Anti-inflammatory drugs, such as ibuprofen, may cause the rash to worsen. The drug dapsone almost always provides relief in 1 to 2 days. Dapsone has many potential side effects, particularly on blood cells, and usually causes anemia. Dermatologists monitor the blood cell levels of people taking this drug. In most patients, the disease lasts a long time, so they need to take dapsone for many years.

CHAPTER 197

Bedsores

Bedsores (pressure sores, skin ulcers) are skin damage resulting from a lack of blood flow and from irritation to the skin over a bony projection where the skin has been under pressure from a bed, wheelchair, cast, splint, or other hard object for a prolonged period.

Causes

Skin has a rich blood supply that delivers oxygen to all its layers. If that blood supply is cut off for more than 2 or 3 hours, the skin will die, beginning at its outer layer (the epidermis). A common cause of reduced blood flow to the skin is pressure. Normal movement shifts pressure, so that the blood supply isn't stopped for any prolonged period. A layer of fat under the skin, especially over the bony projections, helps pad the skin and keeps the blood vessels from being squeezed shut.

People who cannot move are most at risk for developing bedsores. This group includes people who are paralyzed, very weak, or restrained. Also at risk are people unable to sense discomfort or pain, signals that normally motivate people to move. Nerve damage—from injury, stroke, diabetes, or other causes—diminishes the ability to feel pain. Coma also may diminish the ability to feel pain. Malnourished people don't have the protective fat layer, and their skin doesn't heal well because it lacks essential nutrients. These people also are at increased risk of developing bedsores.

When pressure cuts off blood flow, the skin area

Common Sites for Bedsores

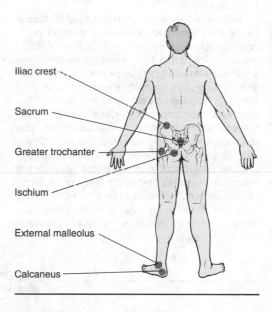

Iliac crest

Sacrum

Greater trochanter

Ischium

External malleolus

Calcaneus

starved for oxygen first becomes red and inflamed, then sore. Even when the blood flow is only partially interrupted, friction and other kinds of damage to the outer skin layer can cause ulcers. Ill-fitting clothing, wrinkled bedding, or shoes rubbing against the skin may contribute to skin injury. Prolonged exposure to moisture—often perspiration, urine, or feces—can damage the skin surface, making bedsores more likely.

Symptoms

In most people, bedsores cause some pain and itching; in people whose senses are dulled, even severe, deep sores may be painless.

Bedsores are categorized by stage. In stage 1, a sore hasn't actually formed; the unbroken skin is simply red. In stage 2, the skin is red and swollen—often with blisters—and the topmost skin layers begin to die. At stage 3, the sore has broken through the skin, exposing deeper levels of skin. By stage 4, the sore extends deeply through the skin and fat and into the muscle. In stage 5, the muscle itself is destroyed. In stage 6, the deepest stage of a bedsore, the bone is exposed, damaged, and sometimes infected.

Once the skin is broken, infection becomes a problem. Infection delays healing of shallow sores and can be life threatening in deeper sores.

Prevention

Established bedsores are painful and life threatening. They lengthen the time spent in hospitals or nursing homes and increase the cost of care.

Prevention is the top priority, and deep bedsores can almost always be prevented with intensive nursing care. Preventing sores often involves the participation of attendants and family members in addition to nurses. Careful daily inspection of a bedridden person's skin can detect early redness. *Any sign of redness is a signal that immediate action is needed to prevent skin breakdown.*

Bony projections can be protected with soft materials, such as cotton or fluffy wool. Beds, chairs, and wheelchairs can be padded to reduce pressure. People who can't move themselves should be repositioned frequently; the usual recommendation is to turn them every 2 hours and keep their skin clean and dry. People who have to spend a lot of time in bed can use special mattresses (water or air-filled mattresses). For people who already have bedsores on several body sites, air-filled mattresses or sponge rubber "egg-crate" mattresses can shift pressure and offer extra relief. An air-suspension mattress may be needed for people with many deep bedsores.

Treatment

Treating a bedsore is much more difficult than preventing one. Fortunately, in the early stages, bedsores usually heal by themselves once pressure is removed. Improving general health by taking protein and calorie supplements may help speed healing.

When the skin is broken, protecting it with a gauze covering can help it to heal. Teflon-coated or petroleum jelly-impregnated gauze has the advantage of not sticking to the healing wound. For deeper sores, special dressings that contain a gelatin-like material can help new skin grow. If the sore appears infected or oozes, rinsing, washing gently with soap, or using disinfectants such as povidone-iodine can remove the dead and infected material. However, cleansing too harshly slows healing. Sometimes a doctor needs to remove (debride) the dead material with a scalpel. Chemical agents can be used instead, but they are generally less thorough than a scalpel.

Deep bedsores are difficult to treat. Sometimes they require transplanting healthy skin to the damaged area. Unfortunately, this type of surgery is not always possible, especially for frail older people who are malnourished. Often when infections develop deep within a sore, antibiotics are given. When bones beneath a sore become infected, the bone infection (osteomyelitis) is extremely difficult to cure and may spread through the bloodstream, requiring many weeks of treatment with an antibiotic.

CHAPTER 198

Sweating Disorders

Sweat is made by sweat glands in the skin and carried to the skin's surface by ducts. Sweating helps keep the body cool. Thus, people sweat more when it's warm. They also sweat when they're nervous or under stress.

Sweat is mostly water, but it also contains salt

(sodium chloride) and other chemicals. When a person sweats a lot, the lost salt and water must be replaced.

Prickly Heat

Prickly heat is an itchy skin rash caused by trapped sweat.

When the narrow ducts carrying sweat to the skin surface get clogged, the trapped sweat causes inflammation, which produces irritation (prickling) and itching. Prickly heat usually consists of a rash of very tiny blisters but also can appear as large, reddened areas of skin.

Prickly heat is most common in warm, humid climates, but people who wear too much clothing in cold weather also can develop the condition. The most common areas for prickly heat are the trunk and thighs.

Reducing sweating usually controls the problem. Keeping the skin cool and dry and avoiding conditions that increase sweating are important; air conditioning is ideal. Often, lotions are used that contain corticosteroids, sometimes with a bit of menthol added; however, these topical treatments are not as effective as modifying the environment and dressing appropriately.

Excessive Sweating

Excessive sweating (hyperhidrosis) may affect the entire surface of the skin, but often it's limited to the palms, soles, armpits, or groin. The affected area is often pink or bluish white, and in severe cases the skin may be cracked, scaly, and soft, especially on the feet. Sometimes the affected area gives off a foul odor (bromhidrosis), which is caused by bacteria and yeasts that break down the sweat and the wet skin.

Clammy hands and feet are a normal response to anxiety, and heavy sweating is normal when a person has a fever. However, frequent heavy sweating all over the body warrants medical attention because it can be a sign of an overactive thyroid, a low blood sugar level, or an abnormality in the part of the nervous system that controls sweating. Blood tests can determine if thyroid function or blood sugar is abnormal.

Treatment

Heavy sweating of the palms, soles, or armpits can be controlled to some degree with a nighttime application of aluminum chloride solution. A per-

What Causes Prickly Heat?

Prickly heat results when sweat glands are blocked and ruptured, and sweat is trapped below the skin.

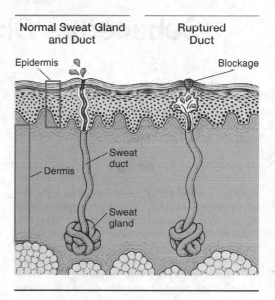

Normal Sweat Gland and Duct

Ruptured Duct

Epidermis

Blockage

Dermis

Sweat duct

Sweat gland

son first dries the sweaty area, then covers it with the solution, and then covers it with a thin plastic film. In the morning, the person removes the film and washes the area. Some people need two applications daily; this regimen usually gives relief in a week. If the solution irritates the skin, the plastic film should be left off.

A solution of methenamine also may help control heavy sweating. Tap water iontophoresis, a process in which a weak electric current is applied to the sweaty area, is sometimes used. If medications aren't effective, a more drastic measure for severe sweating is surgical removal of the sweat glands in the armpits. Psychologic counseling or antianxiety medication may relieve sweating caused by anxiety.

To control odor, a person needs to keep the affected area scrupulously clean; doing so eliminates the microbes that cause odor. A daily bath with a liquid soap containing chlorhexidine or another antiseptic and an application of an aluminum chlorhydroxy preparation (found in most commercial antiperspirants) are effective in stopping odor; shaving the hair in the armpits helps some people. Some people may need to use antibacterial creams or lotions that include antibiotics (such as clindamycin or erythromycin) to eliminate the odor.

CHAPTER 199

Sebaceous Gland Disorders

The sebaceous glands, which secrete oil onto the skin, lie in the dermis, the skin layer just below the surface layer (epidermis). Sebaceous gland disorders include acne, rosacea, perioral dermatitis, and sebaceous cysts.

Acne

Acne is a common skin condition in which the skin pores become clogged, leading to pimples and inflamed, infected abscesses (collections of pus).

Acne tends to develop in teenagers because of an interaction among hormones, skin oils, and bacteria that live on and in the skin and in the hair. During puberty, the sebaceous glands in the skin become more active and produce excessive oil (sebum). Often, dried sebum, flaked skin, and bacteria collect in skin pores, forming a comedo, which blocks sebum from flowing from the hair follicles up through the pores. If the blockage is incomplete, a blackhead appears; if the blockage is complete, a whitehead appears. Bacteria grow in the plugged pores and break down some of the fats in the sebum, further irritating the skin. The irritated blackheads and whiteheads produce the skin eruptions that are commonly known as acne pimples. If the infection and irritation in the pimple get worse, an abscess may form.

When a person has comedones, pimples, and pustules (pus-filled blisters) without abscesses, the condition is called superficial acne; when inflamed pimples project down into the underlying skin and pus-filled cysts appear that may rupture and develop into larger abscesses, the condition is called deep acne.

Symptoms

Acne is often worse in the winter and better in the summer, probably because of the beneficial effects of the sun. Diet has little or no effect on acne, though some people think they're sensitive to certain foods. Eliminating these foods for several weeks and then adding them back into the diet may help determine if the foods really affect the acne. Acne may also appear with each menstrual period in young women and may clear up or substantially worsen during pregnancy. Teenagers who use anabolic steroids are likely to make their acne worse. Certain cosmetics may aggravate acne by clogging the pores.

In deep acne, the infection can spread, producing larger red, raised inflamed areas, pus-filled cysts, and abscesses—all of which may rupture and leave scars. Superficial acne usually doesn't leave scars. Squeezing pimples or trying to open them in other ways can make superficial acne worse by increasing infection, inflammation, and scarring.

Treatment

Washing affected areas several times a day has little effect except to improve the appearance of an oily face. Any good soap may be used. Antibacterial soaps provide no added benefit, and abrasive soaps may enhance drying but may also irritate the skin. Hot water compresses help soften comedones, making them easier to remove. A doctor can show either the person with acne or a family member how to remove comedones carefully once or twice a week, preferably with a sterile needle or a Schamberg loop extractor. A pimple should be opened with a sterile needle only after a pustule has formed. Other treatments depend on the severity of the acne.

Superficial Acne

To clear up pimples, a person can apply the antibiotic clindamycin or erythromycin to the skin with or without an irritant such as tretinoin (retinoic acid). Other antibiotics taken orally,

Comparing Superficial Acne and Deep Acne

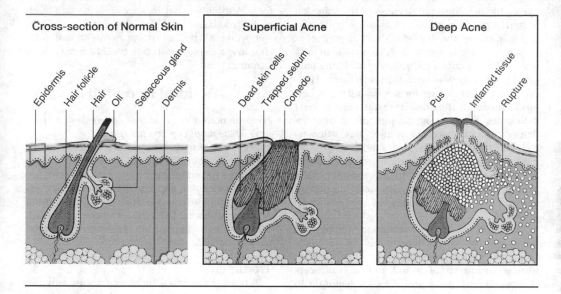

Cross-section of Normal Skin	Superficial Acne	Deep Acne
Epidermis, Hair follicle, Hair, Oil, Sebaceous gland, Dermis	Dead skin cells, Trapped sebum, Comedo	Pus, Inflamed tissue, Rupture

such as tetracycline, minocycline, erythromycin, or doxycycline, can reduce or prevent superficial acne, but a person may have to take the drug for months or years to control acne.

Sunlight can help because it dries the skin and causes slight scaling, which accelerates healing. However, in people using tretinoin, exposure to sunlight can cause severe irritation. Tretinoin applied as a cream, liquid, or gel dries the skin, but it must be used cautiously. If irritation develops, tretinoin should be applied only nightly or every other night. Also, a person should apply it lightly over the face, avoiding the eyes, the creases of the mouth, and the folds just around the nose. The acne may appear worse during the first few days of tretinoin treatment and take 3 to 4 weeks to improve.

Other helpful topical drugs are benzoyl peroxide—the best nonprescription topical drug—and various preparations containing sulfur resorcinol. These drugs are usually applied twice a day, at night and in the morning.

Deep Acne

Doctors do what they can to prevent scarring from deep acne, usually prescribing an oral anti-biotic such as tetracycline, minocycline, or erythromycin. People with deep acne may need to take one of these medications for weeks, months, or even years to prevent a relapse. However, a teenage girl who uses these antibiotics can develop a vaginal yeast infection (candidal vaginitis) that may need to be treated with other drugs. If controlling the yeast infection proves difficult, oral antibiotic therapy for the acne may be impractical.

When antibiotics don't work, isotretinoin taken by mouth is the best treatment. This drug has revolutionized the treatment of acne, but it can have very serious side effects. *Isotretinoin can harm a developing fetus, and women taking it must use strict contraceptive measures so they don't become pregnant.* A sexually active woman should have a pregnancy test before she starts taking isotretinoin and at monthly intervals while she's taking it; contraception or sexual abstinence should begin 1 month before she starts taking the drug and should continue while she takes it and for 1 month after she stops taking it. Blood tests are necessary to make sure the drug isn't affecting blood cells, the liver, or fat (triglyceride and cholesterol) levels. These tests are performed before starting treatment, 2 weeks after starting treatment, and then monthly during treatment. Most people who use isotretinoin develop dry eyes, chapped lips, and dryness of the thin skin lining the penis or vagina. Petroleum jelly can usually help relieve the dry skin. About 15 percent of people who use isotretinoin develop pain or stiffness of large joints and the lower back; the pain often goes away when the dose is reduced. Therapy generally continues for 20 weeks. If more therapy is needed, it shouldn't be restarted for at least 4 months. Dermatologists sometimes treat inflamed cysts or abscesses by injecting corticosteroids into them. Occasionally, a doctor may also cut a cyst or abscess open to drain it. Dermabrasion, a procedure in which the surface of the skin is rubbed with an abrasive metal instrument to remove the top layer, may help remove small scars.

X-ray therapy isn't recommended for treating acne, and topical corticosteroids may actually worsen it. For a woman who develops severe acne during her menstrual period, an oral contraceptive may help, but therapy takes 4 to 6 months to produce results.

Rosacea

Rosacea is a persistent skin disorder that produces redness, tiny pimples, and broken blood vessels, usually on the central area of the face.

The skin may thicken, particularly around the nose, making it look red and bulbous, a condition called rhinophyma. Occasionally, rosacea appears on the torso, arms, and legs rather than on the face.

The cause of rosacea isn't known. The condition usually appears during or after middle age and is most common in people with fair complexions. Some alcoholics develop rosacea, particularly rhinophyma. Corticosteroids applied to the skin tend to make rosacea worse. Although usually easy for doctors to recognize, rosacea sometimes looks like acne and certain other skin disorders.

Treatment

People with rosacea should avoid foods that cause the blood vessels in the skin to dilate—for example, spicy foods, alcohol, coffee, and sodas containing caffeine. Certain antibiotics taken by mouth improve rosacea; tetracyclines are usually most effective and produce the fewest side effects. Antibiotics that are applied to the skin, such as metronidazole gel, are also effective. Severe rhinophyma is unlikely to improve with antibiotic therapy; a person with this condition may need surgery.

Perioral Dermatitis

Perioral dermatitis is a red, often bumpy rash around the mouth and on the chin.

Perioral dermatitis may look a lot like acne or rosacea. However, an area of normal skin usually separates the edge of the lips from the rash.

Corticosteroids and some oily cosmetics, especially moisturizers, tend to cause the condition or make it worse. Often, the cause isn't known. The condition mainly affects women between ages 20 and 60.

Treatment

Tetracyclines taken by mouth are usually the best treatment. If these antibiotics don't clear up the rash and the condition is particularly severe, isotretinoin, an acne medication, may help.

Sebaceous Cysts

A sebaceous cyst (keratinous cyst) is a slow-growing bump containing dead skin, skin excretions, and other skin particles.

These cysts may be tiny and can appear anywhere, most commonly on the scalp, ears, face, back, or scrotum. They tend to be firm and easy to move within the skin. Usually, they aren't painful. Sebaceous cysts may be yellowish or flesh colored; when they're punctured, a cheesy, greasy material comes out. Occasionally, they become infected.

Treatment

A doctor can almost always treat a sebaceous cyst by either puncturing the top with a needle or cutting the top with a scalpel, then squeezing out the contents. However, unless a doctor completely removes large cysts, they may reappear. Infected cysts are treated with an antibiotic and then surgically removed.

Hair Disorders

The hair originates in the dermis, the skin layer just below the surface layer (epidermis). Hair disorders include excessive hairiness, baldness, and ingrown beard hairs.

Excessive Hairiness

Both men and women may develop excessive hair (hirsutism) on parts of the skin that usually aren't very hairy. The trait often runs in families, particularly among people of Mediterranean descent. In women and children, excessive hairiness may result from a disorder of the pituitary or adrenal glands that causes overproduction of masculinizing (virilizing) steroids. Excessive hairiness is common after menopause and in people who use anabolic steroids or corticosteroids. The condition may also develop in people using certain other medications, such as the blood pressure drug minoxidil. People with porphyria cutanea tarda▲ also may have excessive hair.

Treatment

A doctor first determines the cause of the excessive hair growth. Often, laboratory tests aren't needed, but if an endocrine disorder is suspected, blood tests may be ordered.

As a temporary solution, the hair can be shaved. Other common temporary measures include plucking, waxing, and using depilatories. A hair bleach may mask the condition if the person has fine hair.

The hair follicles must be destroyed to permanently remove hair. The only safe permanent treatment is electrolysis.

Baldness

Baldness (alopecia) is much more common in men than in women. It can result from genetic factors, aging, local skin conditions, and diseases that affect the body generally (systemic diseases). Some medications, such as those used to treat cancer, also cause hair loss.

Male-pattern baldness is the most common type of hair loss affecting men. It's rare in women and children because it depends on the presence of the male hormones (androgens), and levels of these hormones are high in males after puberty. Baldness runs in families. The hair loss usually begins on the sides, near the front, or on the top of the head toward the back. The hair loss can begin at any age, even in the middle teen years. Some people lose only some hair and develop a bald spot in the back or a receding hairline; others, especially people whose hair loss begins at a young age, may go completely bald.

Female-pattern baldness is less common than male-pattern baldness. Usually, this condition causes the hair to thin in the front, on the sides, or on the crown. It rarely progresses to total hair loss.

Toxic baldness (toxic alopecia) may follow a severe illness with a high fever. In excessive doses, some drugs—especially thallium, vitamin A, and retinoids—can cause baldness. Many cancer drugs cause baldness. It may also result from an underactive thyroid gland or pituitary gland or even from pregnancy. The hair may fall out as long as 3 or 4 months after the illness or other condition. Usually, the hair loss is temporary, and the hair grows back.

Alopecia areata is a condition in which hair is lost suddenly in a particular area, usually in the scalp or beard. Rarely, all body hair may be lost, a condition called alopecia universalis. The hair usually grows back in several months, except in people with widespread hair loss, for whom regrowth is unlikely.

Hair pulling (trichotillomania) is most common in children, but the habit may persist throughout life. The habit may not be noticed for a long time, making doctors and parents think that an illness such as alopecia areata is causing the hair loss. A biopsy (removal of a skin specimen and examination under a microscope) sometimes helps a doctor pin down the diagnosis.

Scarring alopecia is hair loss that occurs at scarred areas. The skin may be scarred from burns, severe injury, or x-ray therapy. Less obvious causes of scarring include lupus erythematosus, lichen planus, persistent bacterial or fun-

▲ see page 688

gal infections, sarcoidosis, and tuberculosis. Skin cancers also may scar the skin.

Diagnosis and Treatment

Determining the type of baldness simply by observation is sometimes difficult, so a doctor may need a biopsy to make a diagnosis. A biopsy helps determine if the hair follicles are normal; if they're not, the biopsy may indicate possible causes.

Most types of baldness have no cure. A person with male-pattern or female-pattern baldness may undergo hair transplantation, in which hair follicles are removed from one part of the body and transplanted. Some medications, such as topical minoxidil, may promote hair growth in a small percentage of people. The oral drug finasteride may also promote hair growth.

Corticosteroids injected under the skin may help people with alopecia areata, but the results may not last. Another treatment for alopecia areata involves inducing a mild allergic reaction or irritation to promote hair growth. Scarring alopecia is particularly difficult to treat. When possible, the cause of the scarring is treated, but after an area of skin has fully scarred, hair growth is unlikely.

Ingrown Beard Hairs

A hair that curls so the tip punctures the skin can cause inflammation (pseudofolliculitis barbae). This most often happens with the curly hairs of the beard, especially in black men. The best treatment is to grow the beard: When the hairs are longer, they don't curl back and puncture the skin. A man who doesn't want a beard can use a depilatory made of thioglycolate or tretinoin (retinoic acid), but it often irritates the skin.

CHAPTER 201

Bacterial Skin Infections

The skin provides a remarkably good barrier against bacterial infections. Although many bacteria live on the skin, they're normally unable to establish an infection. Bacterial skin infections may affect a single spot, appearing as a pimple, or may spread within hours, affecting a large area. Skin infections can range in seriousness from minor acne to a life-threatening condition, such as staphylococcal scalded skin syndrome.

Many types of bacteria can infect the skin. The most common are *Staphylococcus* and *Streptococcus*. Infections from less common bacteria may develop in hospitals or nursing homes or while gardening or swimming in a pond, lake, or ocean.

Some people are at particular risk of contracting skin infections—for example, people with diabetes because they have poor blood flow to the skin, especially of the hands and feet, and people with AIDS because they have a depressed immune system. Skin damaged by sunburn, scratching, or other irritation also is more likely to get infected. In fact, any break in the skin predisposes a person to infection.

For the most part, keeping the skin undamaged and clean prevents infections. When the skin is cut or scraped, washing the area with soap and water helps prevent infection. Although most antibiotic creams and ointments do little to prevent or treat skin infections, some newer creams such as mupirocin are effective for some skin infections. Warm soaks can increase the blood supply to an infected area and help clear up an infection confined to a small area. Once an infection spreads, antibiotics must be taken internally—by mouth or injection.

Impetigo

Impetigo is a skin infection, caused by Staphylococcus *or* Streptococcus, *leading to the formation of small pus-filled blisters (pustules).*

Affecting mostly children, impetigo can appear anywhere on the body but frequently appears on the face, arms, and legs. The blisters can vary from pea-sized to large rings. Impetigo may follow an injury or a condition that causes a break in the skin, such as a fungal infection, sunburn, or insect bite. Impetigo may also affect normal skin, especially on children's legs.

Early treatment can prevent impetigo from infecting the deeper skin (ecthyma). An antibiotic such as penicillin or a cephalosporin is usually taken by mouth. Rarely, impetigo caused by *Streptococcus* may lead to kidney failure.

Folliculitis, Boils, and Carbuncles

Folliculitis is an inflammation of the hair follicles caused by infection with Staphylococcus.

A small amount of pus develops in the hair follicles, and they become irritated and reddened. The infection damages the hairs, which can be easily pulled out. Folliculitis tends to become a long-term problem where the hair follicles are deepest in the skin, such as the beard area. Stiff hairs may curl and reenter the skin, producing irritation even without substantial infection.

Boils (furuncles) are large, tender, swollen, raised areas caused by staphylococcal infection around hair follicles.

They most frequently form on the neck, breasts, face, and buttocks but are particularly painful when they form around the nose or ears or on the fingers. Boils usually have pus in the center. Often a white, slightly bloody substance oozes from the boil. Some people develop recurrent and troublesome boils (furunculosis), and occasionally epidemics of boils break out among teenagers who live in crowded quarters and have poor hygiene.

Carbuncles are clusters of boils that result in extensive sloughing of skin and scar formation.

Carbuncles develop and heal more slowly than single boils and may lead to fever and fatigue because they are a more serious infection. They appear most frequently in men and most commonly on the back of the neck. Older people, people with diabetes, and those with serious medical conditions are more prone to carbuncles.

Treatment

Keeping the skin clean, preferably with liquid soap containing an antibacterial agent, is the best way to prevent these infections or their spread to others. Moist heat helps collect the pus and can make a single boil drain spontaneously. When a boil appears near the nose, doctors usually prescribe oral antibiotics because the infection can spread quickly toward the brain. When boils or carbuncles emerge, doctors usually collect a sample of the pus for laboratory evaluation and prescribe an oral antibiotic. People with recurring boils may need to take antibiotics for months or even years.

Erysipelas

Erysipelas is a skin infection caused by Streptococcus.

Most commonly, the infection appears on the face, arm, or leg; sometimes, it begins where the skin is broken. A shiny, red, slightly swollen, tender rash develops, often with small blisters. Lymph nodes around the infected area may become enlarged and painful, and people with particularly bad infections develop a fever and chills.

Taking penicillin or erythromycin by mouth for 2 weeks usually cures mild infections. When the infection is severe, usually a doctor first gives an antibiotic by injection.

Cellulitis

Cellulitis is a spreading infection in, and sometimes beneath, the deep layers of the skin.

Cellulitis most often results from a streptococcal infection or, particularly after a wound occurs, a staphylococcal infection. However, many other bacteria can cause cellulitis, especially after bites by humans or animals or after injuries in the water.

The infection is most common on the legs and often begins with skin damage from a minor injury, a sore, or a fungal infection between the toes. Cellulitis produces swelling, tenderness, warmth, and redness. Some areas may look bruised, and small blisters may develop. Symptoms of the infection may include fever, chills, headache, and more serious complications such as confusion, low blood pressure, and rapid heartbeat.

Cellulitis is usually easy for doctors to recognize, but identifying the bacteria causing the infection is more difficult. Doctors usually take blood samples (and sometimes skin samples) and send them to the laboratory, where the bacteria is grown in a culture and identified.

Treatment

Prompt treatment can prevent the infection from spreading rapidly and reaching the blood and other organs. Cellulitis is often treated with penicillin or a penicillin-type drug, such as dicloxacillin. People with mild cellulitis may take oral antibiotics; older people and people with rapidly spreading cellulitis, high fever, or other evidence of serious infection usually receive an antibiotic injection before beginning the oral antibiotics. If the legs are infected, keeping them elevated and applying cool, wet cloth dressings relieves the discomfort and reduces the swelling.

If cellulitis recurs, an underlying condition— such as athlete's foot—that predisposes a person to cellulitis is likely and must also be treated.

Paronychia

Paronychia is an infection around the edge of a fingernail or toenail.

The infection often starts because of a break in the skin from a hangnail, vigorous manicuring, or chronic irritation. Because the nail area has little room to swell, the infection tends to be quite painful. Unlike most other skin infections, paronychia can be caused by many different bacteria, including *Pseudomonas* and *Proteus,* and by fungi, such as *Candida.*

Treatment

Hot compresses and warm soaks help relieve pain and often help drain pus. The warm soaks also increase blood circulation, which in turn helps fight the infection. Sometimes, a doctor drains the infection by making a small cut into the pocket of infection (abscess) with a scalpel. Infections that can be drained adequately may not need to be treated with antibiotics. If the infection appears to be spreading, a doctor may prescribe oral antibiotics.

If paronychia is caused by a fungus, a doctor drains the infection and prescribes an antifungal cream containing ketoconazole, ciclopirox, or miconazole and warm soaks. In severe cases, a doctor prescribes an oral antifungal drug.

Staphylococcal Scalded Skin Syndrome

Staphylococcal scalded skin syndrome is a widespread skin infection in which the skin peels off as though burned.

Certain types of staphylococci produce a toxic substance that causes the top layer of skin (epidermis) to split from the rest of the skin. Skin infections from *Staphylococcus* can sometimes lead to toxic shock syndrome, a potentially life-threatening condition.▲

Staphylococcal scalded skin syndrome almost always affects infants, young children, and people with depressed immune systems. Hospital personnel can carry staphylococci, the infecting bacteria, on their hands and transmit the bacteria from baby to baby, sometimes causing epidemics in hospital nurseries.

Symptoms

The syndrome usually begins with an isolated, crusted infection that may look like impetigo. The infection may appear in the diaper area or around the stump of the umbilical cord during the first few days of life. In children ages 1 to 6, the syndrome may start with a crusted area on the nose or ears. Within a day, scarlet-colored areas appear around the crusted area. These areas may be painful. Other, large areas of skin may redden and develop blisters that break easily.

The top layer of the skin then begins peeling off, often in large sheets, even with slight touching or soft pushing. Within another 1 to 2 days, the entire skin surface may be involved, and the child becomes very ill with a fever, chills, and weakness. With the loss of the protective skin barrier, other bacteria and infective organisms can easily penetrate the body. Also, critical amounts of fluid can be lost because of oozing and evaporation.

Diagnosis

By performing a biopsy (removing a skin specimen and examining it under a microscope) or obtaining a skin specimen and sending it to the laboratory to be cultured, doctors can distinguish staphylococcal scalded skin syndrome from diseases that look similar, such as toxic epidermal necrolysis, which is usually caused by medication.

▲ see page 875

Treatment

Often, a doctor prescribes an intravenous penicillin-type antibiotic, such as cloxacillin, dicloxacillin, or cephalexin. However, if the syndrome is diagnosed early, the oral form of one of these drugs may be given. This therapy continues for at least 10 days. With early treatment, healing takes 5 to 7 days.

The skin must be handled gently to help prevent further sloughing; it should be treated as if it were burned. A doctor may apply a protective covering. Children who are severely affected may be treated in hospital burn units.

Erythrasma

Erythrasma is an infection of the top layers of the skin by the bacterium Corynebacterium minutissimum.

Erythrasma affects mostly adults and those with diabetes; it's most common in the tropics. Like a fungal infection, erythrasma often appears in areas where skin touches skin, such as under the breasts and in the armpits, webs of the toes, and genital area, especially in men, where the thighs touch the scrotum. The infection can produce irregularly shaped pink patches that may later turn into fine brown scales. In some people, the infection spreads to the torso and anal area.

Doctors can easily diagnose erythrasma because *Corynebacterium* glows coral red under an ultraviolet light. An oral antibiotic, such as erythromycin or tetracycline, can eliminate the infection. Antibacterial soaps may also help. Erythrasma may recur in 6 to 12 months, necessitating a second treatment.

CHAPTER 202

Fungal Skin Infections

Fungi that infect the skin (dermatophytes) live only in the dead, topmost layer (stratum corneum) and don't penetrate deeper. Some fungal infections cause no symptoms or produce only a small amount of irritation, scaling, and redness. Other fungal infections cause itching, swelling, blisters, and severe scaling.

Fungi usually make their homes in moist areas of the body where skin surfaces meet: between the toes, in the groin, and under the breasts. Obese people are more likely to get these infections because they have excessive skinfolds.

Strangely, fungal infections on one part of the body can cause rashes on other parts of the body that aren't infected. For example, a fungal infection on the foot may cause an itchy, bumpy rash on the fingers. These eruptions (dermatophytids or id eruptions) represent allergic reactions to the fungus.

Doctors may suspect fungi when they see a red, irritated rash in one of the commonly affected areas. A doctor can usually confirm the diagnosis by scraping off a small amount of skin and having it examined under a microscope or placed in a culture medium that will grow the fungi so they can be identified.

Ringworm

Ringworm is a fungal skin infection caused by several different fungi and generally classified by its location on the body.

Athlete's foot (foot ringworm) is a common fungal infection that usually appears during warm weather. It's usually caused by either *Trichophyton* or *Epidermophyton,* fungi that can grow in the warm, moist areas between the toes. The fungus can produce very mild scaling without other symptoms or more severe scaling with an itchy, raw, painful rash between the toes and over the sides of the feet. Fluid-filled blisters can also form. Because the fungus may cause the skin to crack, athlete's foot can lead to bacterial infection, especially in the elderly and in people with inadequate blood flow to the feet.

Jock itch (groin ringworm) can be caused by a variety of fungi and yeasts. It's much more common in men than in women and develops more frequently in warm weather. The infection produces red, ring-like areas, sometimes with small blisters in the skin around the groin and over the upper, inner thighs. The condition can be quite itchy and even painful. Recurrence is common because the fungi can survive indefinitely on the skin. Even with proper treatment, a susceptible person may have repeated infections.

Scalp ringworm is caused by *Trichophyton* or *Microsporum,* another fungus. Scalp ringworm is highly contagious, especially among children. It may produce a red scaly rash that may be somewhat itchy, or it may produce a patch of hair loss without a rash.

Nail ringworm is an infection of the nail caused by *Trichophyton*. The fungus gets into the newly forming part of the nail, producing a thickened, lusterless, and deformed nail. Infection is much more common on the toenails than on the fingernails. An infected toenail may separate from the toe, crumble, or flake off.

Body ringworm also results from *Trichophyton*. The infection generally produces a pink to red rash that sometimes forms round patches with clear areas in the centers. Body ringworm can develop anywhere on the skin.

Beard ringworm is rare. Most skin infections in the beard area are caused by bacteria, not fungi.

Treatment

Most fungal skin infections, except those of the scalp and nails, are mild, and antifungal creams usually cure them. Many effective antifungal creams can be purchased without a prescription. Antifungal powders are generally not as good for treating fungal infections. The active ingredients in antifungal medications include miconazole, clotrimazole, econazole, and ketoconazole.

Usually, creams are applied twice a day, and treatment should continue for 7 to 10 days after the rash completely disappears. If the cream is stopped too soon, the infection may not be eradicated, and the rash will return.

Several days may pass before antifungal creams take effect. In the meantime, corticosteroid creams are often used to help relieve itching and pain. Low-dose hydrocortisone is available over the counter; more potent corticosteroids require a prescription.

▲ see page 910

For more serious or stubborn infections, a doctor may prescribe several months of therapy with griseofulvin, sometimes together with antifungal creams. Griseofulvin, which is taken by mouth, is very effective, but it may cause side effects such as headache, upset stomach, sensitivity to light, rashes, swelling, and reduced numbers of white blood cells. After treatment with griseofulvin stops, the infection may return. A doctor may also prescribe ketoconazole for fungal skin infections. Like griseofulvin, oral ketoconazole can have serious side effects, including liver disease.

Keeping the infected areas clean and dry helps thwart further fungal growth and promote skin healing. Infected areas should be washed frequently with soap and water, then dusted with talcum powder. Doctors often recommend avoiding powders containing cornstarch because it can promote fungal growth.

If a fungal skin infection oozes, a bacterial infection also may have developed. Such an infection may require treatment with antibiotics. Some doctors prescribe antibiotics that can be applied to the skin; others prescribe antibiotics that must be taken by mouth. Dilute Burow's solution or Whitfield's ointment (both available without a prescription) also may be used to help dry the oozing skin.

Candidiasis

Candidiasis (yeast infection, moniliasis) is an infection by the yeast Candida, *formerly called* Monilia.

Candida usually infects the skin and mucous membranes, such as the lining of the mouth and vagina. Rarely, it invades deeper tissues as well as the blood, causing life-threatening systemic candidiasis.▲ This more serious infection is most common in people with poor immunity—for example, people with AIDS or those receiving chemotherapy.

Candida is a normal resident of the digestive tract and vagina that usually causes no harm. When environmental conditions are particularly favorable (for example, in warm, humid weather) or when a person's immune defenses are impaired, the yeast can infect the skin. Like dermatophytes, *Candida* grows well in warm, moist conditions. Sometimes people taking antibiotics get *Candida* infections because the antibiotics kill the bacteria that normally reside in the tissues, allowing the *Candida* to grow unchecked. Corticosteroids or immunosuppressive therapy after organ transplantation can also lower the body's defenses against yeast infections. Pregnant women, obese people, and people with diabetes also are more likely to be infected by *Candida*.

Symptoms

Symptoms vary, depending on the location of the infection.

Infections in skinfolds (intertriginous infections) or in the navel usually cause a red rash, often with patchy areas that ooze small amounts of whitish fluid. Small pustules may appear, especially at the edges of the rash, and the rash may itch or burn. A *Candida* rash around the anus may be raw, white or red, and itchy.

Vaginal *Candida* infections (vulvovaginitis) are common, especially in women who are pregnant, have diabetes, or are taking antibiotics. Symptoms of these infections include a white or yellow discharge from the vagina and burning, itching, and redness along the walls and external area of the vagina.

Penile *Candida* infections most often affect men with diabetes or men whose female sex partners have vaginal *Candida* infections. Usually the infection produces a red, scaling, sometimes painful rash on the underside of the penis. However, an infection of the penis or vagina may not cause any symptoms.

Thrush is a *Candida* infection inside the mouth. The creamy white patches typical of thrush cling to the tongue and sides of the mouth and often are painful. The patches can be scraped off easily with a finger or spoon. Thrush in otherwise healthy children isn't unusual, but in adults it may signal impaired immunity, possibly caused by diabetes or AIDS. The use of antibiotics that kill off competing bacteria increases the chances of getting thrush.

Perlèche is a *Candida* infection at the corners of the mouth, creating cracks and tiny cuts. It may stem from ill-fitting dentures that leave the corners of the mouth moist enough so that yeast can grow.

Candidal paronychia, *Candida* growing in the nail beds, produces painful swelling and pus. Nails infected with *Candida* may turn white or yellow and separate from the finger or toe.

Diagnosis

Usually, a doctor can identify a *Candida* infection by observing its distinctive rash or the thick, white, pasty residue it generates. To make a diagnosis, a doctor may scrape off some of the skin or residue with a scalpel or tongue depressor. Then the sample is examined under a microscope or placed in a culture medium to identify the cause of the infection.

Treatment

Generally, *Candida* skin infections are easily cured with medicated creams and lotions. Doctors often recommend nystatin cream for skin, vaginal, and penile infections; the cream is usually applied twice daily for 7 to 10 days. Yeast medications for the vagina or anus also are available as suppositories. Thrush medications may be taken as a liquid that is swished around the mouth and spit out or as a lozenge that dissolves slowly in the mouth. For skin infections, sometimes corticosteroid ointments, such as hydrocortisone, are used along with antifungal creams because the ointments quickly reduce itching and pain (although they don't help cure the infection itself).

Keeping the skin dry helps clear up the infection and prevents the fungus from returning. Plain talcum powder or powder that contains nystatin can help keep the surface area dry.

Tinea Versicolor

Tinea versicolor is a fungal infection that causes white to light brown patches on the skin.

The infection is quite common, especially in young adults. It rarely causes pain or itching, but it prevents areas of the skin from tanning, producing patches. People with naturally dark skin may notice pale patches; people with naturally fair skin may get dark patches. The patches are often on the chest or back and may scale slightly. Over time, small areas can join to form large patches.

Diagnosis and Treatment

Doctors diagnose tinea versicolor by its appearance. A doctor may use an ultraviolet light to show the infection more clearly or may examine scrapings from the infected area under a microscope. Dandruff shampoos, such as 1 percent selenium sulfide, usually cure tinea versicolor. These shampoos are applied full-strength to the affected areas (including the scalp) at bedtime, left on overnight, and washed off in the morning.

Treatment is usually continued for 3 or 4 nights. People who develop skin irritations from this treatment may have to limit the time the shampoo is in contact with their skin to 20 to 60 minutes, or they may need to turn to prescription medications.

The skin may not regain its normal pigmentation for many months after the infection is gone. The condition commonly comes back after successful treatment because the fungus that causes it normally lives on the skin. When the condition does come back, treatment must be repeated.

CHAPTER 203

Parasitic Skin Infections

Most skin parasites are tiny insects or worms that burrow into the skin and make their home there. Some parasites live in the skin for part of their life cycles; others are permanent residents that lay their eggs and reproduce there.

Scabies

Scabies is a mite infestation that produces tiny reddish pimples and severe itching.

Scabies is caused by the itch mite *Sarcoptes scabiei*. The infestation spreads easily from person to person on physical contact, often spreading through an entire household. The mites, just barely big enough to be seen, often spread when people sleep together. Mites can rarely be spread on clothing, bedding, and other shared objects; their survival is brief, and normal laundering destroys them.

The female itch mite tunnels under the topmost layer of the skin and deposits her eggs in burrows. Young mites (larvae) then hatch in a few days. The infection causes intense itching, probably from an allergic reaction to the mites.

Symptoms

The hallmark of scabies is intense itching, which is usually worse at night. The burrows of the mites appear as wavy lines up to half an inch long, sometimes with a tiny pimple at one end. The burrows are most common and the itching is most intense in the webs between the fingers, on the wrists, at the elbows, in the armpits, around the nipples of women's breasts, on men's genitals (penis and scrotum), along the belt line, and over the lower part of the buttocks. The face is rarely infected, except in small children where lesions may appear as water-filled blisters. Over time, the

burrows may become difficult to see because they're obscured by inflammation induced by scratching.

Diagnosis and Treatment

Usually, the combination of itching and the burrows is all a doctor needs to make a diagnosis of scabies. However, a doctor can take a scraping from the burrows and look at it under a microscope to confirm the presence of mites.

Scabies can be cured by applying a cream containing permethrin or a solution of lindane. Both are effective, but lindane tends to irritate the skin, is more toxic, and isn't appropriate for young children. Some scabies mites have become resistant to permethrin treatment.

Sometimes, a cream containing corticosteroids, such as hydrocortisone, is used for a few days after treatment with permethrin or lindane to reduce the itching until all the mites are gone.

Family members and people with skin-to-skin contact, such as sexual contact, should be treated at the same time. Extensive cleaning or fumigating of bedding or clothing isn't warranted.

Lice Infestation

Lice infestation (pediculosis) causes intense itching and can affect almost any area of the skin.

Lice are barely visible, wingless insects that spread easily from person to person by body contact and shared clothing and other personal items. Lice found on the head look very much like those found on the body, but they are actually a different species. Lice found in the pubic area have a wider, shorter body shape than the other two species. The rounder shape makes them resemble crabs—the source of the popular name for these parasites. Head lice and pubic lice live directly on the person; body lice are also often found in garments that are in contact with skin.

Head lice are spread by personal contact and by shared combs, brushes, hats, and other personal items. The infestation sometimes extends into the eyebrows, eyelashes, and beard. Head lice are a common scourge of school children of all social strata. Such lice are less common in blacks.

Body lice aren't as easily transmitted as head lice. Body lice usually infest people who have poor hygiene and those living in close quarters or crowded institutions. These lice can carry diseases such as typhus, trench fever, and relapsing fever.

Pubic lice, which infest the genital area, are typically spread during sexual relations.

Symptoms

Lice infestation causes severe itching. Intense scratching often breaks the skin, which can lead to bacterial infections.

Sometimes the lymph glands in the back of the neck become swollen from a scalp infection. Children may hardly notice head lice or may have only a vague scalp irritation. Itching from body lice is generally most intense on the shoulders, buttocks, and abdomen. Pubic lice cause itching around the penis, vagina, and anus.

Diagnosis

Female lice lay shiny grayish-white eggs (nits) that can be seen as tiny globules firmly stuck to hairs. Adult body lice and their eggs are found not only on body hairs but also in the seams of clothing worn close to the skin. Pubic lice leave a scattering of minuscule, dark brown specks (louse excrement) on underwear where they come into contact with the genitals and anus. Pubic lice are particularly difficult to find and may appear as tiny bluish spots on the skin. Unlike other lice, the nits appear at the base of hairs, very close to the skin.

Treatment

Of the medications for lice, permethrin is the safest, most effective, and most pleasant to use. Lindane—which can be applied as a cream, lotion, or shampoo—also cures lice infestation but isn't appropriate for children because in rare instances it can cause neurologic complications. Pyrethrin is also sometimes used. All these med-

---

A Look at Lice

These illustrations show the distinct appearances of the three types of lice. Lice measure up to one eighth of an inch across (3 millimeters).

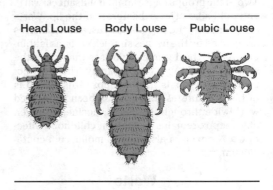

Head Louse   Body Louse   Pubic Louse

---

ications can be irritating, and all require a second application after 10 days to kill newly hatched lice.

Infestation of eyelashes and eyelids is difficult to treat; the parasites usually are removed with tweezers. Plain petroleum jelly may kill or weaken the lice on eyelashes. If sources of infestation (combs, hats, clothing, and bedding) aren't decontaminated by vacuuming, laundering, steam pressing, or dry cleaning, the lice can live on them and reinfect the person.

Creeping Eruption

Creeping eruption (cutaneous larva migrans) is a hookworm infection transmitted from warm, moist soil to exposed skin.

The infection is caused by a hookworm that normally inhabits dogs and cats. The eggs of the parasite are deposited on the ground in dog and cat feces. When bare skin touches the ground, which happens when a person walks barefoot or sunbathes, the hookworm gets into the skin.

Starting from the site of infection—usually the feet, legs, buttocks, or back—the hookworm burrows along a haphazard tract leaving a winding, threadlike rash. The infection itches intensely.

A liquid preparation of thiabendazole applied to the area effectively treats the infestation.

Viral Skin Infections

Many types of viruses invade the skin, but most medical concern focuses on only three groups. Two of the groups cause familiar nuisances: warts and cold sores (fever blisters) on the lip. Warts are caused by the papillomavirus, and cold sores are caused by the herpes simplex virus, as is shingles.▲ The third group of viruses that infect the skin is part of the poxvirus family. The most notorious poxvirus is the smallpox virus, which is of historic interest only; it has been eliminated worldwide through the use of vaccine. However, chickenpox remains a common childhood infection.■ A poxvirus also causes molluscum contagiosum.

Warts

Warts (verrucae) are small skin growths caused by any of 60 related human papillomavirus types.

Warts can develop at any age, but they are most common in children and least common in the elderly. Although warts on the skin are easily spread from one area of the body to another, most are not very contagious from one person to another. Genital warts, however, are contagious.

The overwhelming majority of warts are harmless. The most common types don't become cancerous. Only rare types and some that infect the uterine cervix and the penis very rarely become cancerous.

A wart's ultimate size and shape depend on the particular virus that caused it and its position on the body. Some warts are painless; others cause pain by irritating nerves. Some warts grow in clusters (mosaic warts); others appear as isolated, single growths. Warts often disappear without treatment. However, some persist for many years, and others disappear and then come back.

▲ see page 916

■ see page 1270

★ see page 948

Diagnosis

When doctors examine a growth on the skin, they try to determine whether it's a wart or some other growth. Some growths that may look like warts are actually skin tags, moles, corns, calluses, or even skin cancer. Warts are classified by their position and shape.

Almost everyone gets **common warts** (verrucae vulgaris). These firm growths usually have a rough surface; are round or irregular; are grayish, yellow, or brown; and are usually less than half an inch across. Generally, they appear on areas that are frequently injured, such as the fingers, around the nails (periungual warts), knees, face, and scalp. They may spread, but common warts are never cancerous.

Plantar warts develop on the sole of the foot, where they are usually flattened by the pressure of walking and are surrounded by thickened skin. They may be extremely tender. Unlike corns and calluses, plantar warts tend to bleed from many tiny spots, like pinpoints, when a doctor shaves or cuts the surface away with a knife.

Filiform warts are long, narrow, small growths that usually crop up on the eyelids, face, neck, or lips.

Flat warts, which are more common in children and young adults, usually appear in groups as smooth, yellow-brown spots, most frequently on the face.

The virus that causes moist warts (**venereal warts,** condylomata acuminata) on the genitals is transmitted sexually.★

Treatment

Treatment for warts depends on their location, type, and severity as well as how long they've been on the skin.

Most **common warts** disappear without treatment within 2 years. Daily applications of a solution or plaster containing salicylic and lactic acids soften the infected skin, which can be peeled off to make the wart disappear faster. A doctor can freeze the wart using liquid nitrogen but may have to repeat the freezing process in 2 or 3 weeks to eliminate the wart completely. Electrodesiccation (a treatment that uses an electric current) or laser surgery can destroy the wart, but each may cause scarring. Regardless of the treatment method, about a third of the time the wart comes back. A doctor also can treat common warts with chemicals such as trichloroacetic acid or cantharidin, which destroy the wart; however, new warts sometimes crop up around the edges of the old one.

Plantar warts are usually softened with strong salicylic acid applied as a solution or plaster. This chemical process is used in addition to paring the wart with a knife, freezing it, or applying other acids. Doctors may use additional techniques, such as injecting the wart with chemicals to destroy it. However, plantar warts are difficult to cure.

Flat warts are often treated with peeling agents such as retinoic or salicylic acid, which make the wart come off with the scaly skin.

Molluscum Contagiosum

Molluscum contagiosum is an infection of the skin by a poxvirus that causes skin-colored, smooth, waxy bumps.

The bumps are usually less than half an inch in diameter and have a tiny dimple in the center. Sometimes a single bump may grow to an inch and a half. The virus that causes molluscum is contagious; it spreads by direct skin contact and is often transmitted sexually.

Most common in the groin and pubic areas (though not usually on the penis or in the vagina), the virus can infect any part of the skin. The bumps usually aren't itchy or painful and may be discovered only coincidentally during a physical examination. They often develop a central dimple filled with pasty white material that makes them easy for doctors to identify.

The growths can be treated by freezing or removing their core with a needle.

CHAPTER 205

Sunlight and Skin Damage

The skin shields the rest of the body from the sun's rays—a source of ultraviolet (UV) radiation that can damage cells. Brief overexposure causes sunburn. With long-term exposure to sunlight, the skin's uppermost layer (epidermis) thickens, and pigment-producing skin cells (melanocytes) increase the production of pigment (melanin), which gives the skin its color. Melanin, a naturally protective substance, absorbs the energy of ultraviolet rays and prevents the rays from penetrating deeper into the tissues.

Sensitivity to sunlight varies according to race, previous exposure, and complexion, but everyone is vulnerable to some extent. Because dark-skinned people have more melanin, they have more resistance to the sun's harmful effects, which include sunburn, premature aging of the skin, and skin cancer. Albinos have no melanin in their skin, can't tan at all, and burn severely with even a little sun exposure. Unless albinos protect themselves from the sun, they develop skin can-

cers at an early age. People with vitiligo have patches of skin that don't produce melanin and thus may become severely sunburned.

Sunburn

Sunburn results from an overexposure to ultraviolet B (UVB) rays. Depending on the type of skin pigment a person has and the amount of sun exposure, the skin becomes red, swollen, and painful one hour to one day after exposure. Later, blisters may form, and the skin may peel. Some sunburned people develop a fever, chills, and weakness, and those with very bad sunburns even may go into shock—low blood pressure, fainting, and profound weakness.

Prevention

The best—and most obvious—way to prevent sun damage is to stay out of strong, direct sunlight. Clothing and ordinary window glass filter

Dangers of Unseen Sunlight

The sun radiates energy of different wavelengths; for example, yellow light has a longer wavelength than blue light. Ultraviolet (UV) wavelengths are shorter than wavelengths of visible light and can damage living tissue. Fortunately, the ozone layer of the earth's upper atmosphere filters out the most damaging UV wavelengths, but some UV light, chiefly in the A (UVA) and B (UVB) wavelength bands, penetrates to the earth and can cause skin damage.

The character and amount of UV light varies according to season, weather, and geographic location. Because of the way light slants through the atmosphere at different times of the day in temperate zones, skin exposure is less hazardous before 10 A.M. and after 3 P.M.. The potential for damage is greater at higher altitudes where the protective atmosphere is thinner.

One more consideration: The amount of UV light reaching the earth's surface is increasing, especially in the northern latitudes. That's because chemical reactions between ozone and chlorofluorocarbons (chemicals in refrigerants and spray can propellants) are depleting the protective ozone layer, creating a thinner atmosphere with some holes.

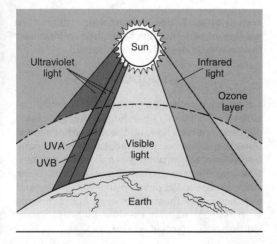

on a cloudy or foggy day. Snow, water, and sand reflect sunlight, magnifying the amount of UV light that reaches the skin.

Before exposure to strong, direct sunlight, a person should apply a sunscreen, an ointment or cream containing chemicals that protect the skin by filtering out UVA and UVB rays. Many sunscreens are either waterproof or water resistant. One common, effective type of sunscreen contains para-aminobenzoic acid (PABA). Because it takes 30 to 45 minutes to bind strongly to the skin, swimming or sweating soon after applying PABA will wash it off. Occasionally, sunscreens containing PABA irritate the skin, and they can cause allergic reactions in some people.

Another type of sunscreen contains a chemical called benzophenone. Many sunscreens contain both PABA and benzophenone or other chemicals; these combinations provide protection from a broader range of UV rays. Other sunscreens contain physical barriers such as zinc oxide or titanium dioxide; these thick, white ointments block sunlight from the skin and can be used on small, sensitive areas, such as the nose and lips. People who are concerned with appearance can tint these ointments with cosmetics to match their skin color.

In the United States, sunscreens are rated by their sun protection factor (SPF) number—the higher the SPF number, the greater the protection. Sunscreens with an SPF of 15 or more block most UV rays, but no see-through sunscreen blocks all UV rays. Most sunscreens tend to block only UVB rays, but UVA rays also can cause skin damage. Some newer sunscreens are somewhat effective at blocking UVA rays.

Treatment

The first tingling or redness is a signal to get out of the sun quickly. Cold tap water compresses can soothe raw, hot areas, as can lotions or ointments without anesthetics or perfumes that might irritate or sensitize the skin. Corticosteroid tablets can help relieve the inflammation and pain within hours.

Sunburned skin begins healing by itself within several days, but complete healing may take weeks. Sunburned lower legs, particularly sunburned shins, tend to be particularly uncomfortable and slow to heal. Skin surfaces rarely exposed to the sun can get badly sunburned because they contain little pigment. Such areas include the skin normally covered by a bathing

out virtually all damaging rays. Water is not a good UV filter: UVA and UVB rays can penetrate a foot of clear water, as snorkelers and barefoot waders may discover. Neither clouds nor fog is a good UV filter either; a person can get sunburned

suit, the tops of the feet, and the wrist normally protected by a watch.

Sun-damaged skin makes a poor barrier against infection, and if an infection develops, healing may be delayed. A doctor can determine the severity of an infection and prescribe antibiotics if necessary.

After burned skin peels, the newly exposed layers are thin and initially very sensitive to sunlight. These areas may remain extremely sensitive for several weeks.

Long-term Effects of Sunlight

Years of exposure to sunlight age the skin, but exposure before age 18 is probably the most damaging. Although fair-skinned people are most vulnerable, with enough exposure, anyone's skin will change.

Damage to the deep skin layers causes wrinkling and yellow discoloration. Sunlight also thins the skin and may induce precancerous growths (actinic keratoses, solar keratoses). These growths appear as flaky, scaly areas that don't heal; they may also be darkened or gray and feel hard. People who are in the sun a lot have an increased risk of skin cancers, including squamous cell carcinoma, basal cell carcinoma, and to some degree, malignant melanoma.

Treatment

The key to treatment is avoiding further sun exposure; however, any damage that's already done can't be reversed. Moisturizing creams and makeup help hide wrinkles. Sometimes, chemical peels, alpha-hydroxy acids, and tretinoin are used in attempts to undo long-term damage, especially very thin wrinkles and irregular pigmentation. Even though the benefits of such treatments have been touted, little convincing evidence exists that deep wrinkles can be smoothed out permanently or that skin damage can be reversed.

Precancerous growths may progress to skin cancer. Solar or actinic keratoses usually can be removed by freezing them with liquid nitrogen; however, if a person has too many growths, a liquid or an ointment containing fluorouracil may be applied. Often, during such treatment, the skin looks worse because fluorouracil causes redness, scaling, and burning of the keratoses and the surrounding sun-damaged skin.

Are Tans Healthy?

In a word—No. Although a suntan is often considered an emblem of good health and an active, athletic life, tanning for its own sake is actually a health hazard. Any exposure to UVA or UVB light can alter or damage the skin. Long-term exposure to natural sunlight or the artificial sunlight in tanning parlors may cause long-term skin damage. Quite simply, there's no "safe tan."

Skin Photosensitivity Reactions

Although sunburn and sun damage take time to show up, some people have unusual reactions after only a few minutes of sun exposure. These reactions include redness, peeling, hives, blisters, and thickened, scaling patches. Many factors may contribute to such sensitivity to the sun (photosensitivity).

The most common cause is the use of certain drugs—such as some antibiotics, diuretics, and antifungal agents. Photosensitivity reactions can also result from soaps, perfumes such as scented toilet waters (especially the ones that contain bergamot and smell like mint or citrus), coal tars used to treat dandruff and eczema, and substances found in plants like meadow grass and parsley. Certain diseases, such as systemic lupus erythematosus and porphyria, also may cause photosensitivity reactions.

Some reactions to light (polymorphous light eruptions) seem to be unrelated to diseases or drugs. For some people, even brief exposure to sun causes hives (red, raised patches) or erythema multiforme on sun-exposed areas. Skin reactions to light are most common in people from temperate climates when they're first intensely exposed to the sun in the spring or summer; such reactions are uncommon in people who are exposed to the sun year-round.

Prevention and Treatment

Extreme sensitivity to sunlight calls for wearing protective clothes, avoiding sunlight as much as possible, and using sunscreens. A careful review of any diseases, drugs taken by mouth, or substances applied to the skin (such as drugs or cosmetics) may help a doctor pinpoint the cause of the photosensitivity. However, pinpointing the cause is difficult and sometimes impossible.

Sometimes long-term treatment with hydroxychloroquine may prevent photosensitivity reactions, and often oral corticosteroids can speed recovery from such reactions. For certain types of photosensitivity, treatment can consist of giving psoralens (drugs that sensitize the skin to sunlight) and exposing the skin to UVA light; people with systemic lupus erythematosus can't tolerate this treatment.

CHAPTER 206

Pigment Disorders

Skin color is determined by a combination of the pigments produced in the skin and the natural colors of the upper layers of the skin. Without pigmentation, the skin would be pale white with varying shades of pink caused by the blood flowing through it. The main skin pigment is melanin, a dark brown pigment made by cells (melanocytes) that are interspersed among the other cells in the upper layer of the skin, the epidermis.

Hypopigmentation, an abnormally low amount of pigment, is usually restricted to small areas of skin. It usually results from a previous inflammatory condition of the skin or, in rare instances, may represent a hereditary condition.

When the skin is exposed to sunlight, melanin production increases, causing tanning. Increased amounts of melanin (hyperpigmentation) can be a response to hormonal changes, like those that may take place in Addison's disease, in pregnancy, or with oral contraceptive use. The skin also can darken in diseases such as hemochromatosis or hemosiderosis or in response to many medications that are applied to the skin, swallowed, or injected.

Albinism

Albinism is a rare, inherited disorder in which no melanin is formed.

People with albinism (albinos) have white hair, pale skin, and pink eyes. Often, they also have abnormal vision and involuntary eye movements (nystagmus).

Because melanin protects the skin from the sun, albinos are prone to sunburn and, therefore, to skin cancers. They can minimize these problems by staying out of direct sunlight, wearing sunglasses, and applying sunscreen with a sun protection factor (SPF) rating higher than 15 to uncovered areas of the skin.

Vitiligo

Vitiligo is a condition in which a loss of melanocytes results in smooth, whitish patches of skin.

In some people, one or two sharply demarcated patches appear; in others, patches of vitiligo appear over a large part of the body. The changes are most striking in darkly pigmented people. As in albinism, the unpigmented skin is extremely prone to sunburn. The areas of skin affected by vitiligo also produce white hair because the melanocytes are lost from the hair follicles.

Vitiligo may occur after unusual physical trauma, especially head injury, and tends to occur with certain other diseases, including Addison's disease, diabetes, pernicious anemia, and thyroid disease. Vitiligo may be devastating psychologically because of the extreme disfigurement that results from the pigmentary change.

Tinea versicolor is a fungal infection of the skin that may appear similar to vitiligo, though sometimes it results in hyperpigmentation.▲

Treatment

No cure is known for vitiligo. Small areas can be camouflaged with various dyes that won't soil clothing and may last for several days. Psoralens (light-sensitive drugs) plus ultraviolet A light

▲ see page 981

(PUVA) treatment is sometimes effective, but the treatment takes a long time and must be continued indefinitely. Sunscreen and coverings that protect against sun exposure can prevent sunburn.

Pigment Loss After Skin Damage

Skin sometimes loses its pigment after certain skin diseases such as blisters, ulcers, burns, and skin infections heal. The skin is usually not as ivory white as in vitiligo, and pigmentation may return eventually. Cosmetics can hide this type of blemish.

Melasma

Melasma appears on the face (usually the forehead, cheeks, temples, and jaws) as a roughly symmetric group of dark brown patches of pigmentation that are often clearly delineated.

Melasma is most likely to appear during pregnancy (mask of pregnancy) and also may appear in women who take oral contraceptives. The darkening usually fades somewhat after a woman gives birth or stops using oral contraceptives.

People with melasma can use sunscreens on the dark patches and avoid sun exposure to prevent the condition from getting worse. If applied regularly for a long time, prescription ointments can lighten the dark patches.

CHAPTER 207

Noncancerous Skin Growths

Skin growths, which are abnormal accumulations of different types of cells, may be present at birth or develop later. When the growth is controlled and the cells don't spread to other parts of the body, the skin growths (tumors) are noncancerous (benign). When the growth is uncontrolled and the cells invade normal tissue and even spread (metastasize) to other parts of the body, the tumors are cancerous (malignant).

Moles

Moles (nevi) are small, usually dark, skin growths that develop from pigment-producing cells in the skin (melanocytes).

Moles vary in size, may be flat or raised, may be smooth or rough (wart-like), and may have hairs growing from them. Although they're usually dark brown or black, moles can be flesh-colored or yellow-brown. Almost everyone has about 10 moles, which commonly develop in childhood or adolescence. Like all cells, pigment cells respond to changes in hormone levels, so moles may appear, enlarge, or darken during pregnancy.

Depending on their appearance and location, moles may be considered either blemishes or beauty marks. Moles that are unattractive or located where clothing can irritate them can be removed by a doctor using a scalpel and a local anesthetic.

Most moles are harmless and don't have to be removed. However, some moles closely resemble malignant melanoma, a skin cancer, and can be difficult to distinguish from it. Also, noncancerous moles can develop into malignant melanoma. In fact, nearly half of all malignant melanomas begin in moles, so a mole that looks suspicious should be removed and examined under a microscope. *Changes in a mole—such as enlargement (especially with an irregular border), darkening, inflammation, spotty color changes, bleeding, broken skin (sore), itching, and pain—are warnings of malignant melanoma.* If a mole proves to be cancerous, additional surgery may be needed to remove skin surrounding it.

Atypical Moles

Atypical moles (dysplastic nevi) are flat or raised dark skin growths, but they are bigger than ordinary moles (larger than a half inch across) and are not necessarily round. They vary in color from tan to dark brown, usually on a pink background.

Some people have more than 100 atypical moles, and new ones may keep appearing even after middle age. Atypical moles may appear anywhere on the body, although they're more common on covered areas, such as the buttocks, breasts, and scalp—a considerably different distribution than that of ordinary moles.

The tendency to grow atypical moles is hereditary, though some people without a family history can develop them. A person who has atypical moles and two or more close family members who have had many atypical moles and melanoma (dysplastic nevus syndrome) has a high risk of developing malignant melanoma. Whether the risk of melanoma is high in people who have atypical moles but no family history of melanoma is unknown.

People with atypical moles—particularly those with a family history of melanoma—must look for any changes that might indicate malignant melanoma. They should have their skin checked yearly by their primary care doctor or dermatologist. Dermatologists observe atypical moles to monitor subtle changes, such as a change in color or size; to help monitor such changes, dermatologists often use full-body color photographs. Any such change in an atypical mole means that the mole should be removed.

Some experts think that sunlight accelerates the development of and changes in atypical moles. People with atypical moles should avoid sun exposure. When in the sun, they should always use a sunscreen with a sun protection factor (SPF) rating of at least 15. These sunscreens can provide a shield against cancer-producing ultraviolet (UV) rays.▲

Skin Tags

Skin tags are soft, small, flesh-colored or slightly darker skin flaps that appear mostly on the neck, in the armpits, or in the groin.

Usually, skin tags cause no trouble, but they may be unattractive, and clothing or nearby skin may rub and irritate them. A doctor can easily remove a skin tag by either freezing it with liquid nitrogen or cutting it off with a scalpel or scissors.

▲ see page 985

Lipomas

Lipomas are soft deposits of fatty material that grow under the skin, causing round or oval lumps.

Some people develop only one lipoma, while others develop many. Lipomas are more common in women than in men, and although lipomas can develop anywhere on the body, they are particularly common on the forearms, torso, and back of the neck. Lipomas rarely cause problems, though they may occasionally be painful.

Usually, a doctor can easily recognize lipomas, and no tests are required for diagnosis. These growths aren't cancers and rarely become cancerous. If a lipoma begins to change in any way, a doctor may perform a biopsy (removal of a specimen and examination under a microscope). Treatment usually isn't required, but bothersome lipomas may be removed by surgery or liposuction.

Angiomas

Angiomas are collections of abnormally dense blood or lymph vessels that are usually located in and below the skin and that cause red or purple discolorations.

Angiomas often appear at birth or soon afterward and may be referred to as birthmarks. (Other types of growths present at birth are also called birthmarks.) About a third of all newborns have angiomas, which vary in appearance from person to person and generally cause only cosmetic problems. Many disappear by themselves. Examples of angiomas are port-wine stains, strawberry marks, cavernous hemangiomas, spider angiomas, and lymphangiomas.

PORT-WINE STAINS

Port-wine stains (nevi flammeus) are flat, pink, red, or purplish discolorations present at birth.

Port-wine stains are usually permanent, but small ones on the face may disappear within a few months. Most port-wine stains are physically harmless, but may be psychologically devastating. Occasionally, they can appear in conjunction with Sturge-Weber syndrome, a rare genetic disorder that leads to mental retardation. Small port-wine stains can be covered with cosmetic cream. If the stain is bothersome, it can be removed with a laser.

STRAWBERRY MARKS

Strawberry marks (capillary hemangiomas) are raised, bright red areas that vary from $1/2$ inch to 4 inches across.

Strawberry marks usually develop soon after birth and tend to enlarge slowly during the first several months of life. More than three quarters of them completely disappear by age 7, but some leave a wrinkled, brownish area. Strawberry marks don't usually need treatment unless they appear near the eyes or other vital organs, where they can interfere with body functions. The corticosteroid drug prednisone may be taken orally to shrink the marks; it's most effective when taken soon after the marks start enlarging. Strawberry marks are rarely removed surgically because extensive scarring is likely.

CAVERNOUS HEMANGIOMAS

Cavernous hemangiomas are raised red or purplish areas made up of abnormal, enlarged blood vessels that are present at birth.

Cavernous hemangiomas sometimes become sore and bleed, after which they may partially disappear. They rarely disappear entirely without treatment. In children, oral prednisone may eliminate cavernous hemangiomas. Small cavernous hemangiomas can sometimes be eradicated by electrocoagulation, a procedure in which a local anesthetic is administered and then a hot electric probe is used to destroy the abnormal tissue. Sometimes, surgical removal is needed, especially when the increased blood flow of the cavernous hemangioma causes an arm or leg to enlarge.

SPIDER ANGIOMAS

Spider angiomas are bright red areas that usually have a central reddish to purplish spot with slender projections resembling spider legs.

Putting pressure on the central spot (the blood vessel that is the source of blood in a spider angioma) can temporarily make the color fade. Spider angiomas often occur in small numbers. People with cirrhosis of the liver often develop many spider angiomas, as do many women who are pregnant or who are using oral contraceptives. Spider angiomas generally cause no symptoms in any of these conditions; the marks disappear without treatment 6 to 9 months after childbirth or after stopping oral contraceptive use. If treatment is desired for cosmetic reasons, the central

blood vessel can be destroyed by electrocoagulation (therapy using a local anesthetic and a heated electric probe).

LYMPHANGIOMAS

Lymphangiomas are skin bumps caused by a collection of enlarged lymphatic vessels—the channels that carry lymph (a clear fluid related to blood) throughout the body.

Most lymphangiomas are yellowish-tan, but a few are reddish. When injured or punctured, they release a colorless fluid. Although treatment isn't usually needed, lymphangiomas can be removed surgically. However, such surgery requires the removal of much dermal and subcutaneous tissue because lymphangiomas grow deep beneath the surface.

Pyogenic Granulomas

Pyogenic granulomas are scarlet, brown, or blue-black slightly raised areas caused by increased growth of capillaries (the smallest blood vessels) and swelling of the surrounding tissue.

The condition develops rapidly, usually after injury to the skin. Pyogenic granulomas may bleed easily because the skin covering them is often thin. For unknown reasons, large pyogenic granulomas may develop during pregnancy, appearing even on the gums (pregnancy tumors). Pyogenic granulomas sometimes disappear by themselves, but if they persist, a doctor may perform a biopsy (removal of a specimen and examination under a microscope) to make sure they aren't melanoma or another cancer. When necessary, pyogenic granulomas can be removed surgically or by electrocoagulation (therapy using a local anesthetic and a heated electric probe), but they may come back after treatment.

Seborrheic Keratoses

Seborrheic keratoses (sometimes called seborrheic warts) are flesh-colored, brown, or black growths that can appear anywhere on the skin.

These keratoses most often appear on the torso and the temples; in blacks, especially women, they often appear on the face. They are most common in middle-aged and older people; their cause isn't known.

Seborrheic keratoses vary in size and grow very slowly. They may be round or oval, appear to be stuck on the skin, and often have waxy or scaly surfaces. These growths aren't cancerous and don't become so. Treatment isn't needed unless the keratoses become irritated or itchy or are cosmetically undesirable. They can be removed by freezing them with liquid nitrogen or by cutting them out with a scalpel while the area is anesthetized; either procedure leaves little or no scarring.

Dermatofibromas

Dermatofibromas are small, red-to-brown bumps (nodules) that result from an accumulation of fibroblasts, the cells that populate the soft tissue under the skin.

The cause of dermatofibromas isn't known. They are common and usually appear as single, firm bumps, often on the legs; some people develop many dermatofibromas. They may cause itching. Usually, dermatofibromas aren't treated unless they become bothersome or enlarge. They can be surgically removed while the area is anesthetized.

Keratoacanthomas

Keratoacanthomas are round, firm, usually flesh-colored growths that have an unusual central crater containing a pasty material..

Commonly, keratoacanthomas appear on the face, forearm, and back of the hand and grow quickly. In 1 or 2 months, they can grow up to 2 inches wide. In a few months, they often begin to disappear but may leave scars.

Keratoacanthomas aren't cancerous, but they can closely resemble squamous cell carcinoma, a type of skin cancer; therefore, doctors often perform a biopsy (removal of a specimen and examination under a microscope). Keratoacanthomas can be treated surgically or with injections of corticosteroids or fluorouracil; both techniques get rid of the keratoacanthomas and usually leave much less scarring than if the growths were left to disappear by themselves.

Keloids

Keloids are smooth, shiny, slightly pink, often dome-shaped, proliferative growths of fibrous tissue that form over areas of injury or over surgical wounds.

These growths can even result from severe acne. Sometimes, they form without any injury. They are much more common in blacks than in whites.

Keloids respond poorly to therapy, but monthly injections of corticosteroid drugs may flatten them somewhat. A doctor may try surgical or laser removal followed by corticosteroid injections, but the results are rarely perfect. Some doctors have applied silicone patches to keloids and have had some success in flattening them.

CHAPTER 208

Skin Cancers

Skin cancer is the most common form of cancer, but most types of skin cancers are curable. The more common forms of skin cancer usually develop on sun-exposed areas. People who have had a lot of sun exposure, particularly people with fair complexions, are most likely to develop skin cancer.

Basal Cell Carcinoma

Basal cell carcinoma is a cancer that originates in the lowest layer of the epidermis.

Basal cell carcinoma usually develops on skin surfaces that are exposed to sunlight. The tumors begin as very small, shiny, firm, raised growths on the skin (nodules) and enlarge very slowly, sometimes so slowly that they go unnoticed as new growths. However, the growth rate varies greatly from tumor to tumor with some growing as much as $\frac{1}{2}$ inch in a year. Basal cell carcinomas may ulcerate or form scabs in the center. They sometimes grow flatter and look somewhat like scars. The border of the cancer sometimes takes on a pearly white appearance. The cancer may alternately bleed and form a scab and heal, leading a person to think that it's a sore rather than a cancer. Actually, this alternate bleeding and healing is often a significant sign of basal cell carcinoma or squamous cell carcinoma.

Rather than spread (metastasize) to distant parts of the body, basal cell carcinomas usually invade and destroy surrounding tissues. When basal cell carcinomas grow near the eye, mouth, bone, or brain, the consequences of invasion can be serious. Yet, for most people, they simply grow slowly into the skin. Nonetheless, removing the carcinomas early can prevent extensive damage to the underlying structures.

Diagnosis and Treatment

A doctor can often recognize a basal cell carcinoma simply by looking at it. A biopsy (removal of a tissue specimen and examination under a microscope) is the standard procedure for confirming the diagnosis.

In the office, a doctor can usually remove all the cancer by scraping and burning it with an electric needle (curettage and electrodesiccation) or by cutting it out. Before performing these procedures, the doctor anesthetizes the area. Rarely, radiation treatment is used. For recurrent tumors and scar-like basal cell carcinomas, microscopically controlled surgery (Mohs' surgery) may be required.

Creams used to treat the cancer, such as fluorouracil, aren't considered appropriate therapy because they sometimes allow the cancer to spread under the healed surface of the skin.

Squamous Cell Carcinoma

Squamous cell carcinoma is cancer that originates in the middle layer of the epidermis.

Squamous cell carcinoma usually develops on sun-exposed areas but may grow anywhere on the skin or in places such as the tongue or the lining of the mouth. It may develop on skin that appears normal or skin that has been damaged—even many years earlier—by sun exposure (actinic keratosis).

Squamous cell carcinoma begins as a red area with a scaly, crusted surface that doesn't heal. As it grows, the tumor may become somewhat raised and firm, sometimes with a wart-like surface. Eventually, the cancer becomes an open sore and grows into the underlying tissue.

Most squamous cell carcinomas affect only the area around them, penetrating deep into nearby tissues. But some spread (metastasize) to distant parts of the body and can be fatal.

Warning Signs of Melanoma

Enlarging pigmented (especially black or deep blue) spot or mole

Changes in color of an existing mole, especially the spread of red, white, and blue pigmentation to surrounding skin

Changes in characteristics of skin over the pigmented spot, such as changes in consistency or shape

Signs of inflammation on skin surrounding an existing mole

Bowen's disease is a form of squamous cell carcinoma that's confined to the epidermis and hasn't yet invaded the underlying dermis. The affected skin is red-brown and scaly or crusted and flat, sometimes looking like a patch of psoriasis, dermatitis, or a fungal infection.

Diagnosis and Treatment

When doctors suspect squamous cell carcinoma, they perform a biopsy (removal of a tissue specimen and examination under a microscope) to differentiate this skin cancer from similar-looking diseases.

Squamous cell carcinoma and Bowen's disease are treated by removing the tumor using the same methods described for basal cell carcinoma. Actinic keratosis, a warty irregularity on the skin surface that may turn into squamous cell carcinoma, is often treated by destroying it with liquid nitrogen or by applying fluorouracil cream that kills the rapidly dividing skin cells.

Melanoma

Melanoma is a cancer that originates in the pigment-producing cells of the skin (melanocytes).

Melanoma can begin as a new, small, pigmented skin growth on normal skin, most often on sun-exposed areas, but nearly half of the cases develop from existing pigmented moles.▲ Unlike other forms of skin cancer, melanoma readily

---

▲ see page 989

spreads (metastasizes) to distant parts of the body, where it continues to grow and destroy tissue.

The less a melanoma has grown into the skin, the greater the chance of curing it. If a melanoma has grown deep into the skin, it's more likely to spread through the lymph and blood vessels and can cause death within months or a few years. The course of the disease varies greatly and appears to depend on the strength of the body's immune defenses. Some people survive in apparent good health for many years despite the spread of the melanoma.

Diagnosis and Treatment

When melanoma is suspected, a biopsy (removal of a tissue specimen and examination under a microscope) is performed. Small growths are removed entirely, but only a small piece is removed from larger growths. In either case, a pathologist examines the tissue microscopically to determine if the growth is a melanoma.

Surgery can remove the entire melanoma; if the melanoma hasn't spread, the cure rate approaches 100 percent. However, anyone who has had a melanoma is at risk of developing others. Therefore, such people need regular skin examinations.

Although chemotherapy is used to treat melanomas that have spread, cure rates are low, and the condition is often fatal. However, experimental treatment with interleukin-2 immunotherapy has yielded promising results.

Kaposi's Sarcoma

Kaposi's sarcoma is a cancer that originates in the blood vessels, usually of the skin.

Kaposi's sarcoma takes two forms. One is a disease of older people, usually of European, Jewish, or Italian heritage, in whom the cancer grows very slowly on the skin and rarely spreads. The second form occurs in children and young men in equatorial Africa and in people with AIDS. This form of Kaposi's sarcoma grows much more quickly and often involves blood vessels in internal organs.

▲ see page 1107

In older men, Kaposi's sarcoma usually appears as a purple or dark brown spot on the toes or leg. The cancer may grow to several inches or more, as a deeply colored, flat, or slightly raised area that tends to bleed and ulcerate. The cancer may spread slowly up the leg.

In Africans and people with AIDS, Kaposi's sarcoma usually first appears as a pink, red, or purple spot that may be round or oval. These spots may appear anywhere on the body, often on the face. In several months, the spots may appear in several areas of the body, including the mouth; they may also develop in internal organs and lymph nodes, where they can cause internal bleeding.

Treatment

Elderly men with slow-growing Kaposi's sarcoma and no other symptoms may not need treatment at all. However, the spots can be treated by freezing, x-ray therapy, or electrocautery (tissue destruction using an electric probe).

In people with AIDS and others with the more aggressive form, treatment hasn't been very successful. Chemotherapy using drugs such as etoposide, vincristine, vinblastine, bleomycin, and doxorubicin has produced disappointing results. Interferon-alfa may slow the progression of the early skin growths, and an injection of vincristine into the growths may make them regress. Treating Kaposi's sarcoma doesn't appear to prolong the lives of people with AIDS. Improvement of immune status may lead to a regression of Kaposi's sarcoma.

Paget's Disease

Paget's disease is a rare type of skin cancer that looks like an inflamed, reddened patch of skin (dermatitis); it originates in glands in or under the skin. (The term Paget's disease also refers to an unrelated metabolic bone disease; these distinct diseases shouldn't be confused with each other.)

Because Paget's disease usually stems from a cancer of the breast milk ducts, the cancer commonly forms around the nipple.▲ Paget's disease can also appear as a red, oozing, crusting rash in the groin or around the anus; the tumor may originate in nearby sweat glands. Paget's disease is treated by surgically removing the entire growth.

Ear, Nose, and Throat Disorders

CHAPTER 209

Ears, Nose, and Throat

The ears, nose, and throat are closely related, both in location and function. Disorders of these organs are diagnosed and treated by specialists called otolaryngologists.

Ears

The ear, the organ of hearing and balance, consists of the outer, middle, and inner ear. The outer ear captures sound waves, which are converted into mechanical energy by the middle ear. The inner ear converts the mechanical energy into nerve impulses, which then travel to the brain. The inner ear also helps maintain balance.

Outer Ear

The outer ear consists of the external part of the ear (pinna or auricle) and the ear canal (ex-

A Look Inside the Ear

Pinna

Ear canal

Eustachian tube

Middle and Inner Ear

Semicircular canals

Stirrup (stapes)

Anvil (incus)

Hammer (malleus)

Eardrum

Tympanic cavity

Oval window

Auditory nerve

Cochlea

Vestibule

ternal auditory meatus). Consisting of cartilage covered by skin, the pinna is rigid yet flexible. Sounds captured by the pinna travel through the ear canal to the eardrum, a thin membrane covered by skin that separates the outer from the middle ear.

Middle Ear

The middle ear consists of the eardrum (tympanic membrane) and a small air-filled chamber containing a chain of three tiny bones (ossicles) that connect the eardrum to the inner ear. The ossicles are named for their shapes: the hammer (malleus) is attached to the eardrum; the anvil (incus) connects the hammer and stirrup; and the stirrup (stapes) is attached to the oval window at the entrance to the inner ear. Vibrations of the eardrum are amplified mechanically by the ossicles and transmitted to the oval window.

The middle ear also contains two tiny muscles. The tensor tympani, which is attached to the hammer, keeps the eardrum taut; the stapedius muscle, which is attached to the stirrup, stabilizes the connection between the stirrup and the oval window. In response to loud noise, the stapedius muscle contracts, making the chain of ossicles more rigid so that less sound is transmitted. This response, called the acoustic reflex, helps protect the delicate inner ear from sound damage.

The eustachian tube, a small tube that connects the middle ear with the back of the nose, allows outside air to enter the middle ear. This tube, which is opened by swallowing, helps maintain equal air pressure on both sides of the eardrum, which is important for normal hearing and comfort. This is why swallowing can relieve pressure on the eardrum caused by a sudden drop in air pressure, as often occurs when riding in an airplane. The eustachian tube's connection with the middle ear explains why upper respiratory infections (such as the common cold), which inflame and block the eustachian tube, can lead to middle ear infections or to increased pressure in the middle ear, resulting in pain.

Inner Ear

The inner ear (labyrinth) is a complex structure consisting of two major parts: the cochlea, the organ of hearing; and the semicircular canals, the organ of balance.

The cochlea, a hollow tube coiled in the shape of a snail's shell, contains thick fluid and the organ of Corti, consisting of thousands of tiny cells (hair cells) with small hairlike projections that extend into the fluid. Sound vibrations transmitted from the ossicles in the middle ear to the oval window in the inner ear cause the fluid and the hairlike projections to vibrate. Different hair cells respond to different sound frequencies and convert them to nerve impulses. The nerve impulses are transmitted along fibers of the auditory nerve, which take them to the brain.

Despite the protective effect of the acoustic reflex, loud noise can damage hair cells. Once a hair cell is destroyed, it doesn't appear to regrow. Continued exposure to loud noise causes progressive damage and hearing loss.

The semicircular canals, which help maintain balance, are three fluid-filled tubes at right angles to one another. Any movement of the head causes the fluid in the canals to move. Depending on the direction of head movement, the fluid movement may be greater in one of the canals than in another. The canals contain hair cells that respond to movement of the fluid. The hair cells initiate nerve impulses that tell the brain which way the head is moving, so appropriate action can be taken to maintain balance.

If the semicircular canals become inflamed, as happens in a middle ear infection or the flu, a person may lose the sense of balance or develop vertigo (a whirling sensation).▲

Nose

The nose is the organ of smell and the main passageway for airflow into and out of the lungs. The nose also adds resonance to the voice, and the paranasal sinuses and tear ducts drain into it.

The upper part of the nose consists of bone and the lower part of cartilage. Inside is a hollow cavity (nasal cavity) divided into two passages by the nasal septum, which extends from the nostrils to the back of the throat. Bones called nasal conchae project into the nasal cavity, forming a series of folds. The folds greatly increase the surface area that air passes over. Lining the nasal cavity is a mucous membrane with many blood vessels. The increased surface area and the many blood vessels enable the nose to warm and moisten incoming air quickly. Cells in the mucous membrane produce mucus and have tiny hairlike projections (cilia). Usually, the mucus traps incoming dirt particles, which are then moved by the cilia toward the front of the nose or down the throat to be removed from the airway. This action helps clean the air before it goes to the lungs. Sneezing automatically clears the nasal passages in response to irritation, as coughing clears the lungs.

Smell receptor cells are located in the upper part of the nasal cavity. These cells have hairlike projections (cilia) that extend downward into the nasal cavity and nerve fibers that extend upward

A Look Inside the Nose and Throat

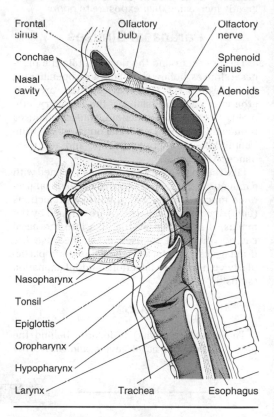

Frontal sinus — Olfactory bulb — Olfactory nerve — Conchae — Sphenoid sinus — Nasal cavity — Adenoids — Nasopharynx — Tonsil — Epiglottis — Oropharynx — Hypopharynx — Larynx — Trachea — Esophagus

to the olfactory bulb, a swelling at the end of each olfactory nerve. The olfactory nerves (nerves of smell) extend directly into the brain.■

The sense of smell, which is not fully understood, is much more sophisticated than the sense of taste. Distinct smells are far more numerous than tastes. The subjective sense of taste while eating involves both taste and smell. That's why food is often somewhat tasteless when a person has a cold and can't smell. Because the smell re-

▲ see page 298

■ see box, page 343

ceptors are located in the upper part of the nose, normal breathing doesn't draw much air over them; however, sniffing draws more air over them, greatly increasing their exposure to odors.

Paranasal Sinuses

The bones around the nose contain the paranasal sinuses, hollow chambers with openings for drainage into the nasal cavity. There are four groups of paranasal sinuses: the maxillary, ethmoid, frontal, and sphenoid sinuses. Sinuses reduce the weight of the facial bones while maintaining bone strength and shape and add resonance to the voice.

Like the nasal cavity, the sinuses are lined with a mucous membrane composed of cells that produce mucus and have tiny hairlike projections (cilia). Incoming dirt particles are trapped by the mucus, then moved by the cilia into the nasal cavity, where the sinuses drain. Because the drainage can be blocked, the sinuses are particularly vulnerable to infections and inflammation (sinusitis).▲

Throat

The throat (pharynx) is located behind the mouth, below the nasal cavity, and above the esophagus and windpipe (trachea). It consists of an upper part—nasopharynx, a middle part—oropharynx, and a lower part—hypopharynx. The throat is a muscular passageway through which food is carried to the esophagus and air to the lungs. Like the nose and mouth, the throat is lined with a mucous membrane composed of cells that produce mucus and have hairlike projections. Dirt particles caught in the mucus are carried by these projections toward the esophagus and are swallowed.

The tonsils are located at the back of the mouth, and the adenoids at the back of the nasal cavity. Tonsils and adenoids consist of lymph tissue and help fight off infections. They are largest during childhood and gradually shrink throughout life.

At the top of the trachea is the voice box (larynx), which contains the vocal cords and is responsible for producing the sounds used in speech. When relaxed, the vocal cords form a V-shaped opening that air can pass through freely. When contracted, they vibrate, generating sounds that can be modified by the tongue, nose, and mouth to produce speech.

The epiglottis, a flap composed mainly of cartilage, is located above and in front of the larynx. During swallowing, the epiglottis closes to prevent food and fluids from entering the trachea.

CHAPTER 210

Hearing Loss and Deafness

Hearing loss is deterioration in hearing; deafness is profound hearing loss.

Hearing loss may be caused by a mechanical problem in the ear canal or middle ear that blocks the conduction of sound (conductive hearing loss) or by damage to the inner ear, auditory nerve, or auditory nerve pathways in the brain (sensorineural hearing loss). The two types of hearing loss can be distinguished by comparing how well a person hears sounds conducted by air with how well the person hears sounds conducted by bones.

Sensorineural hearing loss is categorized as sensory when the inner ear is affected or as neural when the auditory nerve or auditory nerve pathways in the brain are affected. Sensory hearing loss may be hereditary, or it may be caused by very loud noise (acoustic trauma), a viral infection of the inner ear, certain drugs, or Meniere's disease.■ Neural hearing loss may be caused by brain tumors that also damage nearby nerves and the brain stem. Other causes include infections,

---

▲ see page 1016

■ see page 1009

various brain and nerve disorders such as stroke, and some hereditary diseases such as Refsum's disease. In childhood, the auditory nerve can be damaged by mumps, German measles (rubella), meningitis, or inner ear infections. Auditory nerve pathways in the brain can be damaged by demyelinating diseases (diseases that destroy the nerve covering).

Diagnosis

Hearing tests with tuning forks can be conducted in a doctor's office, but hearing is best tested in a soundproof booth by an audiologist (a specialist in hearing loss) using an electronic device that produces sounds at specific pitches and volumes. Hearing by air conduction in adults is tested by placing a vibrating tuning fork near the ear so that sound has to travel through the air to reach the ear. A hearing loss or a subnormal auditory threshold (the faintest sound that can be heard) can indicate a problem in any part of the hearing apparatus—the ear canal, middle ear, inner ear, auditory nerve, or auditory nerve pathways in the brain.

In adults, hearing by bone conduction is tested by placing the base of a vibrating tuning fork against the head. The vibration spreads throughout the skull, including through the bony cochlea in the inner ear. The cochlea contains hair cells that convert the vibrations to nerve impulses, which then travel along the auditory nerve.▲ This test bypasses the outer and middle ear, evaluating only the inner ear, auditory nerve, and auditory nerve pathways in the brain. Tuning forks with a variety of pitches (frequencies) are used because a person may be able to hear sounds at some pitches but not others.

If hearing by air conduction is reduced but hearing by bone conduction is normal, the hearing loss is conductive. If hearing by air and bone conduction is reduced, the hearing loss is sensorineural. Occasionally, hearing loss is both conductive and sensorineural.

Audiometry measures hearing loss precisely with an electronic device (an audiometer) that produces sounds at specific pitches (pure tones) and specific volumes. The auditory threshold for a range of tones is determined by decreasing the volume of each tone until a person can no longer hear it. Each ear is tested separately. Earphones are used to measure air conduction hearing, and a vibrating device is held against the bone behind the ear (mastoid process) to measure bone conduction hearing. Because loud tones presented to one ear may also be heard by the other ear, the test tone is masked by presenting a different sound, usually noise, to the ear not being tested. This way, the person hears the test tone only in the ear being tested.

Speech threshold audiometry measures how loudly words have to be spoken to be understood. A person listens to a series of two-syllable, equally accented words—such as railroad, staircase, and baseball—presented at specific volumes. The volume at which the person can correctly repeat half of the words (spondee threshold) is recorded.

Discrimination, the ability to hear differences between words that sound similar, is tested by presenting pairs of similar one-syllable words. The discrimination score (the percentage of words correctly repeated) is usually in the normal range when hearing loss is conductive, below normal when hearing loss is sensory, and far below normal when hearing loss is neural.

Tympanometry, a type of audiometry, measures the impedance (resistance to pressure) of the middle ear. It's used to help determine the cause of conductive hearing loss. This procedure doesn't require the active participation of the person being tested and is commonly used in children. A device containing a microphone and a sound source that produces continuous sound is placed snugly in the ear canal. The device detects how much sound passes through the middle ear and how much is reflected back as pressure changes in the ear canal. The results of this test indicate whether the problem is a blocked eustachian tube (the tube that connects the middle ear and back of the nose), fluid in the middle ear, or a disruption in the chain of three bones (ossicles) that transmit sounds through the middle ear.

Tympanometry also detects changes in the contraction of the stapedius muscle, which is attached to the stirrup (stapes), one of the three bones in the middle ear. This muscle normally contracts in response to loud noises (acoustic reflex), reducing the transmission of sound and thus protecting the inner ear. The acoustic reflex changes or decays if the hearing loss is neural.

▲ see box, page 996

When the acoustic reflex is decayed, the stapedius muscle can't remain contracted during continuous exposure to loud noise.

Auditory brain stem response is another test that can distinguish between sensory and neural hearing loss. It measures nerve impulses in the brain resulting from stimulation of the auditory nerves. Computer enhancement produces an image of the wave pattern of the nerve impulses. If the cause of hearing loss appears to be in the brain, magnetic resonance imaging (MRI) of the head may be performed.

Electrocochleography measures the activity of the cochlea and the auditory nerve. This test and the auditory brain stem response can be used to measure hearing in people who can't or won't respond voluntarily to sound. For example, these tests are used to find out whether infants and children have profound hearing loss and whether a person is faking or exaggerating hearing loss (psychogenic hypacusis). Sometimes the tests can help determine the cause of sensorineural hearing loss. Auditory brain stem response also can be used to monitor certain brain functions in people who are comatose or in those undergoing brain surgery.

Some hearing tests can detect disorders in the auditory processing areas of the brain. These tests measure the ability to interpret and understand distorted speech, to understand a message presented to one ear when a competing message is presented to the other ear, to fuse incomplete messages to each ear into a meaningful message, and to determine where a sound is coming from when sounds are presented to both ears at the same time.

Because the nerve pathways from each ear cross to the other side of the brain, an abnormality on one side of the brain affects hearing in the ear on the other side. Brain stem lesions can impair the ability to fuse incomplete messages into a meaningful message and to pinpoint where sounds are coming from.

Treatment

Treatment of hearing loss depends on the cause. For example, if fluid in the middle ear or wax in the ear canal is causing a conductive hearing loss, the fluid is drained or the wax removed. Often, no cure is available. In these cases, treatment involves compensating for the hearing loss as much as possible. Most people use a hearing aid. Rarely, a cochlear implant is used.

Hearing Aids

Sound amplification with a hearing aid helps people who have conductive or sensorineural hearing loss, particularly if they have trouble hearing the frequencies of normal speech. Hearing aids also can help people who have predominantly high-frequency sensorineural hearing loss and those who have hearing loss in only one ear. Hearing aids have a microphone to pick up sounds, an amplifier to increase their volume, and a speaker to transmit the amplified sounds.

Air conduction hearing aids, which are generally superior to bone conduction hearing aids, are most commonly used. Usually, they're fitted into the ear canal with an airtight seal or a small open tube. Types of air conduction hearing aids include body aids, aids that fit behind the ear, aids that fit in the ear, canal aids, CROS aids, and BICROS aids.

The body aid, used by people who have profound hearing loss, is the most powerful hearing aid. It's kept in a shirt pocket or a body harness and connected by a wire to the earpiece, which has a plastic ear mold that fits into the ear canal. Infants and young children with hearing loss often wear body aids because they're easier to handle and less likely to break, and they eliminate the problems caused by poorly fitting ear molds.

For moderate to severe hearing loss, an aid that fits behind the ear and is connected to an ear mold by flexible tubing may be used. For mild to moderate hearing loss, a less powerful aid contained entirely within the ear mold may be used. It fits in the outer ear and is relatively inconspicuous. An aid that fits entirely within the ear canal (canal aid) is even less conspicuous and is used by people who might otherwise refuse to wear one.

The CROS (contralateral routing of signals) aid is used by people who have hearing in only one ear. The microphone is placed in the nonfunctioning ear, and sound is routed to the functioning ear through a wire or a miniature radio transmitter. This aid enables a person to hear sounds from the nonfunctioning ear's side and, to some extent, locate sounds. If the functioning ear also has some hearing loss, the sound from both sides can be amplified with the BICROS (bilateral CROS) aid.

A **bone conduction hearing aid** may be used by people who can't use air conduction hearing aids—for example, a person who was born without an ear canal or who has an ear discharge (otorrhea). The device is placed in contact with the head, usually just behind the ear, with a spring band over the head. The aid conducts sound through the skull to the inner ear. Bone conduction hearing aids require more power, cause more distortion, and are less comfortable to wear than air conduction hearing aids. Some bone conduction aids can be implanted surgically in the bone behind the ear.

A hearing aid should be selected by a doctor or an audiologist, who matches the characteristics of the aid with the type of hearing loss, including the degree of loss and the frequencies affected. For example, high frequencies can be enhanced by vents in the ear mold that facilitate the passage of sound waves into the ear. An aid with a vented ear mold benefits many people whose sensorineural hearing loss is greater in high frequencies than in low frequencies. People who can't tolerate loud sounds may need hearing aids with special electronic circuitry that keeps the volume of sound at a tolerable level.

Several types of devices are available for people who have a significant hearing loss. Light alerting systems enable them to know when the door bell is ringing or a baby is crying. Special sound systems help them hear in theaters, churches, or other places where there is competing noise. Telephone communication devices are also available.

Cochlear Implants

A profoundly deaf person who can't hear sounds even with a hearing aid may benefit from a cochlear implant. The implant consists of electrodes inserted into the cochlea and an internal coil implanted in the skull; they are supplemented by an external coil, a speech processor, and a microphone located outside the body. The microphone picks up sound waves and the processor converts them to electrical impulses, which are transmitted by the external coil through the skin to the internal coil and then to the electrodes. The electrodes stimulate the auditory nerve.

A cochlear implant doesn't transmit sounds as well as a normal cochlea but provides different benefits to different people. It helps some people read lips. Others can distinguish some words without reading lips. Some people can hear on the telephone.

A cochlear implant also helps deaf people hear and distinguish environmental and warning signals, such as doorbells, telephones, and alarms.

Cochlear Implant: Aid for the Profoundly Deaf

A cochlear implant, a type of hearing aid for profoundly deaf people, consists of an internal coil, electrodes, an external coil, a speech processor, and a microphone. The internal coil is surgically implanted in the skull behind and above the ear, and the electrodes are implanted in the cochlea. The external coil is held in place by magnets on the skin over the internal coil. The speech processor, connected to the external coil by a wire, may be worn in a pocket or special holster. The microphone is placed in a hearing aid worn behind the ear.

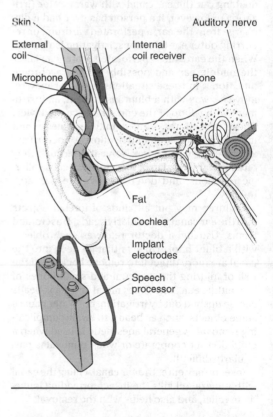

Skin
External coil
Microphone
Auditory nerve
Internal coil receiver
Bone
Fat
Cochlea
Implant electrodes
Speech processor

It helps them modulate their own voices to make their speech easier for others to understand. A cochlear implant is more effective in a person whose hearing loss is recent or who had successfully used a hearing aid before the implant.

Outer Ear Disorders

The outer ear consists of the external part of the ear (pinna or auricle) and the ear canal (external auditory meatus).▲ Disorders of the outer ear include blockages, infections, injuries, and tumors.

Blockages

Earwax (cerumen) may block the ear canal and cause itching, pain, and a temporary loss of hearing. A doctor may remove the earwax by gently flushing out the ear canal with warm water (irrigation). However, if a person has ever had a discharge from the ear, a perforated eardrum, or recurring outer ear infections, irrigation isn't used. When the eardrum is perforated, water can enter the middle ear and possibly worsen a chronic infection.■ In these situations, a doctor may remove earwax with a blunt instrument, an instrument with a loop at the end, or a vacuum device. These procedures are generally less messy and more comfortable than irrigation. A doctor usually doesn't use earwax solvents because they often irritate the skin of the ear canal, cause allergic reactions, and don't dissolve the wax adequately.

Children may put all kinds of foreign objects into the ear canal, particularly beads, erasers, and beans. Usually, a doctor removes such objects with a blunt hook. Objects that go deep into the canal are more difficult to remove because of the risk of injuring the eardrum and small bones of the middle ear. Sometimes metal and glass beads can be flushed out by irrigation, but water causes some objects, such as beans, to swell, complicating removal. A general anesthetic is used when a child doesn't cooperate or when removal is particularly difficult.

Insects may enter the ear canal. Filling the canal with mineral oil kills the insect, providing immediate relief, and also helps with the removal.

▲ see box, page 996

■ see page 1008

External Otitis

External otitis is an infection of the ear canal.

The infection may affect the entire canal, as in generalized external otitis, or just one small area, as a boil (furuncle). External otitis, often called swimmer's ear, is most common during the summer swimming season.

Causes

A variety of bacteria, or rarely, fungi, can cause generalized external otitis; the bacterium *Staphylococcus* usually causes boils. Certain people, including those who have allergies, psoriasis, eczema, or scalp dermatitis, are particularly prone to external otitis. Injuring the ear canal while cleaning it or getting water or irritants such as hair spray or hair dye in the canal often leads to external otitis.

The ear canal cleans itself by moving dead skin cells from the eardrum out through the canal as if they were on a conveyor belt. Attempting to clean the canal with cotton swabs interrupts this self-cleaning mechanism and can push debris toward the eardrum, where it accumulates. Accumulated debris and earwax tend to trap water that gets into the ear canal during a shower or while swimming. The resulting wet, softened skin in the ear canal is more easily infected by bacteria or fungi.

Symptoms

Symptoms of generalized external otitis are itching, pain, and a malodorous discharge. If the ear canal swells or fills with pus and debris, hearing is impaired. Usually, the canal is tender and hurts if the external ear (pinna) is pulled or if pressure is placed on the fold of skin in front of the ear canal. To a doctor looking into the ear canal through an otoscope (a device for viewing the canal and eardrum), the skin of the canal appears red, swollen, and littered with pus and debris.

Boils cause severe pain. When they rupture, a small amount of blood and pus may leak from the ear.

Treatment

To treat generalized external otitis, a doctor first removes the infected debris from the canal with suction or dry cotton wipes. After the ear canal is cleared, hearing frequently returns to normal. Usually, a person is given antibiotic ear drops to instill in the ear several times a day for up to a week. Some ear drops also contain a corticosteroid to reduce swelling. Sometimes ear drops containing diluted acetic acid are prescribed to help restore the acidity of the ear canal. Analgesics such as acetaminophen or codeine may help reduce pain for the first 24 to 48 hours, until the inflammation begins to subside. An infection that has spread beyond the ear canal (cellulitis) may be treated with an antibiotic given by mouth.

Boils are allowed to drain on their own because cutting them open can spread the infection. Antibiotic ear drops are not effective. A heating pad applied for a short time and analgesics can help relieve pain and speed healing.

Perichondritis

Perichondritis is an infection of the cartilage of the external ear.

Injury, insect bites, or an incised boil on the ear may cause perichondritis. Pus accumulates between the cartilage and the layer of connective tissue around it (perichondrium). Sometimes the pus cuts off the blood supply to the cartilage, destroying it and leading eventually to a deformed ear. Although destructive and long lasting, perichondritis tends to produce only mild symptoms.

A doctor makes an incision to drain the pus, allowing blood to reach the cartilage again. Antibiotics are given by mouth for milder infections and intravenously for severe infections. The choice of antibiotic depends on how severe the infection is and which bacteria are causing it.

Eczema

Eczema of the ear is an inflammation of the skin in the external ear and ear canal, characterized by itching, redness, peeling, cracking, and a discharge from the ear.

This condition can lead to an infection of the external ear and ear canal. Treatment consists of applying a solution containing aluminum acetate (Burow's solution) directly to the area. A corticosteroid cream or ointment may reduce the itch-

Irrigating the Ear Canal

The tip of a water-filled syringe is placed just inside the ear canal, and a stream of warm water is instilled into the canal to remove earwax. This procedure should be performed by a doctor or nurse.

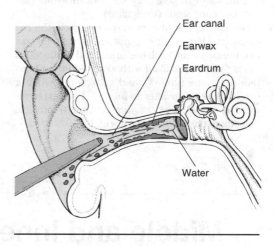

ing and inflammation. If the inflamed area becomes infected, antibiotics may be applied directly to the affected skin. This condition tends to recur.

Injury

An injury such as a blunt blow to the external ear can cause bruising between the cartilage and the layer of connective tissue around it (perichondrium). When blood collects in this area, the external ear becomes a misshapen, reddish purple mass. The collected blood (hematoma) can cut off the blood supply to the cartilage, leading to a deformed ear. This deformity, called a cauliflower ear, is common among wrestlers and boxers. Usually, a doctor uses suction to remove the hematoma, and suction is continued until all evidence of the hematoma is gone, usually 3 to 7 days. Treatment causes the skin and perichondrium to return to their normal positions, allowing blood to reach the cartilage again.

If a cut (laceration) goes all the way through the ear, the skin is sewn back together and a splint is attached to the cartilage to allow healing.

A forceful blow to the jaw may fracture the bones surrounding the ear canal and distort the canal's shape, often narrowing it. The shape can be corrected surgically; general anesthesia is required.

Tumors

Tumors of the ear may be noncancerous (benign) or cancerous (malignant).

Noncancerous tumors may develop in the ear canal, blocking it and causing a buildup of earwax and hearing loss. Such tumors include sebaceous cysts (small sacs filled with skin secretions), osteomas (bone tumors), and keloids (growths of excess scar tissue after an injury). The best treatment is removal of the tumor. After treatment, hearing usually returns to normal.

Ceruminoma (cancer of the cells that produce earwax) develops in the outer third of the ear canal and can spread. Treatment consists of surgical removal of the cancer and the surrounding tissue.

Basal cell and squamous cell cancers▲ are common skin cancers that often develop on the external ear after repeated and prolonged exposure to the sun. When these cancers first appear, they can be successfully treated by excising them or by applying radiation therapy. More advanced cancers may require surgical removal of a larger area of the external ear. When the cancer has invaded the cartilage of the ear, surgery is more effective than radiation therapy.

Basal cell and squamous cell cancers also may develop in or spread to the ear canal. Their treatment consists of surgically removing the cancer and a wide margin of the surrounding tissue, followed by radiation therapy.

CHAPTER 212

Middle and Inner Ear Disorders

The middle ear consists of the eardrum (tympanic membrane) and an air-filled chamber containing a chain of three bones (ossicles) that connect the eardrum to the inner ear.■ The fluid-filled inner ear (labyrinth) consists of two major parts: the cochlea (the organ of hearing) and the semicircular canals (the organ of balance). Middle and inner ear disorders produce many of the same symptoms, and a disorder of the middle ear may affect the inner ear and vice versa.

Middle Ear Disorders

Middle ear disorders produce symptoms such as discomfort, pain, and a sense of fullness or pressure in the ear, as well as a discharge of fluid

or pus, hearing loss, tinnitus (noise in the ear), and vertigo (a whirling sensation).★ These symptoms may be caused by an infection, injury, or pressure in the middle ear resulting from a blocked eustachian tube (the tube that connects the middle ear and back of the nose). When an infection is the cause, additional symptoms such as fever and weakness may affect the whole body.

Perforation of the Eardrum

The eardrum may be perforated (punctured) by objects placed in the ear, such as a cotton-tipped swab, or by objects entering the ear accidentally, such as a low-hanging twig or a thrown pencil. The eardrum also can be perforated by a sudden increase in pressure—such as that caused by an explosion, a slap, or a swimming or diving accident—or a sudden decrease in pressure. An object that penetrates the eardrum can dislocate the chain of small bones (ossicles) in the middle ear or may fracture the stirrup, one of the ossicles. Pieces of the broken ossicles or the object may penetrate the inner ear.

▲ see page 992

■ see page 996

★ see page 298

Tinnitus

Tinnitus is noise originating in the ear rather than in the environment. Why tinnitus occurs isn't known, but it can be a symptom of almost any ear disorder, including the following:

- Ear infections
- Blocked ear canal
- Blocked eustachian tube
- Otosclerosis
- Tumors of the middle ear
- Meniere's disease
- Damage to the ear caused by drugs (such as aspirin and some antibiotics)
- Hearing loss
- Blast injury from a blast or explosion

Tinnitus may also occur with other disorders, including anemia, heart and blood vessel disorders such as hypertension and arteriosclerosis, low thyroid hormone levels in the blood (hypothyroidism), and a head injury.

The noise may be a buzzing, ringing, roaring, whistling, or hissing in the ears. Some people hear more complex sounds that vary over time. The sounds may be intermittent, continuous, or pulsating in time with the heartbeat. A pulsating sound may result from a blocked artery, an aneurysm, a tumor in a blood vessel, or other blood vessel disorders. Because a person who has tinnitus usually has some hearing loss, thorough hearing tests are performed as well as magnetic resonance imaging (MRI) of the head and computed tomography (CT) of the temporal bone (the skull bone that contains part of the ear canal, the middle ear, and the inner ear).

Attempts to identify and treat the disorder causing tinnitus are often unsuccessful. Various techniques can help make tinnitus tolerable, although the ability to tolerate it varies from person to person. Often a hearing aid helps suppress tinnitus. Many people find relief by playing background music to mask the tinnitus. Some people use a tinnitus masker, a device worn like a hearing aid that produces pleasant sounds. For the profoundly deaf, a cochlear implant may reduce tinnitus.

Symptoms

Perforation of the eardrum causes sudden severe pain, followed by bleeding from the ear, hearing loss, and tinnitus (noise in the ear). The hearing loss is more severe if the chain of ossicles has been disrupted or the inner ear has been injured. Injury to the inner ear also can cause vertigo. Pus may begin to drain from the ear in 24 to 48 hours, particularly if water enters the middle ear.

Treatment

An antibiotic usually is given by mouth to prevent infection. The ear is kept dry. Ear drops containing an antibiotic may be used if the ear becomes infected. Usually, the eardrum heals without further treatment, but if it doesn't heal within 2 months, surgery to repair the eardrum (tympanoplasty) may be needed.

A persistent conductive hearing loss▲ suggests a disruption of the ossicles, which can be repaired surgically. A sensorineural hearing loss or vertigo that persists for more than a few hours after the injury suggests that something has penetrated the inner ear. In this case, a surgical procedure called tympanotomy is usually performed to inspect the area and repair the damage.

Barotitis Media

Barotitis media (aerotitis) is damage to the middle ear caused by unequal air pressure on the two sides of the eardrum.

The eardrum separates the ear canal and the middle ear. If air pressure in the ear canal from outside air and air pressure in the middle ear are unequal, the eardrum can be damaged. Normally, the eustachian tube, which connects the middle ear and the back of the nose, helps maintain equal pressure on both sides of the eardrum by allowing outside air to enter the middle ear. When outside air pressure suddenly increases—for instance, during the descent of an airplane or a deep-sea

---

▲ see page 998

Pressure in the Middle Ear

The eustachian tube helps maintain equal air pressure on both sides of the eardrum by allowing outside air to enter the middle ear. If the eustachian tube is blocked, air can't reach the middle ear, so the pressure there falls. When air pressure is lower in the middle ear than in the ear canal, the eardrum bulges inward. The pressure difference can cause pain and can bruise or rupture the eardrum.

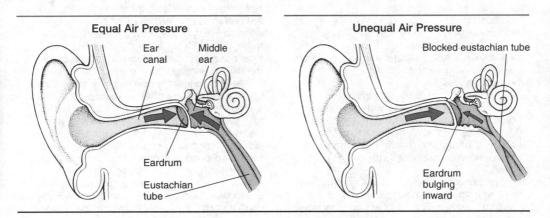

Equal Air Pressure

Ear canal   Middle ear

Eardrum

Eustachian tube

Unequal Air Pressure

Blocked eustachian tube

Eardrum bulging inward

dive—air must move through the eustachian tube to equalize the pressure in the middle ear.▲

If the eustachian tube is partly or completely blocked because of scarring, an infection, or an allergy, air can't reach the middle ear, and the resulting pressure difference may bruise the eardrum or even cause it to rupture and bleed. If the pressure difference is very great, the oval window (the entrance into the inner ear from the middle ear) may rupture, allowing fluid from the inner ear to leak into the middle ear. Hearing loss or vertigo occurring during descent in a deep-sea dive suggests that such leakage is taking place. The same symptoms occurring during ascent suggest that a bubble of air has formed in the inner ear.

When sudden changes in pressure during an airplane flight cause a sense of fullness or pain in the ear, often the pressure in the middle ear can be equalized and the discomfort relieved by breathing with the mouth open, chewing gum, or swallowing. People who have an infection or an allergy affecting the nose and throat may experience discomfort when they fly in a plane or dive. However, if either activity is necessary, a decongestant such as phenylephrine nose drops or nasal spray relieves congestion and helps open the eustachian tubes, equalizing pressure on the eardrums.

Infectious Myringitis

Infectious myringitis is an inflammation of the eardrum resulting from a viral or bacterial infection.

Small, fluid-filled blisters (vesicles) develop on the eardrum. Pain begins suddenly and lasts for 24 to 48 hours. If a person has a fever and any hearing loss, the infection is probably bacterial.

The infection is often treated with antibiotics. Analgesics are given, or the vesicles are ruptured to relieve the pain.

Acute Otitis Media

Acute otitis media is a bacterial or viral infection of the middle ear.

Although this disorder can develop in people of all ages, it's most common in young children,

▲ see page 1351

particularly those between the ages of 3 months and 3 years. Usually, this disorder develops as a complication of the common cold. Viruses or bacteria from the throat can reach the middle ear through the eustachian tube or occasionally through the bloodstream. Viral otitis media is usually followed by bacterial otitis media.

Symptoms

Usually, the first symptom is a persistent, severe earache. Temporary hearing loss may occur. Young children may have nausea, vomiting, diarrhea, and a temperature of up to 105 F. The eardrum becomes inflamed and may bulge. If the eardrum ruptures, discharge from the ear may be bloody at first, then change to clear fluid and finally to pus.

Serious complications include infections of the surrounding bone (mastoiditis or petrositis), infection of the semicircular canals (labyrinthitis), paralysis of the face, hearing loss, inflammation of the covering of the brain (meningitis), and brain abscess. Signs of an impending complication include a headache, sudden profound hearing loss, vertigo, and chills and fever.

Diagnosis and Treatment

A doctor examines the ear to make a diagnosis. If pus or some other discharge is draining from the ear, a sample is sent to a laboratory and examined to identify the organism causing the infection.

The infection is treated with antibiotics given by mouth. Amoxicillin is often the first choice of antibiotics for people of all ages, but penicillin in large doses may be prescribed for adults. Other antibiotics can also be used. Taking cold medications containing phenylephrine can help keep the eustachian tube open, and antihistamines are useful to people who have allergies. If a person has severe or persistent pain, fever, vomiting, or diarrhea, or if the eardrum is bulging, a doctor may perform a myringotomy, in which an opening is made through the eardrum to allow fluid to drain from the middle ear. The opening, which doesn't affect hearing, heals on its own.

Secretory Otitis Media

Secretory otitis media is a disorder in which fluid accumulates in the middle ear from acute otitis media that hasn't completely cleared or from a blocked eustachian tube.

Earache

An earache is a pain that originates or appears to originate in the outer or middle ear. Earaches may result from inflammation caused by infections or from tumors or other growths in the outer or middle ear. Even a mild inflammation of the outer ear canal can be very painful, and inflammation of the external ear's cartilage (perichondritis) can produce severe pain and tenderness.

Infection of the middle ear (otitis media), the most common cause of earaches in children, produces painful inflammation. Blockage of the eustachian tube (the tube that connects the middle ear and back of the nose) leads to pressure in the middle ear, putting pressure on the eardrum, which results in pain. Rapid pressure changes during an airplane flight cause a transient version of this type of earache; swallowing relieves the pressure and pain.

Pain that feels like an earache may actually come from a nearby structure that shares the same nerves to the brain; this type of pain is called referred pain. Structures that share nerves with the ear include the nose, sinuses, teeth, gums, jaw joint (temporomandibular joint), tongue, tonsils, throat (pharynx), voice box (larynx), windpipe (trachea), esophagus, and salivary glands in the cheek (parotid glands). Often, the first symptom of cancer in any of these structures is pain that feels like an earache.

Treatment depends on the cause of the pain. Otitis media is treated with antibiotics to prevent the infection from becoming serious. If the ear doesn't seem to be affected, a doctor examines the structures that share nerves with the ear and treats them as needed. Analgesics such as acetaminophen can reduce the pain.

The fluid usually, though not always, contains bacteria. This disorder is common in children because their narrow eustachian tubes can be blocked easily by allergic reactions, enlarged adenoids, or inflammation of the nose and throat. Normally, pressure in the middle ear is equalized three or four times a minute as the eustachian tube opens during swallowing. If the eustachian tube is blocked, pressure in the middle ear tends to decrease, because although oxygen is absorbed into the bloodstream from the middle ear as usual, it's not replaced. As the pressure decreases, fluid accumulates in the middle ear, reducing the eardrum's ability to move. Conductive hearing loss results.

A doctor examines the ear to make the diagnosis. Often, tympanometry, a simple hearing test, is used to measure the pressure on both sides of the eardrum.

Treatment

Treatment usually begins with antibiotics. Other drugs, such as phenylephrine, ephedrine, and antihistamines (for example, chlorpheniramine), are taken by mouth to reduce congestion and help open the eustachian tube. Low pressure in the middle ear can be temporarily increased by forcing air past the blockage in the eustachian tube. To do this, the person may breathe out with the mouth closed and the nostrils pinched shut. A doctor may perform a myringotomy, in which an opening is made through the eardrum to allow fluid to drain from the middle ear. A tiny tube can be inserted into the opening in the eardrum to help fluid drain and allow air to enter the middle ear.

The condition causing blockage of the eustachian tube, such as an allergy, is treated. In children, the adenoids may have to be removed.

Acute Mastoiditis

Acute mastoiditis is a bacterial infection in the mastoid process, the prominent bone behind the ear.

This disorder usually occurs when untreated or inadequately treated acute otitis media spreads from the middle ear into the surrounding bone—the mastoid process.

Symptoms

Usually, symptoms appear 2 or more weeks after acute otitis media develops, as the spreading infection destroys the inner part of the mastoid process. An abscess may form in the bone. The skin covering the mastoid process may become

red, swollen, and tender, and the external ear is pushed sideways and down. Other symptoms are fever, pain around and within the ear, and a creamy, profuse discharge from the ear, all of which usually worsen. The pain tends to be persistent and throbbing. Hearing loss is progressive.

Computed tomography (CT) scans show that the air cells (spaces in bone that normally contain air) in the mastoid process are filled with fluid. As mastoiditis progresses, the spaces enlarge. Inadequately treated mastoiditis can result in deafness, blood poisoning (sepsis), meningitis, brain abscess, or death.

Treatment

Treatment usually begins with an antibiotic given intravenously. A sample of ear discharge is examined to identify the organism causing the infection, and the antibiotics most likely to eliminate the organism are determined. Then, antibiotic treatment is adjusted accordingly and continued for at least 2 weeks. If an abscess has formed in the bone, it's drained surgically.

Chronic Otitis Media

Chronic otitis media is a long-standing infection caused by a permanent hole (perforation) in the eardrum.

Perforation of the eardrum can be caused by acute otitis media, blockage of the eustachian tube, injury from an object entering the ear or from sudden changes in air pressure, or burns from heat or chemicals.

Symptoms depend on which part of the eardrum is perforated. If the eardrum has a **central perforation** (a hole in the middle), chronic otitis media may flare up after an infection of the nose and throat, such as the common cold, or after water enters the middle ear while bathing or swimming. Usually, flare-ups are caused by bacteria and result in a painless discharge of pus, which may be malodorous, from the ear. Persistent flare-ups may result in the formation of protruding growths called polyps, which extend from the middle ear through the perforation and into the ear canal. Persistent infection can destroy parts of the ossicles, the small bones in the middle ear that conduct sounds from the outer ear to the inner ear, causing conductive hearing loss.▲

Chronic otitis media caused by **marginal perforations** (holes near the edge) in the eardrum also may result in conductive hearing loss and worsening ear discharge. Serious complications such as inflammation of the inner ear (labyrinthitis), facial paralysis, and brain infections are more likely to occur with marginal perforations than with central perforations. Marginal perforations are frequently accompanied by cholesteatomas (accumulations of white skinlike material) in the middle ear. Cholesteatomas, which destroy bone, greatly increase the likelihood of a serious complication.

Treatment

When chronic otitis media flares up, a doctor thoroughly cleans the ear canal and middle ear with suction and dry cotton wipes, then instills a solution of acetic acid with hydrocortisone in the ear. Severe flare-ups are treated with an antibiotic, such as amoxicillin, given by mouth. After the bacteria causing the infection are identified, antibiotic treatment is adjusted accordingly.

Usually, the eardrum can be repaired in a procedure called a tympanoplasty. If the ossicle chain has been disrupted, it may be repaired at the same time. Cholesteatomas are removed surgically. If a cholesteatoma isn't removed, repair of the middle ear may not be possible.

Otosclerosis

Otosclerosis is a disorder in which the bone surrounding the middle and inner ear grows excessively, immobilizing the stirrup (the middle ear bone attached to the inner ear) so that it can't transmit sounds properly.

Otosclerosis, a hereditary disease, is the most common cause of progressive conductive hearing loss in adults whose eardrums are normal. It also can cause a neural hearing loss if the bone's growth pinches and damages the nerves connecting the inner ear with the brain. About 10 percent of white adults have some evidence of otosclerosis, but only about 1 percent develop conductive hearing loss as a result. The disorder first becomes evident in late adolescence or early adulthood.

Removing the stirrup by microsurgery and replacing it with an artificial stirrup restores hearing in most cases. Some people may decide to use a hearing aid instead of undergoing surgery.

Inner Ear Disorders

Inner ear disorders produce symptoms such as hearing loss, vertigo (a whirling sensation), tinnitus (noise in the ear), and congestion. These disorders can have many causes, such as infection, injury, tumors, and drugs; sometimes the cause is unknown.

Meniere's Disease

Meniere's disease is a disorder characterized by recurrent attacks of disabling vertigo, hearing loss, and tinnitus.

Its cause is unknown. Symptoms include sudden attacks of vertigo, nausea, and vomiting that last for 3 to 24 hours and subside gradually. Periodically, a person may feel a fullness or pressure in the affected ear. Hearing in the affected ear tends to fluctuate but progressively worsens over the years. Tinnitus, which may be constant or intermittent, may be worse before, after, or during an attack of vertigo. The disorder affects only one ear in most people and both ears in 10 to 15 percent of the people.

In one form of Meniere's disease, hearing loss and tinnitus precede the first attack of vertigo by months or years. After the attacks of vertigo begin, hearing may improve.

Treatment

Vertigo may be relieved temporarily with drugs given by mouth, such as scopolamine, antihistamines, barbiturates, or diazepam. Scopolamine is also available in skin patches.

Several surgical procedures are available for people who are disabled by frequent attacks of vertigo. Cutting the nerves connected to the semicircular canals (the part of the inner ear involved in balance) relieves the vertigo, usually without

▲ see page 998

damaging hearing. This procedure is called vestibular neurectomy. When the vertigo is disabling and hearing has already deteriorated greatly, the cochlea (the part of the inner ear involved in hearing) and the semicircular canals can be removed in a procedure called labyrinthectomy.

Vestibular Neuronitis

Vestibular neuronitis is a disorder characterized by a sudden severe attack of vertigo, caused by inflammation of the nerve to the semicircular canals.

This disorder is probably caused by a virus. The first attack of vertigo is severe, is accompanied by nausea and vomiting, and lasts for 7 to 10 days. The eyes flicker involuntarily toward the affected side (a symptom called nystagmus). The disorder clears up on its own. It may occur as a single, isolated attack or as several attacks over 12 to 18 months. Each subsequent attack is shorter and less severe than the previous one. Hearing is not affected.

Diagnosis involves hearing tests and tests for nystagmus using electronystagmography, a method of electronically recording eye movements. One test for nystagmus consists of instilling a small amount of ice water into each ear canal and recording the person's eye movements. Magnetic resonance imaging (MRI) of the head may be performed to make sure the symptoms aren't caused by another disorder.

Treatment of vertigo is the same as in Meniere's disease. If vomiting continues for a long time, a person may need to be given fluids and electrolytes intravenously.

Postural Vertigo

Postural vertigo (positional vertigo) is violent vertigo that lasts less than 30 seconds and is triggered by certain head positions.

This type of vertigo can be caused by conditions that damage the semicircular canals (the part of the inner ear involved in balance). For example, postural vertigo may be caused by injury to the inner ear, otitis media, ear surgery, or blockage of the artery to the inner ear.

Vertigo develops when a person lies on one ear or tilts the head back to look up. Abnormal involuntary eye movement (nystagmus) also occurs. Usually, postural vertigo subsides in several weeks or months but may return after months or years.

Diagnosis and Treatment

A doctor tries to trigger an attack by asking the person to lie flat on the examination table with the head turned to one side and hanging over the edge of the table. After several seconds, the person develops severe vertigo, usually for 15 to 20 seconds, and nystagmus.

The person should avoid the position that causes vertigo. If postural vertigo persists for as long as a year, cutting the nerve connected to one of the semicircular canals in the affected ear usually relieves symptoms.

Herpes Zoster of the Ear

Herpes zoster of the ear (Ramsay Hunt's syndrome) is an infection of the auditory nerve by the herpes zoster virus, producing severe ear pain, hearing loss, and vertigo.

Small fluid-filled blisters (vesicles) form on the outer ear and in the ear canal. Blisters also may form on the skin of the face or neck supplied by the infected nerves. If the facial nerve is compressed because it's infected and swollen, the muscles of one side of the face may become paralyzed temporarily or permanently. Hearing loss may be permanent, or hearing may return partially or completely. Vertigo lasts from a few days to several weeks.

The preferred treatment is the antiviral drug acyclovir. Analgesics are given to relieve pain, and diazepam to suppress vertigo. When the facial nerve is compressed, surgery to enlarge the opening through which the facial nerve leaves the skull (surgical decompression) may be performed. This procedure occasionally relieves facial paralysis.

Sudden Deafness

Sudden deafness is severe hearing loss, usually in only one ear, that develops over a period of a few hours or less.

Every year, about 1 out of every 5,000 people develop sudden deafness. It's usually caused by a viral disease such as mumps, measles, influenza, chickenpox, or infectious mononucleosis. Less commonly, strenuous activities such as weight lifting place severe pressure on the inner ear, damaging it and resulting in sudden or fluctuating hearing loss and vertigo. An explosive sound may be heard in the affected ear when the damage first occurs. Sometimes no cause is identified.

Usually, the hearing loss is severe. However, most people completely recover their hearing, usually within 10 to 14 days, and others partially recover it. Tinnitus and vertigo may accompany sudden deafness. Vertigo usually subsides in several days, but tinnitus often persists.

No treatment has proved to be valuable. Corticosteroids by mouth are frequently prescribed, and bed rest is usually advised. In certain cases, surgical procedures may be useful.

Hearing Loss Caused by Noise

Exposure to loud noises, such as those produced by woodworking equipment, chain saws, gasoline engines, heavy machinery, gunfire, or airplanes may cause hearing loss by destroying the hearing receptors (hair cells) in the inner ear.▲ Other common causes include using headphones to listen to loud music and standing near amplified speakers at dances and concerts. Although people vary greatly in their sensitivity to loud noise, almost everyone loses some hearing if exposed to sufficiently loud noise long enough. Any noise above 85 decibels is damaging. Blast injuries after explosions (acoustic trauma) cause the same type of hearing loss.

This type of hearing loss is permanent. Usually, it's accompanied by high-pitched tinnitus.

Prevention and Treatment

Hearing loss can be prevented by limiting exposure to loud noise, reducing noise levels whenever possible, and staying away from the source of the noise. The louder the noise, the less time should be spent near it. Wearing ear protectors, such as plastic plugs in the ear canals or glycerin-filled muffs over the ears, can help reduce exposure to noise.

For people who have severe noise-induced hearing loss, a hearing aid usually is useful.

Age-Associated Hearing Loss

Age-associated hearing loss (presbycusis) is the sensorineural hearing loss ■ that occurs as a part of normal aging.

This type of hearing loss begins after age 20, first affecting the highest pitches and gradually affecting lower pitches. However, the degree of hearing loss varies considerably. Some people are

How Ear Disorders Affect the Facial Nerve

Because the facial nerve winds through the ear, disorders of the ear can affect it. For example, herpes zoster of the ear may affect the facial nerve as well as the auditory nerve. The facial nerve then swells and presses against the opening in the skull that it passes through. The pressure on this nerve can cause temporary or permanent facial paralysis.

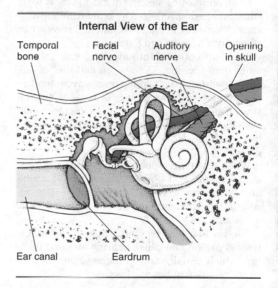

Internal View of the Ear

Temporal bone · Facial nerve · Auditory nerve · Opening in skull · Ear canal · Eardrum

almost completely deaf at age 60, whereas others have excellent hearing at age 90. Men are affected more often and more severely than women. Hearing loss appears to be partly related to the extent of exposure to noise.

No treatment can prevent or reverse age-associated hearing loss. However, such loss can be compensated for by lipreading, learning to recognize nonauditory clues such as body language, and amplifying sounds with a hearing aid.

▲ see page 996

■ see page 998

Drug-Induced Ear Damage

Some drugs—such as certain antibiotics, diuretics (particularly ethacrynic acid and furosemide), aspirin and aspirin-like substances (salicylates), and quinine—can damage the ear. Such drugs affect both hearing and balance, but most affect hearing more.

Almost all of these drugs are eliminated from the body through the kidneys. So any deterioration in the kidneys' functioning increases the likelihood that the drugs will accumulate in the blood and reach levels that can cause damage.

Of all antibiotics, neomycin has the most toxic effect on hearing, followed by kanamycin and amikacin. Viomycin, gentamicin, and tobramycin can affect both hearing and balance.

The antibiotic streptomycin affects balance more than hearing. The vertigo and loss of balance resulting from taking streptomycin tend to be temporary. However, loss of balance may be severe and permanent, causing difficulty when walking in the dark and a feeling that the environment is bouncing with each step (Dandy's syndrome).

When given intravenously to people who have kidney failure and who are also receiving antibiotics, ethacrynic acid and furosemide have resulted in permanent or transient profound hearing loss.

Aspirin taken in very high doses over an extended period can cause hearing loss and tinnitus, which usually are temporary. Quinine can cause permanent hearing loss.

Precautions

Drugs that can damage the ear aren't applied directly to the ear when the eardrum has been perforated because they can be absorbed into the fluids of the inner ear.

Antibiotics that damage hearing aren't prescribed for pregnant women. Neither are they prescribed for the elderly or those who have pre-existing hearing loss unless no other effective drugs are available. Although susceptibility to these drugs varies somewhat from person to person, hearing loss usually can be avoided if blood levels of the drugs are kept within the recommended range. Therefore, blood levels of these drugs usually are monitored. If possible, hearing is measured before and during treatment.

Usually, the first sign of damage is the inability to hear high pitches. High-pitched tinnitus or vertigo may develop.

Temporal Bone Fracture

The temporal bone (the skull bone containing part of the ear canal, the middle ear, and the inner ear) may be fractured by a blow to the skull. Bleeding from the ear or patchy bruising of the skin behind the ear after a head injury suggests that the temporal bone is fractured. If clear fluid drains from the ear, cerebrospinal fluid may be leaking from the brain, indicating that the brain is exposed to infection. Temporal bone fractures frequently rupture the eardrum, causing facial paralysis and profound sensorineural hearing loss. Usually, a computed tomography (CT) scan can detect the fracture.

An antibiotic is given intravenously to prevent infection of the covering of the brain (meningitis). Sometimes, persistent facial paralysis caused by pressure on the facial nerve can be relieved by surgery. Damage to the eardrum and structures of the middle ear is repaired weeks or months later.

Auditory Nerve Tumors

An auditory nerve tumor (acoustic neuroma, acoustic neurinoma, vestibular schwannoma, eighth nerve tumor) is a benign tumor that originates in the Schwann cells (cells that wrap around a nerve).

Auditory nerve tumors account for about 7 percent of all tumors that develop within the skull.

Hearing loss, tinnitus, dizziness, and unsteadiness are early symptoms. Other symptoms may develop if the tumor grows larger and compresses other parts of the brain, the facial nerve, or the trigeminal nerve, which connects the brain with the eye, mouth, and jaw. Early diagnosis is based on a magnetic resonance imaging (MRI) scan and hearing tests, including the auditory brain stem response, which assesses nerve impulses traveling to the brain.

Small tumors are removed by microsurgery to avoid damaging the facial nerve. Large tumors require extensive surgery.

Disorders of the Nose and Sinuses

The upper part of the nose consists of bone and the lower part of cartilage. Inside is a hollow cavity (nasal cavity) divided into two passages by the nasal septum. The bones of the face contain sinuses, which are hollow cavities that open into the nasal cavity.▲

Because of its prominent position, the nose is particularly vulnerable to injury. In addition, disorders such as infections, nosebleeds, and polyps affect the nose. The sinuses may become infected, resulting in inflammation (sinusitis).

Fractures of the Nose

The bones of the nose are broken (fractured) more frequently than other bones of the face. When nasal bones break, the mucous membrane lining the nose usually tears, resulting in a nosebleed. Because the mucous membrane and other soft tissues swell quickly, the break may be difficult to find. Most commonly, the bridge of the nose is pushed to one side, with the nasal bones pushed in on the other side. If blood collects in the cartilage of the nasal septum (the structure that divides the nose), the cartilage may become infected and die, resulting in a saddle deformity, in which the bridge of the nose sags in the middle.

Diagnosis and Treatment

A person whose nose bleeds and hurts after a blunt injury may have a broken nose. Ordinarily, a doctor diagnoses a broken nose by gently feeling the bridge of the nose for irregularities in shape, unusual movement of bones, the rough sensation of broken bones moving against one another, and tenderness. The diagnosis is confirmed with x-rays.

When a broken nose is set, adults are usually given a local anesthetic, and children a general anesthetic. Blood that has collected in the septum is drained to prevent infection and loss of cartilage. After the nose is manipulated into its normal position, it's stabilized with gauze packing inside and splinting outside. Fractures of the septum are difficult to set and often require surgery later.

Deviated Septum

Usually, the nasal septum (the structure that divides the nose) is straight, but it may be bent (deviated) because of birth defects or injuries. A deviated septum, which is common, usually causes no symptoms and requires no treatment. However, it may block the nose, making a person prone to sinusitis (inflammation of the sinuses), particularly if the deviated septum blocks drainage from a sinus into the nasal cavity. Also, a deviated septum may make a person prone to nosebleeds because excess airflow through the unblocked side dries the mucous membrane. A deviated septum that causes problems can be surgically repaired.

Perforations of the Septum

Ulcers and holes (perforations) in the nasal septum may be caused by nasal surgery, repeated injury such as that resulting from picking the nose, infections such as tuberculosis and syphilis, and the use of cocaine in the nose. Symptoms may include crusting around the nostrils and repeated nosebleeds. People who have small perforations in the septum may make a whistling sound when they breathe. Bacitracin ointment reduces the crusting. Perforations can be repaired with a person's own tissue from inside the cheek or another part of the nose or with an artificial membrane made of a soft, pliable plastic, which usually is better. However, most perforations don't need to be repaired unless bleeding or crusting is a major problem.

Nosebleeds

Nosebleeds (epistaxis) have a variety of causes. Most often, the blood comes from Kiesselbach's area, which is located in the front part

▲ see box, page 1016

Causes of Nosebleeds

Localized infections
• Vestibulitis
• Sinusitis

Dried mucous membrane in the nose

Injury
• Repeated injury from picking the nose
• Fracture of the nose

Narrowing of the arteries (arteriosclerosis)

High blood pressure

Disorders causing a tendency to bleed
• Aplastic anemia
• Leukemia
• Low platelet count (thrombocytopenia)
• Liver disease
• Hereditary blood disorders such as hemophilia
• Hereditary hemorrhagic telangiectasia

of the nasal septum and contains many blood vessels. Bleeding usually can be controlled by pinching the sides of the nose together for 5 to 10 minutes. If this technique doesn't stop the bleeding, a doctor looks for the source of the bleeding. Bleeding can be stopped temporarily by applying pressure inside the nose with a piece of cotton wool saturated with a drug that causes blood vessels to constrict, such as phenylephrine, and a local anesthetic, such as lidocaine. After the bleeding has stopped and the site is numb, the doctor seals (cauterizes) the bleeding source with silver nitrate or electrocautery (a device that uses an electric current to produce heat).

If a person has a disorder causing a tendency to bleed, the bleeding source isn't cauterized because it might begin to bleed again. Instead, a doctor gently presses gauze saturated with petroleum jelly against the bleeding source. After the bleeding has stopped, the doctor tries to identify and correct the disorder.

In people who have narrowing of the arteries (arteriosclerosis) and high blood pressure, the bleeding source is likely to be further back in the nose, where bleeding is more difficult to stop.

Sometimes a doctor must close off (ligate) the artery supplying blood to the area or pack the back of the nasal cavity with gauze. Usually, the packing is left in place for 4 days, and an antibiotic such as ampicillin is given by mouth to prevent an infection of the sinuses or middle ear.

People who have hereditary hemorrhagic telangiectasia (a disease in which blood vessels are malformed) may have many severe nosebleeds, resulting in severe, persistent anemia that isn't easily corrected with iron supplements. A skin graft onto the nasal septum reduces the number of nosebleeds so that the anemia can be corrected.

People who have extensive liver disease, which can result in a tendency to bleed, often have severe nosebleeds. Large amounts of blood may be swallowed and broken down into ammonia by bacteria in the intestine. Ammonia can be absorbed into the bloodstream and can make a person sick or become comatose, so enemas and cathartics are given to remove the blood from the intestine as soon as possible. In addition, an antibiotic such as neomycin is given to prevent the breakdown of blood into ammonia. If a large amount of blood is lost, a blood transfusion may be given.

Nasal Vestibulitis

Nasal vestibulitis is an infection of the nasal vestibule (the area just inside the opening of each nostril).

This area becomes infected frequently. Minor infections, such as those affecting hair follicles (folliculitis), produce crusts around the nostrils. Nosebleeds occur as the crusts detach. Bacitracin ointment can usually cure these infections.

Boils (furuncles) in the nasal vestibule usually are caused by the bacterium *Staphylococcus.* Boils may develop into a spreading infection under the skin (cellulitis) of the tip of the nose. A person usually takes an antibiotic and applies moist hot cloths three times a day for about 15 to 20 minutes at a time. Boils in this area are allowed to drain on their own because if they are cut open, the infection could spread to the veins, enabling the bacteria to travel to the brain. The spread of bacteria to the brain can cause a life-threatening condition called cavernous sinus thrombosis.

Nonallergic Rhinitis

Nonallergic rhinitis▲ is an inflammation of the mucous membrane of the nose, characterized by a runny nose and stuffiness and usually caused by an infection.

The nose is the most commonly infected part of the upper airways. Rhinitis may be acute (short-lived) or chronic (long-standing).

Acute rhinitis is the usual sign of a cold.■ It can be caused by a variety of viruses and by bacteria. If it's caused by bacteria, a doctor identifies the bacteria and prescribes an appropriate antibiotic. If the rhinitis is caused by a virus, antibiotics are not effective. In either case, symptoms can be relieved by taking phenylephrine as a nasal spray or pseudoephedrine by mouth. These drugs, available over the counter, cause the blood vessels of the nasal mucous membrane to constrict. Nasal sprays should be used for only 3 or 4 days.

Chronic rhinitis is usually caused by smoking, air pollution, or allergies. It may also result from infections such as syphilis, tuberculosis, rhinoscleroma, rhinosporidiosis, leprosy, leishmaniasis, blastomycosis, and histoplasmosis. These infections destroy soft tissue, cartilage, and bone. Symptoms of chronic rhinitis include blocked nasal passages and a runny nose. When the rhinitis is caused by an infection, discharges of pus and frequent nosebleeds are typical. A doctor tries to identify the microorganism causing the infection by performing a biopsy (removing a small piece of tissue for microscopic examination) or taking a sample of the nasal discharge for culture (growing microorganisms in a laboratory). Treatment depends on the microorganism identified.

Atrophic rhinitis is chronic rhinitis in which the mucous membrane thins (atrophies) and hardens, causing the nasal passages to widen—the major difference between atrophic and other forms of chronic rhinitis. The cause is unknown, although a bacterial infection is probably involved. Crusts form inside the nose, and an offensive odor develops. The cells normally found in the mucous membrane of the nose—cells that secrete mucus and have hairlike projections to move dirt particles out—are replaced by cells like those normally found in the skin. A person loses the sense of smell (anosmia) and may have recurring severe nosebleeds. Treatment is aimed at reducing the crusting and eliminating the odor. Antibiotics, such as bacitracin sprayed into the nose, kill bacteria; estrogens and vitamins A and

Polyp Formation in the Nose

Polyps usually develop in the area where the sinuses open into the nasal cavity and may block drainage from the sinuses. Fluid may accumulate in the blocked sinuses, causing a sinus infection.

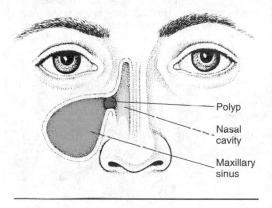

Polyp

Nasal cavity

Maxillary sinus

D sprayed into the nose or taken by mouth may help by promoting mucosal secretions. Blocking or narrowing the nasal passages, by surgery or with a pad of lamb's wool, reduces the crusting because it decreases airflow, which dries the thinned mucous membrane.

Vasomotor rhinitis is chronic rhinitis marked by swollen blood vessels in the mucous membrane of the nose, sneezing, and a runny nose. Its cause is unknown but doesn't appear to be an allergy. The condition comes and goes but is worsened by dry air. The swollen mucous membrane varies from bright red to purple. No crusts form and no pus is discharged. Treatment is aimed at relieving symptoms but isn't always effective. Increased humidity from a humidified central heating system or a vaporizer at home and work may be beneficial.

Nasal Polyps

Nasal polyps are fleshy outgrowths of the mucous membrane of the nose.

▲ see page 825

■ see page 913

Locating the Sinuses

The sinuses are hollow cavities in the bones around the nose. The two frontal sinuses are located just above the eyebrows; the two maxillary sinuses, in the cheekbones; and the two groups of ethmoid sinuses, on either side of the nasal cavity. The two sphenoid sinuses (not shown) are located behind the ethmoid sinuses.

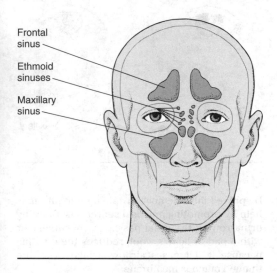

Frontal sinus

Ethmoid sinuses

Maxillary sinus

People who have allergies affecting the nose (allergic rhinitis) tend to develop nasal polyps. Polyps also may develop during infections and may disappear after the infection subsides. Polyps usually grow in areas where the mucous membrane has swollen because of fluid accumulation, such as the area around the openings of the sinuses into the nasal cavity. A polyp is shaped like a teardrop when it's developing and resembles a peeled, seedless grape when it's mature.

Using an aerosol nasal spray containing corticosteroids sometimes shrinks or eliminates polyps. Surgery is needed if polyps block the airway, frequently cause sinus infections by blocking drainage from the sinuses, or are associated with tumors. Polyps tend to grow back unless the un-

derlying allergy or infection is controlled, but using an aerosol corticosteroid spray may slow or prevent recurrence. In severe, recurrent cases, surgery is performed to improve sinus drainage and remove infected material.

Sinusitis

Sinusitis is an inflammation of the sinuses caused by an allergy or a viral, bacterial, or fungal infection.

Sinusitis may develop in any of the four groups of sinuses: maxillary, ethmoid, frontal, or sphenoid.

Causes

Sinusitis may be acute (short-lived) or chronic (long-standing). Acute sinusitis may be caused by a variety of bacteria and often develops after a viral infection of the upper airways, such as the common cold. Occasionally, chronic sinusitis of the maxillary sinus results from a tooth infection.

During a cold, the swollen mucous membrane of the nasal cavity tends to block the openings of the sinuses. When this happens, air in the sinuses is absorbed into the bloodstream, and the pressure inside the sinuses decreases, resulting in negative pressure that's painful—a condition called vacuum sinusitis. If the vacuum remains, fluid is drawn into and fills the sinuses, creating a breeding ground for bacteria. White blood cells and more fluid enter the sinuses to fight the bacteria; this influx increases the pressure and causes more pain.

Symptoms and Diagnosis

Acute and chronic sinusitis produce similar symptoms, such as tenderness and swelling over the affected sinus, but the precise symptoms depend on which sinus is affected. For example, maxillary sinusitis produces pain over the cheeks just below the eyes, toothache, and headache. Frontal sinusitis produces headache over the forehead. Ethmoid sinusitis produces pain behind and between the eyes and headache, often described as splitting, over the forehead. The pain produced by sphenoid sinusitis doesn't occur in well-defined areas and may be felt in the front or back of the head.

A person also may feel generally sick (malaise). Fever and chills suggest that the infection has spread beyond the sinuses. The nasal mucous membrane is red and swollen, and yellow or green pus may be discharged from the nose.

In sinusitis, the sinuses appear opaque on an x-ray, so a computed tomography (CT) scan may be used to determine the extent and severity of sinusitis. If a person has maxillary sinusitis, the teeth are x-rayed to check for tooth abscesses.

Treatment

Treatment of acute sinusitis is aimed at improving sinus drainage and curing the infection. Steam inhalation helps blood vessels in the mucous membrane constrict and improves sinus drainage. Drugs that cause blood vessels to constrict, such as phenylephrine, can be used as nasal sprays but for only a limited time. Similar drugs, such as pseudoephedrine, taken by mouth aren't as effective.

For both acute and chronic sinusitis, antibiotics such as amoxicillin are given, but people who have chronic sinusitis take antibiotics longer. When antibiotics aren't effective, surgery may be performed to improve sinus drainage and remove infected material.

SINUSITIS AND AN IMPAIRED IMMUNE SYSTEM

In people who have poorly controlled diabetes or an impaired immune system, fungi can cause severe and even fatal sinusitis.

Mucormycosis (phycomycosis) is a fungal infection that may develop in people who have poorly controlled diabetes. It results in black, dead tissue in the nasal cavity and blocks the blood supply to the brain, leading to neurologic symptoms such as headaches and blindness. A doctor makes the diagnosis by removing the infected tissue and examining a sample under the microscope. Treatment includes controlling the diabetes and giving the antifungal drug amphotericin B intravenously.

Aspergillosis and candidiasis are often fatal fungal infections that may develop in the sinuses of people whose immune system is impaired by anticancer treatment or by diseases such as leukemia, lymphoma, multiple myeloma, or AIDS. In aspergillosis, polyps develop in the nose and sinuses. A doctor makes the diagnosis by removing and analyzing the polyps. Attempts to control these infections include performing sinus surgery and giving amphotericin B intravenously.

CHAPTER 214

Throat Disorders

Disorders of the throat and voice box include inflammation and infections, noncancerous growths such as vocal cord polyps and nodules, contact ulcers, cancer, vocal cord paralysis, and laryngoceles.

Pharyngitis

Pharyngitis is an inflammation of the throat (pharynx), usually caused by a virus but also commonly caused by bacteria.

Pharyngitis can occur in viral infections such as the common cold, influenza, and infectious mononucleosis and in bacterial infections such as streptococcal infections (strep throat)▲ and sexually transmitted diseases (gonorrhea, for example).

Symptoms, which include a sore throat and pain when swallowing, are similar in viral and bacterial pharyngitis. In both, the mucous membrane that lines the pharynx may be mildly or severely inflamed and may be covered by a whitish membrane or a pus discharge. Fever, enlarged lymph nodes in the neck, and a high white blood cell count typify both viral and bacterial pharyngitis but may be more pronounced in the bacterial form.

Treatment

Common analgesics, throat lozenges, or warm salt-water gargling can relieve throat discomfort,

▲ see page 876

Two Types of Pharyngitis

Viral Pharyngitis	Bacterial Pharyngitis
Usually no discharge of pus in the throat	Discharge of pus in the throat fairly common
Mild or no fever	Mild to moderate fever
Normal or slightly high white blood cell count	Slightly to moderately high white blood cell count
Normal or slightly enlarged lymph nodes	Slightly to moderately enlarged lymph nodes
Throat swab test negative	Throat swab test positive for strep throat
No bacteria grow in laboratory culture	Bacteria grow in laboratory culture

but aspirin must not be taken by children and adolescents under 18 because it can result in Reye's syndrome.▲ Antibiotics don't help if the infection is viral but may be prescribed if a doctor strongly suspects that the infection is bacterial. Otherwise, no antibiotic is given until laboratory tests have confirmed a diagnosis of bacterial pharyngitis. If tests indicate that the pharyngitis is caused by a streptococcal infection (strep throat), a doctor prescribes penicillin, usually in tablet form, to eradicate the infection and prevent complications such as rheumatic fever. People known to have an allergy to penicillin may take erythromycin or another antibiotic instead.

Tonsillitis

Tonsillitis is an inflammation of the tonsils usually caused by a streptococcal or, less commonly, a viral infection.

Symptoms include a sore throat and pain that's aggravated by swallowing. The pain is often felt in the ears because the throat and ears share the same nerves. Very young children may not say

▲ see page 1280

that their throat is sore but may refuse to eat. Fever, a generally sick feeling (malaise), headaches, and vomiting are common.

The tonsils are swollen and bloodshot. A doctor may see pus and a membrane—white, thin, and confined to the tonsil—that can be peeled away without causing bleeding. A throat swab (a sample of pus or mucus taken from the back of the throat with a cotton-tipped applicator) is sent to the laboratory, which cultures any bacteria on the swab and determines which antibiotics are effective against them.

Treatment

Symptoms of viral tonsillitis are relieved in the same ways as those of pharyngitis. For streptococcal tonsillitis, penicillin is taken by mouth for 10 days—considerably beyond the time a person feels well—to ensure that the bacteria have been eradicated. Throat swabs from family members may also be cultured so that those who are infected with the same type of bacteria but have no symptoms (symptomless carriers) can be identified and treated. Removing the tonsils is rarely necessary unless the tonsillitis returns repeatedly or is only briefly controlled by antibiotics.

Tonsillar Cellulitis and Abscess

Cellulitis (inflammation of cells) around the tonsils may occur with or without quinsy (abscess in the area around the tonsils). It's usually caused by a streptococcal infection but can be caused by other bacterial infections. Abscess is rare in children but more common in young adults.

Swallowing causes severe pain. A person feels ill, has a fever, and typically tilts the head toward the side of the abscess to reduce pain. Spasms of the chewing muscles make opening the mouth difficult. The abscess pushes the tonsil forward, and the soft palate at the back of the throat is red and swollen. The uvula (the small, soft projection that hangs down at the back of the throat) is swollen and pushed to the side opposite the abscess.

Penicillin is given intravenously. If no abscess is present, the penicillin usually starts to clear the infection in 24 to 48 hours. If an abscess doesn't rupture and drain spontaneously, a doctor must cut into it and drain it or insert a needle in it to draw out the pus. Treatment with penicillin is continued by mouth. The abscess tends to recur; therefore, the tonsils are usually removed 6 weeks after the infection has subsided or earlier if the infection is controlled with antibiotics.

Parapharyngeal Abscess

Parapharyngeal abscess is a collection of pus within a lymph node located beside the throat (pharynx).

The abscess usually follows pharyngitis or tonsillitis and may occur at any age. The pharynx may not be inflamed. The front part of the neck below the jaw may be noticeably swollen on the affected side. Penicillin is given intravenously at first and by mouth later.

Laryngitis

Laryngitis is an inflammation of the voice box (larynx).

The most common cause is a viral infection of the upper airways, such as the common cold. Laryngitis also may accompany bronchitis, pneumonia, influenza, whooping cough (pertussis), measles, diphtheria, or any inflammation or infection of the upper airways. Excessive use of the voice, allergic reactions, and inhalation of irritants such as cigarette smoke can cause short-lived (acute) or persistent (chronic) laryngitis.

Usually, an unnatural change of voice, such as hoarseness or even loss of voice, is the most noticeable symptom. The throat may tickle or feel raw, and a person may have a constant urge to clear the throat. Symptoms vary with the severity of the inflammation. Fever, a generally sick feeling (malaise), difficulty in swallowing, and a sore throat may occur in severe infections. Swelling (edema) of the larynx may make breathing difficult. Using a small angled mirror such as those used by dentists, a doctor sees a mild to marked reddening of the lining of the larynx, which also may be swollen.

Treatment of viral laryngitis depends on the symptoms. Resting the voice by not speaking, or speaking only in a whisper, and inhaling steam relieve symptoms and help the sore areas heal. Treating bronchitis, if present, may improve the laryngitis. An antibiotic given by mouth is helpful when the infection is caused by bacteria.

Vocal Cord Polyps

Vocal cord polyps are noncancerous growths on the vocal cords that develop from abuse of the voice,

chronic allergic reactions affecting the larynx, or chronic inhalation of irritants such as industrial fumes or cigarette smoke.

Symptoms include chronic hoarseness and a breathy voice.

The diagnosis is made by examining the vocal cords with a mirror and performing a biopsy (removal of a small piece of tissue for examination under a microscope) to make sure the growth isn't cancer.

A surgeon removes the polyp to restore the person's normal voice. The underlying cause is identified and treated to prevent the recurrence of polyps. If abuse of the voice is the cause, voice therapy may be needed.

Vocal Cord Nodules

Vocal cord nodules (singer's nodules) are noncancerous scarlike growths on the vocal cords, similar to vocal cord polyps but firmer, that do not disappear with rest.

Vocal cord nodules are caused by chronic voice abuse, such as repeated yelling, shouting, or strenuous singing. Symptoms consist of hoarseness and a breathy voice. A small sample of tissue is removed from the nodule to make sure the growth isn't cancer. Vocal cord nodules in children usually disappear with voice therapy alone. In adults, the nodules are surgically removed. The only way to prevent more nodules from forming is to stop abusing the voice.

Contact Ulcers

Contact ulcers are raw sores on the mucous membrane covering the cartilages to which the vocal cords are attached.

Contact ulcers are usually caused by abusing the voice with forceful speech, particularly as a person is beginning to speak. These ulcers are typically seen in preachers, sales representatives, and lawyers. Smoking, persistent coughing, and backflow (reflux) of acid from the stomach also may cause contact ulcers.

Symptoms include mild pain while speaking or swallowing and varying degrees of hoarseness. Occasionally, a small tissue sample is removed and examined under a microscope to make sure the ulcer isn't cancerous.

The voice must be rested—by talking as little as possible—for at least 6 weeks so that the ulcers

Vocal Cord Problems

When relaxed, the vocal cords normally form a V-shaped opening to the trachea that air can pass through freely. During speech and swallowing, the cords close.

Holding a mirror in the patient's mouth, a doctor can see the vocal cords and check for problems, such as polyps, nodules, contact ulcers, and paralysis, all of which affect the voice. Paralysis may affect one (one-sided) or both cords (two-sided).

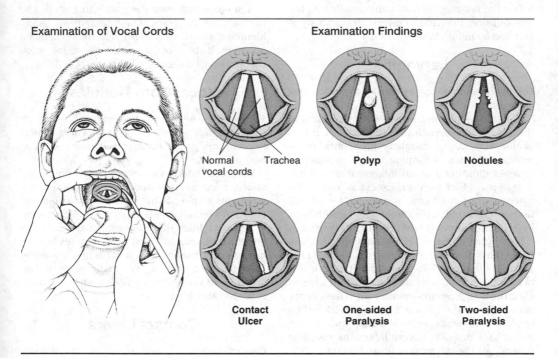

Examination of Vocal Cords

Examination Findings

Normal vocal cords   Trachea

Polyp

Nodules

Contact Ulcer

One-sided Paralysis

Two-sided Paralysis

can heal. To avoid recurrence, people who develop contact ulcers must recognize the limitations of their voice and learn to adjust their vocal activities. Voice therapy may help. If x-rays show acid reflux, treatment includes taking antacids or antiulcer drugs (histamine blockers), not eating within 2 hours of retiring for the night, and keeping the head elevated while sleeping.

▲ see page 318

Vocal Cord Paralysis

Vocal cord paralysis is the inability to move the muscles that control the vocal cords.

Vocal cord paralysis may result from brain disorders, such as brain tumors, strokes, and demyelinating diseases,▲ or damage to the nerves leading to the larynx. Nerve damage may be caused by tumors, injury, a viral infection of the nerves, or neurotoxins (substances that poison or destroy nerve tissue) such as lead or the toxins produced in diphtheria.

Symptoms and Diagnosis

Vocal cord paralysis may affect speaking, breathing, and swallowing. Paralysis may allow food and fluids to be inhaled into the windpipe (trachea) and lungs. If only one vocal cord is paralyzed (one-sided paralysis), the voice is hoarse and breathy. Usually, the airway is not obstructed because the normal cord on the other side opens sufficiently. When both vocal cords are paralyzed (two-sided paralysis), the voice is reduced in strength but otherwise sounds normal. However, the space between the paralyzed cords is very small, and the airway is inadequate so that even moderate exercise causes difficulty in breathing and a harsh, high-pitched sound with each breath.

A doctor tries to find the cause of the paralysis. Endoscopy (direct examination of an organ's interior with a viewing tube) of the larynx, bronchial tubes, or esophagus may be performed. Computed tomography (CT) scans of the head, neck, chest, and thyroid gland and x-rays of the esophagus also may be needed.

Treatment

For one-sided paralysis, injecting Teflon into the paralyzed cord brings it closer to the midline so that the other cord can come into contact with it, thus protecting the airway during swallowing and improving speech. For two-sided paralysis, keeping the airway open adequately is difficult. A tracheostomy (surgery to create an opening into the trachea through the neck) may be performed to allow air to bypass the vocal cords. The tracheostomy opening may be permanent or may be used only during upper airway infections. Arytenoidectomy (an operation in which the vocal cords are permanently separated) widens the airway but may make the voice quality worse.

Laryngoceles

Laryngoceles are outpouchings of the mucous membrane of a part of the voice box (larynx).

Laryngoceles may bulge inward, resulting in hoarseness and airway obstruction, or outward, producing a visible lump in the neck. Laryngoceles are filled with air and can be expanded when a person breathes out forcefully with the mouth closed and the nostrils pinched shut. These pouches tend to occur in musicians who play wind instruments. On a computed tomography (CT) scan, laryngoceles appear smooth and egg-shaped. Laryngoceles may become infected or filled with mucuslike fluid. The usual treatment is to remove them surgically.

Cancer of the Nasopharynx

Cancer of the upper part of the pharynx (nasopharynx) may occur in children and young adults. Although rare in North America, it's one of the most common cancers in the Orient. It's also more common in Chinese who have immigrated to North America than in other Americans and slightly less common in American-born Chinese than in their immigrant parents.

The Epstein-Barr virus, which causes infectious mononucleosis, also plays a role in the development of nasopharyngeal cancer.

Often, the first symptom is persistent blockage of the nose or eustachian tubes. If a eustachian tube is blocked, fluid may accumulate in the middle ear. A person may have a discharge of pus and blood from the nose and nosebleeds. Rarely, part of the face becomes paralyzed. The cancer may spread to lymph nodes in the neck.

A doctor diagnoses the cancer by performing a biopsy (removal of a small tissue sample for examination under a microscope) of the tumor. The tumor is treated with radiation therapy. If the tumor is large or persists, surgery may be needed. Overall, 35 percent of the people survive for at least 5 years after diagnosis.

Cancer of the Tonsil

Cancer of the tonsil occurs predominantly in men and is strongly linked to smoking and alcohol consumption.

Usually, a sore throat is the first symptom. Pain often radiates to the ear on the same side as the affected tonsil. Sometimes, however, a lump in the neck resulting from the cancer's spread to a lymph node (metastasis) may be noticed before any other symptoms. A doctor diagnoses the cancer by performing a biopsy (removal of a tissue sample for examination under a microscope) of the tonsil. Because smoking and alcohol consumption may also be linked to other cancers, laryngoscopy (examination of the larynx), bronchoscopy (examination of the bronchial tubes), and esophagoscopy (examination of the esophagus) also are performed.

Treatment includes both radiation therapy and surgery. Surgery may involve removal of the tumor, lymph nodes in the neck, and part of the jaw. About 50 percent of the people survive for at least 5 years after diagnosis.

Cancer of the Larynx

Cancer of the larynx, the most common cancer of the head and neck except for skin cancer, is more common in men and is linked to cigarette smoking and alcohol consumption.

This cancer commonly originates on the vocal cords, causing hoarseness. A person who has been hoarse for more than 2 weeks should seek medical attention. Cancer in other parts of the larynx causes pain and difficulty in swallowing. Sometimes, however, a lump in the neck resulting from the cancer's spread to a lymph node (metastasis) may be noticed before any other symptoms.

To make the diagnosis, a doctor looks at the larynx through a laryngoscope (a tube used for direct viewing of the larynx) and performs a biopsy (removal of a tissue sample for examination under a microscope) of the tissue suspected to be cancer. Then the cancer is classified by stage, from I to IV, based on how extensively it has spread.

Treatment
Treatment depends on the precise location of the cancer within the larynx. For cancer in an early stage, surgery or radiation therapy is the usual treatment. When the vocal cords are affected, radiation therapy is often preferred because it usually preserves the normal voice. For cancer in an advanced stage, the usual treatment is surgery, which can include removing part or all of the larynx (partial or total laryngectomy), often followed by radiation therapy. When treated, 90 percent of people who have cancer in stage I survive for at least 5 years, compared with 25 percent of those who have cancer in stage IV.

Totally removing the vocal cords leaves a person with no voice. A new voice can be created by one of three methods: esophageal speech, a tracheoesophageal fistula, or an electrolarynx. For esophageal speech, a person is taught to take air into the esophagus while inhaling and gradually expel the air to produce a sound. A tracheoesophageal fistula is a one-way valve surgically inserted between the windpipe (trachea) and the esophagus. The valve forces air into the esophagus while the person inhales, producing a sound. If the valve malfunctions, fluids and food may accidentally enter the windpipe. The electrolarynx is a device that acts as a sound source when it's held against the neck. The sounds produced by all three methods are converted into speech as in normal speech—by using the mouth, nose, teeth, tongue, and lips. However, the voice produced by these methods sounds artificial and is much weaker than the normal voice.

CHAPTER 215

Head and Neck Cancers

The average age of people who have head and neck cancers—excluding cancers of the brain, eyes, and spine—is 59 years. Generally, cancers of the salivary glands,▲ thyroid gland,■ or sinuses affect people under 59, and cancers of the mouth, throat (pharynx), or voice box (larynx) affect those over 59.

Usually, cancers of the head and neck spread to nearby lymph nodes first. These cancers usually don't spread (metastasize) to other parts of the body for 6 months to 3 years. Metastases (cancer that has spread from the original site to other parts of the body) usually come from large or persistent tumors and are more likely to develop in people whose immune system is suppressed.

Causes
About 85 percent of the people who have head or neck cancer are former or current users of al-

▲ see page 477

■ see page 710

cohol and cigarettes. Mouth (oral) cancer may also result from poor oral hygiene, ill-fitting dentures, and use of snuff or chewing tobacco; in India, chewing betel nut is a major cause. The Epstein-Barr virus, which causes infectious mononucleosis, plays a role in the development of cancer in the upper part of the pharynx (nasopharynx).

People who were treated 20 or more years ago with small doses of radiation therapy for acne, excess facial hair, an enlarged thymus gland, or enlarged tonsils and adenoids have a higher risk of developing thyroid and salivary gland cancer. Radiation therapy isn't used for such purposes today.

Staging and Prognosis

Staging is a method of determining the spread of a cancer to help guide therapy and assess prognosis. Head and neck cancers are staged according to the size and location of the original tumor, the number and size of metastases to the lymph nodes in the neck, and evidence of metastases in distant parts of the body. Stage I is the least advanced and stage IV the most advanced.

Tumors that bulge outward tend to respond to treatment better than those that grow into the surrounding structures, form ulcers, or are hard. If the tumor has invaded muscle, bone, or cartilage, a cure is less likely. For people who have metastases, the chance of surviving more than 2 years is poor. A cancer that spreads along the path of a nerve, causing pain, paralysis, or numbness, is likely to be highly aggressive and hard to treat.

Overall, 65 percent of the people who have cancer that hasn't spread survive for at least 5 years, compared with fewer than 30 percent of those who have cancer that has spread to the lymph nodes or beyond. People over age 70 often have longer disease-free intervals (remissions) and better survival rates than younger people.

Treatment

Treatment depends on the stage of the cancer. Stage I cancers, regardless of their location in the head or neck, respond similarly to surgery and to radiation therapy. Usually, radiation is aimed not only at the cancer but also at the lymph nodes on both sides of the neck because more than 20 percent of these cancers spread to the lymph nodes.

Some tumors, including those with a diameter of more than three fourths of an inch and those that have invaded bone or cartilage, are removed by surgery. If cancer is found or suspected in the lymph nodes, surgery is generally followed by radiation therapy. Alternatively, in certain cases, radiation therapy with or without chemotherapy▲ (treatment with anticancer drugs) may be used, resulting in fair survival rates; if the cancer recurs, surgery can usually be performed later. For cancer in an advanced stage, a combination of surgery and radiation therapy usually offers a better prognosis than either treatment alone.

Chemotherapy kills cancer cells at the original site, in the lymph nodes, and throughout the body. Whether combining chemotherapy with surgery or radiation therapy improves the cure rate isn't known, but combined therapy does prolong remission. If the cancer is too advanced for surgery or radiation therapy, chemotherapy can help reduce the pain and the size of the tumor.

Treatment almost always has some adverse effects. Surgery often affects swallowing and speaking; in such cases, rehabilitation is necessary. Radiation may cause skin changes (such as inflammation, itching, and loss of hair), scarring, loss of taste, and dry mouth, and rarely, it destroys normal tissues. Chemotherapy can cause nausea and vomiting, temporary hair loss, and inflammation of the lining of the stomach and intestines (gastroenteritis); it also can reduce the numbers of red and white blood cells and temporarily impair the immune system.

Metastatic Neck Cancers

A doctor may discover an abnormal lump in the neck of a person who has no other symptoms. An abnormal lump may be caused by a birth defect or an enlarged lymph node, which may result from an infection or cancer. Lymph nodes in the neck are a common site for the spread of cancer from all parts of the body. The original cancer may be in the pharynx, larynx, tonsil, base of the tongue, or a more distant site such as the lung, prostate, breast, stomach, colon, or kidney.

▲ see page 799

Diagnosis and Treatment

The cause of a single enlarged lymph node in the neck may be readily apparent to a doctor, or it may be difficult to discover. A doctor examines the ears, nose, pharynx, larynx, tonsils, base of the tongue, and thyroid and salivary glands. Tests may include x-rays of the upper gastrointestinal tract, a thyroid scan, and a computed tomography (CT) scan of the head, neck, and chest. Direct examination of the larynx (laryngoscopy), lungs (bronchoscopy), and esophagus (esophagoscopy) may be needed.

Biopsies (removal of tissue samples for examination under a microscope) are performed if areas suspected to be cancer are seen during these procedures. If the original cancer still can't be located, samples of tissue may also be taken from the pharynx, tonsils, and base of the tongue. A doctor may insert a fine needle into the lump or enlarged lymph node to withdraw cells for analysis, but removal of the whole mass, rather than just a part, is usually preferred for diagnosis.

When cancer cells are found in an enlarged lymph node in the neck and the original cancer can't be found, radiation therapy may be applied to the pharynx, tonsils, base of the tongue, and both sides of the neck. In addition, cancerous lymph nodes and other affected tissue may be surgically removed from the neck.

Eye Disorders

Eyes and Vision

The structure and function of the eye are complex and fascinating. The eye constantly adjusts the amount of light it lets in, focuses on objects near and far, and produces continuous images that are instantly transmitted to the brain.

Structure and Function

The front of the eye's relatively tough white outer layer (sclera or white of the eye) is covered by a thin membrane (conjunctiva). Light enters through the cornea, a transparent dome on the surface of the eye. Besides serving as a protective covering for the front of the eye, the cornea also helps focus light on the retina at the back of the eye. After passing through the cornea, light enters the pupil, the black area in the middle of the iris—the circular, colored area of the eye. The iris controls the amount of light that enters the eye by opening and closing like the aperture of a camera lens. The iris allows more light into the eye when the environment is dark and allows less light into the eye when the environment is bright. The size of the pupil is controlled by the pupillary sphincter muscle, which opens and closes the iris.

Behind the iris sits the lens. By changing its shape, the lens focuses light onto the retina. For the eye to focus on nearby objects, a small muscle called the ciliary muscle contracts, making the lens thicker and thus stronger. For the eye to focus on distant objects, the same muscle relaxes, making the lens thinner and thus weaker. As people age, the lens typically becomes less flexible, less able to thicken, and thus less able to focus on nearby objects, a condition called presbyopia.

The retina contains the nerves that sense light and the blood supply that nourishes them. The most sensitive part of the retina is a small area called the macula, which has hundreds of nerve endings close together. The high density of nerve endings makes the visual image sharp, just as high-resolution film has more tightly packed grains. The retina then converts the image into electrical impulses, which are carried to the brain by the optic nerve.

The optic nerve connects the retina to the brain in a split pathway. Half the fibers of this nerve cross over to the other side at the optic chiasm, an area just below the front of the brain. The bundles of nerve fibers then come together again just before they reach the back part of the brain, where vision is sensed and interpreted.

The eyeball itself is divided into two segments, each filled with fluid. The front (anterior) segment extends from the cornea to the lens; the back (posterior) segment extends from the back edges of the lens to the retina. The anterior segment is filled with a fluid called the aqueous humor that nourishes its internal structures; the posterior segment contains a gel-like substance called the vitreous humor. These fluids help the eyeball maintain its shape. The anterior segment itself is divided into two chambers. The front (anterior) chamber extends from the cornea to the iris; the back (posterior) chamber extends from the iris to the lens. Normally, the aqueous humor is produced in the posterior chamber, passes through the pupil into the anterior chamber, and then drains out of the eyeball through outflow channels at the edge of the iris.

An Inside Look at the Eye

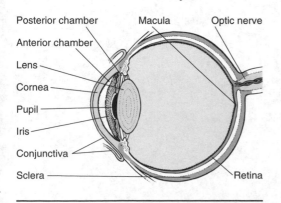

Posterior chamber Macula Optic nerve

Anterior chamber

Lens

Cornea

Pupil

Iris

Conjunctiva

Sclera Retina

Muscles, Nerves, and Blood Vessels

Several muscles working together move the eyes. Each muscle is stimulated by a specific cranial nerve. The bony orbit that protects the eye also contains many other nerves. As mentioned, the optic nerve exits through the back of the eye and carries nerve impulses created in the retina to the brain. The lacrimal nerve stimulates the tear glands to produce tears. Other nerves transmit sensation to other parts of the eye and stimulate the muscles of the orbit.

An ophthalmic artery and a retinal artery provide blood to each eye, and an ophthalmic vein and a retinal vein drain blood from it. These blood vessels enter and leave through the back of the eye.

Protective Features

The structures around the eye protect it while allowing it to move freely in all directions. They protect the eye, which is constantly exposed to dust, wind, bacteria, viruses, fungi, and other potentially injurious substances, while allowing it to remain open enough to catch light rays.

The orbits are bony cavities containing the eyeballs, muscles, nerves, blood vessels, fat, and structures that produce and drain tears. The eyelids, thin folds of skin, cover the eyes. They reflexively close quickly to protect the eye from foreign objects, wind, dust, and very bright light. When blinked, the eyelids help spread liquid over the surface of the eyes, and when closed, they help keep the surface moist. Without such moisture, the normally transparent cornea can become dried, injured, and opaque.

The inner surface of the eyelid is a thin membrane (conjunctiva) that loops back to cover the surface of the eye. The eyelashes are short hairs growing from the edge of the eyelid that help protect the eye by acting as a barrier. Small glands at the edge of the eyelid secrete an oily substance that contributes to the tear film and keeps tears from evaporating.

The lacrimal glands, located at the top outer edge of each eye, produce the watery portion of tears. Tears drain from the eyes into the nose through the two nasolacrimal ducts; each of these ducts has openings at the edge of the upper and lower eyelids near the nose. Tears keep the surface of the eye moist and healthy; they also trap and sweep away small particles that enter the eye. Moreover, tears are rich in antibodies that help prevent infection.

Structures That Protect the Eye

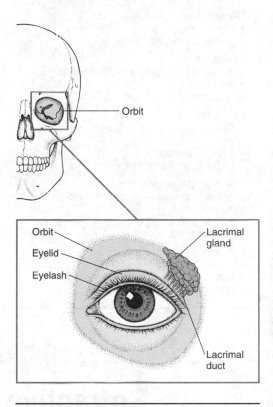

Blindness

Both eye injury and disease can affect vision. The clarity of vision is called visual acuity, which ranges from full vision to no vision. As acuity decreases, vision becomes progressively blurred. Acuity is usually measured on a scale that compares a person's vision at 20 feet with that of someone who has full acuity. Thus, a person who has 20/20 vision sees objects 20 feet away with complete clarity, but a person who has 20/200 vision sees at 20 feet what a person with full acuity sees at 200 feet.

Legal blindness is defined as visual acuity worse than 20/200 even after correction with eyeglasses or contact lenses. Many people who are considered legally blind can distinguish shapes and shadows but not normal detail.

Common Causes of Blindness

Cataract
• Most common cause
• Can be cured with surgery

Infection
• Most common preventable cause in the world
• Not common in United States

Diabetes
• One of most common causes in United States
• Often preventable
• Laser treatment slows vision loss

Macular degeneration
• Affects central vision, not peripheral vision
• Preventable and treatable in fewer than 10 percent of people

Glaucoma
• Highly treatable
• If treated early, should not lead to blindness

Causes

Blindness can occur for any of the following reasons:
• light can't reach the retina
• light rays don't focus properly on the retina
• the retina can't sense light rays normally
• the nerve impulses from the retina aren't transmitted to the brain normally
• the brain can't interpret information sent by the eye.

Several disorders can cause these problems that lead to blindness. A cataract▲ can block light coming into the eye, so that it never reaches the retina. Focusing (refraction) errors■ can usually be corrected with prescription lenses but not always completely. A detached retina and hereditary disorders such as retinitis pigmentosa★ can affect the retina's ability to sense light. Diabetes or macular degeneration● can also damage the retina. Disorders of the nervous system such as multiple sclerosis or inadequate blood supply can damage the optic nerve, which carries impulses to the brain. Tumors in nearby structures, such as the pituitary gland, also can damage this nerve. The areas of the brain that interpret visual impulses may be damaged by stroke, tumor, or other disease.

CHAPTER 217

Refractive Disorders

Normally, the eye creates a clear image because the cornea and lens bend (refract) incoming light rays to focus them on the retina. The shape of the cornea is fixed, but the lens changes shape to focus on objects at various distances from the eye. The shape of the eyeball further helps to create a clear image on the retina.

People who are farsighted (hyperopic) have trouble seeing anything close, and those who are nearsighted (myopic) have trouble focusing on distant objects. As people reach their early 40s, the lens becomes increasingly stiff, so that it can't focus on nearby objects, a condition called presbyopia. If a person has had a lens removed to treat cataracts but hasn't had a lens implant, objects look blurred at any distance; the absence of a lens is called aphakia. An imperfectly shaped cornea may cause visual distortion from astigmatism.

Everyone should have regular eye examinations by a family doctor, internist, ophthalmolo-

▲ see page 1042

■ see below

★ see page 1047

● see page 1045

gist, or optometrist. The eyes are tested together and individually. Vision testing usually also includes assessments unrelated to refractive error, such as a test of the ability to see colors.

Treatment

The usual treatment for refractive errors is to wear corrective lenses. However, certain surgical procedures and laser treatments that change the shape of the cornea also can correct refractive errors.

Corrective Lenses

Refractive errors can be corrected with glass or plastic lenses mounted in a frame (eyeglasses) or with small pieces of plastic placed directly over the cornea (contact lenses). For most people, the choice is a matter of appearance, convenience, and comfort.

Plastic lenses for eyeglasses are lighter but tend to scratch; glass lenses are more durable but more likely to break. Both types can be tinted or treated with a chemical that darkens them automatically on exposure to light. Lenses can also be coated to reduce the amount of potentially damaging ultraviolet light that reaches the eye. Bifocals contain two lenses—an upper lens that corrects nearsightedness and a lower lens that corrects farsightedness.

Many people think contact lenses are more attractive than eyeglasses, and some think that vision is more natural with contact lenses. However, contact lenses require more care than glasses, they may damage the eye, and they can't correct vision for some people as well as eyeglasses can. The elderly and people with arthritis may have trouble handling contact lenses and placing them in their eyes.

Hard (rigid) contact lenses are thin disks made of hard plastic. Gas-permeable lenses, made of silicone and other compounds, are rigid but permit better oxygen transport to the cornea. Soft hydrophilic contact lenses made of flexible plastic are larger and cover the entire cornea. Most soft, nonhydrophilic lenses are made of silicone.

Elderly people generally find soft lenses easier to handle because they're larger. They're also less likely than rigid lenses to fall out or to allow dust and other particles to get trapped underneath. Plus, soft contact lenses are usually comfortable on the first wearing. They do, however, require scrupulous care.

Understanding Refraction

These illustrations show how the cornea and lens focus light on the retina when vision is normal, abnormal, and corrected by eyeglasses or contact lenses.

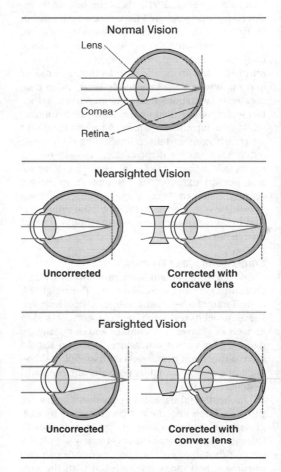

Normal Vision

Lens
Cornea
Retina

Nearsighted Vision

Uncorrected   Corrected with
                               concave lens

Farsighted Vision

Uncorrected   Corrected with
                               convex lens

People need to wear their first pair of rigid contact lenses for up to a week before it feels comfortable for a prolonged period. The lenses are worn for a gradually increasing number of hours each day. Although lenses may be uncomfortable at first, they shouldn't be painful. Pain indicates an improper fit.

Most contact lenses must be removed and cleaned every day. As an alternative, a person can use disposable lenses—some of which are replaced every week or two, others of which are replaced every day. Using disposable lenses avoids the need to clean and store lenses because each lens is regularly replaced with a fresh one.

Wearing any type of contact lenses poses a risk of serious, painful complications, including corneal ulceration from an infection, which can lead to a loss of vision.▲ The risks can be greatly reduced by following the instructions of the manufacturer and the eye doctor and by using common sense. All reusable contact lenses must be sterilized and disinfected; enzyme cleaning is no substitute for sterilizing and disinfecting. The risk of serious infections increases from cleaning contact lenses with homemade saline solution, saliva, tap water, or distilled water and from swimming while wearing contact lenses. A person shouldn't wear soft contact lenses—including daily wear, extended wear, or disposable types—to bed at night, unless there's a special reason for doing so. If a person experiences discomfort, excessive tearing, vision changes, or eye redness, the lenses should be removed immediately. If the symptoms don't resolve quickly, the person should contact an eye doctor.

Surgery and Laser Therapy

Certain surgical and laser procedures (refractive surgery) can be used to correct nearsightedness, farsightedness, and astigmatism. However, these procedures don't usually correct vision as well as glasses and contact lenses do. Before deciding on such a procedure, a person should have a thorough discussion with an ophthalmologist and should carefully consider the risks and benefits.

The best candidates for refractive surgery are people whose vision can't be corrected by eyeglasses or contact lenses and people who can't tolerate wearing them. However, many people undergo this surgery for convenience and cosmetic purposes, and many are satisfied with the outcome.

Radial and Astigmatic Keratotomy: Keratotomy is a surgical procedure used to treat nearsightedness and astigmatism. In radial keratotomy, the

surgeon makes small radial (or wheel spoke) cuts in the cornea. Usually, four to eight cuts are made. In astigmatic keratotomy, which is used to correct naturally occurring astigmatism and astigmatism after cataract surgery or corneal transplant, the surgeon uses perpendicular cuts. Because the cornea is only $\frac{1}{2}$ millimeter in thickness, the depth of the cuts must be determined precisely. The surgeon determines where to make each cut after analyzing the shape of the cornea and the person's visual acuity.

The surgery flattens the cornea, so it can better focus incoming light on the retina. This change improves vision, and about 90 percent of those who have the surgery can function well and drive without their glasses or contact lenses. Sometimes, a second or third touch-up procedure is needed to improve vision sufficiently.

No surgical procedure is risk free, but the risks from radial and astigmatic keratotomy are small. The major risks are overcorrection and undercorrection of the vision problem. Because overcorrection usually can't be treated effectively, a surgeon tries to avoid doing too much correction at any one time. As mentioned, undercorrection can be addressed by a second or third touch-up procedure. The most serious complication is infection, which develops in far less than 1 percent of cases. When it does develop, it must be treated with antibiotics.

Photorefractive Keratectomy: This laser surgical procedure reshapes the cornea. Photorefractive keratectomy uses a highly focused beam of light to remove small amounts of the cornea and thus change its shape. As with the surgical procedures, changing the shape of the cornea better focuses light onto the retina and improves vision.

Although laser surgery appears promising for correcting poor vision, there are problems with it. For example, the recovery period is longer and more painful than with other refractive surgery procedures. However, the risks are similar to those for radial and astigmatic keratotomy.

Laser in situ Keratomileusis (LASIK): LASIK may produce less pain and greater visual recovery than photorefractive keratectomy. However, the possible complications of the LASIK procedure are much greater than with photorefractive keratectomy.

▲ see page 1041

Eye Injuries

The structure of the face and eyes is well suited for protecting the eyes from injury. The eyeball is set into a socket surrounded by a strong, bony ridge. The eyelids can close quickly to form a barrier to foreign objects, and the eye can tolerate a light impact without damage.▲ Even so, the eye and its surrounding structures can be damaged by injury, sometimes so severely that vision is lost, and in rare instances, the eye must be removed. Most eye injuries are minor, but because of extensive bruising, they often look worse than they are. Any injury to the eye should be examined by a doctor to determine whether treatment is needed and whether the eyesight may be affected permanently.

Blunt Injuries

A blunt impact forces the eye back into its socket, possibly damaging the structures at the surface (the lid, conjunctiva, sclera, cornea, and lens) and those at the back of the eye (retina and nerves).■ Such an impact may break bones around the eye as well.

Symptoms

In the first 24 hours after an eye injury, blood leaking into the skin around the eye usually produces a bruise (contusion), commonly called a black eye. If a blood vessel on the surface of the eye breaks, the surface will become red. Such bleeding is usually minor.

Damage to the inside of the eye is often more serious than damage to the surface. Bleeding into the front chamber of the eye (anterior chamber hemorrhage, traumatic hyphema) is potentially serious and requires attention by an eye doctor (ophthalmologist). Recurring bleeding and increased pressure within the eye may lead to blood staining of the cornea, which can reduce vision much as a cataract does,★ and increase the lifelong risk of glaucoma.

Blood can leak into the inside of the eye, the iris (the colored part of the eye) can be torn, or the lens can become dislocated. Bleeding may occur in the retina, which may become detached from its underlying surface at the back of the eye.

Initially, retinal detachment may create images of irregular floating shapes or flashes of light and may make vision blurry, but then vision greatly decreases.● In severe injuries, the eyeball can rupture.

Treatment

Ice packs may help reduce swelling and ease the pain of a black eye. By the second day, warm compresses can help the body absorb the excess blood that has accumulated. If the skin around the eye or on the lid has been cut (lacerated), stitches may be needed. When possible, stitches near the edge of the eyelids should be applied by an eye surgeon to ensure that no deformities develop that will affect the way the lids close. An injury affecting the tear ducts should be repaired by an eye surgeon.

For a laceration of the eye, pain medications may be given along with medications to keep the pupil dilated and to prevent infection. A metal shield is often used to protect the eye from further injury. Serious damage may result in some loss of sight, even after surgical treatment.

Anyone who has internal bleeding in the eye caused by trauma is instructed to rest in bed. A medication to reduce increased eye pressure, such as acetazolamide, may be needed. Sometimes an additional medication, aminocaproic acid, is given to reduce bleeding. Any medication that contains aspirin should be avoided because aspirin can increase internal bleeding in the eye. People taking warfarin or heparin to keep their blood from clotting or aspirin for any reason should tell the doctor immediately. Rarely, recurring bleeding requires surgical drainage by an ophthalmologist.

▲ see page 1027

■ see box, page 1026

★ see page 1042

● see page 1046

Foreign Objects

The most common eye injuries are those to the sclera, cornea, and lining of the eyelids (conjunctiva) caused by foreign objects. Although most of these injuries are minor, some—such as penetration of the cornea or development of an infection from a cut or scratch on the cornea—can be serious.

Perhaps the most common source of surface injuries is the contact lens. Poorly fitting lenses, lenses left in the eyes too long, lenses left in while a person sleeps, inadequately sterilized lenses, and forceful or inept removal of lenses can scratch the surface of the eye. Other causes of surface injuries include glass particles, windborne particles, tree branches, and falling debris. Workers in certain occupations tend to have small particles fly in their faces; these workers should wear protective eyewear.

Symptoms

Any injury to the surface of the eye usually causes pain and a feeling that there's something in the eye. It may also produce a sensitivity to light, redness, bleeding from the surface blood vessels of the eye, or swelling of the eye and eyelid. Vision may become blurred.

Treatment

A foreign object in the eye must be removed. Special eyedrops containing fluorescein dye make the object more visible and reveal any surface abrasions. Anesthetic drops may be instilled to numb the surface of the eye. Using a special lighting instrument to view the surface in detail, the doctor then removes the object. Often the foreign object can be lifted out with a moist sterile cotton swab. Sometimes it can be flushed out with sterile water.

If the foreign object has produced a small, superficial corneal abrasion, an antibiotic ointment applied for several days may be all the treatment needed. Larger corneal abrasions require additional treatment. The pupil is kept dilated with medications, antibiotics are instilled, and a patch is placed over the eye to keep it closed. Fortunately, the surface cells of the eye regenerate rapidly. Under a patch, even large abrasions tend to heal in 1 to 3 days. If the foreign object has pierced the deeper layers of the eye, an ophthalmologist should be consulted immediately for emergency treatment.

Burns

Exposure to strong heat or chemicals makes the eyelids close quickly in a reflex reaction to protect the eyes from burns. Thus, only the eyelids may be burned, although extreme heat can also burn the eye itself. The severity of the injury, the amount of pain, and the appearance of the eyelids depend on the depth of the burn.

Chemical burns can occur when an irritating substance gets into the eye. Even mildly irritating substances can cause substantial pain and damage the eye. Because the pain is so great, there's a tendency to keep the eyelids closed, thereby keeping the substance against the eye for a prolonged period.

Treatment

To treat burns on the eyelids, a health care practitioner washes the area with a sterile solution and then applies an antibiotic ointment or a strip of gauze saturated with petroleum jelly. The treated area is covered with sterile dressings held in place with a plastic bandage or stockinette to allow the burn to heal.

A chemical burn of the eye is treated by immediately flooding the open eye with water. This treatment must be started even before trained medical personnel arrive. Although a person may have difficulty keeping the injured eye open during this painful treatment, quick removal of the chemical is essential. A doctor may begin treatment by instilling anesthetic drops and medication to keep the pupil dilated. Antibiotics are usually used in ointment form. Oral analgesics may also be needed. Severe burns may need to be treated by an ophthalmologist to preserve vision and prevent major complications, such as damage to the iris, perforation of the eye, and deformities of the eyelids. However, even with the best treatment, severe chemical burns of the cornea can lead to scarring, perforation of the eye, and blindness.

Eye Socket Disorders

The eye sockets (orbits) are bony cavities that contain and protect the eyes. Disorders affecting the orbits include fractures, orbital cellulitis, cavernous sinus thrombosis, and exophthalmos.

Fractures

An injury to the face can fracture any of several bones that form the orbits.▲ Although a facial fracture usually doesn't impair vision, certain fractures can.

Blood that accumulates after a fracture can put pressure on the eye or on the nerves and blood vessels going to and from it. The fracture may also impair the function of the muscles that move the eye, producing double vision or inhibiting eye movement to the right, left, up, or down. Rarely, a fragment of broken bone presses on or cuts into a nerve, blood vessel, or muscle, impairing eye movement and vision.

When a fracture traps nerves or muscles or pushes the eyeball backward, a repair of the facial bones—usually a surgical repair—is necessary. After ensuring that the fracture hasn't damaged a vital structure, the surgeon restores the bones to their proper position, using small metal plates and screws or wires.

Orbital Cellulitis

Orbital cellulitis is an infection of the tissues around the eyeball.

The infection may spread from the sinuses, teeth, or bloodstream, or it may develop after an eye injury. Symptoms of orbital cellulitis include extreme pain, bulging eyes, reduced eye movement, swollen eyelids, fever, and a swollen, hazy appearance of the eyeball. If not adequately treated, orbital cellulitis can lead to blindness, infection of the brain and spinal cord, and blood clots in the brain.

Diagnosis and Treatment

Doctors can usually recognize orbital cellulitis without using diagnostic tests. However, determining the cause may require further assessment, including examinations of the teeth and mouth as well as x-rays or computerized tomography (CT)

scans of the sinuses. Often, doctors obtain samples from the lining of the eye and from the skin, blood, throat, or sinuses and send them to the laboratory to be cultured. These tests help determine which type of bacteria is causing the infection and which treatment should be used.

Oral antibiotics are given for mild cases; intravenous antibiotics are given for severe cases. The antibiotic used at first may be changed if the culture results suggest that another one will be more effective. Sometimes surgery is needed to drain a pocket of infection (abscess) or an infected sinus.

Cavernous Sinus Thrombosis

Cavernous sinus thrombosis is the blockage of a large vein at the base of the brain (the cavernous sinus), usually caused by the spread of bacteria from a sinus infection or an infection around the nose.

An infection may spread from a sinus or the area of skin around the nose or eye to the brain either directly or through veins. This infection causes bulging eyes, severe headache, coma, seizures, and other nervous system abnormalities, along with a high fever.

Fortunately, cavernous sinus thrombosis is very rare. About 30 percent of people who have it die, and many who survive are left with serious mental or neurologic handicaps despite medical treatment.

Diagnosis and Treatment

To diagnose cavernous sinus thrombosis and identify the bacteria causing the infection, a doctor takes a blood sample and samples of fluid, mucus, or pus from the throat and nose and sends them to the laboratory to be cultured. Also, a computed tomography (CT) scan of the sinuses, eyes, and brain is usually performed.

High doses of intravenous antibiotics are given immediately. If the condition doesn't improve after 24 hours of antibiotic treatment, the sinus may be drained surgically.

▲ see box, page 1027

Exophthalmos

Exophthalmos is an abnormal bulging of one or both eyes.

All people with protruding eyes don't necessarily have exophthalmos. Some people simply have prominent eyes with more white showing than normal. The extent of the protrusion can be measured in an eye doctor's (ophthalmologist's) office with an ordinary ruler or with an instrument called an exophthalmometer. Further diagnostic tests may include a computed tomography (CT) scan and thyroid function tests.

Many conditions can cause exophthalmos. In some types of thyroid disease, especially Graves' disease, the tissues in the eye socket swell, and deposits of unusual material push the eyeball forward. Exophthalmos can occur suddenly from bleeding behind the eye or from inflammation in the eye socket. Tumors, either cancerous or noncancerous, can form in the eye socket behind the eyeball and push it forward. An unusual growth of tissue (pseudotumor) may produce exophthalmos in 2 to 3 weeks. Cavernous sinus thrombosis causes swelling from the backup of blood in the veins exiting the eye. Abnormal connections of the arteries and veins (arteriovenous malformations) behind the eye may produce a pulsating exophthalmos, in which the eye bulges forward and pulses along with the heartbeat.

Treatment

The treatment depends on the cause. If the problem is an abnormality between arteries and veins, surgery may be needed. If too much thyroid hormone is being produced (hyperthyroidism), the bulging may subside when hyperthyroidism is controlled. Occasionally, however, exophthalmos persists even when the thyroid disease has been controlled. If the optic nerve is being compressed, oral corticosteroids, local radiation therapy, or surgery is needed to ease the pressure. If the eyelids don't properly cover the bulging eyeball, eyelid surgery may be needed to help protect the cornea from drying and infection. Corticosteroids may help in treating pseudotumor and swelling. If tumors threaten the eye by pushing it forward, they may be removed surgically.

CHAPTER 220

Eyelid and Tear Gland Disorders

The eyelids play a key role in protecting the eyes. They help spread moisture (tears) over the surface of the eyes when they close (for example, while blinking); thus, they help prevent the eyes from becoming dry. The eyelids also provide a mechanical barrier against injury, closing reflexively when an object comes too close to the eye. The reflex is triggered by the sight of an approaching object, the touch of an object on the surface of the eye, or the eyelashes being exposed to wind or small particles such as dust or sand.

Tears are a salty fluid that continuously bathes the surface of the eye to keep it moist. This fluid also contains antibodies that help protect the eye from infection. Tears are produced by the lacrimal (tear) glands, located near the outer corner of the eye. The fluid flows over the eye and exits through two small openings in the eyelids (lacrimal ducts); these openings lead to the nasolacrimal duct, a channel that empties into the nose.

If the lacrimal glands don't produce enough tears, the eyes can become painfully dry and can be damaged. A rare cause of inadequate tear production is Sjögren's syndrome.▲ The eyes can also become dry when evaporation causes an excessive loss of tears, for example, if the eyelids don't close properly.

Nasolacrimal Duct Blockage

Blockage of the nasolacrimal duct (dacryostenosis) can result from inadequate development of the nasolacrimal system at birth, a chronic nasal

---

▲ see page 234

infection, severe or recurring eye infections, or fractures of the nasal or facial bones. Blockage can be partial or complete.

Blockage caused by an immature nasolacrimal system usually results in an overflow of tears that runs down the cheek (epiphora) from one eye or, rarely, from both eyes in 3- to 12-week-old infants. This type of blockage usually disappears without treatment by the age of 6 months, as the nasolacrimal system develops. Sometimes the blockage resolves faster when parents are taught to milk the duct by gently massaging the area above it with a fingertip.

Regardless of the cause of the blockage, if inflammation of the conjunctiva (conjunctivitis) develops, antibiotic eyedrops may be needed. If the blockage doesn't clear up, an ear, nose, and throat specialist (otorhinolaryngologist) or an eye specialist (ophthalmologist) may have to open the duct with a small probe, usually inserted through the duct opening at the corner of the eyelid. Children are given general anesthesia for this procedure, but adults need only local anesthesia. If the duct is completely blocked, more extensive surgery may be needed.

Lacrimal Sac Infection

Usually, infection of the lacrimal sac (dacryocystitis) results from a blockage of the nasolacrimal duct. The infection makes the area around the sac painful, red, and swollen. The eye becomes red and watery and oozes pus. Slight pressure applied to the sac may push pus through the opening at the inner corner of the eye, near the nose. The person also has a fever.

If a mild or recurring infection continues for a long time, most of the symptoms may disappear, with only slight swelling of the area remaining. Sometimes, an infection causes fluid to be retained in the lacrimal sac, and a large fluid-filled sac (mucocele) forms under the skin. Recurring infections may produce a thickened, red area over the sac. An abscess may form and rupture through the skin, creating a passage for drainage.

The infection is treated with oral or intravenous antibiotics. Applying frequent warm compresses to the area also helps. If an abscess develops, surgery is performed to open and drain it. For

Viewing the Lacrimal Structures

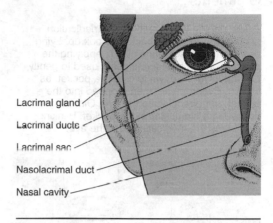

Lacrimal gland
Lacrimal ducts
Lacrimal sac
Nasolacrimal duct
Nasal cavity

chronic infections, the blocked nasolacrimal duct may be opened with a probe or by surgery. In rare instances, surgical removal of the entire lacrimal sac may be necessary.

Eyelid Swelling

Anything that irritates the eyes can also irritate the eyelids and cause swelling (lid edema). The most common irritant is an allergy, which can make one or both lids crinkled and swollen. Allergic reactions may be caused by medications instilled into the eyes, such as eyedrops; other drugs or cosmetics; or pollen or other particles in the air. Insect stings or bites as well as infections from bacteria, viruses, or fungi can also cause the eyelids to swell.

Removing the cause of swelling and applying cold compresses may relieve the swelling. If an allergy is the cause, avoiding the allergen can alleviate the swelling; a doctor may also prescribe drug therapy. If a foreign object such as an insect stinger is lodged in the eyelid, it must be removed.

Eyelid Inflammation

Inflammation of the eyelids (blepharitis) causes redness and thickening; scales and crusts

Using Eyedrops and Eye Ointments

The person who'll receive the medication should lean the head back and look up. Lying down is best if someone else is applying the medication. A clean forefinger is used to gently pull the lower lid down to create a pocket, as shown. Eyedrops are then dropped into the pocket, not directly onto the eye. Ointment is applied in a small strip in the pocket. Blinking distributes the medication over the eye.

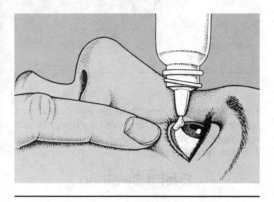

or shallow ulcers often form on the eyelids, as well. Conditions that may occur with eyelid inflammation include staphylococcal infection on the eyelids and in the oil (sebaceous) glands at the edges of the lids, seborrheic dermatitis of the face and scalp, and rosacea.

Blepharitis may produce the feeling that something is in the eye. The eyes and lids may itch, burn, and become red. The eyelid may swell and some of the lashes may fall out. The eyes may become red, teary, and sensitive to bright light. A crust may form and stick tenaciously to the edges of the lid; when the crust is removed, it may leave a bleeding surface. During sleep, dried secretions make the lids sticky.

Blepharitis tends to recur and stubbornly resist treatment. It's inconvenient and unattractive but usually not destructive. Occasionally, it can result in a loss of the eyelashes, scarring of the lid margins, and even damage to the cornea.

Usually, treatment consists of keeping the eyelids clean, perhaps by washing them with baby shampoo. Occasionally, a doctor may prescribe an antibiotic ointment, such as erythromycin or sulfacetamide, or an oral antibiotic, such as tetracycline. When the person's skin is also affected with seborrheic dermatitis, the face and scalp must be treated as well.

Stye

A stye (hordeolum) is an infection, usually a staphylococcal infection, of one or more of the glands at the edge of the eyelid or under it.

An abscess forms and tends to rupture, releasing a small amount of pus. Styes sometimes form simultaneously with or as a result of blepharitis. A person may have one or two styes in a lifetime, but some people develop them repeatedly.

A stye usually begins with redness, tenderness, and pain at the edge of the eyelid. Then a small, round, tender, swollen area forms. The eye may water, become sensitive to bright light, and feel as though something is in it. Usually, only a small area of the lid is swollen, but sometimes the entire lid swells. Often a tiny, yellowish spot develops at the center of the swollen area.

Although antibiotics are used, they don't seem to help much. The best treatment is to apply hot compresses for 10 minutes several times a day. The warmth helps the stye come to a head, rupture, and drain. When a stye forms in one of the deeper glands of the eyelid, a condition called an internal hordeolum, the pain and other symptoms are usually more severe. Pain, redness, and swelling tend to occur in just a very small area, usually at the edge of the eyelid. Because this type of stye rarely ruptures by itself, a doctor may have to open it to drain the pus. Internal styes tend to recur.

Chalazion

A chalazion is an enlargement of a long, thin oil gland in the eyelid that results from an obstruction of the gland opening at the edge of the eyelid.

At first, a chalazion looks and feels like a stye: swollen eyelid, pain, and irritation. However, after a few days the symptoms disappear, leaving a round, painless swelling in the eyelid that grows slowly for the first week. A red or gray area may develop underneath the eyelid.

Most chalazions disappear without treatment after a few months. If hot compresses are applied several times a day, they may disappear sooner. If they remain after 6 weeks, a doctor can drain them or simply inject a corticosteroid.

Entropion and Ectropion

Entropion is a condition in which the eyelid is turned in against the eyeball. Ectropion is a condition in which the eyelid is turned outward and doesn't come in contact with the eyeball.

Normally, the upper and lower eyelids close tightly, protecting the eye from damage and preventing tear evaporation. If the edge of one eyelid turns in (entropion), the lashes rub against the eye, which can lead to ulceration and scarring of the cornea. If the edge of one eyelid turns outward (ectropion), the two eyelids can't meet properly, and tears aren't spread over the eyeball. These conditions are more common in older people and in those who have had an eyelid injury that caused scar formation. Both conditions can irritate the eyes, causing tearing and redness. Both can be treated by surgery, if necessary.

Eyelid Tumors

Noncancerous (benign) and cancerous (malignant) growths can form on the eyelids. One of the most common types of benign tumor is xanthelasma, a yellow-white, flat growth that consists of fatty material. Xanthelasmas needn't be removed unless their appearance becomes bothersome. Because xanthelasmas may indicate elevated cholesterol levels (especially in young people), a doctor will check the person's cholesterol level.

Squamous cell carcinoma and the more common basal cell carcinoma,▲ both cancerous growths, can develop on the eyelid as well as on many other areas of the skin. If a growth on the eyelid doesn't disappear after several weeks, a doctor may perform a biopsy (removal of a specimen and examination under a microscope), and the growth is treated, usually with surgery.

CHAPTER 221

Disorders of the Conjunctiva

The conjunctiva is the thin, tough lining that covers the back of the eyelid and loops back to cover the sclera (the white of the eye).■ The conjunctiva helps protect the eye from foreign objects and infection but can itself become irritated by chemicals or allergic reactions or infected by viruses or bacteria. These conditions generally produce pain, itching, and redness on the surface of the eye.

Conjunctivitis

Conjunctivitis is an inflammation of the conjunctiva, usually caused by viruses, bacteria, or an allergy.

The conjunctiva can be inflamed by an allergic reaction to dust, mold, animal dander, or pollen and can be irritated by wind, dust, smoke, and other types of air pollution. It may also be irritated by a common cold or a bout of measles. The ultraviolet light of an electric welding arc, sunlamp, or even bright sunlight reflected by snow can irritate the conjunctiva.

Sometimes, conjunctivitis can last for months or years. This type of conjunctivitis may be caused by conditions in which an eyelid is turned outward (ectropion) or inward (entropion), problems with the tear ducts, sensitivity to chemicals, exposure to irritants, and infection by particular bacteria—typically chlamydia.

Symptoms and Diagnosis

When irritated, the conjunctiva becomes bloodshot, and a discharge often appears in the

---

▲ see page 992

■ see box, page 1026

eye. In bacterial conjunctivitis, the discharge may be thick and white or creamy. In viral or allergic conjunctivitis, the discharge is usually clear. The eyelid may swell and itch intensely, especially in allergic conjunctivitis.

Usually conjunctivitis is easy to recognize because it commonly occurs with a cold or allergies. Sometimes, however, conjunctivitis resembles iritis, a more severe eye inflammation, or even acute glaucoma—serious conditions that can lead to a loss of vision. A doctor can usually distinguish the diseases. With the more serious eye conditions, the blood vessels closest to the colored part of the eye (iris) are very inflamed. Although conjunctivitis may cause a burning sensation, it's usually less painful than the more serious conditions. Conjunctivitis almost never affects vision unless the discharge temporarily covers the cornea.

Treatment

Treatment for conjunctivitis depends on the cause. The eyelids should be gently bathed with tap water and a clean washcloth to keep them clean and free of discharge. If the cause is a bacterial infection, antibiotic eyedrops or ointment may be prescribed.▲ Sometimes the doctor takes a small sample of discharge with a cotton-tipped applicator for testing in a laboratory, then adjusts the prescription according to the test results. Corticosteroid eyedrops aren't used with antibiotics and should never be used by someone who might have a herpes infection because corticosteroids tend to make herpes worse.

Antibiotics don't help allergic or viral conjunctivitis. Antihistamines taken orally may relieve the itching and irritation. If not, corticosteroid eyedrops can help.

Because infective conjunctivitis is highly contagious, a person should wash the hands before and after bathing the eye or applying medication to it. Also, a person should be careful not to touch the infected eye and then touch the other eye. Towels and washcloths used to clean the eye should be kept separate from other towels and washcloths.

Surgery may be needed to correct the alignment of the eyelids or to open clogged tear ducts.

Gonococcal Conjunctivitis

Newborns can acquire a gonococcal infection of the conjunctiva from their mother while passing through the birth canal. For this reason, most states require that all newborns receive eyedrops—often silver nitrate, povidone iodine, or an antibiotic ointment such as erythromycin—to kill the bacteria that could cause gonococcal conjunctivitis. Adults can contract gonococcal conjunctivitis during sexual activity if, for example, infected semen gets into the eye. Usually only one eye is involved.

Within 12 to 48 hours after the infection starts, the eye becomes red and painful. If the infection isn't treated, ulcers can form on the cornea, an abscess can develop, the eyeball can become perforated, and even blindness can result. Antibiotic tablets, injections, or eyedrops can cure gonococcal conjunctivitis.

Trachoma

Trachoma (granular conjunctivitis, Egyptian ophthalmia) is a prolonged infection of the conjunctiva caused by the bacterium Chlamydia trachomatis.

Trachoma is common in poverty-stricken parts of the dry, hot Mediterranean countries and the Far East. It occurs occasionally among Native Americans and among people in mountainous areas of the southern United States. Trachoma is contagious in its early stages and may be transmitted by eye-hand contact, by certain flies, or by contaminated articles such as towels and handkerchiefs.

Symptoms and Treatment

In the early stages of the disease, the conjunctiva is inflamed, reddened, and irritated, and a discharge appears. In the later stages, the conjunctiva and cornea become scarred, causing the eyelashes to turn inward and vision to become impaired.

When trachoma is suspected, a doctor swabs the eye or scrapes the area to obtain a specimen, which is sent to a laboratory, where the infecting organism is identified. Treatment consists of applying antibiotic ointments containing tetracy-

---

▲ see box, page 1036

cline or erythromycin for 4 to 6 weeks. Alternatively, these antibiotics can be taken orally. If the condition causes deformities of the eyelid, conjunctiva, or cornea, surgery may be needed.

Inclusion Conjunctivitis

Inclusion conjunctivitis is a form of conjunctivitis caused by the bacterium Chlamydia trachomatis.

Newborns may be infected by their mother while passing through the birth canal; adults may be infected by being exposed to genital secretions containing the bacterium.

Symptoms and Treatment

About 5 to 14 days after birth, an infected newborn develops severe conjunctivitis with swelling of the eyelids and conjunctiva. A sticky discharge of pus runs from the eyes. Adults are usually infected in only one eye. The lymph nodes near the ear may swell. Occasionally, the condition damages the cornea, causing cloudy areas and a growth of blood vessels. Antibiotics usually don't reverse such damage, but they may help prevent it if they're given early.

Half of the children who have this condition also have a chlamydial infection of the throat and nose, and about 10 percent develop pneumonia. Regardless of the extent of infection, the antibiotic erythromycin generally cures it. In adults, erythromycin or other antibiotics, such as tetracycline and doxycycline, can be used. The mother of an infected child or the sex partner of an infected adult should also be treated.

Vernal Keratoconjunctivitis

Vernal keratoconjunctivitis is a recurring inflammation of the conjunctiva, usually in both eyes, that may damage the surface of the cornea.

Because the condition is typically caused by allergies, it tends to recur in the spring and summer. Vernal keratoconjunctivitis is most common in children; it usually begins before puberty and resolves before age 20.

Symptoms and Treatment

Symptoms include intense itching; red, watery eyes; sensitivity to sunlight; and a thick, sticky discharge. In one form of the condition, the conjunctiva under the upper lids is most affected, becoming swollen and pale pink to grayish, while the rest of the conjunctiva becomes milky white. In another form, the conjunctiva covering the eyeball is thick and grayish. Sometimes a small area of the cornea is damaged, causing pain and extreme sensitivity to light. All symptoms usually disappear in cold weather and become milder over the years.

Antiallergy eyedrops such as cromolyn, lodoxamide, ketorolac, and levocabastine are the safest treatments. Oral antihistamines may also help. Corticosteroids are more potent but shouldn't be used for more than a few weeks without close monitoring because increased pressure in the eyes, cataracts, and opportunistic infections may result.

Keratoconjunctivitis Sicca

Keratoconjunctivitis sicca is a long-standing dryness of both eyes leading to dehydration of the conjunctiva and cornea.

Dry eyes may be a symptom of diseases such as rheumatoid arthritis, systemic lupus erythematosus, or Sjögren's syndrome. Whether accompanying these diseases or occurring alone, dry eyes are most common in adult women.

Symptoms, Diagnosis, and Treatment

Reduced tear production or a loss of tears by evaporation leads to irritation of the eye, causing a burning sensation. Scattered damage to the surface of the eye increases discomfort and sensitivity to bright light. In the advanced stages of this condition, the surface of the eye can thicken and develop ulcers and scarring, and blood vessel growth can increase. If scarring affects the cornea, it can impair vision.

Although a doctor can usually diagnose dry eyes by the symptoms alone, a Schirmer test—in which a strip of filter paper is placed at the edge of the eyelid—can measure the amount of moisture bathing the eye. Doctors examine the eyes with a slit lamp (a microscope that magnifies the structures of the eye) to determine if damage has developed.

Artificial tears (eyedrops prepared with substances that simulate real tears) applied every few hours can generally control the problem. Surgery can be done to block the flow of tears into the nose, so that more tears are available to bathe

the eyes. In people with very dry eyes, the eyelids may be partially sewn together to decrease tear evaporation.

Episcleritis

Episcleritis is an inflammation of the sclera, a layer of tissue that lies below the conjunctiva.

Usually, the inflammation affects only a small patch of the eyeball and causes a yellow, slightly raised area. The condition isn't usually a sign of any other disease and tends to disappear and recur. Although treatment is often unnecessary, corticosteroid eyedrops can be applied.

Scleritis

Scleritis is a deep, extremely painful inflammation and purple discoloration of the sclera that may severely damage vision.

Scleritis may accompany rheumatoid arthritis and related disorders. In severe cases, this inflam-

mation leads to perforation of the eyeball and loss of the eye.

Scleritis must be treated, usually with nonsteroidal anti-inflammatory drugs or corticosteroids. If the person has rheumatoid arthritis or doesn't respond to corticosteroids, drugs that suppress the immune system, such as cyclophosphamide or azathioprine, may be needed.

Noncancerous Growths

Two kinds of noncancerous (benign) growths can develop on the conjunctiva. A pinguecula, a raised yellowish-white growth next to the cornea, is unsightly but generally doesn't cause any serious problem and needn't be removed. A pterygium, a fleshy growth of the conjunctiva into the cornea, may spread across the cornea and distort its shape, possibly causing astigmatism and other visual changes. Pterygium is more common in hot, dry climates. Either type of growth can be removed by an eye doctor (ophthalmologist).

CHAPTER 222

Corneal Disorders

The cornea, the domed covering in the front of the eye that protects the iris and lens and helps focus light on the retina, consists of cells and fluid and is normally clear.▲ Corneal disease or damage can cause pain and a loss of vision.

Superficial Punctate Keratitis

Superficial punctate keratitis is a condition in which cells on the surface of the cornea die.

The cause may be a viral infection, a bacterial infection, dry eyes, exposure to ultraviolet light (sunlight, sunlamps, or welding arcs), irritation from prolonged use of contact lenses, or irritation from or an allergy to eyedrops. The condition can also be a side effect of certain drugs taken internally, such as vidarabine.

▲ see box, page 1026

■ see box, page 1036

Symptoms and Treatment

The eyes are generally painful, watery, sensitive to light, and bloodshot, and vision may be slightly blurry. When ultraviolet light causes the condition, symptoms usually don't occur for several hours, and they last for 1 to 2 days. When a virus causes the condition, a lymph node in front of the ear may be swollen and tender.

Almost everyone who has this condition recovers completely. When the cause is a virus, no treatment is needed, and recovery usually occurs in 3 weeks. When the cause is a bacterial infection, antibiotics are used. When the cause is dry eyes, treatments such as ointments and artificial tears (eyedrops prepared with substances that simulate real tears) are effective. When the cause is exposure to ultraviolet light or contact lens irritation, an antibiotic ointment, an eyedrop that dilates the pupil,■ and an eye patch may provide relief. And when the cause is a drug reaction, the drug must be stopped.

Corneal Ulcer

A corneal ulcer is a pitting of the cornea, generally from an infection by bacteria, fungi, viruses, or the protozoan Acanthamoeba, *and sometimes from an injury.*

Bacteria (often staphylococci, pseudomonades, or pneumococci) can infect and ulcerate the cornea after the eye is injured, a foreign object lodges in the eye, or the eye is irritated by a contact lens. Other bacteria, such as gonococci, and viruses, such as herpes, can also cause corneal ulcers. Fungi may cause slowly growing ulcers. Rarely, vitamin A or protein deficiency may lead to corneal ulceration.

When the eyelids don't close properly to protect and moisten the cornea, corneal ulcers may develop from dryness and irritation, even without an infection.

Symptoms and Treatment

Corneal ulcers cause pain, sensitivity to light, and increased tear production, all of which may be mild. A whitish yellow spot of pus may appear in the cornea. Sometimes, ulcers develop over the entire cornea and may penetrate deeply. Additional pus may accumulate behind the cornea. The deeper the ulcer, the more severe the symptoms and complications.

Corneal ulcers may heal with treatment, but they may leave a cloudy, fibrous material that causes scarring and impairs vision. Other complications include deep-seated infection, perforation of the cornea, displacement of the iris, and destruction of the eye.

A corneal ulcer is an emergency that should be treated immediately by an eye doctor (ophthalmologist). To see an ulceration clearly, a doctor may apply eyedrops that contain a dye called fluorescein. Antibiotic therapy and surgery may be required.

Herpes Simplex Infection

When a corneal herpes simplex infection▲ (herpes simplex keratoconjunctivitis, keratitis) begins, it may resemble a mild bacterial infection because the eyes are slightly painful, watery, red, and sensitive to light. Corneal swelling makes vision hazy. However, the herpes infection doesn't respond to antibiotics, as a bacterial infection would, and often it continues to worsen.

Most often, the infection produces only mild changes in the cornea and goes away without treatment. Rarely, the virus deeply penetrates the cornea, destroying its surface. The infection may recur, further damaging the surface of the cornea. Several recurrences may result in ulceration, permanent scarring, and a loss of feeling when the eye is touched. The herpes simplex virus can also cause an increased growth of blood vessels, visual impairment, or total loss of vision.

A doctor may prescribe an antiviral drug such as trifluridine, vidarabine, or idoxuridine. These drugs are usually prescribed as an ointment or a solution to be applied to the eye several times a day. However, they're not always effective; sometimes, other drugs must be taken by mouth. Sometimes, to help speed healing, an ophthalmologist may have to gently swab the cornea with a soft cotton-tipped applicator to remove dead and damaged cells.

Herpes Zoster Infection

Herpes zoster is a virus that grows in nerves and may spread to the skin, causing shingles.■ The condition doesn't necessarily threaten the eye, even when it appears on the face and forehead. But if the ophthalmic division of the fifth cranial nerve (trigeminal nerve) becomes infected, the infection is likely to spread to the eye. The infection produces pain, redness, and eyelid swelling. An infected cornea can become swollen and severely damaged and scarred. The structures behind the cornea can become inflamed, a condition called uveitis, and the pressure in the eye can increase, a condition called glaucoma. Common complications of a corneal infection include a lack of feeling when the cornea is touched and permanent glaucoma.

When herpes zoster infects the face and threatens the eye, early treatment with acyclovir taken by mouth for 7 days reduces the risk of eye complications. Corticosteroids, usually in eyedrops, may also help. Atropine drops are often used to keep the pupil dilated and help keep pressure in the eye from increasing. People over age 60 who are in generally good health may find that taking

▲ see page 916

■ see page 918

corticosteroids for 2 weeks helps prevent the pain that may occur after the herpes sores disappear; this pain is called postherpetic neuralgia.

Peripheral Ulcerative Keratitis

Peripheral ulcerative keratitis is an inflammation and ulceration of the cornea that often occurs in people who have connective tissue diseases such as rheumatoid arthritis.

The condition impairs vision, increases sensitivity to light, and produces a sensation of a foreign object trapped in the eye. The condition is probably caused by an autoimmune reaction.▲

Of the people who have rheumatoid arthritis and peripheral ulcerative keratitis, about 40 percent die within 10 years of developing peripheral ulcerative keratitis unless they are treated. Treatment with drugs that suppress the immune system reduces the death rate to about 8 percent in 10 years.

Keratomalacia

Keratomalacia (xerophthalmia, xerotic keratitis) is a condition in which the cornea becomes dry and clouds over because of deficiencies in vitamin A, protein, and dietary calories.

The surface of the cornea dies, and corneal ulcers and bacterial infections may follow. The tear glands and conjunctiva are also affected, resulting in inadequate tear production and dry eyes. Night blindness (poor vision in the dark) may develop because of vitamin A deficiency. Antibiotic eyedrops or ointments can help cure infections, but correcting the vitamin A deficiency with oral vitamin supplements or malnutrition with an improved diet or supplements is more important.

Keratoconus

Keratoconus is a gradual change in the shape of the cornea, causing it to resemble a cone.

The condition begins between ages 10 and 20. One or both eyes may be affected, producing major changes in vision and requiring frequent changes in the prescription for eyeglasses or contact lenses. Contact lenses often correct the vision problems better than glasses, but sometimes the change in corneal shape is so severe that contact lenses either can't be worn or can't correct vision. In extreme cases, corneal transplantation may be needed.■

Bullous Keratopathy

Bullous keratopathy is a swelling of the cornea that's most common in older people.

Occasionally, bullous keratopathy occurs after eye surgery, such as cataract surgery. The swelling leads to fluid-filled blisters on the surface of the cornea that can rupture, causing pain and impairing vision.

Bullous keratopathy is treated by reducing the amount of fluid in the cornea with salty solutions or soft contact lenses. Rarely, corneal transplantation is needed.

CHAPTER 223

Cataracts

A cataract is a cloudiness (opacity) in the eye's lens that impairs vision.

Cataracts produce a progressive, painless loss of vision. Their cause usually isn't known, although they sometimes result from exposure to x-rays (such as high-dose radiotherapy to the eye) or strong sunlight, inflammatory eye diseases, certain drugs (such as corticosteroids), or complications of other diseases such as diabetes. They're more common in older people; babies can be born with cataracts (congenital cataracts).

Symptoms

Because all light entering the eye must pass through the lens, any part of the lens that blocks,

▲ see page 816

■ see box, page 833

distorts, or diffuses light can cause poor vision. How much vision deteriorates depends on where the cataract is and how dense (mature) it is.

In bright light, the pupil constricts, narrowing the cone of light entering the eye, so that it can't easily pass around the cataract. Thus, bright lights are especially disturbing to many people with cataracts, who see halos around lights, glare, and scattering of light. Such problems are particularly troubling when a person moves from a dark to a brightly lit space or tries to read with a bright lamp. People with cataracts who also take glaucoma medication that constricts the pupils may have greater vision loss.

A cataract at the back of the lens (posterior subcapsular cataract) particularly interferes with vision in bright light. It affects vision more than other cataracts because the opacity is at the point where light rays cross.

Surprisingly, a cataract in the central part of the lens (nuclear cataract) may improve vision at first. The cataract causes light to be refocused, improving vision for objects close to the eye. Older people, who generally have trouble seeing things that are close, may discover that they can read again without glasses, a phenomenon often described as gaining second sight.

Although cataracts usually aren't painful, rarely they cause swelling in the lens and increased pressure in the eye (glaucoma), which can be painful.

Diagnosis and Treatment

A doctor can see a cataract while examining the eye with an ophthalmoscope (an instrument used to view the inside of the eye). Using an instrument called a slit lamp, a doctor can see the exact location of the cataract and the extent of its opacity.

Usually, people who have a cataract can determine when to have it surgically removed. When people feel unsafe, uncomfortable, or unable to perform daily tasks, they may be ready for surgery. There's no advantage to having surgery before then.

Before deciding on surgery, a person with a cataract can try other measures. Eyeglasses and contact lenses may improve vision. For certain kinds of cataracts in people who don't have glaucoma, medications that keep the pupil dilated may help. Wearing sunglasses in bright light and using lamps that provide reflected lighting rather than direct lighting decrease glare and aid vision.

How Cataracts Affect Vision

On the left, a normal lens receives light and focuses it on the retina. On the right, a cataract blocks some light that reaches the lens and distorts the light being focused on the retina.

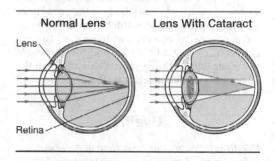

Normal Lens

Lens

Retina

Lens With Cataract

Cataract surgery, which can be performed on a person of any age, usually doesn't require general anesthesia or an overnight hospital stay. During the operation, the lens is removed, and usually a new plastic or silicone lens is inserted; this artificial lens is called a lens implant. Without a lens implant, people usually need a contact lens. If they can't wear a contact lens, they can try eyeglasses, which are very thick and tend to distort vision.

Cataract surgery is common and usually safe. Rarely, after the operation, a person may develop an infection or a hemorrhage in the eye, which can lead to a serious loss of vision. Older people in particular should make arrangements in advance to get extra help at home for a few days after surgery. For a few weeks after surgery, eyedrops or ointment is used to prevent infection, reduce inflammation, and promote healing. To protect the eye from injury, the person wears glasses or a metal shield until healing is complete, usually a few weeks. The person visits the doctor the day after surgery and then typically every week or two for 6 weeks.

Sometimes people develop an opacity behind a lens implant weeks or even years after it is implanted. Usually, such an opacity can be treated with a laser.

Disorders of the Uvea

The uvea, also called the uveal tract, consists of three structures: the iris, the ciliary body, and the choroid. The iris, the colored ring around the black pupil, opens and closes like the aperture of a camera lens. The ciliary body is the set of muscles that makes the lens thicker so the eye can focus on nearby objects and thinner so the eye can focus on distant objects. And the choroid is the inner lining of the eye that extends from the edge of the ciliary muscles to the optic nerve at the back of the eye.

Uveitis

Uveitis is inflammation anywhere in the uvea.

Part or all of the uvea may be inflamed. Inflammation limited to part of the uvea may be referred to by the name of the part—for example, iritis (inflammation of the iris) or choroiditis (inflammation of the choroid). Uveitis has many possible causes—some that are limited to the eye itself and others that affect the entire body. About 40 percent of people with uveitis have a disease that also affects organs elsewhere in the body. Regardless of the cause, uveitis can rapidly damage the eye and produce long-term complications such as glaucoma, cataracts, and detachment of the retina.

A View of the Uvea

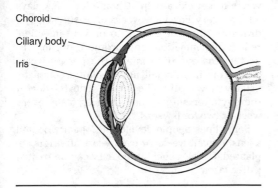

Choroid
Ciliary body
Iris

Symptoms and Diagnosis

The first symptoms of uveitis may be subtle. Vision may become hazy, or the person may see floating black spots. Severe pain, redness in the white of the eye (the sclera), and sensitivity to light are particularly common in iritis. A doctor may be able to see prominent blood vessels at the edge of the iris, subtle changes in the cornea, and clouding of the fluid that fills the eye (vitreous humor). The doctor makes the diagnosis based on the symptoms and the physical examination findings.

Treatment

Treatment must start early to prevent permanent damage and almost always includes using corticosteroids and drugs to dilate the pupils.

Common Causes of Uveitis

Ankylosing spondylitis

Reiter's syndrome

Juvenile rheumatoid arthritis

Pars planitis

Toxoplasmosis

Cytomegalovirus infection

Acute retinal necrosis

Toxocariasis

Birdshot choroidopathy

Histoplasmosis

Tuberculosis

Syphilis

Behçet's syndrome

Sympathetic ophthalmia

Vogt-Koyanagi-Harada syndrome

Sarcoidosis

Sarcoma or lymphoma

Other drugs may be used to treat specific causes; for example, anti-infectives may be given to eliminate bacteria or parasites.

Endophthalmitis

Endophthalmitis is an inflammation possibly resulting from a bacterial or fungal infection and involving all the inner layers of the eye, the fluid of the eye (vitreous humor), and the white of the eye (sclera).

The cause of the infection may be a wound that punctures the eye, surgery, or bacteria that have traveled through the bloodstream to the eye.

Symptoms, often severe, include pain, redness in the white of the eye, extreme sensitivity to light, and loss of vision.

Endophthalmitis is a medical emergency. Treatment must begin immediately; a delay of even a few hours can result in blindness. Antibiotics and often corticosteroids are given at once. Surgery may be needed to drain fluid from inside the eyeball.

Choroid Melanoma

Malignant melanoma▲ in the choroid is the most common cancer originating in the eye; however, it rarely occurs in blacks. In its early stages, the condition usually doesn't interfere with vision, and it may be detected during a routine ophthalmoscopic examination. Early diagnosis is important because the likelihood of curing choroid melanoma is related to the size of the tumor. If it is small, treatment with a laser or an implant of radioactive materials may save the eye and eyesight. If the tumor is large, the eye must be removed. If the cancer isn't removed, it can spread into the eye socket (orbit) and through the bloodstream to other organs, causing death.

CHAPTER 225

Retinal Disorders

The retina is the light-sensitive membrane on the inner surface of the back of the eye. The optic nerve extends from the brain to about the center of the retina and then branches out. The central area of the retina called the macula contains the highest density of light-sensing nerves and thus produces the sharpest visual resolution. The retinal vein and artery reach the retina near the optic nerve and then branch out, following the paths of the nerves. Like the optic nerve and its branches, the retina itself has a rich supply of vessels that carry blood and oxygen.

The cornea and lens near the front of the eye focus light onto the retina. Then the branches of the optic nerve sense the light, and the optic nerve transmits it to the brain, where it's interpreted as visual images.

Macular Degeneration

Macular degeneration is a condition in which the macula, the central and most vital area of the retina, degenerates.

The condition affects older people, is equally common in men and in women, is more common in whites than in blacks, and appears to be more common in those who smoke. The cause is unknown, but the condition tends to run in families.

There are two forms of macular degeneration. In atrophic (dry) macular degeneration, a pigment is deposited in the macula without any evidence of scars, blood, or other fluid leakage. In exudative (wet) macular degeneration, leaked material (exudate) forms a mound, often surrounded by small hemorrhages. Eventually the mound contracts, leaving a scar. Both forms of macular degeneration usually affect both eyes simultaneously.

Symptoms and Treatment

Macular degeneration slowly or suddenly produces a painless loss of vision. Occasionally, the first symptom is a distortion in one eye, so that

▲ see page 993

Viewing the Retina

Side View

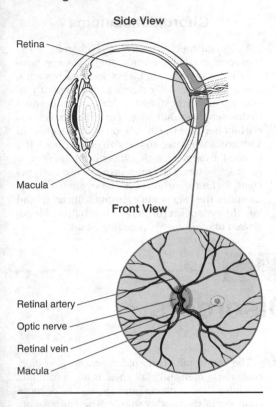

Retina

Macula

Front View

Retinal artery

Optic nerve

Retinal vein

Macula

---

fine, straight lines appear wavy. Sometimes a doctor can see early physical changes near the macula even before symptoms develop. Macular degeneration can severely damage vision but rarely leads to complete blindness. Vision at the outer edges of the visual field (peripheral vision) and the ability to see color generally aren't affected.

Little treatment is available for macular degeneration. However, when new blood vessels grow in or around the macula, laser photocoagulation sometimes can destroy them before they do further harm.

▲ see box, page 1047

Retinal Detachment

Retinal detachment is separation of the retina from its underlying support.

The meshwork of nerves that make up the light-sensitive part of the retina forms a thin film that clings tightly to the supporting tissue beneath it. When these two layers separate, the retina can't function, and unless they're reattached, it can be permanently damaged.

Detachment may begin in a small area, but if it isn't treated, the entire retina can detach. In one form of detachment, the retina actually rips. This form usually occurs in people who are nearsighted (myopic) or who've had cataract surgery or an eye injury. In another form, the retina doesn't rip but separates from the tissue beneath it. The retina separates when fluid movement in the eye pulls the retina or when fluid collecting between the retina and the underlying tissue pushes on the retina.

Symptoms

Retinal detachment is painless but may create images of irregular floating shapes or flashes of light and may make vision blurry. Vision loss begins in one part of the visual field, and as the detachment progresses, the vision loss spreads. If the macular area of the retina becomes detached, vision rapidly deteriorates, and everything becomes blurred.

An eye doctor (ophthalmologist) examines the retina through an ophthalmoscope (an instrument used to view the inside of the eye)▲ and can usually see the detachment. If the detachment isn't visible, an ultrasound scan can reveal it.

Treatment and Prognosis

Anyone who experiences a sudden loss of vision should see an ophthalmologist immediately. In deciding whether to use laser or freezing therapy or an operation, the doctor considers the type of detachment and its cause.

If the macula remains attached, the prognosis is excellent. If the retina is reattached within 48 hours, the prognosis is good. If, however, the retina has been detached for a longer time or if bleeding or scarring has occurred, the prognosis is poor.

Retinitis Pigmentosa

Retinitis pigmentosa is a rare inherited disorder in which the retina slowly, progressively degenerates, eventually causing blindness.

Some forms of retinitis pigmentosa are dominant, requiring only one gene from either parent; others are X-linked, requiring only one gene from the mother. In some people, mostly males, an inherited form of hearing loss also develops.

The light-sensing cells (rods) of the retina, which are responsible for vision when light is low, gradually degenerate, so that vision becomes poor in the dark. The first symptoms often begin in early childhood. Over time, a progressive loss of peripheral vision occurs. In the late stages of the disease, a person has a small area of central vision and a little peripheral vision remaining (tunnel vision).

Examining the retina with an ophthalmoscope, a doctor sees specific changes that suggest the diagnosis. Several tests may help make the diagnosis, and examination of family members may establish the mode of inheritance. No treatment can slow the progression of retinal damage.

Blood Vessel Disorders

Disorders of blood vessels to the eye include bleeding (hemorrhage), inadequate blood supply, and blockage of the vessels. These disorders can have serious consequences, damaging the retina, sometimes permanently, and leading to decreased vision and even blindness. They also indicate that the person is at high risk of other problems, such as stroke.

Arteriosclerotic Retinopathy

In this condition, the small arteries carrying blood to the eye become partially blocked because their walls have thickened. Using an ophthalmoscope, a doctor can see the thickened blood vessels and other indications of decreased blood supply to the retina. Although the thickening itself generally doesn't damage vision, it indicates that the blood vessels here and elsewhere in the body aren't healthy and that prevention and treatment are needed.▲

What's an Ophthalmoscope?

An ophthalmoscope is an instrument that allows a doctor to examine the inside of a patient's eye. The instrument has an angled mirror, various lenses, and a light source. With it a doctor can see the vitreous humor (fluid in the eye), the retina, the head of the optic nerve, and the retinal vein and artery.

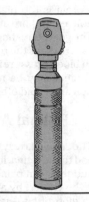

Ophthalmoscopic Examination

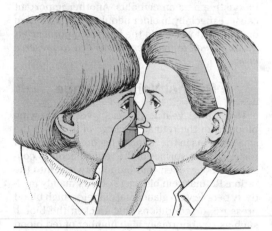

Hypertensive Retinopathy

This condition occurs when blood pressure becomes extremely high, as it does in severe hypertension, malignant hypertension, and toxemia of pregnancy. As the condition progresses, blood leaks into the retina. Patches of the retina become

▲ see page 118

damaged because the blood supply is inadequate, and over years, fat accumulates in the retina. The optic nerve can swell, a condition called papilledema.▲ Such swelling indicates that pressure in the brain is too high. All these changes impair vision and require urgent treatment.

The goal of treatment is to lower the high blood pressure that's the root of the problem. When the high blood pressure is severe and life threatening, treatment may be needed immediately to save vision and avoid other complications.

Retinal Artery Blockage

The retinal artery is the main vessel supplying blood to the retina. If it's blocked, the affected eye is suddenly but painlessly blinded. The blockage may be caused by atherosclerosis, a blood clot, or a glob of fat—usually, fat that escaped from bone marrow after a fracture and traveled in the bloodstream as an embolus. Another important cause, especially in older people, is inflammation of the blood vessels in the head (temporal arteritis). *Immediate treatment is needed to preserve vision.*

Retinal Vein Blockage

The retinal vein is the main vessel carrying blood from the retina. Blockage of it causes the smaller veins in the retina to become swollen and tortuous. The surface of the retina becomes congested and swollen, and blood may leak into the retina. Retinal vein blockage occurs mainly in elderly people with glaucoma, diabetes, high blood pressure, or conditions that thicken the blood, such as an abnormally high number of red blood cells.

Retinal vein blockage causes a painless loss of vision that develops much more slowly than it does in retinal artery blockage. Permanent changes include the growth of new, abnormal blood vessels in the retina and the development of glaucoma. Fluorescein angiography—a procedure in which a doctor injects dye into a vein, waits for it to reach the retina, and then photographs the retina—helps determine the extent of

damage and the plan of treatment. Laser treatment may be used to destroy abnormal blood vessels.

Diabetic Retinopathy

Diabetes can produce two types of changes that are among the leading causes of blindness—nonproliferative and proliferative retinopathy. These changes can occur in diabetics who take insulin and those who don't.

Diabetes affects the retina because high blood sugar (glucose) levels make the walls of small blood vessels thicker but weaker and therefore more prone to deformity and leakage. The extent of retinopathy and vision loss is related to how well blood sugar levels are controlled and, more important, how long the person has had diabetes. In general, retinopathy doesn't develop until at least 10 years after a person becomes diabetic.

In **nonproliferative (background) retinopathy,** small capillaries in the retina break and leak. The area around each break in the capillaries swells, forming small pouches in which blood proteins are deposited. A doctor diagnoses this condition by examining the retina. Fluorescein angiography—a procedure in which a doctor injects dye into a vein, waits for it to reach the retina, and then photographs the retina—helps determine the extent of the condition. In its early stages, nonproliferative retinopathy doesn't cause blindness. Small retinal hemorrhages may distort parts of the field of vision, or if they're near the macula, may blur vision.

In **proliferative retinopathy,** damage to the retina stimulates the growth of new blood vessels. Such growth may seem beneficial, but it isn't. The new blood vessels grow abnormally, leading to scarring and sometimes to retinal detachment. They may grow or bleed into the vitreous cavity. Proliferative retinopathy is much more damaging to the vision than nonproliferative retinopathy and can lead to total or nearly total blindness.

Prevention and Treatment

The best way to prevent diabetic retinopathy is to control diabetes and keep blood pressure at normal levels. People with diabetes should have annual eye examinations starting 5 years after diabetes is diagnosed, so that any necessary treatment can be started early and vision may be saved.

▲ see page 1051

Treatment consists of laser photocoagulation, in which a laser beam is aimed through the eye to destroy the new blood vessels and seal off leaking ones. This treatment is painless because the retina doesn't sense pain. If bleeding from damaged vessels has been extensive, surgery to remove the blood that leaked into the vitreous humor (a procedure called a vitrectomy) may be needed. Vision improves after the vitrectomy, and the vitreous humor is gradually replaced.

CHAPTER 226

Glaucoma

Glaucoma is a disorder in which the pressure in the eyeball increases, damaging the optic nerve and causing a loss of vision.

Both the front (anterior) and back (posterior) chambers of the eye are filled with a thin fluid called the aqueous humor. Normally, the fluid is produced in the back (posterior) chamber, passes through the pupil into the front (anterior) chamber, and then drains from the eye through the outflow channels. If the flow of fluid is interrupted, usually by an obstruction that prevents the fluid from flowing out of the anterior chamber, pressure increases.

Usually, glaucoma has no known cause; however, it sometimes runs in families. If the outflow channels are open, the disorder is called open-angle glaucoma. If the channels are blocked by the iris, the disorder is called closed-angle glaucoma.

An ophthalmologist or optometrist can measure the pressure in the anterior chamber, called intraocular pressure or tension, by using a simple, painless procedure called tonometry. In general, measurements greater than 20 to 22 millimeters indicate increased pressure. Occasionally, glaucoma occurs when pressures are normal. Sometimes a series of measurements must be taken over time to determine that the problem is glaucoma. An examination with an ophthalmoscope (an instrument used to view the inside of the eye) may reveal visible changes in the optic nerve caused by glaucoma. Sometimes, the examiner uses a special lens to observe the outflow channels; this procedure is known as gonioscopy.

Glaucoma produces a loss of peripheral vision or blind spots in the visual field. To find out if such blind spots exist, an examiner asks the person to look straight ahead at a central point and

Normal Fluid Drainage

Fluid is produced in the posterior chamber, passes through the pupil into the anterior chamber, and then drains through the outflow channels.

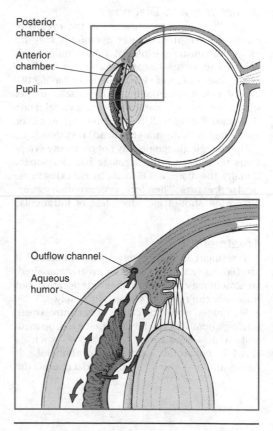

Posterior chamber
Anterior chamber
Pupil

Outflow channel
Aqueous humor

indicate when light can be seen. The test may be done either using a screen and pointer or an automated device that uses spots of light.

Open-Angle Glaucoma

In open-angle glaucoma, fluid drains too slowly from the anterior chamber. Pressure gradually rises—almost always in both eyes—causing optic nerve damage and a slow, progressive loss of vision. Vision loss begins at the edges of the visual field and, if not treated, eventually spreads to all parts of the visual field, ultimately causing blindness.

The most prevalent form of glaucoma, open-angle glaucoma is common after age 35 but occasionally occurs in children. The condition tends to run in families and is most common in people with diabetes or nearsightedness (myopia). Open-angle glaucoma develops more often and may be more severe in blacks than in whites.

Symptoms and Diagnosis

Initially, increased pressure in the eyes produces no symptoms. Later symptoms may include narrowing peripheral vision, mild headaches, and vague visual disturbances, such as seeing halos around electric lights or having difficulty adapting to darkness. Eventually, tunnel vision (an extreme narrowing of the visual fields that makes it difficult to see anything on either side when looking straight ahead) may develop.

Open-angle glaucoma may not cause any symptoms until irreversible damage has developed. Usually, the diagnosis is made by checking intraocular pressure. Therefore, every routine eye examination should include a test of intraocular pressure.

Treatment

Treatment is more likely to be successful if started early. Once vision is greatly impaired, treatment may prevent further deterioration, but it usually can't restore vision completely.

Medicated eyedrops can usually control open-angle glaucoma. Typically, the first eyedrop medication prescribed is a beta-blocker—such as timolol, betaxolol, carteolol, levobunolol, or metipranolol—which probably decreases the production of fluid in the eye. Pilocarpine, which constricts the pupils and increases drainage from the anterior chamber, is also helpful. Other useful medications—such as epinephrine, dipivefrin, and carbachol—work either by improving outflow or decreasing fluid production. A carbonic anhydrase inhibitor, such as acetazolamide, can be taken by mouth, or dorzolamide can be used as eyedrops.

If medication can't control eye pressure or if side effects are intolerable, an eye surgeon can increase drainage from the anterior chamber by using laser therapy to create a hole in the iris or using surgery to cut out part of the iris.

Closed-Angle Glaucoma

Closed-angle glaucoma causes sudden attacks of increased pressure, usually in one eye. In people with this condition, the space between the cornea and iris where fluid filters out of the eye is narrower than normal. Anything that causes the pupil to dilate—dim lighting, eyedrops given to dilate the pupil before an eye examination, or certain oral or injected medications—can result in the iris blocking the fluid drainage. When fluid drainage is blocked, intraocular pressure suddenly increases.

Symptoms

An episode of acute closed-angle glaucoma produces sudden symptoms. It may produce a slight decrease in vision, colored halos around lights, and pain in the eye and head. These symptoms may last only a few hours before an extended attack occurs. The attack itself produces a rapid loss of vision and sudden, severe throbbing pain in the eye. Nausea and vomiting are common and may lead a doctor to think that the problem lies in the digestive system. The eyelid swells, and the eye gets watery and red. The pupil dilates and doesn't close normally in response to bright light.

Although most symptoms disappear after treatment with medication, attacks can recur. Each attack further reduces the field of vision.

Treatment

Several medications can be used to quickly decrease pressure in the eye during an attack of acute closed-angle glaucoma. Drinking a pre-scribed mixture of glycerin and water can reduce increased pressure and stop an attack. Carbonic anhydrase inhibitors, such as acetazolamide, are also helpful if taken early in the attack. Pilocar-pine eyedrops constrict the pupil, which in turn pulls on the iris, thus unblocking the outflow channels. Beta-blocker eyedrops are also used to control the pressure. After an attack, treatment usually continues with both eyedrops and several doses of a carbonic anhydrase inhibitor. In severe cases, mannitol is given intravenously to reduce pressure.

Laser therapy, which creates a hole in the iris to allow drainage, helps prevent further attacks and often cures the disorder permanently. If laser therapy doesn't resolve the problem, surgery is performed to create a hole in the iris. If both eyes have narrow outflow channels, they may both be treated, even if the attacks have affected only one of them.

Secondary Glaucoma

Secondary glaucoma occurs because the eye has been damaged by an infection, inflammation, tumor, an enlarged cataract, or any eye disorder that interferes with fluid drainage from the ante-rior chamber. Inflammatory diseases, such as uveitis, are among the most common of these dis-orders. Other common causes include ophthal-mic vein blockage, eye injury, eye surgery, and bleeding into the eye. Some medications, such as corticosteroids, can also increase pressure in the eye.

Treatment of secondary glaucoma depends on the cause. For example, when the cause is inflam-mation, corticosteroids are often used to de-crease the inflammation along with medications that keep the pupils large. Sometimes surgery is necessary.

CHAPTER 227

Optic Nerve Disorders

The small nerves of the retina (the inner surface at the back of the eye) sense light and transmit impulses to the optic nerve, which carries them to the brain. A problem anywhere along the optic nerve and its branches or damage to the areas at the back of the brain that sense visual stimuli can result in visual changes.

The optic nerves follow an unusual route from the eyes to the back of the brain: Each nerve splits and half of its fibers cross over to the other side at the optic chiasm. Because of this anatomic ar-rangement, damage along the optic nerve path-way causes peculiar patterns of vision loss. If the optic nerve is damaged between an eyeball and the optic chiasm, the person may become blind in that eye. But if the problem lies farther back in the optic nerve pathway, vision may be lost in only half of the visual field of both eyes, a condi-tion called hemianopia. If both eyes lose periph-eral vision, the cause may be damage at the optic

chiasm. If both eyes lose half of the visual field on the same side—for instance, the right side—the cause is usually damage to the optic nerve path-way on the opposite side of the brain caused by a stroke, hemorrhage, or tumor.

Papilledema

Papilledema is a condition in which increased pressure around the brain causes the optic nerve to swell where it enters the eye.

The condition, which almost always occurs in both eyes, is usually caused by a brain tumor or abscess, head injury, bleeding in the brain, infec-tion of the brain or its coverings (meninges), pseudotumor cerebri, cavernous sinus thrombo-sis, or severe high blood pressure. Severe lung disease can also increase pressure in the brain, leading to papilledema.

Tracing the Visual Pathways

The optic nerve from each eye splits, and half of the nerve fibers from each side cross over to the other side at the optic chiasm. Because of this arrangement, the brain receives information via both optic nerves for the left visual field and the right visual field.

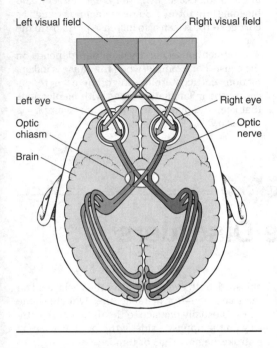

Left visual field

Right visual field

Left eye

Right eye

Optic chiasm

Optic nerve

Brain

At first, papilledema may cause headaches without affecting vision. The treatment depends on what's causing the high pressure in the brain. Medications or surgery may be needed to relieve the pressure. If the high pressure isn't reduced quickly, the optic nerve and the brain can be damaged permanently.

Papillitis

Papillitis (optic neuritis) is inflammation of the tip of the optic nerve where it enters the eye.

Papillitis can result from many causes, though often the exact cause isn't known. In people over age 60, temporal arteritis is a major cause. Papillitis also may result from viral and immunologic disorders.

Although papillitis usually affects only one eye, it can develop in both. The result is a loss of vision, which may vary from a small blind spot to total blindness within a day or two. Sometimes, the loss is permanent. The person may or may not feel pain.

To make the diagnosis, a doctor tests whether vision is normal in all areas, examines the optic nerve with an ophthalmoscope (an instrument used to view the inside of the eye), and tests whether the pupils respond normally to light. Sometimes, a computed tomography (CT) or magtic resonance imaging (MRI) scan is necessary.

The treatment depends on the cause. Often, corticosteroids are given as the first therapy.

Retrobulbar Neuritis

Retrobulbar neuritis is inflammation of the part of the optic nerve just behind the eye; usually it involves only one eye.

Several conditions can inflame and thus damage the area. Often multiple sclerosis is the cause. But several other conditions can also trigger retrobulbar neuritis. Sometimes the cause isn't discovered.

Retrobulbar neuritis rapidly produces a loss of vision, and eye movement becomes painful. An examination with an ophthalmoscope reveals little or no change in the portion of the optic nerve visible at the back of the eye.

About half the episodes of retrobulbar neuritis improve without treatment, often in 2 to 8 weeks. Blurring at the center of the visual field sometimes remains, however, and relapses may occur, especially when multiple sclerosis is the cause. Each relapse may worsen the loss of vision. The optic nerve may be permanently damaged, and in rare cases, repeated attacks lead to total blindness. Treatment depends on the cause and may include corticosteroids. Sometimes, no treatment is given.

Causes of Papillitis and Retrobulbar Neuritis

- Multiple sclerosis
- Viral illness
- Temporal arteritis and other kinds of inflammation of the arteries (vasculitis)
- Poisoning by chemicals, such as lead and methanol
- Tumors that have spread to the optic nerve
- Allergic reactions to beestings
- Meningitis
- Syphilis
- Uveitis
- Arteriosclerosis

Toxic Amblyopia

Toxic amblyopia is a condition similar to retrobulbar neuritis that usually affects both eyes. Alcoholics are particularly susceptible, though the cause of the condition may be malnutrition, not alcohol. Toxic chemicals, such as those in cigarette smoke and lead, methanol, chloramphenicol, digitalis, ethambutol, and many others, may also cause the condition.

Toxic amblyopia produces a small area of vision loss at the center of the visual field that slowly enlarges and can progress to complete blindness. A doctor examining the eye with an ophthalmoscope sees little or no change.

People with toxic amblyopia should avoid tobacco, alcohol, or the responsible toxic chemical. If alcohol use is a contributing cause, the person should eat a well-balanced diet and take a vitamin B complex supplement. If lead is the cause, chelating drugs help remove it from the body.

Men's Health Issues

CHAPTER 228

Male Reproductive System

The external structures of the male reproductive system include the penis, scrotum, and testes (testicles). The internal structures include the vasa deferentia, urethra, prostate gland, and seminal vesicles.

The sperm, which carries the man's genes, is made in the testes and stored in the seminal vesicles. During sexual intercourse, the sperm is transported along with a fluid called semen through the vas deferens and the erect penis.

Structure

The penis consists of the root, which is attached to the abdominal wall; the body, which is the middle portion; and the glans penis, which is the cone-shaped end. The opening of the urethra (the channel that transports semen and urine) is at the tip of the glans penis. The base of the glans penis is called the corona. In uncircumcised males, the foreskin (prepuce) extends from the corona to cover the glans penis.

Most of the body of the penis consists of three cylindrical spaces (sinuses) of erectile tissue. The two larger ones, the corpora cavernosa, are side by side. The third sinus, the corpus spongiosum, surrounds the urethra. When these spaces fill with blood, the penis becomes large, rigid, and erect.

The scrotum is the thin-skinned sac that surrounds and protects the testes. The scrotum also acts as a climate-control system for the testes because they need to be slightly cooler than body temperature to allow normal sperm development. The cremaster muscles in the scrotal wall relax or contract to allow the testes to hang farther from the body to cool or to be pulled closer to the body for warmth or protection.

The testes are oval bodies the size of large olives that lie in the scrotum; usually the left testis hangs a little lower than the right one. The testes have two functions: producing sperm and synthesizing testosterone (the primary male sex hormone). The epididymis, which lies against the testis, is a coiled tube almost 20 feet long. It collects sperm from the testis and provides the space and environment for sperm to mature.

Male Reproductive Organs

Bladder	Seminal vesicle
Pubic bone	Prostate
Vas deferens	Rectum
Urethra	Epididymis
Erectile tissue	Scrotum
Penis	Testis

The vas deferens is a cordlike duct that transports sperm from the epididymis. One such duct travels from each testis up to the back of the prostate and enters the urethra to form the ejaculatory ducts. Other structures, such as blood vessels and nerves, also travel along with each vas deferens and together form a cordlike structure, the spermatic cord.

The urethra serves a dual function in males. This channel is the part of the urinary tract that transports urine from the bladder, and it's the part of the reproductive system through which semen is ejaculated.

The prostate gland lies just under the bladder in the pelvis and surrounds the middle portion of the urethra. Usually the size of a walnut, this gland enlarges with age.▲ The prostate and the seminal vesicles above it produce fluid that nourishes the sperm. This fluid provides most of the volume of semen, the secretion in which the sperm is expelled during ejaculation. Other fluid that makes up the semen comes from the vas deferens and from mucous glands in the head of the penis.

Function

During sexual activity, the penis becomes rigid and erect, enabling penetration during sexual intercourse. An erection results from a complex interaction of neurologic, vascular, hormonal, and psychologic actions. Pleasurable stimuli from the senses cause a reaction in the brain, which sends nerve signals down the spinal cord to the penis. The arteries supplying blood to the corpora cavernosa and corpus spongiosum respond by dilating. The widened arteries dramatically increase blood flow to these erectile areas, which become engorged with blood and expand. Muscles tighten around the veins that normally drain blood from the penis, slowing the outflow of blood. Heightened blood pressure in the penis causes it to increase in length and diameter.

Ejaculation occurs at the climax of sexual excitement when friction on the glans penis and other stimuli send signals to the brain and spinal cord. Nerves stimulate muscle contractions along the ducts of the epididymis and vas deferens, the seminal vesicles, and the prostate. These contractions force semen into the urethra. Contrac-

▲ see page 1059

tion of the muscles around the urethra further propels the semen through and out of the penis. The neck of the bladder also constricts to keep semen from flowing backward into the bladder.

Once ejaculation takes place—or the stimulation stops—the arteries constrict and the veins relax. This reduces blood inflow and increases blood outflow, so that the penis becomes limp.

CHAPTER 229

Disorders of the Penis, Prostate, and Testes

Abnormalities of the penis, prostate, and testes (testicles) can be psychologically disturbing as well as physically damaging. The penis may be affected by injury, inflammation, or infection—including sexually transmitted diseases. Skin cancer can also develop on the penis. Birth defects can cause difficulty in urinating and in performing sexual intercourse.

The most common disorder affecting the prostate is benign prostatic hyperplasia, which makes urination difficult. Other disorders include prostatitis and prostate cancer—one of the most common cancers. Cancer may also develop in the testes, threatening fertility and, if left untreated, causing death. Other disorders affecting the testes include testicular torsion and inguinal hernia.

Penile Injury and Inflammation

Several types of injuries can affect the penis. Catching the penis in a pants zipper is common, but the resulting cut usually heals quickly. A cut or irritation that becomes infected is treated with antibiotics. Excessive bending of an erect penis can cause pain, severely damage the structures that control the erection, and cause difficulty with intercourse. The penis can also be severed either partially or fully. Reattachment may be possible, but full penile sensation and function are rarely recovered.

Balanoposthitis is a generalized inflammation of the head of the penis (glans penis) and foreskin. The inflammation is commonly caused by a yeast or bacterial infection beneath the foreskin of an uncircumcised penis. The inflammation causes pain, itching, redness, and swelling and can ulti-

mately lead to a narrowing (stricture) of the urethra. Men who have balanoposthitis may later develop balanitis xerotica obliterans, phimosis, paraphimosis, and cancer.

In **balanitis xerotica obliterans,** chronic inflammation causes a hardened, whitish area near the tip of the penis. Usually, the cause isn't known, but it can result from an infection or allergic reaction. The opening of the urethra is often surrounded by this hard white skin, which ultimately blocks the flow of urine and semen. Antibacterial or anti-inflammatory creams may cure the inflammation, but often the urethra must be reopened surgically.

Phimosis is a shrinking or tightening of the foreskin. The condition is normal in a newborn or young child, and it usually resolves by puberty without treatment. In older males, phimosis may result from prolonged irritation. Because the tightened foreskin can't be retracted, it may interfere with urination and sexual activity. The usual treatment is circumcision.

In **paraphimosis,** the retracted foreskin can't be pulled back over the head of the penis (glans). Paraphimosis can be cured by circumcision.

Erythroplasia of Queyrat is a clearly defined reddish, velvety area that develops on the skin of the penis, usually on or at the base of the head. This disorder usually occurs in uncircumcised men. If left untreated, the area can become cancerous. To confirm the diagnosis, a doctor may remove a small sample of the skin for microscopic examination (biopsy). Erythroplasia of Queyrat is treated with a cream containing the drug fluorouracil. Because the area may become cancerous, it is examined by the doctor every few months

Drugs That May Cause Priapism

Drugs used to treat impotence

Anticoagulants

Chlorpromazine

Cocaine

Corticosteroids

Marijuana

Prazosin

Tolbutamide

Trazodone

during and after treatment. As an alternative treatment, a doctor may remove the abnormal tissue.

Penile Growths

Although skin cancer can occur anywhere on the penis, the most common site is the head, especially at its base. Circumcised men rarely develop skin cancer of the penis, and such cancer is rare in the United States. Cancer usually appears first as a reddened area with sores that don't heal within a few weeks but are generally painless. Usually, the cancer is squamous cell carcinoma;▲ rarer skin cancers of the penis include Bowen's and Paget's diseases. The cancer is removed surgically, together with a small area of surrounding normal tissue. However, a doctor tries to leave as much penile tissue as possible.

Other growths on the penis may be caused by an infection. For example, a small, painless sore may be a sign of syphilis. Painful, tiny blisters are commonly caused by herpes simplex. Uncommonly, blisters, which later form small ulcers,

▲ see page 993

■ see page 942

may be caused by chancroid.■ One or more raised, firm nodules are usually genital warts, caused by a virus. Small, firm, dimpled growths (molluscum contagiosum) are caused by another virus.

Priapism

Priapism is a painful, persistent erection unaccompanied by sexual desire or excitement.

In most cases, priapism results from drug use, or the cause is unknown. Other possible causes include a blood disorder, such as blood clots, leukemia, or sickle cell disease; a tumor in the pelvis or spine; and an infection of the genitals. The condition probably results because of blood vessel and nerve abnormalities that trap blood in the erectile tissue (corpora cavernosa) of the penis.

The treatment of priapism depends on the cause. If a drug appears to be the cause, it should be stopped at once. If the cause seems to be neurologic damage, continuous spinal anesthesia may help. If a blood clot is the probable cause, the clot must be surgically removed or a shunt must be surgically placed to restore normal circulation in the penis. Most cases of priapism can be treated by draining excess blood from the penis with a needle and syringe and irrigating the blood vessels with fluid to wash out any clots or other blockage. A variety of drugs may also be used, depending on the underlying cause. The likelihood of a man regaining sexual function is poor if the priapism doesn't respond to treatment quickly.

Peyronie's Disease

Peyronie's disease is a fibrous thickening that causes the penis to develop contractures, so that the shape of an erection is distorted.

The cause of Peyronie's disease, which affects adult men, isn't known. The fibrous tissue that forms the contractures causes a curvature in the erect penis that may make sexual penetration difficult or impossible. The condition may make an erection painful. The fibrous tissue may even extend into the erectile tissue (corpora cavernosa), preventing an erection entirely.

Peyronie's disease may resolve by itself over several months. Injections of corticosteroids into the affected area may help. For some men, symptoms can be relieved by ultrasound treatments. More commonly, the fibrous areas must be surgically removed. The surgery may cure the disease, but sometimes it causes further scarring and makes the condition worse. Surgery also may lead to impotence.

Benign Prostatic Hyperplasia

Benign prostatic hyperplasia is a noncancerous (benign) growth of the prostate gland.

Benign prostatic hyperplasia is common in men over age 50. The cause isn't known, but it may involve changes in hormone levels that occur with aging. The prostate gland surrounds the urethra, so a growing gland gradually narrows the urethra. In time, the flow of urine may be obstructed. As a result, the muscles of the bladder grow larger and stronger to push urine through. However, when a man with benign prostatic hyperplasia urinates, the bladder may not empty completely. Consequently, urine stagnates in the bladder, making the man susceptible to infection and stone formation. Prolonged obstruction can damage the kidneys. In a man with benign prostatic hyperplasia, drugs that impair urine flow, such as over-the-counter antihistamines, can bring on an obstruction.

Symptoms

Benign prostatic hyperplasia first causes symptoms when the enlarged prostate begins to block the flow of urine. Initially, a man may have difficulty in starting to urinate. He also may feel that urination has been incomplete. Because the bladder doesn't empty completely each time, he has to urinate more frequently. He needs to urinate at night more frequently (nocturia), and the need becomes more pressing. The volume and force of the urinary flow may become noticeably smaller, and urine may dribble at the end of urination. Eventually, the bladder may overfill, causing urinary incontinence.

Small veins of the urethra and bladder can burst when the man strains to urinate, causing blood to appear in the urine. Complete blockage can make it impossible to urinate, leading to a full feeling and then to severe pain in the lower abdomen.

Bladder infections may cause a burning sensation during urination as well as a fever. The backup of urine also causes increased pressure on the kidneys but rarely leads to permanent kidney damage.

Diagnosis

A doctor who suspects benign prostatic hyperplasia based on the symptoms performs a physical examination. By feeling the prostate during a rectal examination, a doctor can usually determine if it's enlarged. A doctor also feels for nodules, which may indicate cancer, and tenderness, which may indicate infection.

Blood tests that measure kidney function are generally performed, as is a blood test that screens people for prostate cancer. This test measures the levels of prostate-specific antigen (PSA). Results show elevated levels in about 30 to 50 percent of the men with benign prostatic hyperplasia. Such an elevation means that further evaluation should be done to determine if the person has prostate cancer, not that the person has cancer.

Occasionally, further tests are needed. A doctor may use a catheter to measure the amount of urine remaining in the bladder after urination. However, more commonly, a doctor has the person urinate into a uroflometer (a device that measures the urinary flow rate). An ultrasound examination can measure the size of the prostate and help determine whether cancer is a possible cause. Rarely, a doctor passes an endoscope (a flexible viewing tube) up the urethra to determine if the urine flow is blocked for a reason other than enlargement of the prostate.

Treatment

Symptoms may be relieved by alpha-adrenergic drugs that relax the muscles at the bladder outlet, such as terazosin or doxazosin. To shrink the prostate and help delay the need for surgery, drugs such as finasteride may be taken, but symptom relief may take 3 months or more. Additional treatment is needed if the symptoms become unbearable, the urinary tract becomes infected, the kidney starts to lose function, or the urine flow becomes completely blocked. A man who can't urinate at all needs a Foley catheter to drain the bladder. Any infection is treated with antibiotics.

Surgery offers the best relief. The most common procedure is a transurethral resection of the prostate, in which a doctor passes an endoscope up the urethra and removes part of the prostate. This procedure doesn't require a surgical incision, and an anesthetic is usually given by a spinal tap. However, 5 percent or less of the men who undergo the procedure still have some urinary incontinence afterward. Rarely, a man becomes impotent, needs to have the urethra dilated, or needs another transurethral resection within 3 years. Alternatively, an endoscope equipped with a laser can be used to burn away the prostatic tissue, causing less damage to nerves and fewer complications. However, no studies on the long-term consequences of this procedure are available yet. Other recently developed treatments include using a microwave heating element to reduce prostatic tissue and using a balloon to dilate the urethra.

Prostate Cancer

Cancer of the prostate is extremely common, though its exact cause isn't known. When prostatic tissue is examined under a microscope either after prostate surgery or at autopsy, cancer is found in 50 percent of men over age 70 and in virtually all men over age 90. Most of these cancers never cause symptoms because they spread very slowly; however, some prostate cancers do grow more aggressively and spread throughout the body. Although fewer than 3 percent of the men with the disease die of it, prostate cancer is still the second most common cause of cancer death among American men.

Symptoms

Generally, prostate cancer progresses slowly and causes no symptoms until it's in an advanced stage. Sometimes symptoms appear that are similar to those of benign prostatic hyperplasia, including difficulty in urinating and a need to urinate frequently. These symptoms result because the cancer partially blocks the flow of urine through the urethra. Later, prostate cancer may cause bloody urine or sudden urinary retention.

In some cases, prostate cancer isn't diagnosed until it spreads (metastasizes) to the bone—typically the pelvis, ribs, and vertebrae—or the kidneys, producing kidney failure. The bone cancer tends to be painful and may weaken the bone enough to cause fractures. After the cancer spreads, anemia is common. Prostate cancer can also spread to the brain, causing seizures, confusion, and other mental or neurologic symptoms.

Diagnosis

Because prostate cancer is so common, many doctors screen for it, so that a diagnosis can be made at an early stage when the cancer can still be cured. The best way to screen for such cancer is to perform an annual digital rectal examination and blood test. During the digital rectal examination, a doctor feels the prostate. If the person has prostate cancer, a doctor often can feel a nodule. The blood test measures the level of prostate-specific antigen (PSA), a substance that's usually elevated in people with prostate cancer but that also can be elevated (usually to a lesser degree) in people with benign prostatic hyperplasia. This test misses about one third of prostate cancers (a false-negative result), and about 60 percent of the time indicates cancer when there is none (a false-positive result).

Although screening increases the chances of early detection, it also can lead to costly and unnecessary diagnostic tests and treatment performed on the basis of a false-positive result. Some organizations, such as the American Cancer Society and the American Urological Association, recommend annual PSA blood tests to screen for cancer, whereas other organizations, such as the National Cancer Institute, don't endorse the PSA blood test as a screening test.

If a doctor feels a nodule, the prostate can be further examined with an ultrasound scan, a test that uses sound waves. If the ultrasound scan shows a suspicious nodule, a doctor usually obtains several tissue specimens from the prostate. The person receives only a local anesthetic before the specimens are removed, and the procedure doesn't require hospitalization. The tissue specimens are examined under a microscope and may be subjected to biochemical tests. These tests help determine whether the cancer is the aggressive type that is likely to spread quickly or the more typical type that tends to grow and spread slowly. They also indicate how extensive the cancer is within the gland. Metastatic bone tumors can be detected by x-ray examinations or bone scans.

Two features help a doctor determine the likely course of the cancer and the best treatment:

• How far the cancer has spread. If the cancer is confined to a small part of the prostate gland, generally many years will pass before it spreads to areas around the gland and then to bone and other parts of the body.

• How malignant the cells look. Prostate cancer cells that are more distorted under the microscope tend to grow and spread more quickly.

Treatment

Treatment may seriously affect a man's lifestyle. Major surgery, radiation therapy, and drugs for prostate cancer often cause impotence and may cause incontinence. Treatment provides fewer advantages to men over age 70 than to younger men because older men are more likely to die of other causes. Many men with prostate cancer, especially older men with early-stage cancer that's growing slowly, decide that watchful waiting is best.

When a man and his doctor decide that treatment is necessary, the type of therapy depends on the extent of the disease. Cancer that's confined to the prostate often can be cured by surgically removing the prostate or by radiation therapy. In sexually active men with certain types of cancer, a surgical procedure called potency-sparing radical prostatectomy may be used. This procedure, which spares nerves, preserves sexual potency in about 75 percent of patients. Less than 5 percent become incontinent. However, the procedure is less likely to be successful for aggressive types of cancer and has no value for cancers that have spread beyond the prostate.

Radiation therapy can be used to treat cancer that's confined to the prostate. It's also an option when cancer has invaded tissues beyond the prostate but hasn't spread to distant organs. The radiation is given in a beam or in radioactive implants inserted into the prostate.

Advanced metastatic prostate cancer isn't curable, but symptoms often can be alleviated. Because many prostate cancers depend on the person's testosterone, treatments that block the effects of this hormone can slow the growth of

the tumors. About 80 percent of men with prostate cancer have a beneficial response to treatment that blocks these effects. One way to block them is to take certain drugs, such as leuprolide. However, this treatment causes significant changes in a man's body, including reduced libido, impotence, and breast enlargement (gynecomastia). Also, in up to a third of the men with advanced disease, the cancer becomes resistant to such treatment within a year.

Removal of both testes (bilateral orchiectomy) greatly reduces testosterone levels, but the physical and psychologic effects make the procedure unacceptable to some men. Still, it's effective, doesn't require repeated treatments, is less expensive than drug therapy, and doesn't require an overnight hospital stay. Painful bone cancer that doesn't respond to other treatments may be treated with radiation therapy or with drugs that may shrink the tumors, such as mestranol.

Prostatitis

Prostatitis is inflammation of the prostate gland.

Usually, prostatitis isn't caused by an identifiable infection, but sometimes a bacterial infection does spread to the prostate gland from the urinary tract. The infection of the prostate causes pain in the groin, the area between the penis and the anus, and the lower back, as well as chills and a fever. The man also may need to urinate frequently and urgently, and blood may appear in the urine. A bacterial infection may spread to the scrotum, causing intense discomfort, swelling, redness, and extreme pain when the area is touched. The man also may experience impotence because of pain.

Prostatitis also may result from fungal, viral, and protozoal infections.

Diagnosis and Treatment

The diagnosis of prostatitis is usually based on the symptoms and a physical examination. When a doctor performs a rectal examination, the prostate may be swollen and tender to the touch. Sometimes a doctor may obtain a sample of the urine or fluid for culturing by squeezing the prostate during the examination.

When prostatitis isn't caused by an infection, warm sitz baths (baths in which the person sits),

ساه

periodic prostate massage, and frequent ejaculation are recommended to relieve symptoms. An analgesic, such as acetaminophen or aspirin, may be needed to reduce the pain. Taking stool softeners and drinking plenty of fluids can also help relieve symptoms.

When the prostatitis results from a bacterial infection, an oral antibiotic, such as trimethoprim-sulfamethoxazole, is taken for 30 to 90 days. Taking antibiotics for less time may only partially cure the infection and lead to a chronic infection.

Testicular Cancer

Testicular cancer may cause an enlarged testis or a lump in the scrotum. Most lumps in the scrotum aren't caused by testicular cancer, but most lumps in the testes are.

The cause of testicular cancer isn't known, but men whose testes didn't descend into the scrotum by age 3 have a much greater chance of developing testicular cancer than men whose testes descended by that age. Most testicular cancer occurs in men under age 40.

Four types of cancer can develop in the testis: seminoma, teratoma, embryonal carcinoma, and choriocarcinoma.

Symptoms and Diagnosis

Testicular cancer produces a firm, growing lump in the scrotum, which may be painful. Occasionally, blood vessels rupture within the tumor, resulting in a rapidly growing mass that causes severe pain. A firm lump on the testis should always be examined by a doctor without delay.

A physical examination and ultrasound scan help a doctor determine if the lump originated in the testis. If the lump is solid and on the testis, the diagnosis of cancer will usually be obvious in the operating room, but occasionally a piece of tissue is removed first for microscopic examination (biopsy). Surgery can often be performed using a local anesthetic.

Levels of two proteins in the blood, alpha-fetoprotein and human chorionic gonadotropin, tend to be elevated in men with testicular cancers. Blood tests may be used both in screening for cancer and in monitoring treatment. If levels rise after treatment, the cancer may have recurred.

Treatment

The initial treatment for testicular cancer is surgical removal of the entire testis. The other testis isn't removed, so that the man has adequate levels of male hormones and remains fertile. With certain types of tumors, the lymph nodes in the abdomen also may be removed because the cancer tends to spread there first.

Treatment may include radiation therapy as well as surgery, especially for a seminoma. Radiation is usually beamed to the lymph nodes in the abdomen, chest, and neck to try to destroy cancer cells that have spread.

Testicular cancer that has spread is often cured with a combination of surgery and chemotherapy. The prognosis depends on the type and extent of the tumor. More than 80 percent of the men with seminomas, teratomas, or embryonal carcinomas survive 5 years or more. This ability to cure most metastatic testicular cancer is one of the great triumphs of cancer therapy. Very few with rare, highly malignant choriocarcinomas survive even 5 years.

Testicular Torsion

Testicular torsion is the twisting of a testis on its spermatic cord.

Testicular torsion results from an abnormal development of the spermatic cord or the membrane covering the testis. Usually, it occurs in males between puberty and about age 25; however, it can occur at any age. Testicular torsion may occur after strenuous activity, or it may occur for no apparent reason.

Severe pain and swelling in the scrotum along with nausea and vomiting occur immediately. A doctor may diagnose the condition based on only the patient's description of the symptoms and the examination findings. Alternatively, the doctor may use radionucleotide scans to diagnose the condition; however, the results of the test aren't always reliable. Color-flow ultrasound scans, which show both testicular tissue and blood flow, often are preferred.

The twisted cord cuts off the blood supply to the testis. Thus, the only hope of saving the testis is surgery to untwist the cord within 24 hours of the onset of symptoms. During surgery, the other testis is usually better secured to prevent torsion on that side.

Inguinal Hernia

In an inguinal hernia, the intestine pushes through an opening in the abdominal wall into the inguinal

Testicular Torsion

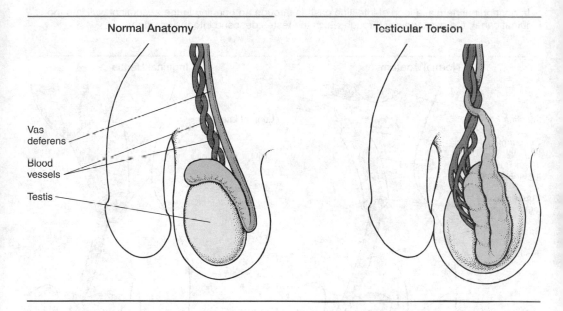

Normal Anatomy	Testicular Torsion

Vas deferens

Blood vessels

Testis

canal (the passageway through which the testes descend from the abdomen into the scrotum shortly before birth).

When the hernia results because the opening is looser or weaker than normal at birth, it's called a congenital or an indirect hernia. When the intestine breaks through a defect in the floor of the inguinal canal, the disorder is called an acquired or direct hernia.

With either type of inguinal hernia, the intestine can push down into the scrotum, usually producing a painless bulge in the groin and scrotum. The bulge may enlarge when the man stands and shrink when he lies down because the contents slide back and forth with gravity. Surgical repair may be recommended depending on the size of the hernia and the discomfort it causes. If a portion of the intestine gets trapped in the scrotum, the blood supply may be cut off, and the portion of intestine may become gangrenous. In this case, emergency surgery is performed to pull the intestine out of the inguinal canal and tighten the opening so the hernia can't recur.

Other Disorders of the Scrotum and Testes

Epididymo-orchitis is inflammation of the epididymis and testis. It may be a complication of a bladder infection, nonspecific urethritis, gonorrhea, prostate surgery, or a procedure such as urinary catheterization. The testis becomes swollen and painful and may be warm. Usually, there's fluid in the scrotal sac. The man also may have a fever. Treatment usually consists of oral antibiotics, bed rest, ice packs applied to the scrotum, and support for the scrotum. Acetaminophen or other pain relievers may be needed. Occasionally, an abscess (accumulation of pus) develops; it feels like a soft lump in the scrotum. The abscess tends to drain on its own, but occasionally surgical drainage is necessary.

Mumps is a viral infection that usually affects children; if an adult contracts mumps, the testes can be affected. The disease causes painful swelling that can permanently damage the ability of the testes to produce sperm.

Inguinal Hernia

In an inguinal hernia, a loop of intestine pushes through an opening in the abdominal wall into the inguinal canal, the passageway through which the testes descend into the scrotum.

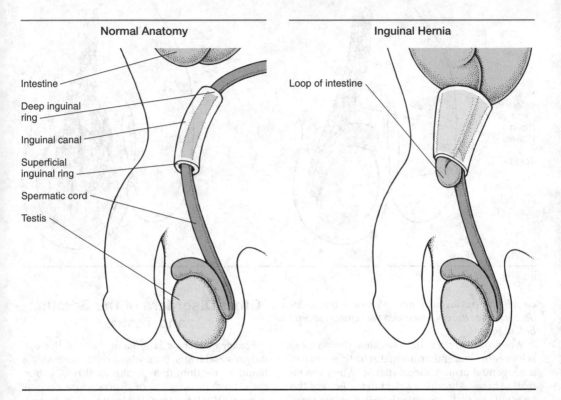

A **hydrocele** is a collection of fluid in the membrane covering the testes that causes a soft swelling of one testis. The condition may be present at birth or develop later in life. A hydrocele often is painless, but it may become so large that surgical removal is recommended to eliminate the annoyance.

A **hematocele** is a collection of blood that usually develops after an injury to the scrotum. Sometimes the blood is reabsorbed without treatment, but large hematoceles often require surgical removal.

A **spermatocele** is a collection of fluid containing sperm that is located adjacent to the epididymis. A spermatocele that becomes large or bothersome is removed surgically.

A **varicocele** is a mass of elongated, widened, wormlike veins in the scrotum, much like varicose veins. A varicocele usually occurs on the left side of the scrotum and feels like a bag of worms. The mass is noticeable when a man is standing but usually disappears when he reclines because blood flow to the enlarged veins decreases. A varicocele may be surgically corrected if it makes the scrotum feel uncomfortably full or impairs fertility.

Impotence

Impotence (erectile dysfunction) is the inability to initiate and maintain an erection in at least 50 percent of the attempts at intercourse or the cessation of attempts at intercourse.

Causes

Impotence usually results from vascular impairment, neurologic disorders, drugs, abnormalities of the penis, or psychologic problems that interfere with sexual arousal.▲ Physical causes are more common in older men; psychologic problems are more common in younger men. Impotence becomes more common with age, though it is not considered a normal part of aging. Instead, it results from underlying problems that commonly occur in older people. About 50 percent of 65-year-old men and 75 percent of 80-year-old men are impotent.

Because the penis needs adequate blood flow to become erect, blood vessel disorders such as atherosclerosis can cause impotence. Impotence can also result from a blood clot or from vascular surgery that impairs arterial blood flow to the penis. In 75 percent of impotent men who have normal neurologic and hormonal function, the blood flows into the penis properly, but it flows out too rapidly.

Damage to the nerves leading to and from the penis also can produce impotence. Such damage may result from many causes, including injury, diabetes mellitus, multiple sclerosis, stroke, and drugs. Diabetes causes peripheral neuropathy,■ a particular pattern of nerve damage that's a very common cause of impotence, especially in the elderly. Alcoholism causes a similar peripheral neuropathy. Lower spinal disease and rectal or prostate surgery can also damage the nerves of the penis.

Drugs are involved in an estimated 25 percent of impotence cases, especially in elderly men, who tend to take more drugs. The drugs that most commonly cause impotence include all antihypertensives, antipsychotics, antidepressants, some sedatives, cimetidine, and lithium. Alcohol also can cause impotence.

Occasionally, impotence results from hormonal disturbances. Low levels of testosterone, for example, can produce impotence. However, low male hormone levels, which tend to occur with aging, are more closely associated with a lowering of the sex drive (libido).

Psychologic factors, such as depression and performance anxiety, can lead to impotence, as can sexual guilt, fear of intimacy, and ambivalence about sexual orientation.★

Diagnosis

Typically, a person tells a doctor about his erection problems. The doctor then asks about the symptoms to be sure that impotence, not another sexual dysfunction (such as a problem with ejaculation), is the problem. A doctor asks if sexual desire is accompanied by the ability to achieve an erection sufficient for sexual intercourse and if the man has erections during sleep or in the morning on awakening. Answers to these questions can help a doctor determine whether the impotence stems from physical or psychologic problems.

A doctor also reviews any history of vascular, pelvic, rectal, or prostate surgery. Any changes in male sex characteristics—such as breast, testicular, and penile size—and changes in the hair, voice, or skin are considered. A doctor can explore the possibility of psychologic problems, such as depression or anxiety. Any new stressful situation, such as a change of sex partners or problems with relationships or work, can also be an important factor. A doctor also asks about the person's use of prescription, nonprescription, and illicit drugs and alcohol.

Blood samples are taken to measure total testosterone levels and the amount of bioavailable (usable) testosterone. Testosterone deficiencies can cause impotence as well as lead to breast enlargement (gynecomastia), loss of pubic hair, and smaller, softer testes. Measurement of blood pressure in the legs may indicate a problem with the arteries in the pelvis and groin that supply

---

▲ see page 422

■ see page 336

★ see box, page 422

blood to the penis. A doctor also can determine if the nerve supply to the penis is normal.

Other blood tests can help identify common diseases that can lead to impotence. For example, a complete blood cell count can identify anemia and infection, a blood sugar (glucose) or glycostatic hemoglobin test can reveal diabetes, and a thyroid-stimulating hormone test can detect an overactive or underactive thyroid gland.

The blood vessels of the penis can be evaluated by an ultrasound examination. Another test involves injecting the penis with drugs that dilate the arteries. If the injection doesn't cause an erection or if the man can't maintain an erection, the penile veins may be leaky and unable to hold blood in the penis.

Treatment

Impotence can usually be treated without surgery. The type of treatment depends on the cause of the impotence and the person's lifestyle.

A specific exercise for those with impotence from psychologic causes is the three-stage sensate focus technique. This technique encourages intimate contact and emotional warmth, putting less emphasis on intercourse than on building a relationship. The first stage consists of caressing; the partners concentrate on giving each other pleasure without touching each other's genital areas. The second stage allows partners to touch the genital areas and other erogenous zones, but intercourse is prohibited. In the third stage, intercourse occurs. Both partners achieve comfort at each level of intimacy before proceeding to the next stage. If this technique isn't successful, psychotherapy or behavioral sex therapy may be appropriate. If the person has depression, drug treatment or counseling may help.

Sildenafil is an oral drug than can relieve some cases by increasing blood flow to the penis. Taken 30 to 60 minutes before sex, it is effective only when sexual arousal occurs. It must not be taken in combination with nitrates because of serious and sometimes fatal side effects. Yohimbine is no better than a placebo (an inactive substance). Testosterone replacement therapy benefits men whose impotence or loss of sex drive stems from abnormally low testosterone levels. The testosterone can be injected, usually weekly, or applied

in a skin patch. This drug may cause side effects, such as prostate growth, and an excess of red blood cells that can lead to a stroke.

Binding and vacuum devices often are used to achieve and maintain an erection, although they aren't appropriate for men with bleeding disorders or those taking anticoagulant drugs. **Binding devices**—such as bands and rings made of metal, rubber, or leather—are placed at the base of the penis to slow the outflow of blood. These medically engineered devices can be purchased with a doctor's prescription in a pharmacy, but inexpensive versions, called cock rings, can be purchased in stores that sell sexual paraphernalia. For mild impotence, a binding device alone can be effective. **Vacuum devices**—consisting of a hollow chamber and a syringe, a pump, or tubing—fit over the limp penis. A gentle vacuum is created by using the syringe or pump or by sucking on the tubing. Vacuum pressure helps draw blood into the arteries of the penis. When the penis is erect, a binding device is applied to prevent the blood from flowing out through the veins. This combination of devices may help an otherwise impotent man maintain an erection for as long as 30 minutes. Occasionally, a binding device causes problems with ejaculation, especially if it's too tight. For safety, the person must remove the device after 30 minutes. Vacuum devices can cause bruises if used too often. However, both devices are considered safe.

Impotence also may be treated with injections of specific drugs self-administered directly into the erectile tissue (corpus cavernosum) of the penis. An erection occurs 5 to 10 minutes after the injection and may last as long as 60 minutes. Side effects may include bruising and aching. Also, injections may cause a painful, persistent erection (priapism).▲

When impotence doesn't respond to other treatments, a permanent penile implant or prosthesis may help. Permanent devices are especially successful for chronic impotence caused by diabetes. A variety of implants and prostheses, all requiring surgical insertion, are available. One device consists of firm rods that are inserted into the penis to create a permanent erection. Another is an inflatable balloon that is inserted into the penis; before having intercourse, the man inflates the balloon. Generally, such surgery requires at least a 3-day hospitalization and a 6-week recovery. Surgical techniques to restore blood flow to the penis are still experimental.

▲ see page 1058

Women's Health Issues

CHAPTER 231

Female Reproductive System

The external female reproductive (genital) organs have two functions—permitting sperm to enter the body and protecting the internal genital organs from infectious organisms. Because the female genital tract has an opening to the outside, disease-producing microorganisms (pathogens) can enter and cause gynecologic infections. These pathogens are usually transmitted during sexual activity.

The internal genital organs form a pathway (the genital tract). This pathway runs from the ovaries, from which eggs are released, through the fallopian tubes (oviducts), where fertilization of an egg can take place, through the uterus, where the embryo can develop into a fetus, to the birth canal (vagina), from which a fully developed baby can ultimately be delivered. Sperm can travel up the tract, and eggs down the tract.

External Genital Organs

The external genital organs (vulva) are bordered by the labia majora (literally, large lips), which are relatively large and fleshy; they are comparable to the scrotum in males. The labia majora contain sweat and sebaceous (oil-secreting) glands; after puberty, they are covered with hair. The labia minora (literally, small lips) can be very small or up to 2 inches wide. They lie just inside the labia majora and surround the openings to the vagina and urethra. The opening to the vagina is called the introitus, and the half-moon–shaped area behind the opening is called the fourchette. Through tiny ducts beside the introitus, Bartholin's glands, when stimulated, secrete a fluid (mucus) that supplies lubrication for intercourse. The opening to the urethra, which carries urine from the bladder to the outside, is in front of the vagina.

The two labia minora meet at the clitoris, a small sensitive protrusion analogous to the penis in the male. The clitoris is covered by a fold of skin (the prepuce) similar to the foreskin at the end of the penis. The clitoris, like the penis, is very sensitive to stimulation and can become erect.

The labia majora meet at the back in the perineum, a fibromuscular area between the vagina and the anus. The skin (epidermis) covering the perineum and the labia majora is similar to that on the rest of the body—it is thick and dry and can become scaly. In contrast, the lining of the labia minora and vagina is a mucous membrane; although its inner layers are structurally similar to epidermis, its surface is kept moist by fluid passing through the tissue from blood vessels in deeper layers. A rich supply of blood vessels gives it a pink color.

The vaginal opening is surrounded by the hymen (maidenhead). In a virgin, the hymen may completely cover the opening, but it usually encircles the opening like a tight ring. Because the degree of tightness varies among women, the hymen may tear at the first attempt at intercourse, or it may be so soft and pliable that no tearing occurs. In a nonvirgin, the hymen usually appears as small tags of tissue surrounding the vaginal opening.

Internal Genital Organs

The front and back walls of the vagina normally touch each other, so that there's no space in the vagina except when it's opened—during an examination or intercourse, for example. In the adult, the vaginal cavity is 3 to 4 inches long. The lower third of the vagina is surrounded by muscles that control its diameter. The upper two thirds of the vagina lies above these muscles and can be easily stretched. The cervix (the mouth and neck of the uterus) is at the top of the vagina. During a woman's reproductive years, the mucosal lining of the vagina has a corrugated appearance. Before puberty and after menopause (if the woman is not taking estrogen), the mucosa is smooth.

The uterus is a pear-shaped organ at the top of the vagina. It lies behind the bladder and in front of the rectum and is anchored in position by six ligaments. The uterus is divided into two parts: the cervix and the main body (the corpus). The cervix, the lower part of the uterus, opens into the vagina. Where the cervix joins the corpus, the corpus is usually bent forward. During the reproductive years, the corpus is twice as long as the cervix. The corpus is a highly muscular organ that can enlarge to hold a fetus. Its muscular walls

External Female Genital Organs

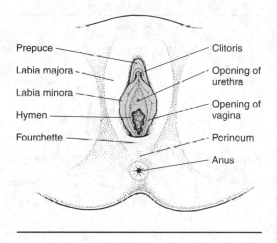

Prepuce — Clitoris
Labia majora — Opening of urethra
Labia minora — Opening of vagina
Hymen —
Fourchette — Perineum
— Anus

contract during labor to push the baby out through the fibrous cervix and the vagina.

A channel through the cervix allows sperm to enter the uterus and menstrual discharges to exit. Except during a woman's menstrual period or ovulation, the cervix is usually a good barrier against bacteria. The channel in the cervix is narrow—too narrow for the fetus to pass through during pregnancy—but during labor it stretches to let the baby through. During a pelvic examination, a doctor can see the part of the cervix that protrudes into the upper end of the vagina. Like the vagina, this part of the cervix is covered by mucosa, but the mucosa of the cervix is smooth.

The canal of the cervix is lined with mucus-secreting glands. This mucus is thick and impenetrable to sperm until just before the ovaries release an egg (ovulation). At ovulation, the consistency of the mucus changes so that sperm can swim through it, allowing fertilization. At the same time, the mucus-secreting glands of the cervix actually become able to store live sperm for 2 or 3 days. These sperm can later move up through the corpus and into the fallopian tubes to fertilize the egg; thus, intercourse 1 or 2 days before ovulation can lead to pregnancy. Because some

Internal Female Genital Organs

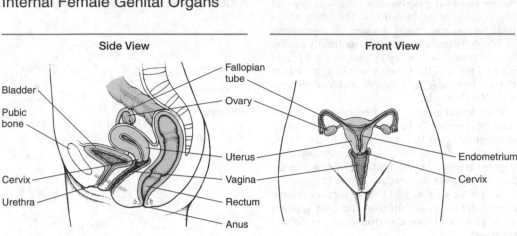

Side View	Front View

Side View labels: Bladder, Pubic bone, Cervix, Urethra, Fallopian tube, Ovary, Uterus, Vagina, Rectum, Anus

Front View labels: Endometrium, Cervix

women do not ovulate consistently, pregnancy can occur at varying times after the last menstrual period.

The inner lining of the corpus (endometrium) thickens each month after the monthly period (menstruation).▲ If the woman doesn't become pregnant during that cycle, most of the endometrium is shed and bleeding occurs, resulting in the monthly period.

The fallopian tubes extend 2 to 3 inches from the upper edges of the uterus toward the ovaries. The end of each tube flares into a funnel shape, providing a larger opening for the egg to fall into when it's released from the ovary. The ovaries aren't attached to the fallopian tubes but are suspended nearby from a ligament. The ovaries are usually pearl colored, oblong, and somewhat smaller than a hard-boiled egg.

Cilia (beating, hairlike extensions on cells) lining the fallopian tube and muscles in the tube's wall propel an egg downward through the tube. If the egg encounters a sperm in the fallopian tube and is fertilized, the fertilized egg begins to divide. Over a period of 4 days, the tiny embryo continues to divide while it moves slowly down the fallopian tube and into the uterus. The embryo attaches to the wall of the uterus, where it becomes embedded; this process is called implantation.■

Each female fetus has 6 to 7 million oocytes (developing egg cells) at 20 weeks of pregnancy and is born with about 2 million oocytes. At puberty, only 300,000 to 400,000 remain to begin to mature into eggs. The many thousands of oocytes that don't complete the maturation process gradually degenerate. All are gone by menopause.

Gynecologic Evaluation

For gynecologic care, a woman should choose a doctor with whom she can comfortably discuss sensitive topics, such as sex, birth control, and pregnancy. A doctor who provides gynecologic care is trained to discuss family problems, such as physical, emotional, and substance abuse, and will keep all information confidential. Some states have laws requiring parental consent for treat-

▲ see page 1075

■ see page 1137

ment of minors (usually under 18 years old). During a gynecologic visit, a doctor—who may be a gynecologist, internist, pediatrician, or general or family practitioner—a nurse practitioner, or a nurse midwife is prepared to answer questions about reproductive and sexual function and anatomy, including safe sex practices.

Gynecologic History

A gynecologic evaluation starts with a series of questions (gynecologic history), which usually focus on the reason for the visit to the doctor's office. A complete gynecologic history includes questions about the age at which menstrual bleeding began (menarche); its frequency, regularity, duration, and amount of flow; and the dates of the last two menstrual periods. A woman can also expect questions about abnormal bleeding—too much, too little, or at times other than normal menstruation. A doctor may ask about sexual activity to assess gynecologic infections, injuries, and the possibility of pregnancy. A woman is asked whether she uses or wants to use birth control and whether she's interested in counseling or other information. The number of pregnancies, dates that they occurred, outcomes, and complications are recorded. The doctor asks the woman whether she has pain during periods, during intercourse, or under other circumstances; how severe it is; and what provides relief. Questions are also asked about breast problems—pain, growths, areas of tenderness or redness, and discharge from the nipples. The woman is asked whether she is performing breast self-examination, how often, and whether she needs any instruction on technique.

The doctor reviews the woman's history of past gynecologic illnesses and usually obtains a full medical and surgical history that includes non-gynecologic health problems. The doctor needs to review all of the drugs a woman is taking, including prescription and over-the-counter drugs, illicit drugs, tobacco, and alcohol, because many of them affect gynecologic function as well as general health. Questions concerning mental, physical, or sexual abuse in the present or the past are important. Some questions focus on urination, to find out whether the woman has a urinary tract infection or is incontinent (can't control urination).

Collecting Cervical Cells for a Pap Test

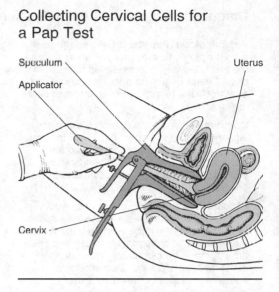

Speculum · Uterus
Applicator
Cervix ·

Gynecologic Examination

Some women are troubled by the gynecologic examination. If a woman lets the doctor know this beforehand, the doctor can take extra time and make sure to answer any questions.

A woman is usually asked to empty her bladder before the physical examination and to collect a urine sample for laboratory evaluation. A breast examination may be performed before or after the pelvic examination.▲ With the woman sitting, the doctor inspects the breasts for irregularities, dimpling, tightened skin, lumps, and a discharge. The woman then either sits or lies down, or both, with her arms akimbo or above her head, while the doctor feels (palpates) each breast with a flat hand and examines each underarm for enlarged lymph nodes. The doctor also feels the neck and the thyroid gland for lumps and abnormalities.

The doctor gently feels the entire area between the rib cage and pelvis (the abdomen), looking for abnormal growths or enlarged organs, especially the liver and spleen. Although the woman may

▲ see page 1099

Diagnostic Procedures in Gynecology

Papanicolaou (Pap) test: Cells are scraped from the cervix to check for possible cancer; the test is usually recommended for women once a year, beginning after first intercourse or at age 18. The procedure is safe and takes only a few seconds.

Colposcopy: A 10-power binocular magnifying lens is used to inspect the cervix for signs of cancer, often as a consequence of an abnormal Pap test result. Colposcopy is painless and requires no anesthetics. It takes several minutes to perform.

Biopsy: A biopsy of the cervix and vagina usually is performed using colposcopy so that tissue samples may be taken from the area that looks most abnormal. A biopsy of a small area of the vulva can usually be performed in the doctor's office with use of a local anesthetic; biopsy of the cervix usually doesn't require use of an anesthetic. In cases of suspected cancer, less than $1/4$ inch of tissue may be removed for microscopic examination.

Endocervical curettage: A small instrument is inserted into the canal of the cervix to scrape tissue. This tissue is examined under a microscope by a pathologist. This procedure is usually performed during colposcopy.

Conization of the cervix (cone biopsy): A cone-shaped piece of tissue, perhaps $1/2$ to 1 inch long and $3/4$ inch across, is taken from the cervix. Cutting may be done with a laser, electrocautery (heat), or a knife; an anesthetic is required. Conization is sometimes performed after abnormal biopsy results to help make the diagnosis or to remove the abnormal area.

Endometrial biopsy: A small tube, either metal or plastic, is inserted through the cervix into the uterine cavity. The tube is moved back and forth and around, with suction applied at the outer end, to dislodge and collect tissue from the lining of the uterus (endometrium). The tissue is sent to a laboratory, usually to determine the cause of abnormal bleeding. Endometrial biopsy can be performed in a doctor's office. It doesn't require an anesthetic and feels like menstrual cramps.

Hysteroscopy: A thin tube about $1/3$ inch in diameter is inserted through the cervix into the uterine cavity. The tube contains fiber optics that transmit light for viewing the dark cavity and may contain a biopsy or electrocautery (heat-sealing) instrument. The source of abnormal bleeding or other abnormalities can usually be seen and either sampled for a biopsy, sealed off, or removed. This procedure may be performed in a doctor's office or in a hospital at the same time as a dilatation and curettage.

---

experience some discomfort when the doctor presses deeply, the examination should not be painful. Tapping with the fingers (percussion) while listening for the border between hollow-sounding and dull-sounding areas helps establish the size of the liver and spleen. To help identify abnormalities that can't be felt, the doctor may listen with a stethoscope for the activity of the intestine and for any abnormal noises made by blood flowing through narrowed blood vessels.

During the pelvic examination, the woman lies on her back with her hips and knees bent and her buttocks moved to the edge of the examining table. Most examining tables have heel or knee stirrups that help a woman hold this position. If a woman wants to observe the pelvic examination while it's being performed, the doctor can provide mirrors as well as explanations or a diagram. The woman should let the doctor know ahead of time that she would like this information. The doctor begins an examination of the pelvis with a visual inspection of the external genital area and notes the distribution of hair and any abnormalities, discoloration, discharge, or inflammation. This examination may confirm that all is well or give clues to hormonal problems, cancer, infections, injury, or physical abuse.

The doctor spreads the labia with gloved fingers to examine the opening of the vagina. Using a warmed, water-lubricated speculum (a metal or

Dilatation and curettage (D and C): The cervix is dilated (stretched open) with metal rods so that a spoon-shaped instrument (curet) can be inserted to scrape the lining of the uterus. This procedure may be used for diagnosis of endometrial abnormalities suggested by biopsy results or for treatment of an incomplete miscarriage. For an incomplete miscarriage, the curet used is a plastic tube with suction applied at the outer end. D and C is often performed in a hospital with use of a general anesthetic.

Hysterosalpingography: X-rays are taken after a dye that can be seen on x-ray film is injected through the cervix to outline the uterine cavity and fallopian tubes, often as part of an examination for causes of infertility. The test is performed in a doctor's office and may cause discomfort, such as cramps. For this reason, a sedative may be given.

Ultrasound scanning (sonography): Sound waves (at a frequency too high to be heard) are directed through the abdominal wall or vagina. The pattern of their reflection off of internal structures can be displayed on a monitor to help determine the condition and size of a fetus and to aid in the diagnosis of fetal abnormalities, multiple pregnancy, tubal pregnancy, tumors, cysts, or other abnormalities in the pelvic organs. Ultrasound scanning is painless. It's also used in amniocentesis and other sampling procedures.

Laparoscopy: A thin viewing tube containing fiber optics is inserted into the abdominal cavity through an incision made at the bottom of the navel. Carbon dioxide is used to inflate the abdomen, so that organs in the entire abdomen and pelvis can be seen clearly. Often, laparoscopy is used to determine the cause of pelvic pain, infertility, and other gynecologic problems. A laparoscope can be used with other instruments to perform biopsies, sterilization procedures, and other types of surgery; it can also help retrieve eggs for in vitro fertilization. This procedure is performed in a hospital and requires an anesthetic; a local anesthetic is used for limited procedures, but a general anesthetic is more commonly used.

Culdocentesis: A needle is inserted through the wall of the vagina just behind the cervix and into the pelvic cavity, usually to look for bleeding when an ectopic pregnancy (a pregnancy that develops outside the uterus) is suspected. Culdocentesis is often performed in the emergency department without use of an anesthetic.

plastic instrument that spreads the walls of the vagina apart), the doctor examines the deeper areas of the vagina and the cervix. The cervix is examined closely for signs of irritation or cancer. To perform a **Papanicolaou (Pap) test,** the doctor scrapes cells from the surface of the cervix with a small wooden applicator much like a tongue depressor. Then, a small bristle brush can be used to obtain a sample of cells from the canal of the cervix. These procedures can be felt but aren't painful. The cells removed with the brush or wooden applicator are placed on a glass slide, sprayed with a preservative, and sent to the laboratory, where they are examined under a microscope for signs of cervical cancer.▲ The Pap test,

the best method for detecting cervical cancer, identifies 80 to 85 percent of such cancers, even in their earliest stages. The test is most accurate if the woman doesn't douche or use vaginal medications for at least 24 hours before the examination.

If the doctor suspects other problems, additional tests may be performed. For example, if an infection is suspected, the doctor wipes the vagina and cervix with a swab and obtains a small

▲ see page 1110

D and C

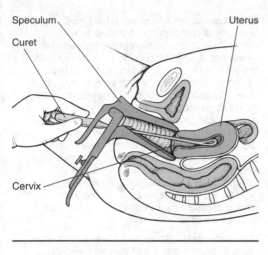

Speculum
Curet
Cervix
Uterus

amount of vaginal discharge to be sent to the laboratory for culture and microscopic evaluation.

The strength and support of the vaginal wall are evaluated. The doctor looks for any protrusion of the bladder into the front part of the wall (cystocele), protrusion of the rectum into the back part of the wall (rectocele), or protrusion of intestine near the very top of the vagina (enterocele).

After removing the speculum, the doctor performs a two-handed examination, inserting the index and middle fingers of one gloved hand into the vagina and placing the fingers of the other hand on the lower abdomen above the pubic bone. Between the two hands, the uterus can usually be felt as a pear-shaped, smooth, firm structure, and its position, size, consistency, and degree of tenderness, if any, can be determined. Then the doctor attempts to feel the ovaries by moving the hand on the abdomen more to the side and exerting slightly more pressure. Because the ovaries are small and much more difficult to feel than the uterus, more pressure is required; the woman may find this part of the examination to be uncomfortable. The doctor determines how large the ovaries are and whether they are tender. The doctor also feels for growths or tender areas within the vagina.

Finally, the doctor performs a rectovaginal examination by inserting the index finger into the vagina and the middle finger into the rectum. In this way, the back wall of the vagina can be examined for abnormal growths or thickness. In addition, the doctor can examine the rectum for hemorrhoids, fissures, polyps, and lumps and can test the stool for unseen (occult) blood. A woman may be given a take-home kit to test for unseen blood in the stool.

Occasionally, more extensive tests are needed. To examine the internal genital organs, doctors use various diagnostic tools, including instruments that apply fiber-optic technology. Fiber optics are thin, flexible strands of plastic or glass that transmit light. A fiber-optic cable attached to a viewing tube called a laparoscope can be used to examine the uterus, fallopian tubes, or ovaries without requiring a large incision. The laparoscope can also help doctors perform surgical procedures in the genital tract.

CHAPTER 232

Hormones and Reproduction

Normal human reproduction involves the interaction of a variety of hormones and organs, orchestrated by the hypothalamus, an area of the brain. In both females and males, the hypothala-

▲ see box, page 697

mus secretes hormones, called releasing factors, that travel to the pituitary, a pea-sized gland located directly below the hypothalamus.▲ These hormones stimulate the pituitary to release other hormones. For example, gonadotropin-releasing hormone, a releasing factor secreted by the hypothalamus, stimulates the pituitary to secrete luteinizing hormone and follicle-stimulating hormone. These hormones stimulate the reproductive glands to mature and to release sex hormones. The ovaries in women release estrogens, and the testes in men release androgens such as testosterone. Sex hormones are also produced by the adrenal glands, located on top of the kidneys.

The patterns of secretion and resulting blood levels of sex hormones determine whether these hormones stimulate or inhibit the release of luteinizing hormone and follicle-stimulating hormone from the pituitary. For example, a decrease in the sex hormone levels stimulates the pituitary to release larger amounts of the two hormones—a negative feedback control mechanism. Virtually all hormones are released in short bursts (pulses) every 1 to 3 hours. As a result, hormone levels in the bloodstream fluctuate.

Puberty

At birth, the levels of luteinizing hormone and follicle-stimulating hormone are high, but they decrease within a few months and remain low until puberty. Early in puberty, these hormone levels increase, stimulating the production of sex hormones. In girls, the increased hormone levels stimulate the breasts, ovaries, uterus, and vagina to mature; menstrual periods to start; and secondary sexual characteristics—such as pubic and underarm hair—to develop. In boys, the testes, prostate, seminal vesicles, and penis mature, and facial, pubic, and underarm hair grows. Normally, these changes occur sequentially during puberty, resulting in sexual maturity.▲

In girls, the first change of puberty usually is breast budding (the breasts start to develop), followed closely by the growth of pubic and underarm hair. The interval from breast budding to the first menstrual period generally is about 2 years. The girl's body shape changes, and the percentage of body fat increases. The growth spurt accompanying puberty typically begins even before the breasts start to develop. Growth is fastest relatively early in puberty, before menstrual periods begin. Then growth slows considerably, usually stopping between ages 14 and 16. In contrast, boys grow fastest between ages 13 and 17 and can continue to grow into their early 20s.

The age at which puberty begins seems to be influenced by a child's general health and nutrition as well as by socioeconomic and hereditary factors. In Western Europe, the average age at which a girl has her first menstrual period de-

How Many Eggs?

A baby girl is born with eggs (oocytes) already in her ovaries. By the time a female fetus is 20 to 24 weeks old, the fetus' ovaries contain 7 to 20 million eggs. The eggs become incorporated into follicles (fluid-filled cavities, each with an egg embedded in its wall). While the follicles are forming, most of the eggs gradually waste away, leaving about 2 million present at birth. No more develop after birth. Fewer than 400,000 remain by the time menstrual periods start—more than enough eggs for a lifetime of fertility.

Only about 400 eggs are released during a woman's reproductive life, usually one during each menstrual cycle. Until released, an egg remains dormant in its follicle—suspended in the middle of a cell division—making the egg one of the longest-lived cells in the body. Because the dormant egg can't perform the usual cellular repair processes, the opportunity for damage increases as a woman ages. A chromosomal or genetic abnormality is thus more likely when a woman conceives a baby later in life.

creased by 4 months for each decade between 1850 and 1950, but the age hasn't decreased in the last four decades. Girls who are moderately obese tend to start menstruating earlier; girls who are severely underweight and malnourished tend to start later. Periods also start earlier among girls who live in urban areas and among those whose mothers started menstruating early.

Menstrual Cycle

Menstruation, the shedding of the lining of the uterus (the endometrium) accompanied by bleeding, occurs in approximately monthly cycles unless a woman is pregnant. It marks the reproductive years of a woman's life, extending from the start of menstruation (menarche) during puberty until its cessation (menopause).

▲ see box, page 1256

Changes During the Menstrual Cycle

A menstrual cycle is regulated by the complex interaction of pituitary hormones (luteinizing hormone and follicle-stimulating hormone) and ovarian sex hormones (estradiol and progesterone).

The menstrual cycle begins with the **follicular phase.** Low levels of estradiol, an estrogen, and progesterone at the beginning of this phase cause the uterine lining (endometrium) to degenerate and be shed in menstruation, which marks the first day of the menstrual cycle. During the first half of this phase, the follicle-stimulating hormone level increases slightly, stimulating the development of several follicles, each containing an egg. Only one follicle continues to develop. During the last part of this phase, the level of estradiol, secreted by the ovaries, increases, stimulating the uterine lining to begin to thicken.

A surge in luteinizing hormone and follicle-stimulating hormone levels begins the **ovulatory phase.** Egg release (ovulation) usually occurs 16 to 32 hours after the surge begins. The estradiol level peaks during the surge, and the progesterone level starts to increase.

During the **luteal phase,** levels of luteinizing hormone and follicle-stimulating hormone decrease. The ruptured follicle closes after releasing the egg and forms a corpus luteum, which secretes progesterone. Progesterone and estradiol cause the uterine lining to thicken. If the egg is not fertilized, the corpus luteum degenerates and no longer secretes progesterone, the estradiol level decreases, and a new menstrual cycle begins.

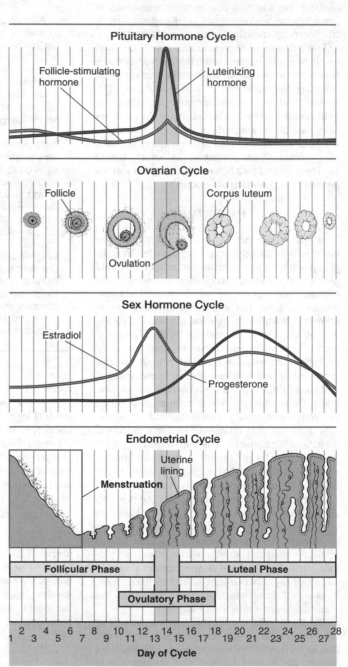

By definition, the first day of bleeding is counted as the beginning of each menstrual cycle (day 1). The cycle ends just before the next menstrual period. Menstrual cycles range from about 21 to 40 days. Only 10 to 15 percent of cycles are exactly 28 days. The intervals between periods are generally longest in the years immediately after menarche and before menopause. The menstrual cycle can be divided into three phases: follicular, ovulatory, and luteal.

The **follicular phase,** which varies in length, extends from the first day of bleeding to immediately before a surge in the level of luteinizing hormone, which causes the egg to be released (ovulation). This phase is so named because the follicles in the ovaries are developing during it. During the first half of the phase, the pituitary gland slightly increases its secretion of follicle-stimulating hormone, stimulating the growth of 3 to 30 follicles, each containing an egg. Only one of these follicles continues to grow. The other stimulated follicles degenerate. The follicular phase tends to become shorter at the end of the reproductive years, near menopause.

In a menstrual period, part of the endometrium is shed in response to a decrease in estrogen and progesterone levels. The endometrium consists of three layers. The top (superficial) layer and most of the middle (intermediate) layer are shed. The bottom (basal) layer remains and produces new cells to rebuild the other two layers. Menstrual bleeding lasts 3 to 7 days, averaging 5 days. Blood loss ranges from $\frac{1}{2}$ to 10 ounces, averaging $4\frac{1}{2}$ ounces. A sanitary pad or tampon, depending on the type, can hold up to an ounce. Menstrual blood usually doesn't clot unless the bleeding is very heavy.

The **ovulatory phase,** during which the egg is released, starts with a surge in the level of luteinizing hormone. The egg is usually released 16 to 32 hours after the surge begins. The one follicle that's growing bulges out from the surface of the ovary, finally rupturing and releasing the egg. Around the time of ovulation, some women feel a dull pain on one side of the lower abdomen, known as mittelschmerz, which may last for a few minutes to a few hours. Although the pain is felt on the same side as the ovary that released the egg, the precise cause of the pain isn't known. The pain may precede or follow the rupture of the follicle and may not occur in all cycles. Egg release doesn't alternate between the two ovaries and appears to be random. If one ovary is removed, the remaining ovary releases an egg every month.

The **luteal phase** follows ovulation. It lasts about 14 days, unless fertilization occurs, and ends just before a menstrual period. In the luteal phase, the ruptured follicle closes after releasing the egg and forms a corpus luteum, which secretes increasing quantities of progesterone.

The progesterone causes body temperature to rise slightly during the luteal phase and remain elevated until a menstrual period begins. This rise in temperature can be used to estimate whether ovulation has occurred.▲

The corpus luteum degenerates after 14 days and a new menstrual cycle begins unless the egg is fertilized. If the egg is fertilized, the corpus luteum begins to produce human chorionic gonadotropin. This hormone maintains the corpus luteum, which produces progesterone, until the growing fetus can produce its own hormones. Pregnancy tests are based on detecting increased levels of human chorionic gonadotropin.

CHAPTER 233

Menopause

Menopause is the time in a woman's life when the cyclic function of the ovaries and menstrual periods cease.

Menopause actually occurs at the end of a woman's last menstrual period. However, that fact is established only later, when a woman has had no periods for at least 12 months. The average age

at which menopause occurs is about 50 years, but menopause may occur normally in women as young as 40. Regular menstrual cycles may con-

---

▲ see page 1116

tinue up to menopause, but usually the last periods tend to vary in duration and amount of flow. Progressively fewer cycles involve the release of an egg.

With age, the ovaries become progressively less responsive to stimulation by luteinizing hormone and follicle-stimulating hormone, which are secreted by the pituitary gland.▲ Consequently, the ovaries secrete smaller and smaller amounts of estrogen and progesterone, and egg release (ovulation) eventually stops.

Premature menopause is menopause occurring before age 40.■ Possible causes include a genetic predisposition and autoimmune disorders, in which antibodies are produced that can damage a number of glands, including the ovaries. Smoking may also cause premature menopause.

Artificial menopause results from a medical intervention that reduces or stops hormone secretion by the ovaries. These interventions include surgery to remove the ovaries or reduce their blood supply and chemotherapy or radiation therapy to the pelvis—including the ovaries—to treat cancer. Surgery to remove the uterus (hysterectomy) ends menstrual periods, but it doesn't affect hormone levels as long as the ovaries are intact and therefore doesn't cause menopause.

Symptoms

During the time before menopause (technically called the climacteric, but more recently called perimenopause), symptoms may be nonexistent, mild, moderate, or severe. Hot flashes affect 75 percent of women. During a hot flash, the skin, especially on the head and neck, becomes red and warm (flushed), and perspiration may be profuse. Most women have hot flashes for more than a year, and 25 to 50 percent have them for more than 5 years. A hot flash lasts from 30 seconds to 5 minutes and may be followed by chills.

Psychologic and emotional symptoms—fatigue, irritability, insomnia, and nervousness—

▲ see page 1074

■ see page 1088

★ see page 218

● see page 679

may be caused by the decrease in estrogen levels. Night sweats may disturb sleep, making fatigue and irritability worse. A woman occasionally may feel dizzy, have tingling sensations (pins and needles), and be unusually aware of her heartbeat, which may seem to be pounding. Loss of bladder control, inflammation of the bladder or vagina, and pain during intercourse because of vaginal dryness may also occur. Sometimes muscles and joints ache.

Osteoporosis (severe thinning of the bones) ★ is a major health hazard of menopause. Slender white women are at highest risk. Women who smoke cigarettes, drink excessive amounts of alcohol, take corticosteroids, have a low intake of calcium, or have a sedentary lifestyle are also at risk. During the first 5 years after menopause, 3 to 5 percent of bone is lost each year. After that, 1 to 2 percent of bone is lost each year. Fractures may result from minor injuries and, in elderly women, even without an injury. The most commonly fractured bones are the vertebrae (leading to stooping and backache), hips, and wrist bones.

Cardiovascular disease progresses more rapidly after menopause, when estrogen levels decrease. A woman whose ovaries have been removed, resulting in premature menopause, and who doesn't take estrogen replacement therapy is twice as likely to have cardiovascular disease as a premenopausal woman of the same age. Postmenopausal women who take estrogen have a much lower rate of cardiovascular disease than those who don't take it. For instance, among postmenopausal women who have coronary artery disease, those who take estrogen survive longer, on the average, than those who don't. These benefits may be partly explained by estrogen's favorable effects on cholesterol levels. A decrease in estrogen levels causes an increase in the so-called bad low-density lipoprotein (LDL) cholesterol levels and a decrease in the so-called good high-density lipoprotein (HDL) cholesterol levels.●

Treatment

Symptoms are treated by restoring estrogen to premenopausal levels. The primary goals of estrogen replacement therapy are the following:

• To relieve symptoms such as hot flashes, vaginal dryness, and urinary problems

- To help prevent osteoporosis
- To help prevent atherosclerosis and coronary artery disease

Estrogen is available in nonsynthetic (natural) or synthetic (laboratory-produced) forms. Synthetic estrogens are a hundred times more potent than natural estrogens and therefore are not routinely recommended for women in menopause. Only very low doses of a natural estrogen are needed to prevent hot flashes and osteoporosis. High doses can cause problems, such as an increased tendency to have migraine headaches.

Estrogen may be given as a tablet or as a skin patch (transdermal estrogen). Estrogen may be applied to the vagina as a cream when the primary reasons for using it are to prevent thinning of the vaginal lining—thereby reducing the risk of urinary infections and incontinence—and to prevent painful intercourse. Some of the estrogen taken this way is absorbed into the bloodstream, particularly as the vaginal lining becomes healthier.

Because estrogen is associated with side effects and long-term risks as well as benefits, a woman and her doctor must weigh the benefits against the risks before deciding whether to use estrogen replacement therapy. Side effects of estrogen include nausea, breast discomfort, headache, and mood changes.

Postmenopausal women who take estrogen without progesterone have an increased risk of endometrial cancer (cancer of the lining of the uterus)▲—from 1 out of 1,000 to 4 out of 1,000 women a year. The increased risk is related to the dose and duration of estrogen therapy. If a woman has abnormal bleeding from the vagina, a biopsy (removal of a tissue sample to be examined under a microscope) of the uterine lining may be performed to determine whether she has endometrial cancer. Women with endometrial cancer who are taking estrogen usually have a good prognosis. About 94 percent of such women survive for 5 years. Taking progesterone in addition to estrogen can almost eliminate the risk of endometrial cancer, reducing it below that for women who don't take estrogen replacement therapy. (A woman whose uterus has been removed has no risk of developing this cancer.) Progesterone doesn't appear to negate estrogen's beneficial effect on cardiovascular disease.

Whether taking estrogen might increase the risk of breast cancer has long been a concern.

Taking Progesterone With Estrogen

Progesterone is taken with estrogen to reduce the risk of endometrial cancer. Commonly, estrogen and progesterone are taken every day. This schedule typically causes irregular vaginal bleeding for the first 2 or 3 months of therapy, but the bleeding usually stops completely within a year. Alternatively, a cyclic schedule may be used: A woman takes estrogen daily for about 2 weeks, progesterone with estrogen for the next few days, then no hormones for the last few days of the month. With this schedule, many women have vaginal bleeding on the days when no hormones are taken.

Synthetic progesterone is available in several forms, which can be taken by mouth or by injection into a muscle. Side effects of progesterone include abdominal bloating, breast discomfort, headaches, mood changes, and acne. It also has some adverse effects on cholesterol levels.

However, no clear-cut association between estrogen replacement therapy and breast cancer has been found. The risk of cancer may be increased when estrogen is taken for more than 10 years. For women who have a high risk of developing breast cancer, estrogen therapy may not be appropriate. However, for women who are prone to osteoporosis and heart disease and who are at low risk for developing breast cancer, the benefit gained from estrogen therapy outweighs the risk.

The risk of developing gallbladder disease is modestly increased during the first year of estrogen replacement therapy.

Generally, estrogen replacement therapy is not prescribed for women who have or have had breast cancer or advanced endometrial cancer or

▲ see page 1108

who have genital bleeding of unknown cause, acute liver disease, or a blood clotting disorder. However, sometimes doctors prescribe estrogen for women who had breast cancer detected and treated in an early stage at least 5 years previously without a recurrence. Usually, estrogen replacement therapy is not prescribed for women who have chronic liver disease or acute intermittent porphyria.▲

Women who can't take estrogen may be given antianxiety drugs, progesterone, or clonidine to reduce the discomfort of hot flashes. Antidepressants may also help some women by relieving depression, anxiety, irritability, and insomnia.

CHAPTER 234

Common Gynecologic Problems

Gynecologic problems are those related to the female reproductive system. Some common problems are caused by such conditions as infections, injuries, or hormonal changes. These common problems include pelvic pain; inflammation of the uterus, fallopian tubes, vagina, or vulva; and noncancerous uterine growths, such as fibroids. Other common problems are related to menstruation—for example, premenstrual syndrome and pain during menstrual periods (dysmenorrhea). Although some problems may be mild and correct themselves, others, such as infections, may be serious and require medical attention.

Pelvic Pain

The pelvis, which contains the uterus, fallopian tubes, ovaries, vagina, bladder, and rectum, is the lowest part of the trunk, below the abdomen and between the hip bones. Women often feel pain in this area. Such pain varies in type and intensity, and the cause can be hard to identify.

Pelvic pain is frequently, but not always, caused by problems related to the reproductive system. Other causes of pelvic pain are related to the intestines or urinary tract. Psychologic factors can make pain seem worse or even cause a sensation of pain where no physical problem exists.

Diagnosis

When a woman suddenly develops very severe pain in the lower abdomen or pelvic area, a doctor must quickly decide whether the situation is an emergency requiring immediate surgery. Examples of emergencies are appendicitis, perforation of the intestine, a twisted ovarian cyst, an ectopic pregnancy, and a ruptured fallopian tube.

The doctor can often determine the cause of the pain from its description, including what it feels like (for example, sharp or dull), under what circumstances and how suddenly it began, how long it has lasted, and where it's located. Additional symptoms, such as a fever, nausea, or vomiting, may help the doctor make the diagnosis. Information about the timing of the pain in relation to eating, sleeping, sexual intercourse, movement, urination, and defecation may also help.

A physical examination is performed. A pelvic (internal) examination,■ always part of an evaluation of pelvic pain, helps the doctor determine which organs are affected and whether an infection is present. Laboratory tests, such as a complete blood cell count, a urinalysis, or a pregnancy test, may indicate internal bleeding, an infection, or an ectopic pregnancy. An ultrasound examination, a computed tomography (CT) scan, or magnetic resonance imaging (MRI) of the internal organs may be needed. Sometimes the doctor performs surgery or laparoscopy (a procedure in which a fiber-optic tube is used to examine the abdominal and pelvic cavities)★ to determine the cause of the pain.

▲ see page 689

■ see page 1071

★ see page 486

Vaginitis and Vulvitis

Vaginitis is an inflammation of the lining of the vagina. Vulvitis is an inflammation of the vulva (the external female genital organs). Vulvovaginitis is an inflammation of the vulva and the vagina.

In these conditions, the tissues are inflamed, sometimes resulting in a vaginal discharge. Causes include infections, irritating substances or objects, tumors or other abnormal tissue, radiation therapy, drugs, and hormonal changes. Poor personal hygiene can contribute to the growth of bacteria and fungi as well as cause irritation. Stool may enter through an abnormal passage (fistula) from the intestine to the vagina, resulting in vaginitis.

During a woman's reproductive years, hormonal changes can result in a normal discharge that's watery, mucous, or milky white, varying in amount and type with the different phases of the menstrual cycle. After menopause, the vaginal lining and vulvar tissues thin, and the normal discharge may decrease because of the lack of estrogen. Consequently, the vagina and vulva are more easily infected and injured.

Newborns may have a vaginal discharge caused by estrogen absorbed from the mother before birth. It usually disappears within 2 weeks.

Symptoms

The most common symptom of vaginitis is an abnormal vaginal discharge. A discharge is considered abnormal if it occurs in large amounts, has an offensive odor, or is accompanied by vaginal itching, soreness, or pain. Often, an abnormal discharge is thicker than a normal discharge and varies in color. For example, it may be the consistency of cottage cheese, or it may be yellow, greenish, or blood-tinged.

A bacterial infection of the vagina tends to produce a white, gray, or yellowish cloudy discharge with a foul or fishy odor. The odor may become stronger after sexual intercourse or washing with soap, both of which reduce vaginal acidity, thus encouraging bacterial growth. The vulva may feel irritated or itch mildly.

A candidal (yeast) infection▲ produces moderate to severe itching and burning of the vulva and vagina. The skin appears red and may feel raw. A thick, cheesy discharge from the vagina tends to cling to the vaginal walls. Symptoms may worsen during the week before a menstrual period. This infection tends to recur in women who

---

What Causes Pelvic Pain?

Related to the reproductive system
- Ectopic pregnancy
- Endometriosis
- Fibroids
- Large ovarian cysts or their rupture
- Mittelschmerz (pain in the middle of the menstrual cycle caused by ovulation)
- Pelvic congestion (vascular engorgement)
- Pelvic inflammatory disease
- Ruptured fallopian tube
- Twisted ovary

Unrelated to the reproductive system
- Appendicitis
- Cystitis (inflammation of the bladder)
- Diverticulitis (inflammation or infection of one or more diverticula, which are small abnormal pouches in the large intestine)
- Gastroenteritis (inflammation of the stomach and intestine)
- Ileitis (inflammation of part of the small intestine)
- Inflammatory bowel disease
- Mesenteric lymphadenitis (inflammation of the lymph nodes in the membrane connecting organs to the abdominal wall)
- Renal colic (pain in the flank, usually caused by an obstruction in the urinary tract)

---

have diabetes that isn't well controlled and in those who are taking antibiotics.

An infection by *Trichomonas vaginalis*, a protozoan, produces a white, grayish-green, or yellowish discharge that may be frothy.■ The discharge often appears shortly after a menstrual period and may have an unpleasant odor. Itching is severe.

A watery discharge, especially if it contains blood, can be caused by cancer of the vagina, cervix, or uterine lining (endometrium). Polyps on the cervix may produce vaginal bleeding after sexual intercourse. If the vulva has been itchy or

---

▲ see page 946

■ see page 945

What Causes an Abnormal Vaginal Discharge?

Infection
- Bacteria, such as chlamydiae and gonococci
- Fungi, such as *Candida* (especially among women who have diabetes, are pregnant, or are taking antibiotics)
- Protozoans, such as *Trichomonas vaginalis*
- Viruses, such as human papillomavirus and herpesvirus

Irritation
- Spermicides, lubricants, condoms, diaphragms, cervical caps, and sponges
- Laundry soaps and fabric softeners
- Deodorant sprays and soaps
- Bathwater additives
- Frequent douching
- Foreign objects in the vagina
- Tight, nonporous, nonabsorbent underpants
- Stool

Tumors or other abnormal tissue
- Cancer of the vulva, vagina, cervix, or uterine lining

Radiation therapy

uncomfortable for some time, causes may include a human papillomavirus infection or carcinoma in situ, a very early cancer that hasn't invaded other areas and can usually be removed easily by a surgeon.

A painful sore on the vulva may be caused by a herpes infection or an abscess. A sore that isn't painful may be caused by cancer or syphilis. Pubic lice can cause itching in the area of the vulva (pediculosis pubis).▲

Diagnosis

The characteristics of the discharge may suggest its cause to a doctor, but additional infor-

mation is needed to make the diagnosis—such as when in the menstrual cycle the discharge occurs, whether the discharge is sporadic or continuous, how it has responded to previous therapy, and whether the woman has vulvar itching, burning, or pain or a vaginal sore. The doctor may ask about birth control, pain after sexual intercourse, previous vaginal infections, sexually transmitted diseases, and the use of laundry detergents that may cause irritation. Questions may include whether the sex partner has symptoms or whether anyone else in the household has itching in the groin.

While examining the vagina, the doctor uses a cotton-tipped swab to take a sample of the discharge, which is examined under a microscope, grown in a laboratory (cultured), or both to identify the infective organism. The cervix is inspected, and a tissue sample is removed for a Papanicolaou (Pap) test,■ which can detect cervical cancer. The doctor also performs a two-handed examination, inserting the index and middle fingers of one gloved hand into the vagina and gently pressing on the outside of the lower abdomen with the other hand to feel the reproductive organs between the hands. When a woman has a long-standing inflammation of the vulva (chronic vulvitis) that doesn't respond to treatment, the doctor usually removes a tissue sample for examination under a microscope (biopsy) to look for cancer cells.

Treatment

For a normal discharge, occasional douching with water may reduce the amount. However, a discharge caused by vaginitis requires specific treatment according to its cause. If the cause is an infection, treatment consists of an antibiotic, antifungal, or antiviral drug, depending on the infective organism. Until the infection has been cured, a premeasured vinegar and water douche can be used briefly to control symptoms. However, douching frequently and using medicated douches are discouraged because they increase the risk of pelvic inflammatory disease. If the labia (folds of skin around the vaginal and urethral openings) are stuck together because of previous infections, applying a vaginal estrogen cream for 7 to 10 days usually opens them.

In addition to an antibiotic, treatment of a bacterial infection may include propionic acid jelly to make the vaginal secretions more acidic—

▲ see page 983

■ see box, page 1071

which discourages bacterial growth. For sexually transmitted infections, both sex partners are treated at the same time to prevent reinfection.

Thinning of the vaginal lining after menopause (atrophic vaginitis) is treated with estrogen replacement therapy.▲ Estrogen can be given by mouth or through a skin patch or applied as a cream directly to the vulva and vagina.

The drugs used to treat vulvitis depend on its cause and are the same as those used to treat vaginitis. Additional measures include wearing loose, absorbent clothing that allows air to circulate, such as cotton or cotton-lined underpants, and keeping the vulva clean. Glycerin soap should be used because many other soaps can irritate the area. Occasionally, placing ice packs against the vulva, sitting in a cool sitz bath, or applying cool compresses may reduce soreness and itching. Corticosteroid creams or ointments, such as those containing hydrocortisone, and antihistamines taken by mouth may also reduce itching that's not caused by an infection. Acyclovir applied as a cream or taken by mouth may reduce symptoms and shorten the course of a herpes infection. Analgesics taken by mouth may help reduce pain.

If chronic vulvitis is caused by poor personal hygiene, instruction in proper hygiene is the first step. A bacterial infection in the area is treated with antibiotics. Skin conditions such as psoriasis may be treated with corticosteroid creams. Substances that may be causing persistent irritation, such as creams, powders, and some brands of condoms, should not be used.

Pelvic Inflammatory Disease

Pelvic inflammatory disease (salpingitis) is an inflammation of the fallopian tubes, usually caused by an infection.

The fallopian tubes extend like arms from the top of the uterus toward each ovary.■

Inflammation of the fallopian tubes occurs mainly in sexually active women. Women using intrauterine devices (IUDs) are especially at risk. An inflammation is usually caused by a bacterial infection, which often enters through the vagina and moves into the uterus and the fallopian tubes. These infections rarely occur before the first menstrual period (menarche), after menopause, or during pregnancy. They are most commonly acquired during sexual intercourse. Less com-

Common Treatments for Vaginal and Vulvar Infections

Type of Infection	Treatment
Candidal (yeast)	Miconazole, clotrimazole, butoconazole, or terconazole (as a cream, vaginal tablets, or suppositories); fluconazole or ketoconazole (by mouth)
Bacterial	Usually, metronidazole or clindamycin (as a vaginal cream) or metronidazole (by mouth); if due to gonococcus, usually ceftriaxone (by intramuscular injection) plus doxycycline (by mouth)
Chlamydial	Doxycycline or azithromycin (by mouth)
Trichomonal	Metronidazole (by mouth)
Viral:	
Human papillomavirus (genital warts)	Trichloroacetic acid (directly on the warts); liquid nitrogen or fluorouracil (directly on the warts) for severe infections
Herpesvirus	Acyclovir (by mouth or as an ointment)

monly, bacteria move into the tubes during a vaginal delivery, a miscarriage, or an abortion.

Less common causes of inflammation include actinomycosis (a bacterial infection), schistosomiasis (a parasitic infection), and tuberculosis. Medical procedures, such as the injection of dye during certain x-ray examinations, may introduce an infection.

Although symptoms may be worse on one side, both tubes are usually infected. The infection can spread into the abdominal cavity, causing peritonitis. The ovaries generally resist infection, unless the infection is severe.

▲ see page 1079

■ see box, page 1070

Symptoms

Symptoms usually begin shortly after a menstrual period. Pain in the lower abdomen becomes increasingly severe and may be accompanied by nausea or vomiting. Particularly at first, many women have only a low fever, mild to moderate abdominal pain, irregular bleeding, and a scant vaginal discharge, making the diagnosis difficult for a doctor. Later, a high fever and a puslike discharge from the vagina are typical, although a chlamydial infection may produce no discharge.

Usually, the infection blocks the fallopian tubes. A blocked tube may become swollen with trapped fluid. Chronic pain, irregular menstrual bleeding, and infertility may result. The infection can spread to surrounding structures, resulting in scarring and abnormal fibrous attachments (adhesions) between organs in the abdomen, causing chronic pain.

Abscesses (collections of pus) may develop in the tubes, ovaries, or pelvis. If antibiotics don't cure the abscesses, surgical drainage may be necessary. If an abscess ruptures—spilling pus into the pelvic cavity—symptoms progress rapidly from severe pain in the lower abdomen to nausea, vomiting, and very low blood pressure (shock). This type of infection may spread to the bloodstream—a condition called sepsis—and can be fatal.▲ A perforated abscess requires emergency surgery.

Diagnosis and Treatment

The symptoms suggest the diagnosis to a doctor. A woman feels considerable pain when the doctor presses on the cervix or surrounding areas during a pelvic examination or palpates the abdomen.

The white blood cell count is usually high. Specimens are generally taken from the cervix, sometimes also from the rectum and throat, and then cultured and examined under a microscope to identify the infective organism. The doctor may perform a culdocentesis, a procedure in which a needle is inserted into the pelvic cavity through the vaginal wall, to obtain a sample of pus. The doctor can also look inside the abdominal cavity with a fiber-optic tube (laparoscope).

Antibiotics are usually given as soon as specimens have been taken to be cultured. Commonly,

a woman is treated at home, but if the infection doesn't improve within 48 hours, she is usually hospitalized. In the hospital, two or more antibiotics are given intravenously to eliminate the infection as quickly and completely as possible. The longer and more severe the inflammation, the higher the risk of infertility and other complications.

Fibroids

A fibroid is a noncancerous growth composed of muscle and fibrous tissue that occurs in the wall of the uterus.

Fibroids occur in at least 20 percent of all women over age 35 and are more common among black women than among white women. The size of fibroids ranges from microscopic to as large as a cantaloupe. The cause is unknown, but fibroids seem to be affected by estrogen levels, often growing larger during pregnancy and shrinking after menopause.

Symptoms

Even when large, fibroids may produce no symptoms. Symptoms depend on the number of fibroids, their size, and their location in the uterus, as well as their status—whether they are growing or degenerating. Symptoms may include heavy or prolonged menstrual bleeding or, less often, bleeding between menstrual periods; pain, pressure, or heaviness in the pelvic area during or between menstrual periods; a need to urinate more frequently; swelling of the abdomen; and rarely, infertility caused by blockage of the fallopian tubes or distortion of the uterine cavity. Menstrual bleeding may be heavy because fibroids increase the surface area of the uterine lining and the amount of tissue shed during menstruation. The heavy bleeding can cause anemia. A fibroid that has previously produced no symptoms occasionally causes problems during pregnancy, such as a miscarriage, early labor, or postpartum hemorrhage (excessive blood loss after delivery).

Diagnosis and Treatment

A doctor can usually make the diagnosis during a pelvic examination. The diagnosis may be confirmed by ultrasound scanning. An endometrial biopsy (removing a tissue sample of the uterine lining for microscopic examination), hysteroscopy (examination of the uterus with a fiber-optic tube), and a Pap test may be performed to make

▲ see page 859

sure the symptoms aren't being caused by other disorders, such as cancer of the uterus.

Most fibroids don't need treatment, but a woman who has them is reexamined every 6 to 12 months. Surgery to remove a fibroid (myomectomy) may be necessary if the fibroid increases in size or produces unacceptable symptoms. A woman may be given hormones for several months before surgery to shrink the fibroid. Generally, surgery is avoided during pregnancy because it can cause a miscarriage and severe blood loss. Removal of the entire uterus (hysterectomy) may be necessary if menstrual bleeding is very severe, symptoms such as pressure or severe pain develop, a fibroid is growing rapidly, or a large fibroid becomes twisted or infected.

Menstrual Disorders

Common menstrual disorders include premenstrual syndrome (PMS) and pain during menstruation (dysmenorrhea). Complex hormonal interactions control the start of menstruation during puberty, the rhythms and duration of cycles during the reproductive years, and the end of menstruation at menopause. Hormonal control of menstruation begins in the hypothalamus (the part of the brain that coordinates and controls hormonal activity) and the pituitary gland, located at the base of the brain, and is ultimately determined by the ovaries.▲ Hormones produced by other glands, such as the adrenal glands, can also affect menstruation.

PREMENSTRUAL SYNDROME
Premenstrual syndrome (PMS, premenstrual dysphoric disorder, late luteal phase dysphoric disorder) is a condition in which a variety of symptoms, including nervousness, irritability, emotional upset, depression, headaches, tissue swelling, and breast tenderness, may occur during the 7 to 14 days before a menstrual period begins.

Premenstrual syndrome may be related to the fluctuations in estrogen and progesterone levels that occur during the menstrual cycle. Estrogen causes fluid retention, which probably explains the weight gain, tissue swelling, breast tenderness, and bloating. Other hormonal and metabolic changes may also be involved.

Symptoms
The type and intensity of symptoms vary, from woman to woman and from month to month in

Menstrual Disorders

Problem	Medical Term
A variety of physical and psychologic symptoms occur before the start of a period	Premenstrual syndrome (PMS)
Periods are painful	Dysmenorrhea
Periods are absent	Amenorrhea
Periods never start	Primary amenorrhea
Periods cease to occur	Secondary amenorrhea
Periods are too long and too heavy	Menorrhagia
Periods are unusually light	Hypomenorrhea
Periods are too frequent	Polymenorrhea
Periods are too infrequent	Oligomenorrhea
Bleeding occurs between periods or is unrelated to periods	Metrorrhagia
Bleeding is heavy and totally irregular in frequency and duration	Menometrorrhagia
Bleeding occurs after menopause	Postmenopausal bleeding

the same woman. The broad range of physical and psychologic symptoms can temporarily upset a woman's life. Women who have epilepsy may have more seizures than usual. Women who have a connective tissue disease, such as systemic lupus erythematosus or rheumatoid arthritis, may have flare-ups at this time.

Usually, symptoms occur a week or two before the menstrual period, last from a few hours to about 14 days, and stop when the next period begins. Women close to menopause may have

▲ see page 1074

Symptoms of Premenstrual Syndrome

Physical Changes
- Backache
- Bloating
- Breast fullness and pain
- Changes in appetite
- Constipation
- Dizziness
- Fainting
- Headaches
- Heaviness or pressure in the pelvic area
- Hot flashes
- Insomnia
- Lack of energy
- Nausea and vomiting
- Severe fatigue
- Skin problems, such as acne and localized scratch dermatitis
- Tissue swelling or joint pain
- Weight gain

Mood Changes
- Agitation
- Anger
- Depression
- Irritability
- Mood swings
- Nervousness

Mental Changes
- Confusion
- Difficulty in concentrating
- Memory loss or forgetfulness

symptoms that persist through and after the menstrual period. The symptoms of premenstrual syndrome are often followed each month by a painful period.

Treatment

Taking combination oral contraceptives, which contain estrogen and progestin, helps reduce the fluctuations in estrogen and progesterone levels. Fluid retention and bloating are often relieved by reducing the intake of salt and taking a mild diuretic, such as spironolactone, just before symp-

toms are expected to begin. Other dietary changes—such as decreasing the amount of sugar, caffeine, and alcohol consumed; eating more carbohydrates; and having more frequent meals—may help. Dietary supplements containing calcium and magnesium may be beneficial. Taking vitamin B supplements, especially B_6 (pyridoxine), may reduce some symptoms, although the benefits of vitamin B_6 have recently been questioned, and a dose that's too high may be harmful (nerve damage has occurred with as little as 200 milligrams a day). Nonsteroidal anti-inflammatory drugs (NSAIDs) may help relieve headaches, pain from uterine cramps, and joint aches.

Nervousness and agitation may be helped by exercise and stress reduction (using meditation or relaxation exercises). Fluoxetine can reduce depression and other symptoms. Buspirone or alprazolam, taken for a short period, may reduce irritability and nervousness and help reduce stress, but drug dependency is a risk of treatment with alprazolam. A woman may be asked to record her symptoms in a diary to help the doctor judge the effectiveness of treatment.

DYSMENORRHEA

Dysmenorrhea is abdominal pain, stemming from uterine cramps, during a menstrual period.

This condition is called primary dysmenorrhea when no underlying cause is found and secondary dysmenorrhea when the cause is identified as a gynecologic disorder. Primary dysmenorrhea is common, possibly affecting more than 50 percent of women; it's severe in about 5 to 15 percent. It usually starts during adolescence and can be severe enough to interfere with everyday activities, resulting in absence from school or work. Primary dysmenorrhea may become less severe with age and after pregnancy. Secondary dysmenorrhea is less common, affecting about one fourth of the women who have dysmenorrhea.

The pain of primary dysmenorrhea is thought to result from contractions of the uterus that occur when the blood supply to its lining (endometrium) is reduced. The pain occurs only during menstrual cycles in which an egg is released. The pain may worsen as endometrial tissue shed during a menstrual period passes through the cervix, particularly when the cervical canal is narrow, as it may be after treatment for cervical disorders. Other factors that may worsen the pain include a uterus that tilts backward (retroverted uterus) instead of forward, lack of exercise, and psychologic or social stress.

One of the most common causes of secondary dysmenorrhea is endometriosis.▲ Others are fibroids and adenomyosis (noncancerous invasion of the muscular wall of the uterus by the uterine lining). Inflammation of the fallopian tubes and abnormal fibrous attachments (adhesions) between organs may cause abdominal pain that's either mild, vague, and continuous or more severe, localized, and short-lived. Either type of pain may be worse during a menstrual period.

Symptoms

Dysmenorrhea causes pain in the lower abdomen, which may extend to the lower back or legs. The pain may consist of cramps that come and go or a dull ache that's constant. Generally, the pain starts shortly before or during the menstrual period, peaks after 24 hours, and subsides after 2 days. Often a woman has a headache, nausea, constipation or diarrhea, and an urge to urinate frequently. Occasionally, vomiting occurs. The premenstrual syndrome symptoms of irritability, nervousness, depression, and abdominal bloating may persist during part or all of the menstrual period. Sometimes clots or pieces of bloody tissue from the lining of the uterus are expelled from the uterus, causing pain.

Treatment

The pain can usually be alleviated most effectively with nonsteroidal anti-inflammatory drugs, such as ibuprofen, naproxen, and mefenamic acid. Such drugs are most effective when begun up to 2 days before a menstrual period and continued through 1 or 2 days of the period. Nausea and vomiting may be alleviated with an antinausea (antiemetic) drug, but these symptoms usually disappear without treatment as cramps subside. Getting enough rest and sleep and exercising regularly may also help reduce symptoms. If pain continues to interfere with normal activity, ovulation can be suppressed with low-dose oral contraceptives containing estrogen and progestin or with long-acting medroxyprogesterone. If these treatments are ineffective, additional tests may be needed, such as laparoscopy (a procedure in which a fiber-optic tube is used to examine the abdominal cavity).

The treatment of secondary dysmenorrhea depends on the cause. A narrow cervical canal can be widened surgically, often providing about 3 to 6 months of relief. When treatment isn't successful and the pain is extreme, severing the nerves to the uterus occasionally helps; complications include injury to other pelvic organs, such as the ureters. Alternatively, hypnosis or acupuncture may be tried.

CHAPTER 235

Absent or Abnormal Uterine Bleeding

Menstruation is normal uterine bleeding. Abnormal uterine bleeding may be caused by physical or hormonal disorders. In amenorrhea, uterine bleeding is absent.

Amenorrhea

Amenorrhea is the absence of menstrual periods—either periods never start (primary amenorrhea) or they cease to occur (secondary amenorrhea).

The absence of menstrual periods is normal only before puberty, during pregnancy, while breastfeeding, and after menopause.

Causes

The absence of periods can result from an abnormality in the brain, pituitary gland, thyroid

---

▲ see page 1092

gland, adrenal glands, ovaries, or virtually any part of the reproductive tract. Normally, the hypothalamus (a small part of the brain just above the pituitary) signals the pituitary gland to release hormones that cause the ovaries to release eggs. In certain disorders, abnormal production of certain pituitary hormones may prevent egg release (ovulation) and may disrupt the sequence of hormonal events that results in periods. High or low levels of thyroid hormones▲ may cause periods to stop, to occur infrequently, or to never start. In Cushing's syndrome,■ excess production of cortisol, a corticosteroid hormone, by the adrenal glands may cause periods to be absent or irregular.

Strenuous exercise can cause periods to stop. Apparently, exercise causes the pituitary to decrease its secretion of the hormones that stimulate the ovaries, so the ovaries produce less estrogen. The absence of periods can also be caused by disorders of the uterus, such as a hydatidiform mole (a tumor of the placenta) and Asherman's syndrome (scarring of the uterine lining resulting from an infection or surgery).

Some women don't undergo puberty; consequently, their periods don't start. Causes include a birth defect in which the uterus or fallopian tubes don't develop normally and chromosomal disorders—for example, Turner's syndrome, in which the cells contain only one X chromosome instead of the usual two.★ A very rare cause is male pseudohermaphroditism, in which a person who is genetically male develops as a female.● A girl who shows no evidence of puberty by age 13, who hasn't had a period by age 16, or who hasn't had a period within 5 years of starting puberty should be examined for possible medical problems.

Symptoms

Symptoms vary, depending on the cause of the absence of periods. For instance, if the cause is failure to undergo puberty, the normal signs of puberty, such as breast development, pubic and underarm hair, and changes in body shape, are absent or only partially present. If the cause is pregnancy, symptoms may include morning sickness and enlargement of the abdomen. If thyroid hormone levels are high, symptoms include a rapid heartbeat, anxiety, and warm, moist skin. Cushing's syndrome produces a moon (round) face, a fat abdomen, and thin arms and legs. Some causes, such as Asherman's syndrome, produce no symptoms other than no periods. Polycystic ovary syndrome produces some masculine characteristics, such as facial hair, and causes periods to be irregular or to stop.

Diagnosis and Treatment

Diagnosis is based on the woman's symptoms and age. During a physical examination, a doctor can determine whether puberty has occurred normally and look for evidence of other causes of amenorrhea. A variety of tests may be performed, depending on the likely cause. For instance, the levels of pituitary hormones, estrogen, thyroid hormones, or cortisol may be measured in a sample of blood. X-rays of the skull may be taken to determine whether the space occupied by the pituitary gland is enlarged because of a pituitary tumor. Computed tomography (CT) or ultrasound scanning may be used to look for a tumor in the ovaries or adrenal glands.

Specific causes are treated whenever possible. For instance, a hormone-producing tumor is removed. However, some causes, such as Turner's syndrome and other genetic abnormalities, can't be cured.

If a girl's periods have never started and all test results are normal, an examination is performed every 3 to 6 months to monitor the progression of puberty. Progesterone and possibly estrogen may be given to start her periods. Estrogen is given to induce the changes of puberty in girls who haven't developed breasts or pubic and underarm hair and who can't develop them spontaneously.

Premature Menopause

Premature (early) menopause is a condition in which the ovaries stop functioning and menstrual periods cease before age 40.

▲ see page 704

■ see page 714

★ see page 1239

● see page 1237

In premature menopause, estrogen levels are low. However, levels of the pituitary hormones that stimulate the ovaries (gonadotropins), especially follicle-stimulating hormone, are high in a vain attempt to stimulate the ovaries. Causes of premature menopause include genetic, usually chromosomal, abnormalities and autoimmune disorders, in which antibodies damage the ovaries. Smoking may cause menopause to begin several months early.

In addition to no longer having periods, a woman with premature menopause often has other symptoms of menopause, such as hot flashes and mood swings.▲

Diagnosis and Treatment

Determining the cause of premature menopause is particularly important for women who want to become pregnant. A physical examination may be helpful. Blood tests may be performed to look for antibodies responsible for damaging the endocrine glands—an example of an autoimmune disease.

For women under age 30, a chromosome analysis is usually performed. If a Y chromosome is present (that is, the person is genetically male), any testicular tissue is surgically removed from the abdomen because the risk of cancer developing in this tissue is 25 percent. Chromosome analysis is probably not needed for women over age 35.

Estrogen replacement therapy can prevent or reverse the symptoms of menopause. However, a woman with premature menopause has less than a 10 percent chance of being able to conceive. She has up to a 50 percent chance of being able to become pregnant by having another woman's eggs (donor eggs) implanted in her uterus after they have been fertilized in the laboratory. Before implantation, artificial menstrual cycles are created by giving the woman estrogen and progesterone, to rejuvenate the lining of the uterus and increase the chances of a successful pregnancy.

Abnormal Uterine Bleeding

Uterine bleeding may be abnormally heavy, light, frequent, or irregular or may occur abnormally after menopause. In about 25 percent of the women who have abnormal bleeding, it's caused by a physical disorder. In the other 75 percent, it's caused by hormonal disorders that affect control of the reproductive system by the hypothalamus and pituitary gland and that are particularly common during the reproductive years; this type of bleeding is called dysfunctional uterine bleeding. Bleeding from the vagina before puberty and after menopause is almost always abnormal.

BLEEDING CAUSED BY A PHYSICAL DISORDER

Bleeding may be caused by an injury to the vulva or vagina, sexual abuse, inflammation of the vagina (for example, from an inserted object), an infection in the uterus, or blood disorders that cause abnormal clotting, such as leukemia or a low platelet count. Other causes include cancer and noncancerous tumors, such as fibroids and cysts in the reproductive tract, as well as adenomyosis (noncancerous invasion of the muscular wall of the uterus by the uterine lining). Tumors of the ovaries occasionally cause bleeding from the vagina, but usually only if they produce hormones. Prolapse of the urethra (a condition in which the channel that transports urine from the bladder to the outside of the body bulges out) may also result in bleeding.

Age is an important factor in determining the likely cause of uterine bleeding. A newborn girl may have some spotting of blood for a few days after birth because of estrogens absorbed before birth from her mother—which is not a cause for concern. Bleeding in childhood may result from puberty that starts very early (precocious puberty).■ Pubic hair and breasts are obvious signs that puberty has begun. Precocious puberty may be caused by certain drugs, brain abnormalities, low thyroid hormone levels, or hormone-producing tumors of the adrenal glands or ovaries. In most cases, however, the cause is unknown.

Bleeding in childhood may also be caused by the overgrowth of glandular tissue in the vagina

---

▲ see page 1078

■ see page 1257

(vaginal adenosis), which most often results from exposure to diethylstilbestrol (DES) taken by the mother before the child's birth.▲ Girls with vaginal adenosis have an increased risk of developing cancer of the vagina and cervix later in life.

During the reproductive years, abnormal bleeding may be caused by birth control methods—such as oral contraceptives, progesterone, or an intrauterine device (IUD)—or by complications of pregnancy—such as placenta previa (an abnormally placed placenta) or an ectopic pregnancy (a pregnancy that develops outside the uterus). Other causes of bleeding include a hydatidiform mole (a tumor of the placenta) and endometriosis. Cancer may cause bleeding in this age group, but not commonly.

The most serious cause of bleeding from the vagina after menopause is cancer, such as cancer of the uterine lining, the cervix, or the vagina. The most common noncancerous causes of bleeding are thinning of the vaginal wall (atrophic vaginitis), thinning or thickening of the uterine lining, and growths on the uterine lining (uterine polyps).

Diagnosis and Treatment

The symptoms and a physical examination help a doctor determine what other procedures are needed for diagnosis. Treatment varies, depending on the cause.

If a doctor suspects vaginal adenosis or cancer in a girl, a sample of cells is removed from the vagina and examined under a microscope. Usually, a girl who has vaginal adenosis doesn't need to be treated—unless cancer is found—but she is reexamined at regular intervals for signs of cancer.

A woman who has abnormal bleeding from the vagina, particularly after menopause, is examined to determine whether she has cancer.

Uterine polyps, fibroids, and cancers may be surgically removed. A postmenopausal woman who has irregular bleeding while taking estrogen may have more regular menstrual periods if a progestin is also taken for about 10 days of each

---

▲ see page 1169

cycle. If a woman doesn't take a progestin with estrogen, she has an increased risk of developing cancer of the uterine lining. If the uterine lining is thickened and contains abnormal cells, which may be precancerous, one common treatment is surgical removal of the uterus (hysterectomy).

DYSFUNCTIONAL UTERINE BLEEDING

Dysfunctional uterine bleeding is abnormal bleeding resulting from hormonal changes, rather than from an injury, inflammation, pregnancy, or a tumor.

Dysfunctional uterine bleeding occurs most commonly at the beginning and end of the reproductive years: 20 percent of cases occur in adolescent girls, and more than 50 percent occur in women over age 45. Most abnormal uterine bleeding is the dysfunctional type, but this diagnosis is made only when all other possibilities have been excluded.

Causes and Symptoms

Dysfunctional uterine bleeding commonly results from sustained levels of estrogen, which cause the uterine lining to thicken. The lining is then shed incompletely and irregularly, causing bleeding. For example, in polycystic ovary syndrome, the overproduction of luteinizing hormone may cause the ovaries to produce large amounts of androgens—some of which are converted to estrogen—rather than to release an egg. Over time, estrogen without sufficient progesterone to counteract its effects can result in abnormal uterine bleeding.

Bleeding is irregular, prolonged, and sometimes heavy. A blood sample is taken and analyzed to determine the extent of the blood loss.

Diagnosis and Treatment

The diagnosis of dysfunctional uterine bleeding is made when no other cause can be found. A biopsy (removal of a tissue sample for examination under a microscope) of the uterine lining is performed before drug treatment is started if a woman is age 35 or older, has polycystic ovary syndrome, or is substantially overweight and hasn't had children. A biopsy is performed because such women have an increased risk of developing cancer of the uterine lining.

Treatment depends on the woman's age, the condition of the uterine lining, and the woman's plans regarding pregnancy.

When the uterine lining is thickened and contains abnormal cells (particularly if a woman is over 35 and doesn't want to become pregnant), often the uterus is removed surgically (hysterectomy), because the abnormal cells may be precancerous.

When the uterine lining is thickened but contains normal cells, heavy bleeding may be treated with high doses of an oral contraceptive containing estrogen and a progestin or with estrogen alone, usually given intravenously, then followed by a progestin given by mouth. Bleeding generally stops in 12 to 24 hours. Low doses of the oral contraceptive may then be given in the usual manner for at least 3 months. Women who have lighter bleeding may be given low doses from the start.

When treatment with oral contraceptives or estrogen is inappropriate,▲ a progestin alone may be given by mouth for 10 to 14 days each month.

If a woman doesn't respond to treatment with these hormones, dilatation and curettage (D and C), in which tissue from the uterine lining is removed by scraping, is usually needed. If she wants to become pregnant, clomiphene may be given by mouth to induce egg release.

CHAPTER 236

Polycystic Ovary Syndrome

Polycystic ovary syndrome (Stein-Leventhal syndrome) is a disorder in which the ovaries are enlarged and contain many fluid-filled sacs (cysts), and levels of male hormones (androgens) may be high, sometimes producing masculine characteristics.

In this syndrome, the pituitary gland commonly secretes large amounts of luteinizing hormone. The excess luteinizing hormone increases the production of androgens, and high levels of androgens sometimes cause a woman to develop such characteristics as acne and coarse hair. If the disorder isn't treated, some of the androgens may be converted to estrogens, and the chronically high levels of estrogens may increase the risk of cancer of the uterine lining (endometrial cancer).

Symptoms and Diagnosis

Symptoms typically develop during puberty, when menstrual periods may or may not begin. Symptoms may include obesity and an increase in body hair growing in a male pattern, such as on the chest and face. Alternatively, irregular, profuse vaginal bleeding may occur, with no increase in weight or body hair.

Often, the diagnosis is made on the basis of the symptoms. Blood levels of luteinizing hormone and male hormones are measured, and ultrasound scanning may be used to view the ovaries. A variety of procedures are used to determine whether the male hormones are being produced by a tumor.

Treatment

No ideal treatment is available. The choice of treatment depends on the type and severity of symptoms, the woman's age, and her plans regarding pregnancy.

A woman who doesn't have increased body hair may be given a synthetic progestin (a progesterone-like drug) or oral contraceptives unless she wants to become pregnant, has reached menopause, or has other significant risk factors for heart or blood vessel disease. A synthetic progestin may also be given to reduce the risk of endometrial cancer from the high estrogen levels. Often, a sample of the uterine lining is removed and examined under a microscope before drug treatment is started to make sure no cancer is present.

A woman who has increased body hair can use a hair removal method, such as electrolysis,

▲ see box, page 1121

plucking, waxing, or hair-removing liquids or creams (depilatories), or bleaching. No drug treatment for removing excess hair is ideal or completely effective. Oral contraceptives may be tried, although they must be taken for several months before any effect, which is often slight, can be seen.

Spironolactone, a drug that blocks the production and action of male hormones, can be effective in reducing unwanted body hair. Side effects include increased urine production, low blood pressure (sometimes to the point of fainting) when sitting up or standing quickly, painful breasts, and irregular vaginal bleeding. Because spironolactone may not be safe for a developing fetus, any sexually active woman taking the drug should use effective birth control methods.

If a woman who has polycystic ovary syndrome wants to become pregnant, she may be given clomiphene, a drug that stimulates the ovaries to release eggs. If clomiphene isn't effective, a variety of hormones may be tried; these include follicle-stimulating hormone and gonadotropin-releasing hormone, which stimulates the release of follicle-stimulating hormone. If drugs aren't effective, the woman may consider having surgery to remove a wedge of ovary (wedge resection) or to cauterize the ovarian cysts (destroy them with an electric current). Although these treatments may induce ovulation for a period of time, surgical procedures are generally considered last because scar tissue can form and may reduce the woman's ability to become pregnant.

CHAPTER 237

Endometriosis

Endometriosis is a disease in which patches of endometrial tissue, which normally is found only in the uterine lining (endometrium), grow outside the uterus.

Usually, endometriosis is confined to the lining of the abdominal cavity or the surface of abdominal organs. The misplaced endometrial tissue (endometrial implant) commonly adheres to the ovaries and the ligaments that support the uterus. Less commonly, it adheres to the outer surface of the small and large intestines, the ureters (tubes leading from the kidneys to the bladder), the bladder, the vagina, surgical scars in the abdomen, or the lining of the chest cavity. Rarely, endometrial tissue is found in the lungs.

Because the misplaced endometrial tissue responds to the same hormones that the uterus responds to, it may bleed during the menstrual period, often causing cramps, pain, irritation, and the formation of scar tissue. As the disease progresses, adhesions (fibrous bands that connect normally unconnected structures) may form. The misplaced endometrial tissue and adhesions can block or interfere with the functioning of organs. Rarely, adhesions block the intestine.

Endometriosis can run in families and is more common in first-degree relatives (mother, sister, daughter) of women who have the disease than in other women. Other factors that increase the risk of endometriosis include giving birth for the first time after age 30, being of Caucasian descent, and having an abnormal uterus.

Endometriosis is estimated to occur in about 10 to 15 percent of menstruating women between the ages of 25 and 44; it can also occur in teenagers. Exactly how many women have this disease is unknown because it usually can be diagnosed only by direct viewing, typically during surgery. As many as 25 to 50 percent of infertile women may have endometriosis, which can physically interfere with conception. Severe endometriosis may cause infertility by blocking the egg's passage from the ovary into the uterus. Mild endometriosis also may cause infertility, but how it does so is less clear.

Causes and Symptoms

The causes of endometriosis haven't been established. Cells from the lining of the uterus may somehow move to places outside the uterus, where they continue to grow. This movement could take place if small pieces of the uterine lining, shed during menstruation, flow backward through the fallopian tubes toward the ovaries into the abdominal cavity, rather than with the menstrual flow through the vagina and outside the body.

Endometriosis can cause pain in the lower abdomen and pelvic area; menstrual irregularities, such as spotting before normal periods; and infertility. Some women with severe endometriosis have no symptoms, whereas some with minimal disease have incapacitating pain. Often, a woman doesn't have menstrual pain from endometriosis until she's had the disease for several years. Some women have pain during sexual intercourse (dyspareunia) before or during menstruation.

Endometrial tissue attached to the large intestine or bladder may cause abdominal swelling, pain during bowel movements, rectal bleeding during menstruation, or lower abdominal pain during urination. Endometrial tissue attached to an ovary or a nearby structure can form a blood-filled mass (endometrioma). Occasionally, an endometrioma ruptures or leaks, causing sudden, sharp abdominal pain.

Diagnosis

A doctor may suspect endometriosis in a woman who has the typical symptoms or unexplained infertility. A physical examination may yield normal findings, but occasionally a woman may feel pain during the examination or the doctor may feel a mass of tissue behind the uterus or near the ovaries. Rarely, endometrial tissue is found in the vulva, cervix, vagina, navel (umbilicus), or surgical scars.

The diagnosis can usually be made only if patches of endometrial tissue are seen. Generally, a doctor inspects the abdominal cavity through a fiber-optic viewing tube (a laparoscope) inserted into the abdominal cavity through a small incision just below the navel. In some cases, endometriosis can't be recognized when viewed, and the diagnosis can only be made by a biopsy (removal of a small sample of tissue for microscopic examination at a laboratory), usually performed during the endoscopy.

Other procedures, such as ultrasound scans, barium enemas with x-ray, computed tomography (CT), and magnetic resonance imaging (MRI),

Endometriosis: Misplaced Tissue

Small pieces of endometrial tissue (shown here as reddish patches) may travel backward from the uterus through the fallopian tubes and move into the abdominal cavity. This tissue may adhere to the ovaries, ligaments supporting the uterus, small and large intestines, ureters, bladder, vagina, surgical scars, or lining of the chest cavity.

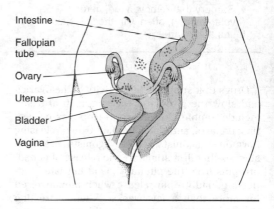

- Intestine
- Fallopian tube
- Ovary
- Uterus
- Bladder
- Vagina

may be used to determine the extent of the disease and follow its course, but their usefulness in diagnosis is limited. Certain blood tests that detect markers for endometriosis, such as CA-125 and antibodies to endometrial tissue, may also help a doctor follow the course of endometriosis. However, because these markers may be elevated in several other diseases, they aren't useful in making the diagnosis.

The American Fertility Society has established criteria for classifying endometriosis based on where the endometrial tissue is located, whether it is on or buried beneath an organ's surface, and whether filmy or dense adhesions are found. Considering all these factors, a doctor may classify the disease as minimal, mild, moderate, or severe. Tests also may be performed to determine if the endometriosis is affecting the woman's fertility.

Treatment

Treatment depends on a woman's symptoms, pregnancy plans, and age, as well as the extent of the disease.

Treatment Choices in Endometriosis

- Drugs that suppress the activity of the ovaries and slow the growth of endometrial tissue

- Surgery that removes as much of the misplaced endometrial tissue as possible

- Combination of drugs and surgery

- Surgery that removes the uterus (hysterectomy), often with the fallopian tubes and ovaries

Drugs Commonly Used to Treat Endometriosis

Drug	Side Effects
Combination estrogen-progestin oral contraceptives	Abdominal swelling, breast tenderness, increased appetite, ankle swelling, nausea, bleeding between periods, deep vein thrombosis
Progestins	Bleeding between periods, mood swings, depression, atrophic vaginitis
Danazol	Weight gain, acne, lowered voice, hair growth, hot flashes, vaginal dryness, ankle swelling, muscle cramps, bleeding between periods, decreased breast size, mood swings, liver malfunction, carpal tunnel syndrome, adverse effects on lipids
GnRH agonists	Hot flashes, vaginal dryness, calcium loss from bone, mood swings

Drugs that suppress the activity of the ovaries and slow the growth of the endometrial tissue include combination oral contraceptives, progestins, danazol, and GnRH (gonadotropin-releasing hormone) agonists. GnRH agonists are substances that first stimulate the release of gonadotropins from the pituitary gland but later suppress gonadotropin release when administered for more than a few weeks. Whether treating women who have minimal or mild endometriosis improves pregnancy rates isn't clear; however, treating women who have more severe disease with drugs or surgery results in pregnancy rates ranging from 40 to 60 percent. Drug treatment doesn't cure endometriosis; the disease usually returns after treatment is stopped.

If a woman has moderate to severe endometriosis, surgery may be necessary. A doctor removes as much misplaced endometrial tissue as possible, generally while preserving the woman's ability to have children. Often, the tissue is removed during laparoscopy when the diagnosis is made. Surgery is usually necessary for patches of endometrial tissue larger than $1\frac{1}{2}$ to 2 inches in diameter, for significant adhesions in the lower abdomen or pelvis, and for endometrial tissue that obstructs one or both fallopian tubes or that's causing extreme lower abdominal or pelvic pain unrelieved by drugs. Sometimes electrocautery (a device that uses an electrical current to produce heat) or a laser (a device that concen-

trates light into an intense beam to produce heat) is used to remove endometrial tissue. However, surgical removal is only a temporary measure; endometriosis recurs in most women. After endometrial tissue has been removed, pregnancy rates range from 40 to 70 percent, depending on the severity of the disease; drug treatment may improve these rates.

Oral contraceptives may slow disease progression after drug treatment or surgical removal of endometrial tissue. However, only surgical removal of both ovaries prevents endometriosis from recurring.

The ovaries and uterus are removed only in women who have lower abdominal or pelvic pain unrelieved by drugs and who aren't planning to become pregnant. After the ovaries and uterus are removed, estrogen replacement therapy is started, because this surgery has the same effects as menopause.▲ This therapy is started either immediately after surgery or, if a lot of endometrial tissue remains, after a delay of 4 to 6 months.

The delay allows the endometrial tissue, which would be stimulated by estrogen replacement therapy, to disappear. During the delay, drugs to suppress endometriosis may be needed.

CHAPTER 238

Breast Disorders

Breast disorders may be noncancerous (benign) or cancerous (malignant). Noncancerous disorders include breast pain, cysts, fibrocystic breast disease, fibrous lumps, nipple discharge, and breast infection. Cancerous disorders include several types of breast cancer and Paget's disease of the nipple. Cystosarcoma phyllodes may or may not be cancerous.

Breast Pain

Women may experience breast pain (mastalgia) or tenderness during or just before their menstrual periods, probably because of the hormonal changes that trigger menstruation. In most cases, breast pain is not a symptom of cancer. Sometimes, cysts in the breasts cause pain. Certain substances in foods or beverages (for example, methylxanthines in coffee) have been suspected of causing breast pain, but avoiding these substances doesn't seem to reduce the pain.

For most women, breast pain isn't severe and goes away on its own after months or years. Severe pain, which is rare, may be treated with drugs. Danazol, a very low potency synthetic hormone related to testosterone, and tamoxifen, a drug that blocks the action of estrogen, may relieve severe breast pain.

Cysts

Cysts are fluid-filled sacs that may develop in the breast and can easily be felt.

The cause of breast cysts is unknown, although injury may be involved. Cysts sometimes cause breast pain. To relieve the pain, a doctor may drain fluid from the cyst with a thin needle. The

fluid is sent to a laboratory to be examined under a microscope. The doctor observes the color and amount of fluid and notes whether the cyst disappears after the fluid has been drained. If the fluid is bloody, brown, or cloudy or if the cyst reappears within 12 weeks after it's drained, the entire cyst is removed surgically because cancer in the cyst wall, although rare, is possible.

Fibrocystic Breast Disease

Fibrocystic breast disease is a common condition in which breast pain, cysts, and noncancerous lumpiness occur together.

Although called a disease, *this condition is not a disease.* Most women have some general lumpiness in the breasts, usually in the upper, outer area. Like breast pain and breast cysts, this kind of lumpiness is very common. Most women with breast cysts do not have an increased risk of developing breast cancer.■ Treatment of the cysts may be all that is needed.

Fibrous Breast Lumps

Fibrous breast lumps (fibroadenomas) are small, noncancerous, solid lumps composed of fibrous and glandular tissue.

These lumps usually appear in young women, often in teenagers. The lumps are easy to move, with clearly defined edges that can be felt during

---

▲ see page 1077

■ see box, page 1098

Inside the Breast

The female breast is composed of milk glands surrounded by fatty tissue and some connective tissue. Milk secreted by the glands flows through ducts to the nipple. Around the nipple is an area of pigmented skin called the areola.

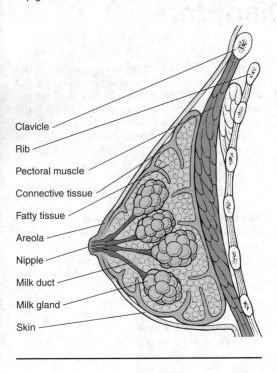

Clavicle

Rib

Pectoral muscle

Connective tissue

Fatty tissue

Areola

Nipple

Milk duct

Milk gland

Skin

self-examination, and may feel like small, slippery marbles. They have a rubbery hardness because they contain collagen (a tough, fibrous protein found in cartilage, bones, tendons, and skin).

Usually, the lumps can be removed surgically with the patient under local anesthesia, but they often recur. After several lumps have been removed and found to be noncancerous, a woman

▲ see page 1107

■ see page 702

and her doctor may decide against removing lumps that recur.

Other types of noncancerous, solid breast lumps include a hardening of glandular tissue (sclerosing adenosis) and scar tissue that replaces injured fatty tissue (fat necrosis). These lumps can be diagnosed only by removing and examining a tissue sample (biopsy).

Nipple Discharge

Fluid leaking from the nipple isn't necessarily abnormal, even in postmenopausal women. Cancer is found in fewer than 10 percent of the women who have a nipple discharge.▲ Nonetheless, a nipple discharge should be evaluated by a doctor.

A bloody discharge is most commonly caused by a small noncancerous lump in a milk duct (intraductal papilloma). Some of these lumps can be felt; others can be located by mammography. If a woman is concerned about the discharge, the lump usually can be removed in a doctor's office, using local anesthetics. A milky discharge (galactorrhea) in a woman who hasn't just given birth often indicates a hormonal problem.■

Breast Infection and Abscess

Breast infections (mastitis) are rare, except around the time of childbirth or after an injury. Occasionally, breast cancer may produce symptoms similar to those of a breast infection.

An infected breast usually appears red and swollen and feels warm and tender. It's treated with antibiotics.

A breast abscess, which is more rare, is a collection of pus in the breast. An abscess may develop if a breast infection isn't treated. It is treated with antibiotics and usually drained surgically.

Breast Cancer

Breast cancer is classified by the kind of tissue in which it starts and by the extent of its spread. Cancer may start in the milk glands, milk ducts, fatty tissue, or connective tissue. Different types of breast cancers progress differently. Generalizations about particular types are based on similarities in how they're discovered, how they progress, and how they're treated. Some grow very

What Are the Risks of Developing or Dying of Breast Cancer?

Age (years)	Risk (%)					
	In 10 Years		In 20 Years		In 30 Years	
	Develop	Die	Develop	Die	Develop	Die
30	0.4	0.1	2.0	0.6	4.3	1.2
40	1.6	0.5	3.9	1.1	7.1	2.0
50	2.4	0.7	5.7	1.6	9.0	2.6
60	3.6	1.0	7.1	2.0	9.1	2.6
70	4.1	1.2	6.5	1.9	7.1	2.0

Based on information from Feuer EJ et al.: "The lifetime risk of developing breast cancer." *Journal of the National Cancer Institute* 85(11):892–897, 1993.

slowly and spread to other parts of the body (metastasize) only after they become very large. Others are more aggressive, growing and spreading quickly. However, the same type of cancer may progress differently in different women. *Only a doctor who has examined a woman and taken her medical history can discuss specific aspects of breast cancer as they apply to her.*

In situ carcinoma, which means cancer in place, is an early cancer that hasn't invaded or spread beyond its point of origin. In situ carcinoma accounts for more than 15 percent of all breast cancers diagnosed in the United States.

About 90 percent of all breast cancers start in the milk ducts or milk glands. **Ductal carcinoma in situ** starts in the walls of milk ducts. It can develop before or after menopause. This type of cancer occasionally can be felt as a lump and may appear as tiny specks of calcium deposits (microcalcifications) on mammograms. Ductal carcinoma in situ is often detected by mammography before it's large enough to be felt. It's usually confined to a specific area of the breast and can be totally removed by surgery. If only the ductal carcinoma in situ is removed, about 25 to 35 percent of women develop invasive cancer, usually in the same breast.

Lobular carcinoma in situ, which starts in the milk glands, usually develops before menopause. This type of cancer, which can't be felt or seen on mammograms, is usually found incidentally on mammography during investigation of a lump or other abnormality that is not lobular carcinoma in situ. Between 25 and 30 percent of women who have it develop invasive breast cancer eventually—sometimes after as long as 40 years—in the same or opposite breast or in both breasts.

Invasive breast cancers, which can spread to and destroy other tissues, may be localized (confined to the breast) or metastatic (spread to other parts of the body). About 80 percent of invasive breast cancers are ductal and about 10 percent are lobular. The prognosis for ductal and lobular invasive cancers is similar. Other, less common types of cancer, such as medullary carcinoma and tubular carcinoma (which start in milk glands), have a somewhat better prognosis.

Risk Factors

Some of the fear about breast cancer is based on misinformation and misunderstanding concerning its risks. For instance, the statement, "One out of every eight women will get breast

Risk Factors for Breast Cancer

Age
Increasing age is an important risk factor. About 60 percent of breast cancers occur in women over age 60. Risk is greatest after age 75.

Previous breast cancer
At highest risk are women who have had in situ or invasive breast cancer. After the diseased breast is removed, the risk of developing cancer in the remaining breast is about 0.5 to 1.0 percent each year.

Family history of breast cancer
Breast cancer in a first-degree relative (mother, sister, daughter) increases a woman's risk by two to three times, but breast cancer in more distant relatives (grandmother, aunt, cousin) increases the risk only slightly. Even a woman whose close relatives had breast cancer has no more than a 30 percent chance of developing breast cancer before age 75.

Breast cancer gene
Recently, two separate genes for breast cancer have been identified in two separate small groups of women. If a woman has one of these genes, her chances of developing breast cancer are very high. However, if such a woman develops breast cancer, her chances of dying of breast cancer are not necessarily greater than those of any other woman with breast cancer. Women likely to have one of these genes are those who have a strong family history of the disease; usually, several women in each of three generations have had breast cancer. For this reason, routinely screening women for these genes doesn't appear necessary, except for women who have an unusual family history. The incidence of ovarian cancer is also increased in families with one of the breast cancer genes.

Previous noncancerous breast disease
Having had noncancerous breast disease seems to increase risk only in women who have an increased number of milk ducts. Even in these women, the risk is moderate unless abnormal tissue structure (atypical hyperplasia) is found during a biopsy or the woman has a family history of breast cancer.

First menstruation before age 12, menopause after age 55, first pregnancy after age 30, or no pregnancies
The relationship between the first three factors and risk is continuous. For example, the earlier menstruation begins, the greater the risk. The risk of developing breast cancer is two to four times greater for women who first menstruated before age 12 than for those who first menstruated after age 14. However, these factors seem to have a very small effect on breast cancer risk.

Prolonged use of oral contraceptives or estrogen replacement therapy
Most studies don't show any relationship between the use of oral contraceptives and the later development of breast cancer, except possibly for women who took them for many years. After menopause, taking estrogen replacement therapy for 10 to 20 years may slightly increase risk. Taking hormone replacement therapy that combines estrogen with progestin may increase the risk, but this isn't certain.

Obesity after menopause
Risk is somewhat higher in obese postmenopausal women, but there is no proof that a particular diet—for example, one high in fat—contributes to the development of breast cancer. Some studies suggest that obese women who are still menstruating actually are less likely to develop breast cancer.

cancer," is misleading. That figure is an estimate based on women from birth to 95 years of age and older; it means that theoretically, one out of every eight women who live beyond age 95 will develop breast cancer. However, the risk is much lower for younger women. A 40-year-old woman has a 1 in 1,200 chance of developing the disease during the next year. Even this figure can be misleading, because it includes all women. Most women have an even smaller risk, but some have a greater risk.

Women who have more risk factors for breast cancer are more likely to develop it, but they can take defensive measures, such as regular breast examinations. The only measure of proven value for reducing the risk of dying of breast cancer is regular mammograms after age 50. However, recent research suggests that regular exercise, particularly during adolescence and young adulthood, and possibly weight control may reduce the risk of developing breast cancer.

Symptoms

Usually, breast pain without a lump is not a sign of breast cancer, although about 10 percent of women who have this cancer have pain without a lump.

At first, a woman who has breast cancer usually has no symptoms. Most commonly, the first symptom is a lump, which usually feels distinctly different from the surrounding breast tissue. In more than 80 percent of breast cancer cases, the woman discovers the lump herself. Scattered, lumpy changes in the breast, especially the upper, outer region, usually aren't cancerous. A firmer, distinctive thickening that appears in one breast but not the other may be a sign of cancer.

In the early stages, the lump may move freely beneath the skin when it's pushed with the fingers. In more advanced stages, the lump usually adheres to the chest wall or the skin over it. In these cases, the lump can't be moved at all or it can't be moved separately from the skin over it. In advanced cancer, swollen bumps or festering sores may develop on the skin. Sometimes, the skin over the lump is dimpled and leathery and looks like the skin of an orange except for the color.

In **inflammatory breast cancer,** a particularly serious but uncommon type of cancer, the breast looks as if it's infected; it's warm, red, and swollen. Often, no lump can be felt in the breast.

Screening

Because breast cancer rarely produces symptoms in its early stages, screening is especially important. Finding the disease early increases the likelihood of successful treatment.

Routine self-examination can allow a woman to detect lumps at an early stage. Although it hasn't yet been proven to reduce the death rate from breast cancer or to detect as many early cancers as does routine screening by mammography,

---

Symptoms That May Indicate Breast Cancer

These symptoms don't necessarily mean that a woman has breast cancer; however, if a woman has them, she should see her doctor.

- A lump that feels distinctly different from other breast tissue or that doesn't go away

- Swelling that doesn't go away

- Puckering or dimpling of the skin

- Scaly skin around the nipple

- Changes in the shape of the breast

- Changes in the nipple, such as turning inward

- Discharge from the nipple, especially if bloody

---

self-examination usually allows for detection of tumors smaller than those found by a doctor or nurse, because it's repeated regularly and a woman becomes more familiar with her breasts. These tumors usually have a better prognosis and are more easily treated with breast-conserving surgery.

A breast examination is a routine part of any physical examination. A doctor inspects the breasts for irregularities, dimpling, tightened skin, lumps, and a discharge. The doctor feels (palpates) each breast with a flat hand and checks for enlarged lymph nodes in the underarm—the area most breast cancers invade first—and also above the collarbone. Normal lymph nodes can't be felt through the skin, so those that can be felt are considered enlarged. However, noncancerous conditions also can cause lymph nodes to enlarge.

Mammography (a test that uses low-level x-rays to find abnormal areas in the breast) is one of the best ways to detect breast cancer early. Mammography is designed to be sensitive enough to detect the *possibility* of a cancer at an early stage. For this reason, the tests may indicate cancer when none is present (false-positive results), and

How to Perform a Breast Self-examination

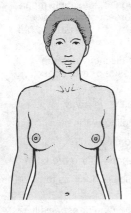

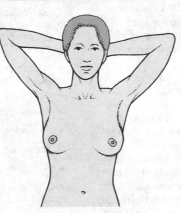

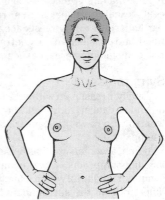

1. While standing in front of a mirror, look at the breasts. The breasts normally differ slightly in size. Look for changes in the size difference between the breasts and changes in the nipple, such as turning inward (inverted nipple) or a discharge. Look for puckering or dimpling.

2. Watching closely in the mirror, clasp the hands behind the head, and press them against the head. This position helps make subtle changes caused by cancer more noticeable. Look for changes in the shape and contour of the breasts, especially the lower part of the breast.

3. Place the hands firmly on the hips and bend slightly toward the mirror, pressing the shoulders and elbows forward. Again, look for changes in shape and contour.

Many women perform the next part of the examination in the shower because the hand moves easily over wet, slippery skin.

usually, more specific follow-up tests are needed to confirm the results.

Having mammograms at intervals of 1 to 2 years can reduce breast cancer deaths by 25 to 35 percent in women aged 50 and over who have no symptoms. No study thus far has shown that having mammograms regularly will reduce breast cancer deaths in women under age 50. However, the evidence may be lacking because breast cancer is uncommon in younger women, so showing a benefit is more difficult. Current evidence is compatible with—but does not prove—the proposition that younger women will benefit from hav-

ing mammograms. For this reason, many authorities recommend that women have mammograms regularly starting at age 40. The American Cancer Society recommends having the first mammogram at age 40. Although a lump is sometimes found, this mammogram also provides a permanent record for comparison with subsequent mammograms. The American Cancer Society also recommends having mammograms at 1- to 2-year intervals between ages 40 and 49 and yearly beginning at age 50. In studies of women without symptoms, mammography detected about 40 percent of cancers missed during physical ex-

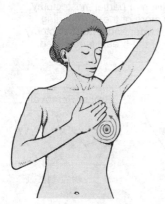

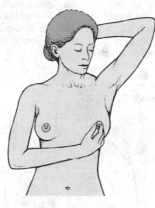

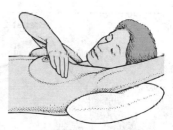

4. Raise the left arm. Using three or four fingers of the right hand, probe the left breast thoroughly with the flat part of the fingers. Moving the fingers in small circles around the breast, begin at the outer edge and gradually move in toward the nipple. Press gently but firmly, feeling for any unusual lump or mass under the skin. Be sure to check the whole breast. Also, carefully probe the area between the breast and underarm, including the underarm, for lumps.

5. Squeeze the left nipple gently and look for a discharge. (See a doctor if a discharge appears at any time of the month, regardless of whether it happens during a breast self-examination.)

Repeat steps 4 and 5 for the right breast, raising the right arm and using the left hand.

6. Lie flat on the back with a pillow or folded towel under the left shoulder and the left arm overhead. This position flattens the breast and makes it easier to examine. Repeat for the right breast. Be sure to examine both breasts.

A woman should repeat this procedure at the same time each month. For menstruating women, 2 or 3 days after their period ends is a good time because the breasts are less likely to be tender or swollen. Postmenopausal women may choose any day of the month that's easy to remember, such as the first.

Adapted from a publication of the National Cancer Institute.

amination. However, mammography isn't infallible and may miss up to 15 percent of breast cancers. If a change that may be cancerous is found, a doctor performs a biopsy, in which a small piece of the lump is removed surgically and examined under a microscope.

Ultrasound scanning (a test that uses high-frequency sound waves) isn't part of routine screening for breast cancer. After a lump is found, ultrasound scanning is sometimes used to help distinguish between a fluid-filled sac (cyst) in the breast and a solid lump. This distinction is important because cysts usually aren't treated if a

woman has no other symptoms, but a solid lump usually requires a biopsy.

Thermography (a test that detects differences in temperature, which cancer sometimes causes) isn't useful to detect or monitor breast cancers because it often misses cancers (false-negative results) or indicates cancer when none is present (false-positive results).

Diagnosis

When a lump that could be cancerous is found, a biopsy is performed—by removing some cells from the lump through a needle attached to a

Surgery for Breast Cancer

Breast cancer may be treated with a variety of surgical options, including removing the whole breast (mastectomy) or removing only the tumor and an area of normal tissue surrounding it (breast-conserving surgery). Types of breast-conserving surgery include lumpectomy, in which a small amount of surrounding normal tissue is removed; wide excision or partial mastectomy, in which somewhat more of the surrounding normal tissue is removed; and quadrantectomy, in which one fourth of the breast is removed.

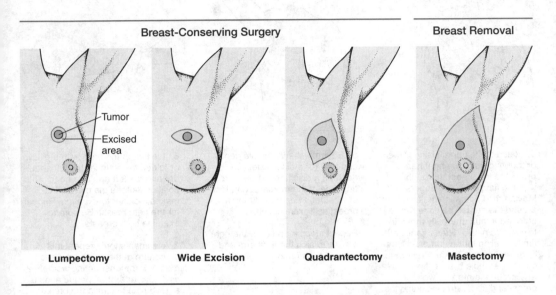

Breast-Conserving Surgery   **Breast Removal**

Tumor
Excised area

Lumpectomy   **Wide Excision**   **Quadrantectomy**   **Mastectomy**

syringe (aspiration biopsy), by removing a small piece of tissue (incisional biopsy), or by removing the entire lump (excisional biopsy). Most women don't need to be hospitalized, and usually only local anesthetics are needed.

If cancer cells are found, more tests are performed because treatment depends on the characteristics of the cancer. One test determines whether the cancer has estrogen or progesterone receptors. Cancer that has estrogen receptors grows more slowly than cancer that doesn't have them, and its treatment with hormone-blocking drugs can be beneficial. This type of cancer is more common among postmenopausal women than among younger women.

A pathologist examines the biopsy samples under the microscope to determine the cancer's potential for rapid spread. Cancers composed of more primitive (undifferentiated) cells or a large number of dividing cells tend to be more serious.

Keeping the cancer's characteristics in mind, the doctor thoroughly examines the woman to determine whether the cancer has spread to the lymph nodes, skin, liver, or elsewhere in the body. If the lymph nodes in the underarm or above the collarbone are matted together or attached to the skin, the cancer probably can't be successfully removed by surgery. A chest x-ray is taken to look for cancer, and blood tests are performed to evaluate liver function and to determine if the cancer has spread. If the tumor is large or the lymph nodes are enlarged, a bone scan (x-ray study of bones throughout the body) may be performed. The doctor keeps these scans to compare with others taken later in the course of the disease.

Treatment

Usually, treatment begins after the woman's condition has been thoroughly evaluated, about

How Lymph Node Status Influences Survival

Lymph Node Status	Chances of Surviving 10 Years	Chances of Surviving 10 Years Without Recurrence
No cancer	Better than 80%	Better than 70%
Cancer in one to three nodes	About 40 to 50%	About 25 to 40%
Cancer in four or more nodes	About 25 to 40%	About 15 to 35%

a week or more after the biopsy. Treatment is complex because the different types of breast cancer differ greatly in their growth rates, tendency to spread (metastasize), and response to treatment. Treatment includes surgery, radiation therapy, chemotherapy, and hormone-blocking drugs. Radiation therapy kills cancer cells at the site from which the tumor was removed and the surrounding area, including nearby lymph nodes. Chemotherapy (combinations of drugs that kill rapidly multiplying cells or suppress their multiplication) and hormone-blocking drugs (drugs that interfere with actions of hormones that support cancer cell growth) are intended to suppress cancer cell growth throughout the body.▲ Often, a woman receives a combination of these treatments.

Because much is still unknown about breast cancer and no single treatment works all the time, doctors may have different opinions about the most appropriate treatment. The preferences of a woman and of her doctor affect treatment decisions. A woman with breast cancer has the right to a clear explanation of what's known about the disease and what's still unknown, as well as a complete description of treatment options. Then, a woman can accept or reject the options offered.

Doctors are continually looking for ways to improve the prognosis of their patients. That is why women who have breast cancer often are asked to participate in research studies that investigate whether a new combination of treatments can improve survival rates or quality of life.

Treatment of Localized Breast Cancer

For cancers that seem to be confined to the breast (localized), treatment almost always includes surgery, performed shortly after diagno-

sis, to remove as much of the tumor as possible. A variety of surgical options are available. The main decision is whether to remove the whole breast (mastectomy) or to remove only the tumor and an area of normal tissue surrounding it (breast-conserving surgery).

Breast-conserving surgery, which leaves as much of the breast intact as possible, can involve removal of the tumor with a small amount of surrounding normal tissue **(lumpectomy),** removal of the tumor and somewhat more surrounding normal tissue **(wide excision or partial mastectomy),** or removal of one fourth of the breast **(quadrantectomy).** Removal of the tumor and some normal tissue gives the best chance of preventing cancer from recurring within the breast. Survival rates for women who have the entire breast removed and for those who have breast-conserving surgery plus radiation therapy appear to be identical for at least the first 20 years after surgery.

The major advantage of breast-conserving surgery plus radiation therapy is cosmetic; this surgery may help preserve body image. However, this advantage may be nonexistent if the tumor is large in relation to the breast, because removing an area of normal tissue, which is necessary for long-term control of breast cancer, results in removing most of the breast. Breast-conserving surgery is usually easier when tumors are small. In about 15 percent of women who undergo breast-conserving surgery, the amount of tissue removed is so small that hardly any difference can be seen between the treated and untreated breasts. More often, however, the treated breast shrinks somewhat and may change in contour.

▲ see page 802

Usually, side effects of the radiation therapy that accompanies breast-conserving surgery are not painful and don't last long. The skin may redden or blister. Fewer than 5 percent of women treated with radiation therapy have rib fractures that cause minor discomfort. About 10 to 20 percent develop mild lung inflammation 3 to 6 months after completing radiation therapy. For up to about 6 weeks, they have a dry cough and shortness of breath during physical activity.

In a **simple mastectomy,** a doctor removes all the breast tissue but leaves the underlying muscle intact and enough overlying skin to cover the wound. The breast can be reconstructed much more easily if the chest muscles and other tissues beneath the breast are left intact. This procedure is commonly used to treat invasive cancer that has spread extensively within the milk ducts, because this type of cancer often recurs within the breast if breast-conserving surgery is used. The lymph nodes in the underarm may also be removed to determine if any cancer cells have spread outside the breast; this procedure is called a **simple mastectomy plus node dissection** or a **modified radical mastectomy.** Follow-up radiation therapy, given after surgery, greatly reduces the risk that cancer will recur on the chest wall or in nearby lymph nodes, but it doesn't seem to improve overall survival rates, probably because the cancer has spread undetected to other parts of the body (metastasized). Women who have had a simple mastectomy live as long as women who have had a **radical mastectomy,** in which the underlying chest muscles and other tissues also are removed.

During surgery, nearby lymph nodes or a tissue sample from the lymph nodes may be removed and examined to determine prognosis. The woman's chances of long-term survival are much better if no cancer cells are found in the lymph nodes.

The size of the tumor and the presence of tumor cells in a lymph node influence the use of chemotherapy and hormone-blocking drugs. Some authorities believe that for tumors smaller than $1/2$ inch in diameter, surgery almost always eliminates the cancer and no other treatment is needed. If the tumor is larger than 2 inches in diameter, chemotherapy is usually given after surgery. If the tumor is 3 inches or larger in diameter, chemotherapy may be given before surgery.

Women who have **lobular carcinoma in situ** may be kept under close observation or may be treated immediately by removing both breasts (bilateral mastectomy). Most doctors don't consider lobular carcinoma in situ to be cancer; instead, they consider it to be a sign that a woman is at greater risk of developing breast cancer. Only about 25 to 30 percent of women who have this condition develop invasive breast cancer and even fewer die of breast cancer, so many women choose to have no treatment. If a woman chooses to have treatment to reduce her risk of developing breast cancer, removal of both breasts is necessary, because cancer doesn't always develop in the same area or same breast as lobular carcinoma in situ. If a woman desires treatment other than mastectomy, tamoxifen is the hormone-blocking drug most often used. The ovaries may be removed in women who are still menstruating, but whether this procedure is as effective or more effective than hormone-blocking drugs isn't clear.

Most women who have **ductal carcinoma in situ** almost never have a recurrence after a simple mastectomy. Many women have only the tumor removed (lumpectomy), sometimes in combination with radiation therapy. These women have a higher chance of developing another cancer in the breast, but there is no evidence that they are more likely to die of breast cancer than those treated with a simple mastectomy.

Women who have **inflammatory breast cancer** usually are treated with both chemotherapy and radiation therapy.

Breast Reconstruction: For breast reconstruction, a silicone or saline implant or tissue taken from other parts of the woman's body may be used. A woman may choose to undergo reconstruction at the same time as the mastectomy, but this choice means that the woman will be under anesthesia for a longer time and the general surgeon and plastic surgeon must cooperate closely. Alternatively, reconstruction may be performed later, but this choice requires anesthesia a second time.

Recently, the safety of silicone implants has been questioned. The silicone occasionally leaks out of its sack. As a result, an implant can become hard, cause discomfort, and appear less attractive. In addition, silicone sometimes enters the bloodstream. However, whether the leaking silicone causes cancer in other parts of the body or rare diseases such as lupus isn't known. There is almost no evidence suggesting that silicone leakage has these serious effects, but because it might, the use of silicone implants has decreased,

Rebuilding a Breast

After a general surgeon removes a breast tumor and the surrounding breast tissue (mastectomy), a plastic surgeon may reconstruct the breast, using a silicone or saline implant or, in a more complex operation, tissue taken from other parts of the woman's body, usually the abdomen.

In many women, a reconstructed breast looks more natural than one that has been treated with radiation therapy, especially if the tumor was large. If a silicone or saline implant is used and enough skin was left to cover it, the sensation in the skin over the implant is relatively normal, but neither type of implant feels like breast tissue to the touch. If tissue from other parts of the body is used, much of the sensation in the skin is lost since the skin is also from another part of the body; however, this type of implant feels more like breast tissue than does a silicone or saline implant.

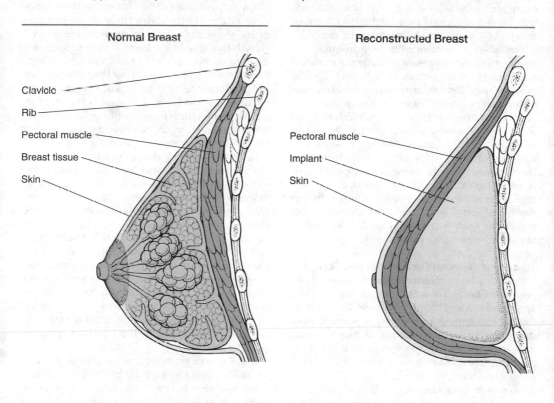

Normal Breast

Clavicle
Rib
Pectoral muscle
Breast tissue
Skin

Reconstructed Breast

Pectoral muscle
Implant
Skin

especially in women who haven't had breast cancer.

Follow-up Chemotherapy and Hormone-Blocking Drugs: Chemotherapy, which kills cancer cells, or hormone-blocking drugs, which interfere with the actions of hormones that support cancer cell growth, are often started soon after breast surgery and are continued for months or years. These treatments delay the return of cancer and prolong survival in most women. These drugs may cure a few women, but this is not yet known with certainty. Treatment with several chemotherapy drugs given together suppresses recurrences more effectively than treatment with a single drug. However, by themselves, without surgery or radiation, these drugs can't cure breast cancer.

Depending on what chemotherapy drugs a woman is taking, she may vomit, feel nauseated or tired, have painful mouth sores, or lose her hair temporarily. Vomiting is relatively uncommon today because of drugs such as ondansetron. If such drugs aren't used, a woman may vomit from one to six times over a period of 1 to 3 days after chemotherapy. The severity and duration of the vomiting varies, depending on the chemotherapy drugs used and the woman. Also, a woman may be unusually prone to infections and bleeding for several months. In most women, these side effects eventually subside, although infections and bleeding are fatal in 1 or 2 out of every 1,000 women receiving chemotherapy.

Tamoxifen is a hormone-blocking drug that may be given as follow-up treatment after a woman has had surgery for breast cancer. In women aged 50 years or over, tamoxifen increases the likelihood of survival in the first 10 years after diagnosis by about 20 to 25 percent. Tamoxifen, which is chemically related to estrogen, has some of the effects of estrogen replacement therapy▲—favorable and unfavorable—such as possibly decreasing the risk of developing osteoporosis or of dying of heart disease and increasing the risk of developing cancer of the uterus. However, unlike estrogen replacement therapy, tamoxifen does not decrease hot flashes or ameliorate the vaginal dryness that occurs after menopause.

Treatment of Breast Cancer That Has Spread

Breast cancer may spread (metastasize) to any area of the body. The most common areas are the lungs, liver, bone, lymph nodes, brain, and skin. Cancer can appear in these areas years or even decades after breast cancer is first diagnosed and treated. If the cancer has spread to one area, it probably has spread to other areas, even if it isn't found right away.

No cure exists for breast cancer that has spread outside the breast, but most women who have it live at least 2 years and a few live 10 to 20 years. Treatment with drugs, in addition to appropriate surgery, extends life slightly, but the main reason for treatment is that drugs, even with their unpleasant side effects, usually relieve symptoms and improve quality of life. In selecting a treatment, a doctor considers whether the cancer's growth is supported by estrogen, how much time has passed since the cancer was first diagnosed and treated, how many organs are involved, and whether a woman is past menopause.

A woman who has cancer that has spread but who has no symptoms usually doesn't benefit from treatment. Consequently, treatment, especially if it has uncomfortable side effects, is often postponed until the woman develops symptoms (pain or other discomfort) or the cancer starts to worsen quickly.

A woman who has pain or other disabling symptoms is usually treated with hormone-blocking drugs or chemotherapy to suppress cancer cell growth throughout the body. However, there are exceptions. For instance, if only one area of cancer is detected in a bone after a long time with no recurrences, the only treatment used might be radiation to that bone. Radiation is the most effective treatment for cancer of the bone, sometimes keeping it in check for years, and also for cancer that has spread to the brain.

Hormone-blocking drugs are prescribed more often than chemotherapy for women whose cancer is supported by estrogen, who have had no evidence of cancer for more than 2 years after diagnosis, or whose cancer is not immediately life threatening. These drugs are especially effective for women in their 40s who are still menstruating and producing a lot of estrogen, as well as for those who are at least 5 years past menopause; however, none of these guidelines is absolute. Because tamoxifen has few side effects, it's usually the first hormone-blocking drug used. Alternatively, surgery to remove the ovaries or radiation to destroy them may be used to stop estrogen production.

If the cancer starts to spread again months or years after being suppressed by a hormone-blocking drug, other hormone-blocking drugs may be tried. Aminoglutethimide is an estrogen-blocking drug widely used for painful cancer in the bone. Hydrocortisone, a steroid hormone, is usually given at the same time because aminoglutethimide suppresses the body's natural production of hydrocortisone, an essential hormone. Newer drugs that are similar to aminoglutethimide but that don't require the use of hydrocortisone have recently been approved to treat breast cancer and appear to be as effective as aminoglutethimide.

▲ see page 1079

Breast Disorders in Men

Breast disorders rarely occur in men. Such disorders include enlargement and, less commonly, cancer of the breast.

Breast Enlargement

Breast enlargement in males (gynecomastia) may occur during puberty. This enlargement is normal and transient, lasting a few months to a few years. Similar changes may take place in old age. Male breast enlargement also may be caused by certain diseases (particularly liver disease); certain drug therapies, such as treatment with female sex hormones; and marijuana use. Less commonly, this condition results from a hormonal imbalance, which can be caused by rare estrogen-producing tumors in the testes or adrenal glands. If this type of tumor is suspected, the testes are examined using ultrasound scanning, and the adrenal glands are examined using computed tomography (CT) or magnetic resonance imaging (MRI).

One or both breasts may become enlarged. The enlarged breast may be tender. If it is, the cause probably isn't cancer. Breast pain in men, as in women, usually isn't a sign of cancer.

Generally, no specific treatment is needed. Breast enlargement usually disappears on its own or after its cause is eliminated by treating the disease or withdrawing the drug that's responsible for it. Whether hormone treatment is beneficial isn't clear. Surgical removal of excess breast tissue is effective but rarely necessary. A new surgical technique, which removes tissue through a suction tube inserted through a small incision, is becoming increasingly popular and sometimes is followed by cosmetic surgery.

Breast Cancer

Men can develop breast cancer, but a man's chances of developing it are only 1 percent of a woman's chances. Because it's uncommon, it's seldom suspected as a cause of symptoms, either by the man who has the cancer or his doctor. As a result, male breast cancer often progresses to an advanced stage before it's diagnosed. The prognosis is the same as that for a woman whose cancer is at the same stage. Treatment is almost the same, except that breast-conserving surgery is rarely used and the value of drug treatment or radiation therapy after surgery hasn't been demonstrated. Spread to other parts of the body is treated with the same hormone-blocking drugs used to treat breast cancer in women or with surgical removal of the testes (orchiectomy) to eliminate hormones that can support cancer growth. Alternatively, a combination of chemotherapy drugs may be used.

The most effective chemotherapy regimens include cyclophosphamide, doxorubicin, paclitaxel, docetaxel, vinorelbine, and mitomycin C. These are often used in addition to hormone-blocking drugs.

Biologic response modifiers are sometimes tried experimentally as treatment for breast cancer.▲ These drugs are natural substances or slightly modified versions of natural substances that are part of the body's immune system. They include interferons, interleukin-2, lymphocyte-activated killer cells, tumor necrosis factor, and monoclonal antibodies. These drugs are given early, before extensive chemotherapy, but their role in treating breast cancer hasn't been established.

Paget's Disease of the Nipple

Paget's disease of the nipple is a type of breast cancer that first appears as a crusty or scaly nipple sore or as a discharge from the nipple.■

Because this disease usually causes little discomfort, a woman may ignore it for a year or more before seeing a doctor. A doctor makes the diagnosis usually by removing and examining a small piece of nipple tissue but sometimes by simply

▲ see page 793

■ see page 994

examining a smear of the nipple discharge under a microscope. Slightly more than half of the women who have this cancer also have a lump in the breast that can be felt. Paget's disease may be in situ or invasive.

Usually, a simple mastectomy with removal of the lymph nodes is performed. Less commonly, removal of the nipple with some surrounding normal tissue is successful. Prognosis depends on how invasive and how large the cancer is as well as whether it has spread to the lymph nodes.

Cystosarcoma Phyllodes

Cystosarcoma phyllodes is a relatively rare type of breast tumor that can be cancerous.

These tumors rarely spread to other areas, but after surgical removal they tend to reappear at the same site. The usual treatment is removal of the tumor and a fairly wide margin of surrounding normal tissue (wide excision). If the tumor is large in relation to the breast, a simple mastectomy may be performed.

CHAPTER 239

Cancers of the Female Reproductive System

Cancers can occur in any part of the female reproductive system—the vulva, vagina, cervix, uterus, fallopian tubes, or ovaries.▲

Cancer of the Uterus

Although commonly called cancer of the uterus, this cancer (endometrial carcinoma) begins in the uterine lining (endometrium). It is the fourth most common cancer among women and the most common cancer of the female reproductive system. This cancer usually develops after menopause, most often in women between the ages of 50 and 60. It can spread (metastasize) either locally or to many other parts of the body— down the uterus to the cervical canal; up from the uterus through the fallopian tubes to the ovaries; into the area surrounding the uterus; through the lymph vessels and lymph nodes (lymphatic system), which transport lymph from all over the body to the bloodstream; or through the bloodstream to distant parts of the body.

▲ see box, page 1070

■ see box, page 1072

Symptoms and Diagnosis

Abnormal bleeding from the uterus is the most common early symptom. Bleeding may occur after menopause, or it may be recurring, irregular, or severe in women who are still menstruating. One out of every three women who develop uterine bleeding after menopause has this type of cancer. *Because of the possibility of cancer, abnormal vaginal bleeding after menopause warrants prompt medical attention.*

Several tests are used to diagnose this cancer.■ A Papanicolaou (Pap) test, which accurately detects cervical cancer cells, may be helpful, but it misses uterine cancer cells about a third of the time. Therefore, doctors also perform an endometrial biopsy or fractional curettage, in which tissue is removed from the uterine lining for examination under a microscope.

If results from a biopsy or fractional curettage confirm the presence of cancer of the uterine lining, additional tests may be performed to determine if the cancer has spread beyond the uterus. Ultrasound scans, computed tomography (CT) scans, cystoscopy (an examination of the bladder through a viewing tube), barium enema, chest x-rays, intravenous urography (an x-ray study to examine the kidneys and ureters), bone and liver scans, sigmoidoscopy (an examination of the rectum through a viewing tube), and lymphangiography (an x-ray study of lymph vessels that have been injected with dye) may provide useful information and help determine the best treatment. Not all of these tests are needed in every case.

Treatment

Hysterectomy, the surgical removal of the uterus, is the mainstay of treatment for women who have this type of cancer. If the cancer hasn't spread beyond the uterus, hysterectomy almost always cures the disease. During the operation, a surgeon usually removes the fallopian tubes and ovaries (salpingo-oophorectomy) and nearby lymph nodes. They are examined by a pathologist to find out whether the cancer has spread, how far it may have spread, and whether the woman needs radiation therapy in addition to surgery.

Even when the cancer doesn't seem to have spread, the doctor may prescribe drug treatment (chemotherapy) after surgery,▲ in case some undetected cancer cells remain. Usually, hormones aimed at stopping the growth of the cancer are used. Progestins (progesterone—a female hormone that blocks the effects of estrogen—and similar drugs) are often effective.

If the cancer has spread beyond the uterus, higher doses of a progestin may be needed. In up to 40 percent of women who have cancer that has spread, a progestin reduces the cancer's size and controls its spread for 2 to 3 years. Treatment may be continued indefinitely if it seems to be working well. Side effects of progestins include weight gain from water retention and occasional feelings of depression.

If the cancer has spread or is not responding to hormone therapy, other chemotherapy drugs—such as cyclophosphamide, doxorubicin, and cisplatin—may be added. These drugs are much more toxic than progestins and cause many side effects. The risks and benefits of cancer chemotherapy are weighed carefully before treatment is chosen.

Overall, almost two thirds of the women who have this type of cancer survive and have no evidence of the cancer 5 years after diagnosis, fewer than one third die of the disease, and nearly one tenth live but still have the cancer. If this cancer is discovered in an early stage, nearly 90 percent of women who have it can expect to live at least

---

Risk Factors for Cancer of the Uterus

• Menopause after age 52

• Menstrual problems (such as excessive bleeding, spotting between menstrual periods, or long intervals without periods)

• Never having had children

• Exposure to high levels of estrogen (the major female hormone) from estrogen-producing tumors or from high doses of estrogen-containing medications, including estrogen replacement therapy without progesterone after menopause

• Tamoxifen therapy

• Obesity

• High blood pressure

• Diabetes

---

5 years, and most are cured. Odds are best for younger women, women whose cancer has not spread beyond the uterus, and women who have slower-growing types of cancer.

Cancer of the Cervix

The cervix is the lower end of the uterus, which extends into the vagina. Of cancers of the female reproductive system, cervical cancer (cervical carcinoma) is the second most common in all women and the most common in younger women. It usually affects women between the ages of 35 and 55. This cancer may be caused by a virus (human papillomavirus), which may be transmitted during sexual intercourse.■

Risk for cervical cancer seems to increase as a woman's age at first sexual intercourse decreases and as the number of sexual partners increases. Failure to have regular Pap tests also increases risk.

▲ see page 802

■ see page 948

Pap Test Results: Stages of Cervical Cancer

- Normal

- Minimal cervical dysplasia (early changes that are not yet cancerous)

- Severe dysplasia (late changes that are not yet cancerous)

- Carcinoma in situ (cancer confined to the outermost layer of the cervix)

- Invasive cancer

About 85 percent of cervical cancers are squamous cell carcinomas, which develop in the scaly, flat, skinlike cells covering the outside of the cervix. Most other cervical cancers develop from gland cells (adenocarcinomas) or a combination of cell types (adenosquamous carcinomas).

Cervical cancer can penetrate deep beneath the surface of the cervix, enter the rich network of small blood and lymphatic vessels that line the inside of the cervix, and then spread to other parts of the body. In this way, the cancer can spread to distant areas as well as to areas near the cervix.

Symptoms and Diagnosis

Symptoms may include spotting between periods or bleeding after intercourse. A woman may not experience any pain or symptoms until the late stages of the disease, but routine Pap tests can detect cervical cancer early. Cervical cancer starts with slow, progressive changes in normal cells and may take several years to develop. The progressive changes can be seen through a microscope on slides containing cells taken during the Pap test. Pathologists have described these changes as stages ranging from normal to invasive cancer.

The Pap test can accurately and inexpensively detect up to 90 percent of cervical cancers, even before symptoms develop. Consequently, the number of deaths from cervical cancer has been reduced by more than 50 percent since Pap tests were introduced. Doctors often recommend that women have their first Pap test when they become sexually active or reach the age of 18 and that the test be performed annually. If their test results have been normal for 3 consecutive years, women may schedule Pap tests every 2 or 3 years as long as they don't change their lifestyle. If all women had Pap tests on a regular basis, deaths from this cancer could be eliminated. However, almost 40 percent of American women aren't tested regularly.

If a growth, sore, or other suspicious area is seen on the cervix during a pelvic examination or if a Pap test shows an abnormality or cancer, the doctor performs a biopsy (removing a sample of tissue for examination under a microscope). The tissue sample is usually removed during colposcopy, in which the doctor uses a viewing tube with a magnifying lens (colposcope) to examine the cervix carefully and to choose the best biopsy site. Two different types of biopsy are performed: punch biopsy, in which a tiny piece of the cervix, viewed and selected with the colposcope, is removed; and endocervical curettage, in which tissue that can't be viewed is scraped from the canal of the cervix. Both types cause little pain and a small amount of bleeding, and the two together usually provide enough tissue for a pathologist to make a diagnosis. If the diagnosis isn't clear, the doctor performs a cone biopsy, in which a larger piece of tissue is removed. Usually, this biopsy is performed with the loop electrosurgical excision procedure (LEEP) in the doctor's office.

If the woman has cervical cancer, the next step is to determine its exact size and locations—a process called staging. Staging begins with a physical examination of the pelvis and a variety of tests (cystoscopy, chest x-ray, intravenous urography, sigmoidoscopy) to find out whether the cervical cancer has spread to adjoining structures or to more distant parts of the body. Other tests, such as a CT scan, barium enema, and bone and liver scans, may be performed, depending on the woman's circumstances.

Treatment

Treatment depends on the stage of the cancer.

If the cancer is confined to the outermost layer of the cervix (carcinoma in situ), a doctor is often able to remove the cancer completely by removing part of the cervix with a knife or with the loop electrosurgical excision procedure. This treatment preserves a woman's ability to have children. But because cancer can recur, doctors advise women to return for examinations and Pap tests every 3 months for the first year and every 6 months after that. If a woman has carcinoma in situ and doesn't plan to have children, removal of the uterus (hysterectomy) may be recommended.

If the cancer is more advanced, hysterectomy plus removal of adjacent structures (radical hysterectomy) and lymph nodes is necessary. Normal, functioning ovaries in younger women are not removed.

Radiation therapy is also highly effective for treating advanced cervical cancer that has not spread beyond the pelvic region. Although radiation therapy usually causes few or no immediate problems, it may irritate the rectum and vagina. Delayed damage to the bladder and rectum may result, and the ovaries usually stop functioning.

When the cancer has spread beyond the pelvis, chemotherapy is sometimes recommended. However, only 25 to 30 percent of those treated can expect any response, and the response is usually temporary.

Cancer of the Ovaries

Cancer of the ovaries (ovarian carcinoma) develops most often in women between the ages of 50 and 70, and about 1 out of 70 women eventually develops this cancer. It is the third most common cancer of the female reproductive system, but more women die of ovarian cancers than of any other cancer of the reproductive system.

Ovaries include a variety of cell types, each of which may give rise to a distinct type of cancer. At least 10 different types of ovarian cancer are recognized; treatment and prospects for recovery differ according to type.

Ovarian cancer cells can spread directly to the surrounding area and through the lymphatic system to other parts of the pelvis and abdomen. The cancer cells can also spread through the bloodstream, eventually appearing at distant places in the body, mainly the liver and lungs.

Symptoms and Diagnosis

An ovarian cancer can grow to considerable size before it causes any symptoms. The first symptom may be vague discomfort in the lower abdomen, similar to indigestion. Uterine bleeding is not a common symptom. Enlarged ovaries in a postmenopausal woman may be an early sign of ovarian cancer, although they can be caused by cysts, noncancerous growths, and other conditions. Fluid may accumulate in the abdomen.

Eventually, the abdomen may swell because of the enlarging ovaries or accumulating fluid. At this stage, a woman may feel pain in her pelvis, may be anemic, and may lose weight. Rarely, ovarian cancers secrete hormones that cause excessive growth of the uterine lining, enlargement of the breasts, or increased hair growth.

Diagnosing ovarian cancer in its early stages is difficult, because symptoms usually don't appear until the cancer has spread beyond the ovaries and because many other less serious diseases cause similar symptoms.

If ovarian cancer is suspected, an ultrasound scan or a computed tomography (CT) scan is needed to provide more information about the enlarged ovary. Sometimes the ovaries are viewed directly with a laparoscope, a small viewing tube inserted through a tiny incision in the abdominal wall. If test results suggest a noncancerous cyst, a woman may be asked to return for periodic pelvic examinations as long as the cyst remains. However, if the test results are inconclusive and ovarian cancer is suspected, abdominal surgery is performed to make the diagnosis and to determine how far the cancer has spread (staging) and how to treat it.

If fluid has accumulated in the abdomen, it can be drawn out (aspirated) through a needle and tested to see whether cancer cells are present.

Treatment

Ovarian cancer is treated with surgery. The extent of surgery depends on the specific type of cancer and its stage. If the cancer hasn't spread beyond the ovary, removing only the single affected ovary and its adjoining fallopian tube may be possible. When cancer has already spread beyond the ovary, both ovaries and the uterus, as well as selected lymph nodes and surrounding structures through which the cancer typically spreads, must be removed.

After surgery, radiation therapy and chemotherapy may be used to destroy any small areas of cancer that may remain. Ovarian cancer that has already spread (metastasized) beyond the ovary is difficult to cure.

Five years after diagnosis, 15 to 85 percent of women who have the most common types of ovarian cancer are still alive. The wide range of survival rates reflects differences in the aggressiveness of particular cancers and in the immune responses of different women against the cancer.

Cancer of the Vulva

The vulva refers to the external female reproductive organs. Cancer of the vulva (vulvar carcinoma) accounts for only 3 to 4 percent of all cancers of the female reproductive system and usually occurs after menopause. As the population ages, this cancer is expected to increase in incidence.

Vulvar cancer is predominantly a skin cancer near or at the opening of the vagina. The same cell types involved in skin cancer (squamous and basal cells)▲ also are involved in most vulvar cancers. About 90 percent of vulvar cancers are squamous cell carcinomas, and 4 percent are basal cell carcinomas. The remaining 6 percent are rare cancers (Paget's disease, cancer of Bartholin's gland, melanomas, and others).

Like other skin cancers, vulvar cancers begin on the surface and at first don't grow much beyond that. Although some may be aggressive, most of these cancers grow relatively slowly. Left untreated, they can eventually invade the vagina, the urethra, or the anus and spread into the network of lymph nodes in the area.

Symptoms and Diagnosis

Vulvar cancers can easily be seen and felt as unusual lumps or sores near or at the opening of the vagina. Sometimes scaly patches or discoloration occurs. The surrounding tissue may contract and pucker. Usually, a woman has little discomfort, although the area may itch. Eventually, bleeding or weeping (watery discharge) may develop. These symptoms warrant prompt medical attention.

To make the diagnosis, a doctor performs a biopsy. After numbing the area with an anesthetic, the doctor removes a small amount of the abnormal skin. The biopsy is needed to determine if the abnormal skin is cancerous and not just infected or irritated. It also identifies the type of cancer, if present, which guides the doctor in developing treatment strategies.

Treatment

Vulvectomy is surgery to remove the large area of tissue at the opening of the vagina. For all but the smallest cancers, vulvectomy is necessary to remove **squamous cell vulvar cancer.** This extensive procedure is performed because this type of vulvar cancer can spread quickly into nearby tissues and lymph nodes. Because vulvectomy may remove the clitoris, doctors work closely with a woman who has vulvar cancer to develop a treatment plan that is best suited to her and takes her other medical problems, age, and sexual lifestyle into account. Intercourse is usually possible after vulvectomy. Radiation therapy may follow surgery for very advanced cases in which a complete cure seems unlikely. If the cancer is detected early, 75 percent of women have no sign of cancer 5 years after diagnosis; if lymph nodes are involved, the survival rate is less than 50 percent.

Because **basal cell vulvar cancer** doesn't tend to metastasize to distant sites, local surgery is usually all that is needed. Removing the whole vulva is not required unless the cancer is extensive.

Cancer of the Vagina

Only about 1 percent of cancers of the female reproductive system occur in the vagina. Cancer of the vagina (vaginal carcinoma) usually affects women between the ages of 45 and 65. More than 95 percent of vaginal cancers are squamous cell carcinomas and are therefore similar to cervical and vulvar cancers. Vaginal squamous cell carcinoma may be caused by human papillomavirus, the same type of virus that causes genital warts■ and cervical cancer. Clear cell carcinoma, a rare vaginal cancer, occurs almost exclusively in women whose mothers took the drug diethylstilbestrol (DES) during pregnancy.

Symptoms and Diagnosis

Vaginal cancer destroys the lining of the vagina and causes sores that may bleed and become infected. A woman may notice a watery discharge or bleeding and pain during sexual intercourse. If the cancer grows large enough, it can also affect the function of the bladder and rectum, so that the woman has a frequent urge to urinate and urinating becomes painful.

When vaginal cancer is suspected, a doctor scrapes cells from the vaginal wall to examine under a microscope and performs a biopsy on any growth, sore, or other suspicious area seen during a pelvic examination. The biopsy is usually performed during colposcopy.

▲ see page 992

■ see page 948

Treatment

Treatment of vaginal cancer depends on both its location and its size. However, all vaginal cancers may be treated by radiation therapy.

For cancer located in the upper third of the vagina, a doctor may perform a hysterectomy and remove the pelvic lymph nodes and the upper part of the vagina, or radiation therapy may be used. Cancer in the middle third of the vagina is treated by radiation therapy, and cancer in the lower part may be treated by surgical removal or radiation therapy.

Intercourse may be difficult or impossible after treatment for vaginal cancer, although sometimes a new vagina can be constructed with skin grafts or part of the intestine. The 5-year survival rate is about 30 percent.

Cancer of the Fallopian Tubes

Cancer also can develop in the fallopian tubes. This cancer is the rarest cancer of the female reproductive system. Symptoms include vague abdominal discomfort and occasionally a watery or blood-tinged discharge from the vagina. Usually, an enlarged mass is found in the pelvis, and the diagnosis is made after removal. A hysterectomy and removal of the ovaries and other surrounding structures, followed by chemotherapy, is almost always necessary. The outlook is similar to that for ovarian cancer.

Hydatidiform Mole

A hydatidiform mole is a tumorous growth of tissue from the placenta or afterbirth.

A hydatidiform mole can develop from cells remaining after a miscarriage or a full-term pregnancy but most often develops from a fertilized egg as an independent abnormal growth (molar pregnancy). Rarely, the placenta becomes abnormal when the fetus is normal. More than 80 percent of hydatidiform moles are not cancerous; however, 15 percent invade the surrounding tissue (invasive mole), and 2 to 3 percent spread throughout the body (choriocarcinoma).

The risk of hydatidiform moles is highest in women who become pregnant in their late 30s and early 40s. These moles occur in about 1 out of every 2,000 pregnancies in the United States and, for unknown reasons, are nearly 10 times more common among Asian women.

Symptoms and Diagnosis

Hydatidiform moles often become apparent shortly after conception. A woman feels as if she's pregnant, but her abdomen gets larger much faster than it does in a normal pregnancy because the mole inside the uterus grows rapidly. Severe nausea and vomiting are common and vaginal bleeding may occur; these symptoms indicate the need for immediate medical attention. Hydatidiform moles can cause serious complications, including infections, bleeding, and toxemia of pregnancy.

If the woman has a hydatidiform mole instead of a normal pregnancy, no fetal movement or fetal heartbeat is detected. Small amounts of a grape-like material may pass through the vagina as parts of the mole decay. A pathologist can examine the discharged material under a microscope to confirm the diagnosis.

A doctor may order an ultrasound scan to be sure that the growth is a hydatidiform mole and not a fetus or amniotic sac (the membranes that contain the fetus and fluid surrounding it). Blood tests to measure the level of human chorionic gonadotropin (a hormone normally produced early in pregnancy) may be performed. If a hydatidiform mole is present, the level is extraordinarily high because the mole produces a lot of this hormone. This test is less useful during early pregnancy, when the level of this hormone is also high.▲

Treatment

The hydatidiform mole must be completely removed. Usually, a doctor is able to remove the mole by dilation and suction curettage (D and C). Only rarely is hysterectomy required.

After surgery, the human chorionic gonadotropin level is measured to determine whether the mole was completely removed. When removal is complete, the level returns to normal, usually within 8 weeks, and remains normal. If a woman who has had a mole removed becomes pregnant, interpretation of a high human chorionic gonadotropin level becomes difficult because it could be caused by the pregnancy or by part of the mole that wasn't removed. Therefore, women who have had a mole removed are advised not to become pregnant for a year.

▲ see page 1139

Noncancerous hydatidiform moles don't require chemotherapy, but cancerous moles do. Drugs used for treatment usually include methotrexate, dactinomycin, or a combination of these drugs.

The cure rate is virtually 100 percent for women whose disease is less advanced and about 85 percent for women whose disease has spread widely. Most women are still able to have children.

CHAPTER 240

Infertility

Infertility is the inability of a couple to achieve a pregnancy after repeated intercourse without contraception for 1 year.

Infertility affects about one of every five couples in the United States. It's increasingly common because people are marrying when they're older and are waiting longer to have a child. Nevertheless, up to 60 percent of the couples who haven't conceived after a year of trying eventually will conceive, with or without treatment. The goal of treatment is to reduce the time needed to conceive.

As a woman gets older, she is less likely to have a successful pregnancy. Particularly after age 35, a woman has a limited time to resolve infertility problems before menopause.

Major causes of infertility include problems with sperm, ovulation, the fallopian tubes, and the cervix as well as unidentified factors. The diagnosis and treatment of these problems require a thorough assessment of both partners.

Problems With Sperm

In an adult male, sperm are being formed continuously (spermatogenesis) in the testes. A nonspecialized cell requires about 72 to 74 days to develop into a mature sperm cell. From each testis, sperm move to the epididymis (a coiled tube located on top and down the back of the testis), where they are stored until ejaculation is about to occur. From the epididymis, sperm move through the vas deferens and the ejaculatory duct. In the ejaculatory duct, fluid produced by the seminal vesicles is added to the sperm to form semen, which moves through the urethra to be ejaculated.▲

To be fertile, a man must be able to deliver an adequate quantity of normal sperm to a woman's vagina. Various factors can interfere with this process, causing infertility.

An increase in the temperature of the testes from a prolonged fever or exposure to excessive heat can greatly reduce sperm count, decrease the vigor of sperm movement, and increase the number of abnormal sperm in semen. Sperm formation is most efficient at about 93.2° F., which is lower than normal body temperature. The testes, where sperm are formed, can be kept at this lower temperature because they are located in the scrotum, which is outside the body cavity.

Complete absence of sperm (azoospermia) results from a serious disorder within the testes or from blocked or missing vasa deferentia (on both sides). Semen that doesn't contain fructose, a sugar produced by the seminal vesicles, indicates that the vasa deferentia or seminal vesicles are missing or the ejaculatory ducts are blocked.

A varicocele, the most common anatomic abnormality in infertile men, is a mass of elongated, widened, snakelike veins in the scrotum, similar to varicose veins. It feels like a bag of worms. This abnormality may prevent proper drainage of blood from the testes, thus raising their temperature and reducing the rate of sperm formation.

More unusually, semen can travel in the wrong direction (retrograde ejaculation)—it backs up into the bladder instead of traveling down the penis. This disorder is more common in men who have had pelvic surgery, particularly prostate removal, and in men who have diabetes. Retrograde ejaculation can also result from abnormal nerve function.

▲ see page 1056

Diagnosis

After obtaining a medical history and performing a physical examination, a doctor orders a **semen analysis,** the main screening test for male infertility. The man is asked not to ejaculate for 2 to 3 days before the analysis. For the analysis, he is asked to ejaculate, usually by masturbation, into a clean glass jar, preferably at the laboratory site. For men who have difficulty producing a semen sample this way, special condoms that have no lubricants or chemicals toxic to sperm can be used to collect semen during intercourse. An analysis based on two or three separate samples is more reliable.

If the semen sample is abnormal, the analysis may be repeated because samples from the same man normally vary greatly. If the semen still seems to be abnormal, the doctor seeks possible causes, such as mumps involving the testes (mumps orchitis), a sudden illness or prolonged fever in the previous 3 months, injury to the testes, exposure to industrial or environmental toxins, use of diethylstilbestrol or anabolic steroids, drug use, and alcohol intake. However, a low sperm count may indicate only that too little time had elapsed since the last ejaculation or that only some of the semen was deposited in the collection jar.

The doctor examines the man for physical abnormalities, such as undescended testes, and for signs of hereditary or hormonal disorders that might explain the infertility. Hormonal disorders that reduce testosterone production (hypogonadism)▲ can originate in the testes or other glands, such as the pituitary.

Infertility centers perform tests of sperm function and quality, often before medically assisted fertilization techniques are considered. One such test detects antibodies to sperm; another determines whether sperm membranes are intact. Still others can determine the sperm's ability to bind to the egg and penetrate it.

Treatment

Treatment depends on the cause of infertility.

Clomiphene, a drug used to induce ovulation in women, can be used to try to increase sperm counts in men. However, clomiphene doesn't seem to improve the sperm's ability to move or to reduce the number of abnormal sperm, and it hasn't been proved to increase fertility.

For men who have few normal sperm, artificial insemination may slightly enhance pregnancy

---

Causes of Infertility

Problem Area	Percentage of Cases
Sperm	30 to 40
Ovulation	15 to 20
Fallopian tubes	25 to 40
Cervix	5
Unidentified factors	5 to 15

---

rates because it uses the first portion of the ejaculated semen, which has the greatest concentration of sperm. A newer technique that selects only the most active sperm (washed sperm) is somewhat more successful. In vitro fertilization and gamete intrafallopian tube transfer (GIFT), which are much more complex and costly procedures, are successful in treating certain types of male infertility.

If a man produces no sperm, inseminating the woman with sperm from another man (a donor) can be considered. Because of the danger of contracting sexually transmitted diseases, including AIDS, fresh semen samples from donors are no longer used. Instead, frozen sperm samples should be obtained from a certified sperm bank, which has tested the donors for sexually transmitted diseases. However, pregnancy is less likely to result when frozen, rather than fresh, sperm samples are used.

Varicoceles can be treated with minor surgery. Studies suggest that pregnancy results in 30 to 50 percent of cases after the male partner has had varicocele surgery, but additional studies are needed for confirmation.

Problems With Ovulation

Ovulation is the release of an egg by the ovary.

A woman who has regular menstrual periods every 26 to 35 days, preceded by breast tender-

---

▲ see page 1298

ness, lower abdominal swelling, and mood changes, usually releases one egg from a follicle (a fluid-filled cavity that contains an egg) in the ovary each month. A woman who has regular menstrual periods without these symptoms also may ovulate. If a woman has irregular periods or no periods (amenorrhea),▲ the cause is determined before treatment to stimulate ovulation is started.

Monitoring Ovulation

Determining whether ovulation actually occurs is an important part of an infertility evaluation. Daily measurements of basal body temperature (temperature of the body at rest), usually taken immediately on awakening, may be used to determine if and when ovulation is occurring. A low point in basal body temperature suggests that ovulation is about to occur, whereas a slight, persistent rise of about 0.5° F. to 1° F. in temperature usually indicates that ovulation has occurred. However, basal body temperature is not a reliable or precise indicator of ovulation. At best, it predicts ovulation only within 2 days. More accurate techniques include ultrasound monitoring and ovulation predictor kits that detect an increase in luteinizing hormone (a hormone that induces ovulation), which peaks in the urine 24 to 36 hours before ovulation. Also, levels of the hormone progesterone in the blood or one of its breakdown products in the urine may be measured; a marked increase indicates that ovulation has occurred.

Whether ovulation occurs also can be determined by performing a biopsy: A small sample is removed from the lining of the uterus 10 to 12 days after ovulation is presumed to have occurred; the sample is examined under a microscope. If changes that normally occur in the uterine lining after ovulation are seen, ovulation has occurred.■

Treatment

A drug to induce ovulation is selected on the basis of the specific problem. For a woman who hasn't ovulated for a long time (chronic anovulation), clomiphene is usually preferred. First, a

menstrual period is induced with another drug, medroxyprogesterone acetate. The woman then takes clomiphene for 5 days. Usually, she ovulates 5 to 10 days (average, 7 days) after clomiphene is stopped and has a period 14 to 16 days after ovulation.

If a woman doesn't have a period after treatment with clomiphene, she takes a pregnancy test. If she isn't pregnant, the treatment cycle is repeated with increasing doses of clomiphene until ovulation occurs or the maximum dose is reached. When the doctor determines the dose that induces ovulation, the woman takes that dose for at least six more treatment cycles. Most women who become pregnant do so by the sixth cycle in which ovulation occurs. Overall, about 75 to 80 percent of women treated with clomiphene ovulate, but only about 40 to 50 percent become pregnant. About 5 percent of pregnancies in women treated with clomiphene are multiple, primarily twins.

Because there is some concern that prolonged use of clomiphene may increase the risk of ovarian cancer, doctors take several precautions: They evaluate the woman before treatment, closely monitor her during treatment, and limit the number of treatment cycles.

Side effects of clomiphene include hot flashes, abdominal swelling, breast tenderness, nausea, vision problems, and headaches. About 5 percent of women treated with clomiphene develop ovarian hyperstimulation syndrome, in which the ovaries become greatly enlarged and a large amount of fluid shifts from the bloodstream to the abdominal cavity. To try to prevent this disorder, the doctor prescribes the lowest effective dose and withholds clomiphene if the ovaries enlarge.

If a woman doesn't ovulate or become pregnant during treatment with clomiphene, hormonal therapy with human menopausal gonadotropins can be tried. Currently, these hormones are extracted from the urine of postmenopausal women, but synthetic versions are being tested. Because human menopausal gonadotropins are expensive and have severe side effects, doctors don't recommend trying this form of therapy until they are sure that ovulation problems, not problems with sperm or fallopian tubes, are the cause of infertility. Even then, treatment cycles are closely supervised by doctors experienced in using these hormones.

▲ see page 1087

■ see box, page 1076

Human menopausal gonadotropins, which are injected into the muscle, stimulate the ovarian follicles to mature. To monitor maturation, a doctor measures blood levels of the hormone estradiol and examines ultrasound scans of the pelvis. Doses are adjusted on the basis of the woman's response to the hormones. After the follicles are mature, the woman is given an injection of a different hormone, human chorionic gonadotropin, to trigger ovulation. Although more than 95 percent of the women treated with these hormones ovulate, only 50 to 75 percent become pregnant. In women treated with human menopausal gonadotropins, 10 to 30 percent of pregnancies are multiple, primarily twins.

A serious side effect of treatment with human menopausal gonadotropins is ovarian hyperstimulation syndrome, which develops in 10 to 20 percent of the women treated. This syndrome can be life threatening but usually can be avoided if the doctor closely monitors the treatment and withholds human chorionic gonadotropin when the woman's response becomes excessive. Human menopausal gonadotropins may increase the risk of ovarian cancer, but current evidence is insubstantial.

Sometimes, ovulation doesn't occur because the hypothalamus (the part of the brain that coordinates and controls hormonal activity) doesn't secrete gonadotropin-releasing hormone, which is necessary for ovulation. In these cases, a synthetic version of gonadotropin-releasing hormone may be used to induce ovulation. The risk of ovarian hyperstimulation is low with this treatment, so intensive monitoring isn't needed.

Problems With the Fallopian Tubes

The fallopian tubes may be abnormal in structure or function. The primary causes of problems are infection, endometriosis, and surgical closure of the fallopian tubes (tubal ligation) as a means of sterilization.

To determine if the fallopian tubes are open, a doctor orders a hysterosalpingogram (a special x-ray of the uterus and fallopian tubes)▲ shortly after the woman's menstrual period ends. This diagnostic test also shows congenital abnormalities (birth defects) of the uterus and fallopian tubes, fibrous masses in the uterus, and adhesions (fibrous bands that connect normally unconnected structures) in the uterus or pelvis. For

---

Causes of Fallopian Tube Problems

Congenital abnormalities

Pelvic inflammatory disease

Ectopic pregnancy

Ruptured appendix

Lower abdominal surgery

Endometriosis

Previous surgical closure (tubal ligation)

---

reasons not clearly understood, fertility appears to be slightly enhanced after a normal hysterosalpingogram. Therefore, the doctor may wait to see if a woman becomes pregnant after this test has been performed before ordering additional tests of fallopian tube function.

If the hysterosalpingogram shows an abnormality such as adhesions in the uterus, the doctor examines the uterus with a hysteroscope (a viewing tube inserted through the cervix into the uterus). The hysteroscope may be manipulated to break adhesions during the procedure, thus increasing the likelihood that the woman will become pregnant. If more diagnostic information is needed, a laparoscope, a small viewing tube, is inserted in the pelvic cavity through a small incision in the abdominal wall.■ This procedure, which is typically performed while the woman is under general anesthesia, enables the doctor to view the uterus, fallopian tubes, and ovaries. The laparoscope also may be used to remove abnormal tissue if the woman has endometriosis or to break adhesions in the pelvic cavity. Drugs can be used to treat endometriosis. For infections, antibiotics must be used. Surgery to repair a damaged fallopian tube, caused by an ectopic (tubal) pregnancy, a tubal ligation, or an infection, can be attempted, but it results in a low rate of normal pregnancies and a high rate of ectopic pregnancies. For these reasons, surgery isn't recommended often.

▲ see box, page 1073

■ see box, page 1073

Problems With the Cervix

Mucus in the cervix (the lower part of the uterus that opens into the vagina) acts as a filter, preventing bacteria in the vagina from entering the uterus; the mucus also enhances sperm survival. This mucus is thick and impenetrable to sperm until the follicular phase of the menstrual cycle, when the egg and follicle are maturing in the ovary. During this phase, the levels of the hormone estradiol increase, making the cervical mucus clear and elastic, so that sperm can move through it into the uterus to the fallopian tubes, where fertilization can take place.

Diagnosis and Treatment

A postcoital test, performed between 2 and 8 hours after intercourse, can determine whether sperm can survive in the cervical mucus. The test is scheduled for the midpoint of the menstrual cycle, when the estradiol level is highest and the woman is ovulating. Normally, the mucus is clear and can be stretched to 3 to 4 inches without breaking. Under a microscope, the mucus has a fernlike appearance, and at the highest magnification, at least five active sperm are visible at one time. Abnormal results include overly thick mucus, no sperm, and sperm clumping together because the mucus contains antibodies to the sperm. However, abnormal results don't always indicate a problem with the mucus. Sperm may be absent only because they were not deposited into the vagina during intercourse, and the mucus may be overly thick only because the test wasn't performed at the proper time in the menstrual cycle. Although this test is widely used, it's not highly accurate.

Treatment of cervical mucus problems includes intrauterine insemination, in which semen is placed directly in the uterus to bypass the mucus, and drugs to thin the mucus, such as guaifenesin—a common ingredient of cough syrups. However, there is no proof that these measures increase the likelihood of pregnancy.

Unidentified Factors

Even when no cause of infertility can be identified, the couple may be able to conceive eventually. Treating the woman with clomiphene or human menopausal gonadotropins and placing washed sperm in her uterus may reduce the time needed to conceive. If the woman hasn't conceived after four to six menstrual cycles, special techniques, such as in vitro fertilization or gamete intrafallopian tube transfer, may need to be considered.

Fertilization Techniques

After all other treatments have failed to result in a pregnancy, more and more infertile couples turn to **in vitro (test tube) fertilization.** This procedure involves stimulating the ovaries, retrieving released eggs, fertilizing the eggs, growing the embryos in a laboratory, and then implanting the embryos in the woman's uterus.

Typically, a combination of clomiphene, human menopausal gonadotropins, and a gonadotropin-releasing hormone agonist (a drug that stimulates the release of gonadotropins from the pituitary gland) is used to stimulate the ovaries so that many eggs will mature. Guided by ultrasound scanning, a doctor inserts a needle through the vagina or abdomen into the ovary and removes several eggs from the follicles. In the laboratory, the eggs are placed in a culture dish and fertilized with washed sperm. After about 40 hours, three or four embryos are transferred from the culture dish into the mother's uterus through the vagina. Additional embryos can be frozen in liquid nitrogen to be used later if pregnancy doesn't occur. Despite the transfer of several embryos, the chances of producing one full-term baby are only about 18 to 25 percent each time eggs are placed in the uterus.

If a woman has unexplained infertility or endometriosis but normal fallopian tube function, **gamete intrafallopian tube transfer (GIFT)** can be performed. Eggs and washed sperm are obtained as for in vitro fertilization, but the eggs aren't fertilized with the sperm in the laboratory. Instead, the eggs and sperm are transferred to the far end of the woman's fallopian tube through the abdominal wall (using laparoscopy) or the vagina (guided by ultrasound scanning), so that the egg can be fertilized in the fallopian tube. At most infertility centers, the success rate for each transfer is about 20 to 30 percent.

Variations of in vitro fertilization and GIFT include the transfer of a more mature embryo (zygote intrafallopian tube transfer), use of donor eggs, and transfer of frozen embryos to a surrogate mother. These techniques raise moral and ethical issues, including questions about the disposal of stored embryos (especially in cases of death or divorce), legal parentage if a surrogate mother is involved, and selective reduction of the number of implanted embryos (similar to abortion) when more than three develop.

Psychologic Aspects

While a couple is undergoing infertility treatment, one or both partners may experience frustration, emotional stress, feelings of inadequacy, and guilt. Feeling isolated and unable to communicate, they may become angry at or resentful toward each other, family, friends, or the doctor. During each month of treatment, the couple may vacillate between hope and despair. The emotional stress can lead to tearfulness, fatigue, anxiety, sleep or eating disturbances, and an inability to concentrate. In addition, the financial burden and time commitment involved in diagnosis and treatment can cause marital strife.

These problems can be lessened if both partners are involved in and are given information about the treatment process, regardless of which one has the diagnosed problem. Knowing what the chances of success are as well as realizing that treatment may not be successful and can't continue indefinitely can help a couple cope with the stress. Information about when to end treatment, when to seek a second opinion, and when to consider adoption is also helpful.

Counseling and psychologic support can help. Support groups for infertile couples, such as RESOLVE, are available at local and national levels.

CHAPTER 241

Family Planning

Family planning is the attempt to control the number and spacing of children.

A couple may use contraception to avoid pregnancy temporarily or sterilization to avoid pregnancy permanently. Abortion may be used to end a pregnancy when contraception has failed.

Contraception

Contraceptive methods include oral contraceptives (birth control pills), condoms, preparations that stop or kill sperm on contact (spermicides—in vaginal foams, creams, gels, and suppositories), withdrawal before ejaculation, diaphragms, cervical caps, rhythm methods, contraceptive implants, injectable contraceptives, and intrauterine devices (IUDs). Contraception may be used by a person who is physically able to conceive a baby and has sexual relations with someone of the opposite sex but doesn't want to have a baby right away. After learning about the advantages and disadvantages of various contraceptive methods, a person can choose the most suitable method.

Contraceptives must be used correctly to be effective. They are more likely to fail when used by people who are younger, have less education, or are less motivated to prevent pregnancy. From 5 to 15 percent of women using contraceptive methods designed for use at the time of sexual intercourse (diaphragm, condom, foam, withdrawal) become pregnant during the first year of use. Generally, these methods are less effective in preventing pregnancy than are oral contraceptives, implants, injectable contraceptives, and intrauterine devices, which provide longer-term protection and don't require last-minute decisions. From 0.1 to 3 percent of women using these longer-term contraceptive methods become pregnant during the first year of use.

ORAL CONTRACEPTIVES

Oral contraceptives, commonly known as the pill, contain hormones—either a combination of progestin and estrogen or progestin alone. They prevent pregnancy by stopping the ovaries from releasing eggs (ovulation) and by keeping the cervical mucus thick so that sperm can't easily pass through it.▲

▲ see page 1137

How Effective Is Contraception?

Method	Percentage of Women Who Become Pregnant During the First Year of Use
Oral contraceptives:	
Combination estrogen-progestin tablets	0.1–3
Progestin-only tablets	0.5–3
Condom:	
Male	3–12
Female	5–21
Diaphragm with spermicide	6–18
Cervical cap with spermicide	11.5–18
Rhythm method	20
Implants (levonorgestrel)	less than 0.1
Injectable medroxyprogesterone	0.3
Intrauterine device	0.6 to 2

Combination tablets are taken once a day for 3 weeks, not taken for a week to allow for the menstrual period, and then started again. Inactive tablets may be included for the week when the combination tablets aren't taken to establish a routine of taking one tablet a day. Progestin-only tablets are taken every day of the month. Missing or forgetting to take tablets may result in pregnancy.

Progestin-only tablets often cause irregular bleeding episodes. They are usually prescribed only when taking estrogen might be harmful—for instance, when a woman is breastfeeding.

The various brands of combination tablets are equally effective. Low-dose estrogen tablets have fewer serious side effects than the older high-

dose estrogen tablets. For women who take certain other drugs, particularly drugs for epilepsy, a doctor may prescribe higher-dose estrogen tablets.

Every woman who is considering oral contraceptives should discuss with her doctor the benefits and risks for her particular situation. Low-dose oral contraceptives pose very few health risks and have many health benefits unrelated to contraception. They reduce the risk of certain types of cancer but may increase the risk of others. A woman's risk of dying from a normal pregnancy or from an abortion is greater than her risk of dying from taking oral contraceptives.

Taking oral contraceptives also reduces the occurrence of menstrual cramps, premenstrual tension, irregular bleeding (in women whose periods have been irregular), anemia, breast cysts, ovarian cysts, tubal pregnancy (pregnancy mislocated in the fallopian tubes, a type of ectopic pregnancy),▲ and tubal infection. Also, women who have taken oral contraceptives are less likely to have rheumatoid arthritis and osteoporosis than women who never took them.

Before starting oral contraceptives, a woman undergoes a physical examination to make sure she has no health problems that would make them risky for her. If she or a close relative has had diabetes or heart disease, usually a blood test is performed to measure cholesterol and glucose (blood sugar) levels. When cholesterol or glucose levels are high, a doctor may prescribe low-dose oral contraceptives but will order more blood tests later to make sure these levels don't rise significantly. Three months after starting oral contraceptives, the woman undergoes another examination to be sure her blood pressure hasn't changed. After that, she undergoes an examination at least once a year.

Some women, such as those over age 35 who smoke, should not use oral contraceptives, because the risks outweigh the benefits. Other women may have a condition in which taking oral contraceptives increases risks. For example, taking oral contraceptives may cause blood pressure to rise in a woman who has high blood pressure. However, when the risks are thought to be balanced by the benefits, a woman can take an oral contraceptive, but a doctor carefully monitors her, so that the drug can be stopped if necessary.

Stopping oral contraceptives occasionally to use other contraceptive methods is unnecessary and has no benefits. Thus a woman doesn't need

▲ see box, page 1155

When Taking Oral Contraceptives Is Restricted

A woman must not take oral contraceptives if any of the following situations apply:

- She smokes and is over age 35
- She has active liver disease or tumors
- She has high triglyceride levels
- She has untreated high blood pressure
- She has diabetes with blockage of the arteries
- She has blood clots
- She has a leg immobilized (as in a cast)
- She has heart disease
- She has had a stroke
- She has had jaundice of pregnancy
- She has breast or uterine cancer

A woman may take oral contraceptives under a doctor's supervision if any of the following situations apply:

- She is depressed
- She frequently has migraine headaches
- She smokes cigarettes but is under age 35
- She has had hepatitis or another liver disease with full recovery

to stop taking the tablets unless she wants to become pregnant, is having intolerable side effects, or has another health problem that makes oral contraceptive use inadvisable. Healthy women who don't smoke can take low-dose oral contraceptives continuously until menopause.

Use After a Pregnancy

The risk of blood clots forming in leg veins increases after a pregnancy and may be further increased by taking oral contraceptives. However, if the pregnancy lasts fewer than 12 weeks from the last menstrual period, a woman can take oral contraceptives right away. She should wait 1 week if the pregnancy lasts 12 to 28 weeks and 2 weeks if the pregnancy lasts more than 28 weeks provided she isn't breastfeeding.

Mothers who breastfeed usually don't ovulate (release eggs) until at least 10 to 12 weeks after delivery. However, they may ovulate and become pregnant before the first menstrual period. Therefore, mothers who breastfeed should use some form of birth control if they don't want to become pregnant. Taking combination oral contraceptives while breastfeeding can reduce both the amount of milk produced and the concentrations of nutritious protein and fat in the milk. Hormones from the contraceptives are transferred to the breast milk and then to the baby. Therefore, mothers who are breastfeeding and want to take oral contraceptives should take progestin-only tablets, which don't affect breast milk production.

Oral contraceptives, if taken right up to conception or early in pregnancy—before a woman realizes she's pregnant—don't harm the fetus.

Side Effects

Bleeding at irregular times during the menstrual cycle is common during the first few months of oral contraceptive use, but abnormal bleeding usually stops as the body adjusts to the hormones. A woman may have no periods for a few months after stopping oral contraceptives, but these drugs don't reduce fertility permanently. Many troubling side effects, such as nausea, breast tenderness, bloating, fluid retention, an increase in blood pressure, and depression, are related to the estrogen in the tablet and are uncommon with the low-dose tablets. Other side effects, such as weight gain, acne, and nervousness, are related to the progestin and are also uncommon with the low-dose tablets. Some women who take oral contraceptives gain 3 to 5 pounds because of fluid retention—and possibly even more because of increased appetite.

Serious side effects are rare. The likelihood of developing gallstones increases during the first few years of oral contraceptive use, then declines. One of every 30,000 to 500,000 women who take oral contraceptives develops a benign liver tumor (adenoma)—a dangerous tumor if it ruptures and bleeds into the abdomen. Adenomas usually disappear on their own after oral contraceptives are stopped.

Blood clots are estimated to have been about three to four times more common in women who took the older high-dose tablets than in women who didn't use oral contraceptives. However, as the estrogen content in the tablets has been reduced, the risk of developing blood clots has also diminished, but it remains higher than that for women who don't use oral contraceptives. If a woman has sudden chest pain or pain in the legs, she must stop taking oral contraceptives and see her doctor immediately, because these symptoms may indicate that blood clots have formed in the leg veins and moved to the lungs or are about to do so. Because both oral contraceptives and surgery increase the risk of developing blood clots, a woman must stop taking oral contraceptives a month before elective surgery and not resume taking them until a month after surgery.

Women taking oral contraceptives may experience nausea and headache, and 1 to 2 percent become depressed and have trouble sleeping. Women should stop taking oral contraceptives and contact their doctor if they have any of the following symptoms, which may indicate an increased risk of a stroke: a problem with headaches, such as a change in their number or severity; tingling in the arms or legs; fainting; or an inability to speak. However, the risk of having a stroke is no greater for healthy women who are taking low-dose estrogen combination tablets than for healthy women of similar age who aren't taking oral contraceptives.

Taking oral contraceptives may change the amounts of some vitamins and other substances in the blood. For instance, the levels of the B vitamins and vitamin C decrease slightly, and the vitamin A level increases. These changes are considered unimportant, so vitamin supplements aren't needed.

In some women, oral contraceptives cause dark patches (melasma)▲ on the face, similar to those that may occur during pregnancy. Sun exposure darkens the patches even more. If the woman stops taking oral contraceptives, the dark patches slowly disappear. No specific treatment exists—other than discontinuing oral contraceptives as soon as the patches are noticed.

▲ see page 989

Using oral contraceptives doesn't change a woman's risk of developing breast cancer regardless of whether that risk was high or low. However, the risk of developing cervical cancer seems to increase among women who take oral contraceptives, particularly those who have taken the tablets for more than 5 years. Therefore, women taking oral contraceptives should have a Papanicolaou (Pap) test at least once a year so that changes in the cervix can be detected early. On the other hand, the risk of developing uterine or ovarian cancer decreases by about half among women who take oral contraceptives compared with women who have never taken them. Furthermore, this effect continues even after women stop taking them.

Interactions With Other Drugs

Oral contraceptives don't interfere with other drugs, but other drugs, particularly some sedatives and antibiotics, can diminish the effectiveness of oral contraceptives. Women taking oral contraceptives may become pregnant if they simultaneously take antibiotics such as rifampin and possibly penicillin, ampicillin, tetracyclines, or sulfonamides. While taking high doses of these antibiotics, women should use a barrier contraceptive, such as a condom or diaphragm, in addition to the oral contraceptive. The anticonvulsants phenytoin and phenobarbital can increase the frequency of abnormal bleeding in women who take oral contraceptives. To counter this effect, women who have epilepsy and take anticonvulsants need to take higher-dose oral contraceptives.

BARRIER CONTRACEPTIVES

Barrier contraceptives physically block the sperm's access to a woman's uterus. They include the condom, diaphragm, cervical cap, and vaginal foams, creams, gels, and suppositories.

Used properly, **condoms** can provide considerable protection against sexually transmitted diseases such as AIDS and can prevent certain precancerous changes in cells of the cervix. Some condoms have a reservoir at the tip to collect semen; if they don't, about half an inch of the condom should be left at the front of the penis. The condom must be removed carefully because if semen is spilled, sperm could enter the vagina,

Barrier Contraceptives

Barrier contraceptives prevent sperm from entering a woman's uterus. They include condoms, diaphragms, and cervical caps. Some condoms contain spermicides; spermicides should be used with condoms and other barrier contraceptives that don't already contain them.

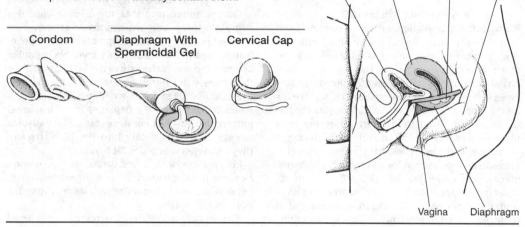

Condom   Diaphragm With Spermicidal Gel   Cervical Cap

Diaphragm in Place Over Cervix

Bladder   Uterus   Cervix   Rectum

Vagina   Diaphragm

resulting in pregnancy. A spermicide, either included in the condom's lubricant or inserted separately into the vagina, may increase the effectiveness of condom use.

The female condom, a newer device, is held in the vagina by a ring. It resembles male condoms but is larger and has a higher failure rate, so the male condom is preferable.

The **diaphragm,** a dome-shaped rubber cup with a flexible rim, fits over the cervix and keeps sperm from entering the uterus. Diaphragms come in various sizes and must be fitted by a doctor or nurse, who also teaches women how to insert them. A diaphragm should cover the entire cervix without causing discomfort. Neither the woman nor her partner should notice its presence. A contraceptive cream or jelly should always be used with a diaphragm, in case the diaphragm is displaced during intercourse. The diaphragm is inserted before intercourse and should remain in place for at least 8 hours but no more than 24 hours afterward. If sexual intercourse is repeated while the diaphragm is in place, additional spermicide should be inserted into the vagina to con-

tinue the protection. If a woman has gained or lost more than 10 pounds, has had a diaphragm for more than a year, or has had a baby or an abortion, she must be refitted for a diaphragm because the vagina's size and shape may have changed.

The **cervical cap,** which is similar to the diaphragm but smaller and more rigid, fits snugly over the cervix. These devices are also available in various sizes and must be fitted by a doctor or nurse. A contraceptive cream or jelly should always be used with a cervical cap, which is inserted before intercourse and left in place for at least 8 hours after intercourse, up to 48 hours at a time.

Vaginal foams, creams, gels, and suppositories are placed in the vagina before sexual intercourse. They contain a spermicide and also provide a physical barrier to sperm. No single type of foam or suppository seems to be more effective than another. As a woman ages, the effectiveness of these preparations typically increases because she becomes more skilled in using them and because her fertility decreases.

WITHDRAWAL BEFORE EJACULATION

In this contraceptive method, also called coitus interruptus, the man withdraws the penis from the vagina before ejaculation, when sperm are released during orgasm. This method isn't reliable because sperm may be released before orgasm. It also requires that the man have a high degree of self-control and precise timing.

RHYTHM METHODS

Rhythm methods depend on abstaining from sexual intercourse during a woman's fertile period. In most women, an egg is released from the ovary about 14 days before the start of a menstrual period. Although the unfertilized egg survives only about 24 hours, sperm can survive for 3 or 4 days after intercourse. Consequently, fertilization can result from intercourse that took place up to 4 days before the release of the egg.

The **calendar rhythm method** is the least effective of these methods, even for women who have regular menstrual cycles. To calculate when to abstain from intercourse, women subtract 18 days from the shortest and 11 days from the longest of their previous 12 menstrual cycles. For example, if a woman's cycles last from 26 to 29 days, she must avoid intercourse from day 8 through day 18 of each cycle.

Other, more effective rhythm methods include the temperature method, mucus method, and symptothermal method.

In the **temperature method,** a woman determines her basal body temperature (temperature of the body at rest) by taking her temperature each morning before getting out of bed. This temperature falls before the egg is released and rises slightly (less than 1° F.) after the egg is released. The couple avoids intercourse from the beginning of the woman's menstrual period until at least 48 to 72 hours after the day her basal body temperature has risen.

In the **mucus method,** the woman's fertile period is established by observing cervical mucus, which usually is secreted in larger amounts and becomes more watery shortly before the egg is released. The woman can have intercourse with a low risk of conception after her menstrual period ends until she observes an increased amount of cervical mucus. She then avoids intercourse until 4 days after the greatest (peak) amount of mucus has been observed.

The **symptothermal method** involves observing changes in both cervical mucus and basal body temperature as well as other symptoms that may be associated with the release of the egg, such as slight cramping pain. Of all the rhythm methods, this one is the most reliable for determining when to abstain from intercourse each month.

CONTRACEPTIVE IMPLANTS

Contraceptive implants are plastic capsules containing progestin, which prevents the ovaries from releasing eggs and keeps sperm from penetrating the thick mucus in the cervix. Six capsules are inserted under the skin of the inner arm above the elbow. After numbing the skin with an anesthetic, a doctor makes a small incision and uses a needle to implant the capsules in a fan-shaped pattern. No stitches are necessary. The capsules release progestin slowly into the bloodstream; they can remain in place for 5 years.

Interactions with other drugs are uncommon because the implants don't contain any estrogen. Otherwise, restrictions are similar to those for oral contraceptives.

The major side effects, irregular menstrual bleeding or no menstrual bleeding at all, may affect up to 40 percent of the women; less common side effects include headaches and weight gain. These side effects may influence women to have the capsules removed prematurely. Because the capsules don't dissolve in the body, a doctor has to remove them. Removal is more difficult than insertion because tissue under the skin thickens around the capsules, making them hard to get out but leaving only a minor scar. As soon as the capsules have been removed, the woman's ovaries return to their normal functioning and she becomes fertile again.

INJECTABLE CONTRACEPTIVES

Medroxyprogesterone, a progestin, is injected once every 3 months into a muscle of the buttock or upper arm. Although extremely effective, medroxyprogesterone can completely disrupt a menstrual cycle. About a third of the women using this contraceptive method have no menstrual bleeding in the first 3 months after the first injection, and another third have irregular bleeding and spotting for more than 11 days each month. As the method is used longer, more women have

Intrauterine Devices

Intrauterine devices (IUDs) are inserted by a doctor into a woman's uterus through the vagina IUDs are made of molded plastic. One type releases copper from a copper wire wrapped around the base; the other type releases progesterone. A plastic string is usually attached, so that a woman can check to make sure the device is still in place.

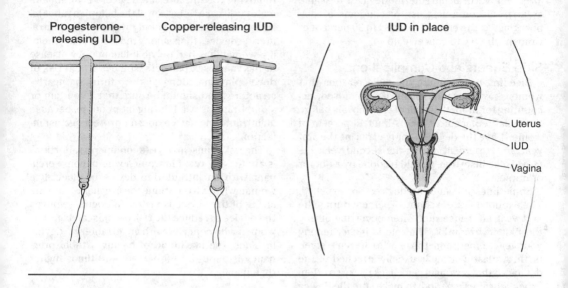

Progesterone-releasing IUD	Copper-releasing IUD	IUD in place

no menstrual bleeding but fewer women have irregular bleeding. After using this method for 2 years, about 70 percent of the women have no bleeding at all. When the injections are stopped, a regular menstrual cycle resumes in about half of the women within 6 months and in about three fourths within 1 year.

Because the drug has long-lasting effects, fertility may not return for up to a year after injections are stopped, but medroxyprogesterone doesn't make women permanently sterile. The drug may cause a slight weight gain. It also may cause temporary thinning of the bones (osteoporosis), but bones return to their previous density after the injections are stopped. Medroxyprogesterone doesn't increase the risk of developing any cancer, including breast cancer, and it greatly reduces the risk of developing cancer of the uterus. Interactions with other drugs are uncommon, and restrictions are similar to those for oral contraceptives.

INTRAUTERINE DEVICES

Only about one million women in the United States use intrauterine devices (IUDs) for contraception, even though they are very effective. These devices have some advantages over oral contraceptives: Side effects are limited to the inside of the uterus, and insertion involves only one birth control decision every year or every 10 years, depending on the type of intrauterine device chosen.

Two types are currently available in the United States. One type, which releases progesterone, must be replaced every year. The other, which releases copper, is effective for at least 10 years.

Although doctors usually insert the device into the uterus during a woman's menstrual period, it can be inserted at any time in the monthly cycle, provided a woman isn't pregnant. If there exists a possibility that the woman's cervix is infected, insertion of the device is postponed until the infection has been treated.

An intrauterine device seems to prevent conception by causing an inflammatory reaction inside the uterus that attracts white blood cells. Substances produced by the white blood cells are toxic (poisonous) to sperm, thus preventing fertilization of the egg. Removing the device halts the inflammatory reaction.

The likelihood of conceiving in the first year after removal of an intrauterine device is the same as after discontinuing use of condoms or diaphragms. At the end of 1 year, 80 to 90 percent of women who try to conceive do so.

Side Effects and Complications

Bleeding and pain are the main reasons that women have intrauterine devices removed, accounting for more than half of all removals before the usual replacement time. About 15 percent of women have the devices removed during the first year and 7 percent during the second year. Removal, like insertion, should be done by a doctor or nurse.

Sometimes intrauterine devices are expelled. The expulsion rate is about 10 percent during the first year after insertion, often occurring during the first few months. The rate is higher among younger women and those who haven't given birth. A plastic string is usually attached to the device so that a woman can check every so often, especially after a period, to make sure the device is still in place. If she can't find the string, she should use another contraceptive method until she can see her doctor to determine if the device is still in place. If a replacement intrauterine device is inserted after one has been expelled, it will probably stay in place. About 20 percent of expulsions aren't noticed and could be followed by pregnancy.

Perforation of the uterus is a potentially serious but uncommon complication that can occur during insertion. The risk is about 1 in 1,000 insertions. Usually, perforation itself doesn't produce symptoms; it's discovered when a woman can't find the plastic string and a doctor locates the intrauterine device with ultrasound scanning or x-ray. A device that perforates the uterus and ends up in the abdominal cavity must be removed to prevent it from injuring and scarring the intestine.

▲ see page 1083

The uterus is briefly infected at the time of insertion, but this infection clears up after 24 hours. Infections of the uterus or nearby structures that start after an intrauterine device has been in place for 30 days or more usually are sexually transmitted diseases, not the result of inserting the device. Unless the infection is severe or the woman is pregnant, these infections can be treated without removing the intrauterine device. Pelvic inflammatory disease (infection of the fallopian tubes)▲ is no more common among women using intrauterine devices than among those not using them. If a woman has had pelvic inflammatory disease or has many sex partners, she has a high risk of developing infections of the uterus or nearby structures and should be sure that a condom or a diaphragm is used during intercourse, because an intrauterine device doesn't protect against infections.

The risk of miscarriage (spontaneous abortion) is about 55 percent in women who become pregnant with an intrauterine device in place. If a woman wishes to continue the pregnancy and the string of the device is visible, a doctor removes the device to reduce the risk of a miscarriage. For women who conceive with an intrauterine device in place, the likelihood of having a tubal pregnancy is about 3 to 9 percent—10 times higher than usual.

Sterilization

About one third of all married couples in the United States who use family planning methods choose permanent sterilization—of either partner. Sterilization is the family planning method most often chosen by couples in which the woman is over 30 years old. In the first 10 years after female sterilization, about 2 percent of women become pregnant. The risk of pregnancy is less that 1 percent after male sterilization.

Sterilization should always be considered permanent. However, an operation that reconnects the appropriate tubes (reanastomosis) can be performed to restore fertility. Reanastomosis is more complex and less likely to be effective in men than in women. In couples, pregnancy rates are 45 to 60 percent after reanastomosis in men and 50 to 80 percent after reanastomosis in women.

Men are sterilized by **vasectomy** (cutting the vasa deferentia, the tubes that carry sperm from the testes). A vasectomy, which is performed by

Sterilization Techniques

Both fallopian tubes (tubes that carry the egg from the ovaries to the uterus) are cut, sealed, or blocked so that sperm can't reach the egg to fertilize it.

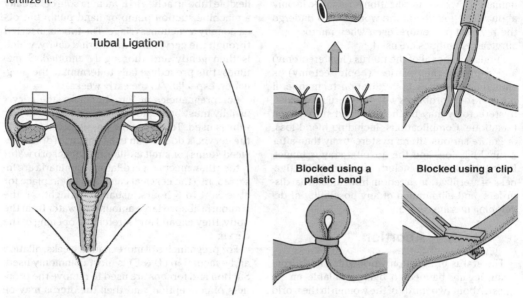

Tubal Ligation

Cut and tied

Sealed using cautery

Blocked using a plastic band

Blocked using a clip

a urologist in the office, takes about 20 minutes and requires only a local anesthetic. Through a small incision in the scrotum, a section of each vas deferens is removed and the open ends of the tubes are closed. A man shouldn't stop using contraception immediately; he usually isn't sterile until about 15 to 20 ejaculations after the operation because many sperm are stored in the seminal vesicles. The man is considered sterile after a laboratory test determines that two ejaculates are free of sperm. Complications of vasectomy include bleeding (in fewer than 5 percent of men), an inflammatory response to sperm leakage, and spontaneous reopening (in fewer than 1 percent), usually shortly after the procedure. Sexual activity, *with contraception*, may resume as soon after the procedure as the man desires.

Women are sterilized by **tubal ligation** (cutting and tying or blocking the fallopian tubes, which carry the egg from the ovaries to the uterus).

More complicated than vasectomy, tubal ligation requires an abdominal incision and a general or regional anesthetic. Women who have just delivered a child can be sterilized immediately after childbirth or on the following day, without staying in the hospital any longer than usual. Sterilization also may be planned in advance and performed as elective surgery.

Sterilization for women is often performed by laparoscopy. Working through a thin tube called a laparoscope inserted through a small incision in the woman's abdomen, a doctor cuts the fallopian tubes and ties off the cut ends. Alternatively, cautery (a device that produces electric current to cut through tissue) may be used to seal off about 1 inch of each tube. The woman usually goes home the same day. About one third of the pregnancies that occur after tubal ligation are tubal pregnancies. Up to 6 percent of women have minor complications after laparoscopy, but fewer than 1 percent have major complications, such as bleeding or punctures of the intestine.

Various mechanical devices, such as plastic bands and spring-loaded clips, can be used to block the fallopian tubes instead of cutting them. Sterilization is easier to reverse when these devices are used because they cause less tissue damage. However, sterilization is reversed in only about three fourths of the women who undergo the reversal procedure, even when microscopic surgical techniques are used.

Surgical removal of the uterus (hysterectomy) and perhaps the ovaries (oophorectomy) is sometimes used as a sterilization technique. If other chronic problems with the uterus also exist, hysterectomy may be the preferred sterilization technique. Complications, including blood loss, are more serious after a hysterectomy than after a tubal ligation, and the hospital stay is longer. Long-term benefits include complete effectiveness of sterilization, freedom from menstrual disorders, and elimination of any possibility of developing uterine cancer.

Abortion

The status of abortion worldwide varies from being legally banned to being available on request. About two thirds of the women in the world have access to legal abortion; about one twelfth live in countries where abortion is strictly prohibited. In the United States, abortion on request is legal during the first 3 months of pregnancy. After that, abortion is regulated by each state. In the United States, about 30 percent of all pregnancies are ended by abortion, which has become one of the most common surgical procedures performed in this country.

In general, contraception and sterilization have much lower complication rates than abortion, especially for young women. Therefore, contraception and sterilization (for a woman who does not wish to become pregnant later) are better choices for preventing an unintended pregnancy, and abortion should be reserved for situations in which safer techniques have failed.

Abortion methods include removing the contents of the uterus through the vagina (surgical evacuation) and using drugs to stimulate contractions of the uterus so that its contents are expelled. The procedure used depends on how many months a woman has been pregnant.

Surgical evacuation through the vagina is used for about 97 percent of abortions and almost always for pregnancies of less than 12 weeks. A technique called suction curettage is used. If it's performed during the first 4 to 6 weeks of pregnancy, the cervix needs to be dilated only a little, if at all. The instrument typically used is a small, flexible tube attached to a vacuum source, usually a machine suction pump or hand pump but occasionally a vacuum syringe. The tube is inserted through the cervix into the uterine cavity, which is then gently and thoroughly emptied. Sometimes, this procedure fails to terminate the pregnancy, especially in the early weeks.

For pregnancies of 7 to 12 weeks, the cervix usually must be dilated because a larger suction tube is used. To reduce the possibility of injuring the cervix, a doctor can use laminaria (dried seaweed stems) or similar dilators that absorb water rather than mechanical dilators. Laminaria are inserted into the cervical canal and left in place for at least 4 to 5 hours, usually overnight. As the laminaria absorb large amounts of water from the body, they expand and stretch the opening of the cervix.

For pregnancies of more than 12 weeks, dilation and evacuation (D & E) is most commonly used. Suction and forceps are used to remove the products of conception, and then the uterus may be gently scraped to make sure all such tissue is removed. Dilation and evacuation is increasingly being used in later pregnancy to induce abortion instead of drugs because its rate of serious complications is lower.

Drugs such as mifepristone (RU 486) and prostaglandins are sometimes used to induce abortions, especially after 16 weeks of pregnancy, because a dilation and evacuation at that stage can cause serious complications, such as damage to the uterus or intestine. RU 486 may also be used shortly after conception. Prostaglandins, drugs that stimulate the uterus to contract, may be given either as vaginal suppositories or injections. Side effects include nausea, vomiting, diarrhea, flushing of the face, and fainting. Prostaglandins may trigger an asthma attack in some women.

Mifepristone, when combined with a prostaglandin, is very effective in ending a pregnancy of less than 7 weeks. This drug blocks the action of progesterone in the uterine lining so that the prostaglandin is more effective. It's currently available (by prescription) only in Europe but may be available in the United States soon. Its effectiveness and safety are being tested in the United States.

High-dose oral contraceptives are sometimes prescribed to prevent pregnancy after a single act of unprotected sexual intercourse, but they aren't always effective. They must be taken within 72 hours. Side effects include nausea and vomiting.

Complications

The risk of complications from an abortion is directly related to the duration of pregnancy and the method used. The longer a woman has been pregnant, the greater the risk. The duration of pregnancy may be hard to estimate if the woman had any bleeding after she conceived, if she is overweight, or if the uterus points backward rather than forward. In these situations, an ultrasound examination is usually performed.

One serious complication is perforation of the uterus by a surgical instrument, which occurs in 1 of every 1,000 abortions. Sometimes the intestine or another organ is also injured. Major bleeding during or immediately after the procedure occurs in 6 of every 10,000 abortions. Especially

during the second 3 months of pregnancy, some procedures can cause a superficial tear or other damage to the cervix.

The most common delayed complications are bleeding caused by part of the placenta remaining in the uterus, infections, and blood clots in the legs. Very rarely, an infection in or near the uterus or scarring inside the uterus (Asherman's syndrome) can cause sterility. Women who have Rh-negative blood may be sensitized to the Rh-positive blood of the fetus—as in any pregnancy, spontaneous abortion, or delivery—unless they are given injections of $Rh_0(D)$ immune globulin.▲

Psychologic Aspects

For most women, abortion is not a threat to mental health and has no long-term adverse psychologic effects. Before abortions became legal, psychologic problems may have been related to the difficulties and stress of obtaining an abortion. Women more likely to be psychologically disturbed after an abortion are adolescents or women who had psychiatric problems before pregnancy, who terminated a desired pregnancy for medical reasons, who were ambivalent about the pregnancy, or who had an abortion late in the pregnancy.

CHAPTER 242

Tests for Genetic Disorders

Genetic disorders may result from defects in genes■ or from chromosomal abnormalities.★ For some people, genetic screening may be possible before they have a baby; others are identified as a carrier for a genetic disorder after they've had a baby or fetus with an abnormality. A genetic abnormality may be diagnosed before or after birth, using different techniques.

Genetic disorders may be apparent at birth (birth defects), or they may not appear until years later. Some defects may result from exposure before birth to drugs, chemicals, or other damaging factors, such as x-rays.

Family History

The first step in considering the possibility of a genetic abnormality is obtaining a family history. A doctor or genetic counselor constructs a family tree by asking about medical problems affecting family members. For an accurate appraisal of genetic risks, information about three genera-

▲ see page 1156

■ see page 8

★ see page 1237

tions is usually needed. The state of health or cause of death of all first-degree relatives (parents, siblings, children) and second-degree relatives (aunts, uncles, grandparents) is noted. Information about ethnic background and intermarriages among relatives is also helpful. If the family history is complicated, information about more distant relatives is needed. Medical records of selected relatives may be requested if they may have had a genetic disorder.

The diagnosis of many genetic disorders is based on a physical examination or laboratory test results. For stillborns or infants who die soon after birth, a detailed record of abnormalities is essential. Photographs and full-body x-rays of such babies, usually taken as part of the medical record, can be invaluable for future counseling. Also, tissues that are frozen and preserved (cryopreservation) can be useful for future genetic studies.

Carrier Screening

A carrier is a person who has a recessive gene for a particular trait but doesn't show it. Tests may be used to screen prospective parents to determine whether they are carriers for certain disorders. Problems can occur in a child whose mother and father carry a recessive gene for the same disease. Although neither parent has the disease, a child who receives the recessive gene from each of the parents will have the disease. The chances of this occurrence are one in four for each pregnancy.

The most common reasons for carrier screening are to provide prospective parents with information about whether a future child could receive two deleterious recessive genes and to help them make decisions about a pregnancy. For instance, parents may decide to have diagnostic tests before the birth (prenatal diagnosis) so that the fetus can be treated or the pregnancy terminated if the fetus has the disease. Alternatively, they may defer having children or use artificial insemination with a donor egg or sperm that does not carry the recessive gene.

Screening everyone for even the most common hereditary disorders is impossible. Whether

screening is performed depends on the following criteria:
• The disease caused by the recessive gene is highly debilitating or lethal
• A reliable screening test is available
• The fetus can be treated or reproductive options are available
• A person is likely to be a carrier because the disease runs in the family or is common in the ethnic, racial, or geographic group

In the United States, the disorders that currently meet these criteria include Tay-Sachs disease, sickle cell anemia, and the thalassemias. Screening may also be performed when a family has a history of hemophilia, cystic fibrosis, or Huntington's disease. A woman who has a brother with hemophilia may have a 50 percent risk of carrying the hemophilia gene. If screening shows that she isn't a carrier, she has virtually no risk of passing on the gene. This information can eliminate the need for more invasive prenatal tests. Several family members, including those who have the disease, are usually screened to determine the family pattern and thus obtain the best estimate of risk.

Sickle cell anemia is the most common hereditary disorder in blacks in the United States, affecting about 1 out of 400.▲ A person who has two recessive sickle cell genes—one from each parent—has **sickle cell disease.** A person who has one sickle cell gene and one normal gene has **sickle cell trait.** In such a person, the normal gene directs the production of normal red blood cells, and the sickle cell gene leads to the production of abnormal cells but not enough to make the person sick. However, these cells can be detected in blood samples. A person with the trait can be identified as a carrier of the disease.

Sickle cell disease can be diagnosed before birth with chorionic villus sampling, in which a sample of the placenta is removed and analyzed, or with amniocentesis, in which a sample of the amniotic fluid surrounding a fetus in the uterus is withdrawn and tested. Newborns can also be screened for the disease. About 10 percent of people born with sickle cell disease die in childhood.

Tay-Sachs disease, an autosomal recessive disorder, occurs in about 1 out of 3,600 infants of Ashkenazi Jewish or French-Canadian parents.■ Testing before or during pregnancy can detect whether a person is a carrier. Amniocentesis or chorionic villus sampling can be used to detect the disease in the fetus.

▲ see page 749

■ see page 684

The thalassemias are a group of hereditary disorders in which the production of normal hemoglobin is reduced, causing anemia.▲ The alpha-thalassemias are most common among people from Southeast Asia; in the United States, they occur most commonly among blacks. The beta-thalassemias are present in all races but are more common among people from Mediterranean countries, the Middle East, and parts of India and Pakistan. Carriers of both types can be identified by performing a routine blood cell count. More sophisticated tests can confirm the diagnosis. The disorder can be diagnosed in a fetus by using molecular biology techniques, which identify both those who have the disorder and those who are carriers.

Prenatal Diagnosis

Tests can be performed before birth (prenatal diagnosis) if the couple has an increased risk of having a baby with a chromosomal or genetic abnormality. Chromosomal abnormalities—in which the number or structure of chromosomes is abnormal—occur in about 1 out of 200 live births. Most fetuses who have chromosomal abnormalities die before birth, usually in the early months of pregnancy. Some of these abnormalities are inherited, but most are random occurrences. Down syndrome (trisomy 21) is the most common and most widely known chromosomal abnormality among liveborn infants, but many others occur. Most can be diagnosed before birth, but diagnostic tests can have very small but real risks, particularly for the fetus. For many couples, the risks outweigh the benefits of knowing whether their child has a chromosomal abnormality, so they choose not to be tested.

The risk of having a child with a chromosomal abnormality is increased in the following circumstances.

Pregnancy after age 35 is the most common risk factor for having a baby with Down syndrome. Although women of all ages have babies with chromosomal abnormalities, the incidence of Down syndrome increases with a woman's age—steeply after age 35, for reasons that aren't known. Testing for chromosomal abnormalities during pregnancy is usually offered to a woman who will be at least 35 years old when she gives birth and may be offered to younger women. The couple's

anxiety, regardless of the woman's age, often justifies prenatal testing.

In a pregnant woman, abnormal blood levels of markers—alpha-fetoprotein (a protein produced by the fetus), human chorionic gonadotropin (a hormone produced by the placenta), and estriol (an estrogen)—may indicate an increased risk of Down syndrome. Amniocentesis should then be considered.

A family history of chromosomal abnormalities also increases the risk. For a couple who has had one baby with Down syndrome, the risk of having another baby with a chromosomal abnormality is increased—to about 1 percent—if the woman is under 30 years old at the time of delivery. However, if the woman is over 30, the risk is the same as that for any woman her age.

For couples who have had a liveborn or stillborn baby with a physical abnormality whose chromosomal status isn't known, the risk of having another baby with a chromosomal abnormality is increased. Chromosomal abnormalities are more common in babies born with physical abnormalities, as well as in apparently normal stillborn babies, 5 percent of whom have chromosomal abnormalities.

A chromosomal abnormality in one or both parents increases the risk. Although carriers may be healthy and unaware of their chromosomal abnormalities, they have an increased risk of having chromosomally abnormal children and may have reduced fertility.

In some people, the genetic material in the chromosomes is rearranged—called a translocation or an inversion. These people may have no physical abnormality yet the risk of having children with chromosomal abnormalities is increased, because their children may receive an extra piece or may be missing a piece of a chromosome.

Prenatal testing is generally offered when a woman or man has an increased risk of having a child with a chromosomal abnormality. Such abnormalities may be found when a woman who has had repeated miscarriages or children born with abnormalities is tested.

In at least half of all miscarriages that occur during the first 3 months of pregnancy, the fetus has a chromosomal abnormality. In half of these,

---

▲ see page 751

How a Mother's Age Affects Her Chances of Having a Baby With a Chromosomal Abnormality

Age of Mother	Risk of Down Syndrome	Risk of Any Chromosomal Abnormality	Age of Mother	Risk of Down Syndrome	Risk of Any Chromosomal Abnormality
20	1 in 1667	1 in 526	35	1 in 385	1 in 192
21	1 in 1667	1 in 526	36	1 in 294	1 in 156
22	1 in 1429	1 in 500	37	1 in 227	1 in 127
23	1 in 1429	1 in 500	38	1 in 175	1 in 102
24	1 in 1250	1 in 476	39	1 in 137	1 in 83
25	1 in 1250	1 in 476	40	1 in 106	1 in 66
26	1 in 1176	1 in 476	41	1 in 82	1 in 53
27	1 in 1111	1 in 455	42	1 in 64	1 in 42
28	1 in 1053	1 in 435	43	1 in 50	1 in 33
29	1 in 1000	1 in 417	44	1 in 38	1 in 26
30	1 in 952	1 in 384	45	1 in 30	1 in 21
31	1 in 909	1 in 384	46	1 in 23	1 in 16
32	1 in 769	1 in 323	47	1 in 18	1 in 13
33	1 in 625	1 in 286	48	1 in 14	1 in 10
34	1 in 500	1 in 238	49	1 in 11	1 in 8

Data based on information in Hook EB: "Rates of chromosome abnormalities at different maternal ages." *Obstetrics and Gynecology* 58:282-285, 1981; and Hook EB, Cross PK, Schreinemachers DM: "Chromosomal abnormality rates at amniocentesis and in live-born infants." *Journal of the American Medical Association* 249(15):2034-2038, 1983.

the abnormality is an extra chromosome (trisomy).▲ If the fetus in a first miscarriage has a chromosomal abnormality, the fetus in subsequent miscarriages is also likely to have one, although not necessarily the same one. If a woman has had several miscarriages, the couple's chromosomes should be analyzed before they try to have another baby. If abnormalities are identified, the couple may choose to have prenatal diagnosis early in the next pregnancy.

Prenatal diagnosis by amniocentesis and ultrasound scanning is recommended for couples who have at least a 1 percent risk of having a baby with a defect of the brain or spinal cord (neural tube defect). In the United States, such birth defects occur in 1 out of 500 to 1,000 births. Some examples are spina bifida (an incompletely enclosed spinal cord) and anencephaly (the absence of a

▲ see box, page 1239

Some Genetic Disorders That Can Be Detected Before Birth

Disorder	Incidence	Inheritance
Cystic fibrosis	1 out of 2,500 white people	Recessive
Congenital adrenal hyperplasia	1 out of 10,000	Recessive
Duchenne's muscular dystrophy	1 out of 3,300 male births	X-linked
Hemophilia A	1 out of 8,500 male births	X-linked
Alpha- and beta-thalassemia	Varies widely, but present in most populations	Recessive
Huntington's disease	4 to 7 out of 100,000	Dominant
Polycystic kidney disease (adult type)	1 out of 3,000 by clinical diagnosis	Dominant
Sickle cell anemia	1 out of 400 black people in the United States	Recessive
Tay-Sachs disease (GM_2 gangliosidosis)	1 out of 3,600 Ashkenazi Jews and French Canadians; 1 out of 400,000 in other populations	Recessive

Adapted from Simpson JL, Elias S: "Prenatal diagnosis of genetic disorders," in *Maternal-Fetal Medicine: Principles and Practice,* ed. 2, edited by RK Creasy and R Resnick. Philadelphia, WB Saunders Company, 1989, pp 99-102; used with permission.

large part of the brain and skull).▲ Most of these defects are caused by abnormalities in several genes (polygenic). A few result from abnormalities in a single gene, chromosomal abnormalities, or exposure to drugs. The risk that the same defect will occur in other babies of a family that has had one such baby depends on the underlying cause. A couple who has had a baby with spina bifida or anencephaly has a 2 to 3 percent risk of having another baby with one of these defects. Couples who have had two children with such abnormalities have a 5 to 10 percent risk. The risk of recurrence also depends on where a person lives. In the United Kingdom, for example, the risk is higher than that in the United States. An increased risk may also be associated with an inadequate diet; therefore, folic acid supplements are now routinely recommended for all women of childbearing age.■ About 95 percent of all cases of spina bifida or anencephaly occur in families in which there is no history of these defects.

Tests for Prenatal Screening and Diagnosis

The most common tests used to screen for or diagnose genetic abnormalities in a fetus include ultrasound scanning, measuring levels of markers such as alpha-fetoprotein in a pregnant woman's blood, amniocentesis, chorionic villus sampling, and percutaneous umbilical blood sampling.

Ultrasound Scanning

Ultrasound scanning during pregnancy is very common and has no known risks for the woman or fetus. Whether all pregnant women should be scanned is controversial, but probably such scanning isn't routinely needed. Ultrasound scans are performed for many reasons throughout preg-

▲ see page 1234

■ see page 1224

nancy. During the first 3 months, an ultrasound scan can detect whether a fetus is alive, how old it is, and how many fetuses are present. After the third month, ultrasound scans can show whether there are any obvious structural birth defects in the fetus, where the placenta is located, and whether an appropriate amount of amniotic fluid is present. The sex of the fetus can usually be determined late during the second trimester.

Often, ultrasound scanning is used to check for abnormalities in the fetus when a pregnant woman has a high alpha-fetoprotein level or a family history of birth defects. However, no test is completely accurate, and a normal scan result doesn't guarantee a normal baby.

Alpha-Fetoprotein Levels

The level of alpha-fetoprotein is measured in a pregnant woman's blood as a screening test, because a high level indicates an increased likelihood of spina bifida, anencephaly, or other abnormalities. A high level may also indicate that the length of the pregnancy was underestimated when the blood sample was taken, more than one fetus is present, a miscarriage is likely (threatened abortion), or the fetus has died.

This test misses 10 to 15 percent of fetuses who have spinal cord defects. The most accurate results can be obtained when a blood sample is taken between 16 and 18 weeks of pregnancy; a sample taken before 14 weeks or after 21 weeks will not give accurate results. Sometimes, the test is repeated 7 days after the first blood sample.

If the alpha-fetoprotein level is high, an ultrasound scan is performed to determine whether an abnormality is present. In about 2 percent of the women screened, an ultrasound scan doesn't determine the reason for the high alpha-fetoprotein level. In these cases, amniocentesis is generally performed to measure the alpha-fetoprotein level in the amniotic fluid, which surrounds the fetus. This test detects neural tube defects more accurately than measuring the alpha-fetoprotein level in the mother's blood. However, the fetus' blood may leak into the amniotic fluid during amniocentesis, causing a falsely high alpha-fetoprotein level. Detecting the enzyme acetyl-

cholinesterase in the amniotic fluid helps support the diagnosis of an abnormality. In virtually all cases of anencephaly and in 90 to 95 percent of cases of spina bifida, the alpha-fetoprotein level is high and acetylcholinesterase can be detected in the amniotic fluid. About 5 to 10 percent of spina bifida cases can't be detected by amniocentesis because skin covers the opening over the spinal cord, thus alpha-fetoprotein can't leak out.

A number of other abnormalities may cause a high level of alpha-fetoprotein in the amniotic fluid, with or without a detectable level of acetylcholinesterase. These include narrowing of the stomach outlet (pyloric stenosis) and abdominal wall defects, such as an omphalocele.▲ Although high-resolution ultrasound scanning can often identify these abnormalities, normal results don't guarantee that the fetus is without abnormalities. Women who have a high alpha-fetoprotein level also are more likely to have complications during pregnancy, such as retarded growth or death of the fetus and early detachment of the placenta (abruptio placentae).

A low level of alpha-fetoprotein, typically with a high level of human chorionic gonadotropin and a low level of estriol, in a mother's blood suggests a different group of abnormalities, including Down syndrome. For example, a doctor can estimate the risk that the fetus has Down syndrome by considering the woman's age and the levels of these markers in her blood. Abnormal levels of these markers may also indicate that the length of the pregnancy has been incorrectly estimated or that the fetus has died.

If ultrasound scanning can't determine the cause of the abnormal marker levels in the blood, amniocentesis and a chromosome analysis are generally performed to check for Down syndrome and other chromosomal abnormalities.

Amniocentesis

One of the most common procedures for detecting abnormalities before birth is amniocentesis, which is best performed between 15 and 17 weeks of pregnancy.

During the procedure, the fetus is monitored by ultrasound scanning. A doctor notes heart motion, the fetus' age, the position of the placenta, the location of the amniotic fluid, and the number of fetuses. Then, guided by ultrasound, the doctor

▲ see page 1231

Detecting Abnormalities Before Birth

Amniocentesis and chorionic villus sampling are used to detect abnormalities in a fetus. In amniocentesis, a doctor uses ultrasound guidance to insert a needle through the abdominal wall into the amniotic fluid. A sample of fluid is withdrawn for analysis. This procedure is best performed between 15 and 17 weeks of pregnancy.

In chorionic villus sampling, a sample of chorionic villi, part of the placenta, is removed by one of two methods. In the transcervical method, a doctor inserts a catheter (a flexible tube) through the vagina and the cervix into the placenta. In the transabdominal method, a doctor inserts a needle through the abdominal wall into the placenta. In both methods, ultrasound guidance is used, and a sample of the placenta is suctioned out with a syringe. Chorionic villus sampling is usually performed between 10 and 12 weeks of pregnancy.

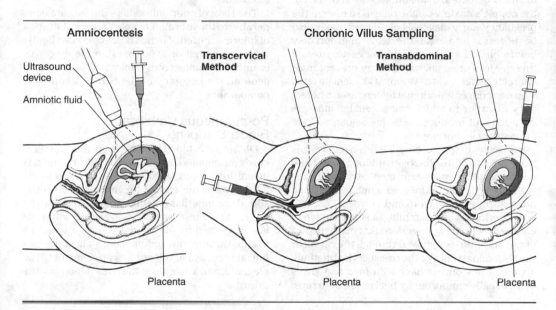

Amniocentesis

Ultrasound device

Amniotic fluid

Placenta

Chorionic Villus Sampling

Transcervical Method

Placenta

Transabdominal Method

Placenta

inserts a needle through the abdominal wall into the amniotic fluid. Fluid is withdrawn for analysis, and the needle is removed. Results are usually available in 1 to 3 weeks. Women who have Rh-negative blood receive $Rh_0(D)$ immune globulin after the procedure to decrease the risk of being sensitized by exposure to the fetus' blood.▲

Amniocentesis poses small risks for the woman and fetus. Brief vaginal spotting or leakage of amniotic fluid occurs in about 1 or 2 percent of the women and usually stops without treatment. After amniocentesis, the risk of miscarriage has been estimated at about 1 in 200, although some studies have found the risk to be lower. Needle injuries to the fetus are extremely rare. Amniocentesis can usually be performed when a woman is pregnant with twins or even more fetuses.

Chorionic Villus Sampling

Chorionic villus sampling is used to diagnose some disorders in the fetus, usually between 10

▲ see page 1155

and 12 weeks of pregnancy. Chorionic villus sampling may be used instead of amniocentesis unless a test specifically requires amniotic fluid—such as measuring the alpha-fetoprotein level in the amniotic fluid. Before the procedure, ultrasound scanning is performed to determine that the fetus is alive, to confirm the fetus' age, and to locate the placenta.

The primary advantage of chorionic villus sampling is that its results are available much earlier in the pregnancy than those of amniocentesis. With earlier results, simpler, safer methods can be used to terminate the pregnancy if an abnormality is detected. If no abnormality is detected, the couple's anxiety can be relieved earlier in the pregnancy. Early diagnosis of a disorder may also be necessary to treat the fetus appropriately before birth. For example, giving corticosteroid therapy to a pregnant woman may prevent male characteristics from developing in a female fetus who has congenital adrenal hyperplasia, a hereditary disorder in which the adrenal glands are enlarged and produce excessive amounts of androgens (male hormones).

If a woman whose blood is Rh-negative has been sensitized to Rh-positive blood, chorionic villus sampling isn't performed because it may worsen her condition. Instead, amniocentesis can be performed between 15 and 17 weeks.

In chorionic villus sampling, a small sample of chorionic villi (tiny projections that make up part of the placenta) is removed through the cervix or the abdominal wall. For the transcervical method, a woman lies on her back with hips and knees bent, usually supported by heel or knee stirrups.

Guided by ultrasound, a doctor inserts a catheter (a flexible tube) through the vagina and the cervix into the placenta. A small sample of the placenta is suctioned into the catheter with a syringe. The transcervical method can't be used if a woman has an abnormality of the cervix or an active genital infection—such as genital herpes, gonorrhea, or a chronic cervical inflammation. For the transabdominal method, the skin over the insertion site is anesthetized, a needle is inserted through the abdominal wall into the placenta, and a sample is suctioned out with a syringe. Neither method is painful. The sample is analyzed in a laboratory.

The risks of chorionic villus sampling are comparable to those of amniocentesis, except the risk of injuring the fetus' hands or feet may be slightly increased (1 out of 3,000 cases). If the diagnosis is unclear, amniocentesis may be necessary. In general, the accuracy of the two procedures is comparable.

Percutaneous Umbilical Blood Sampling

Obtaining a blood sample from the umbilical cord (percutaneous umbilical blood sampling) is useful for rapid chromosome analysis, particularly toward the end of pregnancy when ultrasound scanning has detected abnormalities in the fetus. Often, results can be available within 48 hours. Guided by ultrasound, a doctor inserts a needle through the abdominal wall into the umbilical cord, usually close to its attachment to the placenta, and a sample of the fetus' blood is withdrawn.

CHAPTER 243

Pregnancy

Pregnancy is the condition of carrying a fetus in the body, from conception to delivery.

Conception

Conception (fertilization) is the beginning of pregnancy, when an egg is fertilized by a sperm.

As part of the normal menstrual cycle, one egg (ovum) is released from one of the ovaries about

14 days before the next menstrual period. Release of the egg is called ovulation. The egg is swept into the funnel-shaped end of one of the fallopian tubes, where fertilization may occur, and is transported to the uterus. If fertilization doesn't occur, the egg degenerates and passes through the uterus with the next menstrual period. If, however, the egg is penetrated by a sperm, it is fertil-

From Egg to Embryo

Once a month, an egg is released from an ovary into a fallopian tube. After sexual intercourse, sperm move from the vagina through the cervix and uterus to the fallopian tubes, where one sperm fertilizes the egg. The fertilized egg (zygote) divides repeatedly as it moves down the fallopian tube to the uterus. First, the zygote becomes a solid ball of cells, then a hollow ball of cells called a blastocyst. Inside the uterus, the blastocyst implants in the uterine wall, where it develops into an embryo and a placenta.

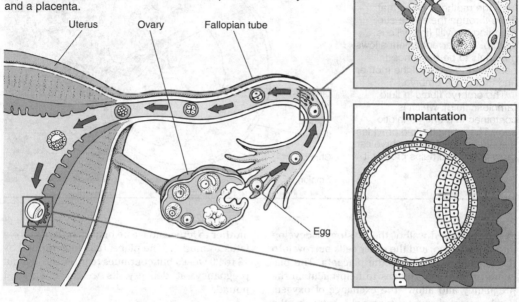

ized and begins to grow into an embryo through a series of cell divisions.

If more than one egg is released and fertilized, a multiple pregnancy—usually twins—occurs. In such a case, the twins are fraternal. Identical twins result when a fertilized egg separates into two independent cells the first time it divides.

At ovulation, the layer of mucus in the cervix (the lower part of the uterus that opens into the vagina) becomes more fluid, allowing sperm to enter the uterus rapidly. Sperm may move from the vagina to the funnel-shaped end of a fallopian tube—the usual site of conception—within 5 minutes. The cells lining the fallopian tube facilitate fertilization and the subsequent development of the fertilized egg (zygote).

The zygote divides repeatedly as it moves down the fallopian tube; it enters the uterus in 3 to 5 days. In the uterus, it becomes a blastocyst, a hollow ball of cells.

Implantation and Development of the Placenta

Implantation is the attachment of the blastocyst to the wall of the uterus, where it becomes embedded.

The blastocyst usually implants near the top of the uterus, on the front or back wall. The blastocyst's wall is one cell thick except in one area where it is three to four cells thick. The inner cells

Placenta and Embryo at 8 Weeks

The developing placenta forms tiny projections (villi) that extend into the wall of the uterus. Blood vessels from the embryo, which pass through the umbilical cord, develop in the villi. A thin membrane separates the embryo's blood in the villi from the mother's blood that flows through the space surrounding the villi (intervillous space). This arrangement allows materials to be exchanged between the blood of the mother and that of the embryo.

The embryo floats in fluid (amniotic fluid), which is contained in a sac (amniotic sac). The amniotic fluid provides a space in which the embryo can grow freely and helps protect it from injury.

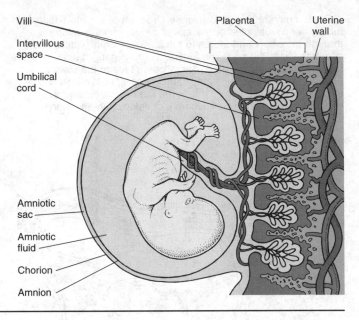

in the thickened wall of the blastocyst develop into the embryo, and the outer cells burrow into the uterine wall to form the placenta. The placenta produces hormones to help maintain the pregnancy and allows the exchange of oxygen, nutrients, and waste materials between the mother and fetus. Implantation begins between 5 and 8 days after fertilization and is completed by 9 or 10 days.

The wall of the blastocyst becomes the outer layer of membranes (chorion) surrounding the embryo. An inner layer of membranes (amnion) develops by about day 10 to 12, forming the amniotic sac. The amniotic sac fills with a clear liquid (amniotic fluid) and expands to envelop the developing embryo, which floats within it.

Tiny projections (villi) from the developing placenta extend into the wall of the uterus and branch and rebranch in a complicated treelike arrangement. This arrangement greatly increases the area of contact between the mother and placenta, allowing more nutrients to pass from

mother to fetus and waste materials to pass from fetus to mother. The placenta is fully formed by 18 to 20 weeks but continues to grow throughout pregnancy; at delivery, its weight is about 1 pound.

Development of the Embryo

The embryo is first recognizable within the blastocyst about 10 days after fertilization. Shortly thereafter, the area that will become the brain and spinal cord (neural crest) begins to develop, and the heart and major blood vessels begin to develop by about day 16 or 17. The heart begins to pump fluid through the blood vessels by day 20, and the first red blood cells appear the next day. After this, blood vessels continue to develop throughout the embryo and in the placenta. Organs are completely formed by 12 weeks of pregnancy (roughly 10 weeks after fertilization), except for the brain and spinal cord, which continue to mature throughout pregnancy. Most malformations occur during the first 12 weeks of pregnancy, the period of organ formation, when the embryo is most vulnerable to the effects of drugs or viruses, such as the one that causes German measles (rubella). Therefore, a pregnant woman shouldn't have any immunizations or take any drugs during the first 12 weeks of pregnancy unless they are considered essential to protect her health. Drugs known to cause malformations must especially be avoided during this period.▲

At first, the developing embryo is situated under the lining of the uterus on one side of the uterine cavity, but by 12 weeks, the fetus—the term used after 8 weeks of pregnancy—has grown so much that the lining on both sides of the uterus meets, because the fetus fills the entire uterus.

Dating a Pregnancy

Pregnancies are conventionally dated in weeks, starting from the first day of the last menstrual period. Because ovulation usually occurs about 2 weeks after a woman's menstrual period starts and fertilization usually occurs shortly after ovulation, the embryo is roughly 2 weeks younger than the number of weeks traditionally assigned to the pregnancy. In other words, a woman who is "4 weeks pregnant" is carrying a 2-week-old embryo. If a woman's periods are irregular, the actual difference may be more or less than 2 weeks. From a practical standpoint, when a woman's period is 2 weeks late, she is considered to be 6 weeks pregnant.

Pregnancy lasts an average of 266 days (38 weeks) from the date of conception or 280 days (40 weeks) from the first day of the last menstrual period. The approximate date of delivery can be calculated by counting back 3 calendar months from the first day of the last menstrual period and adding 1 year and 7 days. Only 10 percent or fewer of pregnant women give birth on the calculated date, but 50 percent give birth within 1 week and almost 90 percent give birth within 2 weeks—before or after the date. Therefore, delivery 2 weeks before or after the calculated date is considered normal.

Pregnancy is divided into three 3-month periods, called the first trimester (weeks 1 to 12), second trimester (weeks 13 to 24), and third trimester (week 25 to delivery).

Detecting a Pregnancy

If a woman who usually has regular menstrual periods is a week or more late, she may be pregnant. In the early months of pregnancy, a woman may experience breast swelling and nausea with occasional vomiting. Breast swelling is caused by increased levels of female hormones—mainly estrogen but also progesterone. Nausea and vomiting may be caused by estrogen and human chorionic gonadotropin (HCG). These two hormones, which help maintain the pregnancy, are produced by the placenta beginning about 10 days after fertilization. Early in pregnancy, many women feel unusually tired, and some experience bloating of the abdomen.

If a woman is pregnant, the cervix is softer than usual and the uterus is irregularly softened and enlarged. Usually, the vagina and cervix become bluish to purple, apparently because they are engorged with blood. A doctor can detect these changes during a pelvic examination.

Usually, a pregnancy test of blood or urine can determine whether a woman is pregnant. An ELISA (enzyme-linked immunosorbent assay) pregnancy test can detect even low levels of human chorionic gonadotropin in the urine quickly and easily. Some of the most sensitive pregnancy tests using this method can detect the extremely low levels of human chorionic gonadotropin that are present about $1\frac{1}{2}$ weeks after fertilization and take only about a half an hour. Other even more sensitive tests, which also detect human chorionic gonadotropin, can determine whether a woman is pregnant several days after fertilization—before a menstrual period is missed. During the first 60 days of a normal pregnancy with one fetus, human chorionic gonadotropin levels double about every 2 days.

The uterus enlarges throughout pregnancy. At 12 weeks, it extends beyond the pelvis into the abdomen and can usually be felt when the lower abdomen is examined. The enlarging uterus extends to the level of the navel by 20 weeks and to the lower edge of the rib cage by 36 weeks.

Other ways of detecting pregnancy include the following:

▲ see page 1167

• Detecting the fetus' heartbeat with a specialized stethoscope or a Doppler ultrasound instrument. The heartbeat can be detected as early as 18 to 20 weeks of pregnancy with this stethoscope and as early as 12 to 14 weeks with the ultrasound instrument.

• Feeling the fetus' movements. The mother always feels the movements before the doctor does, ordinarily at 16 to 20 weeks. Women who have been pregnant before generally feel movements earlier than do women who are pregnant for the first time.

• Detecting the enlarged uterus with ultrasound scanning. The enlarged uterus can be seen at about 6 weeks. The fetus' heart beating may be seen at 6 weeks and is seen at 8 weeks in more than 95 percent of pregnancies.

Physical Changes During Pregnancy

Pregnancy causes many changes throughout the body, most of which disappear after delivery.

Heart and Circulation

During pregnancy, the amount of blood pumped by the heart every minute (cardiac output) increases by 30 to 50 percent. The increase begins by 6 weeks and peaks between 16 and 28 weeks, usually at about 24 weeks. As cardiac output increases, the heart rate at rest speeds up from the normal 70 beats per minute to 80 or 90 beats per minute. After 30 weeks, cardiac output may decrease slightly as the enlarging uterus presses on the veins that carry blood from the legs back to the heart. During labor, however, cardiac output increases by an additional 30 percent. After delivery, cardiac output decreases rapidly at first, to about 15 to 25 percent above the prepregnancy level, then more slowly until it returns to the prepregnancy level—about 6 weeks after delivery.

The increase in cardiac output during pregnancy probably results from changes in the blood supply to the uterus. As the fetus grows, more blood is sent to the mother's uterus. At the end of pregnancy, the uterus is receiving one fifth of the mother's entire blood supply.

During exercise, cardiac output, heart rate, and respiration rate increase more in pregnant women than in nonpregnant women. X-rays and electrocardiograms show a number of changes in the heart, and certain heart murmurs and occasional rhythm irregularities of the heartbeat may appear. All of these changes are normal in pregnancy, but some abnormalities of heart rhythm may require treatment.

Blood pressure usually decreases during the second trimester but may return to normal in the third trimester.

The volume of blood in the circulation increases by 50 percent during pregnancy, but the number of red blood cells, which carry oxygen throughout the body, increases by only 25 to 30 percent. For reasons not clearly understood, the number of white blood cells, which fight infection, increases slightly during pregnancy and markedly during labor and the first few days after delivery.

Kidneys

Like the heart, the kidneys work harder throughout pregnancy. They filter an increasing volume of blood—as much as 30 to 50 percent more—reaching a maximum between 16 and 24 weeks until immediately before delivery, when pressure from the enlarging uterus may slightly decrease their blood supply.

The activity of the kidneys normally increases when a person lies down and decreases when a person stands up. This difference is amplified during pregnancy—which is one reason a pregnant woman feels the need to urinate frequently while trying to sleep. Late in pregnancy, the increase in kidney activity is even greater when a pregnant woman lies on her side rather than on her back. Lying on the side relieves the pressure that the enlarged uterus puts on veins carrying blood from the legs and thus improves blood flow, increasing kidney activity and cardiac output.

Lungs

The space taken up by the enlarging uterus and the increased production of the hormone progesterone cause the lungs to function differently during pregnancy. A pregnant woman breathes faster and more deeply because more oxygen is needed for herself and the fetus. The circumference of the woman's chest enlarges slightly. The lining of the respiratory tract receives more blood and becomes somewhat congested. Occasionally, the nose and throat become partly blocked by this congestion, resulting in a temporary stuffy nose and blockage of the eustachian tubes (tubes that

connect the middle ear to the back of the nose)
The tone and quality of the woman's voice may
change slightly. Virtually every pregnant woman
gets somewhat more out of breath when she ex-
erts herself, especially toward the end of pregnancy.

Digestive System

As pregnancy progresses, pressure from the enlarging uterus on the rectum and the lower part
of the intestine may cause constipation. Constipation may be worsened because the automatic
waves of muscular contractions in the intestine,
which normally move food along, are slowed by
the high levels of progesterone present during
pregnancy. Heartburn and belching are common,
possibly because food remains in the stomach
longer and because the sphincter (a ringlike muscle) at the lower end of the esophagus tends to
relax, allowing the stomach contents to flow back-
wards into the esophagus. Stomach ulcers are uncommon during pregnancy, and those that already exist often improve because less stomach
acid is produced.

The risk of gallbladder disease increases. Even
later in life, women who have been pregnant have
more gallbladder problems than women who
have not been pregnant.

Skin

Mask of pregnancy (melasma) is a blotchy,
brownish pigment that may appear on the skin of
the forehead and cheeks. Pigmentation may also
increase in the skin surrounding the nipples (are-
olae). A dark line commonly appears down the
middle of the abdomen.

Small, spiderlike blood vessels (spider angiomas) may appear in the skin, usually above the
waist, as may thin-walled, dilated capillaries, especially in the lower legs.

Hormones

Pregnancy affects virtually all hormones in the
body. The placenta produces several hormones
that help the body maintain the pregnancy. The
major hormone produced by the placenta, human
chorionic gonadotropin, prevents the ovaries
from releasing eggs and stimulates the ovaries to
continuously produce the high levels of estrogen
and progesterone needed to maintain pregnancy.
The placenta also produces a hormone that

causes the woman's thyroid gland to become
more active. A more active thyroid gland frequently causes a fast heartbeat, an awareness of
heartbeat (palpitations), excessive perspiration,
and mood swings, and the thyroid gland may become enlarged.▲ However, the disorder hyperthyroidism, in which the thyroid gland is truly
overactive, occurs in less than 1 percent of pregnancies.

The placenta also produces a melanocyte-stim-
ulating hormone that causes the skin to darken
and may produce a hormone that increases the
levels of adrenal hormones in the blood. The
increase in adrenal hormone levels probably
causes the pink stretch marks that may appear
on the abdomen.

During pregnancy, more insulin is needed and
is produced by the pancreas. In a pregnant
woman who has diabetes, the disorder may therefore worsen. In addition, diabetes can begin during pregnancy, a condition called gestational diabetes.■

Care During Pregnancy

Ideally, before becoming pregnant, a woman
should see a doctor to be screened for possible
diseases and to discuss the dangers of tobacco,
alcohol, and other substances when used during
pregnancy. Issues such as diet and social or medical problems also can be discussed at this time.

Having an examination between 6 and 8 weeks
of pregnancy (when a menstrual period is 2 to 4
weeks late) is particularly important, so that the
length of the pregnancy can be estimated and the
date of delivery can be predicted as accurately as
possible.

The first physical examination during pregnancy is almost always very thorough. Weight,
height, and blood pressure are measured. The
neck, thyroid gland, breasts, abdomen, arms, and
legs are examined; the heart and lungs are examined with a stethoscope; and the backs of the eyes
are examined with an ophthalmoscope. The doctor also performs a pelvic and a rectal examination, noting the size and position of the uterus
and any abnormalities of the pelvis, such as a

▲ see page 1164

■ see page 1163

deformity resulting from a fracture. Determining the pelvic bone dimensions helps the doctor anticipate how easily the baby will pass through at delivery.

A sample of blood is taken for a complete blood cell count; for laboratory tests for syphilis, hepatitis, gonorrhea, chlamydial infection, and other sexually transmitted diseases; and for blood typing and screening for Rh antibodies. A test for human immunodeficiency virus (HIV) is recommended. The sample is also tested for evidence of previous exposure to German measles (rubella).

Also routine are extensive tests on a sample of the woman's urine and a Papanicolaou (Pap) test▲ for cervical cancer. Black women and women of Mediterranean descent are tested for sickle cell trait or disease. If a woman has a high risk of conceiving a baby with a genetic abnormality, genetic tests are performed.■ Skin tests for tuberculosis are advisable for women from Asia, Latin America, and many urban environments, where the risk of developing the disease is higher than normal. A chest x-ray is performed only when a woman is known to have a heart or lung disorder; otherwise, x-rays should be avoided, especially during the first 12 weeks of pregnancy, because the fetus is extremely sensitive to the harmful effects of radiation. If an x-ray is required, the fetus must be shielded by placing a lead-filled garment over the woman's lower abdomen so that the uterus is covered.

Women who have had large babies or unexplained miscarriages, who have sugar in the urine, or who have a close relative with diabetes should be screened for diabetes soon after 12 weeks of pregnancy. At 28 weeks, all women should be screened for diabetes.

Between 16 and 18 weeks, the level of alphafetoprotein, a protein produced by the fetus, may be measured in the woman's blood. If the level is high, the woman may be carrying a fetus with spina bifida or more than one fetus. A high level also may indicate that the date of conception was miscalculated. If the level is low, the fetus may have chromosomal abnormalities.

Ultrasound scanning is the safest imaging technique. Evidence of pregnancy can be seen as early

as the fourth or fifth week after ovulation, and fetal growth can be followed until the baby's birth. Ultrasound scanning produces high-quality images, including live-action shots that show the fetus in motion. These images give the doctor helpful information and can reassure the mother. Many doctors believe that at least one ultrasound examination should be performed during each pregnancy to make sure the pregnancy is progressing normally and to verify the expected date of delivery.

Before an ultrasound scan of the abdomen is performed, especially early in pregnancy, a woman must drink a lot of water, because a full bladder pushes the uterus out of the pelvis so that a clearer image of the fetus can be obtained. When a vaginal probe is used, the bladder need not be full, and a doctor can detect pregnancy even earlier than with an abdominal scan.

If a woman and her doctor can't pinpoint the date of conception, ultrasound scanning is the most accurate way to establish this date. Dating is most accurate when performed during the first 12 weeks of a pregnancy and again at 18 to 20 weeks.

Ultrasound scanning can determine whether the fetus is growing at a normal rate. It's also used to record fetal heartbeat or breathing movements, to see whether a woman is carrying more than one fetus, and to identify a variety of abnormalities, such as mislocation of the placenta (placenta previa) or an abnormal position of the fetus. Ultrasound scanning helps guide the needle during removal of a sample of amniotic fluid (amniocentesis) for genetic or lung maturity studies of the fetus and during fetal blood transfusion.

Toward the end of pregnancy, a doctor may use ultrasound scanning to identify early (preterm) labor or premature rupture of membranes, when the fluid-filled membranes containing the fetus break before labor begins. Ultrasound scanning can provide information that helps a doctor decide whether to perform a cesarean section.

After the first examination, a pregnant woman should see her doctor every 4 weeks until 32 weeks of pregnancy, then every 2 weeks until 36 weeks, then once a week until delivery. At each examination, the woman's weight and blood pressure usually are recorded, and the size and shape of the uterus is measured to determine whether the fetus is growing and developing normally. A small urine sample is tested for sugar and protein.

▲ see page 1073

■ see page 1129

Sugar in the urine may indicate diabetes, and protein may indicate preeclampsia (high blood pressure, protein in the urine, and fluid accumulation during pregnancy). The ankles are examined for swelling.

If the mother has Rh negative blood, it's tested for Rh antibodies. If the mother has Rh-negative blood and the father has Rh-positive blood, the fetus may have Rh-positive blood.▲ If the fetus' Rh-positive blood enters the mother's bloodstream at any time during pregnancy, the mother may produce Rh antibodies that can pass into the fetus' bloodstream and destroy red blood cells, leading to jaundice, possible brain damage, or death of the fetus.

An average-size woman should gain a total of about 25 to 30 pounds during pregnancy—about 2 or 3 pounds each month. Gaining more than 30 to 35 pounds puts fat on both fetus and mother. Because controlling weight gain is more difficult later in pregnancy, a woman should try to avoid gaining most of the weight during the first months. However, not gaining weight is an ominous sign, especially if the total weight gain is less than 10 pounds, and may indicate that the fetus isn't growing fast enough—a condition called fetal growth retardation.

Sometimes, weight gain is caused by fluid retention resulting from poor blood flow in the legs when a woman stands. Usually, the woman can relieve this problem by lying on one side—preferably the left side—for 30 to 45 minutes two or three times a day.

During pregnancy, most women should add about 250 calories to their daily diet to provide nourishment for the developing fetus. Although protein should supply most of these calories, the diet should be well balanced, including fresh fruits, grains, and vegetables. High-fiber, sugar-free cereals are excellent. Salt, preferably iodized, may be used in moderation, but foods that are excessively salty or that contain preservatives should be avoided. Dieting to lose weight during pregnancy isn't recommended, even for obese women, because some weight gain is essential for proper fetal development and dieting reduces the supply of nutrients to the fetus. Although the fetus has first choice of nutrients, the mother must make sure that the choice involves something worthwhile.

Ultrasound Scanning: Viewing the Fetus

In ultrasound scanning, a transducer (a device that produces sound waves) is placed on the woman's abdomen. The sound waves penetrate the body, reflect off internal structures, and are converted to electric impulses, which are processed to form an image displayed on a monitor.

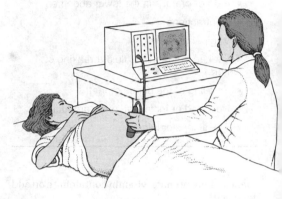

Drugs aren't generally recommended.■ A pregnant woman shouldn't take any drug, including nonprescription (over-the-counter) drugs, such as aspirin, without first checking with her doctor, particularly during the first 3 months. Iron requirements increase greatly during pregnancy to meet the needs of the fetus and mother. Usually, iron supplements are needed—especially by anemic women—because the average woman doesn't absorb enough iron from food to meet the demands of pregnancy, even when combined with iron already stored in her body. Iron supplements may cause mild stomach upset and constipation. Iron requirements become even greater during the second half of the pregnancy. If the diet is adequate, other vitamins and supplements may not be needed, although most doctors recom-

▲ see page 1155

■ see page 1167

Symptoms to Report Immediately to a Doctor

- Persistent headaches
- Persistent nausea and vomiting
- Dizziness
- Disturbances of eyesight
- Pain or cramps in the lower abdomen
- Contractions
- Vaginal bleeding
- Leakage of amniotic fluid (breaking of waters)
- Swelling of the hands or feet
- Reduced or increased urine production
- Any illness or infection

---

mend a daily prenatal vitamin containing iron and folic acid.

Nausea and vomiting may be relieved through dietary changes, such as drinking and eating small portions frequently, eating before getting hungry, and eating bland foods (for example, bouillon, consommé, rice, and pasta) rather than strong or spicy foods. Eating plain soda crackers and sipping a carbonated drink often relieve nausea. Keeping crackers by the bed and eating one or two before getting up is a time-honored solution for morning sickness. No drugs for morning sickness are currently approved by the Food and Drug Administration. If nausea and vomiting are so intense or persistent that the woman becomes dehydrated, loses weight, or develops any other problems, she may have to be hospitalized temporarily and given fluids intravenously.▲

Swelling (edema) is common, especially in the legs. Varicose veins in the legs and the area around the vaginal opening (vulva) also are common and may cause discomfort. Clothing around the waist and legs should be loose. Wearing elastic support hose or resting frequently with the

legs up, preferably lying on the left side, usually reduces leg swelling.

Hemorrhoids (piles), a common problem, can be treated with stool softeners, anesthetic gel, or warm soaks if they hurt.

Backache in varying degrees is common. Eliminating excessive strain on the back and wearing a lightweight maternity girdle may be helpful. Pain in the pelvic bone across the lower abdomen (symphysis pubis) occurs occasionally.

Heartburn, usually caused by the backup of stomach contents into the esophagus, can be relieved by eating smaller meals, avoiding either bending or lying flat for several hours after eating, and taking antacids (except sodium bicarbonate).

Tiredness is common, especially in the first 12 weeks and again in late pregnancy.

Pregnant women commonly have an increased vaginal discharge, which is usually normal. Trichomoniasis (a protozoan infection) and candidiasis (a yeast infection) are common vaginal infections during pregnancy and can be easily treated.■ Bacterial vaginosis, a bacterial infection, may cause preterm labor and must be treated promptly.

Pica, a craving for strange foods or nonfoods, such as starch or clay, may develop. It may represent a subconscious nutritional need. Occasionally, excess salivation may cause distress.

Often, pregnant women are concerned about moderating their activities; however, most women may continue their usual activities and exercises throughout pregnancy. Swimming and other mildly strenuous sports are fine. Pregnant women can engage in vigorous activities, such as horseback riding, if they are cautious. Sexual desire may increase or decrease during pregnancy. Sexual intercourse is permissible throughout pregnancy but should be absolutely avoided if a woman has any vaginal bleeding, pain, or leaking of amniotic fluid, and especially if she has uterine contractions. Several pregnant women have died after air was blown into the vagina during oral sex.

All pregnant women should know what the signs of the beginning of labor are. The principal signs are lower abdominal contractions at regular intervals and back pain. A woman who has had rapid deliveries in previous pregnancies should notify her doctor as soon as she thinks she's going into labor. Toward the end of pregnancy (after 36 weeks), a doctor may perform a pelvic examination to try to predict when labor will start.

▲ see page 1158

■ see pages 945 and 946

High-Risk Pregnancy

A high-risk pregnancy is a pregnancy in which the risk of illness or death before or after delivery is greater than usual for the mother or baby.

To identify a high-risk pregnancy, a doctor evaluates a pregnant woman to determine if she has conditions or characteristics that make her or the fetus more likely to become ill or die during the pregnancy (risk factors). Risk factors can be assigned a score corresponding to the degree of risk. Identifying a high-risk pregnancy ensures that a woman who most needs medical care receives it.

A woman with a high-risk pregnancy may be referred to a perinatal care center; perinatal refers to events immediately before, during, or after delivery. Usually, these centers are linked with an obstetric service and newborn intensive care unit to provide the highest level of care for a pregnant woman and baby. A doctor often refers a woman to a perinatal care center before delivery because early attention greatly reduces the likelihood that the baby will become ill or die. A woman is also sent to a center during labor when unexpected problems occur. The most common reason for referral is the risk of preterm delivery (before 37 weeks), which often occurs when the fluid-filled membranes containing the fetus break before it is ready to be born (premature rupture of the membranes). Treatment at a perinatal care center may reduce the likelihood that the baby will be born prematurely.▲

A pregnant woman dies (maternal mortality) in 6 out of 100,000 births in the United States. The leading cause of death is motor vehicle accidents or other injuries. Next most common are several problems related to pregnancy and delivery: blood clots that travel to the lungs, anesthesia complications, bleeding, infection, and high blood pressure complications.

The baby dies before, during, or after birth (perinatal mortality) in 16 out of 1,000 deliveries in the United States. Slightly more than half of these deaths are stillbirths. The rest occur in babies up to 28 days old. The leading cause of these deaths is birth defects, followed by prematurity.

Some risk factors are present before the woman becomes pregnant. Others develop during pregnancy.

Risk Factors Before Pregnancy

Before a woman becomes pregnant, she may have characteristics or conditions that increase risk during pregnancy. In addition, when a woman has had a problem in a pregnancy, her risk of having the same problem in subsequent pregnancies is increased.

Characteristics of the Mother

The woman's age affects pregnancy risk. Girls aged 15 and under are more likely to develop preeclampsia (a condition in which high blood pressure, protein in the urine, and fluid accumulation develop during pregnancy)■ and eclampsia (seizures resulting from preeclampsia). They are also more likely to deliver underweight or undernourished babies. Women aged 35 and older are more likely to develop high blood pressure, diabetes, or fibroids (noncancerous growths) in the uterus and to have problems during labor. The risk of having a baby with a chromosomal abnormality such as Down syndrome increases rapidly after age 35.★ If an older pregnant woman is concerned about the possibility of abnormalities, chorionic villus sampling or amniocentesis may be performed to assess the fetus' chromosomes.●

A woman who weighs less than 100 pounds when not pregnant is more likely to have a baby who is smaller than expected for the number of weeks she has been pregnant (small for gestational age). If she gains less than 15 pounds during

---

▲ see page 1178

■ see page 1158

★ see box, page 1132

● see box, page 1135

Scoring a High-Risk Pregnancy

A score of 10 or more indicates high risk.

Risk Factors	Score
Before Pregnancy	
Characteristics of the mother	
Age 35 and over or 15 and under	5
Weight less than 100 or more than 200 pounds	5
Events in a previous pregnancy	
Stillbirth	10
Newborn death	10
Premature baby	10
Small for gestational age baby (smaller than expected for number of weeks of pregnancy)	10
Fetal blood transfusion for hemolytic disease	10
Late delivery (beyond 42 weeks)	10
Repeated miscarriages	5
Large baby (more than 10 pounds)	5
Six or more completed pregnancies	5
History of eclampsia (seizures during pregnancy)	5
Cesarean section	5
Epilepsy or cerebral palsy in mother	5
History of preeclampsia (high blood pressure, protein in the urine, and fluid accumulation during pregnancy)	1
Previous baby with birth defects	1
Structural defects	
Double uterus	10
Weak (incompetent) cervix	10
Small pelvis	5

Risk Factors	Score
Before Pregnancy (continued)	
Medical conditions	
Long-standing (chronic) high blood pressure	10
Moderate to severe kidney disease	10
Severe heart disease	10
Insulin-dependent diabetes	10
Sickle cell disease	10
Abnormal results of a Pap test	10
Moderate heart disease	5
Thyroid disease	5
History of tuberculosis	5
Lung disease, such as asthma	5
Positive blood test results for syphilis or human immunodeficiency virus	5
History of bladder infection	1
Family history of diabetes	1
During Pregnancy	
Exposure to drugs and infections	
Use of drugs or alcohol	5
Viral illness, such as German measles	5
Influenza (severe)	5
Smoking	1
Medical complications	
Moderate to severe preeclampsia	10
Mild preeclampsia	5
Kidney infection	5
Diet-controlled diabetes of pregnancy (gestational diabetes)	5

(continued)

Scoring a High-Risk Pregnancy (Continued)

Risk Factors	Score	Risk Factors	Score
During Pregnancy (continued)		**During Pregnancy** (continued)	
Medical complications (continued)		*Pregnancy complications (continued)*	
Severe anemia	5	Rapid labor (less than 3 hours)	5
Bladder infection	1	Cesarean section	5
Mild anemia	1	Induced labor for medical reasons	5
Pregnancy complications		Induced labor by choice	1
Mother:		**Baby:**	
Abnormal location of the placenta (placenta previa)	10	Meconium-stained amniotic fluid (dark green)	10
Premature detachment of the placenta (abruptio placentae)	10	Abnormal presentation (such as breech)	10
Too much or too little amniotic fluid around fetus	10	Breech delivery, assisted throughout delivery	10
Infection of placenta	10	Multiple pregnancy (particularly triplets or more)	10
Ruptured uterus	10	Slow or very fast heart rate	10
Late delivery (beyond 42 weeks or more than 2 weeks late)	10	Umbilical cord in front of fetus (prolapsed cord)	10
Rh sensitization to the fetus' blood	5	Weight less than 5.5 pounds at birth	10
Vaginal spotting	5	Meconium-stained amniotic fluid (light green)	5
Preterm labor	5	Need to use forceps or vacuum extractor	5
Membranes rupture (water breaks) more than 12 hours before delivery	5	Breech delivery, partially or not assisted	5
Cervix stops dilating	5	General anesthesia to mother during delivery	5
Labor lasting more than 20 hours	5		
Pushing more than 2 hours	5		

pregnancy, her risk of having such a baby increases to almost 30 percent. Conversely, an obese woman is more likely to have a very large baby; obesity also increases the risk of developing diabetes and high blood pressure during pregnancy.

A woman shorter than 5 feet is more likely to have a small pelvis. Her risk of having preterm labor and an abnormally small baby whose growth in the uterus has been stunted (growth-retarded) is also greater than usual.

Small Babies

- A **premature baby** is one who is born before 37 weeks of pregnancy.

- A **low-birth-weight (underweight) baby** is any baby weighing 5.5 pounds or less at birth.

- A **small for gestational age baby** is one who is unusually small for the number of weeks of pregnancy. This term refers to weight, not length.

- A **growth-retarded baby** is one whose growth in the uterus has been stunted. This term refers to weight and length. A baby may be growth-retarded or small for gestational age or both.

Events in a Previous Pregnancy

A woman who has had three consecutive miscarriages in the first 3 months of pregnancy has about a 35 percent chance of having another miscarriage. Miscarriage is also more likely for a woman who has had a stillborn baby between the fourth and eighth months of pregnancy or preterm labor in a previous pregnancy. Before trying to become pregnant again, a woman who has had a miscarriage may want to be checked for chromosomal or hormonal abnormalities, structural defects in the uterus or cervix, connective tissue disorders such as lupus, or an immune reaction to the fetus, usually Rh incompatibility. If the cause of the miscarriage is found, the condition may be treatable.

A stillbirth or newborn death may result from chromosomal abnormalities in the baby or from diabetes, long-standing (chronic) kidney or blood vessel disease, high blood pressure, drug abuse, or a connective tissue disorder such as lupus in the mother.

The more preterm deliveries a woman has had, the greater the risk of preterm deliveries in subsequent pregnancies. A woman who has had a baby weighing less than 3 pounds has a 50 percent chance of preterm delivery of her next baby. A woman who has had a baby whose growth in the uterus was stunted (growth-retarded) may do so again. She is evaluated for conditions that can stunt the fetus' growth, such as high blood pressure, kidney disease, inadequate weight gain, infection, cigarette smoking, and alcohol abuse.

If a woman has had a baby weighing more than 10 pounds at birth, she may have diabetes.▲ The risk of miscarriage or death of the woman or baby is increased if the woman has diabetes during pregnancy. Pregnant women are checked for diabetes by measuring blood sugar (glucose) levels between 20 and 28 weeks of pregnancy.

A woman who has had six or more pregnancies is more likely to have weak contractions during labor and bleeding after delivery because of weakened uterine muscles. She may also have rapid labor, which can increase the risk of heavy vaginal bleeding. In addition, she is more likely to have placenta previa (a placenta abnormally located in the lower part of the uterus). This condition may cause bleeding, and because the placenta may block the cervix, a cesarean section is usually necessary.

If a woman has had a baby with hemolytic disease,■ the next baby may be at risk for the same disease, and the severity of the disease in the previous baby predicts its severity in the next. This disease develops when a mother whose blood is Rh-negative has a fetus whose blood is Rh-positive (Rh incompatibility) and the mother produces antibodies against the fetus' blood (Rh sensitization); these antibodies destroy the fetus' red blood cells. In such cases, the blood of both parents is tested. If the father has two genes for Rh-positive blood, all babies will have Rh-positive blood; if he has only one gene for it, a baby has about a 50 percent chance of having Rh-positive blood. This information helps doctors care for the mother and fetus in subsequent pregnancies. Usually, no problems develop in the first pregnancy with a baby whose blood is Rh-positive, but contact between the mother's and baby's blood at delivery causes the mother to produce Rh antibodies. As a result, subsequent babies are at risk. However, after the delivery of a baby

▲ see page 1163

■ see box, page 1211

whose blood is Rh-positive to a mother whose blood is Rh-negative, the mother is usually given $Rh_0(D)$ immune globulin, which destroys Rh antibodies. Consequently, hemolytic disease in babies is rare.

A woman who has had preeclampsia or eclampsia is likely to have it again, particularly if she has chronic high blood pressure when she isn't pregnant.

If a woman has had a baby with genetic disorders or birth defects, genetic analysis of the baby—even if stillborn—and both parents is usually performed before another pregnancy is attempted. If the woman becomes pregnant again, tests such as ultrasound scanning, chorionic villus sampling, and amniocentesis are performed to help determine if the abnormalities are likely to recur.▲

Structural Defects

Structural defects in a woman's reproductive organs, such as a double uterus or a weak cervix that can't support the developing fetus (an incompetent cervix), increase the risk of a miscarriage. Diagnostic surgery, ultrasound scans, or x-rays may be necessary to detect these defects; if a woman is having repeated miscarriages, these tests are performed before she becomes pregnant again.

Fibroids (noncancerous growths) in the uterus, which are more common in older women, may increase the risk of preterm labor, problems during labor, abnormal presentation of the fetus, abnormal location of the placenta (placenta previa), and repeated miscarriages.

Medical Conditions

Certain medical conditions in a pregnant woman may endanger her and the fetus. The most important are chronic high blood pressure, kidney disease, diabetes, severe heart disease, sickle cell disease, thyroid disease, systemic lupus erythematosus (lupus), and blood clotting disorders.■

Family History

A history of mental retardation or other hereditary disorders in the mother's or father's family increases the likelihood that the baby will have such a disorder. The tendency to have twins also runs in families.

Risk Factors During Pregnancy

A pregnant woman at low risk may undergo a change that increases her risk. She may be exposed to teratogens (agents that can produce birth defects), such as radiation, certain chemicals, drugs, and infections, or she may develop a medical condition or a complication related to pregnancy.

Exposure to Drugs or Infections

Drugs known to produce birth defects when taken during pregnancy include alcohol, phenytoin, drugs that oppose the actions of folic acid (such as triamterene or trimethoprim), lithium, streptomycin, tetracycline, thalidomide, and warfarin.★ Infections that may cause birth defects include herpes simplex, viral hepatitis, influenza, mumps, German measles (rubella), chickenpox (varicella), syphilis, listeriosis, toxoplasmosis, and infections with coxsackievirus or cytomegalovirus. Early in pregnancy, a woman is asked if she has taken any of these drugs or has had any of these infections since becoming pregnant. Of particular concern is how smoking cigarettes, drinking alcohol, and abusing drugs during pregnancy affect the fetus' health and development.

Cigarette smoking is the most common addiction among pregnant women in the United States. Despite publicity regarding the health hazards of smoking, the percentage of adult women who smoke or live with someone who smokes has dropped only slightly in 20 years, and the percentage of women who smoke heavily has increased. Smoking among teenage girls has increased substantially and exceeds that among teenage boys.

Although smoking harms both mother and fetus, only about 20 percent of women who smoke quit during pregnancy. The most consistent effect of smoking on the baby during pregnancy is reduction in birth weight: The more a woman smokes during pregnancy, the less the baby is likely to weigh. This effect seems to be greater among older smokers, who are more likely to have babies who weigh less and are shorter. Pregnant

---

▲ see page 1129

■ see page 1160

★ see page 1167

smokers also are more likely to have placental complications, premature rupture of the membranes, preterm labor, and uterine infections. A pregnant woman who doesn't smoke should avoid exposure to secondhand smoke because it may similarly harm the fetus.

Birth defects of the heart, brain, and face are more common in babies of smokers than in those of nonsmokers. Smoking by the mother may increase the risk of sudden infant death syndrome. In addition, children of smoking mothers have slight but measurable deficiencies in physical growth, intellectual development, and behavior. These effects are thought to be caused by carbon monoxide, which may reduce the oxygen supply to the body's tissues, and nicotine, which stimulates the release of hormones that constrict the vessels supplying blood to the placenta and uterus.

Drinking alcohol during pregnancy is the leading known cause of birth defects. Fetal alcohol syndrome, one of the major consequences of drinking during pregnancy, is found in about 2.2 out of 1,000 live births. This condition includes growth retardation before or after birth; facial defects; a small head (microcephaly), probably caused by subnormal brain growth; and abnormal behavioral development. Mental retardation more often results from fetal alcohol syndrome than from any other known cause.▲ In addition, alcohol can cause problems ranging from miscarriage to severe behavioral problems in the baby or developing child, such as antisocial behavior and attention deficit. These problems can occur even when the baby has no obvious physical birth defects.

The risk of miscarriage almost doubles when a woman drinks alcohol in any form during pregnancy, especially if she drinks heavily. Often, the birth weight of babies born to women who drink during pregnancy is below normal. The average birth weight is about 4 pounds for babies exposed to alcohol, compared with 7 pounds for all babies.

Drug abuse and addiction are seen in more and more pregnant women. More than five million people in the United States, many of whom are women of childbearing age, regularly use marijuana or cocaine.

An inexpensive, sensitive laboratory test called chromatography can be used to check a woman's urine for heroin, morphine, amphetamines, barbiturates, codeine, cocaine, marijuana, methadone, or phenothiazines. Women who inject drugs are at greater risk for anemia, infection of the blood (bacteremia) or heart valves (endocarditis), skin abscess, hepatitis, phlebitis, pneumonia, tetanus, and sexually transmitted diseases, including AIDS. About 75 percent of babies who develop AIDS have mothers who injected drugs or were prostitutes. These babies are at risk for other sexually transmitted diseases, hepatitis, and infections. Also, their growth in the uterus is more likely to be retarded, and their birth premature.

About 14 percent of pregnant women use marijuana to some extent. Its main ingredient, tetrahydrocannabinol (THC), can cross the placenta and thus may affect the fetus. Although no specific evidence shows that marijuana causes birth defects or slows growth in the uterus, some studies suggest that heavy use is linked with behavioral abnormalities in babies.

Cocaine abuse during pregnancy causes serious problems for both mother and fetus, and many who use cocaine also abuse other drugs, compounding the problem. Cocaine stimulates the central nervous system, acts as a local anesthetic, and constricts blood vessels. Constricted blood vessels may reduce blood flow so that the fetus sometimes doesn't get enough oxygen. The reduced blood and oxygen supply to the fetus can affect the growth of various organs and commonly results in skeletal defects and abnormally narrow sections of intestine. Nervous system and behavioral problems in babies of cocaine users include hyperactivity, uncontrollable trembling, and substantial learning problems, which may continue through age 5 years or even longer.■

If a pregnant woman suddenly develops severe high blood pressure or bleeding from premature detachment of the placenta (abruptio placentae) or if she has an unexplained stillbirth, her urine is usually tested for cocaine. Among women who use cocaine throughout pregnancy, about 31 percent have a preterm delivery, 19 percent have a growth-retarded baby, and 15 percent have premature detachment of the placenta. If a woman stops using cocaine after the first 3 months of pregnancy, the risks of preterm delivery and premature detachment of the placenta are still in-

▲ see page 1214

■ see page 1214

creased but the fetus' growth will probably be normal.

Medical Conditions

If high blood pressure is first diagnosed when a woman is pregnant, a doctor may have difficulty determining whether it was caused by the pregnancy or by another condition. Treatment of high blood pressure during pregnancy is a problem; benefits for the mother have to be weighed against potential risks to the fetus. However, late in pregnancy, high blood pressure may indicate a serious threat to the mother and fetus and must be treated promptly.

If a pregnant woman has had a bladder infection in the past, a urine sample is evaluated early in the pregnancy. If bacteria are detected, a doctor prescribes antibiotics▲ to try to prevent a kidney infection, which is associated with preterm labor and premature rupture of the membranes.

Bacterial infections of the vagina during pregnancy also may lead to preterm labor or premature rupture of the membranes. Treating the infection with antibiotics reduces the likelihood of these problems.

An illness causing a fever (temperature greater than 103° F.) in the first 3 months of pregnancy increases the likelihood of miscarriage and nervous system defects in the baby. Fever in late pregnancy increases the likelihood of preterm labor.

Emergency surgery during pregnancy increases the risk of preterm labor. Many disorders, such as appendicitis, a gallbladder attack, and intestinal obstruction, are difficult to diagnose because of the normal changes in the abdomen during pregnancy. By the time such a disorder is diagnosed, it may be in an advanced stage, which increases the woman's risk of illness and death.

Pregnancy Complications

Rh Incompatibility: Mother and fetus may have incompatible blood types. The most common is Rh incompatibility,■ which can lead to hemolytic disease of the newborn. This disease can develop only when a mother whose blood is Rh-negative and a father whose blood is Rh-positive have a fetus whose blood is Rh-positive and the mother produces antibodies against the fetus' blood. If an expectant mother's blood is Rh-negative, it's checked for antibodies to the fetus' blood every 2 months. The risk of producing these antibodies is increased after any bleeding episode in which the mother's and fetus' blood may mix, after am-

niocentesis or chorionic villus sampling, and within the first 72 hours after delivery if the baby has Rh-positive blood. At these times and at the 28th week of pregnancy, the mother is given $Rh_0(D)$ immune globulin, which combines with and thereby destroys these antibodies.

Bleeding: The most common causes of bleeding in the last 3 months of pregnancy are abnormal location of the placenta, premature detachment of the placenta from the uterus, and a disease of the vagina or cervix, such as an infection. All women who bleed at this time are considered at risk of losing the baby, bleeding excessively (hemorrhaging), or dying during labor and delivery. Ultrasound scanning, inspection of the cervix, and a Papanicolaou (Pap) test help determine the cause of the bleeding.

Problems With Amniotic Fluid: Too much amniotic fluid in the membranes surrounding the fetus stretches the uterus and puts pressure on the mother's diaphragm. This complication can lead to severe breathing problems in the mother or preterm labor. Too much fluid tends to develop if the mother has uncontrolled diabetes, if more than one fetus is present (multiple pregnancy), if mother and fetus have incompatible blood types, or if the baby has birth defects, especially a blocked esophagus or nervous system defects. About half the time, the cause is unknown. There tends to be too little amniotic fluid when the baby has birth defects in the urinary tract, is growth retarded, or dies.

Preterm Labor: Labor is more likely to be early if the mother has structural defects in the uterus or cervix, bleeding, mental or physical stress, or a multiple pregnancy or if she has had previous uterine surgery. Preterm labor often occurs when the fetus is in an abnormal position such as breech presentation, when the placenta detaches from the uterus prematurely, when the mother has high blood pressure, or when too much amniotic fluid surrounds the fetus. Pneumonia, kidney infection, and appendicitis can also cause preterm labor. About 30 percent of women who have preterm labor have infections of the uterus

▲ see page 1170

■ see page 1155

even though the membranes haven't ruptured. Whether antibiotics help these women isn't known.

Multiple Pregnancy: Having more than one fetus in the uterus also increases the likelihood of birth defects and problems with labor and delivery.

Postterm Pregnancy: In a pregnancy that continues beyond 42 weeks (postterm), death of the baby is three times more likely than that in a normal term pregnancy. Electronic heart monitoring and ultrasound scanning are used to monitor the fetus.

CHAPTER 245

Complications of Pregnancy

Most pregnancies are uneventful, and most complications can be treated. Complications include miscarriage, ectopic pregnancy, anemia, Rh incompatibility, problems with the placenta, excessive vomiting, preeclampsia and eclampsia, and skin rashes as well as preterm labor and premature rupture of the membranes.▲ After a miscarriage, most women are able to have successful pregnancies.

Miscarriage and Stillbirth

A miscarriage (spontaneous abortion) is the loss of a fetus from natural causes before the 20th week of pregnancy. A stillbirth is the loss of a fetus from natural causes after the 20th week of pregnancy.

The term *abortion* is used by doctors to refer both to a miscarriage and to medical termination of pregnancy (induced abortion).

A baby who has spontaneous breathing or a heartbeat after birth is a live birth at any stage of pregnancy. If it subsequently dies, its death is considered a newborn (neonatal) death.

About 20 to 30 percent of pregnant women have some bleeding or cramping at least once during the first 20 weeks of pregnancy. About half of these episodes result in a miscarriage.

About 85 percent of miscarriages occur during the first 12 weeks of the pregnancy and are usually related to abnormalities in the fetus. The remaining 15 percent of miscarriages occur during weeks 13 to 20; about two thirds of them result from

problems in the mother, and one third from no known cause. Many studies have shown that emotional disturbances in the mother are not linked with miscarriages.

Symptoms and Diagnosis

Before a miscarriage, a woman usually has spotting or more obvious bleeding and a discharge from the vagina. The uterus contracts, causing cramps. If the miscarriage continues, the bleeding, discharge, and cramps become more severe. Eventually, part or all of the contents of the uterus may be expelled.

In the early stages of a miscarriage, ultrasound scans can determine whether the fetus is still alive. These scans and other tests may be used after a miscarriage to determine whether all the contents of the uterus have been expelled.

Treatment

No treatment is needed when all of the contents of the uterus are expelled (a complete abortion). When only part of the contents are expelled (an incomplete abortion), suction curettage■ must be performed to empty the uterus.

If the fetus dies but remains in the uterus (a missed abortion), a doctor must remove the fetus and the placenta, usually by suction curettage. A drug, such as oxytocin, that causes the uterus to contract and expel its contents may be used for late missed abortions.

If bleeding and cramping occur during the first 20 weeks of pregnancy (a threatened abortion), bed rest is advised because it often reduces these symptoms. If possible, a woman shouldn't work and should stay off her feet at home. Sexual inter-

---

▲ see page 1178

■ see page 1128

course should be avoided, although it has not been definitely connected with miscarriages. Hormones aren't given because they're almost always ineffective and can cause birth defects, particularly of the heart or reproductive organs. For instance, exposing a female fetus to diethylstilbestrol (DES), a synthetic hormone, at this stage of development may cause vaginal cancer later.

A threatened abortion may result when the cervix opens prematurely because of weak fibrous tissue. Sometimes the cervical opening can be surgically closed (cerclage) with stitches (sutures) that are removed just before delivery.

A septic abortion is a very serious infection. The contents of the uterus must be removed immediately, and the infection must be treated with high doses of antibiotics.

Ectopic Pregnancy

An ectopic (out-of-place) pregnancy is one in which the fetus develops outside the uterus—in the fallopian tubes, the cervical canal, or the pelvic or abdominal cavity.

Normally, an egg is released from one ovary and is swept into the opening of a fallopian tube.▲ Inside the tube, it's propelled by tiny hairlike cilia lining the tube, reaching the uterus after several days. Usually, the egg is fertilized in the fallopian tubes but becomes implanted in the uterus. However, if the tube is blocked—because of a previous infection, for example—the egg may move slowly or become stuck. The fertilized egg may never reach the uterus, and an ectopic pregnancy may result.

One out of 100 to 200 pregnancies is an ectopic pregnancy. For reasons not clearly understood, it's becoming more common. Having had a disorder affecting the fallopian tubes, a previous ectopic pregnancy, exposure to diethylstilbestrol as a fetus, or a failed tubal ligation (a sterilization procedure in which the fallopian tubes are cut or blocked) increases the chances of having an ectopic pregnancy. Ectopic pregnancies are less common among white women than among women of other racial groups. In rare cases when a woman becomes pregnant with an intrauterine device (IUD) in place, the risk of having an ectopic pregnancy is increased.

Ectopic pregnancies usually develop in one of the fallopian tubes (tubal pregnancy). Rarely, they occur in other places, such as the cervical

---

Abortion Terminology

Early
Loss of fetus before 12 weeks of pregnancy

Late
Loss of fetus between 12 and 20 weeks of pregnancy

Spontaneous
Loss of fetus occurring naturally

Induced
Medical termination of pregnancy

Therapeutic
Removal of fetus to save the mother's life or preserve her health

Threatened
Bleeding or cramping in the first 20 weeks of pregnancy, indicating that the fetus is in jeopardy

Inevitable
Intolerable pain or bleeding with opening of the cervix, indicating that the fetus will be lost

Incomplete
Expulsion of only part of the contents of the uterus or rupture of the membranes

Complete
Expulsion of all the contents of the uterus

Habitual
Three or more consecutive miscarriages

Missed
Retention of a dead fetus in the uterus for 4 weeks or longer

Septic
Infection of the contents of the uterus before, during, or after an abortion

---

canal, ovary, or pelvic or abdominal cavity. An ectopic pregnancy is life threatening and must be removed as soon as possible. In the United States, 1 out of 826 women with an ectopic pregnancy dies of complications.

▲ see box, page 1137

Problems in the Mother That Can Cause a Miscarriage
Abnormal uterus
Weak (incompetent) cervix, which may begin to open as the uterus enlarges
Hypothyroidism
Diabetes
Infections, such as a cytomegalovirus infection or rubella
Use of cocaine, especially crack
Injury
Dietary deficiencies

Symptoms

The symptoms of an ectopic pregnancy include spotting and cramping, usually occurring when a period is late. These symptoms occur because once the fetus dies, the uterine lining is shed as in a normal period.

If the fetus dies at an early stage, the fallopian tube isn't damaged. If the fetus continues to grow, however, it may begin to tear the walls of the tube, causing bleeding. If the bleeding is gradual, it causes pain and sometimes a sensation of pressure in the lower abdomen because of the accumulating blood. If the bleeding is rapid, it may lower blood pressure severely and even lead to shock. Typically, after about 6 to 8 weeks, sudden, severe pain is felt in the lower abdomen, followed by fainting. These symptoms usually indicate that the tube has ruptured, causing massive bleeding into the abdomen.

Sometimes an ectopic pregnancy develops partly in one of the tubes and partly inside the uterus. Cramping and spotting are common. In this location, the fetus has more room to grow, so the ectopic pregnancy usually ruptures later, generally between the 12th and 16th weeks of pregnancy. Such a rupture can be catastrophic, with a higher mortality rate.

▲ see page 742

Diagnosis and Treatment

A doctor may suspect that a woman has an ectopic pregnancy if her blood and urine test results are positive for pregnancy, but her uterus is smaller than expected for the length of time she has been pregnant. An ultrasound scan may show that the uterus is empty and that blood is in the pelvic or abdominal cavity. The doctor may then use a laparoscope (a fiber-optic tube inserted through a small incision in the abdomen) to view the ectopic pregnancy directly.

To help confirm the diagnosis, the doctor may insert a needle through the wall of the vagina into the pelvic cavity and remove blood that has accumulated from the bleeding ectopic pregnancy—a procedure called culdocentesis. Unlike blood from a vein or an artery, this blood doesn't clot.

Usually, an ectopic pregnancy must be removed surgically. When it's in a fallopian tube, a doctor usually makes an incision into the tube and removes the fetus and placenta. The tube is left open, allowing it to heal without scar tissue, because scar tissue can make becoming pregnant again more difficult. The procedure is sometimes performed through a laparoscope. Rarely, the tube is so damaged that it can't be repaired and must be removed.

The drug methotrexate, rather than surgery, may be used to treat early tubal pregnancies in which there is no evidence of the fetus' heartbeat.

Anemias

Anemias are conditions in which the number of red blood cells or the amount of hemoglobin (the protein that carries oxygen) in them is below normal.▲

The volume of blood increases during pregnancy, so a moderate decrease in the concentration of red blood cells and hemoglobin (hemodilution) is normal.

During pregnancy, more iron, which is needed to produce red blood cells, is required because the mother must supply the fetus as well as herself. The most common type of anemia during pregnancy is iron deficiency anemia, usually caused by an inadequate amount of iron in the diet. However, this anemia may result from an iron deficiency that already exists because of iron lost during menstrual periods or a previous pregnancy. Less commonly, anemia results from a diet deficient in folic acid (folate), a B vitamin also needed to produce red blood cells.

Locations of Ectopic Pregnancy

- Fallopian tube
- Ovary
- Abdomen
- Cervix

Diagnosis and Treatment

The diagnosis is based on blood tests that determine the red blood cell count, hemoglobin level, and iron level in the blood.

Anemia resulting from iron deficiency is treated with iron tablets. The supplemental iron poses no risk to the fetus but can cause stomach upset and constipation in the mother, especially if the dose is high. Whether all pregnant women should take iron supplements is controversial. However, most pregnant women are advised to take them, even if their red blood cell count and hemoglobin level are normal, to ensure that they have enough iron for themselves and the fetus as the pregnancy progresses. Anemia caused by folic acid deficiency is treated with folate tablets. For pregnant women who have sickle cell anemia ▲ (a hereditary disease in which hemoglobin is abnormal), treatment is more controversial; blood transfusions are sometimes necessary.

Rh Incompatibility

Rh incompatibility is a mismatch of the Rh group in the blood of a pregnant woman with that of her baby.

As a result of Rh incompatibility, the woman may produce antibodies against the baby's red blood cells. The antibodies cause some of these cells to rupture, sometimes producing hemolytic disease, a type of anemia, in the baby.

A person's blood group refers to molecules on the surface of red blood cells that identify the cells as unique to that person. The Rh blood group includes some of these molecules. One of them, $Rh_0(D)$, is the one that usually causes Rh incompatibility problems. If red blood cells have $Rh_0(D)$ molecules, the blood is Rh-positive; if they don't, the blood is Rh-negative.

▲ see page 1162

Problems occur when the mother has Rh-negative blood and the fetus has Rh-positive blood, inherited from the father, who has Rh-positive blood. Some of the fetus' blood may come in contact with the mother's blood through the placenta, particularly in late pregnancy and during delivery. The mother's body may treat the fetus' red blood cells as foreign substances and produce antibodies to destroy them (Rh antibodies). Antibody levels in the mother rise throughout the pregnancy, and antibodies may cross the placenta to the fetus, where they can destroy some of its red blood cells. As a result, hemolytic disease may develop in the fetus (erythroblastosis fetalis) or newborn (erythroblastosis neonatorum).▲ However, during a first pregnancy, the fetus or newborn rarely has problems because usually no significant contact between the fetus' and mother's blood occurs until delivery. In each subsequent pregnancy, however, the mother becomes more sensitized to Rh-positive blood and produces antibodies earlier and earlier in each one.

Red blood cell destruction in the fetus can result in anemia and an increase in the blood level of bilirubin (a waste product from red blood cell destruction). If the bilirubin level becomes too high, the fetus' brain may be damaged.

Among white people in the United States, 85 percent have Rh-positive blood, and in about 13 percent of marriages, the man has Rh-positive blood and the woman has Rh-negative blood. Of babies born to such couples, 1 out of 27 develops hemolytic disease.

Prevention and Treatment

At the first visit to a doctor during a pregnancy, a woman is screened to determine her blood type and group. If she has Rh-negative blood, the father's blood type is determined. If he has Rh-positive blood, the mother's Rh antibody level is measured.

The mother's and baby's blood may come into contact during delivery, causing the mother to produce antibodies. Therefore, as a precaution, Rh antibodies, in the form of $Rh_0(D)$ immune globulin, are given by injection to a mother who has Rh-negative blood within 72 hours after delivery of a baby who has Rh-positive blood, even after a miscarriage or abortion. This treatment destroys any cells from the baby that might sensitize the mother, so that later pregnancies usually aren't endangered. However, in about 1 to 2 percent of the mothers, the injection doesn't prevent sensitization, presumably because the mother was sensitized earlier in the pregnancy. To prevent early sensitization, a doctor gives a mother whose blood is Rh-negative an injection of Rh antibodies at 28 weeks of pregnancy as well as after delivery.

By periodically measuring the changing levels of Rh antibodies in the mother, a doctor can anticipate whether the baby may have problems. If a mother's Rh antibody level becomes too high during pregnancy, amniocentesis may be performed. In this procedure, a needle is inserted through the skin to withdraw fluid from the amniotic sac, which surrounds the fetus inside the uterus. The level of bilirubin is measured in the fluid sample. If this level is too high, the fetus is given a blood transfusion. Additional transfusions generally are given every 10 to 14 days until around 32 to 34 weeks of pregnancy, at which time labor is usually induced. The baby is usually given one or more transfusions after birth. In less severe cases, no transfusions are given until after birth.

Abruptio Placentae

Abruptio placentae is the premature detachment of a normally positioned placenta from the wall of the uterus, occurring during the pregnancy rather than after delivery.

The placenta may detach incompletely, sometimes just 10 to 20 percent, or completely. The cause is unknown. Detachment occurs in 0.4 to 3.5 percent of all deliveries. Women who have high blood pressure, heart disease, diabetes, or a rheumatoid disease■ and women who use cocaine are more likely to develop this complication.

Symptoms and Diagnosis

The uterus bleeds from the site where the placenta was attached. The blood may pass through the cervix and out the vagina (external hemorrhage), or it may be trapped behind the placenta (concealed hemorrhage). Symptoms depend on the degree of detachment and the amount of blood lost and include vaginal bleeding, sudden continuous or crampy abdominal pain, and ten-

---

▲ see box, page 1211

■ see page 1160

Problems With the Placenta

Normally, the placenta is located in the upper part of the uterus, firmly attached to the uterine wall. In abruptio placentae, the placenta detaches from the uterine wall prematurely, causing the uterus to bleed and reducing the fetus' supply of oxygen and nutrients. A woman who has this condition is hospitalized, and the baby may be delivered early. In placenta previa, the placenta is located over or near the cervix, in the lower part of the uterus. Symptoms include painless bleeding starting late in pregnancy, which may become profuse. The baby is usually delivered by cesarean section.

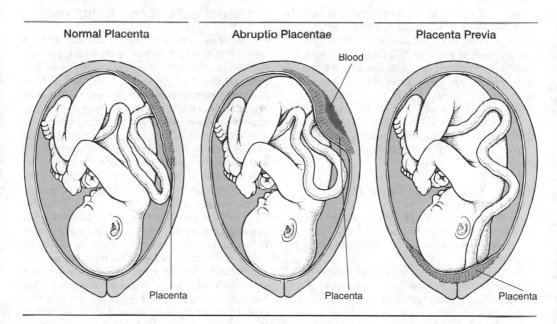

Normal Placenta	Abruptio Placentae	Placenta Previa

Blood

Placenta   Placenta   Placenta

derness when the abdomen is pressed. The diagnosis is usually confirmed with an ultrasound scan.

The detachment reduces the supply of oxygen and nutrients to the fetus and can even cause the fetus' death. Complications for the woman include potentially serious blood loss, widespread clotting inside the blood vessels (disseminated intravascular coagulation), kidney failure, and bleeding into the walls of the uterus. Such complications are more likely in a pregnant woman who has preeclampsia, and they may indicate that the fetus is in distress or has died.

Treatment

Once the diagnosis has been made, a woman is hospitalized. The usual treatment is bed rest un-less the bleeding is life threatening, the fetus is in distress, or the pregnancy is near term. Extended rest may lessen the bleeding. If symptoms lessen, the woman is encouraged to walk around and may even be discharged from the hospital. If bleeding continues or worsens, an early delivery is often best for both the woman and her baby. If vaginal delivery isn't possible, a cesarean section is performed.

Placenta Previa

Placenta previa is implantation of the placenta over or near the cervix, in the lower part of the uterus.

Inside the uterus, the placenta may cover the opening of the cervix completely or partially. Placenta previa occurs in 1 out of 200 deliveries, usually in women who have had more than one pregnancy or have abnormalities of the uterus such as fibroids.

Painless vaginal bleeding begins suddenly in late pregnancy and may become profuse. The blood may be bright red. An ultrasound scan helps a doctor make the diagnosis and distinguish a placenta previa from one that's prematurely detached (abruptio placentae).

Treatment

When bleeding is profuse, repeated blood transfusions may be needed. When bleeding is minor and delivery isn't imminent, bed rest is usually advised. If the bleeding stops, a woman is usually encouraged to walk. If it doesn't recur, she's generally sent home, provided that she can return to the hospital easily. A cesarean section is almost always performed, because if the woman goes into labor, the placenta tends to become detached very early, depriving the baby of its oxygen supply. In addition, there may be massive bleeding in the mother.

Excessive Vomiting

Excessive vomiting during pregnancy (hyperemesis gravidarum), unlike ordinary morning sickness, is extremely severe nausea and vomiting that causes dehydration and starvation.

Its cause is unknown. Psychologic factors may trigger or worsen the vomiting. A woman who has hyperemesis gravidarum loses weight and becomes dehydrated. If a woman has morning sickness but gains weight and isn't dehydrated, she does not have hyperemesis gravidarum.

Dehydration can cause dangerous shifts in the electrolyte levels in the blood, and the blood becomes too acidic.▲ If vomiting persists, the liver may be damaged, sometimes rupturing and bleeding. Another serious complication is bleeding in the retina of the eye (hemorrhagic retinitis), caused by increased blood pressure during vomiting.

Treatment

Because hyperemesis gravidarum can be life threatening to the woman and her baby, the woman is hospitalized and intravenously given

fluids, glucose (a simple sugar), electrolytes, and occasionally vitamins. She may not eat or drink anything for 24 hours; antinausea drugs and sedatives are given as needed. Once dehydration and vomiting have been corrected, she can begin eating frequent, small portions of bland foods. The size of the portions is increased if she can tolerate more food. Usually, vomiting stops within a few days. If symptoms recur, the treatment is repeated.

Preeclampsia and Eclampsia

*Preeclampsia, sometimes called **toxemia of pregnancy**, is high blood pressure accompanied by protein in the urine (proteinuria) or retention of fluid (edema) that develops between the 20th week of pregnancy and the end of the first week after delivery. **Eclampsia** is a more severe form of preeclampsia that results in seizures or a coma.*

Preeclampsia occurs in 5 percent of pregnant women. It's more common in first pregnancies and in women who already have high blood pressure or a blood vessel disorder. Eclampsia develops in 1 out of 200 women who have preeclampsia and is usually fatal unless it's treated promptly. The cause of preeclampsia and eclampsia is unknown. A major risk of preeclampsia is premature detachment of the placenta from the uterine wall.

In preeclampsia, blood pressure is higher than 140/90 mm Hg, the face or hands swell, and abnormally high levels of protein are detected in the urine. A woman whose blood pressure increases markedly but remains below 140/90 mm Hg during pregnancy is also considered to have preeclampsia.

Babies of women who have preeclampsia are four or five times more likely to have problems soon after birth than babies of women who don't have this condition. Babies may be small because the placenta malfunctions or they are premature.

Treatment

Unlike ordinary high blood pressure (hypertension), preeclampsia and eclampsia don't respond to diuretics (drugs that remove excess fluid) and a low-salt diet. A woman is encouraged to consume a normal amount of salt and to drink more water. Bed rest is important. Often, the woman is also encouraged to lie on her left side—which puts less pressure on the large vein in the abdomen (inferior vena cava) that carries blood back to the heart, improving blood flow. Magne-

---

▲ see page 676

sium sulfate may be given intravenously to lower blood pressure and prevent seizures.

For a woman who has mild preeclampsia, bed rest at home may be sufficient, but she should see her doctor every 2 days. If she doesn't improve rapidly, she's usually hospitalized, and if the problem continues in the hospital, the baby is delivered as soon as possible.

A woman who has severe preeclampsia is hospitalized and kept in bed. Fluids and magnesium sulfate given intravenously usually relieve symptoms. In 4 to 6 hours, blood pressure usually decreases to normal levels. Then, the baby can be safely delivered. If blood pressure remains high, additional drugs are given before a delivery is attempted.

A major complication of severe preeclampsia and eclampsia is the HELLP syndrome, which consists of the following:
- *H*emolysis (the breakdown of red blood cells)
- *E*levated *l*iver enzymes, indicating liver damage
- *L*ow *p*latelet count, indicating an impaired blood clotting ability—potentially a major problem during and after labor

The HELLP syndrome is more likely to occur when treatment of preeclampsia is delayed. If the syndrome occurs, the baby is delivered by cesarean section, the fastest available method, unless the cervix is dilated enough to permit a prompt vaginal delivery.

After delivery, the woman is closely monitored for signs of eclampsia. One fourth of the cases of eclampsia occur after delivery, usually in the first 2 to 4 days. As the woman's condition gradually improves, she is encouraged to walk around. She may be given a mild sedative to control blood pressure. Hospitalization may last from a few days to weeks, depending on the severity of the condition and complications. Even after returning home, the woman may have to take drugs to lower blood pressure. Generally, she has a checkup at least every 2 weeks for the first few months after delivery. Her blood pressure may remain high for 6 to 8 weeks. If it remains high longer, its cause may be unrelated to preeclampsia.

Skin Rashes

Some skin rashes occur only during pregnancy. These include herpes gestationis and urticaria of pregnancy.

HERPES GESTATIONIS

Herpes gestationis is an intensely itchy rash of fluid-filled blisters that occurs during pregnancy.

The term *herpes* is misleading, because the rash isn't caused by herpesvirus or any other virus. Herpes gestationis is thought to be caused by abnormal antibodies that react against the body's own tissues (an autoimmune reaction).▲ This uncommon rash can appear at any time after the 12th week of pregnancy or immediately after delivery.

The itchy rash usually includes small fluid-filled blisters (vesicles) and larger, irregularly shaped fluid-filled swellings (bullae). It often starts on the abdomen, then spreads. Sometimes the rash covers a ring-shaped area, with blisters around the outer edge. Typically, it worsens soon after delivery and disappears within a few weeks or months. It often reappears during subsequent pregnancies or with the use of oral contraceptives. The baby may be born with a similar rash, which usually disappears within a few weeks without treatment.

To confirm the diagnosis, a doctor removes a tiny piece of affected skin and sends it to a laboratory to determine whether antibodies are present.

The goal of treatment is to relieve the intense itching and prevent new blisters from forming. For a mild rash, frequent applications of a corticosteroid cream directly to the skin often help. For more widespread rashes, corticosteroids are given by mouth. Taking corticosteroids late in pregnancy doesn't seem to harm the fetus. If the itching worsens or the rash spreads after delivery, a higher dose of a corticosteroid may be needed.

URTICARIA OF PREGNANCY

Urticaria of pregnancy is a common, itchy rash that occurs during pregnancy.

Its cause isn't known. Intensely itchy, red, irregularly shaped, flat or slightly raised hivelike patches—sometimes with tiny fluid-filled blisters in the center—develop on the abdomen. The rash spreads to the thighs, buttocks, and occasionally the arms. Hundreds of itchy patches may de-

---

▲ see page 816

velop. Often the skin around them is pale. The rash usually appears during the last 2 to 3 weeks of pregnancy and occasionally during the last few days. However, it may occur at any time after the 24th week. Itching is bothersome enough to keep a woman awake at night. It usually clears up promptly after delivery and usually doesn't recur during subsequent pregnancies.

No specific test for this rash is available, so a doctor may have difficulty making a definite diagnosis.

The itching and rash may resolve in 2 to 4 days with frequent applications of a corticosteroid cream. Occasionally, if the rash is more severe, corticosteroids are given by mouth. Taken late in pregnancy, they don't seem to harm the fetus.

CHAPTER 246

Diseases That Can Complicate Pregnancy

Diseases such as heart or kidney disease, anemias, infections, or diabetes may cause complications during pregnancy. Such complications may affect only the pregnant woman or both the woman and the fetus.

Heart Disease

In the United States, heart disease has become uncommon in women of childbearing age mainly because of a marked decline in rheumatic fever, a childhood disease that damages the heart.▲ About 1 percent of the women who have severe heart disease before becoming pregnant die as a result of the pregnancy, generally because of heart failure. However, because of improved diagnosis and treatment, most women who have heart disease can give birth safely to healthy children. For them, having a baby doesn't alter heart function permanently or reduce life span.

Normal changes in the blood circulation during pregnancy put an added strain on the heart,■ so a woman who is pregnant or considering pregnancy should tell her doctor if she has or has ever had heart disease.

Pregnancy makes diagnosing heart disease more difficult. During pregnancy, the volume of blood increases, causing murmurs (sounds caused by blood turbulently rushing through the heart) that may suggest heart disease, even when no disease is present. In addition, the veins are dilated, and the heart beats more rapidly and looks different on x-rays.

Heart Failure
Heart failure is the inability of the heart to pump enough blood for the body's needs.

As pregnancy progresses, a woman who has heart failure may become increasingly tired even if she rests sufficiently, avoids stress, eats nutritious foods, takes iron supplements to prevent anemia, and restricts her weight gain. Periods of special concern, when demands on the heart are greatest, are between 28 and 34 weeks of pregnancy, during labor, and immediately after delivery. The mother's heart disease may affect the fetus. A fetus may die during an episode of the mother's heart failure or be born too early (prematurely).

The work of labor and the increased amount of blood returning to the heart from the contracting uterus greatly increase the strain on the heart. During each uterine contraction, the heart pumps about 20 percent more blood. A woman who has severe heart failure may be given an epidural anesthetic to block sensation in the lower spinal cord and prevent her from pushing during labor. Pushing interrupts the absorption of oxygen through the woman's lungs, reducing the oxygen supply to the fetus. The baby is delivered with forceps or by a cesarean section. Forceps delivery involves less risk for the mother than a cesarean

▲ see page 1303

■ see page 1140

section does, although an injury to the baby may be more likely. Usually, such injuries are minor.

After delivery, a new mother's body makes widely varying demands on her heart. A woman who has heart failure isn't out of danger for at least 6 months.

RHEUMATIC HEART DISEASE

Rheumatic heart disease is a common complication of rheumatic fever in which one or more heart valves may become narrowed, particularly the mitral valve (mitral valve stenosis▲).

The problems caused by narrowed heart valves worsen during pregnancy. A narrowed valve compounds the stresses of the more rapid heart rate, increased blood volume, and the heart's increased workload that occur during pregnancy. As a result, fluid may back up into the lungs, causing pulmonary edema—the most dangerous complication of mitral valve stenosis.

A woman who has severe rheumatic heart disease should have surgery to repair the mitral valve before conceiving. If necessary, this surgery can be performed during pregnancy, but open heart surgery increases the risk of losing the fetus or delivering prematurely.

During pregnancy, a woman should limit her physical activity and avoid becoming fatigued and anxious. The best time for labor and delivery is the expected delivery date or a few days before it. Because valves damaged by rheumatic heart disease are more susceptible to infections, antibiotics are given as a preventive measure during labor, 8 hours after delivery, and after any event that increases the risk of infection, such as dental work or premature rupture of the membranes that surround the fetus. Such infections are very serious.

BIRTH DEFECTS OF THE HEART

For most women who have birth defects of the heart (congenital heart disease)■ but have no symptoms before becoming pregnant, the risk of complications during pregnancy is not increased. However, women who have certain disorders affecting the right side of the heart and the lungs, such as Eisenmenger's syndrome and primary pulmonary hypertension, are liable to collapse and die during labor or shortly afterward. The cause of death is unclear, but the risk is great enough to make pregnancy inadvisable. If a woman who has one of these disorders does become pregnant, delivery is performed under the

best conditions possible, with all resuscitative equipment available. Antibiotics may be given to prevent infection of abnormal heart valves. Miscarriage or abortion after 20 weeks of pregnancy is also dangerous for these women.

MITRAL VALVE PROLAPSE

In mitral valve prolapse, the valve leaflets bulge into the left atrium during ventricular contraction, sometimes allowing leakage (regurgitation) of small amounts of blood into the atrium.

Mitral valve prolapse★ is more common in young women and tends to be hereditary. The symptoms are a heart murmur, awareness of the heartbeat (palpitations), and occasionally an irregular heartbeat. Most women who have this disorder don't have complications during pregnancy, but they are usually given antibiotics intravenously during delivery to prevent an infection of the heart valves.

High Blood Pressure

High blood pressure● may be present before pregnancy. It develops during pregnancy in a small percentage of women.

If a woman whose blood pressure is slightly high—140/90 to 150/100 millimeters of mercury (mm Hg)—is trying to become pregnant or finds out she is pregnant, her doctor usually discontinues the drugs she is taking to lower blood pressure (antihypertensive drugs). The risk that the drugs will harm the fetus may be greater than the possible benefit to the woman. The woman may have to restrict salt intake and reduce physical activity to help control her blood pressure.

A pregnant woman who has moderately high blood pressure (150/90 to 180/110 mm Hg) often must continue to take antihypertensive drugs. However, some of the drugs that are safe for the woman may harm the fetus. The antihypertensive drugs usually preferred for a pregnant woman are methyldopa and hydralazine. Drugs that lower blood pressure by removing excess water from

---

▲ see page 96

■ see page 1224

★ see page 95

● see page 112

the body (diuretics) reduce the pregnant woman's blood volume but can inhibit the fetus' growth. If a woman has been taking a diuretic to lower blood pressure, it's usually replaced with methyldopa as soon as the pregnancy is detected. Hydralazine is given in addition, if needed. Every month, the woman has a kidney function test and the fetus' growth is monitored with ultrasound scanning. Labor is usually started (induced) by the doctor at the 38th week of pregnancy.

A pregnant woman who has severe high blood pressure (over 180/110 mm Hg) needs special care. Pregnancy may greatly worsen the high blood pressure, possibly leading to brain swelling, a stroke, kidney failure, heart failure, and death. Early detachment of the placenta from the uterine wall (abruptio placentae) is more common in such women; with detachment, the fetus' supply of oxygen and nutrients is cut off and the fetus may die. Even if the placenta doesn't become detached, high blood pressure can reduce the blood supply to the placenta, slowing the fetus' growth. If a woman wishes to continue the pregnancy, she usually must be given more potent drugs to lower her blood pressure. She is usually hospitalized for the last half—or even more—of the pregnancy to protect herself and the fetus. If her condition deteriorates, the woman may be advised to end the pregnancy to save her life.

Anemias

Anemias are conditions in which the number of red blood cells or the amount of hemoglobin (the protein that carries oxygen) in them is below normal.

Most pregnant women have some degree of anemia that isn't harmful. However, anemias resulting from hereditary abnormalities in hemoglobin can complicate pregnancy. These abnormalities increase the risk of illness and death in the newborn and illness in the mother. Blood tests for hemoglobin abnormalities before delivery are routine for women whose race, ethnic origin, or family history indicates that they are more likely to have such an abnormality. Chorionic villus sampling or amniocentesis may be performed to detect a hemoglobin abnormality in the fetus.

▲ see page 749

Women who have sickle cell disease,▲ the most common hemoglobin abnormality, are particularly at risk of developing infections during pregnancy. Pneumonia, urinary tract infections, and infections of the uterus are the most common. About a third of pregnant women who have sickle cell disease develop high blood pressure during pregnancy. Sickle cell crisis (a sudden, severe attack of pain with a worsening of anemia) is common. Heart failure and life-threatening lung damage from small clots in blood vessels (pulmonary emboli) also may occur. The more severe the disease was before pregnancy, the higher the risk of illness or death during pregnancy.

Regular blood transfusions to maintain the hemoglobin level and other treatments reduce the risk of complications.

Kidney Disease

A woman who has severe kidney disease before becoming pregnant is unlikely to carry the baby to term. However, some women who undergo dialysis regularly for kidney failure and many who have had kidney transplants have given birth to healthy babies.

Pregnant women who have kidney disease usually need care from a kidney specialist (nephrologist) as well as from an obstetrician. Kidney function, blood pressure, and weight are routinely checked. Salt intake is restricted. Taking diuretics helps control blood pressure and excessive water retention (edema). Because early delivery may be necessary to save the baby's life, a woman is often hospitalized after the 28th week of pregnancy and a cesarean section is usually performed.

Infectious Disease

Urinary tract infections are common during pregnancy, probably because the enlarging uterus slows the flow of urine by pressing against the tubes connecting the kidneys to the bladder (ureters). When urine flow is slow, bacteria may not be flushed out of the urinary tract, increasing the chances of an infection. These infections increase the risk of early labor and premature rupture of the membranes that surround the fetus. Sometimes an infection in the bladder or ureters spreads up the urinary tract and reaches the kidney, causing an infection there. Treatment consists of antibiotic therapy.

Some infectious diseases can harm the fetus. German measles (rubella),▲ a well-known viral infection, is a major cause of birth defects, particularly of the heart and inner ear. Cytomegalovirus infection■ can cross the placenta and damage the fetus' liver. Toxoplasmosis, ★ caused by a protozoan, can infect and damage the fetus' brain. Pregnant women should avoid contact with cats and cat feces, which can transmit toxoplasmosis, unless the cats are strictly confined to the home and aren't exposed to other cats. Infectious hepatitis● can cause serious problems during pregnancy, especially in women who are undernourished. The fetus may become infected in the latter part of the pregnancy, making premature delivery more likely.

Sexually transmitted diseases can cause problems during pregnancy. Chlamydial infection may cause premature rupture of the membranes and early labor.

Human immunodeficiency virus (HIV) infection, which causes AIDS, is a major problem in a pregnancy: About one fourth of pregnant women who have the infection transmit it to the fetus. As early as possible in the pregnancy, such women generally are given AZT (zidovudine), which decreases by two thirds the transmission of the virus to the fetus. If infected, a baby can rapidly become very ill and usually dies of complications from AIDS before the age of two. Pregnancy doesn't seem to accelerate the progress of HIV infection in the mother.

Genital herpes◆ can be transmitted to a baby during a vaginal delivery. A baby infected with HIV who contracts herpes can develop a life-threatening brain infection (herpes encephalitis). If a woman has herpes skin sores late in the pregnancy, her doctor generally recommends that she give birth by a cesarean section to prevent transmission of the virus to her baby.

Diabetes

Diabetes is a disorder in which levels of blood sugar (glucose) are abnormally high. ♥

Many changes that take place during pregnancy make controlling blood sugar more difficult for a woman who has diabetes. Changes in the levels and types of hormones produced during pregnancy can cause insulin resistance, increasing the body's requirements for insulin, which for some women results in diabetes.

Diabetes that begins or first becomes apparent during pregnancy (gestational diabetes) occurs in 1 to 3 percent of all pregnancies. It's much more common among certain ethnic groups—particularly Native Americans, Pacific Islanders, and women of Mexican, Indian, and Asian descent—and among obese women. Pregnant women are routinely screened for gestational diabetes. After pregnancy, it usually disappears.

Poorly controlled diabetes may endanger the fetus as well as the woman. With good control, however, the risks are no greater than those for pregnant women who don't have diabetes. During pregnancy, a woman who has diabetes takes insulin by injection rather than oral hypoglycemic drugs, which can be toxic to the fetus. Most women are taught to use blood sugar testing devices and adjust their insulin doses as needed to control blood sugar levels throughout the pregnancy.

Diabetes increases a pregnant woman's risk of infection, early labor, and high blood pressure caused by pregnancy. Treatment of these disorders is the same as that for any other pregnant woman. If high blood pressure is controlled, pregnancy doesn't worsen kidney disease caused by diabetes, and kidney complications during pregnancy are rare.

The baby of a diabetic woman may be unusually large at birth, even when the woman has kept her blood sugar levels normal or nearly normal throughout pregnancy. The risk of birth defects is two times higher in babies of women who have diabetes. Birth defects are most likely to occur when control of diabetes is poor during the period when the fetus' organs are forming, particularly between the sixth and seventh weeks of pregnancy. At 16 to 18 weeks of pregnancy, the level of alpha-fetoprotein, a protein produced by the fetus, is usually measured in a sample of the woman's blood. A high alpha-fetoprotein level sug-

---

▲ see page 1268

■ see page 936

★ see page 899

● **see** page 571

◆ see page 946

♥ see page 717

gests incomplete development of the spine and spinal cord (spina bifida), while a low level suggests Down syndrome.▲ An ultrasound examination is performed at 20 to 22 weeks of pregnancy to look for other birth defects.

During the last 3 months of pregnancy, care focuses on monitoring the fetus' health and assessing the development of the fetus' lungs, as well as controlling the mother's blood sugar levels.

Most women who have diabetes can have vaginal deliveries. However, if a woman's medical care was inadequate or diabetes control was poor during early pregnancy, waiting for a vaginal delivery may be inadvisable. In such cases, amniocentesis may be performed to assess how mature the fetus' lungs are—an indication of whether the fetus can survive delivery—so that the baby can be delivered early by a cesarean section. A cesarean section may also be performed if the baby is too large to exit through the birth canal or if other difficulties occur during labor.

A prolonged pregnancy is particularly harmful for the fetus of a diabetic mother. Labor usually occurs naturally on or before 40 weeks; otherwise, at about 40 weeks, labor is usually induced by rupturing the membranes and giving oxytocin intravenously, or the baby is delivered by cesarean section. The fetus may die before birth if the pregnancy continues beyond 42 weeks.

Immediately after delivery, many women who have diabetes don't need insulin. For those who had diabetes before becoming pregnant, insulin requirements decrease dramatically after delivery, then gradually increase after about 72 hours. Women who developed gestational diabetes are tested after delivery to determine whether the diabetes is persisting or has disappeared.

Babies of women who have diabetes are assessed carefully after birth. These babies are at increased risk of developing breathing difficulties, low blood sugar and calcium levels, jaundice, and a high red blood cell count. These problems are temporary and can be treated.

▲ see page 1134

■ see page 709

★ see page 709

Thyroid Disease

Thyroid problems are common during pregnancy. A high level of thyroid hormone during pregnancy is most commonly caused by Graves' disease or thyroiditis.■ Graves' disease is caused by antibodies that stimulate the thyroid gland to produce too much thyroid hormone. These antibodies can cross the placenta and increase thyroid activity in the fetus, causing the fetus to have a rapid heart rate (more than 160 beats a minute) and slowed growth. Sometimes, Graves' disease produces antibodies that block the production of thyroid hormone. These antibodies can cross the placenta and prevent the fetus' thyroid gland from producing adequate amounts of thyroid hormone (hypothyroidism), which can cause a form of mental retardation called cretinism.

Treatment of Graves' disease varies. Generally, a woman takes the lowest possible dose of propylthiouracil. The woman is monitored carefully because this drug crosses the placenta and may prevent the fetus from producing adequate amounts of thyroid hormone. Often, Graves' disease improves during the last 3 months of pregnancy, so the dose of propylthiouracil can be reduced or stopped. If an experienced thyroid surgeon is available, a woman's thyroid gland may be removed (thyroidectomy) during the second trimester (fourth through sixth months of pregnancy). The woman must begin taking thyroid hormone 24 hours after surgery and take it for the rest of her life. This hormone merely replaces the hormone that the thyroid gland would normally produce and therefore causes no problems in the fetus.

Thyroiditis, an inflammation of the thyroid gland, causes a tender swelling in the neck. During pregnancy, a temporary increase in thyroid hormone levels causes temporary symptoms, which usually don't require treatment. In the first few weeks after delivery, a painless form of thyroiditis with a temporary increase in thyroid hormone production may develop abruptly. This condition may persist or worsen, sometimes with brief, recurring episodes of increased thyroid hormone production.

The two most common causes of low thyroid hormone levels during pregnancy are Hashimoto's thyroiditis,★ which is caused by antibodies that block thyroid hormone production, and previous treatment for Graves' disease. Often, Hashimoto's thyroiditis temporarily becomes less severe during pregnancy. A woman who has a low level of thyroid hormone is given thyroid hormone replacement tablets. After several weeks, blood tests are performed to measure the thyroid hormone level so that the dose can be adjusted if necessary. Modest dose adjustments may be necessary as the pregnancy continues.

In 4 to 7 percent of women, the thyroid gland malfunctions during the first 6 months after delivery. Women who have a family history of thyroid disease or diabetes or who already have a thyroid problem, such as an enlarged thyroid (goiter) or Hashimoto's thyroiditis, are particularly susceptible. A low or high level of thyroid hormone after pregnancy is usually temporary but may require treatment.

Liver Disease

Women with chronic active hepatitis and especially those with cirrhosis (liver damage with scarring)▲ often have difficulty becoming pregnant. Those who do become pregnant are likely to miscarry or give birth prematurely.

Pregnancy may temporarily worsen the blockage of bile flow in primary biliary cirrhosis (scarring of the bile ducts), sometimes producing jaundice or dark urine, but these effects disappear after delivery. For women who have cirrhosis, pregnancy slightly increases the likelihood of massive bleeding in varicose veins around the esophagus, especially during the last 3 months of pregnancy.

Asthma

Pregnancy affects women who have asthma■ in different ways, although the condition is more likely to worsen than improve. Similarly, asthma may have various effects on a pregnancy; it may slow the fetus' growth or trigger early labor.

Treatment of asthma during pregnancy depends on the severity and length of attacks. For mild attacks, a woman inhales a bronchodilator such as isoproterenol, which widens the constricted airways of the lungs. However, pregnant women must not overuse such drugs. For more severe attacks, the bronchodilator aminophylline is given intravenously. Extremely severe attacks (status asthmaticus) are also treated with corticosteroids given intravenously. Antibiotics are given if an infection is present. After an attack, the woman may take sustained action theophylline (a bronchodilator) in tablet form to prevent additional attacks. Bronchodilators and corticosteroids have been widely used during pregnancy without causing any major problems.

Systemic Lupus Erythematosus

Systemic lupus erythematosus (lupus),★ an autoimmune disease that's nine times more common in women than in men, may appear for the first time, worsen, or improve during pregnancy. How a pregnancy will affect the course of lupus can't be predicted, but the most likely time for flare-ups is immediately after delivery.

Women who develop lupus often have a history of repeated miscarriages, midpregnancy stillbirths, fetuses whose growth is slow (intrauterine growth retardation), and premature delivery. A fetus or a newborn may be endangered by complications of the mother's lupus, such as kidney damage, high blood pressure, or heart defects.

The antibodies that produce problems in the mother may cross the placenta and produce a very slow heart rate, anemia, a low platelet count, or a low white blood cell count in the fetus. However, these antibodies gradually disappear over several weeks once the baby is born, and the problems they cause resolve.

Rheumatoid Arthritis

Rheumatoid arthritis is an autoimmune disease that affects women more than twice as often as men.● Rheumatoid arthritis often improves during pregnancy, perhaps because the hydrocortisone level in the blood increases during pregnancy. This disease doesn't affect the fetus, but delivery may be difficult if the arthritis has affected the mother's hip joints or lower (lumbar) spine.

▲ see page 567

■ see page 173

★ see page 231

● see page 227

Myasthenia Gravis

Myasthenia gravis, an autoimmune disease that causes muscle weakness, is more common in women than in men.▲ During labor, a woman who has myasthenia gravis may need help with breathing (assisted ventilation). Because the antibodies that cause this disease can cross the placenta, 20 percent of the babies born to these mothers have myasthenia gravis at birth. However, because the mother's antibodies gradually disappear and the baby doesn't produce antibodies of this type, the muscle weakness is usually temporary.

Idiopathic Thrombocytopenic Purpura

In idiopathic thrombocytopenic purpura, an autoimmune disease, the number of platelets in the blood is greatly reduced, probably because abnormal antibodies destroy them. The result is an increased tendency to bleed. This disease is three times more common in women than in men. If not treated during pregnancy, the disease tends to be more severe. The antibodies may be passed to the fetus, reducing platelets to a dangerously low level before and immediately after birth. The baby may then bleed during labor and delivery, possibly resulting in injury or death, especially if bleeding occurs in the brain. By analyzing a small amount of blood taken from the umbilical cord, a doctor can look for antibodies and a low platelet count in the fetus. If the antibodies have passed to the fetus, a cesarean section can be performed to prevent birth trauma, which can cause bleeding in the baby's brain. The antibodies disappear within 21 days, and the baby's blood then clots normally.

Corticosteroids improve blood clotting in pregnant women who have this disease, but this improvement is long-lasting in only half of them. High doses of gamma globulin may be given intravenously to temporarily improve blood clotting so that labor can be safely induced and a woman can have a vaginal delivery without uncontrolled bleeding. Platelets are transfused only when delivery by a cesarean section is needed to protect

the baby and when the mother's platelet count is so low that severe bleeding may occur. In rare cases in which the platelet count remains dangerously low despite treatment, a woman's spleen, which traps and destroys platelets, is removed. The best time for this surgery is at midpregnancy. Removing the spleen improves blood clotting over the long term in about 80 percent of the people who have immune thrombocytopenic purpura.

Surgery During Pregnancy

Most of the disorders that require surgery during pregnancy are abdominal problems. Pregnancy can make the diagnosis difficult and can complicate any surgical procedure. Because surgery can cause a miscarriage, especially in early pregnancy, surgery is usually delayed as long as possible when the mother's long-term health is not an issue.

Appendicitis may cause cramping pain that resembles uterine contractions. A blood test may detect a high white blood cell count, but because this count normally increases during pregnancy, this test is unreliable for diagnosing appendicitis in a pregnant woman. Furthermore, the appendix is pushed higher in the abdomen as the pregnancy progresses, so that pain in the right lower section of the abdomen, the usual location of appendicitis pain, doesn't reliably indicate appendicitis during pregnancy. If appendicitis seems to be the problem, surgery to remove the appendix (appendectomy) is performed immediately because a ruptured appendix during pregnancy may be fatal. An appendectomy isn't likely to harm the fetus or cause a miscarriage.

Ovarian cysts can develop during pregnancy and may cause painful cramping. Ultrasound scanning can detect ovarian cysts safely and accurately. Unless a cyst is obviously cancerous, surgery is usually postponed until after the 12th week of pregnancy, because the cyst may be producing hormones that are supporting the pregnancy and often disappears spontaneously. However, surgery may be necessary before the 12th week if a cyst or mass continues to enlarge or is tender to the touch, in case the underlying cause is cancer or an abscess.

Gallbladder disorders occur occasionally during pregnancy. A pregnant woman has frequent examinations to monitor the disorder's progress. However, if the condition doesn't improve, surgery may be necessary.

▲ see page 333

Obstruction of the intestine can be extremely serious during pregnancy. If gangrene of the intestine and peritonitis (inflammation of the lining of the abdominal cavity) develop, a woman's life is in jeopardy and she may miscarry. Exploratory surgery is usually performed promptly when a pregnant woman has symptoms of intestinal obstruction, particularly if she has had abdominal surgery or an abdominal infection in the past.

CHAPTER 247

Drug Use During Pregnancy

Most pregnant women take drugs of some kind. The Centers for Disease Control and Prevention and the World Health Organization estimate that more than 90 percent of pregnant women take prescription or nonprescription (over-the-counter) drugs, social drugs such as tobacco and alcohol, or illicit drugs. Drugs cause 2 to 3 percent of all birth defects; most of the others result from hereditary, environmental, or unknown causes.▲

Drugs move from the mother to the fetus primarily through the placenta, the same route taken by nutrients for the fetus' growth and development. In the placenta, drugs and nutrients in the mother's blood cross a thin membrane, which separates the mother's blood from the fetus' blood.

Drugs that a woman takes during pregnancy can affect the fetus in several ways:
• By acting directly on the fetus, causing damage, abnormal development, or death
• By altering the function of the placenta, usually by constricting blood vessels and reducing the exchange of oxygen and nutrients between the fetus and the mother
• By causing the muscles of the uterus to contract forcefully, indirectly injuring the fetus by reducing its blood supply

How a drug affects a fetus depends on the fetus' stage of development and the potency and dose of the drug. Certain drugs taken early in pregnancy—before the 17th day after fertilization—may act in an all-or-nothing fashion, either killing the fetus or not affecting it at all. During this stage, the fetus is highly resistant to birth defects. However, the fetus is particularly vulnerable to birth defects between days 17 and 57 after fertilization, when its organs are developing. Drugs reaching the fetus during this stage may cause a miscarriage, an obvious birth defect, or a permanent but subtle defect noticed later in life, or they may have no noticeable effect. Drugs taken after organ development is complete are unlikely to cause obvious birth defects, but they may alter the growth and function of normally formed organs and tissues.

Anticancer Drugs

Because the fetus' tissues are growing quickly, their rapidly multiplying cells are very vulnerable to anticancer drugs. Many such drugs are teratogens, which are drugs that cause such birth defects as stunted growth in the uterus (intrauterine growth retardation), underdevelopment of the lower jaw, cleft palate, abnormal development of the skull bones, spinal defects, ear defects, clubfoot, and mental retardation. Some anticancer drugs cause birth defects in animals but haven't been shown to do so in humans.

Thalidomide

This drug is no longer prescribed to pregnant women because it causes major birth defects. The drug was first introduced in 1956 in Europe as a remedy for influenza and as a sedative. In 1962, thalidomide taken by pregnant women when the fetus' organs were developing was found to cause

---

▲ see page 1223

How Drugs Cross the Placenta

In the placenta, the mother's blood passes through the space (intervillous space) that surrounds tiny projections (villi) containing blood vessels from the fetus. The mother's blood in the intervillous space is separated from the fetus' blood in the villi by a thin membrane (placental membrane). Drugs in the mother's blood can cross this membrane into blood vessels in the villi and pass through the umbilical cord into the fetus.

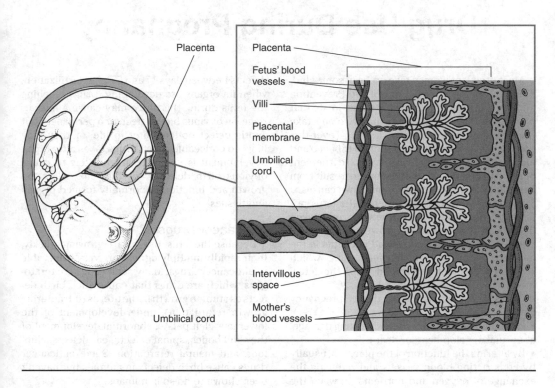

birth defects, including severely underdeveloped arms and legs and defects of the intestine, heart, and blood vessels.

Skin Treatments

Isotretinoin, used to treat severe acne, psoriasis, and other skin disorders, causes major birth defects. Among the most significant are heart defects, small ears, and hydrocephalus—sometimes called water on the brain. The risk of birth defects is about 25 percent. Etretinate, another drug used to treat skin disorders, also causes birth defects in humans. Because this drug is stored in fat beneath the skin and released slowly, it can continue to cause birth defects for 6 months or longer after a woman stops taking it. Therefore, women who use this drug are advised to wait at least 1 year before becoming pregnant.

Sex Hormones

Androgenic (masculinizing) hormones, used to treat various blood disorders, and synthetic progestins taken during the first 12 weeks after fertilization may masculinize a female fetus' genitals. The clitoris, a small protrusion analogous to the penis in the male, may be enlarged—a condition that is permanent unless corrected with surgery—and the labia minora, which surround the openings to the vagina and urethra, may be fused together. Oral contraceptives don't contain enough progestin to produce such effects.

Diethylstilbestrol (DES), a synthetic estrogen, can cause vaginal cancer in adolescent girls whose mothers took this drug during pregnancy. These girls may later suffer from an abnormal uterine cavity, menstrual problems, a weakened (incompetent) cervix that can cause miscarriages, and an increased risk of having an ectopic pregnancy or having a baby who dies shortly before or after birth. Boys exposed to diethylstilbestrol as fetuses may have penis abnormalities.

Meclizine

Meclizine, frequently taken for motion sickness, nausea, and vomiting, causes birth defects in animals, but the same effects haven't been seen in humans.

Anticonvulsant Drugs

Taken during pregnancy by a woman who is epileptic, some anticonvulsant drugs may cause the baby to have a cleft palate and abnormally developed heart, face and skull, hands, or abdominal organs. The baby may also be mentally retarded. Two anticonvulsants are particularly likely to cause birth defects; the risk is about 70 percent with trimethadione and about 1 percent with valproic acid. Carbamazepine, another anticonvulsant, is thought to cause a significant number of minor birth defects. The anticonvulsant phenytoin was previously blamed for a variety of birth defects, but similar defects occurred in babies of epileptic women who didn't take anticonvulsants.

Newborns exposed to phenytoin and phenobarbital (a barbiturate as well as an anticonvulsant) before birth may bleed easily because these drugs can cause a deficiency of vitamin K, which is needed for clotting. This side effect can be prevented if a pregnant woman takes vitamin K by mouth every day for a month before delivery or if the newborn is given an injection of vitamin K soon after birth. During pregnancy, women who have epilepsy are given the smallest effective dose of anticonvulsants and are closely monitored.

Federal Food and Drug Administration Categories of Drug Safety During Pregnancy

Category	Description
A	Human studies have shown no risk.
B	Animal studies have shown no risk but no human studies are available, or animal studies have shown risk but human studies have not.
C	No human or animal studies are available, or animal studies have shown risk but no human studies are available.
D	Human studies have shown risk, but use may be justified in some cases (life-threatening situation or serious disease for which there is no safer drug).
X	The drug should never be taken during pregnancy; known human risk outweighs any benefit.

Women who have epilepsy, even if they don't take anticonvulsants during pregnancy, are more likely to have babies with birth defects than women who don't have epilepsy. The risk is greater in those who have frequent, severe convulsions or complications of pregnancy and in those in low socioeconomic groups, who tend to receive inadequate health care.

Vaccines

Except under special circumstances, vaccines made with a live virus aren't given to women who are or might be pregnant. Rubella vaccine, a live-virus vaccine, can cause infection of both the placenta and the developing fetus. Live-virus vaccines—such as those for measles, mumps, polio, chickenpox, and yellow fever—and other vaccines—such as those for cholera, hepatitis A and B, influenza, plague, rabies, tetanus, diphtheria, and typhoid—are given to a pregnant woman only if she is at substantial risk of becoming infected with one of those microorganisms.

Thyroid Drugs

Radioactive iodine given to a pregnant woman to treat an overactive thyroid gland (hyperthyroidism) can cross the placenta and destroy the fetus' thyroid gland or cause severe underactivity of the thyroid gland (hypothyroidism). Propylthiouracil and methimazole, drugs also used to treat an overactive thyroid gland, cross the placenta and can cause the fetus' thyroid gland to become abnormally enlarged; when needed, propylthiouracil is usually used because it's tolerated better by both the woman and fetus.

Oral Hypoglycemic Drugs

Oral hypoglycemic drugs are given to lower blood sugar (glucose) levels in people who have diabetes, but they often fail to control diabetes in pregnant women and may cause newborns to have very low blood glucose levels (hypoglycemia). Therefore, insulin is preferred for treating diabetes in pregnant women.

Narcotics and Nonsteroidal Anti-inflammatory Drugs

Narcotics and nonsteroidal anti-inflammatory drugs (NSAIDs), such as aspirin, can reach the fetus in significant amounts if taken by a pregnant woman. Babies of women who are narcotic addicts can become addicted before birth and may show withdrawal symptoms 6 hours to 8 days after birth. Taking large doses of aspirin or other NSAIDs during pregnancy may delay the start of labor and may also cause the connection (ductus arteriosus)▲ between the aorta (the large artery that carries blood to the body) and the pulmonary artery (the artery that carries blood to the lungs) in the fetus to close before birth. This connection normally closes immediately after birth. Closure before birth forces blood to flow through the lungs, which haven't expanded yet, overloading the fetus' circulatory system.

When used late in pregnancy, nonsteroidal anti-inflammatory drugs may reduce the amount of amniotic fluid (the liquid surrounding the developing fetus, contained in the amniotic sac)—a potentially dangerous effect. Taking large doses of aspirin may cause bleeding problems in the mother or the newborn. Aspirin or other salicylates may increase bilirubin levels in the fetus'

blood, causing jaundice and occasionally brain damage.

Antianxiety Drugs and Antidepressants

Antianxiety drugs may cause birth defects when taken during the first 3 months of pregnancy, although this effect hasn't been proven. Most antidepressants appear to be relatively safe when used during pregnancy, but lithium can cause birth defects—mainly of the heart. Barbiturates, such as phenobarbital, taken by a pregnant woman tend to reduce the slight jaundice newborns commonly have.

Antibiotics

When taken during pregnancy, antibiotics can cause problems. Tetracycline antibiotics cross the placenta and are stored in the fetus' bones and teeth, where they combine with calcium. As a result, bone growth may be slow, the baby's teeth may be permanently yellow, and the tooth enamel may be soft and abnormally susceptible to cavities. The risk of tooth abnormalities is greatest from the middle to the end of pregnancy. Because several safe alternative antibiotics are available, tetracyclines are avoided during pregnancy.

Taking antibiotics such as streptomycin or kanamycin during pregnancy may damage the fetus' inner ear, possibly resulting in deafness. Chloramphenicol doesn't harm the fetus but can cause a serious illness in the newborn called gray baby syndrome. Ciprofloxacin should not be taken during pregnancy because it has been shown to cause joint abnormalities in animals. Penicillins appear to be safe.

Most sulfonamide antibiotics taken late in pregnancy may cause the newborn to develop jaundice, which can result in brain damage. However, one sulfonamide antibiotic, sulfasalazine, is much less likely to cause this problem.

Anticlotting Drugs

The developing fetus is highly sensitive to warfarin, an anticlotting drug (anticoagulant). Significant birth defects occur in up to one fourth of babies exposed to the drug during the first 3 months of pregnancy. Also, abnormal bleeding may occur in both the woman and fetus. If a pregnant woman is at risk of developing blood clots, heparin is a much safer alternative. However, prolonged use during pregnancy may result in a low

▲ see box, page 1227

platelet count in the mother (platelets are cell-like particles that help blood clot) or in bone thinning (osteoporosis).

Drugs for Heart or Blood Vessel Disorders

Some women need these drugs during pregnancy for disorders that are chronic or that develop during pregnancy, such as preeclampsia (high blood pressure, protein in the urine, and fluid accumulation during pregnancy) and eclampsia (seizures resulting from preeclampsia). Drugs to lower high blood pressure, frequently given to pregnant women with preeclampsia or eclampsia, affect the functioning of the placenta and are used with great care to avoid causing problems in the fetus.▲ In general, these problems result from lowering the mother's blood pressure too rapidly, which markedly reduces blood flow to the placenta. Angiotensin converting enzyme inhibitors and thiazide diuretics usually are avoided during pregnancy because they can cause serious problems in the fetus. Digoxin, used to treat heart failure and some heart rhythm abnormalities, readily crosses the placenta but typically has little effect on the baby before or after birth.

Some drugs, such as nitrofurantoin, vitamin K, sulfonamides, and chloramphenicol, may cause the breakdown of red blood cells in pregnant women and fetuses who have glucose-6-phosphate dehydrogenase (G6PD) deficiency, a hereditary disorder that affects red blood cell membranes. Therefore, these drugs aren't given to women who have this disorder.

Drugs Used During Labor and Delivery

Local anesthetics, narcotics, and other analgesics usually cross the placenta and can affect the newborn—for example, by weakening its urge to breathe.■ Therefore, if drugs are needed during labor, they are given in the smallest effective doses and preferably as late as possible so that they are less likely to reach the fetus before birth.

Social and Illicit Drugs

Smoking during pregnancy can be harmful.★ The average birth weight of babies born to women who smoke during pregnancy is 6 ounces less than that of babies born to women who don't smoke. Miscarriages, stillbirths, premature births, and sudden infant death syndrome (SIDS) are more common among babies of women who smoke during pregnancy.

Drinking **alcohol** during pregnancy can cause birth defects. Babies of women who drink excessive amounts of alcohol during pregnancy may have fetal alcohol syndrome.● Such babies are small, often with small heads (microcephaly), facial abnormalities, and borderline mental deficiency. Less commonly, they have joint abnormalities and heart defects. They don't thrive and are more likely to die soon after birth. Because the amount of alcohol required to cause this syndrome is unknown, pregnant women are advised to abstain from drinking alcohol.

Whether **caffeine** harms the fetus has been debated. Several studies have suggested that drinking more than seven or eight cups of coffee a day may increase the risk of having a stillbirth, premature birth, low-birth-weight baby, or miscarriage. However, these studies were flawed because many of the coffee drinkers also smoked cigarettes. A later study, which accounted for cigarette smoking, concluded that the problems were caused by tobacco, not caffeine. Whether heavy coffee drinking during pregnancy affects the newborn is unclear.

Aspartame, an artificial sweetener, appears to be safe during pregnancy when it's consumed in amounts used for dietary sweetening.

Cocaine use during pregnancy increases the risk of miscarriage; early detachment of the placenta from the uterus (abruptio placentae); birth defects of the brain, kidneys, and genital organs; and less interactive behavior in newborns.◆

No conclusive evidence that **marijuana** causes birth defects or interferes with fetal growth and development has been found. However, studies suggest that heavy use of marijuana during pregnancy may lead to abnormal behavior in newborns.

▲ see page 1161

■ see page 1175

★ see page 1149

● see page 1214

◆ see page 1214

Labor and Delivery

Although each labor and delivery is different, most follow a general pattern. Therefore, an expectant mother can have a general idea of what changes will occur in her body to enable her to deliver the baby and what procedures will be followed to help her. She also has several choices to make—such as whether to have the father present and where to have the baby (hospital, birthing center, or home).

Usually, an expectant mother wants the baby's father to remain with her during labor. His encouragement and emotional support can help her relax so that her need for drugs to relieve pain may be reduced. In addition, sharing the meaningful experience of childbirth has emotional and psychologic benefits, such as creating strong family bonds. Childbirth education classes prepare both father and mother for the entire process. On the other hand, an expectant mother may prefer privacy during labor, the father may not want to be present, or another partner may be more appropriate. The expectant mother and father can decide what is best for them.

Most babies are born in hospitals, but some women want to have their babies at home. Many doctors hesitate to recommend home delivery because they're concerned about unexpected complications, which can include sudden detachment of the placenta, fetal distress (usually caused by lack of oxygen to the fetus during labor), an unexpected multiple pregnancy such as twins, and complications after delivery such as excessive bleeding (postpartum hemorrhage). Home delivery should be considered only by women who have already had at least one uneventful pregnancy and delivery. A doctor or certified nurse midwife, preferably the same person who provided prenatal care, should attend. If possible, a home near a hospital should be used; if a woman's home is too far away, the home of a relative or friend could be considered. A plan for rapid transport from the home to the hospital should be made in case it's needed.

Birthing centers are equipped to handle normal, uncomplicated pregnancies. By providing a homelike atmosphere and allowing family and friends to be present, these centers enable women to have an informal, personal experience of childbirth. If complications develop during labor, centers usually have an arrangement with a nearby hospital to transfer the woman there immediately.

Many hospitals have birthing centers that combine homelike settings and fewer rules—such as those that limit the number of visitors or visiting hours—with the advantage of having a medical staff, emergency equipment, and full hospital facilities, if needed. Some hospitals have private rooms in which a mother stays from labor until discharge; these rooms are called LDRPs for labor, delivery, recovery, and postpartum (after delivery).

Regardless of the choices a woman makes, knowing what to expect is excellent preparation for labor and delivery.

Labor

Labor is a series of rhythmic, progressive contractions of the uterus that gradually move the fetus through the cervix (lower part of the uterus) and vagina (birth canal) to the outside world.

Contractions cause the cervix to open gradually (dilate) and to thin and pull back (efface) until it almost merges with the rest of the uterus. These changes enable the fetus to pass through the birth canal.

Labor usually starts within 2 weeks of (before or after) the estimated date of delivery or confinement. Exactly what causes labor to start is unknown. It may be oxytocin, a hormone that is released by the pituitary gland and causes the uterus to contract during labor, but this hasn't been proved. Labor usually lasts no more than 12 to 14 hours in a woman's first pregnancy and tends to be shorter, averaging 6 to 8 hours, in subsequent pregnancies.

The bloody show (a small amount of blood mixed with mucus from the cervix) usually is a clue that labor is about to begin; however, it may be discharged from the vagina as early as 72 hours before contractions begin. Occasionally, the fluid-filled membranes that contain the fetus rupture before labor begins, and the fluid (amniotic fluid)

Stages of Labor

First Stage

From the beginning of labor to the full opening (dilation) of the cervix—about 4 inches (10 centimeters).

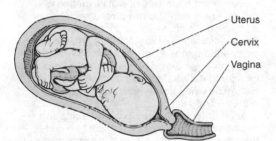

Uterus
Cervix
Vagina

Initial (Latent) Phase

• Contractions become progressively stronger and more rhythmic.
• Discomfort is minimal.
• The cervix thins and opens to about 1½ inches (4 centimeters).
• This phase lasts an average of 8½ hours in a first pregnancy and 5 hours in subsequent pregnancies.

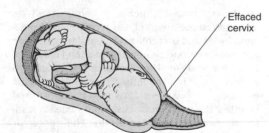

Effaced cervix

Active Phase

• The cervix opens from about 1½ inches (4 centimeters) to the full 4 inches (10 centimeters).
• The presenting part of the baby, usually the head, descends into the mother's pelvis.
• The mother begins to feel the urge to push as the baby descends.
• This phase averages about 5 hours in a first pregnancy and 2 hours in subsequent pregnancies.

Second Stage

From the complete opening of the cervix to delivery of the baby. This stage averages about 60 minutes in a first pregnancy and 15 to 30 minutes in subsequent pregnancies.

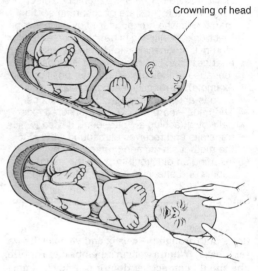

Crowning of head

Third Stage

From delivery of the baby to delivery of the placenta. This stage usually lasts only a few minutes.

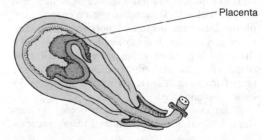

Placenta

Traditionally, labor is divided into three stages; however, the 4 hours immediately after delivery of the placenta, when the risk of bleeding is greatest, is often called the fourth stage of labor.

Fetal Monitoring

Electronic fetal heart monitoring is used to monitor the fetus' heart rate and the contractions of the uterus. Many doctors use it for all deliveries because 30 to 50 percent of babies who develop problems or die during delivery do so without warning. Electronic monitoring may save the life of such a baby. However, women who are monitored electronically have a higher rate of cesarean section than those who are monitored by stethoscope. Electronic monitoring is generally reserved for high-risk pregnancies, for babies whose heartbeat can't be heard with a stethoscope (because of their presentation or position, for example), or for babies whose heartbeat sounds abnormal through the stethoscope. The fetus' heart rate can be monitored externally by attaching an ultrasound device (which transmits and receives ultrasound waves) to the mother's abdomen or internally by inserting an electrode through the mother's vagina and attaching it to the fetus' scalp. The internal approach usually is reserved for high-risk pregnancies.

In a high-risk pregnancy, electronic fetal heart monitoring is sometimes used as part of a **nonstress test,** in which the fetus' heart rate is monitored as the fetus lies still and moves. If the heart rate doesn't increase with movement, a **contraction stress test** may be performed. To start uterine contractions, nipple stimulation or oxytocin (a hormone that causes the uterus to contract during labor) may be used. The fetus' heart rate is monitored during these contractions to determine whether the fetus will be able to withstand labor.

Another test, **fetal scalp blood sampling,** involves removing a small amount of blood from the fetus' scalp to determine how much acid the fetus is producing during labor.

On the basis of such tests, a doctor may allow labor to continue or perform a cesarean section immediately.

---

flows out through the cervix and vagina (the water breaks). When a woman's membranes rupture, she should contact her doctor or midwife immediately. About 80 to 90 percent of women whose membranes have ruptured go into labor spontaneously within 24 hours. If labor hasn't begun after 24 hours and the baby is due, a woman usually is admitted to the hospital, where labor is started (induced) to reduce the risk of infection caused by bacteria from the vagina entering the uterus. Infections may affect mother or fetus. Oxytocin or a similar drug is used to induce labor. If the baby is premature, carefully monitoring the woman may be preferred to inducing labor, and no pelvic examination is performed until after delivery is planned.▲

When a woman in labor—with strong contractions 5 minutes apart or less and the cervix dilated more than 1½ inches (4 centimeters)—is admitted to the hospital, her weight, blood pressure, heart and breathing rates, and temperature are measured, and samples of urine and blood are taken for analysis. Her abdomen is examined to estimate how big the fetus is, whether the fetus is facing rearward or forward (position), and whether the head, buttocks, or shoulder is leading the way out (presentation). The doctor or other health care practitioner listens to the fetus' heartbeat through a stethoscope. The strength, duration, and frequency of contractions are noted. Usually, the vagina is examined to determine if the membranes have ruptured and how dilated and effaced the cervix is, but this examination may be omitted if the woman is bleeding or if the membranes have ruptured spontaneously. A green discoloration of the amniotic fluid after the membranes have ruptured is caused by the fetus' first stool (fetal meconium) and may indicate fetal distress.■ A fetus usually passes meconium before delivery only when in distress or in buttocks-first (breech) presentation.

The fetus' presentation and position affect how the fetus passes through the vagina.★ Head-first

▲ see page 1178

■ see page 1206

★ see box, page 1180

(vertex) presentation, which is by far the most common type, is best for a safe delivery. During the last week or two before delivery, most fetuses turn so that the head presents first. Buttocks-first (breech) presentation makes delivery considerably more difficult for the mother, fetus, and doctor. By delaying the appearance of the fetus' head, breech presentation increases the likelihood of fetal distress. Because the head is wider than the buttocks, fitting the head through the passageway made by the buttocks in the birth canal is harder than the reverse, and the head is more likely to get caught. Shoulder-first presentation also makes the fetus' passage from the uterus more difficult. If the fetus' position is head first and facing rearward (toward the mother's back) rather than facing forward, labor usually is easier.

During labor, a woman usually receives fluids through intravenous tubing to prevent dehydration. Intravenous tubing also provides a way to give drugs immediately, if needed. Receiving fluids intravenously enables a woman to avoid eating and drinking during labor so that she's less likely to vomit and inhale vomit during delivery. Inhaling vomit can cause Mendelson's syndrome, a potentially life-threatening condition in which the lungs are inflamed. Usually, a woman is given an antacid to neutralize stomach acid when she is admitted to the hospital and every 3 hours after that. Antacids reduce the risk of damage to the lungs if vomit is inhaled.

During the first stage of labor, the mother usually is discouraged from pushing, because pushing before the cervix is fully opened wastes energy and may tear the cervix. The heart rate of mother and fetus is checked about every 15 minutes. Monitoring the fetus' heart rate, which is performed with a fetal stethoscope (fetoscope) or electronic fetal heart monitoring, is the easiest way to determine if the fetus is in distress. If the fetus' heart rate becomes too fast or too slow, the doctor may decide to deliver the baby by cesarean section or forceps or to take other corrective measures, such as turning the mother on her left side, increasing the amount of intravenous fluids, or giving oxygen through a nasal tube.

During the second stage of labor, the mother, who is monitored constantly, pushes with each contraction to move the fetus through the vagina. The fetus' heart rate is monitored after every contraction or every 3 minutes, whichever is less.

Pain Relief

With the advice of her doctor or midwife, a woman usually chooses a general approach to pain relief long before labor starts. She may choose natural childbirth, which relies on relaxation and breathing techniques to deal with pain, or she may plan to use analgesics or a particular type of anesthesia, if needed. After labor starts, these plans may be modified, depending on how labor progresses, how the woman feels, and what the doctor or midwife recommends.

A woman's need for pain relief during labor varies considerably, depending to some extent on her level of anxiety. Preparation for labor and delivery as well as emotional support from those attending the labor tends to lessen anxiety and often markedly reduces her need for drugs to relieve pain. Many women take no drugs.

If a woman requests analgesics during labor, they are usually given to her, but as little as possible is used because these drugs can slow (depress) breathing and other functions of the baby after birth. Delivery is a critical time for the baby: Many internal changes take place as the newborn rapidly adjusts from a life of total dependence on the mother to a life of independence. A newborn who is sedated by strong analgesics may be less able to adjust. Most commonly, either meperidine or morphine, given intravenously, is used to relieve pain. Because these drugs can slow the initial phase of labor, they usually are given during the active phase. In addition, because their greatest effect occurs in the first 30 minutes after they're given, these drugs aren't given when delivery is imminent. To counteract the sedating effects of these drugs on the newborn, the drug naloxone can be given immediately after delivery.

If a woman needs more pain relief as delivery is approaching, she may be given a **local anesthetic** at the opening of the vagina. It completely numbs the painful area but allows her to remain awake and doesn't slow the fetus' functions. It may be given as a pudendal block or as regional anesthesia. A **pudendal block,** a commonly used procedure, involves injecting a local anesthetic through the wall of the vagina and anesthetizing the pudendal nerve, which numbs the entire vaginal area except the front of the vulva (the external genital organs). It is useful for uncomplicated deliveries in which a woman wants to push.

Natural Childbirth

Natural childbirth uses relaxation and breathing techniques to control pain during childbirth. An expectant mother and her partner take childbirth classes, usually six to eight sessions over several weeks, to learn how to use these techniques. They also learn what happens in the various stages of labor and delivery.

The relaxation technique involves consciously tensing a part of the body and then relaxing it. This technique helps a woman relax the rest of her body while the uterus is contracting during labor and relax when she isn't having contractions. Several types of breathing can help in the first stage of labor, before the woman begins to push:

• Deep breathing, which helps the woman relax, can be used at the beginning and end of a contraction

• Fast, shallow breathing in the upper chest is used at the peak of a contraction

• A pattern of panting and blowing helps the woman refrain from pushing when she has an urge to push before the cervix is completely dilated

In the second stage of labor, the woman alternates between pushing and panting.

The woman and her partner should practice relaxation and breathing techniques regularly during pregnancy. During labor, the woman's partner can help her by reminding her of what she should be doing at a particular stage and by noticing when she is tense, in addition to providing emotional support. Massage may be used to help the woman relax. Natural childbirth often helps reduce or eliminate the need for analgesics or anesthesia during labor and delivery.

The most well-known method of natural childbirth is probably the Lamaze method. Another method, the Leboyer method, involves birth in a darkened room and immersion of the baby into lukewarm water immediately after delivery.

If a woman doesn't want to feel pushing and wants more pain relief, **regional anesthesia** may be used. Most commonly, a local anesthetic is injected into the space that surrounds the spinal cord (epidural space) in the lower back; this procedure is called a lumbar epidural injection. Alternatively, narcotics such as fentanyl and sufentanil are given by continuous infusion into the epidural space. These procedures are commonly used but may increase the need for cesarean section because the anesthetic can prevent the woman from being able to push adequately. Spinal anesthesia, in which an anesthetic is injected into the central canal of the spinal cord, may be used for a cesarean section or vaginal delivery, but it isn't used often because of the slight risk of headache, sometimes severe, after delivery. When used for vaginal delivery, spinal anesthesia must be given when delivery is imminent because this type of anesthesia prevents a woman from pushing. Because regional anesthesia may cause a dangerous fall in blood pressure, the woman's blood pressure is measured frequently.

General anesthesia, which makes a woman temporarily unconscious, isn't used when it can be avoided because it slows the functioning of the fetus' heart, lungs, and brain as well as the woman's. It may be used for emergency cesarean sections because it's the quickest way to anesthetize the woman.

Delivery

Delivery is the passage of the fetus and placenta (afterbirth) from the uterus to the outside world.

When a woman is about to give birth in the hospital, she may be moved from the labor room to the birthing or delivery room, a small room used only for deliveries, or she may remain in an LDRP. The intravenous tube remains in place. Usually, the father or other support people are encouraged to accompany her.

In the birthing or delivery room, the woman may be placed in a semi-upright position, between lying down and sitting up. Her back can be supported by pillows or a backrest. The semi-upright position makes good use of gravity: The downward pressure of the fetus helps the birth canal and the perineum (the area between the openings of the vagina and anus) stretch gradually with less risk of tearing. This position also puts less strain on the woman's back and pelvis. Some women prefer to deliver lying down; however, delivery in this position may result in a longer delivery and is more likely to require assistance. Also, heart rate abnormalities have been seen less often in babies born to women who were more upright than in babies born to women who were lying down.

As delivery progresses, the doctor or midwife examines the vagina to determine the position of the fetus' head. The mother is asked to bear down and push with each contraction to help move the fetus' head down through her pelvis and to widen the vaginal opening so that more and more of the head appears. When about $1\frac{1}{2}$ to 2 inches of the head appears, the doctor or midwife places a hand over the fetus' head during a contraction to control and, if necessary, slightly slow the fetus' progress. The head and chin are eased out of the vaginal opening to prevent the mother's tissues from tearing. These maneuvers help ease delivery.

Forceps (metal devices, similar to tongs, with rounded edges that fit around the baby's head) allow a doctor to pull the baby out with less risk of injury to the baby and the mother. Rarely used in normal circumstances, forceps are used when the mother is unable to push because she has had an epidural injection, when she is having trouble pushing because labor isn't progressing well, or when the fetus is in distress.

If the vaginal opening isn't stretching enough to let the baby emerge and a tear is likely, a doctor may perform an **episiotomy** (an incision through the perineum and the vaginal wall). This procedure is intended to make delivery easier and to prevent a tear, which is ragged and more difficult to repair than the short, straight cut of an episiotomy. A local anesthetic is used to numb the area. If the sphincter that keeps the anus shut (rectal sphincter) is damaged when the episiotomy is performed or torn during delivery, it generally heals well if the doctor repairs it immediately.

After the baby's head has emerged, the body rotates sideways so that the shoulders can emerge easily, one at a time. The rest of the baby usually slips out quickly. Mucus and fluid are suctioned out of the baby's nose, mouth, and throat. The umbilical cord is clamped in two places▲ and cut between the clamps to prevent bleeding from either end. The baby is then wrapped in a lightweight blanket and placed on the mother's abdomen or in a warmed bassinet.

After delivery of the baby, the doctor or midwife places a hand gently on the mother's abdomen to make sure the uterus is contracting. During the first or second contraction after delivery, the placenta usually detaches from the uterus, and a gush of blood soon follows. Usually, the mother can push the placenta out on her own. If she can't and if she's bleeding excessively, the doctor or midwife applies firm downward pressure on the mother's abdomen, causing the placenta to detach from the uterus and come out. If the placenta is incomplete, the doctor or midwife can remove any remaining pieces by hand.

As soon as the placenta has been delivered, the mother is given oxytocin and her abdomen is periodically massaged to help the uterus contract. Contraction is essential to prevent further bleeding from the area where the placenta was attached to the uterus.

The doctor stitches the episiotomy incision and any tears in the cervix or vagina. The mother is then moved to the recovery room or remains in an LDRP; a baby who doesn't need further medical attention stays with the mother. Typically, mother, baby, and father remain together in a warm, private area for 3 to 4 hours so that bonding can begin. Many mothers wish to begin breastfeeding soon after delivery. Later, the baby may be taken to the hospital nursery. In many hospitals, the mother may choose to have the baby remain with her (rooming-in). Hospitals with LDRPs require it. With rooming-in, the baby usually is fed on demand, and the mother learns how to care for the baby before they leave the hospital. If a mother needs a rest, she may take the baby to the nursery.

Because most complications, particularly bleeding, occur within the first 4 hours after delivery (the fourth stage of labor), the mother is carefully observed during this time.

▲ see box, page 1191

Complications of Labor and Delivery

Labor and delivery is a time of excitement and anxiety, even when no problems occur. A pregnant woman can reduce anxiety and improve the chances of a good outcome by establishing a relationship with a doctor or midwife.

The primary problems in labor are related to timing. Labor may not start when the membranes containing the fetus break (premature rupture of the membranes), or it may start before the 37th week of pregnancy (preterm labor) or more than 2 weeks after the due date (postterm pregnancy). Difficulties may occur if a mother or fetus has a medical problem, if labor progresses too slowly, or if the fetus is in an abnormal position. Other danger signs include excessive vaginal bleeding▲ and an abnormal heart rate in the fetus. Serious problems are relatively rare and often can be anticipated, but problems may appear suddenly and unexpectedly. Ideally, they are detected early so that appropriate treatment can be given to ensure a good outcome.

Premature Rupture of the Membranes

Premature rupture of the membranes is the breaking of the fluid-filled membranes containing the fetus 1 hour or more before labor begins.

Rupture of the membranes, whether premature or not, is commonly referred to as the water breaking. The fluid within the membranes (amniotic fluid) leaks out from the vagina.

In the past, if the membranes ruptured prematurely, every effort was made to deliver the baby promptly to prevent infection, which could affect mother or baby. However, this approach is no longer necessary because the risk of infection can be reduced by performing fewer pelvic examinations. In a single examination with a speculum (an

instrument that spreads the walls of the vagina apart), a doctor can verify the rupture of the membranes, estimate dilation of the cervix, and collect amniotic fluid from the vagina. If analysis of the amniotic fluid indicates that the fetus' lungs are mature enough, labor is artificially started (induced) and the baby is delivered. If the fetus' lungs aren't mature, the doctor tries to delay delivery until they are.

Bed rest and fluids are given intravenously to delay delivery in 50 percent of women, but some also need to take a drug that inhibits contractions of the uterus, such as magnesium sulfate given intravenously, terbutaline given by injection under the skin or by mouth, or rarely, ritodrine given intravenously. The woman is hospitalized and stays in bed but may get up to go to the bathroom. Her temperature and pulse rate are usually recorded at least twice daily. An increase in temperature or pulse rate may be an early sign of infection. If she has an infection, labor is induced and the baby is delivered. If the amniotic fluid stops leaking and the contractions stop, a woman may be able to go home, but she still must stay in bed and should be seen by a doctor at least once a week.

Preterm Labor

Preterm labor is labor that begins early, before the 37th week of pregnancy.

Because babies born prematurely may have health problems, doctors try to stop preterm labor.■ Preterm labor is difficult to stop if vaginal bleeding occurs or the membranes containing the fetus rupture. If vaginal bleeding doesn't occur and the membranes aren't leaking amniotic fluid, bed rest with fluids given intravenously helps 50 percent of the time. However, if the cervix opens (dilates) beyond 2 inches (5 centimeters), labor usually continues until the baby is born.

Magnesium sulfate given intravenously stops labor in up to 80 percent of the women but may

▲ see page 1182

■ see page 1201

produce side effects such as a rapid heartbeat in the woman, baby, or both. Terbutaline given by injection under the skin also can be used to stop labor. While preterm labor is being stopped, a woman may be given a corticosteroid such as betamethasone to help open the baby's lungs and reduce the risk that the baby will have trouble breathing (neonatal respiratory distress syndrome) after birth.

Postterm Pregnancy and Postmaturity

A postterm pregnancy is one that continues beyond 42 weeks. Postmaturity is a syndrome in which the placenta begins to stop functioning normally in a postterm pregnancy, endangering the fetus.▲

Determining when 42 weeks have passed can be difficult, because the precise date of conception can't always be determined. Sometimes the date of conception can't be determined because a woman's menstrual periods are irregular or she isn't sure about the length of time between them. For example, if a woman's menstrual cycles are 35 days or longer, delivery may seem late even though it isn't. Early in pregnancy, an ultrasound examination, which is safe and painless, can help determine the duration of pregnancy. Later, but before 32 weeks (ideally between 18 and 22 weeks), a series of ultrasound examinations to measure the diameter of the fetus' head can help confirm the duration of the pregnancy. After 32 weeks, determining duration by ultrasound examination may be 3 weeks off in either direction.

If the pregnancy continues beyond 42 weeks from the first day of the last menstrual period, mother and fetus are evaluated for signs of postmaturity: shrinkage of the uterus and decreased movement of the fetus. Tests may be started at 41 weeks to evaluate the fetus' movement and heart rate and the amount of amniotic fluid, which decreases markedly in postmature pregnancies. The size of the fetus' head is compared to the size of its abdomen. To confirm a diagnosis of postmaturity, a doctor may perform an amniocentesis (removal and analysis of amniotic fluid). One indication of postmaturity is a green discoloration of the amniotic fluid, caused by the fetus' stool (meconium); this finding indicates fetal distress.

As long as the evaluation doesn't detect signs of postmaturity, a postterm pregnancy can be allowed to continue. However, if the evaluation detects postmaturity, labor is induced and the baby is delivered. If the cervix isn't pliable enough for the fetus to go through, a cesarean section (surgical delivery by incision through a mother's abdomen and uterus) is performed.

Labor That Progresses Too Slowly

Every hour, the cervix should dilate at least four tenths of an inch (1 centimeter), and the fetus' head should descend into the pelvis at least four tenths of an inch. If these things don't happen, the fetus may be too big to move through the birth canal, and forceps delivery or cesarean section is required. If the birth canal is big enough for the fetus but labor isn't progressing fast enough, the mother is given oxytocin intravenously to stimulate the uterus to contract more forcefully. If oxytocin is unsuccessful, a cesarean section is performed.

Abnormal Heart Rate

Throughout labor, the fetus' heart rate is monitored every 15 minutes with a fetal stethoscope (fetoscope) or continuously with electronic fetal heart monitoring.■ Monitoring the fetus' heart rate is the easiest way to determine if the fetus is in distress. If a significant abnormality in the heart rate is heard, corrective measures—such as giving the mother oxygen, increasing the amount of fluids given intravenously, and turning the mother to her left side—are usually effective. If not, the baby is delivered by forceps or cesarean section.

Breathing Problems

Rarely, a newborn doesn't start to breathe, even though no problems were found before delivery. For this reason, medical personnel attending the delivery must be skilled in resuscitating babies.

Abnormal Position of the Fetus

An abnormal position is one in which the fetus takes more space while moving through the birth canal

---

▲ see page 1202

■ see box, page 1174

Position and Presentation of the Fetus

Normally, the position of a fetus is upside down and facing rearward (toward the mother's back) with the neck flexed, and presentation is head first. A less common position is facing forward, and abnormal presentations include face, brow, breech, and shoulder.

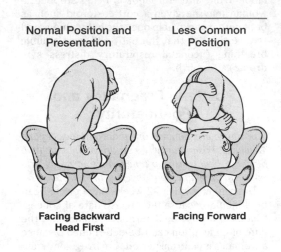

Normal Position and Presentation	Less Common Position

Facing Backward Head First   **Facing Forward**

Abnormal Presentations

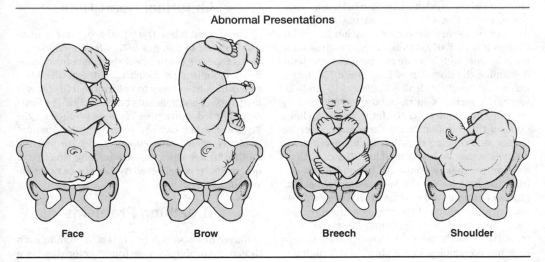

Face   Brow   Breech   Shoulder

than when in the normal position, which is facing rearward with the head leading the way out.

In a description of a fetus in the uterus, position refers to the direction that the fetus is facing, and presentation refers to the body part that leads the way out of the birth canal. The most common and safest combination is facing rearward (toward the mother's back), with the face angled toward the right or left, and head first (vertex presentation), with the neck bent forward, chin tucked in, and arms folded across the chest. If the fetus is in a different position or presentation, labor may be more difficult and vaginal delivery may not be possible.

The fetus may face forward, often with the neck straightened (deflexed). In this position, the head requires more space to pass through the birth canal, so labor may be prolonged and delivery difficult. After evaluating this problem, a doctor decides whether to use forceps or perform a cesarean section. In face presentation, the neck arches back so that the chin presents first. If the chin is at the back and remains that way, vaginal delivery isn't possible. In brow presentation, the neck is moderately arched so that the brow presents first. Usually, fetuses don't stay in this presentation, but if they do, they can't be delivered vaginally.

Breech presentation, in which the buttocks present first, may also occur. Damage, including death, to the baby before, during, or after birth is four times more common with breech presentations than with head-first presentations—largely because breech presentations are much more common when labor is preterm or when the baby has birth defects. Complications can be prevented only if the problem is detected before delivery. Sometimes the doctor can turn the fetus to present head first by pressing on the mother's abdomen before labor begins, usually at the 37th or 38th week of pregnancy.

Because the buttocks are narrower than the head, the passageway made by the buttocks in the birth canal isn't large enough for the head to pass through. In addition, when the head follows the buttocks, it can't be molded to fit through the birth canal. Thus, the baby's body may be delivered and the head may be caught inside the mother. As a result, the spinal cord or other nerves may be stretched, leading to nerve damage. When the baby's navel can first be seen outside the mother, the umbilical cord is compressed between the baby's head and the birth canal, so that very little oxygen can reach the baby. Brain damage from lack of oxygen is more common in fetuses presenting buttocks first than in those presenting head first. In a first delivery, these problems are worse because the mother's tissues haven't been stretched by previous deliveries. Because the baby could die, many doctors advise a cesarean section for most breech presentations in first pregnancies and for all breech presentations in preterm deliveries.

Occasionally, a fetus lying horizontally across the birth canal presents shoulder first. A cesarean section usually is performed, unless the fetus is the second in a set of twins—in which case the fetus may be turned for vaginal delivery.

Twins

Twins occur in 1 out of 70 to 80 deliveries. Before delivery, they can be identified by ultrasound examination—the best way—or by fetal electronic monitoring that shows two distinct heart beats. Twins overstretch the uterus, and an overstretched uterus tends to start contracting before the pregnancy reaches full term. As a result, twins usually are born prematurely and are small. Because twins can be in various positions and presentations, delivery can be complicated. The contraction of the uterus after the first twin is delivered tends to shear away the placenta of the second twin. As a result, the second twin tends to have more problems during delivery and a higher risk of damage or death.

In some instances, the overstretched uterus doesn't contract well after delivery, causing bleeding in the mother. A doctor decides in advance whether to deliver the twins vaginally or by cesarean section and may deliver the first twin vaginally, only to decide that a cesarean section is safest for the second twin.

Shoulder Dystocia

Shoulder dystocia is an uncommon complication, occurring in about 1 out of 1,000 head-first presentations, in which one shoulder of the fetus lodges against the pubic bone and is caught in the birth canal.

When the head comes out, it appears to be pulled back tightly against the vaginal opening. The chest is compressed by the birth canal and the mouth is kept shut by pressure against the vaginal opening, making insertion of a breathing tube difficult for the doctor. As a result, the fetus can't breathe, and oxygen levels fall within 4 to 5 minutes. This complication is more common with large fetuses, particularly when forceps are required before the fetus' head has fully descended in the birth canal. Not all large fetuses have shoulder dystocia.

A doctor quickly tries various techniques to free the shoulder so that the baby can be delivered vaginally. If they fail, the baby rarely can be pushed back into the vagina and delivered by cesarean section.

Prolapsed Umbilical Cord

A prolapsed umbilical cord is a rare complication, occurring in about 1 out of 1,000 deliveries, in which the umbilical cord precedes the baby through the birth canal.

When the baby emerges through the narrow birth canal, the prolapsed cord is compressed so that the baby's blood supply is cut off. This complication may be obvious (overt) or not (occult).

Prolapse is overt when the membranes have ruptured and the umbilical cord protrudes into the vagina before the baby emerges. Overt prolapse usually occurs when a baby emerges buttocks first (breech presentation), but it can occur when the baby emerges head first, particularly if the membranes rupture prematurely or the fetus hasn't descended into the mother's pelvis. If the fetus hasn't descended, the rush of fluid as the membranes rupture can carry the cord out ahead of the fetus. This is one reason that doctors don't rupture the membranes unless the fetus' head has descended into the pelvis. If the cord prolapses, immediate delivery—usually by cesarean section—is necessary to prevent injury to the fetus from having the blood supply cut off. Until surgery begins, a nurse or doctor holds the baby off the cord so that the blood supply through the prolapsed cord isn't cut off.

In occult prolapse, the membranes are intact and the cord is in front of the fetus or trapped in front of the fetus' shoulder. Usually, occult prolapse can be identified by an abnormal pattern in the fetus' heart rate. Changing the mother's position or raising the fetus' head to relieve pressure on the cord usually corrects the problem. Occasionally, a cesarean section is necessary.

Amniotic Fluid Embolism

Amniotic fluid embolism is blockage of a mother's pulmonary (lung) artery by amniotic fluid (the fluid surrounding the fetus in the uterus).

Very rarely, an embolus (a mass of foreign material in the bloodstream) consisting of amniotic fluid enters the mother's bloodstream, usually during a particularly traumatic labor with ruptured membranes. The embolus travels to the

---

▲ see page 1187

mother's lungs and blocks an artery; this blockage is called pulmonary embolism. It may result in a rapid heart rate, irregular heart rhythm, collapse, shock, or even cardiac arrest and death. If the mother survives, widespread blood clotting throughout the bloodstream (disseminated intravascular coagulation) is a common complication, requiring emergency care.

Uterine Bleeding

Excessive bleeding (hemorrhage) from the uterus is a major concern after the baby is delivered.▲ Ordinarily, the mother loses about 1 pint of blood during delivery. Blood vessels are opened when the placenta separates from the uterus. The contractions of the uterus help close these vessels until they can heal. So, blood loss may be greater if the uterus doesn't contract or if a piece of placenta remains inside the uterus after delivery, preventing the uterus from contracting fully. A tear in the vagina or cervix also can cause excessive bleeding.

Procedures

If complications occur during labor and delivery, procedures such as induction of labor or delivery by forceps, vacuum extractor, or cesarean section are used.

Induction of Labor

Induction of labor is the artificial starting of labor. Augmentation of labor uses the same techniques and drugs as induction but is done after labor has started spontaneously.

Usually, induction of labor is considered only when a mother has an obstetric problem or she or the fetus has a medical problem. If the pregnancy is proceeding normally, labor is rarely induced, except when a woman would have difficulty getting to the hospital in time to deliver. Often, such women are admitted to the hospital a short time before the expected date of delivery. Accurate dating is important, and a doctor may perform tests such as amniocentesis to accurately determine the fetus' maturity before inducing labor.

Usually, labor is induced by giving a woman oxytocin, a hormone that makes the uterus contract more forcefully. It is given intravenously

Forceps and Vacuum Extractor

Forceps or a vacuum extractor may be used to assist delivery. Forceps are placed around the baby's head. A vacuum extractor has a small cup made of rubberlike material that adheres to the baby's head when the vacuum is started. With either device, the baby is gently pulled out as the mother pushes.

Forceps	Vacuum Extractor

with an infusion pump, so that the amount of drug given can be controlled precisely. Throughout induction and labor, the fetus' heart rate is monitored electronically. At first this is done with a monitor placed on the woman's abdomen. Then as soon as the membranes can be safely ruptured, a monitor is inserted in the vagina and attached to the fetus' scalp. If induction is unsuccessful, the baby is delivered by cesarean section.

Labor is augmented, by giving oxytocin, when a woman has contractions that aren't effectively moving the fetus through the birth canal. However, if a woman is in the initial phase of labor—when the cervix is barely dilated and contractions are irregular—rest, walking, and general encouragement are better treatment than augmenting labor.

Occasionally, a woman has contractions that are too strong, too close together, or both. This condition, called hypertonic dysfunctional labor, is difficult to control. If these contractions are caused by oxytocin administration, the drug is stopped right away. The woman may be repositioned and given analgesics. Terbutaline or ritodrine, drugs that help stop or slow contractions, may be given.

Forceps and Vacuum Extractor

Forceps are metal surgical instruments, similar to tongs, with rounded edges that fit around the fetus' head. A vacuum extractor is a small cup made of a rubberlike material (Silastic), connected to a vacuum, that is inserted into the vagina and placed on the fetus' head.

Forceps are occasionally used to assist delivery or guide the fetus' head. Forceps are required when the fetus is in distress or in an abnormal position or when labor is prolonged. Occasionally, labor is prolonged when anesthesia prevents the mother from pushing adequately. In all of these cases, a doctor decides between using forceps and performing a cesarean section. If forceps delivery is tried and is too difficult (the doctor can't safely pull any harder), a cesarean section is performed.

An alternative to forceps is a vacuum extractor, a device that applies suction to the fetus' head. With this device, the baby is gently pulled out.

Using forceps can bruise the baby's face or tear the mother's vagina. A vacuum extractor can tear the baby's scalp. All such injuries, however, are uncommon.

Cesarean Section

Cesarean section is surgical delivery of a baby by incision through a mother's abdomen and uterus.

Doctors perform this procedure when they think it's safer than vaginal delivery for a mother, baby, or both. In the United States, about 22 percent of deliveries are cesarean sections. The health care practitioners involved in this surgical procedure are an obstetrician, an anesthesiologist, nurses, and a specialist in disorders of newborns (neonatologist) or a person who can resuscitate the baby if necessary. Cesarean section is safe because of such medical advances as anesthetics, intravenous drugs, antibiotics, and blood transfusions. Having the mother walk around soon after surgery reduces the risk of pulmonary embolism, in which blood clots formed in the legs or pelvis travel to the lungs and block arteries there. Delivery by cesarean section results in more overall pain after the operation than a vaginal delivery and a longer hospital stay.

The incision may be made in the upper part of the uterus (classical incision) or the lower part (lower segment incision). Usually, a classical incision is used only when the placenta is abnormally positioned (a complication called placenta previa)▲ or when the fetus lies horizontally across the birth canal. Blood loss is greater than that with a lower segment incision because the upper part of the uterus has more blood vessels. Also, the scar is weaker, so it's somewhat more likely to open in subsequent pregnancies. A lower segment incision may be horizontal or vertical. In most cases, a horizontal incision is used. Usually, a vertical incision is used when the fetus is in an abnormal position.

The choice of having a vaginal delivery or another cesarean section is usually offered to women who have had a lower segment incision; vaginal delivery is successful in about three fourths of these women. However, vaginal delivery should be performed only at institutions prepared to perform cesarean sections, because there is a very small chance that the incision will open during labor.

CHAPTER 250

Postdelivery Period

After the delivery of a baby, a new mother is monitored and, if needed, treated to relieve pain. She is given information about changes to expect in her body, including those related to breastfeeding, and the type of contraception that can be used in the postdelivery period. She is examined before leaving the hospital and 6 weeks later. Measures are also taken to prevent and treat complications, which are rare. The most common complications are excessive bleeding, urinary tract infections, and problems with breastfeeding.

What to Expect After Delivery

For 6 to 8 weeks after delivery, a new mother may have some mild, temporary symptoms as her body adjusts back to its nonpregnant state. Within the first 24 hours, her pulse rate drops and her temperature may rise slightly. She can expect a bloody vaginal discharge for 3 or 4 days, but it should change over the next 10 to 12 days to pale brown and finally to yellowish-white. Sanitary pads or tampons, changed frequently, may be used to absorb the discharge.

After delivery, the enlarged uterus continues to contract, getting progressively smaller, until it returns to its normal size. These irregular contrac-

▲ see page 1157

tions are often painful and may be treated with analgesics. They last 5 to 7 days and may be intensified by breastfeeding because the hormone oxytocin, released naturally by breastfeeding to start the flow of milk (let-down reflex), also stimulates uterine contractions. After 5 to 7 days, the uterus is normally firm and no longer tender, but a doctor can still feel the uterus through the abdominal wall in its location halfway between the pubic bone and the navel. By 2 weeks after delivery, the uterus can no longer be felt. However, the new mother's abdomen won't become as flat as it was before the pregnancy for several months, even if she exercises. Stretch marks may not lighten for a year.

In the Hospital

The hospital staff makes every effort to minimize a new mother's risk of bleeding, pain, and infection. After delivery of the placenta (afterbirth), she is given oxytocin to stimulate contraction of the uterus, and her abdomen is periodically massaged by a nurse to help the uterus contract. These steps help ensure that the uterus contracts and remains contracted to prevent excessive bleeding. If general anesthesia was used during delivery, the mother is monitored for 2 to 3 hours after delivery, usually in a well-equipped recovery room with access to oxygen, blood that matches the mother's, and intravenous fluids.

After the first 24 hours, recovery is rapid. The mother can have a regular diet as soon as she wants it, sometimes shortly after delivery. She should get up and walk as soon as possible. She can start exercises to strengthen abdominal muscles, often after 1 day; sit-ups with bent knees, done in bed, are effective.

Before the mother leaves the hospital, a complete blood cell count is performed to make sure she's not anemic. If another blood test shows that she has never had German measles (rubella), she's vaccinated on the day she leaves the hospital. If her blood type is Rh-negative and she has a baby whose blood type is Rh-positive, she is given $Rh_0(D)$ immune globulin within 3 days of delivery; this drug combines with and thereby destroys the antibodies produced by the mother against the baby's blood. Such antibodies can endanger future pregnancies.▲

Mild depression (postpartum depression, often called the blues) is common, usually appearing within 3 days of delivery and usually lasting less than 2 weeks. Often, family support is the best treatment. Depression that is combined with lack of interest in the baby, suicidal or violent thoughts, hallucinations, or bizarre behavior is considered abnormal, and treatment usually is needed. Serious depression is more likely to occur in women who had a mental illness before pregnancy.

At Home

A mother and baby commonly leave the hospital within 24 hours after delivery if both are healthy. In fact, many doctors discharge a new mother as early as 6 hours after delivery if she has no complications and if anesthesia wasn't used. Even though major problems are rare, the doctor, hospital staff, or health care plan usually sets up a home visit or close follow-up program.

A new mother may take showers or baths, but she should refrain from vaginal douching for at least 2 weeks after delivery. Washing the area around the vagina with warm water two or three times daily helps reduce tenderness. Pain from an episiotomy can be relieved with warm sitz baths several times daily for as long as needed. If the mother asks for additional pain relievers, she's usually given codeine and aspirin if she isn't breastfeeding or acetaminophen without codeine if she is.

Urine production often increases greatly after delivery, particularly when the administration of oxytocin is stopped. Because bladder sensation may be decreased after delivery, a new mother should urinate regularly, at least every 4 hours. Doing so avoids overfilling the bladder and helps prevent urinary tract infections. She may take laxatives, if needed to avoid constipation, which can cause hemorrhoids (piles). Hemorrhoids can be treated with warm sitz baths.

Breasts become engorged with milk during the early stages of milk production (lactation), and they may become hard and sore.■ If a mother isn't going to breastfeed, drugs can be given to suppress milk production. However, milk produc-

---

▲ see page 1155

■ see page 1195

tion often resumes when she stops taking the drug. Firm support of the breasts helps, since drooping stimulates milk flow. Many mothers who aren't breastfeeding reduce discomfort by binding the breasts tightly and then using firm support for 3 to 5 days, drinking plenty of fluids, and taking aspirin or acetaminophen. Symptoms last only 3 to 5 days.

Mothers who aren't breastfeeding may take drugs to help them sleep or to relieve pain. Those who are breastfeeding are given limited amounts of such drugs because most drugs are secreted in breast milk.

A new mother may resume normal activity when she feels ready. She may resume sexual intercourse as soon as she desires it and it's comfortable. Because pregnancy is possible, contraceptives should be used or intercourse should be avoided. Doctors generally advise a new mother not to become pregnant again for several months after delivery so that she can recover completely. Typically, oral contraceptives▲ are started after the first menstrual period, regardless of whether the mother is breastfeeding. Some doctors recommend starting oral contraceptives even earlier—within the first week after delivery—for mothers who aren't breastfeeding. A new mother can be fitted for a diaphragm after her uterus has returned to its normal size, about 6 to 8 weeks after delivery. In the meantime, foams, jellies, and condoms can be used for contraception if she's not taking oral contraceptives.

Mothers who aren't breastfeeding usually begin to ovulate (release an egg from the ovary) again about 4 weeks after delivery, before their first period. However, ovulation can occur earlier—some women have conceived as early as 2 weeks after delivery. Mothers who are breastfeeding tend to start ovulating and menstruating somewhat later, usually 10 to 12 weeks after delivery. Occasionally, a mother who is breastfeeding ovulates, menstruates, and becomes pregnant as quickly as a mother who isn't breastfeeding. *A woman who has just been immunized against German measles (rubella) must wait at least 3 months before becoming pregnant again to avoid endangering the fetus.*

▲ see page 1119

Postpartum Infections

A doctor presumes a woman has a postpartum infection if she has a temperature of 100.4° F. or higher on two occasions at least 6 hours apart after the first 24 hours following delivery and if no other cause, such as bronchitis, is evident.

Even during the first 12 hours after delivery, a temperature of 101° F. or higher could signal an infection, although it probably doesn't. Infections directly related to delivery occur in the uterus, the area surrounding the uterus, or the vagina. Kidney infections also can develop soon after delivery. Other causes of fever, such as blood clots in the legs or a breast infection, tend to occur 4 or more days after delivery.

UTERINE INFECTIONS

Postpartum infections usually begin in the uterus. An infection of the amniotic sac (the membranes that contain the fetus and the amniotic fluid surrounding it) and fever during labor may result in an infection of the uterine lining (endometritis), uterine muscle (myometritis), or areas surrounding the uterus (parametritis).

Causes and Symptoms

Under certain conditions, bacteria that live in the healthy vagina may cause an infection after delivery. These conditions, which increase a woman's vulnerability to infection, include anemia, preeclampsia (high blood pressure, protein in the urine, and fluid accumulation during pregnancy), repeated vaginal examinations, a delay of longer than 6 hours between rupture of the membranes and delivery, prolonged labor, cesarean section, retention of placental fragments within the uterus after delivery, and excessive bleeding after delivery (postpartum hemorrhage).

Chills, headache, a generally sick feeling, and loss of appetite are common. Usually, a woman looks pale and has a rapid heart rate and an abnormally high number of white blood cells. Her uterus is swollen, tender, and soft. Discharge from the uterus, which can vary in amount, is usually malodorous. When the tissues surrounding the uterus are affected, pain and fever are severe; swollen tissues hold the large, tender uterus rigidly in place.

Complications can include inflammation of the abdominal lining (peritonitis) and blood clots in the pelvic veins (pelvic thrombophlebitis), with the risk of a blood clot traveling to the lung (pulmonary embolus). Poisonous substances (toxins) produced by the infecting bacteria may reach high levels in the bloodstream (endotoxemia), leading to toxic shock, a life-threatening condition in which blood pressure falls dramatically and heart rate is rapid. Toxic shock may result in severe kidney damage and even death.

Diagnosis and Treatment

To diagnose an infection, a doctor examines the woman's lungs and uterus and sends samples of urine and the uterine discharge to a laboratory to be cultured for bacteria.

A doctor tries to prevent or treat conditions that could lead to infections. Vaginal delivery rarely causes an infection. If an infection does develop, a new mother is usually given an antibiotic intravenously until she's had no fever for 48 hours.

KIDNEY INFECTION

A kidney infection (pyelonephritis), caused by bacteria spreading from the bladder, may develop after delivery. An infection sometimes results from a catheter being placed in the bladder to relieve a buildup of urine during and after labor. The infection may begin during pregnancy with bacteria in the urine but with no symptoms. When symptoms occur, they may include a high fever, pain in the lower back or side, a generally sick feeling, constipation, and occasionally painful urination.

Typically, a woman is given an antibiotic intravenously until she's had no fever for 48 hours. Urine specimens are examined for bacteria, and the antibiotic is changed if the bacteria are resistant to it. The woman continues treatment with antibiotics given by mouth for 2 weeks after she leaves the hospital. Drinking plenty of fluids helps maintain good kidney function. Another urine specimen is examined 6 to 8 weeks after delivery, to verify that no bacteria remain.

OTHER POSTPARTUM INFECTIONS

Fever that develops between 4 and 10 days after delivery may indicate a blood clot in the leg (saphenous thrombophlebitis), which is treated with heat, wrapping, and elevation. Anticoagulants may be necessary. Dormant tuberculosis may become activated after delivery; it's treated with antibiotics.

Fever that develops later than 10 days after delivery frequently is caused by a breast infection (mastitis), although a bladder infection (cystitis) is also common. Bladder and breast infections are treated with antibiotics. A mother who has a breast infection should continue breastfeeding, which will decrease the risk of a breast abscess developing. Breast abscesses are rare; they are treated with antibiotics and usually drained surgically.

Postpartum Hemorrhage

Postpartum hemorrhage is the loss of more than 1 pint of blood during or after the third stage of labor, when the placenta is delivered.

This disorder is the third most common cause of maternal death in childbirth, after infection and anesthesia complications. The causes of postpartum hemorrhage vary, and most are avoidable. One cause is bleeding from the area where the placenta detaches from the uterus. Such bleeding can occur when the uterus doesn't contract properly—because it has been stretched too much, the labor was prolonged or abnormal, the woman has had several previous pregnancies, or a muscle-relaxing anesthetic was used during labor and delivery. Postpartum hemorrhage also can be caused by cuts (lacerations) from a spontaneous delivery, by tissue (usually parts of the placenta that didn't separate properly) that wasn't expelled during delivery, or by a low blood level of fibrinogen (an important blood clotting factor). Severe blood loss usually occurs soon after delivery but may occur as late as 1 month afterward.

Prevention and Treatment

Before a woman goes into labor, a doctor takes steps to prevent postpartum hemorrhage. One such step is to treat conditions such as anemia. Another is to gather as much relevant information about the woman as possible. For example, knowing that the woman has an increased amount of amniotic fluid, a multiple pregnancy such as twins, or an unusual blood type or that she has had previous episodes of postpartum hemorrhage can prepare the doctor for possible bleeding problems.

The doctor tries to intervene in the delivery as little as possible. After the placenta has detached from the uterus, the woman is given oxytocin to help the uterus contract and reduce blood loss. If the placenta doesn't detach on its own within 30 minutes after delivery of the baby, the doctor removes it manually. If the expelled placenta is incomplete, the doctor recovers the missing fragments manually. Rarely, infected fragments of the placenta or other tissues need to be removed surgically (by curettage). After delivery of the placenta, the woman is monitored for at least an hour to make sure that the uterus has contracted and to assess vaginal bleeding.

If severe bleeding occurs, the woman's abdomen is massaged to help the uterus contract, and she is given oxytocin continuously through an intravenous tube. If bleeding persists, she may need a blood transfusion. The uterus may be examined for cuts or retained fragments of the placenta and other tissues, and such tissues may be removed surgically; both procedures require use of an anesthetic. The cervix and vagina are also examined. A prostaglandin can be injected into the uterine muscle to help it contract. If the uterus can't be stimulated to contract so that bleeding is reduced, the arteries supplying blood to the uterus may have to be closed off. Because of the abundant blood supply to the pelvis, this procedure has no lasting effect after the bleeding is controlled. Removal of the uterus (hysterectomy) is rarely necessary.

Inverted Uterus

An inverted uterus is a condition in which the body of the uterus turns inside out, protruding through the cervix into or beyond the vagina.

This is an uncommon occurrence. The uterus is inverted usually when an inexperienced medical attendant applies too much pressure to the top of the uterus or pulls too hard on the cord of a placenta that hasn't detached. An inverted uterus is a medical crisis and may lead to shock, infection, and death.

To turn the uterus right side out (reinvert), a doctor pushes it back up into the vaginal canal, passes a tube into the vagina, and holds the entrance of the vagina shut. The doctor then instills a salt solution into the uterus through the tube to inflate the vagina and reinvert the uterus. Surgery is rarely necessary. Usually, the woman recovers fully after this procedure.

Children's Health Issues

CHAPTER 251

Normal Newborns and Infants

The successful transition of a fetus, immersed in amniotic fluid and totally dependent on the placenta for nutrition and oxygen, to a squalling, air-breathing baby is a source of wonder. Healthy newborns need good care to ensure their normal development and continued health.

Initial Care

Immediately after a baby is born, the doctor or nurse gently clears mucus and other material from its mouth, nose, and throat with a suction bulb. The baby then takes its first breath. Two clamps are placed on the baby's umbilical cord, side by side, and the umbilical cord is then cut between the clamps. The baby is dried and laid carefully on a sterile warm blanket or on the mother's abdomen.

The baby is weighed and measured. The doctor examines the baby for any obvious abnormalities; a full physical examination comes later. The ba-

Cutting the Umbilical Cord

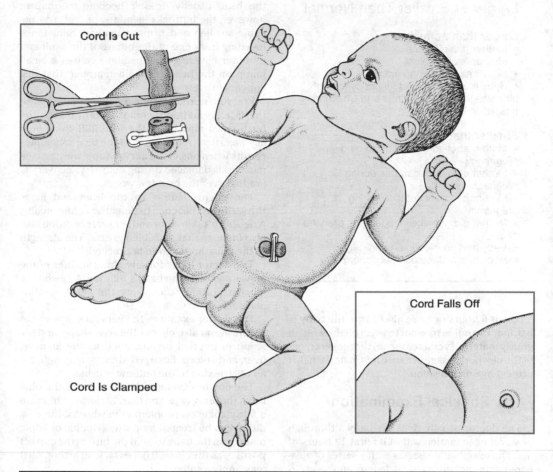

Cord Is Cut

Cord Is Clamped

Cord Falls Off

by's overall condition is recorded at 1 minute and at 5 minutes after birth using the Apgar score. The Apgar score is based on the baby's color (pink or blue), heart rate, breathing, responsiveness, and muscle tone (limp or active).

Keeping the newborn warm is critical. As soon as possible, the baby is wrapped in lightweight clothing (swaddled), and the head is covered to reduce the loss of body heat. A few drops of silver nitrate solution or an antibiotic is placed into the eyes to prevent infection from any harmful organisms that the baby may have had contact with during delivery.

The mother, father, and baby usually recover together in the birthing room. Once transported to the nursery, the baby is placed on its side in a small crib and kept warm. Placing the baby on its side prevents fluid or mucus from blocking the airway and impeding breathing. Because all babies are born with low levels of vitamin K, a doctor or nurse administers an injection of vitamin K to prevent bleeding (hemorrhagic disease of the newborn). An antiseptic solution is usually applied to the newly cut umbilical cord to help prevent infection.

Why a Newborn May Be Larger or Smaller Than Normal

Larger than normal
- Mother has diabetes
- Mother is overweight
- Baby has heart abnormalities
- Baby has an inherited tendency for high birth weight (as in the Crow and Cheyenne Indians in Montana)

Smaller than normal
- Mother abused alcohol or drugs during pregnancy
- Mother smoked cigarettes during pregnancy
- Mother had poor nutrition during pregnancy
- Mother did not receive adequate prenatal care
- Baby had an infection before birth
- Baby has a chromosomal abnormality

About 6 hours or more after birth, the baby is bathed. The nurse tries not to wash off the whitish greasy material (vernix caseosa) that covers most of the newborn's skin, because this material helps protect against infection.

Physical Examination

The doctor usually gives the baby a thorough physical examination within its first 12 hours of life. The examination begins with a series of measurements, including weight, length, and head circumference. The average weight at birth is 7 pounds, and the average length is 20 inches. Then the doctor examines the baby's skin, head and face, heart and lungs, nervous system, abdomen, and genitals.

The **skin** is usually reddish, although the fingers and toes may have a blue tinge because of poor blood circulation during the first few hours.

A normal head-first delivery leaves the **head** slightly misshapen for several days. The bones that form the skull overlap, which allows the head

---

▲ see box, page 1063

to become compressed for delivery. Some swelling and bruising of the scalp is typical. When the baby is delivered buttocks first (breech delivery), the head usually doesn't become misshapen; however, the buttocks, genitals, or feet may become swollen and bruised instead. Sometimes bleeding from one of the bones of the skull and its outer covering (periosteum) causes a small bump on the head (cephalhematoma) that disappears in a few weeks.

Pressure during a vaginal delivery may bruise the **face.** In addition, compression through the birth canal may make the face initially appear asymmetrical. Asymmetry of the face sometimes results when one of the nerves supplying the face muscles is damaged during delivery. Recovery is gradual over the next few weeks.

The doctor listens to the **heart** and **lungs** through a stethoscope to detect any abnormality. A newborn's skin color and general condition may also indicate that a problem exists. The strength of the pulse at the groin is checked.

The doctor looks for any abnormalities of the **nerves** and tests the baby's reflexes. A newborn's most important reflexes are the Moro, rooting, and sucking reflexes.

The doctor examines the general shape of the **abdomen** and also checks the size, shape, and position of internal organs, such as the kidneys, liver, and spleen. Enlarged kidneys may indicate an obstruction to the outflow of urine.

The doctor examines the flexibility and mobility of the **arms, legs,** and **hips.** Dislocated hips are a fairly common problem in newborns; the condition can be treated by putting double or triple diapers on the baby to hold the hips in the correct position as they heal. If necessary, an orthopedist may apply a splint.

The doctor examines the **genitals.** In a boy, the testes should be present in the scrotum. Although rare and apparently not painful in a newborn, the testes can be twisted (a condition called testicular torsion),▲ which requires an emergency operation. In a girl, the labia are prominent; exposure to the mother's hormones causes them to be swollen for the first few weeks.

First Few Days

Immediately after a normal birth, the mother is helped by the delivery room staff to hold her baby. Breastfeeding may be initiated at this time if the mother wishes. The father is also encouraged to hold the baby and share these moments. Some experts believe that early physical contact with the baby helps establish bonding. However, parents can bond well with their babies even when the first hours aren't spent together.

During the first few days after birth, the parents learn to feed, bathe, and dress the baby and become familiar with its activities and sounds. Although mother and baby used to spend a week or more in the hospital, today that period has shrunk to a day or two.

The plastic cord clamp on the umbilical cord is removed 24 hours after birth. The stump that remains should be moistened daily with an alcohol solution. This process speeds drying and reduces the chance that the stump will become infected.

Circumcision, if desired, generally is performed within the first few days of life. However, the procedure should be delayed indefinitely if the penis is abnormal in any way, as the foreskin may be needed for subsequent plastic surgery repair. The decision about having a newborn circumcised usually depends on the parents' religious beliefs or personal preferences. The main medical reason for circumcision is to remove an unusually tight foreskin that is obstructing the flow of urine. Other medical reasons, such as reducing the risk of cancer of the penis, are more controversial. Circumcision can be hazardous if bleeding disorders run in the family. Circumcision must be delayed if, during the pregnancy, the mother had been taking drugs that increase the risk of bleeding, such as anticoagulants or aspirin; the doctor waits until all such drugs have been eliminated from the baby's circulation. The baby is also given vitamin K to counteract the anticoagulant.

Most newborns have a mild skin rash sometime during the first week. The rash usually appears in areas of the body rubbed by clothing—the arms, legs, and back—and rarely on the face. It tends to disappear on its own without treatment. Applying lotions or powders, using perfumed soaps, and putting plastic pants over the diapers are likely to make the rash worse, especially in hot weather. Dryness and some skin peeling often occur after a few days, especially in the creases at the wrists and ankles.

The newborn may have several hard lumps under its skin (subcutaneous fat necrosis) where pressure from bones destroyed some fatty tissue. Such lumps are most common on the head, cheek, and neck when forceps were used during delivery. The lumps may break through to the skin surface,

A Newborn's Reflexes

Reflex	Description
Moro	When the newborn is startled, its arms and legs swing out and forward in a slow movement with fingers outstretched
Rooting	When either side of the mouth is touched, the newborn turns its head toward that side. This reflex enables the newborn to find the nipple
Sucking	When an object is placed in the newborn's mouth, sucking begins immediately

releasing a clear yellow fluid, but they usually heal fairly quickly.

Newborns who are otherwise normal may become slightly jaundiced, beginning after the first day.▲ Jaundice that appears before 24 hours of age is of particular concern.

The first urine produced by a newborn is concentrated and often contains chemicals called urates, which can turn the diaper pink. If a newborn doesn't urinate within the first 24 hours of life, the doctor tries to find out why. Delay in starting to urinate is more common in boys. The delay may be caused by a tight foreskin or by temporary swelling of the penis after circumcision.

The first bowel movement is a sticky greenish-black substance (meconium). Every baby should pass meconium within the first 24 hours after birth. Failure to pass a bowel movement is usually caused by a hardened plug of meconium inside the baby's intestine, which can usually be removed by one or more gentle enemas. A birth defect may cause a more serious blockage.■

A newborn normally loses 5 to 10 percent of its birth weight during the first few days of life. This weight is rapidly regained as the newborn starts to eat.

▲ see page 1212

■ see page 1231

Feeding

A normal newborn has active rooting and sucking reflexes and can start eating immediately after birth. If the baby has not been placed at the mother's breast in the delivery room, feedings are ordinarily begun within 4 hours after birth.

Spitting and regurgitating mucus are common the first day after birth. If mucus is being regurgitated longer than that, the doctor or nurse may gently wash any remaining mucus out of the stomach by gently passing a tube through the nose and down into the stomach.

A newborn who is being bottle-fed may vomit because of a milk allergy. A low-allergy formula may be substituted. If it doesn't help, the doctor tries to find out why the newborn is vomiting. A breastfed newborn who continues to vomit may have a blockage that's preventing the stomach from emptying. Babies aren't allergic to human milk.

Newborns wet at least six to eight diapers a day. In addition, they have bowel movements every day during the first few weeks, cry vigorously, have good skin condition, and exhibit a strong sucking reflex. All these factors indicate that the baby is getting enough milk or formula. Weight gain confirms that point. Sleeping for long periods of time between feedings is usually a sign that the baby is getting enough to eat, although occasionally a breastfed baby may sleep for prolonged periods of time if it isn't receiving enough milk. Therefore, a breastfed baby should be checked early and regularly by the doctor to make sure feedings are adequate.

Bottle-feeding

A bottle-fed baby is often given sterile distilled water for the first feeding to ensure that it can suck and swallow and that its gag reflex is working properly. The water won't harm a baby who has problems feeding. If the baby doesn't spit up the water, formula can be given at the next feeding. In the hospital, babies are usually fed every 4 hours for the sake of efficiency.

Prepackaged formulas containing adequate calories and vitamins are available in sterile 4-ounce bottles. The mother shouldn't urge the baby to finish every bottle, but rather, allow the baby to take as much as it wants. Feeding should be increased gradually during the first week of life, from 1 or 2 ounces to 3 or 4 ounces about 6 times a day.

Commercial infant formulas are preferable to cow's milk, which is not appropriate during the first year of life. Although cow's milk is a well-balanced food for an infant, it lacks iron, which is important for red blood cell development. Multivitamin drops containing vitamins A, C, and D should be given daily to infants receiving formula or breast milk for the first year of life and through a second winter in cold climates, where exposure to the sun and its activation of vitamin D are limited. Fluoride may be added to the formula when fluoridated water isn't available.

The bottle-fed baby should be offered water between feedings, especially when the weather is hot or the environment is hot and dry. Occasionally a baby who isn't feeding properly may need additional intravenous feedings. The doctor will then try to find out what's wrong.

Breastfeeding

Mother's milk is the ideal food for babies. Besides providing the necessary nutrients in the most easily digestible and absorbable form, breast milk contains antibodies and white blood cells that protect the baby against infection. Breast milk favorably changes the pH of the stool and intestinal flora, thus protecting the baby against bacterial diarrhea. Because of the protective qualities of breast milk, infectious diseases occur less often in babies who are breastfed rather than bottle-fed. Breastfeeding offers advantages to the mother as well; for example, it enables her to bond and feel close to her baby in a way that bottle-feeding can't. More than half of all mothers in the United States breastfeed their babies, and this proportion is steadily increasing.

A thin yellow fluid, called colostrum, flows from the nipple before breast milk is produced. Colostrum is rich in calories, protein, and antibodies. The antibodies in colostrum are especially valuable, as they can be absorbed directly into the body from the stomach. In this way, the baby is protected against the illnesses to which its mother has developed antibodies.

The mother's nipples require no special preparation before she can begin breastfeeding. Expressing fluids from the breast manually before delivery may lead to an infection of the breast (mastitis) or even early labor. Nature prepares the areola and nipple for suckling by secreting a lubricant to protect the surface. This lubricant shouldn't be rubbed off. A woman who plans to breastfeed her baby may want to speak with women who have breastfed successfully. Observing other breastfeeding women and asking questions can also be instructive and encouraging.

The mother settles into a comfortable, relaxed position, perhaps lying almost flat, and turns from one side to the other to offer each breast. The baby faces the mother. The mother supports her breast with thumb and index finger on top and other fingers below and brushes her nipple against the baby's lower lip. This stimulates the baby to open its mouth—the rooting reflex—and grasp the breast. As the mother eases the nipple and areola into the baby's mouth, she makes sure the nipple is centered, which helps keep the nipple from becoming sore. Before removing the baby from the nipple, the mother breaks the suction by inserting her finger into the baby's mouth and gently pressing the baby's chin down.

Initially, the baby feeds for several minutes at each breast. The resulting reflex (let-down reflex) in the mother triggers milk production. Excessive suckling should be avoided at first. Sore nipples result from poor positioning and are easier to prevent than to cure. On the other hand, the production of milk depends on sufficient suckling time. Feeding times are gradually increased until milk production has been fully established. About 10 minutes at the first breast and enough time to satisfy the baby at the second are usually adequate. For a first baby, full milk production is usually established in 72 to 96 hours. Less time is needed for subsequent babies. If the mother is particularly tired during the first night, the 2 A.M. feeding may be replaced with water. However, no more than 6 hours should elapse between feeding sessions during the first few days. Feeding should be on demand (the baby's, that is) rather than by the clock. Similarly, the length of each breastfeeding session should be adjusted to meet the baby's needs.

The mother should take the baby, especially a first baby, to the doctor 7 to 10 days after delivery so that the doctor can find out how breastfeeding is going and answer any questions.

The breasts tend to swell uncomfortably (become engorged) during the early days of breastfeeding. Engorgement can be minimized by frequent feeding. Wearing a comfortable nursing bra 24 hours a day can help relieve pain. Expressing milk by hand in a warm shower also relieves the pressure. The mother may have to express her milk manually just before breastfeeding to enable the baby's mouth to reach around the swollen areola. However, excessive expression between feedings tends to cause continued engorgement and should be done only to relieve discomfort.

Poor positioning of the baby can cause the mother's nipples to become sore. Sometimes the baby draws in its lower lip and sucks it, irritating the nipple. In that case the mother can ease the lip out of the baby's mouth with her thumb. After a feeding, she should let the milk dry naturally on the nipples rather than wipe or wash them. She may wish to dry her nipples with a hair dryer set on low. In very dry climates, hypoallergenic lanolin or ointment can be applied to the nipples. Plastic bra liners should be avoided.

The mother needs extra nourishment, especially calcium, while breastfeeding. Dairy products are an excellent source of calcium, but nuts and green leafy vegetables may be substituted if she can't tolerate milk products. Alternatively, oral calcium supplements can be taken. Vitamin supplements aren't necessary if the diet is well balanced, particularly if it includes enough vitamin C and vitamins B_6 and B_{12}. However, the average American diet is low in vitamin B_6, and vegetarian diets are typically low in vitamin B_{12}.

When to stop breastfeeding (wean the infant) depends on the needs and desires of both mother and baby. Breastfeeding for at least 6 months is considered most desirable. Gradual weaning over weeks or months is easier for both the baby and mother than stopping suddenly.

Weaning usually means introducing solids, so that instead of 8 to 10 breastfeeding sessions a day, solids are given up to three times a day and the number of breastfeeding sessions is gradually reduced. One breastfeeding session a day should be replaced by a bottle or cup of fruit juice, expressed breast milk, or formula when the infant is about 7 months old. Learning to drink from a cup is an important developmental milestone, and weaning to a cup can be completed by age 10 months. Some infants cling to one or two breastfeedings daily until the age of 18 to 24 months. When a mother breastfeeds longer, the child should also be eating solid foods and drinking from a cup.

Starting Solid Foods

The time to start solid food depends on the infant's needs and readiness. Generally, infants don't need solids before the age of 6 months, although they can usually swallow food by about 3 or 4 months. They can swallow solids at even

An Infant's First Year: Physical Development

An infant's weight and length are charted at each well-baby visit to make sure that growth is proceeding at a steady rate. Percentiles are a way of comparing infants of the same age. For an infant at the 10th percentile for weight, 10 percent of infants weigh less and 90 percent weigh more. For an infant at the 90th percentile,

Boys

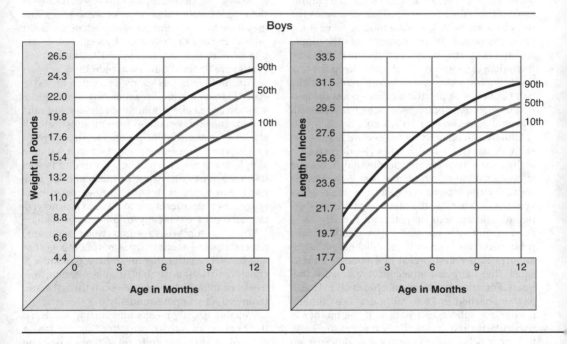

younger ages if the food is placed on the back of the tongue, but they usually refuse it. Some parents coax their infants to eat large amounts of solid food so that they will sleep through the night. This may not work, and forcing an infant to eat early can cause feeding problems later. Many infants take solids after a breastfeeding or bottle-feeding, which both satisfies their need to suck and quickly relieves their hunger.

Single-grain cereals are usually begun first, followed by single-ingredient fruits and vegetables. Allergy or sensitivity to a food is easier to determine if the infant is offered the same single-grain cereal, fruit, or vegetable for several days. The food should be offered on a spoon so that the infant learns the new feeding technique.

Many commercial baby foods, especially desserts and soup mixtures, are high in starch. Starch contains no vitamins or minerals, is high in calories, and is rarely digested by infants. Some commercial baby foods have a high sodium content, over 200 milligrams per jar. Foods with poor nutritional content can be identified by reading labels. Pureed home foods are less expensive than commercial baby foods and offer adequate nutrition.

Meats should be introduced later, after about 7 months, and are preferable to foods that are high

90 percent of infants weigh less and 10 percent weigh more. For an infant at the 50th percentile, half of infants weigh less and half weigh more. Of more significance than the actual percentile is a significant change in percentile between well-baby visits.

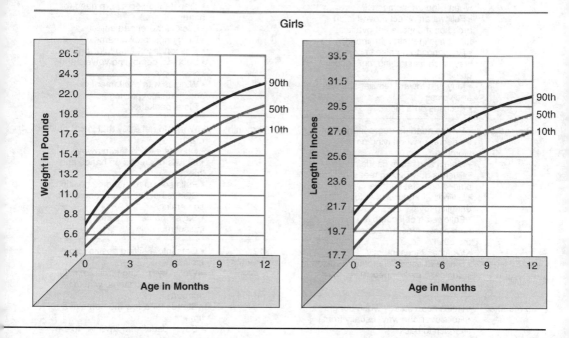

Girls

in carbohydrates, because infants need plenty of protein. However, because many infants reject meat, it should be introduced with great care and attention. Many children are allergic to wheat, eggs, and chocolate, so those foods should be avoided until the child is 1 year old. Eating those foods can cause later allergies to them. Honey must be avoided during the first year because it may contain the spores of *Clostridium botulinum,* which in this form is harmless to older children and adults but can cause botulism in infants.

Physical Development

An infant's physical development depends on heredity, nutrition, and environment. Physical and psychologic abnormalities can also influence growth. Optimal growth requires optimal nutrition and health.

An infant's height increases about 30 percent by age 5 months and more than 50 percent by a year. Birth weight doubles within 5 months and triples within a year.

Different organs grow at different rates. For instance, the reproductive system has a brief growth spurt just after birth, then changes very little until just before puberty. In contrast, the brain grows almost exclusively during the early years of life. At birth, the brain is one fourth of its future adult size. By 1 year, the brain is three fourths of its adult size. The kidneys function at the adult level by the end of the first year.

An Infant's First Year: Developmental Milestones

Age	Milestone	Age	Milestone
1 month	• Brings hands toward eyes and mouth • Moves head from side to side when lying on stomach • Follows an object moved in an arch about 6 inches above face to the midline (straight ahead) • Responds to a noise in some way, such as startling, crying, or quieting • May turn toward familiar sounds and voices • Focuses on a face	7 months	• Sits without support • Bears some weight on legs when held upright • Transfers objects from hand to hand • Looks for dropped object • Responds to own name • Responds to being told "no" • Babbles, combining vowels and consonants • Wiggles with excitement in anticipation of playing • Plays peekaboo
3 months	• Raises head 45 degrees (possibly 90 degrees) when lying on stomach • Opens and shuts hands • Pushes down when feet are placed on a flat surface • Swings at and reaches for dangling toys • Follows an object moved in an arch above face from one side to the other • Watches faces intently • Smiles at sound of mother's voice • Begins to make speechlike sounds	9 months	• Works to get a toy that is out of reach • Objects if toy is taken away • Crawls or creeps on hands and knees • Pulls self up to standing position • Stands holding on to someone or something • Says "mama" or "dada" indiscriminately
5 months	• Holds head steady when upright • Rolls over one way, usually from stomach to back • Reaches for objects • Recognizes people at a distance • Listens intently to human voices • Smiles spontaneously • Squeals in delight	12 months	• Gets into a sitting position from stomach • Walks by holding furniture; may walk one or two steps without support • Stands for a few moments at a time • Says "dada" and "mama" to the appropriate person • Drinks from a cup • Claps hands and waves bye-bye

Lower front teeth appear at the age of 5 to 9 months. Upper front teeth begin to appear at 8 to 12 months.

Behavioral and Intellectual Development

The rate of behavioral and intellectual development varies considerably from child to child.

Some infants develop faster, although certain patterns may run in families, such as late walking or talking. Environmental factors, such as lack of sufficient stimulation, can slow normal development. Physical factors, such as deafness, can also slow development. Although a child's development is usually continuous, temporary pauses may occur in a particular function, such as speech.

At first, a newborn sleeps most of the time. The infant can eat, cough when its airway is blocked, and respond with crying to any discomfort or intrusion. By 6 weeks, the infant looks at objects that are directly in front of him and begins to smile when spoken to. The head still wobbles when the infant is pulled to a sitting position.

By 3 months, the infant smiles at the sound of his mother's voice, makes sounds that sound like the beginnings of speech, and follows a moving object. The head is steady when the infant is held in a sitting position. Objects placed in its hands are grasped. By 6 months, the infant sits with support and rolls over. Most infants can stand with support and transfer an object from one hand to the other. The infant babbles to toys.

By 9 months, the infant sits well and crawls, pulls himself up to a standing position, and says "mama" and "dada" indiscriminately. By 12 months, the infant usually can walk while holding someone's hand and can speak several words.

Testing During the First Year

Screening tests are designed to detect disorders at an early stage. Early diagnosis and prompt treatment can reduce or prevent disorders that may interfere with an infant's healthy development.

Before the newborn leaves the hospital, blood specimens are taken for a number of laboratory tests. For example, one test measures the levels of thyroid hormone in the blood, which is important because low levels can result in cretinism, a chronic thyroid disorder characterized by arrested physical and mental development.▲ A newborn with low thyroid hormone levels should receive thyroid hormone replacement therapy by mouth within the first 7 to 10 days of life. Another disease, phenylketonuria,■ can also cause mental retardation if untreated.

Many other screening tests may be performed. Examples include screening for homocystinuria, maple syrup urine disease, galactosemia, and sickle cell disease. Sometimes the selection of screening tests is guided in part by the ethnic and genetic background of the parents. Cost and technical limitations limit routine screening tests in some states.

Length, weight, and head circumference are measured at each visit to the doctor during the first year of life. At each visit, the doctor listens to the infant's heart through a stethoscope; abnormal sounds may indicate heart disease. Also at every visit, the doctor examines the infant's abdomen, because certain rare cancers, such as Wilms' tumor and neuroblastoma, can be detected only as the infant grows. Hearing and vision are tested. An infant who was born prematurely (after spending less than 37 weeks in the uterus) is regularly examined for retinopathy of prematurity, an eye disease.★

Immunizations

Children should be immunized to protect them against infectious diseases. Vaccines are remarkably safe and effective, although some children occasionally experience minor reactions to them. Most vaccines are given by injection, although a few (such as polio) are given by mouth.

The first vaccine that an infant receives is hepatitis B vaccine, and the first dose of hepatitis B vaccine is given during the first week of life, sometimes when the infant is still in the hospital. Other routine immunizations begin at 6 to 8 weeks, or somewhat later if the infant is ill. Immunization need not be delayed, however, if the infant has a slight fever from a mild infection such as an ordinary cold.

Many vaccines require more than one dose to provide full immunity. Most doctors follow the immunization schedule recommended by the American Academy of Pediatrics. However, the recommended ages for immunizations should not be construed as absolute. For example, 2 months can mean 6 to 10 weeks. Although parents should try to have their children vaccinated according to a schedule, some delay doesn't interfere with the final immunity achieved nor does it entail restarting the series of injections from the beginning. Some vaccines are recommended under special circumstances. For example, hepatitis A

▲ see page 1296

■ see page 1293

★ see page 1207

Immunization Schedule for Infants and Children

Immunization plays an important role in keeping infants and children healthy. Shown are the routinely recommended ages for having an infant or child immunized with specific vaccines. The recommended age for immunization may vary depending on the circumstances. For example, if an infant is born to a woman with the hepatitis B surface antigen in her blood, a doctor will likely recommend immunization with hepatitis B vaccine within 12 hours of birth. However, other infants should receive their first dose of hepatitis B vaccine at first visit and at least by age 1 month. A range of acceptable ages exists for many vaccines, and a child's own doctor will provide specific recommendations. Often, combination vaccines are used, which lessens the number of shots a child will receive.

Key

 Single dose of vaccine

▲ "Catch-up" vaccination for those children not previously immunized (or, in the case of varicella-zoster virus, for those who have not had chickenpox)

▬ Range of acceptable ages for a single dose of vaccine

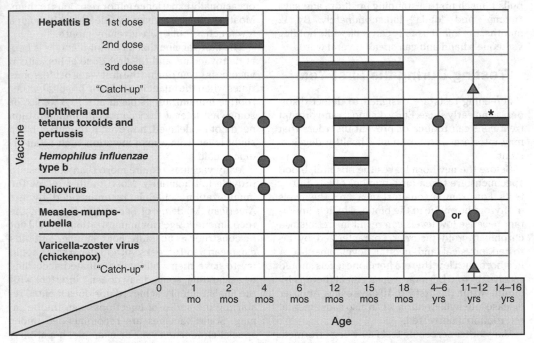

*A booster dose containing just diphtheria and tetanus toxoids (without pertussis vaccine) is recommended between the ages of 11 and 16 if at least 5 years have elapsed since the last dose.

vaccine may be recommended for people going to college or for those traveling overseas.

More than one vaccine may be given during a visit to the doctor's office, but several vaccines are often combined into one injection, for example, pertussis, diphtheria, tetanus, and *Hemophilus influenzae* type b vaccines. A combination vaccine reduces the number of injections needed but doesn't compromise the safety or effectiveness of the vaccines. To help prevent severe gastroenteritis due to rotavirus infection, an oral rotavirus vaccine is available.

Problems in Newborns and Infants

A full-term infant has spent 37 to 42 weeks in the uterus. An infant born earlier than 37 weeks is considered premature; an infant born later than 42 weeks is considered postmature. Different problems are anticipated in infants who are premature, postmature, or full term at birth.

Prematurity

Prematurity is a condition of underdevelopment; it affects infants who have spent less than 37 weeks in the uterus.

Prematurity, especially if extreme, is the greatest single cause of problems and death after delivery. Some of the infant's internal organs may not have developed fully, putting him at greater risk for certain disorders.

Why an infant is born prematurely isn't usually known. However, the risk of a premature delivery is higher in unmarried women and in those who have a low income and a poor education. Having inadequate prenatal care, poor nutrition, or an untreated illness or infection during pregnancy also puts a woman at higher risk of a premature delivery. For reasons that aren't known, black women are more likely than women in other racial groups to have a premature delivery.

Medical care started early in the pregnancy reduces the risk of premature delivery and improves the outcome if a delivery is premature. If premature labor and early delivery seem likely, a doctor can often administer tocolytic drugs to stop labor temporarily and corticosteroids to accelerate maturation of the fetus' lungs.▲

Adequate development of the lungs is critical for the newborn. For the infant to breathe independently, the air sacs (alveoli) in the lungs must be able to fill with air at birth and remain open. The air sacs are able to do so largely because of a substance called surfactant, which is produced in the lungs and lowers surface tension. Premature infants often don't produce enough surfactant, so the air sacs in their lungs do not stay open. Between breaths, the lungs collapse completely. The resulting disease, respiratory distress syndrome,■ can lead to other significant problems and in some cases can even be fatal. Infants with respiratory distress syndrome need treatment with oxygen; if the disease is severe, they need to be placed on a ventilator and treated with a surfactant drug, which can be dripped directly down a tube into the infant's windpipe (trachea).

In addition to underdeveloped lungs, a premature infant has an incompletely developed brain. This can contribute to pauses in breathing (apnea), because the breathing center in the brain may be immature. Drugs can be used to reduce the frequency of apnea episodes, and the infant will outgrow them as the brain matures. The very immature brain is vulnerable to bleeding or injury if its oxygen or blood supply is interrupted. Even if bleeding occurs in the brain, most premature infants develop normally unless they have had a severe brain injury.

Immature development of the brain may initially prevent the infant from sucking and swallowing normally. Many premature infants are fed intravenously at first, then they progress to milk feedings given through a tube passed into the stomach. By around 34 weeks of age, they should be able to breastfeed or take a bottle. Initially, the small size of the stomach may limit the amount that can be given at each feeding; too much milk leads to spitting up.

Premature infants are particularly likely to have swings in blood sugar (glucose) levels—both high and low.

The immune system in premature infants isn't fully developed. They have not received the full complement of the mother's infection-fighting antibodies across the placenta. The risk of developing serious infections, especially infections of the bloodstream (sepsis), is considerably higher in premature infants than in full-term infants. Premature infants are also more susceptible to developing necrotizing enterocolitis (a serious inflammatory disease of the intestines).★

Before birth, waste products produced by the fetus cross the placenta and are excreted by the

---

▲ see page 1178

■ see page 1204

★ see page 1209

Physical Features of a Premature Infant

- Small size
- Low birth weight
- Thin, shiny, pink skin
- Veins visible under the skin
- Little fat under the skin
- Scant hair
- Thin, floppy ears
- Relatively large head
- Underdeveloped breast tissue
- Weak muscles and reduced physical activity (a premature infant tends not to draw up the arms and legs as does a full-term infant)
- Poor sucking and swallowing reflexes
- Irregular breathing
- Small scrotum, with few folds (boys)
- Labia majora not yet covering the labia minora (girls)

---

mother. After delivery, the kidneys and intestine must take over this function. Kidney function in an extremely premature infant is limited, but it improves as the kidneys mature. After delivery, the infant needs normal liver function as well as intestinal function to excrete bilirubin (a yellow pigment resulting from the normal breakdown of red blood cells) in his stools. Most newborns, especially those born prematurely, have a temporary increase in the blood level of bilirubin, which can lead to jaundice. The increase occurs because their liver function is somewhat immature and because they are less able to take feedings and have bowel movements than are older infants. Very high levels of bilirubin can lead to kernicterus, a form of brain damage. However, most infants have mild jaundice, which is not serious; it

---

▲ see page 1206

resolves as the infant's feeding and bowel movements improve.

Because premature infants lose heat quickly and have difficulty maintaining normal body temperature, they are usually placed in an incubator.

Postmaturity

Postmaturity is a condition in which a pregnancy lasts longer than 42 weeks.

What causes a fetus to remain in the uterus for longer than the normal 38 to 42 weeks is usually unknown.

The placenta begins to shrink and its function decreases as a pregnancy comes close to term (40 weeks), even more so several weeks past term. As the placenta becomes less able to provide nutrients, the fetus may need to use its own fat and carbohydrate reserves for energy. As a result, its growth rate slows. If the placenta can't provide enough oxygen during labor, fetal distress may occur, putting the fetus at risk of injury to the brain and other organs. Such injury is probably the greatest risk to a postmature infant, and to prevent such problems, many doctors induce labor if the pregnancy exceeds 42 weeks.

Several problems are typical of postmature infants. They are prone to have low blood sugar (glucose) levels after delivery because energy reserves are low at birth and may be even lower if the oxygen supply during labor was low. These infants are also more prone to develop meconium aspiration syndrome.▲

Small for Gestational Age

A newborn, whether premature, full term, or postmature, who is smaller than normal for the time spent in the uterus is considered small for gestational age.

A newborn may be small at birth because of hereditary factors—small parents or a genetic disorder—or because the placenta functioned poorly, delivering an insufficient supply of nutrients and oxygen to the fetus. The placenta may have functioned poorly if the mother had high blood pressure, kidney disease, or long-standing diabetes during pregnancy. Mothers who are addicted to narcotics or cocaine or who are heavy alcohol users or heavy smokers also tend to have small for gestational age infants. Less commonly, infection of the mother and fetus with cytomegalovirus, rubella virus (German measles), or *Toxo-*

plasma gondii may interfere with the growth of the fetus.

Despite their size, small for gestational age infants usually appear and behave much like normal-sized infants of the same gestational age. Unlike a premature infant, a small for gestational age infant that has reached full term has fully developed internal organs. If the infant's growth was slowed because of inadequate nutrition while in the uterus, his growth may catch up rapidly after delivery when he is provided with adequate nutrition.

A fetus who grew slowly because of poor placental function may not receive enough oxygen during labor. During each contraction, the mother's arteries to the placenta are compressed where they pass through the uterine wall, so that less blood flows through them. If placental function was borderline before labor, the reduced blood supply during labor can jeopardize oxygen delivery and result in injury to the fetus. Normally, the fetus' heart rate slows during labor contractions. A heart rate that is slow to recover (late acceleration) or that doesn't vary as the fetus moves suggests an inadequate oxygen supply. When there is evidence of fetal distress, delivery must be performed quickly, often by cesarean section.

A baby deprived of oxygen during labor may pass stool (meconium) into the amniotic fluid. If the baby inhales the meconium-containing fluid, his lungs are affected.▲ Meconium may plug some of the bronchi, causing areas of the lungs to collapse. Meconium inhaled into the lungs can also lead to inflammation or pneumonitis. Both of these problems impair lung function.

Like the postmature infant, the small for gestational age infant is more likely to develop low blood sugar (glucose) levels—a condition called hypoglycemia■—in the first hours and days after delivery because he hasn't stored much glucose during gestation.

Large for Gestational Age

A newborn, whether premature, full term, or postmature, who weighs more than normal for the time spent in the uterus is considered large for gestational age.

Other than hereditary factors, the main reason an infant may be abnormally large is diabetes in the mother during the pregnancy. Sugar (glucose) in the mother's blood crosses the placenta; in

---

Physical Features of a Postmature Infant

• Full term in length but low in weight, so appears thin

• Mature, alert appearance

• Little fat under the skin, so the skin may hang loosely on the arms and legs

• Dry, peeling skin

• Long fingernails and toenails

• Fingernails, toenails, and umbilical cord may be stained green or brown from meconium (stool passed before birth)

---

response to a high blood level of glucose, the fetus' pancreas produces a large amount of insulin. This causes the fetus to grow excessively large. The poorer the control of the mother's diabetes, the larger the infant is likely to be. The infant's size may make vaginal delivery difficult, increasing the chances of injury. For this reason, a large for gestational age infant may have to be delivered by cesarean section.

At birth, when the umbilical cord is cut, glucose from the mother suddenly stops flowing to the infant, but the infant's insulin levels are still elevated. The infant's blood glucose levels are then likely to fall rapidly, causing hypoglycemia 1 to 2 hours after delivery.★ The infant may not have any symptoms of hypoglycemia, or he may be jittery, listless, limp, or drowsy; may breastfeed poorly; and may even have seizures. Controlling the mother's diabetes helps prevent hypoglycemia in the infant. The infant's blood glucose levels are closely monitored. If necessary, he is given glucose intravenously in the hours just after delivery.

Infants of diabetic mothers have an abnormally high number of red blood cells. Therefore, they are likely to develop high blood levels of biliru-

---

▲ see page 1206

■ see page 1213

★ see page 1213

bin (a yellow pigment formed during the normal breakdown of red blood cells), which results in jaundice. This condition may require treatment with phototherapy (exposure to bilirubin lights▲); rarely, an exchange transfusion is needed.

Infants born to diabetic mothers are more likely to have immature lungs and to develop respiratory distress syndrome, even if delivered fairly late in the pregnancy. Tests of the amniotic fluid performed before elective delivery can determine whether the fetus' lungs have matured.

Birth Injury

The mother's pelvic bones make up the birth canal. Normally, an infant has enough room to pass through the canal. However, if the canal is small or if the fetus is large (as is often true with diabetic mothers), passage through the birth canal may be difficult or may result in injury. When examinations determine that the infant is too large for the mother's birth canal, delivery by cesarean section reduces the chance of injury to the infant more than does a forceps delivery.

Almost any part of the newborn may be injured during delivery. Most injuries are minor and heal quickly. Bruises are common and are of no consequence. The bones of a fetus' skull are not joined together, so that the head can be molded to fit through the birth canal. Molding of the head is normal, and the head shape returns to normal in a few days. Serious injury to the head is rare, and traumatic injury to the brain is now extremely rare. Nerves can be stretched during a difficult delivery, especially nerves to the arms, resulting in temporary or permanent weakness of the arm (Erb palsy). Fractures, especially of the collar bone, occur occasionally and usually heal quickly with no long-term problems.

Respiratory Distress Syndrome

Respiratory distress syndrome (formerly called hyaline membrane disease) is a breathing disorder in which the air sacs (alveoli) in an infant's lungs do not stay open because of high surface tension resulting from insufficient production of surfactant.

▲ see page 1212

For an infant to be able to breathe independently, the air sacs in the lungs must be able to remain open and filled with air after birth. They can do so largely because of a substance called surfactant. Surfactant is produced by cells in the air sacs and lowers surface tension. Surfactant is produced as the fetus' lungs mature, often by 34 weeks and almost always by 37 weeks of gestation.

Respiratory distress syndrome occurs almost exclusively in premature infants—the more premature, the greater the chance of respiratory distress syndrome. The syndrome is also more likely to develop in infants of diabetic mothers.

Symptoms and Diagnosis

Very premature infants may be unable to start breathing, because without surfactant, their lungs are too stiff. Somewhat larger infants may start breathing, but because the lungs tend to collapse, respiratory distress develops. In these infants, breathing is rapid and labored, with flaring of the nostrils; they draw in the chest wall when inhaling and make grunting noises when exhaling. Distress may begin immediately after delivery or within a few hours. If respiratory distress syndrome is severe, the breathing muscles eventually tire, breathing becomes even less effective, and insufficient oxygen is delivered to the tissues, causing the skin to appear bluish. Without treatment, an infant who has respiratory distress syndrome may die.

The diagnosis of respiratory distress syndrome is based on the mother's medical history (for example, premature labor or diabetes), a physical examination of the infant after birth, and a chest x-ray showing that the infant's lungs aren't fully expanded.

Complications

The lungs are stiff, and more pressure, produced by the infant or a ventilator, is needed to expand them. Consequently, a lung may rupture, allowing air to leak into the chest cavity. This air causes the lung to collapse further and impairs ventilation and circulation. Lung collapse (a condition called pneumothorax) usually needs immediate treatment. Treatment involves removing free air in the chest with a syringe and needle, then placing a tube attached to a water seal in the infant's chest so that free air won't reaccumulate.

In addition, infants with respiratory distress syndrome are at increased risk of bleeding in the brain. The risk of bleeding is much less if the mother has been treated with corticosteroids before delivery.

Prevention and Treatment

The risk of respiratory distress syndrome is greatly reduced if delivery can be delayed until the fetus' lungs have produced sufficient surfactant. If a fetus may be born prematurely, amniocentesis may be performed to obtain a sample of amniotic fluid so that surfactant levels can be estimated.

If a doctor anticipates that the fetus' lungs are immature and delivery can't be delayed, a corticosteroid drug may be given to the mother at least 24 hours before the estimated time of delivery. The corticosteroid crosses the placenta to the fetus and stimulates the fetus' lungs to produce surfactant.

After delivery, an infant with mild respiratory distress syndrome may only need to be placed in an oxygen hood. Sicker infants may need support with a ventilator and treatment with a surfactant drug.

A surfactant drug, which closely resembles natural surfactant, can be dripped directly down a tube into the infant's windpipe (trachea). It improves the chance of survival by reducing the severity of respiratory distress syndrome and the risk of complications, such as lung rupture. A surfactant drug may be given immediately after birth to prevent respiratory distress syndrome in a very premature infant who is likely to develop it, or it may be given as soon as signs of the syndrome appear. The infant is monitored closely to make sure that administration of the surfactant drug is being tolerated and that breathing is improving. Treatments may continue for several days, until the infant begins to produce his own surfactant.

Transient Tachypnea

Transient tachypnea (transient rapid breathing, neonatal wet lung syndrome) is a temporary condition of respiratory distress and low blood oxygen levels, which is not as serious as respiratory distress syndrome.

Normally, fluid in the fetus' lungs is rapidly absorbed after birth. Transient tachypnea usually results when absorption is delayed. Infants with transient tachypnea are usually born at or close to full term and often have been delivered by cesarean section. Soon after delivery, the infant begins to breathe rapidly, grunt, and draw in his chest wall while inhaling. The infant's skin may turn blue because of lack of oxygen in the blood. A chest x-ray shows fluid in the lungs.

Oxygen is often the only treatment needed, although some infants may need to receive continuous positive airway pressure (breathing against positive pressure from tubes placed in the nostrils) or the assistance of a ventilator. Most infants recover completely in 1 to 3 days as the fluid in the lungs is absorbed.

Apnea of Prematurity

Apnea of prematurity is a disorder in which a premature infant temporarily stops breathing and is usually defined as cessation of breathing for 15 to 20 seconds.

Apnea of prematurity may occur in infants born before 34 weeks of pregnancy, increasing in frequency among the most prematurely born infants. It is thought to be caused by immaturity of the part of the brain that controls breathing (the respiratory center). An obstruction of the upper airways related to immaturity can also interfere with breathing. Occasionally, gastroesophageal reflux, in which the acidic contents of the stomach flow backward (reflux) into the esophagus, can stimulate a reflex that leads to apnea.

Symptoms

Periods of apnea often begin within the first few days after delivery. The infant may have episodes of regular breathing with brief pauses (periodic breathing). If the pauses last for more than 20 seconds, oxygen levels in the blood may fall, causing the infant to become dusky or blue and the heart rate to slow.

Treatment

Keeping the infant's head and neck straight and placing him on his back or side can help prevent the airway from becoming obstructed. If the episodes of apnea continue, particularly if the infant becomes blue from lack of oxygen or if the heart rate slows, the infant may be given a drug such as aminophylline or caffeine. These drugs stimulate the respiratory center in the brain, leading to more continuous breathing and fewer episodes of apnea. If significant apnea episodes continue, a second drug, doxapram, may be given. If the problem becomes very severe, the infant may need support with continuous positive airway pressure or a ventilator.

Gastroesophageal reflux is treated by thickening the infant's formula with rice cereal and by elevating the head of the bed. Occasionally, drugs may be used to reduce the frequency of reflux.

Most premature infants stop having episodes of apnea before they reach full-term age, often by 34 weeks from the start of the pregnancy, and completely outgrow this problem by the time they are discharged from the hospital. Occasionally, larger premature infants who continue to have apnea episodes may be discharged home on a breathing or heart monitor.

Pulmonary Hypertension

Pulmonary hypertension (high blood pressure in the lungs) is a disorder in which the blood vessels in a newborn's lungs constrict and severely limit the amount of blood flowing through the lungs. As a result, the blood oxygen levels become dangerously low, and the condition may become life threatening.

Because a fetus doesn't breathe air, its blood doesn't need to flow through the lungs to be enriched with oxygen. Instead, much of the fetus' blood flows directly from the right side of the heart to the left side through a passage between the atria (foramen ovale). Of the blood that continues through the right side of the heart, most passes from the pulmonary artery to the aorta through a blood vessel that joins them (the ductus arteriosus). Only a small fraction of the blood from the right side of the heart passes through the lungs. At birth, the foramen ovale and the ductus arteriosus normally close, and the blood from the right side of the heart flows through the lungs. However, in a few newborns, the blood vessels in the lungs constrict, causing the foramen ovale to remain open; the ductus arteriosus may also stay open. When this happens, most of the blood pumped by the right side of the heart bypasses the lungs (as it does in the fetus), resulting in very low blood oxygen levels.

Pulmonary hypertension is more common among infants who are postmature or whose mothers took large doses of aspirin or indomethacin during pregnancy. It frequently occurs in infants with other lung diseases, such as meconium aspiration syndrome or pneumonia, but can develop in infants whose lungs are otherwise normal.

Treatment

An infant with pulmonary hypertension is usually placed in an environment of 100 percent oxygen, often on a ventilator. Sodium bicarbonate may be given intravenously. Both of these treatments help dilate (open) the blood vessels in the lungs. Blood pressure in the rest of the infant's body may need to be maintained by giving fluids or drugs. Otherwise, low blood pressure in the rest of the body results in even less blood flowing to the lungs because it increases the rate of blood flowing from the right to the left side of the heart.

For the most critically ill infants, a technique called extracorporeal membrane oxygenation can be used until the pulmonary hypertension resolves. With this technique, the infant's blood is circulated through a heart-lung machine (membrane oxygenator) that adds oxygen to it and removes carbon dioxide from it; then the blood is returned to the infant. Under investigation is a new treatment in which the infant breathes a very low concentration of nitric oxide gas, which causes the blood vessels in the lungs to dilate.

Meconium Aspiration Syndrome

Meconium aspiration syndrome results when a fetus inhales meconium, which can block the airways and irritate the lungs.

Meconium is the dark green material in the intestine of a full-term fetus. In response to any source of distress, such as inadequate oxygen delivery from the placenta, the fetus passes meconium stools into the amniotic fluid. The distressed fetus also gasps forcefully, inhaling the meconium-contaminated fluid into his lungs. After birth, meconium can block some airways, causing the air sacs (alveoli) supplied by these airways to collapse. Also, inhaled air can become trapped in areas supplied by partially blocked bronchi, causing these areas of the lungs to become overinflated. Overinflation in turn can lead to lung rupture, then collapse (pneumothorax).

Meconium aspiration syndrome is often most severe in postmature infants who are surrounded by a smaller amount of amniotic fluid. Aspirated meconium is therefore thicker and more likely to obstruct the airways.

Treatment

Attempts to prevent meconium aspiration syndrome begin in the delivery room. A doctor immediately suctions the newborn's mouth, nose, and throat to remove any fluid that contains meconium. A tube may then be placed into the newborn's windpipe so that any meconium can be suctioned out.

In the nursery, the infant's lungs are suctioned repeatedly. The infant is treated with oxygen or placed on a ventilator if necessary and is observed closely for serious complications, such as persistent pulmonary hypertension or pneumothorax.

Pneumothorax

Pneumothorax is a collection of air in the chest cavity surrounding a lung that causes the lung to collapse.

In an infant with stiff lungs, especially one whose breathing is being assisted with a ventilator, air can leak from the air sacs into the connective tissue in the lung and then into the soft tissues between the lung and the heart—a condition called pneumomediastinum. This condition usually doesn't affect breathing, and treatment isn't needed. However, pneumomediastinum may progress to pneumothorax.

Pneumothorax develops when air leaks into the chest cavity surrounding a lung (pleural space), where it may then compress the lung. A partially collapsed lung may cause no symptoms and require no treatment. However, if the collapsed lung is severely compressed, the condition may become life threatening, especially in an infant who has severe lung disease. Trapped air may forcibly collapse the lung, making breathing very difficult, and can interfere with the circulation of blood in the chest cavity. In such a case, the air surrounding the lung must be rapidly removed with a needle or a tube.

Bronchopulmonary Dysplasia

Bronchopulmonary dysplasia is lung injury caused by a ventilator.

Infants who stay on a ventilator for a long time, usually for more than 1 week, may develop bronchopulmonary dysplasia. The disorder is more common among premature infants. To prevent bronchopulmonary dysplasia, a doctor places an infant on a ventilator only when necessary and for the shortest time possible.

Injury probably results from stretching of the air spaces by the high pressure needed to inflate the lungs and by the high concentration of oxygen given. These factors can cause the lungs to become inflamed. After many weeks of inflammation, the lungs develop areas of scarring.

Treatment involves gradually weaning the infant from the ventilator. Good nutrition is essential for the lungs to heal and for healthy new lung tissue to grow. Because fluid tends to accumulate in inflamed lungs, some restriction of fluid intake may help, as may diuretics given to increase the excretion of fluid from the body.

Rarely, infants with bronchopulmonary dysplasia die even after months of care. In surviving infants, breathing problems gradually diminish. However, these infants have an increased risk of pneumonia, especially viral pneumonia, in the first few years of life. Immunizations with antibodies to respiratory syncytial virus (RSV) may be given monthly during the late fall and winter. RSV is often serious enough to require rehospitalization and even ventilator support during the first winters. Use of the vaccine reduces that risk by about 50%.

Retinopathy of Prematurity

Retinopathy of prematurity is a disorder in which blood vessels in the back of the eye (retina) develop abnormally in premature infants; these blood vessels may bleed, and in the most severe cases, the retina may detach, leading to visual loss.

In the fetus, the blood vessels supplying the retina grow from the center of the retina and reach the outer edges of the retina only late in pregnancy. Consequently, the blood vessels are incompletely developed in premature infants. Although these vessels continue to grow after birth, sometimes they grow in a disorganized fashion, causing retinopathy of prematurity. The main risk factor for developing retinopathy of prematurity is extreme prematurity; high oxygen levels in the blood from the treatment of breathing problems may increase the risk.

Prevention and Treatment

Good prenatal care reduces the risk that an infant will be born prematurely. If the infant is premature and has breathing problems, oxygen use is monitored carefully to prevent oxygen levels in the blood from becoming too high.

The eyes of premature infants are thoroughly examined about 6 weeks after birth and then every few weeks until growth of the blood vessels in the retina is complete. Mild changes of retinopathy of prematurity often heal spontaneously; nonetheless, a doctor continues to monitor the infant's eyes. Even if the retinopathy heals, the infant has an increased risk of near-sightedness, deviant eyes (squint), and poor vision. Infants with very severe retinopathy have an increased risk of retinal detachment.

For very severe retinopathy of prematurity, cryotherapy—in which the peripheral portions of the retina are frozen—can reduce the risk of retinal detachment and loss of vision. Infants with healed scars from retinopathy must have an eye examination at least every year for the rest of their lives. Treatment of any visual abnormality in the first year of life offers the best chance for good vision later. Retinal detachment sometimes can be corrected if detected early; otherwise, the infant may lose sight in the affected eye.

Feeding and Bowel Problems

Most common feeding and bowel problems in the newborn aren't medically serious. They often resolve spontaneously or can be handled by adjusting the feeding routine.

REGURGITATION AND VOMITING

Infants commonly spit up (regurgitate) small amounts of milk during or soon after feedings, often when being burped. This is normal. Sometimes regurgitation is caused by drinking too fast and swallowing air. For bottle-fed infants, regurgitation may be reduced by using bottles with firmer nipples and smaller holes. Burping the infant more often during the feeding helps both breastfed and bottle-fed infants. Excessive regurgitation may result from overfeeding. Even with optimal feeding methods, many infants continue to spit up a little; this is considered normal.

On the other hand, vomiting large amounts may indicate a problem. Repeated forceful vomiting (projectile vomiting) may indicate a narrowing or blockage at the stomach outlet (pyloric stenosis).

▲ see page 1291

■ see page 1245

★ see box, pages 1196 and 1197

● see page 1222

Blockage of the small intestine may result in bile-stained, greenish-yellow vomit, which should be evaluated by a doctor. Certain disorders of metabolism, such as galactosemia▲ (high blood levels of the sugar galactose), may also cause vomiting. An infant who vomits and has a fever, with or without drowsiness, may have an infection.

UNDERFEEDING

Young infants who have had enough to eat usually become quiet or fall asleep soon after a feeding. An underfed infant, however, often remains restless and awakens 1 to 2 hours after being fed, appearing hungry. A weight gain of less than 6 to 8 ounces a week in an infant under age 4 months is abnormally low and may indicate underfeeding. Sometimes underfeeding is the cause of failure to thrive.■

To determine whether the difficulty is underfeeding or a more serious problem, a doctor reviews the details of the infant's feeding with the parents. Breastfed infants who don't gain enough weight may be weighed before and after several feedings to obtain a more precise estimate of their milk intake. The bottle-fed infant's diet may be changed by increasing the total quantity of formula offered.

OVERFEEDING

Problems with obesity later in life sometimes begin with overfeeding in infancy. Also, an infant is more likely to be obese if his parents are. In fact, an infant has an 80 percent chance of developing obesity if both parents are obese. If weight gain, as plotted on a standard growth chart,★ is too rapid, controlling the rate of weight gain may be valuable.

DIARRHEA

Newborns usually have four to six loose bowel movements a day. Breastfed infants tend to have frequent, frothy bowel movements, especially before they are eating solid foods. The consistency of the bowel movements is not of concern unless the infant has a poor appetite, vomits, loses weight, does not gain weight, or passes blood in the stool.

Infection by bacteria or viruses may cause sudden severe diarrhea. Infection is by far the most common cause of acute diarrhea in young infants.● Mild diarrhea that lasts for weeks or months may be caused by any of several conditions, including celiac disease, cystic fibrosis, the malabsorption of sugar, or an allergy.

Celiac disease is a hereditary disorder in which gluten, a cereal protein found mainly in wheat, triggers an allergic reaction affecting the inner surface of the intestine, causing poor absorption of fats from the diet.▲ Celiac disease causes malnutrition, a poor appetite, and pale, bulky, foul-smelling stools. The disease is treated by excluding all wheat products from the diet.

Cystic fibrosis,■ a hereditary disorder, disturbs the function of several organs, including the pancreas. A pancreas affected by cystic fibrosis doesn't produce enough enzymes to digest proteins and fats. Without the appropriate digestive enzymes, the body loses too much protein and fat in the stools, resulting in malnutrition and slowed growth. Stools are bulky and often foul-smelling. Pancreatic extract may be given orally to control the problem.

Sugar malabsorption occurs if an infant lacks certain intestinal enzymes to digest specific sugars— for example, lactase to digest lactose. The enzymes may be missing temporarily because of an intestinal infection or permanently because of an inherited trait. The problem can be treated by eliminating the specific sugars from the diet.

An **allergy** to milk rarely causes diarrhea, vomiting, and blood in the stools. Symptoms often disappear promptly when a milk formula is replaced with a soybean formula, but they return if the milk formula is restarted. However, some infants intolerant of milk formulas are also intolerant of soy formulas. Infants are almost never allergic to human breast milk.

CONSTIPATION

Recognizing constipation in infants is difficult because the number of bowel movements can vary greatly. An infant who sometimes has a bowel movement four times a day may at other times have one every 2 days.

Most infants have little discomfort when passing a hard, large stool, whereas some cry when passing a soft one. The anus in an infant under 3 months of age may be narrow, causing him to strain persistently and pass thin stools. A doctor can diagnose this condition by gently examining the anus with a gloved finger. Dilating the anus once or twice usually relieves the symptoms.

A large bowel movement may tear the lining of the anus (anal fissure), causing pain during bowel movements and possibly a small amount of bright

red blood in the stools. A doctor may identify a fissure with an anoscope. In infants, most fissures heal quickly without treatment. However, a mild stool softener may help the fissure heal.

Severe constipation that persists, especially if it begins before the first month, may indicate a more serious problem. Such problems include Hirschsprung's disease (an abnormal nerve supply with an oversized large intestine) or an underactive thyroid gland.

Necrotizing Enterocolitis

Necrotizing enterocolitis is a condition in which the inner surface of the intestine becomes injured and inflamed; if severe, a portion of the intestine may die (become necrotic), leading to intestinal perforation and peritonitis.

Necrotizing enterocolitis occurs mainly in premature newborns. Its cause isn't fully understood. An inadequate blood supply to the intestine in a sick premature infant may result in injury to a portion of the intestine. Bacteria can then invade the damaged intestinal wall, producing gas inside the intestinal wall. If the intestinal wall perforates, the intestinal contents can spill into and cause infection of the abdominal cavity (peritonitis); this infection can lead to a bloodstream infection (sepsis) and even death.

Symptoms and Diagnosis

Infants with necrotizing enterocolitis do not tolerate feeding and have a distended abdomen. Eventually, they may vomit bile-stained intestinal contents, and blood may be seen in the stools. A bloodstream infection may cause lethargy and an abnormal, usually low, body temperature. The blood may become acidic, and the infant may have brief periods of apnea, in which breathing stops. X-rays of the abdomen may reveal gas produced by bacteria inside the intestinal wall, which confirms the diagnosis of necrotizing enterocolitis.

Treatment and Prognosis

Some evidence suggests that breast milk may protect premature infants against necrotizing enterocolitis. For tiny or sick premature infants, the

---

▲ see page 536

■ see page 201

risk may be reduced by delaying oral feedings for several days and then slowly increasing the amount of feedings. Feedings are stopped immediately if necrotizing enterocolitis is suspected. Pressure in the intestine is relieved by removing gas and fluid through a suction tube that is passed into the stomach. Fluids are given intravenously, and antibiotics are started immediately.

If the intestine perforates or the abdominal cavity becomes infected, surgery is necessary. Surgery may also be needed if an infant's condition progressively worsens. However, about 70 percent of the infants with necrotizing enterocolitis don't need surgery. During surgery, perforated or dead (necrotic) parts of the intestine are removed. The cut ends of the intestine can be brought to the skin's surface and left open there (ostomy). Sometimes, when the ends of the intestine are healthy, they can be reattached at once. Otherwise, the ends are reattached several weeks or months later, after the intestinal tissue is healthy.

Intensive medical treatment and appropriate surgery have improved the prognosis for infants with necrotizing enterocolitis. More than two thirds of these infants now survive.

Rarely, in infants treated without surgery, part of the large intestine narrows during the following weeks or months, causing a partial blockage of the intestinal tract. Surgery is needed to widen the scarred, narrowed area.

Colic

Colic is a disorder in which an infant has episodes of crying and irritability with what appears to be abdominal pain.

Colic, named for the colon (large intestine), has been blamed on too much gas in the intestine, yet the precise cause of colic isn't known. Colic may begin shortly after an infant comes home from the hospital, but it usually begins a few weeks later. Colic may occur intermittently during the first 3 or 4 months.

Symptoms and Diagnosis

Colic is marked by episodes of uncontrollable crying, which often occur at a predictable time of day or night. However, a few infants cry almost incessantly. Excessive crying causes the infant to swallow air, which results in gas (flatulence) and abdominal swelling. Typically, a colicky infant eats and gains weight well, seems very hungry, and often sucks vigorously on almost anything.

A doctor diagnoses colic by excluding other causes of crying and irritability, including inadequate feeding, overstimulation, sickness, and a milk allergy.

Treatment

A colicky infant may quiet down when held, rocked, or patted gently. An infant with a strong sucking urge who fusses soon after a feeding may need more opportunity to suck. If a bottle-feeding takes less than 20 minutes, different nipples with smaller holes should be tried. A pacifier also may quiet the infant. A very active, restless infant may respond to being swaddled. Very occasionally, a sedative may be given an hour before the anticipated fussy period. In any case, colic usually clears up by 3 months of age.

Anemia

Anemia is a disorder characterized by too few red blood cells (erythrocytes) in the blood.

Anemia in a newborn can result from blood loss, excessive destruction or impaired production of red blood cells, or a combination of these factors.▲ An infant may lose a considerable amount of blood during delivery if the placenta separates prematurely from the wall of the uterus (abruptio placentae)■ or if the umbilical cord tears. In such cases, the infant may be very pale, have low blood pressure (shock), and breathe poorly after delivery.

Anemia in the premature infant is commonly caused by blood loss (through repeated blood sampling for laboratory tests) and lack of production of new red blood cells. Normally, the bone marrow does not produce new red blood cells for 3 or 4 weeks after birth. This anemia is made even more severe because of the rapid rate of growth of the premature infant, who may grow faster than new red blood cells can be produced. However, the premature infant usually does not develop symptoms of anemia, which resolves within a month or two.

Sometimes large numbers of red blood cells are destroyed, as occurs in hemolytic disease of the newborn, because of antibodies produced by the

---

▲ see page 742

■ see page 1156

What is Hemolytic Disease of the Newborn?

Hemolytic disease of the newborn, also called erythroblastosis neonatorum, is a condition in which a newborn's red blood cells are destroyed by antibodies that have crossed the placenta from the mother's blood. Hemolytic disease begins in the fetus, in whom the disease is called erythroblastosis fetalis.

In many cases, severe hemolytic disease results when the fetus has Rh-positive blood and the mother has Rh-negative blood. The fetus' blood is Rh-positive because the father passed along an Rh-positive trait, which is a dominant trait. The mother responds to the incompatible blood by producing antibodies against it. These antibodies cross the placenta into the fetus' circulation, where they attach to and destroy the fetus' red blood cells, leading to anemia. Sometimes other blood type in-

compatibilities are involved. For example, the mother may have type O blood and the fetus has type A or B blood. Rarer incompatibilities include the Kell and Duffy blood groups.

Severe anemia caused by hemolytic disease of the newborn is treated in the same way as are other anemias. The doctor also observes the infant for signs of jaundice, which is likely to occur because hemoglobin from the continued destruction of red blood cells is converted to the bright yellow pigment called bilirubin. If bilirubin accumulates in the body more rapidly than it can be excreted by the liver, the infant's skin appears yellow (jaundice). Jaundice is easily treated by exposing the infant to bright lights; very rarely, it can lead to brain damage (kernicterus) if it becomes extremely severe.

mother against the fetus' red blood cells during pregnancy. Red blood cells may also be destroyed too rapidly if the infant has a hereditary condition in which red blood cells are abnormally shaped. An example is hereditary spherocytosis, in which red blood cells are spherical. Red blood cells may also be destroyed rapidly if they contain an abnormal hemoglobin (the protein in red blood cells that carries oxygen), as occurs in sickle cell anemia▲ or thalassemia.■ An infection acquired before birth, such as toxoplasmosis, rubella, cytomegalovirus disease, herpes simplex, or syphilis, may cause red blood cells to break down rapidly. When red blood cells are destroyed, hemoglobin is metabolized into bilirubin. High bilirubin levels in the blood (hyperbilirubinemia) cause jaundice and, in severe cases, can lead to brain damage (kernicterus).★

Anemia caused by **iron deficiency** can occur in infants at 3 to 6 months of age if they are fed cow's milk or formula that's not supplemented with iron. Untreated infants who have iron deficiency anemia may be lethargic.

Treatment

An infant who has lost a considerable amount of blood during delivery is given a blood transfusion immediately. When anemia is caused by excessive destruction of red blood cells, treat-

ment involves an exchange blood transfusion, in which the infant's blood is slowly exchanged with fresh blood. Damaged red blood cells, bilirubin, and antibodies from the mother are all removed during an exchange blood transfusion. Treatment of iron deficiency anemia consists of iron supplementation. If symptoms of severe anemia develop, a blood transfusion may be required

Polycythemia

Polycythemia, the opposite of anemia, is an abnormally high number of red blood cells.●

Polycythemia increases the thickness of the blood, reducing the rate at which it flows through small blood vessels. If severe, it can lead to blood clots within the blood vessels. An infant who is postmature or one whose mother has hypertension, smokes, has diabetes, or lives at a high altitude is at greater risk of having polycythemia.

▲ see page 749

■ see page 751

★ see box, page 1212

● see page 782

What is Kernicterus?

Kernicterus is a condition in which bilirubin accumulates in the brain, causing brain damage. Kernicterus is now a rare condition most likely to occur in premature or critically ill newborns.

Kernicterus begins with drowsiness, poor feeding, and vomiting. Spasmodic backward arching of the neck and back (opisthotonos), upward rolling of the eyes, seizures, and death may follow. Late effects of kernicterus include mental retardation, abnormal muscle control (cerebral palsy), deafness, and paralysis of upward eye movements.

Polycythemia may also result if the infant receives too much blood from the placenta before the umbilical cord is clamped after delivery.

The infant may have a ruddy red complexion or a blue tinge. The infant may be sluggish, feed poorly, breathe rapidly, and have a rapid heart rate. Seizures occur very rarely.

Although removing blood would help eliminate excess red blood cells, it would also lower the blood volume and worsen the symptoms of polycythemia. Instead, a partial exchange blood transfusion is performed to remove some of the infant's blood and replace it with an equal amount of plasma (the liquid part of blood).

Hyperbilirubinemia

Hyperbilirubinemia is an abnormally high level of bilirubin in the blood.

Aging, damaged, or abnormal red blood cells are removed from the circulation, mainly in the spleen. During the process, hemoglobin (the protein in red blood cells that carries oxygen) is broken down into a yellow pigment called bilirubin. Bilirubin is carried in the circulation to the liver, where it is chemically altered (conjugated), and then excreted into the intestine as a component of bile.

In most newborns, the blood level of bilirubin normally increases temporarily in the first few days after birth, causing the skin to appear yellow (jaundice).

In adults, bacteria normally found in the intestine break down bilirubin. The newborn lacks these bacteria, so that much of the bilirubin is excreted in the stools, typically making them bright yellow. However, the newborn also has an enzyme in the intestine that can alter some of the bilirubin and enables it to be reabsorbed into the blood, contributing to the development of jaundice. As the blood level of bilirubin increases, jaundice becomes visible, advancing in a head-to-foot direction; that is, it is seen first in the face, then the chest, then in the legs and feet. Normally, hyperbilirubinemia and visible jaundice disappear after the first week.

An unusually high blood level of bilirubin may be caused by overproduction or underexcretion of bilirubin or both. Occasionally, in full-term newborns who are breastfed, the blood level of bilirubin increases progressively during the first week of life—a condition called breast milk jaundice. The exact reason for the jaundice is unknown. It is not harmful in most cases. If the bilirubin level becomes extremely high, treatment with bilirubin lights may be needed.

Most increases in bilirubin levels are of no consequence, but in extremely rare circumstances, a very high bilirubin level can produce brain damage. This condition, kernicterus, is most common in very premature and critically ill newborns.

Treatment

Mild hyperbilirubinemia doesn't require treatment. Frequent feedings in a newborn accelerate the passage of intestinal contents, reducing the reabsorption of bilirubin from the intestine and thus the blood level of bilirubin. Higher bilirubin levels can be treated by phototherapy, in which the infant is placed under bilirubin lights. Bright light shined on the infant's skin causes a chemical alteration in the bilirubin molecules in the tissues under the skin. Once altered, the bilirubin can be more rapidly excreted by the liver without first having to be altered (conjugated) by the liver. If the infant's blood contains dangerously high bilirubin levels, it is exchanged with fresh blood (exchange transfusion to remove bilirubin).

Rarely, breastfeeding may need to be discontinued for 1 or 2 days if the bilirubin level becomes extremely high in an infant who has breast milk jaundice. The mother should continue to express breast milk regularly so that she can resume breastfeeding as soon as the infant's bilirubin level starts to decrease. Resuming breastfeeding at this time poses no risk to the infant.

Hypothermia

Hypothermia is an abnormally low body temperature.

The body surface area of a newborn, particularly one who has a low birth weight, is large relative to his body weight, so he can rapidly lose heat. In cool surroundings, a newborn's temperature tends to fall. Heat may also be lost rapidly by evaporation, which can occur when a newborn is wet with amniotic fluid.

An abnormally low body temperature can cause a low blood sugar level (hypoglycemia), high blood acidity (metabolic acidosis), and death. Because the body uses energy rapidly trying to stay warm, an infant needs more oxygen when he becomes cold. Hypothermia may therefore cause the oxygen supply to the tissues to be insufficient.

All newborns should be kept warm to prevent hypothermia. This care begins in the delivery room when a newborn is dried rapidly to avoid heat loss from evaporation and then swaddled in a warm blanket. A cap is placed on the infant's head to help prevent heat loss from the scalp. An infant who must be left uncovered for observation or treatment is placed under a radiant warmer.

Hypoglycemia

Hypoglycemia is an abnormally low blood sugar (glucose) level.

Hypoglycemia usually results when an infant has low reserves of glucose (stored as glycogen) at birth. Other common causes are prematurity, postmaturity, and abnormal placental function during gestation. Infants with low glycogen reserves may become hypoglycemic at any time in the first few days, especially if feedings are too far apart or nutrient intake is low.

Hypoglycemia may also occur in infants who have high insulin levels. Infants born to diabetic mothers often have high insulin levels because their mothers have high blood glucose levels and a large amount of this glucose crosses the placenta from their mother's blood during pregnancy. In response, the fetus produces a large amount of insulin. Severe hemolytic disease in a newborn may also elevate insulin levels. High insulin levels typically cause blood glucose levels to fall rapidly in the first hour after birth, when the continuous supply of glucose from the placenta abruptly ends.

Many newborns with hypoglycemia have no symptoms. Others are listless, feed poorly, have poor muscle tone, are jittery, breathe rapidly, or temporarily stop breathing (apnea). Seizures may occur.

Hypoglycemia is treated with glucose, given orally or intravenously, depending on the seriousness of the problem.

Hyperglycemia

Hyperglycemia is an abnormally high blood sugar (glucose) level.

Hyperglycemia is less common than hypoglycemia in newborns. In very small infants, glucose given intravenously may raise blood glucose levels excessively. Very severely stressed or infected (septic) newborns may also develop high blood glucose levels. If the blood glucose levels are very high, glucose may spill into the urine.

Treatment consists of reducing the amount of glucose given to the infant. If hyperglycemia persists, insulin may be given intravenously.

Hypocalcemia

Hypocalcemia is an abnormally low blood calcium level.▲

Mild hypocalcemia is fairly common in sick newborns in the first day or two. Newborns with a high risk of more severe hypocalcemia include those who are premature, are small for gestational age, received insufficient oxygen during delivery, or have a diabetic mother. The cause of hypocalcemia shortly after delivery isn't well understood but may partly relate to the sudden unavailability of calcium from the mother.

▲ see page 672

High phosphate levels in the blood can also cause hypocalcemia. This type of hypocalcemia can occur in older infants who are fed cow's milk (rather than breast milk or formula), because the phosphate content of cow's milk is too high for them.

Hypocalcemia may cause no symptoms, or it may cause weakness, episodes of apnea in which breathing temporarily stops, poor feeding, jitteriness, or seizures. Infants without symptoms usually don't need treatment. Those with symptoms are treated with calcium solutions, given intravenously or orally.

Hypernatremia

Hypernatremia is an abnormally high blood sodium concentration.▲

Hypernatremia may be caused by excessive sodium (salt) intake or excessive loss of water from the body. Loss of water is particularly common in very premature infants because water readily evaporates from their skin, which is extremely permeable to water. The situation is made worse because their immature kidneys can't absorb water from urine to concentrate it, so the infants continue to lose water through urination.

A newborn who has been given too much sodium often has tissue swelling (edema) and excretes large amounts of sodium in the urine. In contrast, a newborn who has lost too much water is dehydrated. A dehydrated infant has dry skin and mucous membranes in the mouth, urinates little or not at all, and can develop low blood pressure. In severe cases, hypernatremia or dehydration can cause brain damage or death. Dehydration is corrected by giving extra water intravenously.

Fetal Alcohol Syndrome

Fetal alcohol syndrome is a condition that affects some infants born to mothers who drank alcohol during pregnancy.

Alcohol consumption during pregnancy can cause birth defects, especially if the mother consumes large amounts of alcohol or drinks in binges. There is no proof that small amounts of

alcohol are safe; therefore, no alcohol should be consumed during pregnancy. Large amounts of alcohol may cause a miscarriage or fetal alcohol syndrome.

Newborns who have fetal alcohol syndrome are small for gestational age and have a small head, indicating poor brain growth while in the uterus. Small eyes, a flattened midportion of the face, abnormal creases on the palms of the hands, heart defects, and joint abnormalities are among the many malformations that may occur. The most serious consequence is impaired brain development, leading to mental retardation. Alcohol use during pregnancy is the most common preventable cause of mental retardation.

Substance Abuse During Pregnancy

Drug use during pregnancy can have adverse effects on the developing fetus and newborn. Cocaine and opioids are two of the illicit drugs that can cause significant problems.

Cocaine constricts blood vessels and raises blood pressure. Cocaine used by a woman during pregnancy can cause a miscarriage. Rarely, cocaine use early in pregnancy may cause birth defects involving the kidneys, eyes, brain, or extremities. An infant born to a cocaine-addicted mother is more likely to have a low birth weight and a subnormal body length and head circumference.

Opioids, such as heroin, methadone, and morphine, rarely cause birth defects, but because opioids cross the placenta, infants can be born addicted to them. Withdrawal symptoms usually begin within 72 hours of birth. Withdrawal symptoms include irritability with excessive crying, jitteriness, stiff muscles, vomiting, diarrhea, sweating, fast breathing, and seizures. Mild withdrawal symptoms are treated by swaddling the infant and feeding him frequently to reduce restlessness. Severe symptoms may be controlled with small doses of tincture of opium, a narcotic. The dose is very gradually tapered over a period of days to weeks as the symptoms disappear.

Many other drugs have been abused, and often several drugs are abused together during pregnancy. Infants whose mothers abused drugs during pregnancy should be followed closely by health care and social services workers. Some infants have malformations that require special attention, and others, such as those with fetal

▲ see page 669

alcohol syndrome, may be retarded. These infants should be evaluated and receive treatment in an early infant development program. Many will require special education when they reach school age.

An infant whose mother abused drugs should be followed by the local department of social services. The mother's drug abuse or addiction, along with the associated lifestyle, places the infant at serious risk for child abuse or neglect.

Seizure Disorders

Seizures are abnormal electrical discharges in the brain.

Seizures may be caused by any disorder that directly or indirectly affects the brain, such as low blood levels of sugar (glucose), calcium, magnesium, or vitamin B_6 (pyridoxine) and low or high blood levels of sodium. Inflammation of the membranes around the brain (meningitis) may cause seizures. Other causes include brain injury resulting from low levels of oxygen, bleeding within the brain, birth injury, birth defects of the brain, or withdrawal from addictive drugs. Seizures caused by fever occur in older children and are rarely serious.▲

Conditions that cause seizures in newborns are often serious. However, the majority of newborn infants who have seizures survive without disabilities. Seizures caused by low blood glucose or low blood calcium levels are not likely to be associated with disabilities. Seizures resulting from maldevelopment of the brain, injury, or meningitis are more likely to be associated with later neurologic problems.

Seizures may be difficult to recognize. Commonly, the arms and legs jerk rhythmically; chewing movements may occur, or the eyes persistently deviate. Sometimes the breathing or heart rate suddenly changes.

Diagnosis and Treatment

A doctor tries to determine the cause of the seizures by taking a complete history and performing a physical examination. Tests to measure blood glucose, calcium, and electrolyte levels may be indicated. Often an image of the brain is produced by ultrasound scanning, computed tomography (CT), or magnetic resonance imaging (MRI). An electroencephalogram (EEG), which measures electrical activity in the brain, can help diagnose the type of seizure.

Treatment is usually aimed at correcting the cause of the seizure. Persistent seizures may be treated with drugs such as phenobarbital and phenytoin.

Sudden Infant Death Syndrome

Sudden infant death syndrome (SIDS) is the sudden, unexpected death of a seemingly healthy infant.

Sudden infant death syndrome is the most common cause of death in infants between 2 weeks and 1 year of age. It kills 3 of every 2,000 infants, almost always when the infants are sleeping. However, the frequency seems to be decreasing in recent years. Most deaths occur between the second and fourth month of life. The syndrome occurs worldwide. Sudden infant death syndrome is somewhat more common during the winter months, in families with low incomes, among premature infants or those needing resuscitation at birth, among those with brothers or sisters who died of the syndrome, and among those whose mothers smoke. It affects slightly more boys than girls.

The cause of sudden infant death syndrome isn't known, and there may be several factors that result in the sudden, unexpected death of an infant. Recent studies have suggested that sudden infant death syndrome is more common among infants who sleep on their stomach than in those who sleep on their back or side. Putting healthy infants to bed on their back or side is now recommended. Also, there is a risk that infants may suffocate if placed face down on soft bedding, such as a blanket or a soft foam mattress. Therefore, infants should sleep on a firm mattress. No one should smoke in a house with a small infant.

Parents who have lost an infant to sudden infant death syndrome are grief-stricken and unprepared for the tragedy. Because no definite cause can be found for their infant's death, they usually feel excessively guilty. They may be further traumatized by investigations conducted by police, social workers, or others. Counseling and support should be offered by specially trained doctors and nurses. Other parents who have lost an infant to sudden infant death syndrome can also support and comfort the grieving parents.

▲ see page 346

Infections in Newborns and Infants

A newborn may acquire an infection from the mother before or during birth. After birth, the source of a newborn's infection is often the hospital nursery.

At birth, a baby moves from a sterile environment inside the uterus to one teeming with microorganisms. In the normal course of events, some of these microorganisms begin to grow in the infant. Indeed, normal digestion depends on the presence of certain bacteria, which colonize the intestine during early infancy. However, some bacteria in the environment can cause disease. Premature infants are especially vulnerable to harmful bacteria because their immune system isn't mature. In addition, premature infants undergo more treatments and procedures than other infants and so are at greater risk for infection.

Conjunctivitis

Conjunctivitis in a newborn (neonatal conjunctivitis, ophthalmia neonatorum) is an infection of the membrane that lines the eyelid and the exposed part of the eye.▲

In most cases, neonatal conjunctivitis is acquired during passage through the birth canal, and most of the organisms responsible are bacteria that commonly inhabit the vagina. *Chlamydia*—a type of small bacterium—is the most common cause of neonatal conjunctivitis. However, other bacteria, particularly *Streptococcus pneumoniae, Hemophilus influenzae,* and *Neisseria gonorrhoeae* (the bacterium that causes gonorrhea), can also cause neonatal conjunctivitis. So too can viruses. Herpes simplex virus is the most common viral cause.

Symptoms and Diagnosis

Conjunctivitis caused by *Chlamydia* usually develops 5 to 14 days after birth. The infection may

▲ see page 1037

■ see page 916

be mild or severe and may produce small or large amounts of pus. Conjunctivitis caused by other bacteria may begin 4 to 21 days after birth and may or may not produce pus. The herpes simplex virus may infect only the eye, or the eye and other parts of the body may be affected.■ In severe cases, a life-threatening infection may develop throughout the body and the brain. Conjunctivitis caused by the gonorrhea bacterium appears 2 to 5 days after birth or earlier if the membranes ruptured prematurely and the infection had time to start before birth.

Regardless of the cause, the newborn's eyelids and whites of the eyes (conjunctivae) usually become severely swollen. Pus may spurt out when the lids are opened. If treatment is delayed, sores may form on the cornea, permanently impairing vision. To identify the infectious organism, a doctor may take a sample of pus for examination under the microscope or for culture.

Prevention and Treatment

To prevent conjunctivitis, a newborn's eyes are routinely treated with silver nitrate, erythromycin, or tetracycline ointment or drops. None of these medications, however, can always prevent chlamydial conjunctivitis. A newborn whose mother is known to have gonorrhea receives an injection of the antibiotic ceftriaxone, which prevents gonorrheal infection in the eye and elsewhere.

To treat bacterial conjunctivitis, an ointment containing polymyxin plus bacitracin, erythromycin, or tetracycline is applied to the eyes. Because at least half of the infants with chlamydial conjunctivitis also have a chlamydial infection elsewhere, erythromycin is usually given orally. Conjunctivitis caused by the herpes simplex virus is treated with trifluridine drops or ointment and idoxuridine ointment. The infant is also given the antiviral drug acyclovir, because of concerns that the virus has already spread or will spread to the brain and other organs. Corticosteroid ointments aren't used in newborns because they may seriously worsen chlamydial and herpes simplex virus infections.

Sepsis

Sepsis in a newborn (sepsis neonatorum) is a severe bacterial infection that spreads throughout the body in the first month of life.

Sepsis occurs in fewer than 1 percent of newborns but accounts for up to 30 percent of deaths in the first few weeks of life. Bacterial infection is five times more common in newborns weighing less than $5\frac{1}{2}$ pounds than in normal-weight full-term newborns. Sepsis affects twice as many boys as girls. Complications experienced during birth, such as premature rupture of the membranes or bleeding or infection in the mother, put the newborn at increased risk of sepsis.

Symptoms

Sepsis begins within 6 hours of birth in more than half the cases and within 72 hours in the great majority. Sepsis that begins 4 or more days after birth is probably an infection acquired in the hospital nursery (a nosocomial infection).

A newborn with sepsis is usually listless, doesn't suck vigorously, and has a slow heart rate and a fluctuating body temperature (low or high). Other symptoms include difficulty in breathing, seizures, jitteriness, jaundice, vomiting, diarrhea, and a swollen abdomen.

Symptoms depend on where the infection originated and where it has spread. For example, infection of the umbilical cord stump (omphalitis) may cause a discharge of pus or bleeding at the navel. Infection of the lining of the brain (meningitis) or a brain abscess may cause coma, seizures, rigid arching of the back, or bulging fontanelles (the two soft spots between the skull bones). Infection of a bone (osteomyelitis) may restrict movement in the affected arm or leg. Joint infection may cause swelling, warmth, redness, and tenderness over the joint. Infection of the inside lining of the abdomen (peritonitis) may cause a swollen abdomen and bloody diarrhea.

Diagnosis

The organism causing the infection is identified by taking blood samples and culturing any obviously infected part of the body. Antibody tests may help identify the organism. A urine sample is also examined under a microscope and cultured for bacteria. A spinal tap (lumbar puncture) is performed if the doctor suspects meningitis.▲ Samples of fluid from the ears and from the stomach may be taken for examination under a microscope.

Prognosis and Treatment

Sepsis in a newborn is treated with antibiotics given intravenously. Treatment is started even before laboratory results are available; a different antibiotic may later be chosen based on the results of laboratory tests. In rare cases, the infant may also be given a preparation of purified antibodies or white blood cells.

Despite modern antibiotics and intensive care, 25 percent or more of newborns with sepsis die. The death rate is twice as high in small, premature newborns as in normal-weight, full-term newborns.

Pneumonia

Pneumonia is an infection of the lungs, in which the lungs fill with fluid, leading to difficulty in breathing.■

Pneumonia in newborns often starts when premature rupture of the membranes leads to an infection of the amniotic fluid (amnionitis). The fetus is surrounded by the infected amniotic fluid and may inhale the fluid into its lungs. Pneumonia results, sometimes with sepsis. Pneumonia can also occur even weeks after birth, most commonly in infants whose breathing is being assisted by a ventilator.

Symptoms

Symptoms present at birth may range from rapid breathing to respiratory failure and extremely low blood pressure (septic shock). When pneumonia occurs after birth, symptoms may begin gradually. If the infant is breathing with the help of a ventilator, the doctor may find that an increased amount of secretions are being suctioned from the breathing tube in the windpipe and that the infant needs increasingly more help in breathing. Sometimes, however, an infant suddenly becomes ill, with fluctuating high and low temperature.

▲ see box, page 374

■ see page 194

Diagnosis and Treatment

A doctor strongly suspects pneumonia if symptoms appear in an infant born after the membranes ruptured prematurely. Samples of blood and fluid from the airways are sent to the laboratory for culturing. The number of white blood cells and platelets is also determined from a blood sample. Chest x-rays may be taken, and sometimes a sample of cerebrospinal fluid is taken by spinal tap (lumbar puncture) and sent for culture.

Pneumonia is treated with antibiotics given intravenously. Treatment is started as quickly as possible. The choice of antibiotic may be changed after the specific type of bacteria responsible for the pneumonia is determined by laboratory tests.

Meningitis

Meningitis is inflammation of the membranes surrounding the brain as a result of a bacterial infection.▲

Meningitis affects 2 of 10,000 normal-weight, full-term newborns and 2 of 1,000 low-birth-weight newborns. Boys are affected more often than girls. In most cases, meningitis in a newborn is a complication of sepsis—the infection in the blood spreads to the brain.

Symptoms and Diagnosis

The symptoms of meningitis include fever or an abnormally low body temperature, difficulty in breathing, jaundice, drowsiness, seizures, vomiting, and irritability. In about 25 percent of the newborns with meningitis, increased pressure of the fluid around the brain may make the fontanelles (the soft spots between the skull bones) bulge or feel firm. In about 15 percent, the infant's neck may be stiff because head movement is painful. The nerves controlling some eye and facial movements may be damaged, causing an eye to turn inward or outward or the facial expression to become lopsided.

Pockets of pus (abscesses) may form within the infant's brain. As the abscesses grow, pressure on the brain increases, resulting in vomiting, head enlargement, and bulging fontanelles. A sudden worsening of these symptoms suggests that an abscess has ruptured into the space around the brain, causing the infection to spread.

A doctor diagnoses bacterial meningitis by examining a sample of cerebrospinal fluid and sending it to the laboratory for culture. The fluid is obtained by spinal tap (lumbar puncture). Ultrasound examination or computed tomography (CT) may be used to determine if an abscess is responsible for the meningitis.

Prognosis and Treatment

High doses of antibiotics are given intravenously to kill the bacteria in the cerebrospinal fluid as quickly as possible. A doctor chooses an antibiotic based on the type of bacteria causing the meningitis, which is determined by laboratory tests.

Even with modern treatment, as many as 30 percent of the infants with bacterial meningitis die. When a brain abscess occurs, the death rate approaches 75 percent. Of the infants who survive, 20 to 50 percent develop brain and nerve damage, such as enlargement of the ventricles (hydrocephalus), deafness, and mental retardation.

Listeriosis

Listeriosis is an infection with Listeria *bacteria,*■ *which may be acquired before or during birth from the mother or after birth in the nursery.*

Although listeriosis may cause a flulike illness or no symptoms at all in the mother, it can be fatal in a fetus or infant. The amniotic fluid may become infected, and premature delivery, stillbirth, and infection in the newborn's bloodstream (sepsis) are common. Symptoms may start within hours or days of birth or may be delayed for several weeks. Listeriosis is treated with antibiotics, such as ampicillin and gentamycin.

To prevent listeriosis in her baby, a pregnant woman should avoid unpasteurized dairy products or raw vegetables that have been exposed to cattle or sheep manure. These products may be contaminated with *Listeria* bacteria.

Congenital Rubella

Congenital rubella is an infection during pregnancy with the virus that causes German measles, possibly resulting in miscarriage, stillbirth, or birth defects.

Rubella is believed to be transmitted by inhaling viral particles from the air or by having close

▲ see page 373

■ see page 862

physical contact with an infected person.▲ The virus then enters the bloodstream and spreads to other parts of the body, including the placenta in a pregnant woman. If infection occurs during the first 16 weeks of pregnancy, particularly the first 8 to 10 weeks, the woman has a 40 to 60 percent chance of having a miscarriage or a baby born with birth defects. Infection in the early weeks may cause heart or eye defects. Infection during the third month carries a 30 to 35 percent risk of birth defects, such as deafness or heart defects. The risk drops to 10 percent during the fourth month.

Women infected during early pregnancy may be given immune globulin, although its effectiveness is uncertain. Rubella vaccination before pregnancy can prevent congenital rubella. All young women who haven't had German measles should be vaccinated; however, they should then wait 3 months before becoming pregnant. Since 1969, when the rubella vaccine became available, the number of babies born with congenital rubella has fallen considerably.

Herpes

Herpes simplex in the newborn is a serious viral infection that affects major organs (brain, liver, lungs), often causing permanent damage or death.

The herpes simplex virus infects one of every 2,500 to 5,000 newborns. The baby may be infected before or after birth. Mothers of newborns with herpes simplex usually aren't aware of having herpes and don't have any symptoms at the time of delivery.■

Symptoms and Diagnosis

Symptoms generally first appear between the first and second week of life but may not appear until the fourth week. The disease may begin with a skin rash of small fluid-filled blisters; however, up to 45 percent of the infected newborns don't have a skin rash. If treatment isn't started, more serious symptoms often begin within 7 to 10 days. Other symptoms may include a fluctuating temperature, drowsiness or convulsions from a brain infection, poor muscle tone, difficulty in breathing, liver inflammation (hepatitis), and widespread blood clotting within the blood vessels.

A doctor easily recognizes the fluid-filled blisters as symptoms of herpes, but other symptoms aren't as specific. Infection is usually confirmed by sending a sample of fluid from the blisters to the laboratory for culture, which takes 24 to 48 hours. Herpes simplex virus can also be identified in urine specimens, samples of secretions from the eyelids or nostrils, blood samples, or cerebrospinal fluid samples.

Prognosis and Treatment

Without treatment, 85 percent of the newborns with widespread disease die. When the disease is confined to the skin, eyes, and mouth, death is uncommon, but about 30 percent of these infants have some brain or nerve damage, which may not be apparent until they reach 2 to 3 years of age.

Treatment with antiviral drugs, such as acyclovir, given intravenously decreases the death rate by 50 percent and greatly increases the number of infants with herpes who will develop normally. Eye infections are also usually treated with trifluridine drops or ointment and idoxuridine ointment.

Hepatitis

Hepatitis is an infection of the liver, nearly always with the hepatitis B virus.★

In the United States, an infected mother is the usual source of hepatitis B infection in a newborn. The baby is infected during delivery, not usually during pregnancy, because the virus doesn't easily cross into the placenta. Infection from the mother after delivery is rare.

Symptoms and Diagnosis

Most newborns infected with the hepatitis B virus develop a chronic liver infection (chronic hepatitis) that usually doesn't produce symptoms until young adulthood. However, the infection is serious; one fourth of those infected eventually die of liver disease. Occasionally, the liver may enlarge in a child, fluid may accumulate in the abdomen (a condition called ascites), and blood levels of bilirubin may be high, leading to jaundice.

▲ see page 1268

■ see page 916

★ see page 571

Prognosis and Treatment

The long-term prognosis is unknown. Being infected with the hepatitis B virus from infancy increases the risk of liver disease, such as chronic active hepatitis, cirrhosis, and liver cancer, later in life.

Pregnant women are routinely tested for hepatitis B virus infection. Because the baby usually isn't infected until delivery, a baby born to an infected mother can be given an injection of hepatitis B immune globulin within 24 hours of delivery, before the infection has become established. This treatment temporarily protects the baby. At the same time, the baby is immunized with hepatitis B vaccine for long-term protection.▲

Breastfeeding doesn't appear to significantly increase the risk of hepatitis B, particularly if the infant received both immune globulin and the vaccine. However, if a mother has cracked nipples or another breast disorder, breastfeeding could possibly transmit the hepatitis B virus.

No treatment is given to newborns with chronic hepatitis without symptoms. Supportive care is given to infants with symptoms of hepatitis.

Cytomegalovirus Infection

Cytomegalovirus infection is a viral disease that can cause brain damage or death in newborns.

Cytomegalovirus can be acquired before birth or at any age after birth. One in every 50 to 500 newborns is infected with cytomegalovirus before birth. The virus is thought to cross through the placenta from the mother. If the mother becomes infected during the first half of pregnancy, infection of the fetus tends to be more severe.

After delivery, a newborn may become infected with cytomegalovirus by being exposed to infected breast milk or to contaminated blood received in a transfusion. Most full-term infants with infected mothers do not develop symptoms, and infants who are breastfed are protected by antibodies they receive in the milk. Premature infants who aren't breastfed and who receive a contaminated blood transfusion can become severely ill

because they don't have antibodies to cytomegalovirus.

Symptoms and Diagnosis

About 10 percent of the infants born with cytomegalovirus infection have symptoms at birth, including low birth weight, premature birth, a small head, jaundice, small bruises, an enlarged liver and spleen, calcium deposits in the brain, and inflammation of the inside of the eyes. Up to 30 percent of these infants die. More than 90 percent of the survivors and 10 percent of those without symptoms at birth later develop nerve and brain abnormalities, including deafness, mental retardation, and abnormal vision. An infant who becomes infected with cytomegalovirus after birth may develop pneumonia, an enlarged and inflamed liver, and an enlarged spleen.

A doctor can usually diagnose cytomegalovirus infection in the mother by performing an antibody test. Many women who become infected with cytomegalovirus during pregnancy have no symptoms, but some women develop an illness resembling infectious mononucleosis.■ In the infant, the diagnosis is usually made by culturing the virus from a sample of urine or blood.

Prevention and Treatment

Since cytomegalovirus infection is common in children who attend day care centers, pregnant women should always wash their hands thoroughly after being exposed to urine and secretions from the noses and mouths of such children. A vaccine against cytomegalovirus is being developed.

Cytomegalovirus infection in an infant can't be cured. Although the antiviral drug ganciclovir is used to treat cytomegalovirus infections in adults, the drug potentially has serious side effects. It is being studied in newborns.

Congenital Toxoplasmosis

Congenital toxoplasmosis is an infection during pregnancy caused by the parasite Toxoplasma gondii, *which passes from the mother to the fetus.*

The *Toxoplasma gondii* organism exists throughout the world ★ and infects 1 to 8 of every 1,000 newborns. About half of the women infected during pregnancy have a baby with congenital toxoplasmosis. The risk that the fetus will be in-

---

▲ see box, page 1200

■ see page 919

★ see page 899

fected is greater if the woman is infected late in pregnancy, but the disease is generally more severe if the fetus is infected early in pregnancy.

Toxoplasma infects cats, and the parasite's eggs are passed in cat feces. The eggs can remain infectious for many months. Women may become infected by contact with cat litter boxes or other material contaminated with cat feces. Eating undercooked meat (mutton, pork, or beef) can also cause infection.

Symptoms and Diagnosis

Pregnant women and newborns who are infected with toxoplasmosis generally don't have any symptoms. However, a fetus may grow slowly in the uterus and be born prematurely. The infant may have a small head; jaundice; an enlarged liver and spleen; inflammation of the heart, lungs, or eyes; rashes; high spinal fluid pressure from increased fluid around the brain or calcium deposits in the brain; and seizures.

Some infants with these symptoms are severely ill and soon die. Others sustain permanent damage, including inflammation of the inside of the eye (chorioretinitis), mental retardation, deafness, and seizures. Such abnormalities may develop years later in children who appeared healthy at birth.

Blood tests are used to diagnose toxoplasmosis in both the mother and infant. In infants, x-rays of the head, analysis of cerebrospinal fluid, and a thorough eye examination are also performed. At birth, the doctor can examine the placenta to see if it is infected.

Prevention and Treatment

Women who are or may be pregnant should avoid contact with cat litter boxes and other areas contaminated with cat feces. Meat should be thoroughly cooked to destroy possible parasites, and hands should be washed after handling raw meat or unwashed produce.

Transmission of the infection to the fetus may be prevented if the mother takes the drug spiramycin. Pyrimethamine and sulfonamides may be taken later in pregnancy if the fetus is infected. Infected newborns with symptoms are treated with pyrimethamine, sulfadiazine, and folinic acid. Infants with inflammation may also be treated with corticosteroids.

Congenital Syphilis

Congenital syphilis is an infectious disease caused by the bacterium Treponema pallidum *transmitted from mother to fetus.*▲

A pregnant woman infected with syphilis has about a 60 to 80 percent chance of infecting her fetus. Early-stage syphilis that hasn't been treated is usually transmitted, but not latent or late-stage syphilis.

Symptoms and Diagnosis

A newborn with syphilis may have large fluid-filled blisters or a flat copper-colored rash on the palms and soles, with raised bumps around the nose and mouth and in the diaper area. Usually, the lymph nodes, liver, and spleen are enlarged. The infant may not grow well and may have a characteristic "old man" look, with cracks around the mouth. Mucus, pus, or blood may run from the nose. A few infants may develop inflammation of the membranes around the brain (meningitis) or of the eye (choroiditis). These infants may develop convulsions, or the pressure within the brain may increase following enlargement of the fluid-filled spaces (hydrocephalus). Other infants may be mentally retarded. Within the first 3 months of life, inflammation of the bones and cartilages may cause what appears to be paralysis of the arms and legs.

Many children with congenital syphilis remain in the latent stage of the disease throughout their lives and never have any symptoms. Others eventually develop symptoms, such as sores (ulcers) inside the nose and on the roof of the mouth. Knoblike bulges (bosses) may appear in the leg bones and skull. Infection of the brain usually produces no symptoms in childhood, but deafness and blindness may occur. The incisor teeth may be pointed (Hutchinson's teeth).

The characteristic symptoms provide a strong clue to the diagnosis. The doctor confirms the diagnosis by examining a sample from the rash, blister, or nasal mucus under the microscope and by ordering antibody tests.

Prevention and Treatment

Congenital syphilis is almost entirely preventable by giving the mother injections of penicillin

---

▲ see page 938

during pregnancy. However, treatment very late in pregnancy may not totally reverse abnormalities that have already occurred in the fetus. After birth, the infected newborn is also treated with penicillin.

Treatment can cause a severe reaction (the Jarisch-Herxheimer reaction) in the mother and can result in a stillbirth. Such a reaction is usually mild in the newborn.

Tuberculosis

Tuberculosis is a persistent infection by Mycobacterium tuberculosis, *which affects many organs, particularly the lungs.*▲

A fetus may acquire tuberculosis from the mother before birth, before or during birth by breathing in or swallowing infected amniotic fluid, or after birth by breathing in air containing infected droplets. About half of the infants born to mothers with active tuberculosis develop the disease during the first year of life if they aren't treated with antibiotics or vaccinated.

Symptoms and Diagnosis

The symptoms of tuberculosis in a newborn include fever, drowsiness, poor feeding, and difficulty in breathing. Many other symptoms are possible, depending on the extent of the infection. The liver and spleen may be enlarged, because these organs filter tuberculosis bacteria, which cause activation of white blood cells there. The infant may grow poorly and not gain weight (failure to thrive).

Skin testing for tuberculosis (the tuberculin test) is routinely performed on pregnant women. A positive reaction to the tuberculin test should be followed by a chest x-ray.

The tuberculin test is often performed on the infants of mothers who test positive. However, some infants have false-negative test results. If tuberculosis is suspected, a sample of cerebrospinal fluid and fluid from the airway and stomach are sent to the laboratory for culture. A chest x-ray usually can show whether the lungs are infected with tuberculosis. A biopsy of the liver, lymph nodes, or lungs and the surrounding

membrane (pleura) may be necessary to confirm the diagnosis.

Prevention and Treatment

If a pregnant woman has a positive skin test result but no symptoms and normal chest x-ray results, the drug isoniazid taken orally is usually the only treatment needed to cure the disease. However, isoniazid treatment is usually delayed until the last 3 months of pregnancy or until after delivery, because the risk of liver damage in the woman is higher during pregnancy.

If a pregnant woman has symptoms of tuberculosis, she is given the antibiotics isoniazid, pyrazinamide, and rifampin. If a resistant strain of tuberculosis is suspected, additional drugs may be given. These don't seem to harm the fetus. An infected mother is kept isolated from her baby until she is no longer contagious. The baby receives isoniazid as a preventive measure.

The baby may be vaccinated with BCG vaccine. Vaccination doesn't necessarily prevent tuberculosis but usually reduces its severity. Because BCG vaccine isn't 100 percent effective, it isn't routinely given to children or adults in the United States. Once a person is vaccinated, he or she will always have a positive test result for tuberculosis, so a new infection couldn't be detected. In many countries with high rates of tuberculosis, however, the BCG vaccine is routinely used.

An infant with tuberculosis is treated with the antibiotics isoniazid, rifampin, and pyrazinamide. If the brain is involved, corticosteroids may be given at the same time.

Acute Infectious Diarrhea

Infectious diarrhea is the frequent passing of loose and unformed stools as the result of an infection.

Infection by bacteria or viruses is by far the most common cause of acute diarrhea in infants, although diarrhea can have a number of causes.■ A baby may be infected if it swallows organisms while passing through a contaminated birth canal or if it's touched by contaminated hands. Other less common sources are infected household articles and contaminated food or bottles. Occasionally, infection may be caused by inhaling organisms floating in the air, especially during viral outbreaks. Overcrowded hospital nurseries are subject to outbreaks of infectious diarrhea. Diar-

---

▲ see page 885

■ see page 1208

rhea is more likely when hygiene is poor or when a poor family lives in crowded conditions. Infectious diarrhea is also quite common in day care centers.

Symptoms and Diagnosis

Infection may cause sudden diarrhea, vomiting, bloody stools, fever, poor appetite, or listlessness. Diarrhea is frequently accompanied by dehydration. Mild dehydration merely makes the infant's mouth dry. Moderate dehydration causes the skin to lose its firmness. The eyes and a fontanelle (the soft spot on top of the head) may be sunken. Severe dehydration, which can develop rapidly, is life threatening, usually causing a considerable fall in blood pressure (shock).

Diarrhea may lead to the loss of fluid and electrolytes, such as sodium and potassium, which may make the infant drowsy or irritable or, more rarely, cause abnormal heart rhythms or bleeding in the brain.

Electrolyte levels and the number of white blood cells, which is high during a bacterial infection, are measured in a blood sample. The doctor tries to identify the organism that is causing the diarrhea by examining a stool sample under a microscope and sending stool samples to a laboratory for culture.

Prevention and Treatment

To help prevent severe gastroenteritis due to rotavirus infection, an oral rotavirus vaccine is available. Replacing fluid and electrolytes lost by diarrhea and vomiting is the first and most important step in treating the infant. If the infant is very ill, fluids are usually given intravenously in the hospital. Otherwise, the infant can drink any of several commercial preparations that contain electrolytes. Very careful hand washing by anyone handling the infant is important to prevent the spread of infection to others.

Breastfeeding is continued to avoid malnutrition and maintain the mother's milk supply. An infant not being breastfed should be offered a lactose-free formula as soon as the dehydration has been corrected. The usual formula can be offered gradually a few days later, but if diarrhea recurs, the lactose-free formula may be substituted for several weeks.

Although acute infectious diarrhea may be caused by bacteria, antibiotics usually aren't needed, because the infection usually clears without treatment. However, some infections are treated with antibiotics to prevent the infection from spreading beyond the intestine. Nevertheless, giving drugs to stop the diarrhea may actually harm the infant because they prevent the body from flushing out the infectious organisms with the stools.

CHAPTER 254

Birth Defects

Birth defects, also called congenital defects, are physical abnormalities that are present at birth.

About 3 to 4 percent of newborns have a major birth defect. Some birth defects may not be discovered until a child grows. A birth defect is diagnosed in about 7.5 percent of all children by age 5, but many of these are minor. That birth defects are fairly common is hardly surprising, considering the complexities involved in developing a single fertilized egg into the millions of specialized cells that constitute a human being.

Many major abnormalities can be diagnosed before birth.▲ Birth defects range from minor to severe, and many can be treated or repaired. Al-

though some can be treated while the fetus is in the uterus, most are treated after delivery or later. Some abnormalities don't need to be treated at all. Still others can't be treated and leave a child severely and permanently impaired.

Causes and Risks

Although the cause of most birth defects is unknown, certain factors are known to increase the risk of birth defects. These include nutritional de-

▲ see page 1129

ficiencies, radiation, certain drugs, alcohol, certain types of infection and other illnesses in the mother, trauma, and hereditary disorders.

Some risks are avoidable; others are not. Even so, one pregnant woman may do everything that is recommended to produce a healthy infant—such as eating a proper diet, getting sufficient rest, and avoiding drugs—yet have an infant with a birth defect. Another woman may do a number of things that can harm a fetus, yet have an infant with no birth defect.

Teratogens

Any factor or substance that can induce or increase the risk of a birth defect is called a teratogen. Radiation and certain drugs and poisons (toxins) are teratogens. Different teratogens may cause similar defects if exposure to the teratogen occurred at a particular time during fetal development. On the other hand, exposure to the same teratogen at different times in the pregnancy may produce different defects. In general, a pregnant woman should consult with her doctor before taking any drug. She should refrain from smoking or consuming alcohol. She should avoid having x-rays taken unless absolutely necessary. If x-rays are necessary, she should immediately inform the radiologist or technician that she is pregnant, so that the fetus can be protected as much as possible.

Infections contracted during pregnancy may also be teratogenic, especially German measles (rubella).▲ A woman who hasn't had German measles should be vaccinated against it before trying to become pregnant. A pregnant woman who has neither had German measles nor been vaccinated against it should avoid contact with anyone who might have German measles.

A pregnant woman who has been exposed to a teratogen may want to be tested to determine whether her fetus has been affected. However, most pregnant women exposed to such risks have babies without abnormalities.

▲ see page 1218

■ see page 1234

★ see page 1231

● see box, page 1132

◆ see page 68

Nutritional Factors

Keeping a fetus healthy requires not only avoiding possible teratogens but also maintaining a nutritious diet. One substance known to be necessary for proper development is folate (folic acid). Insufficient folate in the diet increases the risk that a fetus will develop spina bifida or other neural tube defects. However, because spina bifida can occur in a developing fetus before a woman knows she is pregnant, women of childbearing age should consume at least 400 micrograms of folate a day. Most doctors advise pregnant women to take supplemental vitamins in appropriate amounts in addition to eating a nutritious diet.

Physical Factors in the Uterus

Amniotic fluid surrounds the fetus in the uterus and protects it from injury. An abnormal amount of amniotic fluid may indicate or cause certain birth defects. Too little amniotic fluid can interfere with normal development of the lungs and limbs or may indicate a kidney abnormality that is slowing urine production. Too much amniotic fluid may accumulate if the fetus has difficulty swallowing, which may be caused by a severe brain disorder, such as anencephaly,■ or by esophageal atresia.★

Genetic and Chromosomal Factors

Some birth defects are inherited by receiving abnormal genes from one or both parents. Other birth defects are caused by spontaneous and unexplained changes (mutations) in genes. Still other defects result from a chromosomal abnormality, such as an extra or a missing chromosome. The older a pregnant woman is—particularly if she's over age 35—the greater the chance that the fetus will have a chromosomal abnormality.● Many chromosomal abnormalities can be detected early in pregnancy.

Heart Defects

One in 120 infants is born with a heart defect, many of which are not severe. Birth defects of the heart may involve abnormal formation of its walls or valves or of the blood vessels that enter or leave it. A defect usually causes the blood to flow in an abnormal path, sometimes bypassing the lungs where enrichment with oxygen occurs.◆ Oxygen-rich blood is necessary for normal

Ventricular and Atrial Septal Defects

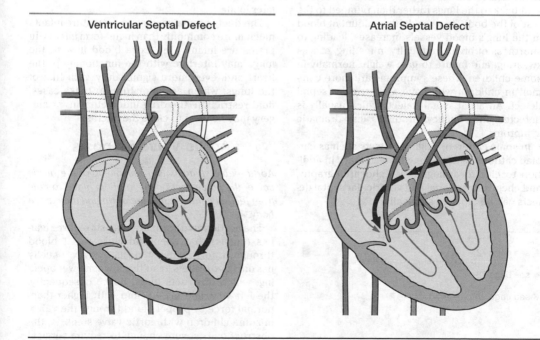

Normal Circulation

Pulmonary artery

Superior vena cava

Right atrium

Right ventricle

Inferior vena cava

Aorta

Pulmonary vein

Left atrium

Left ventricle

Ventricular Septal Defect

Atrial Septal Defect

growth, development, and activity. Some heart defects cause severe problems requiring urgent or emergency treatment, usually surgery.

Diagnosing a heart defect in children involves the same techniques used for adults.▲ In children with a heart defect, the abnormal blood flow usually produces a murmur, an abnormal sound that can be heard through a stethoscope. Electrocardiography (ECG), a chest x-ray, and ultrasound scanning (echocardiography) are usually used to determine the specific nature of the defect. Many heart defects can be corrected surgically. The timing of the operation depends on the specific defect, its symptoms, and its severity.

Atrial and Ventricular Septal Defects

Atrial and ventricular septal defects are holes in the walls (septa) that separate the heart into the left and right sides.

Atrial septal defects occur between the upper chambers of the heart (atria), which receive blood. Ventricular septal defects occur between the lower chambers (ventricles), which pump blood.

In both of these abnormalities, blood returning to the heart from the lungs is short-circuited: It is sent back to the lungs rather than pumped to the rest of the body. As a result, the amount of blood in the lung's blood vessels increases, leading to shortness of breath, difficulty in feeding, excess sweating, and failure to gain weight normally in some children. These symptoms are more common in children who have a ventricular septal defect. An atrial septal defect, which usually is detected after infancy, produces less dramatic symptoms.

In some children, diagnostic tests such as cardiac catheterization■ may be necessary in addition to electrocardiography, echocardiography, and chest x-rays. Atrial and ventricular septal defects can be repaired surgically.

▲ see page 72

■ see page 78

★ see page 97

Patent Ductus Arteriosus

Patent ductus arteriosus is a connection between the aorta (the large artery that carries oxygenated blood to the body) and the pulmonary artery (the artery that carries oxygen-depleted blood to the lungs).

The ductus arteriosus enables blood to bypass the lungs. In the fetus, this function is essential because the fetus doesn't breathe air and thus doesn't need blood to circulate through the lungs to be oxygenated. However, at birth, blood must flow to the lungs to be oxygenated. Normally, the ductus closes very quickly, within a day or two after birth. If the ductus remains open, blood intended for the body may be returned to the lungs, overloading the lung's blood vessels. As a result, some infants develop heart failure, manifested by difficulty in breathing, a fast heart rate, and failure to gain weight.

If the ductus remains open, a full-term infant may develop heart failure at several weeks of age. In such cases, the ductus must be closed surgically. More commonly, the open ductus is detected when the murmur it produces is heard with a stethoscope. In these cases, the ductus is closed in elective surgery when the child is about 1 year of age, primarily to prevent a serious infection later in life.

The ductus remains open in premature infants much more commonly than in full-term infants. In premature infants, the extra blood flow to the lungs may interfere with the functioning of the heart and, even more significantly, with that of the lungs, which are immature. In these cases, fluid restriction, the drug indomethacin, or surgery may be used to close the ductus.

Aortic Valve Stenosis

Aortic valve stenosis is a narrowing of the aortic valve, the valve that opens to allow blood to flow from the left ventricle into the aorta and then to the body. ★

The aortic valve normally consists of three leaflets (cusps) that open and close to let blood through. In aortic valve stenosis, the valve usually has only two leaflets, resulting in a narrower opening, which obstructs blood flow. Consequently, the left ventricle must pump with higher-than-normal force to propel blood through the valve. In some children with aortic valve stenosis, the obstruction is severe enough to require surgical

Patent Ductus Arteriosus

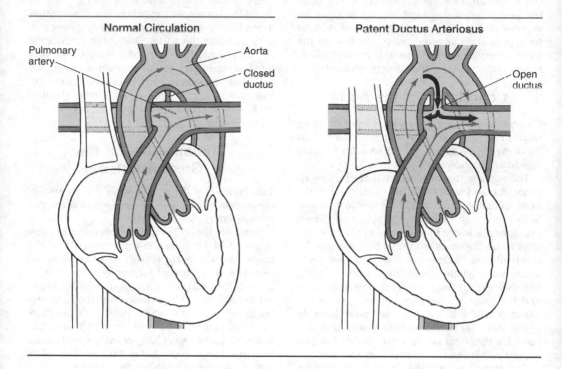

Normal Circulation

Pulmonary artery

Aorta

Closed ductus

Patent Ductus Arteriosus

Open ductus

correction, but such obstruction is more common in adults. In a few infants, heart failure develops, and blood flow to the body is inadequate. Such infants must have emergency treatment, usually including drugs and emergency surgery or a procedure called balloon valvoplasty, in which the valve is stretched and torn with a balloon-tipped tube (catheter). In older children and young adults, the valve may have to be opened surgically or replaced with an artificial one, although other procedures are possible for some patients.

Pulmonary Valve Stenosis

Pulmonary valve stenosis is a narrowing of the pulmonary valve, the valve that opens to allow blood to flow from the right ventricle to the lungs.

In newborns, pulmonary valve stenosis may range in severity from so mild that it requires no treatment to so severe that it is life threatening.

In most children with pulmonary valve stenosis, the valve is mildly to moderately narrowed, making the right ventricle pump harder and at a higher pressure to propel blood through the valve. If the disorder is moderately severe, as confirmed by physical examination, electrocardiography, echocardiography, and occasionally cardiac catheterization, the valve may be opened with a balloon-tipped plastic tube inserted through a vein in the leg. If the valve is not well formed, a surgical procedure to reconstruct the valve may be needed.

When the obstruction is much more severe, very little blood flows to the lungs to be oxygenated. Instead, the pressure in the right ventricle and atrium increases, forcing oxygen-depleted blood, which is blue, through the wall between the right and left atria. The blood then passes into the left ventricle and is pumped into the aorta, which carries it to the body. As a result, the infant appears blue—a condition called cyanosis. When this happens, a prostaglandin drug such as alprostadil is given to keep the ductus arteriosus open until a surgeon can create a connection between the aorta and the pulmonary artery, open the pulmonary valve surgically, or in some instances, do both. These procedures enable blood to bypass the narrowed valve and flow to the lungs for oxygenation. For some of these children, surgery must be repeated when they're older.

Coarctation of the Aorta

Coarctation of the aorta is a narrowing of the aorta, usually at a point where the ductus arteriosus joins the aorta and the aorta turns to descend to the lower chest and the abdomen.

The aorta is the large artery that carries oxygenated blood from the heart to all parts of the body. Coarctation reduces blood flow to the lower half of the body; therefore, the pulses and blood pressure are lower than normal in the legs and tend to be higher than normal in the arms. For most infants, coarctation doesn't cause problems. Some children have headaches or nosebleeds because of high blood pressure in the arms and leg pains during exercise because of low blood pressure in the legs, but most have no symptoms. Most children with coarctation also have an abnormal aortic valve, which has two leaflets rather than the normal three leaflets.

Coarctation is detected during a physical examination because of changes in the pulse and blood pressure, and the diagnosis is confirmed by x-rays, electrocardiography, and echocardiography. This defect should be surgically repaired in early childhood to decrease the workload of the left ventricle, which must pump harder than normal to propel blood into the narrowed aorta, and to prevent problems, such as high blood pressure, later in life. The operation is usually performed when the child is of preschool age (generally 3 to 5 years old).

At a few days to about 2 weeks of age, a few infants with coarctation develop severe heart failure after the ductus arteriosus closes. They develop severe respiratory distress and become extremely pale; blood tests show a marked increase in acid in the blood (metabolic acidosis).▲ This

situation is life threatening and requires immediate medical attention to make the correct diagnosis and begin appropriate treatment. Treatment includes a prostaglandin drug such as alprostadil to reopen the ductus arteriosus, other drugs to support the heart, and emergency surgery to repair the aorta. This surgery may save the life of a newborn; for some children, surgery must be repeated when they're older. Commonly associated problems, such as an aortic valve with two leaflets, aortic stenosis, an abnormal mitral valve, or a ventricular septal defect, may also require treatment.

Transposition of the Great Arteries

Transposition of the great arteries is a reversal of the normal connections of the aorta and the pulmonary artery with the heart.

Normally, the pulmonary artery carries oxygen-depleted blood from the right ventricle to the lungs, and the aorta carries oxygenated blood from the left ventricle to the body. With transposition of the great arteries, oxygen-depleted blood returning from the body flows from the right ventricle to the aorta, which carries the oxygen-depleted blood back to the body, bypassing the lungs. The infant has plenty of oxygenated blood, but this blood recirculates through the lungs rather than traveling to the rest of the body.

Infants with this defect can survive briefly after birth because of a small opening between the right and left atria (foramen ovale) that's normally present at birth. This opening allows a small amount of oxygenated blood from the lungs to cross from the left atrium to the right atrium, then to the right ventricle and aorta, thus supplying enough oxygen to the body to keep the infant alive.

The diagnosis is usually made immediately after birth by physical examination, x-ray, electrocardiography, and echocardiography. Usually, a surgical procedure is performed within the first few days of life. The procedure consists of attaching the aorta and pulmonary artery to the appropriate ventricles and reimplanting the coronary arteries, which supply the heart itself, in the aorta after it has been repositioned. Before surgery, some infants may need to be given a prostaglandin such as alprostadil to keep the ductus arteriosus open. Some may need to have the opening between the atria enlarged with a balloon-tipped

---

▲ see page 676

catheter, allowing more oxygenated blood to reach the aorta.

Underdeveloped Left Ventricle Syndrome

This condition is also called the hypoplastic left heart syndrome. The primary job of the left ventricle is to pump blood to the body. When the left heart chambers and valves are severely underdeveloped or absent, normal blood flow to the body can't be maintained. At birth, the infant appears normal because blood can flow from the right ventricle through the open ductus arteriosus▲ to the body, but when the ductus closes, severe heart failure develops. Most infants who have this condition die.

Tetralogy of Fallot

Tetralogy of Fallot is a combination of heart defects consisting of a large ventricular septal defect, displacement of the aorta that allows oxygen-depleted blood to flow directly from the right ventricle to the aorta, a narrowing of the outflow passage from the right side of the heart, and a thickening of the wall of the right ventricle.

Infants with tetralogy of Fallot usually have a heart murmur heard at birth or very shortly thereafter. They appear blue (a condition called cyanosis) because the blood circulating through the body is not sufficiently oxygenated. This happens because the narrowed passage from the right ventricle restricts blood flow to the lungs, and the oxygen-depleted, blue blood in the right ventricle passes through the septal defect to the left ventricle and into the aorta to be circulated throughout the body. Some infants remain stable with a mild degree of cyanosis, so surgery to repair the defects can be performed later in infancy. Others develop more severe symptoms, interfering with normal growth and development. Such an infant may have attacks, or spells, in which cyanosis suddenly worsens in response to activity, such as crying or having a bowel movement. The infant becomes very blue, is very short of breath, and may lose consciousness. When an infant has a spell, he may be given oxygen and morphine; propranolol may then be used temporarily to prevent other attacks. However, such an infant needs an operation, either to repair the tetralogy or to make a temporary artificial connection between the aorta and pulmonary artery to increase

Tetralogy of Fallot

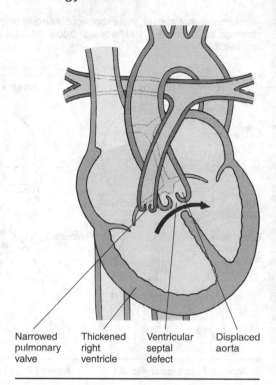

| Narrowed pulmonary valve | Thickened right ventricle | Ventricular septal defect | Displaced aorta |

the amount of blood going to the lungs for oxygenation.

Surgical repair of the problem consists of patching the ventricular septal defect, opening the narrowed passageway from the right ventricle and the narrowed pulmonary valve, and closing any artificial connection made between the aorta and pulmonary artery.

Gastrointestinal Defects

A birth defect can occur anywhere along the length of the gastrointestinal tract—in the esophagus, stomach, small intestine, large intestine, rectum, or anus. In most cases, the defect in-

▲ see box, page 1227

Esophageal Atresia and Fistula

In esophageal atresia, the esophagus narrows or comes to a blind end; it doesn't connect with the stomach as it should. A tracheoesophageal fistula is an abnormal connection between the esophagus and the trachea.

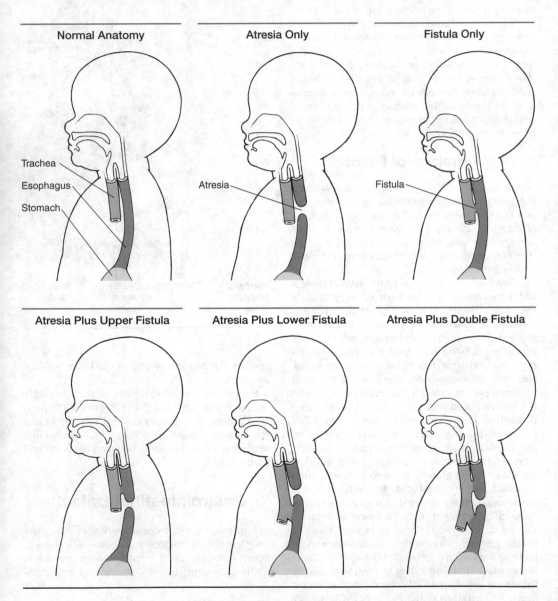

Normal Anatomy

Trachea
Esophagus
Stomach

Atresia Only

Atresia

Fistula Only

Fistula

Atresia Plus Upper Fistula

Atresia Plus Lower Fistula

Atresia Plus Double Fistula

volves incomplete development of an organ, which often causes an obstruction. Generally, gastrointestinal defects must be surgically corrected.

Esophageal Atresia

Esophageal atresia is incomplete development of the esophagus.

In esophageal atresia, the esophagus narrows or comes to a blind end; it doesn't connect with the stomach as it should. Most newborns with esophageal atresia also have a **tracheoesophageal fistula,** an abnormal connection between the esophagus and the trachea.

Characteristically, a newborn with esophageal atresia has excessive saliva, coughs after attempting to swallow, and has cyanosis (a bluish coloration of the skin). The tracheoesophageal fistula allows saliva to enter the lungs when the infant swallows. This puts him at risk for aspiration pneumonia.

When the infant's condition is stable, surgery is performed to repair the esophageal atresia and close the tracheoesophageal fistula. Before correcting the problem surgically, a doctor tries to prevent aspiration pneumonia by withholding oral feedings and placing a continuous suction catheter in the upper esophagus to suction out saliva before it can reach the lungs. The infant is fed intravenously.

Diaphragmatic Hernia

A diaphragmatic hernia is a defect in the diaphragm that allows some of the abdominal organs to protrude into the chest.

A diaphragmatic hernia usually occurs on one side of the body, more often the left side. The stomach, loops of intestine, and even the liver and spleen can protrude through the hernia. If the hernia is large, the lung on the affected side is usually incompletely developed.

After delivery, as the newborn cries and breathes, the loops of intestine quickly fill with air. This rapidly enlarging mass pushes against the heart, compressing the other lung and causing respiratory distress. In severe cases, respiratory distress occurs immediately.

When this defect is diagnosed before birth by ultrasound scanning, the infant is intubated with a breathing tube at birth. Surgery is required to repair the diaphragm.

Hirschsprung's Disease

In Hirschsprung's disease (congenital megacolon), a section of the large intestine is missing the nerve network that controls the intestine's rhythmic contractions.

The large intestine depends on a network of nerves within its wall to synchronize rhythmic contractions and move food along. Without the nerves, the intestine can't contract normally. Fecal matter backs up, resulting in severe constipation and sometimes vomiting.

Severe Hirschsprung's disease must be treated quickly to prevent a potentially fatal complication, toxic enterocolitis, in which severe diarrhea develops. The surgical procedure entails connecting the lower end of the normal part of the intestine to an opening made in the abdominal wall (colostomy). Feces can thus pass through the opening into a collection bag, restoring normal gastrointestinal function. The abnormal section of intestine is left disconnected from the rest of the intestine. When the child is older, the abnormal section of intestine is removed and the normal intestine is connected to the rectum and anus.

Omphalocele

An omphalocele is a defect in the central abdominal wall from which the abdominal organs protrude.

Variable amounts of intestine and other abdominal organs may protrude through an omphalocele, depending on the size of the defect. To prevent injury to the intestine and an infection in the abdomen, a doctor repairs the defect as quickly as possible.

Anal Atresia

Anal atresia is incomplete development of the anus.

A doctor is likely to discover anal atresia during the initial physical examination of the newborn, because the defect is usually obvious. If the diagnosis is missed during routine examination, the defect can usually be detected after the newborn is fed, because signs of intestinal obstruction soon develop.

Most infants with anal atresia develop some type of abnormal connection (fistula) between the anal pouch and either the urethra, perineum, or bladder. Using x-rays, a radiologist can diag-

Facial Abnormalities: Cleft Lip and Cleft Palate

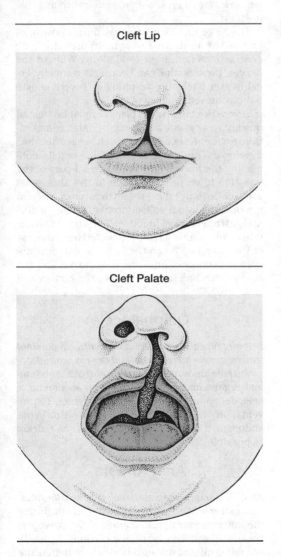

Cleft Lip

Cleft Palate

nose the type of fistula. This information is used to determine the best way to surgically correct the defect.

▲ see page 569

Biliary Atresia

Biliary atresia is a condition in which the bile ducts either failed to develop or developed abnormally.

Bile, a fluid secreted by the liver, carries away the liver's waste products and also helps break down fats in the small intestine. Bile ducts within the liver collect the bile and carry it to the intestine. In biliary atresia, the bile ducts develop only partially or not at all. As a result, the bile can't reach the intestine and instead accumulates inside the liver. Eventually, the accumulated bile escapes into the blood, causing jaundice.

Symptoms and Diagnosis

In infants with biliary atresia, the urine becomes progressively dark, the stools are pale, and the skin becomes increasingly jaundiced. These symptoms and an enlarged liver are usually first noticed about 2 weeks after birth. By the time the infant is 2 to 3 months old, he may have stunted growth, be itchy and irritable, and have high blood pressure in the portal vein (the large blood vessel that carries blood from the stomach, intestine, and spleen to the liver).

To make the diagnosis, a doctor performs a series of blood tests. Ultrasound scans may be helpful. If the diagnosis is still uncertain, an exploratory operation of the abdomen called a laparotomy is performed, usually before the infant is 2 months old. Time is critical because progressive, irreversible scarring of the liver, called biliary cirrhosis, can occur.▲

Treatment

Surgery is needed to relieve the pressure of bile within the liver. Constructing replacement bile ducts that flow into the intestine is the best procedure, but this kind of operation is possible in only 5 to 10 percent of infants with biliary atresia. The prognosis is good for these children, and most of them go on to lead normal lives. The prognosis following various other surgical procedures is not as good, and the infants usually die eventually. One such procedure involves repositioning the liver so that its surface directly touches the intestine, which allows bile to ooze from the liver surface into the intestine despite the lack of bile ducts.

Bone and Muscle Defects

Birth defects can affect any bone or muscle, although the bones and muscles of the skull, face, spine, hips, legs, and feet are most commonly affected. Most of these defects are repaired surgically.

Facial Abnormalities

The most common defects of the skull and face are cleft lip and cleft palate. **Cleft lip** is an incomplete joining of the upper lip, usually just below the nose. **Cleft palate** is an abnormal passageway through the roof of the mouth into the airway of the nose.

Cleft lip is disfiguring and prevents the infant from closing his lips around a nipple. A cleft palate interferes with eating and speech. Cleft lip and cleft palate usually occur together, affecting about 1 in every 600 to 700 births. Cleft lip alone occurs in about 1 in every 1,000 births. Cleft palate alone occurs in about 1 in every 1,800 births.

A dental device can temporarily seal the roof of the mouth so the infant can suckle better. Cleft lip and cleft palate can be permanently corrected with surgery.

Another type of facial defect is a small lower jaw (mandible). If the lower jaw is too small, as occurs in both Pierre Robin syndrome and Treacher Collins' syndrome, the infant may have difficulty eating. Surgery may correct the problem.

Spinal Abnormalities

Congenital torticollis is a condition in which a newborn's neck is twisted to one side and the head is tilted unnaturally toward that side. Usually, injury to the neck muscles during birth is the cause. Other causes include a joining together of the neck vertebrae (Klippel-Feil syndrome) or a joining of the first neck vertebra to the skull (atlanto-occipital fusion).

Congenital scoliosis is an abnormal curvature of the spine in a newborn. Congenital scoliosis is rare; scoliosis usually occurs in older children.▲ Because scoliosis can lead to serious deformity as the child grows, treatment with braces is often started early. Surgery may be needed if the abnormal curvature worsens.

Common Types of Clubfoot

Talipes Varus

Talipes Valgus

Talipes Equinus

Talipes Calcaneus

Hip, Leg, and Foot Abnormalities

Congenital dislocation of the hip is a condition in which a newborn's hip socket and the thighbone (femoral head) that connects to it are separated. The cause of this defect is unknown. Dislocation of the hip is more common in girls, in infants born in a breech (buttocks-first) position, and in infants who have close relatives with the disorder. An ultrasound examination is used to confirm the diagnosis. Putting double or triple diapers on the infant is often sufficient to correct the dislocation. Otherwise, splints or orthopedic surgery may be required.

Femoral torsion is a condition in which the knees point toward (anteversion) or away (retroversion) from each other rather than forward. Femoral torsion often corrects itself when the infant is older and is able to stand and walk.

▲ see page 1300

Knee dislocation is a condition in which the lower leg bends forward at the knee. Dislocation of the knee is rare in newborns, but it must be treated immediately. Gently bending the infant's knee backward and forward into the normal position several times each day and keeping the knee bent with a splint for the rest of the day may help.

Clubfoot (talipes) is a condition in which the foot is twisted out of shape or position. The arch of the foot may be very high, or the foot may be turned inward or outward. True clubfoot is caused by anatomic abnormalities. Sometimes the feet appear abnormal because of the fetus' position in the uterus, but the condition is not a true clubfoot. If no anatomic abnormality is present, the defect can be corrected by casting and physical therapy. Early treatment with casting is beneficial for true clubfoot, but surgery is generally needed.

Missing Limbs

Missing limb (congenital amputation) is a condition in which an arm or a leg or parts of an arm or a leg are missing at birth.

The cause is often unknown. The drug thalidomide, which was taken by some pregnant women in the late 1950s and early 1960s for morning sickness, was removed from the market after being identified as a cause of this type of defect. Thalidomide caused flipperlike appendages to develop in place of arms and legs. Children often become very adept at using a malformed limb, and a prosthesis can often be constructed to make the limb more functional.

Osteogenesis Imperfecta

Osteogenesis imperfecta is a disorder in which the bones are abnormally fragile.

In osteogenesis imperfecta, the bones break so easily that infants with the condition are usually born with many broken bones. During birth, head trauma and bleeding in the brain may occur because the skull is so soft; these children can die suddenly within days or weeks after birth. Most children survive, but the multiple fractures often

cause deformities and dwarfism. Intelligence is normal if the child's brain isn't injured.

Arthrogryposis Multiplex Congenita

Arthrogryposis multiplex congenita is a disorder in which one or more joints become fused together and consequently can't bend.

The cause is unknown. Sometimes the condition is associated with dislocations of the hips, knees, or elbows. Daily physical therapy, in which the stiff joints are carefully manipulated, can improve joint movements.

Muscle Abnormalities

The pectoralis major muscle in the chest may be formed only partially or not at all. Such a defect may be an isolated phenomenon or associated with abnormalities of the hand.

Another muscle defect, called **prune-belly syndrome,** involves the muscles in the abdomen. One or more layers of abdominal muscles may be missing, causing the infant's abdomen to bulge outward. The disorder is associated with severe kidney and urinary abnormalities. The prognosis is best for children whose kidneys function normally.

Brain and Spinal Cord Defects

The brain and spinal cord may develop defects while they are being formed or after they are fully developed. Many brain and spinal cord defects can be detected before birth by ultrasound examination and by tests of amniotic fluid.▲

Brain Defects

Anencephaly is a condition in which most of the infant's brain is missing because it doesn't develop. An infant with anencephaly can't survive and either is stillborn or dies within a few days.

Microcephaly is a condition in which the head is very small. Infants with microcephaly often survive but tend to be mentally retarded and lack muscle coordination. Some also have seizures.

Encephalocele is a condition in which brain tissue bulges through a defect in the skull. Surgery can repair the defect. The prognosis is often good.

▲ see page 1133

Spina Bifida

Spina bifida can vary in severity. In the least severe type, which is also the most common, one or more vertebrae do not form normally, but the spinal cord and the layers of tissue (meninges) surrounding it do not protrude. A tuft of hair, a dimpling, or a pigmented area may be seen over the defect. In a meningocele, a more severe type of spina bifida, the meninges protrude through the incompletely formed vertebrae, resulting in a fluid-filled bulge under the skin. The most severe type is a myelocele, in which the spinal cord protrudes; the affected area appears raw and red, and the infant is likely to be severely handicapped.

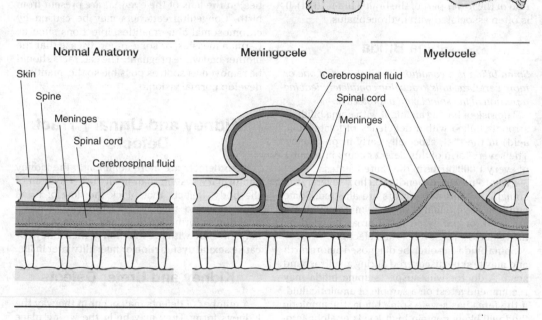

Normal Anatomy	Meningocele	Myelocele

Normal Anatomy: Skin, Spine, Meninges, Spinal cord, Cerebrospinal fluid

Myelocele: Cerebrospinal fluid, Spinal cord, Meninges

Porencephaly is a condition in which an abnormal cyst or cavity exists in a cerebral hemisphere. Porencephaly is evidence of brain damage and is usually associated with abnormalities of brain function. However, some children have normal intelligence.

Hydranencephaly is an extreme form of porencephaly in which the cerebral hemispheres are almost totally missing. Children with hydranencephaly don't develop normally and are severely retarded.

Hydrocephalus (water on the brain) is an enlargement of the ventricles, which are normal spaces in the brain. Cerebrospinal fluid is produced in the ventricles and must drain to the outside of the brain, where it is absorbed into the blood. When the fluid can't drain, pressure inside the brain rises and hydrocephalus occurs. Many things, such as a congenital malformation or bleeding within the brain, can obstruct drainage and cause hydrocephalus. In older children, it is often caused by tumors. Hydrocephalus is the most common reason that a newborn may have an abnormally large head.

Treatment entails providing an alternate drainage path to keep pressure within the brain normal. Drug treatment—with acetazolamide and glycerol—or repeated spinal taps (lumbar punctures) may temporarily reduce the pressure within the brain in some children until a permanent drain (shunt) is inserted. The shunt is placed in the ventricles in the brain and runs under the skin from the head to the abdominal cavity or occasionally to some other site. The shunt contains a valve that allows fluid to leave the brain if the pressure becomes too high. Although some children may eventually be able to do without the shunt as they get older, shunts are rarely removed. The prognosis depends on the cause. Some children can do very well and have normal intelligence. Others may be mentally retarded.

Arnold-Chiari deformity is a defect in the formation of the lower part of the brain (brain stem). It is often associated with hydrocephalus.

Spina Bifida

Spina bifida is a condition in which part of one or more vertebrae fails to develop completely, leaving a portion of the spinal cord unprotected.

The risk of having an infant with spina bifida is strongly linked with a deficiency of folate (folic acid) in the diet, especially early in pregnancy. The severe form of this defect occurs in about 1 of every 1,000 births in the United States.

Symptoms vary depending on how severely the spinal cord and nerve roots are affected. Some children have minimal or no symptoms; others are weak or paralyzed in all areas reached by nerves below the level of the defect.▲

Spina bifida can often be diagnosed before birth and may first be discovered during an ultrasound scan. A doctor who suspects spina bifida may recommend a test on a sample of amniotic fluid. If the fetus has severe spina bifida, the amniotic fluid will likely contain high levels of alpha-fetoprotein.

A child who is born with severe spina bifida needs prolonged, intensive therapy to prevent deterioration in kidney function and physical abilities and to allow for the maximum development possible. Surgery is needed to close the opening and often to treat the associated hydrocephalus, bladder and kidney abnormalities, and physical

deformities. Physical therapy keeps joints mobile and strengthens functioning muscles.

Eye Defects

Congenital glaucoma is a rare eye condition that raises the pressure within the eyeball, usually in both eyes. If the condition isn't treated, the eyeballs enlarge and complete blindness is almost certain. Surgery performed soon after birth gives the best chance of relieving the pressure inside the eye and of preserving the infant's vision.

Congenital cataracts are cloudy areas (opacities) in the lens of the eye that are present from birth. Congenital cataracts may be caused by chromosomal abnormalities, infections such as German measles, or some other disease that the mother had while pregnant. The cataracts should be removed as soon as possible so the infant can develop normal vision.■

Kidney and Urinary Tract Defects

Birth defects are more common in the kidney and urinary system than in any other system of the body. Defects that block the flow of urine cause urine to stagnate, and this can result in infection or formation of kidney stones. A defect may interfere with the function of the kidneys or cause sexual dysfunction or infertility later in life.

Kidney and Ureter Defects

A number of defects may occur in the way the kidneys form. They may be in the wrong place (ectopia), in the wrong position (malrotation), joined together (horseshoe kidney), or missing (kidney agenesis). An infant can't survive when both kidneys are missing (Potter's syndrome). Kidney tissue may also develop abnormally. For instance, a kidney may contain many cysts, as in polycystic kidney disease.★

Possible abnormalities of the ureters, the two tubes that connect the kidneys to the bladder, include extra ureters, misplaced ureters, and narrowed or widened ureters. Urine may flow back from the bladder into the abnormal ureters, making infection in the kidneys (pyelonephritis) more likely. A narrowed ureter prevents urine from passing normally from the kidney to the bladder

---

▲ see box, page 324

■ see page 1043

★ see page 618

and may cause the kidney to become enlarged (hydronephrosis) and lead to kidney damage.

Bladder Defects

A number of defects can affect the bladder. The bladder may not form completely, so that it opens out onto the surface of the abdomen (exstrophy). The wall of the bladder may be abnormal, with outpouchings (diverticula) that allow urine to stagnate and increase the risk of urinary infection. The bladder outlet (the passageway from the bladder to the urethra, which carries urine out of the body) may be narrowed, causing the bladder to empty incompletely. In this case, the urine stream is weak and infections may develop. Most bladder defects can be surgically repaired.

Urethra Defects

The urethra may be abnormal or missing altogether. In boys, the opening of the urethra may be in the wrong place, such as on the underside of the penis (a condition called **hypospadias**). The urethra in the penis may lie open as a channel rather than closed as a tube (a condition called **epispadias**). In both boys and girls, a narrowed urethra may obstruct the flow of urine. Surgery can correct these abnormalities.

Intersex States

An intersex state occurs when a child is born with genitals that aren't obviously male or female (ambiguous genitals).

A child born with genitals that aren't clearly male or female may have normal or abnormal internal reproductive organs (gonads). **True hermaphrodites** have both ovarian and testicular tissue and both male and female internal reproductive organs, but this condition is rare. Most children with ambiguous genitals are **pseudohermaphrodites**—that is, they have ambiguous external genital organs but either ovarian or testicular tissue (not both).

A female pseudohermaphrodite is a genetically normal female (with two X chromosomes) who is born with genitals that resemble a small penis. The internal reproductive organs, however, are female. Female pseudohermaphroditism is caused by exposure to high levels of male hormones before birth. Usually, the fetus has en-

larged adrenal glands (adrenogenital syndrome) that overproduce male hormones, or an enzyme may be missing, so that male hormones can't be converted to female hormones as they normally are. Sometimes, male hormones have entered the placenta from the mother's blood; for example, the mother may have been given progesterone to prevent a miscarriage, or she may have had a hormone-producing tumor.

A male pseudohermaphrodite is a genetically normal male (with one X and one Y chromosome) who is born without a penis or with a very small one. His body fails to produce sufficient male hormones or resists the hormones it does produce (androgen resistance syndrome).

Correctly identifying the child's sex is very important and must be done quickly. Otherwise, bonding by the parents to the child may be made more difficult and the child may develop a gender identity disorder.▲ Surgery to correct the ambiguous genitals can be performed later, usually close to puberty.

Chromosomal Abnormalities

A person normally has 23 pairs of chromosomes. A chromosomal abnormality can affect the number of chromosomes, the size or appearance of certain chromosomes, or the arrangement of parts of chromosomes (genetic material from one chromosome may be attached to another).

Chromosomal analysis may be recommended in a fetus or newborn under the following circumstances:
- A woman over age 35 becomes pregnant
- A fetus has an anatomic abnormality detected by ultrasound
- A newborn has many birth defects or has both male and female genitals

Down Syndrome

Down syndrome (trisomy 21, mongolism) is a chromosomal disorder that results in mental retardation and physical abnormalities

An extra chromosome, making three of a kind, is called trisomy. The most common trisomy in a

▲ see page 418

newborn is trisomy 21, although other trisomies can also occur.

Trisomy 21 is responsible for about 95 percent of the cases of Down syndrome. Other chromosomal abnormalities account for the rest. Down syndrome occurs in 1 of 700 newborns, but the risk varies a great deal with the mother's age.▲ More than 20 percent of the infants with Down syndrome are born to mothers over age 35, yet older mothers bear only 7 to 8 percent of all children. The extra chromosome 21 comes from the father rather than from the mother in one fourth to one third of the cases.

Symptoms

In Down syndrome, both physical and mental development is delayed. Infants with Down syndrome tend to be quiet, rarely cry, and have somewhat floppy muscles. The average intelligence quotient (IQ) in a child with Down syndrome is about 50, compared with a normal average IQ of 100. However, some children with Down syndrome have an IQ above 50.

A child with Down syndrome has a small head. The face is broad and flat, with slanting eyes and a short nose. The tongue is large and often prominent. The ears are small and low set. The hands are short and broad, with a single crease across the palm. The fingers are short; the fifth finger, which often has two instead of three sections, curves inward. A space is visible between the first and second toes. About 35 percent of the children with Down syndrome have heart defects.

Diagnosis

The diagnosis of Down syndrome can often be made before birth, and screening is generally recommended for pregnant women over age 35. Low levels of alpha-fetoprotein in the mother's blood indicate an increased risk of Down syndrome in the fetus; a sample of amniotic fluid can then be taken by amniocentesis for analysis to confirm the diagnosis.■ Using ultrasound scanning, a doctor can often identify physical abnormalities in the fetus.

After birth, an infant with Down syndrome has a physical appearance that suggests the diagno-

sis. A doctor confirms the diagnosis by testing the infant's blood for trisomy 21.

Prognosis

Children with Down syndrome have an increased risk of heart disease and leukemia. Their life expectancy is reduced if these disorders are present; if they are not, most children with Down syndrome survive to adulthood. Many people with Down syndrome develop thyroid problems, which may be difficult to detect unless blood tests are performed. They are prone to hearing problems because of recurrent ear infections and the associated accumulation of inner ear fluid (serous otitis), as well as vision problems because of changes in their corneas and lenses. Both hearing and vision problems can be treated. Many people with Down syndrome develop symptoms of dementia in their 30s, such as memory loss, further lowering of intellect, and personality changes. Death can occur early, but some people with Down syndrome live long lives.

Deletion Syndromes

In some infants, part of a chromosome may be missing. The rare **cri du chat syndrome** (cat's cry syndrome, 5p– syndrome) is an example. Infants with this syndrome have a high-pitched cry that closely resembles the crying of a kitten. The cry is heard immediately after birth, lasts several weeks, and then disappears. An infant with this syndrome is usually underweight at birth and has a small head with an asymmetric face and a mouth that can't close properly. Some infants have a round (moon) face with wide-set eyes. The nose may be wide and the ears low set and abnormally shaped. The neck may be short. Extra skin may be stretched between the fingers (webbed fingers). Heart defects are common. Often the infant seems limp. Mental and physical development is greatly retarded. Despite these abnormalities, many children with cri du chat syndrome survive to adulthood.

Another deletion syndrome, called the **4p– syndrome,** is similar but extremely rare. Mental retardation is profound. A number of physical defects may occur. Many children who have this syndrome die during infancy; the relatively few who

▲ see box, page 1132

■ see page 1134

Trisomy Disorders

Disorder	Incidence	Abnormality	Description	Prognosis
Trisomy 21 (Down syndrome)	1 in 700 births	Extra chromosome 21	Physical and mental development is delayed; many physical abnormalities are present	Generally, affected people live until their 30s or 40s
Trisomy 18 (Edwards' syndrome)	1 in 3,000 births	Extra chromosome 18	Facial abnormalities combine to give the face a pinched appearance. The head is small and the ears are malformed and low set. Other possible defects include cleft lip or cleft palate, missing thumbs, clubfeet, webbed hands, heart defects, and genitourinary defects	Survival for more than a few months is rare; mental retardation is severe
Trisomy 13 (Patau's syndrome)	1 in 5,000 births	Extra chromosome 13	Severe brain and eye defects are common. Other defects may include cleft lip or cleft palate, heart defects, genitourinary defects, and malformed ears	Fewer than 20% survive beyond 1 year of age; mental retardation is severe

survive into their 20s are severely handicapped and are at increased risk of developing infections and epilepsy.

Turner's Syndrome

Turner's syndrome (gonadal dysgenesis) is a condition affecting girls in which one of the two X chromosomes is partially or completely missing.

Turner's syndrome occurs in about 1 in 3,000 female newborns. Many newborns with Turner's syndrome have swelling (lymphedema) on the backs of their hands and tops of their feet. Swelling or loose folds of skin are often evident over the back of the neck.

A girl or woman with Turner's syndrome is short, has a webbed neck (wide skin attachment between her neck and shoulders), and has a low hairline at the back of her neck. She has drooping eyelids, a wide chest with broad-spaced nipples, and many dark moles on her skin. The fourth fingers and toes are short, and the nails are poorly developed. She has no menstrual periods (amenorrhea), and the breasts, vagina, and labia remain immature. The ovaries usually don't contain developing eggs. The lower part of the aorta may be narrowed (coarctation of the aorta), a condition that can cause high blood pressure.▲

Kidney defects and small swellings of blood vessels (hemangiomas) are common. Occasionally, abnormal blood vessels in the intestine cause bleeding. Many girls with Turner's syndrome have difficulty in assessing spatial relationships. They tend to score poorly on certain performance tests and in mathematics, even if they achieve average or above-average scores on verbal intelligence tests. Mental retardation occurs in rare cases.

Triple X Syndrome

Girls who have three X chromosomes have triple X syndrome. About 1 of every 1,000 apparently normal female infants has this disorder. Girls with

▲ see page 1228

three X chromosomes tend to have lower intelligence than their normal brothers and sisters. Sometimes the syndrome causes sterility, although some women with triple X syndrome have given birth to children who had normal chromosomes and who were physically normal.

Rare cases of infants with four or even five X chromosomes have been identified. The risk of mental retardation and physical abnormalities increases with the number of extra X chromosomes, especially with four or more.

Klinefelter's Syndrome

In Klinefelter's syndrome, male infants are born with an extra X chromosome. This relatively common chromosomal abnormality (XXY) affects about 1 in 700 newborn boys.

Although their physical characteristics can vary greatly, most boys with Klinefelter's syndrome are tall but otherwise normal in appearance. They have normal intelligence, but many have speech and reading disabilities. They usually benefit from speech and language therapy and eventually can do well in school. Puberty usually occurs at the normal time, but the testes remain small. Affected boys are usually sterile. Growth of facial hair is often sparse, and the breasts may enlarge somewhat. Some men benefit by taking supplemental male hormones, which improve bone density and help develop a more masculine appearance.

XYY Syndrome

In the XYY syndrome, a male infant is born with an extra Y chromosome. Boys with this chromosomal abnormality tend to be tall and to have difficulties with language. The XYY syndrome was once thought to cause aggressive or violent criminal behavior, but this theory has been disproved.

Fragile X Syndrome

Mental retardation▲ affects boys more often than girls, in part because the X chromosome can have recessive genes for mental retardation (X-linked genes), which in girls is usually balanced by a normal gene on the other X chromosome. One disorder in which such recessive genes exist is called fragile X syndrome. In the fragile X syndrome, the most commonly diagnosed cause of mental retardation after Down syndrome, the X chromosome is abnormal.

The symptoms of fragile X syndrome include mental retardation; large, protuberant ears; a prominent chin and forehead; and large testes (apparent only after puberty). Curiously, some boys with the syndrome are mentally normal, whereas some girls who just carry the recessive genes but who have a normal appearance are mentally retarded. The presence of the fragile X chromosome can be detected by tests before birth, but whether it will cause mental retardation in either sex can't be determined.

CHAPTER 255

Mental Retardation

Mental retardation is subaverage intellectual ability present from birth or early infancy.

People who are mentally retarded have a lower intellectual development than normal and difficulties in learning and social adaptation. About 3 percent of the total population are mentally retarded.

▲ see below

Causes

Intelligence is determined by both heredity and environment. In most cases of mental retardation, the cause is unknown. But several conditions during a woman's pregnancy can cause or contribute to mental retardation in her child. Common ones include the use of certain drugs, excessive consumption of alcohol, radiation therapy, poor nutrition, and certain viral infections, such as German measles (rubella). Chromosomal abnor-

Levels of Mental Retardation

Level	IQ Range	Ability at Preschool Age (Birth–5 years)	Ability at School Age (6–20 years)	Ability at Adult Age (21 years and older)
Mild	52–68	Can develop social and communication skills; muscle coordination is slightly impaired; often not diagnosed until later age	Can learn up to about the 6th-grade level by late teens; can be guided toward social conformity; can be educated	Can usually achieve enough social and vocational skills for self-support, but may need guidance and assistance during times of unusual social or economic stress
Moderate	36–51	Can talk or learn to communicate; social awareness is poor; muscle coordination is fair; profit from training in self-help	Can learn some social and occupational skills; progression beyond 2nd-grade level in schoolwork is unlikely; may learn to travel alone in familiar places	May achieve self-support by performing unskilled or semiskilled work under sheltered conditions; need supervision and guidance when under mild social or economic stress
Severe	20–35	Can say a few words; able to learn some self-help skills; have few or no expressive skills; muscle coordination is poor	Can talk or learn to communicate; can learn simple health habits; benefit from habit training	May contribute partially to self-care under complete supervision; can develop some useful self-protection skills in controlled environment
Profound	19 or below	Extremely retarded; little muscle coordination; may need nursing care	Some muscle coordination; unlikely to walk or talk	Some muscle coordination and speech; may achieve very limited self-care; need nursing care

Adapted from Kenny TJ, Clemmens RL: Mental retardation, in *Primary Pediatric Care,* edited by RA Hoekelman. St. Louis, C.V. Mosby Company, 1997, p. 410; used with permission.

malities, such as Down syndrome,▲ are a common cause of mental retardation. A number of hereditary disorders also can cause mental retardation. Some, such as phenylketonuria■ and cretinism★ (low thyroid levels), can be corrected before mental retardation occurs. Difficulties associated with premature birth, head injury during birth, or very low oxygen levels during birth also may cause mental retardation.

Diagnosis and Prognosis

Once mental retardation has occurred, it is usually irreversible. Diagnosing mental retardation

early makes remedial education and long-term planning possible.

Subaverage intelligence can be identified and measured by standardized intelligence tests. Such tests have a middle-class bias but are rea-

▲ see page 1237

■ see page 1293

★ see page 1296

sonably accurate predictors of intellectual performance, particularly in an older child.

Children with an IQ of 69 to 84 have difficulty in school learning but are not mentally retarded. They are rarely identified before beginning school, when educational and sometimes behavioral problems become evident. With special educational help, they can usually succeed in school and lead normal lives.

All children with mental retardation can benefit from education. Children with **mild retardation** (an IQ of 52 to 68) may attain fourth- to sixth-grade reading skills. Although they have difficulty reading, most mildly retarded children can learn the basic educational skills needed for everyday life. They require some supervision and support and special educational and training facilities. They may later require a sheltered living and work situation. Though usually free of obvious physical defects, people who are mildly retarded may have epilepsy.

The mildly retarded are often immature and unsophisticated, with a poorly developed capacity for social interaction. Their thinking is concrete and they are often unable to generalize. They have difficulty adjusting to new situations and may demonstrate poor judgment, lack of foresight, and gullibility. Although they don't commonly commit serious offenses, the mildly retarded may commit impulsive crimes, often as members of a group and sometimes to achieve peer group status.

Children with **moderate retardation** (an IQ of 36 to 51) are obviously slow in learning to speak and reaching other developmental milestones, such as sitting up and speaking. Given adequate training and support, mildly and moderately retarded adults can live with varying degrees of independence within the community. Some can cope with just a little support in a halfway house, whereas others need greater supervision.

The **severely retarded** child (an IQ of 20 to 35) is trainable to a lesser degree than a child who is moderately retarded. The **profoundly retarded**

▲ see box, page 1135

■ see page 1134

child (an IQ of 19 or below) usually can't learn to walk, talk, or understand very much.

The life expectancy of children with mental retardation may be shortened, depending on the cause and severity. In general, the more severe the retardation, the shorter the life expectancy.

Prevention

Genetic counseling gives parents of a child with retardation knowledge and understanding of the cause of retardation. Counseling helps them assess the risk of having another child who is retarded. Amniocentesis and chorionic villus sampling are diagnostic tests▲ that can detect a number of abnormalities, including genetic abnormalities and spinal cord or brain defects in the fetus. Amniocentesis or chorionic villus sampling is advisable for all pregnant women over 35 years old because of their increased risk of having a baby with Down syndrome. Ultrasound examination may also identify fetal brain defects. The serum alpha-fetoprotein level in the mother's blood can be measured to screen for Down syndrome and spina bifida.■ A diagnosis of mental retardation before birth gives parents the option of abortion and subsequent family planning. The rubella vaccine has dramatically decreased German measles (rubella) as a cause of mental retardation.

Treatment

The primary care doctor, in consultation with a number of specialists, develops a comprehensive, individualized program for the child with retardation. A child with developmental delays should be started in an early intervention program as soon as the diagnosis of mental retardation is suspected. Emotional support of the family is an integral part of the program. A child with retardation usually does best living at home or at a community-based residence and, if possible, attending a normal day care center or preschool program.

The level of social competence is as important as the IQ in determining how limiting the retardation will be. The IQ and social competence are both problems for children at the lower end of the IQ scale. For children with higher IQ scores, other factors—such as physical handicaps, personality problems, mental illness, and social skills—can determine how much care is needed.

Placing a child in a residential facility is rarely indicated, and such a decision requires extensive discussion between the family and the doctors. Although having a mentally retarded child at home can be disruptive, it is rarely the primary cause of family discord. However, the family needs psychologic support and may also need help with the burdens of daily care. Help can be provided by day care centers, housekeepers, child caregivers, and temporary foster homes. A retarded adult can be provided with long-term residence in an apartment cluster, hostel, or nursing home.

CHAPTER 256

Sick Children and Their Families

Everyone who takes care of a sick child—family, friends, doctors, nurses, and other caregivers—is under unusual stress. To see illness in another person is painful, but to see it in a child is particularly upsetting and can lead to worry, anxiety, guilt, anger, and resentment.

Illness in Newborns

A strong psychologic attachment (bonding) begins to develop between parents and their baby in the first hours and days after birth. Bonding is influenced by the parents' own experiences during childhood, their cultural and social attitudes toward child rearing, their personalities, and their desire and psychologic readiness for parenthood. Bonding ensures that the child receives sufficient support from the parents for healthy physical and emotional development.

Bonding becomes much more difficult when a newborn is sick or premature, particularly if the newborn must remain in an intensive care nursery. Parents may be separated from the baby for many days or weeks, and normal bonding may not be possible during this time. Therefore, parents and close relatives should visit the baby frequently, beginning as soon as possible after birth. After washing their hands thoroughly and putting on hospital gowns, they should touch or hold the baby as much as his condition allows. No newborn, even one whose breathing is being assisted by a respirator, is too sick to be visited and touched. Bonding is strengthened if the parents can feed, bathe, and change their baby and if the mother provides breast milk, even if the baby must be fed through a tube at first.

When a newborn has a birth defect, the doctor meets with both parents to discuss the baby's condition, possible treatments, and likely prognosis. The parents should see their baby together, as soon after birth as possible, regardless of his medical condition.

If a newborn dies, parents who have never seen or touched him may feel as though they had never had a baby. The feeling of emptiness can be overwhelming. One or both parents may suffer a prolonged and profound depression because they have difficulty grieving for an infant they have never seen, and their mourning is incomplete. Parents who weren't able to see or hold their baby while he was alive usually benefit from doing so after the baby has died, even though the experience is very painful. Parents also find it helpful to ask questions and have a doctor explain the baby's illness and the care he received. Those who lose an infant often have feelings of guilt, which are usually inappropriate and should be discussed.

If the parents' grief is overwhelming or unusually prolonged, psychologic counseling may help. If hereditary factors were involved, genetic counseling will help the parents understand the risk of having another sick child.

Illness in Children

Chronic illnesses of children include, among many others, asthma, cerebral palsy, cystic fibrosis, heart defects, diabetes, spina bifida, inflammatory bowel disease, kidney failure, epilepsy, cancer, juvenile arthritis, hemophilia, sickle cell disease, and mental retardation. Although each is uncommon, together they affect between 10 and 20 percent of children.

Effects on Children

Despite many differences in the symptoms and severity of these problems, children with chronic illness may share some of the same experiences:
• Pain and discomfort
• Inhibited growth and development
• Frequent visits to doctors and hospitals
• Need for daily medical care (sometimes with painful or embarrassing treatments)
• Fewer opportunities to play with other children
Physical differences may cause a child to be rejected by his peers. A disability can also prevent a child from achieving his goals. The scarcity of adult role models who are disabled (such as television stars) makes it more difficult for a child with a disability to establish an identity.

Effects on Families

For the family, a child's chronic illness can lead to painful disappointment in their dreams for that child. Time spent with the sick child deprives healthy siblings of time with their parents. Other problems include major expenses, a confusing health care system, lost opportunities (for example, when a parent can't return to work), and social isolation. These problems lead to stress that may even cause the parents to separate, especially if they have other problems, such as financial worries. Conditions that disfigure a child, such as a cleft lip or hydrocephalus (a condition in which fluid accumulates in the brain, causing compression of brain tissue and an enlarged head), can interfere with the bonding between child and family.

Parents may grieve on learning that their child has an abnormality. They may also feel shock, denial, anger, sadness or depression, guilt, and anxiety. Such reactions may occur at any time in the child's development, and each parent may react differently, which may strain communication between them. Sympathy for the child and the demands placed on the family may lead to inconsistencies in discipline and behavioral problems. One parent may become overinvolved with the child, disturbing normal family relationships.

A working parent who can't accompany the child on doctor visits may feel distanced from the child.

Effects on the Community

People in the child's neighborhood and community may not understand the disability and the care it entails. Community policies and funding to provide care and schooling may be inconsistent or insufficient, and facilities, such as ramps at sidewalk corners, may be inadequate. Communication and coordination among medical professionals, parents, and health care administrators may be poor.

Solutions

Solutions to most of these problems are often hard to find, partly because the medical system is fragmented. Ideally, one person, typically the family doctor or pediatrician, coordinates all services and plans the treatment program.

This process, which is known as case management, includes the following:
• Assessing the medical, educational, social, and psychologic needs of the child and family
• Arranging for all medical and nonmedical services, with clearly defined roles for each provider
• Coordinating services and providers
• Monitoring the progress made by the child and family, adjusting services and providers as necessary
• Providing the child with training in social skills to help him engage with peers and adults more productively
• Providing the family with appropriate counseling, education, support systems, schools, and respite care to allow occasional relief from child care responsibilities

Because case management is rarely perfect, parents should become thoroughly familiar with their child's illness by reading about it and by talking with doctors and other caregivers. Collaboration among doctors, social workers, teachers, and others—to help provide a team dedicated to the child's support and development—can be very beneficial. If necessary, the family should seek support from family and financial counselors. In addition, parent support groups are found in most communities. These groups can help identify a family that has already faced similar problems with the particular disease or disorder and is willing to speak with and support new parents.

Developmental Problems in Young Children

Developmental problems in young children include, among others, failure to thrive, behavioral problems, eating problems, sleep problems, toilet training problems, phobias, hyperactivity, attention deficit disorder, and learning disabilities.

Failure to Thrive

Failure to thrive refers primarily to a delay in physical growth (size); development (maturation) may also be delayed as a result of either poor physical growth or the problems caused by poor growth.

Causes

Failure to thrive usually applies to young children, especially those under 2 years of age. A child who fails to thrive isn't receiving sufficient nutrition for normal growth and development. The child may have an underlying physical disorder that affects his ability to take in, absorb, process, or retain food. Alternatively, psychologic, social, or economic factors may play a role. The child's appetite may be poor, or he may not be getting enough food. Poor appetite can be caused by depression. Depression may result if a child isn't receiving enough social stimulation, as may happen to an infant isolated in an incubator or to a child who receives insufficient attention from parents or other caregivers.

Diagnosis

Infants and young children are always weighed and measured during their well-child checkups. The doctor compares these measurements with those taken at the last visit and with standard height-weight charts.▲ If the growth rate is adequate, the child may be normal even if small.

To determine why the child is small, the doctor conducts a physical examination and asks the parents detailed questions about feeding, social problems, and illnesses that the child has had or that run in the family. Routine tests, such as a complete blood count, may be performed. More extensive testing is performed only if the doctor suspects an underlying disease.

Prognosis and Treatment

Any disease that seems to be underlying a child's failure to thrive is treated. How well the child responds to treatment depends on the specific problem causing the growth failure. If the child isn't taking in enough food, the doctor addresses possible psychologic, social, or economic factors, in addition to any physical factors. Occasionally, especially in cases in which no underlying cause is found, intervention by a social services agency or psychologic or psychiatric treatment for the parents or caregivers may be needed. In rare instances, foster care for the child may be recommended.

Children who fail to thrive, especially during the first year of life—an important time for brain growth—may never catch up developmentally or socially with their peers, even though their physical growth may improve. The type and extent of developmental or social and emotional problems vary with the individual child. In about one third of these children, mental development, especially verbal skills, remains below normal. About half the children continue to have social and emotional problems or eating problems, such as being picky or slow eaters.

Behavioral Problems

Behavioral problems are behavior patterns so difficult that they threaten normal relationships between the child and others.

Behavioral problems may be the result of the child's environment, health, inborn temperament, or development. A poor relationship with parents, teachers, and caregivers may also be at the root of a behavioral problem.

To diagnose a behavioral problem, a doctor or therapist interviews the parents and asks for a complete chronologic account of the child's activities in a typical day. Discussions focus on the circumstances leading to the problem behavior

---

▲ see box, pages 1196 and 1197

and the details of the behavior itself. The doctor also observes how the child and parents interact.

Behavioral problems tend to worsen with time, and early treatment may help prevent progression. More positive and enjoyable contact between the parents and the child can raise the self-esteem of both child and parents. Improved interaction can help break a vicious circle of negative behaviors causing negative responses.

CHILD-PARENT INTERACTIONAL PROBLEMS

Child-parent interactional problems are difficulties in the relationship between a child and his parents.

Interactional problems may begin during the first few months of life. The relationship between mother and baby may be strained as a consequence of a difficult pregnancy or delivery. Depression after delivery or lack of support from the father, relatives, or friends may also strain a mother's relationship with her baby. Contributing to the strain are the baby's unpredictable feeding and sleeping schedules. Most babies don't sleep through the night until 2 to 3 months of age. During this time, most babies have frequent periods of prolonged, intense crying. The parents' exhaustion, hostility, and guilt may combine with feelings of despair, affecting their relationship with the baby. The poor relationship may slow the child's development of mental and social skills and cause failure to thrive.▲

Treatment

The parents may be offered information on the development of infants and helpful tips for coping. A health care practitioner can also evaluate and discuss the temperament of an individual baby. These measures help the parents develop more realistic expectations and realize that guilt and conflict are normal emotions in early child rearing. This knowledge allows the parents to accept their feelings and try to rebuild a healthy relationship.

SEPARATION ANXIETY

Separation anxiety is anxiety felt by a child when a parent leaves him alone.

▲ see page 1245

Crying when the mother leaves the room or when a stranger approaches is a normal stage of development beginning around age 8 months and lasting until 18 to 24 months. The intensity of this behavior varies with each child. However, some parents, especially first-time parents, think separation anxiety is an emotional problem and respond by becoming protective and avoiding separations or new situations. Such behavior can lead to problems in the child's maturation and development. Fathers may interpret separation anxiety as a sign that the child is spoiled and may criticize the mother or try to modify the child's behavior by scolding and punishment.

Treatment

A doctor or nurse can reassure the parents that the child's behavior is normal and discuss methods of handling it. Parents are encouraged to become gradually less protective and restrictive, allowing the child to develop normally.

DISCIPLINE PROBLEMS

Discipline problems are inappropriate behaviors that develop when discipline is ineffective.

Discipline is a technique of rewards and punishments to enforce desired behavior. Efforts to control a child's behavior through scolding or physical punishments, such as spanking, may work briefly if used sparingly. However, they become ineffective when overused. Scolding or spanking may also reduce the child's sense of security and self-esteem. Failure to adequately discipline a child may lead to socially unacceptable behavior. Threats that the parents will leave or send the child away can be psychologically damaging.

Praise and reward can reinforce good behavior. For bad behavior, a time-out procedure can be helpful. The procedure requires a small, portable kitchen timer and a chair. The chair is placed in a spot without diversions, such as a television or toys. The chair shouldn't be in the child's bedroom or in a place that is dark or scary. Time-outs are a learning process for the child. They are best used for one or just a few types of inappropriate behavior.

Because most children prefer the attention they get for inappropriate behavior to no attention at all, the parents should create special times for pleasant interactions with the child each day. The pleasant interactions also provide an opportunity for rewarding good behavior.

VICIOUS CIRCLE PATTERN

A vicious circle pattern is a cycle of negative (naughty) behavior by the child that causes a negative (angry) response from the parent or caregiver, followed by further negative behavior by the child, leading to a further negative response from the parent.

Vicious circles usually begin when a child is aggressive and resistant. The parents or caregivers respond by scolding, yelling, and spanking. They may be reacting to the typical negative attitude of a 2-year-old or to the back talk of a 4-year-old, or they may be attempting to cope with a child who has had a difficult temperament since birth. Such a child often reacts to stress and emotional discomfort with stubbornness, back talk, aggressiveness, and temper outbursts rather than with crying.

Vicious circles may also result when parents react to a fearful, clinging, or manipulative child with overprotection and overpermissiveness. The parents usually bring the child to a doctor because of "medical" problems that turn out to be problems related to behavior. A typical day includes conflicts at mealtime and difficulties when the parents must leave the child, such as at nap time or bedtime. The parents tend to perform tasks the child could do independently, such as dressing and feeding. The parents often assume incorrectly that the child may be harmed by discipline.

Treatment

The vicious circle pattern may be broken if parents learn to ignore bad behavior that doesn't affect the rights of others, such as tantrums or refusals to eat. For behavior that can't be ignored, distraction or a time-out procedure can be tried. Parents can also reduce friction and encourage good behavior by praising the child appropriately. In addition, the parents and child should spend at least 15 to 20 minutes each day involved in a mutually enjoyable activity.

If these adjustments don't break the vicious circle pattern of behavior within 3 to 4 months, the child may need to be seen by a psychologist or psychiatrist.

Eating Problems

A normal decrease in appetite, caused by a slowing growth rate, is common in children 1 to 8

Time-Out Procedure

• The child misbehaves in a way that has already been agreed to result in a time-out.

• The misbehavior is briefly explained to the child. The child is then calmly told to go to the time-out chair or is led there, if necessary.

• When the child is sitting in the chair, the timer is set to last 1 minute for each year of age, up to a maximum of 5 minutes.

• If the child gets up from the chair before the bell rings, he is put back in the chair and the timer is reset. A child who gets up repeatedly may have to be held in the chair, not in one's lap. Talking and eye contact are avoided. If the child has to be held in the chair for the entire period until the bell rings, the timer is reset.

• If the child stays in the chair but doesn't quiet down before the bell rings, the timer is reset.

• When it's time for the child to get up, the caregiver asks the reason for the time-out without anger and nagging. If the child doesn't recall the correct reason, he is briefly reminded.

• The caregiver should comment on the child's praiseworthy behavior within a short period of time. This behavior may be easier to achieve if the child is started in a new activity far from the scene of the inappropriate behavior.

---

years old. Eating problems may develop if a parent or caregiver tries to coerce the child to eat or shows too much concern about the child's appetite or eating habits. While parents coax and threaten, children with eating problems may sit with food in their mouth. Some children may respond to parental attempts at force-feeding by vomiting.

Treatment

Treatment requires decreasing the tension and negative emotions surrounding mealtimes. Emotional scenes can be avoided by putting food in front of the child and removing it in 15 or 20 minutes without comment. The child should be allowed to eat whatever he chooses at mealtime but is restricted from eating between-meal snacks. With this technique, the balance between appetite, amount eaten, and nutritional needs is quickly restored.

Sleep Problems

Nightmares are frightening dreams that occur during REM (rapid eye movement) sleep. A child having a nightmare usually awakens fully and can vividly recall the details of the dream. An occasional nightmare is normal, and comfort from the parent or caregiver may be all that is needed. Frequent nightmares, however, are abnormal and may indicate an underlying psychologic problem. Frightening experiences, including scary stories or violent television shows, can cause nightmares. This cause is particularly common in children 3 to 4 years of age, who can't readily distinguish fantasy from reality.

Night terrors are episodes of incomplete awakening with extreme anxiety shortly after falling asleep. The child is not able to recall these episodes. **Sleepwalking** is rising from bed and walking around while apparently asleep. Both night terrors and sleepwalking usually take place on incomplete arousal from deep (non-REM) sleep and interrupt the first 3 hours of sleep.▲ Episodes last from seconds to many minutes. Night terrors are dramatic because of the screaming and inconsolable panic of the terrified child during the episode. Night terrors are most common between 3 and 8 years of age.

A sleepwalker walks clumsily but usually avoids bumping into objects. He appears confused but not frightened. A sleepwalking child awakens suddenly with a blank or confused stare. At first, he isn't fully awake or responsive to other people. In the morning, he can't recall the episode. About 15 percent of children between 5 and 12 years of age have at least one episode of sleepwalking. One to 6 percent of children, most commonly school-aged boys, sleepwalk persistently. A stressful event may trigger an episode.

▲ see box, page 301

Resistance to going to bed is a common problem, particularly in children between 1 and 2 years of age. Young children cry when left alone in their cribs, or they climb out and seek their parents. This behavior is related to separation anxiety and to the child's attempts to control more aspects of his environment.

Awakening during the night is another sleep problem in young children. About half of the infants between 6 and 12 months of age awaken during the night. Children with separation anxiety often have episodes of night awakening as well. In older children, night awakening often follows a move, an illness, or another stressful event. Sleeping problems may be exacerbated by long naps late in the afternoon and overstimulating play before bedtime.

Treatment

Both night terrors and sleepwalking almost always stop on their own, though occasional episodes may occur for years. Children in whom these disorders persist into adolescence and adulthood may have an underlying psychologic problem.

Letting the child who resists bedtime get up or staying in the room at length to provide comfort is ineffective. Allowing the child to sleep with parents usually prolongs a night awakening problem. Also counterproductive are playing with or feeding the child during the night, spanking, and scolding. Returning the child to bed with simple reassurances is usually more effective. Settling the child with a brief story, offering a favorite doll or blanket, and using a night-light are often helpful. To fully control the problem, the parent may have to sit quietly in the hallway in sight of the child and make sure the child stays in bed. The child then learns that getting out of bed isn't allowed. The child also learns that the parents can't be enticed into the room for more stories or play. Eventually, the child settles down and goes to sleep.

For a child who gets up and wanders, installing a hook-and-eye lock on the outside of the bedroom door can solve the problem. However, locking the door should be done only after careful consideration, so as not to make the child feel isolated.

Toilet Training Problems

Most children are bowel trained between 2 and 3 years of age and bladder trained between 3 and 4 years. By age 5, the average child can go to the toilet alone, managing all aspects of dressing, undressing, and wiping. However, about 30 percent of normal 4-year-olds and 10 percent of 6-year-olds haven't yet achieved regular nighttime control.

Prevention and Treatment

The best way to avoid toilet training problems is to recognize when the child is ready. Readiness is signaled when the child has dry periods lasting several hours and wants to be changed when wet. The child also shows interest in sitting on a potty chair or toilet and is able to follow simple verbal commands. Children are usually ready between ages 24 and 36 months.

The most common method of toilet training is the timing method. A child who seems ready is introduced to the potty chair and gradually asked to sit on it briefly while fully clothed. The child is then encouraged to practice taking his pants down, sitting on the potty chair for no more than 5 or 10 minutes, and redressing. Simple explanations are given repeatedly, reinforced by placing wet or dirty diapers in the potty bowl. Praise or a reward is given for successful behavior. Anger or punishment for lack of success or accidents may be counterproductive. The timing method works well for children with predictable bowel and urine schedules. Providing the necessary encouragement and rewards is difficult for children with unpredictable schedules. Training for these children is better delayed until they can anticipate the need to visit the bathroom on their own.

A second training method entails the use of a doll. A child who seems ready is taught the steps of toilet training by pretending that the doll is using the toilet. The doll is praised for dry pants and for successful completion of each step of the process. Then the child imitates this process with the doll repeatedly, also praising the doll. Lastly, the child imitates the doll and performs the steps as the parent provides praise and rewards.

A child who resists sitting on the toilet may be allowed to get up and try again after a meal. If resistance continues for days, postponing the training for several weeks is the best strategy.

Behavior Therapy for Bed-wetting

Child's responsibilities
- Keep a calendar to record wet and dry nights
- Refrain from drinking any fluids for 2 to 3 hours before going to bed
- Urinate before going to bed
- Change clothing and bedding when wet

Parents' responsibilities
- Don't punish child for bed-wetting or get angry when bed-wetting occurs
- Give praise and rewards (a star on the calendar or other rewards, depending on child's age) for dry nights

Giving praise or a reward for sitting on the toilet and producing results has succeeded with both normal and retarded children. Once the pattern is established, rewards are given for every other success and then gradually withdrawn. Power struggles are unproductive and may cause a strained parent-child relationship. If a vicious circle of pressure and resistance occurs, the circle may be broken by other techniques.▲

BED-WETTING

Bed-wetting (nocturnal enuresis) is accidental, repeated urination by a sleeping child who is old enough to be expected not to wet the bed.

About 30 percent of children still wet the bed at age 4 years, 10 percent at age 6, 3 percent at age 12, and 1 percent at age 18. Bed-wetting is more common in boys than in girls and seems to run in families. Bed-wetting is usually caused by slow maturation, although it sometimes accompanies such sleep disorders as sleepwalking and night terrors. A physical disorder—usually a urinary tract infection—is found in only 1 to 2 percent of cases. In rare cases, other disorders, such

▲ see page 1247

Causes of Chronic Constipation Leading to Encopresis

- Withholding stool because of fear of using the toilet
- Resistance to toilet training
- A painful tear in the lining of the anus (anal fissure)
- Birth defects, such as a spinal cord abnormality or abnormalities of the anus
- Hirschsprung's disease
- Low thyroid levels
- Poor nutrition
- Cerebral palsy
- Psychiatric disease in the child or family

as diabetes, may cause a child to wet the bed. Bed-wetting occasionally is caused by psychiatric problems, either in the child or in another family member.

Sometimes bed-wetting stops and then begins again. The relapse usually follows a psychologically stressful event or condition, but a physical cause, such as a urinary tract infection, may be responsible.

Treatment

For children younger than age 6, the doctor usually waits to see whether time cures the condition. Each year, in 15 percent of the children older than age 6, bed-wetting stops without intervention. If it doesn't, three different types of treatment may be tried: counseling plus behavior therapy, bed-wetting alarms, and drug therapy.

Counseling plus behavior therapy is probably the most commonly used treatment. Both child and parents receive counseling. They learn that bed-wetting is quite common, that it can be corrected, and that nobody should feel guilty about it.

Bed-wetting alarms are by far the most effective treatment available. They cure bed-wetting in about 70 percent of the children, and only about 10 to 15 percent start bed-wetting again after the alarms are discontinued. Alarms, which are triggered by a few drops of urine, are relatively inexpensive and are easy to set up. The disadvantage is that the treatment works slowly. In the first few weeks of use, the child awakens only after fully urinating. In the next few weeks, the child awakens after urinating a small amount and may wet the bed less often. Eventually, the need to urinate wakes the child before the bed is wet. Most parents find that the alarm can be removed after a 3-week dry period.

Drug therapy is used much less often today than in the past, because bed-wetting alarms are more effective and the drugs may have side effects. However, if other treatments fail and the family strongly wants drug treatment, the doctor may prescribe imipramine. Imipramine is an antidepressant drug that relaxes the bladder and tightens the sphincter that blocks urine flow. If imipramine is going to work, it usually does so in the first week of treatment. This rapid response is the one real advantage of the drug, particularly if the family and child feel they need to cure the problem quickly. After the child goes 1 month without bed-wetting, the drug dose is decreased over 2 to 4 weeks, then stopped. However, about 75 percent of the children treated with imipramine eventually start bed-wetting again. If this happens, a 3-month course of the drug may be tried. Blood samples are taken every 2 to 4 weeks while the child is taking imipramine to ensure that the level of white blood cells has not decreased severely— a rare but serious side effect.

An alternative is desmopressin nasal spray. This drug reduces the output of urine. It has few side effects but is expensive.

ENCOPRESIS

Encopresis is having accidental bowel movements not caused by illness or physical abnormality.

About 17 percent of 3-year-olds and 1 percent of 4-year-olds have accidental bowel movements. Most of these accidents result from resistance to toilet training. However, they are sometimes caused by chronic constipation, which stretches the bowel wall and reduces the child's awareness of a full bowel and impairs muscle control.

A doctor first tries to determine whether the cause is physical or psychologic. If the cause is constipation, a laxative is prescribed and other measures are instituted to ensure regular bowel movements. If this fails, diagnostic tests should be performed. Psychologic counseling may be needed for children whose encopresis is the result of resistance to toilet training.

Phobias

A phobia is an irrational or exaggerated fear of objects, situations, or bodily functions that aren't inherently dangerous.

Phobias are different from the fears that are normal for the child's stage of development or fears caused by conflicts in the home. School phobia is one example of an exaggerated fear. It may cause a child 6 or 7 years of age to refuse to go to school. The child may either directly refuse to go to school or complain of a stomachache, nausea, or other symptoms that justify staying home. Such a child may be overreacting with fear to a teacher's strictness or rebukes, which can frighten a sensitive child. In older children, aged 10 to 14, school phobia may indicate a more serious psychologic problem.

Treatment

The younger child with school phobia should return to school immediately so that he doesn't fall behind in his schoolwork. If the phobia is so intense that it interferes with the child's activity and if the child doesn't respond to simple reassurance by parents or teachers, referral to a psychologist or psychiatrist may be warranted. Some children recover from school phobia, only to develop it again after a real illness or a vacation. Immediate return to school isn't so urgent for an older child, whose treatment may depend on a mental health evaluation.

Hyperactivity

Hyperactivity is a level of activity and excitement in a child so high that it concerns the parents or caregivers.

Generally, 2-year-olds are active and seldom stay still. A high activity and noise level is also common in 4-year-olds. In both age groups, such behavior is normal for the child's stage of development. However, active behavior frequently causes conflicts between parents and child and may worry parents. Whether the activity level is perceived as hyperactivity often depends on how

---

Normal Childhood Fears

Fears of the dark, monsters, bugs, and spiders are common in children 3 to 4 years old. Fears of injury and death are more common in older children. Frightening stories, movies, or television shows are often upsetting to children and can make fears worse. A statement parents may make in anger or jest may be taken literally by preschool children and can be disturbing to them. Shy children may initially react to new situations with fear or withdrawal.

A child can be comforted by his parents' reassurances that monsters don't exist, that spiders aren't harmful, or that what is seen on TV isn't real. If the parents make a disturbing statement in anger or jest, the statement should be explained to alleviate the child's concerns. Parents can help a shy child adapt to a feared situation by repeatedly exposing him to the situation without pressure and by offering him reassurance.

---

tolerant the annoyed person is. However, some children are clearly more active and have shorter attention spans than average. Hyperactivity can create problems for those who supervise such children.

Hyperactivity may have a variety of causes, including emotional disorders or abnormalities of brain function. Alternatively, hyperactivity may be simply an exaggeration of the child's normal temperament.

Treatment

Adults usually deal with a child's hyperactivity by scolding and punishing. However, these responses usually backfire, increasing the child's activity level. Avoiding situations in which the child has to sit still for a long time or finding a teacher skilled in coping with hyperactive children may help.

Attention Deficit Disorder

Attention deficit disorder is a poor or short attention span and impulsiveness inappropriate for the child's age, with or without hyperactivity.

Symptoms of Attention Deficit Disorder

The diagnosis of attention deficit disorder usually requires that the child frequently display at least 8 of the following 14 symptoms:

• Often fidgets with his hands or feet or squirms in his seat (restlessness)

• Has difficulty remaining seated when required to do so

• Is easily distracted by extraneous stimuli

• Has difficulty waiting for his turn in games or group situations

• Often blurts out answers before questions are completed

• Has difficulty following instructions from others, even if he understands them and isn't trying to be contrary

• Has difficulty sustaining attention in tasks or play activities

• Often shifts from one uncompleted task to another

• Has difficulty playing quietly

• Often talks excessively

• Often interrupts or intrudes on others

• Often doesn't seem to listen to what's being said

• Often loses things necessary for tasks or activities at school or home

• Often engages in physically dangerous activities without considering possible consequences

---

Attention deficit disorder affects an estimated 5 to 10 percent of school-aged children and is diagnosed 10 times more often in boys than in girls. Many signs of attention deficit disorder are noticed often before age 4 and invariably before age 7, but they may not interfere significantly until the middle school years.

The disorder is usually inherited. Recent research indicates that the disorder is caused by abnormalities in neurotransmitters (substances that transmit nerve impulses within the brain). Attention deficit disorder is often exaggerated by the child's home or school environment.

Symptoms

Attention deficit disorder is primarily a problem with sustained attention, concentration, and task persistence. A child with attention deficit disorder may also be impulsive and overactive. Many preschool children with attention deficit disorder are anxious, have problems communicating and interacting, and behave poorly. During later childhood, such children often move their legs continuously, move and fidget with their hands, talk impulsively, forget easily, and are disorganized, although they are generally not aggressive. About 20 percent of the children with attention deficit disorder have learning disabilities, and about 90 percent have academic problems. About 40 percent are depressed, anxious, and oppositional by the time they reach adolescence. About 60 percent of young children have such problems as temper tantrums, and most older children have low frustration tolerance. Although impulsiveness and hyperactivity tend to diminish with age, inattentiveness and related symptoms can extend well into adulthood.

Diagnosis

The diagnosis is based on the number, frequency, and severity of symptoms. Often, diagnosis is difficult because it depends on the judgment of the observer. In addition, many symptoms are not unique to children with attention deficit disorder; a child without the disorder may have one or more of the symptoms.

Treatment and Prognosis

Psychostimulant drugs are the most effective treatment. Behavior therapy conducted by a child psychologist is usually combined with drug therapy. Structures, routines, and modified parenting techniques are often needed. However, children who aren't too aggressive and who come from a stable home environment may benefit from drug treatment alone.

Methylphenidate is the drug most often prescribed. It has proved more effective than antidepressants, caffeine, and other psychostimulants and causes fewer side effects than does dextroamphetamine. Common side effects of methylphenidate are sleep disturbances, such as

Insomnia, and appetite suppression; others are depression or sadness, headaches, stomachaches, and high blood pressure. If taken in large doses for a long time, methylphenidate can slow growth.

Children with attention deficit disorder generally don't outgrow their difficulties. Problems that emerge or persist in adolescence and adulthood include academic failure, low self-esteem, anxiety, depression, and difficulty in learning appropriate social behavior. People who have attention deficit disorder seem to adjust better to work than to school situations. If attention deficit disorder is untreated, the risk of alcohol or substance abuse or suicide may be higher among people with this disorder than among those in the general population.

Learning Disabilities

Learning disabilities are inabilities to acquire, retain, or broadly use specific skills or information, resulting from deficiencies in attention, memory, or reasoning and affecting academic performance.

Many types of learning disabilities exist, and no single cause accounts for them. However, the basis of all learning disabilities is believed to be abnormal brain function. An estimated 3 to 15 percent of school children in the United States may need special educational services to compensate for learning disabilities. Boys with learning disabilities outnumber girls five to one.

Symptoms

A young child with a learning disability often has problems coordinating vision with movement and may be clumsy at physical tasks, such as cutting, coloring, buttoning, tying shoes, and running. The child may have problems with visual perception or phonologic processing—for instance, with recognizing sequences or patterns and distinguishing among sounds—or problems with memory, speech, reasoning, and listening. Some children have problems with reading, some with writing, and others with arithmetic. However, most learning disabilities are complex, with deficiencies in more than one area.

The young child may be slow to learn the names of colors or letters, to assign words to familiar objects, to count, and to progress in other early

Common Word and Letter Substitutions in Dyslexia

These letters and words	are substituted for	these letters and words
d		b
m		w
h		n
was		saw
on		no

learning skills. Learning to read and write may be delayed. Other symptoms are a short attention span and distractibility, halting speech, and a short memory span. The child may have difficulty with printing and copying, activities that require fine motor coordination.

A child with a learning disability may have difficulty communicating and controlling impulses and may have discipline problems. He may be easily distracted, hyperactive, withdrawn, shy, or aggressive.

Diagnosis and Treatment

A doctor examines the child for any physical disorders. The child then takes a series of intelligence tests, both verbal and nonverbal, including testing of reading, writing, and arithmetic skills. Psychologic testing is the final step of the evaluation.

Measures such as eliminating food additives, taking large doses of vitamins, and analyzing the child's system for trace minerals are unproved but often tried. No drug treatment has much effect on academic achievement, intelligence, and general learning ability. However, certain drugs, such as methylphenidate, may improve attention and concentration. This improvement enhances the child's ability to learn. The most useful treatment for a learning disability is education that's carefully tailored to the individual child.

DYSLEXIA

Dyslexia is primarily a specific language-based learning disability that interferes with learning words and reading despite average or above-average intelligence, adequate motivation and educational opportunities, and normal eyesight and hearing.

Dyslexia tends to run in families and is identified in more boys than girls. Dyslexia is caused mostly by deficiencies in the processing of sounds and spoken language by the brain. The deficiencies are present from birth, affect word decoding, and may cause spelling and writing problems.

Symptoms and Diagnosis

Preschool children with dyslexia may be very late in speaking, have speech articulation problems, and have difficulty remembering the names of letters, numbers, and colors. Dyslexic children often have difficulty blending sounds, rhyming words, identifying the positions of sounds in words, segmenting words into sounds, and identifying the number of sounds in words. Delays or hesitations in choosing words, making word substitutions, and naming letters and pictures are early indicators of dyslexia. Problems with short-term memory for sounds and with putting sounds in the correct order are common.

Many children with dyslexia confuse letters and words with similar ones. Reversing the letters while writing—for instance, *on* instead of *no*—or confusing letters—for instance, *d* instead of *b*—is common.

Children who aren't progressing in word learning skills by the middle or end of first grade should be tested for dyslexia. So should those who, at any grade level, aren't reading at the level expected for their verbal or intellectual abilities. Any child who is slow in learning to read or in becoming fluent in speaking should also be tested for dyslexia.

Treatment

The best treatment is **direct instruction** that incorporates multisensory approaches. This type of treatment consists of teaching phonics with a variety of cues, usually separately and, when possible, as part of a reading program.

Indirect instruction is also helpful. It usually consists of training to improve word pronunciation or reading comprehension. Children are taught how to process sounds by blending sounds to form words, by separating words into segments, and by identifying the positions of sounds in words.

Indirect treatments may be used but are not recommended. Children are taught to read, read better, or speak in indirect ways, such as by using tinted lenses that allow words and letters to be read more easily, eye movement exercises, or visual perceptual training. Drugs such as piracetam have also been tried. However, the benefits of most indirect treatments haven't been proved.

CHAPTER 258

Puberty and Problems in Adolescents

Adolescence is a time of significant change, including physical growth and psychosocial transition, usually encompassing the second decade of life.

The most common health problems of adolescents relate to growth and development, childhood illnesses continuing into adolescence, and experimentation. As adolescents try new behav-iors, they become vulnerable to certain conditions related to their behaviors, such as sexually transmitted diseases. Heterosexually active adolescent girls are at risk of becoming pregnant.

Adolescence is a time when psychiatric conditions, such as depression and other mood disorders, become apparent, leading to a risk of suicide.▲ Eating disorders, such as anorexia nervosa and bulimia nervosa, are particularly common in adolescents.■

Violence has become a leading cause of illness and death in adolescents. Many factors, including developmental issues, gang involvement, access to firearms, substance use, and poverty, contribute to an increased risk of violence for teenagers. Accidents, particularly car and motorcycle crashes, are the leading cause of death among adolescents. Burns, multiple fractures, and other accidents are responsible for a high rate of severe injuries among teenagers.

Growth and Development

Normal growth during adolescence includes sexual maturation and an increase in body size. The timing and speed of these changes vary with each person and are affected by both heredity and environment. Physical maturity begins at an earlier age today than it did a century ago, probably because of improved nutrition, general health, and living conditions. For example, girls have their first menstrual period at a considerably younger age than did their counterparts 100 years ago. Between 1850 and 1950 in the United States, age at the first period (menarche) declined by 2 months every 10 years. Since 1950, it has leveled off.

During adolescence, the majority of boys and girls reach adult height and weight. Yet, two adolescents who eventually reach the same height may take considerably different amounts of time to do so. The growth spurt in boys occurs between ages 13 and $15\frac{1}{2}$ years; a gain of 4 inches can be expected in the year of maximum growth. The growth spurt in girls occurs between ages 11 and $13\frac{1}{2}$ years; a gain of $3\frac{1}{2}$ inches can be expected in the year of maximum growth. In general, boys become heavier and taller than girls. By age 18, boys have about $\frac{3}{4}$ inch of growth remaining and girls have slightly less. Bones, muscles, and all of the organs grow except the lymphatic system, which decreases in size, and the brain, which reaches its maximum weight during adolescence.

Sexual changes generally proceed in a set sequence. In boys, the first sexual changes are growth of the scrotum and testes, followed by lengthening of the penis and growth of the seminal vesicles and prostate gland. Next, pubic hair appears. Hair grows on the face and in the underarms about 2 years after it starts to appear in the pubic area. The first ejaculation usually occurs between ages $12\frac{1}{2}$ and 14, about 1 year after the penis begins to lengthen. The precise time for first ejaculation is determined by a combination of psychologic, cultural, and physical factors. Breast enlargement (gynecomastia) on one side or both is common in young adolescent boys but usually disappears within a year.

In the majority of girls, the first visible sign of sexual maturation is breast budding, closely followed by the growth spurt.★ Soon afterward, pubic and underarm hair appears. The first menstrual period generally comes about 2 years after the breasts start to enlarge. Height increases most before menstruation begins.

Delayed Sexual Maturation

Delayed sexual maturation is a delay in sexual development.

Some adolescents don't start their sexual development at the usual age. A delay may be perfectly normal; perhaps late development runs in the family. In such adolescents, the growth rate before puberty is usually normal. Although the growth spurt and sexual maturation are delayed, they eventually proceed normally.

Various abnormalities can delay or prevent sexual development. Chromosomal abnormalities can cause Turner's syndrome in girls● and Klinefelter's syndrome in boys.◆ Other genetic disorders can affect hormone production. A tumor that damages the pituitary gland or the part of the brain that is responsible for maturation (hypothalamus) can lower the levels of gonadotropins, the hormones responsible for stimulating the growth of the sex organs, or stop production of the hormones altogether. Chronic illnesses, such as diabetes mellitus, kidney disease, and cystic fibrosis, can also delay sexual maturation.

▲ see page 1319

■ see page 415

★ see page 1075

● see page 1239

◆ see page 1240

Milestones in Sexual Development

During puberty, sexual development usually occurs in a set sequence. When a change begins varies with each person but occurs within a range of ages, indicated by a box in the diagram below. The average age at which a change begins is indicated by a dot.

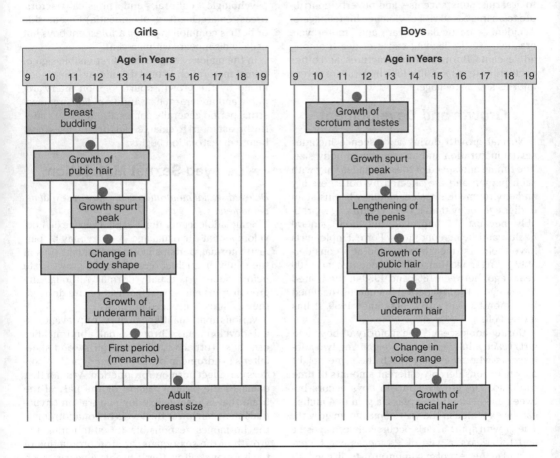

Symptoms and Diagnosis

The symptoms of delayed sexual maturation in boys are lack of testicular enlargement by age 13½, lack of pubic hair by age 15, or more than 5 years from the start to the completion of genital enlargement. In girls, the symptoms are lack of breast development by age 13, more than 5 years from the beginning of breast growth to the first menstrual period, lack of pubic hair by age 14, or failure to menstruate by age 16. A short height (short stature) may indicate delayed maturation in both boys and girls.

To help determine why sexual maturation is delayed, a doctor takes a sample of blood, and in some cases, a chromosomal analysis may be performed. Laboratory tests of these samples may identify abnormal sex chromosomes and hormone levels. The blood is also tested for diabetes mellitus, anemia, and other conditions that can delay sexual development. X-rays, computed tomography (CT) scans, or magnetic resonance imaging (MRI) scans may show abnormalities in the brain. In addition, x-rays of the hand and wrist may be used to estimate bone maturity.

Treatment

The treatment for delayed sexual maturation depends on its cause. Once a chronic underlying disease has been treated, maturation usually proceeds. A naturally late development needs no treatment. A condition resulting from a genetic cause can't be cured, though replacing hormones may help secondary sexual characteristics develop. In some cases, surgery may be needed.

Precocious Puberty

Precocious puberty is sexual maturation that begins before age 8 in a girl or before age 10 in a boy.

In true precocious puberty, the sex glands (ovaries or testes) mature and a child's outward appearance becomes more adult. Pubic hair grows, and the child's body shape changes. In pseudoprecocious puberty, only the outward appearance becomes more adult, while the sex glands remain immature.

True precocious puberty is two to five times more common in girls than in boys.

Causes

True precocious puberty is caused by the early release of sex hormones (gonadotropins) from the pituitary gland; these hormones affect the sex organs. Early hormone release may be caused by an abnormality in the pituitary, such as a hormone-secreting tumor, or by an abnormality in the hypothalamus, the region of the brain that controls the pituitary. About 60 percent of boys with precocious puberty have an identifiable abnormality. In contrast, no abnormality can be found in about 80 percent of girls age 6 or older with this condition, but most girls under 4 years of age with true precocious puberty have a brain abnormality.

In pseudoprecocious puberty, high levels of male sex hormones (androgens) or female sex hormones (estrogens) are produced; the cause may be a tumor in the adrenal gland or in a testis or ovary. These hormones don't cause the sex glands to mature but do cause a child to look more like an adult.

In a rare hereditary disorder that affects boys, a form of pseudoprecocious puberty (testotoxicosis) results directly from maturation of the testes, independent of the hypothalamus or pituitary gland. Similarly, the McCune-Albright syndrome is a condition that causes pseudoprecocious puberty with bone disease, irregular skin pigmentation (café-au-lait spots), and hormonal abnormalities.

Symptoms and Diagnosis

In both true precocious and pseudoprecocious puberty, a boy develops facial, underarm, and pubic hair. His penis lengthens, and his appearance becomes more masculine. A girl may start to have menstrual periods, especially if she has true precocious puberty, or she may develop breasts, pubic hair, and underarm hair. In boys and girls, body odor changes, and acne may appear. Height increases rapidly but stops at an early age. Therefore, the final height is shorter than had been expected. In true precocious puberty, but usually not in pseudoprecocious puberty, the testes or ovaries enlarge to adult size.

Diagnostic tests include measuring blood hormone levels and taking x-rays of the hand and wrist to estimate bone maturity. Ultrasound examination of the pelvis and adrenal glands and computed tomography (CT) or magnetic resonance imaging (MRI) of the brain are performed to see whether tumors have developed in the adrenal glands, hypothalamus, or pituitary gland.

Treatment

In true precocious puberty, taking a drug such as histrelin (a synthetically made gonadotropin-releasing hormone) stops the pituitary gland from producing gonadotropins. When precocious puberty isn't caused by the early release of gonadotropins (pseudoprecocious puberty), a doctor may try to inhibit the action of the sex hormones with various drugs. The antifungal agent ketoconazole reduces the levels of testosterone

Side Effects of Anabolic Steroids

- Mood swings
- Increased aggressiveness
- Worsening acne
- Injuries to muscles and tendons
- Early closure of growth plates, leading to reduced height (if used before an adolescent reaches final height)
- Abnormal liver function or liver tumors, possibly causing jaundice
- High blood pressure
- Increased levels of total cholesterol and a decreased level of high-density lipoprotein (the good cholesterol)
- In boys, no sperm in the semen, reduction in the size of the testes, and breast enlargement
- In girls, male-pattern hair growth, hoarse voice, decreased breast size, thinning of the vaginal lining, and irregular or no menstrual periods
- In both sexes, increased sexual desire

circulating in the blood in boys who have testotoxicosis. A drug called testolactone reduces the levels of estrogen in adolescents who have McCune-Albright syndrome.

When a tumor is responsible for true precocious or pseudoprecocious puberty, removing it may cure the condition.

Contraception and Teenage Pregnancy

Adolescents may experiment sexually. However, many sexually active teenagers are not fully informed about contraception,▲ pregnancy, and sexually transmitted diseases (including AIDS).

▲ see page 1119

■ see page 1128

Problems with contraception include irregular pill taking; unplanned and spontaneous intercourse, which complicates the use of contraceptives; concerns about the pill; and limited choices for birth control methods (for example, the diaphragm requires fitting by a nurse or doctor and must be in place before intercourse). New methods, such as contraceptive implants under the skin, which act continuously over 5 years, are likely to be more successful than other methods.

Teenagers are at a transitional stage in life, and pregnancy or marriage can add significant emotional stress. Pregnant girls and their partners tend to drop out of school or job training, thus worsening their economic problems, lowering their self-esteem, and straining personal relationships.

Pregnant teenagers, particularly the very young who are not enrolled in prenatal care, are more likely to have medical problems during pregnancy, such as anemia and toxemia, than are women in their 20s. With good medical care, however, adolescents have no higher risk of pregnancy problems than adults from similar backgrounds. Infants of young mothers (especially mothers younger than 15 years) are more likely to be born prematurely and to have a low birth weight.

Having an abortion■ does not remove the psychologic problems of an unwanted pregnancy—either for the girl or her partner. Emotional crises may occur when pregnancy is diagnosed, when the decision to have an abortion is made, immediately after the abortion is performed, when the baby would have been born, and on the anniversaries of that date. Family counseling and education about contraceptive methods, for both the girl and her partner, can be very helpful.

Anabolic Steroid Abuse

Anabolic steroid abuse is the use of steroid drugs to enhance bodybuilding or athletic prowess.

Anabolic steroids are very similar to the natural hormone testosterone. Taking these drugs orally or by injection can give a person a competitive advantage in sports—they stimulate the growth of muscles and improve athletic performance. However, they also can produce side effects. Their use, therefore, raises ethical and safety issues. Despite a ban on anabolic steroid use by amateur and professional sports organizations throughout the world, the problem remains in many strength-dependent sports.

Between 6 and 11 percent of high school–aged boys, including a surprising number of nonathletes, use steroids. In a national survey, the largest group of first-time users of steroids comprised boys younger than 15 years old. Of people who use steroids, 95 percent are male, and 65 percent are athletes, typically football players, wrestlers, or weight lifters.

The most common symptom of anabolic steroid use is a dramatic increase in body bulk. The users feel more energetic and often have an increased sexual desire (libido). The side effects are in large part related to the dose used. High doses may produce such psychologic effects as erratic mood swings, irrational behavior, and increased aggressiveness (often called steroid rage).

Acne commonly gets worse and is one of the few side effects of taking anabolic steroids for which an adolescent may visit a doctor. Jaundice may occur if the user has liver damage, which is more likely with tablets than with the injected form of anabolic steroids.

The use of anabolic steroids can be detected up to 6 months after use has stopped. Laboratory tests can measure anabolic steroid breakdown products in the urine.

CHAPTER 259

Bacterial Infections

Most episodes of illness with a fever in children are caused by viral infections, although bacterial infections can also produce a fever. Bacterial infections can be serious but usually are treated readily with antibiotics. Prompt diagnosis of a bacterial infection is thus important to ensure prompt treatment.

A bacterial infection is often hard to distinguish from a viral infection. In general, bacterial infections tend to cause a higher fever—occasionally as high as 106° F.—and result in higher white blood cell counts. Children at particular risk for bacterial infections include infants under 2 months of age, children who have no spleen or who have other immune system disorders, and children who have sickle cell anemia. In temperate climates, many bacterial and viral infections occur in the winter months, perhaps fostered by crowded indoor conditions, but some do occur in the summer.

Diphtheria

Diphtheria is a contagious, sometimes fatal infection caused by the bacterium Corynebacterium diphtheriae.

Years ago, diphtheria was one of the leading causes of death among children. Today, diphtheria is rare in developed countries, primarily because of widespread vaccination against the disease. Fewer than five cases have occurred in the United States each year since 1980, but diphtheria bacteria still exist in the world and can cause outbreaks if vaccination is not used to the fullest extent possible. The largest outbreak in 50 years is currently ongoing in Russia and other countries of the former Soviet Union.

Diphtheria bacteria are usually spread in droplets of moisture coughed into the air. Rarely, bacteria can be spread by contaminated household articles, such as clothing or toys. Usually the bacteria multiply on or near the surface of the mucous membranes of the mouth or throat, where they cause inflammation. Some types of *Corynebacterium diphtheriae* release a potent toxin, which can damage the heart and brain.

Symptoms

The infection begins 1 to 4 days after exposure to the bacteria. Symptoms usually begin with a mild sore throat and pain when swallowing. Generally, the child has a low-grade fever, a fast heart rate, nausea, vomiting, chills, and a headache. The lymph nodes in the neck may swell. The child may have a runny nose, often affecting only one nostril, if the bacteria are localized in the nose. The inflammation may spread from the throat to the voice box (larynx) and may make the throat swell, narrowing the airway and making breathing extremely difficult.

Typically, the bacteria form a pseudomembrane—a sheet of material composed of dead white blood cells, bacteria, and other substances—near the tonsils or other parts of the throat. The pseudomembrane is tough and has a dirty gray color. If the pseudomembrane is forcibly removed, the underlying mucous membranes may bleed. The pseudomembrane may narrow the airway or may suddenly become detached and block the airway completely, preventing the child from being able to breathe—an emergency situation. Some children with mild diphtheria, however, never develop a pseudomembrane.

If the bacteria release a toxin, the toxin travels through the bloodstream and can damage tissues around the body, especially the heart and nerves. Damage to the heart muscle (myocarditis) is usually most severe by day 10 to 14, but it can occur at any time between the first and sixth week. Damage to the heart may be only slight, showing up as minor abnormalities on an electrocardiogram, or very severe, leading to heart failure and sudden death.

The toxin generally affects certain nerves, such as those to the throat, making swallowing difficult. These nerves are often affected during the first week of illness. Between the third and sixth weeks, nerves to the arms and legs may become inflamed, causing weakness. The heart and nerves recover slowly over many weeks.

Diphtheria may also affect the skin (cutaneous diphtheria). Although it is more common in the tropics, cutaneous diphtheria also occurs in the United States, particularly among people with poor hygiene living in crowded conditions (for example, homeless people). In rare instances, diphtheria affects the eye.

Diagnosis and Treatment

A doctor investigates the possibility of diphtheria in a sick child who has a sore throat with a pseudomembrane. The diagnosis may be confirmed by taking a sample of the membrane from the child's throat with a swab and growing the bacteria in a laboratory.

A child with symptoms of diphtheria is hospitalized in an intensive care unit. As soon as possible, the child is given an antitoxin (antibody to neutralize circulating diphtheria toxin). However, the doctor must first make sure that the child isn't allergic to the antitoxin, which is made from horse serum, by performing special skin tests. A child who is allergic must be desensitized first; to do so, a very small dose and then progressively larger doses of antitoxin are given.

In the intensive care unit, doctors and nurses ensure that breathing doesn't become obstructed and that the heart is functioning satisfactorily. Antibiotics, such as penicillin or erythromycin, are given to eradicate the diphtheria bacteria.

Recovery from severe diphtheria is slow, and a child with the infection must avoid resuming activities too soon. Even normal physical exertion may harm an inflamed heart.

Prevention

Children are routinely immunized against diphtheria. The diphtheria vaccine is usually combined with vaccines for tetanus and whooping cough (pertussis), as the DTP (diphtheria-tetanus-pertussis) vaccine.▲ If someone who has been vaccinated against diphtheria is exposed to a person with the infection, a booster dose offers increased protection.

Anyone exposed to a child who is infected with diphtheria should be examined, and a throat swab should be sent to a laboratory for culture. Preventive antibiotics are given for 7 days, and the person is observed for evidence of the disease. A vaccination or booster dose containing the diphtheria bacterium should be given to anyone who is in close contact with an infected child and who has not received a diphtheria vaccination or a booster within the previous 5 years. People with normal throat cultures who have recently been vaccinated against diphtheria don't need treatment and aren't considered a risk to others.

▲ see box, page 1200

However, carriers of diphtheria bacteria (who don't have symptoms) can spread the disease; therefore, these people also require antibiotics and repeated throat cultures for evidence of disease.

Pertussis

Pertussis (whooping cough) is a highly contagious infection caused by the bacterium Bordetella pertussis, *which results in fits of coughing that usually end in a prolonged, high-pitched, deeply indrawn breath (the whoop).*

Pertussis, once rampant in the United States and still a major problem throughout the world, has again become more common in the United States since the late 1980s. Local epidemics occur every 2 to 4 years. A person may develop pertussis at any age, but half the cases occur in children under age 4. One attack of pertussis doesn't always give full immunity for life, but a second attack, if it occurs, is usually mild and not always recognized as pertussis.

An infected person spreads pertussis organisms into the air in droplets of moisture produced by coughing. Anyone nearby may inhale these droplets and become infected. A person with pertussis usually isn't contagious after the third week of the illness.

Symptoms and Diagnosis

Symptoms begin, on the average, 7 to 10 days after exposure to pertussis bacteria. The bacteria invade the lining of the throat, windpipe, and airways, increasing the secretion of mucus. At first the mucus is thin, but later it becomes thick and sticky. The infection lasts about 6 weeks, progressing through three stages: mild coldlike symptoms (catarrhal stage), severe coughing fits (paroxysmal stage), and gradual recovery (convalescent stage).

A doctor who sees a child in the first (catarrhal) stage has to distinguish pertussis from bronchitis, influenza and other viral infections, and perhaps tuberculosis, which have similar symptoms. The doctor takes samples of mucus from the nose and throat with a small swab. The sample is then cultured. If a child is in the early stage, a culture can identify the pertussis bacteria 80 to 90 per-

---

Bacterial Infections Preventable With Routine Immunization*

- Diphtheria
- Infection with *Hemophilus influenzae* type b (meningitis, epiglottitis, some severe eye infections, some types of occult bacteremia)
- Pertussis
- Tetanus

*Note: Many viral infections can also be prevented with routine immunization (see box, page 1200).

---

cent of the time. Unfortunately, the bacteria are difficult to grow later in the illness, even though the cough is at its worst. Results can be obtained faster by analyzing the samples for pertussis bacteria using special antibody stains, but this technique is less reliable.

Complications

The most common complications involve the airway. Infants are particularly at risk for damage that occurs from lack of oxygen after pauses in breathing (apnea) or coughing fits. Children may develop pneumonia, which can be fatal. During coughing fits, air may be driven out of the lungs into the surrounding tissue, or the lungs may rupture and collapse (pneumothorax). Severe coughing fits can cause bleeding in the eyes, the mucous membranes, and occasionally the skin or brain. A sore may develop under the tongue if the tongue is pushed against the lower teeth during coughing fits. Occasionally, coughing may cause an outpouching of the rectum (rectal prolapse) or a hernia at the navel, which may be seen as a bulge.

Convulsions may occur in infants but are rare in older children. Bleeding, swelling, or inflammation in the brain may cause brain damage and mental retardation, paralysis, or other neurologic problems. Ear infections (otitis media) also develop frequently as a result of pertussis.

Stages of Pertussis

First (Catarrhal) Stage	Second (Paroxysmal) Stage	Third (Convalescent) Stage
Onset		
Begins gradually 7 to 10 days (no more than 3 weeks) after exposure	Begins 10 to 14 days after first symptoms	Begins 4 to 6 weeks after first symptoms
Symptoms		
Sneezing, watery eyes, other coldlike symptoms; no appetite; listlessness; a troublesome, hacking cough, first at night, then increasingly during the day as well; fever is rare	Coughing fit of 5 to 15 or more rapid consecutive coughs followed by the whoop (a hurried, deep intake of breath that makes a high-pitched noise). After a few normal breaths, another coughing fit may begin. Large amounts of thick mucus may be coughed up (usually swallowed by infants and children or seen as large bubbles from the nose) during or after the coughing fit. A prolonged fit of coughing or thick mucus may cause vomiting. In infants, choking spells and pauses in breathing (apnea), possibly causing the skin to turn blue, are more common than whoops	Coughing fits become less frequent and severe; vomiting decreases; child looks and feels better. Occasional coughing fits can occur for months, usually triggered by irritation from a respiratory tract infection, such as a cold

Prognosis and Treatment

The vast majority of children with pertussis recover completely, although slowly. About 1 to 2 percent of the children under age 1 die. The disease can be serious in any child under age 2 and is troublesome but rarely serious in older children and adults. However, it is older children and adults with mild disease who most likely transmit pertussis to younger children.

Severely ill infants are usually hospitalized because they need nursing care and oxygen; they may need treatment in an intensive care unit. These infants are generally kept in a darkened, quiet room and are disturbed as little as possible. A disturbance can provoke a coughing fit, which may cause breathing difficulties. Older children who have a mild disease don't need to stay in bed.

During treatment, mucus may be suctioned out of the throat. If needed in severe cases, a tube is placed into the windpipe to deliver oxygen directly to the lungs. Cough medicines are of questionable value and aren't usually used.

Intravenous fluids may be given to replace fluids lost during vomiting and because coughing may prevent infants from being able to feed. Good nutrition is important, and small, frequent meals are best for older children.

The antibiotic erythromycin is usually used to eradicate the bacteria causing pertussis. Antibiotics are also used for infections that accompany the pertussis, such as bronchopneumonia and middle ear infection.

Prevention

Children are routinely immunized against pertussis. The pertussis vaccine is usually combined with vaccines for diphtheria and tetanus as the

DTP (diphtheria-tetanus-pertussis) vaccine.▲ The antibiotic erythromycin is given as a prophylactic measure to those exposed to pertussis.

Occult Bacteremia

Occult (hidden) bacteremia is the presence of bacteria in the bloodstream, although no infection is apparent anywhere else in the body and the child doesn't seem particularly sick.

Occult bacteremia accounts for up to 4 percent of the fevers in infants between the ages of 1 and 24 months. In more than 75 percent of all cases, the infection is caused by the bacterium *Streptococcus pneumoniae*. Sometimes the child has a mild respiratory tract infection or a sore throat, but often the only symptom is a fever (usually 101.3° F. or higher). The only way the diagnosis can be made is by detecting bacteria in a blood sample. Nonspecific tests, such as white blood cell counts, are used to help decide if the risk of bacterial infection (as opposed to viral infection) is such that antibiotics are required before final blood culture tests are available. Occult bacteremia is treated with antibiotics.

Infectious Gastroenteritis

Infectious gastroenteritis is an infection of the gastrointestinal (digestive) tract, causing vomiting and diarrhea.■

A wide variety of bacteria can cause gastroenteritis. Some bacteria cause symptoms by producing toxins; others grow on the intestinal wall. If they grow inside the wall, they can enter the bloodstream. Viruses and parasites, such as *Giardia*, can also cause gastroenteritis. In fact, one virus (the rotavirus) is responsible for almost half of the cases of severe diarrhea that result in hospitalization in the United States and in developing countries. Bacteria and parasites are somewhat less important in the United States than in developing countries, but they cause outbreaks of food poisoning and diarrhea as well. The consequences of severe diarrhea are quite different in industrialized countries and developing countries. For example, despite millions of episodes of diarrhea in children in the United States every year, there are only several hundred deaths,

whereas diarrheal disease kills more than 3 million children younger than 5 years of age every year in developing countries.

Symptoms and Diagnosis

Gastroenteritis normally produces vomiting and diarrhea. To determine the cause, a doctor considers whether a child may have been exposed to a source of infection (such as a particular food, animal, or ill person), how long the child has had symptoms, what the symptoms are, and how often the child vomits or has diarrhea. The doctor also considers the child's age.

As early as 24 hours after the appearance of gastroenteritis, infants under 6 months of age may become dehydrated, losing too much water and salts (electrolytes).★ However, any child may become dehydrated within 24 hours if the vomiting and diarrhea are severe and fluid intake is inadequate. A dehydrated infant may have a poor appetite, a dry mouth, a fever, and a low urine output and may be thirsty and lose weight. More severe dehydration causes the eyes to appear sunken and dry, and the soft spot at the top of the head (fontanelle) also appears sunken. The child may be drowsy. In older infants and overweight young children, symptoms may not appear until the dehydration is critical. These children may be very weak and may have warm, dry skin and sunken, dry eyes.

Treatment

At first, fluids and electrolytes are given—usually in an oral solution but intravenously if the dehydration is severe—to replace fluids and electrolytes lost through vomiting and diarrhea. Older infants and otherwise healthy children are given antibiotics only for certain bacteria and parasites, such as those that cause bloody diarrhea or cholera. Infants under 6 months old and those with an impaired immune system are treated with antibiotics, even when they have no sign of an

---

▲ see box, page 1200

■ see page 514

★ see page 665

infection outside the intestine. Antibiotics are of no value when gastroenteritis is caused by a virus. If the diarrhea is associated with travel and the diarrhea is severe or persistent, antibiotics are often used.

Severe Bacterial Eye Infections

Severe bacterial eye infections cause swelling and redness of the eyelid, the skin surrounding the eye (periorbital cellulitis), *and the area inside the eye socket* (orbital cellulitis).

The area around the eyes can become infected if a child had a wound, insect bite, or sinus infection (sinusitis). An infection can also spread to the eyes from elsewhere in the body by way of the bloodstream. Simple eye infections, such as pinkeye (conjunctivitis), are caused by either bacteria or viruses. Reddened eyes also may be a sign of an allergy.▲ Simple eye infections and eye problems caused by allergies are much more common than the severe eye infections of periorbital and orbital cellulitis.

Symptoms

The first symptom of a severe eye infection is usually swollen, red eyelids. In more than 90 percent of the children who have an eye infection, only one eye is affected. Most children have a fever, about 20 percent have a runny nose, and another 20 percent have an infection of the whites of the eyes (pinkeye, or conjunctivitis). When orbital cellulitis is present, the eye is pushed forward, which paralyzes the eye muscles so that the eye can't move. The eye hurts, and vision is impaired. In periorbital cellulitis especially, but also with orbital cellulitis, the eyelid may be so swollen than an ophthalmologist must open the eye with special equipment.

Orbital cellulitis may cause a blood clot that blocks the main artery or vein supplying the retina. Such a blockage damages the retina and may cause blindness in the infected eye. Sometimes the infection spreads from the eye socket to the brain, causing an abscess, or to the membranes

covering the brain, causing bacterial meningitis. Blood clots may block the veins supplying the brain, causing headaches, loss of consciousness, and even death. Periorbital cellulitis may be associated with a bloodstream infection, but it generally does not spread to the eye socket (orbit) or brain.

Diagnosis and Treatment

A doctor examines the eye for evidence of infection and determines whether the eye can still move, whether it is pushed forward, and whether vision has deteriorated. A blood sample may help identify the bacteria causing the infection. Computed tomography (CT) may help locate the infection and determine how far it has spread.

Children with severe eye infections are hospitalized, and intravenous antibiotic therapy is started immediately. Periorbital cellulitis may require 10 to 14 days of antibiotic treatment (first given intravenously and perhaps later by mouth). Orbital cellulitis may require surgical drainage as well as 2 to 3 weeks of antibiotic treatment (for the most part given intravenously). Some episodes of mild periorbital cellulitis may respond to antibiotics given by mouth. The more common but less severe pinkeye (conjunctivitis) may be treated either with antibiotic eyedrops or ointment or with antibiotics given by mouth for 7 to 10 days, provided the cause is a bacterium rather than a virus.

Epiglottitis

Epiglottitis (sometimes called supraglottitis) is a severe infection of the epiglottis, which can rapidly grow worse and cause respiratory obstruction and death.

The epiglottis is the structure that closes the entrance to the voice box and windpipe (larynx and trachea) during swallowing. An infection of the epiglottis is almost always caused by the bacterium *Hemophilus influenzae* type b. Very rarely, streptococci bacteria are responsible, especially in older children and adults. Epiglottitis is most common in children 2 to 5 years old. It is uncommon in children under age 2 but may affect people of any age, including adults.

The infection usually begins in the upper respiratory tract as inflammation of the nose and

---

▲ see page 826

throat. The infection then moves down into the epiglottis. Often, the infection is associated with bacteria in the bloodstream (bacteremia).

Symptoms

Epiglottitis can quickly become fatal, because swelling of the infected tissue may block the airway and cut off breathing.

The infection usually begins suddenly and progresses rapidly. A previously healthy child develops a sore throat, hoarseness, and often a high fever. Difficulty in swallowing and breathing are common. The child usually drools, breathes rapidly, and wheezes while inhaling. The difficulty in breathing often induces the child to lean forward while stretching the neck backward to try to increase the amount of air reaching the lungs. Labored breathing may lead to a buildup of carbon dioxide and low oxygen levels in the bloodstream. The swollen epiglottis makes coughing up mucus difficult. All these factors may lead to death within a few hours.

Pneumonia may accompany epiglottitis. The infection also sometimes spreads to the joints, the lining of the brain, the sac around the heart, or the tissue beneath the skin.

Diagnosis and Treatment

Epiglottitis is an emergency, and a child is hospitalized immediately when a doctor suspects it. The diagnosis is made by examining the epiglottis with a laryngoscope. However, such an examination can lead to obstruction of the airway, which can cause sudden death. Therefore, this procedure is usually performed by specialists, ideally in an operating room after the child is under general anesthesia. If obstruction occurs, the doctor immediately reopens the airway, either by inserting a rigid tube (endotracheal tube) into the airway or by making an opening through the front of the neck (tracheostomy).

The doctor takes samples of secretions from the upper respiratory tract and from the blood and sends them to the laboratory for culture. However, treatment with antibiotics is started before the results of the culture are available.

Prevention

A vaccine against *Hemophilus influenzae* type b is available. Therefore, epiglottitis may now be preventable by immunizing infants. Fortunately, in the United States, epiglottitis is becoming a rare

disease because of routine immunization. The first in a series of immunizations against *Hemophilus influenzae* type b is generally given at age 2 months.▲

Retropharyngeal Abscess

A retropharyngeal abscess is an infection of the lymph nodes at the back of the throat.

Because the lymph nodes at the back of the throat disappear after childhood, a retropharyngeal abscess is unusual in adults, although other neck and throat abscesses do occur in adults. An abscess is usually caused by a streptococcal infection that has spread from the tonsils, throat, sinuses, adenoids, nose, or middle ear. An injury to the back of the throat from a sharp object, such as a fish bone, occasionally causes a retropharyngeal abscess. Rarely, tuberculosis can also cause a retropharyngeal abscess.

Symptoms and Diagnosis

The main symptoms of a retropharyngeal abscess are pain when swallowing, a fever, and enlargement of the lymph nodes in the neck. The abscess can block the airway, causing difficulty in breathing. The child tends to tilt the head and neck back and raise the chin to facilitate breathing.

Complications include bleeding around the abscess, rupture of the abscess into the airway (which can block the airway), and pneumonia. The larynx may go into spasm and further interfere with breathing. Blood clots may form in the jugular veins of the neck. Infection may spread down into the chest.

After observing the symptoms of a retropharyngeal abscess, a doctor orders x-rays and computed tomography (CT) scans to confirm the diagnosis.

Treatment

Most abscesses need to be drained, which is done surgically by cutting open the abscess and allowing the pus to drain out. Penicillin, clindamycin, or other antibiotics are given, at first intravenously, then orally.

▲ see box, page 1200

Viral Infections

A number of viral infections are common in children. Because most childhood viral infections aren't serious and most children with a viral infection get better without treatment, a doctor usually doesn't need to have a laboratory identify the specific virus involved. Some infections are so distinctive that a doctor can diagnose them based on their symptoms.

Measles

Measles (rubeola, 9-day measles) is a highly contagious viral infection producing various symptoms and a characteristic rash.

People become infected with measles mainly by breathing in small airborne droplets of moisture coughed out by an infected person. A person infected with the measles virus is contagious 2 to 4 days before the rash appears and remains so until the rash disappears.

Before vaccination became widely available, measles epidemics occurred every 2 or 3 years, particularly in preschool-aged and school-aged children, with small localized outbreaks during intervening years. Outbreaks now typically occur in previously immunized teenagers and young adults, as well as in young children (unimmunized preschool-aged children and infants who are too young for the vaccine, that is, 12 months old or younger). A woman who has had measles or been vaccinated passes immunity (in the form of antibodies) to her child; this immunity lasts most of the first year of life. Thereafter, however, susceptibility to measles is high. A single attack of measles makes a person immune for life.

Symptoms and Diagnosis

The symptoms of measles begin about 7 to 14 days after infection. An infected person first develops a fever, runny nose, sore throat, hacking cough, and red eyes. Tiny white spots (Koplik's

spots) appear inside the mouth 2 to 4 days later. A mildly itchy rash appears 3 to 5 days after the start of symptoms. The rash begins in front of and below the ears and on the side of the neck as irregular, flat, red areas that soon become raised. The rash spreads within 1 to 2 days to the trunk, arms, and legs, as it begins to fade on the face.

At the peak of the illness, the person feels very sick, the rash is extensive, and the temperature may exceed 104° F. In 3 to 5 days, the temperature falls, the person begins to feel better, and any remaining rash quickly fades. The diagnosis is based on the typical symptoms and characteristic rash. No special tests are performed.

Prognosis and Complications

In healthy, well-nourished children, measles is rarely serious. However, complicating bacterial infections, such as pneumonia (especially in infants) or a middle ear infection, occur fairly often, and people with measles are especially susceptible to infection with streptococci bacteria. Blood platelet levels may become so low that the child bruises and bleeds easily, but this happens rarely.

Brain infection (encephalitis) complicates about 1 in 1,000 to 2,000 cases. If encephalitis occurs, it often starts with a high fever, convulsions, and coma, usually 2 days to 3 weeks after the rash appears. The illness may be brief, with recovery in about 1 week, or it may be prolonged, resulting in serious brain damage or death. In rare cases, subacute sclerosing panencephalitis—a serious complication of measles—may occur months to years later, resulting in brain damage.

Prevention and Treatment

Measles vaccine is one of the routine immunizations of childhood.▲ The vaccine is usually given in combination with mumps and rubella vaccines and is injected into muscle in the thigh or upper arm.

A child with measles is kept warm and comfortable. Acetaminophen or ibuprofen may be given to reduce fever. If a secondary bacterial infection develops, an antibiotic is prescribed.

▲ see box, page 1200

Some Viral Infections at a Glance

Infection	Period of Incubation	Period of Contagiousness	Site of Rash	Nature of Rash
Measles (rubeola)	7 to 14 days	From 2 to 4 days before the appearance of the rash until 2 to 5 days after the onset	Starts around the ears and on the face and neck, and in more severe cases spreads over the trunk, arms, and legs	Irregular, flat, red areas that soon become raised; begins 3 to 5 days after the onset of symptoms; lasts 4 to 7 days
German measles (rubella)	14 to 21 days	From shortly before the onset of symptoms until the rash disappears; infected newborns are usually infective for many months	Starts on the face and neck; spreads to the trunk, arms, and legs	Fine, pinkish, flat rash; begins 1 or 2 days after the onset of symptoms; lasts 1 to 3 days
Roseola infantum	Probably 5 to 15 days	Unknown	Found on the chest and abdomen, with moderate involvement of the face, arms, and legs	Red and flat, possibly with raised areas; begins on about the 4th day, appearing as body temperature drops suddenly to normal; lasts 1 or 2 days
Erythema infectiosum (fifth disease)	4 to 14 days	From before the onset of the rash until a few days after	Starts on the cheeks; spreads to the arms, legs, and trunk	Red and flat with raised areas, often blotchy and with lacy patterns; begins shortly after the onset of symptoms; lasts 5 to 10 days; may recur for several weeks
Chickenpox (varicella)	14 to 21 days	From a few days before the onset of symptoms until all crops of vesicles have crusted	Usually appears first on the trunk; later on the face, neck, arms, and legs; infrequently on the palms and soles	Small, flat, red spots that become raised and form round, fluid-filled blisters against a red background before finally crusting; appears in crops, so various stages are present simultaneously; begins shortly after the onset of symptoms; lasts a few days to 2 weeks

Subacute Sclerosing Panencephalitis

Subacute sclerosing panencephalitis, a progressive and usually fatal disorder, is a rare complication of measles that appears months or years later and produces mental deterioration, muscle jerks, and seizures.

Subacute sclerosing panencephalitis probably results from brain infection by the measles virus. The virus may enter the brain during a measles infection and remain in the brain without causing problems for a long time. However, the virus can become reactivated for unknown reasons and cause subacute sclerosing panencephalitis. In very rare instances, a person who never had measles but received live measles vaccine may develop subacute sclerosing panencephalitis.

The number of people with subacute sclerosing panencephalitis is declining in the United States and Western Europe. Males are affected more frequently than females.

Symptoms and Diagnosis

The disease usually begins in children or young adults, generally before age 20. The first symptoms may be poor performance in schoolwork, forgetfulness, temper outbursts, distractibility, sleeplessness, and hallucinations. Seizures follow, appearing as sudden muscular jerks of the arms, head, or body. Eventually, seizures may affect the whole body, together with abnormal uncontrollable muscle movements. The intellect continues to deteriorate, and the speech changes. Later, the muscles become increasingly rigid, and swallowing may become difficult. The person may become blind. In the final phases, the body temperature may rise, and the blood pressure and pulse become abnormal.

A doctor makes the diagnosis based on the symptoms. The diagnosis may be confirmed by a blood test that reveals high levels of antibody to the measles virus, by an abnormal electroencephalogram (EEG), or by magnetic resonance imaging (MRI) or computed tomography (CT) scans that show brain abnormalities.

Prognosis and Treatment

The disease is nearly always fatal within 1 to 3 years. Although the cause of death is usually pneumonia, the pneumonia results from the extreme weakness and abnormal muscle control caused by this disease.

Nothing can be done to halt progression of the disease. Anticonvulsant drugs may be taken to control or reduce seizures.

German Measles

German measles (rubella, 3-day measles) is a contagious viral infection that produces mild symptoms, such as joint pain and a rash.

▲ see page 1218

■ see page 1223

German measles is spread mainly by breathing in small virus-containing droplets of moisture that have been coughed into the air by an infected person. Close contact with an infected person can also spread the infection. A person is contagious from 1 week before the rash appears until 1 week after the rash disappears. An infant infected before birth can be contagious for many months after birth.▲

German measles is less contagious than measles, and many children never become infected. Nevertheless, German measles is serious, especially in pregnant women. A woman infected during the first 16 weeks (particularly the first 8 to 10 weeks) of pregnancy may miscarry, give birth to a stillborn baby, or have a baby with birth defects.■ About 10 to 15 percent of young adult women have never had German measles, so they could be at risk of having children with serious birth defects if they become infected during early pregnancy.

Epidemics occur at irregular intervals during the spring. Major epidemics occur about every 6 to 9 years. In the United States, the number of cases of German measles and of infants infected with German measles before birth started to increase in 1988, but this trend peaked in 1991. Now the number of cases is lower than ever. A single attack of German measles gives a person lifelong immunity.

Symptoms and Diagnosis

Symptoms begin about 14 to 21 days after infection. In children, the illness begins with a 1- to 5-day period of feeling mildly ill, with swollen lymph nodes in the neck and back of the head and occasional joint pain. The throat isn't sore but becomes red at the start of the illness. These early symptoms may be very mild or may not occur at all in adolescents and adults. A mild rash also develops and lasts about 3 days. The rash begins on the face and neck and quickly spreads to the trunk, arms, and legs. As the rash appears, a mild reddening of the skin (flush) occurs, particularly on the face. Rose-colored spots appear on the roof of the mouth, later merging with each other into a red blush and extending over the back of the mouth.

The diagnosis is based on the typical symptoms. However, many cases of German measles are misdiagnosed or are mild and go unnoticed. A definite diagnosis, necessary during pregnancy, can be made by measuring blood levels of antibodies to rubella virus.

Prognosis and Complications

Most children with German measles recover fully. Teenage boys or men may experience temporary pain in the testes. Up to one third of women develop arthritis or joint pain with German measles. In rare instances, a middle ear infection (otitis media) develops. Brain infection (encephalitis) is a rare and occasionally fatal complication. German measles in a pregnant woman can be very serious, resulting in possible birth defects, stillbirth, or miscarriage.

Prevention and Treatment

German measles (rubella) vaccine is one of the routine immunizations of childhood.▲ The vaccine is usually injected into muscle in combination with mumps and measles vaccines.

Symptoms of German measles are seldom severe enough to need treatment. A middle ear infection■ can be treated with antibiotics, but no treatment can cure encephalitis.

Progressive Rubella Panencephalitis

Progressive rubella panencephalitis is a very rare progressive brain disorder in children who have birth defects resulting from their mother's exposure to the rubella virus during pregnancy.

A fetus exposed to the rubella virus during gestation may be born with birth defects, such as deafness, cataracts, a small head, and mental retardation. In addition, the virus may lie dormant in the brain and become reactivated, for unknown reasons, when the child is older, particularly in the early teenage years. When this happens, a child may develop progressive worsening muscle stiffness (spasticity), poor coordination, mental deterioration, and seizures. A blood test may show high levels of antibodies against rubella virus, and a computed tomography (CT) or magnetic resonance imaging (MRI) scan may show abnormalities in the brain. No known treatment can cure this disorder.

Roseola Infantum

Roseola infantum is a contagious viral infection of infants or very young children that causes a rash and high fever.

Roseola occurs most often in the spring and fall, sometimes in local outbreaks. The usual cause is herpesvirus 6, one of many herpes viruses.

Symptoms and Diagnosis

Symptoms begin about 5 to 15 days after infection. A fever of 103° to 105° F. begins abruptly and lasts for 3 to 5 days. Convulsions known as febrile seizures are common during the early hours of the infection, particularly as the temperature rises. Despite the high fever, the child is usually alert and active. The lymph nodes at the back of the head, the sides of the neck, and behind the ears may be enlarged. The spleen may also be slightly enlarged. The fever usually disappears on the fourth day.

About 30 percent of children develop a rash, often as the temperature falls. The rash is red and flat, but it may have raised areas, mostly on the chest and abdomen and less extensively on the face, arms, and legs. The rash isn't itchy and may last from a few hours to 2 days.

A doctor makes the diagnosis based on the symptoms. Antibody tests and a culture of the virus are rarely needed.

Treatment

Symptoms are treated as necessary. Reducing the fever is important, particularly if the child has been having febrile seizures. Acetaminophen or ibuprofen, not aspirin, may be used to reduce the fever. Aspirin isn't given to children or teenagers because it increases the risk of Reye's syndrome.★

Erythema Infectiosum

Erythema infectiosum (fifth disease) is a contagious viral infection causing a blotchy or raised red rash with mild illness.

Erythema infectiosum is caused by human parvovirus B19 and occurs most often during the

---

▲ see box, page 1200

■ see page 1006

★ see page 1280

spring months, often in geographically limited outbreaks among children and teenagers. Infection is spread mainly by breathing in small droplets of moisture that have been breathed out by an infected person. The infection can also be transmitted from mother to fetus during pregnancy, possibly causing stillbirth or severe anemia and excess fluid and swelling (edema) in the fetus.

Symptoms, Diagnosis, and Treatment

Symptoms begin about 4 to 14 days after infection. Symptoms can vary, and some people have none. A child with erythema infectiosum typically has a low fever, feels mildly ill, and develops red cheeks that often look like they have been slapped. Within a day or two, a rash appears, especially on the arms, legs, and trunk but not usually on the palms or soles. The rash isn't itchy and consists of raised, blotchy red areas and lacy patterns, particularly on areas of the arms not covered by clothing, because the rash may be worsened by exposure to sunlight.

The illness generally lasts 5 to 10 days. Over the next several weeks, the rash may temporarily reappear in response to sunlight, exercise, heat, fever, or emotional stress. In adults, mild joint pain and swelling may remain or come and go for weeks to months.

A doctor makes the diagnosis based on the characteristic appearance of the rash. Blood tests can help identify the virus. Treatment is aimed at relieving the symptoms.

Chickenpox

Chickenpox (varicella) is a contagious viral infection that produces a characteristic itchy rash, consisting of clusters of small raised or flat spots, fluid-filled blisters, and crusting.

Chickenpox, which is highly contagious, is spread by airborne droplets of moisture containing the varicella-zoster virus. A person with chickenpox is most contagious just after symptoms start but remains contagious until the last blisters have crusted. Isolation of an infected person helps prevent the spread of infection to people who haven't had chickenpox.

A person who has had chickenpox develops immunity and can't contract it again. However, the varicella-zoster virus remains dormant in the body after an initial infection with chickenpox, sometimes reactivating in later life, causing shingles.▲

Symptoms and Diagnosis

Symptoms begin 10 to 21 days after infection. In children over age 10, the first symptoms are mild headache, moderate fever, and a feeling of illness (malaise). Younger children usually don't have these symptoms, and symptoms are usually more severe in adults.

About 24 to 36 hours after the first symptoms begin, a rash of small, flat, red areas (spots) appears. Each spot soon becomes raised; forms an itchy, round, fluid-filled blister (bleb) against a red background; and finally crusts. The whole sequence takes 6 to 8 hours. Successive clusters (crops) of spots continue to develop and crust. New spots usually stop appearing by the fifth day, the majority are crusted by the sixth day, and most disappear in fewer than 20 days.

The face, arms, and legs have relatively few spots, except in severe cases when the entire body surface is affected. When the person has only a few spots, they are usually on the upper trunk. Spots frequently appear on the scalp. Spots in the mouth quickly rupture and form raw sores (ulcers), which often make swallowing painful. Raw sores may also occur on the eyelids and in the upper airways, rectum, and vagina. Spots in the voice box and upper airways may occasionally cause severe difficulty in breathing. Lymph nodes at the side of the neck may become enlarged and tender. The worst part of the illness usually lasts 4 to 7 days.

A doctor is usually certain of the diagnosis of chickenpox because the rash and the other symptoms are so typical. A measurement of the blood levels of antibodies and laboratory identification of the virus are rarely needed.

Complications

Children usually recover from chickenpox without problems. However, the infection may be severe or even fatal in adults and especially in people (children or adults) with an impaired immune system.

▲ see page 918

Pneumonia caused by the virus is a serious complication that may occur, particularly in adults, newborns, or anyone with an impaired immune system. The heart may become inflamed, possibly causing a heart murmur. Joint inflammation may cause joint pain. The liver may become inflamed, but usually there are no symptoms. Occasionally the person has bleeding within the tissues. The skin sores may become infected by bacteria, causing erysipelas,▲ pyoderma, or bullous impetigo.■

Brain infection (encephalitis), which may occur toward the end of the illness or 1 to 2 weeks after, affects less than 1 in 1,000 cases. The encephalitis may cause headaches, vomiting, unsteadiness in walking, confusion, and seizures. Although the encephalitis may be fatal, the chances for complete recovery are generally good. Reye's syndrome, an unusual but very severe complication occurring almost only in those under age 18, may begin 3 to 8 days after the rash begins.★

Prevention and Treatment

A vaccine is available to prevent chickenpox. Antibodies against the varicella virus (zoster immune globulin or varicella-zoster immune globulin) may be given to people who haven't been vaccinated and are at high risk of complications, such as those with an impaired immune system.

Mild cases of chickenpox require only the treatment of symptoms. Wet compresses on the skin help soothe itching, which may be intense, and prevent scratching, which may spread the infection and cause scars. Because of the risk of bacterial infection, the skin is bathed often with soap and water, the hands are kept clean, the nails are clipped to minimize scratching, and clothing is kept clean and dry.

Drugs that relieve itching, such as antihistamines, are sometimes used. If a bacterial infection develops, antibiotics may be needed. Severe cases of chickenpox may be treated with the antiviral drug acyclovir.

Mumps

Mumps is a contagious viral infection causing painful enlargement of the salivary glands. The infection may also affect other organs, especially in adults.

Mumps is caused by a paramyxovirus, a relative of the measles virus. It is spread by breathing in virus-containing droplets of moisture sneezed or coughed into the air or by having direct contact with objects contaminated by infected saliva.

Mumps is less contagious than measles or chickenpox. In heavily populated areas, it occurs year-round but is most frequent in late winter and early spring. Epidemics may occur when susceptible people are crowded together. Although the disease may occur at any age, most cases are in children 5 to 15 years old. The disease is unusual in children under 2 years old. One infection with the mumps virus usually provides lifelong immunity.

Symptoms and Diagnosis

The virus infects the salivary glands. Symptoms begin 14 to 24 days after infection. Chills, headache, poor appetite, a feeling of illness (malaise), and a low to moderate fever may develop 12 to 24 hours before one or more salivary glands begin to swell, but 25 to 30 percent of people don't have these symptoms. The first symptom of salivary gland infection is pain when chewing or swallowing, particularly when swallowing acidic liquids, such as citrus fruit juices. The glands are tender when touched. At this stage, the temperature usually rises to 103° or 104° F. The salivary glands are most swollen around the second day.

Doctors investigate the possibility of mumps when a person has swollen salivary glands. The diagnosis is especially likely if the person has swollen salivary glands during a mumps outbreak. At other times, tests may be needed to rule out other possible causes. Laboratory tests can identify the mumps virus and its antibodies, but such tests are rarely needed to make the diagnosis.

Prognosis and Complications

Almost all children with mumps recover fully without problems, but in rare cases symptoms may worsen again after about 2 weeks.

Complications can involve organs other than the salivary glands, particularly in people who become infected after puberty. Complications may occur before, during, or after swelling of the

---

▲ see page 977

■ see page 976

★ see page 1280

A Child With Mumps

A child with mumps will likely develop a tender swelling between the ear and the angle of the lower jaw.

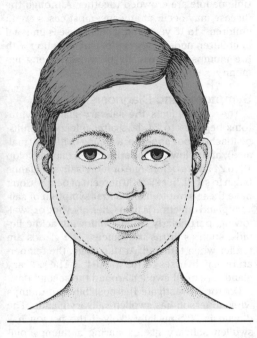

salivary glands, or they may occur without the salivary glands being involved.

About 20 percent of men who become infected after puberty develop painful inflammation of one or both testes (a condition called orchitis). On healing, the affected testis may shrink. In rare cases, the testis is permanently damaged. Sterility may result if both testes are damaged. Inflammation of one or both ovaries in females (oophoritis) is another rare complication. It causes slight abdominal pain and rarely causes infertility.

Mumps can lead to viral inflammation of the brain or its covering (encephalitis or meningitis), causing headache, stiff neck, drowsiness, coma, or convulsions. About 5 to 10 percent of people

▲ see box, page 1200

■ see page 1280

with mumps develop meningitis; most of these people recover completely. About 1 in every 400 to 6,000 people with mumps develops encephalitis; a person who does so is more likely to have permanent nerve or brain damage, such as nerve deafness or paralysis of the facial muscles. Such damage usually affects only one side of the body.

Pancreatitis, inflammation of the pancreas, may occur toward the end of the first week. This condition may cause mild or severe nausea and vomiting with pain in the abdomen. These symptoms disappear in about a week, and the person recovers completely.

Inflammation may affect a number of other organs. For example, if inflammation affects the kidneys, the person may pass large amounts of dilute urine; joint inflammation may cause pain in one or more joints.

Prevention and Treatment

Vaccination against mumps is routine in childhood.▲ Mumps vaccine is usually injected into muscle in combination with measles and rubella vaccines.

Once the infection has started, it just has to run its course. Because chewing may be painful, eating soft foods may be necessary. Acidic foods and fluids, such as citrus fruit juices, cause the salivary gland to secrete saliva, which may be painful. Analgesics such as acetaminophen and ibuprofen may be used for headache and discomfort. Aspirin isn't used for children or teenagers because it may increase the risk of Reye's syndrome.■

Boys or men with testicular swelling require bed rest. The scrotum may be supported by applying cotton to an adhesive tape bridge connected between the thighs. Ice packs may be applied to relieve pain.

If pancreatitis causes severe nausea and vomiting, intravenous fluids may be given.

Respiratory Syncytial Virus Infection

Respiratory syncytial virus infection is a contagious viral disease affecting the lungs.

Respiratory syncytial virus causes outbreaks of lung disease every year in late autumn or in winter. Infection is caused either by inhaling airborne droplets containing the virus or by touching an infected person or objects. Respiratory syncytial virus is the major cause of lung infections, including bronchiolitis and pneumonia, in infants and young children. Infections in infants can be severe and even fatal; elderly people and those with chronic lung disease may also develop severe symptoms. Healthy adults and older children usually develop mild or moderate lung infection. Infection provides only partial immunity, so people can become infected repeatedly. However, subsequent respiratory syncytial virus infections are less severe than the first.

Symptoms and Diagnosis

The symptoms of respiratory syncytial virus infection begin 2 to 8 days after infection. A runny nose and sore throat begin first, followed several days later by breathing difficulties, wheezing, and coughing. Infants may have a fever. Symptoms tend to be milder in older children and adults, in whom the infection may resemble influenza, be no worse than a common cold, or cause no symptoms at all. Symptoms also tend to be milder in those who may have had previous exposure to the virus. The infection is most severe in young children and in people with underlying diseases, especially respiratory conditions.

A doctor usually bases the diagnosis on the symptoms. Laboratory tests can identify the virus or antibodies to the virus in blood samples but are rarely needed.

Prognosis, Prevention, and Treatment

Older children and adults usually get better without treatment in an average of 9 days from the start of symptoms. However, the very young and others with severe disease may be ill for longer and need intensive treatment in the hospital to maintain adequate breathing.

To help prevent infection in premature infants with underlying respiratory disease, passive immunization with antibodies (palivizumab given intramuscularly or respiratory syncytial virus immune globulin given intravenously) may be given monthly during the late fall and winter.

The antiviral drug ribavirin affects the virus' ability to reproduce and can speed recovery but is prescribed only for people with severe infection. Ribavirin is not prescribed for pregnant women because it may harm the fetus.

Croup

Croup is a contagious viral infection of the upper and lower airways that causes difficulty in breathing, especially breathing in.

Croup can be caused by a number of different viruses. In the fall, a parainfluenza virus is the most likely cause. Less commonly, croup can be caused by the measles virus or other viruses, such as the respiratory syncytial virus or an influenza virus, especially in winter and spring. Croup primarily affects children 6 months to 3 years of age, though it occasionally affects those younger or older. Croup caused by an influenza virus may be particularly severe and is more likely to occur in children between 3 and 7 years old. The disease is usually spread by breathing in airborne droplets containing viruses or by having contact with infected objects.

Symptoms and Diagnosis

Croup usually starts with coldlike symptoms. The infection causes swelling of the lining of the airway, so that the airway narrows and breathing becomes difficult. Difficulty in breathing in, together with a barking cough and hoarseness, commonly first occur at night. Difficulty in breathing may awaken the child from sleep. Breathing is rapid and deep, and half of all children have fever. The child's condition may improve in the morning but worsens again at night. The illness usually lasts 3 to 4 days. Croup that keeps coming back is called spasmodic croup. Allergy may be a cause of spasmodic croup, but it usually starts with a viral infection. A doctor distinguishes croup by its characteristic symptoms.

Treatment

A child who is mildly ill with croup may be cared for at home. The child is made comfortable, given plenty of fluids, and allowed to rest because fatigue and crying can worsen the condition. Home humidifying devices (for example, cool-mist vaporizers or humidifiers) may reduce drying of the upper airway and ease breathing. The humidity can be raised quickly by running a hot shower to steam up the bathroom. Increasing or continuing difficulty in breathing, rapid heart rate, fatigue, bluish skin discoloration, or dehydration indicates that the child needs to be hospitalized.

In the hospital, oxygen may be given when blood levels of oxygen are low. High carbon dioxide levels in the blood indicate that the child is becoming exhausted. Mechanical assistance with breathing is then given by inserting a tube into the airway and pumping air in and out of the lungs with a ventilator.

An ultrasonic nebulizer, which is different from a home humidifier, can produce sufficiently small droplets to reach the lower airways and reduce the stickiness of secretions there. These secretions can then be more easily cleared out of the airways by coughing.

Drugs that widen the airway, such as epinephrine, may be breathed as a mist through the nebulizer. These drugs may be used to help the child breathe more easily. A hospitalized child may be given corticosteroids for the early treatment of severe viral croup, but this use is controversial. Antibiotics are used only in the rare situation when a child with croup also develops a bacterial infection.

Bronchiolitis

Bronchiolitis is a contagious viral infection of the airways of infants and young children that causes difficulty in breathing, especially breathing out.

Several different viruses can cause bronchiolitis, including the respiratory syncytial virus▲ and parainfluenza viruses. Bronchiolitis often occurs in epidemics, mostly in children under 18 months of age and most commonly in infants younger than 6 months. During the first year of life, bronchiolitis affects about 11 of every 100 children.

Symptoms and Diagnosis

Bronchiolitis usually follows a cold, which is an infection of the upper airway. Sudden difficulty in breathing, especially in breathing out, develops with rapid breathing, rapid heart rate, and a hacking cough. The child is often very sleepy and may have a fever. The child may tire and start breathing shallowly and ineffectively. Vomiting or decreased drinking may dehydrate the child. A doctor bases the diagnosis on the symptoms.

Prognosis and Treatment

Most children recover at home in 3 to 5 days. During the illness, frequent small feedings of clear

---

▲ see page 1272

liquids may be given. Increasing difficulty in breathing, bluish skin discoloration, fatigue, and dehydration indicate that the child should be hospitalized. Children with conditions such as heart disease or impaired immunity may be hospitalized sooner. With proper care, the chance of dying of severe bronchiolitis is less than 1 percent.

In the hospital, blood levels of oxygen and carbon dioxide are monitored. Oxygen is usually given by an oxygen tent or face mask. A ventilator may be necessary to assist breathing. An ultrasonic nebulizer may be used to open the airways and loosen secretions, and intravenous fluids may be given. The antiviral drug ribavirin may be given to infants who are premature or who have other conditions that put them at high risk.

Polio

Polio (poliomyelitis) is a highly contagious, sometimes fatal, viral infection that can produce permanent muscle weakness, paralysis, and other symptoms.

Poliovirus, an enterovirus, is spread by swallowing material such as water contaminated by infected feces. The infection spreads from the intestine throughout the body, but the brain and spinal cord are the most severely affected.

In the early 20th century, a large portion of health care resources was devoted to people infected with polio. Today, most doctors have never seen a new polio infection. In industrialized countries, polio outbreaks have largely disappeared because of widespread vaccination programs. Before vaccines became available, outbreaks occurred during the summer and autumn months in temperate climates. In developing countries, the virus can be spread through water supplies contaminated by human feces. Children under 5 years of age are particularly likely to become infected with polio from such sources.

Symptoms and Diagnosis

Polio in young children is often mild. Symptoms, which begin 3 to 5 days after infection, include an overall feeling of illness (malaise), a slight fever, headache, a sore throat, and vomiting. The child usually recovers within 24 to 72 hours.

Major illness is more likely in older children and adults. The symptoms, which usually appear 7 to

14 days after infection, include fever, severe headache, a stiff neck and back, and deep muscle pain. Sometimes areas of skin develop odd sensations, such as pins and needles or unusual sensitivity to pain. Depending on which parts of the brain and spinal cord are affected, the disease may progress no further, or weakness or paralysis may develop in certain muscles. The person may have difficulty in swallowing and may choke on saliva, food, or fluids. Sometimes fluids go up into the nose, and the voice may develop a nasal quality.

A doctor can diagnose polio from its symptoms. Diagnosis is confirmed by identifying poliovirus in a stool sample and detecting high levels of antibodies to the virus in the blood.

Complications

The most severe complication of polio is permanent paralysis. Although paralysis develops in less than 1 in every 100 cases, permanent weakness of one or more muscles is common.

Sometimes the part of the brain responsible for breathing may be affected, causing weakness or paralysis of the chest muscles. During the epidemics in the 1940s and 1950s, this complication led to the use of the iron lung, a cumbersome mechanical device that assisted breathing. Today, death from polio is rare.

Some people develop further complications 20 to 30 years after an attack of polio. This condition (postpoliomyelitis syndrome) consists of progressive muscle weakness, often resulting in severe disability.

Prevention and Treatment

Polio vaccine is included among the routine childhood immunizations.▲ Two types of vaccine are available: an inactivated poliovirus vaccine (Salk vaccine) given by injection and a live poliovirus vaccine (Sabin vaccine) taken orally. The live oral vaccine provides better immunity and is usually preferred. However, in very rare cases, the live vaccine can cause polio, especially in people who have an impaired immune system. Therefore, the live vaccine isn't given to people who have an impaired immune system or to those who have close contact with such people, because the live virus is excreted in the stool for some time after vaccination.

A first vaccination of people over 18 years old isn't routinely recommended because the risk of acquiring polio as an adult is extremely low in the United States. Adults who have never been immunized and who are traveling to an area where polio is still a health risk should be vaccinated.

Polio can't be cured, and antiviral drugs don't affect the course of the disease. However, a ventilator may be used if the muscles used in breathing are weakened.

CHAPTER 261

Human Immunodeficiency Virus Infection

Human immunodeficiency virus infection is a viral disorder that progressively destroys the white blood cells and causes acquired immunodeficiency syndrome (AIDS).

Infection by the human immunodeficiency virus (HIV) eventually results in progressive deterioration of the body's immune system, allowing opportunistic infections and, especially in adults, certain cancers to develop. AIDS is the late stage of HIV infection and is, at present, a fatal illness.

HIV infection and AIDS affect primarily young adults;■ only about 2 percent of the people infected with HIV in the United States are children or adolescents. However, the number of young adults with HIV infection who presumably ac-

---

▲ see box, page 1200

■ see page 926

Common Early Symptoms of HIV Infection in Young Children

• Poor growth, weight loss, prolonged or recurring fever, persistent or recurring bouts of diarrhea, swollen lymph nodes, enlarged liver and spleen, swollen and inflamed salivary glands in the cheeks

• Persistent or recurring fungal infection (thrush) in the mouth or diaper area

• Recurring bacterial infections, such as middle ear infections, pneumonia, and meningitis

• Various unusual opportunistic viral, fungal, and parasitic infections

• Delayed or regressed development of the nervous system

quired infection during adolescence is increasing rapidly. In 1995, more than 3,000 children in the United States were living with AIDS, and at least 1,200 more were known to be infected with the virus; about 800 to 1,000 new cases are reported each year. About 90 percent of HIV-infected children were infected before, during, or shortly after birth; about 61 percent of them were black, 23 percent were Hispanic, and 15 percent were white.

Causes

HIV infection is caused by the virus HIV-1 or, less commonly, by a closely related virus called HIV-2.▲ Young children with HIV infection almost always acquired the virus from their mother before or during birth, although more than two thirds of children born to women with HIV infection will not become infected. Because the virus can be transmitted in breast milk, breastfed in-

▲ see page 926

■ see page 759

fants may acquire the infection from their mother after birth.

Mother-to-child transmission of the virus isn't the only way that children can become infected. Although rare, another route of infection is sexual contact through sexual abuse. Finally, a child may have become infected through a blood transfusion if the transfusion was given before 1985. Boys with hemophilia■ who received clotting factor concentrates before the mid-1980s may have become infected if the blood products were contaminated with HIV. Since 1985, all donated blood has been screened for the HIV antibody, and major improvements have been made in the safety of clotting factor concentrates. Today, acquiring HIV infection through transfusion of blood or blood products is extremely rare in the United States.

In adolescents, the means of infection are the same as in adults: sexual intercourse, sharing of infected needles while injecting drugs, and, less commonly, blood transfusions received before 1985. Both homosexual and heterosexual activity can spread the virus. Male homosexual activity is responsible for 33 percent of recent HIV cases among adolescent males; heterosexual activity accounts for about 54 percent of recent cases among adolescent females. Sharing infected needles accounts for about 11 percent of recent cases among all adolescents.

The virus is *not* transmitted through food, water, household articles, or social contact in a home, workplace, or school. In very rare cases, HIV has been transmitted by contact with infected blood on the skin. In almost all such instances, the skin surface was broken by scrapes or open sores, or other factors were involved. Although saliva may contain the virus, transmission by kissing or biting has never been confirmed.

Symptoms and Complications

Infection before, during, or shortly after birth isn't immediately apparent. For about 10 to 20 percent of children, problems start during the first or second year of life; for the remaining 80 to 90 percent of children, problems may not appear until years later. About half of the children infected with HIV are diagnosed with AIDS by their third birthday. If the disease begins after infancy, periods of illness may alternate with periods of relatively normal health. HIV infection acquired during adolescence often remains dormant or causes very few symptoms for months or even years, which is similar to the course of HIV infection acquired during adulthood.

A variety of symptoms and complications can appear as the child's immune system deteriorates. About a third of the HIV-infected children develop lung inflammation (lymphocytic interstitial pneumonitis), usually during the first several years of life. Cough and swelling of the ends of the fingers (clubbing) may result, depending on how severely the lungs are affected.

Pneumonia caused by the microorganism *Pneumocystis carinii* is a serious threat to children with AIDS. Children born with HIV infection commonly have at least one episode of pneumocystis pneumonia in the first 15 months of life. More than half of the children infected with HIV develop the pneumonia at some time. Pneumocystis pneumonia is a major cause of death among children and adults with AIDS.

In a significant number of HIV-infected children, progressive brain damage prevents or delays developmental milestones, such as walking and talking. These children also may have impaired intelligence and a head that is small in relation to their body size. Up to 20 percent of infected children progressively lose social and language skills and muscle control. They may become partially paralyzed or unsteady on their feet, or their muscles may become somewhat rigid.

Some children develop inflammation of the liver (hepatitis) and damage to the heart (heart failure) or kidneys (kidney failure). Cancers are uncommon in children with AIDS, but non-Hodgkin's lymphoma and lymphoma of the brain may occur. Kaposi's sarcoma, a cancer that affects the skin and internal organs, is extremely rare in children.

Diagnosis

HIV infection is suspected in children of mothers known to have the infection or in children with symptoms of HIV infection or with immune system problems. In newborns, the standard blood test for HIV antibodies isn't diagnostic, because their blood almost always contains HIV antibodies if the mother is HIV-infected (even if they themselves are not). Most infants routinely retain these maternal antibodies for 12 to 15 months or more, but the antibodies eventually disappear from the bloodstream in infants not infected with HIV. Therefore, to definitively diagnose HIV infec-

tion in children younger than 18 months of age, special blood tests (a polymerase chain reaction test or HIV virus culture) are used. Through repeated use of such tests, many HIV-infected infants, if not most, can be diagnosed with HIV infection by 6 months of age.

Standard blood tests for HIV antibodies are used to diagnose HIV infection in children older than 18 months and in adolescents.

Treatment and Prognosis

An increasing number of drugs are being used to treat HIV infection in adults and adolescents.▲ Many, but not all, of these drugs have been tested in children and have been found to be useful. Many experts believe that combinations of drugs may be more useful than single drugs. Drugs used in children include zidovudine (AZT), didanosine (ddI), stavudine (d4T), lamivudine (3TC), and zalcitabine (ddC). Some drugs used in adults are just being tested in children; these include saquinavir, ritonavir, and indinavir. Some drugs, such as nevirapine and delavirdine, are being tested in both adults and children.

To prevent pneumocystis pneumonia, infants over 1 month old born to HIV-infected women and children with a significantly impaired immune system are given antibiotics. Trimethoprim-sulfamethoxazole is generally given, but some children may be treated with pentamidine or dapsone. With current drug therapy, 75 percent of children with HIV infection born today are alive at 5 years, and 50 percent are alive at 8 years. The average age at death is still about 10 years for HIV-infected children, but more and more children are surviving well into adolescence.

Intravenous immunoglobulin is occasionally given to boost a child's immunity against infection. The routine childhood vaccinations are given to most HIV-infected children, whether or not they have symptoms of HIV infection. In general, live viral and bacterial vaccines aren't used. However, measles-mumps-rubella vaccine (which contains live virus) is given, since measles can cause a severe or fatal illness in HIV-infected children, and no adverse effects from the vaccine have been reported.

▲ see page 932

For children who need foster care, day care, or schooling, a doctor can help assess the child's risk of exposure to infectious diseases. In general, transmission of infections, such as chickenpox, to the HIV-infected child (or to any child with an impaired immune system) is more of a danger than is transmission of HIV from that child to others. A young child with HIV infection who has open skin sores or who engages in potentially dangerous behavior, such as biting, may not be suitable for a day care center. However, in general, there is no need for anyone other than the parents, the doctor, and perhaps the school physician to be aware of the child's HIV status.

HIV-infected children need close medical supervision as their condition worsens, but treatment is best given in the least restrictive environment possible. If home health care and social services are available, the children can spend more time at home rather than in a hospital.

Prevention

Prevention depends on being aware of how HIV is transmitted and putting the knowledge into practice. Teaching the importance of abstention or safe sex practices is essential to stopping the spread of AIDS among teenagers and adults.

The most effective means of preventing infection in newborns is for HIV-infected women to avoid pregnancy. Some research shows that delivery by cesarean section may reduce the baby's risk of acquiring HIV infection, but this isn't standard practice.

One of the most significant advances in HIV research is the prevention, in many cases, of HIV transmission from mothers to babies by using anti-HIV drugs. Pregnant women known to be infected with HIV are given zidovudine (AZT) by mouth during the second and third trimesters (last 6 months) of pregnancy, along with intravenous zidovudine during labor and delivery. Zidovudine is given to the newborn for 6 weeks. These measures have reduced the rate of transmission from the mother to the child by more than two thirds (from 25 percent to 8 percent). More research is under way to see if other drugs can lower the transmission rate even further. Therefore, all pregnant women should strongly consider being tested for HIV infection early in pregnancy, so that zidovudine therapy can be given in time if needed.

Although the risk of acquiring HIV infection through breast milk is relatively low, HIV-infected mothers should avoid breastfeeding, especially in the United States, where good infant formulas and clean water are readily available. In countries where the risks of malnutrition or infectious diarrhea from unclean water are high, the benefits of breastfeeding more than outweigh any additional risk of HIV transmission.

Since a child's HIV status may not be known, all schools and day care centers should adopt special procedures for handling accidents, such as nosebleeds, and for cleaning and disinfecting surfaces contaminated with blood. During cleanup, personnel are advised to avoid having their skin come in contact with blood. Gloves should be made routinely available, and hands should be washed after the gloves are removed. Contaminated surfaces should be cleaned and disinfected with a freshly prepared bleach solution containing 1 part of household bleach to 10 to 100 parts of water.

CHAPTER 262

Pinworm Infection

Pinworm infection is a condition in which the small roundworm Enterobius vermicularis *grows and reproduces within the intestines.*

The pinworm is the most common parasite in children who live in temperate climates. At least 20 percent of all children, and as many as 90 percent of children in institutions, have pinworms.

Causes

Infection usually occurs in a two-step process. Eggs are first transferred from the area around the anus to clothing, bedding, or toys. The eggs are then transferred, often by the fingers, to the mouth of another child, who swallows them. Eggs may also be inhaled from the air and then swallowed. Children may reinfect themselves by transferring eggs from the area around the anus to the mouth.

Pinworms mature in the lower intestine within 2 to 6 weeks. The female worm moves to the area around the anus, usually at night, to deposit her eggs within the child's anal skinfolds. The eggs are deposited in a sticky, gelatinous substance. This substance and the movements of the mother pinworm cause itching.

Eggs can survive outside the body for as long as 3 weeks at normal room temperature. However, the eggs may hatch quickly and the young worms can migrate back to the rectum and lower intestine.

Symptoms

Most children who carry pinworms have no symptoms. Some children, however, feel itching around the anus and continually scratch the area. The skin around the anus can become raw. In girls, pinworm infection may cause vaginal itching and irritation. Abdominal pain, sleeplessness, convulsions, and other unproven consequences have been falsely blamed on pinworm infection. In rare cases, appendicitis may be caused by pinworms blocking the appendix.

Diagnosis

The diagnosis of pinworm infection is made by finding the worms. The search is best conducted by examining the child's anus about 1 to 2 hours after the child has been put to bed for the night. The worms are white and hair-thin, but they wiggle and are visible to the naked eye. Eggs or worms can be obtained by patting the skinfolds around the anus with the sticky side of a strip of transparent tape in the early morning before the child wakes up. The tape can be folded on itself sticky side down and taken to the doctor. The eggs and worms on the tape can be identified under a microscope.

Prognosis and Treatment

Treatment isn't usually needed. The parasite rarely causes any harm and is extremely common. However, most parents are upset by the idea of pinworm infection and often want to get rid of the worms. A single dose of the drug mebendazole or pyrantel cures about 90 percent of cases. All family members must take the medicine because reinfection can spread from one family member to another. Anti-itching creams or ointments applied directly to the area around the anus two to three times daily may relieve itching.

Despite drug therapy, reinfection is common after treatment because live eggs continue to be shed in the feces for up to a week after treatment. Clothing, bedding, and toys should be machine-washed frequently to try to eliminate any eggs.

CHAPTER 263

Disorders Likely Caused by Infection

With several disorders that affect children, the cause is either unknown or an infectious cause is suspected. Such disorders include fever of unknown origin, Reye's syndrome, and Kawasaki syndrome.

Fever of Unknown Origin

Fever of unknown origin in children is a rectal temperature of at least 101.3° F. on at least four occa-sions over at least 2 weeks, for which no cause can be found.

Short-lived fevers, often from upper respiratory tract infections, are common in children; fever of unknown origin is of longer duration. Because such fever may indicate a serious disease, it requires an extensive medical evaluation.

Causes

In the United States, about 50 percent of children with fever of unknown origin are ultimately

---

Symptoms of Fever of Unknown Origin

General symptoms
- Loss of appetite
- Weight loss
- Fatigue
- Chills
- Sweats

Specific symptoms
- Skin symptoms, such as itchiness, rash, changes in pigment
- Chest pain
- Shortness of breath
- Significant heart murmur
- Joint disease
- Enlarged lymph nodes

---

diagnosed as having an infection. The infection differs depending on the age of the child. In 65 percent of those up to age 6, the cause is a viral infection, typically of the upper respiratory tract (sinuses, nose, and throat). Children over 6 years of age are somewhat more likely to have an infection of the lining of the heart (endocarditis) or infectious mononucleosis.

Typically in children older than age 6, autoimmune diseases▲ cause about 20 percent of cases of fever of unknown origin. Examples of autoimmune diseases that can cause fever of unknown origin include juvenile rheumatoid arthritis, inflammatory bowel disease, and systemic lupus erythematosus.

Cancer, most commonly leukemia or lymphoma, causes about 10 percent of cases of fever of unknown origin in children. Miscellaneous causes, which account for about 10 percent of cases, include drug allergies, Kawasaki syndrome, genetic diseases, and inflammation of various organs, such as the bones, thyroid gland, pancreas, or brain and spinal cord. In about 15

▲ see page 816

percent of children, the cause of fever of unknown origin is never known despite extensive testing.

Symptoms and Diagnosis

Fever of unknown origin is distinguished from other fevers by its persistence. Often, the fever comes and goes over at least a 2-week period. Vague symptoms, such as loss of appetite, weight loss, fatigue, chills, and sweats, are common. These general symptoms are not always helpful in identifying the cause. However, the careful documentation of symptoms, past illnesses, and exposures to medicines, foods, pets, wild animals, travel, and ill people—in conjunction with careful, repeated physical examinations—is often very helpful to the doctor in diagnosing the cause of the fever. The duration, height, and pattern of the fever can also be helpful in making the diagnosis. Skin problems, such as itchiness, rash, or increased pigmentation (darkening), may indicate either an infection or an underlying illness, such as cancer or an autoimmune disease. Chest pain or a heart murmur may also indicate a serious underlying disease, such as an infection of the lining of the heart (endocarditis). Blood tests, urine tests, and x-rays, guided by the results of the history and physical examination, may need to be obtained repeatedly before the final diagnosis is made, and often the child is hospitalized for evaluation.

Prognosis and Treatment

The prognosis depends on the cause. The majority of cases of fever of unknown origin are traced to a common childhood disease. These children recover with appropriate therapy, which may or may not include antibiotics. A drug such as acetaminophen is usually given to lower the temperature.

Reye's Syndrome

Reye's syndrome is a rare but very serious and often life-threatening disorder that causes inflammation of the brain and rapid accumulation of fat in the liver.

Although the cause of Reye's syndrome is unknown, certain viruses, such as influenza A or B or varicella (chickenpox) virus, may be involved, perhaps in combination with the ingestion of aspirin. Taking aspirin during an influenza or chickenpox illness may increase the risk of developing Reye's syndrome by as much as 35-fold. Because of the risk of Reye's syndrome, the use of aspirin or similar compounds (called salicylates) by children and teenagers is considered potentially dangerous. However, the use of such drugs may be warranted in a few specific diseases.

Reye's syndrome was discovered in 1963. It occurred in 200 to 550 children in the United States each year between 1974 and 1984. Reye's syndrome has now become very rare, affecting fewer than 20 children each year in the United States, at least in part because children are now being given drugs other than aspirin when a pain reliever or fever reducer is needed.

Reye's syndrome usually affects children and adolescents. Very rarely, however, it affects adults. In the United States, most cases occur in late fall and winter. Widespread outbreaks have occurred among people with influenza and chickenpox. A sibling of a person who has had Reye's syndrome is slightly more likely to be affected as well. It isn't known whether this tendency occurs because an infection passes from one sibling to the other, whether the siblings share a common exposure to a toxin, or whether heredity plays a part.

Symptoms and Diagnosis

The severity of Reye's syndrome varies greatly. Usually, there is first a viral infection, such as an upper respiratory tract infection, influenza, or chickenpox. Then, typically about 4 or 5 days later, the child has very severe nausea and vomiting. As the vomiting diminishes after about one more day, the child becomes confused. Confusion may be followed by disorientation, agitation, and later, seizures and coma. When the syndrome follows chickenpox, the symptoms usually start about 4 to 5 days after the rash appears. Death can come quickly—an average of 4 days after being admitted to the hospital—but some cases remain mild.

A doctor suspects Reye's syndrome in any child who has severe vomiting and evidence of sudden brain swelling without any reasonable explanation. To make the diagnosis of Reye's syndrome, the doctor will likely perform a liver biopsy▲ and spinal tap (lumbar puncture).■

Prognosis

The child's prognosis depends on the severity of the mental changes and their rate of progression. The prognosis also depends on how high the pressure becomes within the skull and the amount of ammonia in the blood (high ammonia levels indicate abnormal liver function). The chances that the child will die are about 20 percent, but range from less than 2 percent among children with mild disease to more than 80 percent among those in a deep coma.

Children who survive the acute phase of the illness usually have a full recovery. Those who develop convulsions may later show some evidence of brain damage, such as mental retardation, a seizure disorder, abnormal muscle movement, or damage to specific nerves. Reye's syndrome rarely affects a child twice.

Treatment

No specific treatment can stop Reye's syndrome from running its course. Early diagnosis and intensive care to support vital functions, including blood circulation and breathing, are critical. Fluids are given intravenously, along with electrolytes and glucose. Vitamin K is also given to help prevent bleeding. Drugs such as mannitol, corticosteroids (such as dexamethasone), or glycerol may be given to reduce the pressure within the brain. The child's breathing may need to be assisted by a respirator. Hospital staff will likely place tubes (catheters) in the child's arteries and veins to monitor blood pressure and blood gases.

Kawasaki Syndrome

Kawasaki syndrome is an illness primarily of children younger than age 5 that causes skin rash, fever, enlarged lymph nodes, and sometimes heart and joint inflammation.

The cause of Kawasaki syndrome is unknown, but some evidence suggests a virus or other infectious agent. Kawasaki syndrome was first described in Japan in the late 1960s. Since then, thousands of cases have been diagnosed world-

▲ see page 560

■ see box, page 374

Complications of Kawasaki Syndrome

Complications involving the heart
- Inflammation of the arteries that carry blood to the heart (coronary arteries)
- Widening of a section of coronary artery (aneurysm)
- Inflammation of the sac around the heart (pericarditis)
- Inflammation of the heart muscle (acute myocarditis)
- Heart failure
- Death of heart muscle (infarction)

Other complications
- Unusual rashes
- Inflammation of the interior of the eye (anterior uveitis)
- Painful or inflamed joints (mainly small joints)
- Noninfectious inflammation of the lining of the brain (aseptic meningitis)
- Inflammation of the gallbladder
- Diarrhea

wide in a variety of racial and ethnic groups, although the syndrome remains most common in Japan. Several thousand cases of Kawasaki syndrome are estimated to occur in the United States every year.

Most children with Kawasaki syndrome range in age from 2 months to 5 years, although the syndrome has occurred in teenagers. Roughly twice as many boys as girls are affected. Rarely, the disorder can affect several members of the same household.

Symptoms
The illness begins with fever, which rises and falls but is usually above 102.2° F. The child is irritable, is often drowsy, and occasionally has crampy abdominal pain. Within a day, a red, patchy rash usually appears over the trunk and around the diaper area. Within several days, the rash appears on mucous membranes, such as the lining of the mouth or vagina. The child has a red throat; reddened, dry, cracked lips; and a strawberry-red tongue. Both eyes become red but with-

out any discharge. Also, the palms and soles turn red or purplish-red, and the hands and feet often swell. The skin on the fingers and toes begins to peel 10 to 20 days after the illness starts. The lymph nodes in the neck are often swollen and slightly tender.

The most serious complication of Kawasaki syndrome is heart disease; the other symptoms of the illness do not lead to chronic problems in the skin, eyes, or lymph nodes. About 5 to 20 percent of children with Kawasaki syndrome develop complications involving the heart. These complications usually begin 2 to 4 weeks after the onset of illness. The most serious heart problem is abnormal widening (dilation) of the coronary arteries. Although slight widening of the arteries may resolve, severe widening (aneurysm) can cause heart attack and sudden death.

Other complications of Kawasaki syndrome, such as inflammation of the tissues lining the brain (meninges), joint inflammation, and gallbladder inflammation, eventually resolve without causing permanent damage.

Diagnosis
A doctor bases the diagnosis on the symptoms rather than on the results of specific laboratory tests. Fever that lasts at least 5 days and the appearance of four of the five bodily changes (a rash; red, swollen extremities; reddened eyes; changes in the lips and mouth; and swollen lymph nodes) lead to the diagnosis. Blood tests first reveal high numbers of white blood cells and low numbers of red blood cells (anemia); the tests later reveal high numbers of platelets. Results of other laboratory tests may be abnormal as well, depending on the organ systems affected.

Prognosis
Children usually recover completely if their coronary arteries aren't affected. About 1 to 2 percent of children with Kawasaki syndrome die, usually of heart complications. Of these, more than 50 percent die within the first month, 75 percent within 2 months, and 95 percent within 6 months, but death can occur as late as 10 years afterward, sometimes suddenly and unexpectedly. Smaller coronary aneurysms tend to disappear within a year, but the coronary arteries may remain weakened, causing heart problems years later.

Treatment

Early treatment significantly reduces the risk of coronary artery damage and speeds the resolution of fever, rash, and discomfort. For 1 to 4 days, high doses of immunoglobulin are given intravenously, and high doses of aspirin are given by mouth. Once the fever is gone, a lower dose of aspirin is usually continued for several months to reduce the risk of coronary artery damage and blood clots.

A doctor will perform frequent echocardiograms to check for heart complications. Large coronary aneurysms may be treated with anti-clotting drugs, such as warfarin, in addition to aspirin. Small aneurysms may be treated with aspirin alone. If the child contracts influenza or chickenpox, dipyridamole is sometimes used temporarily instead of aspirin to lessen the risk of Reye's syndrome.

CHAPTER 264

Childhood Cancers

Cancer is a rare disease among children, occurring in only one in 5,000 children every year. Cancer in children is different than cancer in adults; many childhood cancers occur only rarely in adults. Additionally, in contrast to many adult cancers, cancers in children are much more curable. Three relatively common childhood cancers are Wilms' tumor, neuroblastoma, and retinoblastoma. Other cancers, such as leukemia,▲ lymphoma,■ and brain tumors,★ also are relatively common in children.

Wilms' Tumor

Wilms' tumor (nephroblastoma) is a cancer of the kidneys that can develop in a fetus but may not cause symptoms for years after birth.

Wilms' tumor usually occurs in children under 5 years of age, although it appears occasionally in older children and rarely in adults. The cause of Wilms' tumor isn't known, although a genetic abnormality may be involved in some cases. Children with certain birth defects, such as absence of the irises or excessive growth of one side of the body, both of which may be caused by a genetic abnormality, have an increased risk of developing Wilms' tumor.

Symptoms and Diagnosis

Symptoms include a large abdomen (for example, a rapid change to a larger diaper size), abdominal pain, fever, poor appetite, nausea, and vomiting. Blood appears in the urine in 15 to 20 percent of cases. Wilms' tumor may cause high blood pressure. This cancer can spread to other parts of the body, especially the lungs, producing a cough and shortness of breath.

A doctor is usually able to feel a lump (mass) in the child's abdomen. If the doctor suspects Wilms' tumor, an ultrasound, a computed tomography (CT) scan, or a magnetic resonance imaging (MRI) scan may be performed to determine the nature and size of the lump.

Prognosis and Treatment

The prognosis depends on the microscopic appearance of the tumor, its spread at the time of diagnosis, and the age of the child. Younger children, children with smaller tumors, and children whose tumor has not spread tend to fare better. Wilms' tumor is very curable. Even older children and children with widespread tumors have a very good prognosis.

If doctors think the tumor can be removed, surgery is performed soon after the diagnosis. During the operation, the other kidney is examined as a precaution to determine whether it also has a tumor. In about 4 percent of the cases, nephroblastoma occurs simultaneously in both kidneys. The anticancer drugs actinomycin D, vincristine,

---

▲ see page 765

■ see page 770

★ see page 379

and doxorubicin may be used, as may radiation therapy,▲ depending on how far the cancer has spread.

Neuroblastoma

A neuroblastoma is a common childhood cancer that grows in parts of the nervous system.

A neuroblastoma may develop in a certain kind of nerve tissue anywhere in the body. It usually originates in nerves in the chest or abdomen, most commonly in the adrenal glands (located above each kidney). Very rarely, a neuroblastoma originates in the brain.

About 75 percent of all neuroblastomas occur in children under 5 years of age. Although its cause isn't known, this cancer sometimes runs in families.

Symptoms and Diagnosis

The symptoms depend on where the neuroblastoma originated and how far it has spread. The first symptoms in many children include a large abdomen, a sensation of fullness, and abdominal pain. Symptoms may also relate to spread of the tumor. For example, cancer that has invaded the bones causes pain. Cancer that has reached the bone marrow may reduce the number of red blood cells, causing anemia; the number of platelets, causing bruising; or the number of white blood cells, lowering the resistance to infection. The cancer can spread to the skin, where it produces nodules, or to the spinal cord, where it may cause weakness of the arms or legs. About 90 percent of neuroblastomas produce hormones, such as epinephrine, which can increase heart rate and cause anxiety.

Early diagnosis of a neuroblastoma isn't easy. If the cancer grows large enough, the doctor may be able to feel a lump (mass) in the abdomen. A doctor who suspects a neuroblastoma may suggest an ultrasound examination, computed tomography (CT), or magnetic resonance imaging (MRI) of the chest and abdomen. A urine sample can be tested for excessive production of epinephrine-like hormones. If the cancer has spread, the doctor may find clues from x-rays or from tissue samples of the liver, lung, skin, bone marrow, or bone taken for biopsy (examination under a microscope).

Prognosis and Treatment

The prognosis for children with neuroblastoma depends on the age of the child, the size of the tumor, and whether the tumor has spread. Children under 1 year of age and children with small tumors have a very good prognosis. Early treatment offers the best hope of cure. If the cancer hasn't spread, it usually can be removed by surgery. If the cancer is large or has spread, anticancer drugs such as vincristine, cyclophosphamide, doxorubicin, and cisplatin may be used, as may radiation therapy. In older children, the cure rate is low for cancer that has spread.

Retinoblastoma

A retinoblastoma is a cancer of the retina, the light-sensing area at the back of the eye.

Retinoblastomas represent about 2 percent of childhood cancers. About 10 percent of children with retinoblastomas have relatives with this type of cancer and inherit the gene for it from their parents. An additional 20 to 30 percent of children have the cancer in both eyes, which indicates they have acquired the gene as a new mutation. A combined total of about 30 to 40 percent of children with retinoblastoma thus have the gene for retinoblastoma, which they can pass on to their children.

Symptoms and Diagnosis

Symptoms of a retinoblastoma can include a white pupil or strabismus (cross-eyes). However, other causes of a white pupil or strabismus are far more common. Retinoblastomas tend to produce few other symptoms. If a doctor suspects a retinoblastoma, the child is given general anesthesia and both eyes are examined. General anesthesia is necessary because small children aren't able to cooperate for the careful, time-consuming examination required to diagnose retinoblastoma. The cancer can also be identified by computed tomography (CT).

Because retinoblastomas can spread to the brain through the optic nerve (the nerve that leads from the eye to the brain), a sample of cere-

---

▲ see page 800

brospinal fluid is examined for cancer cells. Because the tumor can spread to the bone marrow, a sample of bone marrow is obtained for examination.

Prognosis and Treatment

Retinoblastomas that are confined to the eye are cured more than 90 percent of the time. When the cancer affects only one eye, the entire eyeball is removed, along with part of the optic nerve. When the cancer affects both eyes, special microsurgical techniques are used to remove or destroy the tumor, so that both eyes don't have to be removed. Alternatively, one eye may be removed and other techniques, such as radiation therapy and microsurgery, may be used to control the tumor in the other eye. Anticancer drugs (chemotherapy) may be given, especially if the tumor

has spread beyond the eye. The eyes are reexamined every 2 to 4 months. Chemotherapy may be repeated if the cancer returns.

Children with the hereditary type of retinoblastoma have a high risk of having the cancer recur. Furthermore, within 30 years from the time of diagnosis, as many as 70 percent of those with a hereditary retinoblastoma develop a second cancer.

A doctor may recommend that immediate family members of any child with a retinoblastoma have at least one eye examination. Other young children in the family need to be examined for a retinoblastoma, and adults need to be examined for a retinocytoma, a noncancerous tumor caused by the same gene. Family members who have no evidence of cancer can have their DNA analyzed to see if they carry the retinoblastoma gene.

CHAPTER 265

Gastrointestinal Disorders

Most gastrointestinal disorders in children cause pain. Many, such as celiac disease▲ and lactose intolerance,■ also cause malnutrition and diarrhea.

Pain may begin suddenly and may be severe, as in acute appendicitis,★ or it may be less severe and may come and go. Gastrointestinal disorders in which pain typically comes and goes include recurring abdominal pain, peptic ulcer, and Meckel's diverticulum.

Recurring Abdominal Pain

Recurring abdominal pain is three or more episodes of abdominal pain occurring over a period of at least 3 months.

More than 10 percent of all school-aged children have recurring abdominal pain. It is most common between the ages of 8 and 10 and is rare in children under age 4. Recurring abdominal pain is slightly more common in girls than in boys and is fairly common among girls in early adolescence.

Causes

In only 5 to 10 percent of the children with recurring abdominal pain, the pain is caused by a physical disease. The diseases that can cause recurring abdominal pain vary widely and include genitourinary disorders, intestinal disorders, and general illnesses.

Sometimes recurring abdominal pain is caused by the abnormal functioning of internal organs. For instance, the bowel may function abnormally if the child's diet is inappropriate, especially if the child can't tolerate certain foods, such as milk and dairy products.● Another reason for abnormal bowel function is constipation resulting from diminished activity of the colon, sometimes as a reaction to inappropriate toilet training. In teen-

▲ see page 536

■ see page 535

★ see page 547

● see page 535

Some Physical Causes of Recurring Abdominal Pain

Intestinal disorders
- Hiatal hernia
- Hepatitis (inflammation of the liver)
- Cholecystitis (inflammation of the gallbladder)
- Pancreatitis (inflammation of the pancreas)
- Peptic ulcer disease
- Infestation with parasites (for example, giardiasis)
- Meckel's diverticulum
- Crohn's disease
- Tuberculosis of the intestine
- Ulcerative colitis
- Chronic appendicitis

Genitourinary disorders
- Birth defects
- Urinary tract infection
- Pelvic inflammatory disease (in girls)
- Ovarian cyst (in girls)
- Endometriosis (in girls)

General illnesses
- Lead poisoning
- Henoch-Schönlein purpura
- Sickle cell disease
- Food allergy
- Porphyria
- Familial Mediterranean anemia
- Hereditary angioedema
- Migraine

age girls, abdominal pain may be caused by muscle cramps in the uterus during a painful menstrual period (dysmenorrhea).▲ Occasionally, the release of an egg from the ovary during the menstrual cycle is accompanied by pain.

In 80 to 90 percent of the cases, recurring abdominal pain has a psychologic rather than a physical or functional cause. Pain with a psychologic cause appears to be triggered or worsened by stress, anxiety, or depression.

Symptoms

The symptoms of recurring abdominal pain differ depending on the cause. Pain caused by physical disease usually doesn't go away, or it may come in cycles, often brought on by certain activities or by certain foods. The pain tends to occur in a specific site in the abdomen, not usually around the navel, and may penetrate to the back. A urinary tract infection may cause pain in the abdomen or lower pelvis, rather than in the back as it does in adults. Frequently, pain may awaken the child from sleep.

Depending on the underlying physical disease, the child may have any of the following symptoms: loss of appetite, weight loss, recurring or persistent fever, jaundice, changes in the form and color of bowel movements, constipation or diarrhea, blood in the stools, vomiting of food or blood, swelling of the abdomen, and pain or swelling of joints.

The symptoms of recurring abdominal pain caused by abnormal organ functioning vary with its underlying cause. For instance, if the child has a lactose intolerance, pain may occur within a few minutes or up to 2 hours after drinking milk or eating a milk product. If the child has gallbladder disease, abdominal pain may begin shortly after eating fatty foods.

Pain caused by psychologic factors may occur every day or sporadically. Occasionally, a child has no pain for weeks or months. The pain usually isn't sharp; it is more often described in vague terms but sometimes as cramps. This type of pain seldom wakes a child during the night, but the child may awaken earlier than usual.

Abdominal pain with a psychologic cause is most often felt around the navel. The farther the pain is from the navel, the more likely it has a physical cause. Psychologic pain sometimes resembles that caused by a physical disorder, but generally it doesn't change or worsen. A significant change in the nature of the pain may indicate that the child has a physical disorder as well.

Diagnosis

To determine the cause of the pain, a doctor asks the child or parents certain questions: What

▲ see page 1086

is the pain like? When does it occur? Where is it? What brings it on? What makes it worse or better? The doctor asks about other symptoms, such as nausea, vomiting, fever, or rash, that occur with the pain.

Diagnosing a psychologic cause for the pain can be difficult. The doctor first makes sure that a physical disorder isn't causing the pain. The child may be affected by stress at home because of a recent illness in the family, financial problems, or separation from or loss of a loved one. Children under stress are as likely to become physically ill as anyone else.

Prevention and Treatment

The treatment of recurring abdominal pain with a physical or functional cause depends on the underlying problem. For example, a change of diet may help if pain is provoked by eating certain foods. Pain relievers such as ibuprofen may help relieve menstrual cramps.

Recurring abdominal pain with a psychologic cause isn't imagined pain; it is a form of pain caused by such factors as stress and tension. Parents can help by reducing stress and tension as much as possible, helping the child cope with unavoidable stress, and encouraging the child to attend school despite the pain. Teachers can help by resolving conflicts related to school.

At school, a child who needs to take a 15- to 30-minute break from class should be allowed to go to the school nurse's office to rest or lie down. With the parents' permission, the nurse can give the child a mild pain reliever, such as ibuprofen or acetaminophen, if necessary. In some instances, the nurse may allow the child to call a parent, who can then encourage the child to stay in school. Typically, a child will request time in the nurse's office one or more times a day during the first week or two of treatment. This behavior usually stops quickly. Generally, when the parents stop treating the child as different or ill, pain with a psychologic cause initially worsens but then improves.

A doctor usually evaluates a child who has abdominal pain with a psychologic cause at regular intervals—weekly, monthly, or every other month, depending on the child's needs. After the problem has resolved, the doctor may want to monitor the child regularly for a few months. Treatment is not always successful. Some children develop a variety of other physical symptoms or emotional difficulties. If the pain persists despite all efforts, especially if the child is depressed or if there are marital or psychologic problems at home, the child may need to see a mental health professional.

Peptic Ulcer

A peptic ulcer is a well-defined round or oval sore where the lining of the stomach or duodenum has been damaged or eroded by stomach acid and digestive juices.

In a newborn, the first symptom of a peptic ulcer may be blood in the stool. If the ulcer perforates the stomach or small intestine, the infant may show signs of pain. The infant is likely to develop a fever. In older infants and young children, blood in the stool may be accompanied by repeated vomiting or abdominal pain. Often, the pain is worsened or improved by eating. Pain may also awaken the child during the night. About 50 percent of the children with an ulcer in the duodenum, the part of the small intestine near the stomach, have close relatives with the same disorder.

Many children with chronic ulcer disease are infected with a type of bacterium called *Helicobacter pylori*. It isn't clear whether the bacteria cause the ulcer or just prevent it from healing, but eradication of the bacteria has been found to result in healing and cure of recurrent ulcers.

Diagnosis and Treatment

Peptic ulcers in infants and young children are difficult to diagnose, possibly because young children can't describe their symptoms precisely. School-aged children may be better able to indicate the location of the pain, describe it, and explain whether the pain occurs at a specific time of day and whether it is related to eating.

If a doctor suspects a child has a peptic ulcer, a barium x-ray study can confirm the diagnosis. In this procedure, the child drinks a liquid containing barium, a substance that outlines the stomach when viewed on an x-ray.▲ If the x-ray study is normal and the doctor still suspects an ulcer, an endoscopic examination of the stomach

---

▲ see page 486

may be performed. To minimize movement and pain during the procedure, a child under 8 years old is usually given general anesthesia.

The treatment for a peptic ulcer is the same for children as for adults.▲ It usually consists of H_2 blockers, such as ranitidine, famotidine, and cimetidine. Rather than subject the child to the trauma and discomfort of diagnostic procedures, a doctor may assume the child has a peptic ulcer and begin treatment with H_2 blockers. If the symptoms disappear after treatment, then the diagnosis is confirmed.

For children found to have *Helicobacter pylori*, several weeks of dual therapy with amoxicillin and metronidazole or with amoxicillin and bismuth should eradicate the organism. In some cases, triple therapy with amoxicillin, metronidazole, and bismuth is used.

Meckel's Diverticulum

Meckel's diverticulum, a birth defect, is a saclike outpouching of the wall of the small intestine.

Meckel's diverticulum is a fairly common birth defect. The condition is noticed incidentally in about 2 percent of adult patients undergoing abdominal surgery for other reasons.

Symptoms and Diagnosis

Meckel's diverticulum usually doesn't cause symptoms, but the outpouching may secrete acid and cause ulcers, resulting in painless rectal bleeding. Children with Meckel's diverticulum typically have brick, currant jelly–colored, or black stool. In adolescents and adults, the diverticulum is more likely to cause intestinal obstruction, resulting in cramps and vomiting. At any age, sudden inflammation may develop in the diverticulum, a condition called acute diverticulitis.■ The inflammation causes a person to have severe pain and abdominal tenderness, often with vomiting.

The diagnosis of Meckel's diverticulum is difficult. Laboratory tests aren't always helpful, and only rarely can Meckel's diverticulum be seen on a barium x-ray of the small intestine. The best test is a Meckel radionuclide scan, which can help the doctor make the diagnosis in about 90 percent of suspected cases. Many times the diagnosis is made during surgery performed for other reasons.

Treatment

No treatment is needed for a diverticulum that doesn't cause symptoms. A bleeding diverticulum is surgically removed, together with any nearby area of damaged intestine. In people who have symptoms but no nearby intestinal damage, only the diverticulum is removed. If a small diverticulum is found during an operation that is being performed for other reasons, it often isn't removed unless it is causing symptoms.

CHAPTER 266

Nutritional Disorders

From a worldwide perspective, malnutrition is one of the leading causes of death and poor health among children. Malnutrition may be caused by improper or inadequate food intake or an inability to absorb or metabolize nutrients. Malnutrition may occur when requirements for essential nutrients are increased—for example, during stress, an infection, an injury, or a disease.

Protein-energy malnutrition is one of the most serious forms of malnutrition.★ It occurs in infants because breastfeeding or weaning diets are inadequate. This type of malnutrition is relatively common in developing countries; in industrialized countries, mild forms occur among families living in poverty.

▲ see page 498

■ see page 539

★ see page 649

As a part of routine child care, a doctor asks the parent or child about the child's diet and food intolerances and examines the child for signs of a nutritional deficiency or disorders that interfere with nutrition, such as malabsorption, kidney disease, diarrhea, and metabolic or genetic diseases. A doctor evaluates the child's growth by observing changes in height and weight and comparing them to normal growth curves. If malnutrition is suspected, the diagnosis may be confirmed by performing blood or urine tests to measure nutrient levels.

Most vitamin deficiencies are rare among infants and children in industrialized countries. The most common ones are deficiencies of vitamin E, vitamin K, vitamin C (infantile scurvy), or essential fatty acids.

Vitamin E Deficiency

Vitamin E deficiency▲ is relatively common in premature infants because the placenta doesn't transmit fat-soluble vitamins, such as vitamin E, very well and because prematurity worsens the deficiency that results from poor transmission. A formula high in polyunsaturated fatty acids increases the vitamin E requirement, particularly for premature infants who absorb vitamin E poorly. Vitamin E deficiency may also occur in children who have disorders that interfere with fat absorption, such as cystic fibrosis and certain genetic abnormalities. Administering excessive amounts of iron may also aggravate vitamin E deficiency.

Premature infants who are deficient in vitamin E may have muscle weakness together with hemolytic anemia at 6 to 10 weeks of age, associated with reduced blood levels of vitamin E. These problems can be corrected by giving vitamin E supplements. Vitamin E deficiency plays a role in the development of retinopathy of prematurity,■ an eye problem that's aggravated by exposure to high oxygen levels in incubators. Children with intestinal malabsorption may develop severe vitamin E deficiency, which produces a variety of neurologic symptoms, such as reduced reflexes, difficulty in walking, double vision, loss of position sense, and muscle weakness. These symptoms worsen progressively but may be reversed with treatment. The diagnosis is established by measuring the blood level of vitamin E.

Vitamin K Deficiency

Vitamin K is necessary for normal blood clotting.★ In newborns, the principal form of vitamin K deficiency is **hemorrhagic disease of the newborn.** It develops because the placenta doesn't transmit fats, including the fat-soluble vitamin K, very well; because the newborn's liver is too immature to produce enough prothrombin (one of the blood clotting factors), which requires vitamin K; because breast milk is low in vitamin K, containing only 1 to 3 micrograms a liter, whereas cow's milk contains 5 to 10 micrograms a liter; and because the bacteria that produce vitamin K in the intestine aren't present during the first few days of life. Hemorrhagic disease of the newborn generally occurs 1 to 7 days after birth. Symptoms include bleeding into the skin, in the stomach, or in the chest. In the worst cases, bleeding may occur within the brain.

Late hemorrhagic disease occurs 1 to 3 months after birth and produces the same symptoms as hemorrhagic disease of the newborn. It is usually associated with malabsorption or liver disease. The incidence of both types of hemorrhagic disease is increased among infants of mothers who took hydantoin anticonvulsants, such as phenytoin; cephalosporin antibiotics; or coumarin anticoagulants, such as warfarin, during pregnancy.

The American Academy of Pediatrics advises giving newborns an injection of vitamin K intramuscularly within 1 hour of birth to prevent hemorrhagic disease of the newborn. Giving vitamin K by mouth is not recommended because it is variably absorbed and unpredictably retained.

Infantile Scurvy

Infantile scurvy is a condition caused by an inadequate intake of vitamin C (ascorbic acid), usually resulting from receiving cow's milk formulas, which are deficient in this vitamin and need sup-

---

▲ see page 656

■ see page 1207

★ see page 657

plementation. This disease usually occurs between 6 and 12 months of age. Early symptoms include irritability, poor appetite, and failure to gain weight. The infant may scream when moved and may not move his legs because of pain caused by bleeding under the thin layer of tissue covering bones. In older children, bleeding may occur under the skin, and the gums around emerging teeth may bleed easily. Because vitamin C is necessary for the formation of connective tissue (the tissue that holds the body's structures together), scurvy may cause bone abnormalities in the rib cage and in the long bones of the legs. In the rib cage, the junctions between the cartilage and bone enlarge, forming a row of bumps called scorbutic rosary. Scurvy also results in poor wound healing.

A diet adequate in vitamin C can prevent scurvy; citrus fruits and juices are excellent sources. Formula-fed infants should receive 35 milligrams of vitamin C daily (equivalent to 3 ounces of orange or lemon juice). Breastfeeding mothers should take 100 milligrams of vitamin C by mouth daily. For the treatment of scurvy, the infant is given 100 to 200 milligrams of vitamin C by mouth daily for 1 week followed by 50 milligrams daily thereafter.

Essential Fatty Acid Deficiency

Essential fatty acids must be consumed in the diet. They include linoleic, linolenic, arachidonic, eicosapentaenoic, and docosahexaenoic acids. In the body, arachidonic acid can be made from linoleic acid, and eicosapentaenoic and docosahexaenoic acids can be made from linolenic acid. Vegetable oils, such as corn oil, cottonseed oil, and soybean oil, are sources of linoleic and linolenic acids; fish oils are sources of eicosapentaenoic and docosahexaenoic acids. Essential fatty acids are needed for many physiologic processes, including maintaining the integrity of the skin and the structure of cell membranes and synthesizing important biologically active compounds, such as prostaglandins and leukotrienes. Some animal studies suggest that essential fatty acids may be necessary for the development of normal vision in infants.

Linoleic acid deficiency may occur in infants whose formula is deficient in polyunsaturated fatty acids. Symptoms of this deficiency include dry, scaly skin followed by peeling. A puslike fluid may seep from areas around the skinfolds, especially around the anus. An essential fatty acid deficiency also causes significant changes in metabolism, affecting the lipid (fat) content of blood, platelet function, inflammatory responses, and certain immune responses. Similar symptoms may occur in patients who receive all nutrients intravenously for an extended time (long-term total parenteral nutrition) but who are not given essential fatty acids. When long-term total parenteral nutrition doesn't include linolenic acid, neurologic complications including numbness, weakness, an inability to walk, leg pain, and blurred vision may occur along with very low blood levels of linolenic acid. Symptoms resolve when linolenic acid is given.

CHAPTER 267

Metabolic Disorders

Disorders may affect metabolism, which is how the body processes substances needed to carry out its functions. Such disorders are often caused by genetic abnormalities that result in the absence of a specific enzyme needed to stimulate a metabolic process. Depending on the disorder, the effects may be serious or harmless.

Carbohydrate Metabolism Disorders

Carbohydrates are sugars. Many sugars besides the well-known glucose, sucrose, and fructose are present in foods. Some sugars, such as sucrose, must be processed (metabolized) by enzymes in the body before they can be used as a source of energy. If the enzymes needed to process them are missing, these sugars can accumulate, causing problems.

Galactosemia (a high blood level of galactose) is usually caused by the lack of galactose 1-phosphate uridyl transferase, one of the enzymes necessary for metabolizing galactose. This disorder is present from birth.

About 1 out of 50,000 to 70,000 babies is born without this enzyme. The newborn seems normal at first, but within a few days or weeks, he loses his appetite, vomits, becomes jaundiced, and stops growing normally. The liver becomes enlarged, excess amounts of protein and amino acids appear in the urine, tissues swell, and the body retains water. If treatment is delayed, affected children remain short and become mentally retarded. Many of them develop cataracts. The cause of these symptoms is unknown in most cases.

Galactosemia is suspected when laboratory tests detect galactose and galactose 1-phosphate in the urine. The diagnosis is confirmed by the absence of galactose 1-phosphate uridyl transferase in blood and liver cells. If the doctor or parents are concerned about galactosemia because someone in the family has had the disorder, it can be diagnosed at birth by analyzing a blood sample.

Milk and milk products—the source of galactose—must be completely eliminated from an affected child's diet. Galactose is also found in some fruits, vegetables, and sea products such as seaweed, which should also be avoided. However, whether the small amounts in these foods cause problems in the long term is not known. A woman known to carry a gene for the disorder should completely eliminate galactose from her diet during pregnancy. A pregnant woman who has the disorder must also avoid galactose. If she has high galactose levels, the galactose can cross to the fetus and cause cataracts. Those who have the disorder must restrict galactose intake throughout life.

If galactosemia is adequately treated, most children do not become mentally retarded. However, their intelligence quotient (IQ) is lower than that of their siblings, and they frequently have speech problems. Girls often have ovarian failure during puberty and adulthood, and only a few are able to conceive naturally.

Glycogen storage diseases (glycogenoses) are a group of hereditary disorders caused by the absence of one or more of the many enzymes needed to convert sugar into its storage form, glycogen, or glycogen back into glucose for use as energy. In glycogen storage diseases, abnormal types or amounts of glycogen are deposited in the body tissues, mostly the liver.

Symptoms result from the accumulation of glycogen or its by-products or from an inability to produce glucose when needed. The age at which symptoms start and their severity vary considerably among these diseases because different enzymes are affected in each disease.

The diagnosis is made when an examination of a sample of tissue, usually muscle or liver, determines that a specific enzyme is missing.

Treatment depends on the type of glycogen storage disease. For many people, eating several small carbohydrate-rich meals every day helps prevent blood sugar levels from dropping. For some young children, giving uncooked cornstarch every 4 to 6 hours around the clock can also relieve the problem. Sometimes carbohydrate solutions are given through a stomach tube all night.

Glycogen storage diseases tend to cause uric acid, a waste product, to accumulate—which can cause gout ▲ and kidney stones.■ Drug treatment to prevent this accumulation is often necessary. In some types of glycogen storage disease, the amount of exercise children do must be limited to reduce muscle cramps.

Hereditary fructose intolerance is a hereditary disorder in which the body cannot use fructose because the enzyme phosphofructaldolase is absent. As a result, fructose 1-phosphate, a by-product of fructose, accumulates in the body, blocking the formation of glycogen and its conversion to glucose for use as energy.

Ingesting more than minute amounts of fructose or sucrose (table sugar), which is broken down in the body to fructose, causes low blood sugar levels (hypoglycemia) with sweating, involuntary trembling (tremor), confusion, nausea, vomiting, abdominal pain, and sometimes convulsions and coma. Kidney and liver damage and mental deterioration can develop if a person continues to eat foods containing fructose.

▲ see page 244

■ see page 627

Types and Characteristics of Glycogen Storage Diseases

Name	Affected Organs	Symptoms	Missing Enzyme
Type O	Liver, muscle	Enlarged liver with accumulation of fat inside the liver cells (fatty liver); episodes of low blood sugar levels (hypoglycemia) when fasting	Glycogen synthetase
von Gierke's disease (Type IA)	Liver, kidney	Enlarged liver and kidney; slowed growth; very low blood sugar levels; abnormally high levels of acid, fats, and uric acid in blood	Glucose-6-phosphatase
Type IB	Liver, white blood cells	Same as in von Gierke's disease but may be less severe; low white blood cell count; recurring mouth and intestinal infections	Glucose-6-phosphatase translocase
Pompe's disease (Type II)	All organs	Enlarged liver and heart	Lysosomal glucosidase (various types)
Forbes' disease (Type III)	Liver, muscle, heart, white blood cells	Enlarged liver; low blood sugar levels; muscle damage in some people	Debrancher enzyme system
Andersen's disease (Type IV)	Liver, muscle, most tissues	Cirrhosis in juvenile type; muscle damage and heart failure in adult (late-onset) type	Brancher enzyme system
McArdle's disease (Type V)	Muscle	Muscle cramps during physical activity	Muscle phosphorylase
Hers' disease (Type VI)	Liver	Enlarged liver; episodes of low blood sugar when fasting; often no symptoms	Liver phosphorylase
Tarui's disease (Type VII)	Skeletal muscle, red blood cells	Muscle cramps during physical activity; red blood cell destruction (hemolysis)	Phosphofructokinase

The diagnosis is made when an examination of a sample of liver tissue determines that the enzyme is missing. Doctors also test the body's response to fructose and glucose given intravenously. Carriers (people who have one gene for a disorder but don't have the disorder) can be identified by analyzing DNA (genetic material) and comparing it with the DNA of people who have the disorder and with those who do not.

Treatment involves excluding fructose (generally found in sweet fruits), sucrose, and sorbitol (a sugar substitute) from the diet. Attacks of hypoglycemia are treated with glucose tablets, which should be carried by everyone who has hereditary fructose intolerance.

Fructosuria is a harmless condition in which fructose is excreted in the urine. It is caused by an inherited deficiency of the enzyme fructokinase. About 1 out of 130,000 people in the general population has fructosuria. The condition produces no symptoms, but the high level of fructose in the blood and urine can lead to a misdiagnosis of diabetes mellitus. No treatment is necessary.

Pentosuria is a harmless condition characterized by the excretion of the sugar xylulose in the urine, because the enzyme needed to process this sugar is missing.

The condition occurs almost exclusively in Jews; 1 out of 2,500 American Jews has it. Pentosuria causes no problems, but the presence of xylulose in the urine may lead to a misdiagnosis of diabetes mellitus. Treatment is not needed.

Pyruvate Metabolism Disorders

Pyruvate is formed in the processing of carbohydrates, fats, and proteins. Hereditary problems with the processing of pyruvate can cause a wide variety of disturbances.

Pyruvate is an energy source for mitochondria, the energy-generating components of a cell.▲ A problem with pyruvate metabolism can disturb the functioning of the mitochondria, causing any of a variety of symptoms, such as muscle damage, mental retardation, seizures, a buildup of lactic acid leading to excess acid in the body (acidosis),■ or failure of organ function, including that of the heart, lungs, kidneys, or liver. Such problems may develop any time between early infancy and late adulthood. Exercise, infections, or alcohol consumption can worsen symptoms, leading to severe lactic acidosis with muscle cramping and weakness.

A **deficiency of the pyruvate dehydrogenase complex**, a group of enzymes needed to process pyruvate, results in insufficient levels of acetyl coenzyme A, which is essential for energy production. The major symptoms include slowed muscle action, poor coordination, and a severe balance problem that makes walking nearly impossible. In addition, seizures, mental retardation, and brain malformation may occur. This disorder cannot be cured, but some people are helped by a diet high in fat.

Absence of pyruvate carboxylase, an enzyme, interferes with or blocks the production of glucose in the body. Lactic acid and ketones★ build up in the blood, causing nausea and vomiting. Often this disease is fatal. The synthesis of amino acids, the building blocks of proteins, also depends on pyruvate carboxylase. When this enzyme is miss-

ing, the production of neurotransmitters (substances that transmit nerve impulses) is reduced, leading to a variety of neurologic symptoms, including severe mental retardation. Low blood sugar levels (hypoglycemia) and the buildup of acids in the blood (acidosis) may be relieved by eating frequent carbohydrate-rich meals, but no replacements for the missing neurotransmitters are available to treat the neurologic symptoms. A diet restricted in protein may help some people who have milder disease.

Amino Acid Metabolism Disorders

Amino acids, the building blocks of proteins, have many functions in the body. Hereditary disorders of amino acid processing can be defects in either the breakdown of amino acids or their transport into cells. Many of these disorders, including phenylketonuria, have been identified. In all states in the United States, newborns are screened for phenylketonuria as well as for other metabolic disorders.

PHENYLKETONURIA

Phenylketonuria (PKU, phenylalaninemia, phenylpyruvic oligophrenia) is a hereditary disorder in which the enzyme that processes the amino acid phenylalanine is missing, resulting in a dangerously high level of phenylalanine in the blood.

Phenylalanine is normally converted to tyrosine, another amino acid, and eliminated from the body. Without the enzyme that converts it, phenylalanine builds up in the blood and is toxic to the brain, causing mental retardation. Phenylketonuria occurs in most geographic groups but is rare in Jews of Eastern European ancestry and in blacks. In the United States, the incidence is about 1 in 16,000 live births.

Symptoms

The symptoms of phenylketonuria are usually absent in newborns. Rarely, an infant is sleepy or

---

▲ see box, page 3

■ see page 676

★ see page 718

eats poorly. Affected infants tend to have lighter skin, hair, and eyes than family members who don't have the disorder. Some infants develop a rash that looks like eczema.▲ If not treated, affected infants soon develop some degree of mental retardation, usually severe.

Symptoms in children who have undiagnosed or untreated phenylketonuria include seizures, nausea and vomiting, aggressive or self-injurious behavior, hyperactivity, and sometimes psychiatric symptoms. Affected children often give off a "mousy" body odor caused by a by-product of phenylalanine (phenylacetic acid) in their urine and sweat.

Phenylketonuria in a pregnant woman has profound effects on the developing fetus, often causing mental and physical retardation in the infant. Many infants have microcephaly (an abnormally small head, leading to mental retardation) and heart disease. Strict control of the mother's phenylalanine level during pregnancy usually results in a normal outcome for the fetus.

Diagnosis and Treatment

Early diagnosis is made when a high phenylalanine level and a low tyrosine level are detected during the screening of a newborn. If phenylketonuria runs in the family and DNA is available from the affected family member, amniocentesis or chorionic villus sampling■ with DNA analysis can be performed to determine whether the fetus has the disorder.

Treatment consists of limiting but not entirely eliminating the intake of phenylalanine. Because all natural sources of protein contain about 4 percent phenylalanine, consuming enough protein without exceeding the acceptable amount of phenylalanine is impossible. Consequently, instead of milk and meat, a person must eat a variety of synthetic foods that supply the other amino acids. Low-protein natural foods, such as fruits, vegetables, and restricted amounts of certain grain cereals, can be eaten. Phenylalanine-free products are available; they help control phenylalanine intake, giving the person a little more freedom to eat natural foods.

Phenylalanine intake must be restricted beginning in the first few weeks of life to prevent mental retardation. A restricted diet, started early and well maintained, makes normal development possible and prevents brain damage. However, if very strict control of diet is not maintained, affected children may have difficulties in school. Dietary restrictions started after 2 to 3 years of age may control only extreme hyperactivity and seizures. Discontinuing the special diet when brain development is nearly complete was once thought safe, but reports indicating the development of learning and behavioral problems and a decrease in intelligence have caused this recommendation to be reconsidered. Most doctors now believe that a phenylalanine-restricted diet should continue for life.

CHAPTER 268

Hormonal Disorders

The endocrine system consists of a group of glands and organs that secrete hormones into the bloodstream.★ The major glands are the pituitary gland (controlled by the hypothalamus), the thyroid gland, the parathyroid glands, the islets of the pancreas (which produce insulin), the adrenal glands, the testes in males, and the ovaries in females. Hormones secreted by these glands control physical growth, sexual function, metabolism, and other functions. Many of the endocrine disorders that affect adults also affect children but may produce different symptoms.

Pituitary Gland Disorders

The pituitary gland, a pea-sized gland at the base of the brain, produces a number of hor-

▲ see page 959

■ see box, page 1135

★ see box, page 694

mones.▲ Several of these hormones, such as corticotropin, thyroid-stimulating hormone, follicle-stimulating hormone, and luteinizing hormone, control the function of other endocrine glands and stimulate these glands to produce other hormones. Growth hormone, another pituitary hormone, ensures growth during childhood.

Inadequate pituitary function is called **hypopituitarism.** In children, hypopituitarism may be caused by a noncancerous pituitary tumor (craniopharyngioma), an injury, or an infection, or it may have no identifiable cause (idiopathic hypopituitarism). Rarely, hypopituitarism (and diabetes insipidus ■) occurs as part of Hand-Schüller-Christian disease, ★ which affects small areas of bone and lungs and the function of the pituitary gland.

If the pituitary gland malfunctions before puberty, growth is delayed, sexual characteristics do not develop, and the thyroid and adrenal glands function inadequately. After puberty, pituitary malfunction can cause decreased sex drive, impotence, and shrinking of the testes.

In **panhypopituitarism,** the production of all pituitary hormones decreases or stops. This disorder can result when the entire pituitary gland is damaged.

Sometimes only one pituitary hormone is missing. For example, if only luteinizing hormone is missing **(isolated luteinizing hormone deficiency),** the testes develop and produce sperm, because these functions are controlled by follicle-stimulating hormone, but the testes do not produce enough testosterone. Testosterone is the hormone that stimulates the development of male secondary sexual characteristics, such as deepening of the voice, growth of facial hair, and maturation of the penis. Consequently, boys who have isolated luteinizing hormone deficiency do not develop these characteristics. Abnormally long arms and legs may be another symptom of this deficiency.

Growth hormone may also be deficient. In **pituitary dwarfism,** the pituitary gland produces inadequate amounts of growth hormone, which cause abnormally slow growth and short stature with normal proportions. Most short children, however, have normally functioning pituitary glands and are short because their growth spurt is late or their parents are relatively short.

Symptoms and Diagnosis

The symptoms of inadequate pituitary function vary depending on which hormone is deficient. For example, growth may be impaired and mental development may be poor in children who lack thyroid-stimulating hormone.

The age at which the deficiencies start also influences which symptoms develop. The effects on a fetus are different from those on a newborn or an older child.

If inadequate pituitary function seems likely, a doctor orders blood tests to measure hormone levels. Measuring the level of growth hormone is not always useful or indicative of a deficiency because the body produces the hormone in short bursts that cause its level to rise and fall quickly. To look for a deficiency of growth hormone, a doctor can measure the level of insulin-like growth factor I (IGF-I). Some pituitary hormones are measured directly; others are measured repeatedly over 1 to 2 hours after a specific stimulus is given by mouth or by injection. X-rays of the hand may be performed to determine bone age, which indicates whether the bones are still growing and how much longer they are likely to grow. A computed tomography (CT) scan or magnetic resonance imaging (MRI) of the head may detect a tumor or other structural abnormality in or near the pituitary gland.

Treatment

Children deficient in a particular pituitary hormone can be given an identical synthetic hormone as replacement. For instance, children who are short because of a deficiency of growth hormone can be given synthetic growth hormone. They may grow 4 to 6 inches in the first year of treatment; subsequent growth is slower. Growth hormone replacement is not appropriate for short children who have normal levels of growth hormone. New treatments that stimulate the body's natural production of growth hormone are being investigated.

▲ see box, page 697

■ see page 703

★ see page 101

Goiter: An Enlarged Thyroid Gland

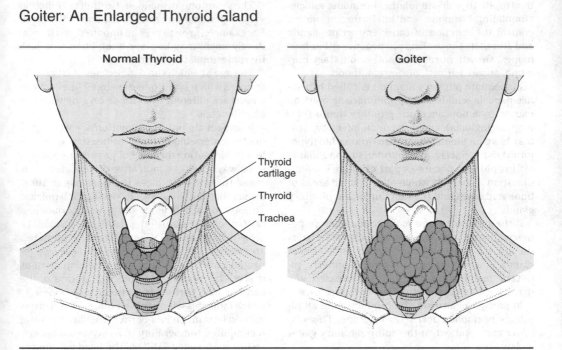

Normal Thyroid	Goiter

Thyroid cartilage

Thyroid

Trachea

Either the missing pituitary hormone or the hormone that is dependent on the pituitary hormone can be replaced. The latter approach is generally preferred. For example, a child who cannot produce thyroid-stimulating hormone is given thyroid hormone. Testosterone is given to a boy who cannot produce follicle-stimulating hormone and luteinizing hormone, and estrogen is given to a girl who cannot produce these two hormones.

Thyroid Gland Disorders

The thyroid gland is located in the front of the neck. It produces thyroid hormone, which controls the speed at which the body's chemical functions proceed (metabolic rate).

Some problems that affect the thyroid gland may also cause the gland to enlarge—a condition called goiter. A goiter may exist if the thyroid

▲ see page 708

gland is underactive (producing too little thyroid hormone) or overactive (producing too much). An enlarged thyroid gland that is present at birth is called **congenital goiter.** Some children have **Pendred's syndrome,** a hereditary condition that combines deaf-mutism and congenital goiter.

Hypothyroidism results when the thyroid gland cannot produce adequate amounts of thyroid hormone for the body's needs. Symptoms of hypothyroidism in children and adolescents differ from those in adults.▲ In newborns, hypothyroidism causes **cretinism** (neonatal hypothyroidism), which is characterized by jaundice, poor appetite, constipation, a hoarse cry, outpouching of the navel (umbilical hernia), and slowed bone growth. If not diagnosed and treated within a few months of birth, hypothyroidism results in mental retardation. Hypothyroidism that begins in childhood (juvenile hypothyroidism) slows growth, sometimes resulting in disproportionately short limbs. Tooth development is delayed. Hypothyroidism that begins in adolescence (adolescent hypothyroidism) is similar to that in adults, except that it may delay puberty. Symptoms include a hoarse voice, slowed speech, droopy eyelids, a puffy face, hair loss, dry skin, a slow pulse, and weight gain.

In all newborns, the thyroid hormone level in the blood is routinely measured within 2 days of birth. A newborn who has hypothyroidism is promptly given thyroid hormone as replacement. This treatment prevents brain damage. Hypothyroidism that begins in childhood or adolescence is also treated with a replacement hormone.

Hyperthyroidism results from overactivity of the thyroid gland.▲ In newborns, the most common cause of hyperthyroidism is **neonatal Graves' disease,** a potentially life-threatening illness that can occur in infants whose mothers have or have had Graves' disease. Graves' disease, a form of hyperthyroidism, is an autoimmune disorder in which the body produces antibodies that stimulate the thyroid gland. In pregnant women, these antibodies cross the placenta and stimulate the fetus' thyroid gland. Graves' disease in the mother may result in stillbirth, miscarriage, or premature birth. In a newborn, symptoms of an overactive thyroid gland—poor weight gain, fast heart rate, high blood pressure, nervousness or irritability, vomiting, and diarrhea—may start within several days after birth. The enlarged thyroid gland (goiter) can press on the windpipe and interfere with breathing. The high thyroid hormone levels cause the fast heart rate, which can lead to heart failure. Bulging eyes, common in the adult form of the disorder, also occur in newborns. Graves' disease is potentially fatal if not recognized and treated appropriately.

Infants who receive treatment recover within weeks, although they may remain at risk of recurring illness for 6 months to a year. Persistently high levels of the thyroid-stimulating antibodies can also lead to premature closure of the bones of the skull (fontanelles), mental retardation, hyperactivity later in childhood, and slowed growth.

Hyperthyroidism is treated with a drug, such as propylthiouracil, that blocks the formation of thyroid hormones. Infants may also need treatment for heart failure. For severely affected newborns who have very high blood levels of thyroid-stimulating antibodies, an exchange blood transfusion (in which some of the newborn's blood is removed and exchanged with donated blood) may be needed to decrease the antibody levels.

Adrenal Gland Disorders

The two adrenal glands, located above the kidneys in the lower back,■ produce several types of hormones. The inner part (medulla) of each gland produces epinephrine and norepinephrine, which are responsible for the fight-or-flight reaction to danger and emotional stress. The outer part (cortex) produces aldosterone, which regulates the salt balance in the body; cortisol, which is essential for processing protein, fat, and carbohydrate; and certain male sex hormones (androgens).

In some adrenal gland disorders, cortisol and aldosterone cannot be produced, most commonly because enzymes needed for their production are missing. The hypothalamus detects the low levels of these hormones and stimulates the pituitary gland, which then tries to stimulate the adrenal glands to produce enough cortisol and aldosterone. The adrenal glands enlarge by as much as 10 to 20 times their normal weight because of the constant stimulation by the hypothalamus and pituitary gland, yet they remain unable to produce cortisol and aldosterone. However, they may produce large amounts of other hormones, such as androgens, which lead to masculinization.

Symptoms and Diagnosis

A deficiency of adrenal hormones causes various symptoms, depending on which hormone is deficient. If aldosterone production is low, too much sodium is excreted in the urine, resulting in low blood pressure and increased blood levels of potassium. If cortisol production is severely deficient, especially if aldosterone production is blocked, life-threatening adrenal failure can occur within days to weeks of birth, along with low blood pressure, a rapid heartbeat, and malfunction of many organs.

A deficiency of androgens before birth leads to inadequate growth of the genitals in male infants—an abnormal urethral opening, a small penis, and small testes—a condition called male pseudohermaphroditism.★ Girls who are defi-

---

▲ see page 705

■ see box, page 713

★ see page 1237

cient in adrenal hormones appear normal at birth but do not undergo puberty or menstruate.

An overabundance of adrenal hormones also produces symptoms. When a female fetus is exposed to high levels of androgens early in pregnancy, the genitals develop abnormally. The external genitals are masculinized (female pseudohermaphroditism).▲ If a female fetus is exposed to high androgen levels before the 12th week of pregnancy, the labia may fuse, and a single opening for the urethra and vagina develops. After the 12th week of pregnancy, the main effect is enlargement of the clitoris, giving the appearance of a penis. The ovaries, uterus, and other internal reproductive organs develop normally. Male fetuses are essentially unaffected by high androgen levels.

In young boys, high androgen levels cause accelerated growth. However, because the bones mature faster than normal and stop growing too soon, final height is shorter than normal.

Adrenal gland disorders can be diagnosed by measuring levels of adrenal hormones in blood or urine samples.

Treatment

Treatment requires giving a synthetic hormone to replace the one the adrenal glands cannot produce. Once the deficient hormone is replaced, the hypothalamus and pituitary gland stop stimulating the adrenal glands, which then stop producing excessive amounts of other hormones. Cortisol deficiency is treated with a corticosteroid, such as hydrocortisone or prednisone; for a severe deficiency, which is an emergency, treatment with fluids, sodium, and other minerals may also be required. Aldosterone is used to treat aldosterone deficiency, and testosterone is used to treat androgen deficiency. Blood pressure is measured frequently because if the levels of these hormones are too high or too low, they can disrupt salt and water regulation in the body and thus affect blood pressure. Growth is checked twice a year, and bone age is determined every year by taking an x-ray of the hand. With sufficient

▲ see page 1237

■ see page 1237

amounts of hydrocortisone, growth is normal. Girls who have been exposed to high androgen levels often need to have surgical reconstruction of the external genitals to create a normal vaginal opening for functional and cosmetic reasons.

Testicular Disorders

The testes have two main functions: synthesizing testosterone, the primary male sex hormone (androgen), and producing sperm. The testes may be underactive—a condition called male hypogonadism—because the pituitary gland does not secrete the hormones that stimulate the testes or because there is a problem within the testes. When the testes are underactive, androgen production is deficient. Growth and sexual development may be retarded, sperm production is low, and the penis may be small.

Symptoms

The symptoms vary depending on the age at which the androgen deficiency begins. In a male fetus, an androgen deficiency before the 12th week of pregnancy causes incomplete development of the genitals. The urethra may open on the underside of the penis instead of at its end, or a male infant may develop female genitals (male pseudohermaphroditism).■ If an androgen deficiency develops later in pregnancy, a male fetus may have an abnormally small penis (microphallus) or testes that do not descend fully into the scrotum.

Androgen deficiency in childhood results in incomplete sexual development. An affected boy retains a high-pitched voice and has poor muscle development for his age. The penis, testes, and scrotum are underdeveloped. Pubic and underarm hair is sparse, and the arms and legs are abnormally long.

Androgen deficiency after puberty can cause a weak sex drive, impotence, and subnormal strength in boys. The testes may be shriveled, the skin around the eyes and lips may be finely wrinkled, body hair may be sparse, and bones may be weak. If the androgen deficiency is caused by a problem within the testes, breasts may develop (gynecomastia).

Klinefelter's syndrome occurs in about 1 out of 700 male births. It is caused by a chromosomal abnormality. Boys with Klinefelter's syndrome usually have two X chromosomes and one Y chromosome (XXY instead of the normal XY), although some have even more copies of the X chromosome. Generally, this syndrome is not detected until puberty, when an affected child does not undergo normal sexual maturation.

Boys with Klinefelter's syndrome have small testes (less than $^3/_4$ inch across the scrotum) that are firm and filled with fibrous tissue. The breasts are usually somewhat enlarged, and the skeletal proportions are abnormal, with the legs longer than the torso and head. Antisocial behavior may occur. Also, the risk of diabetes mellitus, chronic lung disease, varicose veins, hypothyroidism, and breast cancer is increased. The diagnosis is made by analyzing chromosomes in cells from a blood sample.

The **vanishing testes syndrome** (bilateral anorchia) occurs in about 1 out of 20,000 males. The testes are presumably present during early development but are resorbed by the body before or after birth. Without testes, these children cannot produce testosterone or sperm and therefore do not develop male secondary sexual characteristics at puberty and are infertile.

Congenital absence of Leydig's cells (cells in the testes that normally produce testosterone) leads to the development of ambiguous genitals (male pseudohermaphroditism), because not enough testosterone is produced to stimulate the fetus to develop normal male genitals. Affected children are genetically male.

Cryptorchidism is a condition in which one or both testes remain in the abdomen, where they are formed in the fetus. Usually, the testes descend into the scrotum shortly before birth. At birth, about 3 percent of boys have cryptorchidism, but in most of them, the testes descend on their own by 1 year of age. If the testes do not descend, surgery is necessary to reposition the testes in the scrotum to prevent infertility or torsion (painful twisting of the testis on its spermatic cord)▲ and to reduce the risk of testicular cancer. This surgery should be performed before a boy is 5 years old.

Noonan's syndrome results in small testes that produce too little testosterone. Other symptoms may include webbing of the neck, low-set ears,

Undescended Testis

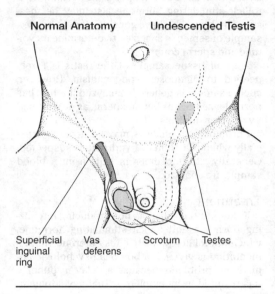

Normal Anatomy	Undescended Testis

Superficial inguinal ring   Vas deferens   Scrotum   Testes

droopy eyelids, short stature, shortened fourth (ring) fingers, a high-arched palate, and heart and blood vessel abnormalities. Blood tests detect low levels of testosterone and high levels of two pituitary hormones, luteinizing hormone and follicle-stimulating hormone.

Myotonic dystrophy is a muscle disease that includes testicular failure in 80 percent of the cases. The testes are replaced by fibrous tissue and usually do not produce sperm. Other symptoms are muscle weakness and wasting, balding, mental retardation, cataracts, diabetes mellitus, hypothyroidism, and abnormally thick skull bones.

Diagnosis

Various tests are used to identify which testicular disorder is present. First, a doctor examines the boy's penis and testes to see if they are nor-

▲ see page 1062

mally developed for his age. Blood levels of testosterone are measured. Because the function of the testes is regulated by the pituitary gland and hypothalamus, levels of luteinizing hormone and follicle-stimulating hormone also may be measured. In boys who have gone through puberty, a sample of semen is analyzed to determine its volume and sperm count.

A small tissue sample of the testis is rarely needed to diagnose hypogonadism. However, such a sample is generally analyzed if a boy has normal-sized testes but no sperm, as determined by a semen analysis.

Chromosomal analysis may be needed, especially when Klinefelter's syndrome is suspected. Generally, chromosomes in cells from a blood sample are analyzed.

Treatment

If the pituitary gland is not producing luteinizing hormone and follicle-stimulating hormone, which stimulate the testes, testosterone supplementation is given. If a boy has psychologic adjustment problems because a delay in puberty has resulted in incomplete sexual development,

he can be given testosterone injections for 3 months. This treatment causes some masculinization without stunting growth.

Testosterone deficiency can be treated with injections of testosterone once or twice a month. The hormone is given by injection because this method is safer than taking it by mouth and fewer doses are needed. Testosterone can also be given in a skin patch applied daily. Treatment with testosterone restores the balance in the body and stimulates growth, sexual development, and fertility. Major side effects include fluid retention, acne, and, occasionally, temporary breast development (gynecomastia).

No cure is available for chromosomal abnormalities, but testosterone may be helpful in treating the symptoms.

Surgery to repair an abnormally developed penis is often possible. Artificial testes can be inserted into the scrotum for cosmetic purposes, but they do not produce sperm or hormones. Surgery to move undescended testes into the scrotum usually enables the testes to function normally.

CHAPTER 269

Musculoskeletal Disorders

In children, a wide variety of disorders affect the muscles, joints, and bones.▲ These disorders may be caused by heredity, injury, inflammation, or infection.

Some Common Skeletal Problems

In developing children, bones may be misaligned. Such problems include scoliosis, in which the spine is curved abnormally, and a variety of problems affecting the hipbones,

thighbones, knees, and feet. Often, the problem resolves on its own, but sometimes it is caused by a disorder that must be treated.

Scoliosis

Scoliosis is an abnormal curvature of the spine.

About 4 percent of all children aged 10 to 14 years have detectable scoliosis. About 60 to 80 percent of all cases occur in girls. Scoliosis may occur as a birth defect. When it develops later, no cause can be found in 75 percent of the cases; the rest are caused by polio, cerebral palsy, juvenile osteoporosis, or other diseases.

Symptoms and Diagnosis

Mild scoliosis usually produces no symptoms. Fatigue in the back may be felt after prolonged

▲ see page 214

sitting or standing. It may be followed by muscular pain in the back and eventually by more severe pain.

Most curves are convex to the right in the upper back and to the left in the lower back, so that the right shoulder is higher than the left. One hip may be higher than the other.

Mild scoliosis may be discovered during a routine physical examination at school. A parent, teacher, or doctor may suspect scoliosis when a child has one shoulder that seems higher than the other or when the child's clothes don't hang straight. To diagnose the condition, a doctor asks the child to bend forward and views the spine from behind, because the abnormal spinal curve can be seen more easily in this position. X-rays help confirm the diagnosis.

Prognosis and Treatment

The prognosis depends on where the abnormal curve is, how severe it is, and when symptoms begin. The more severe the curve, the greater the likelihood that it will worsen.

Half of the children with detectable scoliosis need to be treated or closely monitored by a doctor. Prompt treatment may prevent further deformity.

Usually, a child who has scoliosis is treated by an orthopedic specialist. A brace or plaster cast may be worn to hold the spine straight. Sometimes electrospinal stimulation is performed. In this treatment, the spinal muscles are stimulated by tiny electrical currents that allow the spine to straighten. Sometimes surgery in which the vertebrae are fused together is needed; a metal rod may be inserted during surgery to keep the spine straight until the vertebrae have fused.

Scoliosis and its treatment can cause psychologic problems, threatening an adolescent's self-image. Wearing a brace or a cast can cause concern about appearing different from peers, and hospitalization and surgery may threaten an adolescent's independence. However, the alternative could be an obvious, permanent deformity. Counseling and support can help.

Hipbone and Thighbone Problems

In a young child, the thighbones may turn inward, so that the knees partially face each other

Scoliosis

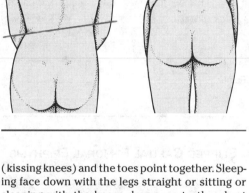

| Standing | Bending Over |

(kissing knees) and the toes point together. Sleeping face down with the legs straight or sitting or sleeping with the knees drawn up to the chest may make the problem worse. If the condition persists after age 8, a child should see an orthopedic surgeon.

In very young children, the thighbones commonly turn outward. Sleeping face down with the feet pointing away from each other and legs rotated outward can prolong the condition. Rotating the legs inward with every diaper change may be helpful, but in most cases, the condition corrects itself when the child learns to walk.

In adolescents, limping and pain in the hip, or occasionally in the knee or thigh, may be caused by a slipped capital femoral epiphysis, in which the upper growing end (epiphysis) of the thighbone is dislocated. In younger children, the same symptoms can be caused by loss of the blood supply to the neck of the thighbone (Legg-Calvé-Perthes disease).

Slipped Capital Femoral Epiphysis

Normal Hip   Slipped Epiphysis

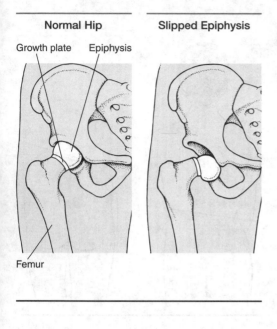

Growth plate   Epiphysis

Femur

SLIPPED CAPITAL FEMORAL EPIPHYSIS

A slipped capital femoral epiphysis is a dislocation of the upper growing end (epiphysis) of the thighbone (femur).

This disorder usually occurs in overweight adolescents, most commonly boys. Although the cause isn't known, the disorder may result from a thickened growth plate (the part of a bone where growth occurs), which is affected by levels of growth hormone and estrogen in the blood.

The first symptom may be stiffness in the hip that improves with rest. Later, a limp develops, followed by hip pain that extends down the inner thigh to the knee. The affected leg is usually twisted outward. The head of the femur may decay, causing the growth plate to collapse. X-rays of the affected hip show a widening of the growth

---

▲ see page 656

plate or an abnormal position of the head of the femur.

Diagnosing the disorder early is important because treatment becomes more difficult as the disorder progresses.

Corrective surgery may be needed to move the growth plate back into its correct position and to secure it with metal pins. The adolescent is immobilized in a cast for several weeks to 2 months.

Knee Problems

Either bowlegs or knock-knees, if not treated, can cause osteoarthritis in the knees later in life.

Bowlegs are common in toddlers and usually correct themselves by age 18 months. If bowlegs persist or worsen, the cause may be osteochondrosis of the tibia (Blount's disease) or rickets, an abnormality of bone development caused by a vitamin D deficiency.▲ Vitamin D is necessary for the normal incorporation of calcium into bones. Blount's disease can sometimes be treated by a splint worn at night, but surgery is often needed. Rickets can usually be treated with vitamin D supplements.

Knock-knees are less common. Even in severe cases, the condition usually corrects itself by age 9. If it persists after age 10, surgery may be needed.

In adolescents, the cartilage under the kneecap (patella) may soften because of unexplained degeneration of the cartilage or minor injury resulting from misalignment of the kneecap. The resulting condition is called chondromalacia patellae. It causes knee pain when climbing, especially going up or down stairs. Treatment consists of performing exercises to strengthen the muscles around the knees, avoiding activities that produce pain, and taking aspirin.

Foot Problems

One out of every 100 newborns has an apparent foot abnormality; most resolve without treatment. An infant may appear falsely flat-footed because of a fat pad in the arch of the foot. The arch usually can be seen when the infant stands on tiptoe. If an older child has pains or cramps in the feet because of flatfeet, corrective shoes may be needed.

Inflammatory Disorders

Some disorders are caused by inflammation of joints or connective tissue, the tissue that binds the body's structures together and provides support. Connective tissue forms a large part of muscles, bones, cartilage, and tendons and is also found in other parts of the body, such as the skin and the membranes surrounding the heart and lungs.

Rheumatic Fever

Rheumatic fever is inflammation of joints (arthritis) and the heart (carditis) resulting from a streptococcal infection, usually of the throat.

Although rheumatic fever may follow a streptococcal infection,▲ it is not an infection. Rather, it is an inflammatory reaction to an infection, affecting many parts of the body, such as the joints, heart, and skin. Poor nutrition and overcrowded living conditions seem to increase the risk of rheumatic fever, and heredity seems to play a part.

In the United States, rheumatic fever rarely develops before age 4 or after age 18 and is much less common than in developing countries, probably because antibiotics are widely used to treat streptococcal infections at an early stage. Recently, however, the incidence of rheumatic fever has been increasing for unknown reasons. In the United States, a child who has a mild streptococcal infection—usually a sore throat—but isn't treated has a 1 in 1,000 chance of developing rheumatic fever. The chances increase to 3 in 100 if the infection is more severe.

Symptoms

Symptoms of rheumatic fever vary greatly, depending on which parts of the body become inflamed. Typically, symptoms begin several weeks after the disappearance of a streptococcal sore throat. The major symptoms of rheumatic fever are joint pain (arthritis), fever, chest pain or palpitations caused by heart inflammation (carditis), jerky uncontrollable movements (Sydenham's chorea), a rash (erythema marginatum), and small bumps (nodules) under the skin. A child may have one symptom or several, although the rash and nodules are rarely the only symptoms.

Joint pain and fever are the most common first symptoms. One or several joints suddenly become painful and feel tender when touched. They may also be red, hot, and swollen and may contain fluid. Ankles, knees, elbows, and wrists are commonly affected; the shoulders, hips, and small joints of the hands and feet also may be affected. As pain in one joint improves, pain in another starts, particularly if the child isn't promptly put to bed and given an anti-inflammatory drug. Sometimes joint pains are very mild. The fever begins suddenly with the joint pain and may go up and down. Joint pains and fever often disappear within 2 weeks and seldom last more than a month.

Inflammation of the heart often starts at the same time as the joint pain and fever. At first, heart inflammation produces no symptoms. It may be discovered by a doctor who hears a heart murmur through a stethoscope. The heart may beat rapidly. The sac around the heart may become inflamed, causing chest pain. Heart failure may develop.■ The symptoms of heart failure in children are different from those in adults: A child may have shortness of breath, nausea, vomiting, stomachache, and a hacking cough. Heart inflammation may cause a child to tire easily. However, the symptoms of heart inflammation are often so mild that the child is not taken to a doctor, and the heart damage may not be discovered until long after the other symptoms of rheumatic fever have disappeared.

Heart inflammation disappears gradually, usually within 5 months. However, it may permanently damage the heart valves, resulting in rheumatic heart disease. The valve between the left atrium and ventricle (mitral valve) is most commonly damaged. The valve may become leaky (mitral valve regurgitation),★ abnormally narrow (mitral valve stenosis),● or both. Valve damage

---

▲ see page 875

■ see page 87

★ see page 93

● see page 96

causes the characteristic heart murmurs that enable a doctor to diagnose rheumatic fever. Later in life, usually in middle age, the damage may cause heart failure and atrial fibrillation, an abnormal heart rhythm.▲

Jerky uncontrollable movements (Sydenham's chorea) may begin gradually. A month may go by before the movements become so intense that the child is taken to a doctor. By then, the child typically has rapid, purposeless, sporadic movements that disappear during sleep. The movements may involve any muscle except those of the eyes. Facial grimacing is common. In mild cases, the child may seem clumsy and may have slight difficulties in dressing and eating. In extreme cases, the child may have to be protected from injuring himself with his flailing arms or legs. The chorea may end gradually after 4 months, but occasionally it lasts 6 to 8 months.

A flat painless rash with a wavy edge may appear as the other symptoms subside. It lasts for only a short time, sometimes less than a day. Small, hard nodules may form under the skin, usually in children with heart inflammation. The nodules are usually painless and disappear without treatment.

Occasionally, a child has a poor appetite and abdominal pain so severe that it's confused with appendicitis.

Diagnosis

The diagnosis of rheumatic fever is based mainly on the characteristic combination of symptoms. Blood tests may detect a high white blood cell count and a high erythrocyte sedimentation rate. Most children with rheumatic fever have antibodies to streptococci, which can be measured in a blood test. Abnormal heart rhythms caused by heart inflammation can be seen on an electrocardiogram (a recording of the heart's electrical activity). An echocardiogram (an image of structures in the heart produced by ultrasound waves) may be used to diagnose abnormalities of the heart valves.

▲ see page 82

■ see page 227

Prevention and Treatment

The best ways to prevent rheumatic fever are good nutrition and prompt antibiotic treatment of any infection thought to be streptococcal.

Treatment of rheumatic fever has three goals: curing a streptococcal infection and preventing its return; reducing inflammation, particularly in the joints and heart; and limiting physical activity that might aggravate the inflamed structures.

If a streptococcal infection such as strep throat is diagnosed, penicillin is given by mouth for 10 days. A child who has rheumatic fever is given an injection of penicillin to eliminate any remaining infection. Aspirin or other nonsteroidal anti-inflammatory drugs (NSAIDs) are given in high doses to reduce inflammation and pain, particularly if inflammation has reached the joints. Stronger analgesics such as codeine are sometimes needed. If heart inflammation is severe, corticosteroids such as prednisone may be given to further reduce inflammation.

Bed rest is important. A child's activity must be limited to avoid stressing the inflamed joints. When the heart is inflamed, more rest is needed.

If the heart valves become damaged, the risk of developing a valve infection (endocarditis) remains throughout life. Through at least age 18, children who have had rheumatic fever should be given penicillin by mouth or by monthly injections into the muscle to help prevent infection. Those who have heart damage must always take an antibiotic before undergoing any surgery, including dental surgery, even in adulthood.

Juvenile Rheumatoid Arthritis

Juvenile rheumatoid arthritis is persistent inflammation of the joints (arthritis) that is similar to rheumatoid arthritis■ in adults but begins before 16 years of age.

The cause is unknown. Hereditary factors may increase the risk of developing it.

Symptoms

This disorder affects only a few joints in about 40 percent of the children who have it; it affects many joints in another 40 percent. In the remaining 20 percent, it is systemic; that is, it affects the whole body, not just the joints, and is accompanied by fever—a condition called Still's disease.

Inflammation in only a few joints typically appears before age 4 (usually in girls) or after age 8 (usually in boys). The child has pain, swelling, and stiffness, most commonly in a knee, an ankle, or an elbow. Occasionally, one or two other joints, such as a single toe or finger, a wrist, or the jaw, become stiff and swollen. The joint symptoms may persist, or they may come and go.

Girls are particularly likely to have inflammation of the iris (chronic iridocyclitis), which often produces no symptoms and is detected only during an eye examination. Inflammation of the iris can cause blindness; therefore, the child must be examined for this condition and treated immediately.

Inflammation in many joints may occur in a child of any age, affecting girls more than boys. Joint pain, swelling, and stiffness may begin gradually or suddenly. The joints usually affected first include the knees, ankles, wrists, and elbows. Later, both hands, the neck, the jaw, and the hips may be affected. The inflammation is usually symmetric, affecting the same joint on both sides of the body—for example, both knees or both hips.

Systemic juvenile rheumatoid arthritis affects boys and girls equally. Fever is intermittent, usually highest in the evening (often 103° F. or higher), then returns rapidly to normal. During the fever, a child may feel very ill. A flat, pale pink or salmon rash—mainly on the trunk and the upper part of the legs or arms—appears for a short while (often in the evening), migrates and disappears, then returns. The spleen and some lymph nodes may become enlarged. Joint pain, swelling, and stiffness may be the last symptoms to appear.

Any type of juvenile rheumatoid arthritis can interfere with growth. When it interferes with growth of the jaw, it can result in a receding chin (micrognathia).

Rheumatoid factor,▲ an antibody that's usually found in the blood of adults who have rheumatoid arthritis, is rarely present in children who have juvenile rheumatoid arthritis. Rheumatoid factor is most likely to occur in girls who have many affected joints.

Prognosis and Treatment

Symptoms of juvenile rheumatoid arthritis completely disappear in up to 75 percent of the children. The prognosis is worse for those who have many affected joints and also have rheumatoid factor.

Large doses of aspirin can usually suppress pain and joint inflammation. Other nonsteroidal anti-inflammatory drugs, such as naproxen and tolmetin, are often used instead because taking aspirin increases the risk of Reye's syndrome.■ The child may be given corticosteroids by mouth if the disease is severe and affects the whole body, but these drugs can slow the growth rate and are avoided if possible. Corticosteroids can also be injected directly into affected joints to relieve inflammation. A child who doesn't respond to aspirin or other anti-inflammatory drugs may be given injections of gold compounds.★ Penicillamine, methotrexate, and hydroxychloroquine may be used when gold compounds are ineffective or cause side effects.

Exercises keep the joints from stiffening. Splints can prevent a joint from becoming locked in an awkward position.

The eyes are examined every 6 months to look for inflammation of the iris. Inflammation is treated with corticosteroid eyedrops or ointment and drugs that widen (dilate) the pupil. Occasionally, eye surgery is needed.

Hereditary Disorders of Connective Tissue or Bone

Some disorders that affect connective tissue are inherited. These include Ehlers-Danlos syndrome, Marfan's syndrome, pseudoxanthoma elasticum, cutis laxa, and mucopolysaccharidoses. Osteochondrodysplasias affect bone or cartilage, and osteopetroses affect bone.

Ehlers-Danlos Syndrome

Ehlers-Danlos syndrome is a very rare hereditary connective tissue disorder that results in unusually flexible joints, very elastic skin, and fragile tissues.

▲ see page 228

■ see page 1280

★ see page 229

This syndrome has several variations, which are caused by abnormalities in the different genes that control the production of connective tissue. Many children have very flexible joints (benign hypermobility) without the other symptoms; flexibility tends to decrease over time.

Symptoms and Diagnosis

The skin can be stretched several inches but returns to its normal position when released. Joints may be extremely flexible. Often, wide scars form over bony parts of the body, particularly the elbows, knees, and shins. Small, hard, round lumps may develop under the skin and may be seen on x-rays.

Minor injuries may cause wide gaping wounds, usually with little bleeding. However, a minority of people with Ehlers-Danlos syndrome have a tendency to bleed easily. Repairing wounds may be difficult because the stitches tend to tear out of the fragile tissue. Organs inside the body may also be fragile, causing problems during surgery. Sprains and dislocations are common. About 25 percent of the children develop a humpback with an abnormal curve of the spine (kyphoscoliosis), and 90 percent develop flatfeet. Hernias and abnormal outpouchings (diverticula) of the intestine are common. Rarely, a fragile intestine bleeds or ruptures (perforates).

A pregnant woman with the syndrome may have a premature delivery because her body tissues stretch easily. If the fetus has the syndrome, the membranes containing the fetus may rupture early. In addition, surgery on the pregnant woman, such as a cesarean section or an incision at the vaginal opening (episiotomy) to facilitate the baby's delivery, may be more difficult because of the fragile tissues. Severe bleeding may occur before, during, or after delivery.

Prognosis and Treatment

Despite the many and varied complications, the life span of people who have Ehlers-Danlos syn-

drome is usually normal. However, in a few people, complications (such as a ruptured blood vessel) are fatal.

No cure is available. Injury should be avoided because of tissue fragility. Wearing protective clothing and padding may be helpful. If people with Ehlers-Danlos syndrome want to have children, genetic counseling to determine the risk of their children inheriting the syndrome is advisable.

Marfan's Syndrome

Marfan's syndrome is an uncommon hereditary connective tissue disorder that results in abnormalities of the eyes, bones, heart, and blood vessels.

Symptoms

The gene for Marfan's syndrome is dominant,▲ but not everyone who inherits it is equally affected. People who have this syndrome are taller than average for their age and family, with an arm span (the distance between fingertips when the arms are outstretched to the side) greater than their height. Their fingers are long and thin. Frequently, the breastbone (sternum) is deformed and pushed either outward or inward. The joints may be very flexible. Flatfeet and a humpback with an abnormal curve of the spine (kyphoscoliosis) are common, as are hernias. Usually, the person has little fat under the skin. The roof of the mouth is often high.

Both lenses of the eyes may be dislocated. A doctor, using an ophthalmoscope, can often see the edge of the dislocated lens in the pupil. The person may be severely nearsighted, and the retina (the light-sensitive area at the back of the eye) may become detached.

Weakness in the wall of the aorta may cause this main artery to widen gradually, forming an aneurysm (a bulge in a blood vessel wall).■ Blood may seep between the layers of its wall (aortic dissection), or the aneurysm may rupture, causing massive bleeding. As the aorta widens, the aortic valve, which leads from the heart into the aorta, may begin to leak (aortic regurgitation).★ The mitral valve, which is located between the left atrium and ventricle, may leak or become prolapsed (bulge backward into the left atrium).● Fluid-filled sacs (cysts) may develop in the lungs. The cysts may rupture, causing pneumothorax◆

▲ see page 9

■ see page 137

★ see page 96

● see page 95

◆ see page 208

(air in the space that surrounds the lungs), which makes breathing difficult.

The risk of complications depends largely on how severe the abnormalities are. The main danger is sudden rupture of the aorta, which can be rapidly fatal. Rupture is more likely during active sports.

Diagnosis and Treatment

If an unusually tall, thin person has any of the characteristic symptoms, a doctor may suspect Marfan's syndrome. However, many people who have the syndrome never experience any unusual illness and aren't recognized as having an abnormality.

The main goal of treatment is to prevent problems with the blood vessels and eyes. The eyes are examined once a year. If any problems with vision develop, a person who has Marfan's syndrome should see a doctor at once.

Reserpine or propranolol may be used to help prevent widening (dilation) and dissection of the aorta by reducing the force of the blood flow. If the aorta widens, the affected section can sometimes be repaired or replaced surgically.

Children who have Marfan's syndrome tend to grow very tall. A doctor may therefore recommend hormone therapy (estrogen and progesterone) for very tall girls. This therapy is usually given by age 10 to induce early puberty and thus stop growth.

People with Marfan's syndrome who wish to have children should seek genetic counseling to determine the risk that their children will inherit it.

Pseudoxanthoma Elasticum

Pseudoxanthoma elasticum is a hereditary connective tissue disorder affecting the skin, eyes, and blood vessels.

Pseudoxanthoma elasticum affects mainly the elastic fibers, which enable tissue to stretch and then spring back into place. The skin of the neck, underarms, and groin and around the navel is thick, grooved, inflexible, and loose. Yellowish pebbly bumps give the skin a plucked chicken appearance. Changes at the back of the eye (retina) can result in severe loss of vision and even

blindness. Arteries may become narrowed, which may result in chest pain and intermittent claudication (leg pain during exercise caused by an inadequate blood supply). Nosebleeds and bleeding in the brain, uterus, and intestine may occur. High blood pressure is common.

The prognosis depends on how severe the disorder is and which arteries are affected. Complications usually cause death between ages 30 and 70.

Cutis Laxa

Cutis laxa is a rare connective tissue disorder in which the skin stretches easily and hangs in loose folds.

Cutis laxa affects mainly elastic fibers. It is usually inherited; however, in rare cases and for unknown reasons, this disorder develops in a person who has no family history of it. Some hereditary forms are fairly mild, some cause mental retardation, and others can be fatal.

Symptoms

In the hereditary forms, the skin may be very loose at birth or it may become loose later. The loose skin is particularly obvious on the face, so that affected children look mournful or Churchillian. A hooked nose is typical. Hernias and outpouchings (diverticula) of the intestine are common. A widening of the air spaces in the lungs may cause high blood pressure in the lungs (cor pulmonale).

The nonhereditary (acquired) form has different symptoms from the hereditary form. It begins later and affects additional areas of the skin. The affected skin looks different from the skin in the hereditary forms, and the nose isn't hooked. Particularly in children or adolescents, cutis laxa may begin as a severe illness with a fever, widespread inflammation of body membranes, and a severe skin rash (erythema multiforme). In adults, the disorder may develop gradually. It sometimes results in lung complications or in death caused by rupture of the aorta.

Diagnosis and Treatment

A doctor can usually diagnose cutis laxa by examining the skin.

No cure is known. For people who have a hereditary form, plastic surgery can improve appearance considerably. However, the skin may become loose again. Plastic surgery is less successful in the acquired form. Lung problems, such as emphysema or high blood pressure in the lungs, are treated as needed.

Mucopolysaccharidoses

The mucopolysaccharidoses are hereditary disorders that result in a characteristic facial appearance and abnormalities of the bones, eyes, liver, and spleen, sometimes accompanied by mental retardation.

The underlying cause of this group of disorders is an inability to break down and store mucopolysaccharides, which are major components of connective tissue. As a result, excess mucopolysaccharides enter the blood and are deposited throughout the body; some are excreted in the urine. There are many different types of mucopolysaccharides and many different enzymes needed to break them down. Therefore, there are many types of mucopolysaccharidosis, each caused by a specific genetic abnormality affecting a particular enzyme.

Symptoms and Diagnosis

Usually, the symptoms are not present at birth. During infancy and childhood, short stature, abnormal bone growth, hairiness, and abnormal development become obvious. The face may have a coarse appearance, with thick lips, an open mouth, and a flattened nose. Depending on the type of mucopolysaccharidosis, some affected children have normal intelligence, and others seem normal at birth but gradually become mentally retarded over several years. In some types, the eyes are affected, causing clouding of the cornea and visual difficulties. Other members of the family may have mucopolysaccharidosis.

A doctor bases the diagnosis on the symptoms. Mucopolysaccharidoses can also be diagnosed

---

▲ see box, page 1135

■ see page 836

before birth using amniocentesis or chorionic villus sampling,▲ in which samples are removed and screened for abnormal enzyme activity. After birth, urine samples can be screened. However, urine test results are often inaccurate, so blood and other tests are needed to confirm the diagnosis. X-rays taken to look for bone abnormalities also help in making the diagnosis.

Prognosis and Treatment

The prognosis depends on the type of mucopolysaccharidosis. Some types cause early death.

No cures are currently available. Attempts at replacing the abnormal enzyme have had limited, temporary success. Bone marrow transplantation■ may produce some small improvements but often causes death or disability, and the treatment remains controversial.

Osteochondrodysplasias

The osteochondrodysplasias are a group of hereditary disorders in which bone or cartilage grows abnormally, so that the skeleton develops abnormally.

Many types of osteochondrodysplasia cause short stature (dwarfism). Achondroplasia is the most common of the many types of short-limbed dwarfism. It occurs in 1 out of 25,000 to 40,000 live births, affecting both sexes and all racial groups.

Symptoms

Each type produces different symptoms. For instance, the symptoms of achondroplasia are short limbs, bowlegs, a bulky forehead, a saddle nose, and an arched back.

Disorders of the skeleton, such as a dislocated hip, are typical of all the osteochondrodysplasias. In some types, an abnormality of the second spinal vertebra (hypoplasia of the odontoid process) allows it to become dislocated from the first vertebra and compress the spinal cord, which can be immediately fatal.

Diagnosis and Treatment

A doctor tries to make a precise diagnosis because each type is caused by a different genetic abnormality, progresses differently, and has a different prognosis. Diagnosis before birth is possible in some cases by directly viewing the fetus with a fiber-optic scope (fetoscopy) or by performing an ultrasound scan. If a person with an osteochondrodysplasia or with close relatives who have one of these disorders wants to have children, genetic counseling is useful in determining the risk of having an affected child.

When joint problems severely affect function, the joint can sometimes be replaced with an artificial one. An abnormal second vertebra must be stabilized surgically to prevent damage to the spinal cord.

Osteopetroses

The osteopetroses (marble bones) are hereditary disorders that increase the density of bones and cause abnormalities of the skeleton.

Some of the osteopetroses cause little disability; others are progressive and fatal. Some types don't produce symptoms right away (delayed onset); in other types, symptoms begin in infancy (early onset).

Most types have no specific treatment. Surgery may be needed to relieve high pressure within the brain caused by skull abnormalities. Bone around the opening through which nerves leave the skull may grow excessively; if this bone compresses the nerves, surgery may be needed to free them. The teeth may be displaced, preventing proper closure of the mouth (malocclusion); orthodontic treatment can correct this condition. The face may be severely distorted by the overgrowth of bone, sometimes causing psychologic problems.

Delayed-Onset Type

Symptoms appear in childhood, adolescence, or young adulthood. **Albers-Schönberg disease,** a mild form of the delayed-onset type, may produce no symptoms. This form is relatively common, occurring in many countries and many ethnic groups. Usually, the skeleton is normal at birth; bone density increases as a child ages. The diagnosis is often made by chance, when x-rays taken for an unrelated purpose detect high bone density. The facial appearance, physique, mentality, and life span are normal, and general health is good. Occasionally, facial paralysis or deafness may result from compression of a nerve by the overgrowth of bone. Mild anemia may develop.

Early-Onset Type

Osteopetrosis with early onset of symptoms is an uncommon, potentially fatal disorder in infants. Symptoms include poor growth and poor weight gain (failure to thrive),▲ easy bruising, abnormal bleeding, and anemia. The liver and spleen may become enlarged, and nerves supplying the eye and face may become damaged. Death from anemia, overwhelming infection, or bleeding usually occurs in the first year of life. X-ray films show a general increase in bone density, which worsens with time. Bone marrow transplantation has apparently been successful in some infants, but the long-term prognosis after this treatment is unknown.

Osteochondroses

Osteochondroses are a group of diseases that affect the growth plate (the part of a bone where growth occurs) during childhood, resulting in abnormal bone growth and deformity. Their cause is not known. Different diseases affect different bones: The affected bone is the thighbone in Legg-Calvé-Perthes disease, the shinbone in Osgood-Schlatter disease, the spine in Scheuermann's disease, and one of the small bones (the navicular bone) of the foot in Köhler's bone disease.

Legg-Calvé-Perthes Disease

Legg-Calvé-Perthes disease is destruction of the growth plate in the neck of the thighbone.

This disease affects 1 in 1,000 to 5,000 children between the ages of 5 and 10 years and is more common in boys than in girls. It usually affects only one hip. It is caused by a poor blood supply to the neck of the thighbone, but the reason for the poor blood supply isn't known.

The main symptoms are hip pain and problems with walking. Symptoms begin gradually and progress slowly. Joint movement becomes limited, and the thigh muscles may become wasted from lack of use. On x-ray films, the head of the thighbone appears flattened at first; later, it appears fragmented.

Treatment includes prolonged bed rest, traction, slings, plaster casts, and splints. Some authorities recommend orthopedic surgery to correct any remaining abnormality in the hip.

▲ see page 1245

Kyphosis: A Humpback

Normal Anatomy	Kyphosis

Without treatment, the disorder may take 2 to 3 years to heal. If any abnormality remains, the risk of developing osteoarthritis in the hip joint is increased. Osteoarthritis is much less likely to develop if the disease is properly treated.

Osgood-Schlatter Disease

Osgood-Schlatter disease is inflammation of the bone and cartilage at the top of the shinbone.

This disease develops between the ages of 10 and 15 years, more commonly in boys. The cause

is thought to be an injury that occurs when the tendon of the kneecap (patellar tendon) pulls excessively on its point of attachment at the top of the shinbone (tibia). This point of attachment is called the tibial tubercle.

The disease usually affects only one shin. Major symptoms are pain, swelling, and tenderness at the top of the shin, where the tendon from the kneecap is attached. X-ray films of the knee may show fragmentation of this part of the tibia.

The only treatment measures needed are pain relief with analgesics and abstinence from sports and excessive exercise, especially deep knee bending. The symptoms usually disappear after several weeks or months. Occasionally, the leg must be immobilized in a plaster cast. In some instances, a doctor may inject hydrocortisone into the abnormal area, surgically remove loose pieces of bone, drill into the bone to generate healing, or perform bone grafting.

Scheuermann's Disease

Scheuermann's disease is a relatively common condition in which backache and humpback (kyphosis) are caused by changes in the vertebrae.

This disease first begins in adolescence, affecting boys more commonly than girls. Scheuermann's disease is probably not a single disease but rather a group of similar diseases. The causes aren't known.

Often, mild cases are diagnosed during routine screening of schoolchildren for spinal deformity. Symptoms usually include rounded shoulders and persistent mild backache. The curve of the upper spine is greater than normal. The disease may continue for a long time—often several years—but is frequently mild. The spine may remain slightly misaligned after symptoms disappear.

Mild nonprogressive cases can be treated by losing weight, which reduces back strain, and by avoiding strenuous activity. Occasionally, when the humpback is more severe, wearing a spinal brace or sleeping on a rigid bed may be necessary. Surgery for misalignment of the spine is occasionally needed if the condition progresses.

Köhler's Bone Disease

Köhler's bone disease is a rare form of inflammation of bone and cartilage (osteochondritis) affecting one of the small bones (the navicular bone) in the foot.

The disease affects children, most commonly boys, between the ages of 3 and 5 years.

The foot swells and becomes painful and tender, especially the inner side of the arch. Putting weight on the foot or walking increases the pain. Limping is common. The disease tends to last many months but rarely more than 2 years.

Taking analgesics and keeping weight off the foot relieve the symptoms. A few weeks in a below-the-knee plaster cast that allows walking while providing good support under the arch may be helpful in the early stages of the disease.

CHAPTER 270

Cerebral Palsy

Cerebral palsy is a condition characterized by poor muscle control, spasticity, paralysis, and other neurologic deficiencies resulting from brain injury that occurs during pregnancy, during birth, after birth, or before age 5.

Cerebral palsy isn't a disease, and it isn't progressive. The parts of the brain that control muscle movements are particularly vulnerable to injury in premature and young infants. Cerebral palsy affects 1 or 2 of every 1,000 infants but is 10 times more common in premature infants and is particularly common in very small infants.

Causes

Many different types of injury can cause cerebral palsy, but most often the cause is unknown.

Birth injuries and poor oxygen supply to the brain before, during, and immediately after birth cause 10 to 15 percent of cases. Premature infants are particularly vulnerable, possibly in part because the blood vessels of the brain are poorly developed and bleed easily or can't supply sufficient oxygen to the brain. High blood levels of bilirubin, common in newborns, can lead to a condition called kernicterus and brain damage.▲ However, the jaundice that results from having high blood levels of bilirubin is now easily treated in newborns, and the incidence of kernicterus has de-

---

▲ see box, page 1212

creased dramatically. During the first years of life, severe illness, such as meningitis, sepsis, trauma, and severe dehydration, can cause brain injury and result in cerebral palsy.

Symptoms

The symptoms of cerebral palsy can range from barely noticeable clumsiness to severe spasticity that contorts the arms and legs and confines the child to a wheelchair. Cerebral palsy is of four main types:

• Spastic—in which the muscles are stiff and weak—occurs in about 70 percent of children with cerebral palsy

• Choreoathetoid—in which the muscles spontaneously move slowly and without normal control—occurs in about 20 percent of children with cerebral palsy

• Ataxic—in which coordination is poor and movements are shaky—occurs in about 10 percent of children with cerebral palsy

• Mixed—in which two of the above types, most often spastic and choreoathetoid, are combined—occurs in many children

In spastic cerebral palsy, stiffness may affect all the arms and legs (quadriplegia), mainly the legs (diplegia), or only the arm and leg on one side (hemiplegia). The affected arms and legs are poorly developed, stiff, and weak.

In choreoathetoid cerebral palsy, movements of the arms, legs, and body are slow, writhing, and uncontrollable, but they may also be abrupt and jerky. Strong emotion makes the movements worse; sleep makes them disappear.

In ataxic cerebral palsy, muscle coordination is poor, and muscle weakness and trembling occur. Children with this disorder have difficulty making rapid or fine movements and walk unsteadily, with legs widely spaced.

In all forms of cerebral palsy, speech may be difficult to understand because the child has difficulty controlling the muscles involved in speech. Most children with cerebral palsy have other disabilities, such as below-normal intelligence; some have severe mental retardation. However, about 40 percent of children with cerebral palsy have normal or near-normal intelligence. About 25 percent of children with cerebral

palsy—most often those with the spastic type—have seizures (epilepsy).

Diagnosis

Cerebral palsy usually can't be diagnosed during early infancy. When such muscle problems as poor development, weakness, spasticity, or lack of coordination are noticed, the doctor tries to monitor the child to determine whether the problem is cerebral palsy or a progressive disorder, particularly one that could be treated. The specific type of cerebral palsy often can't be distinguished before the child is 18 months old.

Laboratory tests can't identify cerebral palsy. However, to rule out other disorders, a doctor may perform blood tests, electrical studies of muscle, a muscle biopsy, and computed tomography (CT) or magnetic resonance imaging (MRI) of the brain.

Treatment

Cerebral palsy can't be cured; its problems are lifelong. However, much can be done to give a child as much independence as possible. Physical therapy, occupational therapy, braces, and orthopedic surgery may improve muscle control and walking. Speech therapy may make speech much clearer and help with eating problems. Seizures can be prevented with anticonvulsant drugs.▲

Many children with cerebral palsy grow normally and attend regular schools if they don't have severe intellectual and physical deficiencies. Other children require extensive physical therapy, need special education, and are severely limited in activities of daily living, requiring some type of lifelong care and assistance. Even severely affected children can benefit from education and training.

Information and counseling are available to parents to help them understand their child's condition and potential and to assist with problems as they arise.■ To help a child reach his highest potential, loving parental care can be combined with assistance from public and private agencies, such as community health agencies and vocational rehabilitation organizations.

The prognosis usually depends on the type of cerebral palsy and on its severity. More than 90 percent of children with cerebral palsy will survive into adulthood. Only the most severely affected—those incapable of any self-care—have a substantially shortened life expectancy.

▲ see box, page 349

■ see page 1243

Ear, Nose, and Throat Disorders

In children, various disorders can affect the ears, nose, and throat. Hearing is tested shortly after birth and regularly thereafter.▲ Deafness is present at birth in 1 out of 1,000 live births and may be caused by the rubella virus, lack of oxygen or an injury during birth, certain drugs given to the mother during pregnancy, hemolytic disease of the fetus, infections, or hereditary diseases. Early detection and treatment, if possible, are important because language is best learned at a young age. Ear infections ■ are common in young children, especially those between the ages of 3 months and 3 years. Children may also develop infections affecting the nose and throat.★ Young children may place a foreign object in the ear ● or nose, which can cause pain, an infection, or a discharge. Noncancerous tumors may develop in the nose of boys at puberty (juvenile angiofibromas) or in the voice box of younger children of either sex (juvenile papillomas).

Objects in the Nose

Young children often put objects in their nose. Although some objects are easy to see and remove, others may be pushed up so high that they can't be seen. Objects lodged high in the nose may cause a malodorous, bloody discharge from one nostril. Over time, an object lodged in the nose may become covered by mineral salts from nasal secretions, producing a lump inside the nose (rhinolith). Rhinoliths are difficult to remove because their shape tends to follow the shape of the inside of the nose. For removal, a general anesthetic is usually needed.

Juvenile Angiofibromas

Juvenile angiofibromas, which occur almost exclusively in boys at puberty, are noncancerous tumors that grow at the back of the nose.

Although this tumor isn't cancerous, it can destroy tissue in the lining of the nose and commonly causes nosebleeds (epistaxis). The tumor may also obstruct air flow. As the tumor grows, it may extend into the nearby sinuses, the eye socket, or the area containing the brain (cranial cavity).

A doctor may suspect an angiofibroma when a child has recurring nosebleeds and obstructed breathing. The tumor may be detected by computed tomography (CT) or by magnetic resonance imaging (MRI). The blood vessels supplying the tumor and its possible extension into the eye socket or cranial cavity can be detected by angiography, a type of x-ray in which a radiopaque substance, visible on x-rays, is injected into blood vessels to outline the tumor.

Although an angiofibroma sometimes shrinks as a child gets older, treatment is virtually always necessary. The best treatment is to block the artery supplying the tumor (angiographic embolization) and then remove the tumor surgically. However, radiation therapy is sometimes given if the tumor extends into the cranial cavity and can't be removed.

Juvenile Papillomas

Juvenile papillomas are noncancerous tumors of the voice box (larynx).

Papillomas are caused by a virus. Papillomas may appear in children as young as 1 year old. A papilloma may cause hoarseness, sometimes severe enough to prevent speaking, and may obstruct the airway.

The diagnosis is made by using a laryngoscope to view the voice box and is confirmed by performing a biopsy of the papilloma.

Papillomas at several sites may become so big that a surgical procedure to create an opening in the windpipe (trachea) may be needed to make breathing possible. Treatment consists of either surgical removal or laser vaporization of the papillomas. Recurrence is common, but at puberty, the papillomas usually disappear on their own.

▲ see page 999

■ see page 1006

★ see page 1265

● see page 1002

Eye Disorders

The eyes of a newborn are examined for such problems as congenital glaucoma and congenital cataracts.▲ Strabismus may be present at birth or may develop later. Conjunctivitis (inflammation of the conjunctiva, which covers the back of the eyelid and the white of the eye) is common in children.■ Children can also develop other types of eye infections.★

Strabismus

Strabismus (squint, cross-eyes) is a wandering or misalignment of one eye so that its line of vision isn't parallel with that of the other eye and both eyes aren't pointed at the same object at the same time.

Normally, both eyes move together so that a single, fused image from both eyes is produced by the brain. Because each eye has a slightly different viewpoint, this image is three-dimensional. If the eyes aren't aligned properly, the brain may receive images from each eye that are too different to be fused, resulting in double vision (diplopia). To avoid double vision, the brain may suppress the image from the deviating eye. If the brain must constantly suppress images from one eye, the vision in that eye gradually will be lost. Because the image produced by a single eye isn't three-dimensional, depth perception is also lost.

Causes and Symptoms

Strabismus is usually caused either by unequal pull of one or more of the muscles that move the eyes (nonparalytic strabismus) or by paralysis of one or more of these muscles (paralytic strabismus).

Unequal pull of one or more of the eye muscles is usually caused by an abnormality in the brain. Regardless of the direction in which the person is looking, the degree of strabismus usually stays constant; that is, the position of the eyes relative to one another doesn't change. In a mild form of

strabismus called phoria, the misalignment is minor and the brain is able to fine-tune the muscle imbalance. As a result, the eyes are aligned and the images from each eye can be fused. Because phoria usually doesn't produce symptoms, it can be detected only by specific tests conducted by an ophthalmologist.

Paralysis of the eye muscles may be caused by damage to the nerve supplying those muscles. As a result, the ability to move the affected eye is reduced, and the degree of strabismus varies as the eyes move. Double vision doesn't occur if the paralysis was present at birth because vision in the affected eye is suppressed by the brain.

Another form of strabismus occurs in farsighted children. Normally, to look at a nearby object, the eyes accommodate by focusing the lenses and turning inward (converging). Farsighted eyes must accommodate in these ways even when looking at distant objects, causing the eyes to turn inward (accommodative esotropia).

Diagnosis and Treatment

Strabismus is usually noticed first by parents or a doctor because the child's eyes appear to be positioned abnormally. An eye examination confirms the diagnosis and identifies the type of strabismus.

Strabismus should never be ignored on the assumption that a child will outgrow it. Unless treated before age 9 years, strabismus may lead to permanent loss of sight (amblyopia) in the deviating eye. Amblyopia develops more quickly in younger children and takes longer to correct in older children. Thus, the earlier treatment is begun, the less severe the initial visual defect and the faster the response. Also, strabismus is sometimes an early indicator of a serious nerve disorder.

Covering the normal eye with a patch may improve poor vision in the deviating eye by forcing the brain to receive an image from that eye without producing double vision. Improving vision gives a child a better chance of eventually developing normal, three-dimensional vision. Once the vision is equal in each eye, surgery can be performed to adjust the strength of the eye muscles so that they pull equally in each eye.

▲ see page 1236

■ see pages 1037 and 1216

★ see page 1264

Strabismus: A Deviating Eye

There are several types of strabismus. An eye may turn inward (esotropia or cross-eye) or outward (exotropia or walleye), or it may turn upward (hypertropia) or downward (hypotropia). In this illustration, the child's right eye is affected.

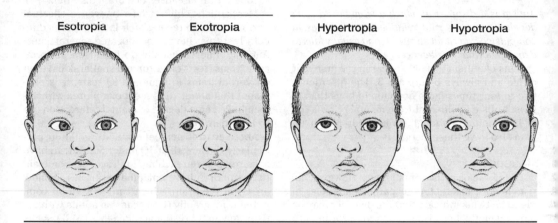

| Esotropia | Exotropia | Hypertropia | Hypotropia |

Accommodative esotropia in farsighted children can be treated early with glasses, so that accommodation is not required when viewing distant objects. In some cases, bifocal glasses are helpful. Other treatments include drugs such as echothiophate drops, which help the eye focus on nearby objects.

Paralytic strabismus may be treated with glasses containing prism lenses that bend the light so that both eyes receive nearly the same image, or it may be treated with surgery.

Periodic follow-up examinations are needed until at least age 10.

CHAPTER 273

Mental Health Disorders

A number of mental health disorders may occur in childhood. Among them are autism, childhood disintegrative disorder, childhood schizophrenia, depression, mania and manic-depressive illness, suicidal behavior, conduct disorder, separation anxiety disorder, and somatoform disorders. In addition, gender identity disorder first becomes apparent during childhood,▲ and substance abuse disorders are becoming more prevalent among both children and adolescents.■ Other important mental health disorders in children include attention-deficit disorder,★ obsessive-

▲ see page 418

■ see page 440

★ see page 1251

compulsive disorder,▲ and Tourette's syndrome.■ Because mental health disorders in children and adolescents tend to be chronic, many families benefit from family therapy and support groups.

Autism

Autism is a disorder in which a young child can't develop normal social relationships, behaves in compulsive and ritualistic ways, and usually fails to develop normal intelligence.

Signs of autism usually appear in the first year of life and always before age 3. The disorder is two to four times more common in boys than in girls. Autism is different from mental retardation or brain injury, although some children with autism also have these disorders.

Causes

The cause of autism isn't known. However, autism is *not* caused by poor parenting. Studies of identical twins indicate that the disorder may be partly genetic, because it tends to occur in both twins if it occurs in one. Although most cases have no obvious cause, some may be related to a viral infection (for example, congenital rubella or cytomegalic inclusion disease), phenylketonuria (an inherited enzyme deficiency), or the fragile X syndrome (a chromosomal disorder).

Symptoms and Diagnosis

An autistic child prefers to be alone, doesn't form close personal relationships, won't cuddle, avoids eye contact, resists change, becomes excessively attached to familiar objects, and continually repeats certain acts and rituals. The child may begin speaking later than other children, may use language in a peculiar way, or may be unable or unwilling to speak at all. When spoken to, the child often has difficulty understanding what is said. He may repeat words as they are spoken to

him (echolalia) and reverse the normal use of pronouns, particularly using *you* instead of *I* or *me* when referring to himself.

Symptoms of autism in a young child lead the doctor to the diagnosis, which is made by close observation. Although no specific tests for autism are available, a doctor may perform certain tests to look for other causes of a brain disorder.

Most autistic children have uneven intellectual performance, so testing their intelligence is difficult. Tests may have to be repeated several times. Autistic children usually do better on performance items (tests of motor and spatial skills) than on verbal items in standard IQ tests. It is estimated that about 70 percent of children with autism have some degree of mental retardation (an IQ less than 70).

About 20 to 40 percent of autistic children, particularly those with an IQ under 50, start to have seizures before reaching adolescence. Some autistic children have enlarged ventricles (hollow areas) in the brain, which can be seen on computed tomography (CT) scans. In adults with autism, magnetic resonance imaging (MRI) scans may show additional brain abnormalities.

A variant of autism, sometimes called **childhood-onset pervasive developmental disorder** or **atypical autism,** can begin later, up to age 12. As with autism that starts in infancy, a child with childhood-onset pervasive developmental disorder doesn't develop normal social relationships and often has bizarre mannerisms and unusual speech patterns. Such children may also have Tourette's syndrome,★ obsessive-compulsive disorder,● or hyperactivity.◆ Because of this, a doctor may find it difficult to distinguish the symptoms of one disorder from those of another.

Prognosis and Treatment

The symptoms of autism generally persist throughout life. Many experts believe the prognosis is strongly determined by how much usable language the child has acquired by age 7. Autistic children with subnormal intelligence—for example, those who score below 50 on standard IQ tests—are likely to need full-time institutional care as adults.

Autistic children in the near-normal or higher IQ range often benefit from psychotherapy and special education. Speech therapy is started

---

▲ see page 400

■ see page 312

★ see page 312

● see page 400

◆ see page 1251

early, as is physical and occupational therapy. Sign language is sometimes used to communicate with mute children, although its benefits are unknown. Behavioral therapy can help severely autistic children learn to manage at home and at school. This therapy is useful when an autistic child tries the patience of even the most loving parents and the most devoted teachers.

Drugs are sometimes helpful, although they can't change the underlying disorder. Haloperidol is used mainly to control severely aggressive and self-destructive behavior. Fenfluramine, buspirone, risperidone, and the selective serotonin reuptake inhibitors (fluoxetine, paroxetine, and sertraline) are all used to treat the various symptoms and behaviors of autistic children.

Childhood Disintegrative Disorder

In childhood disintegrative disorder, an apparently normal child begins to act younger (regress) after age 3.

In most children, physical and psychologic development occurs in spurts. Sometimes a normal child seems to take a step backward; for example, a toilet-trained child occasionally wets himself accidently. Childhood disintegrative disorder, however, is a serious disorder and may be responsible when a child over age 3 stops developing normally (shows signs of arrested development) or regresses. Usually no cause can be found, although sometimes the child has a degenerative brain disorder.

Symptoms and Diagnosis

The typical child with childhood disintegrative disorder develops normally until age 3 or 4, learning speech, becoming toilet trained, and displaying appropriate social behavior. After a period of vague illness and mood change, in which the child is irritable and sickly, the child undergoes obvious regression. He may lose previously acquired language, motor, or social skills, and he may no longer have control over his bladder or bowels. The child gradually deteriorates to a severely retarded level. A doctor makes the diagnosis from the symptoms and searches for an underlying disorder.

Prognosis and Treatment

The prognosis is poor, and a severely retarded child will need lifelong care. However, the child's

---

Symptoms of Childhood Schizophrenia

Thought blocking: Sudden blockage of a train of thought

Perseveration: Repeating the same response to different questions

Ideas of reference: A conviction that the words or actions of others refer to oneself

Hallucinations: The perception (sight, sound, taste) of things that aren't there

Delusions: False beliefs held despite clear evidence to the contrary

Blunted emotions: A flat mood; neither the voice nor the facial expressions change in response to emotional situations

Paranoia: A mental state in which one has a delusion of being persecuted

Thought control: A conviction that other people or powers are controlling one's thoughts

---

life span may be normal if he has no underlying disorder. Childhood disintegrative disorder can't be treated or cured.

Childhood Schizophrenia

Childhood schizophrenia is a disorder involving abnormal behavior and thought, beginning between age 7 and the start of adolescence.

The cause of childhood schizophrenia is unknown. Speculation continues about which chemical abnormalities in the brain are involved and what role heredity plays. Why some children develop schizophrenia at an early age when most don't show symptoms until late adolescence is also unknown. What is known is that schizophrenia is *not* caused by poor parenting.

Symptoms and Diagnosis

Childhood schizophrenia usually appears after age 7. The child becomes withdrawn, loses interest in his usual activities, and develops distorted thinking and perception. Childhood schizophrenia is similar to the schizophrenia that begins in

Symptoms of Depression

- A sad expression
- Apathy
- Withdrawal from friends and social situations
- Reduced capacity for pleasure
- Feeling rejected and unloved
- Sleep problems
- Headaches
- Abdominal pain
- Episodes of clowning or foolish behavior
- Persistent self-blame
- Poor appetite
- Weight loss
- Despondency
- Thoughts of suicide

late adolescence or early adulthood;▲ as with adults, a child with schizophrenia is likely to develop hallucinations, delusions, and paranoia, fearing that others are planning to harm him or are controlling his thoughts. Children with schizophrenia will also likely have blunted emotions— neither their voice nor facial expressions change in response to emotional situations. Events that would normally make them laugh or cry may produce no response.

A doctor bases the diagnosis on the symptoms. No diagnostic tests are available, but the doctor searches for evidence of drug abuse, exposure to toxic substances, and brain injury.

Treatment

Schizophrenia can't be cured, although some symptoms may be controlled with drugs and psychotherapy. Antipsychotic drugs can help correct some of the chemical abnormalities in the brain.

▲ see page 435

Thiothixene and haloperidol are commonly used, although newer drugs, such as risperidone, may produce greater improvement. However, children are particularly susceptible to the adverse effects of antipsychotic drugs, such as tremors, slowed movements, and muscle spasms, and the drugs are used with great caution.

A child with schizophrenia may need to be hospitalized temporarily when the symptoms worsen, so that drug doses can be adjusted and he can be kept from harming himself or others. Some children must remain institutionalized.

Depression

Depression is a feeling of intense sadness; it may follow a recent loss or other sad event but is out of proportion to that event and persists beyond an appropriate length of time.

Severe depression is relatively rare among children but common in adolescents. Nonetheless, some degree of depression can be a problem in school-aged children.

Depression in children and adolescents can be triggered by events or problems such as the following:

- The death of a parent
- A friend moving away
- Difficulty in adjusting to school
- Difficulty making friends
- Drug or alcohol abuse

However, some children become depressed even without profoundly unhappy experiences. Often, family members of such children have experienced depression; studies have found that depression tends to run in families.

Symptoms and Diagnosis

The symptoms of depression in children relate to feelings of overwhelming sadness and worthlessness. Like adults, depressed children may have suicidal thoughts. A doctor can usually diagnose depression by its symptoms. However, depression is sometimes masked by seemingly contradictory symptoms, such as overactivity and aggressive, antisocial behavior.

Treatment

A doctor tries to find out whether family or social stresses may have precipitated the depression and determines whether a physical disorder is the cause.

The doctor may prescribe an antidepressant drug, which works by correcting chemical imbalances in the brain.▲ However, few studies have been conducted to document the effectiveness of antidepressant drugs in children. The drugs prescribed most often are the selective serotonin reuptake inhibitors, such as fluoxetine, sertraline, and paroxetine. Another group of antidepressants, the tricyclic antidepressants such as imipramine, have significant adverse effects and, therefore, are used with extreme caution in children. To find the optimal dose of an antidepressant drug, the doctor monitors any improvement in the child's mental health and observes him for signs of adverse effects.

Treatment of depression in children and adolescents requires more than drug therapy. Individual psychotherapy, group therapy, and family therapy may all be beneficial. Family members and school staff are asked to reduce stress on the child and to make efforts to enhance his self-esteem. A brief hospitalization may be needed in a crisis to prevent a suicide attempt.

Mania and Manic-Depressive Illness

Mania is a mood disorder in which a child is overly elated, excited, and active and thinks and speaks very quickly. A less intense form of mania is called hypomania. In manic-depressive illness, periods of mania or hypomania alternate with periods of depression.

Mania and hypomania are rare in children. Manic-depressive illness is very rare before puberty and unknown in early childhood. Some children have marked mood swings, but these swings usually aren't indicative of manic-depressive illness.

The symptoms and diagnosis of manic-depressive illness in children and adolescents are similar to those in adults.■ However, the treatment is complex and usually involves a combination of mood-stabilizing drugs, such as lithium, carbamazepine, and valproic acid. Children and adolescents with manic-depressive illness should be treated by a child psychiatrist.

Suicidal Behavior

Suicidal behavior encompasses suicide gestures (suicidal actions that aren't intended to be fatal), suicide attempts (actions that are intended to be

Behavioral Changes That Signal Potential Suicide
Despondent mood
Low self-esteem
Sleep and appetite disturbances
Inability to concentrate
Truancy from school
Physical symptoms such as headaches
Preoccupation with suicide and death

fatal but don't succeed), and completed suicide (an act that results in the taking of one's own life).

Suicidal behavior is common among older children, especially among adolescents. Suicide rates in children, especially among boys and particularly adolescents 15 to 19 years old, increased by 50 percent between 1970 and 1990. Suicide is the second leading cause, after accidents, of death in adolescents. Nearly 14 out of every 100,000 adolescents attempt suicide, boys four times more often than girls. In addition, many deaths attributed to accidents, such as from motor vehicles and firearms, are actually suicides.

Causes

A suicide attempt is a clear sign of mental illness, usually depression. Suicidal behavior is often sparked by a loss. Examples of losses include the loss of a boyfriend or girlfriend, the loss of familiar surroundings (school, neighborhood, friends) after a geographic move, and the loss of self-esteem after a family argument. Anguish over an unplanned pregnancy may contribute to suicidal behavior. Another factor may be an overwhelming lack of direction, structure, and boundaries set by parents or other authority figures. Some families apply intense pressure to succeed; the child's belief that he is falling short of expectations may lead to a suicide attempt. A humiliating disciplinary episode may also trigger a sui-

▲ see page 406

■ see page 409

Effects of Extreme Stress on Children

Children and adolescents experience stress just as adults do. A child experiencing extreme stress may show symptoms of depression, anxiety, or suicidal behavior. Adjustment disorder and posttraumatic stress disorder are two other ways that extreme stress can become apparent in children.

A stressful change in a child's life, such as a geographic move, divorce of the parents, or the death of a family member or pet, can trigger an **adjustment disorder.** Adjustment disorder is an acute response to environmental stress. The child may have symptoms of anxiety (for example, nervousness, worries, and fears), symptoms of depression (for example, tearfulness or feelings of hopeless-

ness), or behavioral problems. The symptoms and problems abate as the stress diminishes.

Posttraumatic stress disorder may occur after a natural disaster (such as a hurricane, tornado, or earthquake), after an accident, or after a senseless act of violence. The child usually fails in his attempts to avoid remembering the event and suffers a persistent state of anxiety, with extreme and even bizarre symptoms and behavior. Crisis intervention is usually necessary. Even with prompt displays of empathy and support, an extended period of individual, group, or family therapy may be needed to alleviate the child's anxiety and distress.

---

cide attempt. A common motive is the desire to manipulate or punish others with the fantasy that "they'll be sorry after I'm dead."

Sometimes suicide results when a child imitates the actions of others. For instance, a well-publicized suicide, such as that of a celebrity, is often followed by other suicides. Similarly, a cluster of suicides may take place over a short time among young people in a high school or a college dormitory.

Prevention

Parents, doctors, teachers, and friends may be in a position to identify children or teenagers who might attempt suicide. They may notice recent changes in behavior. Any suicide gesture must be taken seriously. Statements such as "I wish I'd never been born" or "I'd like to go to sleep and never wake up" may indicate a possible intent to commit suicide. A child is at increased risk of suicide if a family member, close friend, or peer has committed suicide, a family member has died recently, or the child has a substance abuse problem or conduct disorder.

▲ see box, page 414

Directly asking a child about suicidal thoughts and plans reduces rather than increases the risk that the child will attempt suicide. Community intervention programs that support young people who have suicidal thoughts can also be helpful. Crisis hot lines, offering 24-hour assistance, are available in many communities.▲

Treatment

Every suicide attempt is an emergency. Once the immediate threat to life has been removed, the doctor decides whether the child should be hospitalized. The decision depends on the degree of risk in remaining at home and the family's capacity to provide support. The seriousness of a suicide attempt can be gauged by a number of factors, for example, whether the attempt was carefully planned rather than spontaneous, what type of method was used (a gun indicates a more serious intent than does a drug overdose), and whether any injury was actually inflicted.

A better outcome is likely if the family shows love and concern. A negative or unsupportive response by the parents tends to worsen the situation. In some cases, hospitalization offers the best protection. Hospitalization is recommended especially if the child is severely depressed or has another mental health disorder, such as schizophrenia. A psychiatrist and the family doctor usually work together in caring for the child. Recovery involves rebuilding morale and restoring emotional calm within the family.

Conduct Disorder

A conduct disorder is characterized by repeatedly disruptive behavior.

Several types of conduct disorder have been identified. Children and adolescents with **solitary aggressive conduct disorder** are selfish, don't relate well to others, and lack an appropriate sense of guilt. Those with **group conduct disorder** are loyal to their peers (such as a gang), often at the expense of outsiders. Some children and adolescents show signs of both solitary aggressive conduct disorder and group conduct disorder. Those with **oppositional defiant disorder** display negative, angry, defiant behavior without actually violating the rights of others. They know the difference between right and wrong and feel guilty if they do anything that is seriously wrong. Although not initially a conduct disorder, oppositional defiant disorder often evolves into a mild one.

Treatment

Psychotherapy may help improve the child or teenager's self-esteem and control, in turn improving his behavior. Moralizing and threatening don't work. Often the most successful treatment is to separate the child from a damaging environment and to administer strict discipline.

Separation Anxiety Disorder

Separation anxiety disorder is characterized by excessive anxiety about being away from home or separated from people to whom the child is attached.

Some degree of separation anxiety is normal and occurs in almost all children, especially in infants and toddlers.▲ In contrast, separation anxiety disorder is excessive anxiety that goes beyond that expected for the child's developmental level. Some life stress, such as the death of a relative, friend, or pet or a geographic move or change in schools, usually triggers the disorder.

Symptoms

Separation anxiety disorder lasts at least a month and causes significant distress or impairment in functioning. The duration of the disorder reflects its severity. Children with this disorder experience great distress when separated from home or people to whom they are attached. They often need to know the whereabouts of these people and are preoccupied with fears that something terrible will happen to them. Traveling by themselves makes them uncomfortable, and they may refuse to attend school or camp or to visit or sleep at friends' homes. Some children are unable to stay alone in a room, clinging to a parent or shadowing the parent around the house.

Difficulty at bedtime is common. A child with separation anxiety disorder may insist that someone stay in the room until he falls asleep. Nightmares may disclose the child's fears, such as destruction of the family through fire or another catastrophe.

Treatment

Because a child who has this disorder often avoids school, an immediate goal of treatment is enabling the child to return to school. Supportive therapy, especially when facilitated by the parents and teachers, is often sufficient for this purpose. In more severe cases, antianxiety drugs and antidepressants can be effective. A small proportion of children develop severe symptoms, requiring hospitalization.

Somatoform Disorders

Somatoform disorders are a group of disorders in which an underlying psychologic problem causes distressing or disabling physical symptoms.

A child with a somatoform disorder may have a number of symptoms without evidence of a physical cause, including pain, difficulty in breathing, and weakness. Often, a child develops symptoms of illnesses he has observed in family members. The child isn't usually aware of a connection between the symptoms and the underlying psychologic problem.

The main types of somatoform disorders are conversion disorder, somatization disorder, and hypochondriasis. In **conversion disorder,** the child converts a psychologic problem into a physical symptom. For example, the child may seem to have a paralyzed arm or leg, may become deaf or blind, or may have simulated seizures. A **somatization disorder** is similar to conversion disorder,

---

▲ see page 1246

but the child develops many symptoms that are more vague. In **hypochondriasis,** the child is obsessed with bodily functions, such as heartbeat, digestion, and sweating, and is convinced that he has a serious disease when nothing is actually wrong. These three types of somatoform disorders also occur in adults.▲

Conversion disorder and hypochondriasis are equally common in young boys and young girls, but they're more common in adolescent girls than in adolescent boys. Somatization disorder occurs almost exclusively in girls.

Diagnosis

Before establishing that a child has a somatoform disorder, the doctor makes sure that the child doesn't have a physical illness that could account for the symptoms. However, extensive laboratory tests are generally avoided because they may further convince the child that a phys-

ical problem exists. If no physical illness can be found, the doctor then talks to the child and family members to try to identify underlying psychologic problems or abnormal family relationships.

Treatment

A child may balk at the idea of visiting a psychotherapist because such treatment threatens to uncover hidden psychologic conflicts. However, relatively short visits to a therapist, with reassurance and inquiries into nonmedical areas, may gradually break the child's pattern of behavior. Reassurance and support by family members help minimize physical symptoms, which are the child's means of receiving continued medical attention and attention in general. If these measures fail, the doctor will likely refer the child to a pediatric psychiatrist.

CHAPTER 274

Child Abuse and Neglect

Child abuse is the maltreatment, physical or mental injury, or sexual abuse of a child. Child neglect is the failure to provide adequate food, clothing, shelter, or love to a child.

More than a million children are abused or neglected every year in the United States. About 20 percent of those who are physically abused are permanently injured, and about 1,200 die each year. Most of these children are under 5 years old, and almost 50 percent are younger than 1 year. An estimated 200,000 children are sexually abused or molested every year. An adult who sexually abuses or molests a child often is related to the child, usually a close family member. Sexual contact between a child and a close blood relative is incest.

About 25 percent of the cases of abuse and neglect occur in children under age 2. Boys and girls are affected equally. Neglect is probably 10 to 15

times more common than abuse, although abuse and neglect often occur together. Neglect is 12 times more common in children living in poverty.

Causes

Abuse may occur when parents or guardians can't control their impulses. Four factors make such loss of control more likely.
• The parent may have psychiatric problems, such as a personality disorder or low self-esteem, or may abuse drugs or alcohol.
• The child may be different from others (irritable, demanding, hyperactive, or handicapped).
• Emotional support from family, neighbors, or friends may be inadequate.
• A crisis may occur, such as loss of money or a job.

Neglect often occurs in families that have many problems. Drug or alcohol abuse or a chronic medical condition may cause financial hardships, leading to the inadequate feeding, care, and attention of a child. Desertion by one parent may result in neglect by the other.

▲ see page 392

Symptoms and Diagnosis

Abuse may lead to recognizable behavioral changes in both the child and the abuser. For instance, a parent may seem unconcerned, even when a child has obviously been injured. The parent may be reluctant to describe to the doctor or friends how the injury occurred, and the description may change each time the story is told. The injury may be unusual for the age of the child.

A child who is repeatedly physically abused may show signs of new and old injuries. Bruises, burns, welts, or scrapes are often evident. Cigarette or scald burns may be visible on the arms or legs. Severe injuries to the mouth, eyes, brain, or other internal organs may be present but not visible. The child may also have evidence of broken bones.

A young child who has been sexually abused may have difficulty in walking or sitting because of a physical injury. A urinary tract infection, vaginal discharge, or sexually transmitted disease may develop. Often, however, no physical injury is apparent. Rather, the child may be irritable or fearful or may sleep fitfully. Because children may be threatened with further abuse if they tell anyone what has happened to them, doctors, police, or relatives may not have an easy time learning the facts from the child.

A neglected child may be malnourished, tired, or dirty or may lack appropriate clothing. In extreme cases, a child may live alone or with siblings without adult supervision. Neglected children may die of starvation or exposure.

A parent may fail to obtain preventive dental or medical care for the child, such as immunizations and routine physical examinations. The parent may also delay seeking medical care when the child is ill.

A neglected or abused infant often fails to develop physically or emotionally at a normal rate.▲ Infants deprived of parental love may seem unemotional or uninterested in their surroundings. They may be misdiagnosed as being mentally retarded or having a physical illness. Social and language skills may be impaired because of insufficient attention. A young child may be distrustful, unassertive, and extremely anxious to please adults. Older children may not attend school regularly or may not perform well when they do. They may have trouble forming relationships with other classmates or with teachers.

Treatment

An abused or neglected child may need to be hospitalized. Social service professionals assess the family situation. In many communities, a health care team consisting of, among others, a social worker, a psychiatrist, and a pediatrician plans and provides care for the child and family.

Doctors and nurses are required by law to promptly report cases of suspected child abuse or neglect to a local child protective service. Prompt reporting is also required by all those who are responsible in their employment for the welfare of children under age 18, such as teachers, day care workers, police, and legal services personnel. Individual citizens are encouraged to make a report when they know of or suspect abuse or neglect, but they are not required to do so.

CHAPTER 275

Poisoning

Poisoning is the most common cause of nonfatal accidents in the home.■ In children, the most common serious poisonings result from ingesting acetaminophen, aspirin, caustic substances, lead, iron, and hydrocarbons. Most poisonings are accidental in young children, but they may result from a suicide attempt in older children. *When a child or an adult is exposed to a poison, the first step is to call the regional Poison Center for advice.* Its telephone number is listed in the local directory or can be obtained from directory assistance.

▲ see page 1245

■ see page 1358

Ways to Prevent Poisoning

- Use safety caps and containers

- Store dangerous substances in locked cabinets

- Do not store household products on lower shelves or leave them out on the floor

- Keep drugs and dangerous substances in their original containers

- Teach children about the dangers of eating or touching drugs and household products

---

Acetaminophen Poisoning

More than 100 products that contain acetaminophen are available without a prescription. Many children's preparations are available in liquid, tablet, and capsule form.

Acetaminophen is a very safe drug, but it isn't harmless. Large amounts of acetaminophen overwhelm the liver, so that it can no longer break down the drug into harmless by-products. As a result, a toxic substance that can seriously damage the liver is produced. Acetaminophen poisoning is rarely fatal in children who haven't reached puberty, for reasons that aren't entirely understood. Children over age 12, like adults, are at risk of developing liver damage from an overdose.

Symptoms

The symptoms of an acetaminophen overdose occur in four stages:
- Stage 1 (first few hours): Few if any symptoms develop, even when large amounts are consumed. The person doesn't seem ill.
- Stage 2 (after 24 hours): Nausea and vomiting are common. Tests show that the liver isn't functioning normally.

▲ see page 565

■ see page 738

★ see page 1280

- Stage 3 (3 to 5 days later): Vomiting continues. Tests show that the liver is barely functioning. Symptoms of liver failure appear.▲
- Stage 4 (after 5 days): The person either recovers or dies of liver failure.

Treatment

The Poison Center should be called to determine whether treatment is needed. If it is, emergency treatment can be started at home. The child may be given syrup of ipecac immediately to induce vomiting and empty the stomach. In the emergency department, a tube may be placed in the stomach through the nose to wash the stomach out with water. Activated charcoal may be given through this tube to absorb any remaining acetaminophen before it can enter the bloodstream. The blood level of acetaminophen is measured 4 to 6 hours after ingestion and may need to be measured again.

If the child has swallowed a large amount of acetaminophen, particularly if the blood level is high, acetylcysteine is generally given to reduce the toxicity of the acetaminophen, usually after the charcoal is removed.

Because liver failure may interfere with the blood's ability to clot, vitamin K_1 (phytonadione) may be injected to counter this effect. The child may need transfusions of fresh plasma or clotting factors.■

In previously healthy children, the liver usually isn't permanently damaged after recovery from an acetaminophen overdose. However, the effects of chronic excessive use or repeated overdoses aren't known.

Aspirin Poisoning

The use of aspirin or similar drugs (salicylates) by children and teenagers is generally considered dangerous because of the risk of Reye's syndrome.★ However, the use of such drugs may be warranted in the treatment of a few specific diseases, such as juvenile rheumatoid arthritis.

Aspirin overdose (salicylism) is a common cause of accidental poisoning, despite safety packaging laws that require safety caps on all medications containing aspirin and that limit the size of a bottle of infant aspirin to 36 tablets. Children who have been ill with a fever or who have been taking aspirin are at greater risk. Poisoning is more severe in a child who has been taking high doses of aspirin for several days.

The most toxic form of salicylate is oil of wintergreen (methyl salicylate). Any exposure to methyl salicylate, a component of products such as liniments and solutions used in hot vaporizers, is potentially lethal to young children. A young child can die from swallowing less than one teaspoonful of pure methyl salicylate.

Symptoms

The early symptoms of aspirin overdose are nausea and vomiting, followed by rapid breathing, hyperactivity, increased temperature, and sometimes convulsions. The child quickly becomes drowsy, has difficulty breathing, and collapses. A high blood level of aspirin greatly increases urination, which can cause severe dehydration, especially in young children.

Diagnosis and Treatment

If a child is exposed to methyl salicylate, the Poison Center should be called immediately for instructions.

Aspirin can be detected in urine or blood using chemically treated test strips. A blood sample can then be taken to measure the precise level. Tests are repeated to monitor treatment.

The stomach must be emptied as soon as possible, but even as late as 6 to 8 hours after the child has swallowed aspirin, emptying the stomach may be helpful. Unless unconscious, the child is given activated charcoal by mouth or through a stomach tube.

For mild dehydration, the child is given plenty of fluids, such as milk or fruit juice. For more severe cases, giving the appropriate fluids is critical, so the precise types and amounts of fluid are given intravenously. Fever is controlled by sponging the child with tepid water. Vitamin K_1 may be given to treat bleeding problems. Kidney failure is rare; if it occurs, hemodialysis may be needed.

Poisoning With Caustic Substances

Swallowing caustic substances (strong acids and alkalies) burns and directly damages the mouth, esophagus, and stomach. Some common

household products containing caustic substances are drain and toilet bowl cleaners and dishwasher detergents; some contain the most damaging caustic substances, such as sodium hydroxide and sulfuric acid. Such products are available as solids and as liquids, the more dangerous form. With the solid products, the burning sensation of a particle sticking to a moist surface prevents a child from consuming much of the product. Because the liquid products don't stick, more is easily consumed and the entire esophagus can be damaged.

Symptoms

Pain is immediate and may be severe. The burned areas swell, and swallowing becomes painful. Breathing is shallow, and the pulse is often rapid and weak. Sometimes swelling obstructs the airway. Excessively low blood pressure (shock) is common.

The caustic substance may eat through the wall of the esophagus or stomach. The damaged esophagus or stomach may become perforated a week or more after the poisoning, possibly resulting from such events as vomiting or severe coughing. Children who survive the initial damage may eventually die of an infection as material from the esophagus leaks into the chest cavity. Even if the early effects are mild, the esophagus can narrow weeks later, resulting in a stricture. In severe cases involving strong substances, death can result from excessively low blood pressure, obstruction of the airway, perforation of the esophagus, destruction of tissue, or inflammation of the lungs.

Diagnosis and Treatment

The Poison Center should be called immediately. Most children need to be taken to an emergency department promptly.

The damage is usually obvious when a child has swallowed a caustic substance. However, the presence or absence of mouth burns doesn't reliably predict whether the esophagus has been burned. Serious burns are likely to be present if a child refuses to swallow and begins to drool. A doctor may look inside the esophagus with a flexible fiber-optic endoscope to determine whether the esophagus is still intact. Assessing the

Sources of Lead

A person can become exposed to relatively large amounts of lead in the following ways:

• Repeatedly swallowing chips of lead-based paint

• Allowing a metallic lead object, such as shot, a curtain weight, a fishing weight, or a bauble, to remain in the stomach or a joint, where the lead slowly dissolves

• Drinking acidic beverages or eating acidic foods—fruits, fruit juices, cola drinks, tomatoes, tomato juice, wine, cider— contaminated by being stored in improperly lead-glazed ceramic ware

• Burning lead-painted wood or battery casings in home fireplaces or stoves

• Taking folk medicines containing lead compounds

• Using lead-glazed ceramic ware or leaded glass to store or serve food

• Drinking home-brewed or illegally imported lead-contaminated whiskey or wine

• Inhaling fumes of leaded gasoline

• Being exposed to work-related sources of lead without being protected by respirators, ventilation, or dust suppression

Exposure to smaller amounts, mainly in lead-contaminated dust and soil, may increase the levels of lead in children, making treatment necessary even though no symptoms develop.

---

amount of damage through the endoscope helps the doctor determine the immediate treatment and predict the risk of subsequent narrowing and the possible need for surgical repair of the esophagus.

Any child who has swallowed a caustic substance should be seen by a doctor immediately. Treatment should be started at once by having the child drink water or milk to dilute the caustic substance. Milk is best for children. It not only coats and soothes the mucous membranes but also substitutes for tissue protein as the caustic substance's target of destruction. Contaminated clothing is removed immediately, and the contaminated area of skin is washed. *Vomiting should not be induced and the stomach should not be washed out* because doing so can cause further damage.

An antibiotic is given if the child has a fever or evidence of a perforated esophagus. In mild cases, the child may be encouraged to begin drinking fluids fairly soon after the poisoning. Otherwise, fluids are given intravenously until they can be taken by mouth. A surgical opening (tracheostomy) may be made into the airway if the airway is obstructed by swelling in the throat. If strictures develop, a tube may be placed in the esophagus surgically to prevent it from closing completely, so that dilation therapy can be performed later. Corticosteroids may be given to reduce inflammation. Dilation therapy may be required for months or years, but surgical reconstruction may also be necessary.

Lead Poisoning

Lead poisoning (plumbism) is usually a chronic disorder. Sometimes symptoms flare up periodically. Damage, such as intellectual deficits in children and progressive kidney disease in adults, may be permanent.

The risk of symptoms from lead poisoning increases as the blood level of lead increases. At a high blood level, the risk of brain damage is great but unpredictable. Lower sustained levels increase the risk of long-term intellectual deficits.

Symptoms

In adults, a characteristic sequence of symptoms may develop over several weeks or longer: personality changes, headaches, a metallic taste in the mouth, poor appetite, and vague abdominal discomfort ending with vomiting, constipation, and crampy abdominal pain. Brain damage is rare in adults.

In young children, symptoms may start with several weeks of irritability and decreased play activity. Then more serious symptoms occur abruptly and worsen over 1 to 5 days. They include persistent forceful vomiting, uncoordinated walking, seizures, confusion, sleepiness, and finally, uncontrollable seizures and coma. These symptoms of brain damage are caused mainly by swelling of the brain. Both children and adults may become anemic.▲ Some symptoms may diminish spontaneously if exposure to lead is stopped, only to worsen again if the exposure is resumed. However, stopping the exposure does not remove all the risks of brain damage, and treatment is needed.

Diagnosis

Most cases of lead poisoning are diagnosed during routine screening of children who are at risk for lead poisoning, such as those living in older houses likely to have peeling lead-based paint. However, a doctor may recognize the symptoms and perform a test to confirm that the blood level of lead is high. Measuring the amount of lead excreted in the urine during the first day of treatment also confirms the diagnosis. Additional diagnostic information can be obtained from analyzing bone marrow samples and, in a child, from abdominal and long-bone x-rays.

Treatment

The most important part of treatment is aggressively removing lead from the child's environment.

In children who have severe symptoms, treatment must often be started before test results are available to confirm the diagnosis. Removing the accumulated lead from the body is difficult. All treatments for lead poisoning take time and must be carefully monitored; even then, they can produce many adverse effects. Succimer, given by mouth, binds with lead and helps it dissolve in body fluids so that it can be excreted in the urine. Common side effects of succimer include a rash, nausea, vomiting, diarrhea, loss of appetite, a metallic taste in the mouth, and abnormalities in blood tests of liver function (transaminase levels).

When the lead level is so high that brain damage is likely, *emergency hospitalization is required.* Dimercaprol and edetate calcium disodium are given in a series of injections. Treatment is given for 5 to 7 consecutive days to avoid depleting the body's stores of other essential metals, particularly zinc. The patient is given fluids intravenously or clear liquids by mouth to avoid the vomiting that dimercaprol often causes. Treatment may need to be repeated after a rest period from it.

After treatment with these drugs is stopped, the blood level of lead usually rises again as lead still stored in body tissues is released. Often, penicillamine, given by mouth, can help remove this lead; it is administered 2 days after treatment with edetate calcium disodium. By reducing the time that the developing brain is exposed to excess lead, edetate calcium disodium followed by penicillamine may help some children who have very high levels of lead. Iron, zinc, and copper supplements are often given to compensate for depletion of these metals during long-term treatment with penicillamine.

Side effects of edetate calcium disodium are probably caused by the depletion of zinc. They include kidney damage, a high blood calcium level, fever, and diarrhea. Kidney damage, more likely at higher doses of this drug, is usually reversible. Penicillamine may cause rashes, protein in the urine, and a low white blood cell count. These reactions are reversible if penicillamine is stopped promptly. Dimercaprol can cause the breakdown of red blood cells (hemolysis) in some people.

None of these drugs should be given for preventive purposes to lead workers or anyone exposed to high levels of lead, because these drugs can increase lead absorption. For such people, a long-term approach—reducing their exposure to lead—is needed. When children have a lead level of 10 micrograms per deciliter (μg/dL) or higher, their exposure to lead should be reduced.

Iron Poisoning

Because vitamin supplements containing iron are commonly used and are found in many households, mild cases of iron overdose are common. However, an iron overdose can be serious or fatal. Iron is included in multiple vitamins for adults and children. Children's chewable vitamins containing iron have a remarkable safety record because of the limited number of tablets in the container.

▲ see page 742

However, all iron supplements are not the same. Taking a few iron tablets formulated for adults can harm a child. The Poison Center should be called immediately to determine if a dangerous amount has been ingested.

Symptoms

A large overdose of iron can cause diarrhea, vomiting, a high white blood cell count, and a high blood glucose level. If no symptoms develop in the first 6 hours and the iron level is low, the risk of poisoning is small.

The symptoms of iron overdose typically occur in the following stages:

• Stage 1 (within 6 hours): Symptoms may include vomiting, irritability, explosive diarrhea, abdominal pain, seizures, drowsiness, and unconsciousness. Irritation of the lining of the digestive tract may cause bleeding in the stomach (hemorrhagic gastritis). Rapid breathing and heart rate, low blood pressure, and increased blood acidity may also result when the blood level of iron is high. Very low blood pressure or unconsciousness during the first 6 hours indicates that the condition is very serious.

• Stage 2 (within 10 to 14 hours): Apparent but deceptive improvement may occur and last for up to 24 hours.

• Stage 3 (between 12 and 48 hours): Very low blood pressure (shock) may develop, blood flow to the tissues may be poor, and the blood glucose level may be low. Blood iron levels may be normal, but tests may indicate that the liver has been damaged. Other symptoms may include fever, an increased white blood cell count, bleeding disorders, abnormal electrical conduction in the heart, disorientation, restlessness, drowsiness, convulsions, and unconsciousness. Death may occur.

• Stage 4 (after 2 to 5 weeks): Complications of the iron poisoning, such as intestinal obstruction, cirrhosis,▲ or brain damage, may occur.

Diagnosis and Treatment

The Poison Center should be called. Giving the child syrup of ipecac immediately at home may be recommended.

▲ see page 567

■ see page 200

At the hospital, the blood level of iron is measured between 2 and 4 hours after the overdose. If it is low, the child is observed for 6 hours but doesn't have to be hospitalized unless symptoms develop. If the blood iron level is high or if symptoms are present, hospitalization is necessary.

A vigorous effort is made to remove any iron remaining in the stomach. In the hospital emergency department, the stomach may be washed out using a stomach tube. Activated charcoal may be used even though it doesn't absorb much iron. The intestine may be washed out (irrigated) to flush the iron out of the body. Several injections of deferoxamine, which binds iron in the blood, are given to a child who has a high blood level of iron or symptoms.

Anemia may develop later because of iron deficiency resulting from the treatment and from bleeding. X-rays of the stomach or upper intestine may be taken 6 weeks or more after the overdose to look for narrowing in these organs caused by irritation of the lining of the digestive tract.

The prognosis is usually good. Overall, about 1 percent of children hospitalized for iron poisoning die, but a child who goes into shock and becomes unconscious has about a 10 percent chance of dying.

Hydrocarbon Poisoning

Hydrocarbons (organic compounds composed of only hydrogen and carbon) are often found in petroleum, natural gas, and coal. Every year, more than 25,000 children under age 5 are poisoned as a result of swallowing petroleum distillates, such as gasoline, kerosene, and paint thinners, and halogenated hydrocarbons, such as carbon tetrachloride (found in dry-cleaning fluids and solvents) and ethylene dichloride (found in paint strippers). However, most of the deaths from hydrocarbon poisoning occur in teenagers who deliberately sniff volatile substances. Small quantities of these substances, especially liquids that flow easily, can get into the lungs and damage them directly. Of the thicker liquids, mineral seal oil, which is used in products such as furniture polish, is the most dangerous because it is extremely irritating and can cause severe aspiration pneumonia.■

Symptoms

The symptoms affect chiefly the lungs and intestine; in extreme cases, the brain is also affected. At first, a child coughs and chokes, even after taking only one small taste. Breathing becomes rapid. The skin may become bluish because of reduced oxygen levels. Gasping, vomiting, and persistent coughing may follow. Older children may complain of a burning sensation in the stomach before vomiting. Neurologic symptoms include drowsiness, stupor or coma, and convulsions. These effects are usually worse with larger amounts and are most severe in children who have swallowed lighter fluid, mineral seal oil, or halogenated hydrocarbons such as carbon tetrachloride.

The kidneys and bone marrow may be damaged. In severe cases, the heart may enlarge; heartbeats may become irregular, as in atrial fibrillation;▲ and cardiac arrest may even occur. Lung inflammation that's severe enough to cause death usually does so within 24 hours. Recovery from pneumonia typically takes about a week. An exception is pneumonia caused by ingesting mineral seal oil, which usually requires 5 to 6 weeks for recovery.

Diagnosis and Treatment

A chest x-ray is the single most important diagnostic test. Evidence of pneumonia can be seen on x-rays within 2 hours in severe cases and within 6 to 8 hours in 90 percent of the people who develop pneumonia as a result of hydrocarbon poisoning. If signs of pneumonia don't develop within 24 hours, they will not. A white blood cell count and urinalysis may identify an infection or kidney damage. Measuring the levels of oxygen and carbon dioxide in arterial blood helps in the diagnosis and treatment of pneumonia.

As soon as the poisoning is discovered, the Poison Center should be called, contaminated clothing should be removed, and the skin should be washed. A child who is awake and alert may drink a small glass of milk to dilute the swallowed material and reduce stomach irritation. A child who has any symptoms involving the lungs, such as rapid breathing, a rapid heart rate, or a cough, should be taken to the hospital. A child without any of these symptoms can usually be treated at home after the Poison Center has been consulted.

Because the pneumonia that may develop is caused by chemical irritation rather than bacteria, antibiotics aren't useful for prevention. If pneumonia develops, treatment may include oxygen therapy, ventilator support, intravenous fluids, and careful monitoring.

CHAPTER 276

Injuries

In the United States, injury is the most common cause of death among children, killing more children than cancer, birth defects, pneumonia, meningitis, and heart disease combined. Even among infants under 1 year of age, almost 1,000 deaths a year are caused by falls, burns, drowning, and suffocation. Injuries are also the leading cause of disability in children: For every child who dies of an injury, 1,000 children survive but become disabled.

Injuries are frequently triggered by a child's curiosity, and most are preventable. They are more common when a child is hungry or tired (before meals or naps), very active, being cared for by a baby-sitter, or living in new surroundings, such as a new home or a vacation site. Injuries are most likely when parents are rushed and busy or when they don't anticipate how risks change as their child grows older.

Motor Vehicle Accidents

Injury from motor vehicle accidents is a major cause of death among all age groups, claiming 4 out of every 100,000 infants under 1 year of age, 7

▲ see page 82

Preventing Injuries

Preventive education is important for parent and child. The child must be protected from hazards and taught how to handle those that are unavoidable. Situations that increase the risk of injuries should be avoided. Preventive measures include the following:

• Using appropriate safety restraints and car seats for children in automobiles

• Using smoke or heat detectors in homes

• Using electrical outlet safety devices

• Adjusting tap water temperatures to less than 120° F.

• Not using infant walkers

• Keeping drugs, poisons, and other hazardous substances out of the reach of children by storing them in cabinets that have childproof latches or that are locked

• Making sure that children wear a life vest or flotation device when by the water (pools, beaches, docks)

• Making sure that children wear a helmet while bicycle riding

• Making sure that children wear appropriate protective clothing when participating in sports—for example, knee pads, elbow pads, and a helmet for roller blading or skateboarding

• Making sure children sled in areas where there are no trees

Parents must set a good safety example—such as by wearing seat belts and bicycle helmets—because children mimic their parents' actions.

out of every 100,000 children aged 1 to 14 years, and up to 40 out of every 100,000 people aged 15 to 24 years. A child who isn't wearing a seat belt or strapped into a correctly installed child safety

▲ see page 357

seat may be the only casualty of a sudden stop that causes no property damage or injury to others in the car.

To reduce the possibility and severity of injuries in a crash, all occupants of a motor vehicle should use seat belts or, for young children (weighing less than 40 pounds), properly installed child safety seats. Children should sit only in the back seat to avoid injury from air bags. Such restraints reduce fatalities by 40 to 50 percent and serious injuries by 45 to 55 percent. Most states have laws requiring that children use safety restraints. A child who is held by an adult, even if the adult is wearing a seat belt, is extremely vulnerable. In the event of a crash, the adult will be unable to hold onto the child, who will be thrown with tremendous force even at low speed. For instance, restraining a 10-pound child during a sudden stop in a car traveling 30 miles an hour would require the strength to lift 300 pounds 1 foot off the ground. An adult not wearing a seat belt may be thrown forward, possibly crushing the child against the interior of the car with a force many times the adult's weight.

The child must be strapped into a restraint appropriate for his age and weight. An infant safety seat should face the back of the vehicle and can be used for children weighing up to 20 pounds. A rear-facing infant seat should be placed only in the back seat of a car; this placement is especially important when the car has air bags. Safety seats for children who weigh 21 to 40 pounds should face forward, be equipped with shoulder restraints and lap guards, and provide stability for the head. The safety seat must be secured to the car according to manufacturer's instructions, or the risk of injury to the child may be increased. An older child should be secured by a seat belt.

A number of child safety seat designs have been approved by the National Highway Traffic Safety Administration. Those that meet federal crash standards are so labeled.

Head Injuries

In children, a high percentage of deaths from injury are caused by head injuries and their complications.▲ Severe head injuries may also seriously damage the developing brain, interfering with the child's physical, intellectual, and emotional development and resulting in long-term disabilities. However, most head injuries are minor.

Head injuries are most common in children under age 1 and in adolescents over age 15. Boys are injured more often than girls. Major head injuries are usually caused by motor vehicle and bicycle accidents. Minor head injuries are predominantly caused by falls in and around the home. Because any head injury is potentially serious, every child who has had a head injury should be evaluated carefully.

Symptoms

A minor head injury may cause vomiting, paleness, irritability, or drowsiness without loss of consciousness or any immediate evidence of brain damage. If symptoms continue for more than 6 hours or worsen, a health care practitioner should evaluate the child further to determine whether the injury is severe.

A concussion is a temporary loss of consciousness immediately after a head injury.▲ It should be evaluated promptly, even if it lasts no more than a minute. Often, the child can't remember the injury itself or the events just before it but has no other symptoms of brain damage.

Head injuries may bruise or tear brain tissue or blood vessels in or around the brain, causing bleeding and swelling inside the brain. The most common brain injury is diffuse (widespread) injury to brain cells. A diffuse injury causes brain cells to swell, increasing pressure inside the skull. As a result, a child may lose strength or sensation and become drowsy or unconscious. These symptoms suggest a severe brain injury, likely to result in permanent damage and the need for rehabilitation. As the swelling worsens, the pressure increases, so that even uninjured tissue can be compressed against the skull, causing permanent damage or death. Swelling with its dangerous results usually occurs in the first 48 to 72 hours after the injury.

If the skull is fractured, a brain injury may be more severe. However, a brain injury commonly occurs without a skull fracture, and a skull fracture often occurs without a brain injury. Fractures at the back or base (bottom) of the skull usually indicate a forceful impact, because these parts of the skull are relatively thick. Such fractures often can't be seen on x-rays or computed tomography (CT) scans. However, the following symptoms suggest this type of fracture:
• Cerebrospinal fluid (the clear fluid that surrounds the brain) draining from the nose or ears

Symptoms of Severe Head Injury

A child who has any of the following symptoms should be evaluated promptly:
• Loss of consciousness
• Inability to move or feel part of the body
• Inability to recognize people or the environment
• Inability to speak or see
• Inability to maintain balance
• Clear fluid (cerebrospinal fluid) draining from the nose or mouth
• Severe headache

• Blood collecting behind the eardrum or bleeding from the ear if the eardrum is ruptured
• Bruising behind the ear (Battle's sign) or around the eyes (raccoon's eyes)
• Blood collecting in the sinuses (can only be seen on x-rays)
In an infant, the membranes surrounding the brain may protrude through a skull fracture and become trapped by it, forming a fluid-filled sac called a growing fracture. The sac develops over 3 to 6 weeks and may be the first evidence that the skull was fractured.

In depressed skull fractures, one or more fragments of bone press inward on the brain. The resulting bruising of the brain may cause seizures.

Seizures occur in about 5 percent of children over age 5 years and in 10 percent of those under age 5 during the first week after a serious head injury. Seizures that start soon after the injury are less likely to result in a long-term seizure problem than those that start 7 or more days later.

A serious but relatively uncommon complication of head injuries in children is bleeding between the layers of membranes surrounding the brain or in the brain itself.■ An **epidural hema-**

▲ see page 359

■ see box, page 356

toma—a collection of blood between the skull and the membrane that lines it (dura mater)—may exert pressure on the brain. It results from damage to arteries or veins that line the skull. In an adult, symptoms of an epidural hematoma are an initial loss of consciousness; a regaining of consciousness, called a lucid interval; and then a worsening of symptoms of pressure on the brain, such as drowsiness and loss of sensation or strength. However, in a young child, there is no lucid interval but rather a gradual loss of consciousness over a period of minutes to hours because of increasing pressure on the brain.

In a **subdural hematoma,** blood collects beneath the dura mater, usually in association with a significant injury to brain tissue. Drowsiness to the point of unconsciousness, loss of sensation or strength, and abnormal movements including seizures usually develop rapidly, although symptoms occasionally develop more gradually when the injury is mild.

Bleeding may occur inside the internal spaces (ventricles) of the brain (intraventricular hemorrhage), within the brain tissue itself (intraparenchymal hemorrhage), or within the membranes covering the brain's surface (subarachnoid hemorrhage). These types of bleeding are evidence of very severe brain injury and are associated with long-term brain damage.

Diagnosis

In evaluating a child who has a head injury, a doctor considers the way the injury occurred as well as the resulting symptoms and performs a thorough physical examination. Special attention is paid to the level of consciousness, the ability to feel and move, any abnormal movements, reflexes, the eyes and ears, pulse, blood pressure, and breathing rate. The size of the pupils and their reaction to light are important; the interior of the eyes is examined with an ophthalmoscope to determine whether pressure within the brain is increased. Infants who have been shaken (shaken baby syndrome, shaken impact syndrome) often develop areas of bleeding in the back of the eyes (retinal hemorrhages). If a significant brain injury is likely, a CT scan of the head is usually obtained.

If a depressed skull fracture without brain injury is possible, the skull may be x-rayed.

Treatment

Most children who have had mild head injuries are sent home, and their parents are instructed to observe them for persistent vomiting or increasing drowsiness. If the child goes home at night, keeping the child awake during the night is not necessary; parents need only to wake the child periodically (as instructed by the doctor—for example, every 2 to 4 hours) to make sure the child can be aroused. Children are observed in the hospital if they are drowsy, were unconscious even briefly, have any abnormality of feeling (numbness) or muscle strength, or are at high risk of worsening. Children who have a skull fracture without evidence of a brain injury need not be routinely hospitalized. In contrast, *infants* with a skull fracture, especially if it is depressed, are almost always observed in the hospital; for a depressed skull fracture, surgery may be needed to lift up the bone fragments and prevent further injury to the brain. Children are also kept in the hospital if child abuse is suspected.▲

In the hospital, children are observed closely for changes in the level of consciousness and in breathing, heart rate, and blood pressure. Doctors also look for evidence of increased pressure within the skull by frequently examining the pupils of the eyes and by watching for changes in sensation or strength and for seizures. A CT scan of the head may be performed or repeated if seizures occur, vomiting continues, drowsiness increases, or the condition deteriorates in any other way.

Nothing can reverse damage that has already occurred. However, further damage may be prevented by ensuring that enough blood containing sufficient oxygen is reaching the brain. Pressure within the brain is kept as normal as possible by immediately treating any brain swelling and reducing any pressure on the brain. For an **epidural hematoma,** emergency surgery must be performed to remove the pooled blood and thus prevent it from pressing on the brain and causing damage. With appropriate treatment, most children who have a simple epidural hematoma recover fully. A **subdural hematoma** also may need to be removed surgically. Brain swelling is usually

▲ see page 1322

evaluated with an intracranial pressure monitor, which measures pressure in the brain. A drain may also be inserted into one of the ventricles to drain cerebrospinal fluid and thus relieve pressure. The head of the bed is raised to reduce pressure within the brain, and various drugs, such as mannitol or furosemide, may be used to reduce this pressure.

Seizures are treated, usually with phenytoin. In children who have seizures after a head injury, an electroencephalogram (EEG) may be performed to assist with diagnosis and treatment.

Prognosis

How much brain function is recovered depends on how severe the injury is, how old the child is, how long he was unconscious, and which part of the brain was most injured. Of the nearly 5 million children who sustain a head injury each year, 4,000 die and 15,000 require prolonged hospitalization. Of those with a severe injury who are unconscious for longer than 24 hours, 50 percent have long-term complications, including significant physical, intellectual, and emotional problems; 2 to 5 percent remain severely handicapped. Young children, especially infants, who have had a severe head injury are more likely to die than older children.

For those who survive, a prolonged period of rehabilitation, particularly in intellectual and emotional development, is often required. Common problems during recovery include loss of memory from the time immediately before the injury (retrograde amnesia), changes in behavior, emotional instability, sleep disturbances, and decreased intellectual ability.

Accidents and Injuries

CHAPTER 277

Burns

*A burn is an injury to tissue resulting from heat,
chemicals, or electricity.*

Most people think heat is the only cause of
burns, but some chemicals and electrical current
can burn as well. Although the skin is usually the
part of the body that's burned, the tissues under
it also can be burned, and internal organs can be
burned even when the skin is not. For example,
drinking a very hot liquid or caustic substance
such as acid can burn the esophagus and stomach. Inhaling smoke and hot air from a fire in a
burning building can burn the lungs.

Tissues that are burned may die. When tissues
are damaged by a burn, fluid leaks from blood
vessels, causing swelling. In an extensive burn,
loss of a large amount of fluid from abnormally

leaky blood vessels can cause shock.▲ In shock,
blood pressure decreases so much that too little
blood flows to the brain and other vital organs.

Electrical burns may be caused by a temperature of more than 9,000° F., generated by an electric current when it passes from the electrical
source to the body; this type of burn, sometimes
called an electrical arc burn, usually completely
destroys and chars the skin at the current's point
of entry into the body.■ Because the resistance
(the body's ability to stop or slow the current's

▲ see page 111

■ see page 1338

flow) is high where the skin touches the current's source, much of the electrical energy is converted to heat there, burning the surface. Most electrical burns also severely damage the tissues under the skin. These burns vary in size and depth and may affect an area much larger than that indicated by the area of injured skin. Large electrical shocks can paralyze breathing and disturb heart rhythm, causing dangerously irregular heartbeats.

Chemical burns can be caused by various irritants and poisons, including strong acids and alkalis, phenols and cresols (organic solvents), mustard gas, and phosphorus. Chemical burns can cause tissue death that can slowly spread for hours after the burn.

Symptoms

The severity of a burn depends on the amount of tissue affected and the depth of the injury, which is described as first, second, or third degree.

First-degree burns are the least severe. The burned skin becomes red, painful, very sensitive to the touch, and moist or swollen. The burned area whitens (blanches) when lightly touched, but no blisters develop.

Second-degree burns cause deeper damage. The skin blisters. The base of the blisters may be red or whitish and filled with a clear, thick fluid. The burn is painfully sensitive to the touch and may blanch when touched.

Third-degree burns cause the deepest damage. The surface of the burn may be white and soft or black, charred, and leathery. Because the burned area may be pale, it can be mistaken for normal skin in light-skinned people, but it doesn't blanch when touched. Damaged red blood cells in the injured area may make the burn bright red. Occasionally, the burned area blisters, and hairs in the burn can easily be pulled from their roots. The burned area has no feeling when touched. Generally, third-degree burns aren't painful, because the nerve endings in the skin have been destroyed.

Distinguishing between deep second-degree burns and third-degree burns is difficult until days after the injury.

Prognosis

Healing depends on the depth and location of the burn. In superficial burns (first-degree and superficial second-degree burns), the dead layers of skin slough off, and the top layer of skin (epidermis) regrows to cover the layers below. A new layer of epidermis can grow quickly from the base of a superficial burn with little or no scarring. These burns don't destroy the deeper layer of skin (dermis), which can't regenerate.

Deep burns injure the dermis. A new layer of epidermis grows slowly from the edges of the burned area and from any remnants of the epidermis in the burned area. Consequently, healing is very slow and scarring is considerable. The burned area also tends to contract, distorting the skin and interfering with its functioning.

Mild burns of the esophagus, stomach, and lungs generally heal without problems. More severe burns, however, can lead to scarring and narrowing, called contractures. Scarring can block the passage of food in the esophagus and prevent the normal transfer of oxygen from the air to blood in the lungs.

Treatment

About 85 percent of burns are minor and can be treated at home, in a doctor's office, or in a hospital's emergency department. Removing all clothing—especially any that's smoldering (such as melted synthetic shirts), covered with hot tar, or soaked with chemicals—helps stop the burning and prevents further injury. Chemicals, including acids, alkalis, and organic compounds, are washed off the skin as soon as possible with large amounts of water.

Hospitalization is more likely to be needed in the following situations:

- The face, hands, genitals, or feet are burned
- The person would have difficulty caring for the wound adequately at home
- The person is under 2 or over 70 years old
- Internal organs are burned

Minor Burns

Minor burns should be immersed immediately in cool water, if possible. Chemical burns should be washed with large amounts of water for a long time. At a doctor's office or emergency department, a burn is cleaned carefully with soap and water to remove all debris. If dirt is deeply embedded, a doctor can anesthetize the area and scrub it with a brush. Any blisters that are broken or could break easily are usually removed. Once the area is clean, an antibiotic cream such as silver sulfadiazine may be applied.

A bandage, usually made of gauze, is applied to protect the burned area from dirt and further injury. Keeping the area clean is extremely important, because once the top layer of skin (epidermis) is damaged, infections can start and spread easily. Antibiotics may help prevent infection but aren't always needed. A tetanus booster is given if immunization isn't up-to-date.

A burned arm or leg is usually kept in a position higher than the level of the heart to reduce swelling. Maintaining this position may be possible only in the hospital, where part of the bed can be raised or traction can be used. If the burn affects a joint and is of second or third degree, the joint may have to be immobilized with a splint because movement may worsen the injury. Many people who have been burned need to take an analgesic, often a narcotic, for at least a few days.

Severe Burns

More severe, life-threatening burns require immediate care, preferably at a hospital equipped to treat burns. Rescue or ambulance personnel usually administer oxygen to fire victims through a face mask to help overcome the effects of carbon monoxide, a poisonous gas often formed in fires. In the emergency department, doctors and nurses make sure that a person can breathe well, check for other life-threatening injuries, and start treatment to replace lost fluids and prevent infection. Hyperbaric oxygen therapy, in which the patient is placed in a special chamber with oxygen at increased pressure, is sometimes used to treat severe burns. However, it must be started within 24 hours of the burn and isn't widely available.

If the airways and lungs have been injured in a fire, a tube may be inserted in the throat to assist breathing. The decision to insert the tube (intubate) depends on such factors as the rate of breathing; breathing too fast or too slowly keeps the lungs from filling with enough air and transferring enough oxygen to the blood. A tube may be needed when the face is directly injured or swelling in the throat threatens breathing. Sometimes a tube is inserted when a doctor suspects airway damage before it's obvious—for example, when a person was exposed to a type of fire that's likely to damage the airway (especially a fire in an enclosed space or an explosion), when soot is found in the nose or mouth, or when the nasal hairs are singed. If breathing is normal, oxygen given through a face mask may be all that's needed.

After the area has been cleaned, an antibiotic cream or ointment is often applied; then the area is covered with sterile bandages. The bandages are usually changed two or three times a day. Because extensive burns are extremely susceptible to severe infections, antibiotics may be given intravenously. A tetanus booster may also be given, depending on the person's previous immunizations.

Extensive burns can lead to a life-threatening loss of body fluids. Therefore, fluids are given intravenously to replace those lost. Deep burns can cause myoglobulinuria, a condition in which the protein myoglobulin is released from damaged muscles and damages the kidneys. Kidney failure may follow unless sufficient fluids are replaced.

Burned skin develops a thick, crusty surface called eschar, which can become taut and restrict blood flow to the area. Restricted blood flow can be dangerous if the burn completely surrounds an arm or a leg. A doctor may need to cut through the eschar (escharotomy) to relieve the tension on the healthy tissue under it.

Even a deep burn can heal itself if the area is small (no larger than a 50-cent piece) and is kept meticulously clean. However, if the underlying dermis is damaged extensively, a skin graft is usually needed to cover the burned area. A skin graft is a piece of healthy skin taken from unburned areas of the burn victim's body (autografts), from another living or dead person (allografts), or from another species (xenografts)—usually pigs because their skin is most similar to human skin. Autografts are permanent, but skin grafts from other people or animals are temporary, protecting the area while the body heals itself and rejected by the body 10 to 14 days later.

Usually, physical and occupational therapy is needed to minimize the amount of scarring and to retain as much function as possible in the burned areas. As soon as possible, splints are applied to keep joints extended so that muscles and skin do not become tight and contracted. The splints are left in place until the area is largely healed.

Before skin grafting is performed, the affected joints are exercised in ways that increase their ability to move through a normal range of motion. After the graft has been applied, a doctor usually immobilizes the area for 5 to 10 days to ensure that the graft is secure before exercises are resumed.

Burn victims need to consume an adequate amount of calories and nutrients for burns to heal. Those who can't eat enough may drink nutritional supplements or receive them by way of a tube inserted through the nose into the stomach (a nasogastric tube). If the intestines aren't functioning because of an injury or repeated operations, nutrients can be given intravenously.

Because severe burns take a long time to heal, sometimes years, a burn victim can become severely depressed. Most burn centers provide psychologic support for their patients through social workers, psychiatrists, and others.

CHAPTER 278

Electrical Injuries

An electrical injury is damage that occurs when electricity passes through the body, either burning tissue or interfering with the function of an internal organ.

Electrical current passing through body tissues generates heat, which can severely burn and destroy tissues. An electrical jolt can short-circuit the body's own electrical systems, causing the heart to stop (cardiac arrest).

Causes

Electrical injury can result from being struck by lightning or touching household wires, downed electrical lines, or something that conducts electricity from a live electrical wire, such as a pool of water. The severity of the injury, which can range from a minor burn to death, is determined by the type and strength of the current, the body's resistance to the current at the point of entry, the pathway of the current through the body, and the duration of exposure to the current.

In general, direct current (DC) is less dangerous than alternating current (AC). The effects of alternating current on the body depend largely on the speed with which the current alternates (frequency), measured in cycles per second (hertz). Low-frequency currents of 50 to 60 hertz, commonly used in the United States, are more dangerous than high-frequency currents and three to five times more dangerous than direct current of the same voltage and strength (amperage). Direct current tends to cause strong muscle contractions that often force the victim away from the current's source. Alternating current at 60 hertz causes muscles to freeze in position, often preventing victims from releasing their grip on the current's source. As a result, exposure may be prolonged, causing severe burns. Generally, the higher the voltage and amperage, the greater the damage from either type of current.

The strength of electrical current is measured in amperes. A milliampere (mA) is 1/1,000 of an ampere. The body can perceive direct current entering the hand at about 5 to 10 milliamperes; it can perceive common household current, which is 60-hertz alternating current, at about 1 to 10 milliamperes. The maximum current that causes arm muscles to contract but still allows the hand to let go of the electric source is appropriately called the let-go current. This value is about 75 milliamperes for direct current and about 2 to 5 milliamperes in children, 5 to 7 milliamperes in women, and 7 to 9 milliamperes in men for alternating current, depending on the muscle mass of a person's arm.

At currents as low as 60 to 100 milliamperes, a low-voltage (110 to 220 volts), 60-hertz alternating current traveling through the chest for a split second can cause life-threatening irregular heart rhythms. About 300 to 500 milliamperes of direct current is required to have the same effect. If the current travels directly to the heart, for instance through a pacemaker, a much lower current (less than 1 milliampere) can cause irregular heart rhythms.

Resistance is the ability to stop or slow the flow of electrical current. Most of the body's resistance is concentrated in the skin and depends directly on the skin's condition. The average resistance of dry, healthy skin is 40 times greater than that of thin, moist skin. When the skin is punctured or scraped or when current is applied to moist mucous membranes such as the mouth, rectum, or vagina, the resistance is only half that of moist, intact skin. The resistance of a thick, callused palm or sole may be 100 times greater than that of thinner areas of skin. As electrical current passes through the skin, much of its energy may be released at the surface because it encounters resistance there. If skin resistance is high, large surface burns can occur at the entrance and exit points, with charring of tissues in between. Internal tissues are also burned, depending on their resistance.

The path that the current takes through the body can be crucial in determining the extent of injury. The most common entry point for electricity is the hand; the second most common is the head. The most common exit point is the foot. Because current that travels from arm to arm or from arm to leg can go through the heart, it's much more dangerous than current that travels between a leg and the ground. Current traveling through the head may cause seizures, brain hemorrhages, paralyzed breathing, psychologic changes (such as short-term memory problems, personality changes, irritability, and sleep disturbances), and irregular heartbeats. Damage to the eyes may lead to cataracts.

The duration of exposure is important. The longer the exposure, the greater the amount of tissue damaged. A person who freezes to a current's source can have severe burns. On the other hand, a person struck by lightning rarely has severe external or internal burns because the event happens so fast that the current tends to flash over the body without causing extensive internal tissue damage. However, a lightning strike may short-circuit the heart and lungs, paralyzing them, and may damage the nerves or brain.

Symptoms

Symptoms depend on the complex interactions of all the characteristics of electrical current. A shock from an electrical current may startle a person, causing a fall, or may trigger powerful muscle contractions. Either can result in dislocations, fractures, and blunt injuries. A person may lose consciousness. Breathing and heartbeat can be paralyzed. Electrical burns may be distinctly outlined on the skin and may extend into deeper tissues.

High-voltage current can kill tissues between its entry and exit points, resulting in large areas of burned muscle. As a result, large amounts of fluids and salts (electrolytes) are lost, sometimes leading to dangerously low blood pressure, as in other severe burns. Damaged muscle fibers release myoglobin, which can injure the kidneys, causing kidney failure.

A person who is wet may come into contact with an electrical current—for example, when a hair dryer falls into a bathtub or a person steps in a puddle that's in contact with a downed electrical line. In such situations, the skin's resistance may be lowered to such an extent that the person may not be burned but may go into cardiac arrest and die if not promptly resuscitated.

Lightning rarely causes entry and exit burns and seldom causes muscle damage or myoglobin in the urine. Loss of consciousness, sometimes followed by coma, or temporary confusion may occur at first but usually disappears within hours or days. The most common cause of death by a lightning strike is heart and lung paralysis (cardiac and respiratory arrest).

Toddlers who suck on extension cords can be burned on the mouth and lips. These burns may not only cause facial deformities but also lead to growth problems of the teeth, jaw, and face. The child should be examined by an orthodontist or oral surgeon as well as by a burn surgeon. An added danger is that severe bleeding from an artery in the lip may occur when the scab falls off, usually 7 to 10 days after the injury.

Prevention

Education about electricity and respect for it are essential. Making sure that all electrical devices are properly designed, installed, and maintained can help prevent electrical injuries at home and work. Any electrical device that touches or may be touched by the body should be properly grounded and plugged into circuits containing protective circuit-breaking equipment. Circuit breakers that interrupt (trip) the circuit when current as low as 5 milliamperes leaks are excellent safety devices and are readily available.

Preventing lightning strikes depends on taking sensible precautions, such as avoiding open fields, baseball diamonds, and golf courses during thunderstorms and seeking shelter—but not under an isolated tree or metal-topped pavilion, which attracts lightning. People should leave a pool, pond, or lake. Inside an automobile is a safe place to be.

Treatment

Treatment consists of separating the person from the current's source, restoring heartbeat and breathing with cardiopulmonary resuscitation (CPR) if needed, and treating burns and related injuries.

The safest way to separate the victim from the current's source is to shut off the current rapidly—for example, by throwing a circuit breaker or switch or by disconnecting the device from an electrical outlet. *If the lines could be high voltage, no one should touch the victim until the current has been shut off.* Many well-meaning rescuers have been injured by electricity when trying to free a victim. High-voltage and low-voltage lines are difficult to distinguish, especially outdoors.

Once the victim can be safely touched, the rescuer should check to see if the victim is breathing and has a pulse. If the victim isn't breathing and has no discernible pulse, cardiopulmonary resuscitation should be started immediately. Emergency or hospital personnel should check the victim for fractures, dislocations, and blunt or spinal cord injuries. If muscle damage is extensive, myoglobin may damage the kidneys, so large amounts of fluids are given to help prevent kidney damage.

Often, victims of lightning strikes can be revived by cardiopulmonary resuscitation. Quick action is crucial, but resuscitation should be attempted even for victims who appear to be dead, because those who can be stimulated to breathe on their own almost always recover.

Electrocardiograms are taken to monitor the victim's heartbeat. If the heart could have received an electric shock, the victim is monitored for 12 to 24 hours. If the victim was unconscious or received a head injury, a computed tomography (CT) scan may be performed to check for damage to the brain.

CHAPTER 279

Radiation Injury

Radiation injury is damage to tissues caused by exposure to radiation.

In general, radiation refers to waves or particles of high energy emitted by naturally occurring or man-made sources. Injury to tissues can be caused by brief exposure to high levels of radiation or long-term exposure to low levels. Some adverse effects of radiation last only briefly; others produce chronic disease. The early effects of large doses of radiation become obvious within minutes or days after exposure. Late effects may not become obvious for weeks, months, or even years. Mutations in the genetic material of cells in the sex organs may become apparent only if a person exposed to radiation has children: The children may be born with genetic defects.

Causes

Harmful sources of radiation once included only x-rays and naturally occurring radioactive materials such as uranium and radon. X-rays used in diagnostic procedures today produce much less radiation than those used in the past. The most common sources of high-level radiation exposure are man-made radioactive materials used in many medical treatments, scientific laboratories, industry, and nuclear power reactors.

Large amounts of radiation have accidentally escaped from nuclear power plants, including the Three Mile Island plant in Pennsylvania in 1979 and the Chernobyl plant in the Ukraine in 1986. The Three Mile Island accident didn't result in major radiation exposure; in fact, a person living within 1 mile of the plant received slightly less radiation than the average person receives from x-rays in 1 year. However, people living near the Chernobyl plant were exposed to considerably more radiation. More than 30 people died and many more were injured. Radiation from that accident reached Europe, Asia, and the United States.

In total, radiation exposure from reactors in the first 40 years of nuclear energy use, excluding Chernobyl, has resulted in 35 serious exposures with 10 deaths, but none was associated with power plants. In the United States, nuclear power reactors must meet stringent federal standards that limit the amount of released radioactive material to extremely low levels.

Radiation is measured in several different units. The roentgen (R) measures the amount of radiation in the air. The gray (Gy) is the amount of energy actually absorbed by any tissue or substance from exposure to radiation. Because some types of radiation can affect biological organisms more than others, the sievert (Sv) is used to describe the strength of the effects on the body for equivalent amounts of absorbed energy.

The damaging effects of radiation depend on the amount (dose), duration of exposure, and rate of exposure. A single, rapid dose of radiation can be fatal, but the same total dose given over a period of weeks or months may have little measurable effect. The total dose and the rate of exposure determine the immediate effects on the genetic material of cells.

The dose rate is the amount of radiation a person is exposed to during a given period of time. The dose rate of unavoidable background radiation in the environment is low—about 1 to 2 milligrays (1 milligray equals 1/1,000 gray) a year, which has no detectable effect on the body. The effects of radiation are cumulative; each exposure adds to the previous ones to determine the total dose and its likely effect on the body. As the dose rate or total dose increases, the likelihood of detectable effects increases.

The effects of radiation also depend on how much of the body is exposed. For example, more than 6 grays generally causes death when the radiation is distributed over the entire surface of the body; however, when beamed to a small area, as in radiation therapy for cancer, three or four

Yearly Radiation Exposure in the United States

Source	Average Dose (millisieverts)
Naturally occurring sources	0.82
Medical procedures (such as x-rays)	0.77
Fallout from weapons testing	0.04–0.05
Nuclear industry	less than 0.01
Research	0.01 or less
Consumer products	0.03–0.04
Airline travel	0.005
Transport of radiation therapy materials	0.0001
Other	0.15
TOTAL	**1.84**

times this amount can be given without serious harm to the body. The distribution of radiation within the body is also important. The parts of the body in which cells are multiplying quickly, such as the intestines and bone marrow, are harmed more easily by radiation than parts in which cells multiply more slowly, such as muscles and tendons. During radiation therapy for cancer, every attempt is made to shield the more vulnerable parts of the body from radiation so that high doses can be used.

Symptoms

Radiation exposure produces two types of injury: acute (immediate) and chronic (delayed). Acute radiation syndromes can affect many different organs.

The **cerebral (brain) syndrome** occurs when the total dose of radiation is extremely high (more than 30 grays). It's always fatal. The first symptoms, nausea and vomiting, are followed by listlessness, drowsiness, and sometimes coma. These symptoms are very likely caused by inflammation of the brain. Tremors (shaking), convulsions, inability to walk, and death occur within a few hours.

The **gastrointestinal syndrome** results from smaller but still high total doses of radiation (4 grays or more). The symptoms are severe nausea, vomiting, and diarrhea, leading to severe dehydration. Initially, the syndrome is caused by the death of cells lining the gastrointestinal tract. Symptoms are perpetuated by the progressive wasting away of the tract's lining and by bacterial infections. Ultimately, the cells that absorb nutrients are completely destroyed, and blood, often in large amounts, leaks from the diseased area into the intestines. New cells may grow, usually 4 to 6 days after exposure to radiation. But even if they do, people who have this syndrome are likely to die of bone marrow failure, which usually occurs 2 or 3 weeks later.

The **hematopoietic syndrome** affects the bone marrow, spleen, and lymph nodes—the primary sites of blood cell production (hematopoiesis). It develops after exposure to 2 to 10 grays of radiation and begins with loss of appetite (anorexia), apathy, nausea, and vomiting. These symptoms are most severe 6 to 12 hours after exposure and may subside completely by 24 to 36 hours after exposure. During this symptom-free period, the blood-producing cells in the lymph nodes, spleen, and bone marrow begin to waste away, leading to a severe shortage of red and white blood cells. A shortage of white blood cells, which fight infections, often leads to severe infections.

If the total dose of radiation is more than 6 grays, the hematopoietic and gastrointestinal malfunctions are usually fatal.

Acute radiation sickness develops after radiation treatment, especially to the abdomen, in a small proportion of patients. Symptoms include nausea, vomiting, diarrhea, loss of appetite, headache, a generally sick feeling (malaise), and an increased heartbeat. The symptoms usually subside within a few hours or days. The cause is not understood.

Prolonged or repeated exposure to low doses of radiation from radioactive implants or external sources may cause cessation of menstrual periods (amenorrhea), decreased fertility in men and women, decreased sex drive (libido) in women, cataracts, and a decreased number of red blood cells (anemia), white blood cells (leukopenia), and platelets (thrombocytopenia). Very high doses to limited areas of the body cause hair loss, skin wasting, and the formation of open sores (ulcers), calluses, and spider veins (small reddened areas of dilated blood vessels just beneath the skin's surface). Over time, such exposure may cause squamous cell skin cancer. Bone tumors may develop years after the ingestion of certain radioactive compounds, such as radium salts.

Occasionally, severe injuries to organs exposed to radiation develop long after the completion of radiation therapy for cancer. Kidney function may decline following a delay (latent period) of 6 months to a year after a person has received extremely high doses of radiation; anemia and high blood pressure may also result. Large accumulated doses to muscles may cause a painful condition that includes muscle wasting (atrophy) and calcium deposits in the irradiated muscle. Very rarely, these changes result in a malignant muscle tumor. Radiation to lung tumors can cause lung inflammation (radiation pneumonitis), and large doses may cause severe scarring (fibrosis) of lung tissue, which can be fatal. The heart and its protective sac (pericardium) can become inflamed after extensive radiation to the breastbone and chest. Large accumulated doses of radiation to the spinal cord can cause catastrophic damage, leading to paralysis. Extensive radiation to the abdomen (for lymph node, testicular, or ovarian cancer) can lead to chronic ulcers, scarring, and perforation of the intestines.

Radiation alters the genetic material in dividing cells. In cells outside the reproductive system, these alterations may cause abnormalities of cell growth, such as cancer or cataracts.

When the ovaries and testes are exposed to radiation, the chance that offspring will have genetic abnormalities (mutations) increases in laboratory animals, but this effect has not been proved in people. Some researchers believe that radiation isn't harmful below a certain dose (threshold), while others believe that any radiation of the ovaries and testes can be harmful. Because the facts aren't yet known, most authorities recommend that all medical and occupational radiation exposure be kept to a minimum. In any case, the chance of developing a radiation-related illness or genetic mutation is estimated at 1 in 100 for every 1 gray of exposure, and the average person receives only about 0.002 gray of radiation in a year.

Diagnosis and Prognosis

A radiation injury is suspected when a person becomes ill after receiving radiation therapy or being exposed to radiation in an accident. No specific tests are available to diagnose the condition, although many different tests may be used to detect swelling or organ malfunction. The prognosis depends on the dose, dose rate, and distribution over the body. Repeated sampling of blood and bone marrow can provide additional information about the severity of the injury.

When a person has the cerebral or gastrointestinal syndrome, the diagnosis is clear and the prognosis is very poor. The cerebral syndrome is fatal within hours to a few days, and the gastrointestinal syndrome generally is fatal within 3 to 10 days, although some people survive for a few weeks. The hematopoietic syndrome often causes death in 8 to 50 days; death may result from an overwhelming infection in 2 to 4 weeks or from massive bleeding (hemorrhage) in 3 to 6 weeks after exposure to radiation.

Chronic radiation injury in which the exposure is either unknown or overlooked is difficult or even impossible to diagnose. If a radiation injury is suspected, a doctor searches for possible occupational exposures, perhaps consulting the files of federally or state-licensed institutions that keep records of radiation exposures. The doctor may periodically examine the chromosomes, which contain the genetic materials in cells, for the kinds of abnormalities likely to occur after significant radiation exposure. However, the results of these examinations may be inconclusive. If exposed to radiation, the eyes are examined periodically for cataracts.

Treatment

Skin contaminated by radioactive materials should be washed immediately with large amounts of water and a solution designed for this purpose, when available. Small puncture wounds should be cleaned vigorously to remove all radioactive particles, even though such scrubbing may cause pain. If a person has recently swallowed radioactive material, vomiting should be induced. People who have been exposed to excessive radiation may be monitored with breath and urine tests for radioactivity.

Because the acute cerebral syndrome is always fatal, treatment is geared toward providing comfort: relieving pain, anxiety, and breathing difficulties. Sedatives are given to control convulsions.

The symptoms of acute radiation sickness caused by radiation therapy to the abdomen can be reduced by taking antinausea and antivomiting drugs (antiemetics) before radiation treatments.

The gastrointestinal syndrome can be relieved with antiemetics, sedatives, and a bland diet. Fluids are replaced as needed. Repeated blood transfusions and antibiotics are given to help keep people alive for the first 4 to 6 days after radiation exposure, until new cells begin to grow in the gastrointestinal tract.

For the hematopoietic syndrome, blood cells are replaced through transfusions. Efforts to prevent infection include treatment with antibiotics and isolation to keep the person away from people who may have microorganisms that cause disease. Sometimes a bone marrow transplantation is performed,▲ but the success rate is low unless an identical twin is available as a donor.

In treating the later effects of chronic exposure, the first step is to remove the source of radiation. Certain radioactive substances, such as radium, thorium, and radiostrontium, can be removed from the body with drugs that adhere to these substances and are then excreted in the urine. However, such drugs are most helpful when they're given soon after the exposure. Sores and cancers are removed or repaired surgically. The treatment of radiation-induced leukemia is the same as that for any case of leukemia—chemotherapy.■ Blood cells can be replaced through transfusions, but this measure is only temporary because bone marrow damaged by radiation is unlikely to grow again. No treatment can reverse sterility, but abnormal ovarian and testicular functioning that leads to low levels of sex hormones can be treated with replacement hormones.

▲ see page 836

■ see page 765

Heat Disorders

By sweating, breathing, shivering, and shifting the flow of blood between the skin and internal organs, the body can usually keep its temperature within a narrow range in hot or cold weather. However, overexposure to high temperatures can result in heat disorders such as heat exhaustion, heatstroke, and heat cramps.

The risk of heat disorders is increased by high humidity, which decreases the cooling effect of sweating, and by prolonged strenuous exertion, which increases the amount of heat produced by the muscles. The elderly, the very obese, and chronic alcoholics are especially susceptible to heat disorders, as are those taking certain drugs, such as antihistamines, antipsychotic drugs, alcohol, and cocaine.

Using common sense is the best way to prevent heat-related illnesses. For example, strenuous exertion in a very hot environment or a poorly ventilated space should be avoided, and appropriate clothing should be worn. Fluids and salts lost through sweating can be replaced by consuming lightly salted foods and beverages, such as salted tomato juice or cool bouillon. Many commercially available drinks, such as Gatorade, include extra salt. When exertion in a hot environment can't be avoided, drinking plenty of liquids and cooling the skin by misting it with cool water are important.

Heat Exhaustion

Heat exhaustion is a condition resulting from exposure to heat for many hours, in which excessive loss of fluids from heavy sweating leads to fatigue, low blood pressure, and sometimes collapse.

Exposure to high temperatures can cause the loss of too much fluid through sweating, particularly during hard physical labor or exercise. Salts (electrolytes) are lost with the fluids, disturbing the circulation and the brain's functioning. As a result, heat exhaustion may develop. Heat exhaustion seems serious but seldom is.

Symptoms and Diagnosis

The major symptoms are increasing fatigue, weakness, anxiety, and drenching sweats. A person may feel faint when standing still because blood collects (pools) in blood vessels of the legs, which are dilated by the heat. The heartbeat becomes slow and weak; the skin becomes cold, pale, and clammy; and the person becomes confused. The loss of fluids reduces the volume of blood, lowers blood pressure, and may cause the person to collapse or faint. Usually, heat exhaustion can be diagnosed on the basis of the symptoms.

Treatment

The main treatment is replacing fluids (rehydration) and salt. Lying flat or with the head lower than the rest of the body and sipping cool, slightly salty beverages every few minutes are generally all that's needed. Sometimes, fluids are given intravenously. Moving to a cool environment helps. After rehydration, a person often recovers rapidly and fully. If blood pressure remains low and the pulse remains slow for more than an hour despite this treatment, another condition should be suspected.

Heatstroke

Heatstroke is a life-threatening condition resulting from long, extreme exposure to heat, in which a person can't sweat enough to lower body temperature.

This condition often develops rapidly and requires immediate intensive treatment. If a person becomes dehydrated and can't sweat enough to cool the body, body temperature may rise to dangerously high levels, causing heatstroke. Certain illnesses, such as scleroderma and cystic fibrosis, decrease the ability to sweat, thus increasing the risk of heatstroke.

Symptoms and Diagnosis

Heatstroke may develop rapidly and is not always preceded by warning signs such as a headache, vertigo (a whirling sensation), or fatigue. Sweating usually but not always decreases. The skin is hot, flushed, and usually dry. The heart rate increases and may quickly reach 160 to 180 beats per minute, in contrast to the normal rate of 60 to 100 beats per minute. The breathing rate usually increases, but blood pressure rarely changes. Body temperature, which should be measured rectally, rises rapidly to 104° F. to 106° F., causing a feeling of burning up. A person may become disoriented and confused and can quickly lose consciousness or have convulsions.

Heatstroke can cause permanent damage or death if not treated immediately. A temperature of 106° F. is very serious; a temperature just one degree higher is often fatal. Permanent damage to internal organs, such as the brain, can occur quickly, often resulting in death. Very old people and those with a debilitating disease, including alcoholics, tend to have the worst outcomes. Usually, the diagnosis of heatstroke is based on symptoms.

Treatment

Heatstroke is an emergency, and lifesaving measures should be started immediately. A person who can't be taken to a hospital quickly should be wrapped in wet bedding or clothing, immersed in a lake, stream, or cool bathtub, or even cooled with ice while waiting for transportation. At the hospital, body temperature is monitored constantly to avoid overcooling. A person may need to be given drugs intravenously to control convulsions. After severe heatstroke, bed rest is advised for a few days. Body temperature may fluctuate abnormally for weeks.

Heat Cramps

Heat cramps are severe muscle spasms resulting from heavy sweating during exertion in extreme heat.

Heat cramps are caused by the excessive loss of fluids and salts (electrolytes)—including sodium, potassium, and magnesium—resulting from heavy sweating, as occurs during strenuous exertion. Heat cramps are common among manual laborers such as engine-room personnel, steel workers, and miners. Many layers of clothing, as worn by mountain climbers or skiers, may hide heavy sweating.

Heat cramps often begin suddenly in the hands, calves, or feet; they are often painful and disabling. The muscles become hard, tense, and difficult to relax.

Heat cramps can be prevented or treated by drinking beverages or eating foods that contain salt. Rarely, a person has to be given fluids and salts intravenously. Salt tablets can help prevent heat cramps but often cause stomach upset. Consuming too much salt can cause fluid retention (edema).

CHAPTER 281

Cold Injuries

The skin and the tissues under it are kept at a constant temperature by the circulating blood. The blood gets its heat from the energy given off by cells when they burn food—a process that requires a steady supply of food and oxygen.

Body temperature falls when the skin is exposed to colder surroundings, which increases heat loss; when the flow of blood is impeded; or when the supply of food and oxygen decreases. The risk of cold injuries increases when nourishment is inadequate or when insufficient oxygen is available, as occurs at high altitudes.

Cold injuries usually don't occur, even in extremely cold weather, if the skin, fingers, toes, ears, and nose are well protected and not exposed for more than a brief time. When exposure is longer, the body automatically narrows the small blood vessels in the skin, fingers, toes, ears, and nose to direct more blood to vital organs such as the heart and brain. However, this self-protective measure comes at a price: As less warm blood reaches these parts of the body, they cool more rapidly.

Preventing a cold injury is simple: Know where the dangers lie and be prepared. Many layers of clothing—preferably made of wool—or hooded jackets filled with down or a synthetic fiber plus a light windproof cover protect people under the harshest conditions. Because a great deal of heat is lost from the head, a warm hat is essential. Eating enough food and drinking enough fluids also help.

Cold injuries include hypothermia, in which the whole body cools to a potentially dangerous temperature; frostnip, in which parts of the body are superficially damaged; and frostbite, in which some body tissues are actually destroyed. Chilblains and immersion foot are also caused by overexposure to cold.

Hypothermia

Hypothermia is an abnormally low body temperature.

The very old and the very young are the most vulnerable. Particularly at risk are elderly people who live alone and sit for hours or days in a cold room, slowly becoming confused and helpless. Half of the elderly people who develop hypothermia die before or soon after being found. However, even strong, young, healthy people are not immune to hypothermia.

Causes

Hypothermia occurs when the body loses heat faster than it can burn fuel to replace it. Cold air, often as wind, can carry heat away from the body by convection. Sitting still for a time on the cold ground or a metal surface or in wet clothing drains heat from the warm body to the colder surface by conduction. Heat can be lost from exposed skin, especially on the head, through radiation and the evaporation of sweat.

Hypothermia frequently occurs when a person is immersed in cold water—the colder the water, the faster hypothermia develops. The onset of hypothermia is easy to ignore during a long period of immersion in water that doesn't seem very cold yet takes away body heat. The dangers of immersion for even a few minutes in icy water or for much longer in temperate water must be recognized, especially since the victim often becomes disoriented.

Symptoms

The onset of hypothermia is usually so gradual and subtle that neither the victim nor others realize what's happening. Movement becomes slow and clumsy, reaction time is longer, the mind is blurred, judgment is impaired, and hallucinations occur. A person who has hypothermia may fall, wander off, or simply lie down to rest and perhaps die. If the person is in water, he will flounder, soon surrender, and drown.

Treatment

In the early stages, changing into warm dry clothing, drinking hot beverages, or snuggling in a sleeping bag with a companion can bring about recovery. If the victim is found unconscious, further heat loss must be prevented by wrapping the victim in a warm dry blanket and, if possible, moving the victim to a warm place while arrangements are made for immediate transportation to a hospital. Often, no pulse can be felt and no heartbeat can be heard. The victim must be handled gently because a sudden jolt may cause an irregular heart rhythm (arrhythmia) that could be fatal. For this reason, cardiopulmonary resuscitation isn't recommended outside of a hospital, unless the victim has been immersed in cold water and is unconscious. Because the risk of an unconscious victim dying is high, such people must be treated and monitored at a hospital to have a chance of survival. People who have hypothermia should not be considered dead until they have been warmed and still have no signs of life.

Frostnip

Frostnip is a cold injury in which parts of the skin are chilled but not permanently damaged.

In frostnip, the chilled areas of skin become white and firm, then swollen and painful. Later, the skin may peel, as it does when sunburned, and the ears or cheeks occasionally are sensitive to cold for months or even years, although they have no obvious damage.

The only treatment needed is warming the area for a few minutes, unless the area is severely chilled. In such cases, treatment is the same as for frostbite.

Frostbite

Frostbite is a cold injury in which one or more parts of the body are permanently damaged.

Frostbite is more likely to occur in people who have poor circulation because of arteriosclerosis (thickening and hardening of the artery walls), spasm—which may be caused by smoking, some neurologic disorders, and certain drugs—or constriction of blood flow by gloves or boots that are too tight. Exposed hands and feet are most vulnerable. The damage from frostbite is caused by a combination of decreased blood flow and the formation of ice crystals in the tissues.

In frostbite, the skin becomes red, swollen, and painful, then black. Cells in the chilled areas die. Depending on the extent of the frostbite, the affected tissue may eventually recover or gangrene may develop.

Treatment
A person who has frostbite should be covered with a warm blanket. The frostbitten hand or foot should be warmed slowly in water that's no hotter than can be comfortably tolerated by the caregiver (100° to 104° F.). The victim should not be warmed in front of a fire nor rubbed with snow. Once the victim is safely sheltered, hot beverages are helpful. The frostbitten area should be gently washed, dried, wrapped in sterile bandages, and kept meticulously clean to prevent infection. As soon as frostbite is diagnosed, an antibiotic should be given. Some authorities recommend an antitetanus injection also. Reserpine given by mouth or injection may be used to dilate blood vessels and improve blood flow to the frostbitten part.

Most people slowly improve over several months, although sometimes surgery is needed later to remove the dead tissues. Because a frostbitten area may appear larger and more severe than it will be weeks or months later, the decision to amputate is usually postponed until the area has had time to heal.

Often, a person who has frostbitten feet must walk to safety. In most cases, if the feet can be protected from further freezing, walking on frozen feet is better than walking on feet that have been thawed. Thawed feet are more vulnerable to damage from walking, especially on rough ground.

Chilblains

Chilblains (sometimes called pernio) are painful chilling or burning sensations in parts of the body that were previously frostbitten.

They are caused by exposure to cold, even slight cold. Chilblains are difficult to treat and persist for years.

Immersion Foot

Immersion foot is a cold injury that develops when a foot is kept in moist, cold socks and boots for several days.

The foot is pale, clammy, and cold, and the circulation becomes weak. Infection can develop if immersion foot isn't treated. The treatment consists primarily of gently warming, drying, and cleaning the foot, elevating it, and keeping it dry and warm. Antibiotics should be given, and possibly a tetanus booster. Rarely, this type of injury occurs in the hands.

CHAPTER 282

Mountain Sickness

Mountain sickness (high-altitude illness) is a disorder caused by lack of oxygen at high altitudes; the disorder takes several forms, first one form dominating and then another.

As altitude increases, the atmospheric pressure decreases and fewer oxygen molecules are available in the thinner air. This decrease in available oxygen affects the body in many ways: The rate and depth of breathing increase, disturbing the balance between gases in the lungs and blood, increasing the alkalinity of the blood, and changing the distribution of salts such as potassium and sodium in the cells. As a result, water is distributed differently between the blood and tissues.

These changes are the principal cause of mountain sickness. At high altitudes, the blood contains less oxygen, resulting in a bluish tinge to the skin, lips, and nails (cyanosis). Over a period of a few weeks, the body responds by producing more red blood cells to carry more oxygen to the tissues.

The effects of high altitude depend on how high and how fast a person ascends. Noticeable effects are few below 7,000 feet but are common above 9,000 feet after a rapid ascent. Most people adjust (acclimatize) to altitudes of up to 10,000 feet in a few days, but adjusting to much higher altitudes takes many days or weeks.

Symptoms

Acute mountain sickness develops in many people who live at sea level when they ascend to a moderate altitude (8,000 feet) in 1 or 2 days. They are short of breath, have a rapid heartbeat, and fatigue easily. About 20 percent also have a headache, nausea or vomiting, and sleep disturbances. Strenuous exertion worsens the symptoms. Most people improve in a few days. This benign condition, which is seldom more than unpleasant, is more common in younger people and is less common with increasing age.

High-altitude pulmonary edema, a more serious condition in which fluid accumulates in the lungs, may follow acute mountain sickness. The risk of developing high-altitude pulmonary edema is somewhat increased in residents of high altitudes, especially children, when they return to a high altitude after spending 7 to 10 days near sea level. People who have had a previous episode are more likely to have another, and even a mild respiratory infection, such as a head or chest cold, seems to increase the risk. High-altitude pulmonary edema is much more common in men than in women. It usually develops 24 to 96 hours after ascent and is uncommon below 9,000 feet.

Shortness of breath is more severe in high-altitude pulmonary edema than in acute mountain sickness; even slight effort causes severe breathlessness. A cough is common, dry and tickling at first but often becoming loose and bubbling. A large amount of phlegm, often pink or even bloody, may be coughed up. The person may have a slight fever. High-altitude pulmonary edema may worsen rapidly and within a few hours progress from a moderate illness to a life-threatening one.

High-altitude cerebral edema, the most serious form of mountain sickness, may develop on its own within 24 to 96 hours after arrival at a high altitude, or it may be preceded by acute mountain sickness or high-altitude pulmonary edema. In high-altitude cerebral edema, fluid accumulates within the brain. Difficulty in walking (ataxia), possibly accompanied by clumsy finger or hand movements, is an early warning sign. Headaches are more severe than in acute mountain sickness. Hallucinations appear somewhat later but often are not recognized as such. The higher the altitude, the greater the impairment of judgment and perception. Symptoms may resemble the effects of drinking alcohol. High-altitude cerebral edema can progress from mild to life-threatening within a few hours. A person thought to have high-altitude cerebral edema should immediately descend to a lower altitude.

Altitude edema (swelling of the hands and feet and, on awakening, the face) often develops in hikers, climbers, and skiers. In part, it's caused by the changing distribution of salts that occurs in the body at high altitudes, but strenuous exertion causes changes in salt and water distribution even at sea level.

High-altitude retinal hemorrhage (small spots of bleeding in the retina at the back of the eye) may develop after ascent to even a moderate altitude. This condition rarely produces symptoms and disappears spontaneously, except in the unusual case when the hemorrhage occurs in the part of the eye that's responsible for central vision (the macula). Then, a small blind spot is noticeable. Rarely, blurred vision in one or both eyes or even blindness develops; such episodes are apparently a form of migraine and disappear promptly after descent.

Subacute mountain sickness is an unusual condition that's been reported in infants of Chinese parents born at or brought to a moderate altitude and in soldiers stationed for many weeks or months at altitudes above 20,000 feet. This condition is caused by heart failure, resulting in a large accumulation of fluid in the lungs, abdomen, and legs. Descent to a lower altitude cures the condition and is necessary to save a life.

Chronic mountain sickness (Monge's disease) develops gradually in some residents of high altitudes after many months or years. Symptoms include shortness of breath, lethargy, and many aches and pains. Blood clots may form in the legs and lungs, and the heart fails. Chronic mountain sickness develops when the body overcompensates for the lack of oxygen by forming too many red blood cells. The person becomes disabled and will die if not taken to a lower altitude.

Prevention

The best way to prevent mountain sickness is to ascend slowly, taking 2 days to reach 8,000 feet and another day for each 1,000 to 2,000 additional feet. Climbing at an individualized pace is more helpful than following a rigid schedule. An overnight stay halfway up also decreases the risk. Physical fitness may help but does not ensure wellness at a high altitude. Avoiding strenuous exertion for a day or two after arrival is advisable. Drinking extra fluids and avoiding salt or salty foods may help, although these measures haven't been proved. Caution should be exercised when drinking alcohol at high altitudes. One alcoholic drink consumed at a high altitude seems to have the effect of two at sea level, and the effects of too much alcohol are similar to some forms of mountain sickness.

Acetazolamide or dexamethasone taken in small doses at the start of the ascent and for a few days after arrival minimizes acute mountain sickness. Doctors may prescribe nifedipine for people who have had several episodes of high-altitude pulmonary edema. Ibuprofen is more effective than other drugs in relieving headaches caused by high altitudes. Eating frequent small high-carbohydrate meals rather than fewer large meals is somewhat beneficial.

Treatment

Mild acute mountain sickness usually goes away in a day or two, with no treatment other than drinking additional fluids to replace those lost through sweating and rapidly breathing the dry air. Taking ibuprofen and drinking extra fluids help relieve headaches. If the condition is more severe, acetazolamide, dexamethasone, or both usually help.

Because high-altitude pulmonary edema is sometimes life-threatening, the person should be watched closely. Often, bed rest and oxygen are effective, but if not, the person should be taken to a lower altitude without delay. Nifedipine is effective immediately, but its effects last only a few hours and it's not a substitute for taking a severely affected person to a lower altitude.

High-altitude cerebral edema, which may also be life-threatening, is treated with a corticosteroid such as dexamethasone, but in severe cases, only while preparing to take the person to a lower altitude. If high-altitude pulmonary edema or high-altitude cerebral edema is worsening, delaying the descent may be fatal.

After descent, people who have any form of mountain sickness improve rapidly. If they don't, another cause for the condition should be sought.

If a prompt descent is not possible, a device that increases pressure, simulating a descent of several thousand feet, can be used to treat a person who is severely ill. The device (a hyperbaric bag) consists of a lightweight fabric bag or tent and a manually operated pump. The person is placed in the bag. After the bag is tightly sealed, the pressure in it is increased with the pump. The person remains in the bag for 2 or 3 hours. This procedure is a valuable temporary measure—as beneficial as supplemental oxygen, which often isn't available when mountain climbing.

CHAPTER 283

Near Drowning

Near drowning is severe oxygen deprivation (suffocation) caused by being under water for a long time but not resulting in death.

Remaining under water for a long time leads to a severe deficiency of oxygen in the blood. The larynx, the first part of the airways, goes into severe spasm, blocking the flow of air. Eventually, water gets past the larynx and fills the lungs. When filled with water, the lungs can't transfer oxygen to the blood. Areas of the lungs collapse, further impairing the lungs' ability to oxygenate the blood.

The **diving reflex**, first identified in seagoing mammals, enables people to survive after long periods of submersion in cold water. The impact of cold water on the lungs stimulates this reflex, which slows the heartbeat and redirects the flow of blood from the hands, feet, and intestines to the heart and brain, helping preserve these vital organs. Furthermore, cold water cools body tissues. Because cool tissues require less oxygen than warm ones, underwater survival time can be extended.

Near drowning can severely injure the lungs, so impaired breathing—which reduces the amount of oxygen delivered to vital organs—is the greatest problem in the hours and days after the episode. Near drowning may also change the volume and content of the blood. Salt water in the lungs draws fluid from the bloodstream into the lungs; freshwater damages the lungs, allowing fluid to pass into the lungs from the bloodstream. Inhaling freshwater can also increase the volume of blood and cause chemical imbalances and destruction of red blood cells.

Treatment

The key factors that influence the chances of survival without permanent brain, heart, and lung damage are the duration of submersion, the water temperature, the victim's age (the diving reflex is more active in children), and the speed of resuscitation. Survival depends on promptly restoring breathing and lung function so that oxygen can reach the vital organs.

If the victim isn't breathing, mouth-to-mouth resuscitation should be started immediately—in the water, if necessary. If a heartbeat can't be detected, cardiopulmonary resuscitation (CPR) should be started.

Because the diving reflex may have reduced the need for oxygen during submersion, vigorous attempts should be made to revive the victim, even when the time under water exceeds an hour. The victim is placed with the head lower than the feet so that water can drain out. Any foreign matter, such as sand or leaves, that is blocking the upper airways and can be extracted from the victim's

mouth should be removed. If the water is cold, the victim may have a low body temperature (hypothermia), requiring treatment.▲

All near-drowning victims must be hospitalized. Resuscitation efforts should continue during transportation to the hospital. Hospitalization is required even if the person regains consciousness because the effects of oxygen deprivation may not appear immediately. The person should be monitored closely so that if a problem develops, treatment is not delayed.

In the hospital, treatment initially focuses on intensive care of the lungs to ensure that enough oxygen gets into the blood. Some people need only a face mask to deliver extra oxygen; others need a mechanical ventilator. A respirator is frequently used to reinflate collapsed sections of the lungs. Drugs are given to prevent airway spasms. Treatment may include solutions given intravenously to help restore the chemical balance of the blood, corticosteroids to reduce lung inflammation, and antibiotics to treat an infection. Blood transfusions may be needed to replace the destroyed red blood cells. In some cases, treatment with oxygen in a high-pressure (hyperbaric) chamber may be needed. Although various maneuvers may be performed to minimize brain damage, some people still sustain permanent brain damage.

CHAPTER 284

Diving Injuries

Deep-sea diving or diving with a self-contained underwater breathing apparatus (scuba) can cause medical problems such as air embolism and decompression sickness that can be fatal if not treated promptly. These problems are caused by the high pressure under water and can also affect people who work in tunnels or caissons (watertight enclosures for construction work under water) in which compressed air is used.

High pressure under water is caused by the weight of the water above, just as barometric (atmospheric) pressure on land is caused by the weight of the air above. In diving, underwater pressure is often expressed in units of depth (feet or meters) or atmospheres absolute. Pressure in atmospheres absolute includes the weight of the water, which at 33 feet is 1 atmosphere, plus the atmospheric pressure at the surface, which is 1 atmosphere. So a diver at a depth of 33 feet in seawater is exposed to a total pressure of 2 atmospheres absolute, or twice the atmospheric pressure at the surface. With each additional 33 feet of depth, the pressure increases by 1 atmosphere.

▲ see page 1346

Effects of High Pressure

When pressure outside the body increases, pressure in the blood and body tissues increases correspondingly, but not necessarily in spaces that contain air, such as the lungs and airways. Pressure in the lungs and airways is automatically equalized with outside pressure when a supply of air is available at depth, as from a diving helmet or scuba.

Air spaces inside a face mask or goggles worn for diving are also subject to pressure changes. Pressure in a face mask is equalized by air from the nose. But the pressure inside goggles can't be equalized; the lower inside pressure causes them to act like suction cups applied to the eyes. The difference in pressure causes blood vessels near the surface of the eyes to dilate, leak fluid, and finally burst and bleed. Divers use the term squeeze for the effects of such differences in pressure.

Pressure differences also occur in the middle ear. If the tube connecting the middle ear and the back of the throat (eustachian tube) doesn't open normally—that is, the ears don't pop when yawning or swallowing—pressure in the middle ear remains lower than pressure in the outer ear.▲ The increased pressure on the eardrum, which separates the middle and outer ear, causes it to bulge inward and, if the pressure becomes high enough, to rupture, resulting in pain and impaired hearing. A ruptured eardrum usually heals but often not before a middle ear infection has developed.

If the eardrum ruptures when a diver is bareheaded in cold water, the rush of cold water into the middle ear produces vertigo (severe dizziness with a spinning sensation),■ disorientation, and nausea. Vomiting could follow, causing the diver to drown. The vertigo diminishes as the water in the ear reaches body temperature.

Pressure differences in the middle ear can affect the inner ear, which is responsible for hearing and balance. This unequalized pressure may explain why divers sometimes experience vertigo (alternobaric vertigo) when they begin their ascent. Rarely, a rupture occurs between the inner and middle ear, allowing fluid to escape. A rupture may require prompt surgical repair to prevent permanent effects.

Wearing earplugs creates a closed space between the earplug and the eardrum in which pressure can't be equalized. Therefore, earplugs must not be used during diving.

Pressure differences have similar effects on the sinuses (air-filled pockets in the bones around the nose), causing facial pain or headaches. When congestion prevents pressure in the ears and sinuses from being equalized, decongestants may temporarily unclog blocked nasal passages, eustachian tubes, or sinuses. However, repeated diving without being able to readily equalize pressure usually causes some injury.

Air Compression and Expansion

Changes in the volume of air inside the body can also lead to medical problems. As pressure increases, air is compressed into less space—its volume decreases. Conversely, as pressure decreases, air expands—its volume increases. For example, when pressure doubles (as when diving from the surface to 33 feet), the volume of air is halved, and when pressure is halved (as when ascending from 33 feet), the volume of air doubles. So if a diver fills his lungs with air at 33 feet and ascends without freely exhaling, the volume of air doubles, causing the lungs to overinflate, sometimes causing death. That's why divers using an air supply such as a scuba tank must not hold their breath during the ascent. Any air inhaled at depth—even the depth of a swimming pool—must be exhaled freely during the ascent.★

Because air is compressed at higher pressures, each breath taken at depth contains many more molecules than a breath taken at the surface. At 66 feet (3 atmospheres absolute), for example, each breath contains three times as many molecules as a breath taken at the surface and therefore depletes an air tank three times as rapidly. Consequently, the deeper a diver descends, the more rapidly the air supply is depleted.

Because the compressed air at depth is denser (it contains more molecules) than air at the surface, greater effort is needed to move it through a diver's airways and breathing apparatus. Therefore, breathing is harder at depth. Some people are unable to exhale carbon dioxide sufficiently, causing carbon dioxide levels in the blood to increase—which can result in blackouts.

▲ see page 1005

■ see pages 298 and 1010

★ see page 1353

Partial Pressure Effects

Air is a mixture of gases, mainly nitrogen and oxygen with very small amounts of other gases. Each gas has a partial pressure, based on its concentration in the air and on the atmospheric pressure. For instance, the concentration of oxygen in the air is about 21 percent; therefore, oxygen's partial pressure is 0.21 atmosphere at the surface. As depth increases, the concentration of oxygen remains the same, but its partial pressure increases because the atmospheric pressure increases. The partial pressure of oxygen at 2 atmospheres absolute is twice that at the surface.

The effects of most gases on the body depend on their partial pressure. For example, high partial pressures of oxygen can have harmful effects (oxygen toxicity). Breathing oxygen at a partial pressure of more than 0.5 atmosphere (as when breathing air that's more than 50 percent oxygen at 1 atmosphere absolute) for a day or more can damage the lungs. Breathing oxygen at higher partial pressures is toxic to the brain. If the partial pressure of oxygen approaches 2 atmospheres, especially during exertion, a diver may have a convulsion resembling an epileptic seizure.

Breathing nitrogen at a high partial pressure produces nitrogen narcosis—a condition that resembles alcohol intoxication. This effect becomes noticeable at 100 feet or less in most divers breathing compressed air and can be incapacitating at 300 feet (about 10 atmospheres absolute). Because helium doesn't have this effect, it's used (rather than nitrogen) to dilute oxygen in air supplies for very deep dives, in which the percentage of oxygen must be reduced to keep its partial pressure below toxic levels.

Divers who hold their breath rather than use a breathing apparatus often breathe vigorously (hyperventilate) before a dive, breathing out a large amount of carbon dioxide but adding little oxygen to the blood. This maneuver allows them to hold their breath and swim under water longer because their carbon dioxide levels are low. However, this maneuver is also hazardous because a diver can run out of oxygen and lose consciousness before the carbon dioxide reaches a level high enough to signal the need to return to the surface and breathe.

The risks of prolonged breath-holding are greater for deeper dives, because the oxygen in the lungs is used up more completely. As a diver comes up from a deep dive, the partial pressure of the oxygen remaining in the blood decreases drastically, so the diver may lose consciousness before inhaling enough oxygen. This sequence of events is probably responsible for many unexplained drownings among spearfishing competitors and others who hold their breath while diving.

Rebreathing types of scuba gear conserve the gas supply, allowing a diver to remain under water longer. One example is a closed-circuit oxygen rebreather, which supplies fresh oxygen to the diver; the rest of the gas is rebreathed. The amount of fresh oxygen needed is only about one twentieth of the total amount of air breathed and doesn't increase with greater depth, so a smaller gas supply is sufficient for most dives. A major disadvantage of rebreathing devices is that a diver's carbon dioxide output, nearly equal to oxygen consumption, must be absorbed by chemical means. If absorption doesn't occur or is inadequate, the carbon dioxide level of the rebreathed gas increases. A diver who doesn't sense this development—for example, by noticing an increase in breathing or shortness of breath—may lose consciousness.

Abnormally high levels of carbon dioxide (carbon dioxide poisoning) can cause blackouts or impaired consciousness. Some people have carbon dioxide buildup because they don't increase their breathing adequately during exertion. High carbon dioxide levels increase the likelihood of convulsions from oxygen toxicity and worsen the severity of nitrogen narcosis. Divers who frequently have headaches after diving or who pride themselves on using air at a low rate may be retaining carbon dioxide.

Diving may be complicated by poor visibility, water currents that demand strenuous physical exertion, and cold. Hypothermia▲ (lowered body temperature) can develop rapidly in water, producing clumsiness and poor judgment. Cold water can trigger fatal heartbeat irregularities in susceptible people. Carbon monoxide poisoning from contaminated air can cause incapacitation or even death in divers. Symptoms of carbon monoxide poisoning may include nausea, a headache, weakness, clumsiness, and mental changes. Prescribed medications as well as alcohol and other abused drugs also may have unanticipated effects at depth.

Air Embolism

Air embolism (gas embolism) is the blockage of blood vessels by bubbles in the bloodstream, usually from the expansion of air held in the lungs as pressure decreases during an ascent from a dive.

In air embolism, the expanding air held in the lungs overinflates the lungs, causing air to leak into the bloodstream in the form of bubbles. If the bubbles block blood vessels in the brain, they can cause damage similar to that resulting from a severe stroke. Air embolism is an extreme emergency and a leading cause of death among divers.

The most common cause of air embolism is breath-holding during an ascent from a scuba dive, typically resulting from running out of air at depth. In panic, a diver may forget to exhale freely as air in the lungs expands during the ascent. Air embolism can occur even in a swimming pool if a person has any external source of air, takes a breath under water, and doesn't exhale while coming up.

Symptoms

Sudden loss of consciousness, with or without convulsions, is the most typical symptom. Sometimes less severe symptoms develop, ranging from confusion or agitation to partial paralysis.

Overinflation of the lungs also can force air out of the lungs into the tissues surrounding the heart (mediastinal emphysema) and even under the skin (subcutaneous emphysema). Sometimes the overinflated lungs burst, releasing air into the space between the lungs and the chest wall (pneumothorax). The lungs then collapse, leading to marked shortness of breath and chest pain. Coughing up blood or developing bloody froth at the mouth indicates a lung injury.

Emergency Treatment

A diver who loses consciousness during an ascent or very shortly afterward probably has air embolism and must be treated promptly. A person who has air embolism must be returned at once to a high-pressure environment, so that the air bubbles are compressed and forced to dissolve in the blood. A number of medical centers have high-pressure (recompression or hyperbaric) chambers for this purpose. The person must be transported to the chamber as quickly as possible while being given oxygen through a close-fitting face mask. Flying, even at a low altitude, reduces atmospheric pressure and allows bubbles to expand, but it can be justified if it saves a substantial amount of time in getting the person to a suitable chamber.

Decompression Sickness

Decompression sickness (decompression illness, caisson disease, the bends) is a condition in which gases dissolved in the blood and tissues form bubbles that block the flow of blood or otherwise produce pain and other symptoms.

Bubbles can form when a person moves from a high-pressure environment to a low-pressure environment, which occurs when ascending from a dive.

Causes and Prevention

A diver or person working in a compressed-air environment who breathes air under high pressure takes in increased amounts of oxygen, nitrogen, and other gases from the air. Because oxygen is used continuously by the body, it usually doesn't accumulate. However, nitrogen and other gases dissolve in the blood and tissues and do accumulate. The only way they can leave the body is through the bloodstream and out the lungs—the reverse of the way they came in—and this process takes time. As the external pressure decreases, which happens during an ascent from a dive, the pressure may not be sufficient to keep the gases dissolved, so bubbles may form in the blood and tissues.

A diver can usually prevent the formation of dangerous bubbles by restricting the total amount of gas the body absorbs. The amount can

---

▲ see page 1346

be restricted by limiting the depth and duration of dives to a range that doesn't require decompression stops during ascent (called no-stop limits by divers) or by ascending with decompression stops as specified in authoritative guidelines such as a decompression table in the *United States Navy Diving Manual.* The table provides a pattern for ascent that usually allows excess nitrogen to escape without causing harm.

Decompression sickness rarely occurs when divers observe no-stop limits or follow a decompression table precisely. However, a diver's perception of the depth, duration, and decompression time of a dive isn't necessarily accurate. Many divers, believing incorrectly that a large margin of safety is built into the Navy diving tables, don't follow them precisely. Newer guidelines for rate of ascent, no-stop limits, tables, and decompression computers carried by divers are claimed to have a greater margin of safety, but they can also be misused. Because most decompression tables and computers haven't been tested adequately in women or older divers, these people should use them with caution. Besides following a table or computer guidelines for ascent, many divers make a safety stop of a few minutes at about 15 feet below the surface.

Repeated dives may cause decompression sickness. Because excess gas remains in the body after each dive, the amount of excess gas increases with each dive. If the interval between dives is less than 12 hours, divers should follow guidelines such as the tables for repeated dives in the *United States Navy Diving Manual* to account for the extra gas.

Diving at high altitudes and flying after diving require special precautions. For example, after several days of diving, a period of 24 hours at the surface is commonly recommended before flying or going to a higher altitude.

Symptoms

Pain, often called the bends, is the most common symptom. Usually, it occurs in or near an arm or leg joint, but it's often hard to pinpoint. The pain may also be hard to describe—"deep" and "like something boring into bone" are descriptions sometimes used. In other cases, the

pain is sharp and the location is clear. At first, the pain may be mild or intermittent, but it may steadily grow stronger and can become severe. Usually, the painful area isn't tender, inflamed, or affected by movement.

Neurologic symptoms range from mild numbness to abnormal brain function. The spinal cord is especially vulnerable, and seemingly minor symptoms such as weakness or tingling in an arm or leg may precede irreversible paralysis unless the condition is treated promptly with oxygen and recompression. The inner ear may be affected, causing severe vertigo.▲

Less common symptoms include itching, skin rash, and extreme fatigue. Mottling (marbling) of the skin, a very uncommon symptom, may precede or accompany serious conditions that require recompression. Abdominal pain may be caused by abdominal bubble formation, but pain that encircles the body near the belt line (girdle pain) may indicate spinal cord damage.

Late effects of decompression sickness include the destruction of bone tissue (dysbaric osteonecrosis, aseptic bone necrosis), especially in the shoulder and hip, producing persistent pain and severe disability. These injuries are much more common among people who work in a compressed-air environment than among divers, probably because the exposures to high pressure are prolonged and the bends isn't always treated. Just one improper decompression can cause such injuries, which gradually worsen over months or years. By the time symptoms appear, it is too late for preventive measures.

Permanent neurologic problems, such as partial paralysis, usually result from delayed or inadequate treatment of spinal cord damage. However, sometimes the damage is too severe to correct, even with appropriate treatment. Repeated treatments with oxygen in a high-pressure chamber seem to help some people recover from spinal cord damage. A spinal cord injury caused by decompression is much more likely to heal than such injury from other causes.

Respiratory decompression sickness (the chokes) is a rare but dangerous condition, caused by widespread blockage by bubbles of blood vessels in the lungs. In some people, this condition resolves without treatment, but it can progress rapidly to circulatory collapse and death unless recompression is performed promptly. Early symptoms consist of chest discomfort and coughing after breathing deeply or inhaling tobacco smoke.

▲ see page 1010

Fitness for Diving

A number of physical and mental conditions can increase the risk of mishaps and injury during diving. Therefore, prospective divers should be evaluated for fitness by a doctor who is familiar with diving. Professional divers may undergo additional medical tests, such as those for heart and lung function, exercise stress, hearing, and vision, as well as bone x-rays. In addition, adequate diver training is absolutely necessary.

Cardiovascular fitness
Needed for heavy exertion—for example, carrying air tanks and strenuous swimming

Irregular heart rhythms
Type and cause should be determined; possible risk of sudden death

Open foramen ovale (a heart defect)
Increased risk of air bubbles reaching the brain (air embolism)

Lung problems such as asthma, lung cysts, emphysema, a history of pneumothorax
Risk of air getting trapped in body spaces and air embolism

Chronic congestion of nose and sinuses, ruptured eardrum
Difficulty in equalizing pressure, increased risk of infection

Nasal congestion from colds or allergy
Diving should be avoided until person is recovered

Epilepsy, fainting spells, insulin-dependent diabetes
Increased risk of loss of consciousness or impaired alertness

Physical handicaps
Should be considered in terms of ability to care for self and to help other divers

Impulsive behavior; prone to accidents
Increased risk of injury to diver and companions

Obesity
Associated with poor fitness and increased risk of decompression sickness

Older age
Should be tested for health risks, especially heart and lung problems; may be more susceptible to decompression sickness

Pregnancy
Risk of causing birth defects or miscarriage

Sex
Women may be more susceptible to decompression sickness

Drugs that can cause drowsiness
Impaired alertness; worsening of nitrogen narcosis

Alcohol or drug abuse
Impaired judgment and skill

Treatment

Decompression sickness requires recompression in a high-pressure chamber, in which the pressure is gradually increased so that bubbles are compressed and forced to dissolve. Consequently, normal blood flow and oxygen supply to affected tissues are restored. After recompression, pressure is reduced gradually, with designated stops, allowing time for excess gases to leave the body harmlessly.

Transport to a suitable chamber takes precedence over any procedure that can be conducted during transport or postponed without serious risk to life. Transport should not be delayed even if symptoms appear mild, because more serious problems may develop. Regardless of distance or time, recompression is likely to be beneficial. Unnecessary recompression involves far less risk than any measure that may be tried in the hope that the problem will subside without recompression. During transport, oxygen should be administered with a close-fitting mask, fluid intake should be ensured, and input and output need to be recorded along with the vital signs. Shock may develop, especially in severe cases with delayed treatment.

Wherever they dive, divers themselves and rescue and police units in popular diving areas should know the location of the nearest recompression chamber, the means of reaching it most rapidly, and the most appropriate source of consultation by telephone. In the absence of such local forethought, the Divers Alert Network number (919-684-8111) can be lifesaving.

Failure to provide prompt and appropriate treatment of air embolism or decompression sickness entails totally unacceptable risk of serious and lasting injury.

Divers reporting only itching, skin rash, and extreme fatigue usually don't need to undergo recompression, but they should be kept under observation because more serious problems may follow. Breathing 100 percent oxygen from a close-fitting face mask may provide relief.

When the chokes occurs at a high altitude, returning to a lower altitude doesn't always cure the condition. Prompt recompression in a high-pressure chamber may be needed.

CHAPTER 285

Air Travel and Medical Problems

Traveling by air can cause or worsen a variety of medical conditions, although very few conditions would prevent a person from flying. Those that may prevent flying include a pneumothorax, lung damage from tuberculosis, diseases that could be spread to other passengers, and conditions in which even a small expansion of air would damage tissues, such as intestinal surgery in the previous 10 days. Some conditions require planning and taking precautions before a flight. For example, people who have had a colostomy should wear a large bag and anticipate frequent filling.

Air travel poses problems related to changes in air pressure, reduced amounts of oxygen, turbulence, disruptions of the body's internal 24-hour (circadian) clock (jet lag), and psychologic or physical stress.

Changes in Air Pressure

Modern jet airplanes maintain air pressure inside the cabin (cabin pressure) at low levels, equivalent to the atmospheric pressure at 5,000 to 8,000 feet. At such levels, air trapped in pockets within the body—such as in the lungs, inner ear, sinuses, and intestinal tract—expands by about 25 percent. This expansion sometimes aggravates certain medical conditions, such as emphysema, blocked eustachian tubes, chronic sinusitis, and chronic gas pains. Problems may be particularly severe when an airplane accidentally loses cabin pressure or when the cabin isn't pressurized, as is the case with some smaller airplanes.

A sensation of pressure in the ears is common during airplane flights. It develops as the difference between pressure outside the ear and inside the ear increases, causing the eardrum to bulge. Eventually, the pressure equalizes when the eustachian tube (a passage that connects the middle ear with the back of the nose) allows air to flow in and out of the middle ear. Head colds or allergies may produce fluid and swelling that block the eustachian tube, and repeated infections may result in scarring that partially blocks it. Then air becomes trapped in the middle ear, producing pressure (barotitis media) and pain.▲ Rarely, the eardrum ruptures. Similarly, air may be trapped in the sinuses (barosinusitis), causing facial pain.

Swallowing frequently or yawning during the airplane's descent and taking decongestants before or during the flight can prevent or relieve these conditions. Because children are particularly susceptible to barotitis media, they should chew gum, suck hard candy, or drink something during ascent and descent to encourage swallowing; babies can be nursed or given a bottle or pacifier.

▲ see page 1005

Reduced Oxygen

The relatively low air pressure inside an airplane also causes problems because of its effect on oxygen levels. Low oxygen levels are particularly troublesome for people who have a severe lung disease such as emphysema or cystic fibrosis, heart failure, severe anemia, severe angina, sickle cell disease, or certain congenital heart diseases. Usually, such people can fly safely if provided with oxygen. Airlines can handle a request for oxygen if notified 72 hours in advance of a flight. People generally may fly 10 to 14 days after a heart attack. During flight, people who have breathing problems should not smoke or drink alcohol—which aggravates the effects of reduced oxygen. In general, anyone who can walk 100 yards or climb one flight of stairs should be able to tolerate normal cabin conditions without additional oxygen.

Turbulence

Turbulence can cause air sickness or an injury. People who are prone to air sickness may benefit from dimenhydrinate taken as a tablet or scopolamine applied to the skin as a patch. However, these drugs may cause adverse effects, particularly in the elderly. The patches cause fewer adverse effects. To prevent injuries, passengers should keep their seat belts fastened while seated.

Jet Lag

Rapid travel across several time zones produces many physical and psychologic stresses known as jet lag (circadian dysrhythmia). A gradual shift in eating and sleeping patterns before departure may alleviate the problem. Some medication schedules may have to be adjusted, for example, the intervals between drugs normally taken at precise times throughout the day should be based on elapsed time—such as every 8 hours—rather than on local time. People who have diabetes and who use long-acting insulin may switch to regular insulin until they've adjusted to the new time zone, food, and activity level, or they may make up the difference in time zone changes over several days. They should work out a medication and eating schedule with their doctor before departure and take with them a device to monitor blood sugar (glucose) levels.

Melatonin, a hormone that regulates the sleep-wake cycle, is reported to help with sleep disturbances caused by jet lag. Its effectiveness depends on taking the doses on a precise schedule.

Because melatonin products are nutritional supplements rather than prescription drugs, the claims made by the manufacturers have not undergone rigorous scrutiny, and the quality of each formulation may vary.

Psychologic Stress

Fear of flying and claustrophobia can cause distress. Hypnosis and behavior modification help some people. Taking a sedative may relieve fears before and during a flight.

Because the behavior of some mentally ill people worsens during airplane flights, those with violent or unpredictable tendencies must be accompanied by an attendant, and they may need to take a sedative before the flight.

General Precautions

Cardiac pacemakers and metal artificial limbs, plates, or pins are affected by airport metal detectors used to scan for concealed weapons; however, newer models of pacemakers can withstand potential interference from such detectors. To avoid security problems, people who wear such devices should carry a doctor's note explaining the situation.

The risk of developing blood clots in the legs is increased in anyone who sits in one place for a long time.▲ Pregnant women and people who have poor circulation are at particular risk. Walking around the airplane cabin every hour or two and contracting and relaxing the leg muscles while sitting help keep the blood flowing.

Dehydration, resulting from the low humidity (about 5 percent) in the cabin, can be prevented by drinking enough liquids and avoiding alcohol, which makes dehydration worse. People who wear contact lenses should apply rewetting solution to their lenses frequently to combat the effects of dry air.

Special foods, including low-salt, low-fat, and diabetic diets, are usually available from an airline by advance request.

Travelers should pack drugs in a carry-on bag rather than in a suitcase checked at the airport, in case their luggage is lost, stolen, or delayed. Drugs should be kept in their original containers. Travelers who must carry narcotics, large amounts of any drug, or syringes should have a

▲ see page 166

doctor's note to avoid being detained by security or customs officers. Travelers may wish to carry a summary of their medical records, including electrocardiogram results, in case they become ill while away from home. Those who have a potentially disabling condition, such as epilepsy, should wear a Medic Alert identification bracelet or necklace.

Women with normal pregnancies can travel by air through the eighth month. Women with high-risk pregnancies should discuss their travel plans with their doctor and obtain approval before flying. Generally, air travel during the ninth month requires a doctor's note dated within 72 hours of departure and indicating the woman's anticipated date of delivery. Seat belts should be worn low across the thighs, not over the abdomen, to prevent injury to the uterus.

Infants under 7 days old aren't permitted to fly. Children with chronic diseases, such as congenital heart or lung diseases or anemia, have the same restrictions as adults with those conditions. There's no upper age limit for travel.

Airlines make reasonable efforts to accommodate the handicapped. Often, wheelchairs and stretchers can be accommodated on commercial flights; otherwise, air ambulance service is necessary. Some airlines accept people who need special equipment such as intravenous lines and mechanical respirators as long as trained personnel accompany them and arrangements have been made at least 72 hours in advance.

Information and advice about air travel can be obtained from the medical departments of major airlines or from the Federal Aviation Administration Regional Flight Surgeon.

Foreign Travel

Of the millions of people who travel or work abroad every year, about 1 out of 30 needs medical attention for an illness or injury. Gastrointestinal infections may result from drinking contaminated water, including ice, and beverages or eating uncooked or improperly cooked foods. Casual sexual contacts produce a high risk for contracting the human immunodeficiency virus (HIV), which exists worldwide, as well as other sexually transmitted diseases. Motor vehicle accidents, especially at night, and drowning are the leading causes of death or injury for travelers in foreign countries. Health risks vary according to country and region; the Centers for Disease Control and Prevention provides up-to-date health advisories.

In foreign countries, many insurance plans, including Medicare, are not valid, and hospitals often require a substantial cash deposit, regardless of health insurance held in the United States. A variety of travel insurance plans, including some that arrange for emergency evacuation, are available through travel agents and some credit card companies. Directories listing English-speaking doctors in foreign countries are available from several organizations, and United States consulates may help secure emergency medical services.

Vaccinations

People planning a trip to another country should have the appropriate vaccinations, depending on their destination. In general, more preparation is needed when the trip lasts longer than 3 weeks, has several destinations in developing countries, or involves travel in rural areas or working with resident populations. Requirements for vaccinations change frequently. Some vaccinations must be given 2 to 12 weeks before the trip, so a traveler should inquire about vaccinations in advance. Information about vaccination requirements is available from various sources.

CHAPTER 286

Poisoning

Poisoning is the harmful effect that occurs when a toxic substance is swallowed, is inhaled, or comes in contact with the skin, eyes, or mucous membranes such as those of the mouth, vagina, or penis.

Fewer than 3,000 of the more than 12 million known chemicals cause most accidental and deliberate poisonings. However, almost any substance ingested in large quantities can be toxic.

Common sources of poisons include drugs, household products, agricultural products, plants, industrial chemicals, and food substances.▲ Identifying the poison and accurately assessing its danger are crucial to successful treatment. Information on treating poisoning from various substances is available from the nearest Poison Control Center, whose telephone number is listed in the local directory or can be obtained from directory assistance.

Poisoning can be an accident or a deliberate attempt to commit murder or suicide. Children, especially those under age 3, are particularly vulnerable to accidental poisoning, as are the elderly (from confusion about their medications), hospitalized patients (from medication errors), and industrial workers (from exposure to toxic chemicals).

Symptoms

The symptoms of poisoning depend on the poison, the amount ingested, and certain characteristics of the person who takes it. Some poisons aren't very potent and require prolonged exposure or repeated ingestion of a large amount to cause a problem. Others are so potent that just a drop on the skin can cause severe damage. Genetic makeup may affect whether a substance is poisonous to a particular person. Some normally nonpoisonous substances are poisonous for people who have a certain genetic makeup. Age may affect how much of a substance can be ingested before poisoning occurs. For example, a young child can ingest larger amounts of acetaminophen before becoming ill from it than an adult can. A benzodiazepine, a sedative, may be toxic to an elderly person at doses that a middle-aged adult could ingest without a problem.

Symptoms may be minor but bothersome—such as itching, dry mouth, blurred vision, and pain—or they may be serious—such as confusion, coma, abnormal heart rhythms, difficulty in breathing, and severe agitation. Some poisons produce symptoms within seconds, while others produce symptoms only after hours or even days. Some poisons produce few obvious symptoms until they have permanently damaged the function of vital organs such as the liver or kidneys. Thus, the symptoms of poisoning are as myriad as the poisons themselves.

Diagnosis and Treatment

After calling the Poison Control Center, family members or coworkers of poisoning victims can start first aid while waiting for professional help. They should determine whether the victim is breathing and has a heartbeat and should begin cardiopulmonary resuscitation (CPR), if needed. Because treatment is best accomplished when the poison is known, containers and samples of vomit should be saved and given to the doctor.

When the poison isn't known, doctors try to identify it with laboratory tests. A blood test may help, but analysis of a urine sample is usually more helpful. Doctors may remove material from the stomach by suctioning and send it to the laboratory to be analyzed and identified.

When a person has swallowed a poison, vomiting should be induced quickly, unless the poison could cause further damage if vomited. Examples of substances that should not be vomited are sharp objects, petroleum products, lye, and acids. If the person is very drowsy, unconscious, or having seizures, vomiting should not be induced because the person may choke. Syrup of ipecac is commonly used to induce vomiting; dosage instructions are printed on the bottle's label. If ipecac isn't available, soapy water can be used.

At a hospital, medical personnel use other techniques to clear the stomach of poisons. They may pump out the stomach by inserting a tube through the mouth or nose into the stomach and washing the stomach with water (gastric lavage). They may give activated charcoal through the stomach tube or may have the patient swallow it. This compound binds with a significant amount of the poison, preventing its absorption into the bloodstream.

Anyone who has been exposed to a toxic gas should be removed from the area as quickly as possible, preferably into fresh air. Emergency medical personnel usually give oxygen to the victim as soon as they arrive.

In chemical spills, all contaminated clothing, including shoes and socks, is usually removed immediately. The skin should be thoroughly washed and the eyes flushed with water if they have been exposed. Rescuers should be careful to avoid contaminating themselves.

▲ see pages 516 and 519

Common Poisons*

Household and agricultural products
Alcohol (rubbing)
Ammonia
Antifreeze
Bleach, chlorine
Cleaning fluids
DDT
Deodorizers
Depilatories
Dishwasher detergents
Drain cleaners
Fuel, solid canned
Gasoline
Glues and cements, model airplane
Herbicides
Kerosene
Lye
Mothballs
Mouthwashes
Nail adhesive, cosmetic
Nail polish and nail polish remover
Paint containing lead
Paint solvents (mineral spirits, turpentine)
Perfumes, colognes, aftershave lotions
Pesticides (ant, rat, and roach poison)
Shampoos
Toilet bowl cleaners
Varnish

Drugs
Any drug taken in large amounts

Plants
Daffodil bulbs
Dieffenbachia
English nightshade
Foxglove
Hemlock

Industrial chemicals
Arsenic
Mercury
Solvents
Strychnine
Syrup of wild cherry (cyanide)

Food substances
Alcoholic beverages (ethanol)
Contaminated foods (food poisoning)
Iron supplements
Some mushrooms

Other
Carbon monoxide (automobile exhaust, coal gas, furnace gas, marsh gas)

*Almost any substance ingested in large quantities can be toxic. A Poison Control Center should be contacted for up-to-date information.

Once poison has been absorbed through the gastrointestinal tract, skin, or lungs, it quickly spreads throughout the body. Eventually, most poisons are detoxified by the liver or excreted in the urine. Doctors try to accelerate the detoxification and elimination of poisons while simultaneously trying to reverse their toxic effects.

Fluids are usually given intravenously to keep the poison victim well hydrated and to maintain urine production. Mild acids or bases may be added to these fluids to increase the amount of poison excreted into the urine. Chemicals that bind to certain poisons, particularly heavy metals such as lead, may be given intravenously to help

neutralize and eliminate the poison. Dialysis▲ may be needed to remove poisons that aren't readily neutralized or eliminated from the blood.

If a specific antidote is available, it's given as quickly as possible. Examples are antidigoxin antibodies for an overdose of digoxin and the drug naloxone for an overdose of morphine or heroin.

Poisoning often requires additional treatment, depending on the symptoms and the substance ingested. A respirator may be needed if breathing stops, as may happen after an overdose of morphine, heroin, or barbiturates. The brain often swells after poisoning from sedatives, carbon monoxide, lead, or other chemicals that depress the nervous system. Drugs given to reduce the swelling include corticosteroids and mannitol. Poisoning can cause kidney failure, which may be severe enough to require dialysis.

▲ see page 597

Venomous Bites and Stings

Certain animals can inject venom (poison) through mouth parts or a stinging apparatus. These animals usually do not bite or sting a person unless they are provoked or otherwise disturbed in some way.

Poisonous Snake Bites

About 25 species of venomous ('poisonous) snakes are native to the United States. They include pit vipers (rattlesnakes, copperheads, and cottonmouths), coral snakes, and a few species of rear-fanged snakes (colubrids). Although more than 45,000 people are bitten by snakes in the United States each year, fewer than 8,000 bites by venomous snakes are reported, and fewer than 15 people die. Most deaths occur in children, the elderly, people who are untreated or treated inappropriately, and people belonging to religious sects in which members handle poisonous snakes. Rattlesnakes account for about 70 percent of poisonous snake bites in the United States and for almost all of the deaths. Copperheads, and to a lesser extent cottonmouths, account for most other poisonous snake bites. Coral snakes inflict less than 1 percent of all bites. Imported snakes found in zoos, snake farms, and amateur or professional collections account for about 15 bites a year.

A poisonous snake bite doesn't always result in snake venom poisoning. Venom is not injected in about 25 percent of all pit viper bites and about 50 percent of cobra and coral snake bites. Snake venom is a complex mixture containing many proteins that trigger harmful reactions. Snake venom can affect every major organ system in the body directly or indirectly.

The venom of rattlesnakes and other pit vipers damages tissue around the bite, produces changes in blood cells, prevents blood from clotting, and damages blood vessels, causing them to leak. These changes can lead to internal bleeding and heart, respiratory, and kidney failure. The venom of coral snakes affects nervous system activity but causes little damage to tissue around the bite.

Symptoms and Diagnosis

The symptoms of pit viper poisoning vary widely, depending on the size and species of snake, the amount and toxicity of the venom injected, the bite's location, the victim's age and size, and the presence of other medical problems. Most bites occur on the hand or foot. Usually, bites by rattlesnakes, cottonmouths, and copperheads cause pain immediately after the venom is injected; swelling follows within 10 minutes. These symptoms are rarely delayed more than 20 to 30 minutes. The pain can vary from mild to severe. A poisonous bite can be diagnosed on the basis of fang marks, redness, pain, swelling, and tingling and numbness in the fingers or toes or around the mouth, among other symptoms. A metallic or rubbery taste in the mouth has been noted after bites by some species of rattlesnakes.

If untreated, the swelling can progress, affecting the entire leg or arm within several hours. The lymph nodes in the area may also swell and may be painful. Other symptoms include fever; chills; general weakness; a rapid, weak heartbeat; faintness; sweating; nausea; and vomiting. Breathing difficulties can develop, particularly after Mojave rattlesnake bites. The victim may have a headache, blurred vision, drooping eyelids, and a dry mouth.

Moderate and severe pit viper poisoning commonly causes bruising of the skin, which may appear 3 to 6 hours after the bite. The skin around the bite appears tight and discolored; blisters may form in the bite area within 8 hours and often fill with blood. Without treatment, tissue destruction around the bite may occur, with blood clots forming in the surrounding blood vessels.

The venom of many pit vipers, particularly rattlesnakes, prevents blood from clotting; the gums may bleed and blood may appear in the vomit, stools, and urine. The results of blood tests that assess clotting may be abnormal, and the number of platelets (the blood components responsible for clotting) may be markedly reduced.

Coral snake bites usually cause little or no pain and swelling. The main symptoms are caused by changes in the nervous system. The area around the bite may tingle, and nearby muscles may become weak. Muscle incoordination and severe general weakness may follow. Other symptoms include visual disturbances and increased saliva production, with speech and swallowing difficulties. Breathing problems, which may be extreme, may follow.

Treatment

Poisonous snake bites are medical emergencies requiring immediate attention. Before starting treatment, emergency medical personnel must try to determine whether the snake was poisonous and whether venom was injected. If no venom was injected, treatment is the same as for a puncture wound—thorough cleaning and a tetanus booster.

Anyone bitten by a pit viper should be kept as calm and still as possible, kept warm, and taken to the nearest medical facility immediately. The bitten limb should be loosely immobilized and kept positioned below heart level. Rings, watches, and tight clothing should be removed, and no stimulants should be given. A Sawyer's extractor (a device that suctions venom from the site of the bite, designed for first aid) should be applied over the bite within 5 minutes and kept in place for 30 to 40 minutes during transportation to the hospital for further treatment.

Venom antidote (antivenom), which neutralizes the venom's toxic effects, is an important part of treatment for most bites. Antivenom is given intravenously. A tetanus booster is also given, and antibiotics are occasionally needed.

The general treatment of coral snake bites is the same as for pit viper bites. If breathing problems develop, respiratory assistance may be needed. Antivenom may be needed; one that's specific for coral snake bites is used.

In all cases of snake bite poisoning, particularly in children and the elderly, a Poison Control Center should be contacted. The local zoo or poison center should be the first place to call for advice on treating a bite by an imported poisonous snake. Personnel at these locations know where to obtain antivenom and have a directory of doctors who specialize in treating these bites.

Poisonous Lizard Bites

The only two lizards known to be poisonous are the beaded lizard of Mexico and the Gila monster, found in Arizona and Sonora, Mexico, and adjacent areas. The venom of these lizards is somewhat similar in content and effect to that of some pit vipers.

Common symptoms include pain, swelling, and discoloration in the area around the bite as well as swollen lymph nodes. Weakness, sweating, thirst, a headache, and ringing in the ears (tinnitus) may develop. In severe cases, blood pressure may fall.

Treatment is similar to that of pit viper bites. A specific antivenom is not available.

Spider Bites

Almost all spiders are poisonous. Fortunately, the fangs of most species are too short or too fragile to penetrate human skin. Nevertheless, at least 60 species in the United States have been implicated in biting people. Species not native to the United States may be brought into the country on fruits, vegetables, or other materials. Although tarantulas native to the United States are considered dangerous, their bites do not seriously harm people. On the average, spider bites cause fewer than three deaths a year in the United States, usually in children.

Only a few spider venoms have been studied in detail. The venoms studied are complex, containing enzymes and other proteins that cause various reactions in the body.

Symptoms

The bite of a black widow spider usually causes a sharp pain, somewhat like a pinprick, followed by a dull, sometimes numbing, pain in the area around the bite. Cramping pain and muscular stiffness in the abdomen or the shoulders, back, and chest also develop. Other symptoms may include restlessness, anxiety, sweating, headaches, dizziness, drooping and swelling of the eyelids, skin rash and itching, severe breathing problems, nausea, vomiting, increased saliva production, and weakness. The skin around the bite may feel warm.

The bite of a brown recluse spider may cause little or no immediate pain, but some pain develops in the area around the bite within an hour or so. Pain may be severe and may affect the entire injured area. The area around the bite becomes red and bruised and may itch. The rest of the body may also itch. A blister forms, surrounded by either an irregular bruised area or a more distinct targetlike red zone. The area appears first as a bull's-eye. Then the blister enlarges, fills with blood, and ruptures, forming an open sore (ulcer) that may leave a large craterlike scar. Nausea, vomiting, aches, fatigue, chills, sweats, blood disorders, and kidney failure may develop, but the bite is rarely fatal.

Treatment

The only first-aid measure of any value for a black widow spider bite is placing an ice cube on the bite to reduce pain. People under 16 or over 60 years of age and those who have high blood pressure and heart disease are usually hospitalized for treatment. Antivenom, which neutralizes the effects of the toxin, is given for severe poisoning. Other measures may be needed to treat breathing difficulties and extremely high blood pressure. Muscle pain and spasms can be relieved by muscle relaxants. Pain can be relieved in mild cases by hot baths and in severe cases by narcotic analgesics.

For brown recluse spider bites, ice placed on the bite helps reduce pain. Corticosteroids are usually given to reduce inflammation. An antivenom is not yet commercially available.

Skin sores are cleaned daily with hydrogen peroxide and soaked three times a day; dead tissue is trimmed away as needed. For most bites, this treatment is all that's needed.

Bee, Wasp, Hornet, and Ant Stings

Stings by bees, wasps, hornets, and ants are common throughout the United States. The average person can safely tolerate 10 stings for each pound of body weight. This means that the average adult could withstand more than 1,000 stings, whereas 500 stings could kill a child. However, one sting can cause death from an anaphylactic reaction▲ in a person who is allergic to such stings. In the United States, three or four times more people die of bee stings than of snake bites every year. The few fatalities from multiple bee stings are usually caused by heart malfunction and collapse of the circulatory system. A more aggressive type of honeybee, called the Africanized killer bee, has reached some southern states as these bees travel north from South America. By attacking their victim in swarms, these bees cause a more severe reaction than do other bees.

Dangerous Spiders

Black widow spiders and related species

Brown or violin spiders, sometimes called brown recluse, and related species

Jumping spiders

Tarantulas (not native to the United States)

Trap-door spiders

Banana spiders (Central America)

Wolf spiders

Orb weavers

Running or gnaphosid spiders

Green lynx spiders

Comb-footed or false black widow spiders

Orange argiopes

Giant crab spiders

Crab spiders

Dysderids

Amaurobiids

Hunting spiders (Central and South America)

In the South, particularly in the Gulf region, fire ants inflict thousands of stings each year. Up to 40 percent of the people who live in infested urban areas may be stung each year, and at least 30 deaths have been attributed to these insect bites. The fire ant sting usually produces immediate pain and a red, swollen area, which disappears within 45 minutes. A blister then forms, rupturing in 30 to 70 hours, and the area often becomes infected. In some cases, a red, swollen, itchy patch develops instead of a blister. Anaphylaxis (a life-threatening allergic reaction in which blood pressure falls and the airways close) occurs in less than 1 percent of the people stung by fire ants. Isolated nerves may become inflamed, and seizures may occur.

▲ see page 828

Treatment

A bee, wasp, hornet, or fire ant may leave its stinger in the skin. The stinger should be removed by gentle scraping or teasing rather than pulling or tweezing, which can inject additional venom into the body. An ice cube placed over the sting reduces the pain. A cream containing a combination of an antihistamine, an analgesic, and a corticosteroid is often useful. People who are allergic to stings should always carry a kit with antihistamine tablets and a preloaded syringe of epinephrine, which block anaphylactic or allergic reactions.

People who have had a severe allergic reaction to a bee sting may undergo desensitization, which may help prevent such reactions in the future. Desensitization is a process of repeatedly exposing the body to small amounts of the substance that causes an allergic response (allergen) until that response is muted.

Insect Bites

Among the more common biting and sometimes bloodsucking insects in the United States are sand flies, horseflies, deerflies, mosquitoes, fleas, lice, bedbugs, kissing bugs, and certain water bugs. The bites of these insects may be irritating because of the components of their saliva. The bites cause a variety of reactions, from small bumps to large sores (ulcers) with swelling and pain. The most severe reactions occur in people who are allergic to the bites or who develop an infection after being bitten. For those who are allergic, bites are sometimes fatal.

The insect should be removed quickly. The bite should be cleaned, and an ointment containing a combination of an antihistamine, an analgesic, and a corticosteroid may be applied to relieve itching, pain, and inflammation. People who are allergic to the bite should seek medical attention immediately or use their emergency allergy kit containing antihistamine tablets and a preloaded syringe of epinephrine.

Tick and Mite Bites

Ticks carry many diseases (for example, deer ticks may carry the bacteria that cause Lyme

▲ see page 880

disease ▲) and a few ticks are poisonous. In North America, some species cause tick paralysis, which results in loss of appetite, listlessness, muscle weakness, incoordination, involuntary sideways twitching of the eyes (nystagmus), and a progressive paralysis, moving up from the legs. The muscles that control breathing may also become paralyzed. The bites of pajaroello ticks, which are found in Mexico and the southwestern United States, produce pus-filled blisters that break, leaving open sores that develop scabs. The area around the sores may be swollen and painful.

Mite infestations are common and are responsible for chiggers (an intensely itchy rash caused by mite larvae under the skin), scabies, and a number of other diseases. The effects on the tissues around the bite vary in severity.

Treatment

Ticks should be removed as soon as possible. Removal is best accomplished by applying petroleum jelly or some other irritant to the tick or by slowly withdrawing it while twisting it slowly with tweezers. The tick's head, which may not come out with the body, should be removed because it can cause prolonged inflammation or move to deeper tissues.

Tick paralysis may require no treatment, but if breathing is impaired, oxygen therapy or a respirator may be needed. Pajaroello tick bites are cleaned and soaked in a cleansing solution, and dead skin is removed, if necessary. Corticosteroids help reduce inflammation in severe cases. Infections of the sores are common but usually can be cured with an antibiotic ointment.

Mite infestations are treated by applying a cream containing permethrin or a solution of lindane. After treatment with permethrin or lindane, a cream containing a corticosteroid is sometimes used for a few days to reduce the itching until all the mites are gone.

Centipede and Millipede Bites

Some of the larger centipedes can inflict a painful bite, with swelling and redness around the bite. Lymph nodes near the bite area may also swell, but usually no tissue damage or infection results. Symptoms rarely persist for more than 48 hours. Millipedes don't bite but may secrete a toxin that can irritate the skin and, in severe cases, damage tissue.

An ice cube placed on a centipede bite usually alleviates the pain. Toxic secretions of millipedes should be washed from the skin with copious amounts of soap and water; alcohol should not be used. If a skin reaction develops, a corticosteroid cream should be applied. Eye injuries should be flushed with water (irrigated) immediately, and a corticosteroid-analgesic ointment appropriate for the eye should be applied.

Scorpion Stings

Almost all North American scorpions are relatively harmless. Usually, the only symptoms of their stings are pain with some swelling, increased tenderness, and warmth at the sting site. However, sculptured centruroides (*Centruroides exilicauda*), which is found in Arizona and New Mexico and on the California side of the Colorado River, is much more toxic. The sting is immediately painful, sometimes causing numbness or tingling in the area around the sting. Swelling is rare. Children become tense and restless and have involuntary, random movements of the head, neck, and eyes. In adults, the heart rate, breathing rate, and blood pressure increase. Muscles may become weak and uncoordinated. Breathing difficulties complicated by increased saliva production can develop in children and adults.

The stings of most North American scorpions require no special treatment. Placing an ice cube on the wound reduces pain, as does an ointment containing a combination of an antihistamine, an analgesic, and a corticosteroid. Muscle spasms and high blood pressure resulting from the sting may require the use of drugs. Complete bed rest is important. No food should be eaten for the first 8 to 12 hours. Antivenom should be given to all people who are unresponsive or have a severe reaction, particularly children.

Marine Animal Stings and Bites

Stingrays have caused about 750 stings a year along North American coasts. A stingray's venom is contained in the one or more spines located on the back of the tail. Injuries usually occur when an unwary person steps on a stingray while wading in ocean surf or a bay. The stingray thrusts its tail upward and forward, driving the spine or spines into the victim's foot or leg. The spine's

covering is ruptured and venom is released, causing immediate severe pain.

The pain may be limited to the area around the sting but often spreads rapidly, reaching its greatest intensity in less than 90 minutes. If untreated, the pain often continues, gradually diminishing over 6 to 48 hours. Fainting spells, weakness, nausea, and anxiety are common. Swollen, tender lymph nodes; vomiting; diarrhea; sweating; generalized cramps; pain in the armpit or groin; and breathing difficulties are less common. The wound from the spine is usually jagged and bleeds freely. Fragments of the spine's covering may remain in the wound, increasing the risk of infection. The wound's edges are often discolored, with some tissue destruction. Swelling around the wound is common.

Injuries to an arm or leg resulting from stings by stingrays and most other fish should be rinsed with salt water. Fragments of the spine's covering left in the wound should be removed if they can be seen. The injured limb should be immersed in water as hot as the person can tolerate for 30 to 90 minutes. If these first-aid measures are delayed, the pain may be severe. In such cases, a doctor can numb the wound with local anesthetics and give the person analgesics. Seeking medical care is important so that the wound can be cleaned and examined thoroughly, a tetanus booster given, antibiotics started if necessary, and the wound closed with stitches.

A few **mollusks,** which include snails, octopuses, and bivalves (such as clams, oysters, and scallops), are poisonous. The California cone (*Conus californicus*) is the only dangerous snail found in North American waters. Its sting produces pain, swelling, redness, and numbness around the sting site. The bites of North American octopuses are rarely serious. Paralytic shellfish poisoning is caused by eating certain bivalves, such as clams and mussels, that have consumed poisonous dinoflagellates (single-celled marine animals).▲

First-aid measures seem to provide little benefit for injuries from *Conus* stings and octopus bites. Severe *Conus* stings may cause shock, requiring intensive medical support of breathing and circulation.

▲ see page 520

Sea urchins and several related creatures are venomous, although the venom itself rarely injures people. More commonly, the spines that cover a sea urchin's shell break off in the skin, causing tissue damage and inflammation. If not removed, the spines move to deeper tissues, causing chronic inflammation, or become wedged against a bone or nerve. Joint and muscle pain and skin rashes may develop.

Sea urchin spines should be removed immediately. A bluish discoloration at the site of entry may help locate a spine. Because vinegar dissolves most sea urchin spines, several vinegar soaks or compresses may be all that's needed to remove the spines. The area around the sting is washed and an ointment containing a combination of an antihistamine, an analgesic, and a corticosteroid is applied. Occasionally, a doctor must make a tiny incision to remove a spine, which is fragile.

Many coelenterates, which include corals, sea anemones, jellyfish, and the Portuguese man-of-war, have highly developed stinging units that can penetrate the skin. These units are particularly abundant on the animal's tentacles; a single tentacle can fire thousands of them into the skin. The resulting damage depends on the type of animal. Generally, a small, raised rash appears in a series of lines, sometimes surrounded by a red area. Pain may be severe; itching is common. The rash may develop into blisters that fill with pus and then rupture. Other symptoms include weakness, nausea, headache, muscle pain and spasms, runny eyes and nose, excessive sweat-

ing, changes in heart rate, and chest pain that worsens with breathing. Stings from the Portuguese man-of-war, including those that occur in North American waters, have caused death.

Various treatments for coelenterate stings have been suggested, although most stings need little more than cleansing. In some parts of the world, ammonia or vinegar is applied to the wound. In the United States, meat tenderizers (such as papain), baking soda, boric acid, lemon or fig juice, alcohol, and many other substances have been used to relieve pain. The following treatment is suggested:

1. Pour ocean (not fresh) water over the injured area.
2. Remove the tentacles with an instrument or a gloved hand.
3. Soak the injured area in a solution of half water and half vinegar for 30 minutes.
4. Pour flour or baking soda over the wound and carefully scrape the powder off with a sharp knife.
5. Soak the area in vinegar again.
6. Apply an ointment containing a combination of an antihistamine, an analgesic, and a corticosteroid.

More serious reactions may require oxygen therapy or other assistance in breathing. Painful muscle spasms and severe pain are treated with drugs given intravenously. An antivenom is available for the stings of certain Australian species, but it doesn't relieve the symptoms caused by the stings of North American species.

Appendixes

APPENDIX I

Legal Issues

Poor health can jeopardize anyone's legal rights; safeguarding those rights requires advance thinking and planning. Sudden illness can cause profound weakness and confusion, while chronic illness can affect the ability to think clearly, making a person vulnerable and perhaps leading to the unwilling forfeiture of control. Conducting personal or business affairs, making wishes known, and making sure those wishes are respected may be impossible for a person who is physically or mentally impaired. Nevertheless, adults of any age can take steps to protect themselves against losing control over their lives, and such steps are especially important for older people. A durable power of attorney, a will, or a living trust can help direct the legal system so that decisions affecting health care and property management and distribution are made in accordance with a person's wishes.

The legal system in the United States operates on federal, state, and local levels. In general, federal law affects how property is taxed when it's given away, either while the owner is alive or after death. Federal law also controls Medicare, a program that provides health care coverage for people aged 65 and older. In general, state laws determine how people can direct their own care if they become incapacitated. State laws also determine who is qualified for benefits under Medicaid,

a program that provides health care coverage for the poor. In addition, state laws control property distribution if a person dies without a will or living trust. Because state laws differ significantly, seeking an attorney's advice is important. However, people can take many steps on their own. For example, simple powers of attorney can be prepared on a standardized form. More complex documents, such as a will or trust, should be written by an attorney.

Competency and Capacity

Laws recognize that adults—in most states people over age 18—have the right to manage their own affairs, conduct business, and make health care decisions. This legal status is called **competency.** Competency and all the rights that go with it remain in effect until death, unless a court of law determines that a person can no longer manage personal affairs in his own best interest (a status called **incompetency**) or unless the person willingly transfers those rights to someone else.

Only a court of law can declare a person incompetent. Doctors may testify about a patient's capacity to understand concepts and make decisions, but a court has the authority to take away a person's right to make decisions by declaring the person incompetent. Then the court must find

Legal Terms Related to Health Care

Competency: The right to manage one's own affairs (bestowed at age 18 in most states).

Incompetency: The inability to manage one's own affairs because of illness, injury, or impending death; declared by a court of law.

Advance Directives

Living will: A document, sometimes called a directive to doctors, that expresses a person's wishes regarding medical intervention when very ill or near death.

Durable power of attorney for health care: A document that allows a person to designate someone else to make medical treatment decisions on his behalf.

someone else to act in the person's best interests. People who have planned ahead will have named such a person by preparing the proper documentation (for example, a durable power of attorney or a living trust document). Otherwise, the court must choose someone.

Incapacity means that a person is physically or mentally unable to make appropriate decisions or to carry them out. A person in a coma can't make *any* decisions, whereas a person with a broken leg may be able to make decisions but be unable to carry them out. People with mild dementia may think clearly enough to understand discussions with their doctors and make decisions about their medical care but may be unable to make decisions about their business affairs. These people must depend on their doctors, lawyers, and bankers to evaluate their judgment before proceeding with medical care or conducting major legal and business transactions.

The issues of incompetency and incapacity come up frequently when older people become ill. Before performing any invasive tests or providing medical treatment, doctors must obtain permission from a person who is able to understand the risks and benefits involved. If a person isn't capable of understanding those risks, the doctor must either turn to the person named in a durable power of attorney for health care or seek advice from the courts. Often, however, doctors simply turn to the next of kin.

Advance Directives

Two types of legal documents extend control over medical care when a person becomes incapacitated or is declared incompetent: a living will and a durable power of attorney for health care. Both documents are called advance directives because they direct, in advance, decisions about aspects of medical care to be carried out during any period when the person can no longer effectively communicate those decisions. An advance directive becomes effective only after incapacity or incompetency has been determined.

If no advance directive has been prepared, someone must be appointed to take control of medical care decisions. Generally, courts tend to assign control to a family member. If no appropriate family member can be found, the court appoints a guardian or conservator, who may be a friend or a stranger, to oversee care. An advance directive can eliminate the need for the courts to get involved.

Living Will

A living will expresses a person's preferences for medical care (it's called a living will because it's in effect while a person is alive). In some states, the document is called a directive to doctors. State laws vary greatly regarding living wills. For example, in some states, only a terminally ill person can create a legally effective living will.

Many people believe that extreme heroic measures and technology should be used to extend life as long as possible, regardless of the degree of medical intervention required or the quality of life that results. Others feel just as strongly that death is preferable to being perpetually dependent on medical equipment or having no hope of returning to a certain quality of life. A living will allows a person to express either of these preferences (or any intermediate measure that the person finds acceptable).

To be valid, a living will must comply with state law. Some states require that living wills be written in a standardized way. Others are more lenient, permitting any language as long as the document is appropriately signed and witnessed.

Medical Terms Related to Life-Sustaining Treatment

Cardiopulmonary resuscitation (CPR): An action taken to revive a person in cardiac or respiratory arrest.

Code: The summoning of professionals trained in cardiopulmonary resuscitation to revive a person in cardiac or respiratory arrest.

No code: An order signed by a patient's doctor stating that cardiopulmonary resuscitation should not be performed if cardiac or pulmonary arrest occurs.

Irreversibly and terminally ill: The state of being near death with no hope of cure.

Life-sustaining treatment: Any treatment given to postpone the death of a terminally ill person who is near death.

Advance directive: A document (a durable power of attorney for health care or living will) that indicates a person's wishes regarding medical treatment.

Supportive care: Measures taken to keep a terminally ill person who is near death as comfortable as possible while closely monitoring his condition.

To indicate preferences for aggressive medical treatment, the document might state: "I want my life to be prolonged to the greatest extent possible without regard to my condition, the chances I have for recovery, the burdens of the treatment, or the cost of the procedures."

To prevent heroic attempts to extend life, the document might state: "I do not want my life to be prolonged and I do not want life-sustaining treatment (including artificial feeding and hydration) to be provided or continued if the burdens of treatment would outweigh the expected benefits. I want the relief of suffering and the quality of my life to be considered in determining whether life-sustaining treatment should be started or continued."

To express a preference for an intermediate position, the document might state: "I want my life to be prolonged and I want life-sustaining treatment to be provided unless I am in a coma that my doctors reasonably believe to be irreversible. After my doctors have reasonably concluded that I am in an irreversible coma, I do not want life-sustaining treatment, including artificial feeding and hydration, to be provided or continued."

Durable Power of Attorney for Health Care

A power of attorney for health care is a document in which one person (the principal) names another person (the agent or the attorney-in-fact)

to make decisions about health care and *only* health care. A power is *durable* if it remains legally in force, even when the principal becomes incapacitated or is declared incompetent.

A durable power of attorney for health care differs from a living will. A living will states a person's preferences regarding medical treatment. A durable power of attorney for health care designates an agent to make health care decisions. The agent is granted the power to discuss medical alternatives with the doctors and make a decision if an accident or illness incapacitates the person. The durable power of attorney for health care can include a living will provision—a description of health care preferences.

Selecting an agent should be done with great care. For example, a person who strongly wishes to avoid aggressive medical treatment shouldn't designate as agent an adult child who believes that every possible medical intervention should be used to prolong life. Similarly, a spouse who is under enormous emotional stress may be unable to make rational decisions. A better choice might be a trusted business associate or a longtime friend.

A principal who is mentally competent can withdraw a durable power of attorney at any time. The choice of agent doesn't have to be permanent. If circumstances change, the person can create a new durable power of attorney naming a new agent.

Checklist for Preparing Advance Directives

An advance directive must meet certain basic requirements to be legally binding. The document should state exactly what is to be done to carry out the intended wishes. The following checklist may help to ensure that these requirements are met:

Living Will
- Form should be dated and signed
- Form should be witnessed or notarized
- Degree of medical intervention desired for a terminal condition should be specified
- Information should be kept current
- Additional instructions about specific treatment (for example, intubation, dialysis, surgery, antibiotics, mechanical ventilation, do-not-resuscitate orders) should be included

Durable Power of Attorney for Health Care
- Form should be dated and signed
- Form should be witnessed or notarized
- Information should be kept current
- Power of attorney should be durable, that is, should stay in effect if the author of the document becomes incapacitated
- Document should specify the powers and limitations of the agent

---

Discussing the details of a durable power of attorney with the person named as agent is important. Since a person named in the document isn't obliged to act and may refuse to do so, the principal should find out whether that person is willing to act before action becomes necessary. The document should name an alternate or successor in case the first-named person is unable or unwilling to serve as agent. Two or more people may be named to serve together (jointly) or alone (severally). A **jointly held power** requires that all agents agree and act together. In this arrangement, all named agents must be contacted and must agree on every decision. A **severally held power** allows any named agent to act alone.

Special circumstances may have to be addressed in drawing up a durable power of attor-

ney for health care. For instance, family members have priority as visitors in a hospital under most circumstances. Unmarried couples may need special protection to preserve such privileges. A durable power of attorney for health care can stipulate visitation rights for people who aren't legally considered family members.

Ideally, a person should give copies of his living will and durable power of attorney for health care to every doctor providing care for him and to the hospital on admission. Copies should also be placed in the person's permanent medical record. A person should also give a copy of the durable power of attorney for health care to his appointed agent and place another copy with important papers. The person's lawyer should hold a copy as well.

Management of Property

People should have contingency plans to deal with injury or illness. Even if an accident or illness doesn't affect a person's ability (capacity) to control assets, serious illness or injury may make it difficult to pay bills, manage finances, take care of property, and handle business affairs. Having plans to turn over legal authority to a trusted decision maker can minimize disruption and expenses.

Three principal mechanisms allow a person to arrange in advance for property and business to be overseen by someone else: a power of attorney, a revocable trust, and joint tenancy. These arrangements are best made with the help of an attorney.

A **power of attorney** is a document in which one person (the principal) appoints another person (the agent or attorney-in-fact) to perform specific actions—such as handling bank accounts, investments, or other property—if the principal is too ill or too severely injured to handle them personally. Usually it's wise to draw up separate powers of attorney for health care and business matters, even if the same person is named as agent.

A **revocable trust (living trust)** places legal title to property in the hands of a trustee, who holds the property for the use and benefit of the beneficiary. The trustee can't legally use the trust property for any purpose not specifically described in the trust document.

Joint tenancy is a form of ownership that gives all named owners the right to manage the property. Many people hold their bank accounts and homes in joint tenancy. In joint tenancy, an owner's share passes automatically after death to the other joint tenants. For example, if a parent has a checking account in joint tenancy with an adult child, both parent and child can write checks from the account. If the parent dies, the child then owns the account. A house owned in joint tenancy becomes fully owned by the surviving joint tenants.

APPENDIX II

Weights and Measures

In medicine, precise measurements are necessary—for example, when various substances are measured in laboratory tests to evaluate health or make a diagnosis. Different units of measure may be used depending on the substance. Usually, the metric system, based on multiples of 10, is used to measure mass, volume, and length. Grams measure mass, the amount of matter in an object; mass is similar to weight, but weight is affected by gravity. Liters measure volume, the amount of space an object occupies. Meters measure length.

Prefixes, indicating which multiple of 10 is meant, can be attached to the basic unit, such as meter (m), liter (L), or gram (gm), to help make a number more readable. Commonly used prefixes include kilo (k), deci (d), centi (c), milli (m), and micro (μ).

Other units measure different properties of a substance. For example, a mole (mol) is the number of particles (molecules or ions) in a substance. Regardless of the substance, 1 mole always equals the same number of particles. However, the number of grams in 1 mole varies greatly from substance to substance. One mole equals the molecular (atomic) weight of a substance in grams. For example, the molecular weight of calcium is 40, and 1 mole of calcium equals 40 grams. Osmoles (Osm) and milliosmoles (mOsm) refer to the number of particles in a specific amount of liquid. Equivalents (Eq) and milliequivalents (mEq) measure a substance's ability to combine with another substance. A milliequivalent is roughly equivalent to a milliosmole.

Formulas are used to convert a measurement from one unit to another. The same amount can be expressed in terms of different units. For example, the concentration of calcium in the blood is normally about 10 milligrams in a deciliter (mg/dL), 2.5 millimoles in a liter (mmol/L), or 5 milliequivalents in a liter (mEq/L).

Prefixes in the Metric System

Prefix	Multiple of 10	Comparison	
kilo (k)	1000	1 kilometer (km) = 1000 meters (m)	1 m = 0.001 km
deci (d)	0.1	1 deciliter (dL) = 0.1 liter (L)	1 L = 10 dL
centi (c)	0.01	1 centimeter (cm) = 0.01 m	1 m = 100 cm
milli (m)	0.001	1 milliliter (mL) = 0.001 L	1 L = 1000 mL
micro (μ)	0.000001	1 microliter (μL) = 0.000001 L	1 L = 1 million μL

Nonmetric Equivalents

Weight	1 lb	= 16 oz
Volume	1 gal	= 4 qt
	1 qt	= 2 pt
	1 pt	= 16 fl oz
	1 cup	= 8 fl oz = 16 tbsp
	1 tbsp	= ½ fl oz = 3 tsp
Length	1 mi	= 1,760 yd
	1 yd	= 3 ft
	1 ft	= 12 in

Metric Equivalents for Weight, Volume, and Length

Weight

1 pound (lb) = 0.454 kilogram (kg)	1 kg = 2.2 lb
1 ounce (oz) = 28.35 grams (gm)	1 gm = 0.035 oz

Volume

1 gallon (gal) = 3.785 liters (L)	1 L = 1.057 qt
1 quart (qt) = 0.946 L	1 cL = 0.338 fl oz
1 pint (pt) = 0.473 L	1 mL = 0.0338 fl oz
1 fluid ounce (fl oz) = 29.573 mL	

Length

1 mile (mi) = 1.609 kilometers (km)	1 km = 0.62 mi
1 yard (yd) = 0.914 meter (m)	1 m = 39.37 in
1 foot (ft) = 30.48 centimeters (cm)	1 cm = 0.39 in
1 inch (in) = 2.54 cm	1 millimeter (mm) = 0.039 in

Metric Equivalents for Height and Weight

Height		Weight	
Ft/in	**Cm**	**Lb**	**Kg**
4'10"	147.3	100	45.4
4'11"	149.9	110	49.9
5'0"	152.4	120	54.5
5'1"	154.9	130	59.0
5'2"	157.5	140	63.6
5'3"	160.0	150	68.1
5'4"	162.6	160	72.6
5'5"	165.1	170	77.2
5'6"	167.6	180	81.7
5'7"	170.2	190	86.3
5'8"	172.7	200	90.8
5'9"	175.3	210	95.3
5'10"	177.8	220	99.9
5'11"	180.3	230	104.4
6'0"	182.9	240	109.0
6'1"	185.4	250	113.5
6'2"	188.0		
6'3"	190.5		
6'4"	193.0		

Centigrade-Fahrenheit Equivalents

To convert Fahrenheit to centigrade: Subtract 32, then multiply by $5/9$ or 0.555.

To convert centigrade to Fahrenheit: Multiply by $9/5$ or 1.8, then add 32.

	Degrees	
	Centigrade (C.)	**Fahrenheit (F.)**
Freezing	0	32.0
Body temperature range	36.0	96.8
	36.5	97.7
	37.0	98.6
	37.5	99.5
	38.0	100.4
	38.5	101.3
	39.0	102.2
	39.5	103.1
	40.0	104.0
	40.5	104.9
	41.0	105.8
	41.5	106.7
	42.0	107.6
Boiling	100.0	212.0

Common Medical Tests

A large number of laboratory tests are widely available. Many tests are specialized for a particular group of diseases. Generally, specialized tests are described with the appropriate diseases in this book. However, many tests are used commonly in many specialties and in general practice.

Screening tests are used to try to detect a disease when there is little or no evidence that a person has the disease. For example, measuring cholesterol levels helps identify the risk of cardiovascular disease, but these tests are performed for people who have no symptoms of cardiovascular disease. To be useful, screening tests must be accurate, be relatively inexpensive, pose little risk, and cause little or no discomfort.

Diagnostic tests, on the other hand, are used when a disease is suspected. For example, a doctor who suspects serious heart disease might recommend cardiac catheterization. This test would not be a good screening test because it is expensive, can produce side effects, and is uncomfortable. However, all of these drawbacks are outweighed by the need for this test when disease must be evaluated.

Every test, whether used for screening or diagnosis, has some risk. The risk may be only the need for further testing if the result is abnormal, or it may be the possibility of injury during the test. Doctors weigh the risk of a test against the usefulness of the information it will provide.

No test is completely accurate. Sometimes a test result is incorrectly abnormal in a person who doesn't have the disease (a **false-positive** result). Sometimes a test result is incorrectly normal in a person who has the disease (a **false-negative** result). Tests are rated in terms of their **sensitivity** (the probability that their results will be positive when a disease is present) and their **specificity** (the probability that their results will be negative when a disease is not present). A very sensitive test is unlikely to miss the disease in people who have it. However, it may falsely indicate disease in healthy people. A very specific test is unlikely to indicate disease in healthy people. However, it may miss the disease in some who have it. Problems with sensitivity and specificity can be largely overcome by using several different tests. For example, a person who tests positive for AIDS with a very sensitive test is retested with another more specific one.

Routine blood testing is often misleading and may cause unnecessary anxiety and expense. When automated analyzers such as the Sequential Multiple Analyzer (SMA) are used to perform several blood tests, false-positive results are very common. By chance alone, at least one false-positive result is expected in almost half the people having 12 tests (SMA-12) and in two thirds of those having 20 tests (SMA-20). Because a doctor can't be sure whether a result in a particular person is false or true, a person with an abnormal result may need to be retested or undergo other tests.

Normal test result values are expressed as a range, which is based on the average values in a healthy population; 95 percent of healthy people have values within this range. These values vary somewhat among laboratories.

Blood Tests

Test	Reference Range (conventional units*)	Test	Reference Range (conventional units*)
Acidity (pH)	7.35–7.45	Electrolytes	*See individual tests:* electrolytes routinely tested include calcium, chloride, magnesium, potassium, sodium
Alcohol (ethanol)	0 mg/dL (more than 0.1 mg/dL usually indicates intoxication)		
Ammonia	15–50 μg of nitrogen/dL	Erythrocyte sedimentation rate (ESR)	*Male:* 1–13 mm/hr *Female:* 1–20 mm/hr
Amylase	53–123 units/L		
Ascorbic acid	0.4–1.5 mg/dL	Glucose	*Fasting:* 70–110 mg/dL
Bicarbonate (carbon dioxide content)	18–23 mEq/L	Hematocrit	*Male:* 45–52% *Female:* 37–48%
Bilirubin	*Direct:* up to 0.4 mg/dL *Total:* up to 1.0 mg/dL	Hemoglobin	*Male:* 13–18 gm/dL *Female:* 12–16 gm/dL
Blood volume	8.5–9.1% of body weight	Iron	60–160 μg/dL (higher in males)
Calcium	8.5–10.5 mg/dL (slightly higher in children)	Iron-binding capacity	250–460 μg/dL
Carbon dioxide pressure	35–45 mm Hg	Lactate (lactic acid)	*Venous:* 4.5–19.8 mg/dL *Arterial:* 4.5–14.4 mg/dL
Carbon monoxide	Less than 5% of total hemoglobin	Lactic dehydrogenase	50–150 units/L
CD4 cell count	500–1500 cells/μL	Lead	40 μg/dL or less (much lower in children)
Ceruloplasmin	15–60 mg/dL		
Chloride	98–106 mEq/L	Lipase	10–150 units/L
Complete blood cell count (CBC)	*See individual tests:* hemoglobin, hematocrit, mean corpuscular hemoglobin, mean corpuscular hemoglobin concentration, mean corpuscular volume, platelet count, white blood cell count	Lipids: Cholesterol	Less than 225 mg/dL (for age 40–49 yr; increases with age)
		Triglycerides	40–200 mg/dL (higher in males)
Copper	*Total:* 70–150 μg/dL	Liver function tests	Include bilirubin (total), phosphatase (alkaline), protein (total and albumin), transaminases (alanine and aspartate), prothrombin
Creatine kinase (CK or CPK)	*Male:* 38–174 units/L *Female:* 96–140 units/L		
Creatine kinase isoenzymes	5% MB or less	Magnesium	1.5–2.0 mEq/L
Creatinine	0.6–1.2 mg/dL	Mean corpuscular hemoglobin (MCH)	27–32 pg/cell
			(continued)

Blood Tests (Continued)

Test	Reference Range (conventional units*)	Test	Reference Range (conventional units*)
Mean corpuscular hemoglobin concentration (MCHC)	32–36% hemoglobin/cell	Sequential multiple analyzer (SMA):	
		SMA-6 (6 tests)	See individual tests: bicarbonate, chloride, glucose, potassium, sodium, urea nitrogen
Mean corpuscular volume (MCV)	76–100 cu μm	SMA-12 (12 tests)	See individual tests: bicarbonate, calcium, chloride, cholesterol, creatinine, glucose, phosphatase (alkaline), potassium, sodium, transaminases (alanine and aspartate), urea nitrogen
Osmolality	280–296 mOsm/kg water		
Oxygen pressure	83–100 mm Hg		
Oxygen saturation (arterial)	96–100%	SMA-20 (20 tests)	See individual tests: protein (albumin), bicarbonate, bilirubin (direct and total), calcium, chloride, cholesterol, creatinine, gamma-glutamyltransferase, glucose, lactic dehydrogenase, magnesium, phosphatase (alkaline), potassium, protein (total), sodium, transaminases (alanine and aspartate), urea nitrogen, uric acid
Phosphatase (acid), prostatic	0–3 units/dL (Bodansky units)		
Phosphatase (alkaline)	50–160 units/L (higher in infants and adolescents)		
Phosphorus (inorganic)	3.0–4.5 mg/dL		
Platelet count	150,000–350,000/mL		
Potassium	3.5–5.0 mEq/L		
Prostate-specific antigen (PSA)	0–4 ng/mL (increases with age)	Sodium	135–145 mEq/L
Protein: Total Albumin Globulin	6.0–8.4 gm/dL 3.5–5.0 gm/dL 2.3–3.5 gm/dL	Thyroid-stimulating hormone (TSH)	0.5–5.0 μ units/mL
		Transaminase: Alanine (ALT) Aspartate (AST)	1–21 units/L 7–27 units/L
Pyruvic acid	0.3–0.9 mg/dL	Urea nitrogen (BUN)	7–18 mg/dL
Red blood cell (RBC) count	4.2–5.9 million/μL/cu mm	Uric acid	3.0–7.0 mg/dL
		Vitamin A	30–65 μg/dL
		White blood cell (WBC) count	4,300–10,800 cells/μL/cu mm

*Conventional units can be converted to international units by using a conversion factor.

Diagnostic Procedures

Procedure	Body Area Tested	Description	More Information (page number)
Amniocentesis	Fluid from the sac surrounding the baby	Analysis of fluid to detect an abnormality in the fetus	1134, 1135 (box)
Arteriography (angiography)	Any artery in the body; commonly in the brain, heart, kidneys, aorta, or legs	X-ray study to detect a blockage or defect of an artery	78, 161, 287, 592
Audiometry	Ears	Assessment of the ability to hear and distinguish sounds at specific pitches and volumes	999
Auscultation	Heart	Listening with a stethoscope for abnormal heart sounds	72
Barium x-ray studies	Esophagus, stomach, duodenum, intestine	X-ray study to detect ulcers, tumors, or other abnormalities	484, 486
Biopsy	Any tissue in body	Examination of tissue specimen under a microscope for cancer or another abnormality	162, 560, 593, 796 (box), 1072 (box)
Blood pressure measurement	Usually an arm	Test for high or low blood pressure	115
Blood tests	Usually a blood sample from an arm	Measurement of substances in the blood to evaluate organ function and to help diagnose and monitor various disorders	558, 591, 736, 1134, 1375
Bone marrow aspiration	Hipbone or breastbone	Examination of marrow under a microscope for abnormalities of blood cells	737
Bronchoscopy	Airways of the lungs	Direct visual inspection for a tumor or other abnormality	162
Cardiac catheterization	Heart	Study of heart function and structure	78
Chorionic villus sampling	Placenta	Examination of a sample under a microscope for an abnormality in the fetus	1135
Chromosomal analysis	Blood	Examination under a microscope to detect a genetic disease or to determine a fetus' sex	1131
Colonoscopy	Large intestine	Direct visual inspection for a tumor or other abnormality	485

(continued)

Diagnostic Procedures (Continued)

Procedure	Body Area Tested	Description	More Information (page number)
Colposcopy	Cervix	Direct visual examination of the cervix with a magnifying lens	1072 (box)
Computed tomography (CT)	Any part of body	Computer-enhanced x-ray study to detect structural abnormalities	76, 161, 286, 559, 592
Conization	Cervix	Removal of a cone-shaped piece of tissue for biopsy	1072 (box)
Dilatation and curettage (D and C)	Cervix and uterus	Examination of a sample under a microscope for an abnormality of the uterine lining	1073 (box), 1074 (box)
Echocardiography	Heart	Study of heart structure and function using sound waves	76
Electrocardiography (ECG)	Heart	Study of the heart's electrical activity	73, 74 (box)
Electroencephalography (EEG)	Brain	Study of bain electrical function	287
Electromyography	Muscles	Recording of a muscle's electrical activity	287
Electrophysiologic testing	Heart	Test to evaluate rhythm or electrical conduction abnormalities	75
Endoscopic retrograde cholangiopancreatography (ERCP)	Biliary tract	X-ray study of the biliary tract after injection of a radiopaque substance using a fiber-optic tube	559 (box), 560
Endoscopy	Digestive system	Direct visual examination of internal structures using a fiber-optic tube	485
Fluoroscopy	Digestive system, heart, lungs	A continuous x-ray study that allows a doctor to see the inside of an organ as it functions	76, 484
Hysteroscopy	Uterus	Direct visual examination of the inside of the uterus with a fiber-optic tube	1072 (box)
Intravenous urography	Kidneys, urinary tract	X-ray study of the kidneys and urinary tract after intravenous injection of a radiopaque substance	591

(continued)

Diagnostic Procedures (Continued)

Procedure	Body Area Tested	Description	More Information (page number)
Laparoscopy	Abdomen	Direct visual inspection for diagnosis and treatment of abnormalities in the abdomen	486, 1073 (box)
Magnetic resonance imaging (MRI)	Any part of body	Magnetic imaging test for any structural abnormality	77, 161, 286, 593
Mammography	Breasts	X-ray study for breast cancer	1099
Mediastinoscopy	Chest	Direct visual examination of the area of the chest between the lungs	163
Myelography	Spinal column	X-ray or CT of the spinal column after injection of a radiopaque substance	287
Occult blood test	Stool	Test for blood in the stool	487
Ophthalmoscopy	Eyes	Direct visual inspection to detect abnormalities at the back of the eye	1047 (box)
Papanicolaou (Pap) test	Cervix	Examination under a microscope of cells scraped from the cervix to detect cancer	1071 (box), 1073
Paracentesis	Abdomen	Insertion of a needle into the abdominal cavity to remove fluid for examination	486
Percutaneous transhepatic cholangiography	Liver, biliary tract	X-ray study of the liver and biliary tract after injection of a radiopaque substance into the liver	559 (box), 560
Positron emission tomography (PET)	Brain and heart	Radioactive imaging to detect abnormality of function	77, 287
Pulmonary function tests	Lungs	Tests to measure the lungs' capacity to hold air, to move air in and out of the body, and to exchange oxygen and carbon dioxide	159
Radionuclide imaging	Many organs	Radioactive imaging to detect abnormalities of blood flow, structure, or function	77
Reflex tests	Tendons	Tests for abnormalities of nerve function	285

(continued)

Diagnostic Procedures (Continued)

Procedure	Body Area Tested	Description	More Information (page number)
Retrograde urography	Bladder, ureters	X-ray study of the bladder and ureters after direct insertion of a radiopaque substance	592
Sigmoidoscopy	Rectum and lower intestine	Direct visual inspection to detect polyps or cancer	485
Skin allergy tests	Usually an arm or the back	Tests for allergies	823
Spinal tap	Spinal canal	Test for abnormalities of spinal fluid	286, 374 (box)
Spirometry	Lungs	Test of lung function involving blowing into a measuring device	160 (box)
Stress test (exercise tolerance)	Heart	Test of heart function with exertion	73
Thoracentesis	Pleural fluid	Removal of fluid from the chest with a needle to detect abnormalities	161
Thoracoscopy	Lungs	Examination of the lungs through a viewing tube	163
Tympanometry	Ears	Measurement of the impedance (resistance to pressure) of the middle ear, which helps in determining the cause of hearing loss	999
Ultrasonography (ultrasound scanning)	Any part of body	Ultrasound imaging to detect structural or functional abnormalities	161, 287, 486, 557, 592, 1133, 1143 (box)
Urinalysis	Urine	Chemical analysis of urine specimen to detect protein, sugar, ketones, and blood cells	590
Venography	Veins	X-ray study to detect blockage of a vein	592

Some Trade Names of Generic Drugs

Most prescription drugs placed on the market are given trade names (also called proprietary, brand, or specialty names) to distinguish them as being produced and marketed exclusively by a particular manufacturer. In the United States, these names are usually registered as trademarks with the Patent Office; this gives the registrant certain legal rights with respect to the names' use. A trade name may be registered for a product containing a single active ingredient, with or without additives, or for one containing two or more active ingredients.

A drug marketed by several companies may have several trade names. A drug manufactured in one country and marketed in many countries may have different trade names in each country.

Throughout this book, generic (nonproprietary) names have been used whenever possible. However, because trade names are used commonly and may be more readily recognized, most of the generic drugs mentioned in this book are listed below in alphabetic order along with many of their trade names.

With few exceptions, the trade names in this list are limited to those marketed in the United States. This list is by no means all-inclusive, and no effort has been made to list every trade name

in current use for each drug. A few drugs in this list are investigational and may subsequently be released as approved new drugs. The inclusion of a drug in this list does not indicate approval of a drug's use, nor does it imply that a drug is effective or safe. Many drugs are marketed almost exclusively under their generic name. Including a trade name of such a drug in this list does not indicate an endorsement or preference for the trade name version over the generic version.

When choosing a drug, doctors must use their own judgment because each patient must be evaluated individually. Also, new research and clinical experience are constantly providing new information that may influence the choice of treatment, and authorities do not always agree on what is the best treatment.

A person fares best when well informed about the drugs he is taking and should not hesitate to ask doctors, nurses, or pharmacists questions about drugs. When using a nonprescription drug, a person should always read the information on the package and any additional information inside the package. A person who has questions about this information should talk to a pharmacist or his doctor, who should be told about any nonprescription drugs being taken.

Drug Names

Generic Name	Trade Names
Acarbose	PRECOSE
Acebutolol	SECTRAL
Acetaminophen	TYLENOL
Acetazolamide	DIAMOX
Acetohexamide	DYMELOR
Acetohydroxamic acid	LITHOSTAT
Acetophenazine	TINDAL
Acetylcysteine	MUCOMYST

Generic Name	Trade Names
ACTH	See Corticotropin
Acyclovir	ZOVIRAX
Adenosine	ADENOCARD
Albuterol	PROVENTIL, VENTOLIN
Allopurinol	LOPURIN, ZYLOPRIM
Alprazolam	XANAX
Amantadine	SYMMETREL
Amikacin	AMIKIN

(continued)

Drug Names (Continued)

Generic Name	Trade Names
Amiloride	MIDAMOR
Aminocaproic acid	AMICAR
Aminophylline	PHYLLOCONTIN
Amiodarone	CORDARONE
Amitriptyline	ELAVIL, ENDEP
Amlodipine	NORVASC
Amoxapine	ASENDIN
Amoxicillin	AMOXIL, POLYMOX
Amoxicillin/clavulanate	AUGMENTIN
Amphotericin B	FUNGIZONE
Ampicillin	OMNIPEN, POLYCILLIN, PRINCIPEN
Anisindione	MIRADON
Anthralin	ANTHRA-DERM
Asparaginase	ELSPAR
Astemizole	HISMANAL
Atenolol	TENORMIN
Atovaquone	MEPRON
Auranofin	RIDAURA
Azathioprine	IMURAN
Azithromycin	ZITHROMAX
Aztreonam	AZACTAM
Baclofen	LIORESAL
Beclomethasone	BECLOVENT, VANCERIL
Benazepril	LOTENSIN
Benzonatate	TESSALON
Benztropine	COGENTIN
Bepridil	VASCOR
Beractant	SURVANTA
Betamethasone	CELESTONE, UTICORT, VALISONE
Betaxolol	BETOPTIC, KERLONE
Bethanechol	URECHOLINE
Bisacodyl	DULCOLAX
Bisoprolol	ZEBETA
Bitolterol	TORNALATE
Bleomycin	BLENOXANE
Bretylium	BRETYLOL
Bromocriptine	PARLODEL
Brompheniramine	DIMETANE

Generic Name	Trade Names
Budesonide	RHINOCORT
Bumetanide	BUMEX
Bupropion	WELLBUTRIN
Buspirone	BuSPAR
Busulfan	MYLERAN
Butoconazole	FEMSTAT
Butorphanol	STADOL
Calcifediol	CALDEROL
Capsaicin	ZOSTRIX
Captopril	CAPOTEN
Carbamazepine	TEGRETOL
Carbenicillin	GEOCILLIN
Carmustine	BiCNU
Carteolol	CARTROL, OCUPRESS
Cefaclor	CECLOR
Cefadroxil	DURICEF, ULTRACEF
Cefazolin	ANCEF, KEFZOL, ZOLICEF
Cefixime	SUPRAX
Cefoperazone	CEFOBID
Cefprozil	CEFZIL
Ceftazidime	FORTAZ, TAZICEF, TAZIDIME
Ceftriaxone	ROCEPHIN
Cefuroxime	CEFTIN
Cephalexin	KEFLEX
Cephapirin	CEFADYL
Cephradine	ANSPOR, VELOSEF
Chlorambucil	LEUKERAN
Chloramphenicol	CHLOROMYCETIN
Chlordiazepoxide	LIBRIUM
Chlormezanone	TRANCOPAL
Chlorotrianisene	TACE
Chlorpheniramine	CHLOR-TRIMETON, TELDRIN
Chlorpromazine	THORAZINE
Chlorpropamide	DIABINESE
Chlorthalidone	HYGROTON
Cholestyramine	QUESTRAN
Cimetidine	TAGAMET
Ciprofloxacin	CILOXAN, CIPRO

(continued)

Drug Names (Continued)

Generic Name	Trade Names
Cisapride	PROPULSID
Cisplatin	PLATINOL
Clarithromycin	BIAXIN
Clemastine	TAVIST
Clindamycin	CLEOCIN
Clofazimine	LAMPRENE
Clofibrate	ATROMID-S
Clomiphene	CLOMID
Clomipramine	ANAFRANIL
Clonazepam	KLONOPIN
Clonidine	CATAPRES
Clorazepate	TRANXENE
Clotrimazole	LOTRIMIN, MYCELEX
Cloxacillin	TEGOPEN
Clozapine	CLOZARIL
Colestipol	COLESTID
Corticotropin (ACTH)	ACTHAR
Cortisol	CORTEF, HYDROCORTONE, SOLU-CORTEF
Cosyntropin	CORTROSYN
Co-trimoxazole	See Trimethoprim-sulfamethoxazole
Cromolyn	CROLOM, INTAL, NASALCHOM
Cyclandelate	CYCLOSPASMOL
Cyclizine	MAREZINE
Cyclobenzaprine	FLEXERIL
Cyclopentolate	CYCLOGYL
Cyclophosphamide	CYTOXAN
Cyclosporine	SANDIMMUNE
Cyproheptadine	PERIACTIN
Cytarabine	CYTOSAR-U
Dacarbazine	DTIC
Dactinomycin	COSMEGEN
Danazol	DANOCRINE
Dantrolene	DANTRIUM
Daunorubicin	CERUBIDINE
Deferoxamine	DESFERAL
Demeclocycline	DECLOMYCIN
Desipramine	NORPRAMIN, PERTOFRANE

Generic Name	Trade Names
Desmopressin	DDAVP, STIMATE
Dexamethasone	DECADRON, HEXADROL
Dexchlorpheniramine	POLARAMINE
Dextromethorphan	BENYLIN DM, DELSYM
Diazepam	VALIUM
Diazoxide	HYPERSTAT, PROGLYCEM
Diclofenac	CATAFLAM, VOLTAREN
Dicloxacillin	DYCILL, DYNAPEN, PATHOCIL
Dicyclomine	BENTYL
Didanosine	VIDEX
Diethylpropion	TENUATE, TEPANIL
Diflunisal	DOLOBID
Digoxin	LANOXIN
Dihydrotachysterol	HYTAKEROL
Diltiazem	CARDIZEM, DILACOR
Dinoprost	PROSTIN F2 ALPHA
Diphenhydramine	BENADRYL, NYTOL, SOMINEX
Diphenidol	VONTROL
Diphenoxylate with atropine	LOMOTIL
Dipivefrin	PROPINE
Dipyridamole	PERSANTINE
Disopyramide	NORPACE
Disulfiram	ANTABUSE
Divalproex	DEPAKOTE
Docusate	COLACE
Dopamine	INTROPIN
Dornase alfa	PULMOZYME
Dorzolamide	TRUSOPT
Doxazosin	CARDURA
Doxepin	SINEQUAN, ZONALON
Doxorubicin	ADRIAMYCIN
Doxycycline	VIBRAMYCIN
Dronabinol	MARINOL
Droperidol	INAPSINE
Echothiophate	PHOSPHOLINE
Edrophonium	TENSILON
Enalapril	VASOTEC

(continued)

Drug Names (Continued)

Generic Name	Trade Names	Generic Name	Trade Names
Enoxacin	PENETREX	Gentamicin	GARAMYCIN
Enoxaparin	LOVENOX	Glipizide	GLUCOTROL
Epoetin alfa	EPOGEN, PROCRIT	Glyburide	DIABETA, MICRONASE
Ergocalciferol	DRISDOL	Gold	MYOCHRYSINE
Erythromycin	E-MYCIN, ERYTHROCIN, ILOSONE	Granisetron	KYTRIL
Estazolam	PROSOM	Griseofulvin	FULVICIN, GRIFULVIN V, GRISACTIN
Estrogens	PREMARIN	Guaifenesin	ROBITUSSIN
Ethacrynic acid	EDECRIN	Guanabenz	WYTENSIN
Ethambutol	MYAMBUTOL	Guanadrel	HYLOREL
Etidronate	DIDRONEL	Guanfacine	TENEX
Etodolac	LODINE	Halazepam	PAXIPAM
Etretinate	TEGISON	Haloperidol	HALDOL
Famciclovir	FAMVIR	Haloprogin	HALOTEX
Famotidine	PEPCID	Hydralazine	APRESOLINE
Felodipine	PLENDIL	Hydrochlorothiazide	ESIDRIX, HydroDIURIL, ORETIC
Fenfluramine	PONDIMIN	Hydrocortisone	See Cortisol
Fenoprofen	NALFON	Hydromorphone	DILAUDID
Fentanyl	SUBLIMAZE	Hydroquinone	ELDOQUIN
Filgrastim	NEUPOGEN	Hydroxychloroquine	PLAQUENIL
Finasteride	PROSCAR	Hydroxyprogesterone	DELALUTIN
Flecainide	TAMBOCOR	Hydroxyurea	HYDREA
Fluconazole	DIFLUCAN	Hydroxyzine	ATARAX, VISTARIL
Flucytosine	ANCOBON	Ibuprofen	ADVIL, MOTRIN, NUPRIN
Fludrocortisone	FLORINEF	Idoxuridine	HERPLEX, STOXIL
Flunisolide	NASALIDE	Imipramine	TOFRANIL
Fluocinolone	SYNALAR	Indapamide	LOZOL
Fluocinonide	LIDEX	Indomethacin	INDOCIN
Fluoxetine	PROZAC	Insulin	HUMULIN, NOVOLIN
Fluoxymesterone	HALOTESTIN	Ipratropium	ATROVENT
Fluphenazine	PERMITIL, PROLIXIN	Isoetharine	BRONKOSOL
Flurandrenolide	CORDRAN	Isoniazid	INH, NYDRAZID
Flurazepam	DALMANE	Isoproterenol	ISUPREL
Flurbiprofen	ANSAID, OCUFEN	Isosorbide	ISORDIL, SORBITRATE
Fluvastatin	LESCOL	Isotretinoin	ACCUTANE
Fosinopril	MONOPRIL	Isradipine	DYNACIRC
Furosemide	LASIX	Itraconazole	SPORANOX
Gabapentin	NEURONTIN	Kanamycin	KANTREX
Ganciclovir	CYTOVENE	Ketoconazole	NIZORAL
Gemfibrozil	LOPID		

(continued)

Drug Names (Continued)

Generic Name	Trade Names
Ketoprofen	ORUDIS, ORUVAIL
Ketorolac	TORADOL
Labetalol	NORMODYNE, TRANDATE
Lactulose	CEPHULAC, CHRONULAC
Lamotrigine	LAMICTAL
Lansoprazole	PREVACID
Levamisole	ERGAMISOL
Levarterenol	See Norepinephrine
Levodopa	DOPAR, LARODOPA
Levodopa-carbidopa	SINEMET
Levothyroxine (T_4)	LEVOXYL, SYNTHROID
Lidocaine	XYLOCAINE
Lindane	KWELL
Liothyronine (T_3)	CYTOMEL
Lisinopril	PRINIVIL, ZESTRIL
Lithium	LITHANE, LITHONATE
Lomefloxacin	MAXAQUIN
Lomustine	CeeNU
Loperamide	IMODIUM
Loratadine	CLARITIN
Lorazepam	ATIVAN
Losartan	COZAAR
Lovastatin	MEVACOR
Loxapine	LOXITANE
Mafenide	SULFAMYLON
Maprotiline	LUDIOMIL
Mazindol	MAZANOR, SANOREX
Mebendazole	VERMOX
Mechlorethamine	MUSTARGEN
Meclizine	ANTIVERT, BONINE
Meclofenamate	MECLOMEN
Medroxyprogesterone	PROVERA
Mefenamic acid	PONSTEL
Megestrol	MEGACE
Melphalan	ALKERAN
Menadiol	SYNKAYVITE
Menotropins	PERGONAL
Meperidine	DEMEROL
Mephenytoin	MESANTOIN

Generic Name	Trade Names
Meprobamate	EQUANIL, MILTOWN
Mercaptopurine	PURINETHOL
Mesalamine	ASACOL, ROWASA
Mesoridazine	SERENTIL
Metaproterenol	ALUPENT, METAPREL
Metaraminol	ARAMINE
Metformin	GLUCOPHAGE
Methadone	DOLOPHINE
Methamphetamine	DESOXYN
Methandrostenolone	DIANABOL
Methdilazine	TACARYL
Methenamine	HIPREX, MANDELAMINE
Methicillin	STAPHCILLIN
Methimazole	TAPAZOLE
Methocarbamol	ROBAXIN
Methotrexate	RHEUMATREX
Methotrimeprazine	LEVOPROME
Methoxsalen	OXSORALEN
Methsuximide	CELONTIN
Methyldopa	ALDOMET
Methylphenidate	RITALIN
Methylprednisolone	MEDROL
Methyltestosterone	ORETON
Methysergide	SANSERT
Metoclopramide	REGLAN
Metolazone	MYKROX, ZAROXOLYN
Metoprolol	LOPRESSOR
Metronidazole	FLAGYL
Mexiletine	MEXITIL
Mezlocillin	MEZLIN
Miconazole	MICATIN, MONISTAT
Milrinone	PRIMACOR
Minocycline	MINOCIN
Minoxidil	LONITEN, ROGAINE
Misoprostol	CYTOTEC
Mitomycin	MUTAMYCIN
Mitotane	LYSODREN
Moexipril	UNIVASC
Molindone	MOBAN
Morphine	MS CONTIN

(continued)

Drug Names (Continued)

Generic Name	Trade Names
Nabumetone	RELAFEN
Nadolol	CORGARD
Nafcillin	UNIPEN
Nalbuphine	NUBAIN
Nalidixic acid	NegGRAM
Naloxone	NARCAN
Naltrexone	REVIA
Nandrolone	DURABOLIN
Naproxen	ALEVE
Nedocromil	TILADE
Nefazodone	SERZONE
Neostigmine	PROSTIGMIN
Nicardipine	CARDENE
Niclosamide	NICLOCIDE
Nicotine	NICORETTE, NICOTROL
Nifedipine	ADALAT, PROCARDIA
Nimodipine	NIMOTOP
Nitrofurantoin	FURADANTIN, MACRODANTIN
Nitroprusside	NIPRIDE
Nizatidine	AXID
Norepinephrine	LEVOPHED
Norfloxacin	NOROXIN
Nortriptyline	AVENTYL
Nystatin	MYCOSTATIN, NILSTAT
Octreotide	SANDOSTATIN
Ofloxacin	FLOXIN
Olsalazine	DIPENTUM
Omeprazole	PRILOSEC
Ondansetron	ZOFRAN
Oxacillin	PROSTAPHLIN
Oxamniquine	VANSIL
Oxandrolone	OXANDRIN
Oxaprozin	DAYPRO
Oxazepam	SERAX
Oxybutynin	DITROPAN
Oxymetazoline	AFRIN
Oxymetholone	ANADROL
Oxytocin	PITOCIN, SYNTOCINON
Paclitaxel	TAXOL
Pamidronate	AREDIA

Generic Name	Trade Names
Pancrelipase	PANCREASE, VIOKASE
Papaverine	PAVABID
Paromomycin	HUMATIN
Paroxetine	PAXIL
Penbutolol	LEVATOL
Penicillamine	CUPRIMINE
Pentamidine	NEBUPENT, PENTAM 300
Pentazocine	TALWIN
Pentobarbital	NEMBUTAL
Pentoxifylline	TRENTAL
Pergolide	PERMAX
Perphenazine	TRILAFON
Phenacemide	PHENURONE
Phenazopyridine	PYRIDIUM
Phenelzine	NARDIL
Phenobarbital	LUMINAL
Phenoxybenzamine	DIBENZYLINE
Phensuximide	MILONTIN
Phentermine	IONAMIN
Phentolamine	REGITINE
Phenylephrine	NEO-SYNEPHRINE
Phenytoin	DILANTIN
Phytonadione	KONAKION, MEPHYTON
Pindolol	VISKEN
Piperacillin	PIPRACIL
Pipobroman	VERCYTE
Piroxicam	FELDENE
Plicamycin	MITHRACIN
Pravastatin	PRAVACHOL
Prazepam	CENTRAX
Praziquantel	BILTRICIDE
Prazosin	MINIPRESS
Prednisolone	DELTA-CORTEF, HYDELTRASOL
Prednisone	DELTASONE, METICORTEN
Primidone	MYSOLINE
Probenecid	BENEMID
Probucol	LORELCO
Procainamide	PROCAN SR, PRONESTYL

(continued)

Drug Names (Continued)

Generic Name	Trade Names
Procaine	NOVOCAIN
Procarbazine	MATULANE
Prochlorperazine	COMPAZINE
Procyclidine	KEMADRIN
Promazine	SPARINE
Promethazine	PHENERGAN
Propafenone	RYTHMOL
Propantheline	PRO-BANTHINE
Proparacaine	OPHTHAINE, OPHTHETIC
Propiomazine	LARGON
Propoxyphene	DARVON, DOLENE
Propranolol	INDERAL
Protriptyline	VIVACTIL
Pseudoephedrine	AFRINOL, SUDAFED
Pyrantel	ANTIMINTH
Pyridostigmine	MESTINON
Pyrimethamine	DARAPRIM
Quazepam	DORAL
Quinacrine	ATABRINE
Quinapril	ACCUPRIL
Quinethazone	HYDROMOX
Quinidine	CARDIOQUIN, QUINAGLUTE
Ramipril	ALTACE
Ranitidine	ZANTAC
Ribavirin	VIRAZOLE
Rifabutin	MYCOBUTIN
Rifampin	RIFADIN, RIMACTANE
Rimantadine	FLUMADINE
Risperidone	RISPERDAL
Ritodrine	YUTOPAR
Salmeterol	SEREVENT
Salsalate	DISALCID, SALFLEX
Sargramostim	LEUKINE
Secobarbital	SECONAL
Selegiline	ELDEPRYL
Selenium	SELSUN
Sertraline	ZOLOFT
Silver sulfadiazine	SILVADENE
Simethicone	MYLICON, PHAZYME

Generic Name	Trade Names
Simvastatin	ZOCOR
Somatrem	PROTROPIN
Somatropin	HUMATROPE
Sotalol	BETAPACE
Spectinomycin	TROBICIN
Spironolactone	ALDACTONE
Stanozolol	WINSTROL
Stavudine	ZERIT
Streptokinase	STREPTASE
Sucralfate	CARAFATE
Sulfamethoxazole	GANTANOL
Sulfasalazine	AZULFIDINE
Sulfinpyrazone	ANTURANE
Sulfisoxazole	GANTRISIN
Sulindac	CLINORIL
Sumatriptan	IMITREX
Suprofen	PROFENAL
Tacrine	COGNEX
Tacrolimus	PROGRAF
Tamoxifen	NOLVADEX
Temazepam	RESTORIL
Terazosin	HYTRIN
Terbutaline	BRETHINE, BRICANYL
Terfenadine	SELDANE
Testolactone	TESLAC
Testosterone	DELATESTRYL, DEPO-TESTOSTERONE
Tetanus immune globulin (human)	HYPER-TET
Tetracycline	ACHROMYCIN V, TETRACYN, TETREX
Theophylline	ELIXOPHYLLIN, THEO-DUR
Thiabendazole	MINTEZOL
Thiethylperazine	TORECAN
Thioridazine	MELLARIL
Thiothixene	NAVANE
Thyrotropin	THYTROPAR
Ticarcillin	TICAR
Ticlopidine	TICLID
Timolol	BLOCADREN, TIMOPTIC

(continued)

Drug Names (Continued)

Generic Name	Trade Names
Tobramycin	NEBCIN, TOBREX
Tocainide	TONOCARD
Tolazamide	TOLINASE
Tolazoline	PRISCOLINE
Tolbutamide	ORINASE
Tolmetin	TOLECTIN
Tolnaftate	TINACTIN
Torsemide	DEMADEX
Tramadol	ULTRAM
Tranylcypromine	PARNATE
Trazodone	DESYREL
Tretinoin	RETIN-A
Triamcinolone	ARISTOCORT, KENACORT, KENALOG
Triamterene	DYRENIUM
Triazolam	HALCION
Trifluoperazine	STELAZINE
Triflupromazine	VESPRIN
Trifluridine	VIROPTIC
Trihexyphenidyl	ARTANE
Trimeprazine	TEMARIL

Generic Name	Trade Names
Trimethadione	TRIDIONE
Trimethobenzamide	TIGAN
Trimethoprim	PROLOPRIM, TRIMPEX
Trimethoprim-sulfamethoxazole	BACTRIM, SEPTRA
Trimipramine	SURMONTIL
Tromethamine	THAM
Tropicamide	MYDRIACYL
Valacyclovir	VALTREX
Valproic acid	DEPAKENE
Vancomycin	VANCOCIN
Vasopressin	PITRESSIN
Venlafaxine	EFFEXOR
Verapamil	CALAN, ISOPTIN
Vidarabine	VIRA-A
Vinblastine	VELBAN
Vincristine	ONCOVIN
Warfarin	COUMADIN
Zalcitabine	HIVID
Zidovudine	RETROVIR
Zolpidem	AMBIEN

APPENDIX V

Resources for Help and Information

The following list is selective and restricted largely to national organizations in the United States, many of which have local chapters. Sites chosen are generally not-for-profit and usually offer information or support rather than advocacy. Telephone numbers, e-mail addresses, and web sites are included as appropriate; however, such information changes frequently. Additional information is available through health care practitioners, local libraries, telephone listings, and the Internet.

ation on Aging
80 (information on Alzheimer's disease)
25 (information on other publications)
oa.gov/aoa/resource

ociation of Retired People
W
C 20049
02-434-2277
rg

on of Area Agencies on

00
36
m

ng

00

itizens

on

);

ER

tion

on Deficit

e 101

n of America

ch

CDC National AIDS/HIV Hotline
800-342-AIDS
http://sunsite.unc.edu/asha

Gay Men's Health Crisis
129 West 20 Street
New York, NY 10011-3629
212-337-3519 (Development); 212-337-3505
(Volunteer)
http://noah.cuny.edu/providers/gmhc.html

National Association for People with AIDS
1413 K Street, NW
Washington, DC 20005
202-898-0414
e-mail: napwa@thecure.org
http://www.thecure.org

Project Inform
1965 Market Street, Suite 220 (at Duboce)
San Francisco, CA 94103
800-822-7422; 415-558-9051; 415-558-8669
http://www.projinf.org

**Universal Fellowship of Metropolitan
Community Churches AIDS Ministry**
5300 Santa Monica Boulevard, Suite 304
Los Angeles, CA 90029
213-464-5100
e-mail: ufmcchq@aol.com
http://www.thebody.com/ufmcc/ufmcc.html

Women Alive
1566 S Burnside Avenue
Los Angeles, CA 90019
213-965-1564
e-mail: womenalive@aol.com
http://www.thebody.com/wa/wapage.html

ALCOHOLISM (see also Drug Abuse)

Al-Anon Family Group Headquarters
1600 Corporate Landing Parkway
Virginia Beach, VA 23454
800-356-9996; 757-563-1600
http://www.al-anon.alateen.org

Alcoholics Anonymous
PO Box 459, Grand Central Station
New York, NY 10163
212-870-3400
http://www.alcoholics-anonymous.org

**National Clearinghouse for Alcohol &
Information**
PO Box 2345
Rockville, MD 20847
800-729-6686; 301-468-2600
http://www.health.org

**National Council on Alc
Dependence**
12 West 21st Street
New York, NY 100
800-NCA-CALL
http://www.nc

Secular Organizations for Sobriety
National Clearinghouse
The Center for Inquiry – West
5521 Grosvenor Boulevard
Los Angeles, CA 90066
310-821-8430
e-mail: sosla@loop.com; cfiflynn@aol.com

ALLERGY & ASTHMA

Allergy and Asthma Network/Mothers of Asthmatics, Inc.
3554 Chain Bridge Road, Suite 200
Fairfax, VA 22030
800-878-4403; 703-385-4403
http://www.podi.com/health/aanma

Asthma & Allergy Foundation of America
1125 15th Street NW, Suite 502
Washington, DC 20005
800-7ASTHMA; 202-466-7643
http://www.aafa.org

ALZHEIMER'S DISEASE & OTHER DEMENTIAS

Alzheimer's Association
919 N Michigan Avenue, Suite 1000
Chicago, IL 60611-1676
800-272-3900; 312-335-8700
http://www.alz.org

Alzheimer's Disease Education & Referral Center
PO Box 8250
Silver Spring, MD 20907-8250
800-438-4380; 301-495-3311
e-mail: adear@alzheimers.org
http://www.alzheimers.org

AMPUTATION
(see also Disabilities & Rehabilitation)

The American Amputee Foundation, Inc.
Executive Assistant
PO Box 250218
illcrest Station
e Rock, AR 72225
66-2523

s' Service Association
ng Park Road
0618

on Foundation

AMYLOIDOSIS

Amyloidosis Network International, Inc.
c/o Jim Lang
7118 Cole Creek Drive
Houston, TX 77092-1421
713-466-4351

AMYOTROPHIC LATERAL SCLERO

The ALS Association
National Office
21021 Ventura Boulevard, Suite 321
Woodland Hills, CA 91364
800-782-4747 (patients only); 818-340-75
e-mail: eajc27b@prodigy.com
http://www.alsa.org

ANKYLOSING SPONDYLITIS

Ankylosing Spondylitis Association
PO Box 5872
Sherman Oaks, CA 91413
800-777-8189
http://www.spondylitis.org

ARTHRITIS

American Juvenile Arthritis Organizat
1314 Spring Street NW
Atlanta, GA 30309
800-283-7800; 404-872-7100

Arthritis Foundation
1330 W Peachtree Street
Atlanta, GA 30309
800-283-7800; 404-872-7100
http://www.arthritis.org

ASTHMA (see Allergy & Asthma)

ATTENTION DEFICIT DISORD

Attention Deficit Disorder Associa
PO Box 972
Mentor, OH 44061
216-350-9595
http://www.add.org

Children and Adults With Attenti Disorders
499 Northwest 70th Avenue, Suit
Plantation, FL 33317
800-233-4050
http://www.chadd.org

Learning Disabilities Associatio
4156 Library Road
Pittsburgh, PA 15234
412-341-1515
http://www.ldanatl.org

AGING

Administration on Aging
800-438-4380 (information on Alzheimer's disease)
800-222-2225 (information on other publications)
http://www.aoa.gov/aoa/resource

American Association of Retired People
601 E Street NW
Washington, DC 20049
800-424-3410; 202-434-2277
http://www.aarp.org

National Association of Area Agencies on Aging
1112 16th Street NW
Washington, DC 20036
202-296-8130
e-mail: jbn4a@erols.com

National Council on Aging
409 Third Street SW
Washington, DC 20024
800-867-2755; 202-479-1200
e-mail: library@ncoa.org
http://www.n4a.org

National Council of Senior Citizens
1331 F Street NW
Washington, DC 20004
202-347-8800

National Institute on Aging
Public Information Office
Building 31, Room 5C27, 31
Center Drive, MSC 2292
Bethesda, MD 20892-2292
800-222-2225, 800-222-4225 (TTY);
301-496-1752
http://www.nih.gov/nia

Older Women's League
666 11th Street NW, Suite 700
Washington, DC 20001
202-783-6686

AIDS

AIDS Action Council
1875 Connecticut Avenue NW, #700
Washington, DC 20009
202-986-1300
http://www.thebody.com/aac/aacpage.html

AIDS National Interfaith Network
110 Washington Avenue NE, Suite 504
Washington, DC 20002
202-546-0807
http://www.thebody.com/anin/aninpage.html

The American Foundation for AIDS Research
733 Third Avenue, 12th Floor
New York, NY 10017
212-682-7440
http://www.thebody.com/amfar/amfar.html

CDC National AIDS/HIV Hotline
800-342-AIDS
http://sunsite.unc.edu/asha

Gay Men's Health Crisis
129 West 20 Street
New York, NY 10011-3629
212-337-3519 (Development); 212-337-3505 (Volunteer)
http://noah.cuny.edu/providers/gmhc.html

National Association for People with AIDS
1413 K Street, NW
Washington, DC 20005
202-898-0414
e-mail: napwa@thecure.org
http://www.thecure.org

Project Inform
1965 Market Street, Suite 220 (at Duboce)
San Francisco, CA 94103
800-822-7422; 415-558-9051; 415-558-8669
http://www.projinf.org

Universal Fellowship of Metropolitan Community Churches AIDS Ministry
5300 Santa Monica Boulevard, Suite 304
Los Angeles, CA 90029
213-464-5100
e-mail: ufmcchq@aol.com
http://www.thebody.com/ufmcc/ufmcc.html

Women Alive
1566 S Burnside Avenue
Los Angeles, CA 90019
213-965-1564
e-mail: womenalive@aol.com
http://www.thebody.com/wa/wapage.html

ALCOHOLISM (see also Drug Abuse)

Al-Anon Family Group Headquarters
1600 Corporate Landing Parkway
Virginia Beach, VA 23454
800-356-9996; 757-563-1600
http://www.al-anon.alateen.org

Alcoholics Anonymous
PO Box 459, Grand Central Station
New York, NY 10163
212-870-3400
http://www.alcoholics-anonymous.org

National Clearinghouse for Alcohol & Drug Information
PO Box 2345
Rockville, MD 20847
800-729-6686; 301-468-2600
http://www.health.org

National Council on Alcoholism & Drug Dependence
12 West 21st Street
New York, NY 10010
800-NCA-CALL; 212-206-6770
http://www.ncadd.org

(continued)

Secular Organizations for Sobriety
National Clearinghouse
The Center for Inquiry – West
5521 Grosvenor Boulevard
Los Angeles, CA 90066
310-821-8430
e-mail: sosla@loop.com; cfiflynn@aol.com

ALLERGY & ASTHMA

Allergy and Asthma Network/Mothers of
Asthmatics, Inc.
3554 Chain Bridge Road, Suite 200
Fairfax, VA 22030
800-878-4403; 703-385-4403
http://www.podi.com/health/aanma

Asthma & Allergy Foundation of America
1125 15th Street NW, Suite 502
Washington, DC 20005
800-7ASTHMA; 202-466-7643
http://www.aafa.org

ALZHEIMER'S DISEASE
& OTHER DEMENTIAS

Alzheimer's Association
919 N Michigan Avenue, Suite 1000
Chicago, IL 60611-1676
800-272-3900; 312-335-8700
http://www.alz.org

Alzheimer's Disease Education & Referral
Center
PO Box 8250
Silver Spring, MD 20907-8250
800-438-4380; 301-495-3311
e-mail: adear@alzheimers.org
http://www.alzheimers.org

AMPUTATION
(see also Disabilities & Rehabilitation)

The American Amputee Foundation, Inc.
Executive Assistant
PO Box 250218
Hillcrest Station
Little Rock, AR 72225
501-666-2523

Amputees' Service Association
3953 W Irving Park Road
Chicago, IL 60618
773-583-3949

National Amputation Foundation
38-40 Church Street
Malverne, NY 11565
516-887-3600

AMYLOIDOSIS

Amyloidosis Network International, Inc.
c/o Jim Lang
7118 Cole Creek Drive
Houston, TX 77092-1421
713-466-4351

AMYOTROPHIC LATERAL SCLEROSIS

The ALS Association
National Office
21021 Ventura Boulevard, Suite 321
Woodland Hills, CA 91364
800-782-4747 (patients only); 818-340-7500
e-mail: eajc27b@prodigy.com
http://www.alsa.org

ANKYLOSING SPONDYLITIS

Ankylosing Spondylitis Association
PO Box 5872
Sherman Oaks, CA 91413
800-777-8189
http://www.spondylitis.org

ARTHRITIS

American Juvenile Arthritis Organization
1314 Spring Street NW
Atlanta, GA 30309
800-283-7800; 404-872-7100

Arthritis Foundation
1330 W Peachtree Street
Atlanta, GA 30309
800-283-7800; 404-872-7100
http://www.arthritis.org

ASTHMA (see Allergy & Asthma)

ATTENTION DEFICIT DISORDER

Attention Deficit Disorder Association
PO Box 972
Mentor, OH 44061
216-350-9595
http://www.add.org

Children and Adults With Attention Deficit
Disorders
499 Northwest 70th Avenue, Suite 101
Plantation, FL 33317
800-233-4050
http://www.chadd.org

Learning Disabilities Association of America
4156 Library Road
Pittsburgh, PA 15234
412-341-1515
http://www.ldanatl.org

AUTISM

Autism Research Institute
4182 Adams Avenue
San Diego, CA 92116

Autism Society of America
7910 Woodmont Avenue, Suite 650
Bethesda, MD 20814
800-328-8476; 301-657-0881
http://www.autism-society.org

National Autism Hotline/Autism Services Center
605 Ninth Street
PO Box 507
Huntington, WV 25710-0507
304-525-8014

BALDING

National Alopecia Areata Foundation
710 C Street, Suite 11
San Rafael, CA 94901
415-456-4644
e-mail: naaf@compuserve.com

BEREAVEMENT (see Death & Bereavement)

BIRTH DEFECTS
(see also Cleft Palate; Spina Bifida)

Association of Birth Defect Children
3526 Emerywood Lane
Orlando, FL 32806
305-859-2821

Federation for Children With Special Needs
95 Berkeley Street, Suite 104
Boston, MA 02116
617-482-2915 (Voice/TTY)
e-mail: fcsninfo@bitwise.net
http://www.tcsn.org

March of Dimes/Birth Defects Foundation
1275 Mamaroneck Avenue
White Plains, NY 10605
888-663-4637; 914-428-7100
e-mail: resources@modimes.org
http://grove.ufl.edu/~kryton/mod/mod.html

National Association for Jewish Genetic Diseases
250 Park Avenue, Suite 1000
New York, NY 10177
212-682-5550

BLINDNESS & VISION PROBLEMS

American Association of the DeafBlind
814 Thayer Avenue, Suite 302
Silver Spring, MD 20910
301-588-6545 (TTY)

American Council of the Blind
1155 15th Street NW, Suite 720
Washington, DC 20005
800-424-8666
http://www.acb.org

American Foundation for the Blind
11 Penn Plaza, Suite 300
New York, NY 10001
800-232-5463; 212-502-7600
e-mail: newyork@fab.org
http://www.igc.apc.org/afb

Association for the Education & Rehabilitation of the Blind & Visually Impaired
206 North Washington Street
Alexandria, VA 22314
703-548-1884
e-mail: aernet@laser.met

Association for Macular Diseases
210 East 64th Street
New York, NY 10021
212-605-3719

Fight for Sight
160 East 56th Street, 8th Floor
New York, NY 10022
212-751-1118

The Foundation Fighting Blindness
1401 Mount Royal Avenue, 4th Floor
Baltimore, MD 21217-4245
800-683-5555; 800-683-5551 (TTY);
410-785-1414
http://www.blindness.org

Glaucoma Research Foundation
490 Post Street, Suite 830
San Francisco, CA 94102
800-826-6696; 415-986-3162
http://www.glaucoma.org

National Association for Visually Handicapped
22 West 21st Street, 6th Floor
New York, NY 10010
212-889-3141
http://www.navh.org

National Family Association for DeafBlind
111 Middle Neck Road
Sands Point, NY 11050
800-255-0411, ext. 275; 516-944-8637 (TTY)
http://www.helenkeller.org

National Retinitis Pigmentosa Foundation
Executive Plaza 1, Suite 800
11350 McCormick Road
Hunt Valley, MD 21031-1014
800-683-5555; 410-771-9470
http://www.blindness.org

Prevent Blindness America
500 East Remington Road
Schaumburg, IL 60173
800-331-2020; 312-843-2020
e-mail: 74777.100@compuserve.com
http://www.prevent-blindness.org

BLOOD DISORDERS

Leukemia Society of America
600 Third Avenue
New York, NY 10016
800-955-4LSA; 212-573-8484
http://www.leukemia.org

National Association for Sickle Cell Disease
200 Corporate Pointe, Suite 495
Culver City, CA 90230
800-421-8453; 310-216-6363

National Hemophilia Foundation
110 Greene Street
New York, NY 10012
212-219-8180
http://www.hemophilia.org

Thalassemia Action Group
129-09 26th Avenue
Flushing, NY 11354
800-522-7222; 718-321-CURE (2873)
http://www.infinet.com/~bzeidman/thal/thal.html

BRAIN DISORDERS (see also Cancer & Other Tumors; Alzheimer's Disease & Other Dementias; Epilepsy)

Brain Injury Association
1776 Massachusetts Avenue NW, Suite 100
Washington, DC 20036
800-444-NHIF; 202-296-6443

National Institute of Neurological Disorders & Stroke
Office of Scientific & Health Reports
PO Box 5801
Bethesda, MD 20824
800-352-9424; 301-496-5751
http://www.ninds.nih.gov

CANCER & OTHER TUMORS

American Cancer Society
1599 Clifton Road NE
Atlanta, GA 30329-4251
800-ACS-2345; 404-320-3333
http://www.cancer.org

Cancer Care, Inc.
1180 Avenue of the Americas
New York, NY 10036
212-302-2400
http://www.cancercareinc.org

National Cancer Institute
Cancer Information Service
9000 Rockville Pike
Bethesda, MD 20892
800-4-CANCER; 301-496-5583

National Coalition for Cancer Survivorship
1010 Wayne Avenue, Suite 300
Silver Spring, MD 20910
301-650-8868
http://www.pageup.com/~partner/rev3

Patient Advocates for Advanced Cancer Treatments
PO Box 141695
Grand Rapids, MI 49514-1695
616-453-1477

Brain

Acoustic Neuroma Association
PO Box 12402
Atlanta, GA 30355
404-237-8023
e-mail: ana usa@aol.com
http://www.anausa.org

American Brain Tumor Association
2720 River Road, Suite 146
Des Plains, IL 60018-4110
800-886-2282; 847-827-9910
e-mail: abta@aol.com
http://www.abta.org

Brain Tumor Foundation for Children
2231 Perimeter Park Drive, Suite 9
Atlanta, GA 30341
770-458-5554

Brain Tumor Hotline
University of Chicago
5841 S Maryland Avenue, Room J331
Chicago, IL 60637
312-684-1400

Brain Tumor Society
84 Seattle Street
Boston, MA 02134
800-770-8287; 617-783-0340
e-mail: info@tbts.org
http://www.tbts.org/welcome.htm

The Children's Brain Tumor Foundation
42 Memorial Plaza
Pleasantville, NY 10570
914-747-0301

National Brain Tumor Foundation
785 Market Street, Suite 1600
San Francisco, CA 94103
800-934-CURE
e-mail: sstf39b@prodigy.com
http://www.braintumor.org

Pituitary Tumor Network Association
16350 Ventura Boulevard, #231
Encino, CA 91436
800-642-9211; 805-499-9973
e-mail: ptna@pituitary.com
http://www.pituitary.com

Breast

**National Alliance of Breast Cancer
Organizations**
9 East 37th Street, 10th Floor
New York, NY 10016
800-719-9154
http://www.nabco.org

**The Susan G. Komen Breast Cancer
Foundation**
National Headquarters
5005 LBJ Freeway, Suite 370
Dallas, TX 75244
800-I'M AWARE (462-9273); 972-233-0351
http://www.breastcancerinfo.com

Y-ME: National Breast Cancer Organization
212 W Van Buren Street
Chicago, IL 60607-3908
800-221-2141; 312-986-8228; 312-986-8338

Prostate

US-TOO International
930 N York Road, Suite 50
Hinsdale, IL 60521-2993
603-323-1002
http://www.ustoo.com

Skin

Skin Cancer Foundation
245 Fifth Avenue, Suite 1403
New York, NY 10016
212-725-5176

CARDIOVASCULAR DISORDERS

American Heart Association
7272 Greenville Avenue
Dallas, TX 75231
214-373-6300
http://www.amhrt.org

Coronary Club
9500 Euclid Avenue, EE37
Cleveland, OH 44195
800-478-4255; 216-444-3690

National Heart, Lung, & Blood Institute
Information Center
PO Box 30105
Bethesda, MD 20824-0105
301-251-1222

National Stroke Association
96 Inverness Drive East, Suite I
Englewood, CO 80112
800-787-6537; 303-649-9299
e-mail: info@stroke.org
http://www.stroke.org

Sister Konny Institute
Division of Abbott-Northwestern Hospital
800 East 28th Street
Minneapolls, MN 55407
612-863-4457

CEREBRAL PALSY

United Cerebral Palsy Associations, Inc.
1660 L Street NW
Washington, DC 20036-5602
800-USA-5-UCP; 202-776-0406; 202-973-7197
(TTY)
e-mail: ucpanatl@ucpa.org
http://www.ucpa.org

CHILD ABUSE & NEGLECT

**American Humane Association, Children's
Division**
63 Inverness Drive East
Englewood, CO 80112-5117
800-227-4645; 303-792-9900
http://www.amerhumane.org

Kempe Children's Center
1205 Oneida Street
Denver, CO 80220
303-321-3963
http://www.hsc.colorado.edu/ctrsinst/clininst/
kempe.html

CHILDBIRTH/PREGNANCY
(see also Family Planning; Infertility)

America's Crisis Pregnancy Helpline
2121 Valley View Lane
Dallas, TX 75234
800-67-BABY6; 972-241-BABY
e-mail: acph@dallas.net
http://www.thehelpline.org

Maternity Center Association
281 Park Avenue South, 5th Floor
New York, NY 10010
212-777-5000

The National Coalition for Birthing Alternatives
4755 West Avenue, L-13
Quartz Hill, CA 93536
e-mail: heathert@ptw.com
http://www.ptw.com/~troytash

CLEFT PALATE

Cleft Palate Foundation
104 South Estes Drive, Suite 204
Chapel Hill, NC 27514
919-933-9604
e-mail: cleftline@aol.com
http://www.cleft.com

(continued)

Wide Smiles
PO Box 5153
Stockton, CA 95205-0153
209-942-2812
e-mail: widesmiles@aol.com
http://www.widesmiles.org/index.html

CONTRACEPTION (see Family Planning)

CYSTIC FIBROSIS

National Cystic Fibrosis Foundation
6931 Arlington Road
Bethesda, MD 20814
800-344-4823
http://www.cff.org

DEAFNESS & HEARING DISORDERS

Alexander Graham Bell Association for the
Deaf
3417 Volta Place NW
Washington, DC 20007
800-432-7543; 202-337-5220 (Voice/TTY)
e-mail: agbell2@aol.com
http://www.agbell.org

American Association of the DeafBlind
814 Thayer Avenue, Suite 302
Silver Spring, MD 20910
301-588-6545 (TTY)

American Society for Deaf Children
2848 Arden Way, Suite 210
Sacramento, CA 95825-1373
800-942-ASDC; 916-482-0120 (Voice/TTY)
e-mail: asdci@aol.com
http://www.deafchildren.org

American Tinnitus Association
PO Box 5
Portland, OR 97207
503-248-9985
e-mail: tinnitus@ata.org

Deafness Research Foundation
15 West 39th Street
New York, NY 10018
800-535-3323; 212-768-1181 (Voice/TDD)

Helen Keller National Center for DeafBlind
Youths and Adults
111 Middle Neck Road
Sands Point, NY 11050
800-255-0411; 516-944-8637 (TTY)

National Association of the Deaf
814 Thayer Avenue
Silver Spring, MD 20910
301-587-1788; 301-587-1789 (TTY)
http://www.nad.org

National Information Center on Deafness
Gallaudet University, 800 Florida Avenue NE
Washington, DC 20002-3695
202-651-5051; 202-651-5052 (TTY)
e-mail: nicd@gallux.gallaudet.edu
http://www.gallaudet.edu\~nicd

DEATH & BEREAVEMENT

AMEND (Moms Experiencing Neonatal Death)
43224 Berrywick Terrace
St. Louis, MO 63128
314-487-7582; 203-746-6518

Choice in Dying
200 Varick Street
New York, NY 10014-4810
800-989-9455; 212-366-5540
e-mail: cid@choices.org
http://www.choices.org

Compassionate Friends, National
Headquarters
PO Box 3696
Oak Brook, IL 60522-3696
630-990-0010
http://www.compassionatefriends.org

Dying Well Network
PO Box 880
Spokane, WA 99210-0880
509-926-2457
e-mail: Rob.Neils@ior.com
http://www.ior.com/~jeffw/dwnflyer.htm

Hemlock Society USA
PO Box 101810
Denver, CO 80250
800-247-7421
e-mail: hemlock@privatei.com
http://www.irsociety.com/hemlock.htm

Hospice Education Institute
190 Westbrook Road
Essex, CT 06426
800-331-1620; 860-767-1620
e-mail: hospiceall@aol.com

National Council on Aging
409 Third Street SW
Washington, DC 20024
800-867-2755; 202-479-1200
e-mail: info@ncoa.org
http://www.ncoa.org

National Hospice Organization
1901 N. Moore Street, Suite 901
Arlington, VA 22209
800-658-8898; 703-243-5900
e-mail: drsnho@cais.com
http://www.nho.org

DEMENTIA
(see Alzheimer's Disease & Other Dementias)

DEPRESSION

National Depressive and Manic-Depressive Association
730 N Franklin, Suite 501
Chicago, IL 60010
800-826-3632; 312-642-0049

Recovery, Inc.
802 N. Dearborn
Chicago, IL 60610
312-337-5661
e-mail: viscam@aol.com
http://www.ed.psu.edu/~recovery

DIABETES

American Diabetes Association
1600 Duke Street
Alexandria, VA 22314
800-232-3472; 703-549-1500
http://www.diabetes.org

Juvenile Diabetes Foundation International
120 Wall Street, 19th Floor
New York, NY 10005
800-223-1138
http://www.jdfcure.com

National Diabetes Information Clearinghouse
One Information Way
Bethesda, MD 20892-3560
301-654-3327
http://www.niddk.nih.gov

DIGESTIVE DISORDERS

Crohn's & Colitis Foundation of America
386 Park Avenue South, 17th Floor
New York, NY 10016
800-343-3637
http://www.ccfa.org

Digestive Disease National Coalition
507 Capitol Court NE, Suite 200
Washington, DC 20002
202-544-7497

International Foundation for Gastrointestinal Function Disorder
PO Box 17864
Milwaukee, WI 53217
888-964-2001; 414-964-1799
http://www.execpc.com\iffgd

Intestinal Disease Foundation
1323 Forbes Avenue, Suite 200
Pittsburgh, PA 15219
412-261-5888

National Digestive Diseases Information Clearinghouse
Two Information Way
Bethesda, MD 20892-3570
301-654-3810

United Ostomy Association
19772 MacArthur Blvd., Suite 200
Irvine, CA 92614
800-826-0826; 714-660-8624
e-mail: uoa@deltanet.com
http://www.uoa.org

DISABILITIES & REHABILITATION
(see also Amputation; Mental Retardation)

Disabled American Veterans
National Headquarters
3725 Alexandria Park
Cold Springs, KY 41076
606-441-7300
http://www.dav.org

Federation of the Handicapped
211 West 14th Street
New York, NY 10011
212-206-4200

Human Resources Center
IU Willets Road
Albertson, NY 11507
516-747-5400

National Easter Seal Society
230 W Monroe Street, Suite 1800
Chicago, IL 60606-4802
800-221-6827; 312-726-6200
e-mail: nessinfo@seals.com
http://www.seals.com

National Organization on Disability
2100 Pennsylvania Avenue NW
Washington, DC 20037
202-293-5960
http://www.nod.org

National Rehabilitation Information Center
8455 Colesville Road, Suite 935
Silver Spring, MD 20910
800-346-2742
http://www.naric.com\naric

National Rehabilitation Institute
633 South Washington Street
Alexandria, VA 22314
800-420-1500; 703-836-0850
http://www.nationalrehab.org

Paralyzed Veterans of America
801 18th Street NW
Washington, DC 20006
202-872-1300
http://www.pva.org

(continued)

People-to-People Committee for the
Handicapped
PO Box 18131
Washington, DC 20036
301-774-7446

DOWN SYNDROME

Association for Children With Down Syndrome
2616 Martin Avenue
Bellmore, NY 11710
516-221-4700
http://macroserve.com/acds/publist.htm

National Down Syndrome Congress
1605 Chantilly Drive, Suite 250
Atlanta, GA 30324
800-232-6372
e-mail: ndsc@charitiesusa.com
http://www.carol.net/~ndsc

National Down Syndrome Society Hotline
666 Broadway
New York, NY 10012
800-221-4602
http://www.ndss.org

Parent Assistance Committee on Down
Syndrome
208 Lafayette Avenue
Peekskill, NY 10566
914-739-4085

DRUG ABUSE (see also Alcoholism)

Cocaine Anonymous World Service Office, Inc.
PO Box 2000
Los Angeles, CA 90049-8000
800-347-8998; 310-559-5833
http://www.ca.org

Drug Abuse Warning Network
Substance Abuse and Mental Health Services
Administration
Parklawn Building, Room 16C-09
5600 Fishers Lane
Rockville, MD 20857
301-443-4404

Hazelden
CO 3, PO Box 11
Center City, MN 55012-0011
800-257-7810; 612-257-4010
e-mail: info@hazelden.org
http://www.hazelden.org

Narcotics Anonymous
PO Box 9999
Van Nuys, CA 91409
818-997-3822
http://www.wsoinc.com

EAR (see Deafness & Hearing Disorders)

EATING DISORDERS

The American Anorexia/Bulimia Association,
Inc.
293 Central Park West, Suite 1R
New York, NY 10024
212-501-8351
http://members.aol.com/amanbu/index.html

Overeaters Anonymous
PO Box 44020
Rio Rancho, NM 87174
505-891-2664

ENDOCRINE DISORDERS (see also Diabetes)

National Adrenal Diseases Foundation
505 Northern Boulevard
Great Neck, NY 11021
516-487-4992
e-mail: nadf@aol.com
http://medhlp.netusa.net/www/nadf.htm

National Cushing's Association
c/o Andrea Hecht
4620½ Van Nuys Boulevard
Sherman Oaks, CA 91403

Thyroid Foundation of America
Ruth Sleeper Hall, Room RSL350
40 Parkman Street
Boston, MA 02114
617-726-8500
http://www.mssm.edu/medicine/endocrinology/
tfa.html

EPILEPSY

Epilepsy Foundation of America
4351 Garden City Drive
Landover, MD 20785
800-EFA-4050; 301-459-3700
e-mail: postmaster@efa.org
http://www.efa.org

EYE
(see Blindness & Vision Problems)

FAMILY PLANNING
(see also Childbirth/Pregnancy; Infertility)

The Alan Guttmacher Institute
120 Wall Street
New York, NY 10005
212-248-1111
http://www.agi/usa.org

Association for Voluntary Sterilization
125 Park Avenue
New York, NY 10017
212-557-6600

Planned Parenthood Federation of America
810 Seventh Avenue
New York, NY 10017
212-541-7800
http://www.igc.apc.org/ppfa

GAUCHER'S DISEASE

National Gaucher Foundation
11140 Rockville Pike, Suite 350
Rockville, MD 20852-3106
800-925-8885; 800-GAUCHER (426-2437);
301-816-1515

GENERAL

The American Medical Association
515 North State Street
Chicago, IL 60610
312-464-5000
http://www.ama-assn.org

The Centers for Disease Control and Prevention
1600 Clifton Road NE
Atlanta, GA 30333
404-639-3311
http://www.cdc.gov

The Merck Manuals
Merck & Co., Inc.
PO Box 4
West Point, PA 19486
http://www.merck.com

National Institutes of Health
9000 Rockville Pike
Bethesda, MD 20892
301-496-4000
http://www.nih.gov

Parents of Chronically Ill Children
1527 Maryland Street
Springfield, IL 62702
217-522-6810

US Department of Health and Human Services
200 Independence Avenue SW
Washington, DC 20201
202-619-0257
http://www.os.dhhs.gov

US Food and Drug Administration
Office of Consumer Affairs Inquiry Information Line
301-827-4420
http://www.fda.gov

GENETIC DISEASES (see also Birth Defects)

Alliance of Genetic Support Groups
35 Wisconsin Circle, Suite 440
Chevy Chase, MD 20015
800-336-GENE; 301-652-5553
http://medhlp.netusa.net/www/agsg.htm

HEADACHE

American Council for Headache Education
875 Kings Highway, Suite 200
Woodbury, NJ 08096
800-255-ACHE
http://www.achenet.org

National Headache Foundation
428 W St. James Place
Chicago, IL 60614
800-843-2256; 312-388-6399
http://www.headaches.org

HEAD INJURY (see Brain Disorders)

HEARING (see Deafness & Hearing Disorders)

HEART DISORDERS
(see Cardiovascular Disorders)

HEMOCHROMATOSIS

Hemochromatosis Foundation, Inc.
PO Box 8569
Albany, NY 12208
518-489-0972

Iron Overload Diseases Association
433 Westwind Drive
North Palm Beach, FL 33408-5123
407-840-8512
e-mail: starlady@emi.net
http://www.emi.net/~iron_iod

HOME CARE

National Association for Home Care
228 7th Street SE
Washington, DC 20003
202-547-7424
http://www.nahc.org

HOSPICES (see Death & Bereavement)

IMPOTENCE

Impotents Anonymous
119 South Ruth Street
Maryville, TN 37803-5746
615-983-6092

INCONTINENCE

Help for Incontinent People
PO Box 544
Union, SC 29379
800-BLADDER; 803-579-7900

National Association for Continence
PO Box 8310
Spartanburg, SC 29305
800-BLADDER; 864-579-7900
e-mail: sbrewer@globalvision.net

Simon Foundation, Inc.
Box 835
Wilmette, IL 60091
800-23-SIMON; 708-864-3913

INFERTILITY
(see also Childbirth/Pregnancy; Family Planning)

Ferre Institute, Inc.
258 Genesee Street, Suite 302
Utica, NY 13502
315-724-4348
e-mail: ferreinf@aol.com

Resolve
1310 Broadway
Somerville, MA 02144
617-623-0744 (National HelpLine); 617-643-2424
e-mail: resolveinc@aol.com
http://www.resolve.org

IRON OVERLOAD (see Hemochromatosis)

KIDNEY DISORDERS

American Association of Kidney Patients
100 S Ashley Drive, Suite 280
Tampa, FL 33602
800-749-2257
e-mail: aakpnat@aol.com
http://cybermart.com/aakpaz/aakp.html

American Kidney Fund
6110 Executive Boulevard, Suite 1010
Rockville, MD 20852
800-638-8299; 301-881-3052
http://www.arbon.com/kidney

National Kidney Foundation
30 East 33rd Street, Suite 1100
New York, NY 10016
800-622-9010; 212-889-2210
http://www.kidney.org

National Kidney and Urologic Diseases
Information Clearinghouse
Three Information Way
Bethesda, MD 20892-3580
301-654-4415
http://www.niddk.nih.gov

LEARNING DISABILITIES
(see also Attention Deficit Disorder)

American Association on Mental Retardation
444 N Capitol Street NW, Suite 846
Washington, DC 20001
800-424-3688; 202-387-1968
e-mail: aamr@access.digex.net
http://www.aamr.org

Learning Disabilities Association
4156 Library Road
Pittsburgh, PA 15234
412-341-1515
http://www.nlld.org

National Center for Learning Disabilities
381 Park Ave South, Suite 1420
New York, NY 10016
212-545-7510

LEPROSY

American Leprosy Foundation
11600 Nebel Street, Suite 210
Rockville, MD 20852
301-984-1336
http://www.charity.org/alf.html

LIVER DISORDERS

American Liver Foundation
1425 Pompton Avenue
Cedar Grove, NJ 07009
800-223-0179; 201-256-2550
http://sadieo.ucsf.edu/alf/alffinal/
homepagealf.html

LUNG DISORDERS (see Respiratory Disorders)

LUPUS

Lupus Foundation of America
1300 Piccard Drive, Suite 200
Rockville, MD 20850
800-558-0121; 301-670-9292
http://internet-plaza.net/lupus

MEDIC ALERT

Medic Alert Foundation International
PO Box 1009
Turlock, CA 95381
800-432-5378

MENTAL HEALTH (see Psychiatric Disease)

MENTAL RETARDATION
(see also Learning Disabilities)

ARC (formerly Association for Retarded
Citizens of the United States)
500 E Border Street, Suite 300
Arlington, TX 76010
817-261-6003
http://thearc.org/welcome.html

FRAXA Research Foundation
PO Box 935
West Newbury, MA 01985-0935
508-462-1990
e-mail: fraxa@seacoast.com
http://www.worx.net/fraxa

Joseph P. Kennedy Foundation
1325 G Street NW, Suite 500
Washington, DC 20005
202-393-1250
http://www.family village.wisc.edu/jpkf/

National Association of Developmental
Disabilities Councils
1234 Massachusetts Avenue NW, Suite 103
Washington, DC 20005
202-347-1234
http://www.igc.apc.org/naddc

Voice of the Retarded (VOR)
5005 Newport Drive, Suite 108
Rolling Meadows, IL 60008
847-253-6020

MULTIPLE SCLEROSIS

National Multiple Sclerosis Society
733 Third Avenue
New York, NY 10017
800-344-4867; 212-986-3240
e-mail: nat@nmss.org
http://www.nmss.org

MUSCULAR DYSTROPHY

Muscular Dystrophy Association of America
10 E 40th Street, Suite 4110
New York, NY 10016
212-689-9040
http://www.mdausu.org

MYASTHENIA GRAVIS

Myasthenia Gravis Foundation
222 S Riverside Plaza, Suite 1540
Chicago, IL 00006
800-541-5454; 312-258-0522
e-mail: mgfa@aol.com
http://www.med.unc.edu/mgfa

NUTRITION

American Dietetic Association
216 West Jackson Boulevard
Chicago, IL 60606
312-899-0040
http://www.eatright.org

OSTEOPOROSIS

National Osteoporosis Foundation
1150 17th Street NW, Suite 500
Washington, DC 20036
202-223-2226
http://www.nof.org

PAGET'S DISEASE

The Paget's Disease Foundation
200 Varick Street, Suite 1004
New York, NY 10014
800-23-PAGET; 212-229-1582
e-mail: pagetfdn@aol.com
http://healthanswers.com/pagnet

PAIN RELIEF

American Chronic Pain Association
PO Box 850
Rocklin, CA 95677
916-632-0922
e-mail: acpa@ix.netcom.com
http://www.members.tripod.com/~widdy/ACPA

National Chronic Pain Outreach Association
7979 Old Georgetown Road, Suite 100
Bethesda, MD 20814
301-652-4948
e-mail: mcp04@aol.com

PARKINSON'S DISEASE

American Parkinson Disease Association
60 Bay Street, Suite 401
Staten Island, NY 10301
800-223-2732; 718-981-8001
e-mail: apda@admin.con2.com
http://www.apdaparkinson.com

(continued)

National Parkinson Foundation
1501 NW Ninth Avenue
Miami, FL 33136
800-327-4545; 800-433-7022 (in FL)
http://www.parkinson.org

Parkinson's Action Network
822 College Avenue, Suite C
Santa Rosa, CA 95404
800-820-4716; 707-544-1994
e-mail: parkactnet@aol.com

Parkinson's Disease Foundation
650 West 168th Street
New York, NY 10032
800-457-6676; 212-923-4700
http://www.parkinsonsfoundation.org

Parkinson Support Groups of America
11376 Cherry Hill Road, #204
Beltsville, MD 20705
301-937-1545

United Parkinson Foundation
833 W Washington Boulevard
Chicago, IL 60607
312-733-1893
e-mail: upf_itf@msn.com

PRADER-WILLI SYNDROME

Prader-Willi Syndrome Association (USA)
2510 S Brentwood Boulevard, Suite 220
St Louis, MO 63144
800-926-4797; 314-962-7644
e-mail: pwsa usa@aol.com
http://www.athenet.net/~pwsa_usa

PREGNANCY (see Childbirth/Pregnancy)

PROSTATE DISORDERS
(see also Cancer & Other Tumors)

The Prostatitis Foundation
Information Distribution Center
2029 Ireland Grove Park
Bloomington, IL 61704
309-664-6222
e-mail: TCapstone@aol.com
http://www.prostate.org

PSORIASIS

National Psoriasis Foundation
6600 SW 92nd Avenue, Suite 300
Portland, OR 97223-7195
800-723-9166; 503-297-1545
e-mail: 76135.2746@compuserve.com
http://www.psoriasis.org/npf.html

Psoriasis Research Association
107 Vista del Grande
San Carlos, CA 94070
415-593-1394

PSYCHIATRIC DISEASE (see also Depression)

The Alliance for the Mentally Ill/Friends and
Advocates of the Mentally Ill
432 Park Avenue South
New York, NY 10016
800-950-NAMI; 212-684-FAMI
http://www.schizophrenia.com/ami

National Alliance for the Mentally Ill
200 N Glebe Road, Suite 1015
Arlington, VA 22203-3754
800-950-6264; 703-524-7600
e-mail: namiofc@aol.com
http://www.nami.org

National Institute of Mental Health
Public Inquiries Section
5600 Fishers Lane, Room 7C-02
Rockville, MD 20857
800-64-PANIC (for panic disorder);
800-421-4211 (for depression); 301-443-4513
e-mail: nimhinfo@nih.gov
http://sis.nlm.nih.gov/aids/nimh.html

National Mental Health Association
1021 Prince Street
Alexandria, VA 22314
800-969-NMHA; 703-684-7722
http://www.worldcorp.com/dc-online/nmha

RARE DISORDERS

National Organization for Rare Disorders
PO Box 8923
New Fairfield, CT 06812-8923
800-999-NORD; 203-746-6518; 203-746-6927
(TTY)
e-mail: orphan@nord-rdb.com
http://www.pcnet.com/~orphan

RESPIRATORY (LUNG) DISORDERS

American Lung Association
1740 Broadway
New York, NY 10019
800-586-4872; 212-315-8700
e-mail: info@lungusa.org
http://www.lungusa.org

Asthma & Allergy Foundation of America
1125 15th Street NW, Suite 502
Washington, DC 20005
800-7ASTHMA; 202-466-7643
http://www.housecall.com/sponsors/nhc/1996vha/
aafa.html

REYE'S SYNDROME

National Reye's Syndrome Foundation
PO Box 829
Bryan, OH 43506-0829
800-233-7393; 419-636-2679
e-mail: reyessyn@mail.bright.net
http://www.bright.net/~reyessyn

SJÖGREN'S SYNDROME

National Sjögren's Syndrome Association
PO Box 42207
Phoenix, AZ 85080
800-395-6772; 602-516-0787
e-mail: nssa@aol.com
http://www.sjogrens.org

SLEEP DISORDERS

American Sleep Apnea Association
2025 Pennsylvania Avenue NW, Suite 905
Washington, DC 20006
202-293-3650
e-mail: asaa@nicom.com
http://www.sleepnet.com/asaa.htm

American Sleep Disorders Association
1610 14th Street NW, Suite 300
Rochester, MN 55901
507-287-6006
e-mail: asda@millcomm.com
http://www.asda.org

SPINA BIFIDA

Spina Bifida Association of America
4590 MacArthur Boulevard NW, Suite 250
Washington, DC 20007-4226
800-621-3141; 202-944-3285
e-mail: spinabifida@aol.com
http://www.infohiway.com/spinabifida

SPINAL CORD INJURY

National Spinal Cord Injury Association
8300 Colesville Road
Silver Spring, MD 20910
800-962-9629; 301-588-6959
email: nscia2@aol.com

Spinal Cord Injury Hotline
2200 Kernan Drive
Baltimore, MD 21207
800-526-3456
e-mail: scihotline@aol.com
http://www.users.aol.com/scihotline

STUTTERING & OTHER SPEECH DISORDERS

National Aphasia Association
PO Box 1887
Murray Hill Station
New York, NY 10156-0611
800-922-4622

National Council on Stuttering & Foundation for Fluency
9242 Gross Point Road, #305
Skokie, IL 60077-1338
804-677-8280

National Stuttering Project
5100 East La Palma Avenue, Suite 208
Anaheim Hills, CA 92807
800-364-1677; 714-693-7480
http://www.member.aol.com/ncphone

Stuttering Foundation of America
PO Box 11749
3100 Walnut Grove Road, Suite 603
Memphis, TN 38111-0749
800-992-9392; 901-452-7343; 901-452-0995
e-mail: stuttersfa@aol.com

SUDDEN INFANT DEATH SYNDROME

SIDS Network
9 Gonch Farm Road
Ledyard, CT 06339
e-mail: sidsnet@q.continuum.net
http://sids-network.org

Sudden Infant Death Syndrome Alliance
1314 Bedford Avenue, Suite 210
Baltimore, MD 21208
800-221-SIDS; 410-653-8226
http://www.circsol.com/sids

Sudden Infant Death Syndrome (SIDS) Clearinghouse
2070 Chain Bridge Road, Suite 450
Vienna, VA 22182
703-821-8955, ext. 249

TAY-SACHS DISEASE

National Tay-Sachs & Allied Diseases Association
2001 Beacon Street, Suite 204
Brookline, MA 02146
800-90-NTSAD; 617-277-4463

TRAVEL HEALTH

Immunization Alert
PO Box 406
Storrs, CT 06268
800-584-1999
e-mail: 73314.3624@compuserve.com
http://www.quikpage.com/I/immuni

International Association for Medical Assistance to Travelers
417 Center Street
Lewiston, NY 14092
716-754-4883

International SOS Assistance
PO Box 11568
Philadelphia, PA 19116
800-523-8930; 215-244-1500
http://www.intsos.com

International Travelers Hotline
Centers for Disease Control and Prevention
404-332-4559

WOMEN'S HEALTH (see also Aging)

American College of Obstetricians and Gynecologists
Resource Center
PO Box 96920
Washington, DC 20090-6920
202-863-2518
http://www.acog.org

National Women's Health Network
514 10th Street NW, Suite 400
Washington, DC 20004
202-347-1140

Index

Note: Page numbers in *italics* refer to illustrations or other sidebars.

──────────── H ────────────